W9-CQI-927

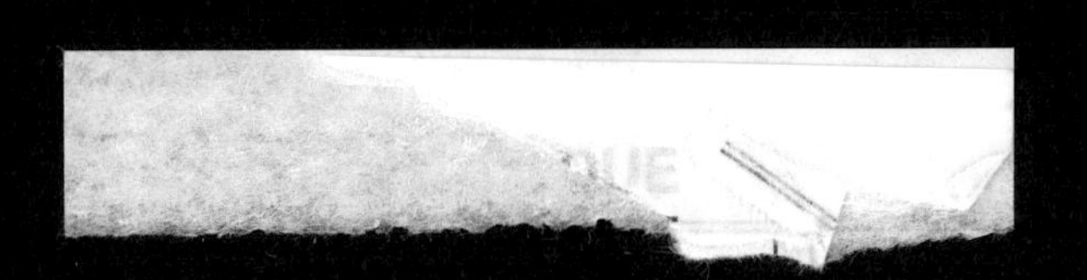

Lever's
Histopathology of the Skin

Lever's
Histopathology of the Skin

EIGHTH EDITION

EDITOR-IN-CHIEF

David Elder, MB, CHB
Professor and Associate Director, Division of Anatomic Pathology
Department of Pathology and Laboratory Medicine
University of Pennsylvania School of Medicine
3400 Spruce Street
Philadelphia, Pennsylvania 19104

ASSOCIATE EDITORS

Rosalie Elenitsas, MD
Department of Dermatology
University of Pennsylvania School of Medicine
415 Curie Boulevard
Philadelphia, Pennsylvania 19104

Christine Jaworsky, MD
Departments of Dermatology and Pathology
Case Western Reserve University
2500 MetroHealth Drive
Cleveland, Ohio 44109

Bernett Johnson Jr., MD
Department of Dermatology
University of Pennsylvania School of Medicine
3600 Spruce Street
Philadelphia, Pennsylvania 19104

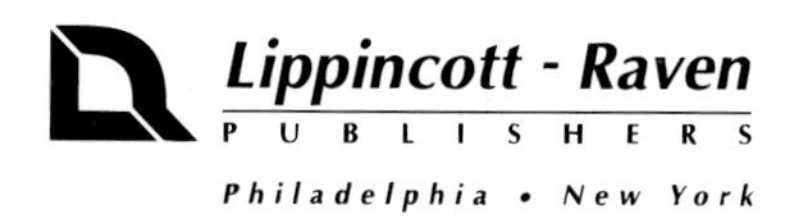

Acquisitions Editor: Richard Winters
Senior Developmental Editor: Delois Patterson
Senior Production Editor: Molly Connors
Production Service: Textbook Writers Associates, Inc.
Compositor: Maryland Composition
Printer/Binder: Quebecor Kingsport
Cover Designer: William T. Donnelly

Eighth Edition

Library of Congress Cataloging-in-Publication Data

Lever's histopathology of the skin. — 8th ed. / editor-in-chief, David Elder ; associate editors, Rosalie Elenitsas, Christine Jaworsky, Bernett Johnson, Jr.
p. cm.
Rev. ed. of: Histopathology of the skin / Walter F. Lever, Gundula Schaumburg-Lever. 7th ed. c 1990.
Includes bibliographical references and index.
ISBN 0-397-51500-6 (hard cover : alk. paper)
1. Skin—Histopathology. I. Lever, Walter F. (Walter Frederick), 1909– Histopathology of the skin. II. Elder, David E.
[DNLM: 1. Skin Diseases—pathology. WR 105 L661 1997]
RL95.L48 1997
616.5′07—dc20
DNLM/DLC
for Library of Congress 96-30912
CIP

9 8 7 6 5 4 3 2 1

In memory of **Walter F. Lever, MD**
(1909–1992)

A pioneer in dermatopathology,
who introduced generations of physicians to the subject,
and whose work lives on in this volume

Contributors

Edward Abell, MD *The Dermatology Laboratory, St. Francis Medical Center, 400 45th Street, Pittsburgh, Pennsylvania 15201-1198*

Zsolt Argenyi, MD *Professor of Pathology and Dermatology, Director of Dermatopathology, Department of Pathology, University of Iowa Hospitals and Clinic, 200 Hawkins Drive, Iowa City, Iowa 52242*

Raymond L. Barnhill, MD *Associate Professor of Pathology, Director of Dermatopathology, Department of Pathology, Brigham and Women's Hospital, Harvard Medical School, 75 Francis Street, MRB 608, Boston, Massachusetts 02115*

Martin M. Black, MD, FRCP, FRCP(Path) *Consultant Dermatologist, Department of Dermatopathology, St. John's Institute of Dermatology, St. Thomas' Hospital, Lambeth Palace Road, London, United Kingdom SE1 7EH*

Walter H. C. Burgdorf, MD *Clinical Lecturer, Department of Dermatology, Ludwig Maximilian University, Munich, Germany*

Klaus J. Busam, MD *Dermatopathology Division, Department of Pathology, Brigham and Women's Hospital, Harvard Medical School, 75 Francis Street, Boston, Massachusetts 02115*

Eduardo Calonje, MD, DIPRCPATH *Consultant Dermatopathologist, Honorary Senior Lecturer in Dermatology, St. John's Institute of Dermatology, St. Thomas' Hospital, Lambeth Palace Road, London, United Kingdom SE1 7EH*

Wallace H. Clark Jr., MD *Professor of Pathology, Harvard Medical School, Beth Israel Hospital, Boston, MA 02115*

Lisa M. Cohen, MD *Beth Israel Hospital, Department of Pathology, Children's Hospital, Department of Dermatology, Instructor in Dermatology and Pathology, Harvard Medical School, 75 Francis Street, Boston, Massachusetts 02115; Pathology Services, Incorporated, 640 Memorial Drive, Cambridge, Massachusetts 02139*

Félix Contreras, MD *Professor of Pathology, Chairman, Department of Pathology, La Paz Hospital, Alcantara 5, Madrid, Spain 28006*

Jacinto Convit, MD *Director, Instituto de Biomedina, Universidad Central de Venezuela, San Nicola's a Providencia, Apartado Postal 4043, Caracas, DF, Venezuela 1010A*

A. Neil Crowson, MD *Misericordia General Hospital, 99 Cornish Avenue, Winnipeg, Manitoba, Canada R3C 1A2*

David Elder, MB, ChB, FRCPA *Professor and Associate Director, Division of Anatomic Pathology, Department of Pathology and Laboratory Medicine, Hospital of the University of Pennsylvania, 3400 Spruce Street, Philadelphia, Pennsylvania 19104-4283*

Rosalie Elenitsas, MD *Assistant Professor of Dermatology, University of Pennsylvania School of Medicine, 415 Curie Boulevard, 217 Clinical Research Building, Philadelphia, Pennsylvania 19104*

Robert J. Friedman, MD, MSc(Med) *Clinical Associate Professor, Department of Dermatology, NYU School of Medicine, 562 First Avenue, New York, New York 10016; DermPath, P.O. Box 1050, Scarsdale, New York 10503-0980*

Thomas D. Griffin, MD *Clinical Assistant Professor, Department of Dermatology, University of Pennsylvania, 137 South Easton Road, Glenside, Pennsylvania 19038*

Allan C. Halpern, MD *Department of Dermatology, University of Pennsylvania, 415 Curie Boulevard, 217 Clinical Research Building, Philadelphia, Pennsylvania 19104*

Terence J. Harrist, MD *Assistant Professor of Pathology, Harvard Medical School, Beth Israel Hospital, Boston, Massachusetts 02115; Medical Director, Pathology Services, Incorporated, 640 Memorial Drive, Fourth Floor, Cambridge, Massachusetts 02139*

John L. M. Hawk, MD *Head, Department of Photobiology, St. John's Institute of Dermatology, St. Thomas' Hospital, Lambeth Palace Road, London, United Kingdom SE1 7EH*

Peter J. Heenan, MB, BS, FRCPath, FRCPA *Associate Professor, Department of Pathology, The University of Western Australia, Queen Elizabeth II Medical Centre, Nedlands, Western Australia 6009*

Edward R. Heilman, MD *Associate Clinical Professor of Dermatology and Pathology, Director of Dermatopathology, Departments of Dermatology and Pathology, SUNY Health Science Center, Brooklyn, 450 Clarkson Avenue, Brooklyn, New York 11203*

Paul Honig, MD *Professor of Pediatrics and Dermatology, Departments of Pediatrics and Dermatology, University of Pennsylvania School of Medicine, Children's Hospital of Philadelphia, 34th Street and Civic Center Boulevard, Philadelphia, Pennsylvania 19104*

Thomas Horn, MD *Associate Professor of Dermatology and Pathology, Department of Dermatology, Johns Hopkins University, 600 North Wolfe Street, Blalock 907, Baltimore, Maryland 21287*

Michael Ioffreda, MD *Department of Dermatology, Allegheny University, Philadelphia, Pennsylvania 19102*

Christine Jaworsky, MD *Assistant Professor, Departments of Dermatology and Pathology, Case Western Reserve University, MetroHealth Medical Center, 2500 MetroHealth Drive, Cleveland, Ohio 44109; Adjunct Assistant Professor, Department of Dermatology, University of Pennsylvania, 3600 Spruce Street, Philadelphia, Pennsylvania 19104*

Bernett Johnson Jr., MD *Professor of Dermatology and Pathology, Department of Dermatology, Hospital of the University of Pennsylvania, 3600 Spruce Street/2 Maloney, Philadelphia, Pennsylvania 19104*

Waine C. Johnson, MD *Chairman and Clinical Professor, Department of Dermatology, The Graduate Hospital, University of Pennsylvania School of Medicine, 137 South Easton Road, Glenside, Pennsylvania 19038*

Hideko Kamino, MD *New York University Medical Center, Dermatopathology Section, Suite 7J, 530 First Avenue, New York, New York 10016*

Gary R. Kantor, MD *Associate Professor, Department of Dermatology, Allegheny University of the Health Sciences, Broad and Vine Streets, Philadelphia, Pennsylvania 19102-1192*

Nigel Kirkham, MD, FRCPath *Consultant Pathologist, Histopathology Department, Royal Sussex County Hospital, Eastern Road, Brighton, United Kingdom BN2 5BG*

Philip E. LeBoit, MD *Associate Professor, Departments of Pathology and Dermatology, University of California, San Francisco, 408 Health Sciences West, San Francisco, California 94143-0506*

B. Jack Longley, MD *Associate Professor of Dermatology and Pathology, Departments of Dermatology and Pathology, Yale University School of Medicine, 333 Cedar Street, New Haven, Connecticut 06510*

Sebastian Lucas, FRCPath *Professor, UMDS Department of Histopathology, St. Thomas' Hospital, Lambeth Palace Road, London, United Kingdom SE1 7EH*

Timothy H. McCalmont, MD *Assistant Clinical Professor, Department of Pathology, University of California, San Francisco, 513 Parnassus Avenue, Room 501 HSW, San Francisco, California 94143-0506*

N. Scott McNutt, MD *New York Hospital—Cornell University Medical Center, Dermatopathology—F309, 525 East 68th Street, New York, New York 10021-4897*

Cynthia Magro, MD *Assistant Professor of Pathology, Department of Pathology, Beth Israel Hospital/Harvard University; Pathology Services, Incorporated, 640 Memorial Drive, Cambridge, Massachusetts 02139*

John Maize, MD *Professor and Chairman, Department of Dermatology, Medical University of South Carolina, 171 Ashley Avenue, Charleston, South Carolina 29425-2215*

John Metcalf, MD *Professor of Pathology and Dermatology, Director of Surgical Pathology, Departments of Pathology and Laboratory Medicine and Dermatology, Pathology and Laboratory Medicine, Medical University of South Carolina, 171 Ashley Avenue, Charleston, South Carolina 29425*

Martin Mihm Jr., MD *Chief, Dermatology and Dermatopathology, Albany Medical College, 47 New Scotland Avenue, A-81, Albany, New York 12208-3478*

Abelardo Moreno, MD *Departamento de Anatomia Patologica, Hospital de Bellvitge "Princeps de Espanya," Feixa Llarga s/n, Hospitalet de Llobregat, Barcelona, Spain 08907*

George F. Murphy, MD *Herman Beerman Professor of Dermatology, Department of Dermatology, University of Pennsylvania, 235B Clinical Research Building, 415 Curie Boulevard, Philadelphia, Pennsylvania 19104*

Neal Penneys, MD, PhD *Department of Dermatology, St. Louis School of Medicine, 1402 South Grand Boulevard, St. Louis, Missouri 63104*

Bruce D. Ragsdale, MD *Lecturer, Department of Dermatology, University of Alabama, Birmingham, Alabama; Central Coast Pathology Consultants, 1010 Murray Street, San Luis Obispo, California 93405*

Richard J. Reed, MD *Director, Department of Pathology, Touro Infirmary, 1401 Foucher Street, New Orleans, Louisiana 70115*

Philip E. Shapiro, MD *Associate Clinical Professor of Dermatology, Yale University School of Medicine, New Haven, Connecticut 06510; Dermatopathology Laboratory of New England, 21 Woodland Street, Suite 210, Hartford, Connecticut 06105*

Debra Karp Skopicki, MD *Pathology Services, Incorporated, 640 Memorial Drive, Cambridge, Massachusetts 02139*

Neil P. Smith, MD *St. John's Institute of Dermatology, St. Thomas' Hospital, Lambeth Palace Road, London, United Kingdom SE1 7EH*

Richard L. Spielvogel, MD *Professor and Chair, Department of Dermatology, Allegheny University of Health Sciences, Broad and Vine Streets, Philadelphia, Pennsylvania 19102*

Sonia Toussaint, MD *New York University Medical Center, Dermatopathology Section, Suite 7J, 530 First Avenue, New York, New York 10016*

Patricia Van Belle, DSN *Department of Pathology and Laboratory Medicine, Hospital of the University of Pennsylvania, 6 Founders, Philadelphia, Pennsylvania 19104*

Edward Wilson-Jones, MD *Professor Emeritus, Institute of Dermatology, St. Thomas' Hospital, Lambeth Palace Road, London, United Kingdom SE1 7EH*

Preface

Lever's "Histopathology of the Skin," currently in its fiftieth year, is a classic work that has been used by several generations of dermatopathologists, pathologists, and dermatologists in their own training, in their current practices, and in the training of their students. The opportunity to participate in its continuing evolution has been an exciting challenge.

Because of the explosion of knowledge that almost precludes the continuing single authorship of a comprehensive dermatopathology text, a cadre of expert contributors has been recruited. These contributors have, for the most part, revised and extended the existing text. Emphasis on discussions of pathogenesis has been increased, and discussion of immunohistochemistry and immunofluorescence as adjuncts to diagnosis have been expanded where appropriate. References have been updated. New information has been added to the text where appropriate, and some of the concepts have been modernized. The emphasis on clinocopathological correlation that made "Lever" so useful to clinicians and pathologists alike has been retained and extended with the use of color photographs of skin diseases, the "gross pathology" of the skin.

An introductory algorithmic classification for differential diagnosis of skin diseases has been added to provide a pattern-based classification that will assist the reader to develop a differential diagnosis for an unknown case and to review relevant descriptive material from elsewhere in the book. A morphologically based pattern classification is optimal for the generation of a differential diagnosis from an unknown slide. However, the organization of diseases into chapters classified according to traditional concepts of pathophysiology and etiology, in addition to morphology, has been retained in order to maintain conceptual links to previous editions and to other literature. This organization also allows for discussion of related entities in proximity to one another and is complemented by the pattern classification in which diseases of diverse etiology may be listed together because of shared morphological features.

The revision process has been coordinated by an Editorial Board that consists of faculty members of the Dermatopathology Programs at the University of Pennsylvania who are not otherwise obligated. The editors have worked closely with the contributors to ensure a coordinated and complete whole work, with value not only as a teaching and learning tool, but also as a diagnostic aid. Thus, the work that was begun and carried on for so long by one man, and then by a couple, has been taken toward the next millennium by a cohort of almost fifty individuals.

David Elder

Preface to the First Edition

This book is based on the courses of dermatopathology that I have been giving in recent years to graduate students of dermatology enrolled at Harvard Medical School and Massachusetts General Hospital. The book is written primarily for dermatologists; I hope, however, that it may be useful also to pathologists, since dermatopathology is given little consideration in most textbooks of pathology.

I have attempted to keep this book short. Emphasis has been placed on the essential histologic features. Minor details and rare aberrations from the typical histologic picture have been omitted. I have allotted more space to the cutaneous diseases in which histologic examination is of diagnostic value than to those in which the histologic picture is not characteristic. In spite of my striving for brevity I have discussed the histogenesis of several dermatoses, because knowledge of the histogenesis often is of great value for the understanding of the pathologic process.

Primarily for the benefit of pathologists who usually are not too familiar with dermatologic diseases, I have preceded the histologic discussion of each disease with a short description of the clinical features.

A fairly extensive bibliography has been supplied for readers who are interested in obtaining additional information. In the selection of articles for the bibliography preference has been given, whenever possible, to those written in English.

I wish to express my deep gratitude to Dr. Tracy B. Mallory and Dr. Benjamin Castleman of the Pathology Laboratory at the Massachusetts General Hospital for the training in pathology they have given me. It has been invaluable to me. Their teaching is reflected in this book. Furthermore, I wish to thank Mr. Richard W. St. Clair, who with great skill and patience produced all the photomicrographs in this book.

Walter F. Lever

Contents

Lever's
Histopathology of the Skin

Lever's Histopathology of the Skin, eighth edition,
edited by David Elder et al. Lippincott–
Raven Publishers, Philadelphia © 1997.

CHAPTER 1

Introduction

David Elder

Readers of this book in its seven previous editions have relied on it to aid them in reaching accurate histologic diagnoses of cutaneous diseases. A histologic diagnosis is a clinical tool that assists in the process of categorizing patients into disease groups, within which patients tend to share a common outcome and a common set of responses to therapy. The histologic diagnosis is then used to aid in the clinical management of patients. The most accurate diagnosis is the one that most closely correlates with clinical outcome and helps direct the most appropriate clinical intervention. By emphasizing certain key observations that have value in identifying particular diseases, this book assists observers in making appropriate histologic diagnoses in the majority of instances. Where applicable, ultrastructural, immunohistochemical, and molecular aids to diagnosis are discussed. These advances have resulted in increased specificity for many diagnoses. For example, an amelanotic dermal tumor composed of large, mitotically active cells that are positive in an immunohistochemical reaction for the HMB-45 antigen is almost certainly a malignant melanoma. In the absence of the immunohistochemical criterion, the specific diagnosis of melanoma cannot be made (Chap. 29).

Although histopathology remains the "gold standard" for most dermatologic diagnoses, it must be recognized that not all lesions are amenable to definitive histologic diagnosis. The histologic features of many inflammatory dermatoses in particular are nonspecific or, at best, only suggestive of specific diagnoses. Even among the more readily characterized papulosquamous dermatoses, such as psoriasis and lichen planus, the histologic picture is more typically "compatible with" rather than "diagnostic of" the clinical process. Sometimes, however, the histopathology can contribute by ruling out an important diagnosis even though an exact diagnosis cannot be made. For example, review of a biopsy of a psoriasiform plaque may rule out mycosis fungoides but may not be able to establish the specific diagnosis of psoriasis. The diagnostic limitations of histology extend to infectious and neoplastic processes as well. For example, infectious granulomas of different etiologies are not readily distinguishable unless the causative organisms can be demonstrated. Similarly, histology may not suffice to distinguish between keratoacanthoma and squamous cell carcinoma or between Spitz nevus and melanoma. In all of these instances, the clinical utility of histology is increased by effective communication between clinician and pathologist with appropriate attention to the clinical and epidemiologic context of the lesion under study.

A major source of difficulty in making an exact diagnosis in pathology, as in clinical medicine, is that the information required to make the diagnosis is frequently incomplete at some level.[1] At the most fundamental level, there may simply be no extant standard for a particular diagnosis. For example, histopathology is often taken to be a "gold standard" for diagnosis of a particular disease, but if the histopathologic parameters that are considered to define that disease have been determined in a clinically defined series of cases, their independence and specificity may be called into question. A histologic study of nummular dermatitis, however complete and accurate it may be, will not glean any information that reliably distinguishes between this diagnosis and that of another spongiotic dermatitis (Chap. 7). Specificity studies to determine the prevalence of criteria in diagnostically challenging cases of other diseases are not always readily available. For example, early marketing of the HMB-45 antibody advertised "100% specificity for melanoma." After the specificity studies were extended, however, it was recognized that this antigen is expressed not only in melanoma but also in dysplastic nevi, blue nevi, and other benign lesions (Chap. 29).

An important element of diagnostic efficacy is prognostication. In some instances, many of them neoplasms, a histologic diagnosis is predictive of biologic behavior, such as the capacity for distant metastasis. Then, follow-up studies of outcome can serve as an appropriate "gold standard" for the diagnosis. Even when such studies are available, however, the prediction of outcome is usually expressed in terms of statistical probabilities, which are not absolute. The information needed to accurately predict outcome in any given individual case is frequently hidden from the observer. For example, the outcome of a viral infection may depend on the presence or absence of antibodies in the patient's serum, which cannot be determined from observation of histologic sections. Similarly, even the most advanced and seemingly lethal primary malignant melanoma has a certain

D. Elder: Department of Pathology and Laboratory Medicine, University of Pennsylvania, Philadelphia, PA

probability of survival, even after utilization of the most sophisticated prognostic models.[2,3]

Foucar has pointed out that the diagnostic process is an example of complex decision making that has intrinsic uncertainty, usually resulting from one or more of the following: (1) the large number of variables that can be evaluated in an attempt to solve the problem results in novel combinations of variables that cannot be managed consistently by problem solvers; (2) one or more key variables lack clear definition; and (3) one or more key variables are hidden from the problem solver.[4] To the uncertainty inherent in these complex problems can be added the uncertainty that may result from deficiencies in the observer's ability to evaluate and categorize histologic findings. Even the most expert observers have inherent and often unrecognized deficiencies that result in less-than-perfect reproducibility of histopathologic observations, and thus of diagnoses.[5] Furthermore, there are limitations on the ability of even the most expert observers to communicate their diagnostic acumen to others.

The diagnostic difficulties that result from uncertainty are compounded when there is also failure to agree on the criteria for diagnosis. Differences in criteria may result from the use of different assumptions for the development of criteria.[1] At the simplest level of diagnosis, an individual pathologist might establish a set of criteria that establishes a diagnosis "by definition." Such a definitional diagnosis reduces uncertainty for that individual to a minimum. At a somewhat more advanced level, criteria are used that are considered likely to be acceptable to other pathologists, constituting a "consensus gold standard." At this level of diagnosis, difficulties in communicating a clear definition of the criteria among pathologists introduce uncertainty resulting from lack of reproducibility, and this uncertainty increases with the number of variables under consideration and the resultant increasing subjectivity of the diagnostic exercise.[4]

The most advanced level of diagnostic problem solving is represented by the attempt to assign a biologically correct label, one that precisely predicts a disease's course.[4] Attempts to resolve fully this more difficult level of prediction are likely in most if not all cases to be frustrated by the uncertainties enumerated above, especially the existence of hidden variables, such as "host resistance," "virulence," "environmental effects," and so on, that are not evident to the observer of a histologic slide, however expert and diligent he or she may be. Efforts to improve on diagnostic efficacy at this level might, for example, pursue information at the ultrastructural or molecular level. However, the accurate and complete prediction of a particular disease outcome is likely to prove an elusive goal.

It is likely that the best approximation to this goal will be achieved by a detailed correlation of findings at the molecular, histologic, and gross anatomic levels with the physical findings and clinical history, interpreted in the context of the whole patient and his or her environment. In the "real world" of clinical medicine, a histologic description and differential diagnosis for a difficult case are often likely to be more useful than a single "specific" diagnosis that may be correct in its own frame of reference but wrong or misleading in the total clinicopathologic context of a particular patient. The former is the traditional method of clinical practice, which should be aided but not supplanted by the tools of histopathology. The information in this book has been designed to assist in this clinical diagnostic process.

REFERENCES

1. Foucar, E. Diagnostic decision-making in surgical pathology. In: Weidner N, ed. Diagnosis of the Difficult Case. Philadelphia: Saunders 1996; 1.
2. Rivers JK, McCarthy SW, Shaw HM et al. Patients with thick melanomas surviving at least ten years: Histological, cytometric and HLA analyses. Histopathology 1991;18:339.
3. Clark WH Jr, Elder DE, Guerry D IV. Model predicting survival in stage I melanoma based on tumor progression. J Natl Cancer Inst 1989;81:1893.
4. Foucar E. Debating "melanocytic tumors of the skin": Does an "uncertain" diagnosis signify borderline diagnostic skill? Am J Dermatopathol 1996;17:626.
5. Farmer EA, Gonin R, Hanna, MP. Discordance in the histopathological diagnosis of melanoma and melanocytic nevi between expert pathologists. Hum Pathol 1996;27:528.

Lever's Histopathology of the Skin, eighth edition,
edited by David Elder et al. Lippincott–
Raven Publishers, Philadelphia © 1997.

CHAPTER 2

Biopsy Techniques

Rosalie Elenitsas and Allan C. Halpern

TECHNIQUE FOR BIOPSY

The technique used for a skin biopsy is of prime importance in the diagnosis of any skin disease. Four techniques can be employed for obtaining a specimen for histologic evaluation: scalpel (incisional and excisional) biopsy, punch biopsy, shave biopsy, and curettage. The choice of technique should be based on the clinical differential diagnosis and a mental review of the pathology of each disorder.

Excisional scalpel biopsy is recommended for removal of atypical pigmented lesions or deep dermal/subcutaneous nodules and when evaluation of margins is necessary. Incisional scalpel biopsy is advisable for the study of panniculitis because it usually is not possible to obtain adequate amounts of subcutaneous tissue by punch biopsy. Diagnosis of connective tissue nevi, anetoderma, atrophoderma, and occasionally of pigmentation disorders where it is important to compare involved and uninvolved skin, may also benefit from incisional biopsy with inclusion of adjacent normal skin.

Punch biopsy is the standard procedure for obtaining samples of inflammatory dermatoses. It is important to select a proper site for biopsy. In most instances, histologic examination of a fully developed lesion will give more information than examination of an early or involuting lesion. Vesicobullous lesions, ulcers, and pustular lesions are exceptions to this rule. For their histologic examination, a very early lesion is required; otherwise, secondary changes, such as regeneration, degeneration, scarring, or secondary infection may obscure essential features and make recognition of the primary pathologic process impossible. Attempts should be made to select a lesion that has not been scratched or traumatized. If possible, it is optimal to submit biopsies that have not been altered by topical or systemic therapy, especially antiinflammatory agents. In scalp biopsies, the punch (6 mm) or scalpel should be inserted into the skin parallel to the direction of hair growth, and the biopsy should be extended well into the subcutis to be certain that the bulbs of terminal follicles are included.[1] In scarring alopecia, it is important that a biopsy be performed in an area of erythema with visible hair shafts; a biopsy of a completely scarred area of alopecia will show only end-stage nonspecific changes.

The biopsy specimen should include subcutaneous fat, because in many dermatoses, characteristic histologic features are found in the lower dermis or in the subcutaneous fat. If there are multiple clinically uncharacteristic lesions, histologic diagnosis may be aided by taking multiple biopsy specimens from lesions in different stages of evolution.

In most instances, a specimen obtained with a 4-mm biopsy punch is adequate for histologic study. A 3-mm punch may be preferable for small lesions or biopsies from the face when cosmesis is a concern. After the skin specimen has been loosened with the biopsy punch, it should be handled very gently and, above all, should not be grasped with forceps. It should be squeezed gently out of its socket, or be carefully speared with the syringe needle that was used for injection of the local anesthetic. Crush artifact, which can occur with almost any technique, makes a specimen of an inflammatory process essentially useless. Lymphoma and leukemic infiltrates are particularly susceptible to crush. Sharp scissors are used to cut through the subcutaneous fat at the base of the specimen.

Shave biopsies should be employed only for lesions in which characteristic histologic changes are expected to be present in the epidermis or the superficial dermis. These include seborrheic keratoses, solar keratoses, verrucae, benign nevi, and basal cell carcinomas. Shave biopsies are inadequate for differentiating between squamous cell carcinoma and keratoacanthoma, and they are contraindicated if there is the slightest suspicion of malignant melanoma because determination of the depth of penetration is of great importance. Because of the thick stratum corneum, a shave biopsy of acral skin may produce a superficial specimen extending only to the midepidermis or papillary dermis. This is especially important when performing a biopsy of an acral pigmented lesion; in this situation a punch biopsy or small excision is the best method.

To carry out a shave biopsy, the skin is raised as a fold and cut with the blade parallel to the skin surface. This method has the advantage of leaving the lower portion of the dermis intact so that, immediately afterwards, lesions such as basal cell carcinomas can be fully removed by curettage with or without electrodesiccation. Aluminum chloride is recommended for

R. Elenitsas: Department of Dermatology, University of Pennsylvania, Philadelphia, PA
A. C. Halpern: Department of Dermatology, University of Pennsylvania, Philadelphia, PA

hemostasis; Monsel's solution and electrocautery are alternatives, but they may affect the interpretation of subsequent biopsies or reexcisions.[2]

Curettage is the least satisfactory method of obtaining material for histologic examination, because the submitted material usually is scanty and superficial; it has lost its architecture and may show crush artifact. Even if this method is performed well, fragmentation and distortion cannot be avoided. Curettage of a melanoma that clinically resembles a seborrheic keratosis or pigmented basal cell carcinoma can be alarming and may prevent accurate diagnosis.

The biopsy specimen should be placed in fixative immediately on removal from the patient to prevent autolysis. It should not be allowed to dry, and the dermatologist should check the specimen bottle to ensure that the tissue has not adhered to the side of the bottle or remained inside the punch. As fixative, 10% buffered formalin can be used in nearly all instances (see Chap. 4). However, if the specimen is mailed in winter, 10% aqueous formalin, which freezes at −11°C, may allow formation of ice crystals in the specimen. This causes damage and distortion in the specimen, particularly in epithelial cells, and makes adequate histologic evaluation impossible. Freezing can be prevented by the addition to the formalin of 95% ethyl alcohol, 10% by volume. An alternative is to let the specimen stand in the formalin solution at room temperature for at least 6 hours before mailing.

Previous biopsies, specific requests (e.g., step sections for a hair follicle), and special handling should be indicated on the requisition sheet sent to the laboratory with the specimen. If, for instance, a stain for lipids is to be carried out, the specimen must not be processed in the automatic processor (see Chap. 4). Handling of biopsies for immunofluorescence is discussed in Chapter 4. The histopathologist's ability to render an accurate diagnosis often depends on the available clinical information. Every specimen submitted for histologic diagnosis should be accompanied by detailed clinical information, including a differential diagnosis. Clinicopathologic correlation is the key to providing optimal patient care.

REFERENCES

1. Headington JT. Transverse microscopic anatomy of the human scalp. Arch Dermatol 1984;120:449.
2. Olmstead PM, Lund HZ, Leonard DD. Monsel's solution: A histologic nuisance. J Am Acad Dermatol 1980;3:492.

Lever's Histopathology of the Skin, eighth edition,
edited by David Elder et al. Lippincott–
Raven Publishers, Philadelphia © 1997.

CHAPTER 3

Histology of the Skin

George F. Murphy

An understanding of the normal histology of the skin is central to an understanding of all that is termed *cutaneous pathology*. The journey to define the normal histology of human skin is a relatively short one in terms of spatial dimensions. From an en face view of the skin surface, characterized by desquamating scale, furrows, and evidence of adnexal growth, to the normal ultrastructure of key organelles within underlying cellular constituents, we span a magnification range of no more than 10^5 (a range of greater than 35 powers of 10 separates the distance from the first celestial impression of our Milky Way Galaxy to the realm of subatomic particles here on planet Earth).[1] And yet, the histology of the skin is amazingly complex. Divided into two seemingly separate but functionally interdependent layers (epidermis and dermis), skin is composed of cells with myriad functions, including mechanical protection and photoprotection, immunosurveillance, nutrient metabolism, and repair.

The epidermal layer is composed primarily of keratinocytes (>90%), with minority populations of Langerhans cells, melanocytes, neuroendocrine (Merkel) cells, and unmyelinated axons. Architecturally, the epidermal layer has an undulant undersurface in two-dimensional sections, with downward invaginations termed *rete*, and interdigitating mesenchymal cones termed *dermal papillae* (not to be confused with follicular papillae of the hair bulb). In actuality, three-dimensional reconstruction reveals that epidermal retia form a honeycomb of interconnected ridges, with dermal papillae representing rounded conical invaginations not dissimilar to the undersurface of an egg carton. Separated from the epidermis by a structurally and chemically complex basement membrane zone, the dermis consists of endothelial and neural cells and supporting elements, fibroblasts, dendritic and nondendritic monocytes and macrophages, and mast cells enveloped within a matrix of collagen and glycosaminoglycan. Adnexa extend from the epidermis into the dermis and consist of specialized cells for hair growth, epithelial renewal (stem cells), and temperature regulation. The subcutis is an underlying cushion formed by cells engorged with lipid and nourished by vessels that grow within thin intervening septa.

G. F. Murphy: Herman Beerman Professor of Dermatology and Professor of Dermatopathology; Director of Dermatopathology, Department of Dermatology, University of Pennsylvania

KERATINOCYTES OF THE EPIDERMIS

Embryology

The developmental anatomy of skin is important not only in understanding the basis for mature structural and functional relationships, but also in terms of certain skin tumors that recapitulate embryologic cutaneous structure. The development of in utero skin biopsy techniques gives practical importance to an understanding of the normal evolutionary histology of fetal skin. The epidermis begins as a single layer of ectodermal cells.[2,3] By 5 weeks of gestational age, this has differentiated at least focally into two layers, the basal layer or statum germinativum and the overlying periderm, and by 10 weeks an intervening layer, the stratum intermedium, develops (Fig. 3-1). Cells forming the periderm are large, bulge from the epidermal surface, and are bathed in amniotic fluid. By 19 weeks, there are several layers of intermediate cells and the periderm has begun to flatten (Figs. 3-1 and 3-2). Keratinization is well developed by 23 weeks within the stratum intermedium, and there are small keratohyaline granules. At this juncture, most of the periderm cells have shed, and the keratinizing cells that remain beneath represent the newly formed stratum corneum.[3]

The ultrastructural histogenesis of the epidermis involves the early formation of immature desmosomes and early hemidesmosomes, and a distinct basement membrane (6 to 7 weeks of gestational age).[4,5] Anchoring filaments are observed several weeks later, and the basement membrane appears structurally mature by the end of the first trimester.[6] The surface cells of the periderm display numerous microvilli and cytoplasmic microvesicles, increasing the area in contact with amniotic fluid and suggesting active interchange between the periderm cells and the amniotic fluid.[2] Tonofilaments are sparse until 16 weeks, when dense accumulations are observed in cells of the intermediate layer, evidence of beginning keratinization.[3]

Normal Microanatomy

Two types of cells constitute the epidermis: keratinocytes and dendritic cells. The keratinocytes differ from the dendritic cells, or clear cells, by possessing intercellular bridges and

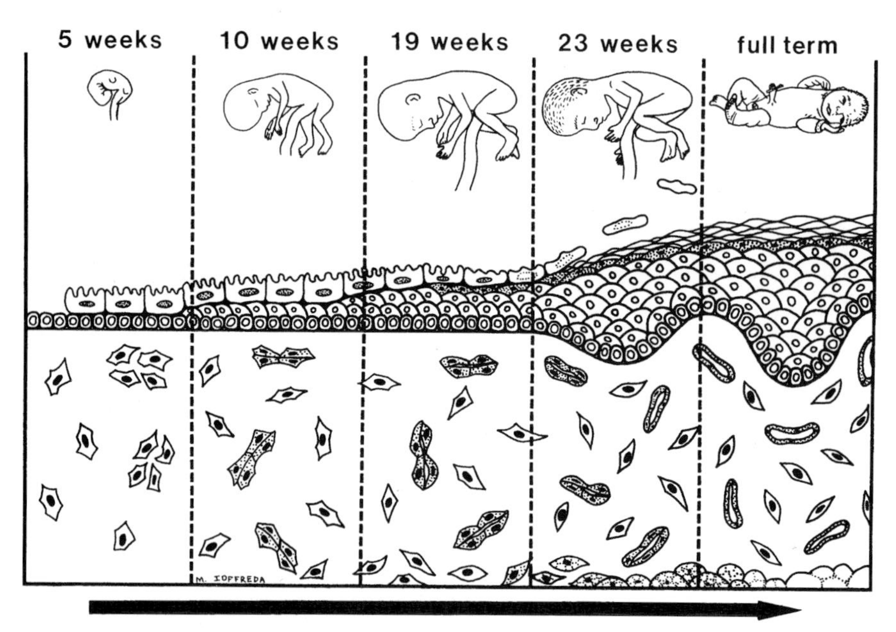

FIG. 3-1. Schematic overview of embryonic development of human skin
(Courtesy of Dr. Michael Ioffreda.)

ample amounts of stainable cytoplasm. As they differentiate into horny cells, the keratinocytes are arranged in four layers: the basal cell layer (stratum basalis), the squamous cell layer (stratum spinosum), the granular layer (stratum granulosum), and the horny layer (stratum corneum) (Fig. 3-3). The terms *stratum malpighii* and *rete malpighii* are often applied to the three lower layers, which contain the basal, squamous, and granular cells and constitute the nucleated, viable epidermis. An additional layer, the stratum lucidum, can be recognized in areas that have a thick stratum granulosum and corneum forming the lowest portion of the horny layer, especially on the palms and soles.

Stratum Basalis

The basal cells form a single layer, are columnar, and lie with their long axes perpendicular to the dividing line between the epidermis and the dermis. They have a more basophilic cytoplasm than cells of the stratum spinosum that parallels skin color, and contain a dark-staining oval or elongated nucleus. They often contain melanin pigment transferred from adjacent melanocytes. The extent and distribution of this pigment correlates with skin color (Fig. 3-4). Basal cells are connected with each other and with the overlying squamous cells by intercellu-

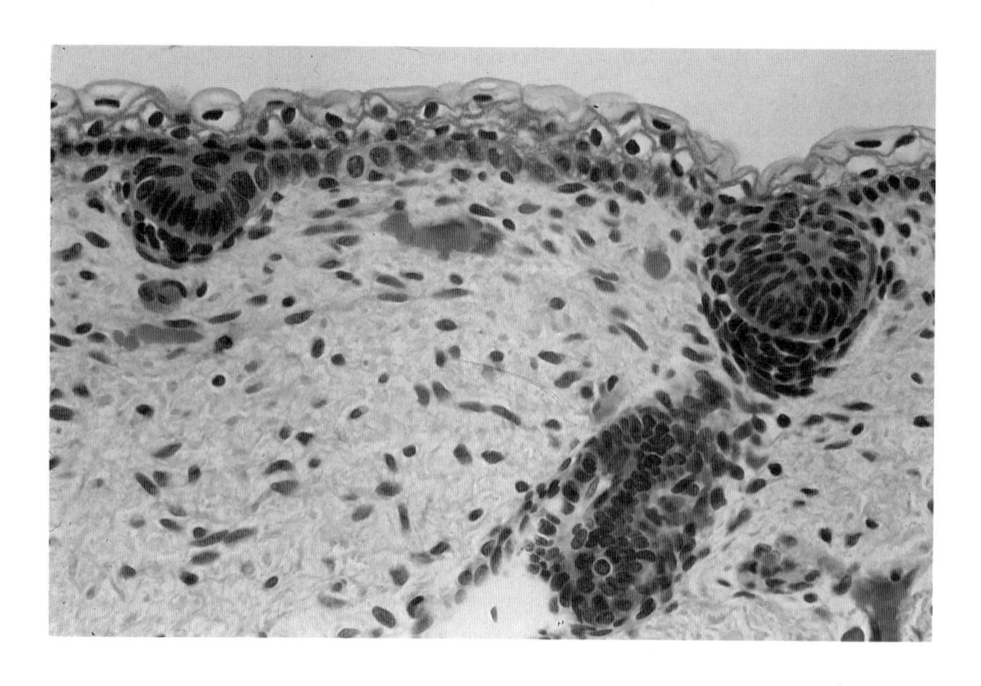

FIG. 3-2. Histology of epidermis, dermis, and forming follicles of 18-week normal human fetal skin

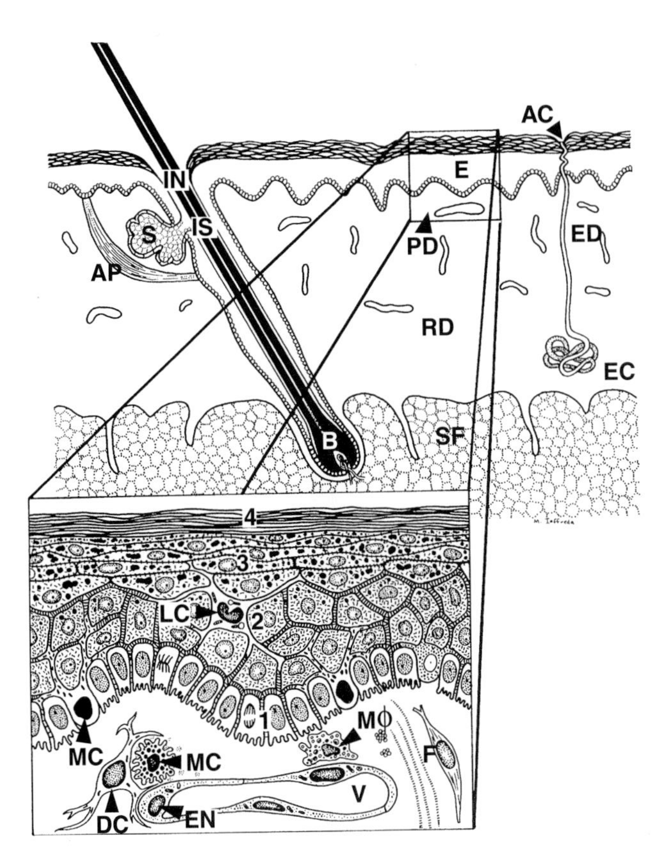

FIG. 3-3. Schematic overview of the architecture and cytologic constituents of normal human skin
Projection demonstrates cellular components of epidermis and superficial dermis in greater detail, with epidermal strata denoted numerically *(1,* stratum basalis; *2,* stratum spinosum; *3,* stratum granulosum; *4,* stratum corneum). *E,* epidermis; *PD,* papillary dermis; *RD,* reticular dermis; *SF,* subcutaneous fat; *LC,* Langerhans cell; *M,* melanocyte; *IN,* follicular infundibulum; *IS,* follicular isthmus; *B,* follicular bulb; *AP,* arrector pili muscle; *S,* sebaceous gland; *AC,* eccrine acrosyringium; *ED,* dermal eccrine duct; *EC,* coil of eccrine gland; *V,* vessel; *EN,* endothelial cell; *MC,* mast cell; *Mϕ,* macrophage; *DC,* perivascular dendritic cell; *F,* fibroblast with adjacent extracellular matrix. (Courtesy of Dr. Michael Ioffreda.)

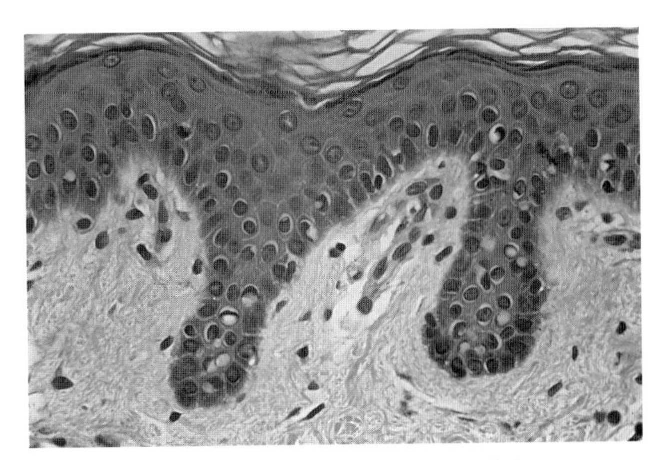

FIG. 3-4. Histology of normal human epidermis and upper dermis (arm skin)

lar bridges or desmosomes (discussed in detail later). At their base, the basal cells are attached to the subepidermal basement membrane zone by modified desmosomes, termed *hemidesmosomes.* Basal cells and overlying squamous cells contain keratin intermediate filaments termed *tonofilaments,* which form the developing cytoskeleton.

Most of the mitotic activity in normal epidermis occurs in the basal cell layer. Even mitoses that appear to be located at a level above the basal cell layer often are found on serial sectioning to be in juxtaposition with a dermal papilla and thus to represent basal cells.[6] A more efficient method of determining the location of proliferating cells in the human epidermis consists of either the intradermal injection of tritiated thymidine in vivo or the incubation of skin slices with tritiated thymidine in vitro (Fig. 3-5). This method labels all cells in the S phase of DNA synthesis, which is approximately 7 times longer than the mitotic or M phase. Thus many more tritiated-thymidine–labeled cells can be visualized than mitoses. With the labeling method, 45% of the labeled cells in normal human epidermis were found in one study to be suprabasal in location; however, after the examination of tracings of serial sections, the corrected value was 32%.[7] Accordingly, the germinative cell population in normal human epidermis is not exclusively within the stratum basalis. In palm skin of nonhuman primates, populations of mitotically quiescent basal cells have been described that retain pulsed thymidine labels in contrast to actively dividing cells, where dilution of label occurs. These cells reside at tips of epidermal rete ridges and have characteristics of stem cells.[8] Recent studies have defined similar populations in the bulge region of the hair follicle.[9]

Stratum Spinosum

The polyhedral cells of the stratum overlying the basal cell layer form a mosaic usually 5 to 10 layers thick. They become flattened toward the surface, with their long axes arranged par-

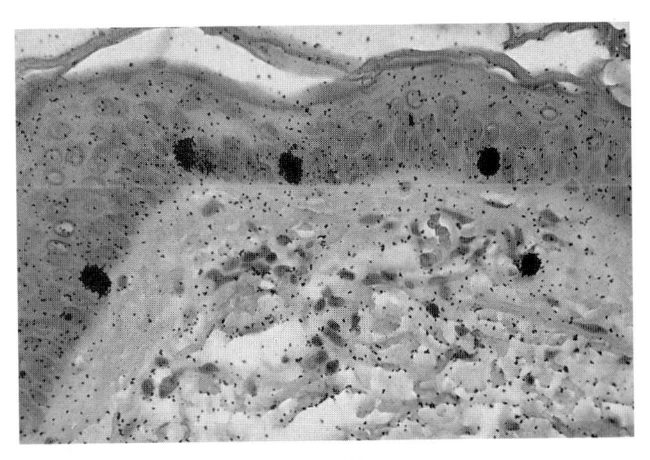

FIG. 3-5. Autoradiogram of skin
Note incorporation of tritiated thymidine into nuclei exhibiting S-phase activity within the basal cell layer as well as within a single dermal cell. (Courtesy of Robert Lavker, Ph.D.)

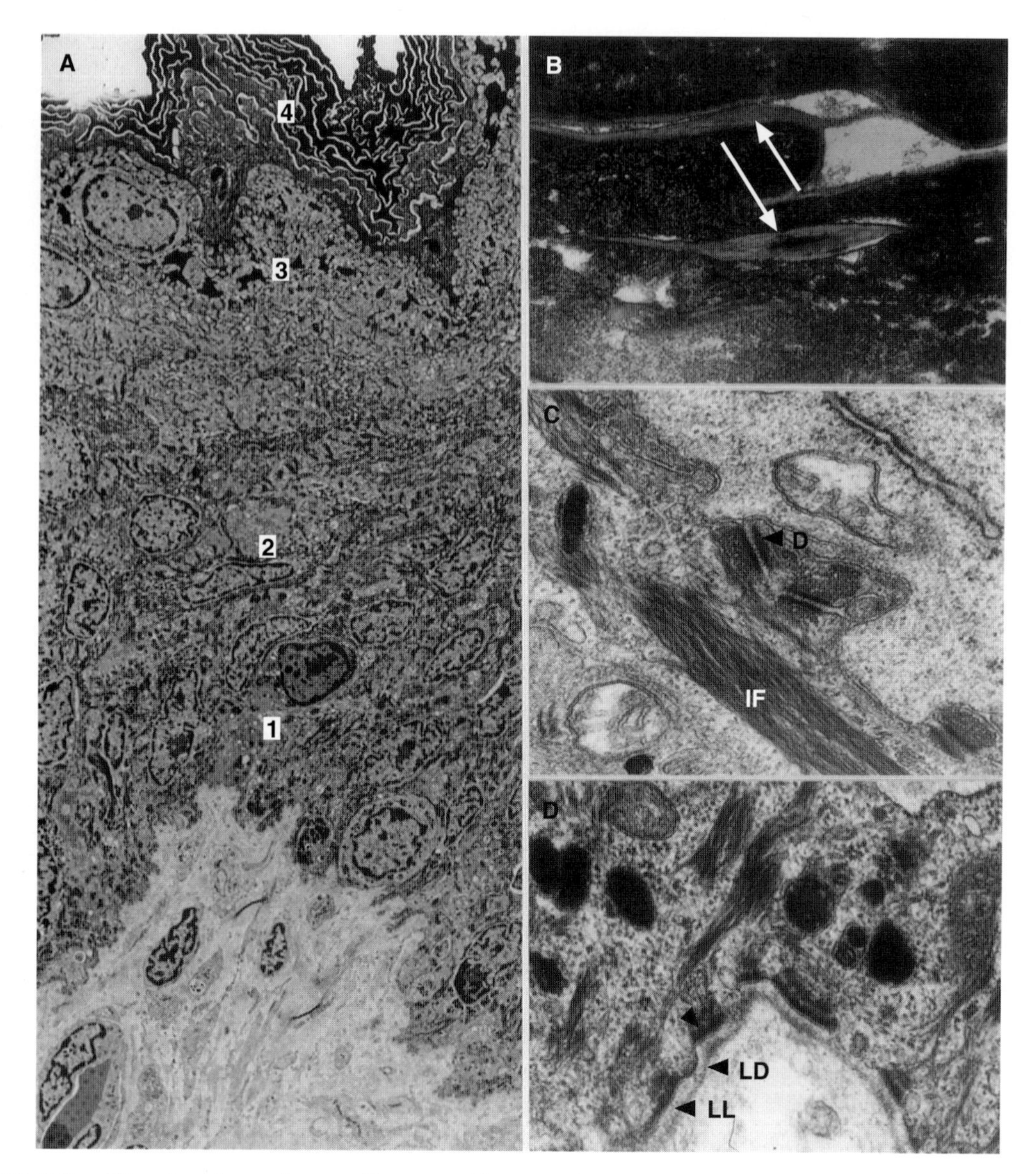

FIG. 3-6. Ultrastructure of normal human skin
(**A**) Overview of full-thickness epidermis and superficial papillary dermis, showing progressive accumulation of tonofilaments with upward maturation and keratohyaline granules within the layer directly beneath the stratum corneum (*1,* stratum basalis; *2,* stratum spinosum; *3,* stratum granulosum; *4,* stratum corneum). (**B**) Stratum corneum with lamellar granules (*arrows*). (**C**) Stratum spinosum with intermediate filaments (*IF*) and desmosomes (*D*). (**D**) Stratum basalis with transferred melanosomes (*M*) within keratinocyte cytoplasm, hemidesmosomes (*HD*), and basement membrane zone showing lamina lucida (*LL*), and lamina densa (*LD*).

allel to the skin surface (Figs. 3-4 and 3-6). The cells are separated by spaces that are transversed by intercellular bridges. These intercellular spaces stain slightly with the PAS stain and with alcian blue and colloidal iron, suggesting that they contain neutral mucopolysaccharides and acid mucopolysaccharides (glycosaminoglycans). Pretreatment with hyaluronidase largely prevents staining with colloidal iron, indicating that hyaluronic acid is an important component of the glycosaminoglycans.[10]

The tonofilaments within the cytoplasm of the keratinocytes of the stratum spinosum are loose bundles of electron-dense filaments (see Fig. 3-6), each filament measuring 7 to 8 nm in diameter. The tonofilaments at one end are attached to the attachment plaque of a desmosome, and the other end lies free in the cytoplasm near the nucleus. The desmosomes correlate with the intercellular bridges. Each desmosome possesses two electron-dense attachment plaques, one at either end, that are located in the cytoplasm of the two keratinocytes connected by the desmosome (see Fig. 3-6). Next to each attachment plaque lies the trilaminar plasma membrane of the two keratinocytes. Each trilaminar plasma membrane is 8 nm thick and consists of two electron-dense lines, called the *inner* and the *outer leaflets*, enclosing an electron-lucent line. In the center of the desmosome lies the intercellular cement substance, which shows greatest electron density in the portion directly adjoining the outer leaflet of the trilaminar plasma membrane representing the cell surface coat.[11] The cell surface coat often cannot be separated visually from the outer leaflet, and the two components have been referred to also as the *intermediate dense layer*.[12] The remaining central portion of the intercellular cement appears electron-lucent, except for a thin electron-dense line exactly in the center of the intercellular cement and the desmosome called the *intercellular contact layer*.[11] The irregular location of the desmosomes shows that the plasma membrane of keratinocytes is remarkably convoluted.

The intercellular cement substance between two adjacent keratinocytes, referred to also as *glycocalyx*, contains glycoproteins, which are stainable in vivo and in vitro with ruthenium red and with lanthanum. Staining with either of these agents often results in greater electron density along the cell surface than in the center of the intercellular space because of a higher concentration of cement substance there as cell surface coat.[13] The fact that the intercellular cement substance has a gel-like consistency explains why it on the one hand provides cohesion between the epidermal cells and on the other hand allows the rapid passage of water-soluble substances such as ruthenium red through the intercellular spaces and, furthermore, allows the opening up of desmosomes and individual cell movement.[14]

Recent studies have begun to establish the molecular basis for keratinocyte-keratinocyte adhesion within the stratum spinosum and other epidermal layers. A key family of molecules is the cadherins, derived from multiple genes and representing Ca^{++} dependent cell adhesion molecules with a characteristic single-spanning transmembrane structure.[15] Desmosomal cadherins are desmogleins and desmocollins[16] that localize to desmosomes and are linked to intracytoplasmic intermediate filaments by plakoglobin and desmoplakin. Within the desmosome complex, desmogleins within the cell membrane bind to plakoglobin through their cytoplasmic domain. Intermediate keratin filaments anchor at the desmosomal plaque, possibly by way of the carboxy-terminal domain of plakoglobin. The structural importance of these molecules in uniting keratinocyte cytoskeletons within the epidermis is indicated by the disorders pemphigus vulgaris and pemphigus foliaceus, where autoantibodies to members of the desmoglein subfamily of the cadherin supergene family result in clinical blisters due to loss of cell-cell adherence (acantholysis).[17,18]

Stratum Granulosum

The cells of the granular cell layer are flattened and their cytoplasm is filled with keratohyaline granules that are deeply basophilic and irregular in size and shape. These granules are also obvious by electron microscopy in the uppermost epidermal layers of panel A of Fig. 3-6. The thickness of the granular layer in normal skin is generally proportional to the thickness of the horny layer: it is only one to three cell layers thick in areas in which the horny layer is thin but measures up to ten layers in areas with a thick horny layer, such as the palms and soles (Fig. 3-7). There often is an inverse relationship between the presence and thickness of the granular cell layer and parakeratosis (e.g., psoriasis, where extensive parakeratosis is associated with a markedly attenuated to absent stratum granulosum).

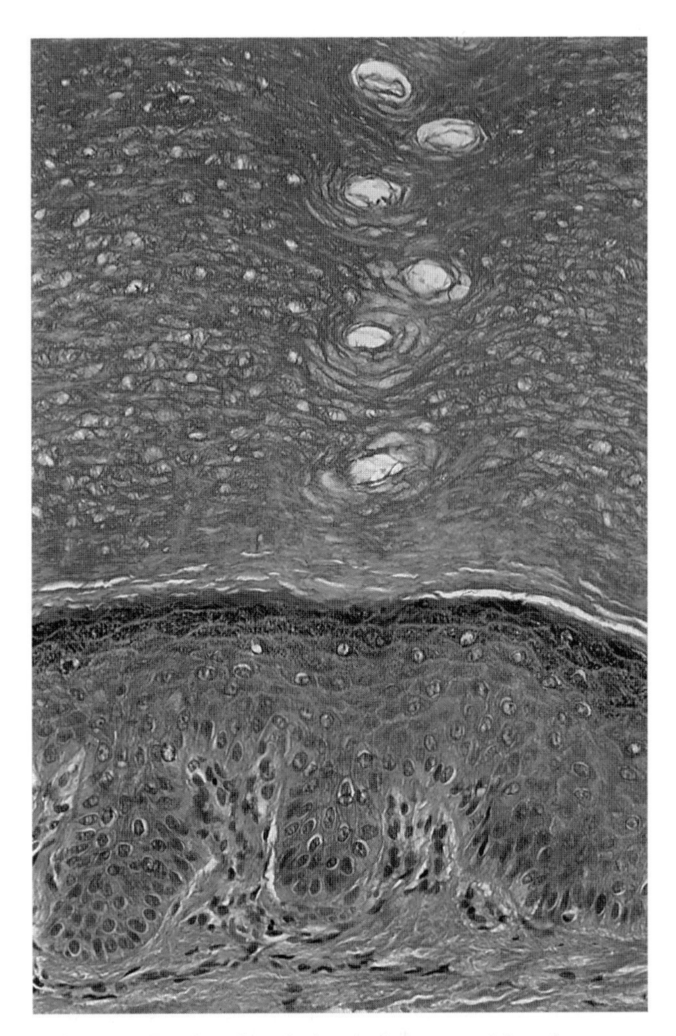

FIG. 3-7. Regional variation in human epidermis
Skin from plantar aspect of foot.

In the process of keratinization, the keratohyaline granules form two structures: the interfibrillary matrix or filaggrin, which cements the keratin filaments together, and the inner lining of the horny cells, the so-called marginal band. Whereas the tonofibrils contain only small amounts of sulfur as sulfhydryl groups, the interfibrillary matrix and the marginal band contain about 10 times the amount of sulfur that is present in the tonofibrils, predominantly as disulfide bonds of cystine.[19,20] Consequently, the tonofibrils are soft and flexible, while the matrix and marginal band provide necessary strength and stability.[20] Thus, the keratin of the epidermis represents "soft" keratin, in contrast to the "hard" keratin of the hair and nails, in which keratohyaline granules are lacking and the tonofibrils themselves harden through the incorporation of disulfide bonds.[21] "Soft" keratin desquamates as the result of enzymatic action, but the "hard" keratin of the hair and nails does not, thus requiring periodic cutting.

The granular cell layer represents the keratogenous zone of the epidermis, in which the dissolution of the nucleus and other cell organelles is prepared. In contrast to the stratum basalis and stratum spinosum, in which lysosomal enzymes, such as acid

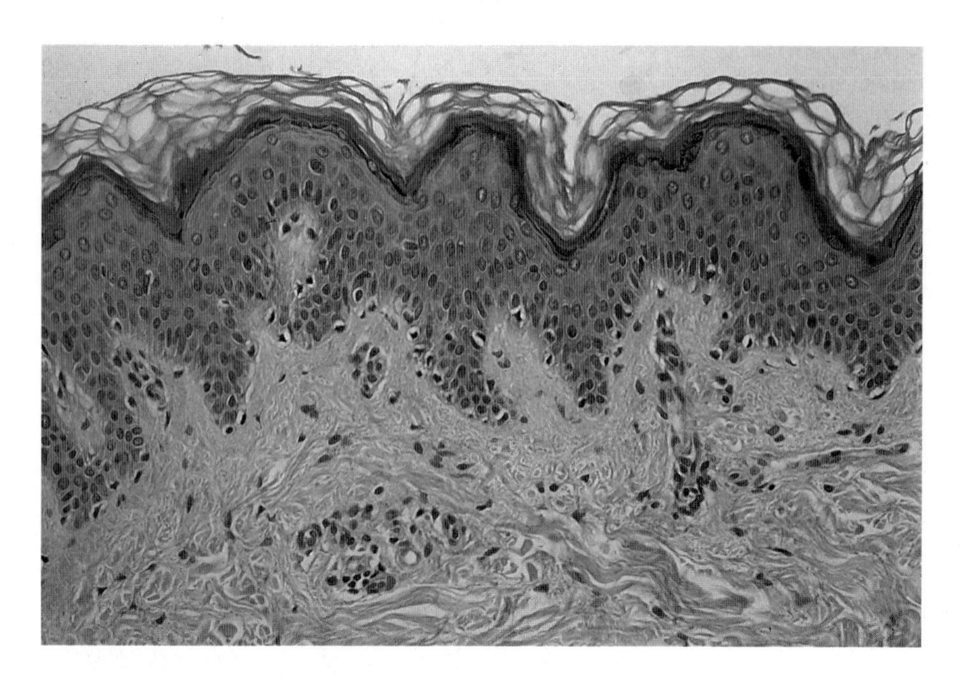

FIG. 3-8. Regional variation in human epidermis
Skin from elbow region.

phosphatase and arylsulfatase, are present as only a few granular aggregates, there is diffuse staining for lysosomal enzymes in the granular cell layer. These diffusely staining lysosomal enzymes probably play an important role in the autolytic changes occurring in the granular layer.[22]

Stratum Corneum

Unlike the nucleated cells of the other epidermal layers that have been discussed, the cells of the normal stratum corneum are anucleate, and thus are technically dead. Thus the horny layer stains eosinophilic as a result of omission of basophilic nuclei. The thickness of the horny layer is often difficult to ascertain in formalin-fixed specimens because some of the outer cell layers frequently detach themselves. Most of the horny layer is apt to show a basket-weave pattern in formalin-fixed specimens because of the presence of large intracellular spaces. These spaces are the result of inadequate fixation of soluble constituents within the horny cells by the formalin and the subsequent removal of these constituents by water, ethanol, and xylene during histologic processing. Thus the portion of the cytoplasm that contains disulfide bonds of cystine has shrunk to form a shell along the cell membrane.[23] In contrast, glutaraldehyde fixation used for electron microscopy causes precipitation of the formalin-soluble substances within the horny cells and allows staining of the contents of the horny cells with stains such as uranyl acetate and lead citrate. With a fluorescent stain it can be shown that the cells of the horny layer are arranged in orderly vertical stacks.[24]

In certain formalin-fixed sections the lowest portion of the stratum corneum appears after processing and staining as a thin homogeneous eosinophilic zone, referred to as the *stratum lucidum*. This zone is most pronounced in areas in which the horny layer is thick, especially on the palms and soles. The stratum lucidum differs histochemically from the rest of the horny layer by being rich in protein-bound lipids contained in the Odland bodies (see text following). It also has been called the stratum conjunctum, in contrast to the overlying stratum disjunctum with its basket-weave pattern.[23]

Regional Variation

The epidermal layer may vary considerably from one body site to the next. Whereas the epidermis of the eyelid, axilla, knee, and elbow all show a slightly verrucous architecture (Fig. 3-8), eyelid epidermis gives rise to numerous vellus hair follicles, and axilla to apocrine glands. Acral skin demonstrates progressive thickening and compaction of the stratum corneum with progression from dorsal to ventral surfaces; nose skin displays prominent, closely packed sebaceous lobules; and scalp skin gives rise to anagen follicles with bulbs that descend deeply into subcutaneous fat. Recognition of these regional variations is essential to avoiding a misdiagnosis of pathology in otherwise normal skin.

Mucosal Epithelium

Skin shows considerable variation among different body sites, and appreciation of such normal differences is critical to accurate diagnostic assessment. Perhaps the most profound differences exist at mucosal and paramucosal sites. For example, with the exception of the dorsum of the tongue and the hard palate, the mucous membrane of the mouth possesses neither a granular nor a horny layer. Where these layers are absent, the epithelial cells in their migration from the basal layer to the surface first appear vacuolated, largely as a result of their glycogen content, then shrink, and finally desquamate. Electron microscopic examination reveals poor development of tonofilaments. The number of tonofilaments diminishes in the upper layers, and they become dispersed. Large aggregates of glycogen are present in the cells. The epithelial cells of the oral mucosa show only few well-developed desmosomes. Instead, they show numerous microvilli at their borders. They are held together by an amorphous, moderately electron-dense intercellular cement substance, the resolution of which causes the detachment of the uppermost cells.[25]

Specialized Structure and Function

Superficial Cellular Cohesion

The number of tonofilaments increases in the upper protion of the squamous layer. The earliest formation of keratohyaline granules consists of the aggregation of electron-dense ribonucleoprotein particles largely along tonofilaments (see Fig. 3-6). The keratohyaline granules increase in size through peripheral aggregation of ribonucleoprotein particles, and they surround more and more tonofilaments.[26] By extending along numerous tonofilaments, the keratohyaline granules assume an irregular, often star-shaped outline and may reach a size of 1 to 2 μm. After ultimately ensheathing all tonofilaments, they form in the horny cells the electron-dense interfilamentous protein matrix of mature epidermal keratin. Keratohyaline granules are biochemically complex. One component is a histidine-rich protein called *filaggrin precursor*.[27] When granular cells are converted to cornified cells, filaggrin precursor is broken down into many units of filaggrin. Filaggrin then aggregates with keratin filaments and acts as a "glue" for keratin filaments.

Terminal Differentiation

The transformation of granular cells into horny cells usually is abrupt. Fixation with glutaraldehyde and osmium tetroxide as used for electron microscopy preserves the internal structure of horny cells (see Fig. 3-6B), in contrast to formalin fixation for light microscopy. By electron microscopy, the cytoplasm of the cells in the lower portion of the horny layer shows relatively electron-lucent tonofilaments, about 8 nm thick, embedded in an interfilamentous substance having the same high degree of electron density as the keratohyaline granules.[28] In the upper portions of the horny layer, however, the cells lose their filamentous structure. Together with the sudden keratinization of the horny cells, an electron-dense, homogeneous marginal band forms in their peripheral cytoplasm in close approximation to the trilaminar plasma membrane. When fully developed, the marginal band measures 16 nm thick, compared with 8 nm for the trilaminar plasma membrane. In the lowermost horny layer the trilaminar plasma membrane is preserved outside the marginal band; in the midportion of the horny layer it becomes discontinuous and then desquamates so that the marginal band serves as the real cell membrane.[25] In the uppermost portion of the horny layer, even the marginal band often disappears concomitant with the degeneration and desquamation of the horny cells. Immunohistochemistry reveals that involucrin, a structural component of mature squamous epithelium, is incorporated into the marginal band as part of the formation of the protein envelope that characterizes squamous cells immediately prior to terminal differentiation.[29] Desmosomal contacts are at first still present in the horny layer but disappear before desquamation of the horny cells.

Barrier Function

Odland bodies, also called membrane-coating granules, lamellar granules, and keratinosomes, are small organelles that are discharged from the granular cells into the intercellular space. They have two important functions: they establish a barrier to water loss, and they mediate stratum corneum cell cohesion. Lamellar granules appear first in the perinuclear cytoplasm in the stratum spinosum. Higher up in the epidermis, they rapidly increase in number and size.[30] Both within and outside the granular cells, lamellar granules are round or oval, measure approximately 300 to 500 nm in diameter, and possess a trilaminar membrane and a laminated interior. The lamellar granules fuse with the plasma membrane of a granular cell, secreting their contents into the intercellular spaces.[31] They contain neutral sugars linked to lipids and/or proteins; hydrolytic enzymes, possibly charged with degrading intercellular materials; and free sterols. The stratum granulosum interstices contain free sterols and sugars; the stratum corneum intercellular spaces stain as a pure neutral lipid mixture with abundant free sterols but no sugars.[31] Sugars are cleaved at the granular-cornified layer interface by sugar-specific glycosidases.

An indication that the lamellar granules contribute to the physiologic water barrier was observed by Schreiner and Wolff in 1969.[32] When these investigators injected intradermally in vivo a solution of horseradish peroxidase as an electron microscopic tracer protein, they found that it penetrated the basement membrane and the intercellular spaces of the epidermis up to the upper portion of the granular layer, where lamellar granules block the intercellular spaces. Conclusive evidence was provided by Elias and colleagues,[33] who showed by freeze-fracture techniques that the lamellar granules fuse and completely fill the intercellular spaces at the level of the granular layer. They concluded that the lipids formed in these organelles act as hydrophobic material, which is important to the barrier function. A similar permeability barrier exists in the oral mucosa. Lamellar granules may also contribute to cohesion between the cells of the lower stratum corneum as a result of the lipids that they contain. The action of enzymes, such as steroid sulfatase, removes the lipids from the upper stratum corneum and brings about desquamation of the cells there.[34]

Enzyme Activity

Primary lysosomes that are membrane-bound and contain a variety of hydrolytic enzymes, such as acid phosphatase, arylsulfatase, and β-galactosidase, are seen in small numbers within keratinocytes, largely but not exclusively in the basal cell layer and lower squamous cell layer.[13] These primary lysosomes are seen in the Golgi area, where they arise, and elsewhere in the cytoplasm. A great number of lysosomal enzymes is demonstrable in the granular layer and in the lowermost horny layer. However, on electron microscopic examination, only a very small proportion of these lysosomal enzymes is seen inside of primary lysosomes; most of the lysosomal enzymes are found free in the cytoplasm as irregularly shaped aggregates that are not membrane-bound.[35] Lysosomal enzymes are found also in the lamellar granules, both while located within granular cells and after their discharge into the intercellular space.[36] In addition to primary lysosomes, some secondary lysosomes, also called *phagolysosomes*, are present in the lower epidermis, especially in the basal cells. They digest phagocytized melanosomes, usually as melanosome complexes (see text following). In cases of epidermal injury, such as sunburn or contact dermatitis, numerous phagosomes containing cellular organelles are present in the keratinocytes, which, as the result of the influx of lysosomal enzymes from primary lysosomes, become phagolysosomes.[36]

Immune Functions of Keratinocytes

In recent years, the epidermal keratinocyte has been recognized as a potent source of immunogenic molecules. Although the list is ever increasing, keratinocytes are capable of producing interleukins (IL-1α, IL-1β, IL-6, IL-8); colony-stimulating factors (IL-3, GM-CSF, G-CSF, M-CSF); interferons (IFN-α, IFN-β); tumor necrosis factors (TNF-α); transforming growth factors (TGF-α, TGF-β); and growth factors (platelet-derived growth factor, fibroblast growth factor).[37] Some of these substances are expressed constitutively, whereas others are synthesized only after signal transduction initiated by external or systemic cues.[38] Accordingly, keratinocytes may play an active role in the elaboration of molecular signals that facilitate leukocyte homing and local activation, enabling certain dermal cells to mature, and in regulating synthesis of extracellular matrix molecules. Because basal keratinocytes may be more potent producers and secretors of certain immunogenic molecules than more superficial epidermal cells, one must rethink the concept of keratinocyte maturation generally derived from efficiency of keratin synthesis.

MELANOCYTES

Embryology

The appearance of melanocytes in the epidermis takes place in a craniocaudal direction, in accordance with the development of the neural crest, from which the melanocytes are derived. By use of light microscopy on sections that have been treated with impregnation by Masson's ammoniated silver nitrate technic or exposed to the dopa reaction, melanocytes can be identified in the epidermis of the head region during the latter part of the third fetal month; in the more caudal body regions, the earliest formed melanin can be observed only in the latter part of the fourth month. Because melanocytes are functionally immature during their migration through the fetal dermis, they cannot be identified by histochemical methods until they have reached the epidermis.[39] Electron microscopy allows an earlier recognition of melanocytes in the epidermis than is possible by light microscopy. Melanocytes with recognizable melanosomes may be seen in the fetal epidermis at a gestational age of 8 to 10 weeks,[40] and using immunohistochemistry for HMB-45 protein, by 50 days estimated gestational age.[41] Synthesis of melanin within the melanosomes occurs on the head in the latter part of the third month and elsewhere in the fourth month.

Normal Microanatomy

In sections stained with hematoxylin-eosin, melanocytes appear as randomly dispersed cells within the basal cell layer having a small, dark-staining nucleus and, largely as the result of shrinkage, a clear cytoplasm. They are found wedged between the basal cells of the epidermis. Although the number of melanocytes in relation to basal cells varies with the body region and increases with repeated exposure to ultraviolet light, the average number of clear cells in hematoxylin-eosin–stained vertical sections is 1 of 10 cells in the basal layer.[42] However, not all clear cells seen in routine sections necessarily are melanocytes; occasionally, basal keratinocytes show the same shrinkage artifact and are indistinguishable from melanocytes.[43] Melanin is transferred by means of the dendritic processes from the melanocytes to the basal keratinocytes, where it is first stored and later degraded. As a rule, a greater amount of melanin is present in the basal keratinocytes than in the melanocytes, and often basal cells at the tips of rete ridges are preferentially more melanized (see Fig. 3-4). Because only about 10% of the cells in the basal layer are melanocytes, each melanocyte supplies several keratinocytes with melanin, forming with them an epidermal melanin unit.[44]

In persons with a light skin color, staining with hematoxylin-eosin may reveal few or no melanin granules in the basal cell layer. In persons with a dark skin color, especially individuals of African heritage, melanin granules are present in the basal cell layer as well as throughout the epidermis, including the horny layer, and in some instances in the upper dermis within macrophages, called melanophages. Accordingly, ethnic background and body site are critical in separating normal variations from true pathology.

Special Stains

There are several special stains that facilitate the light microscopic visualization of melanocytes and their products. Silver stains indicate the presence of melanin, which is both argyrophilic and argentaffin. Argyrophilia is based on the ability of melanin to be impregnated with silver nitrate solutions, which, upon reduction with hydroquinone to silver, stains black. Because melanin is argentaffin, ammoniated silver nitrate may be reduced by phenolic groups in the melanin in the absence of an external reducing agent, forming black silver precipitate (Fontana-Masson method). Neither of these methods is entirely specific for melanin, however. Melanin may be bleached by strong oxidizing agents, such as hydrogen peroxide or potassium permanganate, a method that permits more specific identification[45] and is of use in heavily melanized tumors where pigment may obscure nuclear detail. The dopa reaction[46] is not of practical importance in routine diagnostic dermatopathology, but is instructive with regard to the biochemistry of melanization. Briefly, fresh, unfixed tissue sections or enzymatically separated epidermal sheets are incubated in a 0.01% solution of

3,4-dihydroxyphenylalanine (dopa),[47] staining melanocytes dark brown to black. The reaction imitates physiologic melanin formation, which begins by tyrosinase-dependent hydroxylation of tyrosine to dopa and the oxidation of dopa to dopaquinone, which is subsequently polymerized into melanin. Thus the dopa reaction is in essence an assay for tyrosine activity in melanosomes. Immunohistochemical detection of melanocytes is most commonly accomplished by antibodies to S-100 protein. This protein, originally isolated from bovine brain extract, is present in the cytoplasm of a variety of cells, including those of neural and melanocytic lineage. Specialized macrophages, some epithelial cells, and a variety of nonmelanocytic cell types contain S-100 protein. In human epidermis, only melanocytes, which tend to reside within the basal layer, and Langerhans cells, with cell bodies mostly within the midepidermis, are reactive. HMB-45 protein is a cytoplasmic antigen in cells of most but not all melanomas, in the junctional component of most nevi, and in the dermal component of some nevi (see Chap. 29). Activated and fetal melanocytes may be positive, but normal "resting" melanocytes are most often negative.

Ultrastructure

Melanocytes differ from keratinocytes by possessing no tonofilaments or desmosomes (Fig. 3-9). Typically they "hang" down into the superficial dermis, but like basal keratinocytes, they are separated from the extracellular dermal matrix by the basement membrane zone. At their base, where they lie in close apposition to the lamina densa, melanocytes show structures resembling the half-desmosomes of basal keratinocytes.[48] Each of these structures consists of a cytoplasmic dense plate attached to the inner leaflet of the trilaminar plasma membrane and, except for being slightly smaller, has the same appearance as the attachment plaque of a half-desmosome. Anchoring filaments extend from the outer leaflet of the plasma membrane to the lamina densa. However, there is no sub–basal cell dense plaque as in basal keratinocytes. Melanosomes are the most characteristic organelles of the melanocyte, and although they are commonly transferred to adjacent keratinocytes, identification of various stages of their formation within a cell assist in its ultrastructural identification as a melanocyte (see Fig. 3-9, inset). Melanosomes in their development from stage I to stage IV gradually move from the cytoplasm of the melanocyte into the dendritic processes. However, even in the dendritic processes, stage II melanosomes may be seen. As melanosomes mature, their content of melanin increases, and their concentration of melanogenic enzyme decreases.[49]

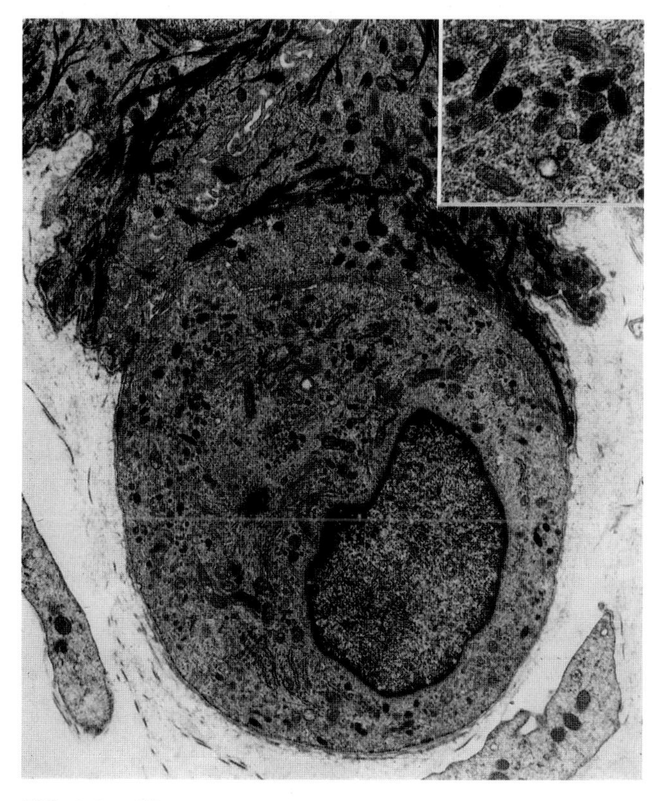

FIG. 3-9. Ultrastructure of human melanocyte
Inset depicts melanosomes in various stages of formation and melanization.

Stage I melanosomes are round, measure about 0.3 μm in diameter, and possess very intense enzyme activity concentrated along filaments. They contain no melanin.[50] Stage II melanosomes are ellipsoid and measure approximately 0.5 μm in length, as do the melanosomes of stages III and IV. They contain longitudinal filaments that are cross-linked with one another. Enzyme activity is present both on the enveloping membrane and on the filaments. Melanin deposition on the cross-linked filaments begins at this stage. Stage III melanosomes have only little tyrosinase activity but show continued melanin deposition, partially through nonenzymatic polymerization. Stage IV melanosomes no longer possess tyrosinase activity. Melanin, which is formed entirely by nonenzymatic polymerization, fills the entire organelle and obscures its internal structure.

Regional Variation

The density of melanocytes has been most precisely determined on biopsy specimens 4 mm in diameter where the epidermis is separated from the dermis by incubation of the specimen in a 2N solution of sodium bromide. The resultant epidermal sheet is treated with 1 : 1000 solution of dopa for 2 to 4 hours and then is fixed in formalin, cleared, and mounted.[47,51] It has thus been determined that the concentration of melanocytes in such epidermal sheets varies in different areas but is quite constant for any particular region. The highest concentration of melanocytes has been found on the face and the male genitals, about 2000/mm^2 melanocytes, and the lowest on the trunk, about 800/mm^2 melanocytes.[51,52] No significant difference in the density of distribution of melanocytes for any given area of the skin exists between darkly and lightly pigmented skin. In the former, the melanocytes are uniformly highly reactive, whereas the melanocytes of the latter, when not exposed to sunlight, are highly variable in dopa-reactivity.[53] In addition, African-American skin contains larger and more highly dendritic melanocytes than white skin.[51,52]

Regional variation of melanocyte number and morphology may also be influenced by environmental factors, such as sun exposure. After a single exposure to ultraviolet light in vivo, the skin of whites, when examined with the dopa reaction, shows no increase in the density of the melanocyte population but does show an increase in the size and functional activity of the exisiting melanocytes.[54] Repeated exposure to ultraviolet light, however, causes an increase in the concentration of dopa-positive melanocytes, as well as an increase in their size and functional activity.[53,55] Thus examination of habitually exposed and of unexposed skin from adjacent anatomic sites, such as the lateral and medial aspects of the upper arm, has shown a twofold higher concentration of melanocytes in the habitually exposed skin.[47] These studies are potentially relevant to the use of S-100 immunohistochemistry in determining subtle increases or decreases in melanocyte populations as compared to age- and site-matched normal skin.

Specialized Structure and Function

Melanogenesis

Enzymatic melanogenesis[52,56,57] involves tyrosinase as the melanogenic enzyme. Tyrosinase is a copper-containing enzyme that catalyzes the hydroxylation of tyrosine to dihydroxyphenylalanine (dopa) and the oxidation of dopa to dopaquinone. However, before tyrosinase can act on tyrosine, two cupric atoms present in tyrosinase must be reduced to cuprous atoms. It is believed that, in addition to being a substrate, dopa activates this reduction, thereby acting as a cofactor in the reaction. The conversion of tyrosine to melanin by tyrosinase is characterized by a variable lag period. When tyrosinase is present in low concentrations, as in epidermal melanocytes of nonirradiated skin, this lag period is markedly prolonged, and no use of tyrosine by tyrosinase is detectable. In contrast, in skin exposed in vivo to ultraviolet light,[44] as well as in epidermal sheets[58] and in hair bulbs,[57] tyrosinase activity is detectable with tyrosine as substrate. Because there is no lag period with dopa as substrate, tyrosinase in epidermal melanocytes can be readily demonstrated even in nonirradiated skin when skin sections are incubated in dopa rather than in tyrosine. The enzyme acting on dopa is therefore thought to be tyrosinase, rather than dopa-oxidase.

The melanogenic enzyme tyrosinase is synthesized in the Golgi-associated endoplasmic reticulum, in which tyrosinase condenses in membrane-limited vesicles. This process has been observed by electron microscopy in epidermal melanocytes after in vivo ultraviolet irradiation with either dopa or tyrosine as substrate.[59] Subsequently, these tyrosinase units are transferred to dilated tubules of the smooth endoplasmic reticulum. There, tyrosinase is incorporated into a structural protein matrix containing filaments that have a distinctive periodicity. This then represents a stage I melanosome.[60] Few stage I and II melanosomes have acid phosphatase activity, but the proportion of acid phosphatase–positive melanosomes increases in stage III, reaching a maximum in stage IV.[61] This enzyme may play a role in the degradation or transfer of melanosomes. Detailed analysis of nonmelanosomal regulatory factors in melanogensis has revealed coated vesicles to be richest in tyrosinase and catalase, whereas premelanosomes have the highest concentrations of peroxidase.[62] Among relevant metal ions, premelanosomes contain higher amounts of copper, zinc, and iron than coated vesicles.

Melanin Transfer

The transfer of melanosomes from melanocytes to epidermal keratinocytes and to hair cortex cells is the result of active phagocytosis of the tips of melanocytic dendrites by keratinocytes and hair cortex cells as demonstrated in tissue cultures[63] and in epidermal constructs seeded with melanocytes.[64] With electron microscopy, one can observe that pseudopod-like cytoplasmic projections of keratinocytes or hair cortex cells are wrapped around the tips of dendrites. After such a projection has completely enveloped the tip of a dendrite, it is pinched off. At first, the melanosomes in the pinched-off dendrite are separated from the cytoplasm of the keratinocyte by the plasma membranes of the dendrite and of the keratinocyte.[65] After the breakdown of these two plasma membranes, the melanosomes are dispersed throughout the cytoplasm of the keratinocyte. In the nonexposed skin of lightly pigmented individuals, such transferred melanosomes are found almost exclusively in the basal cell layer and, to a slight degree, in the layer of keratinocytes above the basal cell layer (see Fig. 3-9). However, in individuals of African heritage, in whom melanosomes are also principally seen in the basal cell layer, moderate quantities of melanosomes are found throughout the epidermis, including the stratum corneum.[66]

The melanosomes present in keratinocytes of white skin lie largely aggregated within membrane-bound melanosome complexes containing two or three melanosomes, and only a small proportion of melanosomes are singly dispersed. The melanosomes present within complexes often show signs of degeneration.[66,67] In contrast, in skin of African and Australian aborigine heritage, the great majority of melanosomes lie singly dispersed, and relatively few melanosome complexes are found.[66–68] The reason for the lack of aggregation of melanosomes in the latter racial groups seems to be their larger size. In whites, melanosomes range in length from 0.3 to 0.5 μm; in African Americans, they range in length from 0.5 to 0.8 μm.[69] Because the membrane-bound melanosome complexes show considerable acid phosphatase activity, it is clear that they represent phagolysosomes in which the melanosomes are being degraded.[70] Thus melanosomes appear to be removed more rapidly in white people than in individuals of African descent. It may be concluded that the difference in skin color is due to the following five factors: in racially heavily pigmented skin, (1) there is greater production of melanosomes in melanocytes, (2) individual melanosomes show a higher degree of melanization, (3) melanosomes are larger, as a consequence of which, (4) there is a higher degree of dispersion in the keratinocytes, and (5) there is a slower rate of degradation.[69] However, the predominant size of the melanosomes does not depend only on racial factors. Thus topical treatment of the skin with trimethylpsoralen followed by irradiation with ultraviolet A light leads to an increase in the size of melanosomes in whites.[71]

MERKEL CELLS

Embryology

Merkel cells arise between weeks 8 and 12 of gestational age from precursor stages of epithelial cells of early fetal epidermis that still express simple epithelial cytokeratins. In situ differentiation from epidermal ectoderm versus immigration of cells from the neural crest is supported by studies of fetal skin without Merkel cells transplanted to nude mice and subsequently found to contain mature Merkel cells within the engrafted tissue.[72] Some Merkel cells detach from the epidermis and migrate temporarily into the upper dermis, where some of them associate with small nerves. The numerous dense-cored neurosecretory granules that they contain are formed within them.

Normal Microanatomy

Merkel cells are present within the basal cell layer of the epidermis, in the oral mucosa, and in the bulge region of hair follicles.[73] They are quite scarce, are irregularly distributed, and are occasionally arranged in groups.[74] It is assumed that the Merkel cell is a touch receptor.[75] The Merkel cell cannot be recognized in light microscopic sections; however, in silver-impregnated sections, the meniscoid neural terminal that covers the basal portion of each Merkel cell can be seen as a Merkel disk.[76] A sensory nerve fiber terminates at the disk. Immunohistochemistry for cytokeratin species more typical of simple epithelial cells than keratinocytes permits a differential identification of Merkel cells in tissue sections.[77]

On electron microscopic examination, Merkel cells usually are located directly above the basement membrane (Fig. 3-10). They are quite easily recognized by electron microscopy, since they possess electron-dense granules, strands of intermediate filaments, and occasional desmosomes on their cell membranes connecting them with neighboring keratinocytes.[75] The electron-dense granules vary in size between 80 and 200 nm and are membrane-bound (see Fig. 3-10, inset). The filaments resemble tonofilaments and, like tonofilaments, are seen in some areas that converge upon desmosomes. In some sections, the Merkel disk can be seen above the basement membrane as a cushion on which the Merkel cell rests. It consists of a mitochondria-rich, nonmyelinated axon terminal.[74]

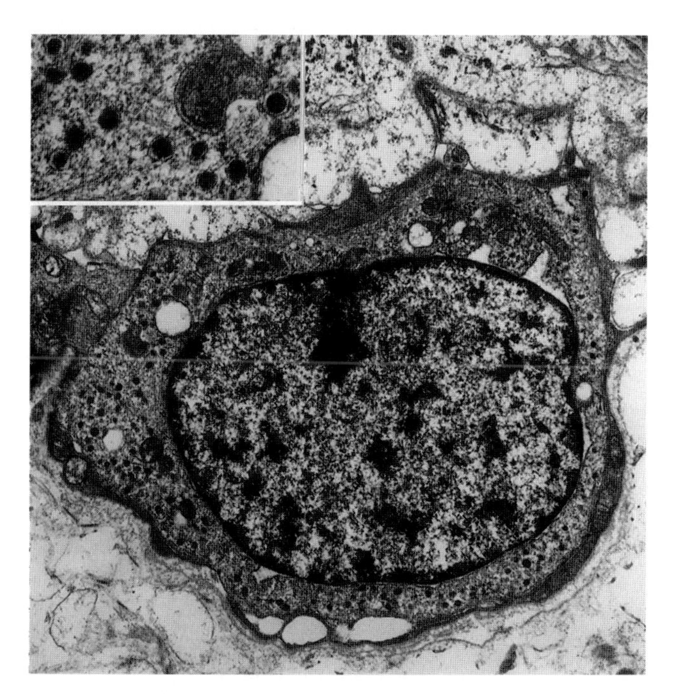

FIG. 3-10. Ultrastructure of human Merkel cell Inset depicts characteristic membrane-bound neurosecretory-type granules.

Regional Variation

Merkel cells are most heavily concentrated in skin with high hair density and in glabrous epithelium of the digits and lips, regions of the oral cavity, and in the outer root sheath of the hair follicle. These cells are present in mammals as so-called touch-domes, also known as *Haarscheiben,* a form of type I mechanoreceptor that surrounds tylotrich hairs and the rete ridge collars about external root sheaths of hair follicles.

Specialized Structure and Function

Merkel cells are specialized epithelial cells that react for the intermediate filament cytokeratin and desmosomal proteins.[78,79] They also express a synaptophysin-like immunoreactivity similar to neuroendocrine carcinoma of the skin, referred to also as Merkel cell carcinoma. The presence of synaptophysin-like immunoreactivity in Merkel cells supports the view that they are epithelial neuroendocrine cells and that they may possess a neurosecretory function.[80] Merkel cells also contain neuron-specific enolase in their cytoplasm,[81] but no neurofilaments.[78]

LANGERHANS CELLS

Embryology

Langerhans cells are bone marrow–derived cells that begin to appear in the epidermis by 7 weeks of gestation, recognizable as such by their positive staining for adenosine triphosphatase (ATPase). At this stage, they are fewer, smaller, and less dendritic than at a later fetal stage. Although all Langerhans cells at this stage are ATPase-positive, they are negative for their characteristic cell surface glycoprotein, CD1a. At a gestational stage of 60 days, Langerhans cells begin to express CD1a reactivity. By 80 to 90 days, the number of CD1a-positive cells increases abruptly, and after 90 days, the expression of CD1a is approximately equivalent to the number of ATPase-positive Langerhans cells.[82] S-100 protein is not found in the Langerhans cells of fetal epidermis, but it can be demonstrated within 1 day after delivery.[83] By electron microscopy, Langerhans cells can be identified by 10 to 11 weeks of gestation on the basis of the presence of Langerhans granules (see text following).

Normal Microanatomy

Langerhans cells are seen in histologic sections stained with hematoxylin-eosin as clear cells in the suprabasal epidermis. However, they cannot be reliably distinguished from occasional intraepidermal T lymphocytes and macrophages, and their dendritic cytoplasmic processes cannot be resolved. Occasionally, focal hyperplasia of Langerhans cells results in an aggregate of these specialized histiocytes. The nuclei within such cellular clusters exhibit pallor and characteristic infoldings typical of Langerhans cells. In 1-μm, plastic-embedded sections, Langerhans cells are visualized as cells with (1) bodies generally situated in the midportion of the stratum spinosum, (2) nuclei with reniform to cleaved contours, and (3) delicate dendrites often extending to the level of the stratum corneum.

Because Langerhans cell detection is difficult in conventional sections, special stains are generally required for their identification and enumeration. Several enzyme histochemical stains may be used for identifying Langerhans cells and differentiating them from melanocytes. Among them are adenosine triphosphatase and aminopeptidase.[84] Langerhans cells are also positive for HLA-DR antigen and S-100 protein, although the former also reacts with cells forming the acrosyringium,[85] and the latter is found in melanocytes. Langerhans cells can be demonstrated more specifically with monoclonal antibody to the prothymocyte differentiation cell surface glycoprotein, CD1a, when the antibody is labeled with either peroxidase or fluorescein (Fig. 3-11A).[86–88]

By electron microscopic examination, Langerhans cells show a markedly folded nucleus and no tonofilaments or desmosomes. Melanosomes are only rarely found in them, and, if they are, they always are located within lysosomes, indicating that they have been phagocytized.[89] Of great interest is the regular presence of an organelle, called the Langerhans or Birbeck granule, in the cytoplasm of Langerhans cells (see Fig. 3-11B).

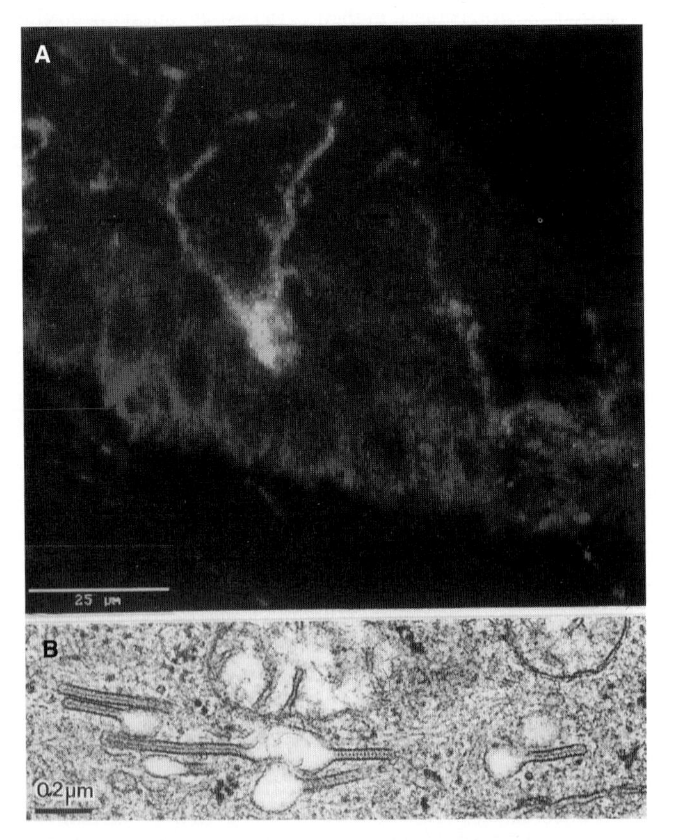

FIG. 3-11. Anatomy of human Langerhans cell (**A**) Typical dendritic architecture (immunofluorescence detection of CD1a glycoprotein by confocal scanning laser microscopy). (**B**) Transmission electron micrograph of characteristic cytoplasmic granules (Birbeck granules).

The two-dimensional profile of these granules varies considerably, from 100 nm to 1 μm.[90] The granule has the three-dimensional shape of a disk and often shows a vesicle at one end and occasionally at both ends. A cross section of the central portion has the appearance of a rod, and, if a vesicle is attached to the rod at one end, the Langerhans granule has the highly characteristic appearance of a tennis racquet. Viewed in rod-shaped cross sections, the central portion has a parallel lamella showing cross striations with a periodicity of 6 nm.[90] Langerhans granules form as a consequence of endocytotic, clathrin-associated invaginations of the cell membrane of Langerhans cells. This was first recognized on the basis of the presence of intradermally injected peroxidase within the granules of Langerhans cells even though the peroxidase molecule cannot cross the cell membrane.[91] Also, when Langerhans cells were incubated with a gold-labeled antibody directed against the CD1a glycoprotein of the cell membrane of the Langerhans cell, it was found that the labeled CD1a was internalized and appeared within Langerhans granules.[92] Cells that have the ultrastructural features of Langerhans cells but lack the Langerhans granule have been called *indeterminate cells*. They also react with the monoclonal antibody to CD1a.[93,94]

Regional Variation

Langerhans cells are present in the epidermis in a concentration slightly less than that of melanocytes, between 460/mm^2 and 1000/mm^2. In contrast to melanocytes, their number does not increase, but rather may decrease with repeated exposure to ultraviolet light.[84] CD1a-positive Langerhans cells have been found to be less plentiful in trunk skin as compared to extremity skin.[95] However, there appears to be considerable site variation among individuals, and the best comparison for determination of site-matched normal Langerhans cell numbers may be uninvolved skin directly adjacent or contralateral to the lesion under study.[95] The number of Langerhans cells may vary in contact allergic reactions because they are involved in the processing of antigen and its conveyance to lymphocytes subsequent to migration from skin to draining lymph nodes. Their number in the epidermis is increased in mycosis fungoides, where they are seen in contact with T-helper lymphocytes.[96] Langerhans cells are present not only in the skin but also in the oral mucosa, the vagina, the lymph nodes, and the thymus; occasionally they are seen in the dermis.[97]

Specialized Structure and Function

Langerhans cells originate in the bone marrow and are functionally and immunologically related to the monocyte-macrophage-histiocyte series.[98] Langerhans cells constitute 2% to 4% of the total epidermal cell population.[99] A few Langerhans cells are present in the dermis of normal skin. The histiocytes present in the cutaneous and visceral lesions of histiocytosis X contain Langerhans granules. These granules are indistinguishable in their electron microscopic appearance from those seen in epidermal Langerhans cells.[100,101] Langerhans cells express immune response–associated antigens class II (HLA-DR in humans, Ia in mice),[102,103] Fc and C3 receptors,

CD1a antigen,[86–88] CD1c (M241) antigen,[104] leukocyte common antigen,[105] a membrane-bound ATPase,[99] S-100 protein, and actin-like and vimentin filaments. These markers are compatible with an active role in cutaneous immunity.

Langerhans cells have antigen-presenting capacity. The recognition of soluble proteins and haptenized antigens by T lymphocytes requires the initial uptake and processing by an HLA-DR–positive cell like the Langerhans cell, which then presents immunologically relevant moieties to the T lymphocyte. Because of their antigen-presenting capacity, Langerhans cells play a crucial role in contact sensitization and in immunosurveillance against viral infections and neoplasms of the skin.

Ultraviolet (UV) radiation interferes with the antigen-presenting capacity of Langerhans cells. After UV irradiation fewer Langerhans cells can be demonstrated in the skin.[106] It is likely that this inital decrease in Langerhans cells is due to a temporary loss of membrane markers, rather than to a destruction of the cells. Chronic repeated exposure to UV light may result in actual depletion of cells, possibly contributing to the potential for carcinogenesis. Similar depletion of Langerhans cells may result from application of potent topical corticosteroids[107] and in the setting of acquired immunodeficiency syndrome.[108] With respect to the latter, viral particles have been identified in Langerhans cells[109] that interestingly express one of the HIV receptors, CD4.[110]

BASEMENT MEMBRANE ZONE

Normal Microanatomy and Ultrastructure

A subepidermal basement membrane zone, not visible in sections stained with hematoxylin-eosin, is seen on staining with the periodic acid–Schiff (PAS) stain (Fig. 3-12). It appears as a homogeneous band 0.5 to 1.0 μm thick at the epidermal-dermal junction.[111] Its positive PAS reaction indicates a relatively large number of neutral mucopolysaccharides in this zone.[112] Furthermore, impregnation with silver nitrate reveals in the uppermost dermis a meshwork of reticulum fibers. Staining with alcian blue, which stains the band of polysaccharides and the reticulum meshwork, reveals that the band of polysaccharides is located above the reticulum layer .[113]

The light microscopic PAS-positive subepidermal basement membrane zone appears heterogeneous on electron microscopy (see Fig. 3-6D). It must be differentiated from the electron microscopic basement membrane, or lamina densa, which is a true membrane and, being only 35 to 45 nm thick, is submicroscopic. Thus the light microscopic PAS-positive basement membrane zone is on the average 20 times thicker than the electron microscopic basement membrane, or lamina densa.[111] A basement membrane zone similar to that seen at the epidermodermal border is present also around the cutaneous appendages.

The plasma membrane at the undersurface of basal cells shows half-desmosomes possessing only one intracytoplasmic attachment plaque to which tonofilaments from the interior of the basal cell are attached (see Fig. 3-6D). Beneath the plasma membrane of the basal cells, a rather electron-lucent zone called the *lamina lucida* separates the trilaminar plasma membrane, about 8 nm wide, from the medium electron-dense basement membrane, or lamina densa.[111] Within the electron-lucent zone, beneath each half-desmosome attachment plaque and extending parallel to it, a plaque 7 to 9 nm thick, the sub–basal cell dense plate, lies about 10 nm from the outer leaflet of the basal cell plasma membrane.[114,115] Filaments 5 to 7 nm thick, called *anchoring filaments,* extend from the basal cell plasma membrane to the lamina densa, traversing the lamina lucida. Filaments arising from the plasma membrane beneath the attachment plaque of a half-desmosome extend vertically to the underlying sub–basal cell dense plaque and from there to the lamina densa, whereas filaments not attached to sub–basal cell dense plaques show an irregular "criss-crossing" course from the basal cell plasma membrane to the lamina densa.

Anchoring fibrils are short, curved structures with an irregularly spaced cross-banding of their central portions.[116] They

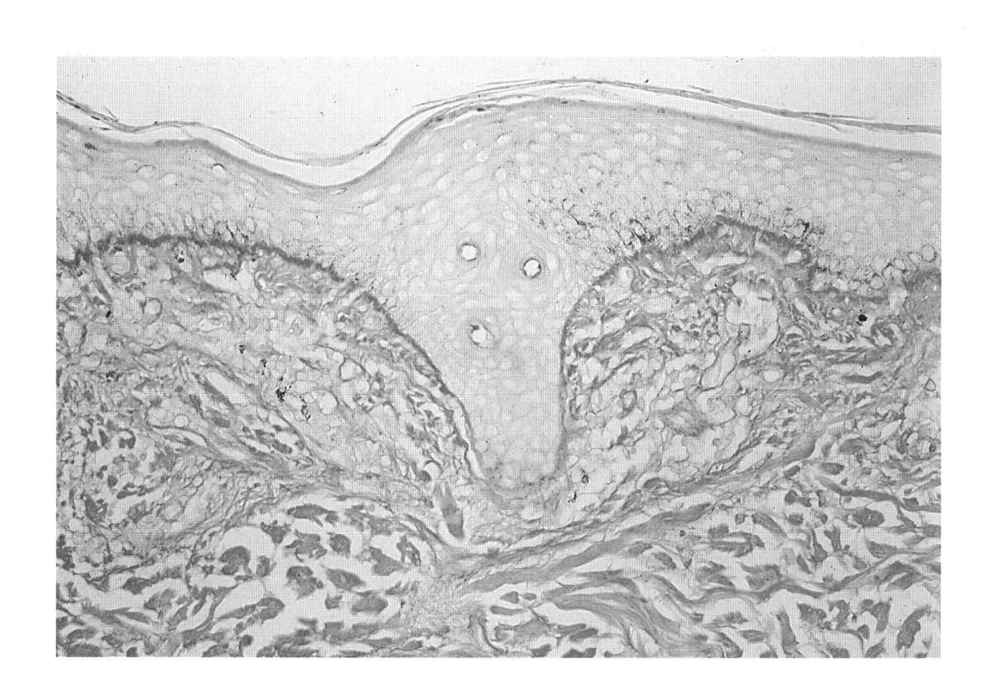

FIG. 3-12. Demonstration of normal basement membrane zone separating epidermal and dermal layers by PAS stain

fan out at either end, the distal part inserting into the lamina densa and the proximal part terminating in the papillary dermis or looping around and merging in the lamina densa. They insert into amorphous patches containing type IV collagen, which is the main component of the lamina densa.[116,117] Anchoring fibrils derive, at least in part, from the dermis and contain type VII collagen, as shown by immunoelectron microscopic localization of type VII collagen antibodies to anchoring fibrils.[118] Besides anchoring fibrils, elastic fibers consisting of microfibril bundles and individual microfibrils approximately 10 nm in diameter are attached to the undersurface of the lamina densa. Three varieties of elastic tissue exist: oxytalan, elaunin, and elastic fibers.[119] The oxytalan fibers consisting of microfibrils form a thin, superficial network perpendicular to the dermoepidermal junction. They originate from a plexus of elaunin fibers located parallel to the dermoepidermal junction in the upper dermis. The elaunin fibers are connected with the thicker elastic fibers of the middle and deep dermis. Effective anchoring of the epidermis to the dermis is a function largely of the anchoring fibrils; anchoring of the basement membrane by oxytalan fibers is quite sparse.[120] Also, the diminution and ultimate disappearance of oxytalan fibers in aging skin indicates that they are of minor importance in the coherence between epidermis and dermis.[119]

Molecular Anatomy

Immunoelectron microscopy has greatly assisted in correlating molecular composition and basement membrane zone ultrastructure (Fig. 3-13). The cytoskeletal intermediate filaments within basal keratinocytes that insert into hemidesmosomes are composed predominantly of keratins 14 and 5 (see ref. 121 for review). Hemidesmosomes contain bullous pemphigoid antigen 1 (BPAG1; 230 kD), bullous pemphigoid antigen 2 (BPAG2; 180 kD), integrin $\alpha6\beta4$ (Fig. 3-14), and other molecules not as yet fully characterized. Both BPAG2 and $\alpha6\beta4$ integrin extend from the basal cell membrane into the lamina lucida, where anchoring filaments are observed by electron microscopy. Proteins associated with these anchoring filaments include laminin 5 (also called kalinin, nicein, epiligrin), and the surrounding lamina lucida is composed of laminin 1 and nidogen (entactin). The lamina densa is composed primarily of type IV collagen. Although the molecular binding interactions are undoubtedly complex, it is known that $\alpha6\beta4$ integrin is a receptor for laminin 1 and 5, and that laminin 5 (epiligrin) is a ligand for $\alpha3\beta1$ integrin, also expressed by basal keratinocytes. Such adhesive interactions are likely to contribute to the anchoring of basal cells to underlying lamina lucida. Nidogen within the lamina lucida is a 150-kd protein that facilitates adhesion between specific do-

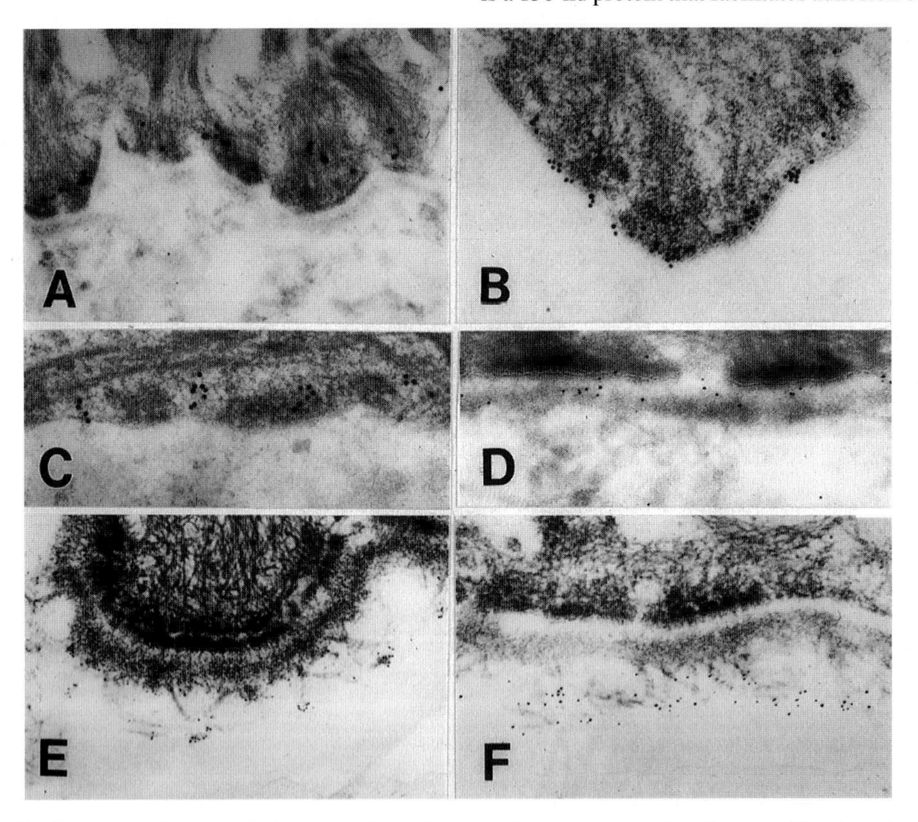

FIG. 3-13. Immunoultrastructural mapping of molecular components of normal human basement membrane zone
(**A**) 230-kDa bullous pemphigoid antigen in the intracellular portion of hemidesmosomes, where keratin filaments insert. (**B**) 180 kDa bullous pemphigoid antigen, a transmembranous molecule along the plasma membrane of hemidesmosomes. (**C**) Desmoyokin, a nonhemidesmosomal and nondesmosomal plasma membrane protein here localizing to the basal cell membrane region adjacent to the basement membrane. (**D**) Laminin 5 (kalinin/nicein/epiligrin) within the lamina lucida. (**E**) Epidermolysis bullosa acquisita antigen showing localization to both ends of anchoring fibrils corresponding to the NC1 domain of type VII collagen. (**F**) Type VII collagen, collagenous domain, with typical central reactivity pattern within anchoring fibrils. (Courtesy of Hiroshi Shimizu, MD, PhD.)

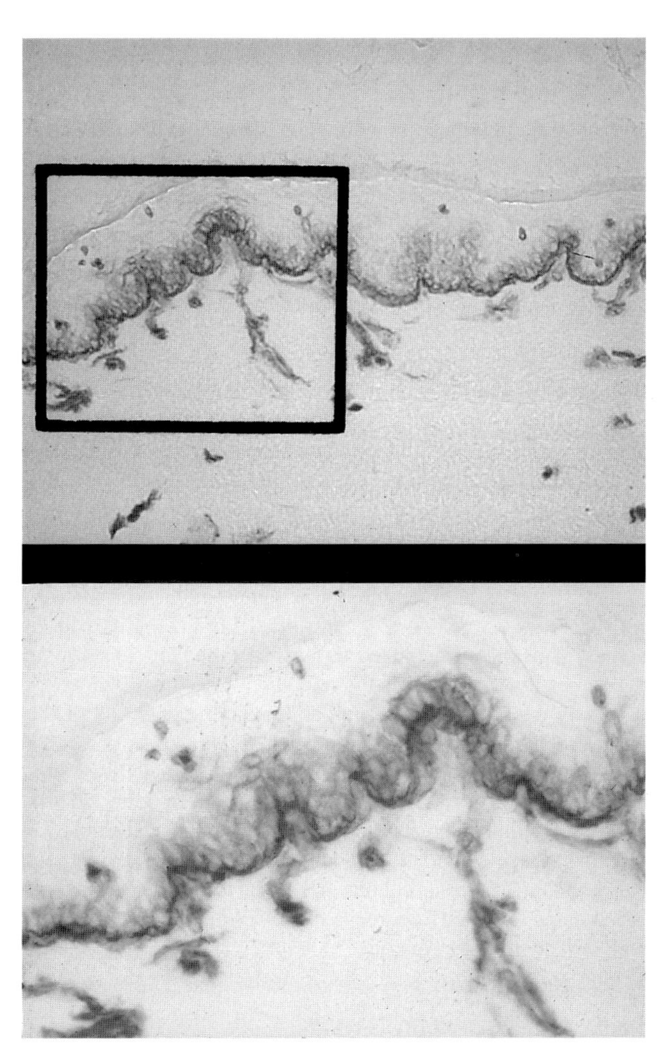

FIG. 3-14. Immunohistochemical detection of integrin α6β4, important in anchoring skin cells to adjacent basement membranes

mains of laminin and type IV collagen within the adjacent lamina densa. The lamina densa itself is anchored to the underlying dermis in part by anchoring fibrils composed of type VII collagen. Defects in basement membrane zone adhesive molecules due to autoantibodies or gene defects may result in disorders characterized by dermoepidermal separation, as in bullous pemphigoid (BPAG1 and 2), cicatricial pemphigoid and Herlitz-type junctional epidermolysis bullosa (laminin 5), and epidermolysis bullosa acquisita and dystrophic epidermolysis bullosa (type VII collagen).

HAIR FOLLICLES

Embryology

Hair germs, or primary epithelial germs, are first observed in embryos in the eyebrow region and the scalp during the third month of gestation.[122] The general development of hair begins in the fourth fetal month in the face and scalp and gradually extends in a cephalocaudal direction. Thus, during the fourth month, whereas some hair follicles on the head are already well matured and are producing hair, most of those on the trunk are barely differentiated.[123] In addition, new primary epithelial germs keep developing between earlier ones so that, in any section obtained from the beginning of the fifth month up to birth, hair structures in different stages of development are found.[124]

Hair germs, or primary epithelial germs, in their earliest stage of development consist of an area of crowding of deeply basophilic cells in the basal cell layer of the epidermis. Subsequently, the areas of crowding develop into buds that protrude into the dermis (Figs. 3-2 and 3-15). Beneath each bud lies a

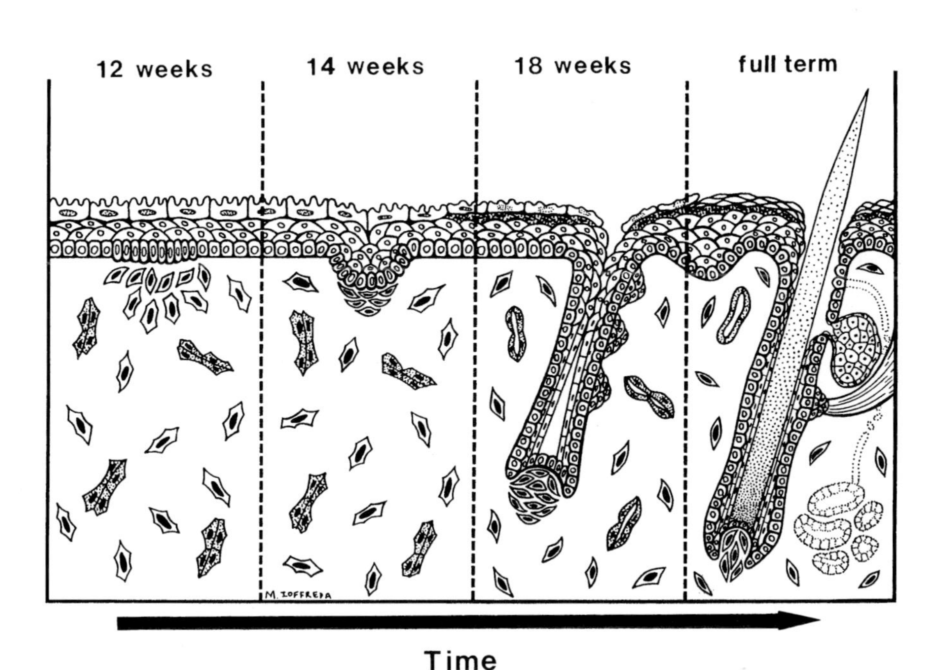

FIG. 3-15. Schematic overview of embryonic trichogenesis in human skin
(Courtesy of Dr. Michael Ioffreda.)

group of mesenchymal cells from which the follicular papilla is later formed. As the primary epithelial germ grows deeper into the dermis under induction by the underlying mesenchymal cells, it forms first the hair peg and then, as the hair matrix cells and the dermal hair papilla develop, the bulbous hair peg.[125] Electron microscopic examination of hair germ buds and hair pegs of the embryo has revealed that relatively large cytoplasmic processes extend like pseudopodia from their basal cells through breaks in the basement membrane into the dermal mesenchyme. The mesenchymal cells that are concentrated beneath the hair germs are in contact with the basement membrane of the hair germs either directly or indirectly through various types of fibrils. Also, the mesenchymal cells are connected to each other through desmosome-like cell-to-cell contacts.[122] These morphologic findings suggest that the "hair germ mesenchymal cells" pull down the hair germ as they move deeper in the dermal mesenchyme.

As the bulbous peg stage is reached, differentiation occurs in the lower and upper portions of the hair follicle and in the overlying epidermis. Differentiation in the lower portion of the follicle leads to the formation of the hair cone and subsequently to the formation of the hair, the cuticle, and the two inner root sheaths. The hair canal in the upper portion of the hair follicle, located at the level of the upper dermis, is formed by the premature death of the central core cells before they have become keratinized. In contrast, the intraepidermal portion of the hair canal is produced by means of premature keratinization and subsequent dissolution of the matrix cells of the cordlike hair canal extending obliquely through the epidermis. By the time the hair cone has reached the upper portion of the hair follicle, the hair canal is already open within the dermis and epidermis.[126]

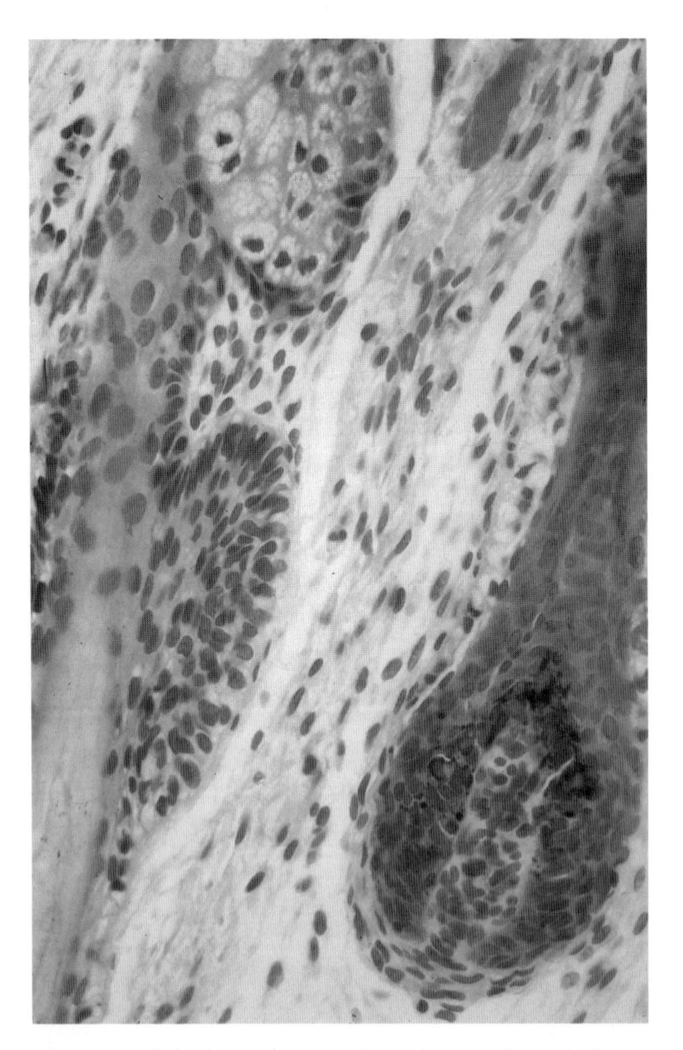

FIG. 3-16. Skin from human fetus of 18-week gestational age
Note prominent bulge (stem cell region) (follicle to left) adjacent to bulb of lanugo hair (follicle to right).

The hair follicles grow at a slant and, in the late hair peg or early bulbous stage, develop two or three bulges on their undersurface (Figs. 3-15 and 3-16). The lowest of the three bulges develops into the attachment for the arrector pili muscle; the middle bulge differentiates into the sebaceous gland. The uppermost bulge, if present, either involutes or develops into an apocrine gland. Apocrine glands develop only in certain regions.[127] Formation of the intraepidermal portion of the hair canal through cellular destruction is found on electron microscopy to be associated with the presence of lysosome-like dense bodies. Thus the intraepidermal portion of the hair canal seems to form by lysosomal digestion of cellular cytoplasm analogous to the formation of the intraepidermal eccrine duct and of the intrafollicular apocrine duct.[126]

In sections treated with the dopa reaction or stained with ammoniated silver nitrate, melanocytes are distributed at random in primary epithelial germs and in hair pegs. During the bulbous peg stage, the melanocytes concentrate in the so-called pigment matrix region (the basal cell layer lying on top of the dermal hair papilla) and to a lesser degree in the lower hair bulb located lateral to the dermal hair papilla.[124]

Normal Microanatomy

General Anatomic Features

The hair follicle, with its hair in longitudinal sections, consists of three parts: the lower portion, extending from the base of the follicle to the insertion of the arrector pili muscle; the middle portion, or isthmus, a rather short section, extending from the insertion of the arrector pili to the entrance of the sebaceous duct; and the upper portion, or infundibulum, extending from the entrance of the sebaceous duct to the follicular orifice. The lower portion of the hair follicle is composed of five major portions: the dermal hair papilla; the hair matrix; the hair, consisting inward to outward of medulla, cortex, and hair cuticle; the inner root sheath, consisting inward to outward of inner root sheath cuticle, Huxley layer, and Henle layer; and the outer root sheath (Figs. 3-17 and 3-18).

Cycles of Hair Growth

The histologic appearance of the hair follicle changes considerably during the hair cycle, which causes the hair to turn from an anagen hair into a catagen hair, then into a telogen hair, and finally into a new anagen hair. In the adult scalp, the anagen stage, the phase of active growth, lasts at least 3 years; catagen, the phase of regression, lasts about 3 weeks; and telogen, the

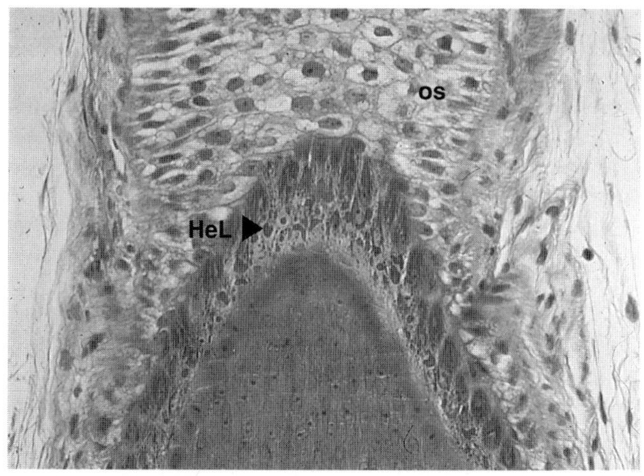

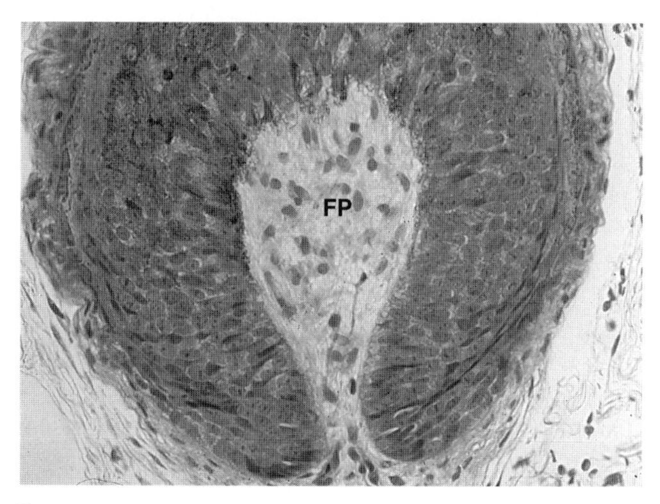

FIG. 3-17. Histology of human hair
Lower portion of human hair follicle (**A**) and underlying bulb (**B**) showing matrix cells, follicular papilla (*FP*), and well-glycogenated clear cells of the outer root sheath (*OS*). Note the prominence of Henle's layer in the tangential section (*HeL*) containing numerous trichohyaline granules.

resting period, lasts about 3 months. At any one time, approximately 84% of scalp hairs are in anagen stage, 2% in catagen, and 14% in telogen.[128] These ratios are important in evaluating abnormalities in the hair cycle in biopsies of partially alopecic scalp. The daily hair growth rate averages about 0.4 mm on the scalp.

During its active growth, or anagen stage, the hair follicle shows at its lower pole a knoblike expansion, the hair bulb, composed of matrix cells and melanocytes. A small, egg-shaped dermal structure, the follicular papilla, protrudes into the hair bulb (see Fig. 3-17). The papilla induces and maintains the growth of the hair follicle.[129] Because of the presence of large amounts of acid mucopolysaccharides in its ground substance, the follicular papilla stains positively with alcian blue and metachromatically with toluidine blue. Because positive staining with alcian blue takes place at pH 2.5 and 0.5, it can be concluded that the ground substance of the hair papilla contains nonsulfated acid mucopolysaccharides, such as hyaluronic acid, and sulfated acid mucopolysaccharides, such as chondroitin sulfate.[130] In addition, there is considerable alkaline phosphatase activity in the hair papilla during the anagen stage as a result of the presence of large numbers of capillary loops.[131,132] In persons with dark hair, large amounts of melanin can be seen in the follicular papilla situated within melanophages.

Bulb and Lowest Portion of the Hair Follicle

The pluripotential cells of the hair matrix present in the hair bulb give rise to the hair and to the inner root sheath. In contrast, the outer root sheath represents a downward extension of the epidermis. The cells of the hair matrix have large vesicular nuclei and a deeply basophilic cytoplasm. Dopa-positive melanocytes are interspersed mainly between the basal cells of the hair matrix lying on top of the dermal hair papilla and, to a lesser degree, between the basal cells of the hair matrix located lateral to the hair papilla.[124] Melanin, varying in quantity in accordance with the color of the hair, is produced in these melanocytes and is incorporated into the future cells of the hair through phagocytosis of the distal portion of dendritic processes by future hair cells. This transfer of melanin is analogous to that observed from epidermal melanocytes to keratinocytes.

As they move upward, the cells arising from the hair matrix differentiate into six different types of cells, each of which keratinizes at a different level (see Fig. 3-18). The outermost layer of the inner root sheath, the Henle layer, keratinizes first, thus establishing a firm coat around the soft central parts. The two

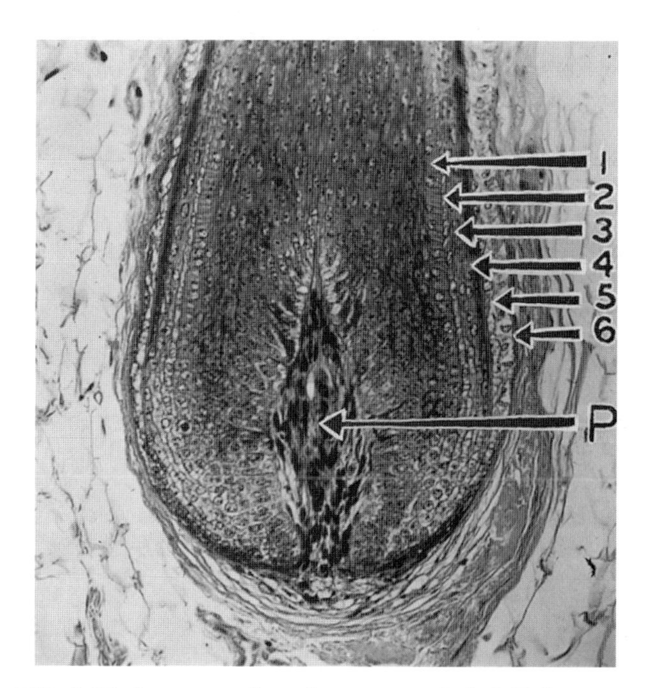

FIG. 3-18. Lower portion of an anagen hair follicle
The follicular papilla (*P*), composed of connective tissue, protrudes into the hair bulb. The various linings of the hair can be recognized. They are, from inside to the outside: (1) the hair cuticle; (2) the inner root sheath cuticle; (3) the Huxley layer; (4) the Henle layer; (5) the outer root sheath; and (6) the glassy or vitreous layer.

apposed cuticles covering the inside of the inner root sheath and the outside of the hair keratinize next, followed by Huxley's layer. The hair cortex then follows, and the medulla is last.[133]

The hair medulla of human hair is often difficult to find by routine light microscopy because it may be discontinuous or even absent.[134] It is more readily recognizable by polariscopic examination, because, unlike the cortex, the only partially keratinized medulla contains hardly any doubly refractile structures.[135] If the medulla is seen by light microscopy in human hairs, it appears amorphous because of partial keratinization.

The hair cortex consists of cells that, during their upward growth from the hair matrix, keratinize gradually by losing their nuclei and becoming filled with keratin fibrils. The process of keratinization takes place without the formation of keratohyaline granules, as seen in the keratinizing epidermis, or of trichohyaline granules, as seen in the inner root sheath. Thus the keratin of the hair cortex represents hard keratin, in contrast to the keratin of the inner root sheath, which, like that of the epidermis, represents soft keratin.[136]

The hair cuticle (1 in Fig. 3-18), located peripheral to the hair cortex, consists of overlapping cells arranged like shingles and pointing upward with their peripheral portion. The cells of the hair cuticle are tightly interlocked with the cells of the inner root sheath cuticle, resulting in the firm attachment of the hair to its inner root sheath. The hair and the inner root sheath move upward in unison.[137]

The inner root sheath is composed of three concentric layers: from the inside to the outside, these are the inner root sheath cuticle (2 in Fig. 3-18), the Huxley layer (3 in Fig. 3-18), and the Henle layer (4 in Fig. 3-18). None of these three layers contains melanin. All three layers keratinize, unlike the cells of the hair cortex and of the hair cuticle, by means of trichohyaline granules. These granules resemble the keratohyaline granules of the epidermis, although they stain eosinophilic, in contrast to the basophilic-staining keratohyaline granules of the epidermis. Closest to the hair is the single-layered inner root sheath cuticle, consisting of flattened overlapping cells that point downward in the direction of the hair bulb. Because the cells of the hair cuticle point upward, these two types of cells interlock tightly. Trichohyaline granules are few in the inner root sheath cuticle cells. The Huxley layer, which usually consists of two rows of cells, develops numerous trichohyaline granules at the level of the keratogenous zone of the hair. The Henle layer, only one cell layer thick and the first layer to undergo keratinization, already has many trichohyaline granules at its emergence from the hair matrix.[138] After having become fully keratinized, the cells of all three layers composing the inner root sheath disintegrate when they reach the isthmus of the hair follicle, which extends from the area of attachment of the arrector pili muscle to the entrance of the sebaceous duct. The cells of the inner root sheath thus do not contribute to the emerging hair.[139]

The outer root sheath (see Fig. 3-17, 5 in Fig. 3-18) extends upward from the matrix cells at the lower end of the hair bulb to the entrance of the sebaceous duct, where it changes into surface epidermis, which lines the upper portion, or infundibulum, of the hair follicle. The outer root sheath is thinnest at the level of the hair bulb, gradually increases in thickness, and is thickest in the middle portion of the hair follicle, the isthmus. In its lower portion, below the isthmus, the outer root sheath is covered by the inner root sheath and does not undergo keratinization. The outer root sheath cells have a clear, vacuolated cytoplasm because of the presence of considerable amounts of glycogen. In contrast to the surface epidermis lining the infundibulum, which contains active, melanin-producing melanocytes in its basal layer, the basal layer of the outer root sheath contains only inactive, amelanotic melanocytes demonstrable with toluidine blue. However, these inactive melanocytes can become melanin-producing cells after skin injuries, such as dermabrasion, when they increase in number and migrate upward into the regenerating upper portion of the outer root sheath and into the regenerating epidermis.[140]

The glassy or vitreous layer (6 in Fig. 3-18) forms a homogeneous, eosinophilic zone peripheral to the outer root sheath. Like the subepidermal basement membrane zone, it is PAS-positive and diastase-resistant, but it differs from the subepidermal basement membrane zone by being thicker and visible with routine stains. It is thickest around the lower third of the hair follicle. Peripheral to the vitreous layer lies the fibrous root sheath, which is composed of thick collagen bundles.

Follicular Isthmus and Infundibulum

In the middle portion of the hair follicle, the so-called isthmus, which extends upward from the attachment of the arrector pili muscle (so-called bulge region) to the entrance of the sebaceous duct, the outer root sheath is no longer covered by the inner root sheath, which by then has keratinized and disintegrated. The outer root sheath therefore undergoes keratinization. This type of keratinization, referred to as trichilemmal keratinization,[141] produces large, homogeneous keratinized cells without the formation of keratohyaline granules. Trichilemmal keratinization is found also in catagen and telogen hairs and in trichilemmal cysts and trichilemmal tumors. The bulge region at the site of the arrector pili muscle insertion is poorly defined in human follicles and difficult to detect in routine sections. When it is visualized, it consists of several knobby protruberances and ridges composed of relatively undifferentiated follicular keratinocytes with putative stem cell capability.[9]

The upper portion of the hair follicle above the entrance of the sebaceous duct, the infundibulum, is lined by surface epidermis, which, like the sebaceous duct, undergoes keratinization with the formation of keratohyaline granules. The infundibulum contains a number of dendritic nonkeratinocytes upon ultrastructural examination, and immunohistochemistry reveals numerous CD1a-positive Langerhans cells within the infundibula of normal adult anagen hairs.

Sebaceous Glands

The sebaceous glands are well developed at birth, most likely because of maternal hormones. After a few months, they undergo considerable atrophy. At puberty, as a result of increased androgen output, the sebaceous glands become greatly enlarged.[142]

A sebaceous gland may consist of only one lobule but often has several lobules leading into a common excretory duct composed of stratified squamous epithelium (Fig. 3-19). Sebaceous glands, being holocrine glands, form their secretion by decomposition of their cells. In sebaceous glands of the skin, the pilosebaceous follicle into which the sebaceous duct leads may possess a large hair or a vellus hair that may be too small to reach

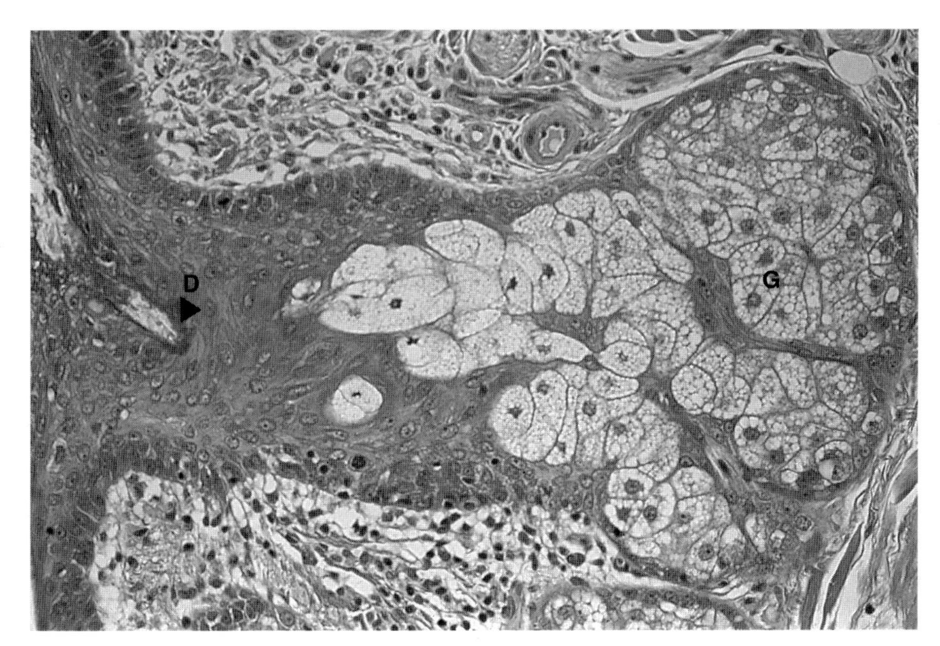

FIG. 3-19. Human anagen hair follicle
Sebaceous duct (*D*) and gland (*G*) budding from human anagen hair follicle.

the skin surface. There is no relationship between the size of the sebaceous gland and the size of the associated hair. In the center of the face and on the forehead, where the sebaceous glands are very large, the associated hairs are of the vellus type.

Each sebaceous lobule possesses a peripheral layer of cuboidal, deeply basophilic cells that usually contain no lipid droplets. The more centrally located cells contain lipid droplets, which can be detected if lipid stains are used on formalin-fixed frozen sections; but in routinely processed sections in which the lipid has been extracted, the cytoplasm of these cells appears as a delicate network. The nucleus is centrally located. In the portion of the lobule located closest to the duct, the cells disintegrate. One sees coalesced lipid droplets in the excretory duct in lipid stains and amorphous material in routine stains.

The composition of lipids in the sebaceous glands is not uniform. Thus, under polarized light, doubly refractile lipids may be present in small to moderate amounts or may be absent.[143] Histochemical examination reveals the presence of triglycerides and small amounts of phospholipids. Esterified cholesterol is present, but there is no free cholesterol. Waxes are also present, but they are not identifiable by histochemical means.[143]

Electron microscopic studies have confirmed that the cells of the peripheral layer usually contain no lipid vacuoles. Analogous to the basal cells of the epidermis, they are attached to a basement membrane by half-desmosomes.[144] In the cells located further inside, one can observe a marked increase in the volume of cytoplasm, the appearance of smooth endoplasmic reticulum, and the formation of fine lipid material within its cisterns. This indicates that the smooth endoplasmic reticulum synthesizes the lipid.[144,145] In the Golgi region, the synthesized lipid material aggregates as lipid droplets. Toward the center of the sebaceous lobules, the cells, as a result of continued lipid synthesis, are almost completely filled with lipid droplets. A true limiting membrane is present around the lipid droplets in the incipient stages, but none is detectable in mature droplets.[146]

Lysosomal enzymes bring about the physiologic autolysis that occurs in the holocrine secretion. Histochemical staining of electron microscopic sections for lysosomal enzymes, such as acid phosphatase and arylsulfatase, reveals an increasing number of lysosomes as the sebaceous cells become more lipidized. In the disintegrating cells located in the preductal region, the acid phosphatase and arylsulfatase activity is most pronounced, but this activity is largely outside of lysosomes, because the lysosomes have released their contents in their function as "suicide bags."[147,148] Prior to the sudden disintegration of the sebaceous cells, an abrupt conversion of – SH to S – S linkages of proteins occurs in sebaceous glands just as in epidermis and hair.[149]

Regional Variation

Hair follicles vary considerably in different anatomic regions and according to age and sex. In adults, deep anagen hairs (extending into subcutaneous fat) are typically found on the scalp and male beard area, whereas vellus hairs typify the female face and nonbeard area facial regions of men. Hair of extremities and trunk generally can be differentiated from scalp by the more superficial location of the bulbs and diminished density. Sebaceous glands are present everywhere on the skin except on the palms and soles. On the skin, they are found in association with hair structures. In addition, free sebaceous glands that are not associated with hair structures occur in some areas of modified skin, such as the nipple and areola of both male and female breasts. There, they occur over the entire surface of the nipple and in Montgomery's areolar tubercles, each of which contains several sebaceous lobules in association with a lactiferous duct. Free sebaceous glands are found also on the labia minora and the inner aspect of the prepuce. Sebaceous glands occur only very rarely on the glans of the penis.[150] The not infrequent presence of free sebaceous glands on the vermilion border of the lips and on the buccal mucosa is known as Fordyce's condition. The meibomian glands of the eyelids are modified sebaceous glands.

Specialized Structure and Function

Hair Cycle

The hair cycle ensures that periodically entirely new hair shafts are produced; the cycle also serves as an intrinsic regulator of maximum hair length. The hair cycle consists of the involutionary stage (catagen) and the end stage (telogen) of the old hair and its replacement by a young, new hair (early anagen). At the onset of the catagen stage, mitotic activity and melanin production in the hair bulb cease. Next, the bulb shrinks, setting the follicular papilla free.[138] As the hair moves upward, the lower portion of the follicle involutes. The reduction in follicle size results from cell deletion by apoptosis, or programmed cell death.[151] The lower follicle thus becomes a thin cord of epithelial cells surrounded by the fibrous root sheath, which is wrinkled in thick folds. Also, as the hair moves upward, growth of the inner root sheath ceases, so that the lower end of the hair shaft becomes surrounded by dense keratin, referred to as trichilemmal keratin, that is formed by the outer root sheath without the interposition of keratohyaline granules.[141] This then represents the club hair of the catagen stage.

Next, the thin cord of epithelial cells retracts upward, faithfully followed by the underlying follicular papilla, which thus also moves upward. The cord of epithelial cells shortens until it forms only a small nipplelike downward protrusion from the club hair, called the secondary hair germ. Under it lies the dermal hair papilla. With the hair follicle decreased to about one third of its former length, the lowest portion of the hair follicle lies at the level of the attachment of the arrector pili. The lower portion of the hair is encased in trichilemmal keratin and completely surrounded by the outer root sheath. Folds of the fibrous root sheath extend downward from the hair follicle. At this point, the hair has reached the telogen stage.[152]

When regrowth of the hair begins, the secondary hair germ begins to elongate by cell division and grows down as an epithelial column together with the follicular papilla inside of the old, collapsed fibrous root sheath of the previous hair. As it is growing down, the lower end of the epithelial column becomes invaginated by the follicular papilla. A new hair bulb is formed, representing the early anagen stage. By subsequent differentiation, a new hair arises. Thus the formation of an active hair follicle from the secondary germ recapitulates the embryonic pattern of development of the hair from the primary hair germ.[152] Recent experimental data in rodents suggest that the primary site that gives rise to new hair germ during follicular regrowth is the bulge region of the follicle where a population of normally slow-cycling, relatively undifferentiated cells with features of stem cells reside.[9] Stimulation of the bulge region, which persists throughout telogen, then gives rise to new hair germ and the developing anagen follicle (bulge activation hypothesis).

Hair Color

Three types of melanosomes are present in hair. Erythromelanin granules, seen in red hair, are polymorphous and have an irregular internal structure. The other two types of granules, homogeneous eumelanin granules and lamellated pheomelanin granules, are found in varying proportions in blond and dark hair and are round to oval. Dark hair contains more melanosomes than light hair, and the melanosomes are largely of the homogeneous eumelanin type; in light hair, lamellated pheomelanin melanosomes predominate.[153]

In grey and white hair, the melanocytes in the basal layer of the hair matrix are greatly reduced in number or are absent. The melanocytes that are present show degenerative changes, especially of their melanosomes.[154] The hair shafts contain only detritus of melanin or none at all.[153]

Follicular Immunity

The number of CD1a-positive Langerhans cells in normal follicular infundibula raises questions concerning their role in follicular immunity. Such populations could be appropriately sequestered from harmful environmental agents, such as ultraviolet light, and thus serve as a reservoir of antigen-presenting cells as well as an evolutionary rationale for preservation of hair follicles in *Homo sapiens* no longer in need of the thermal or protective benefits of hair shafts. Such follicle-associated immune tissue has been evidenced in clinical settings of primarily follicular pathology in certain forms of contact dermatitis, as well as in sequential studies of human experimentally induced contact allergy where the first sentinel lymphocytes selectively home to follicular infundibula.[155]

ECCRINE AND APOCRINE GLANDS

The apocrine glands differ from eccrine glands in origin, distribution, size, and mode of secretion. The eccrine glands primarily serve in the regulation of heat, and the apocrine glands represent scent glands.

Embryology

Eccrine glands are present in mammals, with the exception of anthropoids, only on the soles. Their presence in other parts of the skin in humans is a late development from the phylogenetic point of view. Accordingly, the eccrine glands develop in humans earlier on the palms and soles than elsewhere. On the palms and soles, eccrine gland germs are first seen early in the fourth gestational month.[156] In the early part of the fifth fetal month, they develop in the axillae, and near the end of the fifth month, they begin to appear over the remainder of the body.[123] The eccrine gland germs begin as areas of crowding of deeply basophilic cells in the basal layer of the epidermis. They differ from primary epithelial germs only slightly by being narrower and by showing fewer mesenchymal cells at their base. Like hair follicles, eccrine glands may be seen at one time in different stages of development. In embryos 16 weeks old, some eccrine glands are already beginning to form coils on the palms and soles, while new eccrine gland germs are still forming in the epidermis.[157]

At the time of lumen formation, the intradermal duct and the secretory segment show a wall composed of two layers of cells, an inner layer of luminal cells and an outer layer of basal cells. Although the dermal duct continues to consist of these two layers of cells throughout life, the two layers in the secretory segment undergo differentiation: The luminal cells differentiate into tall, columnar secretory cells extending from the basement membrane to the luminal border, and the basal cells differentiate into secretory cells or into myoepithelial cells, which appear as pyramidal, relatively small cells wedged at the base between secretory cells.[156] The differentiation into secretory and myoepithelial cells in the secretory segment is well advanced on the palms and soles of embryos 22 weeks old. At the time of birth, the appearance of the eccrine glands resembles that of adult eccrine glands.

On electron microscopic examination, the embryonic lumen formation occurring in the eccrine dermal duct and in the secretory segment differs from the lumen formation occurring in the intraepidermal portion of the eccrine duct. (This difference exists also in the apocrine gland.) In the eccrine dermal duct, lumen formation results from a separation of desmosomes between apposing luminal cells and the subsequent formation of microvilli at the luminal surfaces. In the secretory portion, lumen formation also begins with the separation of luminal cells from one another and is followed by the appearance of numerous small secretory vesicles and dense secretory granules in the secretory cells.[156]

In the intraepidermal portion of the eccrine duct, intracytoplasmic vacuoles form through lysosomal action within the inner cells of the intraepidermal eccrine duct units. These vacuoles enlarge, coalesce, and break through the plasma membrane. Through coalescence with similarly produced vacuoles from adjoining inner cells, a patent extracellular lumen is formed. After formation of the lumen, the intraepidermal eccrine duct unit undergoes keratinization—the outer cells at the level of the midsquamous layer and the inner cells at the level of the stratum granulosum.[156]

In contrast to eccrine glands, apocrine glands develop only in certain areas. Wherever they form, they develop from the upper bulge of hair follicles that are in the early bulbous peg stage and show a hair cone. The formation of apocrine glands begins late in the fourth month and continues until late in embryonic life, as long as new hair follicles develop. In the earliest stage, a solid epithelial cord projects into the perifollicular mesenchyme at a right angle to the long axis of the hair follicle and then grows downward past the developing sebaceous gland and arrector pili bulge. By the time the tip of the epithelial cord has reached the level of the sebaceous gland, the intradermal ductal lumen begins to form, as does the intrafollicular lumen.[127] At the time of birth, there is as yet no recognizable myoepithelial layer of cells around the secretory portion of the apocrine glands.[123]

Electron microscopic examination shows that the apocrine dermal duct, like the eccrine duct, forms through separation of apposing luminal cells. In contrast, the intrafollicular lumen forms through lysosomal formation of intracytoplasmic vacuoles in neighboring cells and subsequent extracytoplasmic coalescence of these vacuoles.[127] The formation of the intrafollicular portion of the apocrine duct is analogous to the formation of the intraepidermal portion of the eccrine duct.

Normal Microanatomy

Eccrine glands are composed of three segments: the intraepidermal duct, the intradermal duct, and the secretory portion. The secretory portion makes up about one half of the basal coil, the other half being composed of duct. The basal coil lies either at the border between the dermis and the subcutaneous fat or in the lower third of the dermis. When located in the lower dermis, it is surrounded by fatty tissue that connects with the subcutaneous fat. Eccrine glands are highlighted by immunohistochemical stains for S-100 protein and carcinoembryonic antigen.

The intraepidermal eccrine duct extends from the base of a rete ridge to the surface and follows a spiral course (Fig. 3-20). The cells composing the duct are different from the cells of the surrounding epidermis in that they are derived from dermal duct cells through mitosis and upward migration.[158] For this reason, the intraepidermal eccrine duct has been referred to as the *acrosyringium* or the *epidermal sweat duct unit.* The intraepidermal eccrine duct consists of a single layer of inner or luminal cells and two or three rows of outer cells. The ductal cells begin to keratinize, as evidenced by the presence of keratohyaline granules, at a lower level than the cells of the surrounding epidermis, in the middle squamous layer, and are fully keratinized at the level of the stratum granulosum of the surrounding epidermis.[159] Before keratinization, the intraepidermal lumen is lined by an eosinophilic cuticle.

The intradermal eccrine duct is composed of two layers of small, cuboidal, deeply basophilic epithelial cells. Unlike the secretory portion of the eccrine gland, the eccrine duct has no peripheral hyaline basement membrane zone, but the lumen of the duct is lined with a deeply eosinophilic, homogeneous cuticle that is PAS-positive and diastase-resistant.

The secretory portion of the eccrine gland shows only one

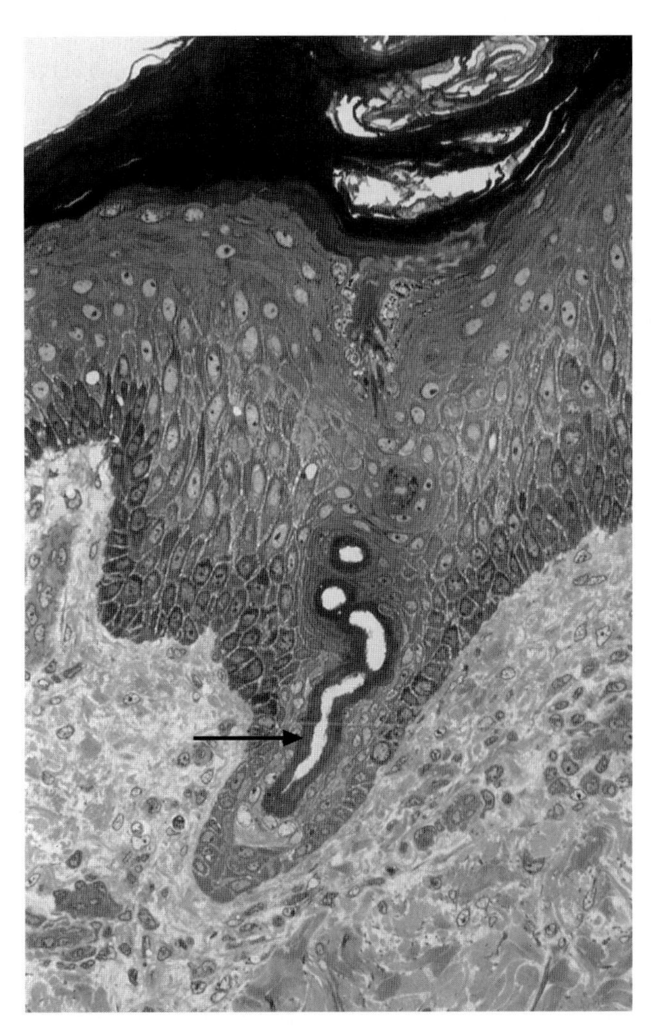

FIG. 3-20. Acrosyringium
Note characteristic spiraling course within the epidermis and acellular lining cuticle (*arrow*).

distinct layer composed of secretory cells (Fig. 3-21). The presence of only one distinct layer is due to the fact that the cells of the outer layer have become differentiated into either secretory or myoepithelial cells during the sixth to eighth months of embryonic life. The secretory cells lining the lumen consist equally of two types, clear cells and dark cells. The clear cells generally are broader at the base than they are near the lumen, appear somewhat larger than the dark cells, and contain very faint, small granules. The dark cells are broadest near the lumen and contain numerous basophilic granules.[160] The clear cells contain PAS-positive, diastase-labile glycogen, and the dark cells contain PAS-positive, diastase-resistant mucopolysaccharides. The clear cells secrete-abundant amounts of aqueous material together with glycogen; the dark cells secrete sialomucin.[161] This substance contains both neutral and nonsulfated acid mucopolysaccharides, is positive for PAS and for alcian blue at pH 2.4, and is resistant to diastase and hyaluronidase. Prolonged sweating leads to a depletion of glycogen in the clear cells.[162] The myoepithelial cells possess a small spindle-shaped nucleus and long contractile fibrils. The fibrils run in a spiral, their long axes aligned obliquely to the direction of the secretory tubule. Delivery of sweat to the skin surface is greatly aided by myoepithelial contraction.[163] Peripheral to the myoepithelial cell lies a hyaline basement membrane zone containing collagen fibers. The transition from the secretory to the ductal epithelium is abrupt (see Fig. 3-21). The lumen of the secretory portion of the eccrine gland, measuring approximately 20 μm in diameter, is small in comparison with that of the apocrine gland (Fig. 3-22). The lumen of the eccrine duct measures about 15 μm across.

The ultrastructure of the secretory portion of the eccrine gland reveals an admixture of clear cells containing glycogen granules, and dark cells containing large electron-dense granules situated within the luminal cytoplasm. The luminal membranes display short microvilli. Adjacent clear cells show prominent villous membrane folds that interdigitate, as well as intercellular canaliculi lined by microvilli.

Apocrine glands are tubular glands, the secretory cells of which pass through various stages. Schiefferdecker, who in 1917 first described these glands, observed that, during secretion, part of the cell was pinched off and released into the lumen.[164] He referred to this process as *decapitation secretion*. He chose the name *apocrine* for these glands to indicate that part of the cytoplasm of the secretory cells was pinched off (*apo* = off).

Apocrine glands, like eccrine glands, are composed of three segments: the intraepithelial duct; the intradermal duct; and the secretory portion. Because apocrine glands originate from the hair germ, or primary epithelial germ, the duct of an apocrine gland usually leads to a pilosebaceous follicle, entering it in the infundibulum above the entrance of the sebaceous duct. An occasional apocrine duct, however, opens directly on the skin surface close to a pilosebaceous follicle. In contrast to eccrine glands, the basal coil of apocrine glands, which is located in the subcutaneous fat, is composed entirely of secretory cells and contains no ductal cells.

The ductal portion of the apocrine glands has the same histologic appearance as the eccrine duct, showing a double layer of basophilic cells and a periluminal eosinophilic cuticle. The intrafollicular or intraepidermal portion of the apocrine duct is straight and not spiral in appearance, as is the intraepidermal eccrine duct.

The secretory portion of the apocrine gland shows a single layer of secretory cells, because the outer layer of cells consist of myoepithelial cells, just as in the eccrine gland. The secretory cells vary greatly in height, depending on the stage of secretion. Variation in height may be seen even in the cross section of the same secretory tubule.[165] The secretory cells possess an eosinophilic cytoplasm. Except in the apical portion, they contain in their cytoplasm fairly large, PAS-positive, diastase-resistant granules, which appear much larger than similar granules seen in the dark secretory cells of eccrine glands. In addition, the apocrine granules frequently contain iron. Maturation of the secretory cells is indicated by the formation of a dome-shaped apical cap. Most of the apical cap is nearly free of large granules, but it contains numerous small, smooth vesicles about 50

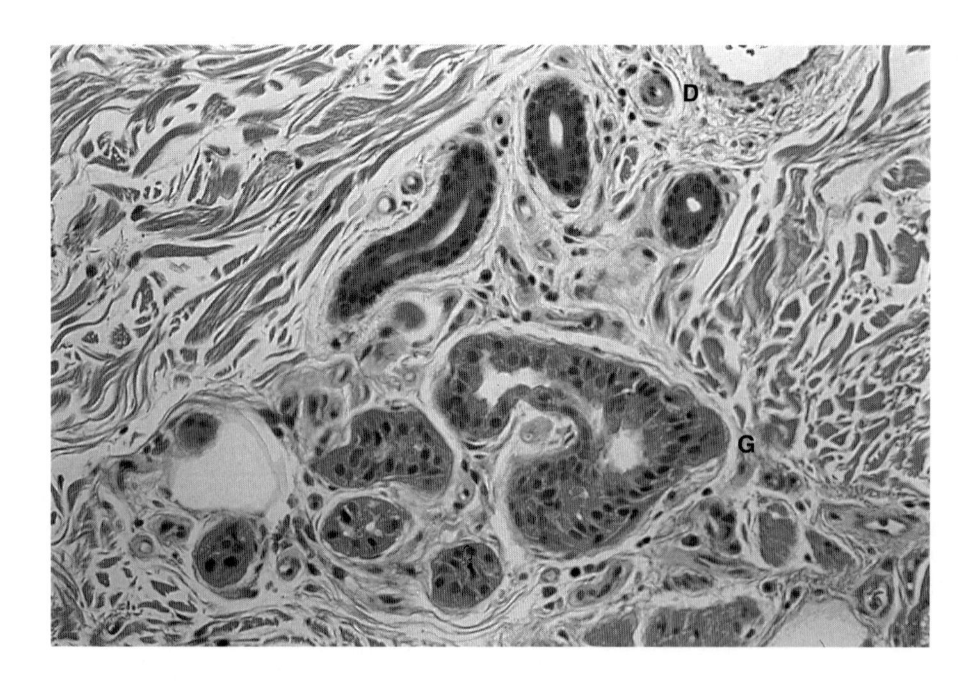

FIG. 3-21. Secretory portion of eccrine gland
Junction between dermal portion of eccrine duct (*D*) and eccrine gland (*G*; secretory coil).

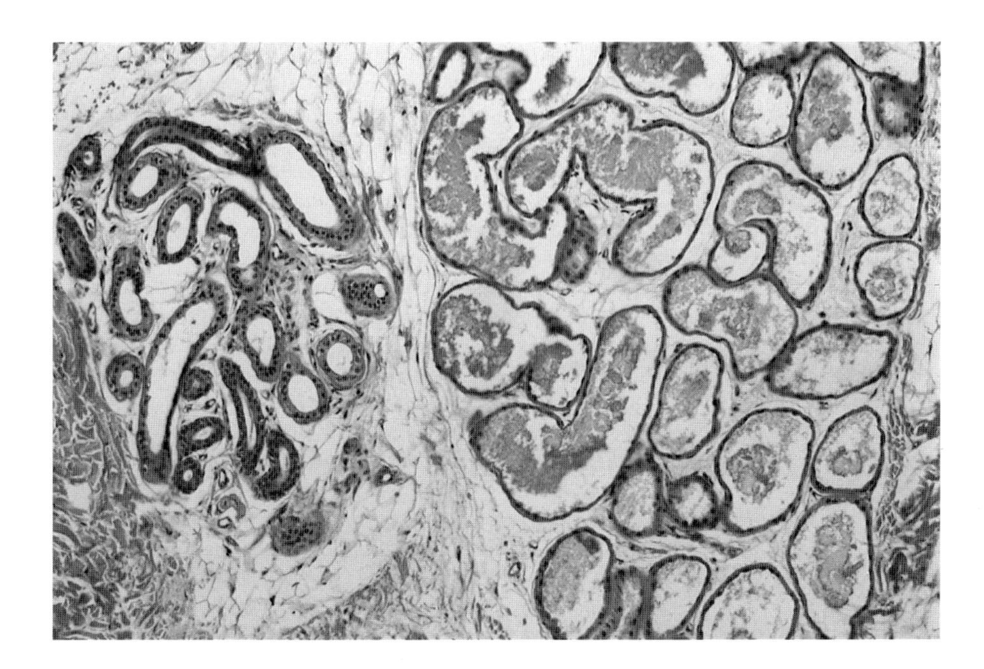

FIG. 3-22. Secretory portion of eccrine and apocrine glands
Comparison of architecture of eccrine gland (*left*) and apocrine gland (*right*).

nm in diameter. Beneath the apical cap, numerous large granules, both of the dark and of the light type, are seen by electron microscopy. The luminal plasma membrane shows a moderate number of microvilli. The lumen of the secretory portion of apocrine glands is large, measuring up to 200 μm in diameter, 10 times the average diameter of the lumen of eccrine glands (see Fig. 3-22). The myoepithelial cells contain numerous contractile fibers extending in a spiral fashion around the secretory tubules. A hyaline basement membrane zone containing collagen is seen peripheral to the myoepithelium.

The type of secretion occurring in apocrine glands consists of the release of portions of cytoplasm into the lumen. Because of this, apocrine secretion, in contrast to eccrine secretion, is visible in histologic sections stained with hematoxylin-eosin (Fig. 3-23). The apocrine secretion contains amorphous, PAS-positive, diastase-resistant material originating from the granules that have dissolved in the apical portion of the secretory cells.[166] This PAS-positive material, like the secretion of the dark cells in eccrine glands, consists of sialomucin.[161]

Regional Variation

Eccrine glands are present everywhere in the human skin; however, they are absent in areas of modified skin that lack all cutaneous appendages, that is, the vermillion border of the lips, the nail beds, the labia minora, the glans penis, and the inner

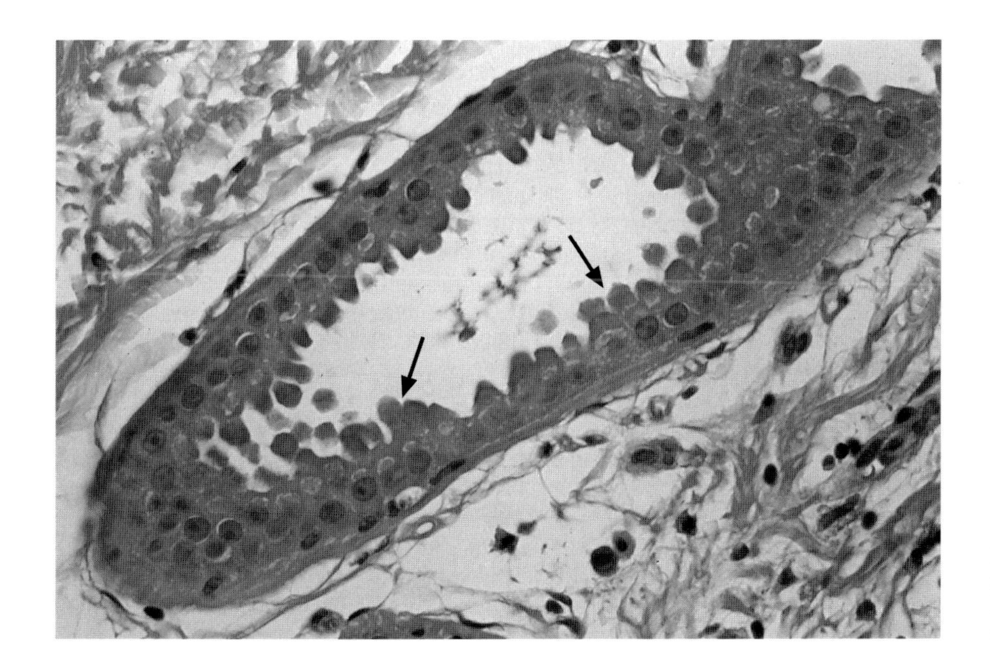

FIG. 3-23. High magnification of apocrine gland segment
Note typical decapitation-type secretion (*arrows*).

aspect of the prepuce. They are found in greatest abundance on the palms and soles and in the axillae.

Apocrine glands are encountered in only a few areas: in the axillae, in the anogenital region, and as modified glands in the external ear canal (ceruminous glands), in the eyelid (Moll's glands), and in the breast (mammary glands). Occasionally, a few apocrine glands are found on the face, in the scalp, and on the abdomen; they usually are small and nonfunctional.[167] Apocrine glands develop their secretory portion and become functional only at puberty. The multiple protuberances present in the areola of the female breast and referred to as *Montgomery's areolar tubercles* each contain a lactiferous duct and several superficially located sebaceous lobules whose ducts lead into the lactiferous duct.[168,169]

Specialized Structure and Function

The eccrine sweat gland is engineered for temperature regulation.[170] With approximately 3 million glands in the human integument weighing 35 μg per gland, the average human boasts about 100 g of eccrine glands capable of producing a maximum of approximately 1.8 L of sweat per hour. The eccrine secretory coil is richly invested in a stroma rich in unmyelinated nerve fibers that are believed to play an important role in regulation of sweat production. Cholinergic stimulation of eccrine clear cells has been shown to increase cytosolic Ca^{++} in a biphasic manner. This results in stimulation of both K^+ and Cl^- membrane channels, resulting in a net efflux of KCl along with Na^+ from the cell. Such electrolyte shifts, associated with water loss, underscore major metabolic implications of excessive eccrine sweating. Aside from potentially critical temperature regulation, the eccrine gland may contribute to general cutaneous homeostasis. For example, patients with congenital anhidrotic ectodermal dysplasia suffer from heat intolerance that cannot be alleviated by simply adding moisture to the skin surface, suggesting that vasodilatation associated with sweating may in some way be linked to eccrine function.[170] There is abundant biologically active K-1 in sweat[171] as well as numerous proteolytic enzymes, raising the possibility that eccrine sweat may possess proinflammatory or protective functions.

The mechanisms and rationale for apocrine-type secretion remain elusive. Decapitation secretion in apocrine glands comparable to that seen by light microscopy has been found on electron microscopic examination by Kurosumi[172] and associates and by Schaumburg-Lever and Lever.[165] Although Kurosumi and coworkers did not actually observe decapitation, they found detached apical caps. Schaumburg-Lever and Lever found three types of secretion: merocrine, apocrine, and holocrine. In the apocrine type of secretion, three stages were observed: (1) formation of an apical cap; (2) formation of a dividing membrane at the base of the apical cap; and (3) formation of tubules above and parallel to the dividing membrane that supply a new plasma membrane for both the undersurface of the apical cap and the top of the residual cell, bringing about detachment of the apical cap. Convincing proof of the detachment of entire apical caps in apocrine glands has been provided through scanning microscopy by Inoue,[173] who observed on each secretory cell a cytoplasmic luminal protuberance about 2 μm in diameter. In the early stage of secretion, the protuberance was hemispheric, but later increased in height to form a linguiform process.

The raison d'être for apocrine secretion in humans remains an enigma, although it may simply be an evolutionary vestige (musk glands of the deer and scent glands of the skunk are modified apocrine-type structures.) The characteristic odor in human axillary sweat has recently been shown to reside in volitile C_6-C_{11} acids, with the most abundant being 3-methyl-2 hexenoic acid.[174] This initially odorless apocrine secretion is formed at the skin surface from protein precursors or via saponification or bacteriolysis. Such chemical interactions are similar to those in lower mammals, where secreted proteins act as carriers of one or more pheromone signals.

SPECIALIZED KERATINIZATION: NAILS

The nail unit is a region of specialized keratinization of practical importance, since dermatoses, infections, and neoplasms may affect this site, prompting histologic sampling.[175] The nail unit has six main components (Fig. 3-24): (1) the nail matrix, which gives rise to the nail plate; (2) the nail plate; (3) the cuticular system, consisting of the dorsal component, or cuticle, and the distal component, or hyponichium; (4) the nail bed, which includes the dermis and underlying bone and soft tissue beneath the nail plate; (5) an anchoring system of ligaments between bone and matrix proximally and between distal grooves distally; and (6) the nail folds proximally, laterally, and distally.

The dorsal surface proximal nail fold contains eccrine but not pilosebaceous units and undergoes epidermal-type keratinization with an intervening granular cell layer, resulting in the production of soft keratin. Its ventral surface forms the dorsal cuticle or eponychium of the nail. The epidermal layer of the ventral surface is devoid of rete ridges and undergoes onycholemmal keratinization. Keratohyaline granules are present in the epidermis of the ventral proximal nail fold, which produces the semihard keratin of the cuticle.

The nail matrix is responsible for the production of the "hard keratin" of the nail plate. This occurs via a process termed onychokeratinization, and as in trichilemmal keratinization, occurs by accretion of tonofilaments without the formation of intervening keratohyaline granules.[176] This process involves thickening of the cellular envelope of the keratinizing cells to form a marginal band, analogous to similar changes in the surface epidermis.[177] The nail matrix may be divided into two regions, one distal, responsible for the formation of the ventral portion of the nail plate, and clinically visible (the lunula); and the other proximal and responsible for the formation of the dorsal surface of the nail plate. The nail thickness is determined predominantly by the matrix, although the nail bed may contribute up to 20% as the nail grows.[178] Melanocytes are present in the distal portion of the nail matrix,[179] and the Langerhans cells and Merkel cells have also been identified in this region.[180]

The nail bed begins at the distal lunula and ends distally at the hyponychium. It also exhibits onycholemmal-type keratinization. The surface of the bed typically shows parallel longitudinal grooves that correlate with interdigitation of underlying rete ridges and dermal papillae. Clinically, the onychodermal band signifies the separation of the nail plate from the hyponychium where the normal volar epidermis and epidermal-type keratinization resumes.

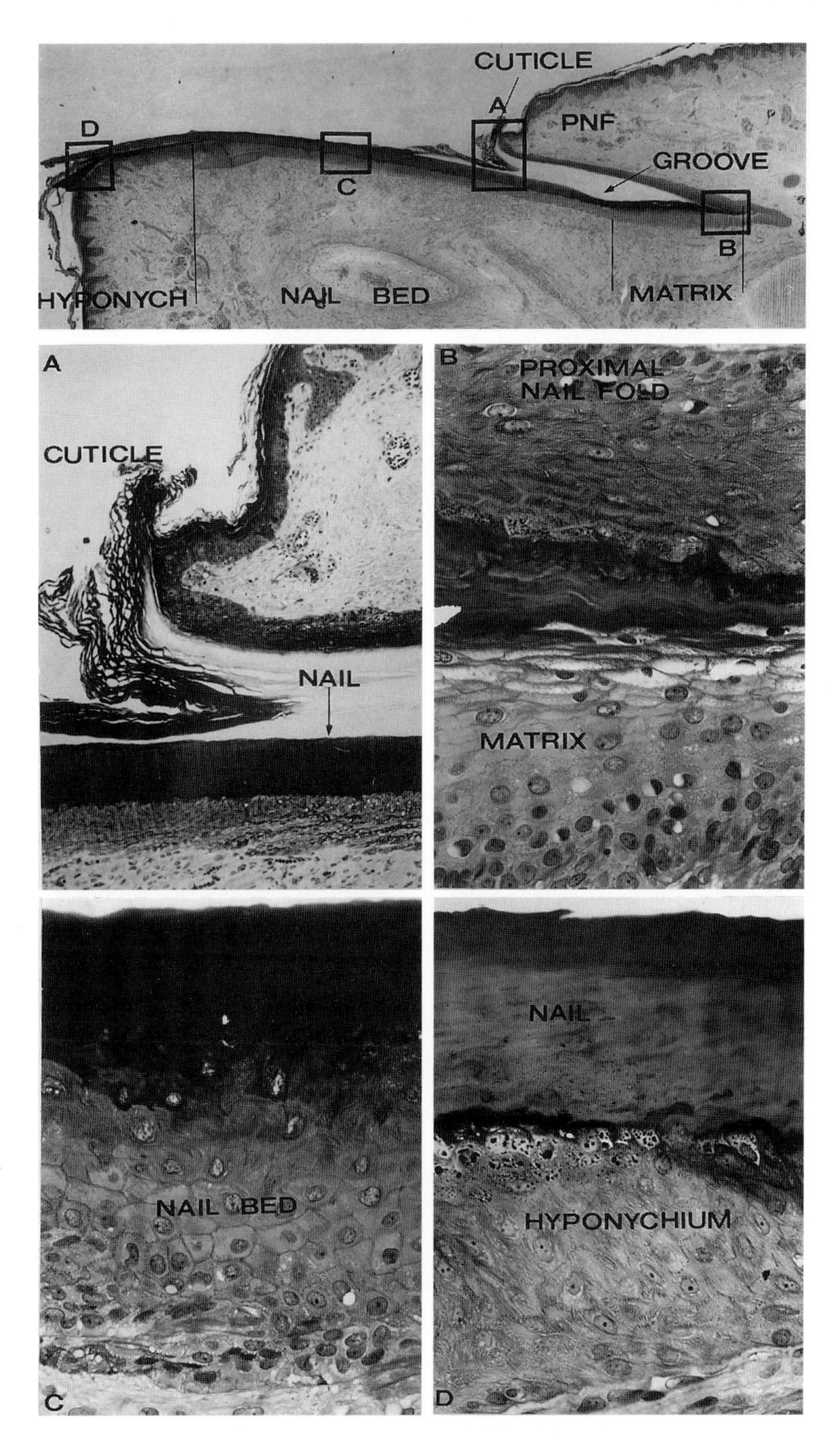

FIG. 3-24. Photomicrograph of a sagittal section through the nail unit
(A to D) Enlargements taken from the indicated areas of the upper figure. The proximal nail fold (*PNF*) is artifactually separated from the nail plate, revealing the upper half of the proximal nail groove (*GROOVE*). In the upper figure, vertical lines indicate the junction between the matrix, nail bed, and hyponychium (*HYPONYCH*). In this nail unit no lunula would be seen, since the matrix–nail bed junction is beneath the proximal nail fold. (**A**) The distal tip of the proximal nail fold. Note the cuticle growing out of the nail plate. (**B**) The proximal margin of the proximal nail groove. Note the transition in the roof (ventral surface) of the proximal nail fold from normal epithelium to nail matrix, with loss of keratohyalin granules. (**C**) The junction of the matrix with the nail bed. Note how thin the epithelium of the nail bed is compared with that of the matrix. Neither epithelium contains keratohyalin granules. (**D**) The junction of the nail bed and the hyponychium. Note the abrupt appearance of keratohyalin granules and a normal, keratinized (orthokeratotic) stratum corneum. (Richardson stain; upper figure original magnification × 18, A–D original magnification × 600.) (Courtesy of Philip Fleckman and Karen Holbrook. Fleckman P. Basic science of the nail unit. In: Scher R, Daniel CR, eds. Nails: Therapy, diagnosis, surgery. Philadelphia: W. B. Saunders 1990;39.)

DERMAL MICROVASCULAR UNIT

Not long ago, the dermis was considered to be a leathery cutaneous layer primarily responsible for housing and protection of vessels that served to nourish the keratinizing epidermis. Today we realize that the dermis is a dynamic microenvironment containing a repertoire of cells and matrix molecules arguably more complex and sophisticated than the epidermis and its appendages. The dermal microvascular unit is the heart of this new concept of the dermis, for it represents an intricate assemblage of cells responsible not only for cutaneous nutrition, but also for immune cell trafficking, regulation of vessel tone, and local hemostasis.

Endothelial Cells

General Microanatomy

The dermal microvasculature is divided into two important strata. The first, the superficial vascular plexus, defines the boundary between the papillary and the reticular dermis and extends within an adventitial mantle to envelop adnexal structures. This plexus forms a layer of anastomosing arterioles and venules in close approximation to the overlying epidermis and is normally surrounded by other cellular components of the dermal microvascular unit (see text following) (Fig. 3-25). Small capillary loops emanate from the superficial vascular plexus and extend into each dermal papilla. The second plexus, the deep vascular plexus, is connected to the first by vertically oriented reticular dermal vessels and separates the reticular dermis from the subcutaneous fat. Many of these vessels are of larger caliber and communicate with branches that extend within fibrous septa that separate lobules of underlying subcutaneous fat.

The small arteries of the deep vascular plexus and the arterioles of the dermis possess three layers: an intima, composed of endothelial cells and an internal elastic lamina which stains for elastic tissue; a media, which contains two or more layers of muscle cells in the small arteries, but only a single layer of muscle cells in the arterioles of the lower dermis, and a discontinuous layer of muscle cells in the arterioles of the upper dermis; and an adventitia of connective tissue.[181] The capillaries that are present throughout the dermis but especially in the papillary dermis are composed of a layer of endothelial cells surrounded by an incomplete layer of pericytes. A basement membrane, which stains positive with PAS, is peripheral to the endothelial cells and surrounds the pericytes. There is alkaline phosphatase activity in the endothelial cells of all capillaries.[131,182] Staining for alkaline phosphatase thus demonstrates well the capillary loop in each subepidermal dermal papilla, with the ascending, arterial limb of the loop staining more heavily than the descending, venous limb.[131] The abundant capillaries present in the hair papilla of anagen hairs also stain heavily.[131]

The walls of veins generally are thinner than those of arteries and less clearly divided into the three classic layers. The postcapillary venules resemble capillaries, because they consist of endothelial cells, pericytes, and a basement membrane. The arteriolar and venous segments can be distinguished from each other on the basis of the basement membrane, which has a homogeneous appearance in the former and is multilaminated in the latter. Furthermore, terminal arterioles have elastin and smooth muscle cells in their walls, whereas postcapillary venules have only pericytes in their walls (see Fig. 3-28).[184] The capillary loops leading from the subpapillary plexus to the dermal papillae and back can be divided into an intrapapillary portion and an extrapapillary portion. The extrapapillary ascending limb and the intrapapillary portion have the characteristics of an arterial capillary, that is, a homogeneous basement membrane, whereas the extrapapillary descending limb has venous characteristics, that is, a multilayered basement membrane.[185] Although some investigators have observed areas of fenestration at the tips of the capillary loops between the endothelial cells,[186] others have failed to find them.[185] Endothelial cells characteristically show a well-developed endoplasmic reticulum, bundles of fairly thick cytoplasmic filaments with a diameter of 5 to 10 nm, and many pinocytotic vesicles at their luminal surface. Frequently, one can observe in endothelial cells a unique structure, the Weibel-Palade body. It is an electron-dense, rod-shaped cytoplasmic organelle measuring approximately 0.1 μm in diameter and up to 3 μm in length. It is composed of a number of small tubules approximately 15 nm thick and arranged in

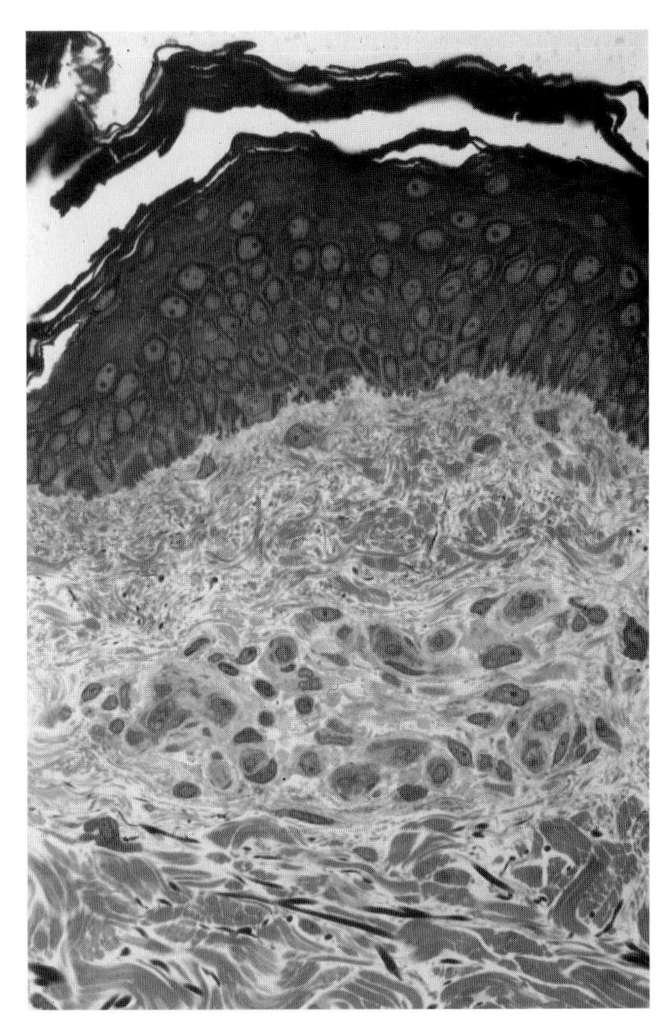

FIG. 3-25. Dermal microvascular unit
Consists of a plexus of central vessels and surrounding cells that form the junction between the papillary and reticular dermis.

the long axis of the rod.[187] Peripheral to the endothelium lies a basement membrane. The peripheral row of cells, the pericytes, have long cytoplasmic processes and form a discontinuous layer. They are completely surrounded by the capillary basement membrane. In larger capillaries, more than one layer of pericytes may be present, and transitional forms between pericytes and smooth muscle cells may be seen.[188]

Endothelial cells of blood capillaries contain α-L-fucose, which can be demonstrated with *Ulex europaeus*,[189] and they contain factor VIII–related antigen. *Ulex* and an antibody against factor VIII–related antigen are used as endothelial markers for the identification of neoplastic endothelial cells. Endothelial cells also express CD31,[190,191] a marker that may be the most sensitive for normal and neoplastic endothelial cells. In addition, endothelial cells of blood capillaries contain class I antigens (HLA-A,B,C) and class II antigen (HLA-DR).[192] HLA-DR is thought to play a role in antigen presentation and elicitation of an immune response,[193] and endothelial cells as well as perivascular dermal dendritic cells are capable of dermal antigen presentation (see text following). Laminin and type IV collagen are present within the vascular basement membranes. Blood capillaries contain vimentin intermediate filaments.

Specialized Structure and Function

Recent evidence indicates that endothelial cells are active participants in transmural shuttling of macromolecules as well as facilitators of normal and pathological trafficking of immune cells. The luminal surface of the endothelial cell that lines the superficial postcapillary venule is the primary site of adhesive interactions that initiate subsequent diapedesis of leukocytes. The outer membrane of the Weibel-Pelade body contains a glycoprotein termed CD62 that is rapidly transported to the luminal endothelial membrane upon exposure to histamine or thrombin.[194,195] This molecule mediates the initial loose rolling adhesion between circulating leukocytes and the endothelial surface. Subsequently, other cytokine-inducible glycoproteins are expressed in a cascade (E-selectin, vascular cell adhesion molecule-1 [VCAM-1], intercellular adhesion molecule-1 [ICAM-1]), on the endothelial surface, resulting in orchestrated and progressively stable leukocyte-endothelial adhesion.[196–200] Some luminal molecules that are constitutively and diffusely expressed (e.g., CD31) redistribute to cell-cell junctions upon endothelial stimulation, thus creating a situation potentially conducive to concentrating adherent leukocytes at sites where transmural diapedesis may occur.[200] Provocative signals for such events may come from inflammatory cells themselves, or from native cells in the perivascular space (see Mast Cells, text following).

Glomus Cells

A special vascular structure, the glomus, is located within the reticular dermis in certain areas. Glomus formations occur most abundantly in the pads and nail beds of the fingers and toes but also elsewhere on the volar aspect of the hands and feet, in the skin of the ears, and in the center of the face. The glomus is concerned with temperature regulation and represents a special arteriovenous shunt that, without the interposition of capillaries, connects an arteriole with a venule. When open, these shunts cause a great increase in blood flow in the area. Each glomus consists of an arterial and a venous segment. The arterial segment, called the Sucquet-Hoyer canal, branches from an arteriole and has a narrow lumen and a thick wall measuring 20 to 40 μm in diameter. The wall shows a single layer of endothelium, surrounded by a PAS-positive, diastase-resistant basement membrane zone, and a media that is densely packed with four to six layers of glomus cells (Fig. 3-26). These are large cells with a clear cytoplasm resembling epithelioid cells. Although myofibrils cannot be recognized within glomus cells with light microscopic staining methods, these cells have generally been regarded as smooth muscle cells.[201] Peripheral to the glomus cells is a zone of loose connective tissue. Staining with silver salts shows many nerve fibers extending to the glomus cells within this zone. The venous segment of the glomus is thin-walled and has a wide lumen. This wide collecting venule functions as reservoir and drains into a dermal venule. As many as four Sucquet-Hoyer canals may be found in a single glomus body, which is encapsulated.[202]

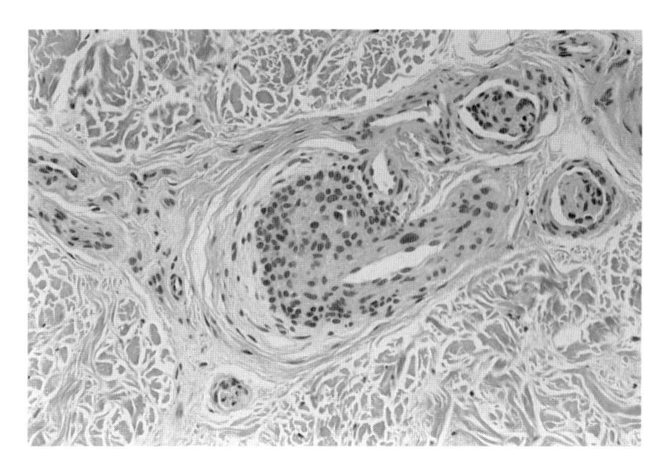

FIG. 3-26. Glomus cells surrounding vessel from acral skin

Electron microscopic study of the Sucquet-Hoyer canal reveals the glomus cells to be vascular smooth muscle cells. As such, each glomus cell is surrounded by a basement membrane. The cytoplasm of the glomus cells is filled with filaments with a diameter of about 5 nm. Cytoplasmic and peripheral dense bodies, 300 to 400 nm in diameter, are present in the glomus cells as a result of condensations of the myofilaments. Numerous nonmyelinated nerves ensheathed by Schwann cells are present peripheral to the glomus cells.[203]

Mast Cells

Mast cells are bone marrow–derived cells that occur in the normal dermis in small numbers as oval to spindle-shaped cells with a centrally located round to oval nucleus. They are generally concentrated about blood vessels, specifically postcapillary venules (1 to 3 cells per cross-sectional vessel profile) (Fig. 3-27). They contain in their cytoplasm numerous granules that do not stain with routine stains like hematoxylin-eosin. Therefore, mast cells in normal skin usually are indistinguishable from other perivascular cells, although one can occasionally recognize in mast cells a small amount of granular cytoplasm

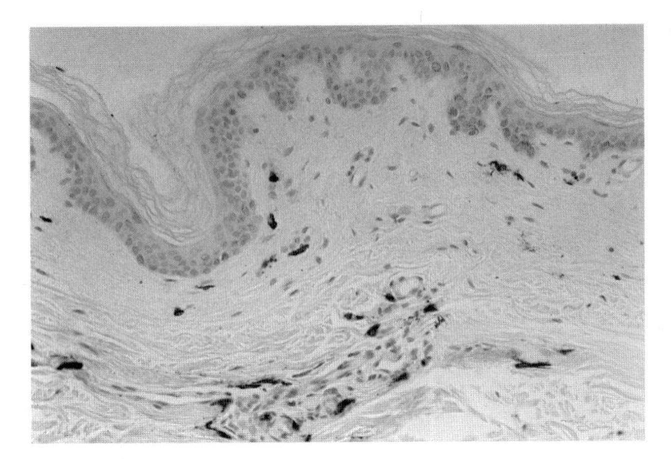

FIG. 3-27. Perivascular mast cells in normal skin Detected immunohistochemically using antibody to chymase, a serine proteinase characteristic of connective tissue-type human mast cells.

and the cell membrane. The granules stain with methylene blue, which is present in the Giemsa stain, with toluidine blue, and with alcian blue. They also stain metachromatically with methylene blue and toluidine blue; that is, they stain in a color different from that possessed by the dye and appear purplish red rather than blue.

Electron microscopic examination of mast cells reveals numerous large and long villi at their periphery (Fig. 3-28). The mast cell granules appear as round, oval, or angular-shaped, membrane-bound structures. Mature granules measure up to 0.8 μm in diameter.[204] They contain two components: lamellae and electron-dense, finely granular material.[205] The lamellae appear in cross sections as thick, curved, parallel filaments forming whorls or scrolls that may resemble fingerprints in their configuration. Each lamella is 7 to 12 nm wide, and their spacing is about 12 nm apart. At high magnification, the lamellae show transverse banding with a periodicity of approximately 6 nm. Tangential sectioning of the lamellae reveals paracrystalline lattices as a result of transverse banding. In some granules, distinct lamellae are not identifiable, and the internal appearance instead is finely granular. Other granules contain both lamellae and finely granular material. Recent immunoultrastructural observations indicate that the various granule subcompartments correlate with distribution of serine proteinases tryptase and chymase within granules.[206] In addition, mast cells that populate connective tissue environments like dermis tend to contain granules with poorly formed scrolls and express both chymase and tryptase, whereas mast cells found primarily in mucosae and associated lamina propria have granules with well-formed scrolls and express tryptase but not chymase.[207,208] Interestingly, one of these two granule types may be preferentially expressed in some cases of mastocytosis.[209]

Degranulation of mast cells occurs after cross-linking of IgE on the cell surface, after exposure to neuropeptides such as substance P, after nonspecific mechanical or thermal stimuli, or after exposure to a variety of exogenous secretagogues (compound 48/80, calcium ionophore, morphine sulfate). Degranulation generally occurs within minutes of exposure of the cell membrane to the secretagogue, and usually consists of the extrusion of entire granules, but some granules may undergo intracellular disintegration.[204,210,211] Initial stages of degranulation consist of granule swelling with loss of internal substructure and electron density. Extrusion of granules takes place through extensive membrane fusion between the plasma membrane and perigranular membranes and is associated with formation of conduits resulting from fusion of the membranes of multiple granules. This results in extensive labyrinthine channels in the cell through which swollen, less electron-dense granules, all of which have lost their individual surrounding membranes, are released into the extracellular space.[205,212] Concomitant with their release into the extracellular space, the granules release their preformed and stored mediators histamine, heparin, serine proteinases, and certain cytokines.

Immediate hypersensitivity reactions can be triggered by mast cells and basophils in "anaphylactically" sensitized persons through the presence on their cell surfaces of specific antibodies of the IgE type. When the specific antigen combines with these antibodies, an anaphylactic reaction is elicited through the

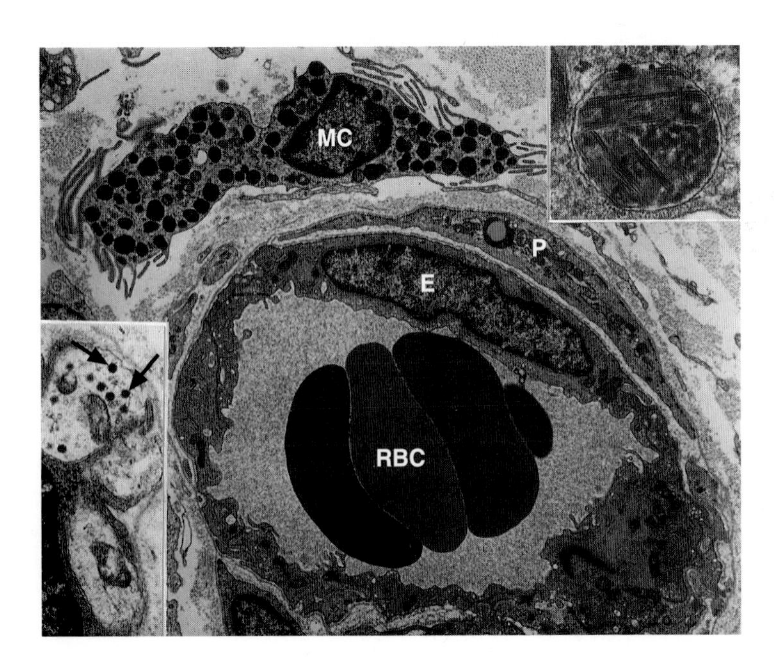

FIG. 3-28. Ultrastructure of human dermal post-capillary venule
(*E,* endothelial cell; *RBC,* intralumenal erythrocyte; *P,* pericyte; *MC,* mast cell). Inset in upper right is high magnification of mast cell granule; inset in lower left is unmyelinated nerve fiber containing neurosecretory granules (*arrows*).

degranulation of mast cells and the release of histamine from the granules.[213] Histamine increases the permeability of postcapillary venules and, if released in sufficient amounts, may produce an anaphylactic shock. In delayed hypersensitivity reactions and in experimental allogeneic cytotoxic reactions, mast cells degranulate early, often preceding the initial influx of pioneer lymphocytes.[214,215] Part of the reason for this lies in the recent discovery that human mast cells contain tumor necrosis factor α (TNF),[216] and local release of TNF as a consequence of mast cell degranulation induces expression of adhesion molecules such as E-selectin in adjacent postcapillary venules,[217] with resultant leukocyte binding to the endothelial luminal membrane.[218] Cooperation between the mast cell and the endothelial cell is also underscored by the observations that mast cells appear to situate in the laminin-rich perivascular space in association with expression of specific laminin receptors on their membranes,[219] and that endothelial cells express mast cell growth factor (c-kit ligand).[220]

Neural Network

In sections stained with routine methods, one can recognize only the larger myelinated nerve bundles and the Meissner and Vater-Pacini end organs. The finer nerves require special staining, and accordingly the potential importance of these structures to cutaneous homeostasis and pathology has been underestimated. Among the staining methods used are impregnation with silver salts,[221] vital staining with methylene blue,[222] and in vitro staining of thick sections with methylene blue.[223] More recently nerves have been identified by the S-100 technique and using antibodies to specific neurofilaments, neuropeptides, and adhesion molecules (neural cell adhesion molecule-1). Nerves are composed of neuraxons, a cytoplasmic process that conducts neural impulses from cell bodies in the central nervous system (see Fig. 3-28, lower inset), and Schwann cells (sheath cells or neurilemmal cells) enveloping the neuraxons. This primary functioning unit may or may not be myelinated and is surrounded by an endoneurium, a mucinous or fibrous matrix containing fibroblasts, which supports the primary functioning unit. A perineurium composed of elongated, flattened cells surrounds several primary functioning units and their endoneurial matrix.[224]

The skin is supplied with sensory nerves and autonomic nerves, which permeate the entire dermis with nerve fibers showing frequent branching. Sensory and autonomic nerves differ in that sensory nerves possess a myelin sheath up to their terminal ramifications, but autonomic nerves do not. The autonomic nerves, derived from the sympathetic nervous system, supply the blood vessels, the arrectores pilorum (Fig. 3-29), and the eccrine and apocrine glands. The sebaceous glands possess no autonomic innervation, and their functioning depends on endocrine stimuli. All autonomic nerves end in fine arborizations. So do the sensory nerves, except in a few areas in which there are, in addition to fine arborizations, special nerve end organs. Hair follicles, especially large hair follicles, are also surrounded below the entry of the sebaceous duct by a network of sensory nerves that lose their myelin sheaths a short distance from the outer root sheath and end in numerous aborizations of fine nonmyelinated fibers.

The papillary dermis is richly endowed with unmyelinated nerve fibers, particularly about the dermal microvascular unit where axons often terminate in close proximity to mast cells.[225] This relationship is of interest inasmuch as small neurosecretory granules within axons contain a variety of mediators, including neuropeptides that may serve as mast cell secretagogues, such as substance P. The development of confocal scanning laser microscopy has permitted the assessment of complicated spatial relationships between axons and skin cells. Recently, superficial dermal axons containing another neuropeptide, calcitonin gene-related peptide (CGRP), were documented to enter the epidermis and to associate selectively with the cell bodies of Langerhans cells.[226] Substance P–induced mast cell degranulation may elicit expression of endothelial-leukocyte adhesion molecules and thus be proinflammatory,[227] and CGRP has been shown to diminish antigen presentation by Langerhans cells.[228]

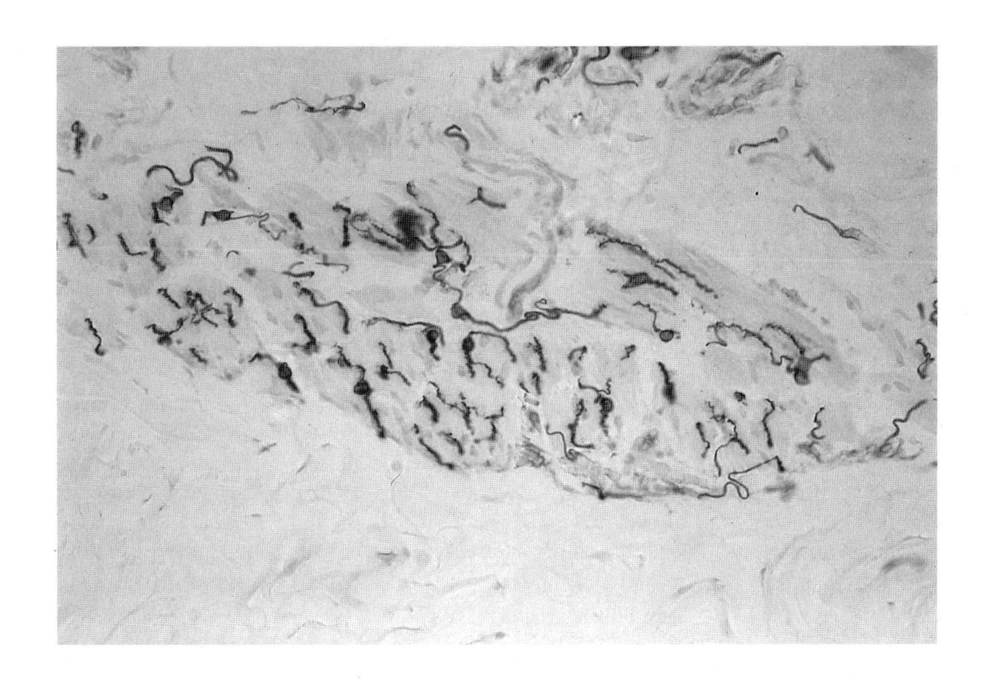

FIG. 3-29. Elaborate plexus of unmyelinated dermal nerve fibers Revealed within arrector pili muscle (immunohistochemical preparation for neural cell adhesion molecule).

Thus the superficial dermal plexus of unmyelinated axons may represent a heretofore unappreciated influence on normal and perturbed cutaneous immunity.

Special Nerve End Organs

In the areas of hairless skin on the palms and the soles and in the areas of modified hairless skin at the mucocutaneous junctions, some of the sensory nerves end in special nerve end organs. They are of three types: mucocutaneous end organs, Meissner corpuscles, and Vater-Pacini corpuscles. Although it is customary to speak of them as end organs, they actually represent starting organs in a functional sense, because nerve impulses start there and are transmitted to the sensory cells of the spinal cord.[229]

The mucocutaneous end organs, on the average 50 μm in diameter, are found in the modified hairless skin at the mucocutaneous junctions, namely, the glans, the prepuce, the clitoris, the labia minora, the perianal region, and the vermilion border of the lip. They are in the papillary dermis. They cannot be recognized in routinely stained sections, in contrast to the Meissner corpuscles in the dermal papillae. Impregnation with silver nitrate reveals that from two to six myelinated nerve fibers enter each mucocutaneous end organ and, after losing their myelin sheaths, form many loops of nerve fibers resembling an irregularly wound ball of yarn. The electron microscopic features of mucocutaneous end organs are similar to those of Meissner corpuscles,[230] despite minor differences in their light microscopic appearance. They show a subdivision into lobules, each containing a complex arrangement of axon terminals. These axon terminals are surrounded by concentric lamellar processes derived from so-called laminar cells, the nuclei of which are situated toward the periphery of the lobules. It is assumed that the laminar cells represent modified Schwann cells. The mucocutaneous end organs are always separated from the basal layer of the epidermis by a band of papillary dermal collagen.

Meissner corpuscles are located in dermal papillae (Fig. 3-30) and mediate a sense of touch. They occur exclusively on the ventral aspects of the hands and feet, their number increasing distally. There are more Meissner corpuscles on the hands than on the feet. At the site of their greatest concentration, the fingertips, approximately every fourth papilla contains a Meissner corpuscle. The size of the Meissner corpuscles averages 30 by 80 μm in diameter. Because of their size and their elongated shape, resembling that of a pine cone, they occupy the greater part of the papilla in which they are located. They possess a capsule composed of several layers of flattened Schwann cells that are arranged transverse to the long axis of the corpuscle. Impregnation with silver salts reveals that several myelinated nerves, as they approach the base or the side of the corpuscle, lose their myelin sheaths and then enter it. Within the corpuscle, the nerves take a meandering course upward. Electron microscopic studies reveal that the principal part of the Meissner corpuscle is made up of irregular layers of flattened, greatly elongated laminar cells. The nuclei of the laminar cells are located largely at the periphery of the corpuscle. The axons terminating within the Meissner corpuscle are surrounded by slender processes of the laminar cells. This enveloping of axons by laminar cells or their lamellar processes is analogous to the enveloping

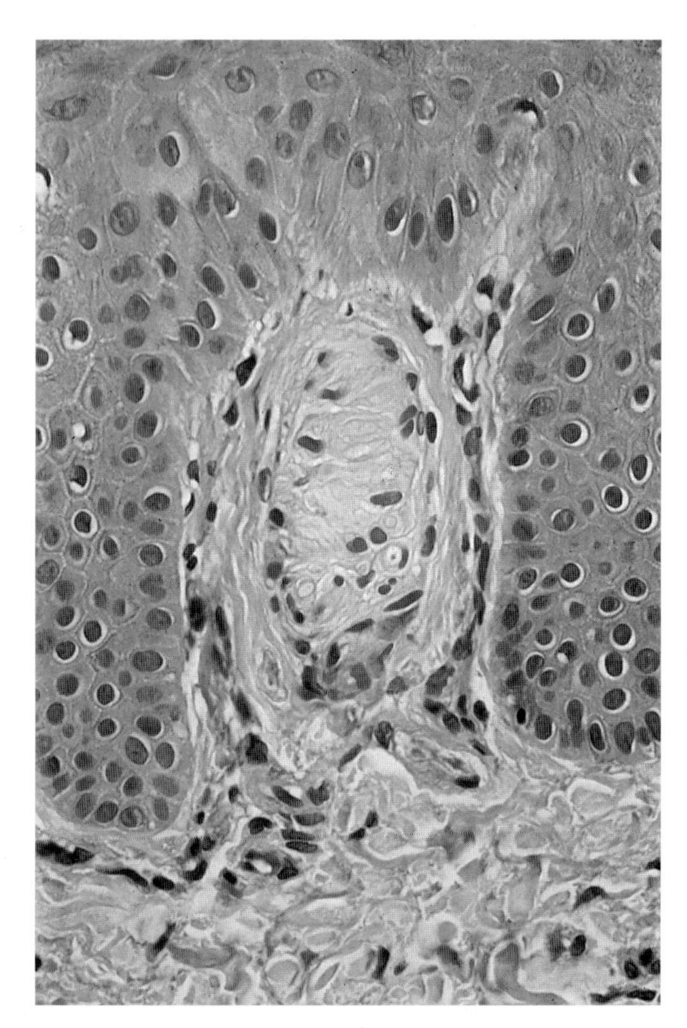

FIG. 3-30. Meissner corpuscle within dermal papilla of human palm skin

of axons by infolding of the plasma membrane of Schwann cells and indicates that the laminar cells are modified Schwann cells.[231] The axon terminals and laminar cells are in direct contact with the epidermal basal cells at the upper end of the Meissner corpuscle without interposition of a basement membrane.[232]

Vater-Pacini corpuscles are large nerve end organs that are located in the subcutis and mediate a sense of pressure. They measure up to 1 mm in diameter and thus are detected easily by light microscopy (Fig. 3-31). They are found most commonly below the skin of the volar aspects of the palms and soles, showing their greatest concentration at the tips of the fingers and toes. In addition, a few Vater-Pacini corpuscles occur in the subcutis of the nipple and of the anogenital region.[230] Vater-Pacini corpuscles vary in shape. Some are ovoid, others have the appearance of a flattened sphere, and still others have an irregular shape. They consist of a stalk and of the body proper, the latter having a small core and a thick capsule. In the stalk, the single thick nerve supplying the Vater-Pacini corpuscle makes several turns and, just after entering the stalk, loses its myelin sheath. The core shows a granular substance surrounding the ascending meandering nerve. The thick capsule consists of 30 or more concentric, loosely arranged lamellae. On electron microscopic

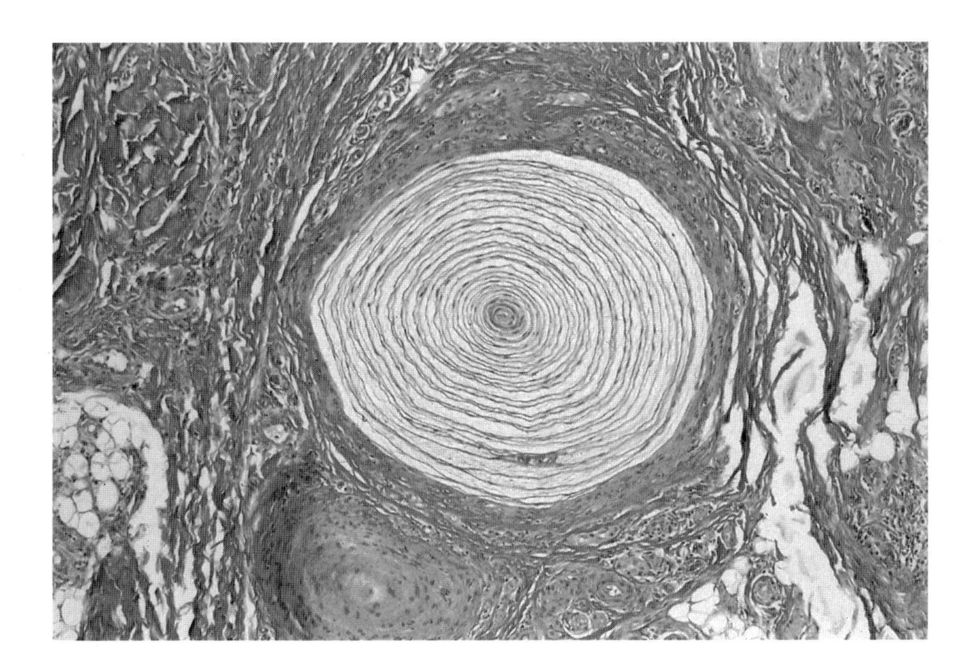

FIG. 3-31. Pacininan corpuscle within deep dermis of human sole skin

examination, the single nerve fiber present in the inner portion of the core retains its Schwann cell cytoplasmic covering for a short distance. The outer portion of the core shows closely packed, greatly elongated laminar cells. The thick capsule consists of at least 30 layers of flattened laminar cells separated from one another by fluid-filled spaces.[233] The laminar cells of the Vater-Pacini corpuscle, analogous to those of the Meissner corpuscle, are modified Schwann cells.

Perivascular Dendritic Cells

In 1986, Headington introduced the term *dermal dendrocyte* to denote newly recognized dendritic cells in the human dermis.[234] These cells were primarily but exclusively perivascular in location and differed from conventional bipolar fibroblasts by their stellate contours. Some of these cells appeared to represent "veil cells" that enshrouded venular walls with thin membrane flaps, as originally described by Braverman et al.[235] Many of these cells were subsequently shown to express the membrane glycoprotein CD1c,[236] HLA-DR, and certain macrophage markers as well as the cytoplasmic transglutaminase, factor XIIIa (Fig. 3-32).[237] Heterogeneity of dermal dendrocytes within different dermal strata with regard to their expression of the hematopoietic progenitor antigen, CD34, and FXIIIa has been described.[238]

Whereas dermal dendrocytes are dendritic only in cross section, three-dimensional reconstructions show elaborate membranous flaps.[238] Truly dendritic cells also do exist in the perivascular space. These cells are Langerhans cell–like, although they generally do not contain Birbeck granules. These cells strongly express HLA-DR, and are believed to be involved in dermal antigen presentation.[239] Considerable plasticity among the various subpopulations of dermal perivascular dendritic cells may exist, and alterations in local microenvironment may induce phenotypic transformation from one subtype to another.[240]

In general, perivascular dendritic cells are not identifiable as

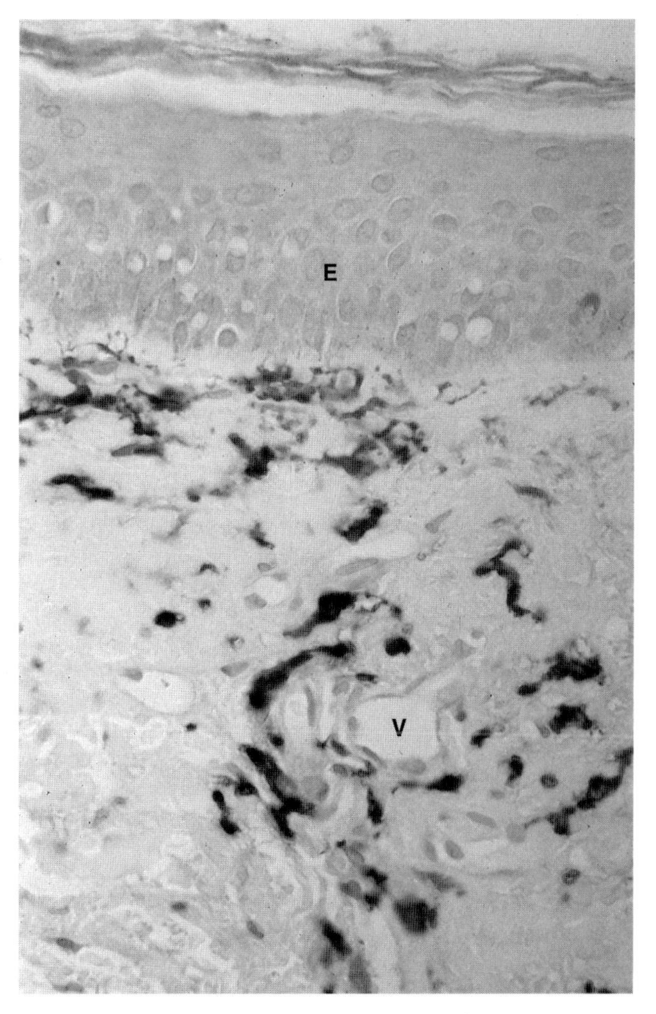

FIG. 3-32. Factor XIIIa–positive "dermal dendrocytes" Concentrated beneath the epidermal layer and about the dermal microvascular unit (*E,* epidermis; *V,* vessel).

such in routinely prepared and stained sections, although immunohistochemistry for the relevant markers permits the ready identification and classification of these cell types (see Fig. 3-32). Dermal dendrocytes may be observed in certain situations where they acquire avid phagocytic potential, taking up hemosiderin, for example. Such phagocytic perivascular dendritic cells have been termed *dendrophages*.[241]

Phagocytic Macrophages

Macrophages, also called histiocytes, are of bone marrow origin, circulate in the blood as precursors, and enter the tissue as monocytes.[242] Upon proper stimulation, monocytes can develop into macrophages in the skin. This process involves a considerable increase in cell size and changes in cellular composition and architecture, including increases in lysosomal enzymes, such as β-glucuronidase, acid phosphatase, lysozyme, and arylsulfatase.[242] Macrophages may develop further into epithelioid histiocytes and foreign-body giant cells. Aggregates of activated macrophages are referred to as *granulomas*. Macrophages are most often concentrated in the perivascular space of normal skin, although, depending on the nature and location of the stimulus for their activation, they may be found anywhere in the dermis (or epidermis).

Macrophages constitute the "mononuclear phagocytic system," a concept that has replaced that of the reticuloendothelial system. The macrophages of the mononuclear phagocytic system, including the alveolar phagocytes in the lungs and the Kupffer cells in the liver, are the "professional" phagocytes, whereas the reticuloendothelial cells, including the dendritic reticulum cells in lymph nodes and the endothelial cells of blood vessels, are merely "facultative" phagocytes and are comparatively inadequate.[243] As "professional" phagocytes, macrophages are capable of ingesting large particles and developing a high concentration of lysosomal enzymes that combine with the particles to form phagolysosomes. In contrast, the facultative phagocytosis carried out by endothelial cells consists merely of pinocytosis of small particles without immune stimulation.[243] Macrophages can be stimulated by immunologic factors, having surface receptors for the Fc portion of IgG, for C3, and for immune-associated HLA-DR antigen (human leukocyte antigen-D subregion of the major histocompatibility complex).[244]

Monocytes are indistinguishable from lymphocytes, because both cells have a small, dark, rounded nucleus and very scanty cytoplasm that cannot be recognized in routine sections. Only slightly larger than lymphocytes, monocytes measure 12 to 15 μm in diameter.[244] Monocytes can be differentiated from lymphocytes in histologic sections through staining for lysosomal enzymes, such as acid phosphatase, which are present in monocytes and absent in lymphocytes. In addition, monocytes but not lymphocytes express intracytoplasmic molecules probably associated with lysosomes, such as CD68, which may be detected immunohistochemically in paraffin sections.[245]

Macrophages, because they are activated monocytes, are larger cells than monocytes and measure from 20 to 80 μm in diameter.[244] They possess a vesicular, lightly staining, elongated nucleus with a clearly visible nuclear membrane. It is often impossible in routinely stained sections to distinguish macrophages from fibroblasts or from endothelial cells except through their respective locations or phagocytic activities. Macrophages that have ingested melanin are referred to as melanophages, and may be observed normally within the papillary dermis of darkly pigmented individuals. Macrophages that have ingested hemosiderin are termed siderophages, and may be suspect because of the characteristic yellow-green color and refractile nature of particulate hemosiderin. Iron stains (e.g., Prussian blue) will be confirmatory.

The origin of the tissue monocytes in human skin from blood monocytes has been established in healthy probands through transfusion of tritiated thymidine–labeled monocytes and their observation 3 hours later in skin window exudates.[246] On the other hand, the dermal infiltrate of monocytes and macrophages in patients with chronic dermatitis is largely self-renewing, because the monocyte recruitment rate from the blood is low in these patients after the autotransfusion of labeled monocytes.[246] Electron microscopic examination reveals in monocytes many primary lysosomes scattered through their cytoplasm as small dense bodies.[247] Macrophages, which represent stimulated monocytes, differ from monocytes in that they are larger, show longer processes, and contain a greater number of lysosomes (Fig. 3-33).[248] Many macrophages contain phagocytized material within phagosomes that, through the influx of the contents of primary lysosomes, have become phagolysosomes.

Emigrant Inflammatory Cells

Various types of cells, largely derived from the bone marrow, infiltrate the dermis and occasionally also the epidermis in the inflammatory dermatoses. Infiltration is initiated at the level of

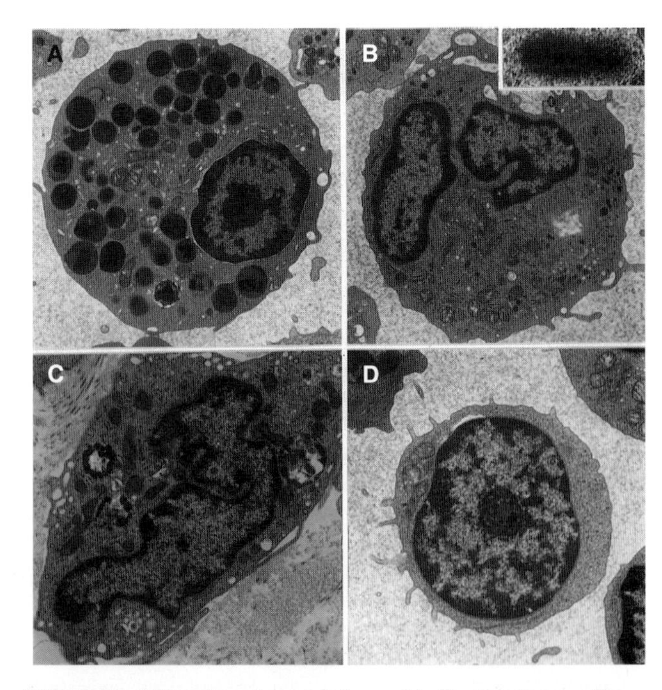

FIG. 3-33. Ultrastructure of dermal inflammatory cells (**A**) Eosinophil. (**B**) Neutrophil (inset represents enlargement of cytoplasmic granule). (**C**) Phagocytic macrophage. (**D**) Lymphocyte.

the dermal microvascular unit, accounting for the observation that upon detection such cells are often partially or exclusively perivascular in location (Fig. 3-34). Such cells may also be present in normal skin in low numbers as part of the skin immune system. It is important for diagnostic purposes to identify the cell types, since many diagnostic algorithms for dermatitis classification and identification depend upon initial categorization by architecture followed by recognition of inflammatory cell type(s) (Chap. 5).[249] Three groups of cells are derived from the bone marrow: the granulocytic group; the lymphocytic group, including plasma cells; and the monocytic or macrophagic group (discussed above).

Neutrophilic Granulocytes

The neutrophilic granulocyte, also called a neutrophil or polymorphonuclear leukocyte, is 10 to 15 μm in diameter and has a lobated nucleus consisting of several segments that are connected only by narrow bridges of nucleoplasm (see Fig. 3-33B). The cytoplasm contains numerous neutrophilic to slightly eosinophilic granules. On histochemical examination, the granules are seen to contain lysosomal enzymes and thus represent primary lysosomes. Two types of membrane-bound cytoplasmic granules or lysosomes are found to be present in neutrophils on electron microscopic examination: azurophilic and specific granules.[250] The azurophilic granules, constituting about 20% of all granules, are relatively dense and large, measuring up to 1 μm in diameter. The more numerous specific granules average 300 nm in diameter. Among other substances, azurophilic granules contain (1) myeloperoxidase, which mediates the formation of hydrogen peroxide, essential for the killing of many microorganisms; (2) acid hydrolases, such as β-glucuronidase and acid phosphatase, capable of degrading dead bacteria and other necrotic material; (3) neutral proteases, such as collagenase and elastase, that may break down collagen and elastin; (4) cationic proteins, which cause an increase in vascular permeability; and (5) lysozyme, an enzyme that degrades and lyses bacterial cell walls. The specific granules also contain lysozyme and, in addition, collagenase, alkaline phosphatase, and lactoferrin, an iron-binding protein with bacteriostatic properties.

Neutrophils are unusual in normal skin but typically occur in a relatively small subset of dermatitides, including urticaria, immune complex–mediated necrotizing vasculitis, the spectrum of neutrophilic dermatosis (e.g., Sweet's syndrome, pyoderma gangrenosum), and in various cutaneous infections. Neutrophils may participate, along with other cell types, in other inflammatory processes, such as psoriasis, seborrheic dermatitis, and pityriasis lichenoides et varioliformis acuta. In tissue sections, neutrophils are often recognized by virtue of their "popcorn"-shaped nuclei within pale pink, faintly granular cytoplasm. Nuclear breakdown due to local necrosis or autodigestion causes fragmentation of the multiple nuclear lobes, resulting in the characteristic "nuclear dust" of vasculitis.

Functionally, neutrophilic granulocytes play an important role (1) in certain inflammatory responses (examples provided in text preceding); (2) in the phagocytosis and killing of microorganisms; and (3) in the immobilization and phagocytosis of antigen-antibody complexes in the presence of complement.[251] Neutrophils fail to kill bacteria in chronic granulomatous disease where they are incapable of oxygen uptake from the surrounding media.[252] Phagocytosis of organisms and antigen-antibody complexes by neutrophils is accompanied by their partial or complete degranulation, with associated discharge of lysosomal enzymes.[253] Endocytotic uptake of microorganisms by neutrophils results in the formation of intracytoplasmic phagolysosomes where high enzyme concentrations result in microbial killing. Immune complexes, after activation of complement, may induce the local accumulation of neutrophils via chemotaxis. Phagocytosis of immune complexes by neutrophils and/or neutrophil degranulation may then occur.[254] Exocytosis of neutrophil granules containing collagenase and elastase may result in local tissue damage, including necrosis of vessels containing immune complexes in their basement membranes.[255]

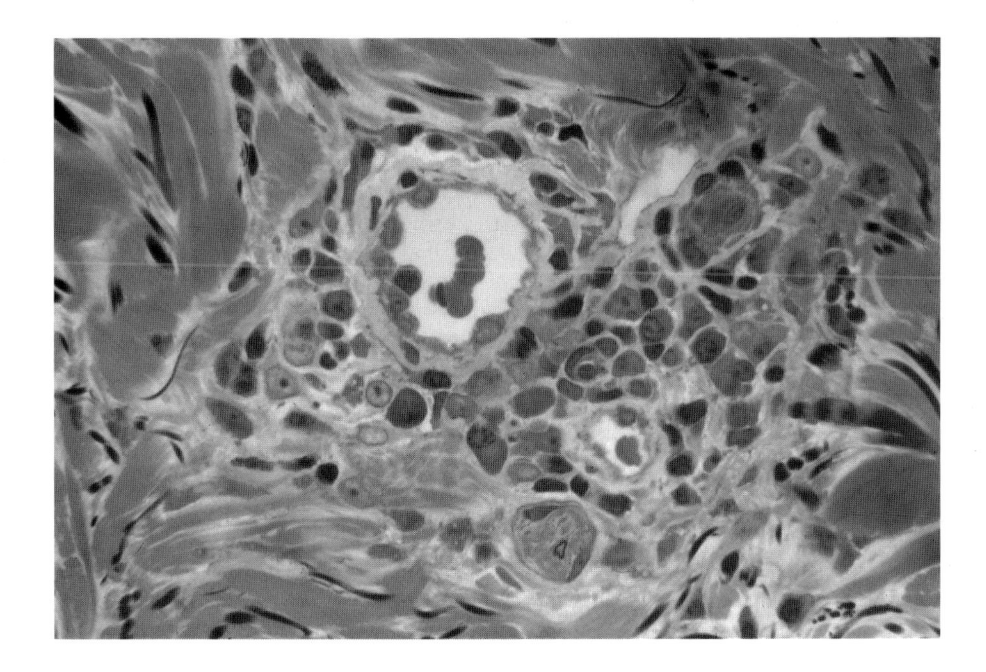

FIG. 3-34. Emigrant inflammatory cells about a postcapillary venule within the superficial dermis
Lymphocytes, monocytes, and plasma cells are represented.

Eosinophilic Granulocytes

The eosinophil, 12 to 17 μm in diameter, is characterized by strongly eosinophilic granules in the cytoplasm and a characteristically bilobed nucleus.[256] Eosinophil granules are larger than the granules of neutrophils. Although visible with routine stains, these granules stand out more clearly in brilliant red when a Giemsa stain is used. On electron microscopic examination, the granules of eosinophils are seen to be round to oval (Fig. 3-33A). They consist of two components, a central, angular-shaped core, often referred to as the *crystalloid,* and a surrounding matrix. In electron microscopic sections stained with lead compounds, the crystalloid is more darkly stained than the matrix.[257] The longer diameter of the granules measures 0.5 to 1.5 μm, and the shorter diameter 0.3 to 1.0 μm.[257] The granules contain a variety of hydrolytic enzymes, particularly peroxidase and arylsulfatase, and therefore can be classified as lysosomes. The phagocytic potential of eosinophils seems to be limited to immune complexes and mast cell granules. During phagocytosis, which is analogous to that seen in neutrophils, the content of the eosinophilic granules is discharged into phagosomes.[258]

Because eosinophils can phagocytize mast cell granules and certain antigen-antibody complexes, tissue eosinophilia in the skin can occur (1) as a result of anaphylactic or atopic hypersensitivity; (2) subsequent to the degranulation of mast cells; and (3) in certain diseases associated with deposits of antigen-antibody complexes in the skin. The tissue eosinophilia appearing in anaphylactic reactions and other forms of "immediate" allergy such as atopy is based on antibodies of the IgE type on the surface of mast cells. The anaphylactic reaction, classified as type I hypersensitivity reaction,[259] occurs after the binding of a specific antigen to a specific antibody on the surface of the mast cells. This leads to degranulation of mast cells and to the release of vasoactive substances, especially histamine. Wherever degranulation of mast cells occurs, eosinophils may appear and phagocytize the released mast cell granules.[253] Eosinophils thus may modify an anaphylactic reaction.[260] Eosinophils are attracted in an anaphylactic reaction by sensitized mast cells, which release an eosinophil chemotactic factor of anaphylaxis (ECF-A). Eosinophils thus attracted to the site of an anaphylactic reaction accumulate around degranulating mast cells and phagocytize the free mast cell granules.[261]

Diseases in which deposition of antigen-antibody complexes is the cause of eosinophilia include pemphigus vulgaris, particularly pemphigus vegetans, pemphigus foliaceus, bullous pemphigoid, and granuloma faciale. The reasons for the occasional presence of tissue eosinophilia in histiocytosis X and in Hodgkin's disease are not fully apparent. Parasitic infestations often are associated with eosinophilia both in the peripheral blood and in the tissue. It is likely that eosinophils function as effector cells in parasite destruction.[258] Destruction of parasites, such as those causing schistosomiasis, is accomplished by means of the major basic protein (MBP) of the eosinophils. The MBP is localized in the crystalloid core of the eosinophil granules and accounts for more than 50% of the protein in the granules and for almost 25% of the total protein in the cell. Its toxicity provides a mechanism by which the eosinophil damages parasites. Release of MBP from degranulating eosinophils is, however, not always beneficial to the host. Release of MBP may partly account for the tissue damage seen in chronic hypersensitivity reactions.[262]

Basophilic Granulocytes

Although basophils and mast cells have similar or identical functions and supplement each other, they are different cells both in microenvironment and in anatomy.[263] Both cells have their origin in the bone marrow, although basophils circulate in the peripheral blood, and mature mast cells are confined to connective tissue and mucosal tissue compartments. Basophils are relatively rare in human dermatitis, although they are active participants in certain forms of dermatitis in rodents.[263] The demonstration of basophils in light microscopic sections requires the use of electron microscopic fixation and processing techniques; biopsy specimens must be embedded in plastic resin and sectioned at 1 μm. The sections then are stained with the Geimsa stain. Basophils possess a multilobed nucleus and large, diffusely arranged metachromatic granules, whereas mast cells have a unilobed nucleus and smaller, peripherally located metachromatic granules.[264]

Lymphocytes

There are two types of peripheral lymphocytes: T and B lymphocytes, both of which arise in the bone marrow. One type migrates to the thymus, where it differentiates to a lymphocyte and then proceeds to the peripheral lymphoid tissues as a thymus-derived or T lymphocyte. In lymph nodes, T lymphocytes are located predominantly in the interfollicular cortex, also called the *paracortical* areas. The other type of lymphocyte, the B lymphocyte, matures in the bone marrow.[265] The term *B lymphocyte,* meaning bursa-derived lymphocyte, originally was given because, in birds, the bursa of Fabricius is held responsible for B-cell maturation.[265] In humans, the term *B lymphocyte* is used to mean bone marrow–derived lymphocyte. In lymph nodes, B lymphocytes largely occupy the lymph follicles, including their germinal centers. Whereas the T lymphocyte is the effector cell for cellular immunity, the B lymphocyte mediates humoral immunity. The lymph nodes and other lymphoid organs share three principal functions: (1) to concentrate within them antigens from all parts of the body; (2) to circulate the lymphocyte population through the lymphoid organs so that every antigen is exposed to antigen-specific lymphocytes; and (3) to carry the products of the immune response, the humoral antibodies and cells mediating cellular immunity, to the blood and tissue.[265] T cells can exert important regulating functions on both T cells and B cells in the form of specific functional subsets termed *helper T cells* and *suppressor T cells.*[266]

Lymphocytes measure on the average 8 μm in diameter and possess a relatively small, round nucleus that appears deeply basophilic because of the presence of numerous chromatin particles (see Fig. 3-34). They have only a very narrow rim of cytoplasm that is hardly recognizable. It is usually impossible by light microscopy to distinguish lymphocytes from monocytes in routinely stained histologic sections; and, in several instances in which it was once assumed that lymphocytes were an important constituent of the dermal infiltrate, such as in contact dermatitis and sarcoidosis, it has been shown through demonstration of the presence of lysosomal enzymes within the cells and through electron microscopy that many of the cells are monocytes rather than lymphocytes. It is therefore preferable to refer to cells with a histologic appearance of lymphocytes as *lymphoid cells*. Ultrastructurally, resting lymphocytes contain relatively few organelles within a thin cytoplasmic rim that surrounds a nucleus with coarsely aggregated heterochromatin (see Fig. 3-33D).

Although T and B cells are indistinguishable by light microscopy, they can be differentiated by in vitro tests. Human T lymphocytes have receptors for sheep erythrocytes, so that, in the E rosette assay, sheep erythrocytes (E) form rosettes around T lymphocytes. Furthermore, T lymphocytes undergo blastic transformation when exposed to mitogens such as phytohemagglutinin or concanavalin A, and anti–T-lymphocyte antisera have a specific cytotoxic effect on them.[267,268] Antibodies are now available for the identification of T cells and B cells in routine paraffin sections (UCHL and L26, respectively). Specific detection of cell surface glycoproteins that correlate with T-cell functional subsets (CD4 for helper, CD8 for suppressor) or with T-cell maturation or activation (CD2, CD3, CD5, and Il-2 receptor, respectively) is most sensitively accomplished in fresh-frozen tissue sections. The same is true for classification of B-cell light chain expression (κ versus λ). It is important to realize that normal skin will contain small numbers of perivascular T cells with the helper subtype predominating as part of the skin immune system.

T cells play an important role in normal cutaneous immunosurveillance and in delayed hypersensitivity reactions. Initial antigen uptake by Langerhans cells occurs during sensitization. After their migration to draining lymph nodes via dermal lymphatics (see text following), Langerhans cells present antigen to naive T cells, which undergo initial clonal expansion to become memory cells. Experimental data suggest that antigen-specific molecules capable of degranulating mast cells upon antigen reexposure may also occur at this step.[269] In the challenge reaction, the dermal microvascular unit is activated (possibly in part because of mast cell degranulation), resulting in a display of leukocyte adhesion molecules on the endothelial luminal surface that facilitate the recruitment of memory T cells. Upon local antigen presentation at the challenge site, these pioneer memory cells, now capable of antigen recognition, respond by elaboration of a cascade of cytokines that results in the recruitment of secondary inflammatory cells.

The B lymphocyte is the effector cell of humoral immunity. On antigenic stimulation, the primary follicles in lymph nodes, composed of small B lymphocytes, develop into secondary follicles, consisting of a germinal center surrounded by a rim of small B lymphocytes.[265] In the germinal centers, small B lymphocytes enlarge through an intermediate stage of centrocytes with cleaved nuclei into centroblasts, which are large cells with noncleaved nuclei.[270] The centroblasts become immunoblasts as a result of antigenic stimulation and produce a clone of daughter cells that mature into immunoglobulin-secreting plasma cells.[271,272] The differentiation of B lymphocytes into plasma cells is aided by helper T cells and is inhibited by suppressor T cells.[273] The plasma cells collect in the medullary cords of lymph nodes without circulating in the bloodstream but secrete immunoglobulins that circulate as "humoral" antibodies. Although these events most commonly occur in lymph nodes, identical alterations may take place in the dermis in response to locally introduced antigen, as is the case in cutaneous lymphoid hyperplasia with prominent germinal center formation.[274,275]

Plasma Cells

Plasma cells have an abundant cytoplasm that is deeply basophilic, homogeneous, and sharply defined (see Fig. 3-34). The round nucleus is eccentrically placed and shows along its membrane coarse, deeply basophilic, regularly distributed chromatin particles, which give the nucleus a cartwheel appearance. The fact that patients with agammaglobulinemia lack plasma cells was responsible for early recognition of the fact that the plasma cell is the site of formation of all immunoglobulins that circulate as humoral antibodies. The synthesis of immunoglobulins takes place in plasma cells located mainly in the lymph nodes, the spleen, and the bone marrow. Because plasma cells are tissue cells and are not seen in the peripheral circulation, it can be assumed that, if they are present in the dermis, they have developed there from B lymphocytes. Intracytoplasmic immunoglobulins may be demonstrated immunohistochemically in paraffin-embedded tissue. Subclassification of cells according to kappa (approximately two thirds of reactive plasma cells) and lambda (approximately one third of reactive plasma cells) is also possible, and may facilitate in some instances detection of a neoplastic clone, where only one of the light chains is produced exclusively. On electron microscopy, plasma cells are characterized by the presence in their cytoplasm of an extensive system of cisternae lined by a rough endoplasmic reticulum. The cisternae usually are flat but may be irregularly dilated. Numerous ribosomes not only line the membranes of the endoplasmic reticulum but are also present in the cytoplasm. The abundant ribosomes and the highly developed endoplasmic reticulum are involved in the synthesis of immunoglobulins. Thus the cisternae are often filled with a homogeneous to granular substance that is released into the extracellular space.

Plasma cells are apt to be present in conspicuous numbers in several infectious diseases, such as early syphilis, rhinoscleroma, and granuloma inguinale. In the presence of many plasma cells, but especially in rhinoscleroma, round, hyaline, eosinophilic bodies called Russell bodies may be found inside and outside of plasma cells. They form within plasma cells as the result of a very active synthesis of immunoglobulins and may ultimately completely replace the plasma cells in which they have formed.[276] They may possess a size twice that of normal plasma cells, measuring up to 20 μm in diameter. They contain varying amounts of glycoproteins and are as a rule Gram-positive as well as PAS-positive and diastase-resistant.[277] Russell bodies are initiated by intracisternal secretion, analogous to the secretion of immunoglobulins. When the plasma cell is overloaded with this material, first the nucleus and ultimately the entire cell lyse.[276] Immunofluorescence staining shows the presence of immunoglobulins within the Russell bodies. Intense staining of Russell bodies is observed when anti–light chain conjugates are used, but not when anti–heavy chain conjugates are used.[278]

DERMAL LYMPHATICS

Dermal lymphatics are often inconspicuous in normal skin because they do not have well-developed walls, as do blood vessels. They are easily detected, however, when they become slightly ectatic as a result of increased lymphatic drainage, as in urticaria. Lymph vessels typically are not rounded in contour, but rather show angulations dictated by the fact that their lining endothelium is buttressed by adjacent collagen bundles (Fig. 3-35). In normal skin, the perilymphatic space is relatively devoid of other cells, and the lumen is lined by relatively flattened endothelial cells. Occasional valves may be observed emanating from the endothelial lining. By electron microscopy, the thin layer of endothelium does not contain Weibel-Palade bodies and is devoid of a basement membrane or surrounding pericytes. Lymphatic vessels show a negative or weakly positive reaction when incubated with *Ulex europaeus* lectin and no reaction with an antibody against factor VIII-related antigen in most instances. They do not contain class I (HLA-A,B,C) or class II (HLA-DR) antigens.[192] Endothelial cells of lymphatic vessels contain cytoplasmic filaments,[279] which probably represent vimentin filaments.

DERMAL FIBROBLASTS

The dermis of a 2-month-old embryo consists of loosely arranged mesenchymal cells that are embedded in ground substance. During the third month, argyrophilic reticulum fibers appear. As these fibers increase in number and in thickness, they arrange themselves in bundles that no longer can be impregnated with silver and, instead, stain with the methods for collagen. Simultaneously, the mesenchymal cells develop into fibroblasts. Electron microscopic examination of the fetal dermis from week 6 to week 14 reveals, apart from Schwann cells identified by their association with neuraxons, three main types of cells: (1) stellate mesenchymal cells with long processes; (2) phagocytic macrophages of probable yolk-sac origin; and (3) cells containing granules, which could be either melanoblasts or mast cell precursors. From week 14 on, fibroblasts become numerous. In the normal adult dermis, fibroblasts appear as inconspicuous bipolar spindle cells with elongated ovoid nuclei. They cannot reliably be distinguished from other dermal spindle-shaped and dendritic cells. By electron microscopy, fibroblasts that actively synthesize collagen have a prominent rough endoplasmic reticulum composed of many membrane-lined cisternae with large numbers of attached ribosomes (Fig. 3-36). The dilated cisternae are filled with an amorphous material produced by the ribosomes lining the cisternae.[280] This apparently amorphous material consists of triple helical procollagen molecules, each molecule being composed of three pro-alpha polypeptide chains. The procollagen molecules pass from the cisternae of the rough endoplasmic reticulum to the Golgi area, on which they are excreted into the extracellular space by means of secretory vesicles.[281,282] Conversion of procollagen molecules into collagen molecules composed of three alpha chains then occurs outside the cell.[283]

DERMAL MUSCLE CELLS

Smooth Muscle

Smooth or involuntary muscle of the skin occurs as arrectores pilorum (Fig. 3-37), as tunica dartos of the external genitals, and in the areola of the nipples. The muscle fibers of the arrectores pilorum arise in the connective tissue of the upper dermis and are attached to the hair follicle below the sebaceous glands (see Fig. 3-15). They are situated in the obtuse angle of the hair follicle. Thus, when contracted, they pull the hair follicle into a vertical position and produce the perifollicular elevations of "gooseflesh."

Smooth muscle is characterized by the absence of striation and by the location of the nucleus in the center of the muscle

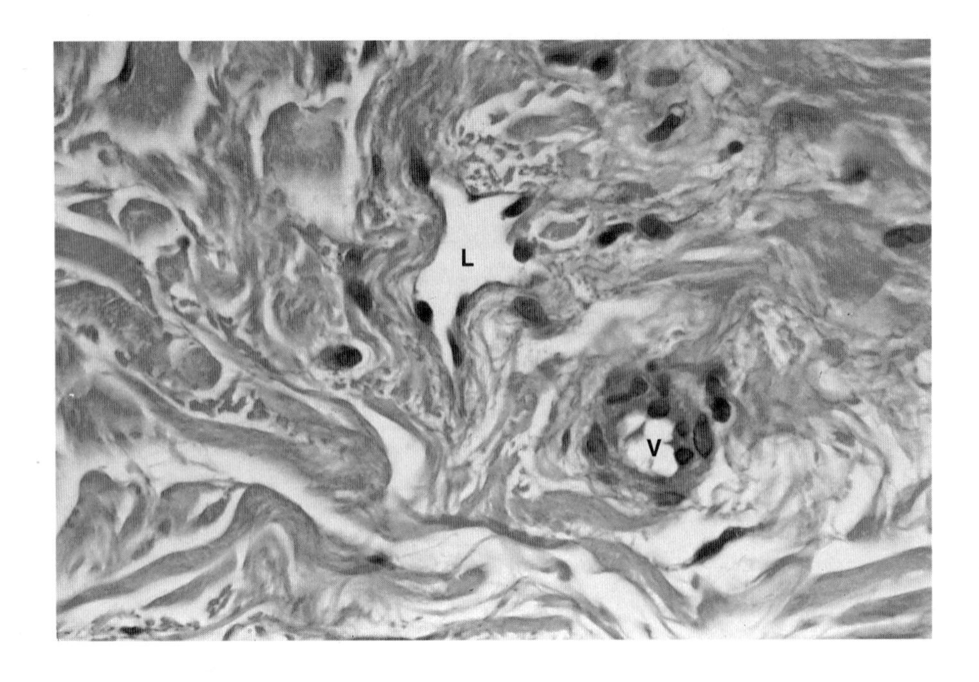

FIG. 3-35. Lymph vessel Dermal lymphatic (*L*) and adjacent blood vessel (*V*); note relative absence of vessel wall defining lymphatic space.

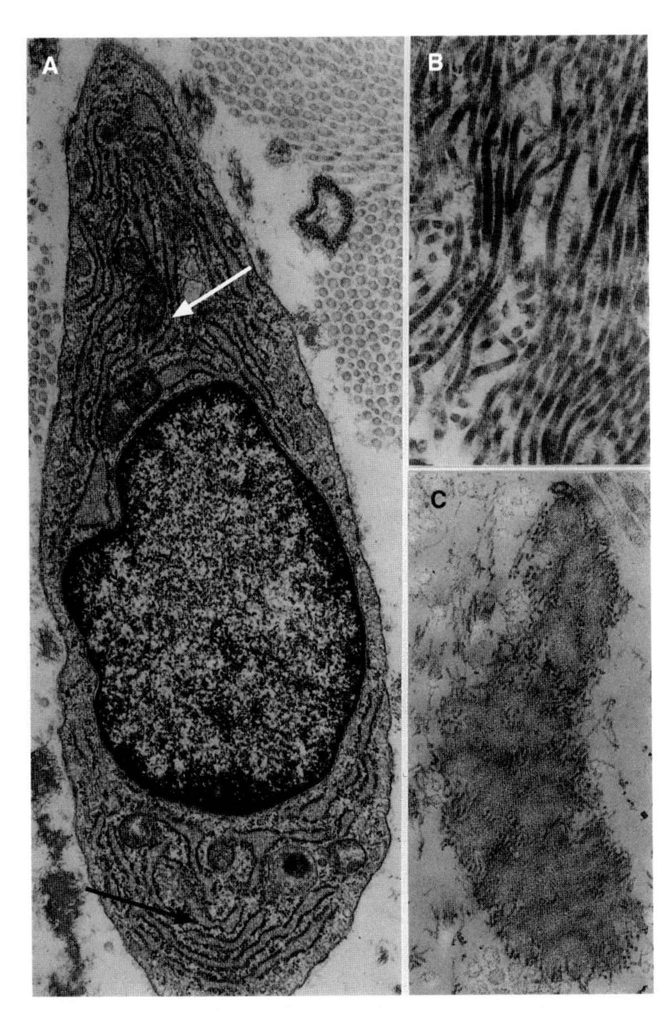

FIG. 3-36. Dermal fibroblast
(**A**) Dermal fibroblast with dilated cisternae of rough endoplasmic reticulum (*arrows*). (**B**) Collagen fibrils. (**C**) Elastic fibrils.

cell. Typically, the nuclei are "cigar-shaped," with rounded ends, a feature that may be diagnostically helpful in assessing dermal spindle cell proliferations and neoplasms. Argyrophilic reticulum fibers surround each muscle cell. Electron microscopic examination reveals that smooth muscle cells possess a basement membrane peripheral to the plasma membrane. The cytoplasm of the cells is filled with myofilaments, 5 nm in diameter, that form cytoplasmic and peripheral dense bodies as a result of condensations, just as the myofilaments do in myoepithelial cells, in vascular smooth muscle cells, and in glomus cells. The rather narrow spaces between the muscle cells are occupied by collagen fibrils and by Schwann cells with associated nonmyelinated axons.

Smooth muscle cells contain vimentin and desmin as intermediate filaments. In addition, they show a positive reaction when incubated with an antibody against actin protein.

Striated Muscle

Striated or voluntary muscle is found in the skin of the neck as platysma and in the skin of the face as muscles of expression. The striated muscle bundles take their origin either from a fascia or from the periosteum, or they form a closed ring, as in the musculus sphincter oris. They extend through the subcutaneous tissue into the lower dermis. The muscle fibers, like skeletal muscle, show characteristic cytoplasmic cross striations (Fig. 3-38). Their nuclei are located at the periphery of the fibers immediately beneath the sarcolemma, the limiting membrane of the fibers.

EXTRACELLULAR MATRIX

The extracellular matrix of the dermis consists of collagenous and elastic fibers embedded into ground substance. All three components are formed by fibroblasts.

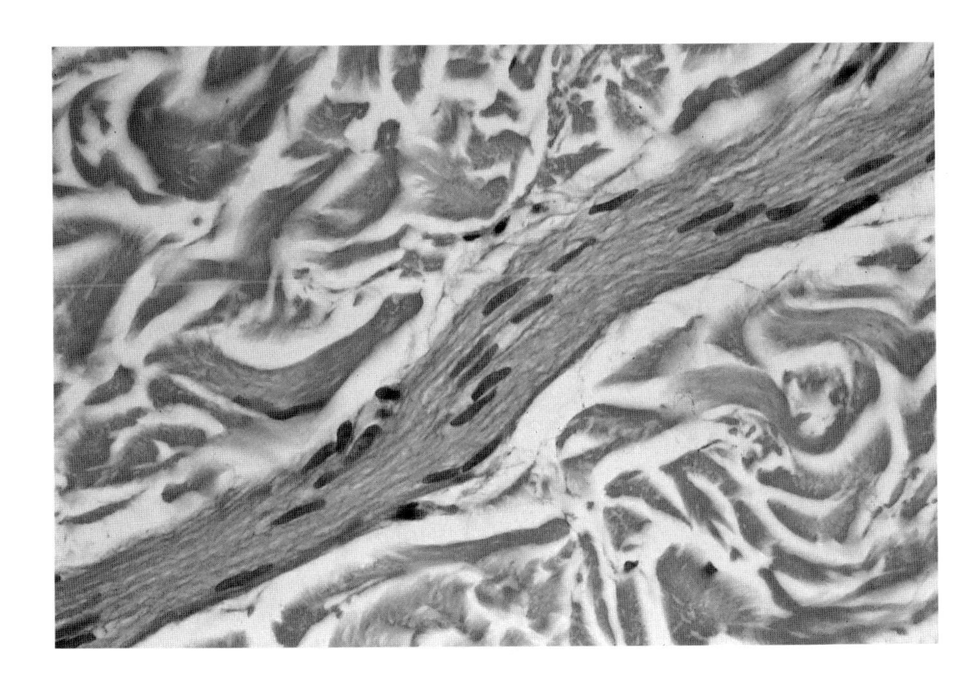

FIG. 3-37. Arrector pili muscle
Surrounded by reticular dermal collagen bundles.

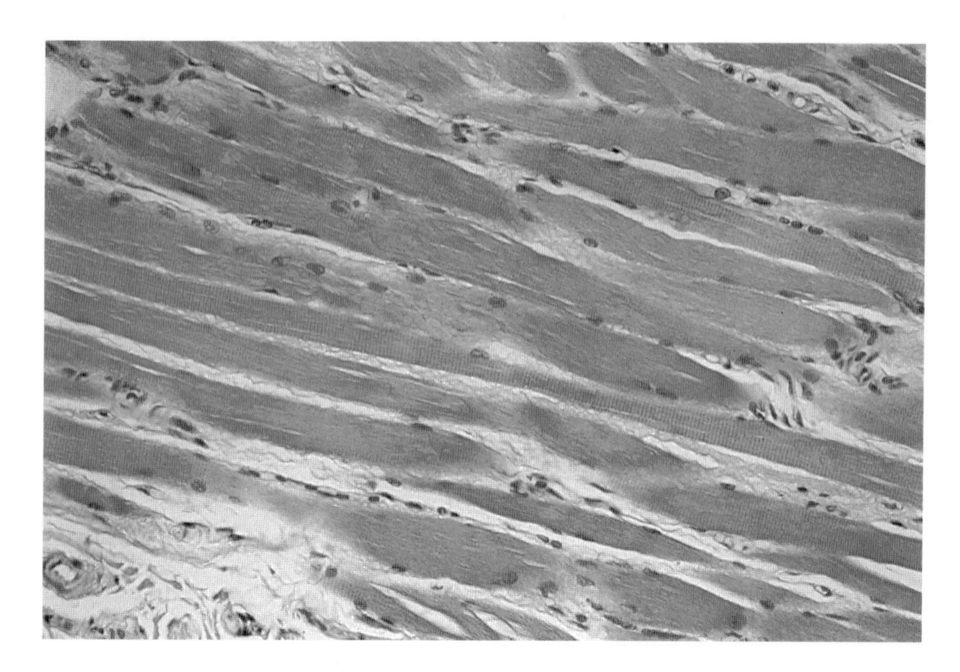

FIG. 3-38. Subcutaneous skeletal muscle with characteristic striations

Collagen Fibers

Collagen represents by far the most abundant constituent of the connective tissue of the dermis. On light microscopy, collagen consists of fibers (Fig. 3-39). The diameter of collagen fibers is quite variable, ranging from 2 to 15 μm. The collagen fibers are present either as a finely woven network or as thick bundles. Collagen as a finely woven meshwork of collagen fibers is found in the papillary layer of the dermis, which includes not only the subepidermal papillae situated between the rete ridges but also the subpapillary layer forming a narrow ribbon between the rete ridges and the subpapillary blood vessels (see Fig. 3-4). This is referred to as the *papillary dermis.* In addition, the pilosebaceous units and the eccrine and apocrine glands are encircled by a thin meshwork of collagen fibers similar to that present in the papillary dermis. Therefore, the papillary and the periadnexal dermis are regarded as a single anatomical unit, the adventitial dermis. The blood vessels of the dermis are also surrounded by a thin layer of fine collagen fibers. Biochemically, the papillary dermis is composed primarily of type III collagen.

The rest of the dermis, constituting by far the largest portion of the dermis and referred to as the *reticular dermis,* shows the collagen fibers united into thick bundles (see Figs. 3-37 and 3-39). These collagen bundles extend in various directions horizontally, and thus some are cut lengthwise and others across in histologic sections. As a rule, collagen bundles that are cut lengthwise appear slightly wavy. Biochemically, reticular dermal collagen is composed primarily of type I collagen.

Reticulum fibers are not recognizable with routine stains,

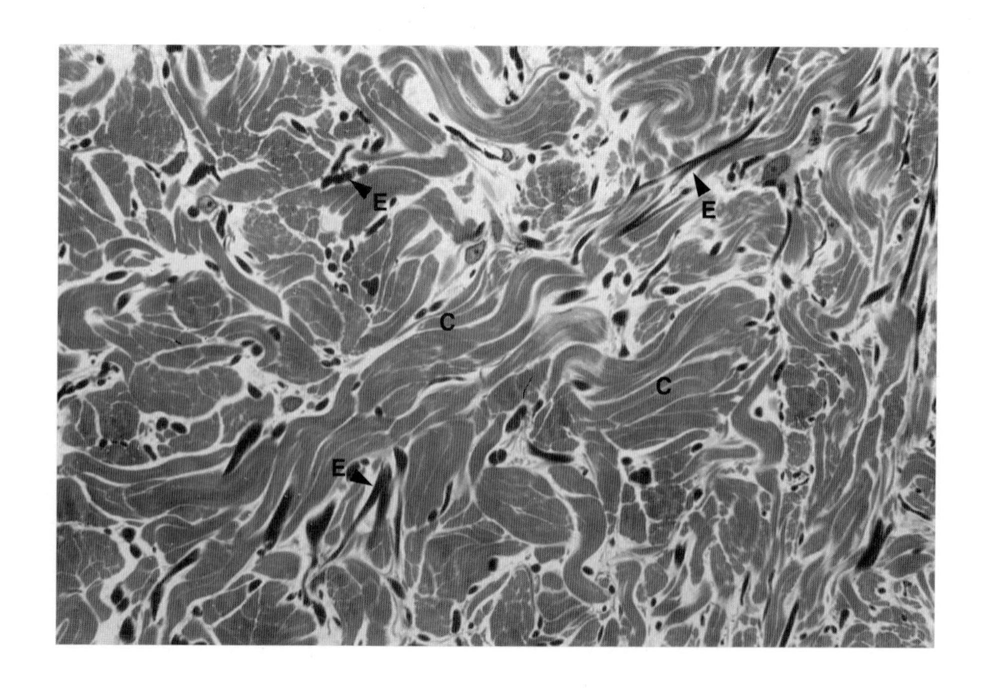

FIG. 3-39. Collagen fibers Plastic-embedded section showing collagen (*C*) and elastin (*E*) within normal human reticular dermis. Normal elastin is often less conspicuous in routinely stained paraffin sections.

but, being argyrophilic, they can be impregnated with silver nitrate, which, by being subsequently reduced to silver, stains black. Reticulum fibers represent a special type of thin collagen fiber that measures from 0.2 to 1.0 μm in diameter. The argyrophilia shown by reticulum fibers, in contrast to collagen fibers, probably is related to the fact that reticulum fibers correspond to the distribution of type III collagen rather than type I collagen.

Argyrophilic reticulum fibers are the first-formed fibers during embryonic life and in various pathologic conditions are associated with increased fibroblastic activity. In normal skin, even though collagen is being continuously replaced, the formation of new collagen is not preceded by an argyrophilic phase. Rather, all newly formed collagen consists of large fibers. However, there are a few areas in which normally small collagen fibers are present as reticulum fibers without transforming into larger, nonargyrophilic collagen fibers. This occurs above all in the basement membrane zone, the region of the adventitial dermis that lies closest to the epidermis and its appendages. In addition, reticulum fibers are present normally around blood vessels and as a basketlike capsule around each fat cell.

The biosynthesis of collagen begins within the fibroblast by the assembly of three pro-alpha polypeptide chains into a triple helical procollagen molecule.[283] After excretion into the extracellular space, the three pro-alpha chains of each procollagen molecule are shortened by 30% to 40% through removal of the carboxy-terminal and amino-terminal peptide extensions brought about by the action of two enzymes produced by the fibroblast: carboxy-terminal peptidase and amino-terminal peptidase.[282] This results in conversion of the procollagen molecule into the collagen molecule. Although the additional peptides present in procollagen keep it soluble and prevent its intracellular polymerization, collagen molecules polymerize readily. The collagen molecule is a rigid rod in which each of the three coiled alpha chains consists of about 1000 amino acids.[283] The collagen molecule is about 300 nm long and 1.5 nm wide.[284,285] Collagen fibrils form by both lateral and longitudinal association of collagen molecules. However, the collagen fibrils vary in diameter as a result of varying degrees of polymerization of collagen molecules, with younger collagen fibrils being thinner than older fibrils. In the normal dermis, the thickness of collagen fibrils ranges from 70 to 140 nm; most of the fibrils are approximately 100 nm thick.[286]

Collagen fibrils possess characteristic cross striations with a periodicity of 68 nm (see Fig. 3-36B). The periodicity of the cross striations in the collagen fibrils can be explained as follows. Each collagen molecule possesses along its length of 300 nm five charged regions 68 nm apart, and although neighboring collagen molecules overlap each other, they always have their charged regions lying side by side. This parallel alignment of the charged regions produces the cross striations.[285] Reticulum fibrils possess the same 68-nm periodicity of their cross striations as collagen fibrils but have a smaller diameter than collagen fibrils, varying between 40 and 65 nm rather than between 70 and 140 nm.[287] Furthermore, reticulum and collagen differ in the number of fibrils present in the cross section of each fiber and in the amount of ground substance present within and around each fiber. The amount of ground substance around the fibrils and on the surface of the fiber may explain the presence of argyrophilia in reticulum fibers and its absence in collagen fibers.[287]

At least seven different types of collagen have been recognized that differ in composition and antigenicity. Type I collagen, the predominant collagen in postfetal skin, is found in the large fiber bundles of the reticular dermis. Reticulum fibers are composed of type III collagen. Although type III collagen is the prevalent type of collagen in early fetal life, in postfetal life it is limited to the subepidermal and periappendageal regions, that is, the basement membrane zones and the perivascular region.[288] Basement membrane collagen (basal lamina collagen) is type IV, and the collagen of cartilage is type II. Type V collagen has been recognized in fetal membranes and vascular tissue.[289] Type VII collagen occurs in different basement membranes, including those of the skin, and forms a major structural component of anchoring fibrils.[290] The skin of the human fetus contains a large percentage of type III collagen, in contrast to the skin of the adult, which contains a large proportion of type I collagen.[291]

Among the differences in compostion are the following. In type I collagen, the three alpha chains in the collagen molecule consist of two different kinds: two identical alpha chains designated as alpha-1(I), and a third chain called alpha-2. In type II collagen, the collagen molecules are composed of three identical, genetically distinct alpha chains, alpha-1(II). Type III collagen is also composed of three identical, distinct alpha chains.[282] Type IV collagen consists of procollagen composed of three identical pro-alpha chains that have retained their nonhelical extensions. Types V and VI collagen have not yet been adequately characterized. Type VII collagen consists of 3 alpha chains, with the terminal regions being noncollagenous.[290]

Elastic Fibers

Elastic fibers appear in the dermis at 22 weeks, much later than the collagenous fibers. At this time, acid orcein stains show elastic tissue in the reticular dermis either as granular material interspersed with occasional short fibers or as a delicate network of branching fibers. As gestation progresses, elastic fibers increase in quantity. At 32 weeks, a well-developed network of elastic fibers indistinguishable from that seen in term infants is present in both the papillary and the reticular dermis.[292] Young elastic fibers, as seen in a 22-week-old fetal dermis, show masses of peripheral microfibrils surrounding a small amorphous electron-lucent core representing elastin, with only a few internal microfibrils. As the embryo matures, the amount of elastin and the number of microfibrils within the elastin increase while the number of perpheral microfibrils decreases.[293]

In light microscopic sections that are routinely stained, elastic fibers are inconspicuous. With special elastic tissue stains, such as orcein or resorcin-fuchsin or in plastic-embedded sections, they are found entwined among the collagen bundles (see Fig. 3-39). Because elastic fibers are thin in comparison with collagen bundles, measuring from 1 to 3 μm in diameter, and are wavy, only a small portion of any fiber is seen in histologic sections, giving even normal elastic fibers a fragmented appearance. The elastic fibers are thickest in the lower portion of the dermis, where they are arranged, like collagen bundles, chiefly parallel to the surface of the skin. Elastic fibers become thinner as they approach the epidermis. In the papillary dermis, they form an intermediate plexus of thinner elaunin fibers running

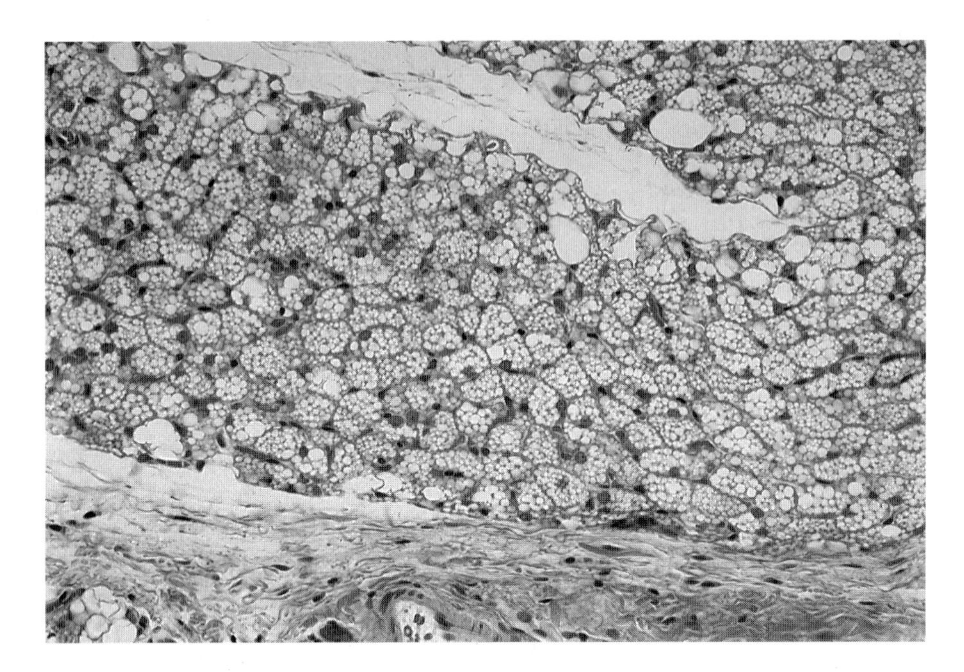

FIG. 3-40. Subcutaneous fat Fetal (brown) adipose tissue.

parallel to the dermoepidermal junction. From this plexus, thin fibers termed oxytalan fibers run upwards in the papillary dermis perpendicular to the dermoepidermal junction and terminate at the PAS-positive basement membrane zone.

The elastic fiber of the dermis consists of two components: the microfibrils and the matrix elastin. The microfibrils are electron-dense and measure 10 to 12 nm in diameter. They are aggregated at the periphery of the elastic fiber, giving the fiber its characteristic frayed appearance by ultrastructure (see Fig. 3-36C). In addition, microfibrils are present within the elastin as strands 15 to 80 nm in diameter, extending in a longitudinal direction.[294] The microfibril component amounts to only 15% of the elastic fiber, whereas the amorphous electron-lucent elastin makes up to 85% of the the fiber.[295] It is the elastin that stains with elastic tissue stains, is removable by elastase, and is markedly extensible, whereas the microfibrils are the elastic resilient component of the elastic fiber.[294]

Elastic fibers undergo significant changes during life. One change, representing aging, is best studied in nonexposed skin. The other change, elastotic degeneration, is the result of chronic sun exposure and will be described elsewhere. In young children up to the age of 10 years, the elastic fibers may not be fully matured, so that microfibrils predominate.[296] Physiologic aging is a gradual process and usually becomes quite apparent by ages 30 to 50. There is a gradual decrease in the number of peripheral microfibrils, so that ultimately there may be none and, instead, the surface of the elastic fiber appears irregular and granular.[296] The microfibrils within the elastin matrix become thicker and show electron-lucent holes of varying sizes.[297] In very old persons, fragmentation and disintegration of some of

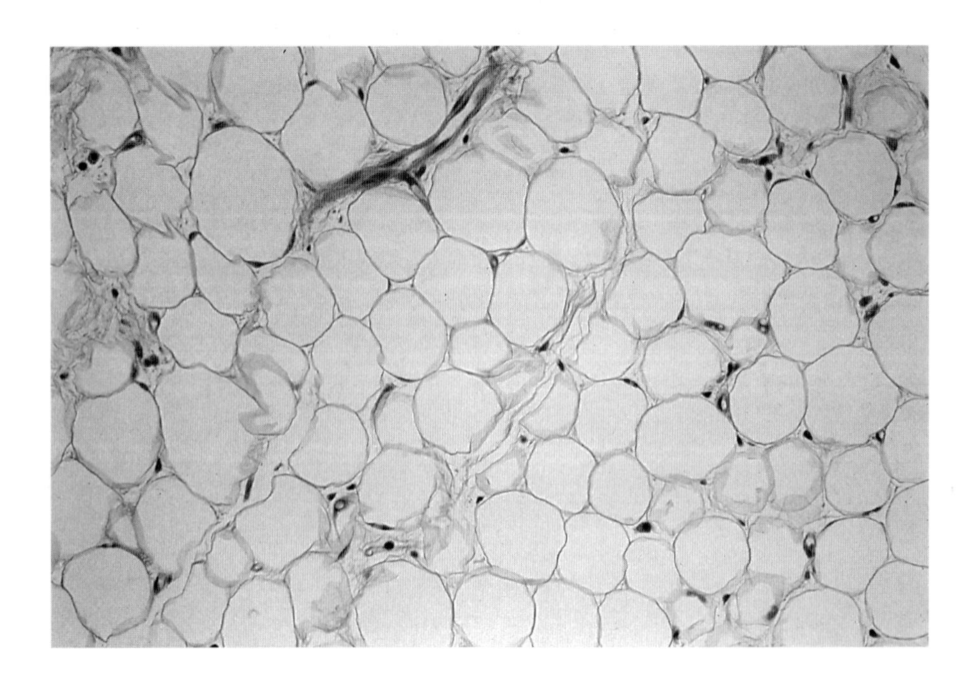

FIG. 3-41. Subcutaneous fat Mature adipose tissue forming the subcutaneous layer.

the elastic fibers may be observed. Oxytalan fibers that consist of microfibrils diminish and ultimately disappear in aging skin.

Ground Substance

The ground substance, an amorphous substance that fills the spaces between collagen fibers and collagen bundles, contains glycosaminoglycans, or acid mucopolysaccharides. These glycosaminoglycans are covalently linked to peptide chains to form high-molecular-weight complexes called proteoglycans.[298] Glycosaminoglycans are present in normal skin in such small amounts that they cannot be demonstrated with either routine or special histologic staining methods except in the hair papilla of anagen hair, which contains both nonsulfated and sulfated acid mucopolysaccharides. However, through the study of tissues with an active growth of fibroblasts, as seen in the papillary dermis in dermatofibroma and in the connective tissue around the tumor islands of basal cell epithelioma, it is known that the dermal ground substance consists largely of nonsulfated acid mucopolysaccharides such as hyaluronic acid.[130] In healing wounds, however, in which new collagen is laid down, the ground substance contains sulfated and nonsulfated acid mucopolysaccharides.[299]

The nonsulfated acid mucopolysaccharides consist largely of hyaluronic acid, are stainable with alcian blue at pH 3.0 but not at pH 0.5, and show metachromasia with toluidine blue at pH 3.0 but not at pH 1.5. The sulfated acid mucopolysaccharides consist largely of chondroitin sulfate, are stainable with alcian blue at pH 0.5 as well as at pH 3.0, and show metachromasia with toluidine blue at pH 1.5 as well as at pH 3.0. Both nonsulfated and sulfated acid mucopolysaccharides stain with colloidal iron. Testicular hyaluronidase hydrolyzes hyaluronic acid but not the sulfated acid mucopolysaccharides.[130]

SUBCUTANEOUS FAT

Fat cells begin to develop in the subcutaneous tissue toward the end of the fifth month. Histologic examination at that time shows (1) spindle-shaped, lipid-free mesenchymal cells as precursor cells; (2) young-type fat cells containing two or more small lipid droplets; and (3) mature fat cells possessing one large central lipid droplet and a peripherally located nucleus, so-called signet-ring cells. Although some of the cells containing multiple small lipid droplets resemble the multivacuolated mulberry cells present in brown fat and in hibernoma (Fig. 3-40), only few such cells occur in embryonic white fat. Brown and white fat are two separate entities incapable of interconversion.[300]

Mature subcutaneous fat consists of lobules composed of adipocytes with cytoplasm markedly expanded by nonvacuolated or membrane-bound lipid that displaces the cell nucleus eccentrically to produce a thin, fusiform contour compressed along the inner plasma membrane (Fig. 3-41). The lipid dissolves in routinely processed specimens, although it is visible in glutaraldehyde-fixed, plastic-embedded specimens. It may be stained histochemically in frozen section obtained from fresh or "wet" tissue retrieved while still in formalin. The lobules that form the subcutis are separated by thin fibrous septa through which small vessels course. The septa provide structural stability to the subcutaneous layer by compartmentalizing it and by connecting the lowermost reticular dermis to the fascial planes that underlie the subcutis.

REFERENCES

1. Morrison P, Morrison P. Powers of Ten. New York: Scientific American Library, 1994.
2. Breathnach AS. Embryology of human skin. J Invest Dermatol 1971; 57:133.
3. Holbrook KA, Odland GF. The fine structure of developing human epidermis: Light scanning and transmission electron microscopy of the periderm. J Invest Dermatol 1975;65:16.
4. Hashimoto K, Gross BG, Dibella RJ et al. The ultrastructure of the skin of human embryos: IV. The epidermis. J Invest Dermatol 1966; 47:317.
5. Matsunaka M, Mishima Y. Electron microscopy of embryonic human epidermis at seven and ten weeks. Acta Derm Venereol (Stockh) 1969;49:241.
6. Van Scott EJ, Ekel TM. Kinetics of hyperplasia in psoriasis. Arch Dermatol 1963;88:373.
7. Penneys NS, Fulton JE Jr, Weinstein GD et al. Location of proliferating cells in human epidermis. Arch Dermatol 1970;101:323.
8. Lavker RM, Sun T-T. Heterogeneity in epidermal basal keratinocytes: Morphological and functional correlations. Science 1982;215:1239.
9. Cotsarelis G, Sun T-T, Lavker RM. Label-retaining cells reside in the bulge area of the pilosebaceous unit: Implications for follicular stem cells, hair cycle and skin carcinogenesis. Cell 1990;61:1329.
10. Cerimele D, Del Forno C, Serri F. Histochemistry of the intercellular substance of the normal and psoriatic human epidermis. Arch Dermatol Res 1978;262:27.
11. Hashimoto K, Lever WF. The cell surface coat of normal keratinocytes and of acantholytic keratinocytes in pemphigus. Br J Dermatol 1970;83:282.
12. Odland GF. The fine structure of the interrelationship of cells in the human epidermis. J Biophys Biochem Cytol 1958;4:529.
13. Wolff K, Schreiner E. An electron microscopic study on the extraneous coat of keratinocytes and the intercellular space of the epidermis. J Invest Dermatol 1968;51:418.
14. Wolff K, Wolff-Schreiner EC. Trends in electron microscopy of skin. J Invest Dermatol 1976;67:39.
15. Amagi M: Adhesion molecules: I. Keratinocyte-keratinocyte interactions; cadherins and pemphigus. Prog Dermatol 1995;104:146.
16. Buxton RS, Magee AI. Structure and interactions of desmosomal and other cadherins. Semin Cell Biol 1992;3:157.
17. Amagai M, Klaus KV, Stanley JR. Autoantibodies against a novel epithelial cadherin in pemphigus vulgaris: A disease of cell adhesion. Cell 1991;67:869.
18. Shimuzu H, Masunaga T, Ishiko A et al. Demonstration of desmosomal antigens by electron microscopy using cryofixed and cryosubstituted skin with silver-enhanced gold probe. J Histochem Cytochem 1994;42:687.
19. Matoltsy AG. Desmosomes, filaments, and keratohyaline granules: Their role in stabilization and keratinization of the epidermis. J Invest Dermatol 1975;65:127.
20. Matoltsy AG. Keratinization. J Invest Dermatol 1976;67:20.
21. Schwarz E. Biochemie der epidermalen keratinisation. In: Marchionini A, ed: Handbuch der hautund geschlectskrankheiten. Vol. 1. Berlin: Springer-Verlag, 1979;1.
22. Lazarus GS, Hatcher VB, Levine N. Lysosomes and the skin. J Invest Dermatol 1975;65:259.
23. Spearman RIC. Some light microscopical observations on the stratum corneum of the guinea pig, man and common seal. Br J Dermatol 1970;83:582.
24. Christophers E. Cellular architecture of the stratum corneum. J Invest Dermatol 1971;56:165.
25. Hashimoto K. Cellular envelopes of keratinized cells of the human epidermis. Arch Klin Exp Dermatol 1969;235:374.
26. Bell RF, Kellum RE. Early formation of keratohyalin granules in rat epidermis. Acta Derm Venereol (Stockh) 1967;47:350.
27. Dale BA. Filaggrin: The matrix protein of keratin. Am J Dermatopathol 1985;7:65.

28. Brody I. An electron microscopic study of the fibrillar density in the normal human stratum corneum. J Ultrastruct Res 1970;30:209.
29. Murphy GF, Flynn TC, Rice RH, Pinkus GS. Involucrin expression in normal and neoplastic human skin: A marker for keratinocyte differentiation. J Invest Dermatol 1884;82:453.
30. Wolff-Schreiner EC. Ultrastructural cytochemistry of the epidermis (review). Int J Dermatol 1977;16:77.
31. Elias PM. Epidermal lipids, barrier function, and desquamation. J Invest Dermatol 1983;80:44.
32. Schreiner E, Wolff K. Die permeabilitüt des epidermalen intercellularraums für kleinmolekulares protein. Arch Klin Exp Dermatol 1969; 235:78.
33. Elias PM, Goerke J, Friend DS. Mammalian epidermal barrier layer lipids: Composition and influence on structure. J Invest Dermatol 1977;69:535.
34. Epstein EH Jr, Williams ML, Elias PM. Editorial: Steroid sulfatase, X-linked ichthyosis, and stratum corneum cell cohesion. Arch Dermatol 1981;117:761.
35. Braun-Falco O, Rupec M. Die verteilung der sauren phosphatase bei normaler und psoriatischer verhornung. Dermatologicia 1967;134: 225.
36. Wolff K, Schreiner E. Epidermal lysosomes: Electron microscopic cytochemical studies. Arch Dermatol 1970;101:276.
37. Bos JD, Kapsenberg ML. The skin immune system: Progress in cutaneous biology. Immunol Today 1993;14:75.
38. Katz SI. The skin as an immunologic organ: Allergic contact dermatitis as a paradigm. J Dermatol 1993;20:593.
39. Becker SW Jr, Zimmermann AA. Further studies on melanocytes and melanogenesis in the human fetus and newborn. J Invest Dermatol 1955;25:103.
40. Sagebiel RW, Odland GF. Ultrastructural identification of melanocytes in early human embryos (abstr). J Invest Dermatol 1970;54:96.
41. Holbrook KA, Underwood RA, Vogel AM. The appearance, density and distribution of melanocytes in human embryonic and fetal skin revealed by the anti-melanoma monoclonal antibody HMB-45. Anat Embryol 1989;180:443.
42. Cochran AJ. The incidence of melanocytes in normal skin. J Invest Dermatol 1970;55:65.
43. Clark WH Jr, Watson MC, Watson BEM. Two kinds of "clear" cells in the human epidermis. Am J Pathol 1961;39:333.
44. Fitzpatrick TB. Human melanogenesis. Arch Dermatol Syph 1952;65: 379.
45. Pearse AGE. Histochemistry: Theoretical and Applied. 3rd ed. Edinburgh: Churchill Livingstone, 1972;1056.
46. Bloch B. Das problem der pigmentbildung in der haut. Arch Dermatol Syph Berlin 1917;124:129.
47. Gilchrest BA, Blog FB, Szabo G. Effects of aging and chronic sun exposure on melanocytes in human skin. J Invest Dermatol 1979;73:141.
48. Tarnowski WM. Ultrastructure of the epidermal melanocyte dense plate. J Invest Dermatol 1970;55:265.
49. Fitzpatrick TB, Miyomato M, Ishikawa K. The evolution of concepts of melanin biology. Arch Dermatol 1967;96:305.
50. Toshima S, Moore GE, Sandberg AA. Ultrastructure of human melanoma in cell culture: Electron microscopic studies. Cancer 1968; 21:202.
51. Staricco RJ, Pinkus H. Quantitative and qualitative data on the pigment cells of adult human epidermis. J Invest Dermatol 1957;28:33.
52. Fitzpatrick TB, Szabo G. The melanocytes: Cytology and cytochemistry. J Invest Dermatol 1959;32:197.
53. Quevedo WC Jr, Szabo G, Virks J et al. Melanocyte populations in UV-radiated human skin. J Invest Dermatol 1965;45:295.
54. Pathak MA, Sinesi SJ, Szabo G. The effect of a single dose of ultraviolet radiation on epidermal melanocytes. J Invest Dermatol 1965;45: 520.
55. Mishima Y, Tanay A. The effect of alpha-methyldopa and ultraviolet irradiation on melanogenesis. Dermatologica 1968;136:105.
56. Lerner AB, Fitzpatrick TB. Biochemistry of melanin formation. Physiol Rev 1950;30:91.
57. Lerner AB. On the etiology of vitiligo and gray hair. Am J Med 1971; 51:141.
58. Szabo G. Tyrosinase in the epidermal melanocytes of white human skin. Arch Dermatol 1967;76:324.
59. Hunter JAA, Mottaz JH, Zelickson AS. Melanogenesis: Ultrastructural histochemical observations on ultraviolet irradiated human melanocytes. J Invest Dermatol 1970;54:213.
60. Jimbow K, Quevedo WC Jr, Fitzpatrick TB et al. Some aspects of melanin biology (review). J Invest Dermatol 1976;67:72.
61. Nakagawa H. Rhodes A, Fitzpatrick TB et al. Acid phosphatase in melanosome formation: A cytochemical study in normal human melanocytes. J Invest Dermatol 1984;83:140.
62. Shibata T, Prota G, Mishima Y. Non-melanosomal regulatory factors in melanogenesis. J Invest Dermatol 1993;100s:274.
63. Cruickshank CND, Harcourt SA. Pigment donation in vitro. J Invest Dermatol 1964;42:183.
64. Valyi-Nagy IT, Murphy GF, Mancianti M-L et al. Phenotypes and interactions of human melanocytes and keratinocytes in an epidermal reconstruction model. Lab Invest 1990;62:314.
65. Mottaz JH, Zelickson AS. Melanin transfer: A possible phagocytic process. J Invest Dermatol 1967;49:605.
66. Olson RL, Nordquist J, Everett MA. The role of epidermal lysosomes in melanin physiology. Br J Dermatol 1970;83:189.
67. Szabo G, Gerald AB, Pathak MA et al. The ultrastructure of racial color differences in man (abstr). J Invest Dermatol 1970;54:98.
68. Mitchell RE. Melanocytes in Australian Aboriginal skin. J Invest Dermatol 1970;94:93.
69. Flaxman BA, Sosio AC, Van Scott EJ. Changes in melanosome distribution in Caucasoid skin following topical application of N mustard. J Invest Dermatol 1973;60:321.
70. Wolff K, Schreiner E. Melanosomal acid phosphatase. Arch Dermatol Forsch 1971;241:255.
71. Toda K, Kathak MA, Parrish JA et al. Alteration of racial differences in melanosome distribution in human epidermis after exposure to ultraviolet light. Nature 1972;236:143.
72. Moll I et al. Intraepidermal formation of Merkel cells in xenografts of human skin. J Invest Dermatol 1990;94:359.
73. Moll I. Merkel cell distribution in human hair follicles of the fetal and adult scalp. Cell Tissue Res 1994;277:131.
74. Hashimoto K. Fine structure of Merkel cell in human oral mucosa. J Invest Dermatol 1972;58:381.
75. Kidd RL, Krawczyk WS, Wilgram GF. The Merkel cell in human epidermis: Its differentiation from other dendritic cells. Arch Dermatol Forsch 1971;241:374.
76. Smith KR Jr. The ultrastructure of the human Haarsheibe and Merkel cells. J Invest Dermatol 1970;54:150.
77. Moll R et al. Identification of Merkel cells in human skin by specific cytokeratin antibodies: Changes in cell density and distribution in fetal and adult plantar epidermis. Differentiation 1984;28:136.
78. Saurat JH, Merot Y, Didierjean L et al. Normal rabbit Merkel cells do not express neurofilament proteins. J Invest Dermatol 1984;82:641.
79. Ortonne JP, Darmon M. Merkel cells express desmosomal proteins and cytokeratins Acta Derm Venereol (Stockh) 1985;65:161.
80. Ortonne JP, Petchot-Bacque JP, Verrando P et al. Normal Merkel cells express a synaptophysin-like immunoreactivity. Dermatologica 1988; 177:1.
81. Masuda T, Ikida S, Tajima K et al. Neuron-specific enolase (NSE): A specific marker for Merkel cells in human epidermis. J Dermatol 1986;13:67.
82. Foster A, Holbrook KA, Farr AG. Ontogeny of Langerhans cells in human embryonic and fetal skin. J Invest Dermatol 1986;86:240.
83. Penneys NS, Stoer C, Buck B et al. Langerhans cells in fetal and newborn skin and newborn thymus (abstr). Arch Dermatol 1984;120: 1082.
84. Wolff K, Winkelmann RK. The influence of ultraviolet light on the Langerhans cell population and its hydrolytic enzymes in guinea pigs. J Invest Dermatol 1967;48:531.
85. Murphy GF, Shepard RS, Harrist TJ et al. Ultrastructural documentation of HLA-DR antigen reactivity in normal human acrosyringeal epithelium. J Invest Dermatol 1983;81:181.
86. Murphy GF, Bhan AK, Sato S et al. A new immunologic marker for human Langerhans cells. N Engl J Med 1981;304:791.
87. Fithian E, Kung P, Goldstein G, et al. Reactivity of Langerhans cells with hybridoma antibody. Proc Natl Acad Sci USA 1981;78:2541.
88. Murphy GF, Bhan AK, Sato S et al. Characterization of Langerhans cells by the use of monoclonal antibodies. Lab Invest 1981;45:465.
89. Breathnach AS, Wyllie LMA. Melanin in Langerhans cells. J Invest Dermatol 1965;45:401.
90. Niebauer G, Krawczyk WS, Wilgram GF. Über die Langerhans-

zellorganelle bei morbus letterer-siwe. Arch Klin Exp Dermatol 1970; 239;125.
91. Hashimoto K. Langerhans cell granule: An endocytic organelle. Arch Dermatol 1971;104:148.
92. Hanau D, Fabre M, Schmitt DA et al. Human epidermal Langerhans cells internalize by receptor-mediated endocytosis T6 (CD1 "NA1/34") surface antigen: Birbeck granules are involved in the intracellular traffic of the T6 antigen. J Invest Dermatol 1987;89:172.
93. Murphy GF, Bhan AK, Harrist TJ, Mihm MC. In situ identification of T6-positive cells in normal human dermis by immunoelectron microscopy. Br J Dermatol 1983;108:423.
94. Chu, A, Eisinger M, Lee JS et al. Immunoelectron microscopic identification of Langerhans cells using a new antigenic marker. J Invest Dermatol 1982;78:177.
95. Horton JJ, Allen MH, MacDonald DM. An assessment of Langerhans cell quantification in tissue sections. J Am Acad Dermatol 1984;11: 591.
96. Mackie RM, Turbitt ML. The use of a double-label immunoperoxidase monoclonal antibody technique in the investigation of patients with mycosis fungoides. Br J. Dermatol 1982;106:379.
97. Kiistala U, Mustakallio KK. The presence of Langerhans cells in human dermis with special reference to their potential mesenchymal origin. Acta Derm Venereol (Stockh) 1968;48:115.
98. Tamaki K, Stingl G, Katz SI. The origin of Langerhans cells. J Invest Dermatol 1980;74:309.
99. Wolff K, Stingl G. The Langerhans cell. J Invest Dermatol 1983;80: 17.
100. Wolff K. The Langerhans cell. In: Mali JWH, ed. Current Problems in Dermatology. Vol 4. Basel: S Karger AG, 1972;79.
101. Nezelof C, Basset F, Rousseau MF. Histiocytosis X: Arguments for a Langerhans cell origin. Biomedicine 1973;18:365.
102. Shimada S, Katz SI. The skin as an immunologic organ. Arch Pathol Lab Med 1988;112:231.
103. Breathnach S, Katz SI. Cell-mediated immunity in cutaneous disease. Hum Pathol 1986;17:161.
104. Murphy GF, Bronstein BR, Knowles RW, Bhan AK. Ultrastructural documentation of M241 glycoprotein on dendritic cells in normal human skin. Lab Invest 1985;52:264.
105. Flotte TJ, Murphy GF, Bhan AK. Demonstration of T200 on human Langerhans cell surface membranes. J Invest Dermatol 1984;82:535.
106. Krueger GG, Emam M. Biology of Langerhans cells: Analysis by experiments to deplete Langerhans cells from human skin. J Invest Dermatol 1984;82:613.
107. Belsito DV, Flotte TJ, Lim HW et al. Effect of glucocorticosteroids on epidermal Langerhans cells. J Exp Med 1982;155:291.
108. Belsito DV, Sanchez MR, Baer RL et al. Reduced Langerhans cell Ia antigen and ATPase activity in patients with acquired immunodeficiency syndrome. N Engl J Med 1984;310:1279.
109. Tschachler E, Groh V, Popovic M et al. Epidermal Langerhans cells: A target for HTLV-III/LAV infection. J Invest Dermatol 1987;88:233.
110. Wood GS, Warner NL, Warnke RA. Leu3/4 antibodies react with cells of monocyte/macrophage and Langerhans cell lineage. J Immunol 1983;131:212.
111. Bourlond A, Vandooren-Deflorenne R. La membrane basale sous-épidermique: Sa structure et son ultrastructure. Arch Belg Dermatol Syphiligr 1968;24:119.
112. Stoughton R, Wells G. A histochemical study on polysaccharides in normal and diseased skin. J Invest Dermatol 1950;14:37.
113. Cooper JH. Microanatomical and histochemical observations on the dermal-epidermal junction. Arch Dermatol 1958;77:18.
114. Hashimoto K, Lever WF. An ultrastructural study of cell junctions in pemphigus vulgaris. Arch Dermatol 1970;101:287.
115. Tarnowski WM. Ultrastructure of the epidermal melanocyte-dense plate. J Invest Dermatol 1970;55:265.
116. Eady RAJ. The basement membrane. Arch Dermatol 1988;124:709.
117. Eady RAJ. Babes, blisters and basement membranes: From sticky molecules to epidermolysis bullosa. Clin Exp Dermatol 1986;12:161.
118. Bruckner-Tuderman L, Ruegger S, Odermatt B et al. Lack of type VII collagen in unaffected skin of patients with severe recessive dystrophic epidermolysis bullosa. Dermatologica 1988;176:57.
119. Frances C, Robert L. Elastin and elastic fibers in normal and pathologic skin. Int J Dermatol 1984;23:166.
120. Kobayasi T. Dermoepidermal junction of normal skin. J Dermatol 1978;5:157.
121. Yancey KB. Adhesion molecules: II. Interactions of keratinocytes with epidermal basement membrane. Prog Dermatol 1995;104:1008.
122. Hashimoto K. The ultrastructure of the skin of human embryos: V. The hair germs and perifollicular mesenchymal cells. Br J Dermatol 1970a;83:167.
123. Serri F, Montagna W, Mescon H. Studies of the skin of the fetus and the child. J Invest Dermatol 1962;39:199.
124. Mishima Y, Widlan S. Embryonic development of melanocytes in human hair and epidermis. J Invest Dermatol 1966;46:263.
125. Pinkus H. Embryology of hair. In: Montagna W, Ellis RA, eds. The biology of hair growth. New York: Academic Press, 1958;1.
126. Hashimoto K. The ultrastructure of the skin of human embryos: IX. Formation of the hair cone and intraepidermal hair canal. Arch Klin Exp Dermatol 1970c;238:333.
127. Hashimoto K. The ultrastructure of the skin of human embryos: VII. Formation of the apocrine gland. Acta Derm Venereol (Stockh) 1970b;50:241.
128. Thiers BH, Galbraith GMP. Alopecia areata. In: Thiers BH, Dobson RL, eds. Pathogenesis of skin diseases. New York: Churchill Livingstone, 1986;57.
129. Kollar EJ. The induction of hair follicles by embryonic dermal papillae. J Invest Dermatol 1970;55:374.
130. Johnson WC, Helwig EB. Histochemistry of the acid mucopolysaccharides of skin in normal and in certain pathologic conditions. Am J Clin Pathol 1963;40:123.
131. Kopf AW, Orentreich N. Alkaline phosphatase in alopecia areata. Arch Dermatol 1957;76:288.
132. Cormia F. Vasculature of the normal scalp. Arch Dermatol 1963;88: 692.
133. Pinkus H. Anatomy and histology of skin. In: Graham JH, Johnson WC, Helwig EB, eds. Dermal Pathology. Hagerstown: Harper & Row, 1972;1.
134. Zaun H. Histologie, histochemie und wachstumsdynamik des haarfollikels. In: Marchionini A, ed. Handbuch der haut- und geschlechtskrankheiten. Ergänzungswerk. Vol 1. Berlin: Springer-Verlag, 1968; 143.
135. Garn SM. The examination of hair under the polarizing microscope. Ann N Y Acad Sci 1951;53:649.
136. Leppard BJ, Sanderson KV, Wells RS. Hereditary trichilemmal cysts. Clin Exp Dermatol 1976;2:23.
137. Bandmann HJ, Bosse K. Histologie und anatomie des haarfollikels im verlauf des haarcyclus. Arch Klin Exp Dermatol 1966;227:390.
138. Montagna W. The structure and function of skin. 2nd ed. New York: Academic Press, 1962;174.
139. Parakkal PF, Matoltsy AG. A study of the differentiation products of the hair follicle cells with the electron microscope. J Invest Dermatol 1964;43:23.
140. Staricco RG. The melanocytes and the hair follicle. J Invest Dermatol 1960;35:185.
141. Pinkus H. "Sebaceous cysts" are trichilemmal cysts. Arch Dermatol 1969;99:544.
142. Strauss JS, Pochi PE. Histology, histochemistry, and electron microscopy of sebaceous glands in man. In: Marchionini A, ed. Handbuch der Haut- und geschlechtskrankheiten, Ergänzungswerk. Vol 1. Berlin: Springer-Verlag, 1968;184.
143. Suskind RK. The chemistry of the human sebaceous gland: I. Histochemical observations. J Invest Dermatol 1951;17:37.
144. Cashion PD, Skobe Z, Nalbandian J. Ultrastructural observations on sebaceous glands of the human oral mucosa: Fordyce's disease. J Invest Dermatol 1969;53:208.
145. Rupec M. Zur ultrastruktur der talgdrüsenzelle. Arch Klin Exp Dermatol 1969;234:273.
146. Niizuma K. Lipid droplets on the sebaceous glands: Some observations from tannic acid fixation. Acta Derm Venerol (Stockh) 1979;59: 401.
147. Rupec M, Braun-Falco O. Zur frage lysosomaler aktivität in normalen menschlichen talgdrüsen. Arch Klin Exp Dermatol 1968;232:312.
148. Rowden G. Aryl sulfatase in the sebaceous glands of mouse skin. J Invest Dermatol 1968;51:41.
149. Ito M, Suzuki M, Motoyoshi K et al. New findings on the proteins of sebaceous glands. J Invest Dermatol 1984;82:381.
150. Hyman AB, Brownstein MH. Tyson's glands. Arch Dermatol 1969; 99:31.
151. Weedon D, Strutton G. Apoptosis as the mechanism of the involution

of hair follicles in catagen formation. Acta Derm Venereol (Stockh) 1981;61:335.
152. Kligman AM. The human hair cycle. J Invest Dermatol 1959;33:307.
153. Mahrle G, Orfanos CE. Haarfarbe und haarpigment. Arch Dermatol Forsch 1973;248:109.
154. Herzberg J, Gusek W. Das ergrauen des kopfhaares. Arch Klin Exp Dermatol 1970;236:368.
155. Waldorf HA, Walsh LJ, Schechter NM, Murphy GF. Early cellular events in evolving cutaneous delayed hypersensitivity in humans. Am J Pathol 1991;138:477.
156. Hashimoto K, Gross BG, Lever WF. The ultrastructure of the skin of human embryos: I. The intraepidermal eccrine sweat duct. J Invest Dermatol 1965;45:139.
157. Hashimoto K, Gross BG, Lever WF. The ultrastructure of human embryo skin: II. The formation of intradermal portion of the eccrine sweat duct and of the secretory segment during the first half of embryonic life. J Invest Dermatol 1966;46:513.
158. Christophers E, Plewig G. Formation of the acrosyringium. Arch Dermatol 1973;107:378.
159. Hashimoto K, Gross BG, Lever WF. Electron microscopic study of the human adult eccrine gland: I. The duct. J Invest Dermatol 1966;46: 172.
160. Montagna W, Chase HB, Lobitz WC Jr. Histology and cytochemistry of human skin: IV. The eccrine sweat glands. J Invest Dermatol 1963; 20:415.
161. Headington JT. Primary mucinous carcinoma of skin: Histochemistry and electron microscopy. Cancer 1977;39:1055.
162. Dobson RL, Sato K. The secretion of salt and water by the eccrine sweat gland. Arch Dermatol 1972;105:366.
163. Hurley HJ, Witkowski JA. The dynamics of eccrine sweating in man. J Invest Dermatol 1962;39:329.
164. Schiefferdecker P. Die hautdrüsen des menschen und der säugetiere, ihre biologische und rassenanatomische bedeutung, sowie die muscularis sexualis. Biol Ztrbl 1917;37:534.
165. Schaumburg-Lever G, Lever WF. Secretion from human apocrine glands. J Invest Dermatol 1975;64:38.
166. Montes LF, Baker BL, Curtis AC. The cytology of the large axillary sweat glands in man. J Invest Dermatol 1960;35:273.
167. Hurley HJ, Shelley WB. The human apocrine sweat gland in health and disease. Springfield, IL: Charles C Thomas, 1960.
168. Montagna W, Yun JS. The glands of Montgomery. Br J Dermatol 1972;86:126.
169. Smith DM Jr, Peter TG, Donegan WL. Montgomery's areolar tubercle. Arch Pathol Lab Med 1982;106:60.
170. Sato K, Kane N, Soos G, Sato F. The eccrine sweat gland: Basic science and disorders of eccrine sweating. Prog Dermatol 1995;29:1.
171. Sato K, Sato F. Interleukin-1α in human sweat is functionally active and derived from the eccrine sweat gland. Am J Physiol 1994;266: 950.
172. Kuroisumi K, Yamagishi M, Sekine M. Mitochondrial deformation and apocrine secretory mechanism in the rabbit submandibular organ as revealed by electron microscopy. Z Zellforsch Mikrosk Anat 1961; 55:297.
173. Inoue T. Scanning electron microscope study of the human axillary apocrine glands. J Dermatol 1979;6:299.
174. Spielman AI, Zeng X-N, Leyden JJ, Preti G. Proteinaceous precursors of human axillary odor: Isolation of two novel odor-binding proteins. Experiential 1995;51:40.
175. Scher R, Daniel CR. Nails: Therapy, diagnosis, surgery. Saunders, Philadelphia: 1990.
176. Hashimoto K. Ultrastructure of the human toenail: II. Keratinization and formation of the marginal band. J Ultrastruct Res. 1971;36:391.
177. Hashimoto K. The marginal band: A demonstration of thickened cellular envelope of the human nail cell with the aid of lanthanum staining. Arch Dermatol 1971;103:387.
178. Johnson M, Shuster S. Continuous formation of a nail along the bed. Br J Dermatol 1993;128:277.
179. Higashi N. Melanocytes of the nail matrix and nail pigmentation. Arch Dermatol 1971;97:570.
180. Hashimoto K. Ultrastructure of the human toenail: I. Proximal nail matrix. J Invest Dermatol 1971;56:235.
181. Moretti G. The blood vessels of the skin. In: Marchionini A, ed. Handbuch der haut- und geschlechtskrankheiten, ergänzungswerk. Vol 1. Berlin: Springer-Verlag, 1968;491.
182. Kopf AW. The distribution of alkaline phosphatase in normal and pathologic human skin. Arch Dermatol 1957;75:1.
183. Klingmuller G. Die darstellung alkalischer phosphatase in capillaren. Hautarzt 1958;9:84.
184. Yen A, Braverman IM. Ultrastructure of the human dermal microcirculation: The horizontal plexus of the papillary dermis. J Invest Dermatol 1976;66:131.
185. Braverman IM, Yen A. Ultrastructure of human dermal microcirculation: II. The capillary loop of the dermal papillae. J Invest Dermatol 1977;68:44.
186. Seifert HW, Klingmuller G. Elektronenmikroskopische struktur normaler kapillaren und das verthalten alkalischer phosphatase. Arch Dermatol Forsch 1972;242:97.
187. Thorgeirsson G, Robertson AL Jr. The vascular endothelium: Pathobiolgic significance. Am J Pathol 1978;93:803.
188. Weber K, Braun-Falco O. Ultrastructure of blood vessels in human granulation tissue. Arch Dermatol Forsch 1973;248:29.
189. Holthofer H, Virtanen I, Kariniemi A-L et al. ULEX europaeus I lectin as a marker for vascular endothelium in human tissues. Lab Invest 1982;47:60.
190. Albelda SM, Oliver P, Romer L, Buck CA. EndoCAM: A novel endothelial cell-cell adhesion molecule. J Cell Biol 1990;110:1227.
191. Berger R, Albelda S, Berd D et al. Expression of platelet-endothelial cell adhesion molecule-1 (PECAM-1) during melanoma-induced angiogenesis in vivo. J Invest Dermatol 1992;98:584.
192. Suzuki Y, Hashimoto K, Crissman J et al. The value of blood group-specific lectin and endothelial associated antibodies in the diagnosis of vascular proliferations. J Cutan Pathol 1986;13:408.
193. Smolle J. HLA-DR antigen-bearing keratinocytes in various dermatologic diseases. Acta Derm Venereol (Stockh) 1985;65:9.
194. Jones DA, Abbasi O, McIntire LV et al. P-selectin mediates neutrophil rolling on histamine-stimulated endothelial cells. Biophys J 1991;65: 1560.
195. Thorlacius H, Raud J, Rosengren-Beezley S et al. Mast cell activation induces P-selectin-dependent leukocyte rolling and adhesion in post-capillary venules in vovo. Biochem Biophys Res Commun 1994;203: 1043.
196. Albelda SM, Smith CW, Ward PA. Adhesion molecules and inflammatory injury. FASEB J 1994;8:504.
197. Butcher EC. Leukocyte-endothelial cell recognition: Three (or more) steps to specificity and diversity. Cell 1991;67:1033.
198. Walsh LJ, Murphy GF. Role of adhesion molecules in cutaneous inflammation and neoplasia. J Cutan Pathol 1992;19:161.
199. McEver RP. Selectins: Novel receptors that mediate leukocyte adhesion during inflammation. Thromb Haemost 1991;65:22.
200. Ioffreda M, Elder DE, Albelda SM et al. TNFa induces E-selectin expression and PECAM-1 (CD31) redistribution in extracutaneous tissues. Endothelium 1993;1:47.
201. Mescon H, Hurley HJ, Moretti G. The anatomy and histochemistry of the arteriovenous anastomosis in human digital skin. J Invest Dermatol 1956;27:133.
202. Pepper M, Laubenheimer R, Cripps DJ. Multiple glomus tumors. J Cutan Pathol 1977;4:244.
203. Goodman TF. Fine structure of the cells of the Suquet-Hoyer canal. J Invest Dermatol 1972;59:363.
204. Hashimoto K, Tarnowski WM, Lever WF. Reifung und degranulierung der mastzellen in der menschlichen haut. Hautarzt 1967;18: 318.
205. Lagunoff D. Contributions of electron microscopy to the study of mast cells. J Invest Dermatol 1972;58:296.
206. Whitaker-Menezes D, Schechter NM, Murphy GF. Serine proteinases are regionally segregated within mast cell granules. Lab Invest 1995; 72:34.
207. Irani AA, Bradford TR, Kepley CL et al. Detection of MCT and MCTC types of human mast cells by immunohistochemistry using new monoclonal anti-tryptase and anti-chymase antibodies. J Histochem Cytochem 1989;37:1509.
208. Craig SS, Schechter NM, Schwartz LB. Ultrastructural analysis of maturing human T and TC mast cells identified by immunoelectron microscopy. Lab Invest 1988;58:682.
209. Mirowski G, Austen KF, Horan RF et al. Characterization of the cellular dermal infiltrates in human cutaneous mastocytosis. Lab Invest 1990;63:52.
210. Kobayasi T, Asboe-Hansen G. Degranulation and regranulation of human mast cells. Acta Derm Venereol (Stockh) 1969;49:369.

211. Kaminer MS, Lavker RM, Walsh D et al. Extracellular localization of human connective tissue mast cell granule contents. J Invest Dermatol 1991;96:1.
212. Uvnas B. Chemistry and storage function of mast cell granules. J Invest Dermatol 1978;71:76.
213. Kaliner MA. Editorial: The mast cell, a fascinating riddle. N Engl J Med 1979;301:498.
214. Lewis RE, Buchsbaum M, Whitaker D, Murphy GF. Intercellular adhesion molecule expression in the evolving cutaneous delayed hypersensitivity reaction. J Invest Dermatol 1989;93:672.
215. Murphy GF, Sueki H, Teuschler C et al. Role of mast cells in early epithelial target cell injury in experimental acute graft-versus-host disease. J Invest Dermatol 1994;102:451.
216. Walsh LJ, Trinchieri G, Waldorf HA et al. Human dermal mast cells contain and release tumor necrosis factor-α which induces endothelial leukocyte adhesion molecule-1. Proc Natl Acad Sci USA 1991;88: 4220.
217. Klein LM, Lavker RM, Matis WL, Murphy GF. Degranulation of human mast cells induces an endothelial antigen central to leukocyte adhesion. Proc Natl Acad Sci USA 1989;86:8972.
218. Christofidou-Solomidou M, Murphy GF, Albelda SM. Induction of E-selectin-dependent leukocyte recruitment by mast cell degranulation in human skin grafts transplanted on SCID mice. Am J Pathol 1996; 148:177.
219. Walsh LJ, Kaminer MS, Lazarus GS et al. Role of laminin in localization of human dermal mast cells. Lab Invest 1991;65:433.
220. Weiss RR, Whitaker-Menezes D, Longley J et al. Human dermal endothelial cells express membrane-associated mast cell growth factor. J Invest Dermatol 1995;104:101.
221. Winkelmann RK. Silver impregnation method for peripheral nerve endings. J Invest Dermatol 1955;24:57.
222. Woollard HH, Weddell G, Harpman JA. Observations on neurohistological basis of cutaneous pain. J Anat 1940;74:413.
223. Arthur RP, Shelley WB. The innervation of human epidermis. J Invest Dermatol 1959;32:397.
224. Reed RJ. Cutaneous manifestations of neural crest disorders. Int J Dermatol 1977;16:807.
225. Wiesner-Menzel L, Schultz B, Vakilzadeh F, Czarnetzki BM. Electron microscopical evidence for a direct contact between nerve fibers and mast cells. Acta Derm Venereol (Stockh) 1981;61:465.
226. Hosoi J, Murphy GF, Egan CL et al. Regulation of Langerhans cell function by nerves containing calcitonin gene-related peptide. Nature 1993;363:159.
227. Matis WL, Lavker RM, Murphy GF. Substance P induces the expression of an endothelial-leukocyte adhesion molecule by microvascular endothelium. J Invest Dermatol 1990;94:492.
228. Ashina A, Hosoi I, Bruvers S et al. Regulation of Langerhans cell protein antigen presentation by calcitonin gene-related peptide, granulocyte-macrophage colony stimulating factor, and tumor necrosis factor α (abstr). J Invest Dermatol 1993;100:489.
229. Orfanos CE, Mahrle G. Ultrastructure and cytochemistry of human cutaneous nerves. J Invest Dermatol 1973;61:108.
230. MacDonald DM, Schmitt D. Ultrastructure of the human mucocutaneous end organ. J Invest Dermatol 1979;72:181.
231. Cauna N, Ross LL. The fine structure of Meissner's touch corpuscles of human fingers. J Biophys Biochem Cytol 1960;8:467.
232. Hashimoto K. Fine structure of the Meissner corpuscle of human palmar skin. J Invest Dermatol 1973;60:20.
233. Pease DC, Quilliam TA. Electron microscopy of the Pacinian corpuscle. J Biophys Biochem Cytol 1957;3:331.
234. Headington JT. The dermal dendrocyte. In: Callen JP et al., eds. Advances in dermatology. Vol. 1. Chicago: Year Book Medical, 1986; 159.
235. Braverman IM, Sibley J, Keh-Yen A. A study of Veil cells around normal, diabetic, and aged cutaneous microvessels. J Invest Dermatol 1986;86:57.
236. Nestle FO, Zheng XG, Thompson CB et al. Characterization of dermal dendritic cells obtained from normal human skin reveals phenotypic and functionally distinctive subsets. J Immunol 1993;151:6535.
237. Cerio R, Griffiths CEM, Cooper KD et al. Characterization of factor XIIIa positive dermal dendritic cells in normal and inflamed skin. Br J Dermatol 1989;121:421.
238. Sueki H, Whitaker D, Buchsbaum M, Murphy GF. Novel interactions between dermal dendrocytes and mast cells in human skin: Implications for hemostasis and matrix repair. Lab Invest 1993;69:160.
239. Meunier L, Gonzalez-Ramos A, Cooper KD. Heterogeneous populations of class II MHC+ cells in human dermal cell suspensions. J Immunol 1993;151:4067.
240. Murphy GF, Messadi D, Fonferko E, Hancock WW. Phenotypic transformation of macrophages to Langerhans cells in the skin. Am J Pathol 1986;123:401.
241. Nickoloff BJ, Griffiths CEM. Not all spindle-shaped cells embedded in a collagenous stroma are fibroblasts: Recognition of the "collagen-associated dendrophage." J Cutan Pathol 1990;17:252.
242. Hirsh BC, Johnson WC. Concepts of granulomatous inflammation. Int J Dermatol 1984;23:90.
243. Wells GS. The pathology of adult-type Letterer-Siwe disease. Clin Exp Dermatol 1979;4:407.
244. Lasser A. The mononuclear phagocytic system: A review. Hum Pathol 1983;14:108.
245. Pulford KAF, Rigney EM, Jones M et al. KP1: A new monoclonal antibody that detects a monocyte/macrophage associated antigen in routinely processed tissue section. J Clin Pathol 1989;42:414.
246. Meuret G, Marwendel A, Brand ET. Makrophagenrekrutierung aus blutmonocyten bei Entzündungsreaktionen der haut. Arch Dermatol Forsch 1972;245:254.
247. Papadimitriou JM, Spector WG. The origin, properties and fate of epithelioid cells. J Pathol 1971;105:187.
248. Spector WG. Epithelioid cells, giant cells, and sarcoidosis. Ann NY Acad Sci 1976;278:3.
249. Murphy GF. Dermatopathology. Philadelphia: Saunders, 1995.
250. Weissmann G, Smolen JE, Hoffstein S. Polymorphonuclear leukocytes as secretory organs of inflammation. J Invest Dermatol 1978;71: 95.
251. Wilkinson DS. Pustular dermatoses. Br J Dermatol 1969;81:38.
252. Wade BH, Mandell GL. Polymorphonuclear leukocytes: Dedicated professional phagocytes. Am J Med 1983;74:686.
253. Parish WE. Investigations on eosinophils. Br J Dermatol 1970;82:42.
254. Henson PM. Pathological mechanisms in neutrophil-mediated injury. Am J Pathol 1972;68:593.
255. Lazarus GS, Daniels JR, Lian J et al. Role of granulocyte collagenase in collagen degradation. Am J Pathol 1972;68:565.
256. Berretty PJM, Cormane RH. The eosinophilic granulocyte. Int J Dermatol 1978;17:776.
257. Poole JCF. Electron microscopy of polymorphonuclear leukocytes. Br J Dermatol 1969;81:1.
258. Zucker-Franklin D. Eosinophilic function related to cutaneous disorders. J Invest Dermatol 1978;71:100.
259. Gell PGH, Coombs RRA. Classification of hypersensitivity reactions. In: Gell PGH, Coombs RRA, eds. Clinical aspects of immunology. 2nd ed. Oxford: Blackwell Scientific Publications, 1968.
260. Berretty PJM, Cormane RH. Eosinophilic granulocytes and skin disorders. Int J Dermatol 1981;20:531.
261. Goetzl EJ, Wasserman SI, Austen KF. Eosinophil polymorphonuclear leukocyte function in immediate hypersenstivity. Arch Pathol 1975; 99:1.
262. Butterworth AE, David JR. Eosinophil function. N Engl J Med 1981; 304:154.
263. Dvorak HF, Dvorak AM. Basophils, mast cells, and cellular immunity in animal and man. Hum Pathol 1972;3:454.
264. Katz SI. Recruitment of basophils in delayed hypersensitivity reactions. J Invest Dermatol 1978;71:70.
265. Weissman IL, Warnke R, Butcher EC et al. The lymphoid system: Its normal architecture and the potential for understanding the system through the study of lymphoproliferative diseases. Hum Pathol 1978; 9:25.
266. Stingl G, Knapp W. Immunological markers for characterization of subpopulations of mononuclear cells. Am J Dermatopathol 1981;3: 215.
267. Claudy AL. The immunological identification of the Sézary cell. Br J Dermatol 1974;91:597.
268. Luckasen JR, Sabad A, Goltz RW et al. T and B lymphocytes in atopic eczema. Arch Dermatol 1974;110:375.
269. Askenase PW. Delayed-type hypersensitivity (DTH) recruitment of T cell subsets via antigen-specific non-IgE antibodies: Relevance to asthma, autoimmunity and immune responses to tumors and parasites. In: Coffman R, ed. The regulation and functional significance

of T cell subsets: Progress in chemical immunology. Basel: S Karger, 1993.
270. Gerard-Marchant R, Hamlin I, Lennert K et al. Classification of non-Hodgkin's lymphoma. Lancet 1974;2:406.
271. Wilson Jones E. Prospectives in mycosis fungicides in relation to other lymphomas. Trans St Johns Hosp Dermatol Soc 1975;61:16.
272. Rywlin AM. Non-Hodgkin's malignant lymphomas: Brief historical review and simple unifying classification. Am J Dermatopathol 1980; 2:17.
273. Aisenberg AC. Cell lineage in lymphoproliferative disease. Am J Med 1983;74:679.
274. Murphy GF, Mihm MC. Benign, dysplastic, and malignant lymphoid infiltrates of the skin: An approach based on pattern analysis. In: Murphy GF, Mihm MC, eds. Lymphoproliferative disorders of the skin. Boston: Butterworth, 1986;123.
275. Murphy GF, Elder D. Non-melanocytic tumors of the skin (Atlas of tumor pathology). Washington, DC: AFIP Fascicles, third series, Vol 1. 155.
276. Erlach E, Gebhart W, Niebauer G. Ultrastructural investigations on the morphogenesis of Russell bodies (abstr). J Cutan Pathol 1976;3:145.
277. Tappeiner J, Pfleger L, Wolff K. Das vorkommen und histochemische verhalten von Russellschen körperchen bei plasmacellulären hautinfiltraten. Arch Klin Exp Dermatol 1965;222:71.
278. Blom J, Wiik A. Russell bodies: Immunoglobulins? Am J Clin Pathol 1983;79:262.
279. Doroczy J. Die struktur der dermalen lymphkapillaren und ihre funktionelle interpretation. Hautarzt 1984;35:630.
280. Scarpelli DG, Goodman RM. Observations on the fine structure of the fibroblast from a case of Ehlers-Danlos syndrome with the Marfan syndrome. J Invest Dermatol 1968;50:214.
281. Ross R, Benditt EP. Wound healing and collagen formation: V. Quantitative electron microscopic radioautographic observations of proline-H3 utilization by fibroblasts. J Cell Biol 1965;27:83.
282. Uitto J, Lichtenstein JR. Defects in the biochemistry of collagen in diseases of connective tissue. J Invest Dermatol 1976;66:59.
283. Nigra TP, Friedland M, Martin GR. Controls of connective tissue synthesis: Collagen metabolism. J Invest Dermatol 1972;59:44.
284. Lazarus GS. Collagen, collagenase and clinicians. Br J Dermatol 1972;26:193.
285. Grant ME, Prockop DJ. The biosynthesis of collagen. N Engl J Med 1972;286:194.
286. Hayes RL, Rodnan GP. The ultrastructure of skin in progressive sclerosis (scleroderma). Am J Pathol 1971;63:433.
287. Schmidt W. Die normale histologie von corium und subcutis. In: Marchionini A, ed. Handbuch der haut-und geschlechtskrankheiten, ergänzungswerk. Vol 1. Berlin: Springer-Verlag, 1968;430.
288. Meigel WN, Gay S, Weber L. Dermal architecture and collagen type distribution. Arch Dermatol Res 1977;259:1.
289. Byers PH, Barsh GS, Holbrook KA. Molecular pathology in inherited disorders of collagen metabolism. Hum Pathol 1982;13:89.
290. Leigh IM, Eady RAJ, Heagerty AHM. Type VII collagen is a normal component of epidermal basement membrane. J Invest Dermatol 1988;90:639.
291. Stenn KS. Collagen heterogeneity of skin. Am J Dermatopathol 1979; 1:87.
292. Deutsch TA, Esterly NB. Elastic fibers in fetal dermis. J Invest Dermatol 1975;65:320.
293. Varadi DP. Study on the chemistry and fine structure of elastic fibers from normal adult skin. J Invest Dermatol 1972;59:238.
294. Hashimoto K, Dibella RJ. Electron microscopic studies of normal and abnormal elastic fibers of the skin. J Invest Dermatol 1967;48:405.
295. Varadi DP. Studies on the chemistry and fine structure of elastic fibers from normal adult skin. J Invest Dermatol 1972;59:238.
296. Stadler R, Orfanos CE. Reifung und alterung der elastischen fasern. Arch Dermatol Forsch 1978;262:97.
297. Marsch WC, Schober E, Nurnberger F. Zur ultrastruktur und morphogenese der elastischen faser und der aktinischen elastose. Z Hautkr 1979;54:43.
298. Winand R. Biosynthesis, organization and degradation of mucopolysaccharides. Arch Belg Dermatol Syphiligr 1972;28:35.
299. Jacques J, Cameron HCS. Changes in the ground-substance of healing wounds. J Pathol 1969;99:337.
300. Seemayer TA, Knaack J, Wang NS et al. On the ultrastructure of hibernoma. Cancer 1975;36:1785.

Lever's Histopathology of the Skin, eighth edition,
edited by David Elder et al. Lippincott–
Raven Publishers, Philadelphia © 1997.

CHAPTER 4

Laboratory Methods

Rosalie Elenitsas, Patricia Van Belle, and David Elder

There are a number of important steps in preparing histologic sections prior to their interpretation by the dermatopathologist. Failure to handle the tissue properly may make it difficult to provide an accurate diagnosis or appropriate margins.

PREPARATION OF SPECIMENS

Fixation

It is important to properly fix a skin biopsy to stabilize proteins and prevent postmortem decay. The specimen should be placed in fixative immediately after it is removed from the patient; artifacts may result if it is allowed to dry. The fixative of choice is a 10% buffered formalin solution. The volume of formalin should be 10 to 20 times the volume of the specimen. During winter, either 95% ethyl alcohol, 10% by volume, should be added to the formalin solution or the specimen should be allowed to stand in the formalin solution at room temperature for at least 6 hours before mailing.

Adequate time should be allowed for fixation. Fixation time is 1 to 2 hours per millimeter thickness. Large specimens, such as excised tumors, should be cut in the laboratory into slices 4 to 5 mm thick for further fixation, generally overnight. These specimens will also require greater volumes of formalin.

Grossing

After fixation, ink should be applied to the deep and lateral margins of an excisional specimen for which examination of margins has been requested. The specimen should be appropriately cut for the examination of margins. Some examples are demonstrated in Fig. 4-1. It is important to remember that these cuts are only representative of the margins, since it is almost impossible to evaluate every marginal cell. If a localizing suture has been placed by the surgeon, a different color ink should be applied to that margin or some other method of labeling should be used to identify the margins. Four-mm and 6-mm punch biopsies are generally bisected, and specimens less than 3 mm in size should be submitted in toto. If a laboratory does not handle many skin specimens, discussion with the embedding technician may be appropriate to facilitate optimal orientation of the blocks.

Demonstration of Enzyme Activities

With few exceptions, specimens should not be placed in formalin for the demonstration of enzyme activities. Instead, they should be delivered to the laboratory wrapped in water-moistened gauze and placed in a clean container, because frozen sections cut on a cryostat are usually used for enzyme staining. Staining for enzyme activities is not routinely done and therefore should not be requested without first checking with the laboratory.

Although immunohistochemistry has largely replaced histochemistry for routine diagnostic use, demonstration of dopa-oxidase activity in melanocytes could potentially aid in distinguishing a malignant melanoma from tumors not composed of melanocytes. Also, the distinction between eccrine and apocrine differentiation in cutaneous appendage tumors is often possible by means of enzyme stains, since certain enzymes, such as succinic dehydrogenase and phosphorylase, are characteristic of eccrine differentiation, whereas acid phosphatase and beta-glucuronidase are characteristic of apocrine differentiation (see Chap. 31). However, these differentials are not usually significant clinically.

Several enzyme reactions can be carried out on formalin-fixed, paraffin-embedded tissue: (1) demonstration of naphthol AS-D chloracetate esterase activity, with naphthol AS-D chloracetate as substrate (present in mature and immature granulocytes, except in myeloblasts[1] and mast cells); and (2) demonstration of lysozyme with the antilysozyme immunohistochemical technique (lysozyme being present in mature and immature granulocytes, even in myeloblasts, and in histiocytes) (see Chap. 32).[1]

In two diseases, scleredema of Buschke and amyloidosis, unfixed frozen sections may show a more conclusive reaction to

R. Elenitsas: Department of Dermatology, University of Pennsylvania, Philadelphia, PA

P. Van Belle and D. Elder: Department of Pathology and Laboratory Medicine, University of Pennsylvania, Philadelphia, PA

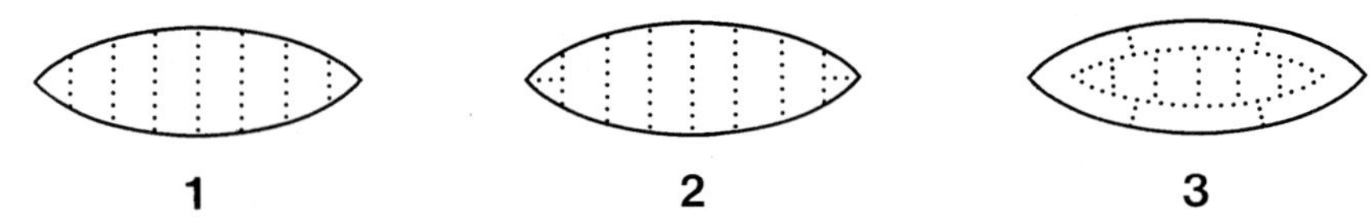

FIG. 4-1. Preparation of blocks from a skin ellipse
After the margins have been painted with ink, the specimen is sectioned for processing and later embedding. In example 1 the tissue is cut as if one is slicing a loaf of bread; this is one of the most common methods used in dermatopathology laboratories. Example 2 allows for better evaluation of the "tips" of the ellipse; however, embedding of these small pieces is more difficult. Often only the center section of the "tips" is embedded, or the tips may be cut in half and embedded flat, especially for smaller specimens (example 3). In example 3, the entire margin is theoretically visualized; however, this method requires the technician to meticulously embed and orient small pieces of tissue and is not recommended for most specimens in most routine laboratories.[30]

specific staining methods than is obtainable with formalin-fixed material. It is therefore recommended that, in these two diseases, only part of the tissue be fixed in formalin and the remainder be used for frozen sections. In scleredema, demonstration of hyaluronic acid with toluidine blue at pH 7.0 may be more intense in unfixed, frozen sections than in formalin-fixed sections; in amyloidosis, the reactions of the amyloid with crystal violet or Congo red may be conclusive only in unfixed, frozen sections (see Chap. 17).

Processing

The purpose of processing is to remove the extractable water from the skin and to provide a supporting matrix (paraffin) so that the tissue can be cut with minimal distortion. After fixation, routine specimens are processed in an automatic processor. An exception is specimens that are to be stained for lipids. Because lipids are extracted by the xylene used for the processing of specimens, frozen sections are cut and postfixed in 10% neutral buffered formalin for lipid staining.

In the automated histology processor, the specimens pass first through increasing concentrations of ethanol for dehydration, then through xylene for lipid extraction and clearing of alcohol. Finally, the tissues are infiltrated with several changes of hot, melted paraffin (or Paraplast), to provide a matrix so that the tissue can be stabilized and cut easily. This processing takes between 4 and 12 hours; in most laboratories, processing is run overnight. The next morning, the specimens are embedded with the cut surface face down into the cassette base mold, in the liquid paraffin, which is allowed to harden. To prevent tangentially oriented sections, it is important that this cut surface be firmly embedded in the base of this mold. The specimens are then cut on a rotary microtome into sections 5 to 7 μm thick.

Staining

Routine sections are usually stained with hematoxylin-eosin, the most widely used routine stain. With this staining method, nuclei stain blue or "basophilic," and collagen, muscles, and nerves stain red or "eosinophilic." Special stains are employed when particular structures need to be demonstrated. (For details, see later and the *Manual of Histologic Staining Methods of the Armed Forces Institute of Pathology.*[2])

HISTOCHEMICAL STAINING

Histochemistry, especially immunohistochemistry, at both the light microscopic and electron microscopic level, has gained increasing importance in recent years and has been largely responsible for the expansion of histopathology from a purely descriptive science to one that is dynamic and functional. Many enzyme histochemical methods are used only for research and have the limitation of usually requiring fresh tissue in the place of formalin-fixed tissue.

Most histochemical "special" stains can be carried out on formalin-fixed, paraffin-embedded material. Their primary uses in dermatopathology are listed in Table 4-1.

The *PAS stain* demonstrates the presence of certain polysaccharides, particularly glycogen and mucoproteins containing neutral mucopolysaccharides, by staining them red. The PAS reaction consists of the oxidation of adjacent hydroxyl groups in 1,2-glycols to aldehydes and the staining of the aldehydes with fuchsin-sulfuric acid. The PAS reaction is of value also in the study of basement membrane thickening, such as in lupus erythematosus or porphyria cutanea tarda. Furthermore, because the cell walls of fungi are composed of a mixture of cellulose and chitin and thus contain polysaccharides, fungi stain bright pink-red with the PAS reaction.

For the distinction of neutral mucopolysaccharides and fungi from glycogen deposits, it is necessary to compare two serial sections, one exposed to diastase before staining and the other not. Because glycogen is digested by the diastase, and thus no longer colored red by the PAS reaction, it can be easily distinguished from neutral mucopolysaccharides and fungi that are diastase-resistant. Because glycogen is present in outer root sheath cells and eccrine gland cells, and neutral polysaccharides are found in eccrine and apocrine gland cells, demonstration of glycogen is of diagnostic value in trichilemmal tumor, in trichilemmoma, in clear cell hidradenoma, and in eccrine poroma. Demonstration of neutral mucopolysaccharides is of value in Paget's disease of the breast, in extramammary Paget's disease, in clear cell hidradenoma, and intraluminally in eccrine spiradenoma and eccrine poroma (see Chaps. 30 and 31).

The *alcian blue reaction* demonstrates the presence of acid mucopolysaccharides by staining them blue. Acid mucopolysaccharides are present in the dermal ground substance, but in amounts too small to be demonstrable in normal skin. However, in the dermal mucinoses, there is a great increase in nonsulfated acid mucopolysaccharides, mainly hyaluronic acid, so that the mucin stains with alcian blue (see Chap. 17). In ex-

TABLE 4-1. *Histochemical stains used in dermatopathology*

Stain	Purpose of stain	Results
Hematoxylin-eosin	Routine	Nuclei: blue Collagen, muscles, nerves: red
Masson trichrome	Collagen	Collagen: blue or green Nuclei, muscles, nerves: dark red
Verhoeff–van Gieson	Elastic fibers	Elastic fibers: black Collagen: red Nuclei, muscles, nerves: yellow
Pinkus acid orcein	Elastic fibers	Elastic fibers: dark brown
Silver nitrate	Melanin, reticulum fibers (argyrophilic)	Melanin, reticulum fibers: black
Fontana-Masson	Melanin (argentaffin)	Melanin: black
Methenamine silver	Fungi, Donovan bodies, Frisch bacilli (rhinoscleroma), basement membranes	Black
Grocott	Fungi	Fungus cell walls: black
Periodic acid-Schiff/diastase (PAS)	Glycogen, neutral MPS*, fungi	Glycogen: red; diastase labile Neutral MPS*, fungi: red; diastase resistant
Alcian blue, pH 2.5	Acid MPS*	Blue
Alcian blue, pH 0.5	Sulfated MPS*	Blue
Toluidine blue	Acid MPS*	Blue
Colloidal iron	Acid MPS*	Blue
Hyaluronidase	Hyaluronic acid	Hyaluronidase labile
Mucicarmine	"Epithelial" mucin	Red
Giemsa	Mast cell granules, acid MPS*, myeloid granules, Leishmania	MCG,† acid MPS*: metachromatically purple Myeloid granules, Leishmania: red
Fite	Acid-fast bacilli	Red
Perls potassium ferrocyanide	Hemosiderin (iron)	Blue
Alkaline Congo red	Amyloid	Pink-red, green birefringence in polarized light
Von Kossa	Calcium	Black
Scarlet red	Lipids	Red
Oil red O	Lipids	Red
Dopa (in unfixed tissue)	Tyrosinase in melanocytes	Black dopa-melanin
Naphthol-AS-D-chloroacetate esterase	Mast cells, neutrophils, myelocytes	Granules stain red
Warthin-Starry	Spirochetes	Black
Dieterle and Steiner	Spirochetes, bacillary angiomatosis	Black

* MPS = mucopolysaccharides.
† MCG = mast cell granules.
Note: All stains except those for lipids, can be carried out on formalin-fixed paraffin-embedded specimens. The stains for lipids require formalin-fixed frozen sections.

tramammary Paget's disease of the anus with rectal carcinoma (see Chap. 30) and in cutaneous metastases of carcinoma of the gastrointestinal tract containing goblet cells (see Chap. 37), tumor cells in the skin, like their parent cells, secrete sialomucin. Sialomucin contains nonsulfated acid mucopolysaccharides staining with alcian blue, as well as PAS-positive neutral mucopolysaccharides. Whereas nonsulfated acid mucopolysaccharides stain with alcian blue at pH 2.5 but not at pH 0.5, strongly acidic sulfated acid mucopolysaccharides, such as heparin in mast cell granules and chondroitin sulfate in cartilage, stain with alcian blue both at pH 2.5 and at pH 0.5.

Several special stains for elastic tissue are available. The most commonly used stains are the Verhoeff–van Gieson (Fig. 4-2) or Weigert resorcin-fuchsin. Additional techniques, such as the Luna stain and Miller stain, may allow better visualization of elastic fibers than traditional methods.[3] These stains are beneficial in the diagnosis of anetoderma, connective tissue nevi, middermal elastolysis, and other alterations of elastic tissue.

POLARISCOPIC EXAMINATION

Polariscopic examination is the examination of histologic sections under the microscope with polarized light, with light from which all rays except those vibrating in one plane are excluded.

For polariscopic examination, two disks made of polarizing plastics are inserted in the microscope. One disk is placed below the condenser of the microscope and acts as the polarizer. The second disk is placed in the eyepiece of the microscope or on top of the glass slide and acts as the analyzer. When one of the two disks is rotated so that the path of the light through the two disks is broken at a right angle, the field is dark. However, when doubly refractile substances are introduced between the two disks, they break the polarization and are visible as bright white bodies in the dark field.

Polariscopic examination is useful in evaluating lipid deposits, certain foreign bodies, gout, and amyloid.

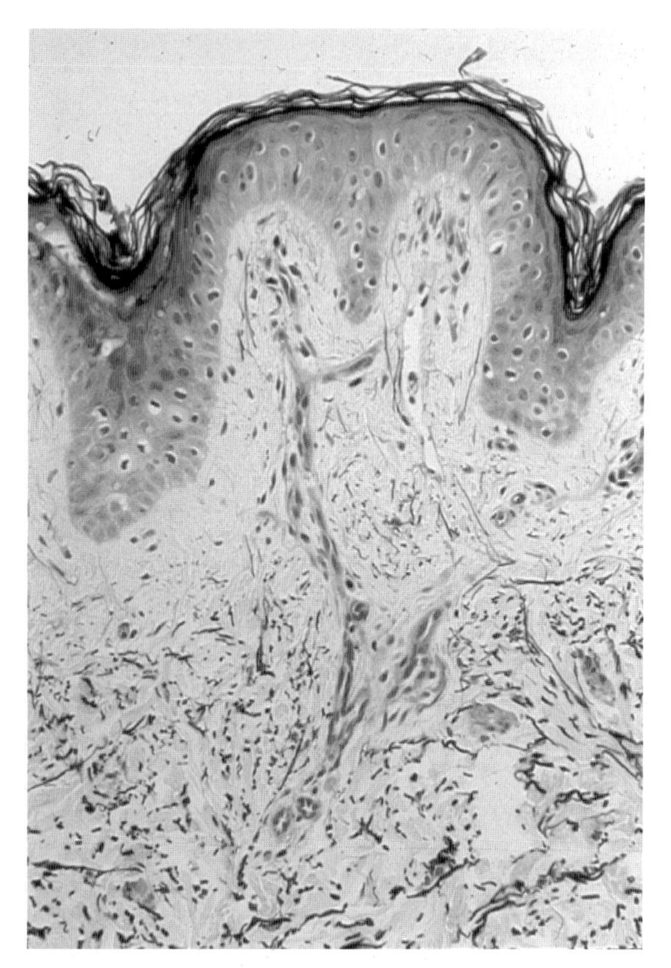

FIG. 4-2. Elastic fibers
This Verhoeff–van Gieson stain demonstrates the darkly staining normal elastic fibers of the skin.

With regard to lipids, it is not fully known why certain lipids are doubly refractile and others are not. In general, cholesterol esters are doubly refractile, but free cholesterol, phospholipids, and neutral fat are not. Only formalin-fixed, frozen sections can be used for a polariscopic examination for lipids.

Doubly refractile lipids are regularly present in the tuberous and plane xanthomas and xanthelasmata (but not always in the eruptive xanthomas) of hyperlipoproteinemia, in the cutaneous lesions of diffuse normolipemic plane xanthoma, and in the vascular walls of angiokeratoma corporis diffusum (Fabry disease) (see Chap. 27). Doubly refractile lipids are present, as long as the cutaneous lesions contain a sufficient amount of lipid, in histiocytosis X (Hand-Schüller-Christian type) (see Chap. 27), in juvenile xanthogranuloma (see Chap. 27), in erythema elevatum diutinum (extracellular cholesterosis) (see Chap. 8), and in dermatofibroma (lipidized "histiocytoma") (see Chap. 33).

Doubly refractile lipids are absent in lipid-containing lesions, as a rule, in necrobiosis lipoidica (see Chap. 14), in hyalinosis cutis et mucosae or lipoid proteinosis (see Chap. 17), and in multicentric reticulohistiocytosis and solitary reticulohistiocytic granuloma (see Chap. 27).

Among foreign bodies, silica causes granulomas showing doubly refractile spicules. These granulomas are caused either by particles of soil or glass (silicon dioxide) or by talcum powder (magnesium silicate) (see Chap. 14). Wooden splinters, suture material, and starch granules are also doubly refractile. An example of polariscopic examination is seen in Fig. 4-3.

Gout tophi show double refraction of the urate crystals if the crystals are sufficiently preserved. They are preserved by the use of alcohol rather than formalin for fixation (see Chap. 17).

Amyloid shows a characteristic green birefringence in polarized light after staining with alkaline Congo red (see Chap. 17).

IMMUNOFLUORESCENCE TESTING

Two methods are in use: direct immunofluorescence testing, which tests for immunoreactants localized in the tissues of the patient's own skin or mucous membrane, and indirect immunofluorescence testing, which tests for circulating antibodies in the patient's blood serum. Direct immunofluorescence testing is a valuable diagnostic procedure in three groups of diseases: the immune-mediated vesiculobullous diseases, lupus erythematosus, and leukocytoclastic vasculitis. Indirect immunofluorescence testing is beneficial in some of the vesiculobullous diseases, such as the various forms of pemphigus and pemphigoid, because of the presence of circulating antibodies. Although indirect immunofluorescence is less sensitive than direct immunofluorescence, it may be used as a supplementary test.

Biopsy Technique

A 3-mm punch biopsy is generally adequate. In the group of vesiculobullous diseases, the biopsy should be taken from perilesional skin because if lesional skin is used, detachment of the roof of the blister from its base may cause a false-negative result. In the various forms of pemphigoid, direct immunofluorescence may be negative when the biopsy specimen is taken from an area far away from active lesions, especially in patients with only a few lesions. False-negative results have also been reported in lower extremity biopsies of patients with pemphigoid.[4,5] As will be described under the headings of the various vesiculobullous diseases, positive direct immunofluorescence is obtained in almost 100% of the cases in the various forms of pemphigus, bullous pemphigoid, and dermatitis herpetiformis, as well as in a very high percentage of cases in cicatricial pemphigoid and herpes gestationis.

In lupus erythematosus, biopsy of a lesion that has been present at least 2 to 3 months is optimum. A positive lupus band test consists of more than one immune reactant (immunoglobulin or complement) in a granular pattern at the dermal-epidermal junction. A positive lupus band test from uninvolved, sun-protected skin may be seen in patients with systemic disease. A false-positive lupus band test may result from a biopsy from sun-exposed skin. Therefore, correlation with routine histology, serology, and clinical findings is essential.

In cases of vasculitis, the granular deposition of immune reactants in vessel walls is transient. The biopsy specimen should be taken from a very early lesion, preferably one less than 24 hours old. Although immune reactants can be detected in biopsies of leukocytoclastic vasculitis, they may also be seen in lesions that show vascular injury without fibrinoid destruction of vessels, such as erythema multiforme and pityriasis lichenoides et varioliformis acuta. Direct immunofluorescence for vasculi-

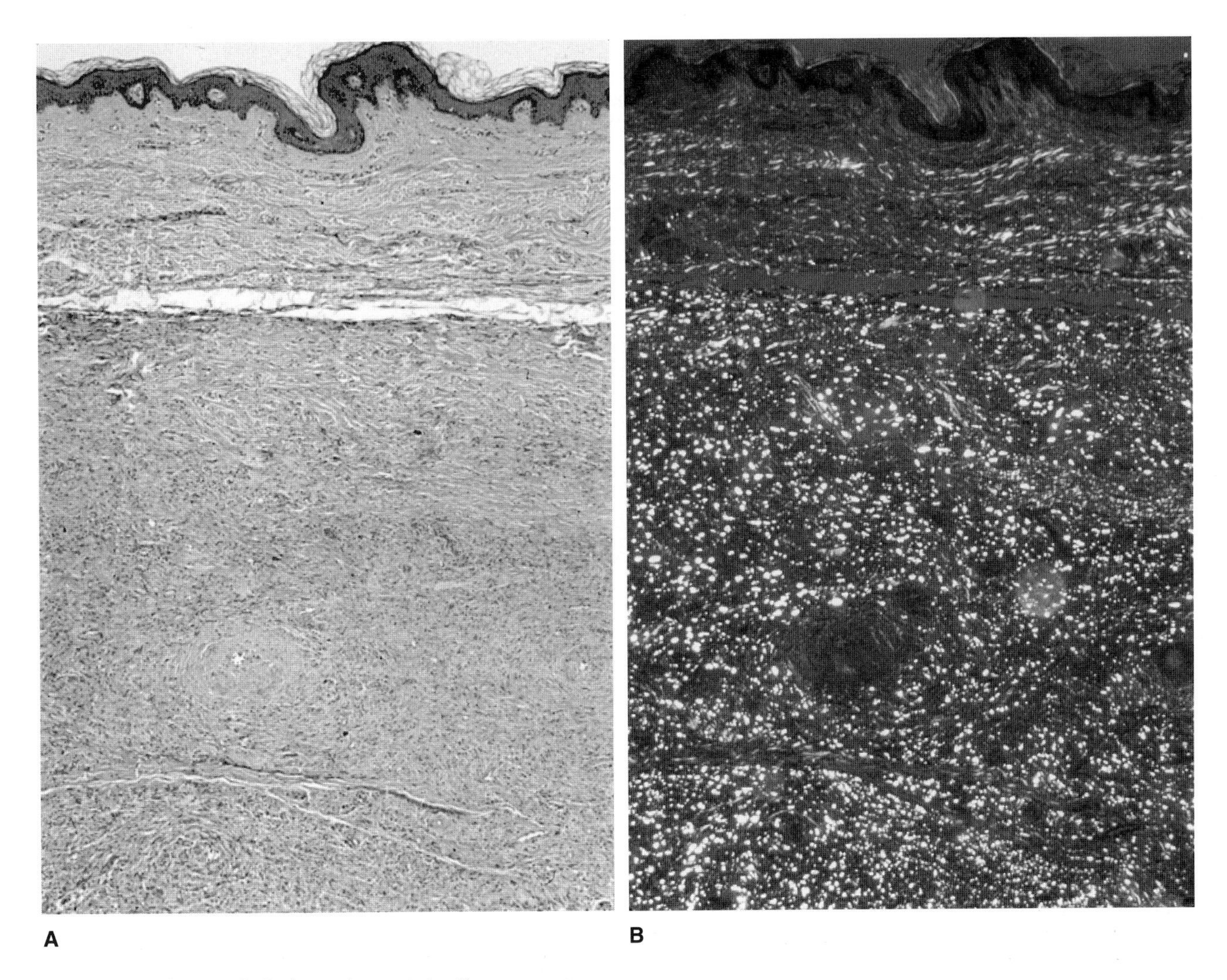

FIG. 4-3. Polariscopic examination
In this talc granuloma (**A**), polaroscopy (**B**) reveals hundreds of refractile foreign bodies within the dermis.

tis is most beneficial in Henoch-Schönlein purpura to detect IgA deposition, and in urticarial vasculitis, where the changes in routine histology may be subtle.

Transport of the Biopsy Specimen

It was originally thought necessary to quick-freeze the biopsy specimen and to keep it in a frozen state up to the time of testing. It has since become evident that specimens can be kept in transport medium (Michel's medium: ammonium sulfate, *N*-ethylmaleimide and magnesium sulfate in a citrate buffer) for 2 weeks and longer without loss of reactivity.[6] This, of course, has made the direct immunofluorescence technique much more readily applicable. A preliminary report suggests that this medium may also be reliable for immunoelectronmicroscopy of basement membrane zone components.[7]

Immunofluorescence Techniques

For direct immunofluorescence, frozen sections are typically incubated with antibodies to complement: IgG, IgA, IgM, and fibrin or fibrinogen. These antibodies are linked to a fluorescent label such as fluoroscein isothiocyanate to allow visualization using a fluorescence microscope. The indirect immunofluorescence method involves incubation of various dilutions of the patient's serum with an epithelial substrate such as monkey esophagus. Circulating antibasement membrane antibodies and cell surface membrane antibodies are detected (Fig. 4-4) and reported as the highest positive dilution.

IMMUNOHISTOCHEMISTRY

Introduction, Techniques

Immunohistochemistry techniques have been available since the early 1970s, but they have been used widely for diagnostic pathology only since the early 1980s. They are mainly used to diagnose poorly differentiated malignant tumors and lymphoma. They can also be beneficial in the diagnosis of bullous diseases.[8] With the refinement of techniques, immunohistochemistry methods have achieved the same sensitivity for many antigens in paraffin-embedded tissues as the direct immunofluorescence method in frozen sections. The paraffin-embedded

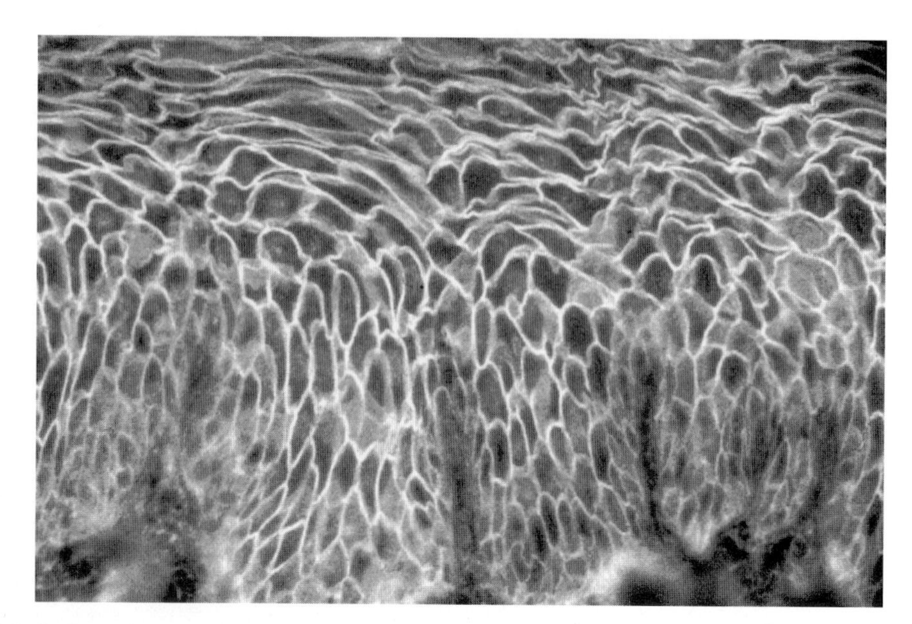

FIG. 4-4. Indirect immunofluorescence
Indirect immunofluorescence of pemphigus using monkey esophagus as the substrate reveals IgG cell surface membrane staining in a "fishnet" pattern.

tissues offer the advantage over frozen sections of better preservation of cellular details and permanency of the reaction, so that the specimens can be preserved and stored. Most monoclonal antibodies, especially those necessary for the diagnosis of lymphoma, have required frozen section studies, but monoclonal antibodies are presently being produced that can be applied to formalin-fixed, paraffin-embedded tissue, such as antibodies for the identification of B cells, T cells, and macrophages.

Sections that will be incubated with polyclonal or monoclonal antibodies should be mounted on glass slides specially coated or charged to ensure better adherence.[9] With the newer Microprobe Slide Staining System (Fisher Scientific, Pittsburgh, PA), slides with a positively charged surface are used.

Certain antibodies, including antibodies against keratins, lysozyme, or chymotrypsin, require protease digestion if formalin-fixed, paraffin-embedded sections are used. Other "antigen retrieval" methods include the use of heat, either by microwaving or steaming the sections, and pretreatment of the sections with acid (HCl).

Immunohistologic Techniques

In most laboratories, immunopathology techniques are well established. Historically, several techniques have been used; the peroxidase-antiperoxidase (PAP) technique has been replaced by more sensitive techniques, namely, the avidin-biotin-peroxidase complex (ABC), the alkaline phosphatase–anti-alkaline phosphatase (APAAP), and the streptavidin peroxidase or alkaline phosphatase techniques. In all of these methods, the antibody is used to localize an enzyme (peroxidase or phosphatase) to sites of antigen expression in tissue sections. An appropriate "chromogen" is then added. A chromogen is a reagent that has the property of developing a color that can be visualized at sites of localization of the enzyme-antibody-antigen complex.

The Alkaline Phosphatase–Anti-Alkaline Phosphatase (APAAP) Technique

This is an unlabeled antibody bridge technique that utilizes three antibodies; the first and third antibodies are from the same species and are monoclonal. The second antibody is polyclonal, from the rabbit, and forms a bridge between the first and third antibody.[10] The third antibody is linked to the enzyme alkaline phosphatase. After applying these antibodies with the linked enzyme, an alkaline phosphatase substrate is added containing a compatible indole chromogen such as INT/BCIP (which yields a red color after the phosphatase-catalyzed reaction), naphthol fast red (red color), or NBT/BCIP (blue). This method may be useful for pigmented tumors since the blue or red reagents can be distinguished easily from melanin.[9]

The Avidin-Biotin-Peroxidase Complex and Streptavidin Peroxidase or Alkaline Phosphatase Techniques

The avidin-biotin technique takes advantage of the strong interaction of avidin with biotin.[11,12] Avidin is a glycoprotein found in egg white that has a strong affinity to biotin, a vitamin of low molecular weight. The streptavidin technique is exactly analogous, but achieves 1 to 2 orders of magnitude greater sensitivity by using streptavidin in place of avidin. This method is now becoming standard. In these techniques, the primary antibody (which may be monoclonal or polyclonal) binds directly with the specific antigen, in or on the cells, to form a stable antigen-antibody complex within the tissue section. A secondary antibody that has been labeled with biotin (biotinylated), and that is directed against the same species and immunoglobulin type, binds to the primary antibody, leaving the biotinylated end available. A peroxidase or an alkaline phosphatase detection system can be used. In a peroxidase method, the biotinylated complex is detected by avidin or streptavidin that has been conjugated to the peroxidase enzyme. A peroxidase-oriented chromogen is then added, such as diaminobenzidine (yielding a brown color) or aminoethylcarbazole (red color and therefore useful for pigmented lesions). The alkaline phosphatase-streptavidin method is analogous to the streptavidin peroxidase method, but in this case the biotinylated complex is detected with an alkaline phosphatase–linked streptavidin, and requires a compatible chromogen such as the indole reagents INT/BCIP (red color), naphthol fast red (red), or NBT/BCIP (blue). This technique in the authors' experience achieves the greatest sensitivity of all immunohistochemical methods.

The origin of an undifferentiated cell can usually be determined with the application of monoclonal or polyclonal antibodies. A "panel approach" using multiple markers is the best method for evaluating problem neoplasms. Positive and negative controls should be used. If tumor cells unexpectedly do not show a positive reaction with a certain antibody, several possibilities exist, including technical difficulties with the assay. One may encounter nonspecific staining as well as aberrant immunoreactivity (observed staining with a particular antibody where it is theoretically unexpected). Caution should be taken not to make a diagnosis based on immunohistochemistry alone. Unfortunately, there is no antibody that distinguishes between benign and malignant cells.

APPLICATIONS OF IMMUNOHISTOPATHOLOGY

Diagnosis of Tumors (Excluding Lymphomas)

The most important antibodies for routine dermatopathology and their occurrence in certain cells and tissues are listed in Table 4-2. The most frequently used antibodies in dermatopathology are discussed below. The list of currently available antibodies is extensive; detailed information is available in literature and text reviews.[13–16]

Antibodies Against Cytoskeletal Antigens

The cytoskeleton of a cell consists of intermediate filaments measuring 7 to 11 nm in diameter, actin-containing microfilaments, and tubulin-containing microfilaments.[17] Intermediate filaments are smaller than microtubules (25 nm) and larger than microfilaments.

Antibodies against cytofilaments help to identify the origin of an anaplastic cell. Malignant tumors retain the intermediate filament-type characteristic of the cell type of origin, and metastases generally continue to express these intermediate filaments.[18] There are five types of intermediate filaments: cytokeratins, characteristic for true epithelia; vimentin, found in mesenchymal cells and melanocytes; desmin, found in most muscle cells; neurofilaments, found in neuronal cells; and glial filaments, found in astrocytes. In dermatopathology, antikeratin antibodies are used to differentiate epithelial from nonepithelial (melanocytic, hematopoietic, mesenchymal) tumors. A mixture of low and intermediate keratins such as AE1 and AE3 is commonly used. An additional antibody to low molecular-weight keratins such as CAM 5.2 may be beneficial in poorly differentiated carcinomas. The keratin marker CK20 has useful specificity for Merkel cell carcinoma (see Chap. 37).

Atypical spindle cell tumors, for example, are difficult to diagnose with routine stains. The differential diagnosis includes spindle cell squamous cell carcinoma, atypical fibroxanthoma, leiomyosarcoma, and spindle cell malignant melanoma. The most important antibodies to use are listed in Table 4-3. Argenyi has comprehensively reviewed the diagnosis of cutaneous spindle cell tumors using immunohistochemistry.[19]

Vimentin

Vimentin is an intermediate filament originally isolated from chick embryo fibroblasts. It is found in fibroblasts, endothelial cells, macrophages, melanocytes, lymphocytes, and smooth muscle cells. Antibodies to vimentin are found in both benign and malignant counterparts of these cells.[20] There have also been reports of positivity in epithelial tumors; however, normal epidermis is negative with this antibody. Because of the nonspecific nature of the antibody, it is useful only as a panel approach to support mesenchymal or melanocytic differentiation.

Antibodies Against Leukocyte Common Antigen (LCA)

This antibody helps to distinguish between undifferentiated lymphomas and carcinomas. Leukocyte common antigen is found on all leukocytes, including granulocytes, lymphocytes, monocytes, macrophages, mast cells, and Langerhans cells. The lymphomas and leukemias react with the antibody against leukocyte common antigen; carcinomas and melanomas are negative. In addition to LCA, lysozyme and chloroacetate esterase aid in the diagnosis of leukemia cutis.[21] LCA is particularly useful in the evaluation of tumors composed of small atypical basophilic cells in the dermis (Table 4-4). Other antigens useful in the analysis of suspected lymphomas include B- and T-cell markers: L-26 (CD-20, B cells) or MB2 (B cells) and UCHL-1 (CD-45RO, T cells) (see Chap. 32).

Carcinoembryonic Antigen and Epithelial Membrane Antigen

Carcinoembryonic antigen (CEA) has been found in normal eccrine and apocrine cells, in benign sweat gland tumors, and in mammary and extramammary Paget's disease of the skin. Incubation with anti-CEA can be helpful in distinguishing Paget cells from atypical melanocytes in malignant melanoma in situ. However, reactivity of melanomas with CEA has been reported (see Chap. 29).[22] Carcinoembryonic antigen typically stains adenocarcinoma of most organ systems. Most epithelial tumors react with antibodies against epithelial membrane antigen (EMA), including squamous cell carcinoma, breast carcinoma, and large cell lung carcinoma. EMA will also stain normal sweat and sebaceous glands, although epidermis is unreactive with this antibody. Epithelioid sarcoma is also stained by EMA (see Chap. 33).

TABLE 4-2. *Common antigens that can be detected in formalin-fixed, paraffin-embedded sections*

Antigen	Location
Cytokeratins, including AE1, AE3, CAM 5.2, CK20	Epidermis and its appendages and their tumors
Vimentin	Mesenchymal cells, melanocytes, lymphomas, sarcomas, melanomas
Desmin	Smooth and skeletal muscle, muscle tumors
Leukocyte common antigen (LCA)	Benign leukocytes, lymphoma, leukemia
UCHL-1	T lymphocytes
L-26	B lymphocytes
Epithelial membrane antigen (EMA)	Sweat and sebaceous glands, carcinoma, epithelioid sarcoma
Carcinoembryonic antigen (CEA)	Eccrine and apocrine glands and their tumors, Paget cells
S-100 protein	Melanocytes, Langerhans cells, eccrine and apocrine glands and their tumors, Schwann cells, nerves, interdigitating reticulum cells, chondrocytes, melanomas, adipose tissue, liposarcomas, histiocytosis X
HMB-45	Melanoma cells, some nevus cells
Chromogranin	Neuroendocrine cells, Merkel cell carcinoma, eccrine gland cells
Synaptophysin	Neuroendocrine cells, Merkel cell carcinoma
Lysozyme	Macrophages, granulocytes, myeloid cells
Alpha$_1$-antitrypsin, alpha$_1$-antichymotrypsin	Macrophages, "fibrohistiocytic" neoplasms including MFH, but nonspecific in most routine practice
Factor VIII–related antigen	Endothelial cells, angiosarcomas, Kaposi's sarcoma
Ulex europaeus agglutinin I	Endothelial cells, keratinocytes, angiosarcomas, Kaposi's sarcoma
CD31	Endothelial cells
CD34	Endothelial cells, bone marrow progenitor cells, cells of dermatofibrosarcoma protuberans

Note: Few if any of these reagents are perfectly specific for their target antigens. Every test must be interpreted in the context of all the available histologic and clinical information.

Neuron-Specific Enolase

Neuron-specific enolase (NSE) is an acidic enzyme found in neuroendocrine cells, neurons, and tumors derived from them. Merkel cell carcinoma contains NSE; however, NSE can be detected in a variety of other tumors, including malignant melanoma, and therefore has low specificity. The keratin marker CK20 has better specificity for Merkel cell tumor than for melanoma and other neuroendocrine tumors.[23]

Chromogranin

The soluble proteins of chromaffin granules are called *chromogranin*.[24] Chromogranins consist of three families of acidic proteins: chromogranin A, B, and C. They are normally found in most endocrine cells (e.g., thyroid, parathyroid, anterior pituitary). In the skin, chromogranin A has been found in Merkel cell carcinoma.[25] In contrast, nevi and melanoma do not contain chromogranin.

Synaptophysin

Synaptophysin is a 38-kD glycoprotein that participates in calcium-dependent release of neurotransmitters.[26] It is a neuroendocrine antigen with a distribution similar to chromogranin. Positive staining with antibodies to synaptophysin is useful in the diagnosis of neuroendocrine tumors such as Merkel cell carcinoma. Interestingly, normal Merkel cells are negative with this antibody. Similar to chromogranin, melanocytic tumors do not stain with synaptophysin.

TABLE 4-3. *Differential diagnosis of malignant spindle cell tumors*

Diagnosis	Keratin	Vimentin	Desmin	S-100	HMB-45	Factor VIII
Squamous cell carcinoma	+	−	−	−	−	−
Atypical fibroxanthoma	−	+	−	−	−	−
Melanoma	−	+	−	+	+	−
Leiomyosarcoma	−	+	+	−	−	−
Angiosarcoma	−	−	−	−	−	+

Note: Few if any of these reagents are perfectly specific for their target antigens. Every test must be interpreted in the context of all the available histologic and clinical information.

TABLE 4-4. *Immunohistochemistry of basophilic small cells in the dermis*

Diagnosis	S-100	Synaptophysin	LCA*	Keratin
Lymphoma	−	−	+	−
Merkel cell carcinoma	−	+	−	+†
Carcinoma	+/−	−	−	+
Melanoma	+	−	−	−

* LCA = Leukocyte common antigen.
† Perinuclear staining.
Note: Few if any of these reagents are perfectly specific for their target antigens. Every test must be interpreted in the context of all the available histologic and clinical information. Poorly differentiated carcinoma may be keratin negative, or only positive with low-molecular-weight keratin antibodies.

S-100 Protein

S-100 protein is an acidic protein that binds Ca^{2+} and Zn^{2+}. It was called S-100 because of its solubility in 100% ammonium sulfate at neutral pH. It is found in the cytoplasm and in the nucleus. S-100 protein can be detected in a large variety of cells: melanocytes, Langerhans cells, eccrine and apocrine gland cells, nerves, muscles, Schwann cells, myoepithelial cells, chondrocytes, and their malignant counterparts. Histiocytes may also stain positively with S-100 protein. The polyclonal antibody against S-100 works well on paraffin sections. Its high sensitivity contrasts a low specificity, a feature that supports the concept of a panel approach to immunohistochemistry.

Useful applications of the antibody against S-100 protein include (1) diagnosing of spindle cell melanoma and desmoplastic melanoma; (2) distinguishing between melanocytes and lymphocytes in halo nevi; (3) differentiating between pigmented actinic keratoses and lentigo maligna; and (4) diagnosing poorly differentiated cutaneous metastases.

HMB-45

HMB-45 is a monoclonal antibody that was initially generated from an extract of metastatic melanoma. Both primary and metastatic melanomas reveal cytoplasmic staining with HMB-45; spindle cell melanomas and desmoplastic melanomas are frequently negative. This antibody reacts with a melanosomal protein, GP-100, which tends to be expressed in immature or proliferating cells. Unfortunately, HMB-45 may react with melanocytes in nevi, including dysplastic nevi and Spitz nevi.[27] Therefore, it should not be used for the differential diagnosis between a malignant melanoma and a benign nevus.

Antibodies Against Lysozyme, α_1-Antitrypsin, α_1-Antichymotrypsin

These antibodies have been regarded as markers of mononuclear phagocytic cells. Although once felt to be markers for "fibrohistiocytic" neoplasms, they have also been identified in carcinomas and melanomas, making them less specific.

Factor VIII–Related Antigen, Ulex Europaeus Agglutinin I, CD31, CD34

Factor VIII–related antigen is a large glycoprotein produced by endothelial cells and therefore is useful in benign and malignant vascular neoplasms.

Ulex europaeus agglutinin I is a lectin that reacts specifically with α-L-fucose present in endothelial cells, keratinocytes, and most eccrine gland cells. Ulex is a reliable marker for endothelial cells of blood vessels and lymphatics in paraffin sections, although it is less specific than factor VIII–related antigen.

CD31 and CD34 are newer markers for endothelial differentiation that are discussed in Chapter 34, Vascular Tumors.

Electron Microscopy

Transmission electron microscopy may be beneficial in the diagnosis of poorly differentiated skin neoplasms for which immunohistochemistry is negative.[28] Using electron microscopy, the identification of intercellular junctions (epithelial tumors), melanosomes (melanocytic tumors) or Weibel-Palade bodies (endothelial cells) can provide an important diagnostic aid. Other uses of diagnostic electron microscopy include the subtype determination of epidermolysis bullosa and the diagnosis of metabolic storage diseases (e.g., Fabry disease) or amyloidosis. For optimum results, fresh tissue should be fixed in Karnovsky medium (paraformaldehyde-glutaraldehyde) and stored in the refrigerator until processing; although electron microscopy rarely can be performed from paraffin-embedded tissue, there may be extensive distortion precluding valuable interpretation.

Diagnosis of Lymphomas

The application of monoclonal antibodies for the diagnosis of lymphomas is expanding. However, there is no antibody that distinguishes between benign and malignant lymphocytes. Hence, the difficult distinction between lymphoma and pseudolymphoma remains.

Although many antibodies are best used on frozen sections, an increasing number of commonly available antibodies can be used on formalin-fixed paraffin-embedded tissue. The quality of certain markers such as kappa and lambda light chains has been variable in paraffin sections, and is more reliable on frozen sections. Monoclonal antibodies can determine the cell types in a lymphoma or pseudolymphoma: helper or suppressor T cells, B cells, plasma cells, or macrophages. A confusing issue is that B-cell lymphomas may contain reactive T-cell infiltrates, which can outnumber the B cells. The predominance of a T-helper lymphocytic infiltrate with epidermotropism of the T-helper subtype is highly suggestive of cutaneous T-cell lymphoma. In contrast, a mixture of T-helper and T-suppressor phenotypes is most consistent with a reactive profile (e.g., spongiotic dermatitis). In dense nodular infiltrates, the presence of germinal center formation with B-lymphocyte aggregates surrounded by a mantle of T cells favors lymphocytoma cutis over lymphoma. A detailed discussion of antibodies helpful in the diagnosis of lymphoma is found in Chapter 32.

Molecular studies can provide additional information in the evaluation of atypical lymphoid infiltrates. Detection of a characteristic gene rearrangement coding for B- and T-cell antigen receptors will identify the presence or absence of a monoclonal population of lymphocytes.[29] These applications are an important supplement to routinely available technology; they are widely available in specialized laboratories in major medical centers.

REFERENCES

1. Neiman RS, Barcos M, Berard C et al. Granulocytic sarcoma. Cancer 1981;48:1426.
2. Luna LG, ed. Manual of histologic staining methods of the Armed Forces Institute of Pathology. 3rd ed. New York: McGraw-Hill, 1968.
3. Roten SV, Bhat S, Bhawan J. Elastic fibers in scar tissue. J Cutan Pathol 1996;23:37.
4. Weigand DA. Effect of anatomic region on immunofluorescence diagnosis of bullous pemphigoid. J Am Acad Dermatol 1985;12:274.
5. Weigand DA, Clements MK. Direct immunofluorescence in bullous pemphigoid: Effects of extent and location of lesions. J Am Acad Dermatol 1989;20:437.
6. Nisengaard RJ, Blaszczyk M, Chorzelski T et al. Immunofluorescence of biopsy specimens: Comparison of methods of transportation. Arch Dermatol 1978;114:1329.
7. Vaughn Jones SA, Palmer I, Vhogal BS et al. The use of Michel's transport medium for immunofluorescence and immunoelectron microscopy in autoimmune bullous diseases. J Cutan Pathol 1995;22:365.
8. Pardo RJ, Penneys NS. Location of basement membrane type IV collagen beneath subepidermal bullous diseases. J Cutan Pathol 1990;17:336.
9. Schaumburg-Lever G. The alkaline phosphatase anti-alkaline phosphatase technique in dermatopathology. J Cutan Pathol 1987;14:6.
10. Cordell JL, Falini B, Erber WN et al. Immunoenzymatic labeling of monoclonal antibodies using immune complexes of alkaline phosphatase and monoclonal anti-alkaline phosphatase (APAAP complexes). J Histochem Cytochem 1984;32:219.
11. Hsu SM, Raine L. Protein A, avidin and biotin in immunohistochemistry. J Histochem Cytochem 1981;29:1349.
12. Elias JM. Immunohistochemical methods. In Elias JM. Immunohistology: A practical approach to diagnosis. Chicago: ASCP Press, 1990;1.
13. Wallace ML, Smoller BR. Immunohistochemistry in diagnostic dermatopathology. J Am Acad Dermatol 1996;34:163.
14. Wick MR, Swanson PE, Ritter JH, Fitzgibbon JF. The immunohistology of cutaneous neoplasia: A practical perspective. J Cutan Pathol 1993;20:481.
15. Googe PB, Bhan AK, Mihm MC. Application of immunohistochemistry in the differential diagnosis of skin tumors: Tumor markers in diagnostic pathology. Clin Lab Med 1990;10:179.
16. True LD. Atlas of diagnostic immunohistopathology. Philadelphia: JB Lippincott, 1990.
17. Murphy GF. Cytokeratin typing of cutaneous tumors: A new immunochemical probe for cellular differentiation and malignant transformation. J Invest Dermatol 1985;84:1.
18. Osborn M. Component of the cellular cytoskeleton: A new generation of markers of histogenetic origin. J Invest Dermatol 1984;82:443.
19. Argenyi ZB. Spindle cell neoplasms of the skin: A comprehensive diagnostic approach. Semin Derm 1989;8:283.
20. Leader M, Collins M, Patel J et al. Vimentin: An evaluation of its role as a tumour marker. Histopathology 1987;11:63.
21. Ratnam KV, Su WPD, Ziesmer SC, Li CY. Value of immunohistochemistry in the diagnosis of leukemia cutis: Study of 54 cases using paraffin-section markers. J Cutan Pathol 1992;19:193.
22. Sanders DSA, Evans AT, Allen CA et al. Classification of CEA-related positivity in primary and metastatic malignant melanoma. J Pathol 1994;172:343.
23. Moll R, Lowe A, Laufer J, Franke WW. Cytokeratin 20 in human carcinomas. Am J Pathol 1992;140:427.
24. Schober M, Fischer-Colbrie R, Schmid KW et al. Comparison of chromogranin A, B, and secretogranin II in human adrenal medulla and phaeochromocytoma. Lab Invest 1987;57:385.
25. Lloyd RV, Cano M, Rosa P et al. Distribution of chromogranin A and chromogranin I (chromogranin B) in neuroendocrine cells and tumors. Am J Pathol 1988;130:296.
26. Weidenmann B, Franke WW. Identification and localization of synaptophysin: an integral membrane glycoprotein of MW 38,000 characteristic of presynaptic vesicles. Cell 1985;45:1017.
27. Wick MR, Swanson PE, Rocamora A. Recognition of malignant melanoma by monoclonal antibody HMB-45: An immunohistochemical study of 200 paraffin-embedded cutaneous tumors. J Cut Pathol 1988;15:201.
28. Murphy GF, Dickersin GR, Harrist TJ, Mihm MC. The role of diagnostic electron microscopy in dermatology. In: Moschella S, ed. Dermatology Update. New York: Elsevier Press, 1981;355.
29. Weinberg JM, Rook AH, Lessin SR. Molecular diagnosis of lymphocytic infiltrates of the skin. Arch Dermatol 1993;129:1491.
30. Rapini R. Comparison of methods for checking surgical margins. J Am Acad Dermatol 1990;23:288.

Lever's Histopathology of the Skin, eighth edition, edited by David Elder et al. Lippincott–Raven Publishers, Philadelphia © 1997.

CHAPTER 5

Algorithmic Classification of Skin Disease for Differential Diagnosis

David Elder, Rosalie Elenitsas, Bernett Johnson Jr., Christine Jaworsky, and Michael Ioffreda

The diagnosis of disease concerns the ability to classify disorders into categories that predict clinically important attributes such as prognosis or response to therapy. This permits appropriate interventions to be planned for particular patients. Understanding this process involves mastering the stages of disease, the mechanisms of changes in morphology over time, and the molecular, cellular, gross clinical, and epidemiologic reasons for the differences among diseases.

The process of cutaneous diagnosis at its simplest level might involve the matching of a large number of attributes contained in classical descriptions of skin diseases with the presence or absence of the same attributes in a particular case under consideration. Since there are hundreds of potential diagnostic categories, each having potentially scores of attributes, it is evident that an efficient strategy must be employed to enable diagnoses to be considered, dismissed, or retained for further consideration. An experienced dermatopathologist can make a rapid and accurate diagnosis that precludes the simultaneous consideration of more than a few variables. Indeed, the process of diagnosis by an experienced observer is quite different from that employed by the novice, and is based on the rapid recognition of combinations or patterns of criteria.[1,2] Just as the recognition of an old friend occurs by a process that does not require the serial enumeration of particular facial features, this process of pattern recognition occurs almost instantly, and is based on broad parameters that do not, at least initially, require detailed evaluation.

D. Elder: Department of Pathology and Laboratory Medicine, University of Pennsylvania, Philadelphia, PA

R. Elenitsas: Department of Dermatology, University of Pennsylvania, Philadelphia, PA

B. Johnson Jr.: Department of Dermatology, University of Pennsylvania, Philadelphia, PA

C. Jaworsky: Cleveland Skin Pathology Laboratory, Cleveland, OH

M. Ioffreda: Department of Dermatology, University of Pennsylvania, Philadelphia, PA

In clinical medicine, patterns may present as combinations of symptoms and signs or even of laboratory values, but in dermatopathology the most predictive diagnostic patterns are recognized through the scanning lens of the microscope, or even before microscopy as the microscopist holds the slide up to the light to evaluate its profile and distribution of colors. Occasionally, a specific diagnosis can be made during this initial stage of pattern recognition by a process of "gestalt" or instant recognition, but this should be tempered with a subsequent moment of healthy analytic scrutiny. More often, the scanning magnification pattern suggests a small list of possible diagnoses, a "differential diagnosis." Then, features that are more readily recognized at higher magnification may be employed to differentiate among the possibilities. Put in the language of science, the scanning magnification pattern suggests a series of hypotheses, which are then tested by additional observations.[1] The tests may be observations made at higher magnification, the results of special studies such as immunohistochemistry, or external findings such as the clinical appearance of the patient or the results of laboratory investigations. For example, a broad plaquelike configuration of small blue dots near the dermal-epidermal junction could represent a lichenoid dermatitis or a lichenoid actinic keratosis. At higher magnification, the blue dots are confirmed to be lymphocytes, and one might seek evidence of parakeratosis, atypical keratinocytes, and plasma cells in the lesion, a combination that would rule out lichen planus and establish a diagnosis of actinic keratosis.

Most diagnoses in dermatopathology are established either by the "gestalt" method or by the process of hypothesis generation and testing (differential diagnosis and investigation) just described, but in either case the basis of the methods is the identification of simple patterns recognizable with the scanning lens that suggest a manageably short list of differential diagnostic considerations. This *pattern recognition method* was first developed for diagnosis of skin disease in a series of lectures given in Boston by Wallace Clark,[3] and has been refined since for inflammatory skin disease by Ackerman,[4] for inflammatory and neoplastic skin disease by Mihm,[5] and most recently by Murphy.[6] The last three authors have published texts based more or less extensively on the pattern classification. The present work, however, has been organized upon more traditional lines, in which diseases are discussed on the basis of pathogenesis (mechanisms) or etiology as well as upon reaction patterns. Such a classification has the advantage of placing disorders such as infections in a common relationship to one another, facilitating the description of their many common attributes. From a histopathologic point of view, however, the novice must learn that some infections, such as syphilis, can resemble disorders as disparate as psoriasis, as lichen planus, as a cutaneous lymphoma, or as a granulomatous dermatitis.

Because there is a limited number of reaction patterns in the skin, morphologic simulants of disparate disease processes are common in the skin, as elsewhere. For this reason, classification methods based on patterns and those based on pathogenesis are incompatible with each other. To partially circumvent this problem, the present section of this book presents a pattern-based classification of cutaneous pathology based on *location in the skin*, on *reaction patterns*, and where applicable on *cell type*, indexed to the more detailed descriptions of the disease entities discussed in other sections of the book. The section has been based (with permission) on the original lecture notes prepared by Wallace H Clark Jr., M.D., in 1965, and on the published works cited above, especially that of Hood, Kwan, Mihm, and Horn.[5]

The classification is presented here in tabular form and is redundant, in that a particular disease entity may appear in several positions in the table because of the morphologic heterogeneity of disease processes, which are often based on evolutionary or involutionary morphologic changes as a disease waxes and wanes. The order of presentation of particular entities in any given position in the table reflects the authors' opinion of the relative frequency of the entities in the list as encountered in a typical dermatopathology practice. For example, lichenoid drug eruption may be more common than lichen planus in most hospital-based practices. However, lichen planus is the "prototypic" lichenoid dermatitis, whereas drug eruptions may adopt any of a number of morphologies as reflected by their appearance in the psoriasiform, lichenoid, perivascular, and bullous categories as well as elsewhere. The "prototypic" member of each category is italicized for easy reference to the detailed descriptions, because such entities constitute the descriptive standard in a given category, and they are also the standard against which other entities are evaluated. For example, a "naked" epithelioid cell granuloma may suggest sarcoidosis, whereas the presence of lymphocytes and necrosis in addition to granulomas might suggest tuberculosis, plasma cells might suggest syphilis, and neuritis might suggest leprosy.

The classification tables may be used as the basis of an algorithmic approach to differential diagnosis or as a guide to the descriptions in the other sections of this book. For example, a psoriasiform dermatitis with plasma cells may represent syphilis or mycosis fungoides, whose descriptions are to be found in Chaps. 22 and 32, respectively. Terms such as *psoriasiform* and *lichenoid* are defined briefly, and appropriate page references are provided in this section so that the reader may review more specific criteria for the distinctions among morphologic simulants. This system of hypothesis generating and testing should not only lead to more efficient use of this book in the evaluation and diagnosis of an unknown case, but should also facilitate the development of pattern recognition skills as more subtle diagnostic clues are absorbed into the diagnostic repertoire to allow for "tempered gestalt" diagnosis in an increasing percentage of cases.

This chapter is intended as a guide to differential diagnosis but should not be construed as an infallible diagnostic tool. Diagnosis should be based not only on the diagnostic considerations presented here but also on those discussed elsewhere in this book and in the literature, all considered in a clinical and epidemiologic context appropriate to the individual patient.

REFERENCES

1. Sackett DL, Haynes RB, Guyatt GH, et al. Clinical Epidemiology. A Basic Science for Clinical Medicine. 2nd ed. Boston: Little Brown, 1991.
2. Foucar E. Diagnostic decision-making in surgical pathology. In: Weidner N. Diagnosis of the Difficult Case.
3. Reed RJ, Clark WH Jr. Pathophysiologic reactions of the skin. In: Fitzpatrick TB, ed. Dermatology in General Medicine. New York: McGraw-Hill, 1971;192.
4. Ackerman AB. Histologic Diagnosis of Inflammatory Skin Diseases: A Method by Pattern Analysis. Philadelphia: Lea & Febiger, 1978.
5. Hood AF, Kwan TH, Mihm MC, Horn TD. Primer of Dermatopathology. Boston: Little, Brown, 1993.
6. Murphy GF. Dermatopathology. Philadelphia: Saunders, 1995.

Part 1: Site Categories of Cutaneous Pathology

In this part, the major categories of cutaneous disease based on their location in the skin and subcutis are briefly discussed.

I. Disorders Mostly Limited to the Stratum Corneum • 84, 87

The stratum corneum is usually arranged in a delicate meshlike or "basket-weave" pattern. It may be shed (exfoliated) or thickened (hyperkeratosis) with or without retention of nuclei (parakeratosis or orthokeratosis, respectively). Usually, alterations in the stratum corneum result from inflammatory or neoplastic changes that affect the whole epidermis and, more often than not, the superficial dermis. Only a few conditions, mentioned in this section, show pathology mostly or entirely limited to the stratum corneum.

II. Localized Superficial, Epithelial, or Melanocytic Proliferations/Neoplasms • 84, 87

Localized proliferations may be reactive but are often neoplastic. The epidermis (keratinocytes) may proliferate without extension into the dermis, may extend into the dermis, and may be squamous or basaloid. Melanocytes within the epidermis may proliferate with or without cytologic atypia (nevi, dysplastic nevi, melanoma in situ) in a proliferative epidermis (superficial spreading melanoma in situ, Spitz nevi) or an atrophic epidermis (lentigo maligna); they can also extend into the dermis as proliferative infiltrates (invasive melanoma with or without vertical growth phase). There may be an associated variably cellular, often mixed, inflammatory infiltrate, or inflammation may be essentially absent.

III. Inflammation of the Superficial Cutaneous Reactive Unit • 84, 90

The epidermis, papillary dermis, and superficial capillary-venular plexus react together in many dermatologic conditions, and have been termed the *superficial cutaneous reactive unit* by Clark. Many dermatoses are associated with infiltrates of lymphocytes, with or without other cell types, around the superficial vessels. The epidermis in pathologic conditions can be thinned (atrophy), thickened (acanthosis), edematous (spongiosis), and/or infiltrated by inflammatory cells (exocytosis). The epidermis may proliferate in response to chronic irritation or infection (bacterial, yeast, deep fungal, or viral). The epidermis may proliferate in response to dermatologic conditions (psoriasis, atopic dermatitis, prurigo). The papillary dermis and superficial vascular plexus may have a variety of inflammatory cells, can be edematous, may have increased ground substance (hyaluronic acid), or may be sclerotic or homogenized.

IV. Acantholytic, Vesicular, and Pustular Disorders • 85, 96

Keratinocytes may separate from each other, resulting in separation and rounding up of keratinocyte cell bodies (acantholysis). This may occur on the basis of immunologic antigen-antibody mediated damage, on the basis of edema and inflammation (spongiosis), or on the basis of structural deficiencies of cell adhesion (Darier's disease). These processes produce spaces within the epidermis (vesicles, bullae, pustules). The adhesion of basal layer keratinocytes to the papillary dermis may be altered, producing spaces that form subepidermally.

V. Inflammation of the Reticular Dermis • 85, 99

The dermis serves as a reaction site for a variety of inflammatory, infiltrative and desmoplastic (fibrogenic) processes. These include infiltrations of a variety of cells (lymphocytes, histiocytes, eosinophils, plasma cells, melanocytes, etc.); perivascular and vascular reactions; infiltration with organisms and foreign bodies; and proliferations of dermal fibers and precursors of dermal fibers as reactions to a variety of stimuli. The infiltrates may be characterized as perivascular, diffuse, or granulomatous.

VI. Neoplastic Nodules and Cysts of the Reticular Dermis • 85, 106

Neoplasms of the reticular dermis may arise from any of the tissues included in the dermis—lymphoreticular tissue, connective tissue, and epithelial tissue of the skin appendages. In addition, metastases commonly present in the dermis.

VII. Inflammatory Disorders of Skin Appendages • 86, 112

The hair, sebaceous glands, eccrine glands, apocrine glands, and nails may be involved in inflammatory processes (hidradenitis, folliculitis). Some neoplasms may masquerade as inflammatory processes.

VIII. Disorders of the Subcutis • 86, 114

The reactions in the subcutis are mostly inflammatory, although neoplastic proliferations of the subcutis do occur (lipoma). Pathologic conditions centered in the dermis may infiltrate the subcutis.

Part 2: Site, Pattern, and Cytologic Categories of Cutaneous Pathology

In the following listings, the categories of cutaneous disease based on location in the skin (categories I, II, III, etc.), architectural pattern (categories A, B, C, etc.), and cytology (categories 1, 2, 3, etc.) are presented. A single example of each disease category is listed, and an example of each major pattern category is illustrated. The disease illustrated is italicized in the listings.

I. DISORDERS MOSTLY LIMITED TO THE EPIDERMIS AND STRATUM CORNEUM

A. Hyperkeratosis With Hypogranulosis

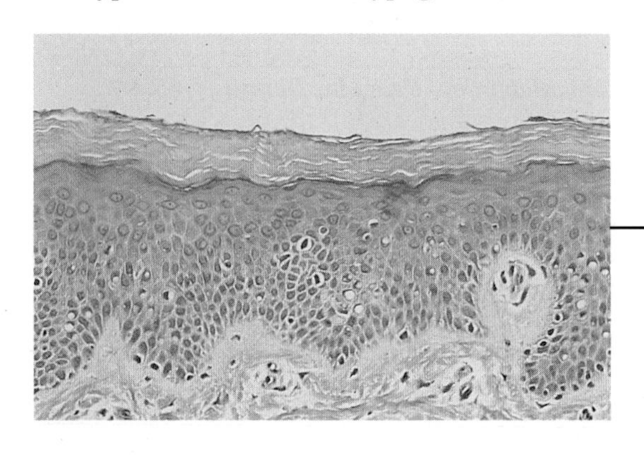

1. No Inflammation
   ichthyosis vulgaris

B. Hyperkeratosis With Normal or Hypergranulosis

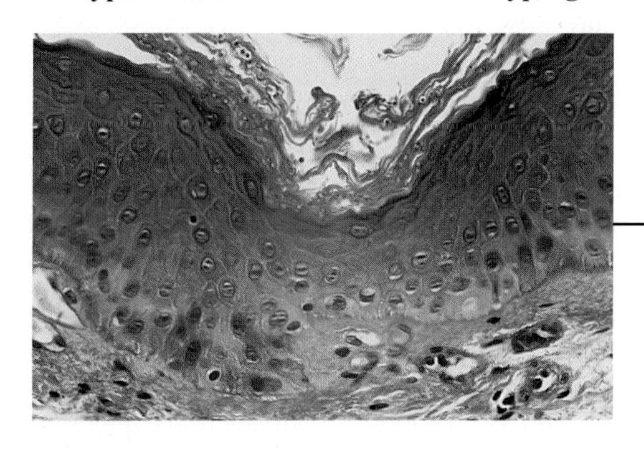

1. No Inflammation
   lamellar ichthyosis
2. Scant Inflammation
   dermatophytosis

C. Hyperkeratosis With Parakeratosis

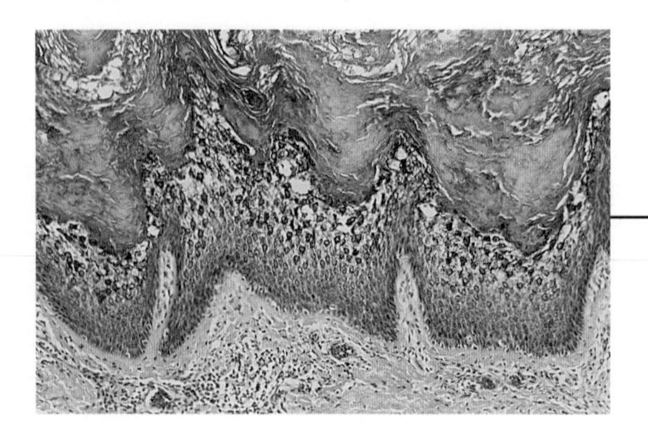

1. No Inflammation
   epidermolytic hyperkeratosis
2. Scant Inflammation
   scurvy

D. Localized or Diffuse Hyperpigmentations

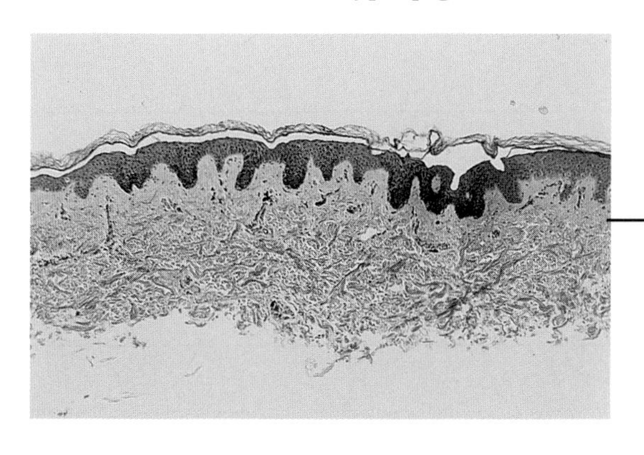

1. No Inflammation
   actinic lentigo

2. Scant Inflammation
   postinflammatory hyperpigmentation

E. Localized or Diffuse Hypopigmentations

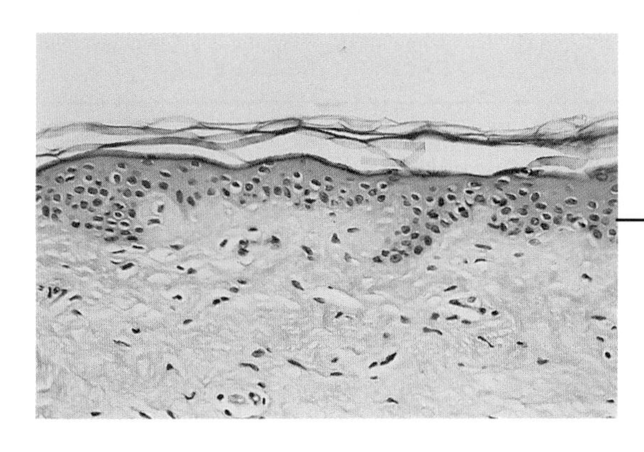

1. With or Without Slight Inflammation
   vitiligo

II. LOCALIZED SUPERFICIAL, EPIDERMAL, OR MELANOCYTIC PROLIFERATIONS/NEOPLASMS

A. Localized Irregular Thickening of the Epidermis

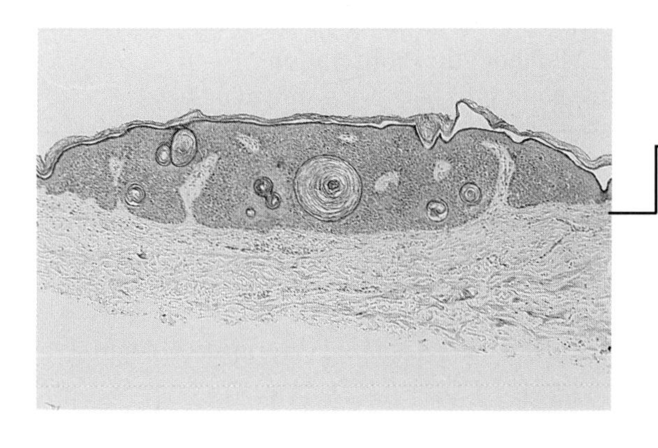

1. Epidermal Proliferation
   seborrheic keratosis

2. Melanocytic Proliferation
   melanoma in situ (superficial spreading type)

B. Localized Lesions with Thinning of the Epidermis

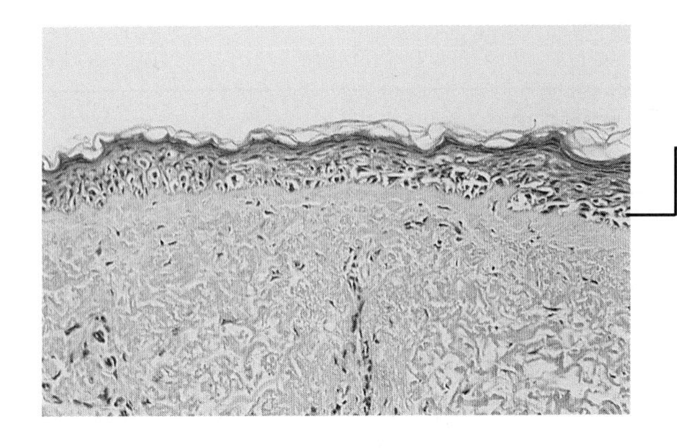

1. With Melanocytic Proliferation
   melanoma in situ (lentigo maligna type)

2. Without Melanocytic Proliferation
   actinic keratosis

C. Localized Lesions With Elongated Rete Ridges

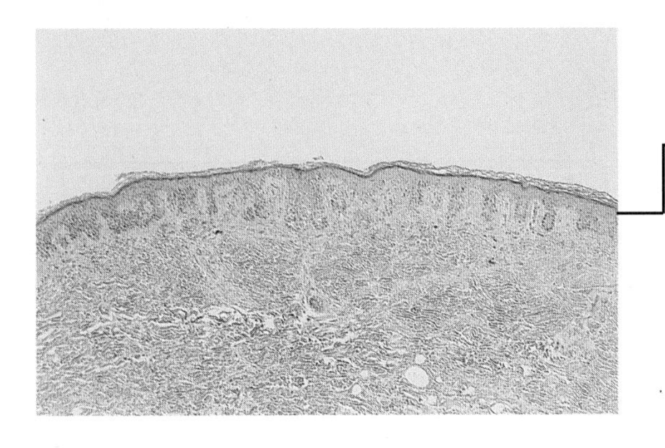

1. With Melanocytic Proliferation
   lentiginous junctional nevus

2. Without Melanocytic Proliferation
   epidermal nevus

D. Localized Lesions With Pagetoid Epithelial Proliferation

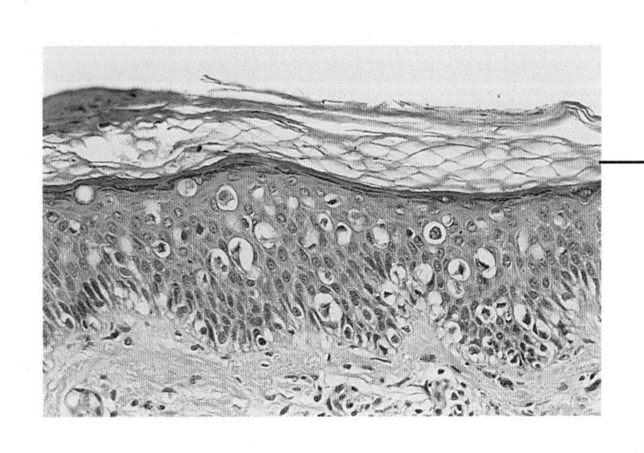

1. Keratinocytic Proliferation
   pagetoid squamous cell carcinoma in situ

2. With Melanocytic Proliferation
   melanoma in situ (superficial spreading type)

3. Glandular Epithelial Proliferation
   Paget's disease (mammary or extramammary)

4. Lymphoid Proliferation
   Pagetoid reticulosis, localized (Woringer-Kolopp)

E. Localized Papillomatous Epithelial Lesions

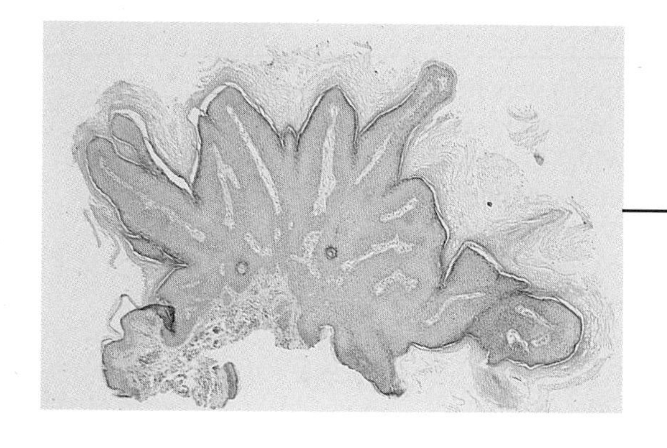

1. With Viral Cytopathic Effect
   verruca vulgaris

2. No Viral Cytopathic Effect
   verruciform xanthoma

F. Irregular Proliferations Extending Into the Dermis

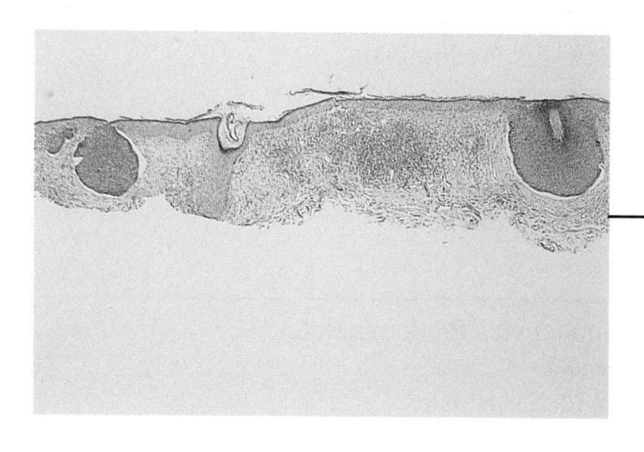

1. Squamous Differentiation
   squamous cell carcinoma, superficial

2. Basaloid Differentiation
   basal cell carcinoma, superficial type

G. Superficial Polypoid Lesions

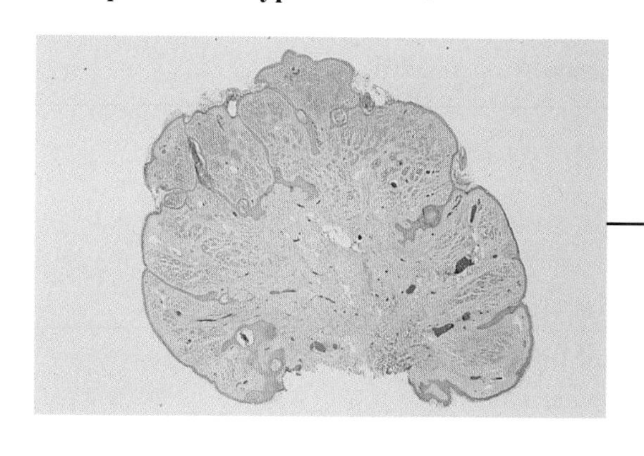

1. Melanocytic Lesions
   polypoid dermal and compound nevi

2. Stromal Lesions
   soft fibroma

III. DISORDERS OF THE SUPERFICIAL CUTANEOUS REACTIVE UNIT

A. Superficial Perivascular Dermatitis

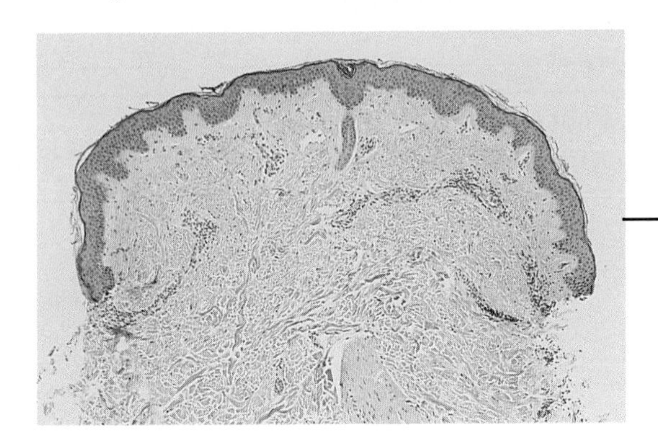

1. Lymphocytes Predominant
   morbilliform viral exanthem
   a. With Eosinophils
      arthropod bite reaction
   b. With Neutrophils
      erysipelas
   c. With Plasma Cells
      secondary syphilis
   d. With Extravasated Red Cells
      pityriasis rosea
   e. Melanophages Prominent
      postinflammatory hyperpigmentation

2. Mast Cells Predominant
   urticaria pigmentosa, nodular type

B. Superficial Perivascular Dermatitis With Spongiosis (Spongiotic Dermatitis)

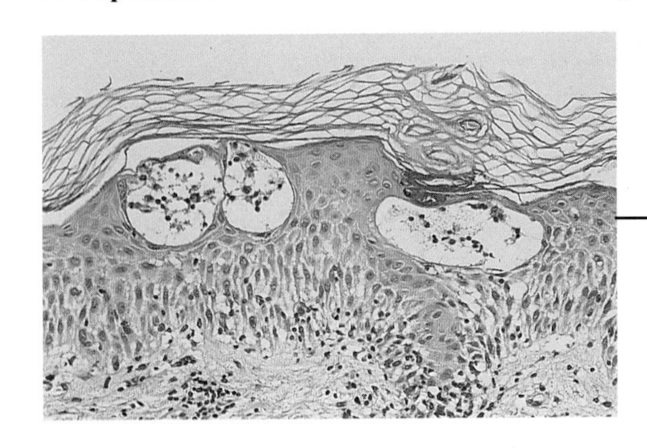

1. Lymphocytes Predominant
   nummular eczema
   a. With Eosinophils
      allergic contact dermatitis
   b. With Plasma Cells
      syphilis, primary or secondary lesions
   c. With Neutrophils
      seborrhcic dermatitis

C. Superficial Perivascular Dermatitis With Epidermal Atrophy (Atrophic Dermatitis)

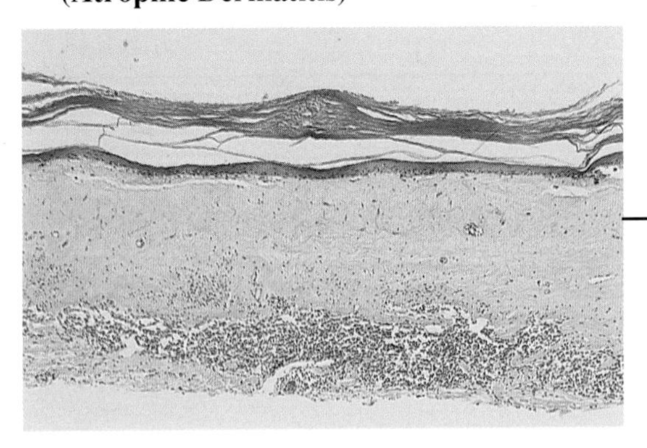

1. Scant Inflammatory Cells
   radiation dermatitis

2. Lymphocytes Predominant
   parapsoriasis/early mycosis fungoides
   a. With Papillary Dermal Sclerosis/Matrix Changes
      lichen sclerosus et atrophicus

D. Superficial Perivascular Dermatitis With Psoriasiform Proliferation (Psoriasiform Dermatitis)

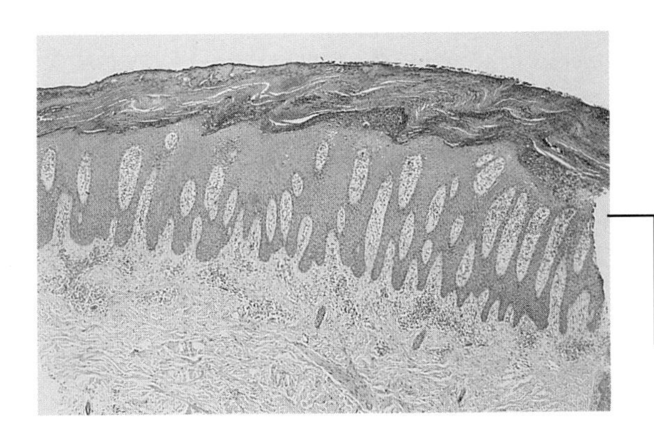

1. Lymphocytes Predominant
   chronic atopic dermatitis
   a. With Plasma Cells
      secondary syphilis
   b. With Eosinophils
      chronic allergic contact dermatitis

2. Neutrophils Prominent
   psoriasis vulgaris

E. Superficial Perivascular Dermatitis With Irregular Epidermal Proliferation (Hypertrophic Dermatitis)

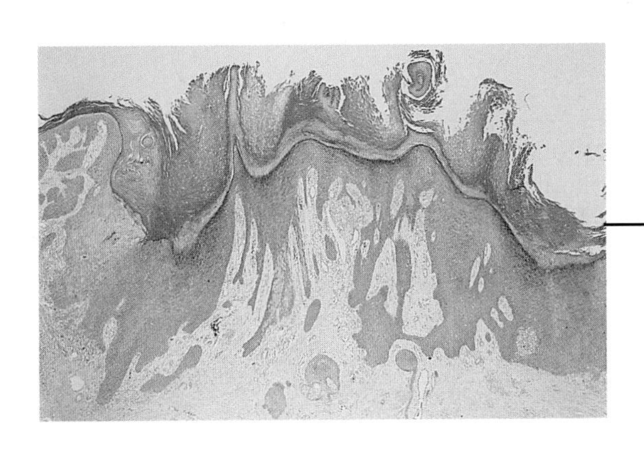

1. Lymphocytes Predominant
   prurigo nodularis
   a. Plasma Cells Present
      rupial secondary syphilis, condyloma lata

2. Neutrophils Prominent
   deep fungal infection

3. Neoplastic
   squamous cell carcinoma

F. Superficial Dermatitis With Lichenoid Infiltrates (Lichenoid Dermatitis)

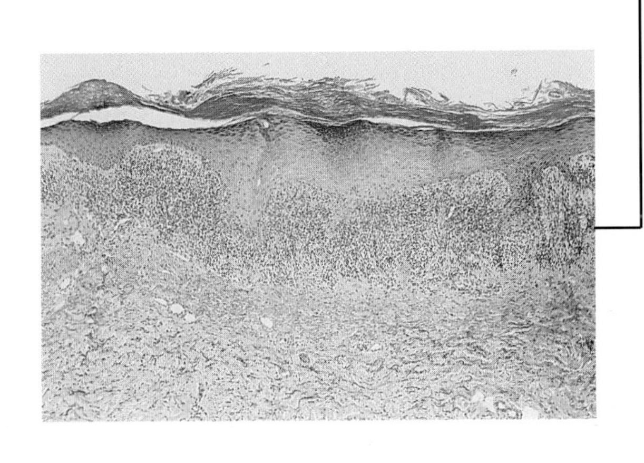

1. Lymphocytes Exclusively
   lichen planus

2. Lymphocytes Predominant
   lichen planus–like keratosis (benign lichenoid keratosis)
   a. Eosinophils Present
      lichenoid drug eruption
   b. Plasma Cells Present
      secondary syphilis
   c. With Melanophages
      postinflammatory hyperpigmentation

3. Histiocytes Predominant
   lichen nitidus

4. Mast Cells Predominant
   urticaria pigmentosa, papulonodular

G. Superficial Vasculitis and Vasculopathies

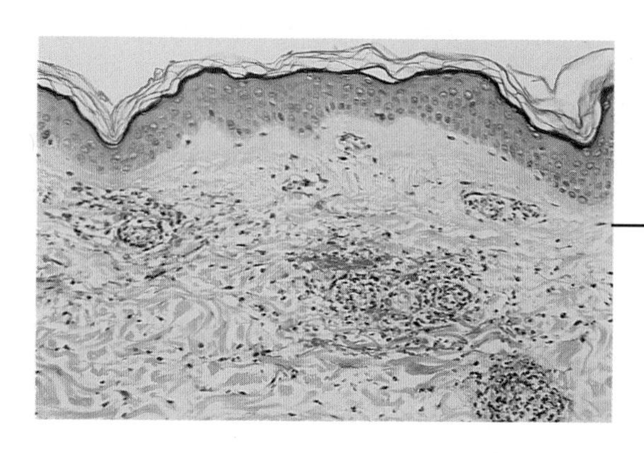

1. Neutrophilic Vasculitis
   cutaneous necrotizing (leukocytoclastic) vasculitis
2. Mixed Cell and Granulomatous Vasculitis
   Churg-Strauss vasculitis
3. Vasculopathies With Scant Inflammation
   malignant atrophic papulosis (Degos)
4. Thrombotic, Embolic, and Other Microangiopathies
   disseminated intravascular coagulation

H. Superficial Perivascular Dermatitis With Interface Vacuoles (Interface Dermatitis)

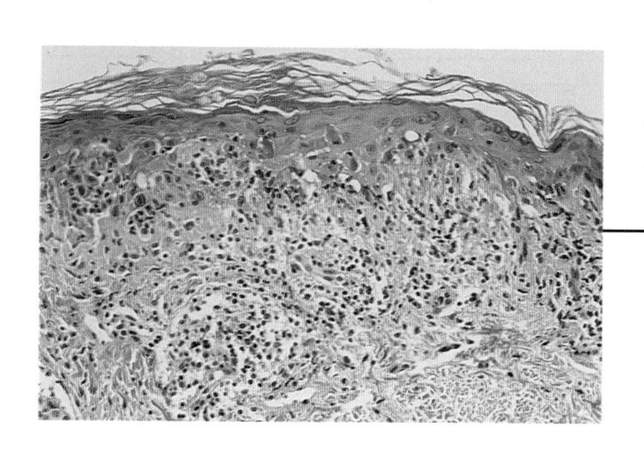

1. Apoptotic Cells Prominent (Cytotoxic Dermatitis)
   erythema multiforme
2. Apoptotic Cells Usually Absent
   dermatomyositis
3. Variable Apoptosis
   cytotoxic drug eruption
4. Basement Membranes Thickened
   lupus erythematosus

IV. ACANTHOLYTIC, VESICULAR, AND PUSTULAR DISORDERS

A. Subcorneal or Intracorneal Separation

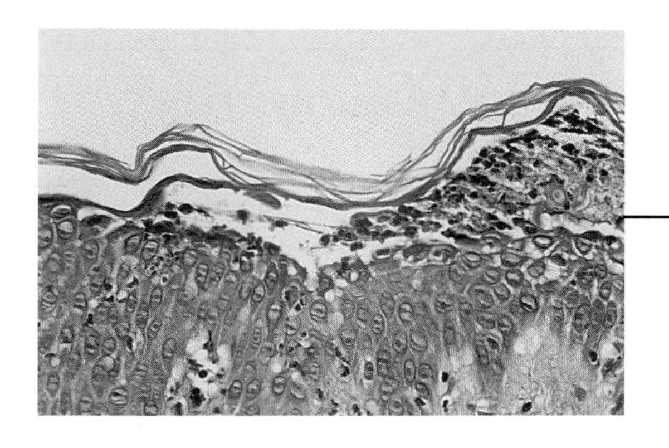

1. Scant Inflammatory Cells
   staphylococcal scalded skin
2. Neutrophils Prominent
   impetigo contagiosa
3. Eosinophils Predominant
   erythema toxicum neonatorum

B. Intraspinous Keratinocyte Separation, Spongiotic

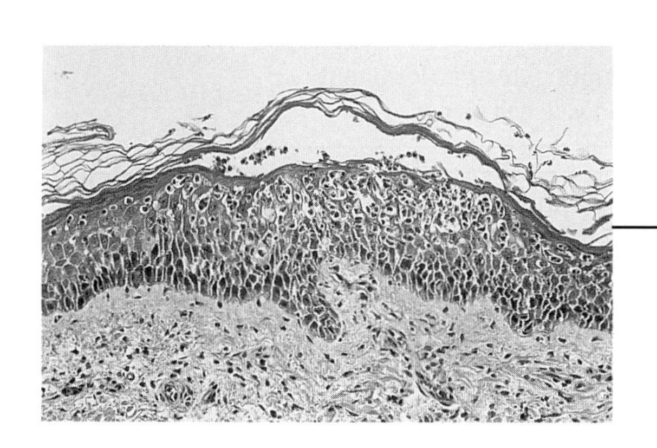

1. Scant Inflammatory Cells
   miliaria rubra
2. Lymphocytes Predominant
   nummular eczema
   a. Eosinophils Present
      allergic contact dermatitis
3. Neutrophils Predominant
   pustular psoriasis

C. Intraspinous Keratinocyte Separation, Acantholytic

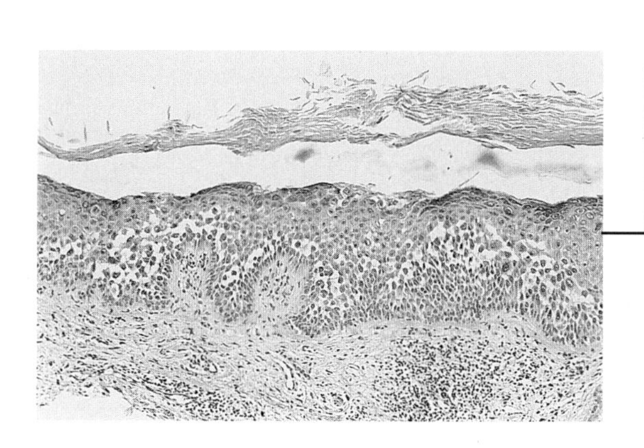

1. Scant Inflammatory Cells
   Hailey-Hailey disease
2. Lymphocytes Predominant
   herpes simplex, varicella-zoster
   a. Eosinophils Present
      pemphigus vegetans
3. Mixed Cell Types
   acantholytic solar keratosis

D. Suprabasal Keratinocyte Separation

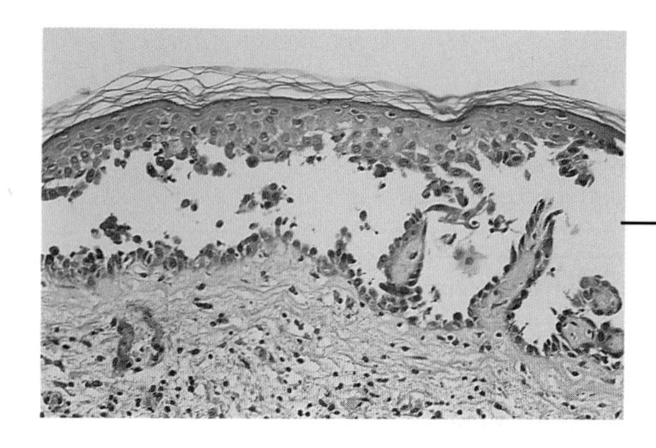

1. Scant Inflammatory Cells
   transient acantholytic dermatosis (Grover)

2. Lymphocytes and Plasma Cells
   acantholytic solar keratosis

3. Lymphocytes and Eosinophils
   pemphigus vulgaris

E. Subepidermal Vesicular Dermatitis

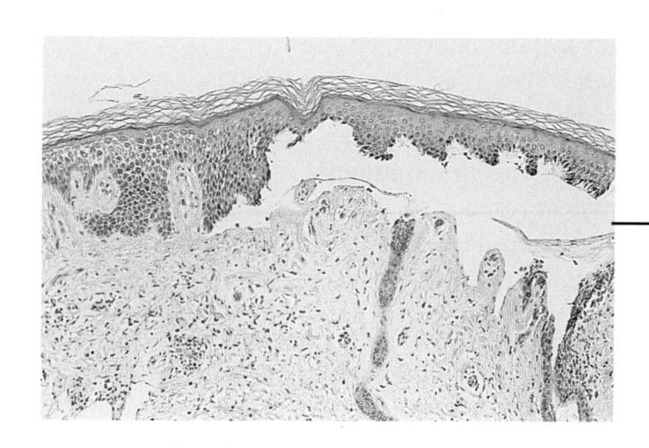

1. Scant/No Inflammation
   porphyria cutanea tarda

2. Lymphocytes Predominant
   bullous lichen planus

3. Eosinophils Prominent
   bullous pemphigoid

4. Neutrophils Prominent
   dermatitis herpetiformis

5. Mast Cells Prominent
   bullous mastocytosis

V. PERIVASCULAR, DIFFUSE, AND GRANULOMATOUS INFILTRATES OF THE RETICULAR DERMIS

A. Superficial and Deep Perivascular Infiltrates Without Vascular Damage or Vasculitis

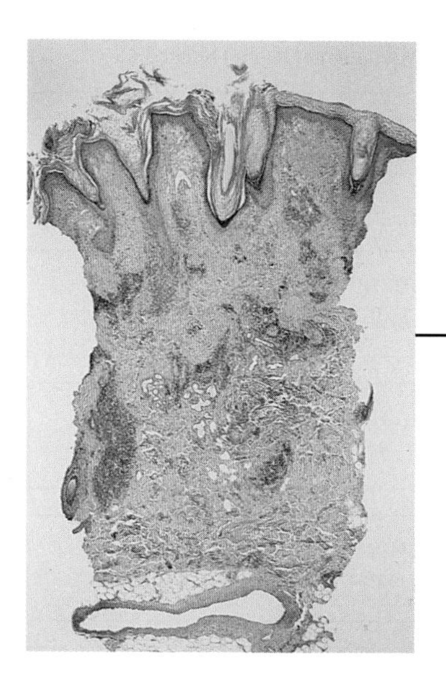

1. Lymphocytes Predominant
   discoid lupus erythematosus (DLE)
2. Neutrophils Predominant
   acute febrile neutrophilic dermatosis (Sweet's)
3. Lymphocytes and Eosinophils
   papular urticaria
4. Plasma Cells Present
   scleroderma/morphea
5. Mixed Cell Types
   erythema chronicum migrans

B. Superficial and Deep Vasculitis and Vasculopathies

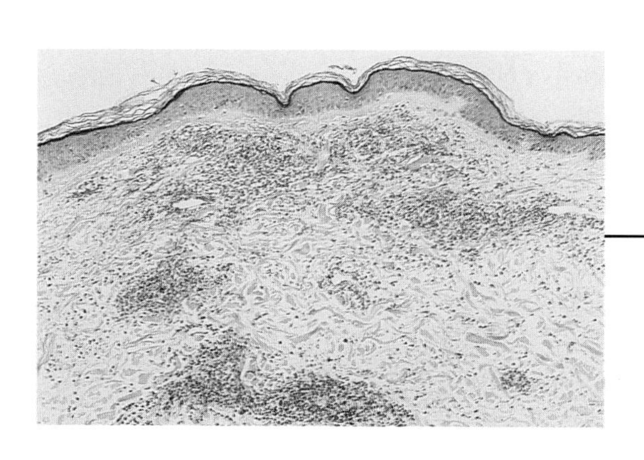

1. Scant Inflammatory Cells
   Degos disease (malignant atrophic papulosis)
2. Lymphocytes Predominant
   "lymphocytic vasculitis"
3. Neutrophils Prominent
   leukocytoclastic vasculitis
4. Mixed Cell Types and/or Granulomas
   allergic granulomatosis (Churg-Strauss)
5. Thrombotic and Other Microangiopathies
   disseminated intravascular coagulation

C. Diffuse Infiltrates of the Reticular Dermis

1. Lymphocytes Predominant
   cutaneous lymphoid hyperplasia/lymphocytoma cutis
2. Neutrophils Predominant
   acute febrile neutrophilic dermatosis (Sweet's)
3. "Histiocytoid" Cells Predominant
   lepromatous leprosy
4. Plasma Cells Prominent
   plasmacytoma, myeloma
5. Mast Cells Predominant
   urticaria pigmentosa
6. Eosinophils Predominant
   eosinophilic cellulitis (Well's syndrome)
7. Mixed Cell Types
   syphilis (primary, secondary, or tertiary)
8. Melanocytic Cells
   nevus of Ota, nevus of Ito
9. Extensive Necrosis
   calciphylaxis

D. Diffuse or Nodular Infiltrates of the Reticular Dermis With Epidermal Proliferation

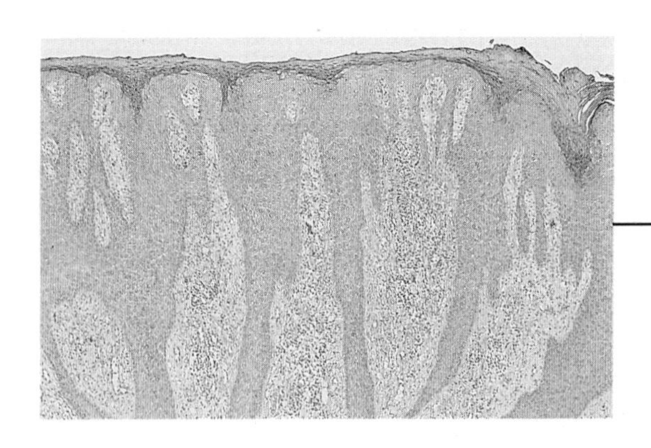

1. With Mixed Cellular Infiltrates
   verruciform xanthoma

E. Nodular Inflammatory Infiltrates of the Reticular Dermis—Granulomas, Abscesses, and Ulcers

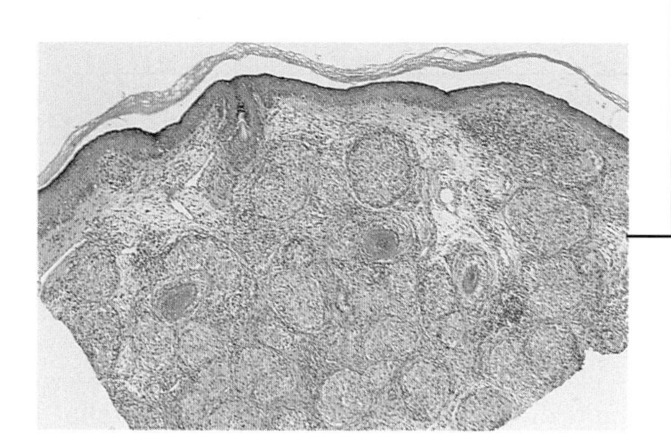

1. Epithelioid Cell Granulomas Without Necrosis
   sarcoidosis (lupus pernio and other types)
2. Epithelioid Cell Granulomas With Necrosis
   tuberculosis (lupus vulgaris and other types)
3. Palisading Granulomas
   granuloma annulare
4. Mixed Cell Granulomas
   keratin granuloma (ruptured cyst)
5. Inflammatory Nodules With Prominent Eosinophils
   angiolymphoid hyperplasia with eosinophils
6. Inflammatory Nodules With Mixed Cell Types
   sporotrichosis
7. Abscesses
   acute or chronic bacterial abscesses
8. Inflammatory Nodules With Prominent Necrosis
   aspergillosis
9. Chronic Ulcers and Sinuses
   pyoderma gangrenosum

F. Dermal Matrix Fiber Disorders

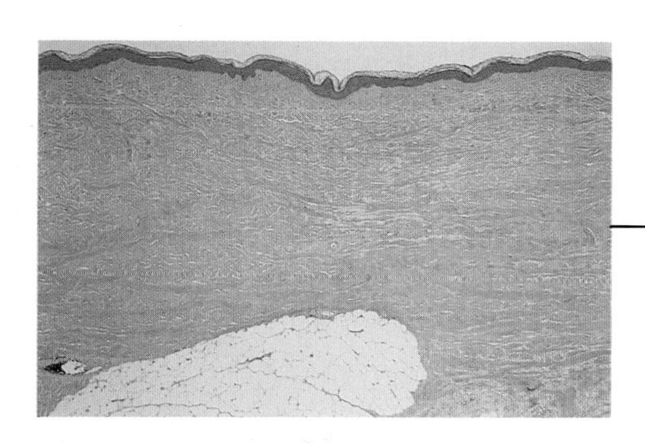

1. Collagen Increased
   scleroderma/morphea
2. Collagen Reduced
   atrophoderma
3. Elastin Altered
   pseudoxanthoma elasticum
4. Elastin Reduced
   cutis laxa
5. Perforating
   elastosis perforans serpiginosa

G. Deposition of Material in the Dermis

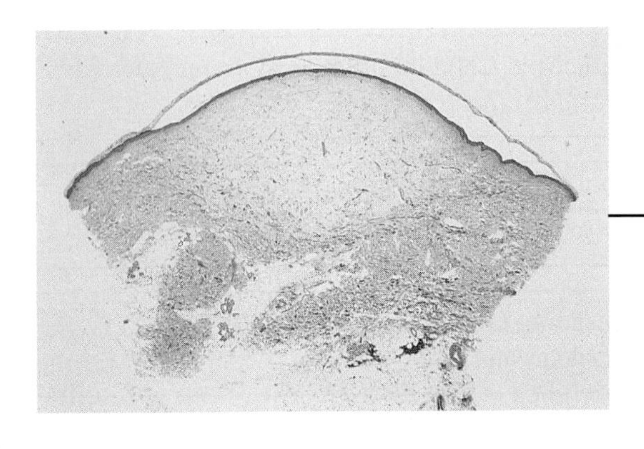

1. Increased Normal Matrix Constituents
   focal dermal mucinosis

2. Material Not Normally Present in the Dermis
   gout

3. Parasitic Infestations of the Dermis and/or Subcutis
   larva migrans (*Ancylostoma*)

VI. TUMORS AND CYSTS OF THE DERMIS AND SUBCUTIS

A. Small Cell Tumors

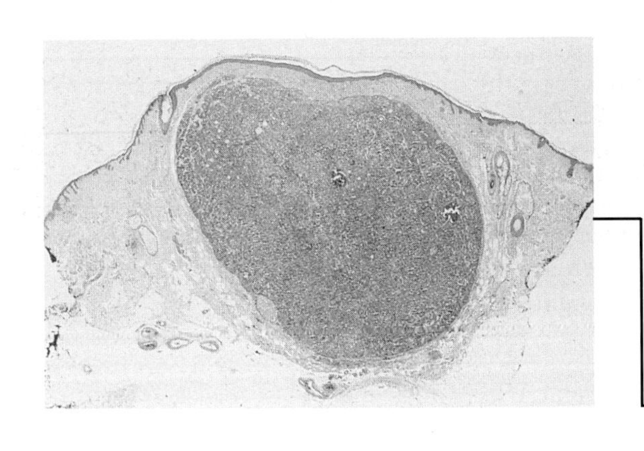

1. Tumors of Lymphocytes or Hemopoietic Cells
   tumor-stage mycosis fungoides

2. Tumors of Lymphocytes and Mixed Cell Types
   cutaneous lymphoid hyperplasia/lymphocytoma cutis

3. Tumors of Plasma Cells
   cutaneous plasmacytoma and myeloma

4. Small Round Cell Tumors
   eccrine spiradenoma

B. Large Polygonal and Round Cell Tumors

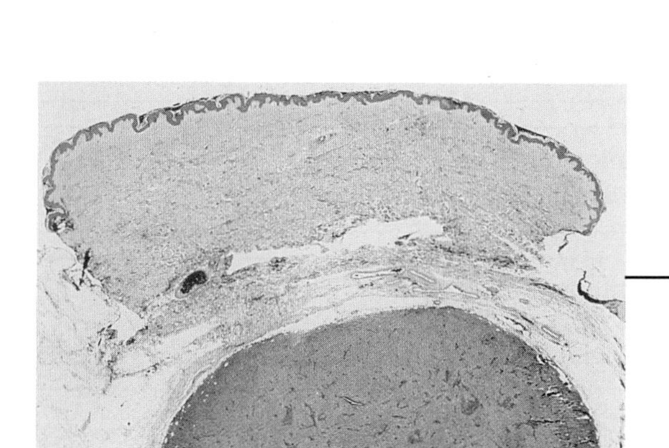

1. Squamous Cell Carcinomas
   primary squamous cell carcinoma

2. Adenocarcinomas
   metastatic adenocarcinoma

3. Melanocytic Tumors
   metastatic melanoma

4. Eccrine Tumors
   nodular hidradenoma

5. Apocrine Tumors
   hidradenoma papilliferum

6. Pilar Tumors
   trichoepithelioma

7. Sebaceous Tumors
   sebaceous adenoma and epithelioma

8. "Histiocytoid" Tumors
   xanthomas (eruptive, plane, tuberous, tendon)

9. Tumors of Large Lymphoid Cells
   cutaneous anaplastic large cell lymphoma (Ki-1)

10. Mast Cell Tumors
    mastocytosis

11. Tumors With Prominent Necrosis
    epithelioid sarcoma

12. Miscellaneous and Undifferentiated Epithelial Tumors
    undifferentiated carcinoma (large cell, small cell)

C. Spindle Cell, Pleomorphic, and Connective Tissue Tumors

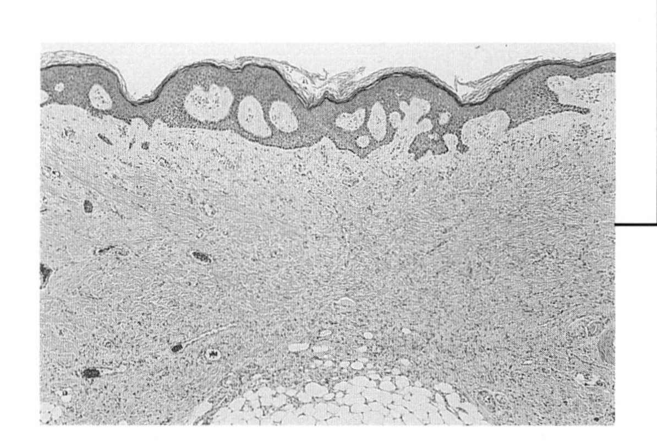

1. Fibrohistiocytic Spindle Cell Tumors
   benign fibrous histiocytoma (dermatofibroma)
2. Schwannian/Neural Spindle Cell Tumors
   neurofibromas
3. Spindle Cell Tumors of Muscle
   leiomyoma
4. Melanocytic Spindle Cell Tumors
   desmoplastic melanoma, including amelanotic
5. Tumors and Proliferations of Angiogenic Cells
   pyogenic granuloma
6. Tumors of Adipose Tissue
   nevus lipomatosus superficialis
7. Tumors of Cartilaginous Tissue
   soft tissue chondroma
8. Tumors of Osseous Tissue
   osteoma cutis

D. Cysts of the Dermis and Subcutis

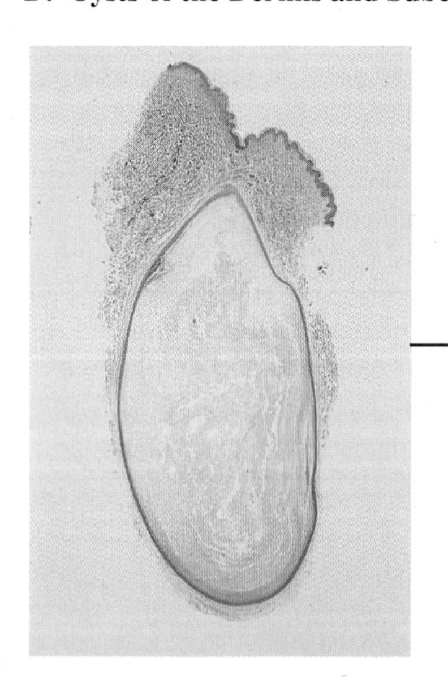

1. Pilar Differentiation
   epidermal cyst
2. Eccrine and Similar Differentiation
   eccrine hidrocystoma
3. Apocrine Differentiation
   apocrine hidrocystoma

VII. INFLAMMATORY AND OTHER DISORDERS OF SKIN APPENDAGES

A. Pathology Involving Hair Follicles

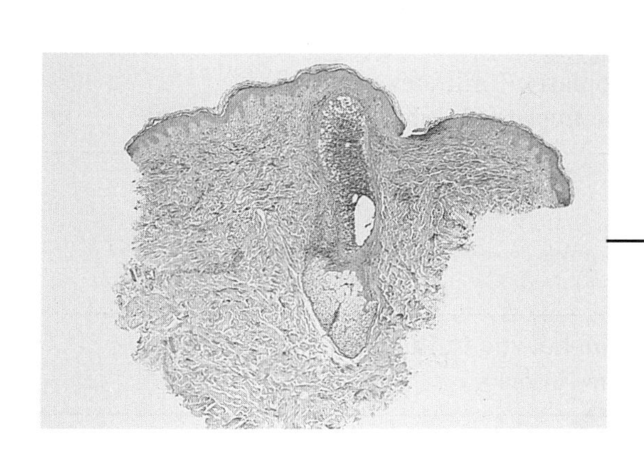

1. Scant Inflammation
   androgenic alopecia
2. Lymphocytes Predominant
   alopecia areata
   a. With Eosinophils Present
      eosinophilic pustular folliculitis
3. Neutrophils Prominent
   acute bacterial folliculitis
4. Plasma Cells Prominent
   acne keloidalis nuchae
5. Fibrosing and Suppurative Follicular Disorders
   hidradenitis suppurativa

B. Pathology Involving Sweat Glands

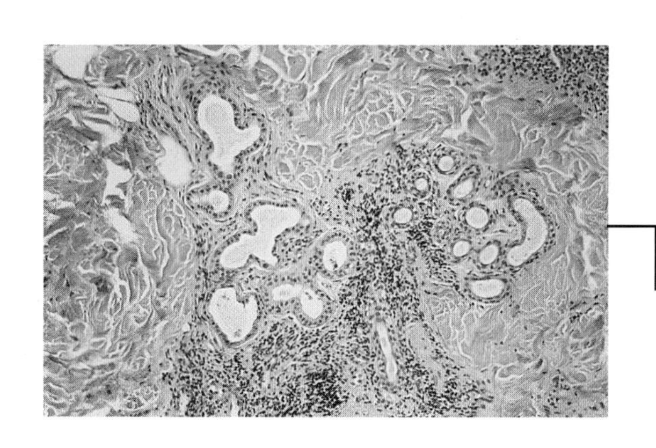

1. Scant Inflammation
   eccrine nevus
2. Lymphocytes Predominant
   lupus erythematosus
   a. With Plasma Cells
      cheilitis glandularis
   b. With Eosinophils
      insect bite reactions
   c. With Neutrophils
      neutrophilic eccrine hidradenitis

C. Pathology Involving Nerves

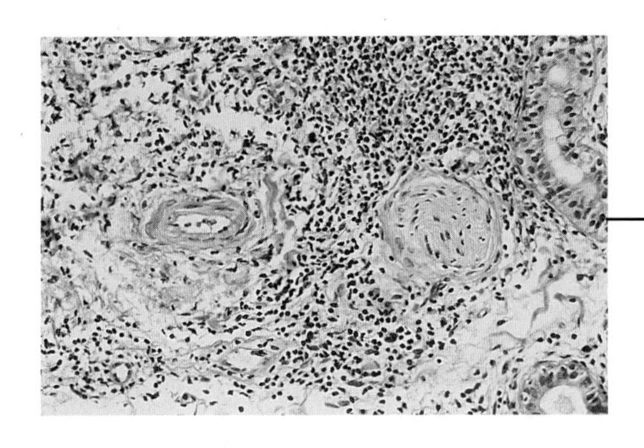

1. Lymphocytic Infiltrates
   herpes zoster
2. Mixed Inflammatory Infiltrates
   leprosy
3. Neoplastic Infiltrates
   neurotropic melanoma

D. Pathology of the Nails

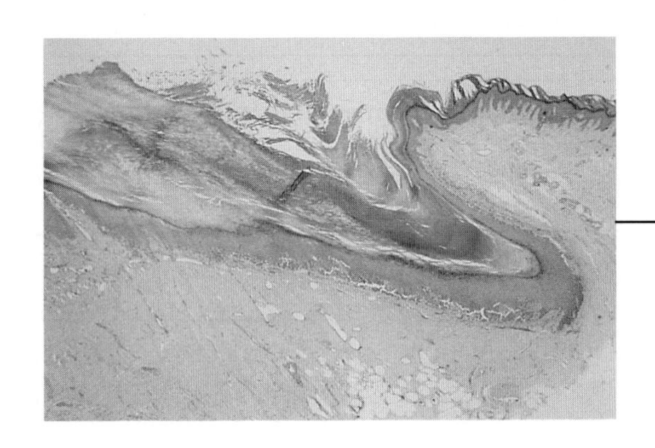

1. Lymphocytic Infiltrates
   lichen planus
2. Lymphocytes With Neutrophils
   tinea unguium, onychomycosis
3. Bullous Diseases
   Darier's disease
4. Parasitic Infestations
   scabies
5. Melanocytic Proliferation
   malignant melanoma, acral-lentigmone type

VIII. DISORDERS OF THE SUBCUTIS

A. Subcutaneous Vasculitis and Vasculopathy (Septal or Lobular)

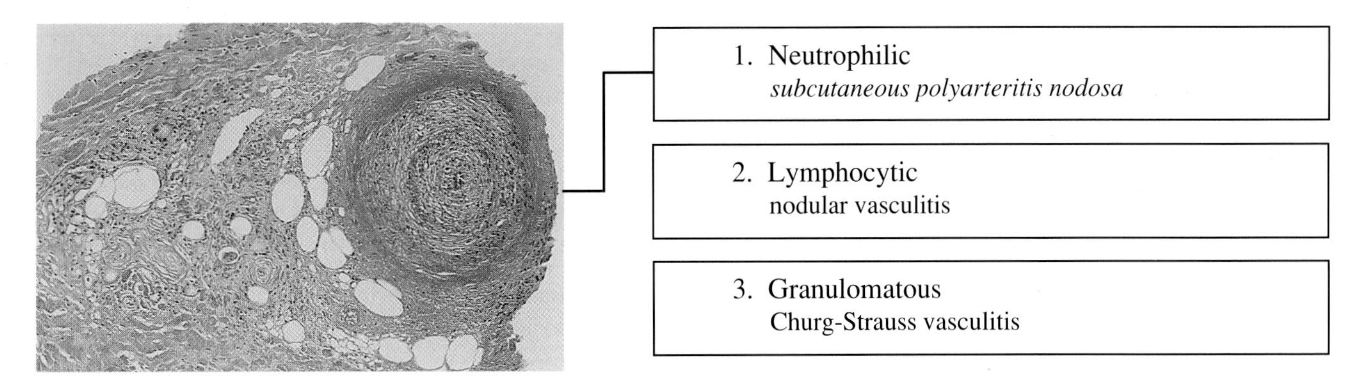

B. Septal Panniculitis Without Vasculitis

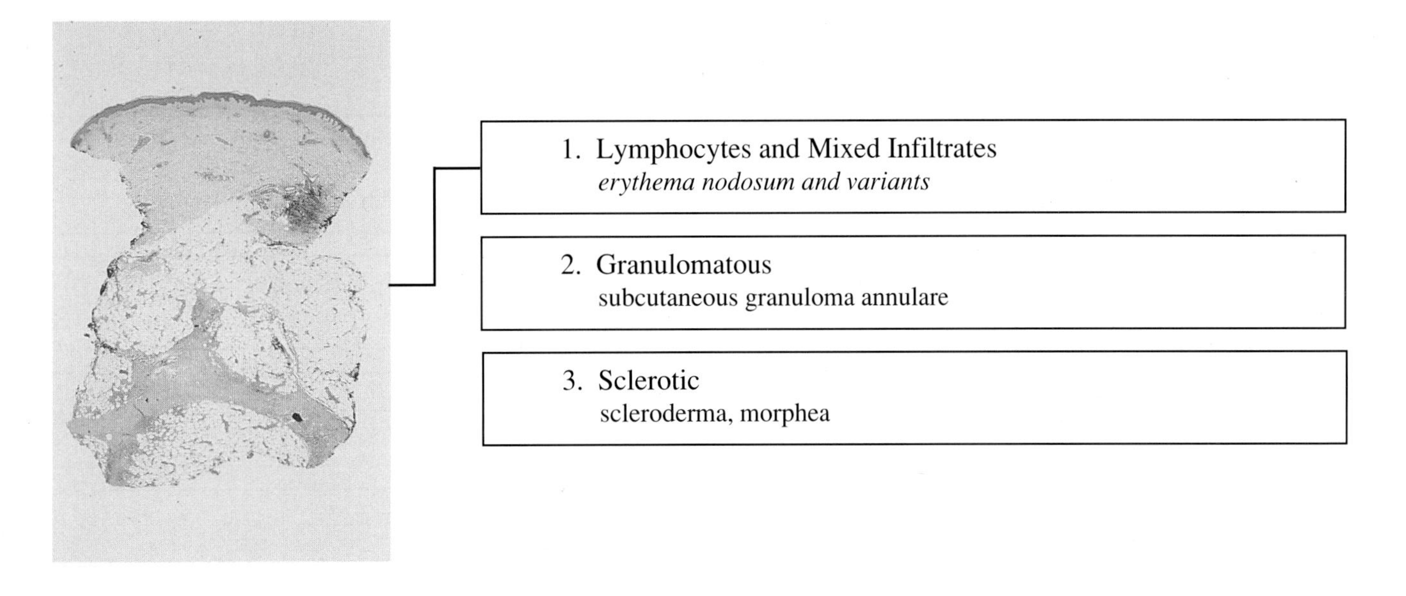

C. Lobular Panniculitis Without Vasculitis

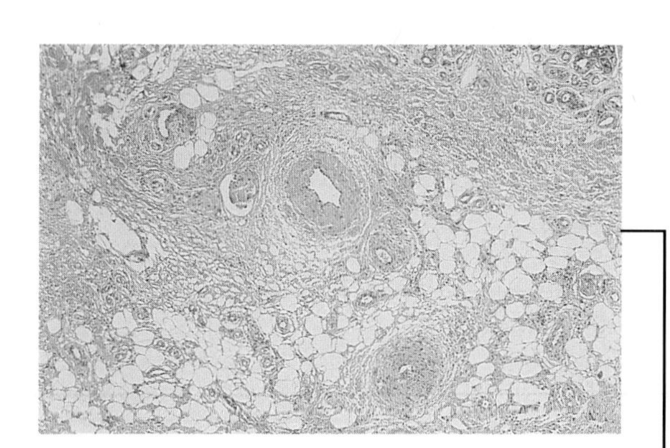

1. Lymphocytes Predominant
   lupus panniculitis
2. Lymphocytes and Plasma Cells
   scleroderma
3. Neutrophilic
   infection (cellulitis)
4. Eosinophils Prominent
   eosinophilic fasciitis
5. Histiocytes Prominent
   cytophagic histiocytic panniculitis
6. Mixed With Foam Cells
   Weber-Christian disease
7. Granulomatous
   subcutaneous sarcoidosis
8. Crystal Deposits, Calcifications
   sclerema neonatorum
9. Necrosis Prominent
   pancreatic panniculitis
10. Embryonic Fat Pattern
    lipoatrophy
11. Miscellaneous
    lipomembranous panniculitis

D. Mixed Lobular and Septal Panniculitis

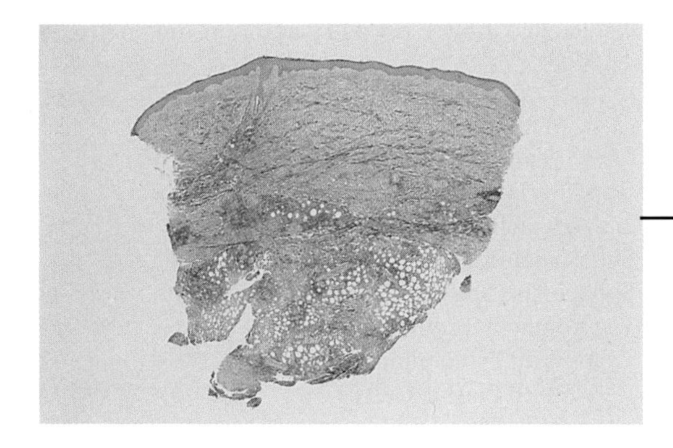

1. With Hemorrhage or Sclerosis
   traumatic panniculitis
2. Prominent Neutrophils
   necrotizing fasciitis (bacterial infection)
3. Prominent Lymphocytes
   nonspecific panniculitis
4. With Cytophagic Histiocytes
   histiocytic cytophagic panniculitis (late lesion)
5. With Granulomas
   mycobacterial panniculitis

E. Subcutaneous Abscesses

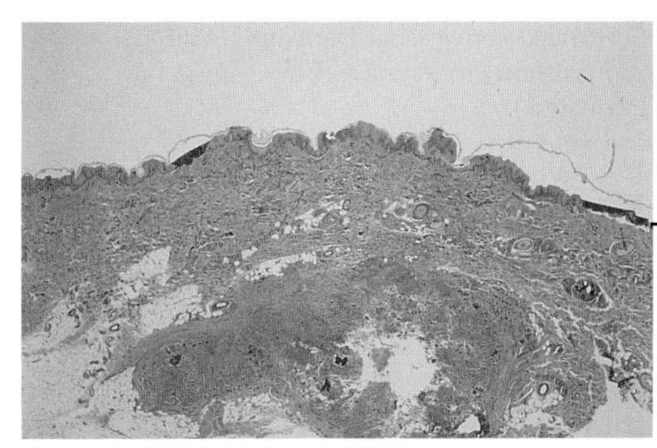

(Courtesy of Waine Johnson, MD.)

1. With Neutrophils
   deep fungus infection

Part 3: Site, Pattern, and Cytologic Categories of Cutaneous Pathology

In the following listings, the categories of cutaneous disease based on location in the skin (categories I, II, III, etc.), architectural pattern (categories A, B, C, etc.), and cytology (categories 1, 2, 3, etc.) are presented with page references for convenient access to the detailed disease listings that follow in Part 4.

Part 4: Disease Listings Categorized by Site, Pattern, and Cytology

In this section, the cutaneous diseases are listed in categories based on their location in the skin, their architectural patterns, and their cytology. The listings may be used as a basis for differential diagnosis generation and for review of material covered elsewhere in this text. The prototype disease in each category is in italics.

I. DISORDERS MOSTLY LIMITED TO THE EPIDERMIS AND STRATUM CORNEUM*

The stratum corneum is usually arranged in a delicate meshlike or "basket-weave" pattern. It may be shed (exfoliated) or thickened (hyperkeratosis) with or without retention of nuclei (parakeratosis or orthokeratosis, respectively). The granular layer may be normal, increased (hypergranulosis), or reduced (hypogranulosis). Usually, alterations in the stratum corneum result from inflammatory or neoplastic changes that affect the whole epidermis and, more often than not, the superficial dermis. Only a few conditions, mentioned in this section, show pathology mostly or entirely limited to the stratum corneum.

A. Hyperkeratosis With Hypogranulosis

1. No inflammation

ichthyosis vulgaris 117

B. Hyperkeratosis With Normal or Hypergranulosis

The stratum corneum is thickened, the granular cell layer is normal or thickened, and the dermis shows only sparse perivascular lymphocytes. There is no epidermal spongiosis or exocytosis.

1. No Inflammation

The upper dermis contains only sparse perivascular lymphocytes.

lamellar ichthyosis 119
X-linked ichthyosis 117
epidermolytic hyperkeratosis 118, 687
epidermolytic acanthoma 687
oculocutaneous tyrosinosis (tyrosinemia) . . 396
acanthosis nigricans 393
large cell acanthoma 693
hyperkeratosis lenticularis perstans (Flegel's disease) 349

2. Scant Inflammation

Lymphocytes are minimally increased about the superficial plexus. There may be a few neutrophils in the stratum corneum.

dermatophytosis 517
lichen amyloidosis 371

C. Hyperkeratosis With Parakeratosis

The stratum corneum is thickened, the granular cell layer is reduced, and there is parakeratosis. The dermis may show only sparse perivascular lymphocytes, although some of these conditions in other instances may show more substantial inflammation. There is no epidermal spongiosis or exocytosis.

1. No Inflammation

The upper dermis contains only sparse perivascular lymphocytes.

epidermolytic hyperkeratosis 687
epidermal nevi 686
porokeratotic eccrine duct nevus 687
cutaneous horn 706
oral leukoplakia 706
leukoplakia of the vulva 711

2. Scant Inflammation

Lymphocytes are minimally increased about the superficial plexus. There may be a few lymphocytes and/or neutrophils in the stratum corneum.

scurvy 353
vitamin A deficiency 353, 396
pellagra (niacin deficiency) 354, 396
Hartnup disease 396
acrokeratosis neoplastica (Bazex syndrome) 365
dermatophytosis 517
epidermal dysmaturation (cytotoxic chemotherapy—variable keratin alterations) 289

* In the lists that follow, the term *predominant* is used to describe an infiltrate in which the majority of the cells are of a certain type, usually lymphocytes or neutrophils. Many dermatoses are composed of infiltrates that are predominantly lymphocytic, with only an occasional other cell; these are listed as, for example, "1. Lymphocytes Predominant." Many other dermatoses contain a diagnostically significant admixture of other cell type(s) as a minority population; these are listed in subsequent sections as "1a. With Eosinophils," "1b. With Plasma Cells," etc., it being understood that lymphocytes predominate in these dermatoses also. Infiltrates in which there is an approximately equal admixture of multiple cell types are listed as "mixed" infiltrates.

D. Localized or Diffuse Hyperpigmentations

Increased melanin pigment is present in basal keratinocytes, without melanocytic proliferation.

1. No Inflammation

The upper dermis contains only sparse perivascular lymphocytes.

simple ephelis 630
melanotic macules 630
café au lait macule 978
actinic lentigo 631
pigmented actinic keratosis 704
melasma 618
Becker's melanosis 631
congenital diffuse melanosis 617
reticulated hyperpigmentations 617
Addison's disease 618
alkaptonuric ochronosis 384
hemochromatosis 395

2. Scant Inflammation

Lymphocytes are minimally increased about the superficial plexus. There may be a few lymphocytes and/or neutrophils in the stratum corneum. Melanophages may be present in the papillary dermis.

tinea versicolor 521
lichen amyloidosis 371
postinflammatory hyperpigmentation 618
erythema dyschromicum perstans 154

E. Localized or Diffuse Hypopigmentations

Melanin pigment is reduced in basal keratinocytes, with (vitiligo) or without (early stages of chemical depigmentation) a reduction in the number of melanocytes.

1. With or Without Slight Inflammation

Lymphocytes may be minimally increased about the dermal-epidermal junction, as in the active phase of vitiligo, or may be absent, as in albinism.

vitiligo 620
chemical depigmentation 619
idiopathic guttate hypomelanosis 619
albinism 619
tinea versicolor 521
piebaldism 620
Chédiak-Higashi syndrome 622
hypopigmented mycosis fungoides 821
postinflammatory hypopigmentation 618

II. LOCALIZED SUPERFICIAL EPIDERMAL OR MELANOCYTIC PROLIFERATIONS/ NEOPLASMS

Localized proliferations may be reactive but are often neoplastic. The epidermis (keratinocytes) may proliferate without extension into the dermis, may extend into the dermis, and may be squamous or basaloid. Melanocytes within the epidermis may proliferate with or without cytologic atypia (nevi, dysplastic nevi, melanoma in situ) in a proliferative epidermis (superficial spreading melanoma in situ, Spitz nevi) or an atrophic epidermis (lentigo maligna); they can also extend into the dermis as proliferative infiltrates (invasive melanoma with or without vertical growth phase). There may be an associated variably cellular, often mixed, inflammatory infiltrate, or inflammation may be essentially absent.

A. Localized Irregular Thickening of the Epidermis

Localized irregular epidermal proliferations are usually neoplastic.

1. Localized Epidermal Proliferations

The epidermis is thickened secondary to a localized proliferation of keratinocytes (acanthosis). The proliferation can be cytologically atypical, as in squamous cell carcinoma in situ, or bland, as in eccrine poroma.

no cytologic atypia
seborrheic keratosis 689
dermatosis papulosa nigra 693
stucco keratosis 693
large cell acanthoma 693
clear cell acanthoma 693
epidermal nevi 685
eccrine poroma 779
hidroacanthoma simplex 780
oral white sponge nevus 688
leukoedema of the oral mucosa 688
verrucous hyperplasia of oral mucosa (oral florid papillomatosis) 707
with cytologic atypia
actinic keratosis 701
arsenical keratosis 711
squamous cell carcinoma in situ 703
Bowen's disease 708
erythroplasia of Queyrat 710
erythroplakia of the oral mucosa 706
Bowenoid papulosis 584
pseudoepitheliomatous hyperplasia
halogenodermas 296
deep fungal infections 526
epidermis above granular cell tumor 993
Spitz nevus 640
verrucous melanoma 670

2. *Superficial Melanocytic Proliferations*

The epidermis may be thickened (acanthosis) and is associated with a proliferation of single or nested melanocytic cells. The proliferation can be malignant as in superficial spreading melanoma or benign as in nevi.

junctional nevi 634
recurrent melanocytic nevi 654
Spitz nevi 640
compound or dermal nevi, papillomatous . . . 633
junctional or superficial compound
dysplastic nevi 648
melanoma in situ 655

B. Localized Lesions With Thinning of the Epidermis

A thinned epidermis is characteristic of aged or chronically sun-damaged skin. The epidermis is thinned secondary to diminished number and to decreased size of keratinocytes.

1. *With Melanocytic Proliferation*

The epidermis is thinned (atrophic) and there is proliferation of single or small groups of atypical melanocytes, resulting in the localization of melanocytes in contiguity with one another in the basal layer of the epidermis.

melanoma in situ (lentigo maligna type) . . . 654

2. *Without Melanocytic Proliferation*

The epidermis is thinned without proliferation of keratinocytes or melanocytes. Each melanocyte is separated from the next by several keratinocytes.

actinic keratosis 701
porokeratosis 122

C. Localized Lesions With Elongated Rete Ridges

Elongation of the rete ridges without melanocytic proliferation is termed *psoriasiform hyperplasia* because this pattern is seen in psoriasis. An elongated rete ridge with melanocytic proliferation and predominance of single cells over nests is termed a *lentiginous* pattern. The prototype of this pattern, also seen in dysplastic nevi and in the "lentiginous" melanomas, is the lentigo simplex.

1. *With Melanocytic Proliferation*

The epidermal rete ridges are elongated and within these retia there is melanocytic proliferation.

lentigo simplex 630
nevus spilus 632
lentiginous junctional nevus 635
junctional nevus 633
dysplastic nevus 648
acral-lentiginous melanoma 663
mucosal-lentiginous melanoma 664

2. *Without Melanocytic Proliferation*

The epidermis is thickened (acanthotic). Melanocytes are normal, as are keratinocytes. The only change is acanthosis.

epidermal nevi 686
psoriasis 156
lichen simplex chronicus 163, 212
acanthosis nigricans 393

D. Localized Lesions With Pagetoid Epithelial Proliferation

A neoplastic proliferation of one cell type distributed as single cells or nests within a benign epithelium is termed *pagetoid* after Paget's disease of the breast (mammary carcinoma cells proliferating in skin of the nipple).

1. *Keratinocytic Proliferation*

The epidermis has atypical keratinocytes scattered within mature epithelium at all or multiple levels; there is loss of normal maturation. Mitoses are increased, and there may be individual cell necrosis.

pagetoid squamous cell carcinoma in situ 728
intraepithelial epithelioma (Borsst-Jadassohn) 728
clonal seborrheic keratosis 728

2. *Melanocytic Proliferation*

Atypical melanocytes are seen at all levels within the otherwise mature but often hyperplastic epidermis.

melanoma in situ (superficial spreading type) 657
recurrent nevus (pseudomelanoma) 654

3. *Glandular Epithelial Proliferation*

Atypical large clear cells with glandular differentiation (mucin production, lumen formation) proliferate in a normally maturing epidermis.

Paget's disease (mammary or extramammary) 734

4. *Lymphoid Proliferation*

Atypical large clear lymphoid cells proliferate in a normally maturing epidermis.

pagetoid reticulosis
  localized (Woringer-Kolopp) 828
  disseminated (Ketron-Goodman) 828

E. Localized Papillomatous Epithelial Lesions

A "papilla" may be likened to a "finger" of stroma with a few blood vessels, collagen fibers, and fibroblasts, covered by a "glove" of epithelium that may be reactive or neoplastic, benign or malignant.

1. With Viral Cytopathic Effects

The epidermis is acanthotic with vacuolated cells (koilocytes), the granular cell layer is usually thickened with enlarged keratohyaline granules, and there is parakeratosis in tall columns overlying the thickened epidermis. Large inclusions are seen in molluscum contagiosum.

verruca vulgaris 579
orf 576
condyloma accuminatum 583
molluscum contagiosum 577
Bowenoid papulosis 584

2. No Viral Cytopathic Effect

The epidermis proliferates. The cells may be basophilic or "basaloid" in type (seborrheic keratoses). There may be increased stratum corneum and elongation of the dermal papillae (squamous papilloma), or there may be basilar keratinocyte atypia (actinic keratosis).

seborrheic keratosis 689
acanthosis nigricans 393
confluent and reticulated papillomatosis ... 395
actinic keratosis, hypertrophic 703
nonspecific squamous papilloma 578
epithelial nevus/epidermal nevus 686
hyperkeratosis of the nipple and areola 687
verruciform xanthoma 606
verrucous melanoma 670

F. Irregular Proliferations Extending Into the Dermis

Irregular or asymmetrical proliferations of keratinocytes extending into the dermis are usually neoplastic. The differential diagnosis includes reactive pseudoepitheliomatous hyperplasia, which may be seen around chronic ulcers or in association with other inflammatory conditions.

1. Squamous Differentiation

The epidermis is irregularly thickened, the maturation is abnormal, and there may be keratinocyte atypia (squamous cell carcinoma). The proliferation is often associated with a thick parakeratotic scale.

lichen simplex chronicus 163, 212
squamous cell carcinoma, superficial 712
prurigo nodularis 155
actinic prurigo 306
inverted follicular keratosis 691
verrucous carcinoma 584, 716
  of oral mucosa 717
  of genitoanal region (giant condyloma of
    Buschke and Lowenstein) 584, 717
  of plantar skin (epithelioma cuniculatum) 717
pseudoepitheliomatous hyperplasia 717
  deep fungal infection 526
  halogenoderma 296
  chronic ulcers 457, 526, 555
  granular cell tumor 993
  Spitz nevus 640
  verrucous melanoma 670

2. Basaloid Differentiation

The proliferation is of basal cells from the epidermis, extending into the dermis. The epidermis can be thickened, normal, or atrophic.

basal cell carcinoma, superficial types 719, 726

G. Superficial Polypoid Lesions

A polyp consists of a "finger" of stroma covered by a "glove" of epithelium. It is to be distinguished from a papilloma, which shows elongated papillae.

1. Melanocytic Lesions

polypoid dermal and compound nevi 633

2. Stromal Lesions

neurofibroma 978
soft fibroma (fibroepithelial polyp,
  acrochordon, skin tag) 872

III. DISORDERS OF THE SUPERFICIAL CUTANEOUS REACTIVE UNIT

The epidermis, papillary dermis, and superficial capillary-venular plexus react together in many dermatologic conditions, and have been termed the *superficial cutaneous reactive unit* by Clark. Many dermatoses are associated with infiltrates of lymphocytes, with or without other cell types, around the superficial vessels. The epidermis in pathologic conditions can be thinned (atrophic), thickened (acanthosis), edematous (spongiosis), and/or infiltrated (exocytosis). The epidermis may proliferate in response to chronic irritation, infection (bacterial, yeast, deep fungal, or viral). The epidermis may proliferate in response to dermatologic conditions (psoriasis, atopic dermatitis, prurigo). The papillary dermis and superficial vascular plexus may have a variety of inflammatory cells, can be edematous, may have increased ground substance (hyaluronic acid), or may be sclerotic or homogenized.

A. Superficial Perivascular Dermatitis

Many dermatoses are associated with infiltrates of lymphocytes, with or without other cell types, around the vessels of the superficial capillary-venular plexus. The vessel walls may be quite unremarkable, or there may be slight to moderate endothelial swelling. Eosinophilic change ("fibrinoid necrosis"), a hallmark of true vasculitis, is not seen. The term *lymphocytic vasculitis* may encompass some of the conditions mentioned here but is of doubtful validity in the absence of vessel wall damage. The epidermis is variable in its thickness, in the amount and type of exocytotic cell, and in the integrity of the basal cell zone (liquefaction degeneration). In some of the entities listed here, the perivascular infiltrate may in some examples also involve vessels of the mid and deep vessels. These conditions are also listed in Section V: Perivascular, Diffuse, and Granulomatous Infiltrates of the Reticular Dermis.

1. Superficial Perivascular Dermatitis, Lymphocytes Predominant

Lymphocytes are seen about the superficial vascular plexus. Other cell types are rare or absent.

morbilliform viral exanthem 569
papular acrodermatitis
(Gianotti-Crosti) 165, 364
stasis dermatitis 215, 914
pityriasis lichenoides et varioliformis acuta
(PLEVA), early 176
Jessner's lymphocytic infiltrate 268
tinea versicolor 521
candidiasis 522
superficial gyrate erythemas 153
lupus erythematosus, acute 261
mixed connective tissue disease 270
dermatomyositis 271
early herpes simplex, zoster 569
morbilliform drug eruption 287
cytomegalovirus inclusion disease 574
polymorphous drug eruption 287
progressive pigmented purpura 202
parapsoriasis, small plaque type (digitate
dermatosis) 164
Langerhans' cell histiocytosis
(early lesions) 597
mucocutaneous lymph node syndrome
(Kawasaki disease) 166
secondary syphilis 503

a. Superficial Perivascular Dermatitis With Eosinophils

In addition to lymphocytes, eosinophils are present in varying numbers, with both a perivascular and interstitial distribution.

arthropod bite reaction 565
allergic urticarial reaction (drug) 287
bullous pemphigoid, urticarial phase 226
erythema toxicum neonatorum 237
Well's syndrome 408
mastocytosis/ telangiectasia eruptiva
macularis perstans 141
angiolymphoid hyperplasia with
eosinophilia 891
Kimura's disease 895
Langerhans' cell histiocytosis
(early lesions) 597

b. Superficial Perivascular Dermatitis With Neutrophils

In addition to lymphocytes, neutrophils are present in varying numbers, with both a perivascular and interstitial distribution.

cellulitis 460
erysipelas 459
urticaria 151
if vasculitis, refer to III.G.

c. Superficial Perivascular Dermatitis With Plasma Cells

Plasma cells are seen about the dermal vessels as well as in the interstitium. They are most often admixed with lymphocytes.

secondary syphilis 503
arthropod bite reaction 808
Kaposi's sarcoma, nonspecific patch stage . 909
actinic keratoses and Bowen's
disease 701, 708
Zoon's plasma cell balanitis
circumscripta 710
erythroplasia of Queyrat 710

d. Superficial Perivascular Dermatitis With Extravasated Red Cells

A perivascular lymphocytic infiltrate is associated with extravasation of lymphocytes, without fibrinoid necrosis of vessels.

pityriasis rosea 164
lupus erythematosus, subacute 259
lupus erythematosus, acute 261
stasis dermatitis 215, 914
Kaposi's sarcoma, patch stage 909
pityriasis lichenoides et varioliformis acuta
(PLEVA) 176
pityriasis lichenoides chronica 176
pigmented purpuric dermatoses
(Schamberg) 202

e. Superficial Perivascular Dermatitis, Melanophages Prominent

There is a perivascular infiltrate of lymphocytes with an admixture of pigment-laden melanophages, indicative of prior damage to the basal layer, and "pigmentary incontinence." Some degree of residual interface damage may also be evident.

postinflammatory hyperpigmentation 618
postchemotherapy hyperpigmentation 290
chlorpromazine pigmentation 293
amyloidosis 369
regressed melanocytic lesion 672
resolved lichenoid reaction including
fixed drug reaction 288

2. *Superficial Perivascular Dermatitis, Mast Cells Predominant*

Mast cells are the main infiltrating cells seen in the dermis. Lymphocytes are also present, and there may be a few eosinophils.

urticaria pigmentosa, nodular type 141
telangiectasia macularis eruptiva perstans,
adult mast cell disease (TMEP) 141

B. Superficial Dermatitis With Spongiosis (Spongiotic Dermatitis)

Spongiotic dermatitis is characterized by intercellular edema in the epidermis. In mild or early lesions, the intercellular space is increased with stretching of desmosomes but the integrity of the epithelium is intact. In more severe spongiotic conditions, there is separation of keratinocytes to form spaces (vesicles). For this reason, the spongiotic dermatoses are also discussed later in Section IV: Acantholytic, Vesicular, and Pustular Disorders.

1. *Spongiotic Dermatitis, Lymphocytes Predominant*

There is marked intercellular edema (spongiosis) in the epidermis. In the dermis, perivascular lymphocytes are predominant.

eczematous dermatitis 210
atopic dermatitis 214
allergic contact dermatitis 212
photoallergic drug eruption 214, 292
irritant contact dermatitis 213
nummular eczema 214
dyshidrotic dermatitis 213
parapsoriasis, small plaque type
(digitate dermatosis) 164
polymorphous light eruption 305
lichen striatus 174
chronic actinic dermatitis
(actinic reticuloid) 308
actinic prurigo, early lesions 306
"id" reaction 214
seborrheic dermatitis 215
stasis dermatitis 215, 914
erythroderma 216
miliaria 216
pityriasis rosea 164
Sézary syndrome 827
papular acrodermatitis
(Gianotti-Crosti) 165, 364

a. *Spongiotic Dermatitis With Eosinophils*

There is marked intercellular edema (spongiosis) within the epidermis. In the dermis, lymphocytes are predominant. Eosinophils can be found in most examples of atopy and allergic contact dermatitis, and are numerous in incontinentia pigmenti.

spongiotic (eczematous) dermatitis 210
atopic dermatitis 214
allergic contact dermatitis 212
photoallergic drug eruption 214, 292
insect bite reaction 565
incontinentia pigmenti, vesicular stage 144
eczematous nevus (Meyerson's nevus) 653
erythema gyratum repens 154
scabies 559
erythema toxicum neonatorum 237

b. *Spongiotic Dermatitis With Plasma Cells*

There is marked intercellular edema (spongiosis) within the epidermis. In the dermis, perivascular lymphocytes are predominant, and plasma cells are present.

syphilis, primary or secondary lesions 503
pinta, primary or secondary lesions 510
seborrheic dermatitis in HIV 215

c. *Spongiotic Dermatitis With Neutrophils*

There is marked intercellular edema (spongiosis) within the epidermis. Lymphocytes are present in the dermis. There is focal and shoulder parakeratosis, with a few neutrophils in the stratum corneum.

dermatophytosis 517
seborrheic dermatitis 215
toxic shock syndrome 464

C. Superficial Perivascular Dermatitis With Epidermal Atrophy (Atrophic Dermatitis)

Most inflammatory dermatoses are associated with epithelial hyperplasia. Only a few chronic conditions exhibit epidermal atrophy.

1. *Epidermal Atrophy, Scant Inflammatory Cells*

The epidermis is thinned, only a few cell layers thick. There is a scanty lymphocytic infiltrate about the superficial capillary-venular plexus.

aged skin 341
chronic actinic damage 341
radiation dermatitis 313
porokeratosis 122

acrodermatitis chronica atrophicans 512
malignant atrophic papulosis 188
poikiloderma atrophicans vasculare 273

2. *Epidermal Atrophy, Lymphocytes Predominant*

The epidermis is thinned, but not as marked as in aged or irradiated skin. In the dermis there are many lymphocytes about the superficial capillary-venular plexus.

parapsoriasis/early mycosis
  fungoides 164, 820
lupus erythematous 253
mixed connective tissue disease 270
pinta, tertiary lesions 510
dermatomyositis 271

a. *Epidermal Atrophy With Papillary Dermal Sclerosis/ Matrix Changes*

The epidermis is thinned, and there can be hyperkeratosis. The dermis is homogenized and edematous; inflammation is minimal.

lichen sclerosus et atrophicus 280
thermal burns 245, 311
parapsoriasis/early mycosis fungoides 164, 820
poikiloderma vasculare atrophicans 273
radiation dermatitis 313

D. Superficial Perivascular Dermatitis With Psoriasiform Proliferation (Psoriasiform Dermatitis)

Psoriasiform proliferation is a form of epithelial hyperplasia characterized by uniform elongation of rete ridges. Although the surface may be slightly raised to form a plaque, the epidermal proliferation tends to extend downwards into the dermis, in contrast to a papillomatous pattern, in which the rete ridges are elongated upwards above the plane of the epidermal surface and a papilloma (such as a wart) is formed. The prototype is psoriasis, in which the suprapapillary plates are thinned. In most other psoriasiform conditions, the suprapapillary plates are thickened, but not as much as the elongated rete. Because of the increased epithelial turnover, there is often associated hypogranulosis and parakeratosis.

1. *Psoriasiform Epidermal Proliferation, Lymphocytes Predominant*

The epidermis is evenly and regularly thickened in a psoriasiform pattern, and spongiosis is variable (rare to absent in psoriasis, common in seborrheic and inflammatory dermatoses). There is an infiltrate of lymphocytes about dermal vessels.

chronic spongiotic dermatitis 211
  atopic dermatitis 214
  seborrheic dermatitis 215
  nummular eczema 214
lichen simplex chronicus 163, 212
prurigo nodularis 155
psoriasis 156
pityriasis rosea 164
exfoliative dermatitis 216
pityriasis rubra pilaris 176
parapsoriasis/early mycosis fungoides .. 164, 820
verrucous hyperkeratotic mycosis
  fungoides 821
inflammatory linear verrucous epidermal
  nevus (ILVEN) 175
pellagra 354, 396
necrolytic migratory erythema
  (chronic lesions) 354
acrodermatitis enteropathica 356
kwashiorkor 356
reticulated hyperpigmentations
  (e.g., Dowling-Degos' disease) 617

a. *Psoriasiform Epidermal Proliferation With Plasma Cells*

The epidermis is evenly thickened and may be spongiotic. There may be exocytosis of lymphocytes. The stratum corneum is variable, often parakeratotic. Plasma cells are found about the superficial vessels in varying numbers, admixed with lymphocytes.

arthropod bite reactions 565
secondary syphilis 503
cutaneous T-cell lymphoma
  (mycosis fungoides) 820
prurigo nodularis 155

b. *Psoriasiform Epidermal Proliferation With Eosinophils*

The epidermis is evenly thickened and may be spongiotic, and there may be exocytosis of inflammatory cells, including eosinophils. Eosinophils are easily identified in the dermis and may be numerous in some conditions (e.g., incontinentia pigmenti).

chronic spongiotic dermatitis
  chronic allergic dermatitis 211
  chronic atopic dermatitis 214
exfoliative dermatitis 216
cutaneous T-cell lymphoma 820
incontinentia pigmenti, verrucous stage 144

2. *Psoriasiform Epidermal Proliferation, Neutrophils Prominent (Neutrophilic/Pustular Psoriasiform Dermatitis)*

The epidermis is evenly thickened, and there is exocytosis (migration of inflammatory cells through the epidermis) of neutrophils. These may collect into abscesses in the epidermis at the level of the stratum corneum (Munro microabscess). The stratum corneum is thickened and parakeratotic and contains neutrophils.

psoriasis vulgaris 156
  pustular psoriasis 156
  Reiter's syndrome, keratoderma
  blennorrhagicum 163
pustular drug eruption 287, 296
geographic tongue (lingua geographica) 163, 688
candidiasis 522
pustular secondary syphilis (rare) 507
dermatophytosis 517

E. Superficial Perivascular Dermatitis With Irregular Epidermal Proliferation (Hypertrophic Dermatitis)

Irregular thickening and thinning of the epidermis is seen in some reactive conditions, but the possibility of squamous cell carcinoma should also be considered. As in other conditions associated with increased epithelial turnover, there may be hypogranulosis and parakeratosis.

1. Irregular Epidermal Proliferation, Lymphocytes Predominant

The epidermis is irregularly thickened, with areas of normal thickness, of acanthosis, and of thinning. Lymphocytes are the predominant inflammatory cell about the dermal vessels.

lichen simplex chronicus 163, 212
inflammatory linear verrucous nevus
  (ILVEN, psoriasiform category) 175
prurigo nodularis 155
incontinentia pigmenti, verrucous stage ... 144
pellagra (niacin deficiency) 354, 396
Hartnup disease 354, 396

a. Irregular Epidermal Proliferation, Plasma Cells Present

The epidermis is irregularly acanthotic. Plasma cells are found about the dermal vessels admixed with lymphocytes.

squamous cell carcinoma in situ
  (Bowen's disease) 708
erythroplasia of Queyrat 710
rupial secondary syphilis, condyloma lata .. 506
yaws, primary or secondary 508
pinta, primary or secondary lesions 510
actinic keratosis 701
pseudoepitheliomatous hyperplasia 717
pemphigus vegetans 221

2. Irregular Epidermal Proliferation, Neutrophils Prominent

The epidermis has focal areas of acanthosis; neutrophils can be seen as exocytotic cells and are found in the dermis in abscesses and about dermal vessels even without a primary vasculitis.

deep fungal infections
  (superficial biopsy, see later) 526
halogenodermas 296
botryomycosis 495
keratoacanthoma 731
impetigo contagiosa 457
granuloma inguinale 491

3. Irregular Epidermal Proliferation, Neoplastic

The epidermis is irregularly acanthotic. There is an associated neoplastic infiltrate in the epidermis or dermis, or in both.

squamous cell carcinoma 712
malignant melanoma
  ("verrucous" pattern) 670
granular cell tumor 993

F. Superficial Perivascular Dermatitis With Lichenoid Infiltrates (Lichenoid Dermatitis)

Lichenoid inflammation is a dense "bandlike" infiltrate of small lymphocytes clustered about the dermal-epidermal junction and obscuring the interface. The epidermis is variable in its thickness, in the amount of exocytotic lymphocytes, and in the integrity of the basal cell zone (liquefaction degeneration). Hypergranulosis due to delayed epidermal maturation is a commonly associated feature. For the same reason, there may be orthokeratotic hyperkeratosis. Apoptotic or necrotic keratinocytes are often present. In lichen planus, these are called Civatte bodies. Pigmentary incontinence (melanin-laden macrophages in the papillary dermis) is common, as in any condition in which there is destruction of basal keratinocytes.

1. Lichenoid Dermatitis, Lymphocytes Exclusively

The bandlike infiltrate is composed almost exclusively of lymphocytes. Eosinophils and plasma cells are essentially absent.

lichen planus–like keratosis
  (benign lichenoid keratosis) 172
lichen planus 166
pityriasis lichenoides chronica 177
lupus erythematosus, lichenoid forms . 171, 253
mixed connective tissue disease 270
acrodermatitis chronica atrophicans 512
poikiloderma atrophicans vasculare 273
pigmented purpuric dermatitis, lichenoid
  type (Gougerot-Blum) 202
graft-versus-host disease, lichenoid stage .. 240
erythema multiforme 239
pityriasis lichenoides et varioliformis acuta
  (PLEVA), early lesions 176
parapsoriasis/mycosis fungoides,
  patch/plaque stage 164, 820
Sézary syndrome 827

2. *Lichenoid Dermatitis, Lymphocytes Predominant*

The bandlike lichenoid infiltrate is composed almost exclusively of lymphocytes. A few plasma cells and eosinophils may also be present.

lichen planus–like keratosis (benign lichenoid keratosis) 172
parapsoriasis/mycosis fungoides, patch/plaque stage 164, 820
paraneoplastic pemphigus 225
Sézary syndrome 827
secondary syphilis 506
halo nevus 652
lichen striatus 174
lichenoid tattoo reaction 322

a. Lichenoid Dermatitis, Eosinophils Present

Eosinophils are found in the lichenoid dermal infiltrate, about the dermal vessels, and in some instances around the adnexal structures.

lichenoid drug eruptions 288
lichenoid actinic keratoses 703
lichen planus, hypertrophic 168
arthropod bite reactions 565
cutaneous T-cell lymphoma, mycosis fungoides, patch/plaque stage 164, 820
histiocytosis X (Letterer-Siwe) 597
mastocytosis/telangiectasia eruptiva macularis perstans (TMEP) 141

b. Lichenoid Dermatitis, Plasma Cells Present

Plasma cells are found in the lichenoid infiltrate; their number is variable, but they do not as a rule constitute the major portion of the dermal infiltrate.

lichenoid actinic keratosis 703
Bowen's disease 708
erythroplasia of Queyrat 710
secondary syphilis 506
pinta, primary or secondary lesions 510
arthropod bite reaction 565
CTCL, mycosis fungoides, patch/plaque stage 164, 820
Zoon's plasma cell balanitis 710
keratosis lichenoides chronica 172

c. Lichenoid Dermatitis, With Melanophages

Most of the conditions listed as lichenoid dermatoses may be associated with release of pigment from damaged basal keratinocytes into the papillary dermis, or "pigmentary incontinence." If a specific dermatosis cannot be identified, the appearances may be classified as postinflammatory hyperpigmentation.

postinflammatory hyperpigmentation 618
regressed melanocytic lesion 672

3. *Lichenoid Dermatitis, Histiocytes Predominant*

Histiocytes are the predominant cell type in the dermal infiltrate.

lichen nitidus 173
actinic reticuloid/chronic actinic dermatitis .. 308
histiocytosis-X (Letterer-Siwe, Hand Schüller-Christian) 597
granulomatous slack skin 829

4. *Lichenoid Dermatitis, Mast Cells Predominant*

Mast cells are the predominant cell type in the dermis. They are frequently accompanied by eosinophils.

urticaria pigmentosa, papulonodular 141

G. Superficial Vasculitis and Vasculopathies

Endothelial swelling, eosinophilic degeneration of the vessel wall ("fibrinoid necrosis"), and infiltration of the vessel wall by neutrophils, with nuclear fragmentation or leukocytoclasis resulting in "nuclear dust," define true vasculitis. There are extravasated red cells in the vessel walls and adjacent dermis. If the vasculitis is severe, ulceration or subepidermal separation ("bullous vasculitis") can occur. *Lymphocytic vasculitis* in which there is no vessel wall damage is a controversial term and is discussed under lymphocytic infiltrates. A *vasculopathy* includes any abnormality of the vessel wall that does not meet the criteria above for vasculitis, such as fibrosis or hyalinization of the vessel wall without inflammation or necrosis.

1. *Neutrophilic Vasculitis*

In the dermis, vessels are necrotic, fibrinoid is present, and there are perivascular and intravascular neutrophils with leukocytoclasis and nuclear dust.

cutaneous necrotizing (leukocytoclastic) vasculitis 194
- Henoch-Schönlein purpura 195
- cryoglobulinemia 196
- connective tissue associated (RA, LE) ... 197
- septicemia, especially meningococcemia/gonococcemia 195, 464, 466
- urticarial vasculitis 151, 196
- erythema elevatum diutinum 198
- miscellaneous 194–198

polyarteritis nodosa 191
vasculitis in exanthemic pustulosis (drug-induced) 287

2. *Mixed Cell and Granulomatous Vasculitis*

There is vessel wall damage, and a mixed infiltrate in the dermis that includes eosinophils, plasma cells, histiocytes, and giant cells.

- *Churg-Strauss vasculitis* 199
- Wegener's granulomatosis 201
- giant cell arteritis 190
- granuloma faciale 207
- Buerger's disease 193

3. *Vasculopathies With Scant Inflammation*

There is fibrosis or hyalinization of the vessel walls, with few inflammatory cells.

- atrophie blanche (segmental hyalinizing vasculitis) 187
- *malignant atrophic papulosis (Degos)* 188
- Mondor's disease 192
- pigmented purpuric dermatoses (Majocchi-Schamberg-Gougerot-Bloom) 202

4. *Thrombotic, Embolic, and Other Microangiopathies*

There are thrombi or emboli within the lumens of small vessels. In other microangiopathies, the vessel walls may be thickened with compromise of the lumen (amyloidosis, calciphylaxis).

- *disseminated intravascular coagulation* 186
- thrombotic thrombocytopenic purpura 186
- cryoglobulinemia/macroglobulinemia 196
- antiphospholipid syndrome 186, 266
- lupus anticoagulant and antiocardiolipin syndromes 186, 266
- connective tissue disease (rheumatoid, mixed) 197, 270
- calciphylaxis 380, 447
- amyloidosis 369
- porphyria cutanea tarda and other porphyrias 376
- cholesterol emboli 187

H. Superficial Dermatitis with Interface Vacuoles (Interface Dermatitis)

1. *Vacuolar Dermatitis, Apoptotic/Necrotic Cells Prominent*

Lymphocytes approximate the dermal-epidermal junction. Vacuolar degeneration is present in the basal cell zone. Apoptotic keratinocytes are found in the epidermis in variable numbers, visualized as round eosinophilic anuclear structures. The dermis usually has perivascular lymphocytes and may show pigment incontinence.

- *erythema multiforme* 239
  - toxic epidermal necrolysis (Lyell) 240
  - Stevens-Johnson syndrome 239
- fixed drug eruption 289
- phototoxic drug eruption 293
- radiation dermatitis 313
- sunburn reaction 311
- thermal burn 311
- pityriasis lichenoides et varioliformis acuta (PLEVA) 176
- graft-versus-host disease, acute 240
- eruption of lymphocyte recovery 244
- lupus erythematosis 253

2. *Vacuolar Dermatitis, Apoptotic Cells Usually Absent*

There is basilar keratinocyte vacuolar destruction; apoptotic cells are rare or absent. The dermis has perivascular lymphocytes and may show pigment incontinence.

- *dermatomyositis* 271
- morbilliform viral exanthem 569
- poikiloderma vasculare atrophicans 273
- paraneoplastic pemphigus 225
- erythema dyschromicum perstans 154
- pinta, tertiary stage 510

3. *Vacuolar Dermatitis, Variable Apoptosis*

Vacuolar degeneration is associated with variable numbers of apoptotic cells in the epidermis. The dermis may have increased ground substance and there may be pigmentary incontinence.

- *cytotoxic drug eruptions* 287
- lupus erythematosus 253
- drug-induced lupus 267, 296

4. *Vacuolar Dermatitis, Basement Membranes Thickened*

Vacuolar degeneration is associated with variable numbers of apoptotic cells in the epidermis. The basement membrane zone is thickened by deposition of eosinophilic hyaline material.

- *lupus erythematosus* 253

IV. ACANTHOLYTIC, VESICULAR, AND PUSTULAR DISORDERS

Keratinocytes may separate from each other on the basis of immunologic antigen-antibody–mediated damage, resulting in separation and rounding up of keratinocyte cell bodies (acantholysis). This may occur on the basis of edema and inflammation (spongiosis), or perhaps on the basis of structural deficiencies of cell adhesion (Darier's disease). These processes produce intraepidermal spaces (vesicles, bullae, pustules).

A. Subcorneal or Intracorneal Separation

There is separation within or just below the stratum corneum. Inflammatory cells may be sparse or may consist predominantly of neutrophils.

1. Sub/Intracorneal Separation, Scant Inflammatory Cells

There is separation within or just below the stratum corneum, associated with scant inflammation, usually lymphocytic.

- *staphylococcal scalded skin* 223, 457
- bullous impetigo 457
- miliaria crystallina 216
- exfoliative dermatitis 216
- pemphigus foliaceus 222
- pemphigus erythematosus 224
- necrolytic migratory erythema 354
- pellagra 354
- acrodermatitis enteropathica 356

2. Sub/Intracorneal Separation, Neutrophils Prominent

There is separation in or just below the stratum corneum. Neutrophils are prominent in the stratum corneum and in the superficial epidermis, and can often be found in the dermis.

- *impetigo contagiosa* 457
- epidermis adjacent to folliculitis 460
- impetiginized dermatitis 457
- candidiasis 522
- pustular psoriasis 160
- subcorneal pustular dermatosis (Sneddon-Wilkinson) 238
- IgA pemphigus 225
- secondary syphilis 503
- acropustulosis of infancy 237
- transient neonatal pustular melanosis 237

3. Sub/Intracorneal Separation, Eosinophils Predominant

There is separation in or just below the stratum corneum, with (pemphigus) or without acantholytic keratinocytes. Eosinophils are present in the epidermis, and occasionally there is eosinophilic spongiosis. The separation is associated with a dermal infiltrate that contains eosinophils.

- *erythema toxicum neonatorum* 237
- pemphigus foliaceus 222
- pemphigus erythematosus 224
- eosinophilic pustular folliculitis 407
- incontinentia pigmenti, vesicular 144
- exfoliative dermatitis, drug-induced 216

B. Intraspinous Keratinocyte Separation, Spongiotic

There are spaces within the epidermis (vesicles, bullae). There may be dyskeratosis or acantholysis, and a few eosinophils may be present in the epidermis.

1. Intraspinous Spongiosis, Scant Inflammatory Cells

The infiltrate in the dermis is scant, and lymphocytic or eosinophilic.

- *early spongiotic dermatitis* 210
- epidermolytic hyperkeratosis 686
- epidermolytic acanthoma 687
- miliaria rubra 216
- transient acantholytic dermatosis 244
- bullous dermatitis of diabetes and of uremia 229, 379
- coma bulla 291
- friction blisters 244

2. Intraspinous Spongiosis, Lymphocytes Predominant

In the dermis, lymphocytes predominate. Eosinophils can be found in most examples of atopy and allergic contact dermatitis and in fewer numbers in the other disorders.

- spongiotic (eczematous) dermatitis 210
  - atopic dermatitis 214
  - allergic contact dermatitis 212
  - photoallergic drug eruption 214, 292
  - irritant contact dermatitis 213
  - *nummular eczema* 214
  - dyshidrotic dermatitis 213
  - "id" reaction 214
- seborrheic dermatitis 215
- stasis dermatitis 215, 914
- erythroderma 216
- miliaria rubra 216
- pityriasis rosea 164

a. Intraspinous Spongiosis, Eosinophils Present

The number of eosinophils seen is variable, from many in incontinentia pigmenti and pemphigus vegetans to few in atopic dermatitis.

- spongiotic (eczematous) dermatitis 210
  - atopic dermatitis 214
  - *allergic contact dermatitis* 212
  - photoallergic drug eruption 214, 292
- incontinentia pigmenti, vesicular stage 144

3. Intraspinous Spongiosis, Neutrophils Predominant

Neutrophils are seen in the epidermis, stratum corneum, and dermis. Aggregations of neutrophils in the superficial spinous layer constitute the spongiform pustules of Kogoj characteristic of psoriasis.

- *pustular psoriasis* 156
  - Reiter's syndrome 163
- IgA pemphigus 225

subcorneal pustular dermatosis
(Sneddon-Wilkinson) 238
exanthemic pustular drug eruptions 287
impetiginized dermatosis 457
dermatophytosis 517
rupial secondary syphilis 506
seborrheic dermatitis 215
epidermis adjacent to folliculitis 460
impetigo contagiosa 457
hydroa vacciniforme 308
mucocutaneous lymph node syndrome
(Kawasaki disease, pustular variant) 166
if vasculitis, refer to III.G. or V.B.

C. Intraspinous Keratinocyte Separation, Acantholytic

There are spaces within the epidermis (vesicles, bullae). The process of separation is acantholysis. Keratinocytes within the spinous layer detach or separate from each other or from basal keratinocytes. There may be dyskeratosis, and a few eosinophils may be present in the epidermis. The infiltrate in the dermis is variable, composed of lymphocytes with or without eosinophils.

1. Intraspinous Acantholysis, Scant Inflammatory Cells

The infiltrate in the dermis is scant, and lymphocytic or eosinophilic.

epidermolytic hyperkeratosis 686
epidermolytic acanthoma 687
Darier's disease 132
isolated keratosis follicularis
(warty dyskeratoma) 700
Hailey-Hailey disease 131
transient acantholytic dermatosis 244
focal acantholytic dyskeratosis 688
acantholytic actinic keratosis 703
pemphigus erythematosus 224
pemphigus foliaceus 222
friction blister (cytolytic blister) 244

2. Intraspinous Acantholysis, Predominant Lymphocytes

In the dermis, lymphocytes are predominant. In erythema multiforme and related lesions there is necrosis of individual cells (apoptosis) that may become confluent.

erythema multiforme (with vacuolar and
apoptotic changes) 239
Stevens-Johnson 239
toxic epidermal necrolysis (TEN) 240
herpes simplex, varicella-zoster 569
hydroa vacciniforme (epidermal necrosis) . . 308
cowpox 574
hand-foot-and-mouth disease
(coxsackie virus) 586
orf 576
paraneoplastic pemphigus 225

a. Intraspinous Acantholysis, Eosinophils Present

The number of eosinophils seen is variable, from many in incontinentia pigmenti and pemphigus vegetans to few in atopic dermatitis.

pemphigus vegetans 221
pemphigus vulgaris 218
drug-induced pemphigus 224, 295
paraneoplastic pemphigus 225

3. Intraspinous Separation, Neutrophils, Mixed Cell Types

Inflammatory cells in the dermis include lymphocytes and plasma cells, with or without eosinophils, neutrophils, mast cells, and histiocytes.

acantholytic actinic keratosis 703
acantholytic squamous cell carcinoma 715
hydroa vacciniforme (epidermal necrosis) . . . 308
IgA pemphigus 225

D. Suprabasal Keratinocyte Separation

There is separation between the keratinocytes of the basal layer and those of the spinous layer.

1. Suprabasal Vesicles, Scant Inflammatory Cells

The suprabasal separation may be associated with scant inflammation, and frequently with dyskeratotic or atypical keratinocytes.

transient acantholytic dermatosis
(Grover) 244
benign familial pemphigus
(Hailey-Hailey) 131
Darier's disease (keratosis follicularis) 132
acantholytic actinic keratosis 703
acantholytic squamous cell carcinoma 715
focal acantholytic dyskeratosis 688

2. Suprabasal Separation, Lymphocytes and Plasma Cells

Suprabasal separation is associated with keratinocyte atypia.

acantholytic actinic keratosis 703
acantholytic squamous cell carcinoma 715

3. Suprabasal Vesicles, Lymphocytes, and Eosinophils

There is suprabasal separation with eosinophils in the epidermis (eosinophilic spongiosis) and in the dermis.

pemphigus vulgaris 218
pemphigus vegetans 221

E. Subepidermal Vesicular Dermatitis

A *subepidermal blister* refers to separation of the epidermis from the dermis. The roof of the blister is composed of an intact or (partially) necrotic epithelium.

1. *Subepidermal Vesicles, Scant/No Inflammation*

The infiltrate in the dermis in most of these conditions is scant (few lymphocytes, eosinophils, neutrophils).

porphyria cutanea tarda and other porphryrias 376
drug-induced pseudoporphyria 300
bullous pemphigoid, cell-poor 226
epidermolysis bullosa simplex 128
epidermolysis bullosa letalis 128
epidermolysis bullosa acquisita (classic) . . . 232
GVHD, acute 240
acute radiation dermatitis 313
bullous dermatosis of diabetes 229
bullous dermatosis of uremia 279
electrical burn (polarized epidermis) 245
thermal burn (epidermal necrosis) 245
suction blister 245
Vibrio vulnificus septicemia (necrotic bullae) 465

2. *Subepidermal Vesicles, Lymphocytes Predominant*

The epidermis is separated from the dermis, predominantly because of liquefaction of the basal cell layer. In polymorphous light eruption (PMLE) massive papillary dermal edema is the cause. The infiltrate in the dermis is primarily lymphocytic.

vesicular lichen planus 169
erythema multiforme 239
fixed drug eruption 289
lichen sclerosus et atrophicus 280
bullous lupus erythematosus, mononuclear type 262
graft-versus-host disease 240
polymorphous light eruption (PMLE) 305
epidermolysis bullosa acquisita (usually neutrophils) 232

3. *Subepidermal Vesicles, Eosinophils Prominent*

The subepidermal blister is associated with a dermal infiltrate rich in eosinophils. Eosinophils may extend into the overlying epidermis.

bullous pemphigoid 226
cicatricial pemphigoid 229
bullous drug eruption 300
herpes gestationis 232
dermatitis herpetiformis (old lesions) 234

4. *Subepidermal Vesicles, Neutrophils Prominent*

A neutrophilic infiltrate is often seen in dermal papillae at the dermal-epidermal junction adjacent to the subepidermal blister, or in the blister.

dermatitis herpetiformis 234
bullous lupus erythematosus, neutrophilic type 262
bullous vasculitis 194
linear IgA dermatosis (adult, childhood, drug-associated) 235
epidermolysis bullosa acquisita (inflammatory) 232
vesiculopustular eruption of hepatobiliary disease 238, 363
toxic shock syndrome 464

5. *Subepidermal Vesicles, Mast Cells Prominent*

The epidermis is separated from the dermis. There is an infiltrate in the superficial dermis composed almost entirely of mast cells, with or without a few eosinophils. This may be associated with separation of the epidermis from the dermis.

bullous mastocytosis 141

V. PERIVASCULAR, DIFFUSE, AND GRANULOMATOUS INFILTRATES OF THE RETICULAR DERMIS

The dermis serves as a reaction site for a variety of inflammatory, infiltrative, and desmoplastic processes. These include infiltrations of a variety of cells (lymphocytes, histiocytes, eosinophils, plasma cells, melanocytes, etc.); perivascular and vascular reactions; infiltration with organisms and foreign bodies; and proliferations of dermal fibers and precursors of dermal fibers as reactions to a variety of stimuli.

A. Superficial and Deep Perivascular Infiltrates Without Vascular Damage or Vasculitis

In some of the diseases considered here, the infiltrates are predominantly in the upper reticular dermis (urticarial eruptions), and others are both superficial and deep (gyrate erythemas). Most of these also involve the superficial plexus. A few diseases are mainly deep (some examples of lupus erythematosus, scleroderma).

1. *Perivascular Infiltrates, Lymphocytes Predominant*

In the dermis there is no vasculitis, only perivascular lymphocytes as the predominant cells.

pityriasis lichenoides et varioliformis acuta (PLEVA) 176
stasis dermatitis 215, 914
acne rosacea 404

2. *Perivascular Infiltrates, Neutrophils Predominant*

Neutrophils are seen in perivascular or perivascular and diffuse patterns in the dermis. Edema is prominent in some instances (Sweet's).

if vasculitis, refer to V.B.

3. *Perivascular Infiltrates, Lymphocytes and Eosinophils*

Lymphocytes and eosinophils are mixed in the infiltrate. Lymphocytes are always seen; eosinophil numbers may vary, being greatest in bite reactions and often (though variable and sometimes very few) in eosinophilic fasciitis.

4. *Perivascular Infiltrates, With Plasma Cells*

In addition to lymphocytes, plasma cells are found in the dermal infiltrate.

5. *Perivascular Infiltrates, Mixed Cell Types*

In addition to lymphocytes, plasma cells and eosinophils are found in the dermal infiltrate.

B. Vasculitis and Vasculopathies

True vasculitis is defined by eosinophilic degeneration of the vessel wall ("fibrinoid necrosis") and infiltration of the vessel wall by neutrophils, with neutrophils, nuclear dust, and extravasated red cells in the vessel walls and adjacent dermis. Some of the conditions mentioned here lack these prototypic findings and may be termed *vasculopathies* (e.g., Degos' disease).

1. *Vascular Damage, Scant Inflammatory Cells*

Although there is significant vascular damage, there is little early inflammatory response.

2. *Vasculitis, Lymphocytes Predominant*

The term *lymphocytic vasculitis* is controversial, but there are some conditions in which perivascular and intramural lymphocytes may be associated with some degree of vasculopathy, not usually including frank fibrinoid necrosis. Most of these conditions are discussed elsewhere as "perivascular lymphocytic infiltrates." In angiocentric lymphomas, the cells infiltrating the vessel walls are neoplastic, but the process may be mistaken for an inflammatory reaction.

3. *Vasculitis, Neutrophils Prominent*

Neutrophils are prominent in the infiltrate, with fibrinoid necrosis and nuclear dust; eosinophils and lymphocytes are also found.

small-vessel leukocytoclastic vasculitis 194
neutrophilic dermatoses 206
 Sweet's syndrome 204
 granuloma faciale 207
 bowel-associated dermatosis-arthrosis
  syndrome 206, 358
septic/embolic lesions of gonococcemia/
 meningococcemia 195, 464, 466
Rocky Mountain spotted fever
 (Rickettsia rickettsii) 490
polyarteritis nodosa 191
erythema elevatum diutinum 198
Behçet's syndrome 359
papulonecrotic tuberculid 472

4. *Vasculitis, Mixed Cell Types and/or Granulomas*

Histiocytes and giant cells are a part of the infiltrate. Lymphocytes and eosinophils can also be found, depending on the diagnosis. Giant cell arteritis is a true inflammation of the artery wall (true arteritis), although there is no fibrinoid necrosis.

allergic granulomatosis (Churg-Strauss) .. 199
Wegener's granulomatosis 201
giant cell arteritis (temporal arteritis) 190
erythema nodosum leprosum 486
some insect bite reactions 565
"secondary vasculitis" at the base of ulcers
 of diverse etiology 185
Behçet's syndrome 359

5. *Thrombotic and Other Microangiopathies*

The dermal vessels contain fibrin, red cells and platelet thrombi, and/or eosinophilic protein precipitates.

septicemia 195
disseminated intravascular coagulation 186
coumarin necrosis 186
amyloidosis 369
porphyria cutanea tarda and other
 porphyrias 376
calciphylaxis 380, 447
thrombophlebitis and superficial migratory
 thrombophlebitis 192
Lucio reaction 486

C. Diffuse Infiltrates of the Reticular Dermis

Diffuse infiltrates of the reticular dermis may show some relation to vessels or to skin appendages, or may be randomly distributed in the reticular dermis.

1. *Diffuse Infiltrates, Lymphocytes Predominant*

Lymphocytes are seen almost to the exclusion of other cell types.

cutaneous lymphoid hyperplasia/
 lymphocytoma cutis 258, 805
Jessner's lymphocytic infiltrate 268
leukemia cutis (chronic lymphocytic
 lymphoma, CLL) 840

2. *Diffuse Infiltrates, Neutrophils Predominant*

Neutrophils are the main infiltrating cell, although lymphocytes can be found.

acute neutrophilic dermatosis (Sweet's) ... 204
erythema elevatum diutinum 198
rheumatoid neutrophilic dermatosis 204
granuloma faciale 207
cutaneous reaction to cytokines,
 especially gamma colony stimulating
 factor (G-CSF) 292
bowel arthrosis dermatosis syndrome . 206, 358
cellulitis 459
pyoderma gangrenosum 206, 357
dermis adjacent to folliculitis 460
abscess 461, 526
Behçet's syndrome 359

3. *Diffuse Infiltrates, "Histiocytoid" Cells Predominant*

Histiocytes or histiocytoid cells are found in great numbers in the dermal infiltrate. Some may be foamy; others may contain organisms. The leukemic cells of myeloid leukemia may be easily mistaken for histiocytes and may have histiocytic differentiation (myelomonocytic leukemia).

xanthelasma, xanthomas
 (usually nodular) 593
atypical mycobacteria
 Mycobacterium avium-intracellulare
  (MAI) 474
deep fungus infection
 cryptococcosis 537
 histoplasmosis 538
paraffinoma 317
silicone granuloma 317
talc and starch granuloma 318, 319
annular elastolytic giant cell granuloma
 (actinic granuloma) 334
lepromatous leprosy 477
histoid leprosy 480
cutaneous leishmaniasis 553
rhinoscleroma (Klebsiella
 rhinoscleromatis) 492
histiocytosis X 597
leukemia cutis (myeloid, myelomonocytic) 840
anaplastic large cell lymphoma (Ki-1) 832

4. *Diffuse Infiltrates, Plasma Cells Prominent*

Plasma cells are found in the diffuse dermal infiltrate, though they may not be the predominant cell.

5. *Diffuse Infiltrates, Mast Cells Predominant*

Mast cells compose almost the entire dermal infiltrate. There may be an admixture of eosinophils.

6. *Diffuse Infiltrates, Eosinophils Predominant*

Eosinophils are prominent although not the only infiltrating cell. Lymphocytes are found, and plasma cells may be present.

7. *Diffuse Infiltrates, Mixed Cell Types*

The diffuse infiltrate contains plasma cells, lymphocytes, histiocytes, and a variety of acute inflammatory cells.

8. *Diffuse Infiltrates, Pigment Cells*

The diffuse infiltrate contains bipolar, cuboidal, or dendritic cells with brown cytoplasmic pigment.

9. *Diffuse Infiltrates, Extensive Necrosis*

Vascular and dermal necrosis are found secondary to vascular occlusion or to destruction by organisms.

D. Diffuse or Nodular Infiltrates of the Reticular Dermis With Epidermal Proliferation

Ill-defined nodules or diffuse infiltrates of inflammatory cells, usually including lymphocytes, plasma cells, and neutrophils, are in the dermis, and the epidermis is irregularly thickened.

1. *Epidermal Proliferation With Mixed Cellular Infiltrates*

E. Nodular Inflammatory Infiltrates of the Reticular Dermis—Granulomas, Abscesses, and Ulcers

A granuloma is defined as a collection of histiocytes that may have abundant cytoplasm and confluent borders ("epithelioid histiocytes"), often with Langhans'-type giant cells. Granulomas may be associated with necrosis, may palisade around areas of necrobiosis, may be mixed with other inflammatory cells, may include foreign-body giant cells, and may contain ingested foreign material or pathogens (acid-fast bacilli, fungi). An abscess is a localized area of suppurative necrosis containing abundant neutrophils mixed with necrotic debris, and usually is surrounded by a reaction of granulation tissue and fibrosis.

1. *Epithelioid Cell Granulomas Without Necrosis*

Large epithelioid histiocytes are common in the infiltrate as well as giant cells. The infiltrate may also contain a few plasma cells as well as lymphocytes.

sarcoidosis (lupus pernio and other types) 322
lichen scrofulosorum 473
granulomatous granuloma annulare 328
foreign-body granulomas 317
syphilis, secondary or tertiary 503
granulomatous rosacea 404
cheilitis granulomatosa (Miescher-Melkersson-Rosenthal) 326
tuberculoid leprosy 482
tuberculosis
  lupus vulgaris 468
Crohn's disease 361
allergic granulomatous reactions
  to chemical agents: silica, zirconium, aluminum, beryllium granulomas 319
collagen implant granuloma 322
granulomatous mycosis fungoides 820
chronic cutaneous leishmaniasis 555
necrobiosis lipoidica 330

2. *Epithelioid Cell Granulomas With Necrosis*

The presence of necrosis in an epithelioid cell granuloma of the skin strongly suggests tuberculosis except in lesions of the face. Epithelioid sarcoma may simulate a necrotizing granuloma.

tuberculosis 468
  tuberculosis verrucosa cutis 468
  miliary tuberculosis 468
  lupus vulgaris (necrosis usually slight or absent) 468
nontuberculosis mycobacteria 474
lupus miliaris disseminatus facei 406
tertiary syphilis 508
epithelioid sarcoma 865
cryptococcosis 537
histoplasmosis 538
sarcoidosis (usually noncaseating) 322

3. *Palisading Granulomas*

There are foci of altered collagen ("necrobiosis") surrounded by histiocytes, and lymphocytes. Histiocytic giant cells are also seen in the infiltrate. The lesions of epithelioid sarcoma are associated with true tumor necrosis but may superficially resemble rheumatoid nodules.

granuloma annulare 328
rheumatoid nodule 333
necrobiosis lipoidica 330
subcutaneous granuloma annulare 328
annular elastolytic giant cell granuloma (actinic granuloma) 334
rheumatic nodule 334
epithelioid sarcoma 865
occasional examples of deep fungus infections 334, 526

4. *Mixed Cell Granulomas*

Lymphocytes and plasma cells are present in addition to epithelioid histiocytes, which may form loose clusters, and giant cells, which may be quite inconspicuous. In many of these granulomatous infiltrates, organisms are found. Keratin granuloma is the most common mixed granuloma. Flakes of keratin may be appreciated as fibers, often gray rather than pink, in the cytoplasm of giant cells.

keratin granuloma
  ruptured cyst 317, 694
  folliculitis 460
sporotrichosis 541
persistent arthropod bite 565
syphilis, secondary and tertiary 503
cryptococcosis 537
candidal granuloma 524
nontuberculosis mycobacteria 474
catscratch disease 494
North American blastomycosis 529
South American blastomycosis 532
chromomycosis 533
phaeohyphomycosis 528
coccidioidomycosis 534

5. *Inflammatory Nodules With Prominent Eosinophils*

The nodular dermal infiltrates contain many eosinophils often admixed with lymphocytes.

angiolymphoid hyperplasia with eosinophils 891
Kimura's disease 895
scabetic nodule 559

6. *Inflammatory Nodules With Mixed Cell Types*

A variety of cells are in the infiltrate, including neutrophils, histiocytes, plasma cells, giant cells, and lymphocytes.

chronic bacterial infections 457
keratin granuloma
  ruptured cyst 694
  folliculitis 460

sporotrichosis 541
rhinoscleroma (Klebsiella
rhinoscleromatis) 492
atypical mycobacteria 474
Mycobacterium avium-intracellulare 474
Mycobacterium marinum 474
nocardiosis 496
lobomycosis 533
protothecosis 546

7. Inflammatory Nodules With Necrosis and Neutrophils (Abscesses)

Inflammatory nodules are characterized by central suppurative necrosis, with neutrophils adjacent to the necrosis, and often with granulation tissue, mixed inflammatory cells including epithelioid histiocytes and giant cells, and fibrosis at the periphery.

acute or chronic bacterial abscesses 457
deep fungal infections 526
phaeohyphomycotic cyst 528
North American blastomycosis 529
chromoblastomycosis 533
cutaneous alternariosis 529
paracoccidioidomycosis 532
coccidioidomycosis 534
sporotrichosis 541
botryomycosis 495
actinomycosis 497
nocardiosis 496
cat scratch disease 494
erythema nodosum leprosum 486
scrofuloderma 471
tuberculous gumma 471
protothecosis 546

8. Inflammatory Nodules With Prominent Necrosis

Necrosis is a striking feature, along with variable but sometimes sparse infiltrates of inflammatory cells that may include plasma cells, epithelioid histiocytes, neutrophils, lymphocytes, and hemorrhage. Organisms may be demonstrable.

tertiary syphilis 508
tertiary yaws 508
aspergillosis 525
zygomycosis (mucormycosis) 525
tuberculosis 468
atypical mycobacteria 474
infarcts 186
deep vasculitis 190
deep thrombi 193
calciphylaxis 186, 380, 448
frostbite 312
necrobiotic xanthogranuloma
with paraproteinemia 605
gangrenous ischemic necrosis 186
epithelioid sarcoma 865

9. Chronic Ulcers and Sinuses Involving the Reticular Dermis

An chronic ulcer is characterized by central suppurative necrosis, with neutrophils adjacent to the necrosis, and often with granulation tissue, fibrosis, and reactive epithelium at the periphery. A sinus extends deeper into the dermis than most ulcers, in a serpentine fashion. A fistula is an abnormal communication between two epithelial-lined surfaces. The histologic architecture of fistulas and sinuses is similar to that of chronic ulcers.

pyoderma gangrenosum 206, 357
ecthyma gangrenosum 465
deep fungal infection
North American blastomycosis 529
eumycetoma 543
tuberculosis cutis orificialis 471
enterocutaneous fistula 361
ecthyma 459
papulonecrotic tuberculid 472
Buruli ulcer (*M ulcerans*) 476
chancroid (*Haemophilus ducreyi*) 490
granuloma inguinale (*Calymmatobacterium granulomatis*) 491
lymphogranuloma venereum (*Chlamydia trachomatis*) 493
follicular occlusion disorder
pilonidal sinus 462
hidradenitis suppurativa 461
acne conglobata 461
perifolliculitis capitis abscedens et suffodiens (dissecting cellulitis of the scalp) 461
anthrax (*Bacillus anthracis*) 488
tularemia (*Francisella tularensis*) 488
cutaneous leishmaniasis 553
necrotizing sialometaplasia of hard palate ... 707
eosinophilic ulcer of the tongue 708

F. Dermal Matrix Fiber Disorders

The dermis serves as a reaction site for a variety of inflammatory, infiltrative, and desmoplastic processes. These may include accumulations or deficiencies of dermal fibrous and nonfibrous matrix constituents as reactions to a variety of stimuli.

1. Fiber Disorders, Collagen Increased

Dermal collagen is increased with production at the dermal-subcutaneous interface. Inflammation is seen at this site. The inflammatory cells are lymphocytes, plasma cells, and eosinophils. Fibroblasts in some instances are increased.

scar, keloid 881
scleroderma/morphea 274
sclerodermoid GVHD 242

- phytonadione-induced pseudoscleroderma ... 301
- necrobiosis lipoidica ... 330
- eosinophilic fasciitis ... 279
- radiation fibrosis ... 313
- acrodermatitis chronica atrophicans ... 512
- facial hemiatrophy ... 513
- chronic lymphedema ... 918
- acro-osteolysis ... 350

2. *Fiber Disorders, Collagen Reduced*

Collagen may be reduced focally or diffusely as part of an inborn error of collagen fiber metabolism or as an acquired phenomenon.

- Ehlers-Danlos syndrome ... 138
- Marfan's syndrome ... 344
- penicillamine-induced atrophy ... 295
- striae distensae ... 349
- aplasia cutis ... 126
- focal dermal hypoplasia (Goltz) ... 125
- *atrophoderma (Pasini and Pierini)* ... 278
- relapsing polychondritis (type II collagen degeneration of cartilage) ... 417

3. *Fiber Disorders, Elastin Altered*

Abnormal elastic fibers are increased focally in the dermis and may become calcified (PXE), or there is diffuse elastosis in the superficial reticular dermis of sun-exposed skin.

- *pseudoxanthoma elasticum (PXE)* ... 135
- penicillamine-induced elastosis perforans serpiginosa ... 295
- solar elastosis ... 341
- erythema ab igne ... 311
- annular elastolytic giant cell granuloma (actinic granuloma) ... 334

4. *Fiber Disorders, Elastin Reduced*

Elastin may be reduced focally or diffusely as part of an inborn error of its metabolism, or as an acquired phenomenon.

- *cutis laxa* ... 139
- anetoderma ... 349
- mid dermal elastolysis ... 349

5. *Fiber Disorders, Perforating*

Abnormal elastin or collagen fibers may be extruded through the epidermis, forming channels that extend into the dermis.

- *elastosis perforans serpiginosa* ... 344
- Kyrle's disease ... 343
- perforating folliculitis ... 343
- reactive perforating collagenosis ... 345
- perforating disorder of renal failure and diabetes ... 345
- perforating calcific elastosis ... 348
- perforating granuloma annulare ... 328

G. Deposition of Material in the Dermis

The dermis serves as a reaction site for a variety of inflammatory, infiltrative and desmoplastic processes, which may include accumulations of matrix molecules that may either be indigenous to the normal dermis or foreign to it.

1. *Increased Normal Nonfibrous Matrix Constituents*

Ground substance (hyaluronic acid) is increased, associated with a varying inflammatory infiltrate that can include lymphocytes, plasma cells, and eosinophils.

- granuloma annulare ... 328
- *pretibial myxedema* ... 387
- generalized myxedema ... 387
- juvenile cutaneous mucinosis ... 390
- papular mucinosis (lichen myxedematosus) ... 388
- scleromyxedema ... 389
- reticulated erythematous mucinosis (REM) ... 390
- scleredema ... 390
- focal dermal mucinosis ... 879
- digital mucous cyst/myxoid cyst ... 879
- cutaneous myxoma ... 878
- mucocoele, mucinous mucosal cyst ... 881
- lupus erythematosus ... 253
- hereditary progressive mucinous histiocytosis ... 612

2. *Increased Material Not Normally Present in the Dermis*

Materials not present in substantial amounts in the normal dermis are deposited as crystals (gout), amorphous deposits (calcinosis), hyaline material (colloid milium, amyloidosis, porphyria), or pigments.

- *gout* ... 382
- colloid milium ... 373
- calcinosis cutis
  - calcinosis universalis, circumscripta (scleroderma, dermatomyositis) ... 381
  - tumoral calcinosis ... 382
  - idiopathic calcification of the scrotum ... 382
  - subepidermal calcified nodule ... 382
- amyloidosis ... 369
- dermal pigments
  - minocycline ... 294
  - argyria ... 298
  - chrysiasis ... 299
  - mercury pigmentation ... 300
  - hemochromatosis ... 395

- alkaptonuric ochronosis ... 384
- calcaneal petechiae (hemoglobin) ... 315
- lipoid proteinosis (hyalinosis cutis et mucosae, Urbach-Wiethe) ... 375
- cryoglobulinemia ... 196
- porphyria cutanea tarda ... 378
- foreign material—dirt, glass, paraffin, grease, etc ... 317
  - tattoo reactions ... 322
  - silicone, talc, starch ... 317
  - cactus, sea urchin, hair granulomas ... 319
  - injected materials ... 443
  - vaccines ... 321
- Hunter's syndrome (lysosomal storage granules) ... 393

3. *Parasitic Infestations of the Dermis and/or Subcutis*

Macroscopically visible parasitic agents may infest the dermis and subcutis.

- *larva migrans (Ancylostoma)* ... 560
- subcutaneous dirofilariasis ... 560
- onchocerciasis ... 562
- strongyloidiasis ... 564
- schistosomiasis ... 564
- subcutaneous cysticercosis ... 565
- myiasis ... 565

VI. TUMORS AND CYSTS OF THE DERMIS AND SUBCUTIS

Neoplasms in the reticular dermis may arise from any of the tissues included in the dermis—lymphoreticular tissue, connective tissue, and epithelial tissue of the skin appendages. In addition, metastases commonly present in the dermis and subcutis.

A. Small Cell Tumors

A neoplastic nodule is a circumscribed collection of neoplastic cells in the dermis. Abscesses, granulomas, and cysts may also present as nodules. Cysts are considered separately. In general, neoplastic nodules can be differentiated from reactive and inflammatory nodules by the presence of a monotonous population of cells consistent with a clonal proliferation, whereas inflammatory nodules are composed of inflammatory cell types (lymphocytes, neutrophils, histiocytes, etc.), generally in a heterogeneous mixture.

1. *Tumors of Lymphocytes or Hemopoietic Cells*

Nodular infiltrates or extensive diffuse infiltrates of normal and/or atypical lymphocytes are found in the dermis.

- cutaneous T-cell lymphoma
  - lymphoblastic lymphoma, T-cell type ... 820
  - *tumor-stage mycosis fungoides* ... 823
  - adult T-cell lymphoma/leukemia ... 829
- cutaneous B-cell lymphoma
  - lymphoblastic lymphoma, B-cell type ... 808
  - small lymphocytic lymphoma ... 808
  - immunocytoma (lymphoplasmacytoid lymphoma) ... 811
  - primary cutaneous follicular lymphoma ... 811
  - diffuse large B-cell lymphoma (centroblastic/immunoblastic) ... 816
- drug-induced pseudolymphoma ... 300
- leukemia cutis ... 840
- aluminum granuloma ... 321
- pseudolymphomatous tattoo reaction ... 322

2. *Tumors of Lymphocytes and Mixed Cell Types*

Nodular infiltrates or extensive diffuse infiltrates of normal lymphocytes are found in the dermis. Other reactive cell types (plasma cells, histiocytes) are admixed.

- *cutaneous lymphoid hyperplasia/lymphocytoma cutis* ... 805, 819
- Lennert's (lymphoepithelial) lymphoma ... 830
- angioimmunoblastic lymphadenopathy ... 831
- Borrelial lymphocytoma cutis ... 514
- chronic myelogenous leukemia ... 840

3. *Tumors of Plasma Cells*

Nodular plasma cell infiltrates, with scattered lymphocytes.

- *cutaneous plasmacytoma and myeloma* ... 814

4. *Small Round Cell Tumors*

Tumors of small cells with scant cytoplasm and with small dark nuclei constitute a group of tumors that can usually be distinguished from one another with appropriate immunohistochemical investigations, in conjunction with light microscopic and clinical information. Some of these tumors arise in the deep soft tissue, but they may rarely present in a deep skin biopsy.

- primitive neuroepithelial tumors (PNET)
  - peripheral neuroblastoma/neuroepithelioma ... 1002
  - Ewing's sarcoma ... 878, 1002
- cutaneous small cell undifferentiated carcinoma (CSCUC/Merkel cell tumor) ... 1000, 1017
- melanotic neuroepithelial tumor of infancy ... 1002
- lymphoma/leukemia ... 805
- rhabdomyosarcoma ... 961
- metastatic neuroendocrine carcinoma ... 1017
- small cell melanoma ... 656
- small cell carcinoma (squamous or adenocarcinoma) ... 1011
- *eccrine spiradenoma* ... 783

B. Large Polygonal and Round Cell Tumors

1. Squamous Cell Carcinomas

Proliferations of atypical cells with more or less abundant cytoplasm, contiguous cell borders, evidence of keratinization, and/or desmosomes occupy the dermis as nodular masses. Most primary squamous cell carcinomas show evidence of epidermal origin, often with associated squamous cell carcinoma in situ.

2. Adenocarcinomas

Proliferations of atypical cells with more or less abundant cytoplasm and with evidence of gland formation and/or mucin production occupy the dermis as nodular masses. The possibility of metastatic adenocarcinoma must be considered and differentiated from the possibility of a primary cutaneous adenocarcinoma of skin appendages (refer to eccrine, apocrine, pilar, sebaceous tumor sections later).

3. Melanocytic Tumors

The proliferations in the dermis are melanocyte-derived, pigmented or amelanotic, benign, atypical, or malignant. Superficial lesions may involve the epidermis (junctional component). There may be a fibrous and inflammatory host response. S-100 and HMB-45 stains may be of value in recognizing melanocytic differentiation in amelanotic tumors.

4. Eccrine Tumors

There are proliferations of eccrine ductal (small dark cells usually forming tubules at least focally) or glandular tissue or both in a hyalinized or sclerotic dermis. The inflammatory infiltrate is mainly lymphocytic.

malignant eccrine spiradenoma 785
malignant eccrine poroma
(porocarcinoma) 780
eccrine adenocarcinoma 791
mucinous eccrine carcinoma 793
adenoid cystic eccrine carcinoma 795
aggressive digital papillary
adenoma/adenocarcinoma 795
syringoid eccrine carcinoma 792

5. *Apocrine Tumors*

Tumors in the dermis are composed of proliferations of apocrine ductal and glandular epithelium (large pink cells with decapitation secretion). The stroma is sclerotic and well vascularized, and the inflammatory cells are mainly lymphocytes.

circumscribed, symmetrical
apocrine nevus 769
tubular apocrine adenoma
("tubulopapillary hidradenoma") 773
cylindroma (some consider eccrine) 775
hidradenoma papilliferum 770
syringocystadenoma papilliferum 771
apocrine hidrocystoma 769
infiltrative, asymmetrical
apocrine adenocarcinoma 795
malignant cylindroma 776
erosive adenomatosis (florid
papillomatosis of the nipple) 773

6. *Pilar Tumors*

The dermal infiltrating tumor is composed of epithelium that differentiates toward hair, or is a proliferation of portions of the follicular structure and its stroma. The inflammatory cell infiltrate is mainly lymphocytic, and the dermis is fibrocellular.

follicular infundibular neoplasms
dilated pore of Winer 750
pilar sheath acanthoma 750
trichilemmoma 761
tumor of the follicular infundibulum 762
branching and lobular pilosebaceous
neoplasms
trichofolliculoma 749
trichoepithelioma 751
tumor of follicular infundibulum 762
top of nevus sebaceous 763
nodular pilosebaceous neoplasms
hair follicle nevus 749
keratoacanthoma 731
trichoepithelioma 751
desmoplastic trichoepithelioma 755
immature trichoepithelioma 757
hair follicle hamartoma 757
pilomatricoma 757
trichoblastoma 753
trichoblastic fibroma 753
trichoadenoma 756
proliferating trichilemmal cyst
(pilar tumor) 759
inverted follicular keratosis 691
tumors of pilosebaceous mesenchyme
trichodiscoma 750
fibrofolliculoma 750
tumors of the erector pilae muscle 959
infiltrative, asymmetrical
pilomatrix carcinoma
(malignant pilomatricoma) 759
trichilemmal carcinoma 763
basal cell carcinoma with follicular
differentiation 729

7. *Sebaceous Tumors*

The dermal masses are proliferations of the germinative epithelium and of mature sebocytes. The admixture of these cell varies from one tumor to the other. The dermis is fibrocellular.

symmetrical, circumscribed
sebaceous hyperplasia 765
Fordyce's condition (ectopic sebaceous
glands in mucosae) 765
rhinophyma 404, 765
nevus sebaceus 763
sebaceous adenoma 766
sebaceous epithelioma 766
sebaceous trichofolliculoma 750
infiltrative, asymmetrical
sebaceous carcinoma 768
basal cell carcinoma with sebaceous
differentiation 723

8. *"Histiocytoid" Tumors*

"Histiocytes" may have foamy cytoplasm reflecting the accumulation of lipids, or they may have eosinophilic or amphophilic cytoplasm surrounding an ovoid nucleus with open chromatin. Some nonhistiocytic lesions whose cells may simulate histiocytes are also included here.

foamy histiocytes
xanthomas—eruptive, plane, tuberous,
tendon 593
verruciform xanthoma 606
xanthelasma 594
cholestanolemia, phytosterolemia 593
xanthoma disseminatum 603
diffuse normolipemic plane xanthoma 604
papular xanthoma 606
eruptive normolipemic xanthoma 596
progressive nodular histiocytoma
(superficial) 612
Langerhans' cell histiocytosis
(rare xanthomatous type) 597
histoid leprosy 480
nonfoamy histiocytes
dermatofibroma/histiocytoma 847
Langerhans' cell histiocytosis 597

congenital self-healing
  reticulohistiocytosis 600
indeterminate cell histiocytosis 601
granuloma annulare 328
eruptive histiocytomas 612
benign cephalic histiocytosis 614
sinus histiocytosis with massive
  lymphadenopathy 602
giant cells prominent
  juvenile xanthogranuloma 607
  multicentric reticulohistiocytosis 610
  giant cell reticulohistiocytoma 610
  necrobiotic xanthogranuloma with
    paraproteinemia 604
  xanthoma disseminatum 603
histiocytic simulants
  pleomorphic large cell lymphoma
    (Ki-1,usually T cells) 832
  epithelioid sarcoma 865

9. Tumors of Large Lymphoid Cells

Large lymphoid cells may be mistaken for carcinoma or melanoma cells, but may be distinguished morphologically by their tendency to have less cohesive growth in large sheets, by the absence of epithelial or melanocytic differentiation, and by immunopathology.

pleomorphic peripheral T-cell lymphoma . . 830
cutaneous anaplastic large cell lymphoma
  CD30 (Ki-1) lymphoma (regressing
    atypical histiocytosis) 832
leukemia cutis 840
cutaneous Hodgkin's disease 837

10. Mast Cell Tumors

Mast cells predominate in a nodular dermal infiltrate, with scattered eosinophils.

mastocytosis 141

11. Tumors With Prominent Necrosis

Necrosis is a striking feature in epithelioid sarcoma, which may in consequence be mistaken for a granulomatous process. In addition, many advanced malignancies, often metastatic, have prominent necrosis.

epithelioid sarcoma 865
metastatic carcinomas, sarcomas,
  melanomas 1011
occasional advanced primary malignant
  tumors 659, 712, 719

12. Miscellaneous and Undifferentiated Epithelial Tumors

Proliferations of atypical cells with more or less abundant cytoplasm and contiguous cell borders occupy the dermis as nodular masses.

undifferentiated carcinoma
  (large cell, small cell) 1000, 1011
granular cell nerve sheath tumor (granular
  cell tumor/schwannoma) 993
  plexiform granular cell nerve sheath
    tumor 994
malignant granular cell tumor 995
neuroendocrine carcinoma 1000
cephalic brain–like hamartoma
  (nasal glioma) 1003
encephalocele 1003
cutaneous meningiomas 1003
epithelial simulants
  pleomorphic large cell lymphoma (Ki-1,
    usually T cells) 832
  epithelioid sarcoma 865
  epithelioid angiosarcoma 921
  cellular neurothekeoma (immature nerve
    sheath myxoma) 992
  ganglioneuroma 1002

C. Spindle Cell, Pleomorphic, and Connective Tissue Tumors

In the dermis is a proliferation of elongated tapered "spindle cells"; these may be of fibrohistiocytic, muscle, neural (Schwannian), melanocytic, or unknown origin. Immunohistochemistry may be essential in making these distinctions.

1. Fibrohistiocytic Spindle Cell Tumors

There is a proliferation of spindle to pleomorphic cells that may synthesize collagen or be essentially undifferentiated. In the absence of specific markers for fibroblasts, immunohistochemistry is of little diagnostic utility except to rule out nonfibrous spindle cell tumors. Morphology is critical for accurate diagnosis.

benign fibrous histiocytoma
  (dermatofibroma) 847
aneurysmal fibrous histiocytoma 853
fibrous papule (angiofibroma) 871
hypertrophic scar, keloid 881
atypical fibroxanthoma 863
juvenile xanthogranuloma, spindle cell
  variant 607
dermatofibrosarcoma protuberans 853
fibromatoses
  desmoid tumor 858
  infantile digital fibromatosis 869
  juvenile hyaline fibromatosis 878
giant cell tumors
  giant cell fibroblastoma 857
  giant cell tumor of tendon sheath 874
proliferative lesions of the fascia
  nodular fasciitis 875
  cranial fasciitis of childhood 875

2. Schwannian/Neural Spindle Cell Tumors

These tumors are composed of elongated, narrow spindle cells that tend to have serpentine S-shaped nuclei and to be arranged in "wavy" fiber bundles. Immunohistochemistry for S-100 is useful, but not specific.

3. Spindle Cell Tumors of Muscle

Smooth muscle cells have more abundant cytoplasm than fibroblasts or Schwann cells. The cytoplasm is trichrome-positive and reacts with muscle markers—desmin, muscle-specific actin. The nuclei tend to have blunt ends. In neoplasms, the cells tend to be arranged in whorled bundles.

4. Melanocytic Spindle Cell Tumors

Melanocytic spindle cell tumors may have many attributes of Schwannian tumors described above. S-100 is positive, and HMB-45 is often negative in the spindle cell melanomas. Diagnosis of melanoma then depends on recognizing melanocytic differentiation (pigment synthesis) or a characteristic intraepidermal in situ or microinvasive component.

5. Tumors and Proliferations of Angiogenic Cells

There is a dermal proliferation of vascular endothelium. Factor VIII staining may be helpful in demonstrating endothelial differentiation. The many variants of benign hemangiomas should be carefully considered in the differential diagnosis of Kaposi's sarcoma and angiosarcoma.

6. *Tumors of Adipose Tissue*

7. *Tumors of Cartilaginous Tissue*

8. *Tumors of Osseous Tissue*

D. Cysts of the Dermis and Subcutis

A cyst is a space lined by epithelium; its contents are usually a product of its lining. Some cysts are inclusion or retention cysts of normal structures (hair follicle–related cysts). Others are benign neoplasms. Some malignant neoplasms may be cystic. These tend to be larger and asymmetric, with a poorly circumscribed and infiltrative border. Their epithelial lining is proliferative, with cytologic atypia.

1. *Pilar Differentiation*

Cystic proliferations are present in the dermis; these show spaces surrounded by epithelium of follicular origin and differentiation. Keratin is usually seen in the cystic cavity. Associated cells may be sparse or may include lymphocytes and plasma cells.

2. *Eccrine and Similar Differentiation*

Cystic proliferations are present in the dermis; these show spaces surrounded by eccrine epithelium (small dark epithelial cells). The epithelium of ciliated and bronchogenic cysts is not eccrine but may resemble that of an eccrine cyst.

3. *Apocrine Differentiation*

Cystic proliferations are present in the dermis; these show spaces surrounded by apocrine epithelium (large pink cells with decapitation secretion). There may be lymphocytes and plasma cells (syringocystadenoma).

VII. INFLAMMATORY AND OTHER DISORDERS OF SKIN APPENDAGES

The hair, sebaceous glands, eccrine glands, apocrine glands, and nails may be involved in inflammatory processes (hidradenitis, folliculitis). Some neoplasms may masquerade as inflammatory processes.

A. Pathology Involving Hair Follicles

Inflammatory processes may present as alopecia, or as follicular localization of inflammatory rashes. Acne and related conditions present as dilatation of follicles that are filled with keratin.

1. *Scant Inflammation*

There is follicular alteration with a sparse infiltrate of cells, mainly lymphocytes.

2. *Lymphocytes Predominant*

There is follicular alteration with an inflammatory infiltrate mainly of lymphocytes.

a. *With Eosinophils Present*

Eosinophils are prominent in the infiltrate and may infiltrate the follicular structures.

3. *Neutrophils Prominent*

There is a follicular alteration with an inflammatory infiltrate containing neutrophils, which may result in disruption of the follicle.

fungal folliculitis
  Majocchi granuloma (*T rubrum*) 521
  favus (*T schoenleinii*) 521
Pityrosporum folliculitis 522
viral folliculitis 588
acne fulminans 403

4. *Plasma Cells Prominent*

Plasma cells are seen in abundance in the infiltrate. In most instances they are admixed with lymphocytes.

acne keloidalis 461
fungal folliculitis 521
alopecia of secondary syphilis 411, 506

5. *Fibrosing and Suppurative Follicular Disorders*

There is extensive fibrosis of the dermis, often with keratin tunnels of follicular origin and with embedded hairs with associated foreign-body inflammation. Neutrophils and plasma cells are seen in abundance in the infiltrate, in addition to lymphocytes.

acne keloidalis 461
follicular occlusion disorders
  pilonidal sinus 461
  hidradenitis suppurativa 461
  acne conglobata 461
  perifolliculitis capitis abscedens et suffodiens (dissecting cellulitis of the scalp) 461
deep folliculitis
  folliculitis barbae, decalvans 461

B. Pathology Involving Sweat Glands

The sebaceous glands, eccrine glands, and apocrine glands may be involved in inflammatory processes (hidradenitis).

1. *Scant inflammation*

Sweat glands are abnormal in color or size and number, but there is little or no inflammation.

argyria 298
syringosquamous metaplasia 290
eccrine nevus 687, 777
eccrine angiomatous hamartoma 777
coma blister 291

2. *Lymphocytes Predominant*

There is a predominantly lymphocytic infiltrate in and around the sweat glands.

lupus erythematosus 253
syringolymphoid hyperplasia
  with alopecia 416
lichen striatus 174
morphea/scleroderma 274

a. *With Plasma Cells*

There is a predominantly lymphocytic infiltrate in and around the sweat glands. Plasma cells are also present as a minority population.

lupus erythematosus 253
secondary syphilis 503
cheilitis glandularis 328
morphea/scleroderma 274

b. *With Eosinophils*

There is an inflammatory infiltrate with eosinophils in and around the sweat glands.

insect bite reactions 565

c. *With Neutrophils*

There is an inflammatory infiltrate with neutrophils in and around the sweat glands.

insect bite reactions 565
neutrophilic eccrine hidradenitis 289
secondary syphilis 503

C. Pathology Involving Nerves

Specific inflammatory involvement of nerves is uncommon in dermatopathology.

1. *Lymphocytic Infiltrates*

Neurotropic spread of neoplasms, especially neurotropic melanoma, may be associated with a dense lymphocytic infiltrate that may tend to obscure a subtle infiltrate of neoplastic spindle cells.

neurotropic melanoma 668
leprosy 477
herpes zoster 573

2. *Mixed Inflammatory Infiltrates*

There is a mixed inflammatory infiltrate involving nerves.

leprosy 477
erythema chronicum migrans 511

3. *Neoplastic Infiltrates*

Many neoplasms may occasionally involve nerves. The involvement by carcinomas (basal cell, squamous cell, metastatic) is commonly in the perineural space, whereas involvement by neurotropic melanoma tends to occupy the endoneurium and to be associated with a dense lymphocytic infiltrate that may tend to obscure a subtle infiltrate of neoplastic spindle cells.

neurotropic melanoma 668
neurotropic carcinoma 1005

D. Pathology of the Nails

Several inflammatory dermatoses more often seen elsewhere in the skin may present incidentally or exclusively in the nails. The reaction patterns may vary from those seen elsewhere because of the unique responses of the nail plate to injury.

1. *Lymphocytic Infiltrates*

spongiotic dermatitis 423
lichen planus 166, 424
melanoma in situ with lichenoid inflammation 663

2. *Lymphocytes With Neutrophils*

psoriasis 156, 424
tinea unguium, onychomycosis 426, 518

3. *Bullous Diseases*

Darier's disease 426
pemphigus 426
erythema multiforme 426
toxic epidermal necrolysis 426
epidermolysis bullosa 426

4. *Parasitic Infestations*

scabies 559

5. *Melanocytic Proliferation*

malignant melanoma, acral-lentiginous type 663

VIII. DISORDERS OF THE SUBCUTIS

The reactions in the subcutis are mostly inflammatory, although tumors (proliferations) of the subcutis do occur (lipoma). Pathologic conditions arising in the dermis may infiltrate the subcutis.

A. Subcutaneous Vasculitis and Vasculopathy (Septal or Lobular)

True vasculitis is defined by the presence of necrosis and inflammation in vessel walls. Other forms of vasculopathy include thrombosis and thrombophlebitis, fibrointimal hyperplasia, and neoplastic infiltration of vessel walls.

1. *Neutrophilic*

Neutrophils and disrupted nuclei are present in the wall of the vessel, with associated eosinophilic "fibrinoid" necrosis.

leukocytoclastic vasculitis 194
subcutaneous polyarteritis nodosa 191
superficial migratory thrombophlebitis 437
erythema nodosum leprosum 486

2. *Lymphocytic*

The concept of "lymphocytic vasculitis" is a controversial one. Many disorders characterized by lymphocytes within the walls of vessels are best classified as lymphocytic infiltrates. The term *vasculitis* may be appropriate when there is vessel wall damage, as in nodular vasculitis, even in the absence of neutrophils and "fibrinoid."

nodular vasculitis 437
perniosis 312, 444
angiocentric lymphomas 199, 836
superficial migratory thrombophlebitis (older lesion) 437

3. *Granulomatous*

The inflammatory infiltrate in the vessel walls is composed of mixed cells, including greater or lesser numbers of epithelioid histiocytes, and giant cells. Other cell types, including lymphocytes and plasma cells and sometimes neutrophils and eosinophils, are commonly present also.

erythema induratum/nodular vasculitis (inconspicuous vasculitis) 437
erythema nodosum leprosum 486
Wegener's granulomatosis 200
Churg-Strauss vasculitis 199
Crohn's disease 326, 361

B. Septal Panniculitis Without Vasculitis

1. *Septal Panniculitis, Lymphocytes and Mixed Infiltrates*

The inflammation predominantly involves the subcutaneous septa, although there may be "spillover" into the fat lobules. The infiltrate is mainly lymphocytic, but other cells can be found, including plasma cells and acute inflammatory cells.

erythema nodosum and variants 431
Crohn's disease 326, 361
morphea 274, 450

2. *Septal Panniculitis, Granulomatous*

Subcutaneous granulomas may present as ill-defined collections of epithelioid histiocytes, as well-formed epithelioid-cell granulomas, and as palisading granulomas in which histiocytes are radially arranged around areas of necrosis or necrobiosis.

palisaded granulomas
subcutaneous granuloma annulare 328
rheumatoid nodules 334
necrobiosis lipoidica 330
sarcoidosis 322
lichen scrofulosorum 473
Crohn's disease 326, 361
subcutaneous infections
syphilis 503
tuberculosis 434, 468

3. Septal Panniculitis, Sclerotic

Sclerosis of the panniculitis may begin as a septal process and extend into the lobules

scleroderma, morphea 450
eosinophilic fasciitis 279
ischemic liposclerosis 448
toxins 443

C. Lobular Panniculitis Without Vasculitis

The inflammation is mainly confined to the lobules, although there may be some septal involvement.

1. Lobular Panniculitis, Lymphocytes Predominant

Lymphocytes are the primary infiltrating cells.

lupus panniculitis 440
nodular vasculitis/erythema induratum, inapparent vasculitis 437
poststeroid panniculitis 447
subcutaneous lymphoma-leukemia 805

2. Lobular Panniculitis, Lymphocytes and Plasma Cells

Lymphocytes and plasma cells are the primary infiltrating cells.

lupus profundus 440
scleroderma 274, 450

3. Lobular Panniculitis, Neutrophilic

Lymphocytes and neutrophils are the primary infiltrating cells.

infection (cellulitis) 457
ruptured follicles and cysts 318
pancreatic fat necrosis 444

4. Lobular Panniculitis, Eosinophils Prominent

Lymphocytes and eosinophils are the primary infiltrating cells.

eosinophilic fasciitis 279
eosinophilic panniculitis 434
arthropod bites 565
parasites 559

5. Lobular Panniculitis, Histiocytes Prominent

Lymphocytes and histiocytes are the primary infiltrating cells.

cytophagic histiocytic panniculitis 448
Rosai-Dorfman disease 430

6. Lobular Panniculitis, Mixed With Foam Cells

Lymphocytes, plasma cells, and a variety of infiltrating cells can be seen, including giant cells and foamy histiocytes.

α_1-antitrypsin deficiency panniculitis 434
Weber-Christian disease 441
traumatic fat necrosis 443
cold panniculitis 443
injection granuloma 444
factitious panniculitis 443
necrobiotic xanthogranuloma with paraproteinemia 604

7. Lobular Panniculitis, Granulomatous

Lymphocytes and histiocytes are the primary infiltrating cells.

erythema induratum/nodular vasculitis (if vasculitis is inapparent) 437
palisaded granulomas
subcutaneous granuloma annulare (pseudorheumatoid nodule) 328
rheumatoid nodules 334
subcutaneous sarcoidosis 322
tuberculosis 434, 468

8. Lobular Panniculitis, Crystal Deposits, Calcifications

Crystalline deposits derived from free fatty acids or other precipitated salts are present in the fat lobules.

sclerema neonatorum 445
subcutaneous fat necrosis of the newborn 446
gout 382
oxalosis 430
calcifying panniculitis 447

9. Lobular Panniculitis, Necrosis Prominent

There is fat necrosis with a resulting infiltrate that is mixed.

pancreatic panniculitis 444
erythema induratum, inapparent vasculitis 437

necrobiotic xanthogranuloma
  with paraproteinemia 604
infarct 185
abscess 457, 526

10. Lobular Panniculitis, Embryonic Fat Pattern

Because of atrophy or failure of normal morphogenesis, immature small fat cells are present in the lobules.

lipoatrophy 444
lipodystrophy 444
postcorticosteroid injection 447

11. Lobular Panniculitis, Miscellaneous

Lymphocytes, plasma cells, and a variety of infiltrating cells can be seen, including giant cells and histiocytes.

lipomembranous panniculitis 448
lipogranulomatosis of Rothmann-Makai 443
early stages of pyoderma gangrenosum 206, 450
necrobiotic xanthogranuloma 604

D. Mixed Lobular and Septal Panniculitis

Neoplastic infiltrates and inflammation due to trauma or infection do not respect anatomic compartments of the subcutis.

1. With Hemorrhage or Sclerosis

Inflammation due to trauma is likely to be associated with hemorrhage, neutrophilic inflammation, and sclerosis in late lesions.

traumatic panniculitis 443
cold panniculitis 443
injections, including factitial panniculitis ... 443
blunt trauma: sclerosing lipogranuloma 443

2. With Many Neutrophils

Neutrophilic inflammation diffusely involves the subcutis.

necrotizing fasciitis (bacterial infection) 459
abscesses 457, 526
North American blastomycosis 529
pyoderma gangrenosum (also involves
  dermis) 206, 450
ecthyma gangrenosum 465
α_1-antitrypsin deficiency 434
infection (*cellulitis*) 459
dissecting cellulitis of the scalp
  (perifolliculitis capitis abscedens et
    suffodiens) 461
hidradenitis suppurativa 461
ruptured follicles and cysts 317, 460, 694

3. With Many Lymphocytes

Lymphocytic infiltrates diffusely involve the subcutis.

lupus panniculitis 259, 440
chronic lymphocytic leukemia 840
subcutaneous T-cell lymphoma 441, 841
histiocytic cytophagic panniculitis
  (early lesion) 450

4. With Cytophagic Histiocytes

Histiocytes with phagocytized erythrocytes diffusely infiltrate the subcutis.

α_1-antitrypsin deficiency (late lesion) 434
histiocytic cytophagic panniculitis
  (late lesion) 448
Rosai-Dorfman disease 430

5. With Granulomas

There is granulomatous inflammation diffusely involving the subcutis.

gummatous tertiary syphilis 508
erythema nodosum leprosum 486
chronic erythema nodosum 431
mycobacterial panniculitis 434, 450
subcutaneous sarcoidosis 322

D. Subcutaneous Abscesses

There is a collection of neutrophils in the subcutis, usually surrounded by granulation tissue and fibrosis.

1. With Neutrophils

The center of the abscess contains pus, which is viscous because of the presence of DNA fragments derived from neutrophils and dead organisms.

acute or chronic bacterial abscesses 457
deep fungal infections 526
  phaeohyphomycotic cyst 528
  North American blastomycosis 529
  chromoblastomycosis 533
  cutaneous alternariosis 529
  paracoccidioidomycosis 532
  coccidioidomycosis 534
  sporotrichosis 541
protothecosis 546
mycobacterial panniculitis 450, 468

Lever's Histopathology of the Skin, eighth edition, edited by David Elder et al. Lippincott–Raven Publishers, Philadelphia © 1997.

CHAPTER 6

Congenital Diseases (Genodermatoses)

Bernett Johnson Jr. and Paul Honig

ICHTHYOSIS

A classification of ichthyosis includes four major and three minor forms. In addition, there are a number of syndromes that are associated with ichthyosis.

Ichthyosis Vulgaris

Ichthyosis vulgaris, which is inherited in an autosomal dominant fashion, is a common disorder. It develops a few months after birth. The skin shows scales that are large and adherent on the extensor surfaces of the extremities, resembling fish scales, and are small elsewhere. The flexural creases are spared. Keratosis pilaris is often present, and the palms and soles may show hyperkeratosis.

A noninherited form of the disease may appear in patients with lymphoma, particularly Hodgkin's disease,[1] but this form has been reported also in association with carcinoma[2] and sarcoidosis.

Histopathology. The characteristic finding is the association of a moderate degree of hyperkeratosis with a thin or absent granular layer (Fig. 6-1). The hyperkeratosis often extends into the hair follicles, resulting in large keratotic follicular plugs. The dermis is normal.

Histogenesis. Labeling with tritiated thymidine shows a normal rate of epidermal proliferation.[3] The hyperkeratosis is regarded as a retention keratosis resulting from increased adhesiveness of the stratum corneum.[3] The reason for this, as seen by electron microscopy, is a delay in the dissolution of the desmosomal disks in the horny layer. Keratohyaline granules are regularly seen on electron microscopy, in contrast to light microscopy. The stratum granulosum, however, consists of only a single layer, and the keratohyaline granules appear small and crumbly or spongy, evidence of defective synthesis. The reason for the inadequate formation of keratohyaline granules lies in a defect in the synthesis of filaggrin, a histidine-rich protein.[4] Defective profilaggrin expression in ichthyosis vulgaris may be a result of selectively impaired post transcriptional control.[5] In noninherited ichthyosis vulgaris associated with neoplasia, the keratohyaline granules have been described as being small but showing a normal structure, indicating a reduced but not an abnormal synthesis.[6]

Differential Diagnosis. Although the noninflamed but dry skin of patients with atopic dermatitis clinically resembles ichthyosis vulgaris, on histologic examination it does not show the features of ichthyosis vulgaris but rather increased epidermal thickness, patchy parakeratosis, and slight hypergranulosis in places, as seen in chronic dermatitis.[7]

X-Linked Ichthyosis

X-linked ichthyosis is recessively inherited, about 90% caused by gene deletion. It is only rarely present at birth. Although female heterozygotes are frequently affected, males have a more severe form of the disorder. The thickness of the adherent scales increases during childhood.[8] In contrast to ichthyosis vulgaris, the flexural creases may be involved.

Histopathology. There is hyperkeratosis. The granular layer is normal or slightly thickened but not thinned as in dominant ichthyosis vulgaris. The epidermis may be slightly thickened.[9]

Histogenesis. X-linked ichthyosis, like ichthyosis vulgaris, shows a normal rate of epidermal proliferation. The disorder is a retention hyperkeratosis characterized by delayed dissolution of the desmosomal disks in the horny layer. In contrast to that of ichthyosis vulgaris, the synthesis of keratohyaline granules in X-linked ichthyosis is not defective, and the rate of synthesis is slightly increased.[10] The cause of the retention hyperkeratosis in X-linked ichthyosis is the virtual absence of steroid sulfatase activity. This was first recognized in skin fibroblasts[11] but was found subsequently also in the entire epidermis and in leukocytes.[12] Steroid sulfatase normally acts on cholesteryl sulfate, a product of the Odland bodies that is discharged with them from the granular cells into the intercellular space and provides cell cohesion in the lower stratum corneum. Failure of steroid sulfatase to remove cholesteryl sulfate results in persistent cell cohesion even in the upper stratum corneum and interferes with the normal process of desquamation.[13]

B. Johnson Jr. and P. Honig: Department of Dermatology, University of Pennsylvania, Philadelphia, PA

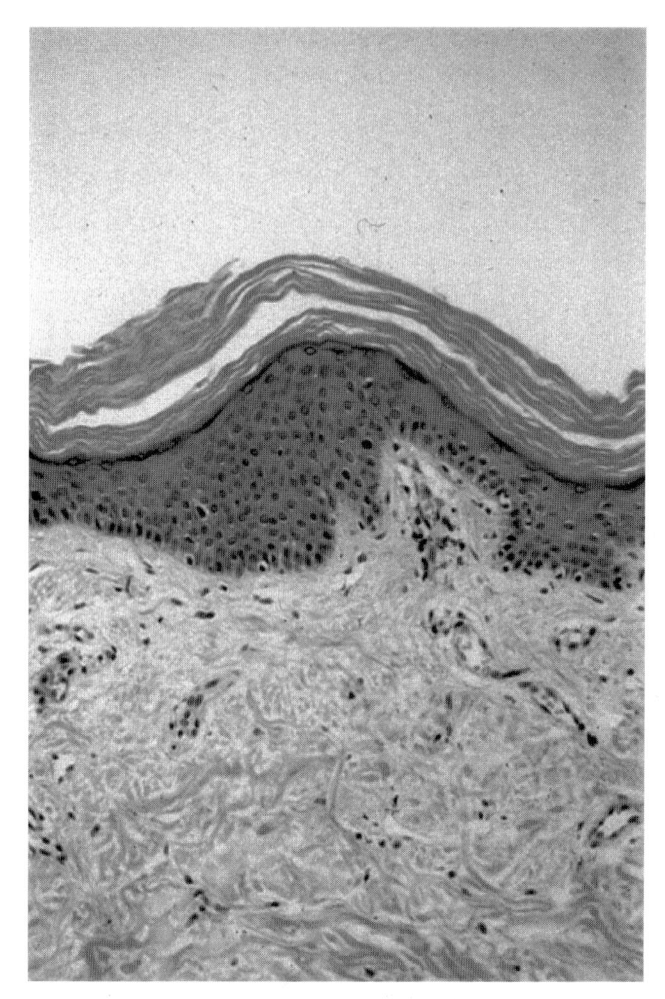

FIG. 6-1. Ichthyosis vulgaris
Hyperkeratosis with a diminished and focally absent granular cell layer (original magnification × 100).

Epidermolytic Hyperkeratosis

Epidermolytic hyperkeratosis, an autosomal dominantly inherited disease also known as *bullous congenital ichthyosiform erythroderma*, shows from the time of birth generalized erythema (Fig. 6-2). Within a few days after birth, there is thick, brown, verrucous scaling (Fig. 6-3). The flexural surfaces of the extremities show marked involvement, often consisting of furrowed hyperkeratosis. Vesicles and bullae are usually encountered only during the first few years.

Histopathology. A characteristic histologic picture is seen in the epidermis (Fig. 6-4) and is referred to either as epidermolytic hyperkeratosis[3] or as granular degeneration.[14] It is present in bullous as well as in nonbullous areas. There are variously sized clear spaces around the nuclei in the upper stratum spinosum and in the stratum granulosum. Peripheral to the clear spaces the cells show indistinct boundaries formed by lightly staining material or by keratohyaline granules. One observes a markedly thickened granular layer containing an increased number of irregularly shaped keratohyaline granules and compact hyperkeratosis.[15] When bullae form, they arise intraepidermally through separation of edematous cells from one another.[16] The upper dermis shows a moderately severe, chronic inflammatory infiltrate. Mitotic figures are five times more numerous than in normal epidermis.[3]

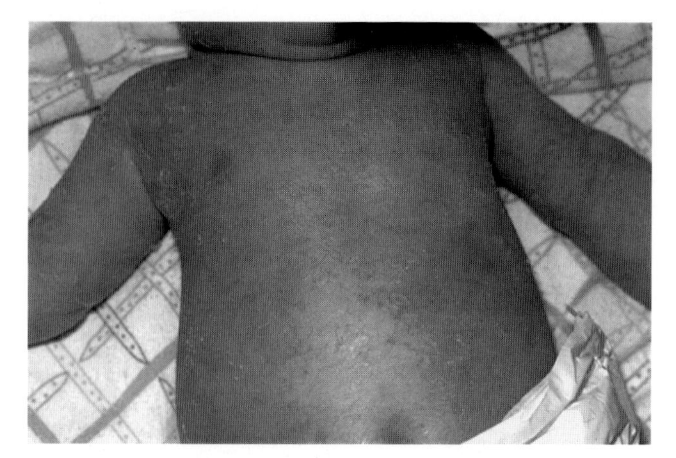

FIG. 6-2. Epidermolytic hyperkeratosis
Infant with generalized erythema, scaling, and a re-epithlialized right axilla (previously denued).

Pathogenesis. Defects in keratin genes (K1 and K10) are now known to be associated with this disorder. Mutations were found in the carboxy terminal of the rod domain of keratin 1 and the aminoterminal of the rod domain of keratin 10.[17] The essential electron microscopic features are excessive production of tonofilaments and excessive and premature formation of keratohyaline granules, so that at the periphery of the cells numerous keratohyaline granules are embedded in thick shells of irregularly clumped tonofilaments.[14,18] The desmosomes appear normal, but the association of tonofilaments and desmosomes is disturbed, so that many desmosomes are attached to only one keratinocyte instead of connecting two neighboring keratinocytes. Because of this disturbance in desmosomal attachment, blister formation takes place and real acantholysis occurs.[19] Labeling with tritiated thymidine reveals greatly increased proliferative activity in the epidermis.[3] It can be concluded that keratinization is both excessive and abnormal.

Differential Diagnosis. Although the histologic picture of epidermolytic hyperkeratosis is diagnostic for the type of

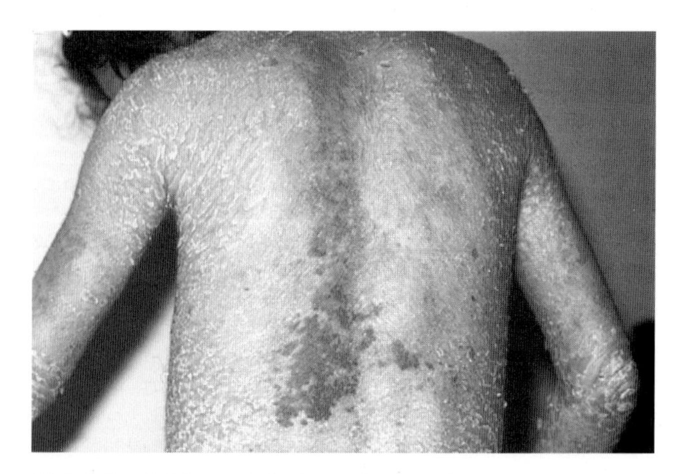

FIG. 6-3. Epidermolytic hyperkeratosis
Erythema and thick "scales" in older child.

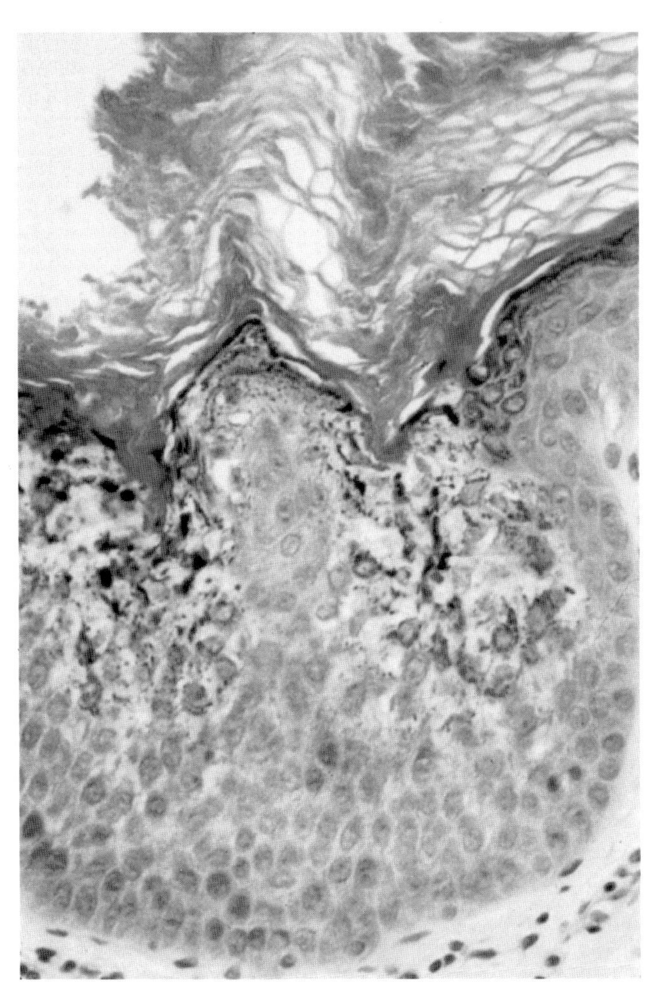

FIG. 6-4. Epidermolytic hyperkeratosis
There is vacuolization of the upper and mid-spinus layer. There is hyperkeratosis with large keratohyaline granules in the vacoulated expanded granular cell layer (original magnification × 100).

ichthyosis called epidermolytic hyperkeratosis, it is not specific for it. Hyperkeratosis is found also in several other seemingly unrelated conditions[20,21]: epidermolytic keratosis palmaris et plantaris, solitary epidermolytic acanthoma, disseminated epidermolytic acanthoma, and linear epidermal nevus, usually of the systematized type. This latter entity was thought to be an entirely different condition than epidermolytic hyperkeratosis but with similar histologic findings. However, it is now known that epidermal nevi of the epidermolytic hyperkeratotic type are a mosaic genetic disorder of suprabasal keratin (i.e., point mutations of 10k alleles of epidermal cells in keratinocytes from lesional skin) that can be transmitted to offspring producing generalized epidermolytic hyperkeratosis.[22] Epidermolytic hyperkeratosis can be an incidental finding in a variety of conditions.

Autosomal Recessive Ichthyosis

In many instances it is possible to subdivide recessive ichthyosis into two types. A less severe type, *congenital ichthyosiform erythroderma*, shows fine white scales with fairly pronounced erythroderma and has a tendency to improve at the time of puberty. The more severe type, *lamellar ichthyosis*, shows large, plate–like scales and severe ectropion but only slight erythroderma. In both forms the flexural surfaces and the palms and soles are involved.[12,23] Several hypotheses have been proposed for this condition, including a transglutaminase acylation defect[24] and/or a defect in lamellar body secretion.[25]

In rare instances, autosomal recessive ichthyosis is associated with storage of neutral lipid in multiple tissues, the Chanarin-Dorfman syndrome.[26] It is easily recognized by the presence of lipid vacuoles in leukocytes.

Histopathology. The histologic findings in both congenital ichthyosiform erythroderma and lamellar ichthyosis are nonspecific. As a rule, however, congenital ichthyosiform erythroderma shows only mild thickening of the stratum corneum with foci of parakeratosis, whereas lamellar ichthyosis has a markedly thickened stratum corneum without areas of parakeratosis.[27]

In the Chanarin-Dorfman syndrome, lipid stains reveal prominent neutral lipid droplets in some of the epidermal cells.[26]

CHILD Syndrome

This rare but clinically striking dermatosis shows from birth unilateral ichthyosiform erythroderma and ipsilateral underdevelopment of the limbs (Fig. 6-5). It is known under the acronym Congenital **H**emidysplasia with **I**chthyosiform erythrodermal and **L**imb **D**efects.[28] Because nearly all published cases have been female, it is likely that the disease is the result of an X-linked dominant gene defect that is lethal in the hemizygote male fetus. Peroxisomal abnormalities have been found in fibroblasts from involved skin in these children.[29]

Histopathology. On a thickened epidermis one observes pronounced hyperkeratosis with prominent parakeratotic foci.[30]

Harlequin Ichthyosis

Harlequin ichthyosis is a rare condition that is frequently but not invariably fatal.[31] It is probably of autosomal recessive inheritance since in one family five siblings had the disease. At

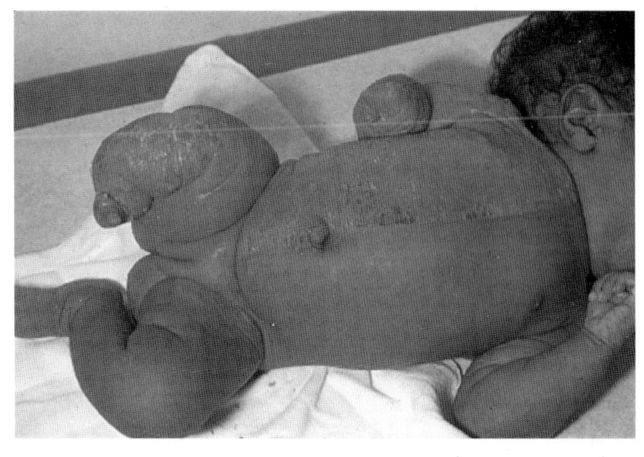

FIG. 6-5. CHILD syndrome
Note unilateral erythema, scaling and underdevelopment of limbs.

birth, the child is encased in a thick, horny cuirass with deep fissures. Marked ectropion and eclabium are present.

Histopathology. There is usually a massive hyperkeratosis, the stratum corneum being 20 to 30 times thicker than the stratum malpighii.[32] The appearance of the stratum granulosum is variable; it may be normal or it may be flattened to absent. A stain for fat has shown small droplets of neutral fat distributed uniformly throughout the cornified cells. Some cases have shown papillomatosis in addition to the massive hyperkeratosis or areas of parakeratosis.

Pathogenesis. An abnormality in lamellar body formation and secretion[33] may exist, which results in inadequate delivery of desmosomal proteases to the stratum corneum,[25] leading to failure to degrade corneodesmosers and, therefore, massive hyperkeratosis.[34]

Erythrokeratodermia Variabilis

A rare, dominantly inherited disorder, erythrokeratodermia variabilis starts in infancy rather than at birth. It has two morphologic components. First, areas of erythema expand centrifugally and coalesce into circinate figures. These lesions fluctuate, sometimes rapidly, in their configuration and extent and thus are "variable." Second, persistent hyperkeratotic plaques develop both within the areas of erythema and in areas of apparently normal skin.[35] In rare cases, referred to as *progressive symmetric erythrokeratodermia*, only persistent erythematous hyperkeratotic plaques are present, and they are limited to the extremities.[36]

Histopathology. The changes are nonspecific. In the hyperkeratotic plaques, they consist of hyperkeratosis with moderate papillomatosis and acanthosis. The granular layer appears normal, being two to three cell layers thick.[35]

Pathogenesis. Labeling with tritiated thymidine shows a normal rate of proliferation. It is likely that the hyperkeratosis is due to decreased shedding of horny cells and is of the retention type.[35]

Ichthyosis Linearis Circumflexa

A recessive disorder that is present at birth or starts shortly thereafter, ichthyosis linearis circumflexa shows extensive migratory polycyclic lesions of erythema and scaling.[37] Some of the areas show at their periphery a distinctive "double-edged" scale. The presence of extensive erythema causes a resemblance to psoriasis. The dermatosis persists through life. In more than half of the reported cases, hair anomalies have been present in the scalp, usually trichorrhexis invaginata, the so-called Netherton's syndrome.[38]

Histopathology. The areas of erythema and scaling show nonspecific changes with some resemblance to psoriasis, such as elongation of the rete ridges and hyperkeratosis, as well as parakeratosis.[39]

The double-edged scale frequently shows in the upper stratum malpighii intracellular edema and irregular spongiosis resulting in multilocular vesicles or vesiculopustules within the horny layer.[40] In other cases, focal accumulations of PAS-positive, diastase-resistant, homogeneous material representing exuded serum protein are seen within a parakeratotic stratum corneum.[41] The presence of such exudative changes, however, is not specific or characteristic for ichthyosis linearis circumscripta, as has been claimed.[42]

Pathogenesis. Electron microscopic examination has shown the presence of multilocular vesicles that are filled with an amorphous substance compatible with serum protein.[43]

Syndromes Associated with Ichthyosis

There is an expanding list of syndromes that combine ichthyosis with neuroectodermal and mesodermal defects.[44] Some of the syndromes described in the literature may be chance associations.[45] Among the well-established syndromes are the *Sjögren-Larsson syndrome,* which is characterized by lamellar ichthyosis in association with mental retardation and spastic paresis[46]; skin fibroblasts and leukocytes from these patients are deficient in activity of the enzyme fatty alcohol, NAD oxidoreductase[47]; *Rud's syndrome,* showing generalized ichthyosis with hypogonadism, mental deficiency, and epilepsy[48]; *Conradi's syndrome,* in which ichthyosis with a whorled pattern is associated with skeletal and ocular abnormalities.[49] Some forms are associated with peroxisome abnormalities.[50] *Netherton's syndrome,* which consists of a combination of either ichthyosis linearis circumflexa or, less commonly, lamellar ichthyosis with trichorrhexis invaginata; IBIDS syndrome, icthyosis associated with brittle hair, impaired intelligence, decreased fertility, and short stature[44]; and PIBIDS syndrome, showing photosensitivity and IBIDS. Patients with these syndromes have sulfur deficient, sparse hair. Also, KID syndrome, keratitis associated with ichithyosis and deafness[51]; neutral lipid storage disease, ichthyosis with cataracts, deafness, ataxia and lipid droplets in many circulating cells[52]; and multiple sulfatase deficiencies, a combination of ichthyosis, neurodegeneration, organomegaly, and skeletal dysplasia (includes steroid sulfatase deficiency). The only syndrome showing specific histologic changes in the skin is *Refsum's syndrome.*

Refsum's Syndrome

An autosomal recessive disorder, Refsum's syndrome is characterized by generalized ichthyosis, cerebellar ataxia, progressive paresis of the extremities, and retinitis pigmentosa.

Histopathology. The skin shows hyperkeratosis, hypergranulosis, and acanthosis. In the basal and suprabasal cells of the epidermis are variably sized vacuoles that, on staining for lipids, are seen to contain lipid accumulations.[53]

Pathogenesis. The primary metabolic defect in Refsum's syndrome is an accumulation of phytanic acid, which results from a deficiency of alpha-phytanic acid alpha-hydroxylase.[54]

KERATOSIS PALMARIS ET PLANTARIS

Three major autosomal dominant forms and two autosomal recessive forms of keratosis palmaris et plantaris exist. The three dominantly inherited forms are:

1. *Keratosis palmaris et plantaris of Unna-Thost,* showing either diffuse or localized, occasionally linear hyperkeratosis of the palms and soles (Fig. 6-6). A division into two types , a cir-

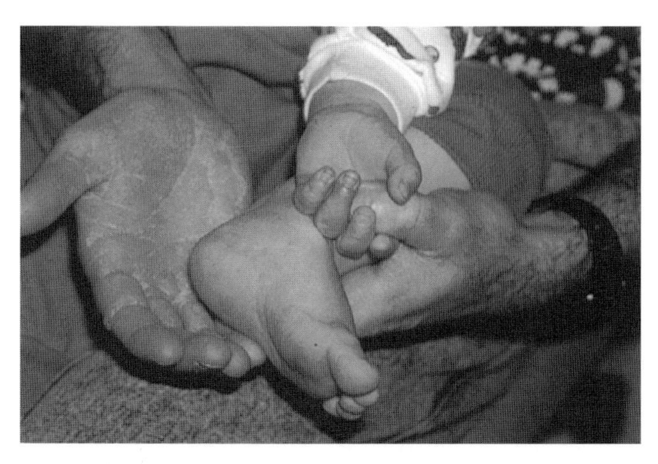

FIG. 6-6. Keratosis palmeris et plantaris of Unna-Thost Thickened palms and soles of child and thickened palms of his father.

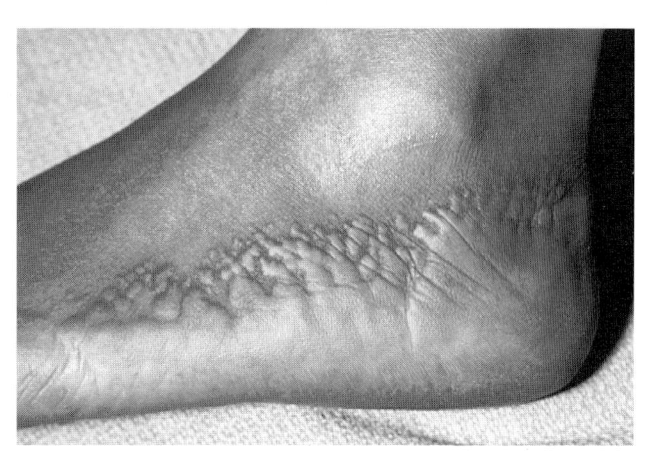

FIG. 6-7. Acrokeratoelastoidosis Firm papules at side of foot.

cumscribed type with limitation to the palms and soles and an extending type with gradual progression to the dorsa of the hands and feet, the ankles and wrists, and the elbows and knees, is not tenable because both types may occur in the same family.[55]

2. *Epidermolytic keratosis palmaris et plantaris,* although clinically indistinguishable from the Unna-Thost type, histologically shows epidermolytic hyperkeratosis. Apparently this form is quite common.[56] This variant has been associated with mutations in keratin type 9 localized within the keratin gene cluster on chromosome 17q.[57]

3. *Keratosis palmo-plantaris punctata* (or *papulosa*) has multiple keratotic plugs.

The two recessively inherited forms are:

1. *Keratosis palmaris et plantaris of the Meleda type*, showing diffuse involvement of the palms and soles and a marked tendency toward progression to the dorsa of the hands and feet, the ankles and wrists, and the elbows and knees.[58]

2. The *Papillon-Lefèvre syndrome* shows the clinical characteristics of the Meleda type in association with periodontosis resulting in the loss first of the deciduous teeth and later of the permanent teeth.[59]

In addition, keratosis palmaris et plantaris occurs in three syndromes: (1) pachyonychia congenita, (2) hidrotic ectodermal dysplasia, and (3) the Richner-Hanhart syndrome associated with tyrosinemia.

Histopathology. In keratosis palmaris et plantaris of the Unna-Thost type and the Meleda type, as well as in the Papillon-Lefèvre syndrome, the histologic picture is nonspecific, consisting of considerable hyperkeratosis, hypergranulosis, acanthosis, and a sparse inflammatory infiltrate of lymphocytes in the upper dermis.[58,59]

In epidermolytic keratosis palmaris et plantaris, the histologic picture is identical with that seen in epidermolytic hyperkeratosis. Many cells in the middle and upper stratum malpighii appear vacuolated, and scattered cavities are present as a result of ruptured cell walls. Keratohyaline granules are numerous and large.[60–62]

In keratosis palmo-plantaris punctata, there is massive hyperkeratosis over a sharply limited area, with depression of the underlying malpighian layer below the general level of the epidermis. There is an increase in the thickness of the granular layer. The dermis is free of inflammation.[63] In two cases reported as punctate keratoderma, a cornoid lamella was seen in the center of the hyperkeratotic plug; these cases represent punctate porokeratosis with the lesions limited to the palms and soles, rather than keratosis palmo-plantaris punctata.[64,65]

ACROKERATOELASTOIDOSIS

Acrokeratoelastoidosis is a rare, autosomal dominantly inherited condition in which firm, shiny papules are seen at the periphery of the palms and soles with extension to the dorsa of the fingers and the sides of the feet (Fig. 6-7).[66,67]

Histopathology. The essential histologic feature in the papules consists of diminution and fragmentation of the elastic fibers, especially in the deeper portions of the dermis.[66,67] Some of the fragmented elastic fibers appear thickened and tortuous.[68]

Histogenesis. On electron microscopic examination, the elastic fibers in the reticular dermis appear disaggregated, with fragmentation of the microfibrils.[67,69]

Differential Diagnosis. In *focal acral hyperkeratosis*, the lesions have the same clinical appearance as in acrokeratoelastoidosis. There may or may not be a familial predisposition, but the elastic tissue stains fail to reveal any abnormalities.[70,71] In *degenerative collagenous plaques of the hands* the lesions develop late in life; there is no involvement of the feet and no familial predisposition. These histologic changes consist of basophilic degeneration of the elastic tissue.[72,73]

PACHYONYCHIA CONGENITA

A disorder with autosomal dominant inheritance, pachyonychia congenita, is characterized by the following triad: (1) subungual hyperkeratosis with accumulation of hard, keratinous material beneath the distal portion of the nails (Fig. 6-8), lifting the nails from the nail bed; (2) keratosis palmaris et plantaris with thick callosities, especially on the soles, that are tender and are often associated with blister formation; and (3) thick white areas on the oral mucosa (Fig. 6-9) that resemble those seen in white sponge nevus and possess no tendency toward malignant

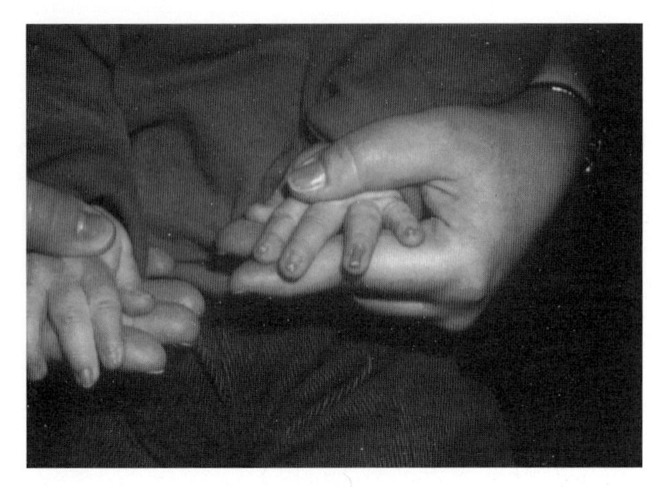

FIG. 6-8. Pachyonychia congenita
Thickened nails in infant with this syndrome.

degeneration.[74] Follicular hyperkeratosis may occur, mainly on the elbows and knees.

Histopathology. The nail bed shows marked hyperkeratosis. As in a normal nail bed, there is no granular layer.[74] The blisters that may be seen beneath and around the plantar callosities arise in the upper layers of the stratum malpighii through increasing intracellular edema and vacuolization. Unlike friction blisters, they show no areas of necrosis.[75] The oral lesions show thickening of the oral epithelium with extensive intracellular vacuolization, exactly as seen in white sponge nevus, and without evidence of dyskeratosis.[76]

Pathogenesis. A defect in keratin synthesis is suggested by mutations of K16 and K17 mapped to the type I keratin cluster on 17q.[77]

DYSKERATOSIS CONGENITA

Dyskeratosis congenita usually is inherited as an X-linked, recessive disorder, most likely location Xq28, occurring only in males; but in some instances it is transmitted in an autosomal dominant fashion, in which case females also may be affected.[78]

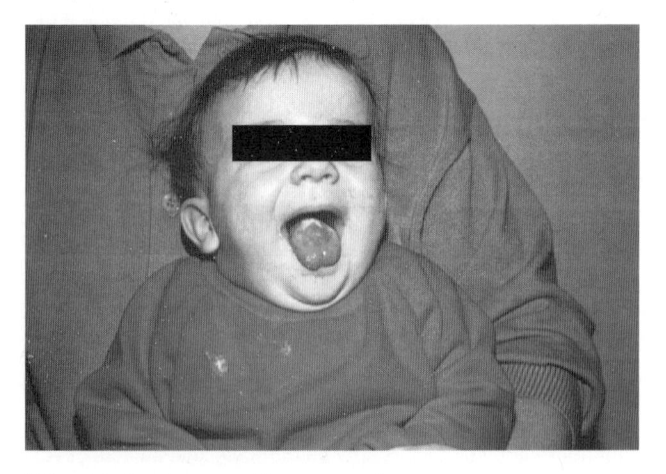

FIG. 6-9. Pachyonychia congenita
Note whitened mucosa at back of tongue.

It is characterized by the following triad: (1) dystrophy of the nails, with failure of the nails to form a nail plate; (2) white thickening (leukokeratosis) of the oral and occasionally also of the anal mucosa; and (3) extensive areas of netlike pigmentation of the skin suggestive of poikiloderma atrophicans vasculare but with less atrophy and telangiectasia. Carcinoma may develop in areas of buccal and anal leukokeratosis. In many cases, a Fanconi type of anemia develops that may begin with leukopenia and thrombocytopenia but ends in severe pancytopenia.[79]

Histopathology. In dyskeratosis congenita, the areas of netlike pigmentation show as their only constant feature melanophages in the upper dermis.[80] In contrast to poikiloderma atrophicans vasculare, atrophy of the epidermis, vacuolization of basal cells, and inflammatory infiltration of the upper dermis are either absent[81] or are mild and thus not diagnostic.[80] Oral biopsies may show squamous cell carcinoma in situ or invasive squamous cell carcinoma.

Pathogenesis. Although the primary defect of this disease remains unknown, it is likely that it predisposes dykeratosis congenita cells to develop chromosomal rearrangements.[82]

POROKERATOSIS

Porokeratosis has a wide variety of manifestations, but with the exception of the punctate type, it is characterized by a distinct peripheral keratotic ridge that corresponds histologically to the cornoid lamella (Fig. 6-10). Porokeratosis is inherited in an autosomal dominant pattern. Five different forms can be distinguished.[83]

The *plaque type,* as originally described by Mibelli, shows a single or a few lesions several centimeters in diameter. Rarely, there are numerous lesions.[84] The border often consists of a raised wall, having on its top a furrow filled with keratotic material. The lesions have a tendency toward peripheral extension.

Disseminated superficial actinic porokeratosis, the most common type, shows lesions that often are most pronounced in sun-exposed areas and may be exacerbated by exposure to the sun.[85] However, the term "actinic" cannot be applied to all cases. In some instances the lesions are distributed mainly in areas not exposed to the sun,[86] and in some cases immunosuppression has been the eliciting factor.[87] The extensor surfaces of the extremities are the most common site of involvement. The lesions in disseminated superficial porokeratosis are small and are surrounded only by a narrow, slightly raised, hyperkeratotic ridge without a distinct furrow.[85]

Linear porokeratosis may involve only a segment of the body or may have a generalized distribution. The lesions clinically resemble those of linear verrucous epidermal nevus.[88,89]

Porokeratosis plantaris, palmaris, et disseminata is characterized by the appearance in adolescence or early adult life of many lesions on the palms and soles and, subsequently, by the involvement of other areas of the body with large numbers of small superficial lesions.[90–92]

Punctate porokeratosis, limited to the palms and soles, shows numerous punctate, 1- to 2-mm seed-like keratotic plugs without tendency to centrifugal enlargement. They may be moderately tender to pressure.[93]

Development of a squamous cell carcinoma or of Bowen's disease within lesions of porokeratosis has been repeatedly re-

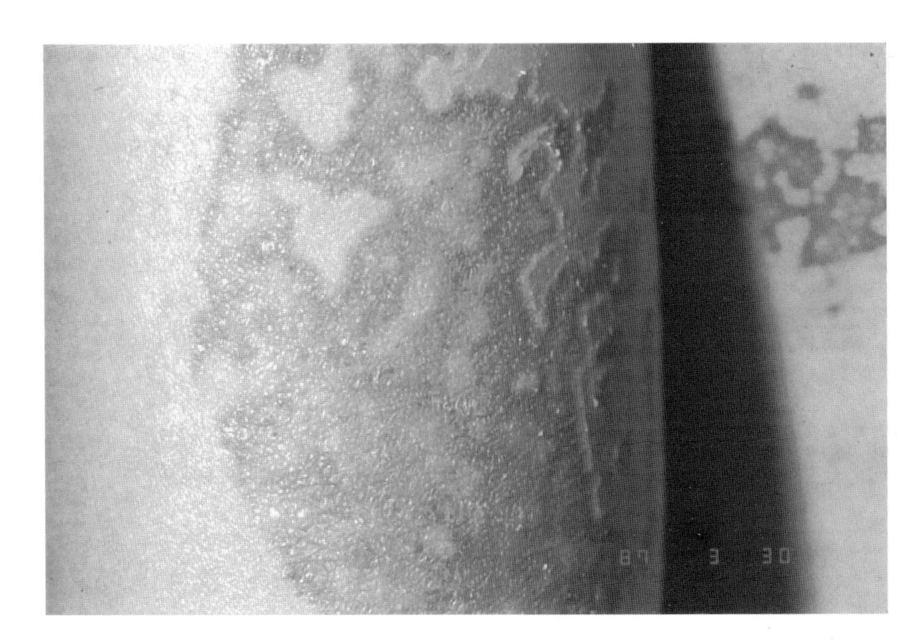

FIG. 6-10. Porokeratosis
Note ridging at periphery of lesions on right side of photograph.

ported in patients with solitary lesions [94] and in persons with disseminated lesions[90] or linear lesions.[95] In one reported instance with many lesions and multiple squamous cell carcinomas, visceral metastases resulted in death.[84]

Histopathology. It is essential that the specimen for biopsy be taken from the peripheral, raised, hyperkeratotic ridge. On histologic examination, the ridge then shows a keratin-filled invagination of the epidermis. In the plaque type of porokeratosis, the invagination extends deeply downward at an angle, the apex of which points away from the central portion of the lesion. In the center of this keratin-filled invagination rises a parakeratotic column, the so-called cornoid lamella, representing the most characteristic feature of porokeratosis of Mibelli (Fig. 6-11).[96] Within the parakeratotic column, the horny cells appear homogeneous and possess pyknotic nuclei. In the epidermis beneath the parakeratotic column, the keratinocytes are irregularly arranged and have pyknotic nuclei with perinuclear edema. In the upper stratum malpighii, some cells possess an eosinophilic cytoplasm as a result of premature keratinization.[97] Usually no granular layer is found at the site at which the parakeratotic column arises, but elsewhere the keratin-filled invagination of the epidermis has a well-developed granular layer.

The histologic changes in the other forms of porokeratosis are similar to those seen in the plaque type but less pronounced, the central invagination being rather shallow, especially in disseminated superficial actinic porokeratosis. The shallow parakeratotic invagination then stands out by showing homogeneous cells rather than the basket-weave pattern seen in the surrounding orthokeratotic stratum corneum (Fig. 6-12).

Because the peripheral raised ridge in porokeratosis slowly moves centrifugally, it stands to reason that the invagination is not bound to a definite structure, such as the sweat pore, as originally assumed by Mibelli. Although the invagination occasionally may be seen within a sweat pore or a pilosebaceous follicle, it is found most commonly in the epidermis independent of these cutaneous appendages.[98] Overexpression of the P53 tumor-supressor protein has been found in porokeratosis.[99] The epidermis overlying the central portion of a lesion of porokeratosis may be either flattened or normal in thickness or, rarely, acanthotic. A nonspecific perivascular infiltrate of chronic inflammatory cells is present in the dermis.

Pathogenesis. The presence of a clone of abnormal epidermal cells located at the base of the parakeratotic column explains the lesions of porokeratosis. As a result of a gradual centrifugal movement of this clone, the furrow is slanted, its apex pointing away from the center of the lesion.[98]

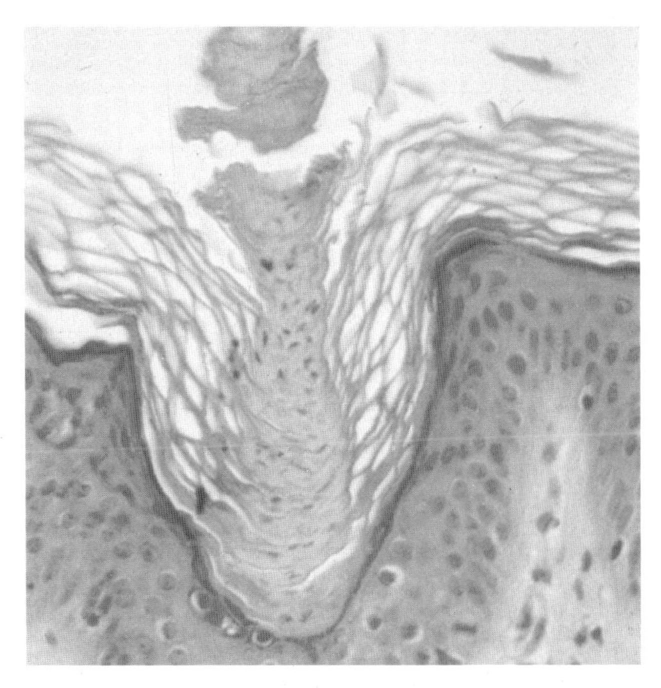

FIG. 6-11. Porokeratosis of Mibelli
Stacked parakeratosis in an area of delled epidermis. The underlying granular cell layer is diminished to absent (original magnification × 200).

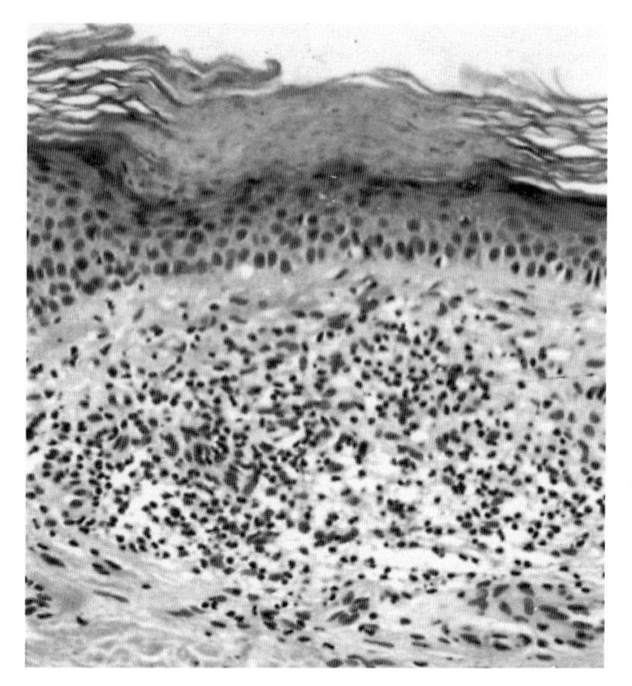

FIG. 6-12. Disseminated actinic porokeratosis
In this type of porokeratosis, the central furrow from which the parakeratotic column arises is quite superficially located and therefore often very shallow (original magnification × 100).

Electron microscopic examination reveals that, in the epidermis beneath the parakeratotic column, many keratinocytes show signs of degeneration. They show a pyknotic nucleus, large perinuclear vacuoles that are separated from one another by cytoplasmic strands, and condensation of tonofilaments at their periphery.[100] At the base of the parakeratotic column, dyskeratotic cells composed of nuclear remnants and aggregated tonofilaments are seen.[101] The parakeratotic column is composed chiefly of cells with a pyknotic nucleus and a cytoplasm possessing high electron density because of the presence of many partially degraded organelles. In addition, a few dyskeratotic cells are present.[101]

Differential Diagnosis. Even though cornoid lamellation is a typical finding for porokeratosis, it is found in a variety of other conditions,[102] especially in verruca vulgaris and solar keratosis. A histologic distinction of punctate porokeratosis from plantar or palmar warts may be impossible, and clinical data, such as age of onset, inheritance, and number and size of lesions may be needed. For discussion of porokeratotic eccrine duct nevus, see section on nevus comedonicus.

XERODERMA PIGMENTOSUM

In xeroderma pigmentosum, an autosomal recessive disorder, excessive solar damage to the skin develops at an early age. Consequently, the lesions occur chiefly in areas of the skin habitually exposed to sunlight. Three stages are recognized. In the first stage, which usually starts when the child is 1 or 2 years old, slight diffuse erythema is associated with scaling and small areas of hyperpigmentation resembling freckles. In the second stage, atrophy of the skin, mottled pigmentation, and telangiectases give the skin an appearance similar to that of a chronic radiodermatitis. Solar keratoses arise in areas of scaling. In the third stage, which usually starts in adolescence but sometimes much earlier in the patient's life, various types of malignant tumors of the skin appear, often causing death. They include squamous cell carcinoma, basal cell epithelioma, and, rarely, fibrosarcoma. In about 3% of the patients with xeroderma pigmentosum, malignant melanomas arise. In some patients they show no tendency to metastasize but in others they metastasize rapidly.[103] Multiple malignant melanomas have been observed.[104] The eyes also are affected, showing conjunctivitis and often keratitis with corneal opacities.

A very rare form of xeroderma pigmentosum is the *De Sanctis-Cacchione syndrome,* which in addition to severe skin lesions shows neurologic manifestations, especially microcephaly, retarded growth, and cerebellar ataxia.[105]

Histopathology. In the first stage, the histopathologic appearance is not specific, but the diagnosis is suggested by a combination of changes that normally are not seen in the skin of young persons. They are hyperkeratosis, thinning of the stratum malpighii with atrophy of some of the rete ridges and elongation of others, a chronic inflammatory infiltrate in the upper dermis, and irregular accumulations of melanin in the basal cell layer, with or without an increase in the number of melanocytes.

In the second stage, the hyperkeratosis and irregular hyperpigmentation already present in the first stage are more pronounced. The epidermis shows atrophy in some areas and acanthosis in others. There may be disorder in the arrangement of the epidermal nuclei, and in some areas the epidermis may show atypical downward growth, so that the histologic picture in such areas is identical with that of solar keratosis. The upper dermis shows basophilic degeneration of the collagen and solar elastosis, as also is seen in solar degeneration.

In the third, or tumor, stage, histologic evidence of the various malignant tumors mentioned earlier is found.

Pathogenesis. In patients with xeroderma pigmentosum (with the exception of those who have the so-called XP variant; see below), cells of the skin in tissue culture show a decrease in their ability to repair the damage induced by sunlight to their deoxyribonucleic acid (DNA). This repair is brought about by *excision repair*, a system whereby damaged single-strand regions of DNA are excised and replaced with new sequences of bases.[106] The reason for the inadequate excision repair is that the DNA–endonuclease that initiates the excision process is deficient. In vitro testing of skin fibroblasts from different patients with xeroderma pigmentosum shows considerable variation in the excision defect, the extent of repair replication varying between 0% and 90% of normal. Affected siblings are usually similar to each other in degree of repair replication. However, no correlation exists between the level of repair replication and the severity of clinical symptoms.[107]

There are at least five patients known in whom excision repair is normal but the cells are defective in a DNA repair mode referred to as postreplication repair. This represents the so-called XP variant form. In cells of this variant form, the rate of conversion from low- to high-molecular-weight DNA is defective.[108]

Electron microscopic examination of the epidermis has revealed in pigmented areas marked pleomorphism and a definite increase in the number of melanosomes. In some cases, very large melanosomes, referred to as giant melanosomes, are present in both melanocytes and keratinocytes.[109] Even epidermis that is protected from light and shows no clinical abnormalities exhibits significant cellular alterations.

ECTODERMAL DYSPLASIA

Two forms of ectodermal dysplasia are recognized: *hidrotic* and *anhidrotic* (now called hypohidrotic).

The *hidrotic* form, which has an autosomal dominant inheritance, is primarily a disorder of keratinization and is characterized by hypotrichosis, dystrophic nails, and palmoplantar hyperkeratosis. It is sometimes associated with dental hypoplasia.[110] The degree of alopecia varies from slight to total.[111]

The *anhidrotic* (hypohidrotic) form is an X-linked recessive disorder (the gene has been localized to Xq11–12) occurring in its full expression only in males. Females, as heterozygotes, may be mildly affected, with reduced sweating and faulty dentition. Males affected with anhidrotic ectodermal dysplasia show the tetrad of anhidrosis or hypohidrosis; hypotrichosis, dental hypoplasia, and a characteristic facies (Fig. 6-13).[112] Frequently, there is also dystrophy of the nails.[113] The greatly reduced or absent function of the eccrine glands results in intolerance to heat. The face shows prominent frontal bosses and a depressed nasal bridge (Fig. 6-14). In addition, the mucous glands of the mouth and respiratory tract may be absent.[114] The lack of mammary glands and nipples has been noted.[113]

Histopathology. Both the hidrotic and the anhidrotic forms show hypoplasia of the hair and the sebaceous glands, with a decrease in their number, size, and degree of maturation.[110,113]

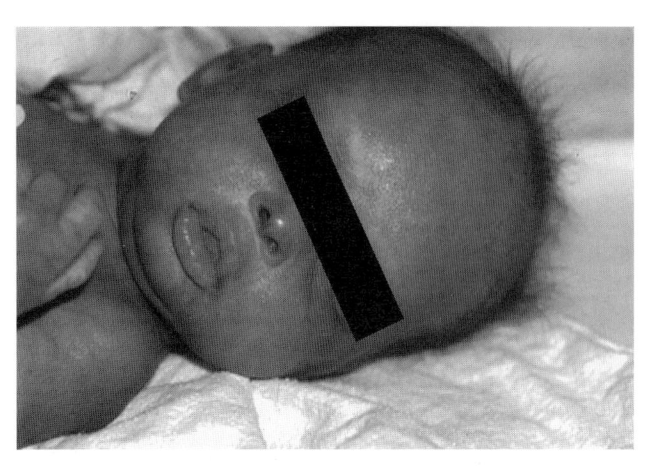

FIG. 6-14. Hypohidrotic ectodermal dysplasia
In addition to frontal bossing and a flat nasal bridge, this infant demonstrates hyperpigmentation of the eyelids and surrounding skin, as well as patulous lips.

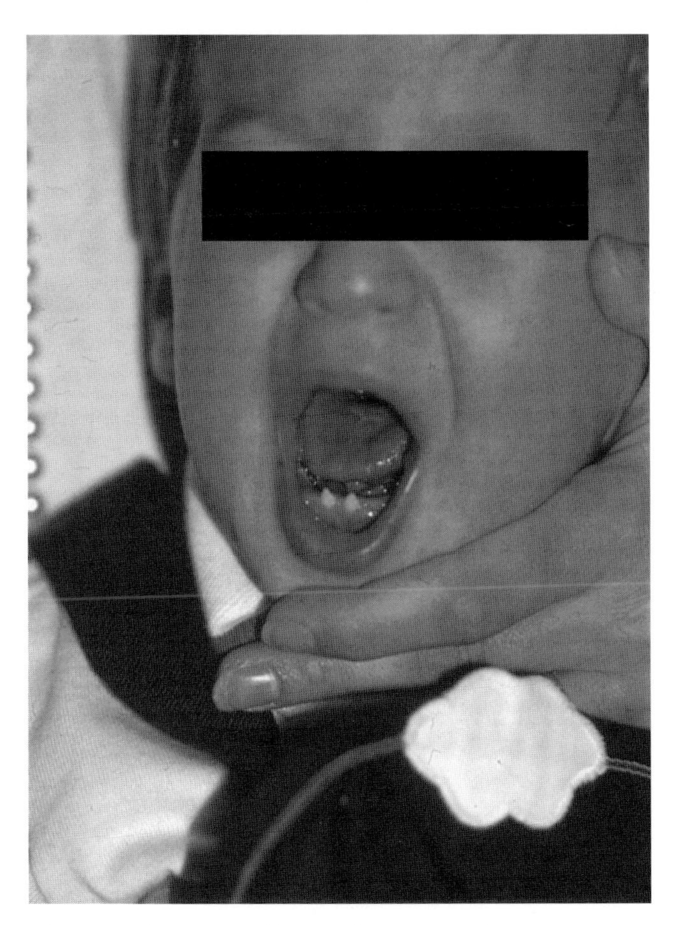

FIG. 6-13. Hypohidrotic ectodermal dysplasia
Characteristic pegged teeth.

In the anhidrotic form, there is, in addition, either a total absence or severe hypoplasia of the eccrine glands. In the case of hypoplasia, eccrine glands are present in only a few areas, especially the axillae and palms, but even in these areas, they are sparse and poorly developed. The secretory cells may be small and flat, so that they resemble endothelial rather than epithelial cells, and the excretory ducts may be composed of a single instead of a double layer of epithelial cells.[115] The apocrine glands of the axillae are present in some patients with the anhidrotic form; in others, these glands are hypoplastic and cannot be distinguished from hypoplastic eccrine glands; in still others, both eccrine and apocrine glands are absent.

FOCAL DERMAL HYPOPLASIA SYNDROME

The focal dermal hypoplasia syndrome, or Goltz's syndrome, is probably due to an X-linked dominant gene lethal in homozygous males. Therefore, the syndrome occurs largely in females. Its occasional occurrence in males may be the result of a new mutation.[116] The mode of inheritance thus is similar to that of incontinentia pigmenti.

The cutaneous manifestations of the focal dermal hyperplasia syndrome include widely distributed linear areas of hypoplasia of the skin resembling striae distensae; soft, yellow nodules, often in linear arrangement; and large ulcers due to congenital absence of skin that gradually heal with atrophy. One must remember that there are varied presentations of this syndrome.[117] Frequent additional abnormalities include lack of a digit, which may be associated with syndactyly and which results in the very characteristic "lobster-claw deformity"; colobomata of the eyes, or microphthalmia, or agenesis of an eye[118]; and hypoplasia of hair, nails, or teeth.[119] The presence of fine, parallel, vertical striations in the metaphysis of long bones on radiography, referred to as osteopathia striata, is a reliable diagnostic marker of Goltz's syndrome.[120]

Histopathology. The linear areas of hypoplasia of the skin show a marked diminution in the thickness of the dermis, the

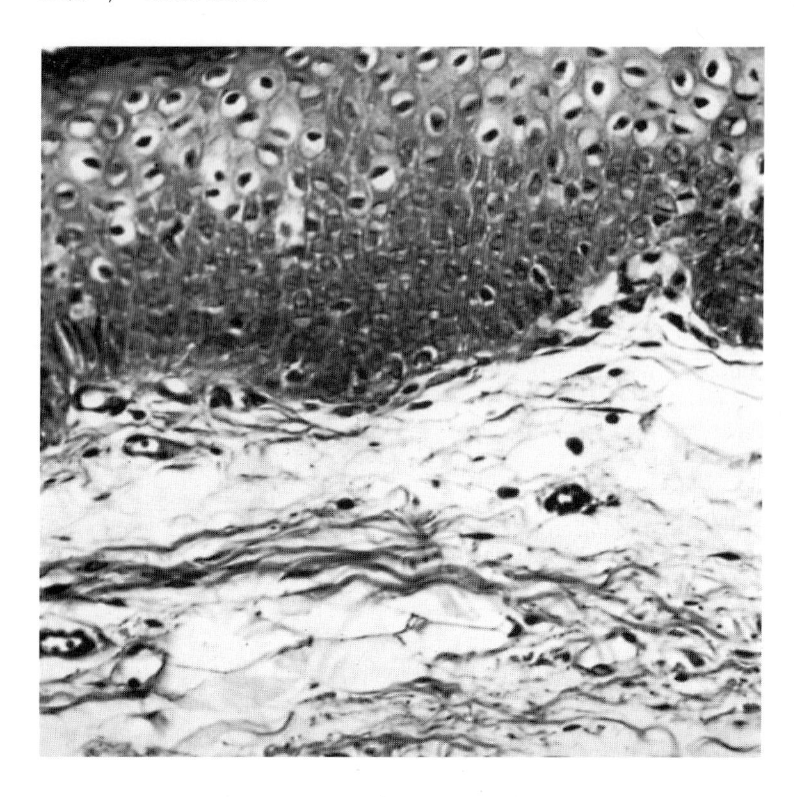

FIG. 6-15. Focal dermal hypoplasia
Adipose tissue is present very near the epidermis, separated from it by only a few collagen fibers (original magnification × 200).

collagen being present as thin fibers not united into bundles.[120] The soft, yellow nodules represent accumulations of fat that largely replace the dermis, so that the subcutaneous fat extends upward to the epidermis in some areas (Fig. 6-15).[119,121] Thin fibers of collagen and even some bundles of collagen resembling those of normal dermis may be located between the subepidermal adipose tissue and the subcutaneous fat.[120]

Pathogenesis. Electron microscopic examination shows, in addition to collagen fibrils 70 nm or more in diameter, many fine filamentous structures measuring 5 to 70 nm in diameter. There are two types of fat cells, one unilocular and the other multilocular, the latter representing young lipocytes.[122]

Differential Diagnosis. Fat cells are seen in the dermis also in the nevus lipomatosus of Hoffmann and Zurhelle, but the extreme attenuation of the collagen that occurs in some areas of the skin in patients with focal dermal hypoplasia syndrome is not seen in nevus lipomatosus. Several females with deletions of the distal short arm of X(Xp22.3–p22.2) have recently been described who have lapping features of this syndrome.

APLASIA CUTIS CONGENITA

Aplasia cutis congenita consists of a localized absence of skin at the time of birth (Fig. 6-16). Most commonly, one observes a single ulcer or several ulcers on the scalp that measure only 1 to 3 cm in diameter and heal uneventfully. In some instances, intrauterine healing has occurred. Occasionally, large defects of the skin are present; but even then, as a rule, healing takes place within several months.[123,124] The condition includes a diverse

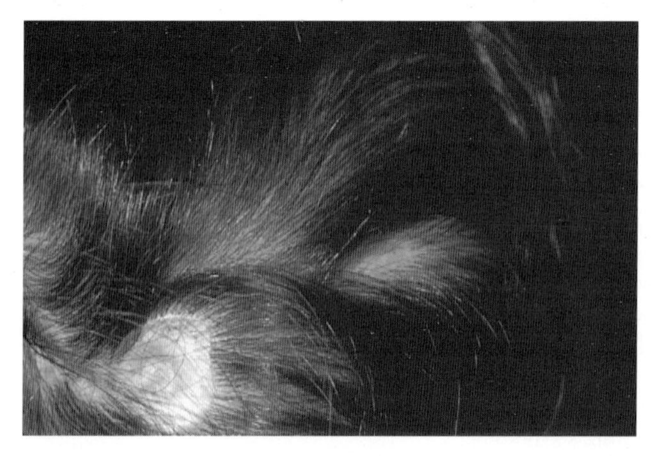

FIG. 6-16. Aplasia cutis congenita
Two areas of congenitally absent skin (scarred and hairless).

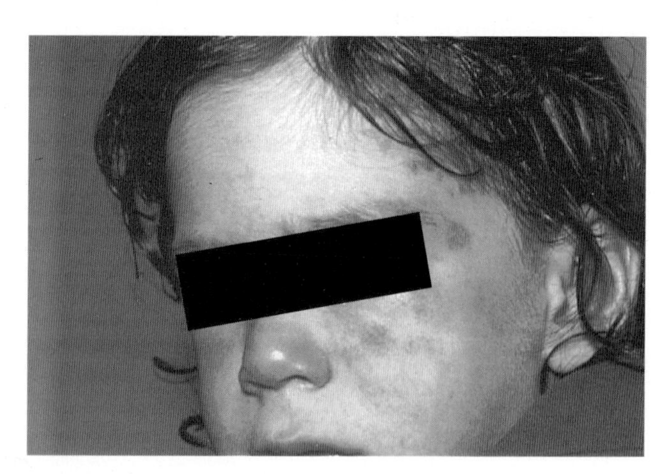

FIG. 6-17. Poikiloderma congenitale
Toddler with facial erythema.

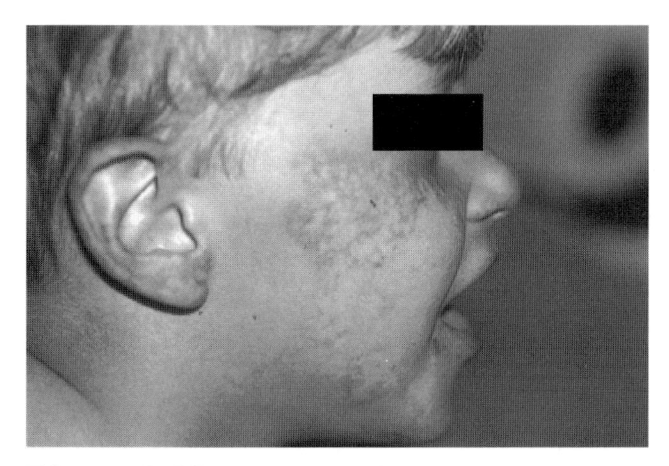

FIG. 6-18. Poikiloderma congenitale
Older child with poikilodermatous changes of the cheek and ear.

group of disorders in which localized absence of skin occurs alone or in association with a wide variety of abnormalities.[125]

Histopathology. Ulcers extend through the entire thickness of the dermis, exposing the subcutaneous fat.[126] Healed areas show, besides a flattened epidermis, fibrosis in the dermis and complete absence of adnexal structures.[123]

Differential Diagnosis. Aplasia cutis should not be confused with congenital absence of the skin, where only epidermis is absent. This is a variant of *epidermolysis bullosa*[127]*(Bart's syndrome).*

POIKILODERMA CONGENITALE (ROTHMUND-THOMSON SYNDROME)

Poikiloderma congenitale is inherited in an autosomal recessive pattern. It begins a few months after birth with erythema on the face (Fig. 6-17) and subsequently extends to the dorsa of the hands and feet and occasionally also to the arms, legs, and buttocks. Later on, slight atrophy develops with telangiectases and mottled hyper- and hypopigmentation, so that the appearance is that of poikiloderma atrophicans vasculare (Fig. 6-18). Exposure to light aggravates the lesions. Most patients show dwarfism and hypogonadism. In about 40% of the patients, cataracts develop between the ages of 4 and 7.[128] Recent evidence suggests children with this syndrome have a reduced DNA repair capacity.[129]

Histopathology. During the early phase occurring in infancy and early childhood, there is hydropic degeneration of the basal layer leading to "pigment incontinence" with presence of melanophages in the upper dermis.[130] A mild chronic inflammatory infiltrate is intermingled with the melanophages and may show a bandlike arrangement close to the flattened epidermis (Fig. 6-19).[128] The histologic changes thus may be identical with those seen in the early stage of poikiloderma atrophicans vasculare. In later childhood and adult life, the epidermis is flattened, and dilated capillaries as well as melanophages are present in the upper dermis, but there is no longer any inflammatory infiltrate.

BLOOM'S SYNDROME (CONGENITAL TELANGIECTATIC ERYTHEMA)

Bloom's syndrome, with autosomal recessive inheritance, resembles poikiloderma congenitale by showing (1) telangiectatic erythema of the face starting in infancy and often extending to the forearms and hands, (2) sensitivity to sunlight, (3) café au lait macules in over 50% of patients,[131] and (4) growth retardation (Fig. 6-20). It differs from poikiloderma congenitale by (1) the lack of netlike hyper- and hypopigmentation[132]; (2) the absence of hypogonadism (testicular atrophy and sterility are common in male patients) and cataracts; (3) the occasional presence of immunoglobulin deficiencies, especially of IgA and IgM[133,134]; (4) a high incidence of nonspecific chromosomal breakage[133] and a great increase in the frequency of another type of chromosome instability, sister chromatid exchanges[135]; and (5) an increased risk for malignant disease, especially leukemia, lymphoma, and carcinoma of the alimentary tract.[136]

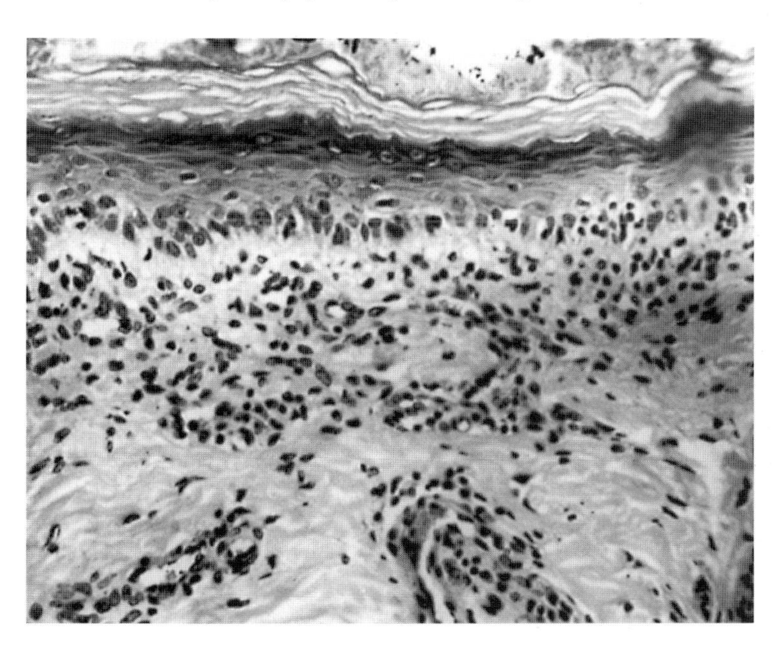

FIG. 6-19. Poikiloderma congenitale (Rothman-Thompson), early
This section from a young child shows flattening of the epidermis, hydropic degeneration of the basal layer, and a bandlike inflammatory infiltrate in the upper dermis (original magnification × 200).

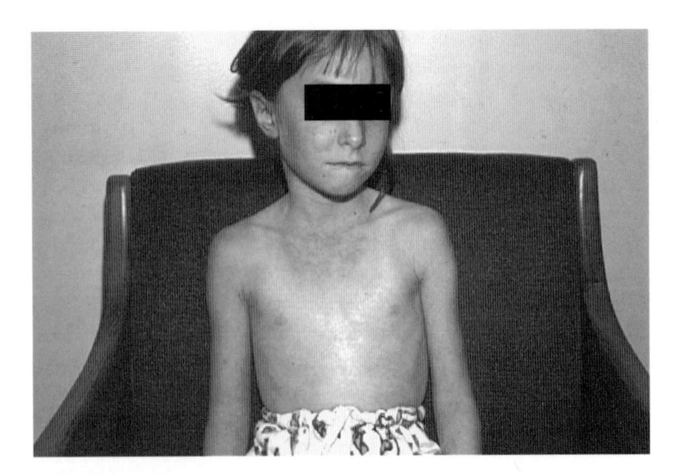

FIG. 6-20. Bloom's syndrome
Erythema of face and photodistributed skin changes.

Histopathology. The epidermis is flattened and may show hydropic degeneration of the basal cell layer.[135] There is dilatation of the capillaries in the upper dermis, which may be associated with a perivascular mononuclear infiltrate[131,135]; however, there may be absence of any infiltrate.[132]

Pathogenesis. Bloom's syndrome shows impairment of both cellular and humoral immunity, although this is not as pronounced as in *ataxia-telangiectasia* (see later). Evidence of impaired cellular immunity is the occasional absence of delayed hypersensitivity reactions[134] and the tendency toward development of malignant disease. Evidence of impaired humoral immunity is the occasional presence of immunoglobulin deficiencies. However, in contrast to ataxia-telangiectasia, susceptibility to infections is not pronounced.

Differential Diagnosis. Pigmentary incontinence is not pronounced in Bloom's syndrome, as it is in poikiloderma congenitale. The presence of hydropic degeneration of the basal cell layer and of a perivascular infiltrate may cause difficulties in differentiation from lupus erythematosus. However, no linear deposits of immunoglobulin are seen at the dermal-epidermal junction in Bloom's syndrome.[135]

ATAXIA-TELANGIECTASIA

Ataxia-telangiectasia is transmitted in an autosomal recessive mode. The ataxia is evident already in infancy, whereas the telangiectases do not appear until childhood. They usually appear first on the bulbar conjuntivae, with subsequent extension to the cheeks, ears, and neck and often also to other areas, such as the buttocks and extremities. A marked susceptibility to infections, particularly sinopulmonary infections, exists. Death from chronic respiratory infection or lymphoma-leukemia is common in the second or third decade of life.[137]

Histopathology. The upper dermis shows numerous markedly dilated vessels that belong to the subpapillary venous plexus.[138]

Pathogenesis. All patients have severe defects in both humoral and cellular immunity. In approximately 75% of the patients there is an absence or extreme deficiency of the serum IgA, and in about 80% a great IgE deficiency.[139] Autopsies have established maldevelopment of the thymus as an integral part of ataxia-telangiectasia.[140] Increased number of T cells with gamma/delta chains in the T-cell receptors rather than alpha/beta chains may produce defects in immunity.[141] Chromosomal breakage is common, but there is no increased rate of sister chromatid exchanges.[138]

PROGERIA OF THE ADULT (WERNER'S SYNDROME)

Werner's syndrome, which has an autosomal recessive mode of inheritance, does not manifest itself until the second or third decade of life. The subcutaneous fat and the musculature of the extremities undergo atrophy, so that the patient exhibits thin arms and legs. The skin of the extremities gradually becomes taut, and ulcers may develop on the legs. As signs of premature senility, patients show graying of the hair, cataracts, and atherosclerosis in early adult life. Diabetes of the late-onset type[142] and hypogonadism due to interstitial fibrosis of the testes[143] are common. Death usually occurs in the fifth decade of life because of atherosclerosis.

Histopathology. On the arms and legs, where the skin is taut, the epidermis is thin and devoid of rete ridges, and the dermis shows fibrosis with or without hyalinization of the collagen. The pilosebaceous structures degenerate. The subcutaneous fatty tissue is largely replaced by newly synthesized, hyalinized collagen that merges with the collagen of the overlying dermis.[144]

Pathogenesis. Poor growth and decreased life span of cultured skin fibroblasts have been found.[145]

Differential Diagnosis. Differentiation from a late lesion of scleroderma may be difficult, because fibrosis and hyalinization of the collagen are seen also in scleroderma.[142] In its late stage, scleroderma may also show no inflammatory infiltrate, so that differentiation has to be made on the basis of the patient's history and clinical manifestations.

EPIDERMOLYSIS BULLOSA

On the basis of clinical, histologic, and electron microscopic findings, three groups of epidermolysis bullosa (EB) are recognized: epidermal, junctional, and dermal (Table 6-1).

In all types of EB, the blisters form as a result of minor trauma. Because of the great differences in prognoses, identification of the type of EB is often very important. In families with the potential of having an infant born with one of the frequently or potentially fatal forms of EB, such as *EB letalis* (Fig. 6-21) or generalized *EB dystrophica-recessive* (Fig. 6-22), a prenatal biopsy at 18 to 20 weeks of gestation is recommended. On electron microscopy EB letalis shows abnormalities of the hemidesmosomes while generalized EB dystrophica-recessive shows absence of anchoring fibrils.

There is more variability in the clinical course in some forms of EB than was previously appreciated.[146] For example, within the epidermal type of EB, which usually has a good prognosis, some cases of *EB herpetiformis*, which is known also as the Dowling-Meara variant, may show generalized blistering that at times is associated with mortality during early infancy (Fig. 6-23).[147] Also, the junctional form of EB can result in scarring as *cicatricial junctional EB*.[148] Occasionally dermal EB may be

TABLE 6-1. *Comparison of the clinical features and prognosis in epidermolysis bullosa*

Type	Epidermolysis bullosa	Distribution	Inheritance	Oral	Scarring	Prognosis
Epidermal	EB simplex	Generalized	Dominant	+	–	Good
	EB Cockayne	Feet, hands	Dominant	–	–	Good
	EB Dowling–Meara (Herpetiform)	Generalized	Dominant	+	Atrophy	Improves by school age
Junctional	EB letalis	Generalized	Recessive	+	–	Usually fatal
	EB benign	Generalized	Recessive	+/–	Atrophy	Good
Dermal	EB dystr-dom	Extremities	Dominant	+/–	+	Good
	EB dystr-rec	Generalized	Recessive	+ +	+ + +	Poor
	EB dystr-rec	Localized	Recessive	+	+	Good
	EB dystr-inversa	Mainly trunk	Recessive	+	+, late	Good
	EB acquisita	Generalized	—	+	+	Good

transient and heal within a few months.[149,150] It is likely that the majority of cases published as Bart's syndrome, which was originally described as congenital absence of the skin,[151] belong in this group.[152,153]

Histopathology. If a fresh blister is available, a specimen for biopsy may be taken from its edge. However, it is advisable to carry out a biopsy also on an induced blister because it will show a blister free of secondary changes. In an existing blister the location of the blister may have changed as the result of regeneration of keratinocytes at the base of the blister or degeneration of the keratinocytes over the blister. The mode of artificially producing a blister depends on the degree of vulnerability of the skin, but in most instances gentle friction with a cotton swab or a pencil eraser is used. The preferred type of biopsy is either a shave or an ellipse. The use of a punch is not recommended because the applied torsion will frequently cause total separation and even loss of the epidermis.[154]

Even though electron microscopic examination (discussed later) is informative, the light microscopic features seen in the various forms of EB are of diagnostic value.

In *epidermal EB,* which includes EB simplex, EB of feet and hands of Weber and Cockayne,[155] and EB herpetiformis (Dowling-Meara),[156,157] the primary separation in experimentally induced blisters always occurs within the basal cell layer. Spontaneously arising blisters may be found subepidermally as the result of complete disintegration of the basal cell layer; in bullae of more than one day's duration the cleavage may be found intraepidermally or subcorneally as a result of epidermal regeneration.[155] In sections stained with the PAS technique, the PAS–positive basement membrane zone is located on the dermal side of the blister.[158]

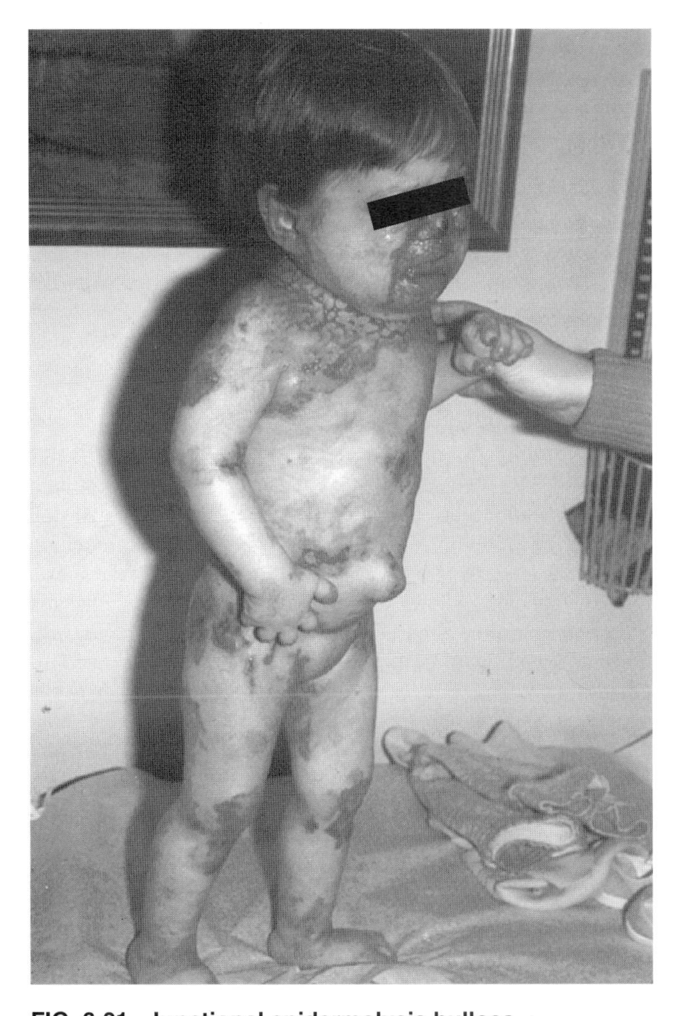

FIG. 6-21. Junctional epidermolysis bullosa
Note significant facial involvement and granulation tissue on neck.

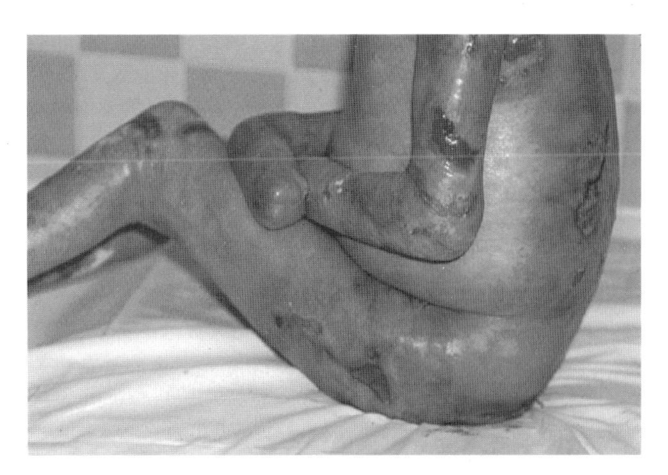

FIG. 6-22. Recessive dystrophic epidermolysis bullosa
Child with mitten deformity of hands, as well as generalized blisters and scarring.

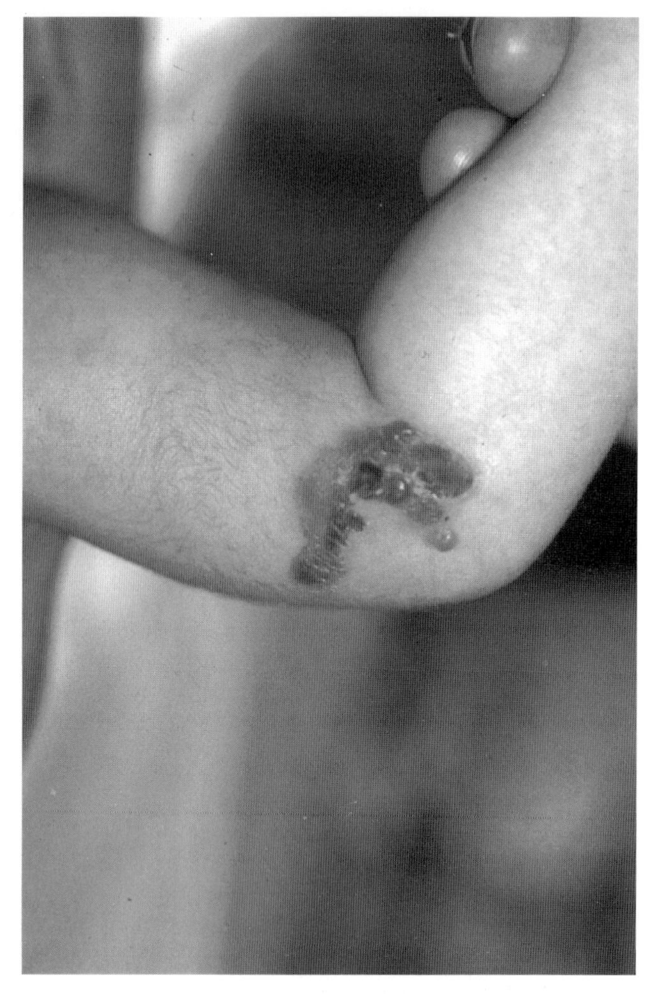

FIG. 6-23. Epidermal epidermolysis bullosa
Herpetiform blistering on arm.

In *junctional EB*, the trauma of having a specimen taken for biopsy generally is sufficient to induce separation. This separation is located between the epidermis and the dermis, with the PAS–positive basement membrane zone usually remaining with the dermis.[159] Autopsy has revealed in some cases of EB letalis extensive subepithelial separation also in the gastrointestinal, respiratory, and urinary tracts.[159,160] There are no morphologic or enzymatic abnormalities to distinguish the atrophic benign form of junctional EB from EB letalis.[162]

In *EB dystrophica-dominant* and *EB dystrophica-recessive*, light microscopy shows dermal-epidermal separation. A PAS stain is of little help in ascertaining the exact level of cleavage because the PAS–positive basement membrane zone often appears hazy.[159] If recognizable, it is seen in contact with the detached epidermis or it appears split. In EB dystrophica-dominant scarring is mild, but in generalized EB dystrophica-recessive extensive erosions may occur, resulting in ulcerations and severe scarring. Severe oral involvement can lead to esophageal stenoses.[163] In especially severe cases, death may occur. The ulcers and scars of the skin, mouth, and esophagus may give rise to squamous cell carcinomas, which tend to metastasize.[164]

EB acquisita is not a genodermatosis but an autoimmune disorder.

Pathogenesis. If possible, all specimens of artificially induced blisters should be subjected to electron microscopic examination and immunofluorescence mapping.[159] The latter procedure consists of exposing cryostat sections to specific antisera against type IV collagen (localized in the lamina densa or basal lamina), against laminin (localized in the lower portion of the lamina lucida), and against bullous pemphigoid antigen (localized in the upper portion of the lamina lucida in the vicinity of the hemidesmosomes). For the latter test, bullous pemphigoid antibodies contained in many bullous pemphigoid sera are used.

In the epidermal types of EB electron microscopic examination shows that cleavage is the result of degenerative cytolytic changes occurring in the lower portion of the basal cells between the dermal-epidermal junction and the nucleus (EM 4). Immunofluorescence mapping shows all three antigens (type IV collagen, laminin, bullous pemphigoid antigen) to be located beneath the cleavage. Studies in several families with the Dowling-Meara form of epidermolysis bullosa revealed point mutations of keratin genes for K5 and K14 on chromosome 12 and 17 respectively.[165]

In the junctional types of EB electron microscopic examination often shows the hemidesmosomes to be abnormal, especially in EB letalis. They may be reduced in size or number, and may lack their sub-basal cell-dense plaque.[166] There are, however, exceptions. In one fatal case of EB letalis, the hemidesmosomes were structurally and numerically normal. Also, one patient with nonlethal junctional EB showed similar abnormalities of the hemidesmosomes as seen in the majority of patients in the lethal group.[167] It is possible that the abnormalities of the hemidesmosomes are a secondary phenomenon and that the basic cause of the junctional types of EB is a biochemical disorder of a lamina lucida constituent. In favor of this theory is the fact that normal skin shows separation at the dermal-epidermal junction when cultured with blister fluid of patients with EB letalis.[168] Immunofluorescence mapping shows type IV collagen and laminin on the floor of the blister; bullous pemphigoid antigen is present mainly on the blister roof, but also in a more spotty distribution and to a much lesser extent on the blister floor.[159] Mutations have been found in a family with atrophic benign junctional epidermolysis bullosa within the LAMB3 gene. The gene is responsible for encoding a portion of Laminin 5. This mutation may have significance in reducing adhesion between the epidermis and dermis.[169] A newly found mutation of the gene encoding $beta_4$ integrin has been found in the subset of EB letalis with pyloric atresia.

The dermal types of EB, on electron microscopy, show abnormalities in regard to their anchoring fibrils. Generalized recessive dystrophic EB shows absence of the anchoring fibrils even in nonlesional unscarred skin. On the other hand, in both dominant dystrophic EB and in localized recessive dystrophic EB structurally normal anchoring fibrils are present but in significantly reduced number.[170] The complete absence of anchoring fibrils in generalized recessive dystrophic EB could be established through the lack of a reaction with monoclonal antibodies to anchoring fibrils.[171] Because type VII collagen is a major structural component of the anchoring fibrils, immunofluorescence staining with polyclonal antibodies to type VII collagen reveals complete absence of staining, even in the unaffected skin of patients with severe dystrophic recessive EB.[172] Similarly, there was no reaction with periodic acid-thiosemicarbazide-silver proteinate, which stains anchoring fibrils selectively.[173] Mutations in the gene encoding type VII collagen (COL 7A1) located at chromosome band 3p21 has been reported to cause these abnormal findings in the dystrophic forms of epidermolysis bullosa.[174,175] Immunofluorescence mapping shows all three basement membrane zone constituents—bullous pemphigoid antigen, laminin, and type IV collagen—on top of the cleavage.[159]

Epidermolysis Bullosa Acquisita

EB acquisita starts in childhood or adult life[176] with blisters at sites of trauma resulting in atrophic scars which in some cases are not pronounced (Figs. 6-24 and 6-25). Milia may not appear until the disorder has been present for many years. Oral lesions are seen occasionally. A significant proportion of patients with EB acquisita have circulating IgG antibodies.[177]

Histopathology. The bullae are located beneath the epidermis and thus are indistinguishable in their location from those seen in bullous pemphigoid. The prevalence of eosinophils in the infiltrate of bullous pemphigoid often helps in distinguishing the two diseases. However, because the findings by light microscopic immunofluorescence are identical in the two diseases, patients with EB acquisita have been misdiagnosed frequently as having bullous pemphigoid before the recognition of the different location of the respective antibodies on immunoelectron microscopy. "Salt split" skin combined with immunofluorescence has proven to be an aid in distinguishing EBA from BP. The early studies demonstrated EB acquisita antibodies on the dermal side (floor) of the salt split skin and BP antibodies on the epidermal side (roof).[178,179] Later studies have found BP as well as EB acquisita antibodies on the floor of the salt split.[180] In spite of these latter studies this technique still has value in differentiating these two conditions.

Histogenesis. Since EB acquisita on direct immunofluorescence shows subepidermal deposits of IgG and C3 and on indirect immunofluorescence often shows circulating antibodies against IgG, a misdiagnosis of bullous pemphigoid has been made in some cases,[181] or in the case of pronounced scarring, a misdiagnosis of cicatricial pemphigoid.[182] Immunoelectron microscopy, however, has shown a different location of the IgG deposits in these two disease groups: in bullous pemphigoid and cicatricial pemphigoid they are located in the lamina lucida[183]; in EB acquisita they are found in the upper dermis just beneath or contiguous to the lamina densa.[177] Similarly, whereas type IV collagen and laminin are located at the floor of the blister in bullous pemphigoid, they are seen on the roof of the blister in EB acquisita. Because antibody to human type IV collagen functions also in formalin fixed, paraffin embedded tissue sections, standard immunoperoxidase methods have revealed type IV collagen to be associated with the blister roof in EB acquisita and with the blister base in bullous pemphigoid and cicatricial pemphigoid.[184]

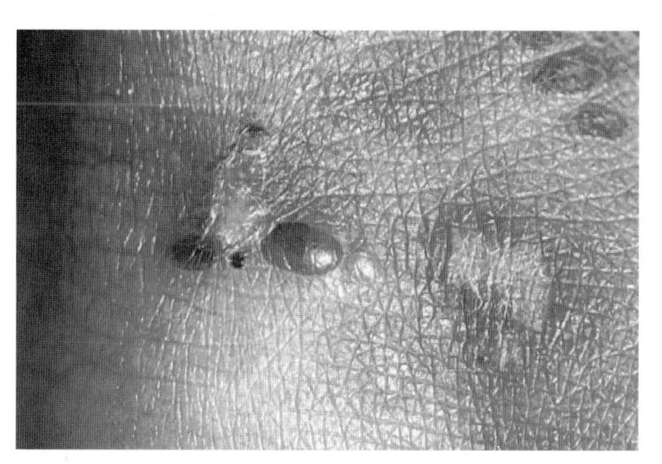

FIG. 6-24. Epidermolysis bullosa acquisita
A blister surrounded by two scars.

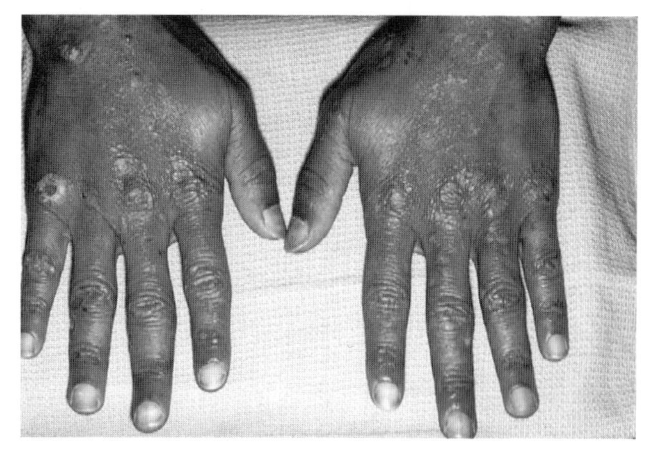

FIG. 6-25. Epidermolysis bullosa acquisita
Blistering and scarring on backs of hands.

FAMILIAL BENIGN PEMPHIGUS (HAILEY-HAILEY DISEASE)

Familial benign pemphigus is inherited as an autosomal dominant trait, with a family history obtainable in about two thirds of the patients.[211] Genetic studies have localized the gene on chromosome 3q.[212] It is characterized by a localized, recurrent eruption of small vesicles on an erythematous base. By peripheral extension, the lesions may assume a circinate configuration. The sites of predilection are the intertriginous areas, especially the axillae and the groin. Only very few instances of mucosal lesions have been reported, of the mouth,[213,214] the labia majora,[214] and the esophagus.[215]

Histopathology. Although, as in *Darier's disease*, early lesions may show small suprabasal separations, so called lacunae, fully developed lesions show large separations, that is, vesicles and even bullae, in a predominantly suprabasal position (Fig. 6-26). Villi, which are elongated papillae lined by a single layer of basal cells, protrude upward into the bulla, and, in some cases, narrow strands of epidermal cells proliferate downward into the dermis. Many cells of the detached stratum malpighii show loss of their intercellular bridges, so that acantholysis affects large portions of the epidermis. Individual cells and groups of cells usually are seen in large numbers in the bulla cavity. In spite of the extensive loss of intercellular bridges, the cells of the detached epidermis in many places show only slight separation from one another because a few intact intercellular bridges still hold them loosely together. This quite typical feature gives the detached epidermis the appearance of a dilapidated brick wall.

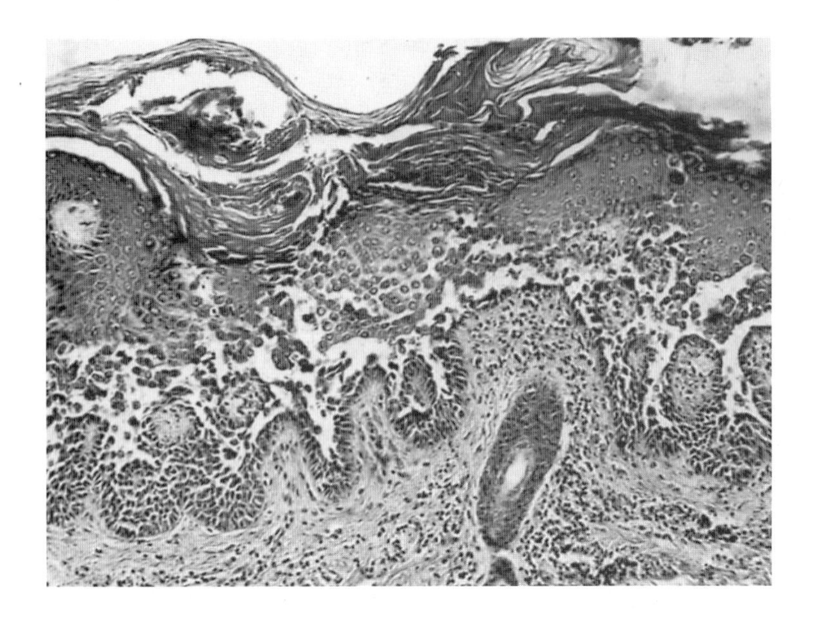

FIG. 6-26. Familial benign pemphigus (Hailey-Hailey)
The bulla is largely in a suprabasal position. The extensive loss of intercellular bridges with partial coherence of cells gives the detached epidermis the appearance of a dilapidated brick wall. On the right side within the granular layer, a corps rond can be seen (original magnification × 200).

Many of the cells of the stratum malpighii that have lost all or most of their intercellular bridges show a fairly normal cytoplasm and a normal nucleus in which mitotic activity has even been observed.[216,217] Some of the acantholytic cells, however, have a homogenized cytoplasm, suggesting premature partial keratinization. In some instances, such acantholytic cells with premature keratinization resemble the grains of Darier's disease. Occasionally, a few corps ronds are present in the granular layer (Fig. 6-26).[218,216,217].

Differential Diagnosis. Histologically, familial benign pemphigus shares certain features with both Darier's disease and pemphigus vulgaris. In all three diseases, one finds predominantly suprabasal separation of the epidermis caused by acantholysis and resulting in lacunae or bullae, and villi formation.

Differentiation of familial benign pemphigus from Darier's disease as a rule is not very difficult, because in Darier's disease (1) the suprabasal separations usually are smaller, thus appearing as lacunae rather than as bullae; (2) acantholysis is less pronounced, being limited to the lower epidermis, especially the suprabasal region; and (3) dyskeratosis consisting of the formation of corps ronds and grains is much more evident.

Pemphigus vulgaris often resembles familial benign pemphigus to a striking degree, and, in some specimens, histologic differentiation of these two diseases may be impossible. As a rule, however, in pemphigus vulgaris there is less extensive acantholysis, limited largely to the suprabasal region, so that the detached epidermis appears normal and lacks the appearance of a dilapidated brick wall, and more severe degeneration of the acantholytic cells within and near the bulla cavity. The presence of eosinophils in the bulla points toward a diagnosis of pemphigus vulgaris, but their absence does not rule it out. In case of doubt immunofluorescence will decide the issue.

There used to be much discussion as to whether familial benign pemphigus represents a vesicular variant of Darier's disease. Two points in favor of the basic unity of the two diseases were stressed: the alleged simultaneous presence of both diseases in the same patient, and the occurrence of corps ronds in both diseases. However, it has become apparent that patients described as having both diseases were either cases of Darier's disease with vesicular lesions[219] or cases of familial benign pemphigus with the presence of corps ronds.[220,221] Evidence against a relationship is also the fact that, in affected families, always only one of the two diseases occurs.

KERATOSIS FOLLICULARIS (DARIER'S DISEASE)

Darier's disease, although usually transmitted in an autosomal dominant pattern, may occur as a mutation (Color Fig. 6-3). In typical cases, there is a more or less extensive, persistent, slowly progressive eruption consisting of hyperkeratotic or crusted papules often showing a follicular distribution. By coalescence verrucous, crusted areas may form. The so-called seborrheic areas are the sites of predilection. The oral mucosa is involved occasionally.[185] In some cases of Darier's disease one finds on the dorsa of the hands and feet keratotic papules that resemble those seen in *acrokeratosis verruciformis of Hopf.*[186]

Special clinical variants of keratosis follicularis are a hypertrophic type, a vesiculobullous type, and a linear or zosteriform type. In the hypertrophic type, widespread, markedly thickened, and hyperkeratotic lesions are seen, especially in the intertriginous areas.[187] In the vesiculobullous type, vesicles and small bullae are seen in addition to papules.[188,189] In the linear or zosteriform type, usually limited to one side, there are either localized or widespread lesions that may be present at birth[190] but in most cases have arisen in infancy, childhood, or adult life.[191] The question has been raised as to whether this type of lesion represents a linear epidermal nevus with acantholytic dyskeratosis rather than Darier's disease,[190] and the designation *acantholytic dyskeratotic epidermal nevus* has been suggested.[191] It is quite likely that some of the cases with scattered papular lesions of limited extent arising in adult life and diagnosed as acute, eruptive Darier's disease[192] or acute adult-onset Darier–like dermatosis in reality represented transient acantholytic dermatosis. A recent review on the clinical aspects of this condition has been written.[193]

Histopathology. The characteristic changes in Darier's disease are: (1) a peculiar form of dyskeratosis resulting in the formation of corps ronds and grains, (2) suprabasal acantholysis

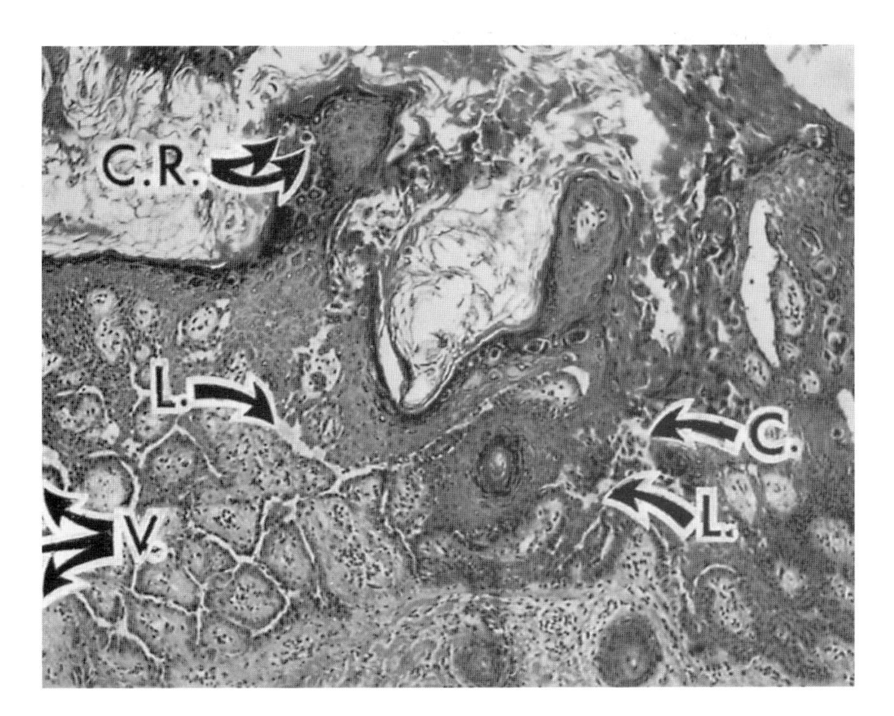

FIG. 6-27. Darier's disease, low magnification
Hyperkeratosis and papillomatosis are evident. Numerous lacunae (*L.*) are present. On the left are elongated papillae lined by a single layer of cells, so-called villi (*V.*). Corps ronds (*C.R.*) are present in the granular layer, and grains are seen in the horny layer. The lacunae contain desquamated cells (*C.*) (original magnification × 100).

leading to the formation of suprabasal clefts or lacunae, and (3) irregular upward proliferation into the lacunae of papillae lined with a single layer of basal cells, so-called villi (Fig. 6-27). There are also papillomatosis, acanthosis, and hyperkeratosis. The dermis shows a chronic inflammatory infiltrate. In some cases, there is downward proliferation of epidermal cells into the dermis.

The corps ronds occur in the upper stratum malpighii, particularly in the granular and horny layers; grains are found in the horny layer and as acantholytic cells within the lacunae. Corps ronds possess a central homogeneous, basophilic, pyknotic nucleus that is surrounded by a clear halo. By virtue of size and the conspicuous halo, corps ronds stand out clearly (Fig. 6-28). Peripheral to the halo lies basophilic dyskeratotic material as a shell.[194] The nonstaining halo in some instances is partially replaced by homogeneous, eosinophilic dyskeratotic material.[195] Compared with the corps ronds, the grains are much less conspicuous. They resemble parakeratotic cells but are somewhat larger. The nuclei of grains are elongated and often grain-shaped and are surrounded by homogeneous dyskeratotic material that usually stains basophilic but may stain eosinophilic. The lacunae represent small, slitlike intraepidermal vesicles most commonly located directly above the basal layer. They contain acantholytic cells and show premature partial keratinization. Because of shrinkage, some of them are elongated, and these then appear identical with the grains in the horny layer. The villi projecting into the lacunae may be quite tortuous, so that, on histologic examination, some of them appear in cross section as rounded dermal structures lined by a solitary row of basal cells (see Fig. 6-27).

Hyperkeratosis and papillomatosis may cause the formation of keratotic plugs, which often fill the pilosebaceous follicles but are found also outside of follicles. That Darier's disease is not exclusively a follicular disorder is also proved by the fact that areas devoid of follicles, such as palms, soles, and the oral mucosa, may be affected.

In hypertrophic lesions of Darier's disease, one can occa-

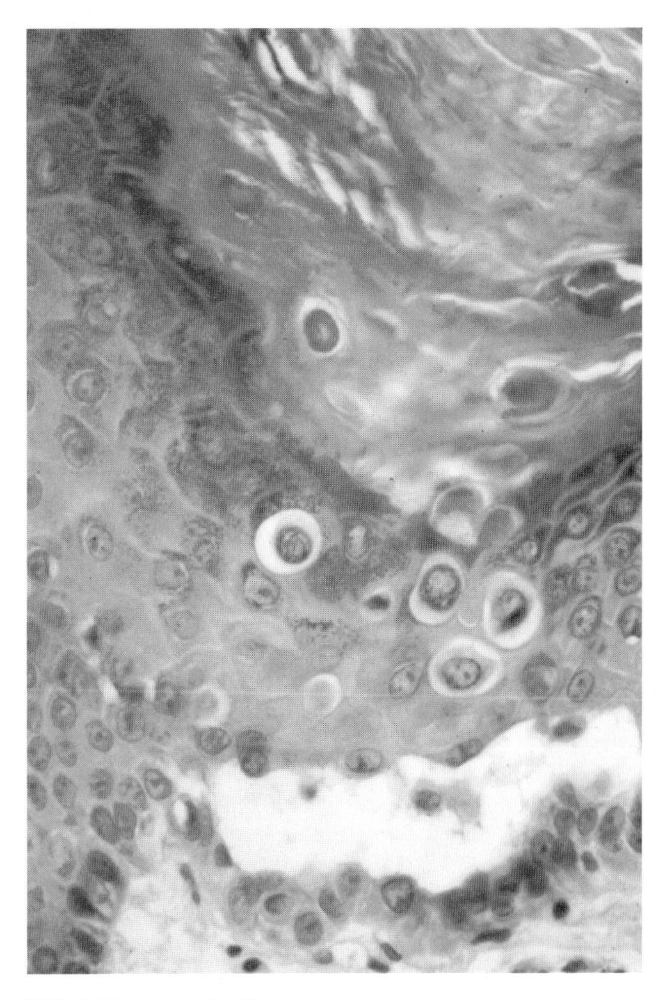

FIG. 6-28. Darier's disease
Hyperkeratosis corps ronds are in the thickened stratum corneum and epidermis. Suprabasalar acantholysis is present.

sionally observe considerable acanthosis, either as proliferations of basal cells or as pseudocarcinomatous hyperplasia. Proliferations of basal cells consist of long, narrow cords composed of two rows of basal cells separated by a narrow lacunar space.[196]

The vesiculobullous lesions, which occur in rare instances, differ from lacunae merely in size; they contain numerous shrunken cells with the appearance of grains.[188,189]

The keratotic papules that may occur on the dorsa of the hands and feet and that clinically resemble those seen in acrokeratosis verruciformis of Hopf in most instances, on serial sectioning, show mild dyskeratotic changes and often suprabasal clefts as well.[186] They are a manifestation of Darier's disease and not of acrokeratosis verruciformis.

The lesions on the oral mucosa are analogous in appearance to those observed on the skin and thus show lacunae and dyskeratosis, although definite well-formed corps ronds generally are absent.[197]

The occasional reports of patients having both Darier's disease and familial benign pemphigus or a transition from one of these two diseases to the other are discussed in the differential diagnosis of familial benign pemphigus.

Pathogenesis. Whereas histologically a distinction between Darier's disease and familial benign pemphigus is generally possible, with dyskeratosis being the predominating factor in Darier's disease and acantholysis in familial benign pemphigus, this distinction is not as clearly evident in electron microscopic examination. The reason for this is that for electron microscopy only a small specimen can be processed, which in either of the two diseases shows predominantly acantholysis in some instances and dyskeratosis in others and only rarely shows both. In both diseases, however, acantholysis precedes dyskeratosis.

Acantholysis has been thought by some authors to be due to the loss of the intercellular contact layer within desmosomes, both in Darier's disease[198,199] and in familial benign pemphigus.[200] The two halves of the desmosomes then pull apart, after which the tonofilaments become detached from them. Another group of authors believes that there is some basic defect in the tonofilament—desmosome complex in Darier's disease[195,210] and in familial benign pemphigus[202]—resulting in separating of tonofilaments from the attachment plaques of desmosomes and subsequently leading to the disappearance of desmosomes and thus to acantholysis. It is likely that both processes take place simultaneously in both Darier's disease[194] and familial benign pemphigus.[203]

The cause for the acantholysis in Darier's disease and familial benign pemphigus is not yet definitely known. The faulty synthesis of the intercellular substance has long been suspected. Recently the existence of a major defect of the intercellular material, the glycocalyx, has been shown by the fact that within the acantholytic lesions of both diseases binding of concanavalin A is absent or markedly reduced.[204] Also, it seems that a proteolytic enzyme, called *epidermal cell dissociating factor,* is discharged from the keratinocytes in lesions of Darier's disease and familial benign pemphigus, causing separation of normal keratinocytes in vitro.[205] Recent data have linked the Darier's disease locus to 12q23–24.1.[206]

In association with the loss of desmosomes, excessive amounts of tonofilaments form within the keratinocytes around the nucleus as thick, electron-dense bundles. A defect of the tonofilaments would best explain the dyskeratotic features of both Darier's disease and familial benign pemphigus. In Darier's disease, in which the dyskeratosis is much more pronounced than in familial benign pemphigus, thick bundles of tonofilaments, often in association with large keratohyaline granules, form large aggregates of homogenized dyskeratotic material. The corps ronds, on electron microscopic examination, are characterized by extensive cytoplasmic vacuolization.[207] They show in their center an irregularly shaped nucleus surrounded by a halo of autolyzed electron-lucid cytoplasm and at their periphery a shell of tonofilaments (EM 16).[194,198] The grains are seen on electron microscopic examination to consist of nuclear remnants surrounded by dyskeratotic bundles of tonofilaments.

In familial benign pemphigus, too, after loss of the desmosomes, excessive amounts of tonofilaments form within the keratinocytes and aggregate around the nucleus as thick, electron-dense bundles, often in a whorling configuration; however, even though dyskeratosis is present, it is less pronounced than in Darier's disease, and most of the keratinocytes keratinize normally, only very few becoming grains or corps ronds as the result of dyskeratotic degeneration.

On intralesional injection of tritiated thymidine one group[208] observed labeling of many acantholytic keratinocytes in familial benign pemphigus but not in Darier's disease, suggesting to them that in familial benign pemphigus the epidermal cells participated in the renewal of the epidermis but did not do so in Darier's disease, probably because these cells were undergoing keratinization. However, another group[209] could not confirm this observation.

Differential Diagnosis. Although acantholytic dyskeratosis in association with corps ronds is highly characteristic of Darier's disease, it occurs also in several other conditions[210]: in warty dyskeratoma, a solitary lesion with a deep central invagination; in transient or persistent acantholytic dermatosis, in which the lesions consist of discrete papules; in focal acantholytic dyskeratoma, manifesting itself as a solitary papule; and as an incidental small focus in a variety of unrelated lesions. Occasionally, a few corps ronds are seen also in familial benign pemphigus (see preceding text).

ACROKERATOSIS VERRUCIFORMIS OF HOPF

In acrokeratosis verruciformis, an autosomal dominant disorder, numerous flat, hyperkeratotic, occasionally verrucous papules are present on the distal part of the extremities, predominantly on the dorsa of the hands (Color Fig. 6-4) and feet.[222]

Histopathology. The papules show considerable hyperkeratosis, an increase in thickness of the granular layer, and acanthosis. In addition, there is slight papillomatosis, which is frequently but not always associated with circumscribed elevations of the epidermis resembling church spires (Fig. 6-29).[223,224] The rete ridges are slightly elongated and extend to a uniform level.

Histogenesis. A possible relationship between acrokeratosis verruciformis and Darier's disease has been repeatedly discussed. On the one hand, there is no question that acrokeratosis verruciformis usually occurs as an independent entity, often in several family members[222] and occasionally even in many family members[225] but also as a solitary incidence.[224] On the other hand, a relationship to Darier's disease is suggested by several observations: (1) Patients with Darier's disease not infrequently

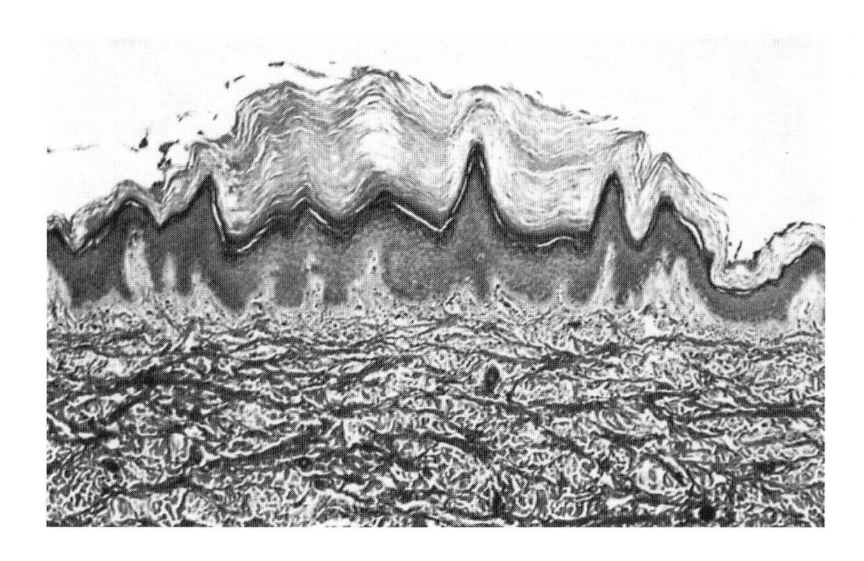

FIG. 6-29. Acrokeratosis verruciformis of Hopf
A well-circumscribed lesion shows hyperkeratosis and papillomatosis. The latter is associated with elevations of the epidermis resembling church spires (original magnification × 100).

show lesions that are indistinguishable from acrokeratosis verruciformis both clinically and histologically[223,226]; (2) some of the lesions of presumed acrokeratosis verruciformis occurring in patients with Darier's disease show dyskeratosis and lacunae as seen in Darier's disease, whereas others do not; and (3) patients with apparent histologic lesions of acrokeratosis verruciformis may later develop histologic lesions of Darier's disease. Admittedly, there can be considerable clinical resemblance between the acral lesions of both diseases, but, if multiple specimens for biopsy are taken and serial sections carried out, clear histologic evidence of Darier's disease is obtained only in those patients who have Darier's disease.[227] It seems that there is only one instance in which both diseases were seen in different members of the same family,[228] and this may well have been coincidence. Rather than taking the view that the two diseases result from a single dominant defect with variable expressivity,[228] it is best to regard acrokeratosis verruciformis as an independent entity.

Differential Diagnosis. Although elevations of the epidermis with the configuration of church spires are quite typical of acrokeratosis verruciformis, they may be absent and are not specific for that disease. Particularly, they are present in the hyperkeratotic type of seborrheic keratosis. Even though seborrheic keratoses usually are larger than the lesions of acrokeratosis verruciformis, clinical data may be necessary for the differentiation of these two conditions. Also, acrokeratosis verruciformis may resemble verrucae clinically, but it differs from verruca plana by the absence of vacuolization in the cells of the upper epidermis and from verruca vulgaris by the absence of parakeratosis.

PSEUDOXANTHOMA ELASTICUM

In this disorder, genetically abnormal elastic fibers with a tendency toward calcification occur in the skin and frequently also in the retina and within the walls of arteries, particularly the gastric mucosal arteries, coronary arteries, and large peripheral arteries. The inheritance is usually autosomal recessive but is occasionally autosomal dominant. It seems that two recessive and two dominant forms exist.[229] The classic disorder in this classification is recessive type 1. In the dominant type 1, the cutaneous and internal manifestations are more severe than in recessive type 1, whereas in dominant type 2 they are less severe. The very rare recessive type 2 shows only cutaneous involvement, which, however, is extensive.[230] The accuracy of the Pope classification has been disputed leading to a new classification.[231]

The cutaneous lesions usually appear first in the second or third decade of life and are generally progressive in extent and severity. They consist of soft, yellowish, coalescing papules, and the affected skin appears loose and wrinkled. The sides of the neck, the axillae, and the groin are the most common sites of lesions (Fig. 6-30). In the eyes, so-called angioid streaks of the fundi may cause progressive impairment of vision. Involvement of the arteries of the gastric mucosa may lead to gastric hemorrhage; involvement of coronary arteries may result in attacks of angina pectoris, although myocardial infarction is rare; involvement of the large peripheral arteries may cause intermittent claudication.[232] Radiologic examination in such cases reveals extensive calcification of the affected peripheral arteries.[233]

In rare instances, the coexistence of pseudoxanthoma elasticum with elastosis perforans serpiginosa has been reported, with perforation and transepidermal elimination present only in the lesions of elastosis perforans serpiginosa.[234] Calcific elastosis, which has been referred to also as perforating pseudoxanthoma elasticum or localized acquired pseudoxanthoma elasticum, is not related to pseudoxanthoma elasticum. The absence of skin lesions should not be used to exclude pseudoxanthoma elasticum in patients with an inherited predisposition and suspicious manifestations, such as angioid streaks or gastric bleeding. In these patients, biopsies of scars or of flexural skin may show the characteristic changes of pseudoxanthoma elasticum in the deep dermis.[231]

Histopathology. Histologic examination of the involved skin reveals in the middle and lower thirds of the dermis considerable accumulations of swollen and irregularly clumped fibers staining like elastic fibers; that is, they stain deeply black with orcein or Verhoeff's stain (Figs. 6-31 and 6-32). Although normally elastic fibers do not stain with routine stains such as hematoxylin-eosin, the altered elastic fibers in pseudoxanthoma elasticum stain faintly basophilic because of their

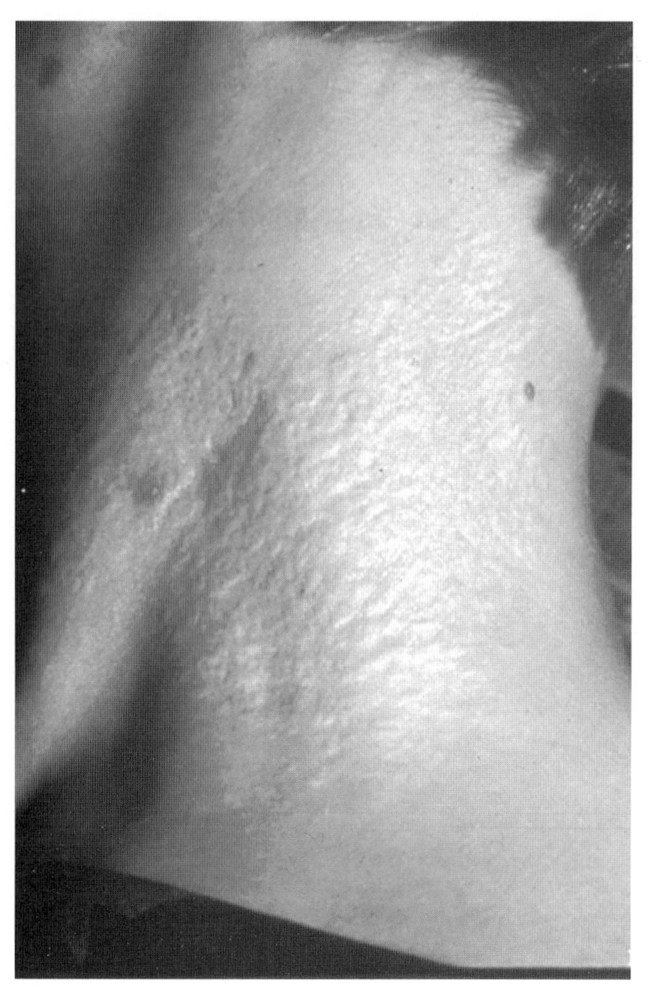

FIG. 6-30. Pseudoxanthoma elasticum
Yellow coalescing papules at the side of neck.

calcium imbibition. Staining for calcium with the von Kossa method also shows these fibers well. In the vicinity of the altered elastic fibers, there may be accumulations of a slightly basophilic mucoid material, which stains strongly positive with the colloidal iron reaction or with alcian blue.[235] The number of collagen bundles is reduced in such areas, and numerous reticulum fibers are seen on impregnation with silver.[236] In some cases with pronounced elastic tissue calcification a macrophage and giant cell reaction may be present.[237]

The angioid streaks occur in Bruch's membrane, which is located between the retina and the choroid and possesses numerous elastic fibers in its outer portion, the lamina elastica. Calcification of these fibers causes fissures to form in the lamina elastica. These fissures result in repeated hemorrhages and exudates, which in turn cause degenerative changes in the retina consisting of scar formation and pigment shifting.[237,238]

Gastric bleeding is the result of calcification of elastic fibers in the thin-walled arteries located immediately beneath the gastric mucosa. The internal elastic lamina is particularly affected. In muscular arteries, such as the coronary arteries and the large peripheral arteries, calcification begins in the internal and external elastic laminae, leading to their fragmentation, and subsequently extends to the media and intima.[232] Calcification of the elastic fibers in the endocardium is a common occurrence but is clinically silent.[239]

Histogenesis. Electron microscopic examination shows that the calcification occurs in normal-appearing elastic fibers.[236,239–242] In some patients, especially in young persons, only some of the elastic fibers in the lower dermis are calcified, and the calcification is variable in degree. In adult patients, however, most elastic fibers show considerable calcification and, as a result, degeneration. Early calcification of elastic fibers consists either of diffuse granular deposits throughout the elastic fiber or of dense aggregates that may be located in the center or near the margin of the fiber (EM 5). With progression of the calcification, the elastic fibers ultimately become fully calcified, showing marked swelling and bizarre distortions. In addition, heavy calcium deposits may be seen in the ground substance adjacent to elastic fibers and free in the ground substance. The presence of calcified material outside of elastic fibers can be explained by the disintegration of completely calcified elastic fibers.[242]

Besides varying numbers of normal collagen fibrils, irregularly twisted collagen fibrils and granulofilamentous aggregates are present. It appears unlikely that the process of calcification

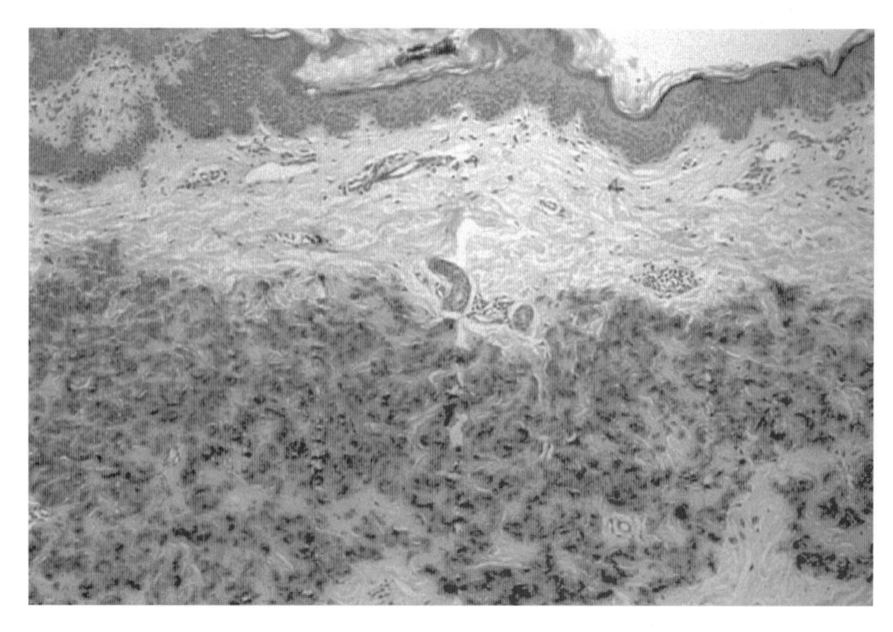

FIG. 6-31. Pseudoxanthoma elasticum
Low magnification, H&E stained tissue showing calcified altered elastic fibers in the midreticular dermis (original magnification × 100).

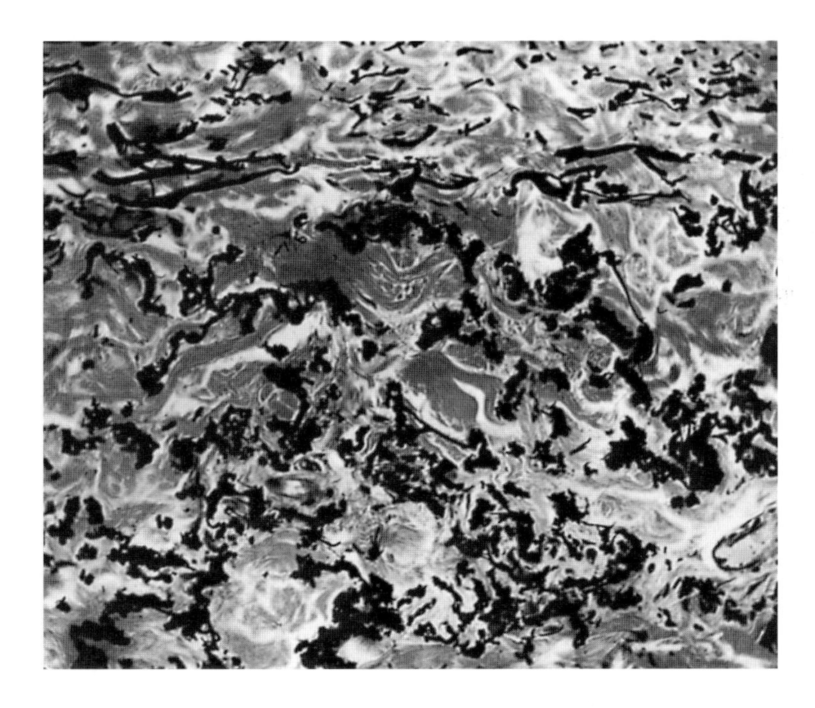

FIG. 6-32. Pseudoxanthoma elasticum, high magnification, elastic tissue stain
The elastic fibers in the upper fourth of the illustration have a normal appearance; those in the lower three fourths show marked degeneration (original magnification × 200).

begins in the granulofilamentous material, as maintained by some authors who regard this material as an abnormal precursor of elastic fibers.[238,243] It is probable that this misinterpretation has resulted from the examination of advanced lesions containing disintegrated calcified elastic fibers within the granulofilamentous material.[239] In favor of a primary location of the calcification within elastic fibers is the important observation that, in decalcified sections of endocardial lesions, the internal structure of the calcified segments of elastic fibers is very similar to that of the adjacent noncalcified segments.

Differential Diagnosis. Solar elastosis, like pseudoxanthoma elasticum, shows abnormal elastic tissue. However, in solar elastosis this material is located in the upper third of the dermis and is present as dense masses rather than as individual altered fibers. Furthermore, these dense masses always show negative staining for calcium. If associated with a perforation, calcific elastosis is easily distinguished from pseudoxanthoma elasticum. In the absence of a perforation the two are indistinguishable, and clinical data are necessary for differentiation.

CONNECTIVE TISSUE NEVUS

The connective tissue nevus represents a hamartoma in which the amount of collagen is increased, but the amount of elastic tissue may be increased, normal or decreased. The lesions consist of slightly elevated, slightly indurated nodules that may be grouped together in one or several plaques or may be widely disseminated (Fig. 6-33). A connective tissue nevus can: occur without alterations in other organs and without being genetically determined[244]; occur without alterations in other organs, being inherited as an autosomal dominant trait[245]; or occur with osteopoikilosis, being inherited in an autosomal dominant pattern.[246] The shagreen patches of tuberous sclerosis do not strictly belong in the category of connective tissue nevi, since they always consist only of excessive amounts of collagen and thus are "collagen nevi" rather than connective tissue nevi.[247]

Connective tissue nevi associated with osteopoikilosis are also referred to as *Buschke-Ollendorff syndrome,* because these authors first recognized the frequent simultaneous occurrence of these two types of lesions. The skin lesions in this syndrome consist of firm, pale papules and plaques in asymmetric distribution with a tendency to grouping.[246] Individual members of affected families may have skin lesions without bone lesions, and vice versa. The bone lesions of osteopoikilosis are asymptomatic and, on x-ray examination, consist of round or oval densities 2 to 10 mm in diameter in the long bones and in the bones of the hands, feet, and pelvis.

Histopathology. A clear separation of collagenoma and elastoma is not always possible, because in many instances both collagenous and elastic fibers are increased, as indicated by the fact that most lesions of connective tissue nevus feel firm to the touch. The increase in the amount of collagen may be difficult to ascertain if the collagen bundles are normal in appearance. In some lesions of collagenoma[245] and lesions of the connective tissue nevus–osteopoikilosis syndrome,[248] the collagen bundles are thickened and homogenized.

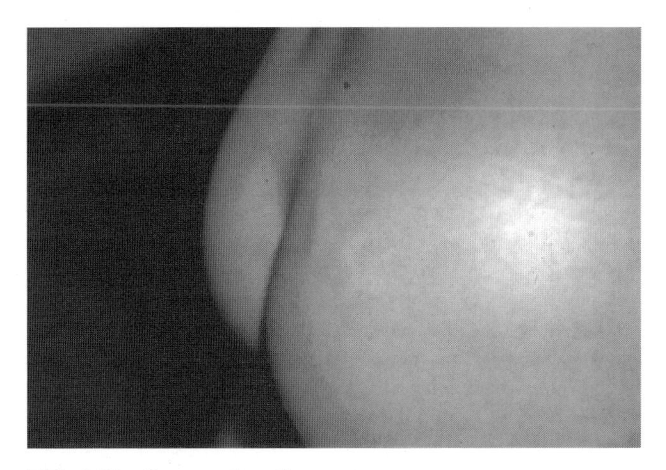

FIG. 6-33. Connective tissue nevus
Grouped slightly raised nodules producing an irregular surface on the buttock.

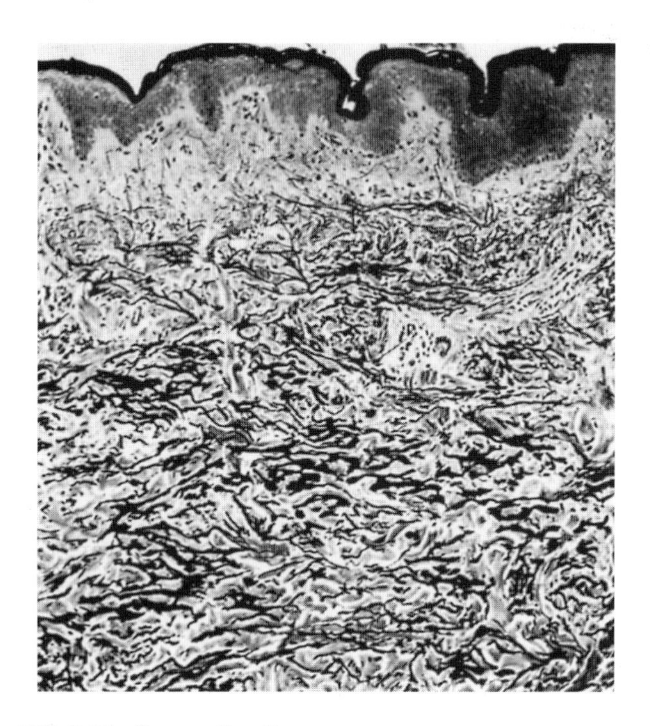

FIG. 6-34. Connective tissue nevus
The elastic fibers are markedly increased in number and size without showing signs of degeneration (original magnification × 100).

Most cases of the connective tissue nevus–osteopoikilosis syndrome clearly show a marked increase in the amount of elastic fibers, which are present as broad, interfacing bands, without showing signs of degeneration (Fig. 6-34).[249,250]

Pathogenesis. On electron microscopic examination connective tissue nevi show a variable picture. In some cases the elastic fibers appear thick and are surrounded by a thready material.[244] In the Buschke-Ollendorff syndrome[251] the elastic fibers lack their microfibrillar component so that only electron-lucent elastin is present.[252]

Differential Diagnosis. Pseudoxanthoma elasticum is the major differential disease. The connective tissue nevus does not show elastic tissue fragmentation and calcification as does pseudoxanthoma elasticum.

LINEAR MELORHEOSTOTIC SCLERODERMA

Melorheostosis is characterized by linear hyperostosis of an extremity. It may be associated with thickening and hypertrichosis of the overlying skin. Although not familial, its start in infancy suggests a congenital disorder.[253]

Histopathology. The skin shows thickening of the dermis caused by the extension of normal-appearing collagen and elastic tissue in strands and lobules into the subcutaneous fat.[254]

Pathogenesis. Hyperplasia of the skin is related to the underlying cortical hyperostosis. The normal appearance of the thickened dermis indicates that the process does not represent localized scleroderma.[254]

WINCHESTER SYNDROME

A rare autosomal recessive disorder described only in the offspring of consanguinous parents, Winchester syndrome is characterized by dwarfism, small-joint destruction, corneal opacities, thickening and hypertrichosis of the skin, and hypertrophic lips and gingivae.[255]

Histopathology. In the early stage, the skin shows proliferation of fibroblasts in the lower portions of the dermis with extension into the subcutaneous tissue. At a later stage, the collagen appears homogenized and contains only few fibroblasts.[256] Some areas may show an increase in both the number of fibroblasts and the density of the collagen bundles.[257]

Pathogenesis. An abnormal function of the fibroblasts is the likely cause for all manifestations. Electron microscopic examination has shown dilated and vacuolated mitochondria in the fibroblasts.[256]

EHLERS-DANLOS SYNDROME

The Ehlers-Danlos syndrome (E-D) has been divided into more than ten types on the basis of clinical, genetic, and biochemical information.[258] The common clinical features are: hyperextensibility of the skin; fragility of the skin with impaired wound healing, resulting in the formation of atrophic scars; and hypermobility of the joints, which may lead to dislocations (Fig. 6-35). Occasionally, one observes at sites of traumatic

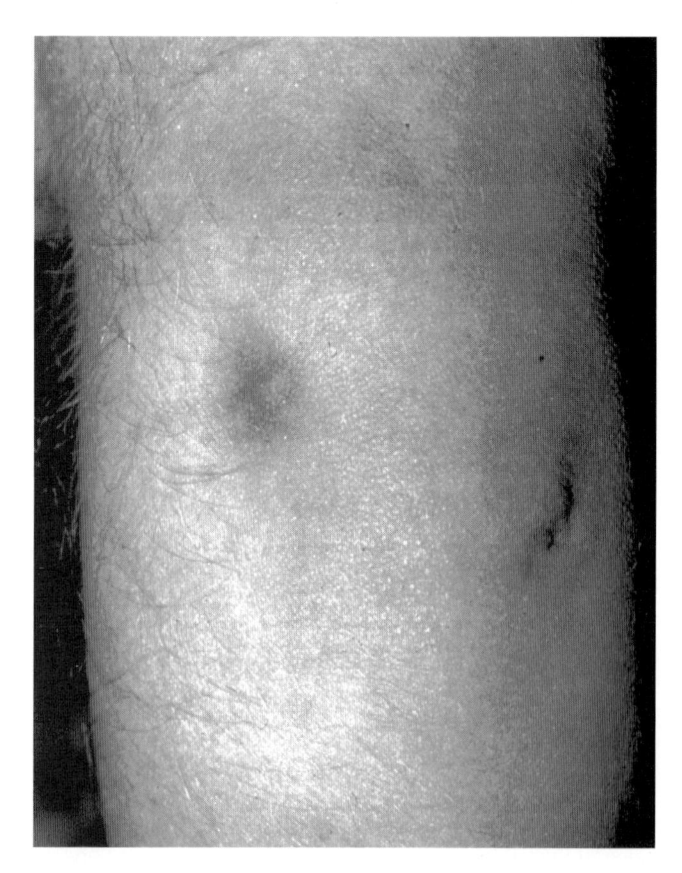

FIG. 6-35. Ehlers-Danlos syndrome
Scarring at the back of elbow.

hematomas raisin-like pseudotumors that are raised and soft and have a wrinkled surface. In some cases, firm, spheroid subcutaneous nodules form at sites of traumatic fat necrosis.

E-D types I, II, and III, the most common forms of this syndrome, are inherited in an autosomal dominant pattern and are distinguished by the extent and severity of the symptoms, type I being the gravis type, type II the mitis form, and type III the benign hypermobile type. No biochemical defect has been detected.[259]

E-D type IV, the arterial form, is inherited as an autosomal dominant or recessive trait. The skin of persons with this disorder is thin and fragile. Ecchymoses are very common. Patients rarely live beyond the second decade of life because of ruptures of large arteries or of the gastrointestinal tract.[260] This tendency toward rupture is explained by the fact that there is a deficiency of type III collagen (COL3A1 gene) in the skin and in other tissues. Even though cultured fibroblasts are capable of normal synthesis of collagen type III, they show poor secretion of it into the medium.[261]

E-D type V has an X-linked recessive inheritance pattern and clinical features similar to those of type I. The fibroblasts produce only 15% to 30% of the normal amount of lysyl oxidase. This deficiency results in deficient intramolecular cross-linking in the collagen molecule.[258]

E-D type VI, the ocular type, with autosomal recessive inheritance, is characterized by severe scoliosis and intraocular bleeding.[262] There is a deficiency in lysyl hydroxylase in this form of the disorder.

E-D type VII, the arthrochalasis type, also with autosomal dominant or recessive inheritance, shows marked looseness of joints resulting in multiple joint dislocations. The skin and tendons of patients with this form of E-D contain collagen polypeptides with a length intermediate between pro-alpha (procollagen) chains and alpha (collagen) chains. This is due to a structural mutation in the pro-alpha 2 chain that prevents the normal enzymatic removal of the aminopropeptide from it.[263]

E-D type VIII, the periodontal type, inherited as an autosomal dominant trait, is characterized by severe periodontitis and moderate skin fragility. Its biochemical defect is thought to be due to decreased production of type III collagen.

E-D type IX, the occipital horn syndrome (X-linked cutis laxa), with X-linked recessive inheritance, shows moderate skin extensibility, joint hypermobility, bladder diverticula, herniae, and rhizomelic limb shortening. The defect is due to abnormal copper metabolism and a decrease in lysyl oxidase. This disorder may be allelic with Menkes' syndrome.

E-D type X, the fibronectin type, with autosomal recessive inheritance, shows stria, moderate skin extensibility, joint hypermobility, and a platelet aggregation defect caused by dysfunction of the plasma fibronectin.[264]

Histopathology. Except for areas of the skin that have been altered secondarily by trauma, most patients with types I to III show no abnormalities either in the thickness of the skin or in the appearance of the collagen or of the elastic fibers. Only an exceptional patient shows thin collagen fibers that are not united to collagen bundles. In these cases, the skin may also be reduced in thickness and show a relative increase in amount of elastic fibers.[265] These changes are more pronounced in the type I (gravis) than in the types II and III and are more evident when a large excision biopsy is carried out, rather than a punch biopsy. They are often seen best in the collagen bundles of the connective tissue septae of the hypodermis, with the collagen bundles appearing thin and rare.[266]

E-D type IV shows the most pronounced degree of dermal thinning of all types, usually to half or three quarters of normal thickness. There is a relative abundance of elastic fibers that appear shortened and fragmented. This probably is secondary to changes in collagen fiber morphology.[267]

The raisin-like pseudotumors that arise at the site of hematomas show fibrosis and numerous capillaries; they may also show accumulations of foreign body giant cells.[268] The spheroid subcutaneous nodules consist of partially necrotic adipose tissue that may contain areas of dystrophic calcification and that is surrounded by a thick layer of dense collagen.[269]

Histogenesis. The enzyme deficiencies observed in the various types of the Ehlers-Danlos syndrome suggest a disturbance in collagen biosynthesis. In several electron microscopic studies, no abnormalities were observed in the normal skin of patients with Ehlers-Danlos syndrome[270,271]; however, other studies have reported abnormalities. In a study comparing healing experimental wounds in a patient with Ehlers-Danlos syndrome with those in normal persons, the fibroblasts of the patient with Ehlers-Danlos syndrome showed a paucity of rough-surfaced endoplasmic reticulum, and the bundles of collagen appeared small and sparse.[273] Similar abnormalities were observed also in the normal-appearing skin of five patients with various types of Ehlers-Danlos syndrome. The fibroblasts were smaller than in the skin of normal control persons, the endoplasmic reticulum was underdeveloped, and ribosome content was diminished. In addition, some collagen fibrils possessed an irregular outline, and lateral aggregation of the fibrils into bundles was reduced.[273] Scanning electron microscopic examination in various types of Ehlers-Danlos syndrome has revealed thinner collagen bundles than normal and, within the bundles, gross disorganization of the collagen fibers.[271] Scanning electron microscopy has shown that the hyperextensibility in the Ehlers-Danlos syndrome is due to defective "wicker work" of the collagen fiber bundles.

CUTIS LAXA (ELASTOLYSIS)

Cutis laxa, also called dermatochalasis and generalized elastolysis, is characterized by loose, pendulous skin resulting in a prematurely aged appearance (Fig. 6-36). There are two types, congenital and acquired. In the congenital type, the usual mode of inheritance is autosomal recessive,[274] although autosomal dominant transmission has been described in a few relatively mild cases.[275] The acquired type has no genetic background.[276]

In both the congenital and the acquired types, internal organs are frequently involved. There may be pulmonary emphysema causing death in infancy in some of the congenital cases[274,277] or later in life in some of the acquired cases.[276] In addition, there may be diverticula in the gastrointestinal tract or in the bladder. Also, rectal prolapse and inguinal, umbilical, and hiatal hernias have been observed.[274] About half of the cases of acquired cutis laxa are preceded or accompanied by a cutaneous eruption showing urticaria,[278] erythematous plaques,[279] or a vesicular eruption.[280]

Histopathology. In cases without an inflammatory infiltrate, the changes are limited to the elastic fibers and depend on the stage and the severity of the disease. In the early stage, the

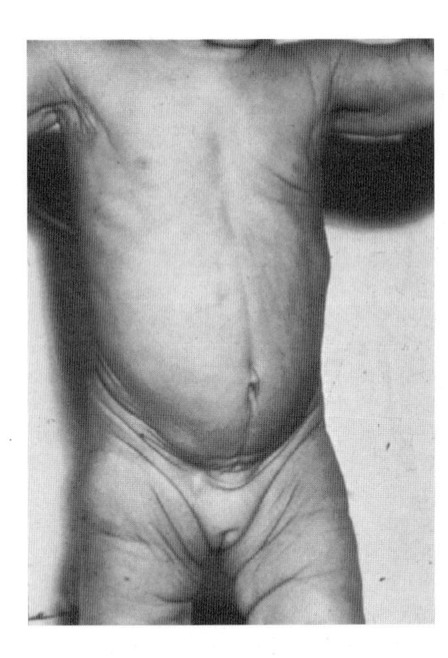

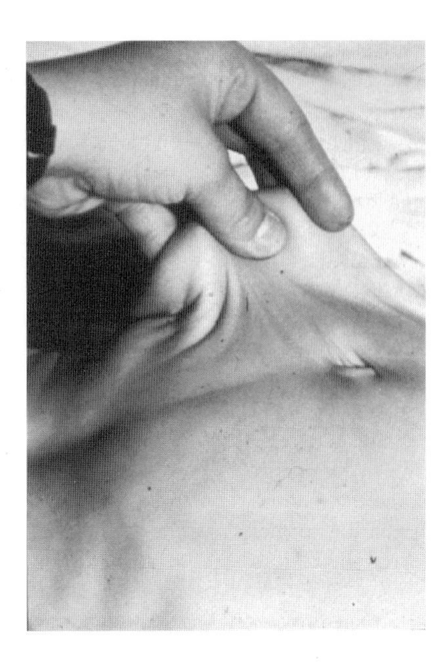

FIG. 6-36. Cutis laxa
Child with pendulous skin.

elastic fibers are diminished either throughout the dermis or largely in the upper dermis or the lower dermis.[281] Those elastic fibers that are present may be considerably thickened in their midportion and may taper to a point at either end. Their borders may be indistinct and they may stain unevenly, showing a granular appearance (Fig. 6-37). Ultimately, no intact elastic fibers may be identifiable. Instead, fine, dustlike orceinophilic granules may be scattered in the dermis.

In cases in which an inflammatory infiltrate is present, it may consist of a nonspecific chronic inflammatory infiltrate of lymphocytes and histiocytes. However, it may also contain neutrophils. If vesicles are present, they are subepidermal in location and may show papillary microabscesses composed of neutrophils and eosinophils suggestive of dermatitis herpetiformis.

In patients with involvement of internal organs, the lungs and gastrointestinal tract show the same granular changes in the elastic fibers as seen in the skin.

Histogenesis. Electron microscopic examination shows degenerative changes in the elastic fibers that vary somewhat from case to case. In some instances, the elastic fibers show normal microfibrils but a deficiency of the amorphous, electron-lucent elastin[277,282]; in other instances, the elastin is preserved and the microfibrils are absent. In most electron microscopic examinations, the most significant finding is the presence of electron-dense amorphous or granular aggregates in the vicinity of the elastic fibers.[283] The presence of this electron-dense material outside of elastic fibers suggests that, instead of a primary elastolysis, as generally assumed, a defect in the synthesis of elastic fibers causes the disease.[277,279]

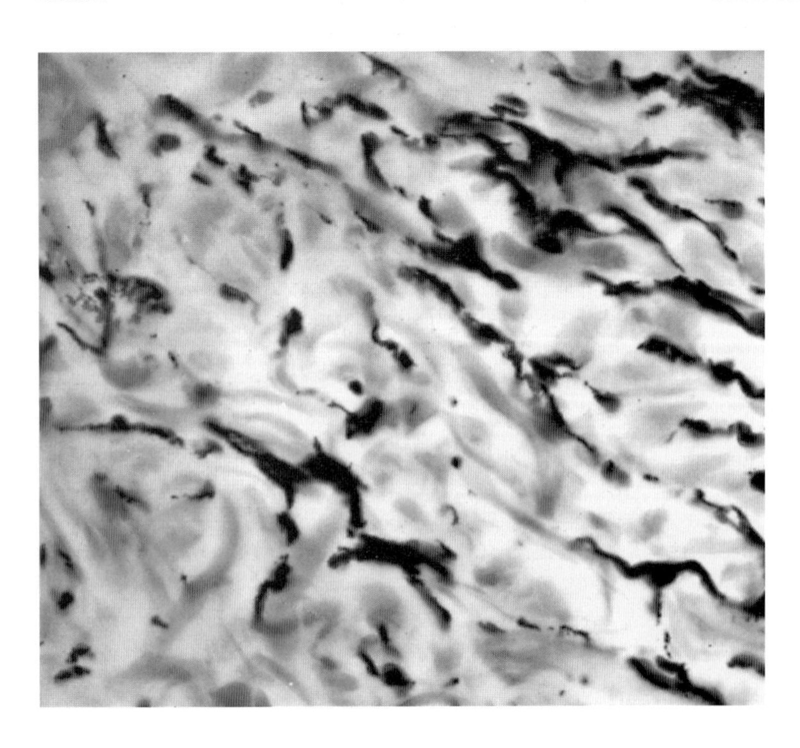

FIG. 6-37. Cutis laxa, elastic tissue stain
The degenerated elastic fibers stain unevenly, resulting in a granular appearance and indistinct border (original magnification × 400). (Courtesy of Dr. Robert W. Goltz.)

Another controversy concerns the role of the cutaneous eruption that precedes or accompanies many of the reported cases of acquired cutis laxa. The traditional view has been that the inflammatory infiltrate is in some way responsible for the damage to the elastic fibers.[284] However, in one reported case, sequential biopsies seemed to indicate that the changes in the elastic fibers induced the inflammatory infiltrate, and the possibility therefore exists that the inflammatory infiltrate is a consequence of changes in the fibers.

PACHYDERMOPERIOSTOSIS

An idiopathic and an acquired form of pachydermoperiostosis exist, the latter being secondary to carcinoma of the lung. The idiopathic form is transmitted as an autosomal dominant trait, males being more severely affected than females.[285] The manifestations include (1) clubbing of the digits, with periosteal proliferation of the bones of the hands and feet; (2) hyperplasia of the soft parts of the forearms and legs, with periosteal proliferation of the corresponding bones; and (3) thickening and furrowing of the skin of the face and scalp (cutis verticis gyrata). In abortive forms, there may be only clubbing of the fingers with periosteal proliferation of the bones of the hands and forearms.[286]

Histopathology. The skin of the face shows thickening of the dermis, with thick fibrous bands extending into the subcutaneous tissue.[287] In addition to an increase in the amount and size of the collagen bundles in the dermis, there is an increase in the number of fibroblasts and in the amount of ground substance. The latter stains with colloidal iron, and because it is composed largely of hyaluronic acid, it stains with alcian blue at pH 2.5 but not at pH 0.45.

URTICARIA PIGMENTOSA

Urticaria pigmentosa, although occasionally showing an autosomal dominant mode of transmission,[288,289] in most instances occurs without a family history. It can be divided into four forms: (1) urticaria pigmentosa arising in infancy or early childhood without significant systemic lesions, [290] (2) urticaria pigmentosa arising in adolescence or adult life without significant systemic lesions,[291] (3) systemic mast cell disease, and (4) mast cell leukemia.

In the first form, the cutaneous lesions often improve or even clear at puberty.[292] Systemic lesions are absent as a rule and, if present, usually are few in number. Progression into systemic mast cell disease is very rare (see later). In the second form, urticaria pigmentosa arising in adolescence or adult life, systemic lesions are often present but as a rule are rather static in their course.[293,294] However, spontaneous regression has never been documented in adults, in contrast to children.[295] In only a few patients is there progression to the third form, systemic mast cell disease, which shows extensive and progressive involvement of internal organs (see section on systemic lesions). The fourth form, mast cell leukemia, is very rare. It is characterized by the presence of cytologically malignant mast cells in many organs of the body, especially in the bone marrow and the peripheral blood, and is a rapidly fatal disease.[296] Usually there are no skin lesions.[297]

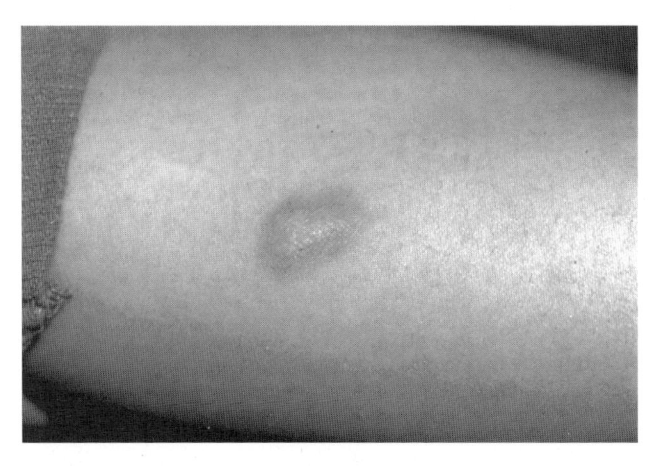

FIG. 6-38. Urticaria pigmentosa
Urtication of a papular lesion following stroking (Darier's sign).

Patients with extensive mast cell infiltration of the skin or the internal organs commonly have attacks of flushing, palpitation, or diarrhea as a result of degranulation of mast cells and the release of histamine.

Five types of cutaneous lesions are seen in urticaria pigmentosa.[292] Two types can occur in both the infantile and the adult forms. One is the maculopapular type, the most common type, consisting usually of dozens or even hundreds of brown lesions that urticate on stroking (Fig. 6-38); the other type exhibits multiple brown nodules or plaques, and, on stroking, shows urtication and occasionally blister formation (Color Fig. 6-5). The third type, seen almost exclusively in infants, is characterized by a usually solitary, large cutaneous nodule, which on stroking often shows not only urtication but also large bullae. In rare instances, solitary nodules have been described as arising in adults without giving rise to bullae.[298] The fourth type, the diffuse erythrodermic type, always starts in early infancy and shows generalized brownish red, soft infiltration of the skin, with urtication on stroking. Multiple blisters may form during the first two years of life on stroking and also spontaneously. If bullae are a predominant clinical feature, the term *bullous mastocytosis* has been applied.[299,300] Although visceral lesions are common in the diffuse erythrodermic type, they usually improve and only very rarely progress to fatal systemic mast cell disease. On rare occasions, death occurs in early infancy, apparently as a result of histamine shock with no or with only insignificant mast cell infiltration of visceral organs.[301] The fifth type of lesion, telangiectasia macularis eruptiva perstans, which usually occurs in adults, consists of an extensive eruption of brownish red macules showing fine telangiectasias, with little or no urtication on stroking.[302]

Histopathology. In all five types of lesions, the histologic picture shows an infiltrate composed chiefly of mast cells, which are characterized by the presence of metachromatic granules in their cytoplasm. These granules are not visible with routine stains but can be seen well after staining with a Giemsa stain or with toluidine blue. Also, the method using naphthol AS-D chloroacetate esterase, often called Leder's method, makes mast cell granules appear red and thus quite conspicuous.[303]

In the maculopapular type and in telangiectasia macularis

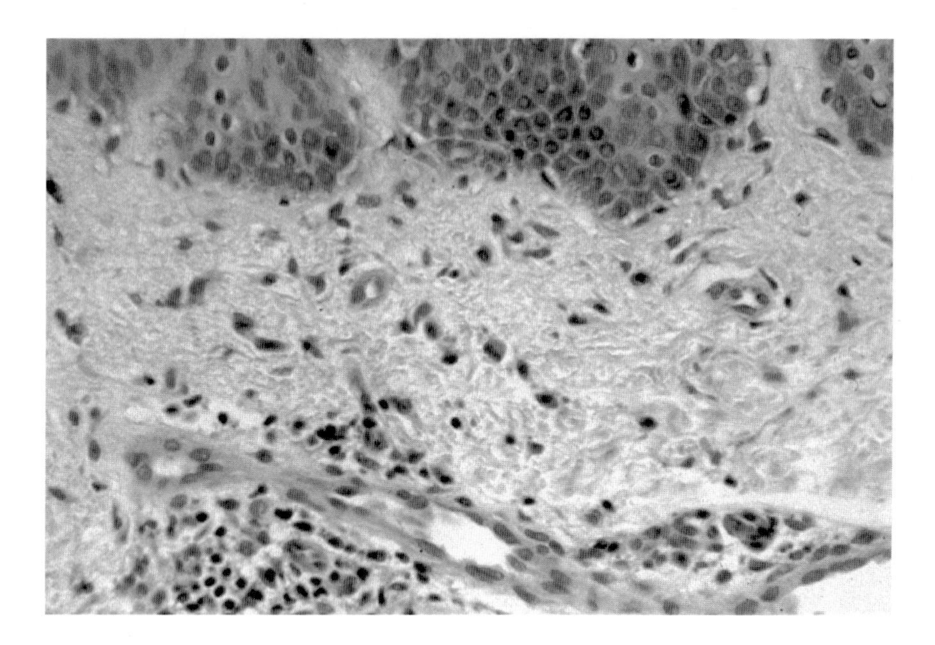

FIG. 6-39. Urticaria pigmentosa, maculopapular (adult type) Scattered mast cells are seen, some cuboidal in shape. The greatest numbers are about dermal vessels. The epidermis is hyperpigmented (original magnification × 100).

eruptiva perstans, the mast cells are limited to the upper third of the dermis and are generally located around capillaries. In some mast cells, the nuclei may be round or oval, but in most mast cells, they are spindle shaped (Fig. 6-39). Because the mast cells may be present only in small numbers, and because in sections stained with hematoxylin-eosin, their nuclei resemble those of fibroblasts or pericytes, the diagnosis may be missed unless special staining is employed.[304]

In cases with multiple nodules or plaques or with a solitary large nodule, the mast cells lie closely packed in tumorlike aggregates (Figs. 6-40 and 6-41). The infiltrate may extend through the entire dermis and even into the subcutaneous fat.[305] Whenever the mast cells lie in dense aggregates, their nuclei are cuboidal rather than spindle shaped, and they show ample eosinophilic cytoplasm and a well-defined cell border. Because of the shape of their nuclei and ample cytoplasm, they have a rather distinctive appearance, so that the diagnosis usually can be made even before special staining has been carried out.

In the diffuse, erythrodermic type, one observes in the upper dermis a dense, band-like infiltrate of mast cells with a rather uniform appearance showing round to oval nuclei and a distinctly outlined cytoplasm.[306]

Eosinophils may be present in small numbers in all types of urticaria pigmentosa with the exception of telangiectasia macularis eruptiva perstans, in which eosinophils are generally absent because of the small numbers of mast cells within the lesions. If a biopsy is taken shortly after the lesion has been stroked, one observes an increased number of eosinophils and extracellular mast cell granules as an indication that granules have been released by the cells.[307]

The bullae that may occur in infants with multiple or solitary nodules or with the diffuse erythrodermic type arise subepidermally.[308] Because of regeneration of the epidermis at the base of the bulla, older bullae may be located intraepidermally. The bullous cavity often contains mast cells as well as eosinophils.[309] The pigmentation of lesions of urticaria pigmentosa is due to the presence of increased amounts of melanin

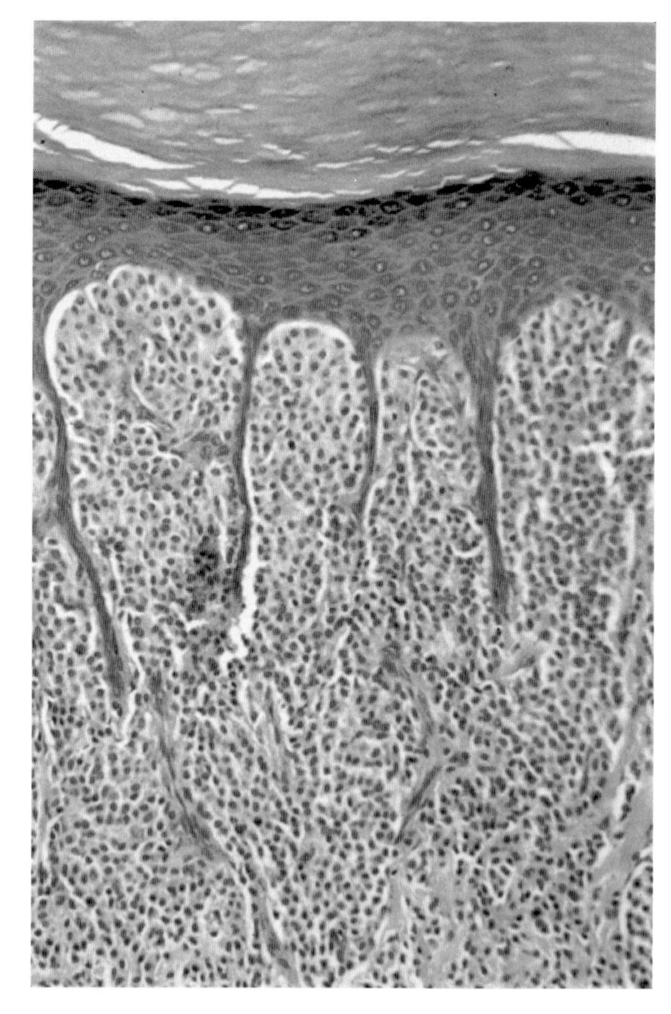

FIG. 6-40. Urticaria pigmentosa, nodular type Mast cells fill the expanded papillary dermis (H&E stain, original magnification × 100).

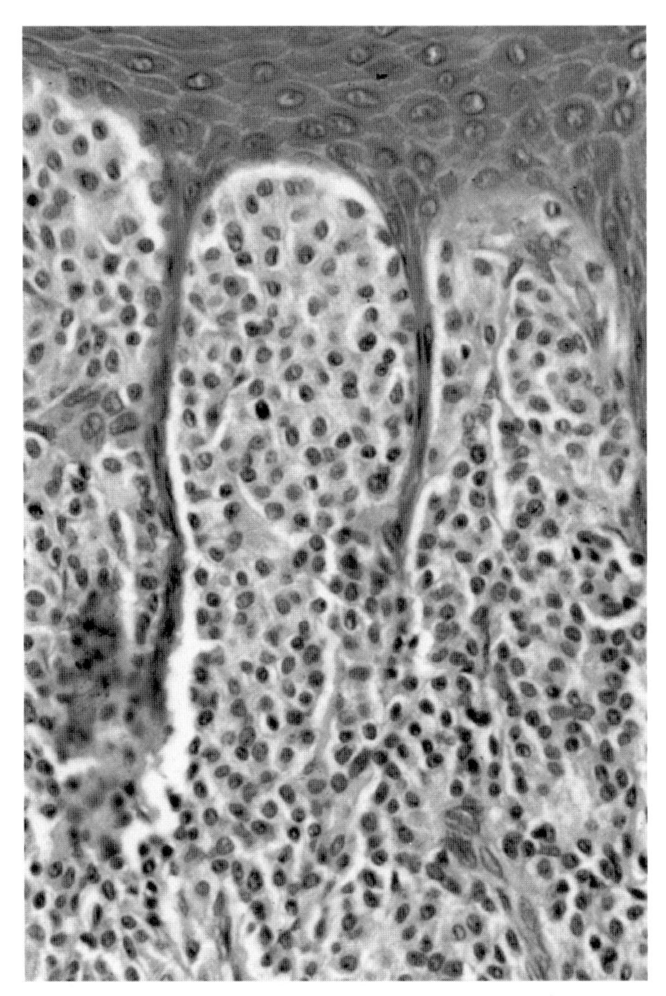

FIG. 6-41. Urticaria pigmentosa, nodular type
Cuboidal mast cells that fill and expand the papillary dermis. These cells closely resemble nevus cells. Special stains will differentiate (original magnification × 400).

in the basal cell layer and occasionally also of melanophages in the upper dermis.

Systemic Lesions

It is important to distinguish between asymptomatic systemic involvement of limited degree and true systemic mast cell disease, in which the lesions are symptomatic, widespread, and progressive.

Asymptomatic systemic involvement of a limited degree may occur in urticaria pigmentosa of children, but it is not common. It occurs most commonly in the erythrodermic and nodular types and consists of bone and bone marrow involvement or of hepatosplenomegaly. In urticaria pigmentosa of adults, systemic lesions are more common. For instance, in routinely carried out bone marrow biopsies, as many as 75% of adult patients show mast cell infiltration of bone marrow, in contrast to only 18% of children; radiologic survey of the skeleton has revealed bone changes in 44% of adult patients with urticaria pigmentosa, but in only 5% of children.[310] On radiologic examination, bones with mast cell infiltration may show areas of increased lucency intermingled with areas of increased density owing to the fact that mast cell aggregates in the bone marrow can cause focal bone resorption as well as reactive bone formation.[311]

In true systemic mast cell disease, massive infiltration of the bones may cause collapse of several vertebrae or a fracture of long bones.[312] Myelofibrosis may occur, resulting in anemia, leukopenia, and thrombocytopenia.[313] Pancytopenia may cause death. Systemic mastocytosis, besides involving the bone marrow and bones, generally involves various groups of lymph nodes and the liver and spleen, resulting in hepatosplenomegaly. In some cases, the gastrointestinal tract, lungs, and meninges are also infiltrated with mast cells.[295] Mature mast cells may be found in the peripheral blood.

Histogenesis. As seen by both light microscopy and electron microscopy, the mast cells of urticaria pigmentosa do not differ from normal mast cells either in structure or in mode of degranulation (EM 18).[314,315] Because mast cells contain histamine and release it during degranulation, chemical analysis of cutaneous lesions of urticaria pigmentosa reveals a considerably higher level of histamine than is found in normal skin.[316]

The increased melanin pigmentation in lesions of urticaria pigmentosa is the result of stimulation of epidermal melanocytes by mast cells. It is not caused by any substance present within the mast cells. In one case of nodular urticaria pigmentosa, however, some mast cells showed dual granulation containing both mast cell granules and melanosomes, as well as granules representing intergrades between mast cell granules and melanosomes.[317]

Differential Diagnosis. Even if numerous mast cells are present, an absolutely reliable diagnosis of urticaria pigmentosa requires the demonstration of mast cell granules with the Giemsa stain, Leder's method, or toluidine blue stain. On routine staining, the mast cells in macular lesions may resemble fibroblasts or pericytes, but those in nodular or erythrodermic lesions may resemble the histiocytes that are seen in Letterer-Siwe disease or in eosinophilic granuloma. Differentiation of urticaria pigmentosa from these two diseases on routine staining can be particularly difficult because, in all three diseases, the infiltrate may contain eosinophils. In contrast with Letterer-Siwe disease, the cells of urticaria pigmentosa have no tendency to invade the epidermis. Occasionally, the cuboidal mast cells in nodular urticaria pigmentosa resemble nevus cells, but they show no tendency to lie in nests and show no junction activity.

The macular type of urticaria pigmentosa, especially telangiectasia maculosa eruptiva perstans, occasionally may be difficult to diagnose even with the Giemsa stain because the number of mast cells may be so small that it does not differ significantly from the number normally present.[310] Some inflammatory dermatoses, such as atopic dermatitis, lichen simplex chronicus, and lichen planus, may contain a high percentage of mast cells in their inflammatory cell infiltrates.[318] In urticaria pigmentosa, however, the infiltrate consists exclusively of mast cells, except for a slight admixture of eosinophils as a result of the degranulation of some of the mast cells.

INCONTINENTIA PIGMENTI

Incontinentia pigmenti is an X-linked dominantly inherited disorder. Females with the abnormal gene on only one of their two X chromosomes are heterozygous for this condition and are not severely affected, but males with the abnormal gene on their single X chromosome are hemizygous for this condition and hence are so severely affected that they die in utero. This explains the predominance of female patients with this disorder.[319] Of 609 reported cases, only 16 have been in boys. The fact that these boys were no more severely affected than their female counterparts suggests that the disease in all living male patients is the result of spontaneous mutation.[320] The familial form of this disorder is localized to the Xq27–q28 region.[321]

The disorder has four stages. The first stage, consisting of erythema and bullae arranged in lines, either is present at birth or starts shortly thereafter. The extremities are predominantly affected. There is also marked blood eosinophilia. In the second stage, which occurs after about 2 months, the vesicular lesions gradually are superseded by linear, verrucous lesions that persist for several months. As the verrucous lesions subside, widely disseminated areas of irregular, spattered, or whorled pigmentation develop. This pigmentation, representing the third stage, is most pronounced on the trunk (Color Fig. 6-6). It diminishes gradually after several years and may even clear completely. The fourth stage is seen in adult females. Subtle, faint, hypochromic or atrophic lesions in a linear pattern are most apparent on the lower extremeties.[322]

In about 80% of the cases, incontinentia pigmenti is associated with various congenital abnormalities, particularly of the central nervous system, eyes, and teeth. Partial alopecia at the vertex is also often seen.[320]

Histopathology. The vesicles seen during the first stage arise within the epidermis and are associated with spongiosis. They are of the type seen in dermatitis.[323] However, they differ from the vesicles of dermatitis by the numerous eosinophils within them and around them in the epidermis (eosinophilic spongiosis) (Color Figs. 6-7 and 6-8). The epidermis between the vesicles often shows single dyskeratotic cells and whorls of squamous cells with central keratinization. Like the epidermis, the dermis shows an infiltrate containing many eosinophils and some mononuclear cells.

The alterations in the second stage consist of acanthosis, irregular papillomatosis, and hyperkeratosis. Intraepidermal keratinization, consisting of whorls of keratinocytes and of scattered dyskeratotic cells, is often more pronounced than in the first stage. The basal cells show vacuolization and a decrease in their melanin content. The dermis shows a mild, chronic inflammatory infiltrate intermingled with melanophages. This infiltrate extends into the epidermis in many places.

The areas of pigmentation seen in the third stage show extensive deposits of melanin within melanophages located in the upper dermis. Usually, this dermal hyperpigmentation is found in association with a diminution of pigment in the basal layer, the cells of which show vacuolization and degeneration.[324] In some cases, however, the cells of the basal layer contain abundant amounts of melanin.[325,326]

A different pattern has recently been described on the skin of the legs of an infant in whom the vesiculation had produced superficial scarring and depigmentation. The light-colored skin lacked melanocytes and appendages as the result of scarring, and the darker skin showed a normal degree of pigmentation without incontinence of pigment.[327]

Pathogenesis. The fact that the first two stages of incontinentia pigmenti are seen predominantly on the extremities and the third stage mainly on the trunk has led to the assumption by some authors that the pigmentary changes of the third stage occur independently of the bullous and verrucous lesions of the first two stages and represent some sort of nevoid anomaly. Electron microscopic studies, however, have revealed common features, albeit to varying extents, in all three stages of incontinentia pigmenti and thus suggest that the three stages are related to each other.[328–330] Even in the first stage, many keratinocytes and melanocytes show degenerative changes resulting in the migration of macrophages to the epidermis, where they phagocytize dyskeratotic keratinocytes and melanosomes. Subsequently, the macrophages return to the dermis (EM 6). The macrophages seen in the dermis in the second and third stages contain many melanosome complexes and thus are easily recognizable as melanophages even by light microscopy, whereas the macrophages in the first stage contain only few melanosome complexes and therefore can be identified as melanophages only in the electron microscope.[328] The phagocytosis of melanin by dermal macrophages in the first stage of the disease [329] and the presence of dyskeratotic keratinocytes in the epidermis during all three stages of the disease have been confirmed.

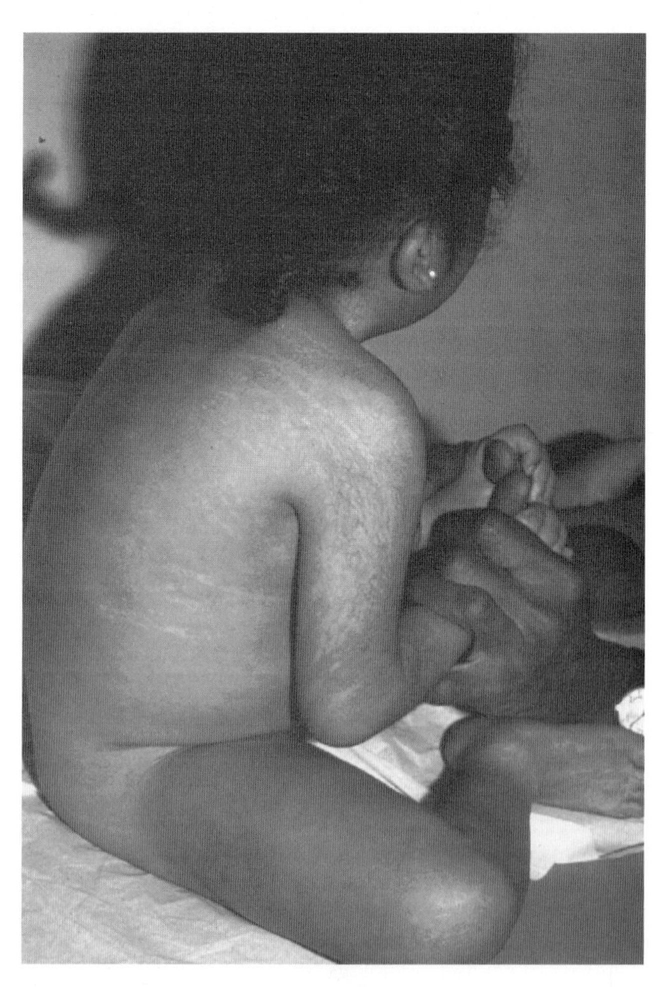

FIG. 6-42. Hypomelanosis of Ito
Streaking hypopigmentation on trunk.

The presence of eosinophils in epidermal and dermal infiltrates can be explained by the presence in the early vesicular stage of basophils, which release eosinophil chemotactic factor of anaphylaxis.[331] Eosinophil chemotactic activity has been demonstrated in patients with incontinentia pigmenti in the blister fluid [332] and in eluates of crusted scales overlying the lesions.[333]

HYPOMELANOSIS OF ITO

Hypomelanosis of Ito was originally called incontinentia pigmenti achromians, but because the disorder shows no pigmentary incontinence, this term has been largely abandoned.

The hypomelanosis seen in this disorder may be present at birth. However, it usually develops during the first year of life. In some instances the loss of pigment does not begin until childhood. There is a tendency for the pigmentary loss to become more pronounced at first but to be followed by partial repigmentation in adult life. The pattern and distribution of the hypopigmentation in hypomelanosis of Ito is similar to the pattern of hyperpigmentation seen in incontinentia pigmenti (Fig. 6-42). Although first reported in Japanese patients, hypomelanosis of Ito has since been observed in many races.

Congenital abnormalities are found in 50% of the cases.[334] Most common are mental retardation and seizure disorders, but there also may be abnormalities of the eyes, hair, teeth, or the musculoskeletal system.[335] Abnormal chromosomal constitutions are common.[336]

Histopathology. In the hypopigmented areas, a Fontana-Masson stain shows a decrease in the amount of melanin granules in the basal cell layer, with a complete absence of melanin in some areas.[337] With the dopa reaction, the hypopigmented areas are seen to contain fewer and smaller melanocytes than normal, with sparse, short dendrites.[338]

Pathogenesis. The electron microscopic findings show a significant decrease in the number of melanosomes within melanocytes and keratinocytes.[335,338] In addition, some melanocytes show degenerative changes and an absence of melanosomes.[339]

REFERENCES

1. Stevanovic DV. Hodgkin's disease of the skin. Arch Dermatol 1960; 82:96.
2. Flint GL, Flam M, Soter NA. Acquired ichthyosis: A sign of nonlymphoproliferative malignant disorder. Arch Dermatol 1975;111:1446.
3. Frost P, Van Scott EJ. Ichthyosiform dermatoses. Arch Dermatol 1966;94:113.
4. Sybert VP, Dale BA, Molbrook KA. Ichthyosis vulgaris: Identification of a defect in synthesis of fillagrin correlated with an absence of keratohyaline granules. J Invest Dermatol 1985;84:191.
5. Nirunsuksiri W, Presland RB, Brumbaugh SG et al. Decreased profillagrin expression in ichthyosis vulgaris is a result of selectively impaired posttranscriptional control. J Biol Chem 1995;270:871.
6. Perrot H, Schmitt D, Thivolet J. Ichtyose paraneoplasique: Étude ultrastructurale. Ann Dermatol Syphiligr 1976;103:413.
7. Finley AY, Nicholls S, King CS et al. The dry non-eczematous skin associated with atopic eczema. Br J Dermatol 1980;103:249.
8. Frost P. Ichthyosiform dermatoses. J Invest Dermatol 1973;60:541.
9. Feinstein A, Ackerman AB, Ziprkowski L. Histology of autosomal dominant ichthyosis vulgaris and X-linked ichthyosis. Arch Dermatol 1970;101:524.
10. Anton-Lamprecht L. Zur ultrastruktur hereditarer verhornungsstorungen: IV. X-chromosomal-recessive ichthyosis. Arch Dermatol Forsch 1974;248:361.
11. Shapiro LJ, Weiss R, Webster D et al. X-linked ichthyosis due to steroid-sulphatase deficiency. Lancet 1978;1:70.
12. Williams ML, Elias P. X-linked ichthyosis: Elevated cholesterol sulfate in pathological stratum corneum (abstr). J Invest Dermatol 1981; 76:312.
13. Epstein EH Jr, Williams ML, Elias PM. Editorial: Steroid sulfatase, X-linked ichthyosis, and stratum corneum cohesion. Arch Dermatol 1981;117:761.
14. Ishibashi Y, Klingmuller G. Erythrodermia ichthyosiformis congenita bullosa Brocq. Arch Klin Exp Dermatol 1968;232:205.
15. Ackerman AB. Histopathologic concept of epidermolytic hyperkeratosis. Arch Dermatol 1970;102:253.
16. McCurdy J, Beare JM. Congenital bullous ichthyosiform erythroderma. Br J Dermatol 1976;79:294.
17. Rothnagel JA, Dominey AM, Dempsy LD et al. Mutations in the rod domains of keratins 1 and 10 in epidermolytic hyperkeratosis. Science 1992;257:1128.
18. Schnyder UW. Inherited ichthyosis. Arch Dermatol 1970;102:240.
19. Anton-Lamprecht I, Schnyder UW. Ultrastructure in inborn errors of keratinization. Arch Dermatol Forsch 1974;250:207.
20. Mehregan AH. Epidermolytic hyperkeratosis. J Cutan Pathol 1978; 5:76.
21. Niizuma K. Isolated epidermolytic acanthoma. Dermatologica 1979; 159:30.
22. Paller AS, Synder AJ, Chan YM et al. Genetic and clinical mosaicism in a type of epidermal nevus. N Engl J Med 1994;331:1408.
23. Hazell M, Marks R. Clinical histology and cell kinetic discriminants between lamellar ichthyosis and nonbullous congenital ichthyosiform erythroderma. Arch Dermatol 1985;121:489.
24. Hohl D, Huber M, Frenk E. Analysis of the cornified cell envelope in lamellar ichthyosis. Arch Dermatol 1993;129:618.
25. Menon GK, Williams ML, Ghadally R, Elias PM. Lamellar bodies as delivery systems of hydrolytic enzymes: Implications for normal cohesion and abnormal desquamation. Br J Dermatol 1992;126;337.
26. Elias PM, Williams ML. Neutral lipid storage disease with ichthyosis. Arch Dermatol 1985;121:1000.
27. Williams ML, Elias PM. Heterogeneity in autosomal recessive ichthyosis. Arch Dermatol 1985;121:477.
28. Happle R. X-chromosomal vererbte dermatosen. Hautarzt 1982;33: 73.
29. Emami S, Rizzo WB, Hanley KP et al. Peroxisomal abnormality in fibroblast from involved skin of CHILD syndrome. Arch Dermatol 1992;128:1213.
30. Christiansen JV, Petersen HO, Søgaard H. The CHILD syndrome: Congenital hemodysplasia with ichthyosiform and limb defects. Acta Derm Venereol (Stockh) 1984;64:165.
31. Roberts LJ. Long term survival of a harlequin fetus. J Am Acad Dermatol 1989;21:335.
32. Luderschmidt C, Dorn M, Bassermann R et al. Kollodiumbaby und harlekinfetus. Hautarzt 1980;31:154.
33. Milner ME, O'Guin WM, Holbrook KA et al. Abnormal lamellar granules in harlequin ichthyosis. J Invest Dermatol 1992;99:824.
34. Williams ML. Ichthyosis: Mechanisms of disease. Pediatr Dermatol 1992;9:365.
35. Vandersteen PR, Muller SA. Erythrokeratodermia variabilis. Arch Dermatol 1971;103:362.
36. Nir M, Tanzer F. Progressive symmetric erythrokeratodermia. Dermatologica 1978;156:268.
37. Judge MR, Morgan G, Harper JI. A clinical and immunological study of Netherton's syndrome. Br J Dermatol 1994;131:615.
38. Mehvorah B, Frenk E, Brooke EM. Ichthyosis linearis circumflexa Comèl. Dermatologica 1974;149:201.
39. Altman J, Stroud J. Netherton's syndrome and ichthyosis linearis circumflexa: Psoriasiform ichthyosis. Arch Dermatol 1969;100:550.
40. Hersle K. Netherton's disease and ichthyosis linearis circumflexa. Acta Derm Venereol (Stockh) 1972;52:298.
41. Thorne EG, Zelickson AS, Mottaz JH et al. Netherton's syndrome: An electron microscopic study. Arch Dermatol Res 1975;253:177.
42. Mehvorah B, Frenk E. Ichthyosis linearis circumflexa Comèl with trichorrhexis invaginata (Netherton's syndrome). Dermatologica 1974; 149:193.

43. Zina AM, Bundino S. Ichthyosis linearis circumflexa Comèl and Netherton's syndrome: An ultrastructural study. Dermatologica 1979; 158:404.
44. Jorizzo JL, Crounse RG, Wheeler CE Jr. Lamellar ichthyosis, dwarfism, mental retardation, and hair shaft anomalies. J Am Acad Dermatol 1980;2:309.
45. Wells RS. Some genetic aspects of dermatology: A review. Clin Exp Dermatol 1980;5:1.
46. Heijer A, Reed WB. Sjögren-Larsson syndrome. Arch Dermatol 1965; 92:545.
47. Rizzo WB, Dammann AL, Craftda et al. Sjögren-Larsson syndrome: Inherited defect in the fatty alcohol cycle. J Pediatr 1989;115:228.
48. Maldonado RR, Tamayo L, Carnevale A. Neuroichthyosis with hypogonadism (Rud's syndrome). Int J Dermatol 1975;14:347.
49. Edidin DV, Esterly NB, Bamzai AK et al. Chondrodysplasia punctata: Conradi-Hunermann syndrome. Arch Dermatol 1977;113:1431.
50. Emami S, Hanley KP, Esterly NB et al. X-Linked dominant ichthyosis with peroxisomal deficiency: An ultrastructural and ultracytochemical study of the Conradi-Hunermann syndrome and its murine homolog, the Bare Patches Mouse. Arch Dermatol 1994;130:325.
51. Skinner BA, Greist MC, Norins AL. The keratins, ichthyosis and deafness (KID) syndrome. Arch Dermatol 1981;177:285.
52. Williams ML, Coleman RA, Placzek D et al. Neutral lipid storage disease with ichthyosis: Evidence for a function defect in phospholipid linked triacylglycerol metabolism in cultured fibroblasts. Biochem Biophys Acta 1991;1096:162.
53. Davies MG, Marks R, Dykes PJ et al. Epidermal abnormalities in Refsum's disease. Br J Dermatol 1977;97:401.
54. Rand RE, Baden HP. The ichthyoses: A review. J Am Acad Dermatol 1983;8:285.
55. Kansky A, Arzensek J. Is palmoplantar keratoderma of Greither's type a separate nosologic entity? Dermatologica 1979;158:244.
56. Hamm H, Happlf R, Butterfass T et al. Epidermolytic keratoderma of Vorner: Is it the most common type of hereditary palmoplantar keratoderma? Dermatologica 1988;177:138.
57. Rothnagel JA, Wojcik S, Leifer KM et al. Mutations in the 1A domain of keratin-9 in patients with epidermolytic palmoplantar keratoderma. J Invest Dermatol 1995;104:430.
58. Salamon T, Bogdanovic B, Lazovic-Tepava CO. Die krankheit von Mljet. Dermatologica 1969;138:433.
59. Bach JN, Levan NE. Papillon-Lefevre syndrome. Arch Dermatol 1968;97:154.
60. Klaus S, Weinstein GD, Frost P. Localized epidermolytic hyperkeratosis: A form of keratoderma of the palms and soles. Arch Dermatol 1970;101:272.
61. Moulin G, Bouchet B. La keratodermie palmo-plantaire familiale avec hyperkeratose epidermolytique. Ann Dermatol Venereol 1977;104: 38.
62. Fritsch P, Honigsmann H, Jaschke E. Epidermolytic hereditary palmoplantar keratoderma. Br J Dermatol 1978;99:561.
63. Buchanan RN Jr. Keratosis punctata palmaris et plantaris. Arch Dermatol 1963;88:644.
64. Brown FC. Punctate keratoderma. Arch Dermatol 1971;104:682.
65. Herman PS. Punctate porokeratotic keratoderma. Dermatologica 1973;147:206.
66. Costa OG. Acrokeratoelastoidosis. Arch Dermatol 1954;70:228.
67. Jung EG, Beil FU, Anton-Lamprecht I et al. Akrokeratoelastoidosis. Hutarzt 1974;25:7.
68. Highet, Rook A, Anderson JR. Acrokeratoelastoidosis. Br J Dermatol 1982;106:337.
69. Johansson EA, Kariniemi AL, Niemi KM. Palmoplantar keratoderma of punctate type: Acrokeratoelastoidosis costa. Acta Derm Venereol (Stockh) 1980;60:149.
70. Dowd PM, Hartman RRM, Black MM. Focal acral hyperkeratosis. Br J Dermatol 1989;109:97.
71. Blum SL, Cruz PD Jr, Siegel DM. Focal acral hyperkeratosis. Arch Dermatol 1987;123:1225.
72. Burks JW, Wise LJ, Clark WH Jr. Degenerative collagenous plaques of the hands. Arch Dermatol 1960;82:362.
73. Ritchie EB, Williams HM Jr. Degenerative collagenous plaques of the hands. Arch Dermatol 1966;93:202.
74. Kelly EW Jr, Pinkus H. Report of a case of pachyonychia congenita. Arch Dermatol 1958;77:724.
75. Schonfeld PHIR. The pachyonychia congenita syndrome. Acta Derm Venereol (Stockh) 1980;60:45.
76. Witkop CJ, Gorlin RJ. Four hereditary mucosal syndromes. Arch Dermatol 1961;84:762.
77. Mc Lean WHI, Rugg EL, Lunny DP et al. Keratin-16 and keratin-17 mutations cause pachyonychia congenita. Nature Genetics 1995; 9:273.
78. Tchou PK, Kohn T. Dyskeratosis congenita: An autosomal dominant disorder. J Am Acad Dermatol 1982;6:1034.
79. Gutman A, Frumkin A, Adam A et al. X-linked dyskeratosis congenita with pancytopenia. Arch Dermatol 1978;114:1667.
80. Bryan HG, Nixon RK. Dyskeratosis congenita and familial pancytopenia. JAMA 1965;192:203.
81. Costello MJ, Buncke CM. Dyskeratosis congenita. Arch Dermatol 1956;73:123.
82. Dokal I, Luzzatto L. Dyskeratosis congenita is a chromosomal instability disorder. Leukemia and Lymphoma 1995;15:1.
83. Chernosky ME. Editorial: Porokeratosis. Arch Dermatol 1986;122: 869.
84. Brodkin RH, Rickert RR, Fuller FW et al. Malignant disseminated porokeratosis. Arch Dermatol 1987;123:1521.
85. Chernosky ME, Freeman RG. Disseminated superficial actinic porokeratosis (DSAP). Arch Dermatol 1967;96:611.
86. Schwarz T, Seiser A, Gschnait F. Disseminated superficial actinic porokeratosis. J Am Acad Dermatol 1984;11:724.
87. Neumann RA, Knobler RM, Metze D et al. Disseminated superficial porokeratosis and immunosuppression. Br J Dermatol 1988;119:375.
88. Rahbari H, Cordero AA, Mehregan AH. Linear porokeratosis. Arch Dermatol 1974;109:526.
89. Nabai H, Mehregan AH. Porokeratosis of Mibelli: A report of two unusual cases. Dermatologica 1979;159:325.
90. Guss SB, Osbourn RA, Lutzner MA. Porokeratosis plantaris, palmaris et disseminata. Arch Dermatol 1971;104:366.
91. Shaw JC, White CR Jr. Porokeratosis plantaris, palmaris et disseminata. J Am Acad Dermatol 1984;11:454.
92. Brasch J, Scheuer B, Christophers E. Porokeratosis plantaris, palmaris et disseminata. Hautarzt 1985;36:459.
93. Himmelstein R, Lynnfield YL. Punctate porokeratosis. Arch Dermatol 1984;120:263.
94. Oberste-Lehn H, Moll B. Porokeratosis Mibelli und stachelzellcarcinom. Hautarzt 1968;19:399.
95. Coskey RJ, Mehregan A. Bowen disease associated with porokeratosis of Mibelli. Arch Dermatol 1975;111:1480.
96. Mibelli V. Contributo allo studio della ipercheratosi dei canali sudoriferi. G Ital Mal Ven 1983;28:313.
97. Braun-Falco O, Balsa RE. Zur histochemie der cornoiden lamelle. Hautarzt 1969;28:543.
98. Reed RJ, Leone P. Porokeratosis: A mutant clonal keratosis of the epidermis. Arch Dermatol 1970;101:340.
99. Magee JW, McCalmont TH, LeBoit PE. Over expression of P53 tumor supressor protein in porokeratosis. Arch Dermatol 1994;130:187.
100. Mann PR, Cort DF, Fairburn EA et al. Ultrastructural studies on two cases of porokeratosis of Mibelli. Br J Dermatol 1974;90:607.
101. Sato A, Anton-Lamprecht I, Schnyder UW. Ultrastructure of inborn errors of keratinization: Vll. Porokeratosis Mibelli and disseminated superficial actinic porokeratosis. Arch Dermatol Res 1976;255:271.
102. Wade TR, Ackerman AB. Cornoid lamellation: A histologic reaction pattern. Am J Dermatopathol 1980;2:5.
103. McGovern VJ. Melanoblastoma, with particular reference to its incidence in childhood. Australas J Dermatol 1962;6:190.
104. Tullis GD, Lynde CW, McLean DI. Multiple melanomas occurring in a patient with xeroderma pigmentosum. J Am Acad Dermatol 1984; 11:364.
105. Reed WB, Sugarman Gl, Mathis RA. DeSanctis-Cacchione syndrome. Arch Dermatol 1977;113:1561.
106. Cleaver JF. Xeroderma pigmentosum. Genetic and environmental influences in skin carcinogenesis. Int J Dermatol 1978;17:435.
107. Akiba H, Kato T, Seiji M. Enzyme defects in xeroderma pigmentosum. J Dermatol 1976;3:163.
108. Friedberg EC. Recent studies on the DNA repair defects. Arch Pathol 1978;102:3.
109. Guerrier CJ, Lutzner MA, Devico V et al. An electron microscopical study of the skin in 18 cases of xeroderma pigmentosum. Dermatologica 1973;146:211.
110. Pierard GE, Van Neste D, Letot B. Hidrotic ectodermal dysplasia. Dermatologica 1979;158:168.

111. McNaughton PZ, Pierson DL, Rodman RG. Hidrotic ectodermal dysplasia in a black mother and daughter. Arch Dermatol 1976;112:1448.
112. Clarke A, Phillips DIM, Brown R, et al. Clinical aspects of x-linked hypohidrotic ectodermal dysplasia. Arch Dis Child 1987;62:989.
113. Martin-Pascual A, De Unamuno P, Aparicio M et al. Anhidrotic (or hypohidrotic) ectodermal dysplasia. Dermatologica 1977;154:235.
114. Reed WB, Lopex DA, Landing B. Clinical spectrum of anhidrotic ectodermal dysplasia. Arch Dermatol 1970;102:134.
115. Malagon V, Taveras JE. Congenital anhidrotic ectodermal and mesodermal dysplasia. Arch Dermatol 1956;74:253.
116. Happle R, Lenz W. Striation of bone in focal dermal hypoplasia: Manifestation of functional mosaicism. Br J Dermatol 1977;96:133.
117. Kilmer SL, Grix AW, Isseroff RR. Focal dermal hypoplasia. Four cases with varying presentations. J Am Acad Dermatol 1993;28:1839.
118. Gottlieb SK, Fisher BK, Violin GA. Focal dermal hypoplasia. Arch Dermatol 1973;108:551.
119. Goltz RW, Henderson RR, Hitch JM et al. Focal dermal hypoplasia syndrome. Arch Dermatol 1970;101:1.
120. Howell JB, Reynolds J. Osteopathia striata. Trans St Johns Hosp Dermatol Soc 1974;60:178.
121. Lever WF. Hypoplasia cutis congenita (case presentation). Arch Dermatol 1964;90:340
122. Tsuji T. Focal dermal hypoplasia syndrome: An electron microscopical study of the skin lesions. J Cutan Pathol 1982;9:271.
123. Harari Z, Pusmanik A, Dvoretsky I et al. Aplasia cutis congenita with dystrophic nail changes. Dermatologica 1976;153:363.
124. Levin DL, Nolan KS, Esterly NB. Congenital absence of skin. J Am Acad Dermatol 1980;2:203.
125. Frieden IJ. Aplasia cutis congenita: A clinical review and proposal for classification. J Am Acad Dermatol 1986;14:646.
126. Deeken JH, Caplan RM. Aplasia cutis congenita. Arch Dermatol 1970;102:386.
127. Bart BJ. Epidermolysis bullosa and congenital localized absence of skin. Arch Dermatol 1970;101:78.
128. Rook A, Davis R, Stevanovic D. Poikiloderma congenitale: Rothmund-Thomson syndrome (review). Acta Derm Venereol (Stockh) 1959;39:392.
129. Venos EM, Collins M, Jane WD. Rothmund-Thomson syndrome: Review of the world literature. J Am Acad Dermatol 1992;27:750.
130. Dick DC, Morley WN, Watson JT. Rothmund-Thomson syndrome and osteogenic sarcoma. Clin Exp Dermatol 1982;7:119.
131. Gretzula JL, Hevia O, Weber PJ. Bloom's syndrome. J Am Acad Dermatol 1987;17:479.
132. Braun-Falco O, Marghescu S. Kongenitales telangiektatisches erythem (Bloom syndrom) mit diabetes insipidus. Hautarzt 1966;17:155.
133. Landau IW, Sasaki MS, Newcomer VD et al. Bloom's syndrome. Arch Dermatol 1966;94:687.
134. Bloom D, German J. The syndrome of congenital telangiectatic erythema and stunted growth. Arch Dermatol 1971;103:545.
135. Dicken CH, Dewald G, Gordon H. Sister chromatid exchanges in Bloom's syndrome. Arch Dermatol 1978;114:755.
136. Sawitsky A, Bloom D, German J. Chromosomal breakage and acute leukemia in congenital telangiectatic erythema and stunted growth. Ann Intern Med 1966;65:487.
137. Swift M, Morrell D, Massey RB et al. Incidence of cancer in 161 families affected by ataxia-telangiectasia. N Engl J Med 1991;325:1831.
138. Gschnait F, Grabner G, Brenner W et al. Ataxia telangiectatica (Louis-Bar syndrom). Hautarzt 1979;30:527.
139. Smith LL, Conerly SL. Ataxia telangiectasia or Louis-Bar syndrome. J Am Acad Dermatol 1985;12:681.
140. McFarlin DE, Strober W, Waldmann TA. Ataxia-telangiectasia (review). Medicine (Baltimore) 1972;51:281.
141. Carbonari M, Cherc M, Paganelli R et al. Relative increase of T cells expressing the gamma/delta rather than the alpha/beta receptor in ataxia-telangiectasia. N Engl J Med 1990;322:73.
142. Epstein CJ, Martin GM, Schultz AL et al. Werner's syndrome (review). Medicine (Baltimore) 1966;45:177.
143. Tritsch H, Lischka G. Werner's Syndrom, kombiniert mit Pseudo-Klinefelter syndrom. Hautarzt 1968;19:547.
144. Fleischmajer R, Nedwich A. Werner's syndrome. Am J Med 1973;54: 111.
145. Bauer EA, Silverman N, Busiek D et al. Diminished response of Werner's syndrome fibroblasts to growth factors PDFG and FGF. Science 1986;234:1240.
146. Fine JD. Editorial: Changing clinical and laboratory concepts in inherited epidermolysis bullosa. Arch Dermatol 1988;124:523.
147. Buchbinder LH, Lucky AW, Dallard E et al. Severe infantile epidermolysis bullosa simplex: Dowling-Meara type. Arch Dermatol 1986; 122:190.
148. Haber RM, Hanna W, Ramsay CA et al. Cicatricial junctional epidermolysis bullosa. J Am Acad Dermatol 1985;12:836.
149. Hashimoto K, Matsumoto M, Iacobelli D. Transient bullous dermolysis of the newborn. Arch Dermatol 1985;121:1429.
150. Fisher GB Jr, Greer KE, Cooper PH. Congenital self-healing (transient) mechanobullous dermatosis. Arch Dermatol 1988;124:240.
151. Bart BJ, Gorlin RJ, Anderson VE et al. Congenital localized absence of skin and associated abnormalities resembling epidermolysis bullosa. Arch Dermatol 1966;93:296.
152. Voss M. Epidermolysis bullosa dystrophica Bart (Bart-Syndrom). Hautarzt 1985;36:351.
153. Smith SZ, Cram DL. A mechanobullous disease of the newborn: Bart's syndrome. Arch Dermatol 1978;114:81.
154. Eady RAJ, Tidman MJ. Diagnosing epidermolysis bullosa (comment). Br J Dermatol 1983;108:621.
155. Haneke E, Anton-Lamprecht I. Ultrastructure of blister formation in epidermolysis bullosa hereditaria: V. Epidermolysis bullosa simplex localisata type Weber-Cockayne. J Invest Dermatol 1982;78:219.
156. Anton-Lamprecht I, Schnyder UW. Epidermolysis bullosa Dowling-Meara. Dermatologica 1982;164:221.
157. Medenic A, Mojsilovic L, Fenske NA, Espinoza CG. Epidermolysis bullosa herpetiformis with mottled pigmentation and an unusual punctate keratoderma. Arch Dermatol 1986;122:900.
158. Hintner H, Stingl G, Schuler G et al. Immunofluorescence mapping of antigen determinants within the dermal-epidermal junction in mechanobullous diseases. J Invest Dermatol 1981;76:113.
159. Pearson RW. The mechanobullous diseases. In: Fitzpatrick TB, Amdt KA, Clark WH Jr et al., eds. Dermatology in general medicine. New York: McGraw-Hill, 1971;621.
160. Schachner L, Lazarus GS, Dembitzer H. Epidermolysis bullosa hereditaria letalis. Br J Dermatol 1977;96:51.
161. Lowe LB. Hereditary epidermolysis bullosa. Arch Dermatol 1967;95: 587.
162. Paller AS, Fine JD, Kaplan S et al. The generalized atrophic benign form of junctional epidermolysis bullosa. Arch Dermatol 1986;122: 704.
163. Bergenholtz A, Olsson O. Die epidermolysis bullosa hereditaria dystrophica mit oesophagusveranderungen. Arch Klin Exp Dermatol 1963;271:518.
164. Reed WB, College J Jr, Prancis MJO et al. Epidermolysis bullosa dystrophica with epidermal neoplasms. Arch Dermatol 1974;110:894.
165. Epstein EH. Molecular basis of epidermolysis bullosa. Science 1992; 256:799.
166. Oakley CA, Wilson N, Ross JA et al. Junctional epidermolysis bullosa in two siblings: Clinical observations, collagen studies, and electron microscopy. Br J Dermatol 1984;111:533.
167. Tidman MJ, Eady RAJ. Hemidesmosome heterogeneity in junctional epidermolysis bullosa revealed by morphometric analysis. J Invest Dermatol 1986;86:51.
168. Matsumoto M, Hashimoto K. Blister fluid from epidermolysis bullosa letalis induces dermal-epidermal separation in vitro. J Invest Dermatol 1986;87:117.
169. McGrath JA, Pulkkinen L, Christiano AM et al. Altered lamin-5 expression due to mutations in the gene encoding the beta-3 chain (LAMB 3) in generalized atrophic benign epidermolysis bullosa. J Invest Dermatol 1995;104:467.
170. Tidman MJ, Eady RAJ. Evaluation of anchoring fibrils and other components of the dermal-epidermal junction in dystrophic epidermolysis bullosa by a quantitative ultrastructural technique. J Invest Dermatol 1985;84:374.
171. Goldsmith LA, Briggaman RA. Monoclonal antibodies to anchoring fibrils for the diagnosis of epidermolysis bullosa. J Invest Dermatol 1983;81:464.
172. Bruckner-Tuderman L, Ruegger S, Odermatt B et al. Lack of type VII collagen in unaffected skin of patients with severe recessive dystrophic epidermolysis bullosa. Dermatologica 1988;176:57.
173. Nanchahal J, Tidman MJ. A study of the dermo-epidermal junction in dystrophic epidermolysis bullosa using the periodic add-thiosemicarbazide-silver proteinate technique. Br J Dermatol 1985;113:397.

174. Uitto J, Christiano AM. Molecular basis for the dystrophic forms of epidermolysis bullosa: Mutations in the type VII collagen gene. Arch Dermatol Res 1994;287:16.
175. Dunhill MGS, Richards AJ, Milana G et al. Genetic linkage to the type VII collagen gene (COL7A1) in 26 families with generalized recessive dystrophic epidermolysis bullosa and anchoring fibril abnormalities. J Med Genet 1994;31:745.
176. Lacour JP, Bernard P, Rostain G et al. Childhood acquired epidermolysis bullosa. Pediatr Dermatol 1995;12:16.
177. Gammon WR, Briggaman RA, Woodley DT et al. Epidermolysis acquisita: A pemphigoid-like disease. J Am Acad Dermatol 1984;11: 820.
178. Woodley DT. Immunofluoresence on *salt-split* skin for the diagnosis of epidermolysis bullosa acquisita. Arch Dermatol 1990;126:229.
179. Valeski JE, Kumar V, Beutner EH et al. Differentation of bullous pemphigoid from epidermolysis bullosa acquisita on frozen skin biopsies. Int J Dermatol 1992;31:37.
180. Pang BK, Lee YS, Ratnam VK. Floor pattern *salt-split skin* cannot distinguish bullous pemphigoid from epidermolysis bullosa acquisita: Use of toad skin. Arch Dermatol 1993;129:744.
181. Gammon WR, Briggaman RA. The incidence of epidermolysis bullosa acquisita among patients diagnosed as bullous pemphigoid (abstr). J Invest Dermatol 1984;2:407.
182. Dahl MGC. Epidermolysis bullosa acquisita: A sign of cicatricial pemphigoid. Br J Dermatol 1979;101:475.
183. Fine JD, Neiser GR, Katz SI. Immunofluorescence and immunoelectron microscopic studies in cicatricial pemphigoid. J Invest Dermatol 1984;82:39.
184. Pardo R, Penneys N. The location of basement membrane type IV collagen in subepidermal bullous diseases (abstr). J Cutan Pathol 1988; 15:334.
185. Ferris T, Lamey PJ, Rennies JS. Darier's disease: Oral features and genetic aspects. Br Dent J 1990;168:71.
186. Panja RK. Acrokeratosis verruciformis (Hopf): A clinical entity? Br J Dermatol 1977;96:643.
187. Wheeland RG, Gilmore WA. The surgical treatment of hypertrophic Darier's disease. J Dermatol Surg Oncol 1985;11:420.
188. Piérard J, Geerts ML, Vandeputte H et al. A propos de quelques cas de dyskeratose folliculaire. Arch Belg Dermatol 1968;24:381.
189. Hori Y, Tsuru N, Niimura M. Bullous Darier's disease. Arch Dermatol 1982;118:278.
190. Demetree JW, Lang PG, St Clair JT. Unilateral, linear, zosteriform epidermal nevus with acantholytic dyskeratosis. Arch Dermatol 1979; 115:875.
191. Starink TM, Woerdeman MJ. Unilateral systematized keratosis follicularis: A variant of Darier's disease or an epidermal nevus (acantholytic dyskeratotic epidermal nevus)? Br J Dermatol 1981;105:207.
192. Fishman HC. Acute, eruptive Darier's disease (keratosis follicularis). Arch Dermatol 1975;111:221.
193. Burge SM, Wilkerson JD. Darier-White disease: A review of the clinical features in 163 patients. J Am Acad Dermatol 1992;27:40.
194. Sato A, Anton-Lamprecht I, Schnyder UW. Ultrastructure of dyskeratosis in Morbus Darier. J Cutan Pathol 1977;4:173.
195. Piérard J, Kint A. Die Dariersche krankheit. Arch Klin Exp Dermatol 1968;231:382.
196. Krinitz K. Tumorose veranderungen bei Morbus Darier. Hautarzt 1966;7:445.
197. Weathers DR, Olansky S, Sharpe LO. Darier's disease with mucous membrane involvement. Arch Dermatol 1969;100:50.
198. Mann PR, Haye KR. An electron microscope study on the acantholytic and dyskeratotic processes in Darier's disease. Br J Dermatol 1970;82:561.
199. Biagini G, Costa AM, Laschi R. An electron microscope study of Darier's disease. J Cutan Pathol 1975;2:47.
200. De Dobbeleer G, Achten G. Disrupted desmosomes in induced lesions of familial benign chronic pemphigus. J Cutan Pathol 1979;6:418.
201. Caulfield JB, Wilgram GF. An electron-microscope study of dyskeratosis and acantholysis in Darier's disease. J Invest Dermatol 1963;41: 57.
202. Wilgram GF, Caulfield JB, Lever WF. An electron microscopic study of acantholysis and dyskeratosis in Hailey and Hailey's disease. J Invest Dermatol 1962;39:373.
203. Gottlieb SK, Lutzner MA. Hailey-Hailey disease: An electron microscopic study. J Invest Dermatol 1970;54:368.
204. Abell E. Immunopathological investigation of glycocalyx material in Darier's and Hailey-Hailey disease (abstr). J Invest Dermatol 1983; 80:355.
205. Ishibashi Y, Kajiwara Y, Andoh I et al. The nature and pathogenesis of dyskeratosis in Hailey-Hailey's disease and Darier's disease. J Dermatol 1984;11:335.
206. Kenney JL, Berg D, Bassett AS et al. Genetic linkage for Darier's disease (keratosis follicularis). Am J Med Genet 1995;55:307.
207. Gottlieb SK, Lutzner MA. Darier's disease. Arch Dermatol 1973;107: 225.
208. Lachapelle JM, De La Brassinne M, Geerts MI. Maladies de Darier et de Hailey-Hailey: Etude comparative de l'incorporation dethymidine tritiee dans les cellules epidermiques. Arch Belg Dermatol 1973;29: 241.
209. Pierard-Franchimont C, Pierard GE. Suprabasal acantholysis. Am J Dermatopathol 1983;5:421.
210. Ackerman AB. Focal acantholytic dyskeratosis. Arch Dermatol 1972; 106:702.
211. Palmer DD, Perry HO. Benign familial chronic pemphigus. Arch Dermatol 1962;86:493.
212. Peluso AM, Bonifast J, Ikeda S et al. Hailey-Hailey disease sublocalization of the gene on chromosome 3Q and identification of a kindred with an apparent deletion. J Invest Dermatol 1995;104:598.
213. Botvinick I. Familial benign pemphigus with oral mucous membrane lesions. Cutis 1973;12:371.
214. Heinze R. Pemphigus chronicus benignus familiaris (Gougerot/Hailey-Hailey) mit schleimhautbeteiligung bei einer diabehkerin. Dermatol Monatsschr 1979;165:862.
215. Kahn D, Hutchinson E. Esophageal involvement in familial benign chronic pemphigus. Arch Dermatol 1974;109:718.
216. Winer LH, Leeb AJ. Benign familial pemphigus. Arch Dermatol 1953;67:77.
217. Herzberg JJ. Pemphigus Gougerot/Hailey-Hailey Arch Klin Exp Dermatol 1955;202:21.
218. Ellis FA. Vesicular Darier's disease (so-called benign familial pemphigus). Arch Dermatol Syph 1950;61:715.
219. Niordson AM, Sylvest B. Bullous dyskeratosis follicularis and acrokeratosis verruciformis. Arch Dermatol 1965;92:166.
220. Nicolis G, Tosca A, Marouli O et al. Keratosis follicularis and familial benign chronic pemphigus in the same patient. Dermatologica 1979;159:346.
221. Schanne R, Burg G, Braun-Falco O. Zur nosologischen beziehung der dyskeratosis follicularis (Darier) und des pemphigus benignus chronicus familiaris (Hailey-Hailey). Hautarzt 1985;36:504.
222. Panja RK. Acrokeratosis verruciformis (Hopf): A clinical entity? Br J Dermatol 1977;96:643.
223. Waisman M. Verruciform manifestations of keratosis follicularis. Arch Dermatol 1960;81:1.
224. Schueller WA. Acrokeratosis verruciformis of Hopf. Arch Dermatol 1972;106:81.
225. Niedelman ML, McKusick VA. Acrokeratosis verruciformis (Hopf). Arch Dermatol 1962;86:779.
226. Penrod JN, Everett MA, McCreight WG. Observations on keratosis follicularis. Arch Dermatol 1960;82:367.
227. Beerman H. In discussion of Waisman M: Verruciform manifestations of keratosis follicularis. Arch Dermatol 1960;81:1.
228. Herndon JH Jr, Wilson JD. Acrokeratosis verruciformis (Hopf) and Darier's disease. Arch Dermatol 1966;93:305.
229. Pope FM. Historical evidence for the genetic heterogeneity of pseudoxanthoma elasticum. Br J Dermatol 1975;92:493.
230. Pope FM. Two types of autosomal recessive pseudoxanthoma elasticum. Arch Dermatol 1974;110:209.
231. Lebwohl M, Nelder K, Pope M et al. Classification of pseudoxanthoma elasticum: Report of a consensus conference. J Am Acad Dermatol 1994;30:103.
232. Mendelsohn G, Bulkley BH, Hutchins GM. Cardiovascular manifestations of pseudoxanthoma elasticum. Arch Pathol 1978;102:298.
233. Eddy DD, Farber EM. Pseudoxanthoma elasticum. Arch Dermatol 1962;86:729.
234. Caro J, Sher A, Rippey JJ. Pseudoxanthoma elasticum and elastosis perforans serpiginosum. Dermatologica 1975;150:36.
235. Huang SN, Steele HD, Iqumar G et al. Ultrastructural changes of elastic fibers in pseudoxanthoma elasticum. Arch Pathol 1967;83:108.
236. Danielsen L, Kohayasi T, Larsen HW et al. Pseudoxanthoma elasticum. Acta Derm Venereol (Stockh) 1970;50:355.
237. Goodman RM, Smith EW, Paton D et al. Pseudoxanthoma elasticum:

A clinical and histopathological study (review). Medicine (Baltimore) 1963;42:297.
238. Kreysel HW, Lerche W, Janner M. Beobachtungen zum Gronblad-Strandberg-Syndrom (angioid streaks, pseudoxanthoma elasticum). Hautarzt 1967;8:24.
239. Akhtar M, Brody H. Elastic tissue in pseudoxanthoma elasticum: Ultrastructural study of endocardial lesions. Arch Pathol 1975;99:667.
240. Hashimoto K, Dibella RJ. Electron microscopic studies of normal and abnormal elastic fibers of the skin. J Invest Dermatol 1967;48:405.
241. Martinez-Hernandez A, Huffer WE. Pseudoxanthoma elasticum: Dermal polyanions and the mineralization of elastic fibers. Lab Invest 1974;31:181.
242. McKee PH, Cameron CHS, Archer DB et al. A study of four cases of pseudoxanthoma elasticum. J Cutan Pathol 1977;4:146.
243. Saito Y, Klingmuller G. Elektronenmikroskopische untersuchungen zur morphogenese elastischer fasern bei der senilen elastose und dem pseudoxanthoma elasticum. Arch Dermatol Res 1977;260:179.
244. Danielsen L, Kobayasi T, Jacobsen GK. Ultrastructural changes in disseminated connective tissue nevi. Acta Derm Venereol (Stockh) 1977;57:93.
245. Uitto J, Santa-Cruz J, Eisen AZ. Familial cutaneous collagenoma: Genetic studies on a family. Br J Dermatol 1979;101:185.
246. Morrison JGL, Wilson Jones E, Macdonald DM. Juvenile elastoma: The Buschke-Ollendorff syndrome. Br J Dermatol 1977;97:417.
247. Kobayasi T, Wolf-Jurgensen P, Danielsen L. Ultrastructure of shagreen patch. Acta Derm Venereol (Stockh) 1973;53:275.
248. Schorr WF, Opitz JM, Reyes CN. The connective tissue nevus: Osteopoikilosis syndrome. Arch Dermatol 1972;106:208.
249. Cole GW, Barr RJ. An elastic tissue defect in dermatofibrosis lenticularis disseminata. Arch Dermatol 1982;118:44.
250. Verbov J, Graham R. Buschke-Ollendorff syndrome: Disseminated dermatofibrosis with osteopoikilosis. Clin Exp Dermatol 1986;11:17.
251. Buschke A, Ollendorff H. Ein fall von dermatofibrosis lenticularis disseminata und osteopathia condensans disseminata. Dermatol Wochenschr 1928;86:257.
252. Reymond JL, Stoebner P, Beani JC et al. Buschke-Ollendorf syndrome: An electron microscopic study. Dermatologica 1983;166:64.
253. Miyachi Y, Hori OT, Yamada A et al. Linear melorheostotic scleroderma with hypertrichosis. Arch Dermatol 1979;115:1233.
254. Wagers LT, Young AW Jr, Ryan SF. Linear melorheostotic scleroderma. Br J Dermatol 1972;86:297.
255. Winter RM. Winchester syndrome. J Med Genet 1989;26:772.
256. Cohen AH, Hollister DW, Reed WB. The skin in the Winchester syndrome. Arch Dermatol 1975;111:230.
257. Nabai H, Mehregan AH, Mortezai A et al. Winchester syndrome: Report of a case from Iran. J Cutan Pathol 1977;4:281.
258. Byers PH. Ehlers Danlos syndrome: Recent advances and current understanding of the clinical and genetic-heterogeneity. J Invest Dermatol 1994;103:47.
259. Uitto J, Lichtenstein JR. Defects in the biochemistry of collagen in diseases of connective tissue. J Invest Dermatol 1976;66:59.
260. McFarland W, Fuller DE. Mortality in Ehlers-Danlos syndrome due to spontaneous rupture of large arteries. N Engl J Med 1964;271:1309.
261. Temple AS, Hinton P, Narcisi P et al. Detection of type III collagen in skin fibroblasts from patients with Ehlers-Danlos syndrome type IV by immunofluorescence. Br J Dermatol 1988;118:17.
262. Pinnell SR, Crane SM, Kenzora JE et al. A heritable disorder of connective tissue. N Engl J Med 1972;286:1013.
263. Prockop DJ, Kivirikko KL, Tuderman L et al. The biosynthesis of collagen and its disorders. N Engl J Med 1979;301:77.
264. Arneson MA, Hammerschmidt DE, Furcht LT et al. A new form of Ehlers-Danlos syndrome. JAMA 1980;244:144.
265. Sulica VL, Cooper PH, Pope FM et al. Cutaneous histologic features in Ehlers-Danlos syndrome. Arch Dermatol 1979;115:40.
266. Pierard GE, Pierard-Franchimont C, Lapiere CM. Histopathological aid at the diagnosis of the Ehlers-Danlos syndrome, gravis and mitis types. Int J Dermatol 1983;22:300.
267. Pope FM, Nicholls AC, Narcisi P et al. Type III collagen mutations in Ehlers-Danlos syndrome type IV and other related disorders. Clin Exp Dermatol 1988;13:285.
268. Ronchese F. Dermatorrhexis. Am J Dis Child 1936;51:1403.
269. Cullin SI. Localized Ehlers-Danlos syndrome: Arch Dermatol 1979; 115:332.
270. Wechsler HL, Fisher ER. Ehlers-Danlos syndrome. Arch Pathol 1964; 77:613.
271. Black CM, Gathercole LJ, Bailey AJ et al. The Ehlers-Danlos syndrome: An analysis of the structure of the collagen fibres of the skin.Br J Dermatol 1980;102:85.
272. Scarpelli DG, Goodman RM. Observations on the fine structure of the fibroblast from a case of Ehlers-Danlos syndrome with the Marfan syndrome. J Invest Dermatol 1968;50:214.
273. Sevenich M, Schultz-Ehrenburg U, Orfanos CE. Ehlers-Danlos syndrome eine fibroblasten-und kollagenkrankheit. Arch Dermatol Res 1980;267:237.
274. Goltz RW, Hult AM, Goldfarb M et al. Cutis laxa. Arch Dermatol 1965;92:373.
275. Schreiber MM, Tilley JC. Cutis laxa. Arch Dermatol 1961;84:266.
276. Reed WB, Horowitz RE, Beighton P. Acquired cutis laxa. Arch Dermatol 1971;103:661.
277. Hashimoto K, Kanzaki T. Cutis laxa. Arch Dermatol 1975;111:861.
278. Scott MA, Kauh YC, Luscome HA. Acquired cutis laxa associated with multiple myeloma. Arch Dermatol 1976;112:853.
279. Nanko H, Jepsen LV, Zachariae H et al. Acquired cutis laxa (generalized elastolysis). Acta Derm Venereol (Stockh) 1979;59:315.
280. Kerl H, Burg G, Hashimoto K. Fatal, penicillin-induced, generalized, postinflammatory elastolysis (cutis laxa). Am J Dermatopathol 1983; 5:267.
281. Reed WB, Horowitz RE, Beighton P. Acquired cutis laxa. Arch Dermatol 1971;103:661.
282. Ledoux-Corbusier M. Cutis laxa, congenital form with pulmonary emphysema: An ultrastructural study. J Cutan Pathol 1983;10:340.
283. Sayers CP, Goltz RW, Mottaz J. Pulmonary elastic tissue in generalized elastolysis (cutis laxa) and Marfan's syndrome. J Invest Dermatol 1975;65:451.
284. Harris RB, Heapy MR, Perry HO. Generalized elastolysis (cutis laxa). Am J Med 1979;65:815.
285. Rimoin DL. Pachydermoperiostosis (idiopathic cubbing and periostosis). N Engl J Med 1965;272:923.
286. Curth HO, Firschein IL, Alpert M. Familial clubbed fingers. Arch Dermatol 1961;83:828.
287. Hambrick GW, Carter DM. Pachydermoperiostosis. Arch Dermatol 1966;94:594.
288. Shaw JM. Genetic aspects of urticaria pigmentosa. Arch Dermatol 1968;97:137.
289. Bazex A, Dupre A, Christol B et al. Les mastocytoses familiales. Ann Dermatol Syphiligra 1971;98:241.
290. Kettelhut BV, Metcalfe DD. Pediatric mastocytosis. Ann Allergy 1994;73:197.
291. Longley J, Duffy TP, Kohn S. The mast cell and mast cell disease. J Am Acad Dermatol 1995;32:545.
292. Klaus SN, Winkelmann RK. Course of urticaria pigmentosa in children. Arch Dermatol 1962;86:68.
293. Iwatsuki K, Tadahiro A, Tagami H et al. Immunofluorescent study in purpura pigmentosa chronica. Acta Derm Venereol (Stockh) 1980;60: 341.
294. Caplan RM. The natural course of urticaria pigmentosa. Arch Dermatol 1963;6.
295. Roberts PL, McDonald HB, Wells RF. Systemic mast cell disease in a patient with unusual gastrointestinal and pulmonary abnormalities. Am J Med 1968;45:638.
296. Friedman BL, Will JJ, Freidman DG et al. Tissue mast cell leukemia. Blood 1958;13:70.
297. Horny HP, Parwaresch MR, Lennert K. Bone marrow findings in systemic mastocytosis. Hum Pathol 1985;16:808.
298. Baraf CS, Shapiro L. Solitary mastocytoma. Arch Dermatol 1969;99: 589.
299. Orkin M, Good RA, Clawson CC et al. Bullous mastocytosis. Arch Dermatol 1970;101:547.
300. Welch EA, Alper JC, Bogaars H et al. Treatment of bullous mastocytosis with disodium cromoglycate. J Am Acad Dermatol 1983;9:349.
301. Allison J. Skin mastocytosis presenting as a neonatal bullous eruption. Australas J Dermatol 1967;9:83.
302. Cramer JH. Telangiectasia macularis eruptiva perstans, eine sonderform der urticaria pigmentosa. Hautarzt 1964;15:370.
303. Wong E, Morgan EW, MacDonald DM. The chloroacetate esterase reaction for mast cells in dermatopathology. Acta Derm Venereol (Stockh) 1982;62:431.
304. Mihm MC, Clark WH, Reed RJ et al. Mast cell infiltrates of the skin and the mastocytosis syndrome. Hum Pathol 1973;4:231.
305. Johnson WC, Helwig EB. Solitary mastocytosis (urtcaria pigmen-

tosa). Arch Dermatol 1961;84:806.
306. Braun-Falco O, Jung J. Uber klinische und experimentelle beobachtungen bei einem fall von diffuser haut-mastocytose. Arch Klin Exp Dermatol 1961;39.
307. Drennan JM. The mast cells in urticaria pigmentosa. J Pathol Bacteriol 1951;63:513.
308. Miller RO, Shapiro L. Bullous urticaria pigmentosa in infancy. Arch Dermatol 1965;91:595.
309. Dewar WA, Milene JA. Bullous urticaria pigmentosa. Arch Dermatol 1955;71:717.
310. Rodermund OR, Klingmuller G, Rohner HG. Interne befunde bei mastozytose. Hautarzt 1980;31:175.
311. Sostre S, Handler HL. Bony lesions in systemic mastocytosis. Arch Dermatol 1977;113:1245.
312. Naveh Y, Ludatscher R, Gellei B et al. Ultrastructural features of mast cells in systemic mastocytosis. Acta Derm Venereol (Stockh) 1970; 55:443.
313. Monheit GD, Murad T, Conrad M. Systemic mastocytosis and the mastocytosis syndrome. J Cutan Pathol 1979;6:42.
314. Freeman RG. Diffuse urticaria pigmentosa. Am J Clin Pathol 1967;48: 187.
315. Hashomoto K, Gross BG, Lever WF. An electron microscopic study of the degranulation of mast cell granules in urticaria pigmentosa. J Invest Dermatol 1966;46:139.
316. Davis MJ, Lawler JC, Higdon RS. Studies on an adult with urticaria pigmentosa. Arch Dermatol 1958;77:224.
317. Okun MR, Bhawan J. Combined melanocytoma-mastocytoma in a case of nodular mastocytosis. J Am Acad Dermatol 1979;1:338.
318. Mixhail GR, Miller-Milinska A. Mast cell population in human skin. J Invest Dermatol 1964;43:249.
319. Gordon H, Gordon W. Incontinentia pigmenti: Clinical and genetical studies of two familial cases. Dermatologica 1961;140:150.
320. Carney RG Jr. Incontinentia pigmenti: A world statistical analysis. Arch Dermatol 1976;112:535.
321. Wijker M, Ligtenberg MJL, Schoute F et al. The gene for hereditary bullous dystrophy: X-linked macular type maps to the XQ27.3 region. Am J Hum Genet 1995;56:1096.
322. Dutheil P, Valpres P, Hors Cayla MC et al. Incontinentia pigmenti late sequelae and genotypic diagnosis: a three generation study of four patients. Pediatr Dermatol 1995;12:107.
323. Epstein S, Vedder IS, Pinkus H. Bullous variety of incontinentia pigmenti (Bloch-Sulzberger). Arch Dermatol Syph 1952;65:557.
324. Sultzberger MB. Incontinentia pigmenti (Bloch-Sulzberger). Arch Dermatol Syph 1938;38:57.
325. Vilanova X, Aguade JP. Incontinentia pigmenti. Ann Dermatol Syphiligra 1959;86:247.
326. Rubin L, Becker SW Jr. Pigmentation in the Bloch-Sulzberger syndrome (incontinentia pigmenti). Arch Dermatol 1956;74:263.
327. Ashley JR, Burgdorf WHC. Incontinentia pigmenti: Pigmentary changes independent of incontinence. J Cutan Pathol 1987;14:248.
328. Schaumburg-Lever G, Lever WF. Electron microscopy of incontinentia pigmenti. J Invest Dermatol 1973;61:151.
329. Gurrier LJW, Wong CK. Ultrastructural evolution of the skin in incontinentia pigmenti (Bloch-Sulzberger). Dermatologica 1974;149: 10.
330. Caputo R, Gianotti F, Innocenti M. Ultrastructural findings in incontinentia pigmenti. Int J Dermatol 1975;14:46.
331. Schmalstieg FC, Jorizzo JL, Tschen J et al. Basophils in incontinentia pigmenti. J Am Acad Dermatol 1984;10:362.
332. Tsuda S, Higushi M, Ichiki M et al. Demonstration of eosinophil chemotactic factor in the blister fluid of patients with incontinentia pigmenti. J Dermatol 1985;12:363.
333. Takematsu H, Terui T, Torinuki W et al. Incontinentia pigmenti: Eosinophil chemotactic activity of the crusted scales in the vesiculobullous stage. Br J Dermatol 1986;115:61.
334. Sultzberger MB. Incontinentia pigmenti (Bloch-Sulzberger). Arch Dermatol Syph 1938;38:57.
335. Cambazard F, Hermier C, Thivol ET Jr et al. Hypomelanose de Ito: Revue de littérature à propos de 3 cas. Ann Dermatol Venereol 1986; 113:15.
336. Sybert VP. Hypomelanosis of Ito: A description not a diagnosis. Acta Derm Venerol (Stockh) 1977;57:216.
337. Grosshans EM, Stoebner P, Bergoend H et al. Incontinentia pigmenti achromians (Ito). Dermatologica 1971;142:65.
338. Nordlund JJ, Klaus SN, Gino J. Hypomelanosis of Ito. Acta Derm Venereol (Stockh) 1977;57:261.
339. Morohashi M, Hashimoto K, Goodman TF Jr et al. Ultrastructural studies of vitiligo, Vogt-Koyanagi syndrome and incontinentia pigmenti achromians. Arch Dermatol 1977;113:755.

Lever's Histopathology of the Skin, eighth edition, edited by David Elder et al. Lippincott–Raven Publishers, Philadelphia © 1997.

CHAPTER 7

Noninfectious Erythematous, Papular, and Squamous Diseases

Sonia Toussaint and Hideko Kamino

URTICARIA

Urticaria is characterized by the presence of transient, recurrent wheals, which are raised, and erythematous areas of edema usually accompanied by itching. When large wheals occur, in which the edema extends to the subcutaneous tissue, the process is referred to as angioedema.

Acute episodes of urticaria generally last only several hours.[1] When episodes of urticaria last up to 24 hours and recur over a period of at least six weeks, the condition is considered chronic urticaria. Urticaria and angioedema may occur simultaneously, in which case the affliction tends to have a chronic course.

In approximately 15% to 25% of patients with urticaria, an eliciting stimulus or underlying predisposing condition can be identified.[2] The various causes of urticaria include soluble antigens in foods, drugs, insect venom, and contact allergens; physical stimuli such as pressure, vibration, solar radiation, cold temperature; occult infections and malignancies; and some hereditary syndromes such as familial cold urticaria and Muckle-Wells syndrome (amyloidosis, nerve deafness, and urticaria).

In *hereditary angioedema,* a rare form of dominantly inherited angioedema, recurrent attacks of edema involve not only the skin but also the oral, laryngeal, and gastrointestinal mucosa. Itching is absent. However, lesions may be painful. In the skin, the edema tends to be circumscribed and nonpitting. Attacks are commonly precipitated by trauma, such as dental extraction, or by emotional stress. Before treatment with the synthetic androgen danazol was available, death from sudden laryngeal edema could occur.[3]

Urticarial vasculitis is a syndrome consisting of recurrent episodes of urticarial lesions often associated with arthralgia and abdominal pain and rarely with glomerulonephritis.[4] The individual skin lesions tend to persist for one to three days and may resolve with purpura or hyperpigmentation.[5] Lesions in urticarial vasculitis are not necessarily acral in distribution. Urticarial vasculitis should be suspected when individual lesions persist for more than 24 hours and produce burning or stinging sensations.[6] Hypocomplementemia was detected in 32% of patients with urticarial vasculitis[7] and organ involvement is much more common in hypocomplementemic urticarial vasculitis than in the normocomplementemic form.[5] A C1q precipitin has been found in hypocomplementemic urticarial vasculitis.[6,8,9] Measurements of CH50 (total hemolytic complement) and C1q binding assays are helpful in the initial evaluation of patients with urticarial vasculitis. Urticarial vasculitis may be associated with infectious mononucleosis, infectious hepatitis, serum sickness, and autoimmume diseases such as systemic lupus erythematosus. Urticarial vasculitis may antedate other symptoms of collagen vascular disease by months or years.[10] Accordingly, the appropriate serologic studies should be performed and periodically monitored.

Histopathology. In *acute urticaria* one observes interstitial dermal edema, dilated venules with endothelial swelling, and a paucity of inflammatory cells. In *chronic urticaria* interstitial dermal edema and a perivascular and interstitial mixed-cell infiltrate with variable numbers of lymphocytes, eosinophils, and neutrophils are present[11] (Figs. 7-1 and 7-2).

In *angioedema* the edema and infiltrate extend into the subcutaneous tissue. In *hereditary angioedema* there is subcutaneous and submucosal edema without infiltrating inflammatory cells.[12]

In *urticarial vasculitis* the dermis shows an early leukocytoclastic vasculitis characterized by (1) an infiltrate predominantly within and around the walls of small blood vessels composed largely of neutrophils, some of which show fragmentation of their nuclei; (2) minimal to absent deposits of fibrin in the vessel walls; and (3) slight to moderate extravasation of erythrocytes.[13]

The existence of intermediate cases suggests that urticaria

S. Toussaint: Dermatopathology Section, New York University Medical Center, New York, NY

H. Kamino: Dermatopathology Section, New York University Medical Center, New York, NY

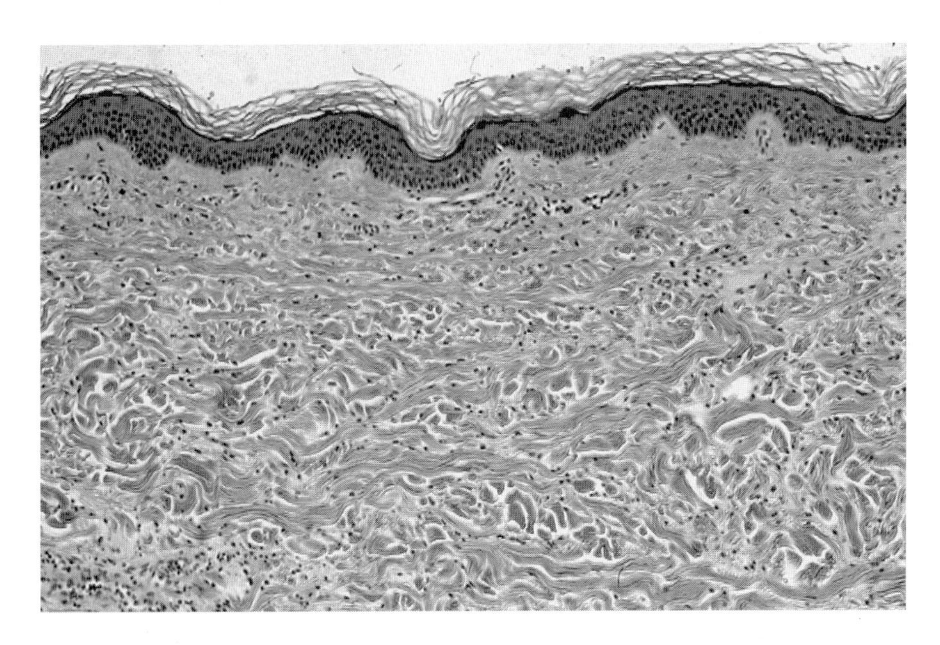

FIG. 7-1. Urticaria
Sparse superficial perivascular and interstitial inflammatory infiltrate.

and urticarial vasculitis form a disease continuum.[14,15] In intermediate cases the perivascular infiltrate is predominantly mononuclear but contains significant numbers of neutrophils and eosinophils. Deposition of fibrinoid material within vessel walls is not seen and leukocytoclasia, if present, is minimal.[16]

Pathogenesis. On electron microscopic examination common urticaria reveals mast cell and eosinophilic degranulation.

Vascular deposits of immunoglobulins, complement, or fibrin are only rarely seen.[12] Autoantibodies to the high-affinity IgE receptor on mast cells have recently been uncovered in chronic urticaria.[14] However, most cases of chronic urticaria are considered idiopathic.

Most patients with hereditary angioedema have a low serum level of the esterase inhibitor of the first component of complement (C1). Exhaustion of this inhibitor allows activation of C1. This leads to activation of C4 and C2, with the generation of a C2 fragment possessing kinin-like activity and causing increased vasopermeability.[2] A smaller proportion of patients with hereditary angioedema have a deficit in functional C1-esterase inhibitor.

In urticarial vasculitis, circulating immune complexes are found in about one half of the patients. By direct immunofluorescence testing, vascular deposits of immunoglobulins, complement, or fibrin are found in about one third.[12] Positive immunofluorescence findings are more common in patients with the hypocomplementemic form of urticarial vasculitis.[6] Renal

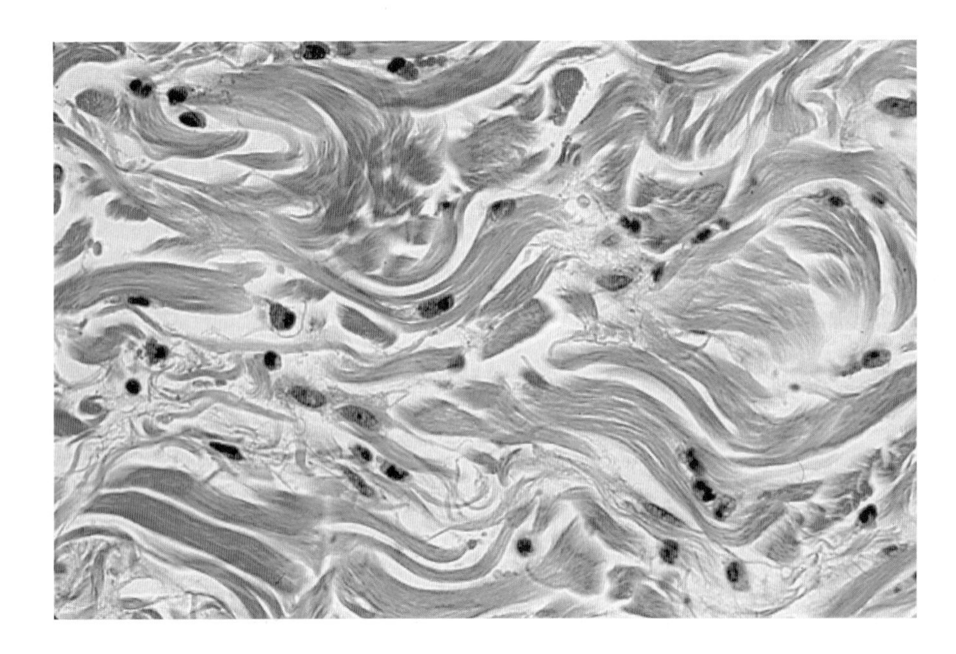

FIG. 7-2. Urticaria
Interstitial infiltrate of eosinophils, neutrophils, and lymphocytes.

biopsy in patients with hypocomplementemia frequently shows glomerulonephritis.[4]

PRURITIC URTICARIAL PAPULES AND PLAQUES OF PREGNANCY

Pruritic urticarial papules and plaques of pregnancy (PUPPP) is a fairly common entity first described in 1979 by Lawley et al.[17] The condition has a predilection for primigravidas in the third trimester of pregnancy. The rash usually starts on the abdomen and is composed of intensely pruritic erythematous urticarial papules, which may be surmounted by vesicles. The proximal parts of the extremities are also affected. There is no increased incidence of the rash in subsequent pregnancies.[18] The rash usually involutes spontaneously after delivery. Fetal outcome appears to be unaffected.

Histopathology. Microscopic findings most commonly show a superficial and middermal perivascular lymphohistiocytic infiltrate with variable numbers of eosinophils and neutrophils together with edema of the superficial dermis. Epidermal involvement is variable and consists of focal spongiosis with exocytosis, parakeratosis, and mild acanthosis.[17–19]

Pathogenesis. A possible correlation has been proposed between susceptibility to PUPPP and higher maternal weight gain and/or twin pregnancies.[20] In addition, a paternal factor hypothetically generated or expressed by the fetal portion of the placenta has been invoked as the cause of PUPPP in two families with unusual conjugal patterns.[21] Direct immunofluorescence findings are negative for deposition of immunoreactants and complement.

ERYTHEMA ANNULARE CENTRIFUGUM

Erythema annulare centrifugum is also known as gyrate erythema and represents a hypersensitivity reaction manifesting as arcuate and polycyclic areas of erythema. The condition has been categorized into superficial and deep variants. The deep form was originally described by Darier and is characterized by annular areas of palpable erythema with central clearing and absence of surface changes.[22] The superficial variant differs only by the presence of a characteristic trailing scale, a delicate annular rim of scale that trails behind the advancing edge of erythema.[23,24] Small vesicles may occur.

The lesions may attain considerable size (up to 10 cm across) over a period of several weeks, may be mildly pruritic, and have a predilection for the trunk and proximal extremities. Most cases resolve spontaneously within six weeks; however, the condition may persist for years.

Histopathology. In the classic deep form or indurated type, a superficial and deep perivascular lymphocytic infiltrate characterized by a tightly cuffed "coat-sleeve–like" pattern is present in the middle and lower portions of the dermis[25] (Figs. 7-3 and 7-4).

In the superficial variant of gyrate erythema, there is a superficial perivascular tightly cuffed lymphohistiocytic infiltrate with endothelial cell swelling and focal extravasation of erythrocytes in the papillary dermis. In addition, there is focal epidermal spongiosis and focal parakeratosis.[23,24]

Pathogenesis. The exact pathogenesis of erythema annulare centrifugum is not clear. Erythema annulare centrifugum has been associated with occult infections, dermatophytosis, medications, and, rarely, underlying malignancy. The rash responds poorly to topical steroids. Treatment of any underlying disorder, if identifiable, is indicated.

Differential Diagnosis. The rather striking coat-sleeve–like perivascular arrangement of the infiltrate seen in the deep form of erythema annulare centrifugum is encountered also in secondary syphilis. However, in secondary syphilis numerous plasma cells and histiocytes are usually present, and the intima and endothelial cells are swollen.

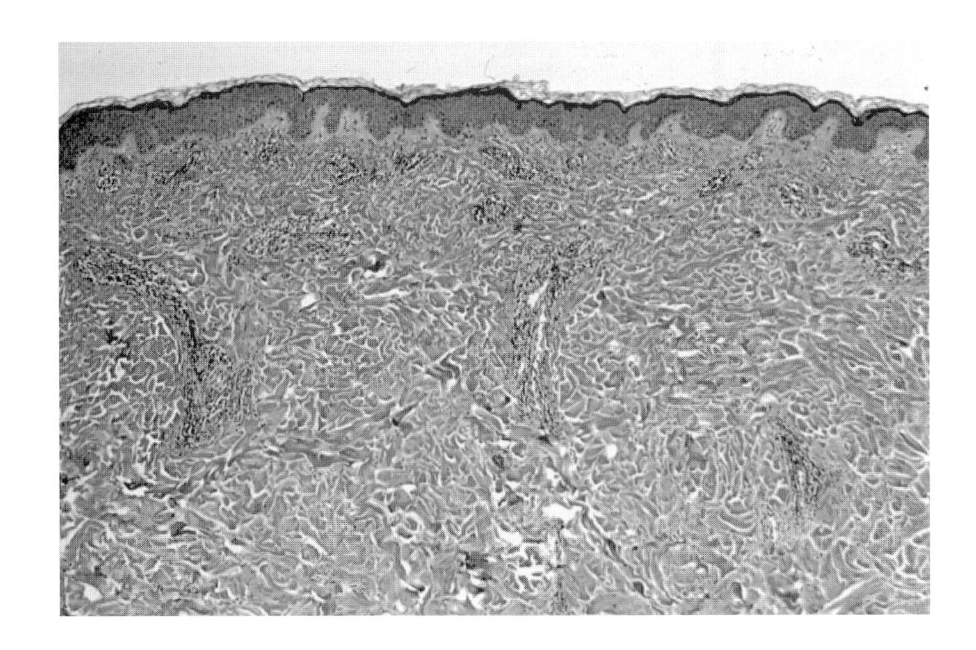

FIG. 7-3. Gyrate erythema, deep form
Superficial and deep, dense perivascular lymphocytic infiltrate.

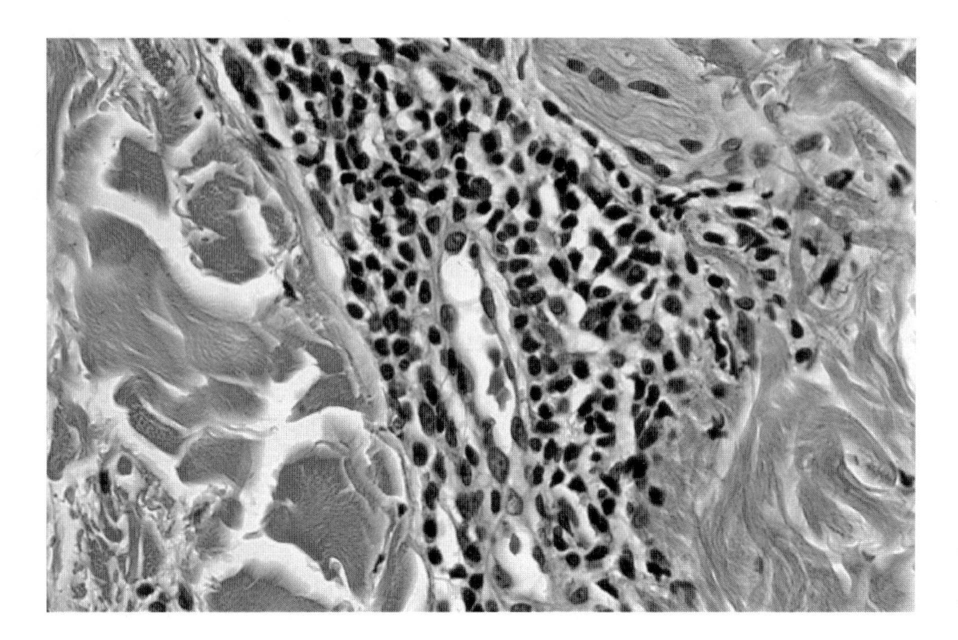

FIG. 7-4. Gyrate erythema, deep form
Dense perivascular lymphocytic infiltrate.

ERYTHEMA GYRATUM REPENS

A very rare, but clinically highly characteristic, dermatosis first reported in 1952 by Gammel,[26] erythema gyratum repens is associated with internal malignancy in up to 28% of cases.[25] The eruption typically is very pruritic and is composed of concentric and parallel bands of erythema and scale producing a "wood-grain" pattern on the skin. The trunk and extremities are preferentially involved; however, the entire integument may be affected. The rash of erythema gyratum repens constantly migrates at a fairly rapid rate (up to 1 cm per day). Ichthyosis and palmar/plantar hyperkeratosis have been observed concomitantly in 16% and 10% of patients, respectively.[27] The most common underlying malignancy is lung cancer. The condition is known to remit with treatment and eradication of the associated malignancy.

Histopathology. The histologic picture usually shows mild epidermal acanthosis with spongiosis, focal parakeratosis, and a superficial perivascular lymphohistiocytic infiltrate that may also include eosinophils and melanophages.[27,28] Exocytosis of neutrophils and eosinophils may be seen.

Pathogenesis. Several authors have described granular deposition of IgG and/or C3 at the basement-membrane zone on direct immunofluorescence suggesting that erythema gyratum repens may have an immunologic basis.[29–31] In particular, Caux et al. noted that the deposits are located in the sublamina densa region using immunoelectron microscopy.[31]

ERYTHEMA DYSCHROMICUM PERSTANS

Erythema dyschromicum perstans, also called ashy dermatosis, is an extensive asymptomatic eruption. It begins with disseminated macules showing an elevated, red active border, which, by peripheral extension and coalescence, form large patches with a polycyclic outline. Although the macules may at first be erythematous before assuming their characteristic bluish gray color, they often appear blue-gray from the very beginning. The disease progresses slowly, and the discoloration persists. The most common areas of involvement are the trunk, arms, and face. Most patients with this disorder are Latin American.[32]

Histopathology. In the early active stage or in the erythematous active border many keratinocytes in the basal layer, but also some keratinocytes in the lower spinous layer, show vacuolization of their cytoplasm leading to liquefaction degeneration. The upper dermis shows a mild to moderate perivascular infiltrate of lymphocytes and histiocytes intermingled with melanophages.[33,34] There may also be exocytosis of the infiltrate into the epidermis, and occasional necrotic keratinocytes or colloid bodies resembling those seen in lichen planus may be present.[35] The only abnormality late lesions show is aggregates of melanophages in the papillary dermis.[33]

Pathogenesis. Electron microscopic examination reveals many vacuoles delimited by a membrane within the affected keratinocytes as the ultrastructural counterpart of the liquefaction degeneration. This is associated with widening of the intercellular spaces and retraction of desmosomes to either one cell or the other. Additional findings include discontinuities in the subepidermal basement membrane and the presence in the dermis of melanophages containing aggregates of melanosomes enclosed by a lysosomal membrane.[36] It can be assumed that the vacuolar alteration of basal keratinocytes is the cause of the incontinence of pigment and of the formation of the colloid bodies.

Direct immunofluorescence studies have shown IgG deposition on necrotic keratinocytes at the dermal-epidermal junction, and immunohistochemical stains revealed that in early lesions the dermal inflammatory infiltrate is composed primarily of T lymphocytes, both $CD4^+$ (helper-inducer) and $CD8^+$ (cytotoxic-suppressor) subtypes.[37]

Damage and necrosis of the basal keratinocytes resulting in formation of colloid bodies and pigmentary incontinence suggests a possible relationship of erythema dyschromicum perstans to lichen planus pigmentosus, also called lichen planus actinicus or subtropicus.[35,38,39] However, lichen planus pigmentosus shows a different clinical presentation characterized by dark brown macules located predominantly on exposed areas and flexural folds; histologically it sometimes has a more pronounced lichenoid, that is, subepidermal, distribution of the infiltrate.[34,40]

Differential Diagnosis. The histologic picture of erythema dyschromicum perstans may show similarities with the inflammatory infiltrate and pigmentary incontinence seen in interface drug eruptions, especially in the late stage of fixed-drug eruption.[33]

PRURIGO SIMPLEX

Prurigo simplex is characterized by intensely pruritic, erythematous urticarial papules that are seen in symmetric distribution, especially on the trunk and extensor surfaces of the extremities of middle-aged patients. Some patients may have an atopic background or may exhibit dermographism.[41] In contrast with dermatitis herpetiformis, which prurigo simplex may resemble in clinical appearance, there is no grouping of lesions.[42] In other cases, prurigo simplex greatly resembles arthropod bites (papular urticaria).

Histopathology. The histologic picture of the early papules shows mild acanthosis, spongiosis with an occasional small spongiotic vesicle, and parakeratosis. The upper dermis contains a mild lymphocytic inflammatory infiltrate in a largely perivascular arrangement.[43] An admixture of eosinophils is present in some cases.[42,44] Excoriated papules show partial absence of the epidermis, and they are covered with a crust containing degenerated nuclei of inflammatory cells.[42] On serial sectioning, most histologic changes may be found to be located around hair follicles, which then show spongiosis and exocytosis of lymphocytes in the follicular infundibulum, and a perifollicular infiltrate.[45] In other instances, there is distinct sparing of the follicular structures.[44]

Differential Diagnosis. The diagnosis of dermatitis herpetiformis is easily excluded by the absence in prurigo simplex of neutrophilic microabscesses at the tips of papillae and of neutrophils, eosinophils, and nuclear dust in the dermal infiltrate. A negative direct immunofluorescence study of perilesional skin confirms the exclusion of dermatitis herpetiformis or urticarial bullous pemphigoid.[41] The histologic picture of prurigo simplex resembles that of a subacute eczematous dermatitis, except that the extent of its papular lesions is much more limited. Histologic differentiation from papular urticaria is not possible.[42]

PRURIGO NODULARIS

Prurigo nodularis is a chronic skin dermatitis characterized by discrete, raised, firm hyperkeratotic papulonodules, usually from 5 to 12 mm in diameter but occasionally larger. They occur chiefly on the extensor surfaces of the extremities and are intensely pruritic. The disease usually begins in middle age and women are more frequently affected than men.[46] Prurigo nodularis may coexist with lesions of lichen simplex chronicus and there may be transitional lesions.[47]

The cause remains unknown but local trauma, insect bites, atopic background, and metabolic or systemic diseases have been implicated as predisposing factors in some cases.[47–50]

Histopathology. One observes pronounced hyperkeratosis and irregular acanthosis. In addition, there may be papillomatosis and irregular downward proliferation of the epidermis and adnexal epithelium[51] approaching pseudocarcinomatous hyperplasia[52] (Fig. 7-5). The papillary dermis shows a predominantly lymphocytic inflammatory infiltrate and vertically oriented collagen bundles. Occasionally, prominent neural hyperplasia may be observed[52]; however, this is an uncommon finding and is not considered by some authors to be an essential feature for the diagnosis of prurigo nodularis.[53] In some cases, silver stains or cholinesterase stains demonstrate the increased number of cutaneous nerves.[46]

Eosinophils and marked eosinophil degranulation may be seen more frequently in patients with an atopic background.[48]

Pathogenesis. It is generally assumed that the neural proliferation in prurigo nodularis is a secondary phenomenon due to

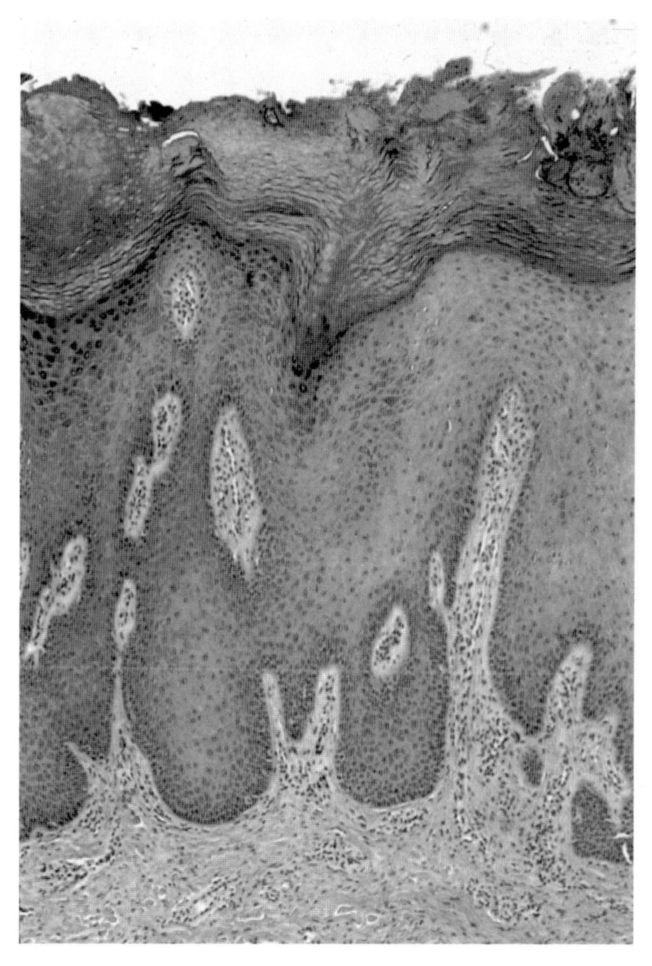

FIG. 7-5. Prurigo nodularis
Marked irregular acanthosis, focal hypergranulosis, and orthokeratosis with parakeratosis.

chronic traumatization by scratching. Still, it may be that the extreme pruritus is related to the increased number of dermal nerves.[52]

On electron microscopic examination it is evident that the neural proliferation involves both axons and Schwann cells.[52] Many nerve fibers are demonstrable also with immunostains for S-100 protein,[54] neurofilament, and myelin proteins.[55] Immunohistochemical analysis has confirmed that they are mostly sensory nerves by demonstrating the presence of sensory neuropeptides.[56] In addition, Merkel's cells are reported to be increased in number in the basal cell layer of the affected interfollicular epidermis, suggesting that these specialized sensory receptors interacting with the neural fibers may participate in the pathogenesis of the disease.[57]

Differential Diagnosis. Lichen simplex chronicus may have a similar histologic picture, although less exuberant and less circumscribed.[53] Multiple keratoacanthomas, which often show less of a central crater than solitary keratoacanthomas, may be difficult to distinguish from prurigo nodularis because both show marked epidermal and epithelial hyperplasia.[58]

PSORIASIS

Psoriasis may be divided into *psoriasis vulgaris, generalized pustular psoriasis*, and *localized pustular psoriasis*.

Psoriasis Vulgaris

Clinical Features

Psoriasis vulgaris is a common chronic inflammatory skin disorder that affects approximately 1.5% to 2% of the population in the western countries. It is characterized by pink to red papules and plaques. The lesions are of variable size, sharply demarcated, dry, and usually covered with layers of fine, silvery scales. As the scales are removed by gentle scraping, fine bleeding points usually are seen, the so-called Auspitz sign. The scalp, sacral region, and extensor surfaces of the extremities are commonly involved, although in some patients the flexural and intertriginous areas (inverse psoriasis) are mainly affected. An acute variant, guttate or eruptive psoriasis, is often seen in younger patients and is characterized by an abrupt eruption of small lesions associated with acute group A β-hemolytic streptococcal infections.[59] Involvement of the nails is common; the most frequent alteration of the nail plate surface is the presence of pits.[60] In severe cases the disease may affect the entire skin and present as generalized erythrodermic psoriasis. Pustules generally are absent in psoriasis vulgaris, although pustules on palms and soles occasionally occur. Rarely, one or a few areas show pustules, and this is referred to as "psoriasis with pustules." Also rarely, severe psoriasis vulgaris develops into generalized pustular psoriasis. Oral lesions such as stomatitis areata migrans (geographic stomatitis) and benign migratory glossitis may be seen in psoriasis vulgaris as well as in generalized pustular psoriasis.[61,62]

Psoriatic arthritis characteristically involves the terminal interphalangeal joints, but frequently the large joints are also affected so that a clinical differentiation from rheumatoid arthritis often is impossible. However, the rheumatoid factor generally is absent.

Generalized Pustular Psoriasis

Clinical Features

Generalized pustular psoriasis includes (1) acute generalized pustular psoriasis (von Zumbusch–type and acute exanthematic type), (2) generalized pustular psoriasis of pregnancy (impetigo herpetiformis), (3) infantile and juvenile pustular psoriasis, and (4) subacute annular or circinate pustular psoriasis.[63]

This cutaneous eruption is characterized by the presence of variable numbers of sterile pustules appearing in erythematous and scaly lesions associated with moderate to severe constitutional symptoms.[64] Several exacerbations may occur, and in the intervals between them, lesions of ordinary psoriasis may be seen.

The four variants of generalized pustular psoriasis show considerable resemblance and overlapping in their clinical picture and also have a similar histologic appearance. They differ mainly in mode of onset and in distribution of the lesions. Frequently, all four diseases show oral pustules, particularly on the tongue.[65]

Acute generalized pustular psoriasis, the *pustular psoriasis of von Zumbusch*, is generally diagnosed when the pustular eruption occurs in patients with preexisting psoriasis, either of the plaque type[66] or of the erythrodermic type.[67] Frequently, the eruption occurs after provocation by external factors such as systemic steroid therapy withdrawal.[63,68] The *exanthematous type of generalized pustular psoriasis* refers to a group of patients with later onset of psoriasis, atypical distribution of the lesions, and a rapid and apparently spontaneous pustular eruption.[69]

Generalized pustular psoriasis of pregnancy is a rare pustular eruption that appears during the last trimester of pregnancy. It starts with flexural lesions of psoriasis followed by a generalized pustular eruption. It may occur repeatedly during successive pregnancies.[70] Some authors have considered it to be the same disease as *impetigo herpetiformis*,[63] but others claim that they stand as separate entities.[71,72]

In some instances of *subacute annular pustular psoriasis* the annular or gyrate lesions show a clinical resemblance to subcorneal pustular dermatosis.[73,74] Figurated lesions are more frequently seen in subacute or chronic forms of generalized pustular psoriasis.[63] Annular pustular psoriasis, though usually generalized, in some instances is localized.[75]

Very rarely, children develop generalized pustular psoriasis also known as *infantile and juvenile pustular psoriasis*. In these patients the disease has a benign course with frequent spontaneous remissions.[76]

Localized Pustular Psoriasis

Clinical Features

There are three types of localized pustular psoriasis: (1) "psoriasis with pustules,"[68,69] in which only one or a few of the areas of psoriasis show pustules and the tendency to change into a generalized pustular psoriasis is not great; (2) localized acrodermatitis continua of Hallopeau, which occasionally evolves into generalized acrodermatitis continua; and (3) pustular psoriasis of the palms and soles, with two variants: the chronic palmoplantar pustulosis, also called pustulosis palmaris et plantaris, and the acute palmoplantar pustulosis or "pustular bacterid." Both are occasionally seen in association with psoriasis vulgaris.[63] The relationship of Reiter's disease to psoriasis will be discussed in the description of Reiter's disease.

Acrodermatitis continua of Hallopeau is the term used if the pustular eruption involves the distal portions of the hands and feet. In the localized type of acrodermatitis continua these are the only areas affected, while in the generalized type of acrodermatitis continua extensive areas of the skin, in addition to the acral portions of extremities are involved.[69] Atrophy of the skin and permanent nail loss may occur on the fingers and toes.

Pustulosis palmaris et plantaris is a chronic, relapsing disorder occurring on the palms, soles, or both. Crops of small, deep-seated pustules are seen within areas of erythema and scaling. In the earliest stage, the lesions may appear as vesicles or vesiculopustules. During the subsiding stage, the pustules appear as brown macules. The sites of predilection are the midpalms and thenar eminences of the hands, and the heels and insteps of the feet.[77] In pustulosis palmaris et plantaris, in contrast to acrodermatitis continua of Hallopeau, the acral portions of the fingers and toes are spared. An acute variant called "pustular bacterid"[78] describes a rare eruption of large and sterile pustules on hands and feet.

Psoriasis and Acquired Immunodeficiency Syndrome (AIDS)

Clinical Features

The association between psoriasis and human immunodeficiency virus (HIV) infection is commonly seen. The prevalence of psoriasis is reported to be 1.3% to 2.5% in the HIV-positive population.[79,80] Clinically, psoriasis may have a more severe course with sudden exacerbations and may be refractile to treatment.[79,81] Extensive erythrodermic psoriasis may occur.[82] Palmoplantar involvement, flexural (inverse) psoriasis, and psoriatic arthritis were found to be more frequent in patients who developed psoriasis after the HIV infection.[80] Although a direct relation between the stage of HIV infection and the severity of psoriasis has not been found, a trend of low peripheral T-cell $CD4^+$ (helper-inducer) counts and a more severe clinical course has been noted.[80]

Psoriasis Vulgaris Histopathology

The histologic picture of psoriasis vulgaris varies considerably with the stage of the lesion and usually is diagnostic only in early, scaling papules and near the margin of advancing plaques.

The earliest pinhead-sized macules or smooth-surfaced papules show a subtle histologic picture with a preponderance of dermal changes.[83,84] At first, there is capillary dilatation and edema in the papillary dermis, with a lymphocytic infiltrate surrounding the capillaries. The lymphocytes extend into the lower portion of the epidermis, where slight spongiosis develops. Then focal changes occur in the upper portion of the epidermis, where granular cells become vacuolated and disappear, and mounds of parakeratosis are formed. The neutrophils usually are seen only at the summits of some of the mounds of parakeratosis and appear scattered through an otherwise orthokeratotic cornified layer (Fig. 7-6). These mounds of parakeratosis with neutrophils represent the earliest manifestation of Munro microabscesses.[84] At this stage, which is characterized clinically by an early, scaling papule, a histologic diagnosis of psoriasis can often be made. In some cases, when there is marked exocytosis of neutrophils, they may aggregate in the uppermost portion of the spinous layer to form small spongiform pustules of Kogoj. Lymphocytes remain confined to the lower epidermis, which, as more and more mitoses occur, becomes increasingly hyperplastic. The epidermal changes at first are focal but later on become confluent, leading clinically to plaques.

In the fully developed lesions of psoriasis, as best seen at the margin of enlarging plaques, the histologic picture is characterized by (1) acanthosis with regular elongation of the rete ridges with thickening in their lower portion, (2) thinning of the supra-

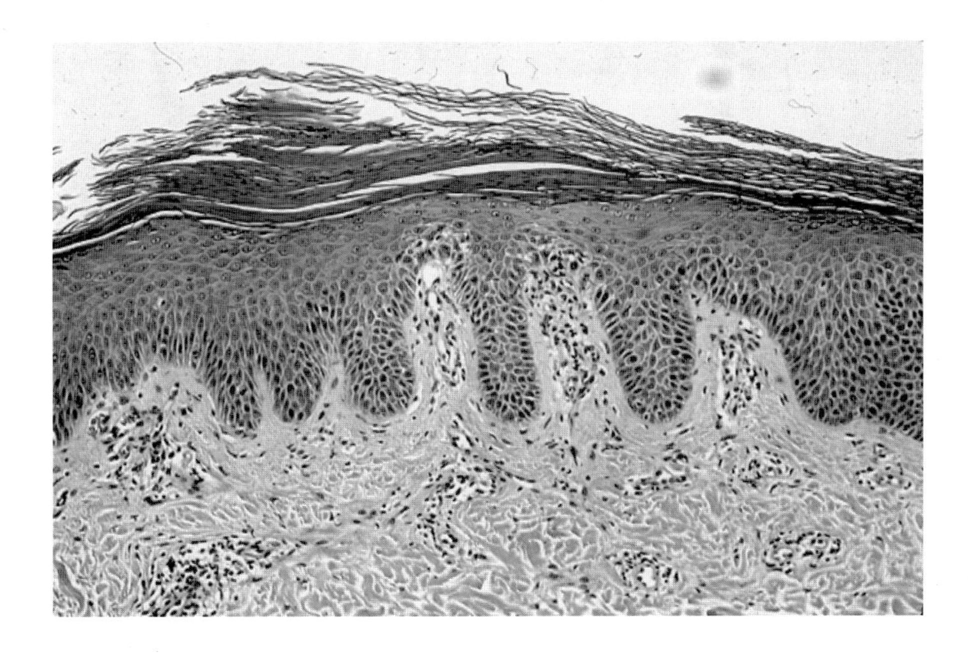

FIG. 7-6. Early psoriasis
Mounds of parakeratosis with neutrophils, thin granular layer, moderate acanthosis, focal spongiosis, increased mitotic figures, dilated blood vessels at the tip of the dermal papillae, and perivascular infiltrate of lymphocytes and a few neutrophils.

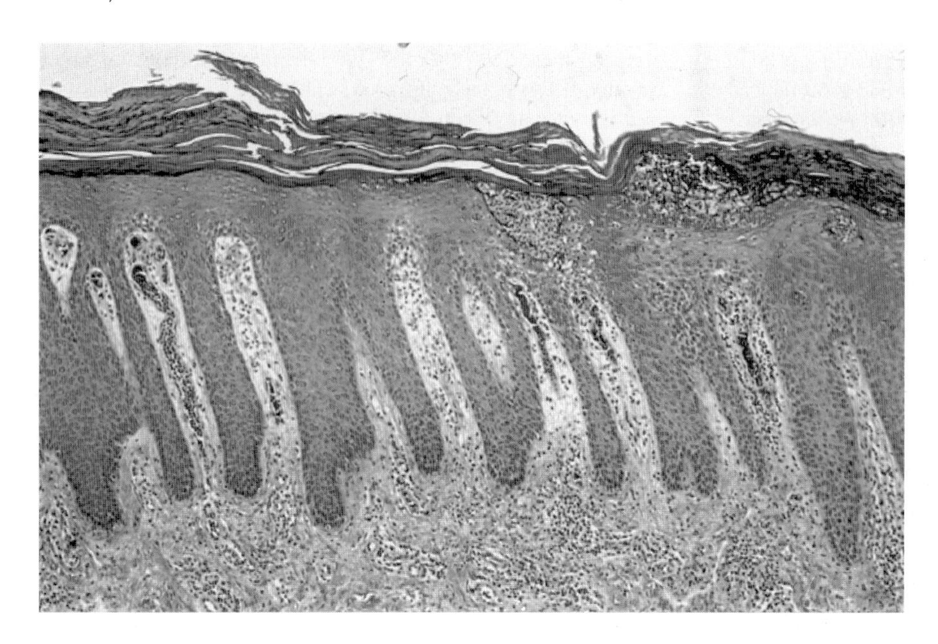

FIG. 7-7. Psoriasis, well-developed plaque
Markedly elongated rete ridges, absent granular layer, small spongiform pustule at the right, parakeratosis with neutrophils, and dilated tortuous vessels in the dermal papillae.

papillary epidermis with the occasional presence of small spongiform pustules, (3) pallor of the upper layers of the epidermis, (4) diminished to absent granular layer, (5) confluent parakeratosis, (6) the presence of Munro microabscesses; (7) elongation and edema of the dermal papillae, and, (8) dilated and tortuous capillaries (Fig. 7-7).

Of all the listed features, only the spongiform pustules of Kogoj and Munro microabscesses are truly diagnostic of psoriasis, and, in their absence, the diagnosis rarely can be made with certainty on a histologic basis. In detail, the changes in active psoriasis are as follows.

The rete ridges show considerable elongation and extend downward to a uniform level, resulting in regular acanthosis (Fig. 7-8). They are often slender in their upper portion but show thickening ("clubbing") in their lower portion. Not infrequently, neighboring rete ridges are seen to coalesce at their bases. Usually, intercellular and intracellular edema are absent in the rete ridges and keratinocytes located well above the basal layer show deep basophilia. In addition, mitoses are not limited to the basal layer as in normal skin, but are also seen above the basal layer. This, together with a considerable lengthening of the basal cell layer due to elongation of the rete ridges, results in a great increase in the number of mitoses. This increase has been calculated to be 27 times the number of mitoses in uninvolved skin.[85]

The suprapapillary epidermis appears relatively thin in comparison with the markedly elongated rete ridges, and the cells in the upper layers of the epidermis may appear enlarged and pale-stained as a result of intracellular edema. The epidermal cells located immediately beneath the parakeratotic cornified layer may be intermingled with neutrophils.[86] The histologic picture is then that of a small spongiform pustule of Kogoj (Fig. 7-9). Although it is only a micropustule, it is nevertheless of the same type as the much larger macropustules seen in pustular psoriasis. Such a spongiform pustule, highly diagnostic for psoriasis and its variants, shows aggregates of neutrophils within the in-

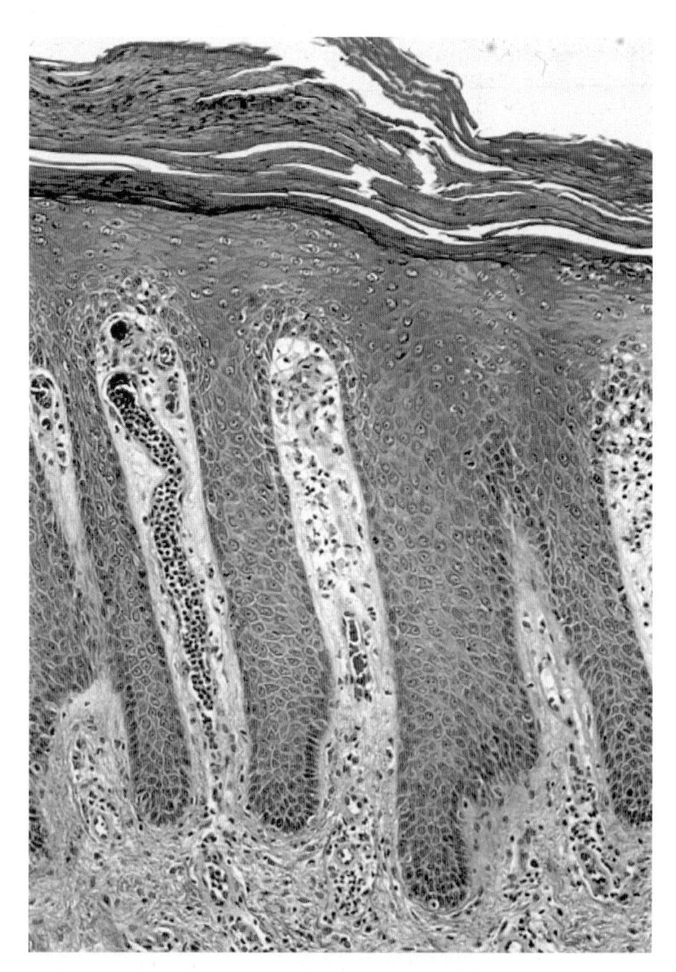

FIG. 7-8. Psoriasis, well-developed plaque
Acanthosis with club-shaped rete ridges of even length, thin suprapapillary epidermal plates, absent granular layer, pallor of the upper epidermis, and confluent parakeratosis.

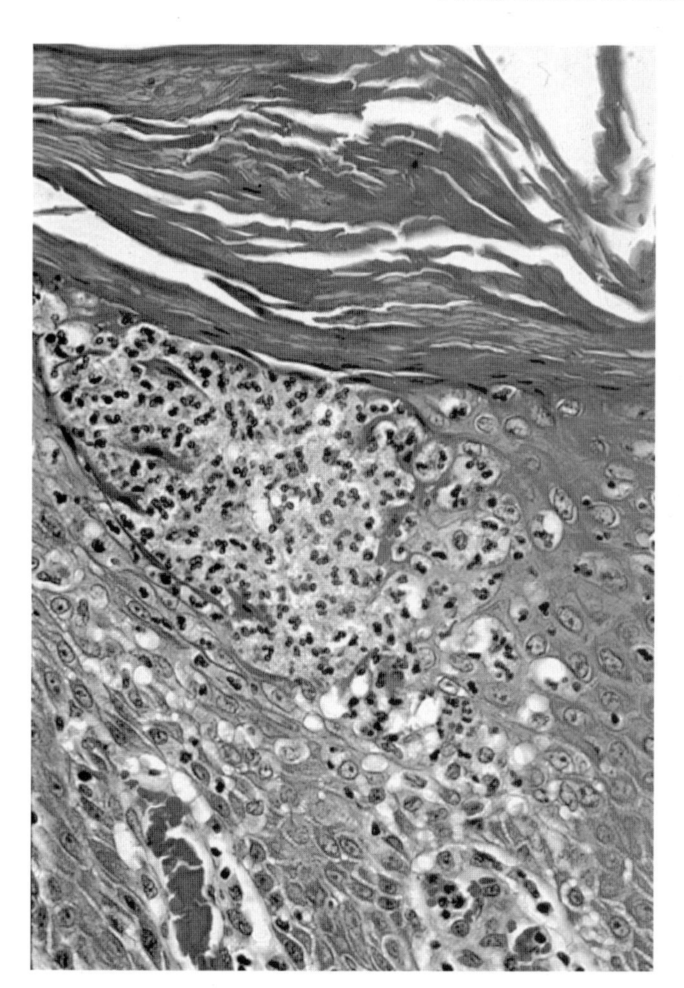

FIG. 7-9. Psoriasis
Closer view of a spongiform pustule of Kogoj formed by collections of neutrophils in the spinous and granular layers.

terstices of a sponge-like network formed by degenerated and thinned epidermal cells.[87]

In some instances the cornified layer consists entirely of confluent parakeratosis forming a plate-like scale with a concomitant absence or diminution of the granular layer. However, occasional focal orthokeratosis with preservation of the underlying granular cells is present.

Munro microabscesses are located within parakeratotic areas of the cornified layer (Fig. 7-10). They consist of accumulations of neutrophils and pyknotic nuclei of neutrophils that have migrated there from capillaries in the papillae through the suprapapillary epidermis. As a rule, Munro microabscesses are found easily in early lesions but are few in number or absent in longstanding lesions.[88]

The dermal papillae, in accordance with the elongation and basal thickening of the rete ridges, are elongated and club shaped. They show edema, and the capillaries within them appear dilated and tortuous. A relatively mild inflammatory infiltrate is present in the upper dermis and the papillae. It consists of lymphocytes, except in early lesions, in which neutrophils are also present in the upper portion of the papillae.[89]

An entirely typical histologic picture as described above is not always found, even if the biopsy specimens are from clinically typical lesions of psoriasis.[90] Orthokeratosis often appears intermingled with parakeratosis. In such cases, one may see vertically adjoining areas of orthokeratosis and parakeratosis, patchy parakeratosis, or occasionally, alternating layers of orthokeratosis and parakeratosis. The latter pattern indicates a fluctuation in the activity of the psoriasis.

The bleeding points that may be produced by gentle scraping of the skin (Auspitz sign) correspond to the tips of papillae. They are attributable to the following histologic changes: parakeratosis, intracellular edema of the keratinocytes in the suprapapillary epidermis, thinning of the suprapapillary plates, and dilatation of the capillaries in the upper portion of the papillae.

Guttate or eruptive psoriasis shows the histologic features of an early or active lesion of psoriasis, where there is more pronounced inflammatory infiltrate and less acanthosis as compared with a well-developed chronic plaque of psoriasis. Because of its acute onset, one may observe the remaining normal orthokeratotic layer overlying the areas of parakeratosis with neutrophils, which, in turn, may appear loosely arranged (Fig. 7-11).

The histologic picture of *erythrodermic psoriasis* in some

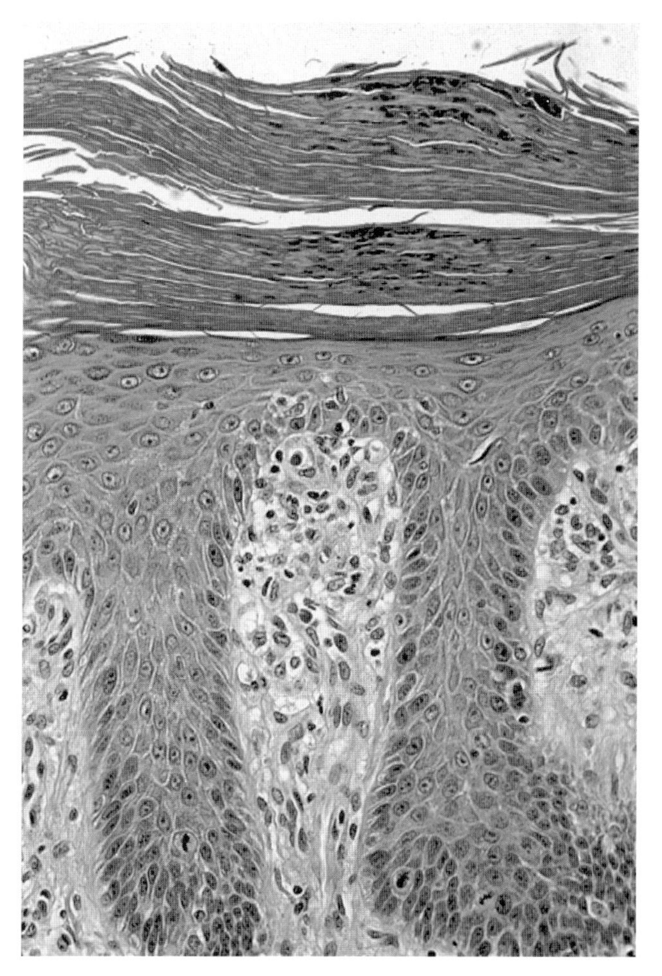

FIG. 7-10. Psoriasis, plaque lesion
Club-shaped rete ridges, suprabasal mitotic figures, thin suprapapillary epidermal plates, parakeratosis with collections of neutrophils (Munro microabscess), and dilated tortuous blood vessels in the dermal papillae.

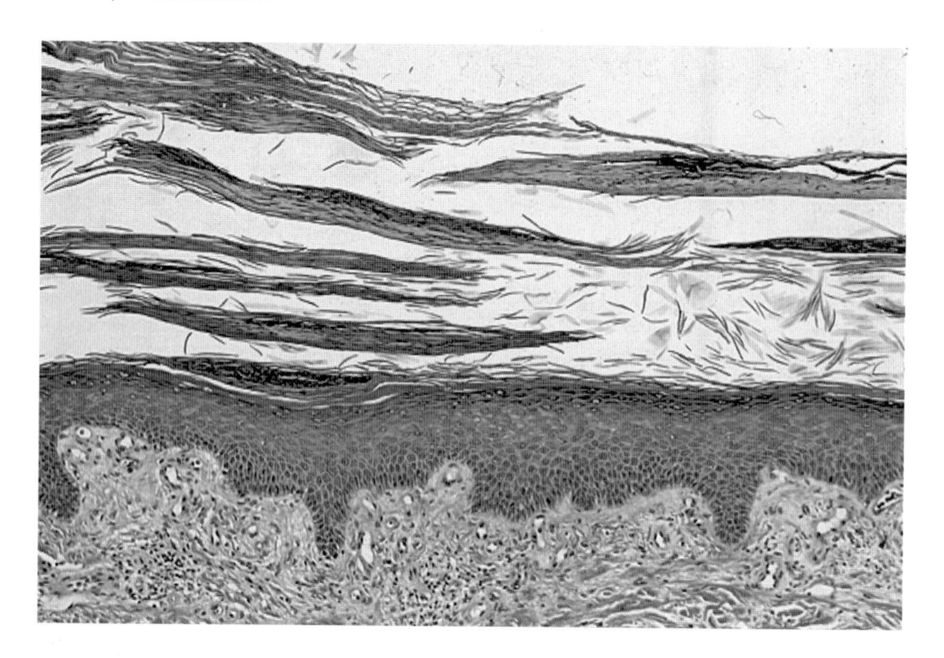

FIG. 7-11. Eruptive psoriasis
Multilayered mounds of parakeratosis admixed with basketweave orthokeratosis, slight acanthosis, and dilated blood vessels in the dermal papillae.

instances shows enough of the characteristics of psoriasis to allow this diagnosis. Frequently, however, the histologic appearance is indistinguishable from that of a chronic eczematous dermatitis.[91]

Generalized Pustular Psoriasis Histopathology

Whereas, in ordinary psoriasis, the spongiform pustule of Kogoj is a very small micropustule and is seen only in early, active lesions, it occurs as a macropustule in all variants of generalized pustular psoriasis and represents their characteristic histologic lesion. The spongiform pustule forms through the migration of neutrophils from the papillary capillaries to the upper layer of epidermis, where they aggregate within the interstices of a sponge-like network formed by degenerated and thinned epidermal cells.[87] As the size of the pustule increases, the epidermal cells in the center of the pustule undergo complete cytolysis so that a large single cavity forms (Fig. 7-12). At the periphery of the pustule, however, the network of thinned epidermal cells persists for a much longer time. As the neutrophils of the spongiform pustule move up into the cornified layer, they become pyknotic and assume the appearance of a large Munro abscess.[66,92]

Besides the large spongiform pustules, the epidermal changes in generalized pustular psoriasis are very much like those seen in psoriasis vulgaris, consisting of parakeratosis and elongation of the rete ridges. The upper dermis contains an infiltrate of mononuclear cells, and neutrophils can often be seen migrating from the capillaries in the papillae into the epidermis.[93] The oral lesions show the same spongiform pustule formation as those seen on the skin.[65]

In the healing stage the lesions of all types of generalized pustular psoriasis may present the same histologic appearance as ordinary psoriasis.[66]

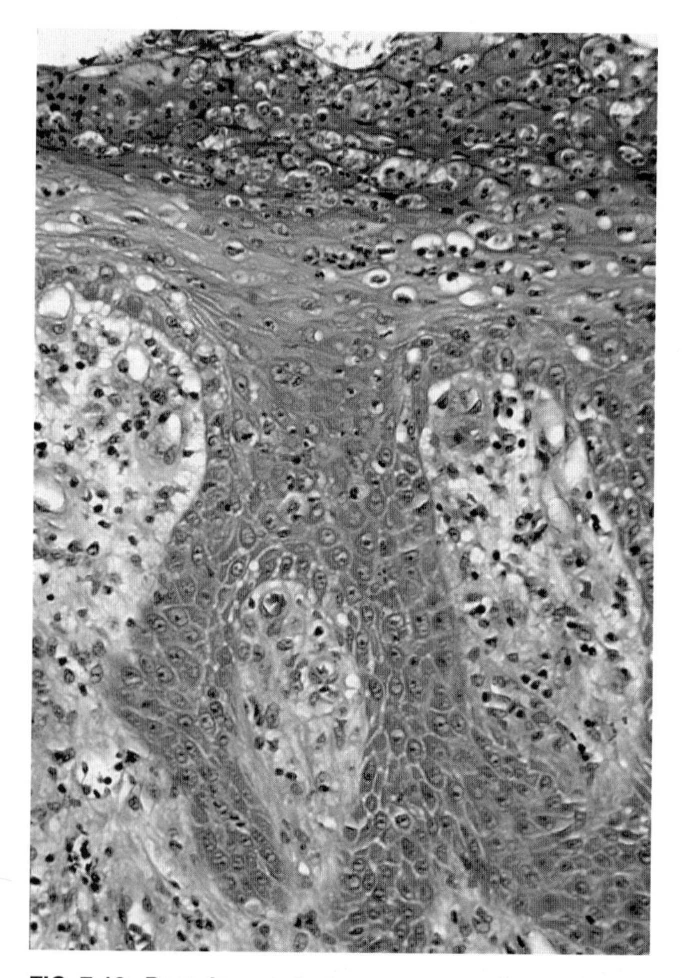

FIG. 7-12. Pustular psoriasis
Large collections of neutrophils with spongiosis in the upper spinous layer and granular layer.

Localized Pustular Psoriasis Histopathology

In the variants of localized pustular psoriasis, "psoriasis with pustules,"[68,69] and localized annular pustular psoriasis, the histologic picture is the same as that described for generalized pustular psoriasis.

In localized acrodermatitis continua of Hallopeau, the nail bed is mainly affected, showing marked epidermal hyperplasia with variable numbers of spongiform pustules, hypergranulosis, and hyperkeratosis with mounds of parakeratosis with neutrophils. The nail matrix is only occasionally involved.[94]

In pustulosis palmaris et plantaris a fully developed pustule is large, intraepidermal in location, unilocular, and rounded on both sides. It is elevated only slightly above the surface but extends into the underlying dermis. Many neutrophils are present within the cavity of the pustule. The epidermis surrounding the pustule shows slight acanthosis, and an inflammatory infiltrate can be seen beneath the pustule.[95] In many instances, one can observe typical, though small, spongiform pustules in the epidermal wall of the pustule, most commonly at the junction of the lateral walls and the overlying epidermis.[95–99] These spongiform pustules are identical with those seen in the walls of the pustules of generalized pustular psoriasis.

Very early lesions may show spongiosis and a mononuclear infiltrate in the lower epidermis overlying the tips of dermal papillae.[98] This may be followed by the formation of an intraepidermal vesicle containing mostly mononuclear cells.[95,98] Subsequently, as the vesicle expands, it becomes a pustule. There is a massive invasion of the cavity by neutrophils, which penetrate the intercellular spaces of the vesicle wall, where the histologic picture of spongiform pustules is then seen.[95] In the acute form, pustular bacterid, leukocytoclastic vasculitis has been described.[100]

Psoriasis and AIDS Histopathology

The histological picture in most cases is similar to that of psoriasis. In others, the histologic sections may show acanthosis without thinning of the suprapapillary epidermis, slight spongiosis, rare necrotic keratinocytes, and a superficial perivascular infiltrate of lymphocytes and histiocytes that occasionally contains some plasma cells.[101] As in other dermatitides related to AIDS, eosinophils may be present in the inflammatory infiltrate.

Pathogenesis of Psoriasis Vulgaris

Although the cause of psoriasis is still unknown, there is increasing evidence of a complex interaction between altered keratinocytic proliferation and differentiation, inflammation, and immune dysregulation.

Electron Microscopy

The earliest recognizable morphologic events in psoriasis have been investigated in lesions cleared with corticosteroid under occlusion and then allowed to relapse. The earliest indications of relapse, as seen by electron microscopy, are swelling and intercellular widening of endothelial cells. This is followed by the appearance around postcapillary venules of mast cells showing degranulation. Hours later, activated macrophages migrate into the lower epidermis, where there is loss of desmosome-tonofilament complexes. Only then lymphocytes and neutrophils are seen.[102]

Ultrastructurally, in well-developed lesions, psoriatic keratinocytes from the suprabasal layers of the epidermis show significant abnormalities. The tonofilaments are decreased in number and in diameter and lack their normal aggregation. The size and number of keratohyaline granules are greatly reduced, and occasionally these are absent.[103,104] The cornified cells possess thin tonofilaments and often retain organelles and a nucleus as parakeratotic cells. They often fail to form a marginal band and to lose their outer plasma membrane.[105] Basal keratinocytes may show cytoplasmic processes protruding into the dermis through gaps in the basal lamina. The presence of these herniations correlates with psoriatic activity. They are more numerous in active and untreated lesions and are absent in completely resolved and uninvolved psoriatic skin.[106] The intercellular spaces between all epidermal cells are widened because of a deficiency in the glycoprotein-rich cell surface coat, so that intercellular adhesion is limited to the desmosomes.[105,107] Electron microscopic studies have confirmed the view that the keratinocytes in psoriasis are defective and not just immature owing to accelerated epidermal proliferation. Although a correlation exists in psoriasis between an increased rate of mitosis and parakeratosis, rapid proliferation of the epidermis does not cause parakeratosis.[108]

Ultrastructural studies of the spongiform pustule of Kogoj, one of the most characteristic histologic structures encountered in psoriasis, reveal that it is located in the uppermost portion of the spinous and granular layers, where neutrophils lie intercellularly in a multilocular pustule in which the sponge-like network is composed of degenerated and flattened keratinocytes.[87]

The ultrastructure of the capillary loops in the dermal papillae shows them to be different from normal capillary loops. Normal skin microvasculature has a homogeneous-appearing basement membrane and no bridged fenestrations between endothelial cells. In psoriasis, however, the capillaries show a wider lumen, bridged fenestrations and gaps between endothelial cells, edematous areas in the cytoplasm of endothelial cells, pericytes and myocytes, extravasation of red blood cells and inflammatory cells and a thickened multilayered basement membrane.[109] This finding may be a result of the deposition of amorphous substances and accumulation of collagen fibrils in the basement membrane zone.[110]

Epidermal Cell Cycle Kinetics

The rate of epidermal cell replication is markedly accelerated in active lesions of psoriasis, as shown by the higher than normal number of basal and suprabasal mitotic figures and the greater number of premitotic cells labeled by tritiated thymidine.[111] The mitotic activity within different lesions of psoriasis and even within the same lesion can vary considerably and seems to correlate with the degree of parakeratosis. Thus, psoriatic epidermis with 91% to 100% parakeratosis shows on the average five times as many mitotic figures as psoriatic epidermis with only 0% to 20% parakeratosis.[90] The frequent finding in psoriasis of alternating layers of orthokeratosis and parakeratosis suggests that epidermal growth activity fluctuates in the lesions.[90] Step sections of early "punctate" papules show a mitotically very active parakeratotic center surrounded by a zone with a thickened granular layer and a relatively low mitotic rate.[112]

Early calculations made it appear likely that, in psoriatic lesions, there was a great acceleration of the transit time of cells from the basal cell layer to the uppermost row of the squamous cell layer, from approximately 53 days in normal epidermis to only seven days in the epidermis of active psoriatic lesions.[111]

Further investigations[113] have found that (1) the germinative cell cycle is shortened from 311 to 36 hours, indicating that psoriatic keratinocytes proliferate approximately eightfold faster than do normal keratinocytes, (2) there is a doubling of the proliferative cell population in psoriasis from 27,000 to 52,000 cells/mm^2 of epidermal surface area, and (3) 100% of the germinative cells of the epidermis enter the growth fraction instead of only 60% for normal subjects. However, in another study,[114] it was shown that the germinative cell cycle time in normal epidermis is around 200 hours and in psoriatic epidermis about 100 hours, a twofold rather than an eightfold acceleration.

The source of the cycling cells in the suprabasal layers of the epidermis is not yet well defined. They could be an expanded population of basal keratinocytes or could be recruited from the transit-amplifying cells (TAC), which refers to suprabasal keratinocytes committed to terminal differentiation, that might undergo rounds of amplifying divisions above the basal layer.[115] Based on keratin studies, it is believed that proliferating keratinocytes may result from recruitment of TAC[115] because they express K1/K10 and K6/K16 keratins and not K5/ K14 as basal keratinocytes do.[116]

Keratinocyte Differentiation

Keratinocytes undergo the process of differentiation as they migrate upward through the epidermis from the basal layer to the cornified layer. During this process, different structural proteins are synthesized. One such protein family is the keratins, which are intermediate filaments found in the cytoplasm of all the epithelial cells. Studies have revealed that the keratin pair K5/K14 is expressed in basal keratinocytes[117] and keratins K1/ K10 are found in the suprabasal layers. Involucrin, one of the major precursor proteins of the cornified cell envelope, is detected higher in the granular and cornified layers.[118] In psoriatic skin, basal keratinocytes continue to express K5/K14; however, keratins K1/K10 are replaced by the so-called hyperproliferation-associated keratins K6 and K16. In addition, involucrin is expressed prematurely in the lower suprabasal layers.[116,119] Keratin 17, normally expressed in the deep outer root sheath of the hair follicle, has been found also in the upper supra-basal keratinocytes within the interfollicular psoriatic epidermis.[116]

Immunopathology

Immunologic factors play a very important role in the pathogenesis of psoriasis. It has been shown that T lymphocytes predominate in the inflammatory infiltrate. They are mainly CD4$^+$ (helper-inducer) lymphocytes and just 25% belong to the CD8$^+$ (suppressor-cytotoxic) subset.[120,121] T lymphocytes in psoriatic lesions are known to be in an activated state because they express HLA-DR and interleukin-2 receptor.[122] The activation of T lymphocytes may be due to bacterial superantigens such as streptococcal enterotoxin B, which may participate in the pathogenesis of poststreptococcal guttate psoriasis.[123] Activated CD4$^+$ T lymphocytes produce a variety of cytokines including interleukin-2 (IL-2), tumor necrosis factor-alpha (TNF-α) and gamma-interferon (γ-IFN).[124]

Keratinocytes stimulated by TNF-α may produce interleukin-8 (IL-8), which is a potent T lymphocyte and neutrophil chemoattractant present in increased amounts in psoriatic epidermis. This cytokine may be involved in the formation of Munro microabscesses.[125]

γ-IFN is thought to play an important role in the initiation of psoriatic lesions as demonstrated by the induction of pinpoint lesions of psoriasis at sites of γ-IFN injection in previously uninvolved skin.[126] γ-IFN induces the expression of the intercellular adhesion molecule-1 (ICAM-1) in keratinocytes and endothelial cells. This molecule mediates the adhesion and trafficking of lymphocytes into the epidermis by binding to its ligand LFA-1 (lymphocyte function-associated antigen-1) expressed on lymphocyte membranes.[125] In addition, γ-IFN inducible protein (IP-10) is overexpressed by keratinocytes in psoriatic lesional skin.[127] IP-10 is detected in epidermis during cellular immune responses and may have chemotactic as well as mitogenic properties. However, it has been shown that keratinocytes from lesional psoriatic skin have altered responses to γ-IFN.[128] In normal skin, γ-IFN induces the expression of HLA-DR in keratinocytes, whereas in psoriatic keratinocytes this expression is infrequently observed.[129] Furthermore, psoriatic keratinocytes are not responsive to the growth inhibition effects of γ-IFN.[129] These findings suggest that decreased responsiveness of keratinocytes to γ-IFN may contribute to the hyperproliferation and altered differentiation of epidermal cells in psoriasis.[130]

Pathogenesis of Localized Pustular Psoriasis

A relationship of pustulosis palmaris et plantaris with psoriasis is not generally accepted, although two facts favor a close relationship: the relatively common occurrence of psoriasis in patients with pustulosis palmaris et plantaris, observed by various observers in 19%, 24%, and 48% of the patients, respectively[131–133]; and the common presence of spongiform pustules in the walls of the pustules of pustulosis palmaris et plantaris. The argument that the primary occurrence of a mononuclear reaction in pustulosis palmaris et plantaris speaks against a relationship with psoriasis[95] can be countered by the fact that a mononuclear infiltrate precedes the appearance of neutrophils in psoriasis as well. Also, a leukotactic factor identical to that noted in psoriasis has been found in pustulosis palmaris et plantaris.[134]

Pathogenesis of Psoriasis and AIDS

T-helper lymphocytes and γ-IFN are known to participate in the pathogenesis of psoriasis in AIDS.[101] Paradoxically, as T-helper lymphocyte counts decline, it appears that psoriatic lesions exacerbate until a preterminal stage when the dermatitis improves. The latter event is probably a consequence of a decreased local production of γ-IFN due to the increasing number of infected T-helper lymphocytes or a diminished number of dermal lymphocytes available to produce this cytokine.[101] In addition, the human immunodeficiency virus has pleiotropic effects on the immune system, vascular endothelium, and cytokine production, which could result in epidermal proliferation as in psoriasis.[135]

Immunohistochemical studies have shown similar proportions of T-lymphocyte subtypes in psoriasis of HIV patients and in psoriasis of immunocompetent hosts.[136] Furthermore, there is evidence of identical keratinocyte expression of γ-interferon–induced protein 10 in both groups.[101] These two findings suggest that the cellular immune reactions involved in the pathogenesis of psoriasis may be similar in AIDS and non-AIDS patients.[136]

Differential Diagnosis

Two histologic features are of great value in the diagnosis of psoriasis vulgaris: (1) mounds of parakeratosis with neutrophils at their summits (Munro microabscesses), and (2) spongiform micropustules of Kogoj in the uppermost layers of the spinous layer. Dilatation and tortuosity of capillaries in the papillae may also be of help in the diagnosis. All other features, such as acanthosis with elongation of the rete ridges and parakeratosis, can be found also in chronic eczematous dermatitis, such as *atopic dermatitis*, *nummular dermatitis*, or *allergic contact dermatitis*, which then may appear to be "psoriasiform." However, the elongation of rete ridges is uneven. Although mild spongiosis may be seen in psoriasis in the lower epidermis, the presence of marked spongiosis and especially of coagulated serum as evidence of crusting in the cornified layer are features speaking against psoriasis. In addition, eosinophils, which are commonly found in allergic contact dermatitis, are rarely seen in the psoriatic infiltrate. Difficulties may arise in treated lesions of psoriasis and in those with superimposed allergic contact dermatitis secondary to topical treatments. *Lichen simplex chronicus* is considered in the differential diagnosis of fully developed psoriatic lesions. In contrast to psoriasis, it shows a prominent granular layer, more irregular acanthosis, and fibrosis of the papillary dermis with collagen bundles aligned perpendicularly to the skin surface.[137] *Seborrheic dermatitis* may be very difficult to distinguish from psoriasis vulgaris, especially if overlap occurs. Accentuated spongiosis, mounds of parakeratosis with neutrophils predominantly at the follicular ostia, and more irregular acanthosis are histologic features suggestive of seborrheic dermatitis. *Pityriasis rubra pilaris* shares some histologic features with psoriasis, namely, acanthosis and parakeratosis. However, it could be differentiated from well-developed lesions of psoriasis by the presence of thick suprapapillary plates, broader and shorter rete ridges, and a prominent granular layer. It lacks Munro microabscesses and neutrophils in the infiltrate.[138] Although the Kogoj spongiform pustule is highly diagnostic of the psoriasis group of diseases, including Reiter's disease, histologically typical spongiform pustules may occur also in *pustular dermatophytosis*, *bacterial impetigo*, *pustular drug eruptions*, and *candidiasis*, particularly if pustules are clinically present.[139] PAS and Gram stains are useful to identify the infectious microorganisms. Aggregates of neutrophils with pyknotic nuclei within areas of parakeratosis may occur in conditions other than psoriasis, but they generally differ from Munro microabscesses by being larger and less well circumscribed and by often showing crusting.

Because of the clinical and, particularly, the histologic, resemblance of the tongue lesions in pustular psoriasis with those seen in geographic tongue, it has been suggested that geographic tongue represents an abortive form of pustular psoriasis.[140]

REITER'S DISEASE

Reiter's disease is a sterile arthritis associated in most cases with a distant infection causing enteritis or urethritis. Reiter's disease predominantly affects young men and consists of the triad of urethritis, arthritis, and conjunctivitis. Although as a rule the arthritis occurs in attacks and is followed by recovery, it progresses in some cases to cause permanent damage to the affected joints.[141,142] Cutaneous lesions occur in about half of affected patients. Lesions have a predilection for the glans penis (balanitis circinata), the palms and soles (keratoderma blennorrhagicum), and the subungual areas.

In uncircumcised men, balanitis circinata presents as superficial crusted erosions forming a serpiginous pattern. In circumcised men the condition presents as erythematous hyperkeratotic and coalescent papules on the glans.[143] Lesions on the palms and soles are erythematous, mollusk-like plaques with central keratotic excrescences. Pustular lesions may also develop. The subungual lesions consist of hyperkeratosis with opacification of the nail plate and eventual shedding of the nail plate may occur. The prevalence of Reiter's disease in HIV-infected individuals is less than 1%; however, the disease appears to be more severe in immunocompromised patients.[143]

Histopathology. Early pustular lesions on the palms or soles show a spongiform macropustule in the upper epidermis.[141,144] In addition, one observes parakeratosis and elongation of the rete ridges.

As the lesions age, the parakeratotic cornified layer overlying the spongiform pustule thickens considerably. This greatly thickened cornified layer is the anatomic substrate for the keratotic excrescences seen clinically. The cornified layer consists of parakeratotic cells intermingled with the pyknotic nuclei of neutrophils. In old lesions, spongiform pustules are no longer seen. The histologic picture shows acanthosis and hyperkeratosis with only a few areas of parakeratosis, but occasionally the histologic picture resembles psoriasis.[141]

Pathogenesis. Most cases of Reiter's disease are probably caused by infection with microorganisms that infect the urogenital or gastrointestinal systems such as *Chlamydia trachomatis*, *Ureaplasma urealyticum*, Shigella, Salmonella, Campylobacter, and Yersinia species. *Chlamydia trachomatis* has been cultured from urethral sections in nearly half of the patients and is thought to be capable of triggering Reiter's syndrome in susceptible men.[145] Although joint cultures are negative for bacteria in Reiter's disease, hybridization studies have detected chlamydial RNA in synovial specimens.[146] Eighty percent of Reiter's disease patients are HLA-B27-positive.[143] However, the precise role of this MHC Class I antigen in the development of this disease remains unclear.

A close relationship to psoriasis has been assumed for the cutaneous lesions because of their clinical resemblance to psoriasis and the presence of spongiform pustules.[141] Similarly, the arthritis of Reiter's disease resembles psoriatic arthritis not only clinically but also because of the absence of the rheumatoid factor.[142]

Differential Diagnosis. The early spongiform pustule seen in Reiter's disease is indistinguishable from the spongiform pustule seen in pustular psoriasis. Slightly older lesions often can be identified as representing Reiter's disease in contradistinction to psoriasis by the presence of a greatly thickened cornified layer.

PARAPSORIASIS

There are still three entities described as parapsoriasis: *small plaque parapsoriasis*, *large plaque parapsoriasis*, and *parapsoriasis variegata*.

Large plaque parapsoriasis and *parapsoriasis variegata* are best considered as early stages of cutaneous T-cell lymphoma.[147] They are discussed in Chapter 32.

The *small plaque parapsoriasis* is known also as xanthoerythrodermia perstans of Crocker[148] and as digitate dermatosis.[149] Pink to yellow, slightly scaling, oval or elongated, often finger print–like patches 1 to 5 cm in diameter are symmetrically distributed over the trunk and the proximal portions of the extremities following the tension lines of the skin.[150] The eruption is usually asymptomatic, has a chronic course, and tends to persist. In some instances, cases diagnosed originally as representing the small plaque type later on show reticulate pigmentation and atrophy, requiring reclassification as the large plaque type.[151]

Histopathology. The *small plaque parapsoriasis* shows focal epidermal involvement consisting of slight spongiosis, exocytosis of lymphocytes, mild acanthosis, and parakeratosis.[149,152] Elongated mounds of parakeratosis with collections of plasma above a basketweave cornified layer is a characteristic finding (Fig. 7-13). In the papillary dermis, there is a mild superficial perivascular lymphocytic infiltrate that in some instances is more pronounced and resembles that seen in the large plaque type; such cases require inclusion in the large plaque category.[151,153] It must be conceded that, in some instances, a clinical or histologic distinction of small plaque parapsoriasis from large plaque parapsoriasis is difficult, so that only the subsequent course decides the issue.[151]

Pathogenesis. The inflammatory infiltrate in small plaque parapsoriasis is dominated by $CD4^+$ (helper-inducer) T lymphocytes with a small proportion of the $CD8^+$ (cytotoxic-suppressor) T lymphocytes subset. Langerhans' cells are found increased in the epidermis and dermis.[154]

Relationship to Lymphoma. Because of the division of parapsoriasis en plaques into a small plaque type and a large plaque type and the gradual acceptance of the term *digitate dermatosis* for the small plaque type, the relationship of parapsoriasis to mycosis fungoides has been greatly clarified. It is now generally accepted that the small plaque parapsoriasis, or digitate dermatosis, is a benign disorder without any potential of transformation into mycosis fungoides.[147,149,151,155,156] However, it has been shown that in some cases there is a dominant clonal rearrangement of the infiltrating T lymphocytes.[154] This finding has led to the hypothesis that small plaque parapsoriasis could be placed into the category of "abortive lymphomas," which includes conditions where clonality can be demonstrated, but which never converts into a systemic lymphoma.[157]

PITYRIASIS ROSEA

Pityriasis rosea is a self-limited dermatitis lasting from four to seven weeks. It frequently starts with a herald patch followed by a disseminated eruption. The lesions, found chiefly on the trunk, neck, and proximal extremities, consist of round to oval

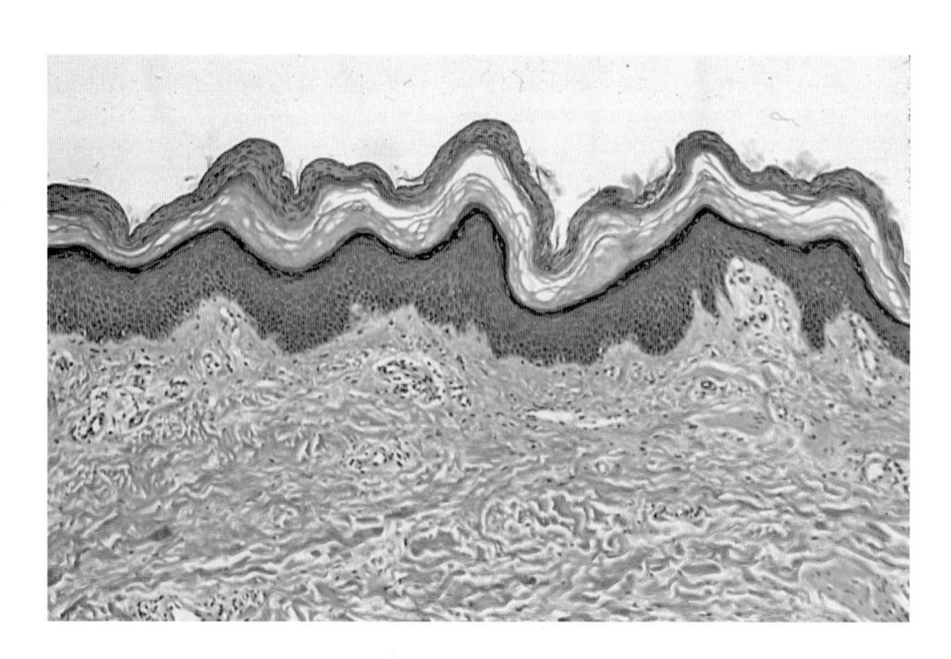

FIG. 7-13. Digitate dermatosis (small plaque parapsoriasis) Characteristic elongated mound of parakeratosis with collections of plasma above a basketweave cornified layer, preserved granular layer, and minimal acanthosis. There is a sparse superficial perivascular lymphocytic infiltrate.

salmon-colored patches following the lines of cleavage and showing peripherally attached, thin, cigarette-paper–like scales. Several typical and atypical clinical variants have been described including papular, vesicular, urticarial, purpuric, and recurrent forms.[158]

Histopathology. The patches of the disseminated eruption show a superficial perivascular infiltrate in the dermis that consists predominantly of lymphocytes, with occasional eosinophils and histiocytes. Lymphocytes extend into the epidermis (exocytosis), where there is spongiosis, intracellular edema, mild to moderate acanthosis, areas of decreased or absent granular layer, and focal parakeratosis with plasma.[159–161] Intraepidermal spongiotic vesicles[159,160] and a few necrotic keratinocytes[162] are found in some cases. A common feature is the presence of extravasated erythrocytes in the papillary dermis, which sometimes extends into the overlying epidermis[162,163] (Fig. 7-14). Occasionally, multinucleated keratinocytes in the affected epidermis can be seen.[163] Late lesions from the disseminated eruption are more likely to have a psoriasiform or lichen planus–like appearance[159] and a relatively increased number of eosinophils in the inflammatory infiltrate.[161]

The herald patch may have, in addition to the histopathologic changes described above, greater acanthosis, deeper and denser perivascular inflammatory infiltrate, and more evident papillary dermal edema.[163]

Pathogenesis. The cause of pityriasis rosea is still unknown, although a viral etiology is suspected. Cell-mediated immune mechanisms may be involved in the pathogenesis of pityriasis rosea due to the presence of activated helper-inducer T lymphocytes ($CD4^+$/HLA-DR^+) in the epidermal and dermal infiltrate[164] in association with a highly increased number of Langerhans' cells ($CD1a^+$)[165,166] and the expression of HLA-DR^+ antigen on the surface of keratinocytes located around the area of lymphocytic exocytosis.[167]

Differential Diagnosis. The differential diagnosis includes superficial gyrate erythema and small plaque parapsoriasis (digitate dermatosis). The histopathologic picture in superficial gyrate erythema could be identical to that seen in milder forms of pityriasis rosea. Focal or diffuse elongated mounds of parakeratotic crusts and occasional collections of lymphocytes in the epidermis with minimal spongiosis are features suggestive of small plaque parapsoriasis.[152]

GIANOTTI–CROSTI SYNDROME (PAPULAR ACRODERMATITIS OF CHILDHOOD AND PAPULOVESICULAR ACROLOCATED SYNDROME)

Papular acrodermatitis of childhood, first described in 1955 by Gianotti[168] is characterized by: (1) a nonpruritic, symmetrical eruption of monomorphic erythematous papules on the face, extremities, and buttocks lasting about three weeks; (2) enlargement of subcutaneous lymph nodes; (3) acute hepatitis, usually anicteric; and (4) hepatitis B surface antigenemia, subtype ayw.[169] In recent years, it has become apparent that similar acral papular eruptions may be associated with several other viruses, such as Epstein-Barr virus, coxsackie virus, parainfluenza virus, vaccine related virus, and cytomegalovirus, among others.[170–173] In such cases, there is often no hepatitis or lymphadenopathy. These eruptions were classified by Gianotti[169] in a separate category as "papular or papulovesicular acrolocated syndrome." However, further studies[173,174] have failed to identify repeatable clinical differences between papular acrodermatitis of childhood and papulovesicular acrolocated syndrome, proposing the term Gianotti-Crosti syndrome to describe all self-limited, acrolocated, papular eruptions that occur in association with an underlying viral infection.[175]

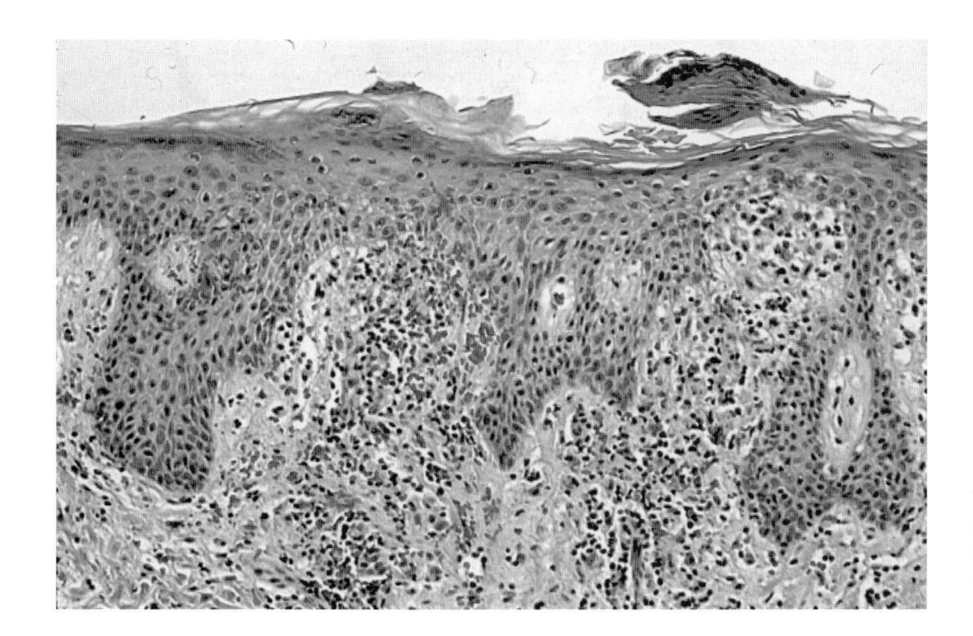

FIG. 7-14. Pityriasis rosea Superficial perivascular infiltrate of lymphocytes and extravasated erythrocytes that extend to the epidermis, where there is moderate acanthosis, spongiosis, decreased granular layer, and mounds of parakeratosis.

Histopathology. There is a mild to moderate infiltrate of lymphocytes and histiocytes in the upper and mid dermis, mainly around capillaries, which exhibit endothelial swelling.[169] In addition, focal spongiosis, exocytosis of lymphocytes, and parakeratosis may be present.[171] In some instances true lymphocytic vasculitis has been described with cellular infiltration of the vessel walls and extravasated erythrocytes into the upper dermis.[170]

Pathogenesis. Immunohistochemical stains have shown that the inflammatory infiltrate of the papules is composed predominantly of $CD4^+$ (helper-inducer) T lymphocytes and about 20% of $CD8^+$ (suppressor-cytotoxic) T lymphocytes. There is also an increased number of Langerhans' cells in the epidermis. A virus-induced type IV hypersensitivity reaction has been proposed.[176] The surface antigen of the hepatitis B virus is detectable in the sera of all cases of papular acrodermatitis of childhood due to hepatitis B virus by radioimmunoassay and in nearly all cases by immunodiffusion. Cases in which serologic studies for hepatitis B virus are negative require studies for other viruses by means of throat swabs and stool samples and by testing for antibodies.[171]

MUCOCUTANEOUS LYMPH NODE SYNDROME (KAWASAKI DISEASE)

The mucocutaneous lymph node syndrome, first reported in 1967,[177] is most common in Japanese or Korean children under 5 years of age, although it can occur in all races[178] either sporadically or epidemically. A definitive diagnosis is established by the presence of unexplained fever lasting five or more days and of at least four out of five clinical criteria: (1) bilateral conjunctivitis; (2) erythematous oral mucosa, injected or dry fissured lips, and "strawberry tongue"; (3) erythema and indurated edema of hands and feet often followed by periungual desquamation; (4) polymorphous skin rash; and (5) cervical nonsuppurative lymphadenopathy.[179] Measles and group A β-hemolytic streptococcal infections may closely resemble Kawasaki disease and must be excluded.[180]

The course of the disease could be divided in three clinical phases: acute, subacute, and convalescent. The first phase is the febrile period in which all the diagnostic signs may be seen.[181] The rash appears around the third to fifth day of illness and may have different morphological patterns such as maculopapular, morbilliform, scarlatiniform, or urticarial.[182] It involves the trunk and extremities and in some cases has a peculiar perineal distribution.[183]

There are many other associated systemic manifestations, but cardiovascular complications account for the death of 2% of the children with the disease.[177] Twenty percent of untreated patients may develop coronary artery aneurysms[184] and myocardial infarction secondary to aneurysmal thrombosis is the principal cause of death.[185] A rare and serious complication is the development of peripheral ischemia and gangrene.[186]

Histopathology. The histologic changes in the skin consist of a sparse perivascular infiltrate of lymphocytes and histiocytes,[177] marked papillary dermal edema, and dilatation of blood vessels.[187] Mild exocytosis of lymphocytes can be seen.[188] An uncommon pustular variant of Kawasaki disease shows sterile intraepidermal spongiform pustules with neutrophils.[189]

Pathogenesis. Electron microscopy studies have revealed swelling and focal degenerative changes of endothelial cells form the superficial and deep vascular plexus of the skin.[187] Immunohistochemical stains have shown that the inflammatory infiltrate has predominantly $CD4^+$ (helper-inducer) T lymphocytes and $CD13^+$ macrophages, with only a few $CD8^+$ (suppressor-cytotoxic) T cells and no $CD20^+$ B cells.[188] There is also expression of HLA-DR by keratinocytes and endothelial cells.[188] In the acute stage of the disease, interleukin-1 alpha (IL-1α) and tumor necrosis factor-alpha (TNF-α) can be detected in the epidermis. TNF-α is also found on blood vessel walls.[188] All these findings support the hypothesis of a cell-mediated immune reaction in the pathogenesis of the disease, possibly triggered by a conventional antigen[190] or superantigen.[191]

LICHEN PLANUS

Lichen planus is a subacute or a chronic dermatosis that may involve skin, mucous membranes, hair follicles, and nails.[192]

In glabrous skin, the eruption is characterized by small, flat-topped, shiny, polygonal, violaceous papules that may coalesce into plaques. The papules often show a network of white lines known as Wickham's striae. Itching is usually pronounced. The disease has a predilection for the flexor surfaces of the forearms, legs, and the glans penis. The eruption may be localized or extensive and Koebner's phenomenon is commonly seen.[193]

The oral lesions of lichen planus are frequently found, either as sole manifestation of the disease or associated with cutaneous involvement.[194] They usually involve the buccal and glossal mucosa and most often consist of a lacy, reticular network of coalescent papules.[195] Besides the reticular type, other lesional patterns have been described, such as plaquelike, atrophic, papular, erosive, and bullous.[192,196]

The nails are involved in about 10% of cases and show roughening, longitudinal ridging, and, rarely, thinning and destruction.[197] Pterygium formation is a frequent finding.

A common variant is *hypertrophic lichen planus*, which is usually found on the shins and consists of thickened, often verrucous plaques. In contrast, *vesicular lichen planus* is rare. It shows vesicles situated only on some of the preexisting lesions.[198,199] It is different from so-called *lichen planus pemphigoides* in which the eruption is more disseminated and the bullae are more extensive,[200] arising from papules of lichen planus and from normal-appearing skin.[199,201–203] At one time, lichen planus pemphigoides was thought to represent a coexistence of lichen planus and bullous pemphigoid. However, the lichen planus pemphigoides antigen differs from that of bullous pemphigoid.[204]

Lichen planopilaris designates lichen planus with a follicular arrangement of some or all of the lesions. This type of lichen planus predominantly affects the scalp. Initially, there may be only follicular papules or perifollicular erythema; however, with progressive hair loss irregularly shaped atrophic patches of scarring alopecia develop on the scalp. The axillae and the pubic region may also be affected and the alopecia in these areas may be cicatricial.[205] Hyperkeratotic follicular papules may also be seen on glabrous skin.[206] The association of scarring alopecia of hair-bearing areas and hyperkeratotic follicular papules on glabrous skin is known as Graham Little syndrome. Lichen planopilaris may also coexist with typical lichen planus lesions on skin, mucous membranes, or nails. Linear lichen planopilaris of the face resolving with scarring has also been described.[207]

Ulcerative lichen planus, a rare but quite characteristic variant of lichen planus, shows bullae, erosions, and painful ulcerations on the feet and toes resulting in atrophic scarring and permanent loss of the toenails. It is usually associated with patches of atrophic alopecia of the scalp and with cutaneous and oral lesions of lichen planus.[208–210]

Lichen planus actinicus, or *pigmentosus,* occurs mainly in Middle Eastern countries, where between 20% and 30% of the cases of lichen planus are of this type.[211,212] The lesions develop in spring and summer on sun-exposed parts, especially the face, and are typically annular plaques with central slate blue to light brown pigmentation and well-defined, slightly raised, hypopigmented borders. A different pattern, resembling melasma, has been described.[213] Pruritus is minimal or absent.

The *overlap syndrome, lichen planus/lupus erythematosus,* refers to a heterogeneous group of patients bearing at the same time, skin lesions with clinical, histological, and/or immunological features typical of both diseases.[214] The cutaneous findings in these unusual cases consist of erythematous to purplish scaly patches and plaques, some of them with central atrophy, with a predilection for photodistributed areas[215] or acral portions of extremities.[214]

Twenty-nail dystrophy may be encountered in adults as well as children. The nails have longitudinal ridging and distal notching and splitting. With time they become thin and roughened. Clinically, the nail changes resemble those seen in lichen planus.[216,217] Other manifestations of lichen planus are usually absent. In children, the nail changes tend to involute spontaneously after a few years. The condition may be familial, in which case it tends to have an unremitting course. Congenital cases have been described.[218] Twenty-nail dystrophy may be idiopathic or may be associated with alopecia areata, atopic dermatitis, lichen planus, or psoriasis.

The coexistence of *lichen nitidus* with lichen planus is frequent enough to have suggested to some authors that they are variants of the same disease.[219]

Malignant transformation of cutaneous lichen planus occurs in less than 1% of cases.[220] In hypertrophic lichen planus of the leg, development of squamous cell carcinoma or keratoacanthoma is an exceptional occurrence.[221,222] There have been reports of squamous cell carcinoma arising occasionally on longstanding lesions of lichen planus situated on mucous membranes or the vermillion border.[223–226] The incidence of carcinoma evolving in oral lichen planus in two large series was about 0.5%.[227–229] Development of carcinoma in ulcers of the feet in ulcerative lichen planus has been reported to occur rarely in lesions that had not been previously grafted.[230,231]

Histopathology. Typical papules of lichen planus show (1) compact orthokeratosis, (2) wedge-shaped hypergranulosis, (3) irregular acanthosis, (4) damage to the basal cell layer, and (5) a band-like dermal lymphocytic infiltrate in close approximation to the epidermis (Figs. 7-15 and 7-16). This constellation of findings is sufficiently diagnostic that a histologic diagnosis can be rendered in more than 90% of cases.[232]

The cornified layer shows compact orthokeratosis and contains very few, if any, parakeratotic cells, a fact that is important for the diagnosis.

The thickening of the granular layer is uneven and wedge shaped. The granular cells appear increased in size and contain coarse and more abundant keratohyaline granules. On step sectioning, the areas of wedge-shaped hypergranulosis are found to be contiguous to intraepidermal adnexal structures, namely acrosyringia and acrotrichia.[233] Wickham's striae are believed to be caused by a focal increase in the thickness of the granular layer and of the total epidermis.[234]

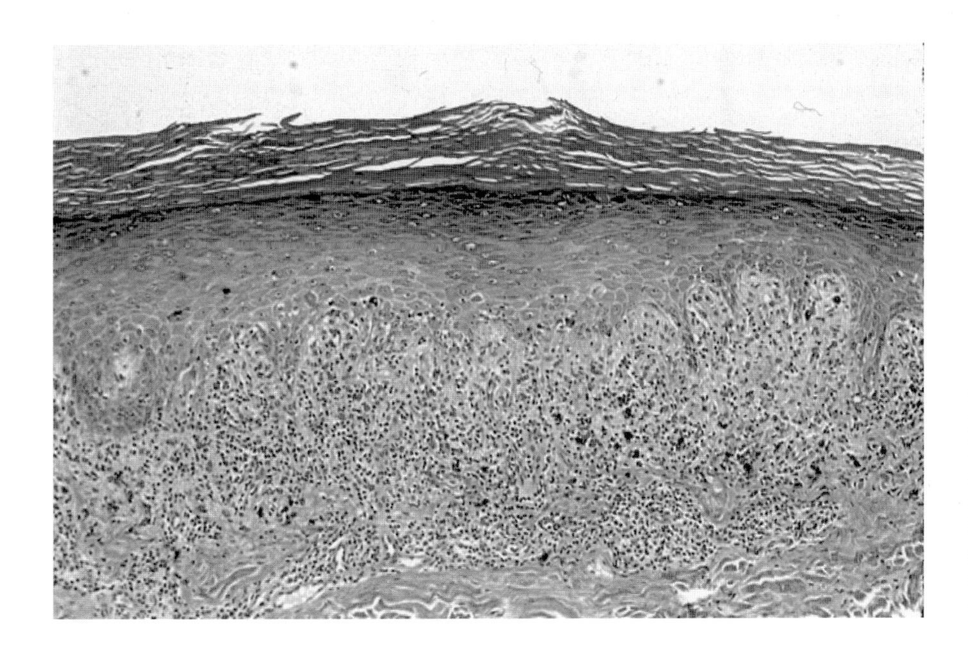

FIG. 7-15. Lichen planus
Dense band-like infiltrate predominantly of lymphocytes in the papillary dermis that extends to the epidermis, where there is vacuolar alteration of the basal layer, necrotic keratinocytes, irregular acanthosis, wedge-shaped hypergranulosis, and compact orthokeratosis.

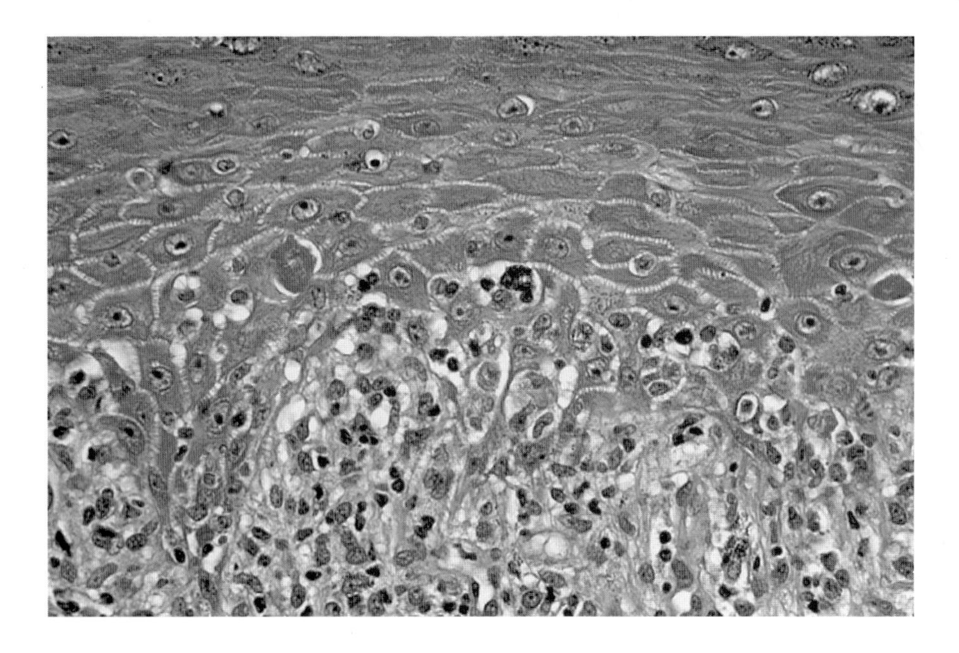

FIG. 7-16. Lichen planus
Closer view shows lymphocytes and melanophages in the papillary dermis, vacuolar alteration of the basal layer, necrotic keratinocytes (Civatte bodies), and enlarged keratinocytes with eosinophilic cytoplasm.

The acanthosis in lichen planus is irregular and affects the spinous layer of the rete ridges as well as the suprapapillary plates. The keratinocytes of the spinous layer often appear eosinophilic, possibly because of advanced keratinization. The rete ridges show irregular lengthening, and some of them are pointed at their lower end, giving them a saw-toothed appearance. The dermal papillae between lengthened rete ridges are often dome shaped.[235]

The cells of the basal layer are not clearly visible in early lesions because the dense dermal infiltrate obscures the dermal-epidermal junction with vacuolar degeneration and necrosis of the basal cells. In fully developed lesions the basal layer has the appearance of flattened squamous cells.

The infiltrate in the upper dermis is band-like and sharply demarcated at its lower border and is composed almost entirely of lymphocytes intermingled with macrophages. A few eosinophils and/or plasma cells may be seen. Melanophages are seen in the upper dermis, often in considerable number, as a result of damage to the basal cells with subsequent pigment incontinence. In some instances, the dermal lymphocytic infiltrate is seen in juxtaposition to the acrosyringium and liquefaction degeneration of the acrosyringeal basal cell layer is a prominent finding (*acrosyringeal lichen planus*).[236]

In old lesions the cellular infiltrate decreases in density, but the number of macrophages increases. In areas in which a basal cell layer has reformed, the dermal infiltrate no longer lies in close approximation to the epidermis. Chronic lesions may show considerable acanthosis, papillomatosis, and hyperkeratosis (*hypertrophic lichen planus*) (Fig. 7-17).

Necrotic keratinocytes are present in most of the cases in the lower epidermis and especially in the papillary dermis. They are also referred to as colloid, hyaline, cytoid, or Civatte bodies. They average 20 μm in diameter and have a homogeneous, eosinophilic appearance (see Fig. 7-16). They are PAS positive and diastase resistant. Even though necrotic keratinocytes are found most commonly in lichen planus, they may occur in any disease in which damage to the basal cells occurs, including graft-versus-host disease, lichen planus–like keratosis (benign

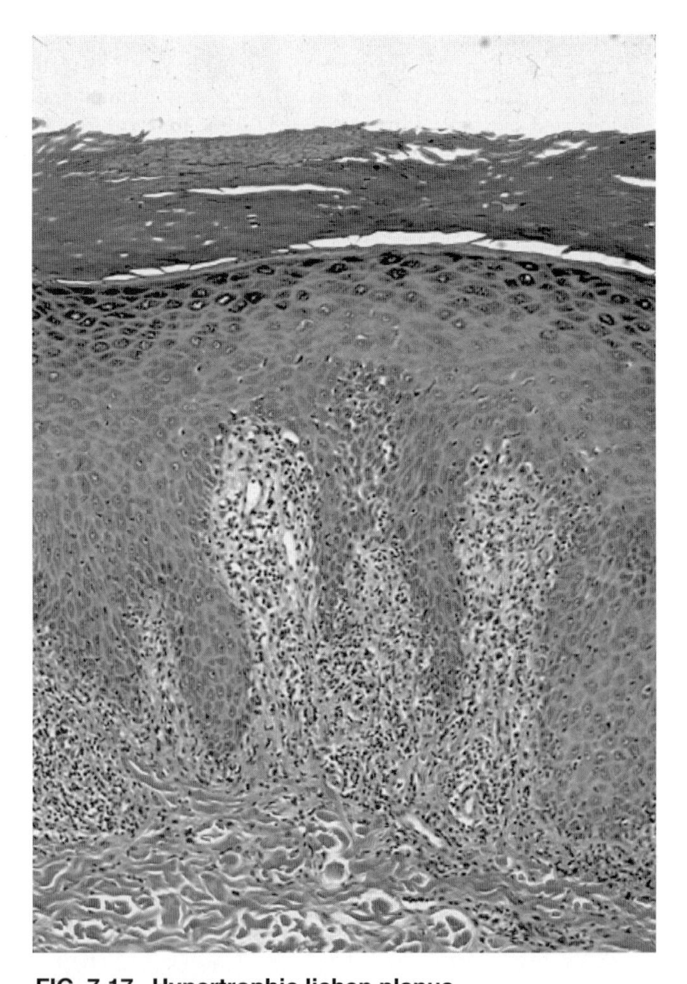

FIG. 7-17. Hypertrophic lichen planus
Marked irregular acanthosis with pointed rete ridges, hypergranulosis, and compact orthokeratosis. The vacuolar alteration and the lymphocytic inflammatory infiltrate is accentuated at the base of the rete ridges.

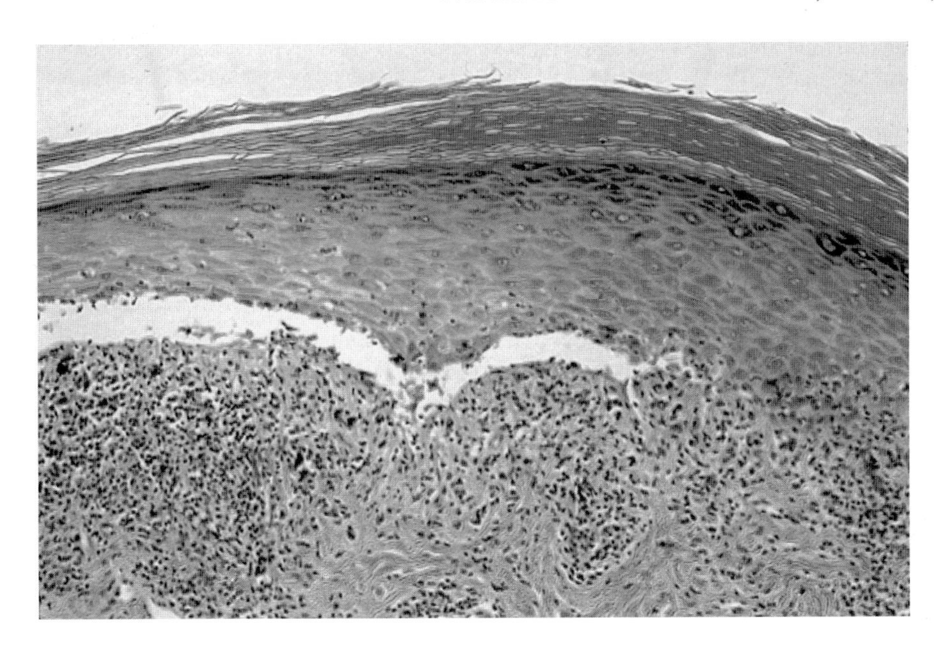

FIG. 7-18. Lichen planus
Artifactual cleft between the epidermis and the lichenoid infiltrate known as a Max-Joseph space.

lichenoid keratosis), lichen nitidus, and lupus erythematosus. They are even seen in normal skin.[237] In lichen planus the number of necrotic keratinocytes may be so large that they are seen lying in clusters in the uppermost dermis.[214] Their aggregation may result in perforation of the epidermis with subsequent transepidermal elimination.[238]

Occasionally, small areas of artifactual separation between the epidermis and the dermis, known as Max-Joseph spaces, are seen (Fig. 7-18).[232] In some instances, the separation occurs in vivo and subepidermal blisters form (*vesicular lichen planus*). These vesicles form as a result of extensive damage to the basal cells.[198,200]

Oral lichen planus. The oral lesions of lichen planus differ in their histologic appearance from those of the skin, as one would expect, since the oral mucosa normally shows parakeratosis without the presence of a granular layer. Thus, the lesions of the mouth often show parakeratosis rather than orthokeratosis, although alternating areas of both types of keratinization with the presence of a granular layer may be observed (Fig. 7-19).[196] Also, rather than showing acanthosis, the epithelium often is atrophic. Ulcerations may develop either through the rupture of vesicles or as a result of necrosis of the epithelium.

Lichen planopilaris. Most early lesions of lichen planopilaris show a focally dense, band-like perifollicular lymphocytic

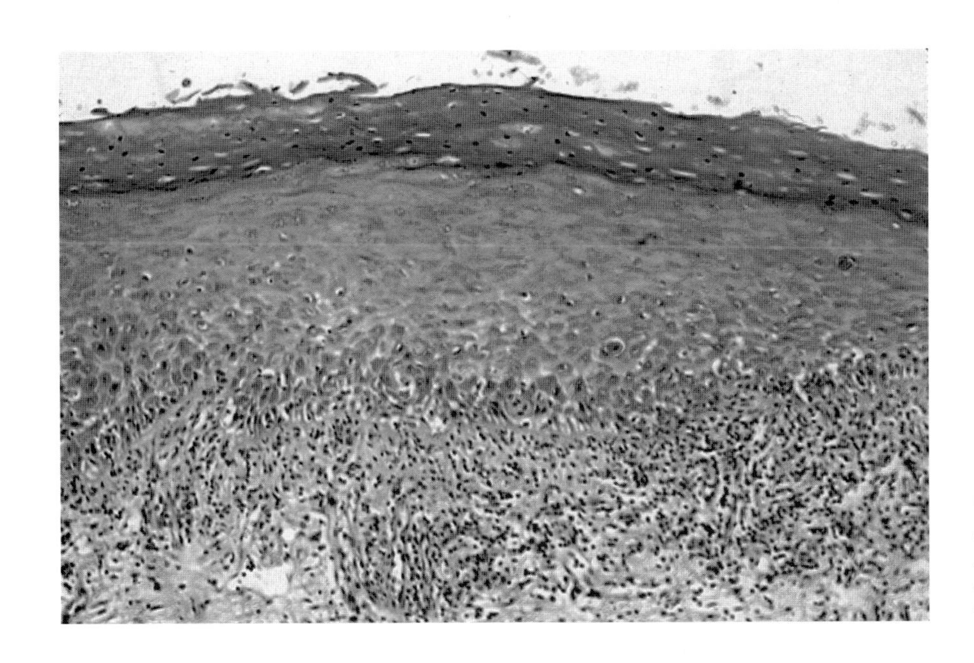

FIG. 7-19. Oral lichen planus
Similar lichenoid inflammatory pattern as seen in the skin, except for an inconspicuous granular layer and confluent parakeratosis.

infiltrate at the level of the infundibulum and the isthmus where the hair "bulge" is located. Initially, the inferior segment of the hair follicle is spared. Vacuolar changes of the basal layer of the outer root sheath and necrotic keratinocytes are often seen. In addition, orthokeratosis and follicular plugging are observed (Fig. 7-20). A few biopsies exhibit simultaneous involvement of the interfollicular epidermis and the hair follicles.[239] In more developed lesions perifollicular fibrosis and epithelial atrophy at the level of the infundibulum and isthmus are characteristic findings. Damage to the hair bulge, the site where stem cells of the hair follicle supposedly reside, results in permanent scarring alopecia. Advanced cases show alopecia with vertically oriented fibrotic tracts containing clumps of degenerated elastic fibers replacing the destroyed hair follicles. This end-stage scarring alopecia in which no visible hair follicles remain is called pseudopelade of Brocq.[240]

The hyperkeratotic follicular papules that are occasionally seen on glabrous skin in association with lichen planopilaris of the scalp exhibit similar changes; however, perifollicular fibrosis is usually slight and the process does not eventuate in scarring.[241]

Ulcerative lichen planus. In ulcerative lichen planus specimens taken from skin situated just outside an ulcer generally show active lichen planus.[208,210,230]

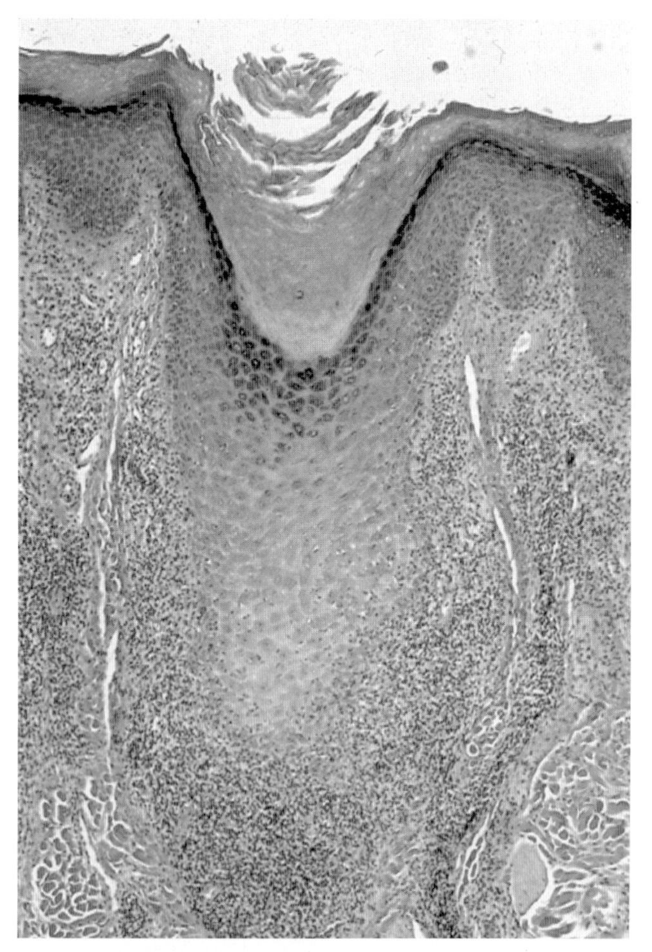

FIG. 7-20. Lichen planopilaris
Follicular plugging, hypergranulosis, and dense band-like perifollicular lymphocytic infiltrate that obscures the infundibular epithelium.

Lichen planus actinicus. In some instances, the histologic picture of lichen planus actinicus is similar to the typical lichen planus but with a tendency toward thinning of the epidermis in the center of the lesion and more evident and numerous melanophages and pigment incontinence in the upper dermis.[34,212] A relationship between lichen planus actinicus and erythema dyschromicum perstans has been postulated[242] because of the histologic resemblance in some cases; however, they have significant clinical differences.[34]

Overlap syndrome—lichen planus/lupus erythematosus. In some cases of the overlap syndrome, the histologic features and direct immunofluorescence findings are more consistent with lichen planus. In others, the immunofluorescence testing favors lupus erythematosus[215] and still in another subset of patients there are lesions of lichen planus that coexist, rather than overlap, with those of lupus erythematosus.[243,244]

Twenty-nail dystrophy. Histologic data on twenty-nail dystrophy are available in only a few cases. Biopsies may show typical lichen planus involving the nail matrix.[216,245] However, spongiosis may be prominent as in cases associated with atopic dermatitis. Twenty-nail dystrophy is a manifestation of diverse underlying processes; therefore, its histology will vary.[217,218]

Lichen planus pemphigoides. In lichen planus pemphigoides, biopsies taken from bullae arising from noninvolved skin show subepidermal bullae with an infiltrate that is not band-like and that contains eosinophils.[199]

Pathogenesis. The eosinophilia of the keratinocytes and the increase in thickness of the granular and cornified layers suggest a decreased epidermal turnover. However, in spite of severely damaged basal cells, measurements of cell proliferation in lichen planus with tritiated thymidine have shown an increase in cell proliferation.[246]

Electron microscopy. On electron microscopy the basal keratinocytes in lichen planus, together with their desmosomes and hemidesmosomes, show degenerative changes.[247] Whereas the tonofilaments in the basal cells are decreased in early lesions, they are increased in later lesions.[248] Because of the presence of degenerated and necrotic keratinocytes on the basal layer, it is assumed that the basal cells in later lesions are largely regenerated cells. The dermal infiltrate, on invading the epidermis, causes damage to the lamina densa such as fragmentation (EM 12). This may be followed by duplication and irregular folding of the lamina densa.[249] The dermal infiltrate contains mainly lymphocytes but also macrophages. Some of the lymphocytes have hyperconvoluted nuclei and appear indistinguishable from Sézary cells.

Necrotic keratinocytes or colloid bodies are located largely in the papillary dermis but also in the lower most epidermis (EM 12). They can be seen to develop from damaged keratinocytes through filamentous degeneration. This is followed by their discharge into the dermis.[250] Necrotic keratinocytes consist of aggregates of filament bundles, with each filament measuring approximately 10 nm in diameter. The use of antikeratin immune sera has resulted in their intense staining.[251] Necrotic keratinocytes often still contain cell organelles, such as melanosomes and mitochondria, but only rarely contain nuclear material.[252] Fibrin deposits in the upper dermis are a common finding under electron microscopy studies (EM 12).

In the vesicular lesions of lichen planus, electron microscopic examination shows cytolysis of basal keratinocytes; the blister cavity is, therefore, situated below the spinous layer.[253]

Immunofluorescence. In lichen planus, fibrinogen deposition can be demonstrated by direct immunofluorescence as shaggy deposits at the dermal-epidermal junction.[254] Only occasionally are there granular deposits of IgM,[255] or linear deposits of C3,[256] or both IgG and C3[257] in the basement membrane zone. Necrotic keratinocytes are demonstrable in lichen planus by direct immunofluorescence staining in about 87% of the cases.[254] They stain mainly for IgM but often also for IgG, IgA, C3, and fibrin. Although necrotic keratinocytes are found occasionally in many other conditions with damage to the basal cell layer, such as lupus erythematosus, they are highly suggestive of lichen planus if they are present in large numbers or arranged in clusters. Their staining for IgM facilitates their recognition.[237]

In lichen planopilaris, direct immunofluorescence in many specimens shows deposition of IgM and/or IgA, IgG, and, rarely, C3 at the level of the infundibulum and isthmus.[258] The necrotic keratinocytes may react with anti-IgM antibody. There is often deposition of fibrinogen in a shaggy pattern surrounding the affected follicles. The dermal-epidermal junction is virtually always negative for deposition of immunoreactants.[239]

In lichen planus pemphigoides, direct immunofluorescence of perilesional skin shows the presence of IgG and C3 in a linear arrangement along the basement membrane zone at the dermal-epidermal border,[199,259] and on immunoelectron microscopy, C3 is seen to be localized within the lamina lucida, analogous to its location in bullous pemphigoid.[201] Circulating antibasement membrane IgG antibodies have also been found.[199,202] Immunoelectron microscopic studies have shown that the lichen planus pemphigoides antigen is located in the same site as the bullous pemphigoid antigen: the basal cell hemidesmosomes on the epidermal side of salt-split skin.[260] However, no immunoprecipitation occurs when the serum of a patient with lichen planus pemphigoides is mixed with bullous pemphigoid antigen, suggesting that another antigen is involved.[261] Furthermore, by western blot analysis, patient's serum reacted with a unique 200-kD antigen and a minor bullous pemphigoid antigen (180-kD) different from the classical 220-kD antigen of bullous pemphigoid.[204]

In the overlap syndrome lichen planus/lupus erythematosus, some patients show immunofluorescence testing consistent with lichen planus; in another group direct immunofluorescence, instead, shows deposition of immunoglobulins and C3 at the dermal-epidermal junction in a linear granular pattern as in cutaneous lupus erythematosus.[215]

Immunohistochemistry. The infiltrating cells in lichen planus are predominantly T lymphocytes with very few B lymphocytes. More than 90% are activated T lymphocytes expressing HLA-DR antigen and some interleukin-2 receptor.[262] The identification of various subtypes of T lymphocytes has given contradictory results in regard to the predominance of helper-inducer T lymphocytes or suppressor-cytotoxic T lymphocytes in the infiltrate.[263–265] It is likely that both subsets participate in the immunologic reaction. It has been shown that suppressor T lymphocytes predominate in later lesions and in the epidermotropic lymphocytes, supporting a cell-mediated cytotoxic mechanism against epithelial cells.[264,266] In the epidermis adjacent to the infiltrate, basal keratinocytes express HLA-DR surface antigen and intercellular adhesion molecule-1 (ICAM-1)[267]; both are implicated to enhance the interaction between lymphocytes and their epidermal targets resulting in keratinocyte destruction.[265] Probably, these surface antigens are induced by cytokines (γ-interferon and tumor necrosis factor) released by lymphocytes from the infiltrate.[268,269] Immunophenotyping studies on T lymphocytes extracted from specimens of lichen planus have shown that the majority of clones had $CD8^+$ cells, displayed suppressor activity, and expressed $\alpha\beta$T-cell receptor[270] or a distinctive $\gamma\delta$T-cell receptor.[271] Clonal expansion of $\alpha2\beta3$T-cell receptor of the V-gene family has been reported, suggesting that a superantigen could be involved in the pathogenesis of the disease.[272]

The number of Langerhans' cells in the epidermis is increased very early in the disease,[233] especially near keratinocytes expressing $HLA\text{-}DR^+$ antigen.[273] Immunoelectron studies have shown close contacts of lymphocytes with Langerhans' cells and macrophages. Specific conjugations between $CD4^+$ (helper-inducer) T lymphocytes and dendritic ($HLA\text{-}DR^+$) cells and between $CD8^+$ (cytotoxic-suppressor) T lymphocytes and degenerated basal keratinocytes have been observed in lesional epithelium of oral mucosa. These cell-to-cell interactions suggest that a cell-mediated immune mechanism is operative.[274]

Differential Diagnosis. It should be borne in mind that parakeratosis is not a feature of lichen planus of the skin and that, if more than focal parakeratosis is present, a diagnosis of lichen planus should not be made on histologic grounds.

Focal parakeratosis and adjacent solar lentigines in an otherwise typical histologic picture of lichen planus should be regarded as lichen planus–like keratosis, even more so if it is a solitary and nonpruritic lesion.[275] Lichenoid drug eruptions may be differentiated from lichen planus by the presence of focal parakeratosis with concomitant absence of the granular layer, necrotic keratinocytes, and exocytosis of lymphocytes within upper layers of the epidermis and a deeper inflammatory infiltrate with numerous eosinophils.[276]

Differentiation from lichenoid lupus erythematosus is based on (1) atrophy of the epidermis in addition to acanthosis, (2) absence of eosinophilia of the keratinocytes in the spinous layer, (3) a superficial band-like infiltrate with a superficial and deep perivascular and periadnexal infiltrate, (4) the presence of a thickened PAS-positive basement membrane, and (5) dermal mucin deposits. Direct immunofluorescence findings may also be helpful; in lupus erythematosus linear deposits of immunoglobulins and C3 predominate in lesional skin, while in lichen planus clusters of necrotic keratinocytes with absorbed immunoglobulins and complement are found. Langerhans' cells ($CD1a^+/S\text{-}100^+$) are decreased in number in discoid and systemic lupus erythematosus; in contrast, they are increased in lichen planus.[265] The epidermal changes in chronic graft-versus-host disease (GVHD) may be similar to lichen planus; however, the inflammatory infiltrate tends to be perivascular instead of band-like. In addition, the number of Langerhans' cells in graft-versus-host disease is decreased and nearly all intraepidermal lymphocytes are cytotoxic-suppressor T cells.[277] In long-standing hypertrophic lichen planus, the basal layer may show hardly any residual damage and the infiltrate may no longer be band-like, rendering differentiation from lichen simplex chronicus at times difficult.[278] However, in the case of lichen planus, deeper sections still may show areas of damage to the basal layer at the base of the rete ridges.

On the lips and in the mouth, the differentiation of lichen planus from early squamous cell carcinoma in situ ("dysplastic leukoplakia") may cause difficulties clinically as well as histologically. Both diseases may show hyperkeratosis and an inflammatory infiltrate close to the epidermis. Yet thorough study of the epidermis reveals more atypical keratinocytes in squamous cell carcinoma in situ. Furthermore, squamous cell carcinoma in situ is more apt than lichen planus to show irregular downward proliferation of the rete ridges and numerous plasma cells.

Lichen planopilaris of the scalp must be differentiated in its early phase from discoid lupus erythematosus, which affects the hair follicles as well as the interfollicular epidermis. Lupus erythematosus shows more prominent vacuolar degeneration of the basal cells both in the epidermis and in the hair follicles without disappearance of basal cells. In addition, it also shows an interfollicular perivascular infiltrate. In their late stages, both lichen planopilaris and lupus erythematosus may result in permanent scarring alopecia, which is known as pseudopelade of Brocq.[240]

LICHEN PLANUS–LIKE KERATOSIS

Lichen planus–like keratosis (LPLK), also known as "benign lichenoid keratosis," was originally described in 1966 as "solitary lichen planus"[279] and as "solitary lichen planus–like keratosis."[280] It is a common lesion that occurs predominantly on the trunk and upper extremities of adults between the fifth and seventh decades.[281–283] LPLK consists of a nonpruritic papule or slightly indurated plaque that is nearly always solitary. It usually measures 5 to 20 mm in diameter and its color varies from bright red to violaceous to brown. Its surface may be smooth or slightly verrucous.[284] Lichen planus–like keratosis probably represents the inflammatory stage of involuting solar lentigines.[285]

Histopathology. Histologic examination shows, at least in a part of the lesion, a lichenoid pattern that may be indistinguishable from lichen planus.[279,280,283] As in lichen planus, there is vacuolar alteration of the basal cell layer and a band-like lymphocytic infiltrate that obscures the dermal-epidermal junction. Necrotic keratinocytes are commonly seen and may be numerous.[284] As in lichen planus, the epidermis often shows increased eosinophilia, hypergranulosis, and hyperkeratosis.[286] In contrast to lichen planus, however, parakeratosis is fairly common[282] (Fig. 7-21). Although usually focal,[283] at times parakeratosis is prominent.[284] In addition, eosinophils and plasma cells in the infiltrate are more frequently found in some cases of LPLK as opposed to lichen planus, in which they are rarely seen.[283,287] A residual solar lentigo at the edge of the lesion supports the diagnosis of LPLK.[288] Immunohistochemistry studies have shown that LPLK has significantly fewer Langerhans' cells in the epidermis compared to lichen planus.[289] Even though some keratinocytes may show pyknotic hyperchromatic nuclei, no definite nuclear atypia is seen. If marked keratinocytic atypia is found in association with a lichenoid inflammatory pattern, a lichenoid actinic keratosis should be considered in the differential diagnosis.[290]

Pathogenesis. LPLK has been noted to involute spontaneously.[291] LPLK may be the inflammatory stage of regressing solar lentigines and reticulated seborrheic keratoses.[285,287,288] These precursor lesions could be the target of an immune cell–mediated reaction.[283]

KERATOSIS LICHENOIDES CHRONICA

A rare asymptomatic dermatosis, keratosis lichenoides chronica was first described by Kaposi in 1895 as "lichen ruber acuminatus verrucosus et reticularis"[292] and received its present name in 1972.[293] It usually begins in adulthood between 20 and 50 years of age, being extremely rare in children.[294,295] It shows an extensive eruption, symmetrically distributed, predominantly on dorsal aspects of extremities and trunk consisting of red to violaceous papulonodules covered with a thick, adherent scale and arranged often in a characteristic linear and occasionally reticular pattern. These lesions may coalesce to form erythematosquamous or hyperkeratotic plaques.[296,297] Very fre-

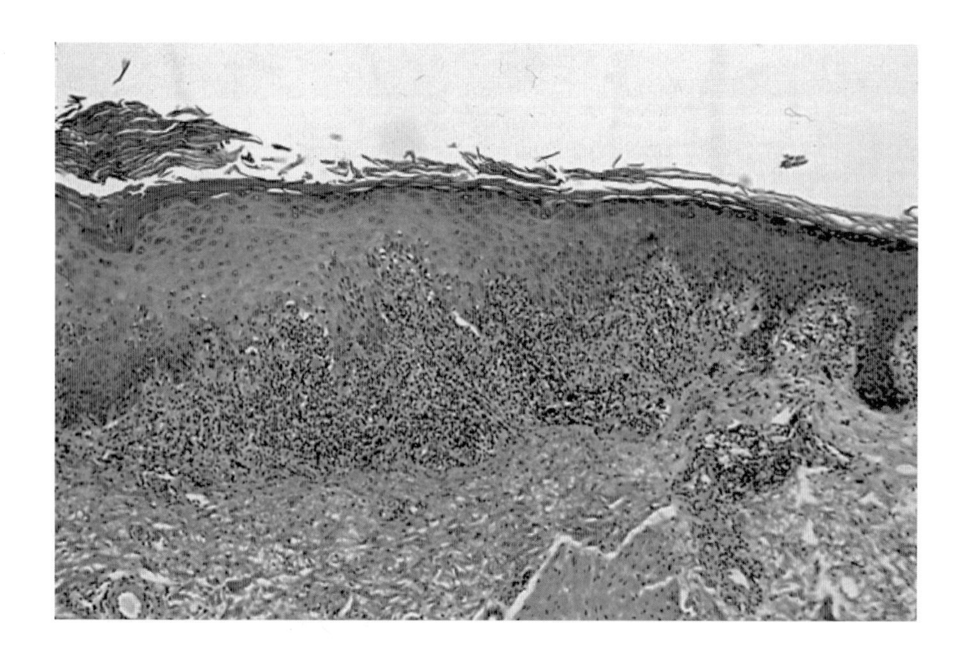

FIG. 7-21. Lichen planus–like keratosis
Lichenoid inflammatory pattern with numerous necrotic keratinocytes, granular layer of uneven thickness, orthokeratosis, and parakeratosis with a residual solar lentigo.

quently there is associated seborrheic dermatitis-like eruption of the face, palmoplantar hyperkeratosis,[296] and, in some cases, nail changes with warty hypertrophy of the periungual tissues, which has been described as a distinctive feature of the disease.[298] Mucosal membrane involvement is common and includes oral ulcers, nodular infiltration of the epiglottis and larynx, blepharitis, and keratoconjunctivitis among others.[293,296,297,299] Although the disease is characterized by a chronic and progressive course, spontaneous resolution has been reported.[300]

Histopathology. In most cases, there is a lichenoid inflammatory pattern with areas of vacuolar alteration of the basal cell layer, necrotic keratinocytes, and a band-like inflammatory infiltrate of lymphocytes, histiocytes, and numerous plasma cells that obscures the dermal-epidermal junction.[296,301] The epidermis shows areas of acanthosis as well as atrophy covered by a hyperkeratotic cornified layer showing focal parakeratosis and follicular plugging.[302] Prominent dilated dermal capillaries are seen in cases with associated telangiectasias.[303]

Differential Diagnosis. Although the histologic picture may closely resemble that of lichen planus, the presence of parakeratosis, alternating areas of atrophy and acanthosis, numerous plasma cells, and a heavier infiltrate than is usually seen in lichen planus may help in the differentiation. In addition, the clinical appearance of keratosis lichenoides chronica is quite different from that of lichen planus.

LICHEN NITIDUS

Lichen nitidus is a chronic dermatitis, usually asymptomatic, which begins commonly in childhood or early adulthood.[304] It is characterized by round, flat-topped, flesh-colored papules 2 to 3 mm in diameter that may occur in groups but do not coalesce. The lesions appear frequently as a localized eruption affecting predominantly the arms, trunk, or penis. In some patients the eruption may become generalized[305] and Koebner's phenomenon may be observed.[306] There are a few cases reported to occur on palms, soles, nails, and mucous membranes.[307] The clinical course is unpredictable and spontaneous resolution may be seen.[304]

Histopathology. Each papule of lichen nitidus consists of a well-circumscribed mixed-cell granulomatous infiltrate that is closely attached to the lower surface of the epidermis and confined to a widened dermal papillae. The infiltrate is composed of lymphocytes, numerous foamy or epithelioid histiocytes, and a few multinucleated giant cells. The dermal infiltrate often extends to a slight degree into the overlying epidermis, which is flattened and shows vacuolar alteration of the basal cell layer, focal subepidermal clefting, diminished granular layer, and focal parakeratosis.[304] Transepidermal perforation of the infiltrate through the thinned epidermis may occur.[308] At each lateral margin of the infiltrate, rete ridges tend to extend downward and seem to clutch the infiltrate in the manner of a "claw clutching a ball" (Fig. 7-22). Follicular involvement in lichen nitidus has been described.[309]

Relationship Between Lichen Planus and Lichen Nitidus. There are controversial facts regarding the relation that might exist between lichen planus and lichen nitidus. The view that lichen nitidus represents a variant of lichen planus has been supported by several authors because both diseases are occasionally present simultaneously,[305] ultrastructural findings are similar,[310] and, in some cases of lichen planus, small miliary papules may have a histologic appearance consistent with lichen nitidus.[311] However, the subsequent evolution is different; in lichen nitidus the papule remains small and develops parakeratosis and epidermal flattening, whereas in lichen planus the papule develops acanthosis and hyperkeratosis.[305] Occasional deposits of fibrinogen can be observed by direct immunofluorescence in lichen nitidus, in contrast to lichen planus, where most of the lesions have globular deposits of immunoglobulins at the dermal-epidermal junction.[312] Furthermore, immunohistochemical studies have revealed different cell populations in the inflammatory infiltrate of each disease.[313] Lichen nitidus has a significantly smaller proportion of $CD4^+$ (helper-inducer) and HECA-452^+ (skin-homing

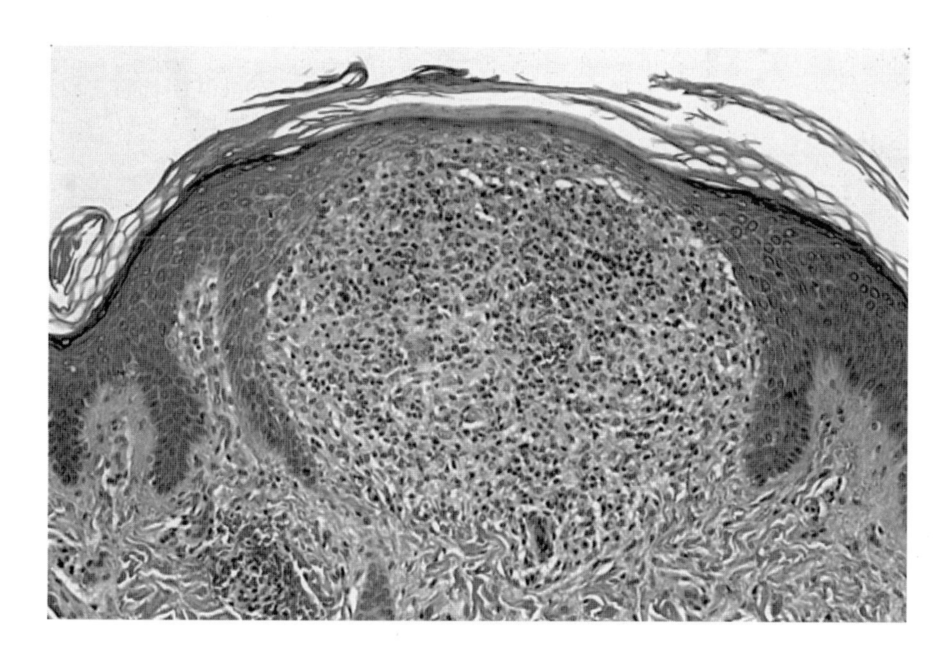

FIG. 7-22. Lichen nitidus
Dense infiltrate of lymphocytes and histiocytes in an expanded dermal papilla, thin suprapapillary epidermis with vacuolar alteration of the basal layer, and focal parakeratosis.

receptor) T lymphocytes, compared to lichen planus, suggesting different immunologic pathways.[313]

LICHEN STRIATUS

Lichen striatus is a fairly uncommon dermatitis that, as a rule, occurs in children from 5 to 15 years of age, but may be seen in adults.[314] It usually manifests itself as a unilateral eruption along Blaschko's lines[315] on the extremities, trunk, or neck as either a continuous or an interrupted band composed of minute, slightly raised, erythematous papules, which may have a scaly surface. The lesions appear suddenly and usually involute within a year. They are occasionally pruritic.[316] Hypopigmented lesions may be seen in dark-skinned patients.[317] A few cases with associated onychodystrophy[318] and rare cases of multiple or bilateral presentations[319] have been reported.

Histopathology. Although lichen striatus has been recognized by its variable histologic picture,[314,317,320] some constant microscopic findings may be present.[321] There is usually a superficial perivascular inflammatory infiltrate of lymphocytes admixed with a variable number of histiocytes. Plasma cells and eosinophils are rarely seen (Fig. 7-23).[314] Focally, in the papillary dermis the infiltrate may have a band-like distribution with extension into the lower portion of the epidermis, where there is vacuolar alteration of the basal layer and necrotic keratinocytes. In these areas the papillary dermis occasionally contains melanophages.[314,320] Additional epidermal changes consist of spongiosis and intracellular edema often associated with exocytosis of lymphocytes and focal parakeratosis (Fig. 7-24). Less frequently, there are scattered necrotic keratinocytes in the spinous layer as well as subcorneal spongiotic vesicles filled with Langerhans' cells.[321] A very distinctive feature is the presence of inflammatory infiltrate in the reticular dermis around hair follicles and eccrine glands.[314,321] An unusual perforating variant of lichen striatus has been described, which shows transepidermal elimination of clusters of necrotic keratinocytes.[322]

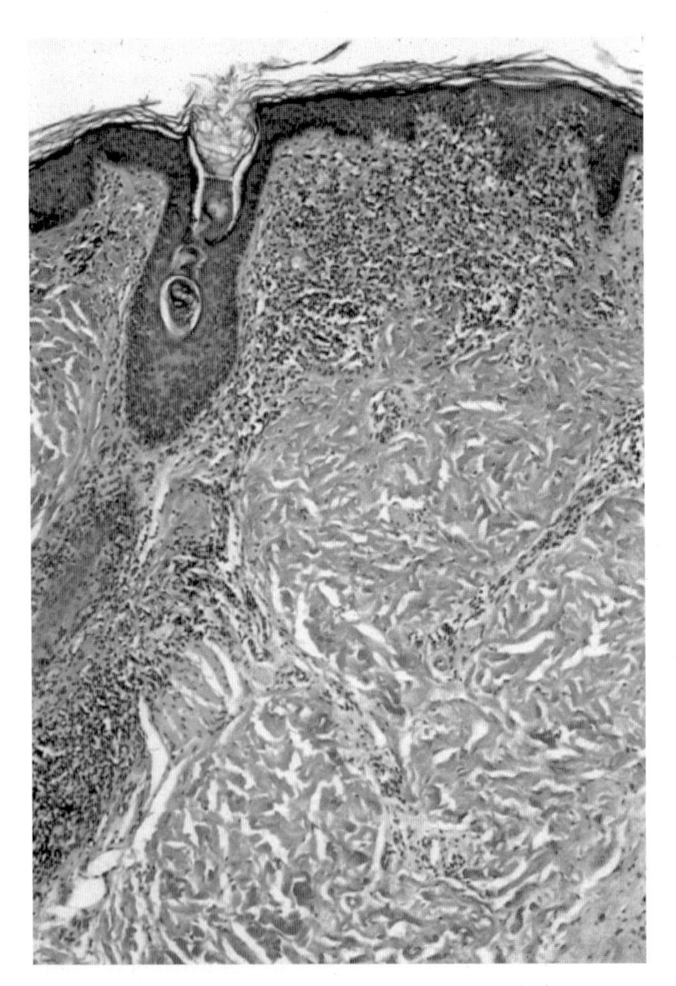

FIG. 7-23. Lichen striatus
Superficial and deep perivascular and perifollicular infiltrate of lymphocytes and histiocytes that extends to the epidermis, which shows acanthosis and spongiosis.

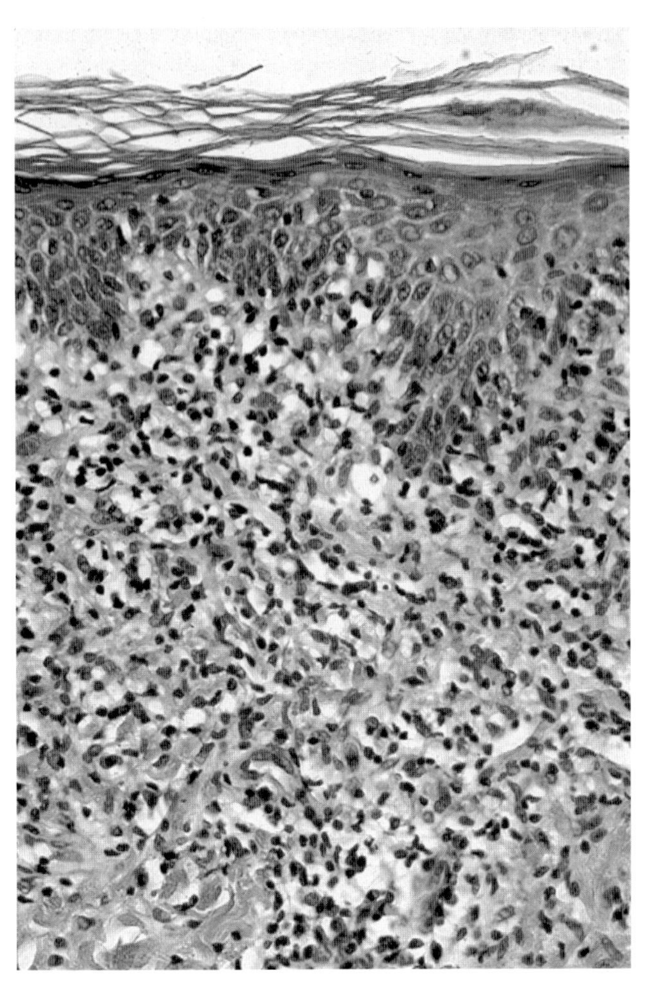

FIG. 7-24. Lichen striatus
Closer view shows an infiltrate of lymphocytes and histiocytes, exocytosis of lymphocytes, acanthosis, spongiosis, and focal parakeratosis.

Pathogenesis. In lichen striatus it has been found that the inflammatory cells reaching the epidermis are a subpopulation of $CD8^+$ (suppressor-cytotoxic) T lymphocytes[321] that express HLA-DR^+ antigen on their surface.[167] These findings suggest a cell-mediated immunologic mechanism where cytotoxic events against keratinocytes could be taking place during the evolution of the disease.[321]

Differential Diagnosis. Lichen striatus may show histologic features similar to other interface dermatitides such as lichen planus, lichen nitidus, or graft-versus-host disease. In contrast to lichen striatus, the inflammatory infiltrate of lichen nitidus is just focally present in a widened dermal papillae and contains more histiocytes. The presence of epidermal spongiosis and a deeper dermal inflammatory infiltrate around adnexal structures are features rarely seen in lichen planus.

INFLAMMATORY LINEAR VERRUCOUS EPIDERMAL NEVUS

Inflammatory linear verrucous epidermal nevus (ILVEN) presents as a persistent, linear, intensely pruritic lesion. It is composed of erythematous, slightly verrucous, scaling papules arranged in one or several lines. Although the usual time of onset is early childhood, the disease may arise in adults.[323] The most common location is one of the lower extremities. On rare occasions the lesions are bilateral.[324]

ILVEN is considered to be a variant of epidermal nevi; however, it is described in the papulo-squamous disorders due to its clinical and histologic similarity to psoriasis.

Histopathology. One observes hyperkeratosis with foci of parakeratosis, moderate acanthosis, elongation and thickening of the rete ridges with a "psoriasiform" appearance, papillomatosis, and, occasionally, slight spongiosis with exocytosis of lymphocytes.[325]

Frequently, a rather characteristic histologic feature is seen, consisting of a sharply demarcated alternation of orthokeratosis and parakeratosis in the cornified layer (Fig. 7-25). The parakeratotic areas are slightly raised, lack a granular layer, and show a compact eosinophilic cornified layer with nuclear remnants. The orthokeratotic areas instead are slightly depressed and show hypergranulosis and a basketweave appearance of the corneocytes.[324,326,327] In the parakeratotic areas, there is mild exocytosis of lymphocytes and the intercellular spaces are slightly widened.[328] The papillary dermis shows a mild to moderate perivascular inflammatory infiltrate of lymphocytes and histiocytes.

Pathogenesis. Electron microscopy and immunohistochemistry studies have shown that keratinocyte differentiation is altered in the parakeratotic areas.

Ultrastructurally, keratinocytes have prominent Golgi apparatuses and vesicles in their cytoplasm. The intercellular spaces in upper layers of the epidermis are widened by deposits of an electron-dense homogeneous substance. The cytoplasm of parakeratotic corneocytes contains remnants of nucleus and membrane structures and a few lipid droplets. The marginal band formation inside the plasma membrane is incomplete, suggesting a deficient keratinization process.[328]

Involucrin expression has a very characteristic pattern in ILVEN. The orthokeratotic epidermis shows increased involucrin expression, whereas, the parakeratotic areas are almost negative for involucrin staining.[328] This pattern differs from that of psoriasis, in which involucrin is expressed prematurely in most of the suprabasal keratinocytes.[329]

In the dermal infiltrate more than 90% of the mononuclear cells are T lymphocytes $CD4^+$ (helper-inducer) subtype; in contrast, the majority of the epidermal infiltrating T lymphocytes are CD4 negative.[330]

Differential Diagnosis. The clinical appearance of lichen striatus and ILVEN may be indistinguishable. However, ILVEN, in contrast to lichen striatus, is pruritic and persistent. Histologically, lichen striatus tends toward a lichenoid pattern, and ILVEN toward a psoriasiform pattern. Furthermore, careful search of step sections will usually reveal in ILVEN alternate areas of hyperkeratosis with a thickened granular layer and of parakeratosis without a granular layer. The view that they are one and the same diseases[331] does not appear warranted.

While alternating orthokeratosis and parakeratosis can be seen in psoriasis and occasionally Munro microabscesses can be found in ILVEN, the differential diagnosis of these two entities

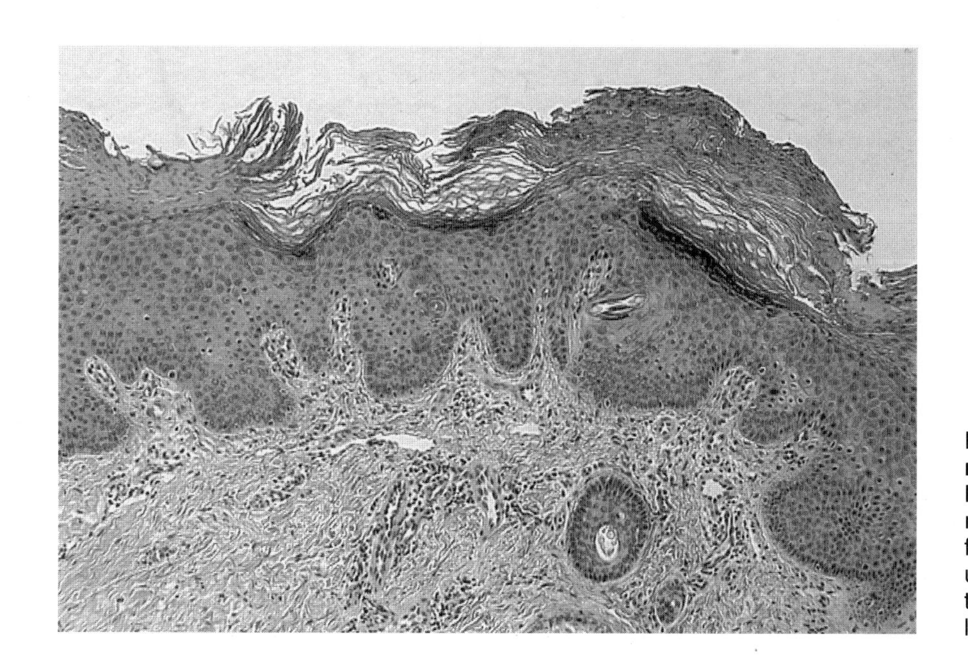

FIG. 7-25. Inflammatory linear verrucous epidermal nevus (ILVEN) Moderate acanthosis with elongated rete ridges and alternating elevated foci of parakeratosis with absent granular layer and depressed foci of orthokeratosis with preserved granular layer.

could be sometimes difficult to assess and clinico-pathological correlation is necessary.[332]

PITYRIASIS RUBRA PILARIS

Pityriasis rubra pilaris is an erythematous squamous disorder characterized by follicular plugging and perifollicular erythema that coalesces to form orange-red scaly plaques that frequently contain islands of normal-appearing skin.[333] As the erythema extends, the follicular component is often lost, but it persists longest on the dorsa of the proximal phalanges. The lesions spread caudally and may progress to a generalized erythroderma.[334] Other clinical findings are palmoplantar keratoderma and scaling of the face and scalp. Five types can be recognized.[334] However, only three types are common enough to deserve mention. *Type I classical adult type* and *type III classical juvenile type* are seen in 55% and 10% of the patients, respectively. They are considered to be the same disease in different age groups.[335] In both groups, the majority of the patients clear on average within three years.[335,336] *Type IV*, the *circumscribed juvenile type*, accounts for approximately one quarter of the patients. It affects children and is characterized by sharply demarcated areas of follicular hyperkeratosis and erythema on the knees and elbows. It may improve in the late teens.[335] There is a familial form of pityriasis rubra pilaris inherited as an autosomal dominant trait.[337]

Histopathology. The histologic picture of a fully developed erythematous lesion shows acanthosis with broad and short rete ridges, slight spongiosis, thick suprapapillary plates, focal or confluent hypergranulosis, and alternating orthokeratosis and parakeratosis oriented in both vertical and horizontal directions[138] (Fig. 7-26). In the dermis there is a mild superficial perivascular lymphocytic infiltrate and moderately dilated blood vessels.[138,338]

Areas corresponding to follicular papules show dilated infundibula filled out with an orthokeratotic plug and often display perifollicular shoulders of parakeratosis and a mild perifollicular lymphocytic infiltrate[339] (Fig. 7-27). Erythrodermic lesions have a thinned or absent cornified layer, plasma exudates, and a diminished granular zone.[138]

Differential Diagnosis. Even though pityriasis rubra pilaris and psoriasis bear a similar clinical appearance, they are not alike histologically. Psoriasis differs from pityriasis rubra pilaris by the presence of neutrophils and Munro microabscesses, more pronounced parakeratosis in mounds, thin suprapapillary plates, elongated rete ridges, and tortuous blood vessels.[338] Pityriasis rubra pilaris has a more prominent granular layer with less epidermal spongiosis and inflammatory infiltrate.[138] Moreover, it has been demonstrated that pityriasis rubra pilaris has a lower keratinocyte proliferation rate compared to psoriasis, suggesting differences in cell kinetic characteristics.[338,340,341]

Pathogenesis. The cause of pityriasis rubra pilaris is unknown. There is recent evidence that suggests an abnormal epidermal differentiation based on the presence of suprabasal staining with monoclonal antibody against AE1 and the detection of cytokeratins K6 and K16, which are not expressed in normal skin.[337]

PITYRIASIS LICHENOIDES

Pityriasis lichenoides is an uncommon cutaneous eruption usually classified in two forms that differ in severity. Simultaneous appearance of the two types[342] and transitions between them often occur, suggesting that they are variants of the same disease.[343,344] Both are rarely pruritic or painful, with crops of self-healing lesions affecting young adults[343] and occasionally children.[342,345]

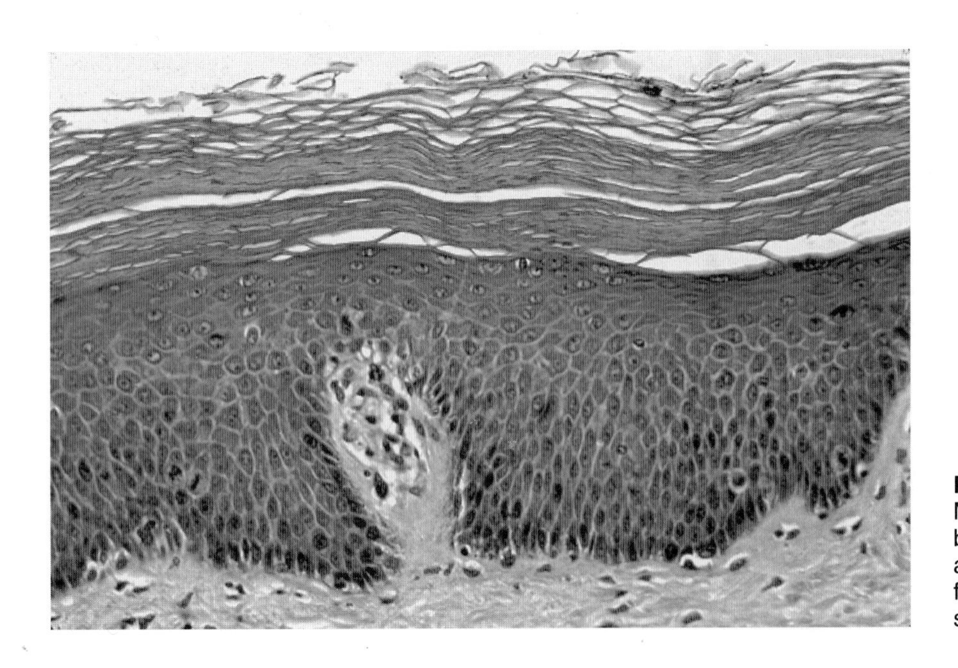

FIG. 7-26. Pityriasis rubra pilaris Moderate acanthosis with short and broad rete ridges, thin granular layer, and alternating vertical and horizontal foci of orthokeratosis and parakeratosis.

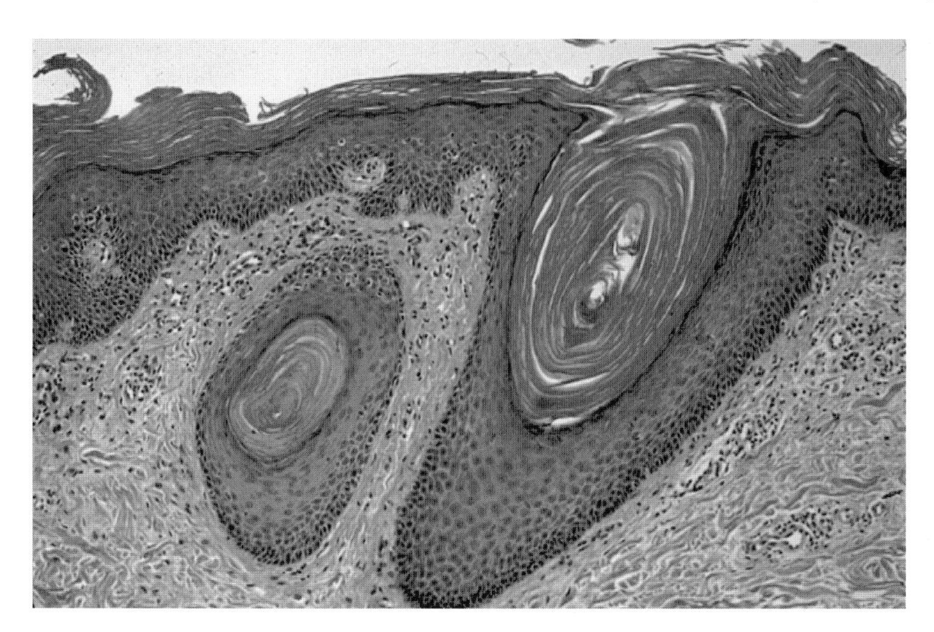

FIG. 7-27. Pityriasis rubra pilaris, follicular papule
Dilated follicular infundibulum with hyperkeratotic plug.

The milder form, called *pityriasis lichenoides chronica,* is characterized by recurrent crops of brown-red papules 4 to 10 mm in size, mainly on the trunk and extremities, that are covered with a scale and generally involute within three to six weeks with postinflammatory pigmentary changes.[152]

The more severe form, called *pityriasis lichenoides et varioliformis acuta* (PLEVA) and referred to also as Mucha-Habermann disease, consists of a fairly extensive eruption, present mainly on the trunk and proximal extremities. It is characterized by erythematous papules that develop into papulonecrotic, occasionally hemorrhagic or vesiculo-pustular lesions that resolve within a few weeks, usually with little or no scarring. In occasional patients, some lesions increase in size to necrotic ulcers of 1 to 2 cm in diameter healing with an atrophic or varioliform scar. Although the individual lesions follow an acute course, the disorder is chronic, extending over several months or even years because of the development of crops of new lesions. Very rarely, patients with PLEVA have a sudden, severe flareup of their disease, characterized by innumerable coalescent necrotic ulcerations associated with high fever and systemic manifestations.[346–348]

Histopathology. In pityriasis lichenoides chronica, the mild form, one observes a superficial perivascular infiltrate composed of lymphocytes that extends into the epidermis, where there is vacuolar alteration of the basal layer, mild spongiosis, a few necrotic keratinocytes, and confluent parakeratosis. Melanophages and small numbers of extravasated erythrocytes are commonly seen in the papillary dermis.[152,343]

In PLEVA, the more severe form, the perivascular (predominantly lymphocytic) infiltrate is dense in the papillary dermis and extends into the reticular dermis in a wedge-shaped pattern (Fig. 7-28). The infiltrate obscures the dermal-epidermal junction with pronounced vacuolar alteration of the basal layer, marked exocytosis of lymphocytes and erythrocytes, and intercellular and intracellular edema leading to variable degree of epidermal necrosis (Fig. 7-29). Ultimately, erosion or even ulceration may occur. The overlying cornified layer shows parakeratosis and a scaly crust with neutrophils in the more severe cases.[343,349]

Variable degrees of papillary dermal edema, endothelial swelling, and extravasated erythrocytes are seen in the majority of cases. Although occasionally small deposits of fibrin are present within vessel walls, severe vascular damage is rarely found[343] except in the severe febrile ulceronecrotic variant of PLEVA where lymphocytic vasculitis with leukocytoclasia is a fairly common feature.[346,348]

Differential Diagnosis. Occasionally, the histologic picture of PLEVA can be mimicked by other diseases such as pityriasis rosea, vesicular insect bites, and subacute eczematous dermatitis. The presence of a deeper inflammatory infiltrate, the extensive epidermal necrosis, and the absence of intraepidermal spongiotic microvesicles may help to distinguish PLEVA from pityriasis rosea and subacute eczematous dermatitis. Numerous eosinophils in a vertically oriented dermal infiltrate is more commonly seen in insect bites.[350] The differential diagnosis with lymphomatoid papulosis is discussed in Chapter 32, Lymphoma and Leukemia in the Skin.

Pathogenesis. Most of the cells in the inflammatory infiltrate are activated T lymphocytes (HLA-DR^+/$CD3^+$)[344,349,351] that uniformly express CD7 and rarely lack other T-cell antigens (CD2, CD5).[344,352] Two constant findings in PLEVA are the predominance of $CD8^+$ (cytotoxic-suppressor) over $CD4^+$ (helper-inducer) T cells at the dermal-epidermal junction, and the expression of HLA-DR on the surrounding keratinocytes,[344,349,351,352] suggesting a direct cytotoxic immune reaction in the pathogenesis of the epidermal necrosis. Sporadic reports of clonal T-cell receptor β gene rearrangement[353] and rare associations with cutaneous lymphomas[354,355] have led to the assumption that PLEVA could be regarded as a lymphoproliferative disorder.

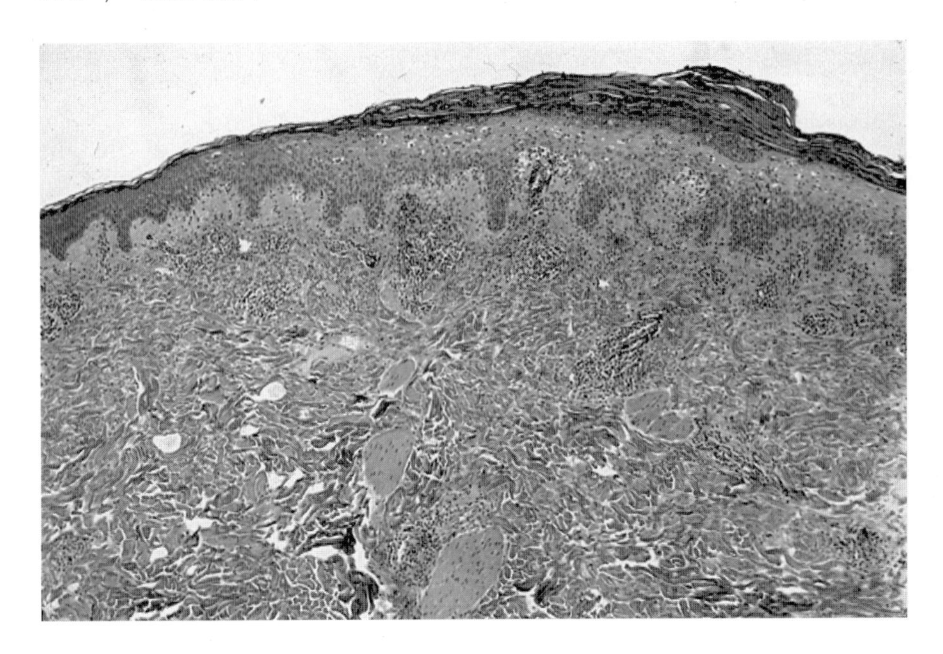

FIG. 7-28. Pityriasis lichenoides et varioliformis acuta
Lichenoid inflammatory pattern with a superficial and deep perivascular lymphocytic inflammatory infiltrate.

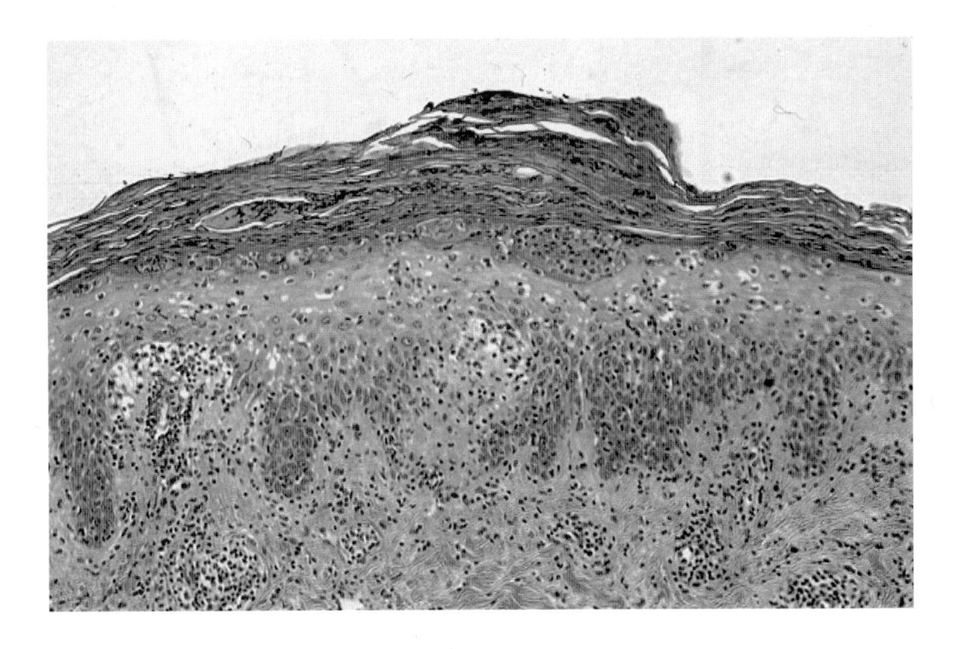

FIG. 7-29. Pityriasis lichenoides et varioliformis acuta
Closer view reveals lichenoid inflammatory pattern with an infiltrate of lymphocytes, extravasated erythrocytes, irregular acanthosis, pallor of the upper layers of the epidermis, spongiosis, necrotic keratinocytes, and confluent mounds of parakeratosis with plasma, neutrophils, and lymphocytes.

ACKNOWLEDGMENT

We thank Dr. Patricia Ceballos for her help in library research, discussion of some entities, and helpful comments in editing the manuscript.

REFERENCES

1. Aoki T, Kojima M, Horiko T. Acute urticaria: History and natural course of 50 patients. J Dermatol 1994;21:73.
2. Cooper KD. Urticaria and angioedema: Diagnosis and evaluation. J Am Acad Dermatol 1991;25:166.
3. Tappeiner G, Hintner H, Glatzl J et al. Hereditary angioedema: Treatment with danazol. Br J Dermatol 1979;100:207.
4. Soter NA. Chronic urticaria as a manifestation of necrotizing venulitis. N Engl J Med 1977;296:1440.
5. Sanchez NP, Winkelmann RK, Schroeter AL. The clinical and histopathologic spectrums of urticarial vasculitis. J Am Acad Dermatol 1982;7:599.
6. Gammon WR. Urticarial vasculitis. Dermatol Clin 1985;3:97.
7. Mehregan DR, Hall MJ, Gibson LE. Urticarial vasculitis: A histopathologic and clinical review of 72 cases. J Am Acad Dermatol 1992;26:441.
8. Wisnieski JJ, Naff GB. Serum IgG antibodies to Clq in hypocomplementemic urticarial vasculitis syndrome. Arthritis Rheum 1989;32:1119.
9. Wisnieski JJ, Jones SM. IgG autoantibody to the collagen-like region of C1q in hypocomplementemic urticarial vasculitis syndrome, systemic lupus erythematosus, and 6 other musculoskeletal or rheumatic diseases. J Rheumatol 1992;19:884.
10. Bisaccia E, Adamo V, Rozan SW. Urticarial vasculitis progressing to systemic lupus erythematosus. Arch Dermatol 1988;124:1088.

11. Huston DP, Bressler RB. Urticaria and angioedema. Med Clin North Am 1992;76:805.
12. Soter NA, Wasserman SI. Urticaria, angioedema (review). Int J Dermatol 1979;18:517.
13. Soter NA, Austen KF, Gigli I. Urticaria and arthralgias as manifestations of necrotizing angiitis (vasculitis). J Invest Dermatol 1974;63:485.
14. Monroe EW, Schulz CI, Maize JC et al. Vasculitis in chronic urticaria. J Invest Dermatol 1981;76:103.
15. Russell Jones R, Bhogal B, Dash A et al. Urticaria and vasculitis: A continuum of histological and immunopathological changes. Br J Dermatol 1983;108:695.
16. Michichiro H, Davis FM, Gratten CEH et al. Autoantibodies against the high-affinity IgE receptor as a cause of histamine release in chronic urticaria. N Engl J Med 1993;328:1599.
17. Lawley TJ, Hertz HC, Wade TR et al. Pruritic urticarial papules and plaques of pregnancy. JAMA 1979;241:1696.
18. Callen JP, Hanno R. Pruritic urticarial papules and plaques of pregnancy (PUPPP). J Am Acad Dermatol 1981;5:401.
19. Yancey KB, Russel RP, Lawley TJ. Pruritic urticarial papules and plaques of pregnancy. J Am Acad Dermatol 1984;10:473.
20. Cohen LM, Capeless EL, Krusinski PA, Maloney ME. Pruritic urticarial papules and plaques of pregnancy and its relationship to maternal-fetal weight gain and twin pregnancy. Arch Dermatol 1989;125:1534.
21. Weiss R, Hull P. Familial occurrence of pruritic urticarial papules and plaques of pregnancy. J Am Acad Dermatol 1992;26:715.
22. Darier J. De l'erytheme annulaire centrifuge. Ann Dermatol Syphilol 1916;6:57.
23. Ackerman AB. Histologic diagnosis of inflammatory skin diseases. Philadelphia: Lea and Febiger, 1978;174:231.
24. Bressler GS, Jones RE Jr. Erythema annulare centrifugum. J Am Acad Dermatol 1981;4:597.
25. Tyring SK. Reactive erythemas: Erythema annulare centrifugum and erythema gyratum repens. Clin Dermatol 1993;11:135.
26. Gammel JA. Erythema gyratum repens. Arch Dermatol 1952;66:494.
27. Boyd AS, Neldner KH, Menter A. Erythema gyratum repens: A paraneoplastic eruption. J Am Acad Dermatol 1992;26:757.
28. Leavell US, Winternitz WW, Black JH. Erythema gyratum repens and undifferentiated carcinoma. Arch Dermatol 1977;95:343.
29. Holt PJA, Davies MG. Erythema gyratum repens: An immunologically mediated dermatosis. Br J Dermatol 1977;96:343.
30. Albers SE, Fenske NA, Glass LF. Erythema gyratum repens: direct immunofluorescence microscopic findings. J Am Acad Dermatol 1993;29:493.
31. Caux F, Lebbe C, Thomine E et al. Erythema gyratum repens. A case studied with immunofluorescence, immunoelectron microscopy and immunohistochemistry. Br J Dermatol 1994;131:102.
32. Dominguez-Soto L, Hojyo-Tomoka T, Vega-Memije E et al. Pigmentary problems in the tropics. Dermatol Clin 1994;12:777.
33. Knox JM, Dodge BG, Freeman RG. Erythema dyschromicum perstans. Arch Dermatol 1968;97:262.
34. Vega ME, Waxtein L, Arenas R et al. Ashy dermatosis and lichen planus pigmentosus: A clinicopathologic study of 31 cases. Int J Dermatol 1992;31:90.
35. Tschen JA, Tschen EA, McGavran MH. Erythema dyschromicum perstans. J Am Acad Dermatol 1980;2:295.
36. Soter NA, Wand C, Freeman RG. Ultrastructural pathology of erythema dyschromicum perstans. J Invest Dermatol 1969;52:155.
37. Miyagawa S, Komatsu M, Okuchi T et al. Erythema dyschromicum perstans: Immunopathologic studies. J Am Acad Dermatol 1989;20:882.
38. Bhutani LK, Bedi TR, Pandhi RK et al. Lichen planus pigmentosus. Dermatologica 1974;149:43.
39. Naidorf KF, Cohen SR. Erythema dyschromicum perstans and lichen planus. Arch Dermatol 1982;118:683.
40. Sanchez NP, Pathak MA, Sato SS et al. Circumscribed dermal melaninoses: Classification, light, histochemical, and electron microscopic studies on three patients with the erythema dyschromicum perstans type. Int J Dermatol 1982;21:25.
41. Sheretz EF, Jorizzo JL, White WL et al. Papular dermatitis in adults: Subacute prurigo, American style? J Am Acad Dermatol 1991;24:697.
42. Braun-Falco O, von Eickstedt UM. Beitrag zur urticaria papulosa chronica. Hautarzt 1957;8:534.
43. Kocsard E. The problem of prurigo. Australas J Dermatol 1962;6:156.
44. Rosen T, Algra RJ. Papular eruption in black men. Arch Dermatol 1980;116:416.
45. Uehara M, Ofuji S: Primary eruption of prurigo simplex subacuta. Dermatologica 1976;153:49.
46. Doyle JA, Connolly SM, Hunziker N et al. Prurigo nodulans: A reappraisal of the clinical and histologic features. J Cutan Pathol 1979;16:392.
47. Rowland Payne CME, Wilkinson JD, McKee PH et al. Nodular prurigo: A clinicopathological study of 46 patients. Br J Dermatol 1985;113:431.
48. Tanaka M, Aiba S, Matsumura N et al. Prurigo nodularis consists of two distinct forms: Early-onset atopic and late-onset non-atopic. Dermatology 1995;190;269.
49. Rien BE, Lemont H, Cohen RS. Prurigo nodularis in association with uremia. J Am Podiatry Assoc 1982;72:321.
50. Fina L, Grimalt R, Berti E, Caputo R. Nodular prurigo associated with Hodgkin's disease. Dermatologica 1991;182:243.
51. Miyauchi H, Uehara M. Follicular occurrence of prurigo nodularis. J Cutan Pathol 1988;15:208.
52. Runne U, Orfanos CE. Cutaneous neural proliferation in highly pruritic lesions of chronic prurigo. Arch Dermatol 1977;113:787.
53. Lindley RP, Rowland P. Neural hyperplasia is not a diagnostic prerequisite in nodular prurigo. J Cutan Pathol 1989;16:14.
54. Harris B, Harris K, Penneys NS. Demonstration by S-100 protein staining of increased numbers of nerves in the papillary dermis of patients with prurigo nodularis. J Am Acad Dermatol 1992;26:56.
55. Aso M, Hashimoto K, Hamzavi A. Immunohistochemical studies of selected skin diseases and tumors using monoclonal antibodies to neurofilament and myelin proteins. J Am Acad Dermatol 1985;13:37.
56. Molina FA, Burrows NP, Jones RR et al. Increased sensory neuropeptides in nodular prurigo: A quantitative immunohistochemical analysis. Br J Dermatol 1992;127:344.
57. Nahass GT, Penneys NS. Merkel cells and prurigo nodularis. J Am Acad Dermatol 1994;31:86.
58. Ereaux LP, Schopflocher P. Familial primary self-healing squamous epithelioma of skin. Arch Dermatol 1965;91:589.
59. Telfer NR, Chalmers RJG, Whale K, Colman G. The role of streptococcal infection in the initiation of guttate psoriasis. Arch Dermatol 1992:128:39.
60. Faber EM, Nall ML. Natural history of psoriasis in 5,600 patients. Dermatologica 1974;148:1.
61. Morris LF, Phillips CM, Binnie WH et al. Oral lesions in patients with psoriasis: A controlled study. Cutis 1992;49:339.
62. Pogrel MA, Cram D. Intraoral findings in patients with psoriasis with a special reference to ectopic geographic tonge (erythema circinata). Oral Surg Oral Med Oral Pathol 1988;66:184.
63. Baker H. Pustular psoriasis. Dermatol Clin 1984;2:455.
64. Zelickson BD, Muller SA. Generalized pustular psoriasis. Arch Dermatol 1991;127:1339.
65. Wagner G, Luckasen JR, Goltz RW. Mucous membrane involvement in generalized psoriasis. Arch Dermatol 1976;112:1010.
66. Shelley WB, Kirschbaum JO: Generalized pustular psoriasis. Arch Dermatol 1961;84:73.
67. Braverman IM, Cohen I, O'Keefe EO. Metabolic and ultrastructural studies in a patient with pustular psoriasis (Von Zumbusch). Arch Dermatol 1972;105:189.
68. Schuppener JH. Ausdrucksformen pustulöser psoriasis. Dermatol Wochenschr 1958;138:841.
69. Baker H, Ryan TJ. Generalized pustular psoriasis. Br J Dermatol 1968;80:771.
70. Katzenellenbogen I, Feuerman EI. Psoriasis pustulosa and impetigo herpetiformis: Single or dual entity? Acta Derm Venereol (Stockh) 1966;46:86.
71. Pierard GE, Pierard-Franchimont C, de la Brassine M. Impetigo herpetiformis and pustular psoriasis during pregnancy. Am J Dermatopathol 1983;5:215.
72. Lotem M, Katzenelson V, Rotem A et al. Impetigo herpetiformis: A variant of pustular psoriasis or a separate entity? J Am Acad Dermatol 1989;20:338.
73. Resneck JS, Cram DL. Erythema annulare-like pustular psoriasis. Arch Dermatol 1973;108:687.
74. Adler DJ, Rower JM, Hashimoto K. Annular pustular psoriasis. Arch Dermatol 1981;117:313.

75. Zala L, Hunziker T. Lokalisierte form der psoriasis von typ des erythema annulare centrifugum mit pustulation. Hautarzt 1984;35:53.
76. Zelickson BD, Muller SA. Generalized pustular psoriasis in childhood: Report of thirteen cases. J Am Acad Dermatol 1991;24:186.
77. Ashhurst PJC. Relapsing pustular eruptions of the hands and feet. Br J Dermatol 1964;776:169.
78. Andrews GC, Machacek GF. Pustular bacterids of the hands and feet. Arch Dermatol Syphilol 1935;32:837.
79. Duvic M, Johnson TM, Rapini RP et al. Acquired immunodeficiency syndrome-associated psoriasis and Reiter's syndrome. Arch Dermatol 1987;123:1622.
80. Obuch ML, Maurer TA, Becker B, Berger TG. Psoriasis and human immunodeficiency virus infection. J Am Acad Dermatol 1992;27:667.
81. Lazar AP, Roenigk HH. AIDS and psoriasis. Cutis 1987;39:347.
82. Johnson TM, Duvic M, Rapini RP et al. AIDS exacerbates psoriasis. N Engl J Med 1985;313:22,1415.
83. Braun-Falco O, Christophers E. Structural aspects of initial psoriatic lesions. Arch Dermatol Forsch 1974;251:95.
84. Ragaz A, Ackerman AB. Evolution, maturation, and regression of lesions of psoriasis. Am J Dermatopathol 1979;1:199.
85. Van Scott EJ, Ekel TW. Kinetics of hyperplasia in psoriasis. Arch Dermatol 1963;88:373.
86. Gordon M, Johnson WC. Histopathology and histochemistry of psoriasis. Arch Dermatol 1967;95:402.
87. Rupec M. Zur ultrastruktur der spongiformen pustel. Arch Klin Exp Dermatol 1970;239:30.
88. Burks JW, Montgomery H. Histopathologic study of psoriasis. Arch Dermatol Syphilol 1943;48:479.
89. Pinkus H, Mehregan AH. The primary histologic lesion of seborrheic dermatitis and psoriasis. J Invest Dermatol 1966;46:109.
90. Cox AH, Watson W. Histologic variations in lesions of psoriasis. Arch Dermatol 1972;106:503.
91. Abrahams J, McCarthy JT, Sanders ST. 101 cases of exfoliative dermatitis. Arch Dermatol 1963;87:96.
92. Muller SA, Kitzmiller KW. Generalized pustular psoriasis. Acta Derm Venereol (Stockh) 1962;42:504.
93. Kingery FAJ, Chinn HD, Saunders TS. Generalized pustular psoriasis. Arch Dermatol 1961;84:912.
94. Piraccini BM, Fanti PA, Morelli R, Tosti A. Hallopeau's acrodermatitis continua of the nail apparatus: A clinical and pathological study of 20 patients. Acta Derm Venereol (Stockh) 1994;74:65.
95. Pierard J, Kint A. La pustulose palmo-plantaire chronique et recidivante. Ann Dermatol Venereol 1978;105:681.
96. Pierard J, Kint A. Les "bacterides pustuleuses" d'Andrews. Arch Belg Dermatol Syphiligr 1966;22:83.
97. Lever WF. In discussion with Pay D: Pustular psoriasis. Arch Dermatol 1969;99:641.
98. Uehara M, Ofuji S. The morphogenesis of pustulosis palmaris et plantaris. Arch Dermatol 1974;109:518.
99. Thorman J, Heilesen B. Recalcitrant pustular eruptions of the extremities. J Cutan Pathol 1975;2:19.
100. Tan RS. Acute generalized pustular bacterid. Br J Dermatol 1974;91: 209.
101. Smoller BR, McNutt S, Gray MH et al. Detection of the interferon-gamma-induced protein 10 in psoriasiform dermatitis of acquired immunodeficiency syndrome. Arch Dermatol 1990;126:1457.
102. Schubert C, Christophers E. Mast cells and macrophages in early relapsing psoriasis. Arch Dermatol Res 1985;277:352.
103. Brody I. The ultrastructure of the epidermis in psoriasis vulgaris as revealed by electron microscopy. J Ultrastruct Res 1962;6:304.
104. Hashimoto K, Lever WF. Elektronenmikroskopische untersuchungen der hautveränderungen bei psoriasis. Dermatol Wochenschr 1966; 152:713.
105. Orfanos CE, Schaumburg-Lever G, Mahrle G et al. Alterations of cell surfaces as a pathogenetic factor in psoriasis. Arch Dermatol 1973; 107:38.
106. Heng MCYL, Kloss SG, Kuehn CD, Chase DG. The significance and pathogenesis of basal keratinocyte herniations in psoriasis. J Invest Dermatol 1986;87:362.
107. Mercer EH, Maibach HI. Intercellular adhesion and surface coats of epidermal cells in psoriasis. J Invest Dermatol 1968;51:215.
108. Christophers C, Braun-Falco O. Mechanisms of parakeratosis. J Dermatol 1970;82:268.
109. Braverman IM, Yen A. Ultrastructure of the human dermal microcirculation: II. The capillary loops of the dermal papillae. J Invest Dermatol 1977;68:44.
110. Mordovtsev VN, Albanova VI. Morphology of skin microvasculature in psoriasis. Am J Dermatopathol 1989:11:33.
111. Weinstein GD, Van Scott EJ. Autoradiographic analysis of turnover times of normal and psoriatic epidermis. J Invest Dermatol 1965;45: 257.
112. Soltani K, Van Scott EJ. Patterns and sequence of tissue changes in incipient and evolving lesions of psoriasis. Arch Dermatol 1972;106: 484.
113. Weinstein GD, McCullough JL, Ross PA. Cell kinetic basis for pathophysiology of psoriasis. J Invest Dermatol 1985;85:579.
114. Gelfant S. The cell cycle in psoriasis: A reappraisal. Br J Dermatol 1976;95:577.
115. McKay IA, Leigh IM. Altered keratinocyte growth and differentiation in psoriasis. Clin Dermatol 1995;13:105.
116. Leigh IM, Navsaria H, Purkis PE et al. Keratins (K16 and K17) as markers of keratinocyte hyperproliferation in psoriasis in vivo and in vitro. Br J Dermatol 1995;133:501.
117. Nelson W, Sun TT. The 50- and 58-kdalton keratin classes as molecular markers for stratified squamous epithelia: Cell culture studies. J Cell Biol 1983;97:244.
118. Hohl D. The cornified cell envelope. Dermatologica 1990;180:201.
119. Stoler A, Kopan R, Duvic M, Fuchs E. Use of monospecific antisera and cRNA probes to localize the major changes in keratin expression during normal and abnormal epidermal differentiation. J Cell Biol 1988;107:427.
120. Cooper KD. Psoriasis: Leukocytes and cytokines. Dermatol Clin 1990;8:737.
121. Nikaein A, Morris L, Phillips C, et al. Characterization of T-cell clones generated from skin of patients with psoriasis. J Am Acad Dermatol 1993;28:551.
122. Christophers E, Mrowietz U. The inflammatory infiltrate in psoriasis. Clin Dermatol 1995;13:131.
123. Leung DYM, Walsh P, Giorno R, Norris DA. A potential role for superantigens in the pathogenesis of psoriais. J Invest Dermatol 1993; 100:225.
124. Baker BS, Fry L. The immunology of psoriasis. Br J Dermatol 1992; 126:1.
125. Griffiths CEM, Voorhees JJ. Immunological mechanisms involved in psoriasis. Springer Semin Immunopathol 1992;13:441.
126. Fierlbeck G, Rassner G, Muller C. Psoriasis induced at the injection site or recombinant interferon gamma. Arch Dermatol 1990;126:351.
127. Gottlieb AB, Luster AD, Posnett DN, Martin Carter D. Detection of gamma interferon-induced protein IP-10 in psoriatic plaques. J Exp Med 1988;168:941.
128. Nickoloff BJ, Griffiths CEM, Barker JNWN. The role of adhesion molecules, chemotactic factors and cytokines in inflammatory and neoplastic skin diseases: 1990 update. J Invest Dermatol 1990;94: 151S.
129. Baker BS, Powles AV, Valdimarsson H, Fry L. An altered response by psoriatic keratinocytes to gamma interferon. Scand J Immunol 1988;28:735.
130. Nickoloff BJ, Mitra RS, Elder JT et al. Decreased growth inhibition by recombinant gamma interferon is associated with increased transforming growth factor-alpha production in keratinocytes cultured from psoratic lesions. Br J Dermatol 1989;121:161.
131. Everall J. Intractable pustular eruption of the hands and feet. Br J Dermatol 1957;69:269.
132. Enfors W, Molin L. Pustulosis palmaris et plantaris. Acta Derm Venereol (Stockh) 1971;51:289.
133. Thomsen K. Pustulosis palmaris et plantaris treated with methotrexate. Acta Derm Venereol (Stockh) 1971;51:397.
134. Tagami H, Ofuji S. A leukotactic factor in the stratum corneum of pustulosis palmaris et plantaris. Acta Derm Venereol (Stockh) 1978;58: 401.
135. Duvic M. Immunology of AIDS related to psoriasis. J Invest Dermatol 1990;95:38S.
136. Ichihashi N, Seishima M, Takahashi T et al. A case of AIDS manifesting pruritic papular eruptions and psoriasiform lesions: An immunohistochemical study of the lesional dermal infiltrates. J Dermatol 1995;22:428.
137. Barr RJ, Young EM. Psoriasiform and related papulosquamous disorders. J Cut Pathol 1985:12:412.

138. Soeprono FF. Histologic criteria for the diagnosis of pityriasis rubra pilaris. Am J Dermatopathol 1986;8:277.
139. Degos R, Garnier G, Civatte J. Pustulose par *Candida albicans* avec lésions psoriasiformes rappelant le psoriasis pustuleux. Bull Soc Fr Dermatol Syphiligr 1962;69:231.
140. Dawson TAJ. Tongue lesions in generalized pustular psoriasis. Br J Dermatol 1974;91:419.
141. Perry HO, Mayne JG. Psoriasis and Reiter's syndrome. Arch Dermatol 1965;92:129.
142. Khan MY, Hall WH. Progression of Reiter's syndrome to psoriatic arthritis. Arch Intern Med 1965;116:911.
143. Altman EM, Centeno LV, Mahal M, Bielory L. AIDS-associated Reiter's syndrome. Ann Allergy 1994;72:307.
144. Weinberger HW, Ropes MW, Kulka JP et al. Reiter's syndrome: Clinical and pathologic observations (review). Medicine (Baltimore) 1962;41:35.
145. Martin DH, Pollock S, Kuo CC et al. *Chlamydia trachomatis* infections in men with Reiter's syndrome. Ann Intern Med 1984;100:207.
146. Rahman MU, Cheema MA, Schumacher HR, Hudson AP. Molecular evidence for the presence of chlamydia in the synovium of patients with Reiter's syndrome. Arthritis Rheum 1992;35:521.
147. Burg B, Dummer R, Nestle FO et al. Cutaneous lymphomas consist of a spectrum of nosologically different entities including mycosis fungoides and small plaque parapsoriasis. Arch Dermatol 1996;132: 567.
148. Radcliffe-Crocker H. Xanthoerythrodermia perstans. Br J Dermatol 1905;17:119.
149. Hu CH, Winkelmann RK. Digitate dermatosis: A new look at symmetrical small plaque parapsoriasis. Arch Dermatol 1973;107:65.
150. Yeager JK, Posnak EJ, Cobb MW. Digitate dermatosis. Cutis 1991; 48:457.
151. Samman PD. The natural history of parapsoriasis en plaques (chronic superficial dermatitis) and prereticulotic poikiloderma. Br J Dermatol 1972;87:405.
152. Benmaman O, Sanchez JL. Comparative clinicopathological study on pityriasis lichenoides chronica and small plaque parapsoriasis. Am J Dermatopathol 1988;10:189.
153. Binazzi M. Some research on papapsoriasis and lymphoma. Arch Dermatol Res 1977;258:17.
154. Haeffner AC, Smoller BR, Zepter K, Wood GS. Differentiation and clonality of lesional lymphocytes in small plaque parapsoriasis. Arch Dermatol 1995;131:321.
155. Bonvalet D, Colau-Gohm K, Belaich S et al. Les differentes formes du parapsoriasis en plaques. Ann Dermatol Venereol 1977;104:18.
156. Heid E, Desvaux J, Brändle J et al. Der verlauf der parapsoriasis en plaques (Brocq'sche Krankheit). Z Hautkr 1977;52:658.
157. Burg B, Dummer R. Small plaque (digitate) parapsoriasis is an "abortive cutaneous T-cell lymphoma" and is not mycosis fungoides. Arch Dermatol 1995;131:336.
158. Parsons JM. Pityriasis rosea update:1986. J Am Acad Dermatol 1986; 15:159.
159. Bunch LW, Tilley JC. Pityriasis rosea. Arch Dermatol 1961;84:79.
160. Aiba S, Tagami H. Immunohistologic studies in pityriasis rosea. Arch Dermatol 1985;121:761.
161. Panizzon R, Bloch PH. Histopathology of pityriasis rosea Gibert: Qualitative and quantitative light- microscopic study of 62 biopsies of 40 patients. Dermatologica 1982;165:551.
162. Okamoto H, Imamura S, Aoshima T et al. Dyskeratotic degeneration of epidermal cells in pityriasis rosea: Light and electron microscopic studies. Br J Dermatol 1982;107:189.
163. Bonafe JL, Icart J, Perpere M et al. Etude histopathologique, ultrastructurale, immunologique et virologique du pityriasis rose de Gibert. Ann Dermatol Venereol 1982;109:855.
164. Yoshiike T, Aikawa Y, Wongwaisayawan H, Ogawa H. HLA-DR antigen expression on peripheral T cell subsets in pityriasis rosea and herpes zoster. Dermatologica 1991;82:160.
165. Baker BS, Lamber S, Powles AV et al. Epidermal DR+T6-dendritic cells in inflammatory skin diseases. Acta Derm Venereol (Stockh) 1988;68:209.
166. Bos JD, Huisman PM , Kreg SR, Fabaer WR. Pityriasis rosea (Gibert): Abnormal distribution pattern of antigen presenting cells in situ. Acta Derm Venereol (Stockh) 1985;65:132.
167. Aiba S, Tabami H. HLA-DR antigen expression on the keratinocyte surface in dermatosis characterized by lymphocytic exocytosis (e.g., pityriasis rosea). Br J Dermatol 1984;3:285.
168. Gianotti F. Rilievi di una particolare casistica tossinfettiva caratterizzata de eruzione eritemato-infiltrativa desquamativa a focolai lenticolari, a sede elettiva acroesposata. G Ital Dermatol 1955;96:678.
169. Gianotti F. Papular acrodermatitis of childhood and other papulovesicular acro-located syndromes. Br J Dermatol 1979;100:49.
170. Spear KL, Winkelmann RK. Gianotti-Crosti syndrome: A review of ten cases not associated with hepatitis B. Arch Dermatol 1984;120: 891.
171. Taieb A, Plantin P, Du Pasquier P et al. Gianotti-Crosti syndrome: A study of 26 cases. Br J Dermatol 1986;115:49.
172. Baldari U, Monti A, Righini MG. An epidemic of infantile papular acrodermatitis (Gianotti-Crosti syndrome) due to Epstein-Barr virus. Dermatology 1994;188:203.
173. Draelos ZK, Hansen RC, James WD. Gianotti-Crosti syndrome associated with infections other than hepatitis B. JAMA 1986;256:2386.
174. Caputo R, Gelmetti C, Ermacora E et al. Gianotti-Crosti syndrome: A retrospective analysis of 308 cases. J Am Acad Dermatol 1992;26: 207.
175. Blauvelt A, Turner ML. Gianotti-Crosti syndrome and human immunodeficiency virus infection. Arch Dermatol 1994;130:481.
176. Margyarlaki M, Drobnitsch I, Schneider I. Papular acrodermatitis of childhood: Gianotti-Crosti disease. Pediatr Dermatol 1991;8:224.
177. Kawasaki T, Kosaki F, Owaka S et al. A new infantile acute febrile. mucocutaneous lymph node syndrome (MLNS) prevailing in Japan. Pediatrics 1974;54:271.
178. Melish ME, Hicks RV. Kawasaki syndrome: Clinical features, pathophysiology, etiology and therapy. J Rheumatol 1990;17:2.
179. Dajani AS, Bisno AL, Chung KJ, et al. Diagnostic guidelines for Kawasaki disease. American Heart Association Committee on Rheumatic Fever, Endocarditis, and Kawasaki Disease. Am J Dis Child 1990;144:1218.
180. Burns JC, Mason WH, Glode MP et al. Clinical and epidemiologic characteristics of patients referred for evaluation of possible Kawasaki disease. J Pediatr 1991;118:680.
181. Wortmann DW. Kawasaki syndrome. Semin Dermatol 1992;11:37.
182. Ducos MH, Taieb A, Sarlangue J et al. Manifestations cutanees de la maladie de Kawasaki: A propos de 30 observations. Ann Dermatol Venereol 1993;120:589.
183. Friter BS, Lucky AW. The perineal eruption of Kawasaki syndrome. Arch Dermatol 1988;124:1805.
184. Suzuki A, Kamiya T, Kuwahara N et al. Coronary arterial lesions of Kawasaki disease: Cardiac catheterization findings of 1100 cases. Pediatr Cardiol 1986;7:3.
185. Kato H, Ichinose E, Kawasaki T. Myocardial infarction in Kawasaki disease: Clinical analyses in 195 cases. J Pediatr 1986;108:923.
186. Tomita S, Chung K, Mas M et al. Peripheral gangrene associated with Kawasaki disease. Clin Infect Dis 1992;14:121.
187. Hirose S, Hamashima Y. Morphological observations on the vasculitis in the mucocutaneous lymph node syndrome: A skin biopsy study of 27 patients. Eur J Pediatr 1978;129:17.
188. Sato N, Sagawa K, Sasaguri Y et al. Immunopathology and cytokine detection in the skin lesions of patients with Kawasaki disease. J Pediatr 1993;122:198.
189. Kimura T, Miyazawa H, Watanabe K, Moriya T. Small pustules in Kawasaki disease: A clinicopathological study of four patients. Am J Dermatopathol 1988;10;218.
190. Shulman ST, De Inocencio J, Hirsch R. Kawasaki disease. Pediatr Clin North Am 1995;42:1205.
191. Leung DY, Meissner HC, Fulton DR et al. Superantigens in Kawasaki syndrome. Clin Immunol Immunopathol 1995;77:119.
192. Boyd AS, Neldner KH. Lichen planus. J Am Acad Dermatol 1991; 2593.
193. Boyd AS, Neldner KH. The isomorphic response to Koebner. Int J Dermatol 1990;29:401.
194. Conklin RJ, Blasberg B. Oral lichen planus. Dermatol Clin 1987; 5:663.
195. Bricker SL. Oral lichen planus: A review. Semin Dermatol 1994;13: 87.
196. Shklar G. Erosive and bullous oral lesions of lichen planus. Arch Dermatol 1968;97:411.
197. Samman PD. The nails in lichen planus. Br J Dermatol 1961;73:288.
198. Sarkany I, Caron GA, Jones HH. Lichen planus pemphigoides. Trans St Johns Hosp Dermatol Soc 1964;50:50.
199. Saurat JH, Guinepain MT, Didierjean L et al. Coexistence d'un lichen plan et d'un pemphigoide bulleuse. Ann Dermatol Venereol 1977; 104:368.

200. Gawkrodger DJ, Stavropoulos PG, McLaren KM, Buxton PK. Bullous lichen planus and lichen planus pemphigoides: Clinico-pathological comparisons. Clin Exp Dermatol 1989;14:150.
201. Hintner H, Tappeiner G, Honigsmann H, Wolf K. Lichen planus and bullous pemphigoid. Acta Derm Venereol Suppl (Stockh) 1979;85:71.
202. Mora RG, Nesbitt LT Jr, Brantley JB. Lichen planus pemphigoides: Clinical and immunofluorescence findings in four cases. J Am Acad Dermatol 1983;8:331.
203. Allen CM, Camisa C, Grimwood R. Lichen planus pemphigoides: Report of a case with oral lesions. Oral Surg Oral Med Oral Pathol 1987; 63:184.
204. Davis AL, Bhogal BS, Whitehead P et al. Lichen planus pemphigoides: Its relationship to bullous pemphigoid. Br J Dermatol 1991;125:263.
205. Silvers DN, Katz BE, Young AW. Pseudopelade of Brocq is lichen planopilaris: Report of four cases that support this nosology. Cutis 1993;51:99.
206. Waldorf DS. Lichen planopilaris. Arch Dermatol 1966;93:684.
207. Kuster W, Kind P, Holzle E, Plewig G. Linear lichen planopilaris of the face. J Am Acad Dermatol 1989;21:1331.
208. Cram DL, Kierland RR, Winkelmann RK. Ulcerative lichen planus of the feet. Arch Dermatol 1966;93:692.
209. Thormann J. Ulcerative lichen planus of the feet. Arch Dermatol 1974;110:753.
210. Weidner F, Ummenhofer B. Lichen ruber ulcerosus (dystrophicans). Z Hautkr 1979;54:1008.
211. Katzenellenbogen I. Lichen planus actinicus: Lichen planus in subtropical countries. Dermatologica 1962;124:10.
212. Dilaimy M. Lichen planus subtropicus. Arch Dermatol 1976;112:125.
213. Salman SM, Kibbi AG, Zaynoun S. Actinic lichen planus: A clinicopathologic study of 16 patients. J Am Acad Dermatol 1989;20:226.
214. Camisa C, Neff JC, Olsen RG. Use of indirect immunofluorescence in the lupus erythematosus/lichen planus overlap syndrome: An additional diagnostic clue. J Am Acad Dermatol 1984;11:1050.
215. Davies MG, Gorkiewicz A, Knight A, Marks R. Is there a relationship between lupus erythematosus and lichen planus? Br J Dermatol 1977; 96:145.
216. Scher RK, Fischbein R, Ackerman AB: Twenty-nail dystrophy: A variant of lichen planus. Arch Dermatol 1978;114:612.
217. Wilkinson JD, Dawber RPR, Bowers RP, Fleming K. Twenty-nail dystrophy of childhood. Br J Dermatol 1979;100:217.
218. Kechijian P. Twenty nail dystrophy of childhood. Cutis 1985;35:38.
219. Kawakami T, Soma Y. Generalized lichen nitidus appearing subsequent to lichen planus. J Dermatol 1995;22:434.
220. Sigurgeirsson B, Lindelof B. Lichen planus and malignancy: An epidemiologic study of 2071 patients and a review of the literature. Arch Dermatol 1991;127:1684.
221. Kronenberg K, Fretzin D, Potter B. Malignant degeneration of lichen planus. Arch Dermatol 1971;104:304.
222. Allen JV, Callen JP. Keratoacanthomas arising in hypertropic lichen planus. Arch Dermatol 1981;117:519.
223. Fowler CB, Rees TD, Smith BR. Squamous cell carcinoma on the dorsum of the tongue arising in a long-standing lesion of erosive lichen planus. J Am Dent Assoc 1987;115:707.
224. Katz RW, Brahim JS, Travis WD. Oral squamous cell carcinoma arising in a patient with long-standing lichen planus: A case report. Oral Surg Oral Med Oral Pathol 1990;70:282.
225. Marder MZ, Deesen KC. Transformation of oral lichen planus to squamous cell carcinoma: A literature review and report of case. J Am Dent Assoc 1982;105:55.
226. Kaplan B, Barnes L. Oral lichen planus and squamous carcinoma: Case report and update of the literature. Arch Otolaryngol 1985;111:543.
227. Fulling HJ. Cancer development in oral lichen planus. Arch Dermatol 1973;108:667.
228. Holmstrup P, Pindborg JJ. Erythroplakic lesions in relation to oral lichen planus. Acta Derm Venereol Suppl (Stockh) 1979;85:77.
229. Murti PR, Daftary DK, Bhonsle RB et al. Malignant potential of oral lichen planus: Observation in 722 patients from India. J Oral Pathol 1986;15:71.
230. Male O, Azambuja R. Diagnostische und therapeutische probleme beim lichen ruber ulcerosus. Z Hautkr 1975;50:403.
231. Crotty CP, Su WP, Winkelmann RK. Ulcerative lichen planus: Follow-up of surgical excision and grafting. Arch Dermatol 1980;116: 1252.
232. Ellis FA. Histopathology of lichen planus based on analysis of one hundred biopsies. J Invest Dermatol 1967;48:143.
233. Ragaz A, Ackerman AB. Evolution, maturation, and regression of lesions of lichen planus. Am J Dermatopathol 1981;3:5.
234. Rivers JK, Jackson R, Orizaga M. Who was Wickham and what are his striae? Int J Dermatol 1986;25:611.
235. Gougerot H, Civatte A. Criteres cliniques et histologiques des lichens planus cutanes et muqueux: Delimitation. Ann Dermatol Syphilol 1953;80:5.
236. Enhamre A, Lagerholm B. Acrosyringeal lichen planus. Acta Derm Venereol (Stockh) 1987;67:346.
237. Grubauer G, Romani N, Kofler H et al. Apoptosic keratin bodies as autoantigen causing the production of IgM-anti-keratin intermediate filament autoantibodies. J Invest Dermatol 1986;87:466.
238. Hanau D, Sengel D. Perforating lichen planus. J Cutan Pathol 1984; 11:176.
239. Mehregan DA, Van Hale HM, Muller SA. Lichen planopilaris: Clinical and pathologic study of forty-five patients. J Am Acad Dermatol 1992;27:935.
240. Dawber PRP. What is pseudopelade? Clin Exp Dermatol 1992;17: 305.
241. Matta M, Kibbi AG, Khattar J et al. Lichen planopilaris: A clinicopathologic study. J Am Acad Dermatol 1990;22:594.
242. Tschen JA, Tschen EA, McGavran MH. Erythema dyschromicum perstans. J Am Acad Dermatol 1980;2:295.
243. Van der Horst JC, Cirkel PKS, Nieboer C. Mixed lichen planus-lupus erythematosus disease: A distinct entity? Clin Exp Dermatol 1983; 8:631.
244. Grabbe S, Kolde G. Coexisting lichen planus and subacute cutaneous lupus erythematosus. Clin Exp Dermatol 1995;20:249.
245. Colver GB, Dawber RPR. Is childhood idiopathic atrophy of the nails due to lichen planus? Br J Dermatol 1987;116:702.
246. Ebner H, Gebhart W, Lassmann H et al. The epidermal cell proliferation in lichen planus. Acta Derm Venereol (Stockh)1977;57:133.
247. Medenica M, Lorincz A. Lichen planus: An ultrastructural study. Acta Derm Venereol (Stockh) 1977;57:55.
248. Clausen J, Kjaergaard J, Bierring F. The ultrastructure of the dermo-epidermal junction in lichen planus. Acta Derm Venereol (Stockh) 1981;61:101.
249. Ebner H, Gebhart W. Epidermal changes in lichen planus. J Cutan Pathol 1976;3:167.
250. Hashimoto K. Apoptosis in lichen planus and several other dermatoses. Acta Derm Venereol (Stockh) 1976;56:187.
251. Gomes MA, Staquet MJ, Thivolet J. Staining of colloid bodies by keratin antisera in lichen planus. Am J Dermatopathol 1981;3:341.
252. Ebner H, Gebhart W. Light and electron microscopic studies on colloid and other cytoid bodies. Clin Exp Dermatol 1977;2:311.
253. Ebner H, Erlach E, Gebhart W. Untersuchungen über die blasenbildung beim lichen ruber planus. Arch Dermatol Forsch 1973;247: 193.
254. Abell E, Presbury DG, Marks R et al. The diagnostic significance of immunoglobulin and fibrin deposition in lichen planus. Br J Dermatol 1975;93:17.
255. Baart de la Faille-Kuyper EH, Baart de la Faille H. An immunofluorescence study of lichen planus. Br J Dermatol 1974;90:365.
256. Varelzidis A, Tosca A, Perissios A et al. Immunohistochemistry in lichen planus. Dermatologica 1979;159:137.
257. Morel P, Perron J, Crickx B et al. Lichen plan avec depots lineaires d'IgG et de C3 a la junction dermo-epidermique. Dermatologica 1981; 163:117.
258. Ioannades D, Bystryn JC. Immunofluorescence abnormalities in lichen planopilaris. Arch Dermatol 1992;128:214.
259. Sobel S, Miller R, Shatin H. Lichen planus pemphigoides. Arch Dermatol 1976;112:1280.
260. Song Y, Naito K, Yaguchi H et al. Lichen planus pemphigoides: Report of a case and binding sites of circulating anti-basement membrane zone antibodies. Nippon Hifuka Gakkai Zasshi 1989;99:1111.
261. Lang PG Jr, Maize JC. Coexisting lichen planus and bullous pemphigoid or lichen planus pemphigoides? J Am Acad Dermatol 1983; 9:133.
262. Sundquist KG, Wanger L. Expression of lymphocyte activation markers in benign cutaneous T cell infiltrates: Discoid lupus erythematosus versus lichen ruber planus. Acta Derm Venereol (Stockh) 1989;69: 292.

263. Buechner SA. T-cell subsets and macrophages in lichen planus. Dermatologica 1984;169:325.
264. Ishii T. Immunohistochemical demonstration of T cell subsets and accessory cells in oral lichen planus. J Oral Pathol 1987;16:356.
265. Shiohara T, Moriya N, Tanaka K et al. Immunopathologic study of lichenoid skin diseases: Correlation between HLA-DR positive keratinocytes or Langerhans' cells and epidermotropic T cells. J Am Acad Dermatol 1988;18:67.
266. Matthews JB, Scully CM, Potts AJ. Oral lichen planus: An immunoperoxidase study using monoclonal antibodies to lymphocyte subsets. Br J Dermatol 1984;3:587.
267. Bennion SD, Middleton MH, David-Bajar KM et al. In three types of interface dermatitis, different patterns of expression of intercelullar adhesion molecule-1 (ICAM-1) indicate different triggers of disease. J Invest Dermatol 1995;105:71S.
268. Griffiths CE, Voorhees JJ, Nickiloff BJ. Characterization of intercellular adhesion molecule-1 and HLA-DR expression in normal and inflamed skin: Modulation by recombinant gamma interferon and tumor necrosis factor. J Am Acad Dermatol 1989;20:617.
269. Dustin ML, Singer KH, Tuck DT, Springer TA. Adhesion of T lymphoblasts to epidermal keratinocytes is regulated by interferon gamma and is mediated by intercellular adhesion molecule-1 (ICAM-1). J Exp Med 1988;167:1323.
270. Surgeman PB, Savage NW, Seymour GJ. Phenotype and suppressor activity of T-lymphocyte clones extracted from lesions of oral lichen planus. Br J Dermatol 1994;131:319.
271. Gadenne AS, Struke R, Dunn D et al. T-cell lines derived from lesional skin of lichen planus patients contain a distinctive population of T-cell receptor gamma delta-bearing cells. J Invest Dermatol 1994; 103:347.
272. Simark-Mattsson C, Bergenholtz G, Jontell M et al. T cell receptor V-gene usage in oral lichen planus: Increased frequency of T cell receptors expressing V alfa2 and V beta3. Clin Exp Immunol 1994;98: 503.
273. Farthing PM, Matear P, Cruchley AT. Langerhans' cell distribution and keratinocyte expression of HLA-DR in oral lichen planus. J Oral Pathol Med 1992;21:451.
274. Hirota J, Osaki T. Electron microscopy study on cell-to-cell interactions in oral lichen planus. Pathol Res Pract 1992;188:1033.
275. Prieto BG, Casal M, McNutt NS. Lichen planus-like keratosis: A clinical and histological reexamination. Am J Surg Pathol 1993;17:259.
276. Van den Haute V, Antoine JL, Lachapelle JM. Histopathological discriminant criteria between lichenoid drug eruption and idiopathic lichen planus: Retrospective study on selected samples. Dermatologica 1989;179:10.
277. Rocken M: Zur pathogenese des lichen ruber planus, ein modernes konzept. Z Hautkr 1988;63:911.
278. Haber H, Sarkany I. Hypertrophic lichen planus and lichen simplex. Trans St Johns Hosp Dermatol Soc 1958;41:61.
279. Lumpkin LR, Helwig EB. Solitary lichen planus. Arch Dermatol 1966;93:54.
280. Shapiro L, Ackerman AB. Solitary lichen planus-like keratosis. Dermatologica 1966;132:386.
281. Laur WE, Posey RE, Waller JD. Lichen planus-like keratosis: A clinicopathologic correlation. J Am Acad Dermatol 1981;4:329.
282. Scott MA, Johnson WC. Lichenoid benign keratosis: J Cutan Pathol 1976;3:217.
283. Prieto VG, Casal M, McNutt NS. Lichen planus-like keratosis: A clinical and histological reexamination. Am J Surg Pathol 1993;17:259.
284. Goette DK. Benign lichenoid keratosis. Arch Dermatol 1980;116:780.
285. Goldenhersh MA, Barnhill RL, Rosenbaum HM, Stenn KS. Documented evolution of a solar lentigo into a solitary lichen planus-like keratosis. J Cutan Pathol 1986;13:308.
286. Frigg AF, Cooper PH. Benign lichenoid keratosis: Am J Clin Pathol 1985;83:439.
287. Berger TG, Graham JH, Goette DK. Lichenoid benign keratosis. J Am Acad Dermatol 1984;11;635.
288. Mehregan AH. Lentigo senilis and its evolution. J Invest Dermatol 1975;65:429.
289. Prieto VG, Casal M, McNutt NS. Immunohistochemistry detects differences between lichen planus-like keratosis, lichen planus, and lichenoid actinic keratosis. J Cutan Pathol 1993;20:143.
290. Tan CY, Marks R. Lichenoid solar keratosis: Prevalence and immunologic findings. J Invest Dermatol 1982;79:365.
291. Berman A, Herszenson S, Winkelmann RK. The involuting lichenoid plaque. Arch Dermatol 1982;118:93.
292. Kaposi M. Lichen ruber acuminatus and lichen ruber planus. Arch Dermatol Syphilol 1895;31:1.
293. Margolis MG, Cooper GA, Johnson SAM. Keratosis lichenoides chronica. Arch Dermatol 1972;105:739.
294. Torrelo A, Mediero IG, Zasmbrano A. Keratosis lichenoides chronica in a child. Pediatr Dermatol 1994:11:46.
295. Patrizi A, Neri I, Passasrini B, Varotti C. Keratosis lichenoides chronica: A pediatric case. Dermatology 1995;191:264.
296. Masouye I, Saurat JH. Keratosis lichenoides chronica: The century of another Kaposi's disease. Dermatology 1995;191:188.
297. Braun-Falco O, Bieber T, Heider L. Chronic lichenoid keratosis: Disease variant or disease entity? Hautarzt 1989;40:614.
298. Baran R, Panizzon R, Goldberg L. The nails in keratosis lichenoides chronica: Characteristics and response to treatment. Arch Dermatol 1984;120:1471.
299. Duperrat B, Carton FX, Denoeux JP et al. Keratose lichenoide striae. Ann Dermatol Venereol 1977;104:564.
300. van der Kerkhof PCM. Spontaneous resolution of keratosis lichenoides chronica. Dermatology 1993;187:200.
301. Nabai H, Mehregan AH. Keratosis lichenoides chronica. J Am Acad Dermatol 1980;2:217.
302. Petrozzi JW. Keratosis lichenoides chronica. Arch Dermatol 1976; 112:709.
303. David M, Filhaber A, Rotem A et al. Keratosis lichenoides chronica with prominent telangiectasia: Response to etretinate. J Am Acad Dermatol 1989;21:1112.
304. Lapins JA, Willoughby C, Helwig EB. Lichen nitidus: A study of forty-three cases. Cutis 1978:21:634.
305. Kawakami T, Soma Y. Generalized lichen nitidus appearing subsequent to lichen planus. J Dermatol 1995;22:434.
306. Maeda M. A case of generalized lichen nitidus with Koebner's phenomenon. J Dermatol 1994;21:273.
307. Munro CS, Cox NH, Marks JM, Natarajan S. Lichen nitidus presenting as palmoplantar hyperkeratosis and nail dystrophy. Clin Exp Dermatol 1993;18:381.
308. Itami A, Ando I, Kukita A. Perforating lichen nitidus. Int J Dermatol 1994;33:382.
309. Madhok R, Winkelmann RK. Spinous, follicular lichen nitidus associated with perifollicular granulomas. J Cutan Pathol 1988;15:248.
310. Fimiani M, Alessandrini C, Castelli A et al. Ultrastructural observations in lichen nitidus. Arch Dermatol Res 1986;279:77.
311. Wilson HTH, Bett DCG. Miliary lesions in lichen planus. Arch Dermatol 1961;83:74.
312. Waisman M, Dundon BC, Michel B. Immunofluorescent studies in lichen nitidus. Arch Dermatol 1973;107:200.
313. Smoller BR, Flynn TC. Immunohistochemical examination of lichen nitidus suggests that it is not a localized papular variant of lichen planus. J Am Acad Dermatol 1992;27:232.
314. Reed RJ, Meek T, Ichinose H. Lichen striatus: A model for the histologic spectrum of lichenoid reactions. J Cutan Pathol 1975;2:1.
315. Taieb A, el Youbi A, Grosshans E, Maleville J. Lichen striatus: A Blaschko linear acquired inflammatory skin eruption. J Am Acad Dermatol 1991;25:637.
316. Vasily D, Bhatia SG. Lichen striatus. Cutis 1981;28:442.
317. Patrone P, Patrizi A, Bonci A, Passacini B. Lichen striatus: Studio clinico ed istologico di 8 casi. G Ital Dermatol Venereol 1990;125: 267.
318. Karp DL, Cohen BA. Onychodystrophy in lichen striatus. Pediatr Dermatol 1993;10:359.
319. Mopper C, Horwitz DC. Bilateral lichen striatus. Cutis 1971;8:140.
320. Stewart WM, Pietrini LP, Thomine E. Lichen striatus: Criteres histologiques. Ann Derm Venereol 1977;104:132.
321. Gianotti R, Restano L, Grimalt R et al. Lichen striatus—a chameleon: An histopathological and immunohistological study of forty-one cases. J Cutan Pathol 1995;22:18.
322. Pujol RM, Toneu A, Moreno A, De Moragas JM. Perforating lichen striatus. Acta Derm Venereol (Stockh) 1988;68:171.
323. Goldman K, Don PC. Adult onset of inflammatory linear verrucous epidermal nevus in a mother and her daughter. Dermatology 1994; 189:170.
324. Landwehr AJ, Starink TM. Inflammatory linear verrucous epidermal naevus. Dermatologica 1983;166:107.

325. Altman J, Mehregan AH. Inflammatory linear verrucose epidermal nevus. Arch Dermatol 1971;104:385.
326. Dupre A, Christol B. Inflammatory linear verrucose epidermal nevus. Arch Dermatol 1977;113:767.
327. Toribio J, Quinones PA. Inflammatory linear verrucose epidermal nevus. Dermatologica 1975;150:65.
328. Ito M, Shimizu N, Fujiwara H et al. Histopathogenesis of inflammatory linear verrucose epidermal naevus: Histochemistry, immunohistochemistry and ultrastructure. Arch Dermatol Res 1991;283:491.
329. Bernard BA, Reano A, Darmon YM, Thivolet J. Precocious appearance of involucrin and epidermal transglutaminase during differentiation of psoriatic skin. Br J Dermatol 1986;114:279.
330. Welch ML, Smith KJ, Skelton HG et al. Immunohistochemical features in inflammatory linear verrucous epidermal nevi suggest a distinctive pattern of clonal dysregulation of growth. J Am Acad Dermatol 1993;29:242.
331. Laugier P, Olmos L. Naevus lineaire inflammatoire (NEVIL) et lichen striatus: Deux aspects d'une meme affection. Bull Soc Fr Dermatol Syphiligr 1976;83:48.
332. De Jong EMGJ, Rulo HFC, Van de Kerkhof PCM. Inflammatory linear verrucous epidermal naevus (ILVEN) versus linear psoriasis: A clinical, histological and immunohistochemical study. Acta Derm Venereol (Stockh) 1991;71:343.
333. Fox BJ, Odom RB. Papulosquamous diseases: A review. J Am Acad Dermatol 1985;12:597.
334. Griffiths WAD. Pityriasis rubra pilaris. Clin Exp Dermatol 1980; 5:105.
335. Griffiths WAD. Pityriasis rubra pilaris: The problem of its classification (letter). J Am Acad Dermatol 1992;26:140.
336. Gelmetti C, Schiuma AA, Cerri D, Gianotti F. Pityriasis rubra pilaris in childhood: A long-term study of 29 cases. Pediatr Dermatol 1986; 2:446.
337. Vanderhooft SL, Francis JS, Holbrook KA et al. Familial pityriasis rubra pilaris. Arch Dermatol 1995;131:448.
338. Braun-Falco O, Ryckmanns F, Schmoeckel C, Landthaler M. Pityriasis rubra pilaris: A clinico-pathological and therapeutic study with special reference to histochemistry, autoradiography, and electron microscopy. Arch Dermatol Res 1983;275:287.
339. Niemi KM, Kousa M, Storgards K, Karvonen J. Pityriasis rubra pilaris. Dermatologica 1976;152:109.
340. Kanitakis J, Hoyo E, Chouvet B et al. Keratinocyte proliferation in epidermal keratinocyte disorders evaluated through PCNA/cyclin immunolabelling and AgNOR counting. Acta Derm Venereol (Stockh) 1993;73:370.
341. Griffiths WAD, Pieris S. Pityriasis rubra pilaris: An autoradiographic study. Br J Dermatol 1982;107:665.
342. Gelmetti C, Rigoni C, Alessi E et al. Pityriasis lichenoides in children: A long-term follow-up of eighty-nine cases. J Am Acad Dermatol 1990;23:473.
343. Willemze R, Scheffer E. Clinical and histologic differentiation between lymphomatoid papulosis and pityriasis lichenoides. J Am Acad Dermatol 1985;13:418.
344. Wood GS, Strickler JG, Abel EA et al. Immunohistology of pityriasis lichenoides et varioliformis acuta and pityriasis lichenoides chronica. J Am Acad Dermatol 1987;16:559.
345. Longley J, Demar L, Feinstein RP et al. Clinical and histologic features of pityriasis lichenoides et varioliformis acuta in children. Arch Dermatol 1987;123:1335.
346. Maekawa Y, Nakamura T, Nogami R. Febrile ulceronecrotic Mucha-Habermann's disease. J Dermatol 1994;21:46.
347. De Cuyper C, Hindryckx P, Deroo N. Febrile ulceronecrotic pityriasis lichenoides et varioliformis acuta. Dermatology 1994;189:50.
348. Lopez-Estebaranz JL, Vanaclocha F, Gil R et al. Febrile ulceronecrotic Mucha- Habermann disease. J Am Acad Dermatol 1993; 29:903.
349. Muhlbauer JE, Bhan AK, Harrist TJ et al. Immunopathology of pityriasis lichenoides acuta. J Am Acad Dermatol 1984;10:783.
350. Hood AF, Mark EJ. Histopathologic diagnosis of pityriasis lichenoides et varioliformis acuta and its clinical correlation. Arch Dermatol 1982;118:478.
351. Giannetti A, Girolomoni G, Pincelli C, Benassi L. Immunopathologic studies in pityriasis lichenoides. Arch Dermatol Res 1988;280:S61.
352. Varga FJ, Vonderheid EC, Olbricht SM, Kadin ME. Immunohistochemical distinction of lymphomatoid papulosis and pityriasis lichenoides et varioliformis acuta. Am J Pathol 1990;136;979.
353. Weiss LM, Wood GS, Ellisen LW et al. Clonal T-cell populations in pityriasis lichenoides et varioliformis acuta: Mucha-Habermann Disease. Am J Pathol 1987;126;417.
354. Fortson JS, Schoroeter AL, Esterly NB. Cutaneous T-cell lymphoma (parapsoriasis en plaque): An association with pityriasis lichenoides et varioliformis acuta in young children. Arch Dermatol 1990;126:1449.
355. Panizzon RC, Speich R, Dassi H. Atypical manifestations of pityriasis lichenoides chronica: Development into paraneoplasia and non-Hodgkin lymphomas of the skin. Dermatology 1992;184:65.

Lever's Histopathology of the Skin, eighth edition,
edited by David Elder et al. Lippincott–
Raven Publishers, Philadelphia © 1997.

CHAPTER 8

Vascular Diseases

Raymond L. Barnhill and Klaus J. Busam

This chapter discusses vasculopathies, vasculitides, and several other disease processes with vascular injury that can affect the skin. The spectrum of clinical manifestations of such diseases is broad and depends on several factors: the number, size, and type of vessels involved (arterial vs. venous); the extent of vascular damage; the presence or absence of inflammation; the type of inflammatory infiltrate (neutrophilic vs. lymphocytic); the infiltrate's distribution (superficial dermis vs. deep dermis or subcutis); and other parameters.

In general, severe vascular damage with vascular occlusion leads to ischemic damage, and may result in necrosis, blister formation, and/or ulceration. Nonocclusive vascular disease may be associated with damage to the structural integrity of the vessel wall and may lead to leakage of blood, resulting in dermal hemorrhage and edema. Dermal hemorrhage is clinically seen as purpura. Lesions less than 3 mm in diameter are called petechiae. Larger lesions are called ecchymoses. If an inflammatory infiltrate is present, purpura may become palpable.

CRITERIA FOR VASCULITIS

Before proceeding further, some discussion concerning the criteria for vasculitis is in order, because there is considerable controversy on this issue. The essence of the problem is that vascular injury is a continuum and the cells involved dynamic. Furthermore, the degree of vascular injury resulting from any given insult is likely to be dose-related. Thus, criteria for recognizing microvascular injury are somewhat arbitrary. The spectrum of vascular reaction to injury ranges from endothelial cell swelling and leakiness to frank fibrinoid necrosis and the attendant changes such as fibrin deposition.

The minimum criteria for vasculitis have remained controversial. In general, vasculitis must have two components: (1) an inflammatory cell infiltrate and (2) evidence of vascular injury (Table 8-1). Vasculitis is an inflammatory process and thus the absence of inflammation precludes the diagnosis even though vascular alterations may be present. However, in the late, healing state, the inflammatory cell infiltrate may be minimal. The cells involved may include neutrophils, lymphocytes, or monocytes/macrophages. The type of infiltrating cell may correlate to some extent with the chronology of the process, but not always.

Another major aspect in defining vasculitis is the indices of vascular injury. Such criteria have included edema or leakiness, extravasation of erythrocytes, infiltration of vascular walls by inflammatory cells, necrosis of endothelium and other cells comprising the vascular wall, deposition of fibrinoid material within the vascular lumina or vessel walls, and leukocytoclasis of the surrounding inflammatory cell infiltrate. As mentioned above, there is a continuum of injury. However, for several years pathologists have required a certain degree of injury, as manifested by deposition of fibrinoid material and/or necrosis of the vessel itself, as a primary indicator of a true vasculitis. It must be emphasized that certain changes, including edema, extravasation of erythrocytes, infiltration of vessel walls, leukocytoclasis, and thrombosis, may occur without fibrinoid necrosis of the vessel. Edema and extravasation of erythrocytes may develop with minimal evidence of vascular injury. Leukocytoclasis also may result from necrosis of the infiltrate itself without fibrinoid necrosis of vessels. Similarly, fibrin thrombi may be present in vessels without other clear evidence of vasculitis as in the setting of hypercoagulable states.

The term *vasculopathy* may be used to describe certain degrees of vascular alteration and injury that fail to satisfy the criteria for vasculitis. Such vascular alterations might include vascular thrombosis with little other evidence of injury, deposition of fibrinoid material with little or no inflammation, and minimal infiltration of vessel walls with little or no leukocytoclasis.

Another major problem in dealing with vasculitis is the question of whether the vascular injury is primary or secondary. Primary vascular injury implies that the vascular insult is the predominant disease process. On the other hand, secondary vascular injury indicates that another disease process outside the vessels is the primary pathologic process. An example of the latter is vascular alteration noted near cutaneous ulceration. In many instances it may not be possible to distinguish clearly between a primary and a secondary vascular insult. However, secondary vascular injury is often variable with sparing of some vessels within the zone of tissue injury. Other indications of

R. L. Barnhill: Department of Pathology, Dermatopathology Division, Brigham and Women's Hospital and Harvard Medical School, Boston, MA

K. J. Busam: Department of Pathology, Dermatopathology Division, Brigham and Women's Hospital and Harvard Medical School, Boston, MA

TABLE 8-1. *Definitions of vascular injury*

Definitions of vascular injury
Primary vascular injury
Vasculopathy
Fibrinoid deposition, thrombosis with limited or no inflammation
Infiltration of vessel wall by inflammatory cells with otherwise minimal alteration
Leukocytoclasis of tissue infiltrate with minimal alteration of vessel—that is, swelling only, absence of fibrinoid necrosis
Vasculitis
Perivascular inflammatory cell infiltrate* (neutrophilic, eosinophilic, lymphocytic, histiocytic, or mixed)
Fibrinoid necrosis*—necrosis of vessel wall with deposition of fibrinoid material
Other changes often present but not essential: edema, extravasation of erythrocytes, leukocytoclasis, infiltration of vessel wall by inflammatory cells, swelling of endothelial cells, luminal thrombosis
Secondary vascular injury†
Vasculopathy or vasculitis
Secondary to another insult such as external trauma or ulceration
Variable vascular alterations with sparing of some vessels
Peripheral perivascular fibrinoid deposition

* Essential for diagnosis.

† Distinguishing between primary and secondary vasculitis is often not possible.

secondary vascular injury include deposition of fibrinoid material at the periphery of the vessel wall and focal thrombosis without significant infiltration by inflammatory cells.

VASCULOPATHIC REACTIONS

A vasculopathic reaction as defined in Table 8-1 refers to the histologic finding of vascular damage in the absence of vasculitis. Vasculopathic reactions may be associated with (1) coagulopathies, (2) metabolic disorders leading to alterations of the vessel wall, (3) structural deficiencies of the perivascular connective tissue, or (4) miscellaneous other disease processes.

Coagulopathies

Any coagulopathy may be accompanied by vasculopathic changes. The extent of vascular damage is variable. Vascular damage may occur in the setting of altered platelet counts, such as in idiopathic thrombocytopenic purpura, in coagulation factor deficiencies (e.g., inherited or acquired protein C and S deficiencies), coagulopathies associated with connective tissue disease (e.g., lupus anticoagulant, antiphospholipid antibody syndrome), calciphylaxis, and platelet thrombosis in heparin necrosis. Extensive vascular damage with luminal occlusion by thrombotic material may develop in coumarin necrosis, in thrombotic thrombocytopenic purpura, and in disseminated intravascular coagulation—specifically in the setting of purpura fulminans.[1]

In mild forms, the clinical manifestations may be subtle and limited to petechiae. In severe forms of coagulopathies, large areas of ecchymosis may be present, typically located on the extremities. Large hemorrhagic bullae may overlie the ecchymoses, and some of the ecchymotic areas may undergo necrosis.

Histopathology. The histologic features are nonspecific for any particular disorder. In mild forms of coagulopathies, the only histologic manifestation may be dermal hemorrhage—that is, extravasation of red blood cells into perivascular connective tissue. With increasing severity of the disease process, intravascular fibrin thrombi may be found (Fig. 8-1). In severe forms (e.g., thrombotic thrombocytopenic purpura, coumarin necrosis, and purpura fulminans), thrombotic vascular occlusion may lead to hemorrhagic infarcts, epidermal and dermal necrosis, or subepidermal bulla formation. In severe systemic intravascular coagulation, internal organs may also show widespread thrombosis of small vessels and hemorrhagic necrosis.

Metabolic Vasculopathies

Vasculopathies may arise also from metabolic disorders. Deposition of endogenously produced material, as in diabetes mel-

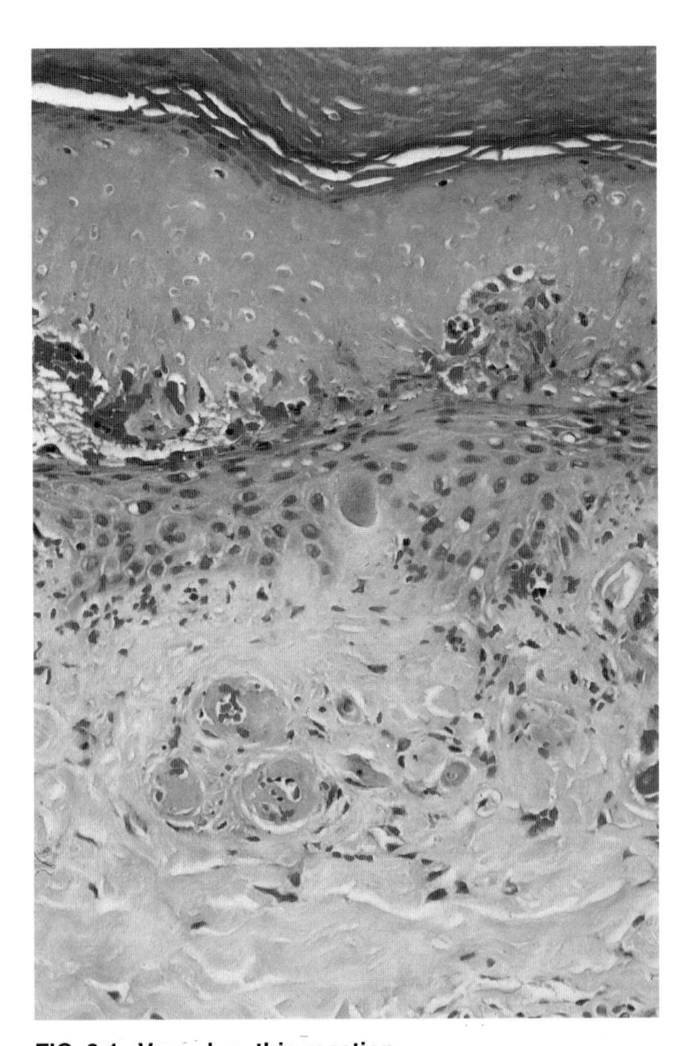

FIG. 8-1. Vasculopathic reaction
Fibrin thrombi in small dermal vessels and ischemic necrosis of the overlying epidermis can be seen.

litus, amyloidosis, or porphyria, may lead to an angiopathy that may cause ischemic damage to the area of skin supplied by the affected vessels. The histopathology of these disorders is discussed in more detail in other chapters of this book. The salient histologic vascular alteration in the above-mentioned disorders is the deposition of amorphous material in the walls of dermal capillaries.

Atherosclerosis is by far the most common form of vasculopathy. However, it is not discussed here in detail because it is primarily a disease of large vessels supplying visceral organs. Cutaneous changes are usually rare and are secondary manifestations of peripheral ischemia. Luminal occlusion may result from intimal thickening and lipid deposition, superimposed thrombosis, or, less frequently, cholesterol emboli. Because cholesterol microemboli can cause cutaneous findings mimicking vasculitis, this phenomenon is discussed in more detail here.

Cutaneous Cholesterol Embolism

Cholesterol crystal embolization is usually a disease of the elderly with significant atherosclerosis.[2] Atheromatous plaque material may detach spontaneously. However, it is more common for plaque material to be dislodged by an invasive procedure, such as arterial catheterization. Microemboli or cholesterol crystals typically lead to ischemic changes. Cutaneous manifestations are common and often affect the lower extremities. There may be livedo reticularis, purple discoloration, gangrene of toes, and small, painful ulcerations on the legs. Occasionally, there are also a few nodules or indurated plaques. A typical feature is adequate distal pulsation, indicating that the ischemia is arteriolar rather than arterial.

Histopathology. Cholesterol emboli may be found as needle-shaped clefts within the lumina of small vessels. The intravascular clefts, which are in effect dissolved crystals, may be single or multiple and are commonly associated with amorphous eosinophilic material, macrophages, or foreign-body giant-cell reactions. Vascular walls exhibit intimal fibrosis and often obliteration of lumina in older lesions. In many instances, only fibrin thrombi are observed. Often a deep biopsy is needed to reveal such emboli, which are distributed focally and therefore are difficult to find.

Vasculopathies Resulting from Deficiencies in Connective Tissue

Lastly, structural deficiencies in the perivascular connective tissue may cause vascular fragility and lead to dermal hemorrhage. Such alterations underlie the hemorrhages that accompany senile purpura and scurvy.

Histopathology. In senile purpura, extravasation of red blood cells is encountered in atrophic skin with solar elastosis and normal-appearing capillaries. In scurvy, dermal hemorrhage is found predominantly in the vicinity of hair follicles without evidence of capillary changes. Hemosiderin-laden macrophages are usually noted.[3] Other findings associated with scurvy include intrafollicular keratotic plugs and coiled hair.

Other Clinical Presentations Associated with Vasculopathic Reactions

Livedo Reticularis

Livedo reticularis is persistent red-blue mottling of the skin in a netlike pattern. It is a nonspecific sign of sluggish blood flow from any cause. It differs from cutis marmorata by not subsiding with warming of the skin. It may occur in association with a vasculitis or a vasculopathy in the context of several different systemic or localized disease processes, such as infection, atrophie blanche, cholesterol emboli, and connective tissue disease. Frequently, however, the condition is idiopathic and limited to the lower extremities. Livedo reticularis in particular, as a generalized presentation, has also been described as part of a potentially severe arterio-occlusive syndrome (Sneddon's syndrome) that is often complicated by cerebrovascular disease.[4]

Histopathology. A biopsy specimen taken from an erythematous area may be normal, whereas a biopsy specimen from a white area may show a vessel with a thickened wall and the lumen occluded by a thrombus. In other cases, deeply situated dermal arterioles have shown obliterative changes. Other changes observed in livedo reticularis are intravascular aggregates of red blood cells, suggesting a low flow state.

Atrophie Blanche

Atrophie blanche is a common condition that usually affects the middle-aged or elderly female.[5] Synonymous terms are *livedoid vasculitis* and *segmental hyalinizing vasculitis.* In its fully developed state, typically located on the lower portions of the legs, particularly on the ankles and the dorsa of the feet, there are irregularly outlined, whitish atrophic areas with peripheral hyperpigmentation and telangiectasia. This is preceded by purpuric macules and papules, which develop into small, painful ulcers with a tendency to recur. Healing of the ulcers results in the white atrophic areas that have given the disease its name. Many of the patients have associated livedo reticularis. The condition also may be seasonal, with the greatest disease activity in the summer and winter months.

Histopathology. The histologic findings are nonspecific and vary with the stage of the lesion. However, in all stages, vascular changes are present. In early lesions, fibrinoid material may be noted in the vessel wall or vessel lumen (Fig. 8-2). Infarction with hemorrhage and an inflammatory infiltrate may be present as well. In late atrophic lesions, the epithelium is thinned and the dermis is sclerotic, with little if any cellular infiltrate. The walls of the dermal vessels may show thickening and hyalinization of the intima. Luminal occlusion by intimal proliferation and/or fibrinoid material and sometimes recanalized thrombotic vessels may be seen. In some cases, the vessels in the superficial dermis are predominantly affected; in others, the vessels in the middle and even deep dermis are mostly affected.

Pathogenesis. The etiology of atrophie blanche is unknown. Immune-complex deposits that have been observed in late lesions are likely secondary changes.[6] A primary disturbance of fibrinolysis in the endothelium of affected microvessels has been postulated.[7]

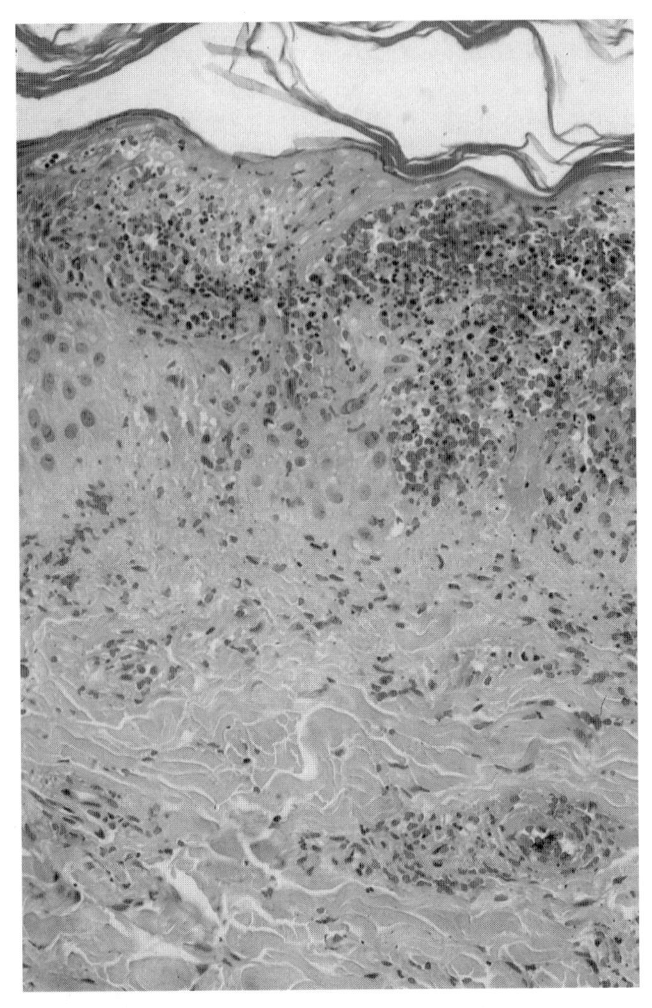

FIG. 8-2. Atrophie blanche
Epidermal atrophy, dermal hemorrhage, and fibrin thrombi are present.

Degos' Syndrome

Although the pathogenesis of Degos' syndrome is poorly understood, a thrombotic vasculopathy is a characteristic associated finding. The clinical manifestations of Degos' syndrome include crops of asymptomatic, slightly raised, yellowish red papules that gradually develop an atrophic porcelain-white center. These papules tend to affect the trunk and proximal extremities. Degos had initially described a cutaneointestinal syndrome, in which distinct skin findings ("drops of porcelain") were associated with recurrent attacks of abdominal pain that often ended in death from intestinal perforations.[8] He chose the name *malignant atrophic papulosis* (MAP) to emphasize the serious clinical course of the disease. Whereas the cutaneous lesions were then thought to be specific and pathognomonic for a unique disease entity (Degos' disease), it is nowadays believed that MAP is a clinicopathologic reaction pattern that can be associated with a number of conditions other than the cutaneointestinal syndrome described by Degos and others.[9] Lesions similar if not identical to MAP have been noted, in particular, in connective tissue diseases such as lupus erythematosus, dermatomyositis, and progressive systemic sclerosis, in atrophie blanche, and in Creutzfeld-Jakob disease.[10]

Histopathology. A typical lesion shows a wedge-shaped area of altered dermis covered by atrophic epidermis with slight hyperkeratosis. Dermal alterations may include frank necrosis. More common, however, are edema, extensive mucin deposition, and slight sclerosis (Fig. 8-3). There may be a sparse perivascular lymphocytic infiltrate. However, the dermis is largely acellular. Typically, vascular damage is noted in the vessels at the base of the "cone of necrobiosis." Vascular alterations may be subtle and manifest as endothelial swelling. However, more characteristically, intravascular fibrin thrombi may be noted. Their presence suggests that the dermal and epidermal changes result from ischemia. Altered vessels usually lack an inflammatory infiltrate.

Pathogenesis. The etiology of Degos' syndrome is unclear. The findings have been ascribed to a coagulopathy, vasculitis, or mucinosis. However, convincing evidence to support any single causal factor is lacking.

VASCULITIS

Clear-cut histologic evidence of vasculitis is present once fibrinoid necrosis of the vascular wall is observed together with an inflammatory infiltrate. However, vascular damage may be less obvious histologically, and it may be difficult to decide whether or not the features are sufficient for vasculitis (see "Criteria for Vasculitis" at beginning of chapter, and Table 8-1).

The classification of inflammatory vascular reactions—specifically that of vasculitides—is difficult for a variety of reasons.[11–14] Clinically different entities lack histologic specificity, and the same disease process may show a spectrum of histologic changes depending on the stage of the disease, its level of activity, and the type of treatment that might have modified its course. Moreover, advances in research have led to redefinitions or expanded definitions of certain disease processes with subsequent loss of what has been thought to be a specific finding.

A major recent advance in our understanding and classification of vasculitides has been the recognition that antineutrophil cytoplasmic antibodies (ANCAs) are associated with certain vasculitides.[15–17] Indirect immunofluorescence assays reveal two staining patterns: cytoplasmic (c-ANCA) and perinuclear (p-ANCA). The majority of c-ANCAs react with proteinase 3, and most p-ANCAs are specific for myeloperoxidase (MPO). Although several different vasculitic processes can be associated with ANCA, these antibodies are especially helpful in the differential diagnosis of Wegener's syndrome (WG), Churg-Strauss syndrome (CSS), and microscopic polyarteritis (MPA). WG is usually associated with c-ANCA and only rarely with p-ANCA, whereas MPA and CSS show the opposite pattern: they are more likely to be positive for p-ANCA and less likely for c-ANCA (see text following and Table 8-2).

In an attempt to standardize nomenclature for vasculitides, an international conference has proposed a system primarily based on vessel size.[13–16] Classification based on vessel size is helpful because there is some correlation with the clinical presentation. Purpura typically reflects small vessel injury. Cutaneous nodules suggest the involvement of medium-sized arteries. However, classification based on vessel size alone is of limited value in dermatopathology, because most cutaneous vasculitides affect primarily small dermal vessels.

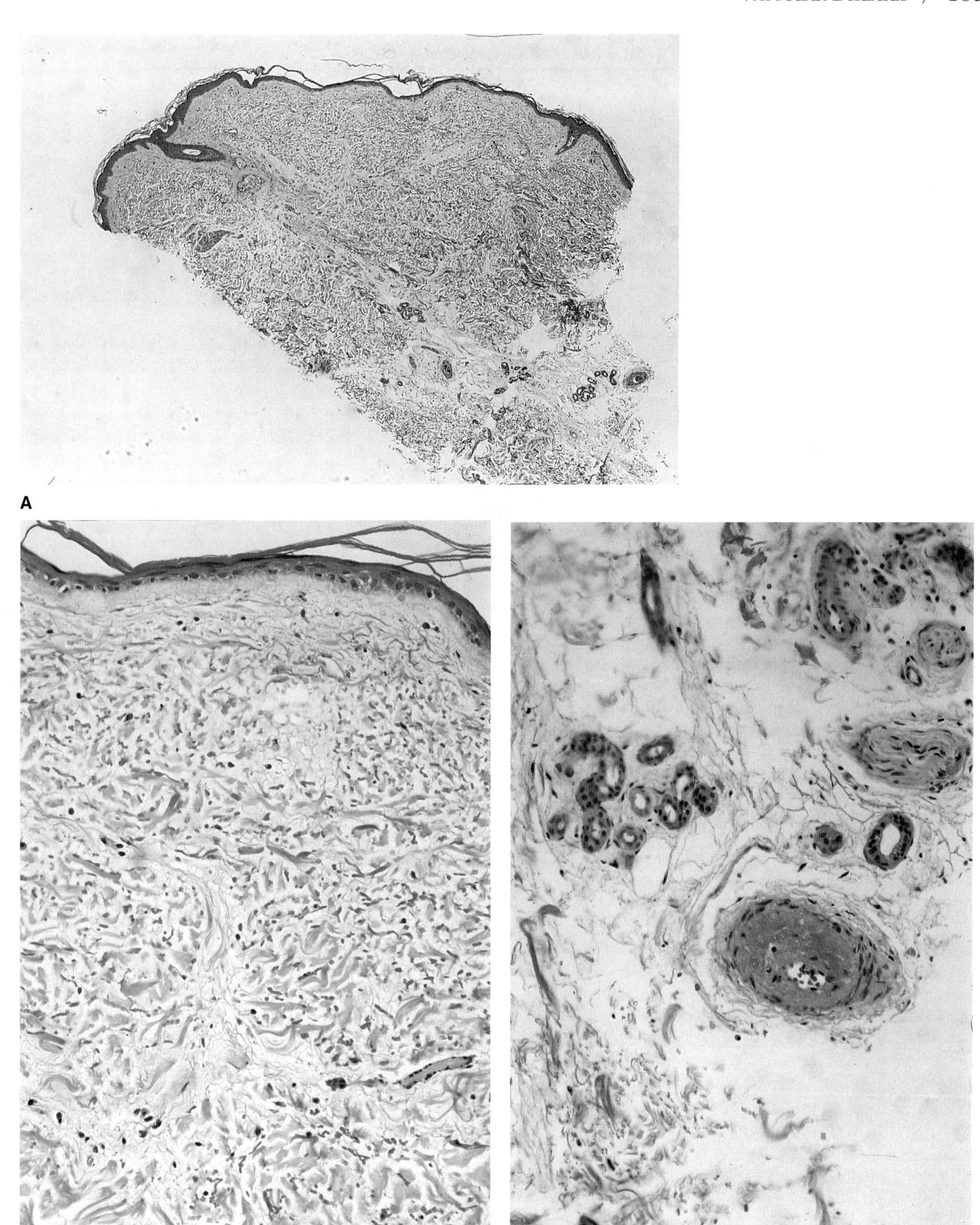

FIG. 8-3. Degos' lesion
Atrophic epidermis overlies a wedge-shaped area of dermis (**A**) with mucin deposition (**B**) and a thrombosed vessel at the base (**C**). This Degos' lesion was observed in a patient with dermatomyositis.

TABLE 8-2. *ANCA-positive vasculitides*

Disease process	Antimyeloperoxidase (p-ANCA)	Antiserine proteinase (c-ANCA)
Wegener's syndrome	Rare (5%)	Common (80%)
Microscopic polyangiitis (polyarteritis)	Common (50–60%)	Common (45%)
Churg-Strauss syndrome	Common (70%)	Rare (7%)

A practical approach (Table 8-3) for the histopathologist in evaluating small-vessel inflammatory reactions is first to decide whether or not clear-cut vascular damage is present and sufficient for a designation as vasculitis, then to assess the composition of the inflammatory infiltrate (neutrophilic/leukocytoclastic vs. eosinophilic vs. lymphocytic vs. granulomatous), its distribution (superficial, superficial and deep, or deep only), and to look for associated findings, such as microorganisms, that might narrow the differential diagnosis. It is important to consider the context of the histologic findings—for example, vasculitic changes may merely be secondary events in the setting of an ulcer resulting from nonvasculitic causes, such as viral infection or trauma. One should also realize that lesions have life spans and a lesion that shows, for example, a leukocytoclastic vasculitis at one point in time may show a predominantly lymphocytic or even granulomatous infiltrate at another point.

The following subsections discuss the histologic features and clinical differential diagnoses of inflammatory vascular reactions affecting the skin. Vasculitides are categorized first by vessel size. The only large-vessel vasculitis with cutaneous findings mentioned here is temporal (giant cell) arteritis. Vasculitis affecting medium-sized and small arteries, and, in particular, small-vessel vasculitides, are discussed in more detail. Small-vessel vasculitides are classified according to the composition of the inflammatory infiltrate: neutrophilic/leukocytoclastic versus lymphocytic versus granulomatous vasculitis.

TABLE 8-3. *Approach to vasculitis*

1. Determine if vasculitis or vasculopathy is present or absent.
2. Primary or secondary
3. Size of vessel and type
   a. Large
   b. Medium
   c. Small
4. Composition of infiltrate
   a. Neutrophilic/leukocytoclastic
   b. Eosinophilic
   c. Lymphocytic
   d. Histiocytic/granulomatous
5. Evaluation for infection
6. Serologic and immunopathologic evaluation
   a. Evaluation for ANCA, ANA, rheumatoid factor, cryoglobulins
   b. Immunofluorescence and other studies for the detection of immune complexes—for example, IgA fibronectin aggregates
7. Clinical context
   a. Cutaneous involvement only
   b. Extent of systemic involvement

Vasculitis of Large and Medium-Sized Vessels: Temporal (Giant Cell) Arteritis

Giant cell arteritis of the elderly primarily affects large or medium-sized arteries in the temporal region. It may be unilateral or bilateral and may be associated with involvement of other cranial arteries—in particular, retinal arteries. The clinical presentation may include pain and tenderness of the forehead and possible sudden visual impairment. There may be erythema and edema of the skin overlying the involved arteries, and occasionally there are ulcerations of the scalp.[19] The involved artery may be palpable. Clinical laboratory data include a significantly elevated erythrocyte sedimentation rate (ESR).

Although the clinical presentation is strongly suggestive of the diagnosis, a biopsy is often performed for confirmation prior to the initiation of systemic steroid therapy. However, results of diagnostic tests are not always positive.

Histopathology. Involved arteries show an inflammatory process that may extend throughout the entire arterial wall and is composed mainly of lymphocytes and macrophages (Fig. 8-4). Some of the macrophages are multinucleated. In some instances, neutrophils may be present, but this finding should not dissuade one from the diagnosis. The inflammatory infiltrate is unevenly distributed, and step sections are often needed for identification. There is fragmentation of the lamina elastica and elastophagocytosis by multinucleated giant cells. An Elastica–van Gieson stain greatly facilitates the evaluation of elastic fibers. However, depending on the stage of the disease process, giant cells may not be present. In late stages, there may be only thickening of the intima by deposits of fibrinlike material and myofibroblastic proliferation with subsequent luminal narrowing. Disruption of the internal elastic lamina is not sufficient for diagnosis, because this is nonspecific.

Differential Diagnosis. Infection-related vasculitis, connective tissue disease, and polyarteritis nodosa might enter into the differential diagnosis. The latter processes often show necrotizing neutrophilic vasculitides (depending on the stage), and diagnosis is dependent on serologic studies, the absence of infection, and clinical findings.

Vasculitis Affecting Medium-Sized and Small Vessels

Vasculitides affecting medium-sized vessels include polyarteritis nodosa, microscopic polyangiitis, Kawasaki syndrome, WG, Churg-Strauss syndrome, rheumatoid vasculitis, giant cell (temporal) arteritis, Takayasu arteritis, infections, and Buerger's disease. This section discusses primarily polyarteritis nodosa, Kawasaki, Mondor's and Buerger's diseases.

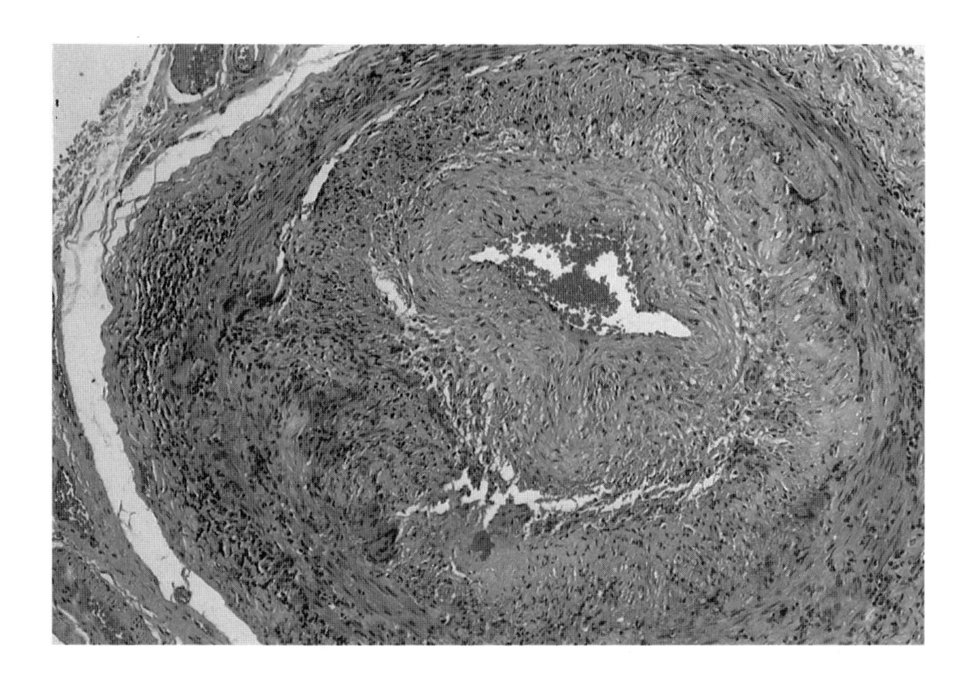

FIG. 8-4. Giant cell arteritis
A biopsy of the temporal artery shows a panmural predominantly mononuclear infiltrate with giant cells and fragmentation of elastic fibers.

Polyarteritis Nodosa and Microscopic Polyangiitis

Kussmaul and Maier reported in 1866 the case of a 27-year-old man with fever, abdominal pain, muscle weakness, peripheral neuropathy, and renal disease.[20] They termed the fatal illness *periarteritis nodosa* (PAN), referring to nodular protuberances along the course of medium-sized muscular arteries, which histologically were characterized by inflammation predominantly at the periphery of the vessel walls, with vessel-wall destruction. Ferrari noted in 1903 the more characteristic presence of inflammatory cells within all levels of the affected vessels and suggested the term *polyarteritis* instead of *periarteritis*.[21]

The term *periarteritis nodosa* was used rather indiscriminately in the early half of the twentieth century for many types of vasculitides until Zeek redefined periarteritis nodosa as a systemic necrotizing vasculitis primarily affecting muscular arteries and resulting in lesions of various ages, often with focal aneurysms.[22] The kidney and gastrointestinal tract were among the organs most frequently affected.

Davson, Ball, and Platt distinguished *classic* and *microscopic polyarteritis nodosa*.[23] *Classic* referred to the form originally described by Kussmaul and Maier, in which ischemic glomerular lesions were common but glomerulonephritis was rare. *Microscopic polyarteritis nodosa*, also termed *microscopic polyangiitis* (MPA), on the other hand, referred to a systemic small-vessel vasculitis primarily affecting arterioles and capillaries that is typically associated with focal necrotizing glomerulonephritis with crescents. Although MPA is predominantly a small-vessel vasculitis, it is discussed here because it is considered part of the spectrum of PAN.

The majority of patients with MPA are male and over 50 years of age. Prodromal symptoms include fever, myalgias, arthralgias, and sore throat. The most common clinical feature is renal disease manifesting as microhematuria, proteinuria, or acute oliguric renal failure. Although in classic PAN cutaneous involvement is rare, 30 to 40% of patients with MPA exhibit skin changes. These changes include palpable purpura, splinter hemorrhages, and ulcerations. The tender erythematous nodules and livedo reticularis that are seen in classic PAN appear exceedingly rarely in MPA. Pulmonary involvement without granulomatous tissue reaction occurs in approximately one-third of all patients. Other organ systems (e.g., gastrointestinal tract, central nervous system, and serosal and articular surfaces) may also be affected, but less commonly. Serious clinical complications usually arise from renal and pulmonary disease.

At present, pathologists continue to distinguish between classic and microscopic polyarteritis, although the rationale for this separation has been challenged by an increasing number of cases with overlapping features. This has led to the introduction of the term *overlapping syndrome of vasculitis*[24] to encompass vasculitis affecting both small and medium-sized arteries.

The advent of ANCA in the 1990s has had a major impact on the concept of PAN. PAN is currently considered to be in the spectrum of pauci-immune ANCA-associated vasculitides ranging from localized forms, such as renal-limited disease (rapidly progressive glomerulonephritis type III), to multisystemic disease with many features overlapping those of WG, CSS, and other vasculitides. Although the relationship of ANCA to classic PAN is still not clearly delineated, the majority of patients with MPA are p-ANCA-positive (serum: approximately 50 to 60% positive for MPO; approximately 40% positive for antiserine proteinase). In contrast to WG, a clear relationship between ANCA titer and disease activity has not been established for MPA.

For patients presenting with cutaneous small-vessel vasculitis only (no arteriolar or arterial involvement) and elevated ANCA titers,[15] Jennette has proposed the term ANCA-positive *leukocytoclastic angiitis*. However, the differential diagnosis of ANCA-positive pauci-immune leukocytoclastic angiitis still includes MPA, because failure to detect arteriolar involvement could be related to sampling error. The differential diagnosis also includes Wegener's vasculitis and other small-vessel vasculitides that are occasionally ANCA-positive, such as certain drug reactions.

A variant of PAN shows cutaneous lesions with little or no visceral involvement (*cutaneous PAN*).[16] However, localization of PAN only to the skin has been questioned.

Histopathology. The characteristic lesion of classic PAN is a panarteritis involving medium-sized and small arteries (Fig. 8-5). Even though in classic PAN the arteries show the characteristic changes in many visceral sites, affected skin often shows only small-vessel disease, and arterial involvement is typically focal. The changes affecting cutaneous small vessels are usually those of a necrotizing leukocytoclastic vasculitis. If there is a clinical presentation of cutaneous nodules, panarteritis similar to visceral lesions is usually detected. In classic PAN, the lesions typically are in different stages of development (i.e., fresh and old). Early lesions show degeneration of the arterial wall with deposition of fibrinoid material. There is partial to complete destruction of the external and internal elastic laminae. An infiltrate present within and around the arterial wall is composed largely of neutrophils showing evidence of leukocytoclasis, although it often contains eosinophils. At a later stage, intimal proliferation and thrombosis lead to complete occlusion of the lumen with subsequent ischemia and possibly ulceration. The infiltrate also may contain a significant number of lymphocytes, histiocytes, and some plasma cells, which may extend far into the surrounding perivascular tissue and may be predominant at a certain stage. In the healing stage, there is fibroblastic proliferation extending into the perivascular area. The small vessels of the middle and upper dermis often exhibit a nonspecific lymphocytic perivascular infiltrate.

Differential Diagnosis. Vasculitis indistinguishable from PAN may be observed in infections (bacterial, e.g., pseudomonas; viral, e.g., hepatitis B or HIV), in connective tissue diseases (lupus erythematosus, rheumatoid arthritis), in WG, in CSS, and in other settings—for example, acute myelogenous leukemia—without explanation. As with all vasculitides, one must systematically evaluate the disease process by ruling out infection (special stains, cultures, other studies) and specific systemic diseases such as lupus erythematosus, and then documenting the extent of systemic involvement as well as other findings (serologic and other laboratory and clinical findings).

Pathogenesis. The pathogenesis of classic PAN is poorly understood. Direct immunofluorescence testing of skin lesions of PAN shows some immune deposits in dermal vessels. However, they may reflect a secondary event after vascular injury from another cause. In MPA, ANCAs may play a role in inducing vasculitis by activating circulating neutrophils and monocytes, causing them to adhere to vessels, degranulate, and release toxic metabolites, thereby causing vascular injury.

Kawasaki Disease

Kawasaki disease is a necrotizing arteritis that usually affects young children, with a peak age incidence at one year old.[25] Mucocutaneous findings are common and include a polymorphous exanthematous macular rash, conjunctival congestion, dry reddened lips, "strawberry tongue," oropharyngeal reddening, and swelling of the hands and feet—especially the palms and soles. There is typically an associated nonpurulent cervical lymphadenopathy. Desquamation of the skin of the fingers typically occurs after 1 to 2 weeks, often followed by thrombocytosis. The most serious clinical complications are related to arteritis and thrombosis of coronary arteries.

Histology. Cutaneous vasculitis is rare. The macular rash is usually accompanied by nonspecific histologic changes. Characteristic arteritis is typically found in visceral sites, such as the coronary arteries.

Mondor's Disease and Other Superficial Thrombophlebitides

Mondor's disease is a thrombophlebitis of the subcutaneous veins of the chest region and is often manifested clinically by a cordlike induration.[26] It is usually not accompanied by general symptoms and tends to resolve within weeks.

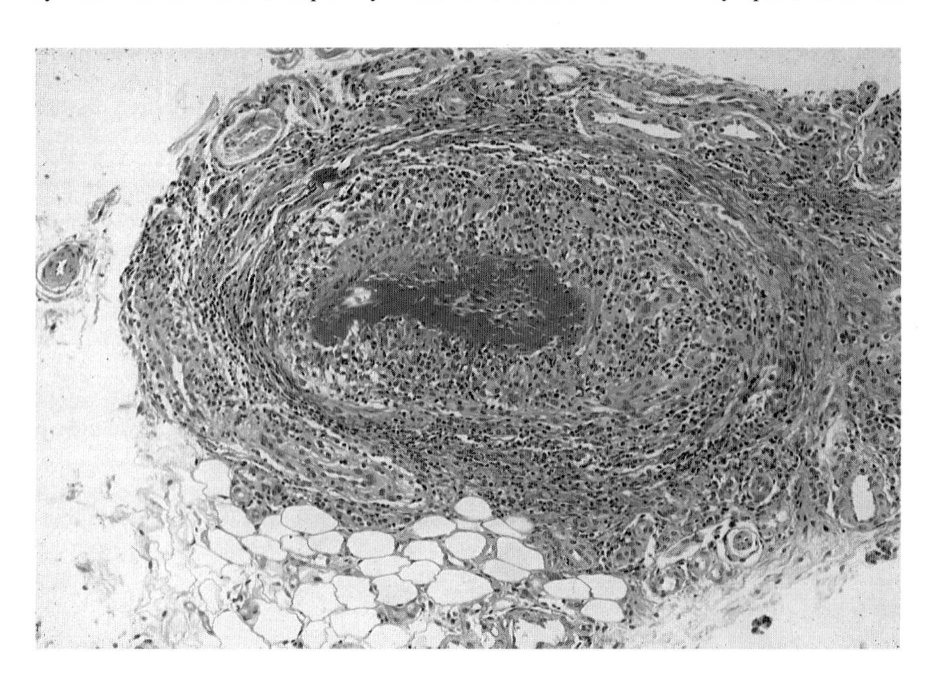

FIG. 8-5. Panarteritis nodosa
A subcutaneous medium-sized artery shows fibrinoid necrosis and a florid inflammatory cell infiltrate.

Histopathology. In early lesions, a polymorphonuclear infiltrate may be present. However, most biopsied lesions show subcutaneous veins with organizing thrombi and fibrous thickened walls that give them a cordlike appearance at scanning magnification.

Pathogenesis. In the majority of cases, the etiology remains unknown. However, it has been associated with trauma, connective tissue disease, and rarely with breast carcinoma and a variety of other conditions.

Superficial thrombophlebitis of small to medium-sized veins may be encountered at other anatomic sites. It most commonly occurs on the lower extremities. It clinically presents with tenderness and erythema of the overlying skin. Histologic changes are nonspecific and typically show organizing thrombi and a variably dense mononuclear cell infiltrate.

Thromboangiitis Obliterans (Buerger's Disease)

Buerger's disease is a distinctive condition characterized by a segmental, thrombosing inflammatory process affecting intermediate and small arteries and sometimes veins. It primarily involves the vessels of the upper and lower extremities. The condition almost exclusively affects smokers. Cutaneous findings are manifestations of ischemic injury.

Histopathology. Active lesions are characterized by luminal thrombotic occlusion and a mixed inflammatory cell infiltrate of the vessel wall, characteristically with microabscesses (Fig. 8-6). A granulomatous reaction may be present as well.

Differential Diagnosis. The histologic findings in Buerger's disease have been thought to be characteristic; however, they are likely to be nonspecific and probably occur in other pro-

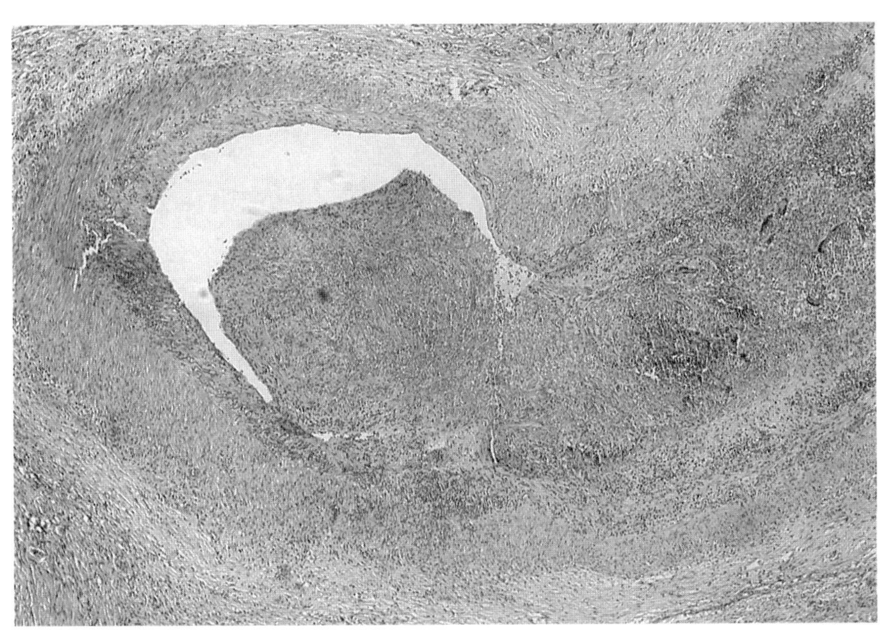

A

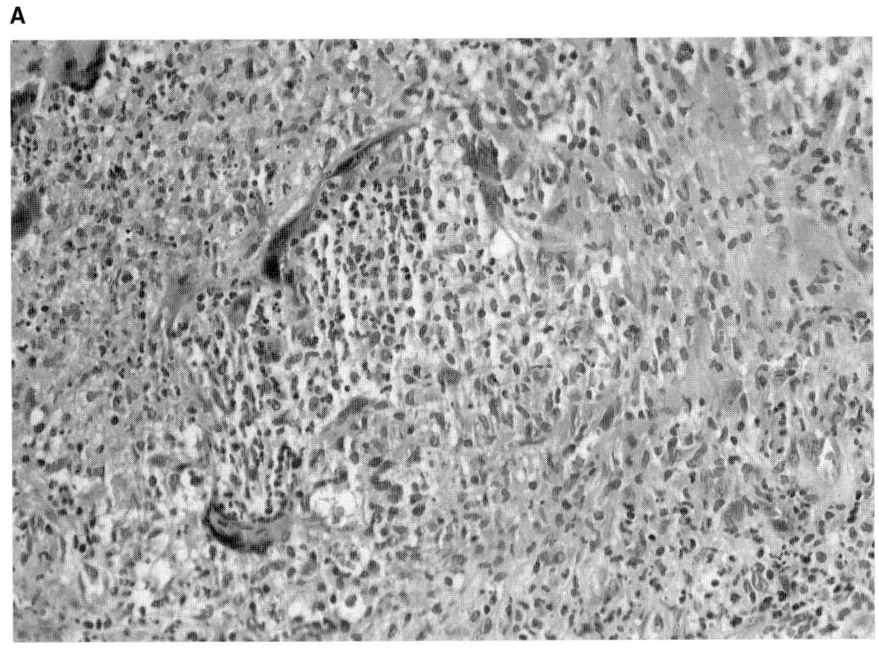

B

FIG. 8-6. Thromboangiitis obliterans
Thrombosis is present (**A**) with focal microabscess formation and giant-cell reaction (**B**).

cesses, including nonspecific thrombosis and inflammation of intermediate-sized arteries and veins.

Small-Vessel Neutrophilic/Leukocytoclastic Vasculitis

A large number of different disease processes can be accompanied by small-vessel vasculitis with predominantly neutrophilic infiltrates. The main diseases to be considered are listed in Table 8-4.[14,15]

Histopathology of Neutrophilic Small-Vessel Vasculitis. Neutrophilic small-vessel vasculitis is a reaction pattern of small dermal vessels, almost exclusively postcapillary venules, characterized by a combination of vascular damage and an infiltrate composed largely of neutrophils (Fig. 8-7). Because there is often fragmentation of nuclei (karyorrhexis or leukocytoclasis), the term *leukocytoclastic vasculitis* (LCV) is frequently used. Depending on its severity, this process may be subtle and limited to the superficial dermis or be pandermal and florid and associated with necrosis and ulceration. If edema is prominent, a subepidermal blister may form. If the neutrophilic infiltrate is dense and there is pustule formation, the term *pustular vasculitis* may be applied (Fig. 8-8). In a typical case of LCV, the dermal vessels show swelling of the endothelial cells and deposits of strongly eosinophilic strands of fibrin within and around their walls. The deposits of fibrin and the marked edema together give the vessel walls a "smudgy" appearance referred to as *fibrinoid degeneration.* Actual necrosis of the perivascular collagen, however, is seen only rarely in conjunction with ulcerative lesions. If the vascular changes are severe, luminal occlusion of vessels may be observed. The cellular infiltrate is present predominantly around the dermal blood vessels or within the vascular walls, so that the outline of the blood vessels may appear indistinct. The infiltrate consists mainly of neutrophils and of varying numbers of eosinophils and mononuclear cells. The infiltrate also is scattered throughout the upper dermis in association with fibrin deposits between and within collagen bundles. Extravasation of erythrocytes is commonly present.

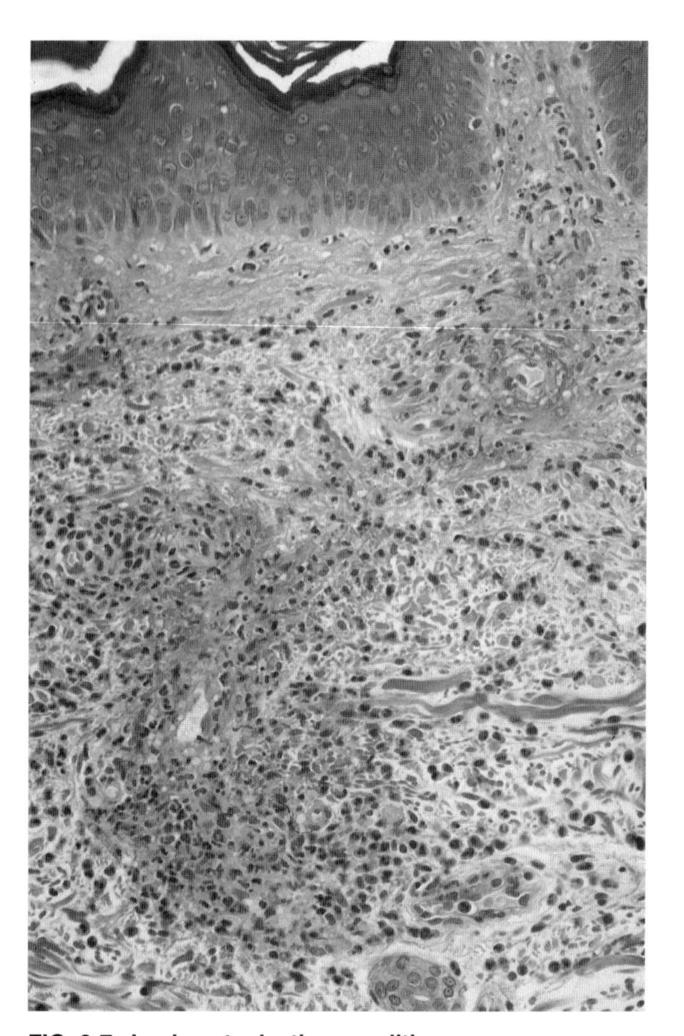

FIG. 8-7. Leukocytoclastic vasculitis
Vascular damage with perivascular neutrophilic infiltrate, eosinophilic fibrinoid change of vessel walls, and nuclear debris can be seen.

TABLE 8-4. *Differential diagnosis of cutaneous neutrophilic small-vessel vasculitis, categorized on the basis of proposed pathogenic mechanisms*

- Infection
  - Bacterial (gram-positive/-negative organisms, mycobacteria, spirochetes)
  - Rickettsial
  - Fungal
  - Viral
- Immunologic injury
  - Immune-complex mediated
    - Henoch-Schönlein purpura
    - Urticarial vasculitis
    - Cryoglobulinemia
    - Serum sickness
    - Connective tissue diseases
  - Autoimmune-diseases
    - Infection-induced immunologic injury (e.g., hepatitis B or C, streptococcal)
  - Drug-induced
  - Paraneoplastic processes
  - Behçet's disease
    - Erythema elevatum diutinum
  - Antineutrophil antibody associated
    - Wegener's granulomatosis
    - Microscopic polyangiitis
    - Churg-Strauss syndrome
    - Some drug-induced vasculitis
  - Unknown
    - Polyarteritis nodosa

As with any inflammatory process, the appearance of the reaction pattern depends on the stage at which the biopsy is taken. In older lesions, the number of neutrophils may be decreased and the number of mononuclear cells increased so that mononuclear cells may predominate and a designation of a lymphocytic or even granulomatous vasculitis or vascular reaction might be made.

Pathogenesis. Many disease processes may exhibit LCV. The major causes of vasculitis are infection and immune-mediated inflammation. Table 8-4 categorizes vasculitides on the basis of suggested pathogenetic mechanisms. Although T-cell mediated inflammation has been implicated in large-vessel vasculitides, antibody-mediated inflammation seems to play a prominent role in small-vessel vasculitis. Its final common pathway typically involves neutrophils and monocyte activation with adherence to endothelial cells, infiltration of the vessel wall, and release of lytic enzymes and toxic radicals. This final pathway of vascular injury may be initiated by (1) the deposition of immune complexes, (2) direct binding of antibodies to antigens in vessel walls, and (3) activation of leukocytes by antibodies with specificity for leukocyte antigens (ANCAs). It must be stressed that an immune-complex etiology has been invoked much too often to explain all forms of vasculitis and particularly small-vessel vasculitis. In many instances, immune complexes are not the primary events in vascular injury but simply epiphenomena.

Diagnostic Approach to Neutrophilic Small-Vessel Vasculitis. As already mentioned, the clinical and histologic manifestations are fairly nonspecific for a particular category of vasculitis. For example, palpable purpura may be the clinical appearance of dermal leukocytoclastic small-vessel vasculitis secondary to infection (e.g., gonococcal sepsis), immune-complex-mediated vasculitis (e.g., cryoglobulinemia or Henoch-Schönlein purpura), ANCA-associated vasculitis (e.g., WG), allergic vasculitis (e.g., reaction to a drug), vasculitis associated with connective tissue, or a paraneoplastic phenomenon. It is important therefore, to interpret the histologic findings only in the context of clinical information to reach an appropriate diagnosis. Often, additional laboratory data, such as from microbiologic cultures, special stains for organisms, or immunofluorescence or serologic studies, are needed. Because the treatment for infectious vasculitides is so radically different from the treatment for immune-mediated diseases, the most important diagnostic step in the evaluation of a vasculitis is to rule out an infectious process. If noninfectious vasculitis is suspected, evidence for systemic vasculitis must be sought. Clinical findings—such as hematuria, arthritis, myalgia, enzymatic assays for muscle or liver enzymes, and serologic analysis for ANCAs, antinuclear antibodies, cryoglobulins, hepatitis B and C antibodies, IgA-fibronectin aggregates, and complement levels—are important to further delineate the disease process. Exposure to a potential allergen, such as a drug, that might have elicited a hypersensitivity reaction should be sought. Evidence of an allergic pathogenesis is reassuring because it suggests that the vasculitic process may be self-limited and not associated with systemic vasculitis. As mentioned previously, it is also important to address the possibility that the histologic findings of vasculitis may be a secondary phenomenon, as, for example, in ulceration from localized trauma.

The following subsections discuss the main clinical settings in which LCV occurs.

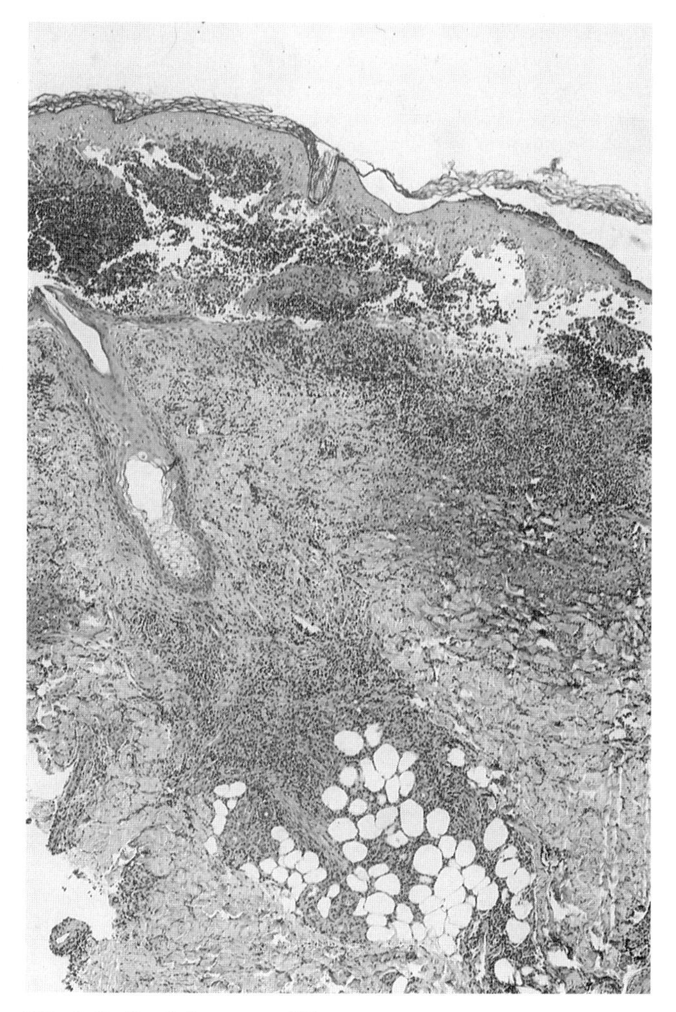

FIG. 8-8. Pustular vasculitis
Subepidermal blister formation with many polymorphonuclear cells and vascular damage are present.

Infectious Vasculitis

An infectious process needs to be ruled out early in the evaluation of an LCV.[11,14] Microorganisms may invade vessels directly or damage them by an immune-mediated mechanism. *Neisseria meningitides* is a common cause of infectious cutaneous leukocytoclastic vasculitis. Meningococci may be found within endothelial cells and neutrophils at sites of vascular inflammation. However, other Gram-positive or Gram-negative bacteria and fungi also may cause cutaneous small-vessel vasculitis. Staphylococcal sepsis can lead to neutrophilic vasculitis with purpura or nodular lesions, which may contain microabscesses (Fig. 8-9). Rickettsial infections, such as Rocky Mountain spotted fever (RMSF), are characterized by invasion of endothelial cells by organisms causing vascular damage. Inflammation, however, is often minimal in RMSF. Direct immunofluorescence microscopy may demonstrate the organism. Clinically, the spectrum of changes ranges from small macules to papules and purpura.

Henoch-Schönlein Purpura

Henoch-Schönlein purpura (H-SP) is clinically characterized by palpable purpura of the buttocks and lower extremities, abdominal pain, and hematuria.[27] It typically affects children following streptococcal upper respiratory tract infections, and is usually self-limited with a resolution expected 6 to 16 weeks after the onset of symptomatology. Complications generally arise from renal involvement.

Histology. Henoch-Schönlein purpura cannot be distinguished histologically from other forms of LCV, although the degree of vascular damage is often not as great as that usually observed in typical LCV. Immunofluorescence studies typically

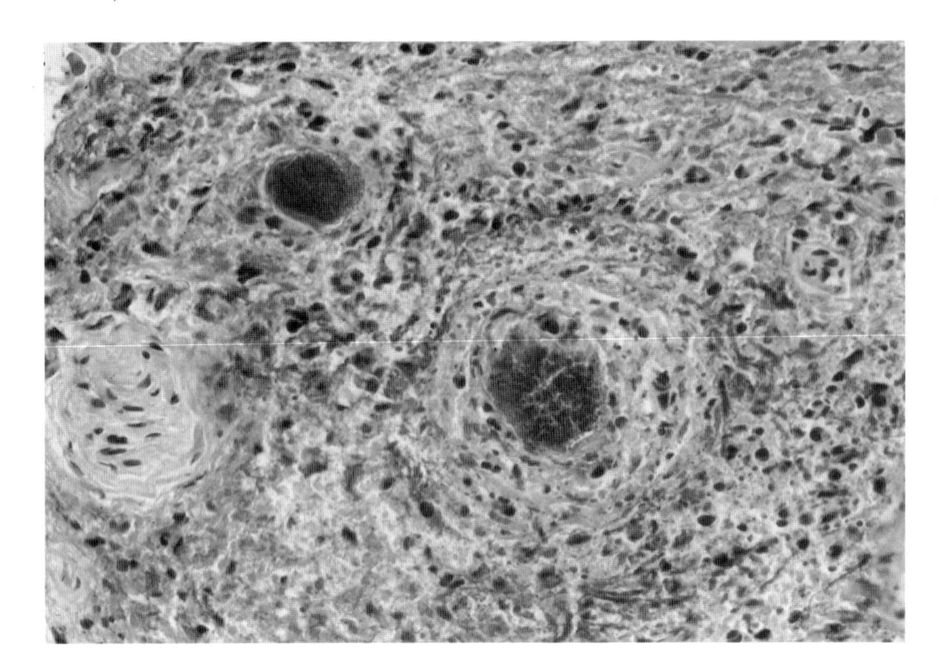

FIG. 8-9. Septic vasculitis
Small dermal vessels are filled with coccal forms and surrounded by a neutrophilic infiltrate.

demonstrate the deposition of IgA in capillaries. Such a limited extent of vascular damage is also commonly observed in urticarial vasculitis (see text following), and clinical findings may be necessary for distinction of H-SP from urticarial vasculitis. Jennette and colleagues have recently reported that serologic detection of IgA-fibronectin aggregates may be associated with greater likelihood of renal or systemic disease in patients with cutaneous LCV.[28]

Urticarial Vasculitis

Urticarial vasculitis shows wheals that persist longer than those in conventional urticaria.[29] Purpura is usually only faint. Urticarial vasculitis is not a specific disease but rather a manifestation of a vasculitis that is associated with increased vascular permeability. Approximately one-third of all patients with vasculitic urticaria have decreased complement levels (hypocomplementemic vasculitis). They may have systemic findings, such as arthralgias and adenopathy. The course of urticarial vasculitis is generally benign and episodic, lasting several months. Urticarial vasculitis sometimes occurs in lupus erythematosus and may be the initial clinical manifestation of that disease.

Histopathology. The histology of urticarial vasculitis ranges from mild to fully developed LCV (Fig. 8-10).

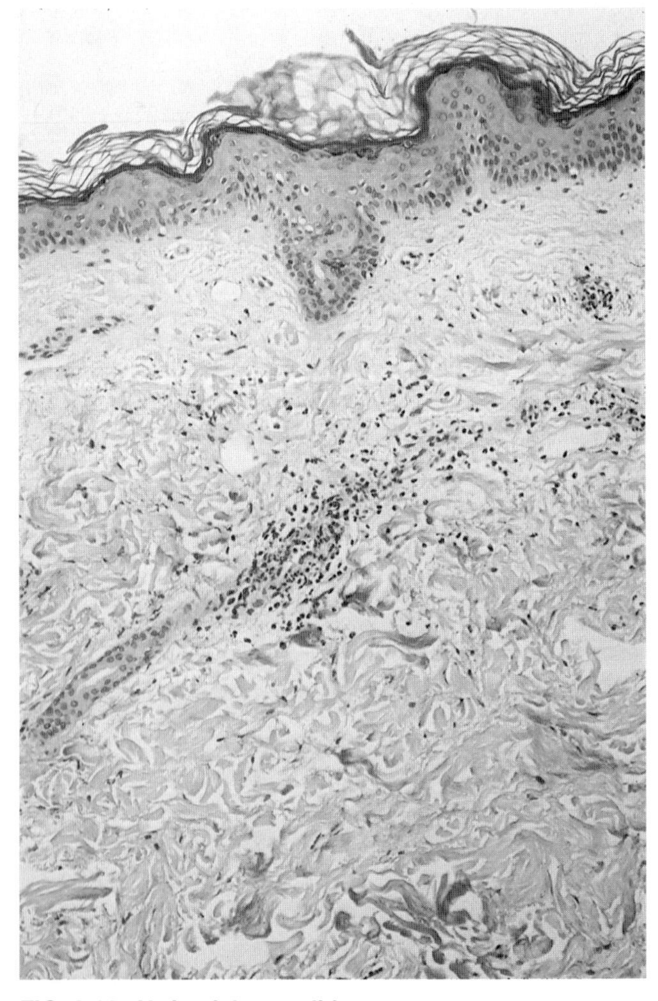

FIG. 8-10. Urticarial vasculitis
Dermal edema and a sparse predominantly polymorphonuclear vascular reaction can be seen.

Cryoglobulinemias and Other Small-Vessel Vasculitides Associated with Paraproteins

Small-vessel vasculitis may be associated with paraproteins—that is, abnormal serum proteins.[11,30] Such paraproteins include cryoglobulins, cryofibrinogens, macroglobulins, and gamma heavy chains. Cryoglobulins are serum immunoglobulins that precipitate when the serum is cooled and redissolve upon rewarming. There are three major types of cryoglobulinemia: in type I cryoglobulinemia, monoclonal IgG or IgM cryoglobulins are found, often associated with lymphoma, leukemia, Waldenstrom's macroglobulinemia, or multiple myeloma, or without known underlying disease. In type II cryoglobulinemia, the cryoprecipitate consists of both monoclonal and polyclonal cryoglobulins, with one cryoglobulin acting as an antibody against the other. These cryoglobulins are circulating immune complexes. The most common combination is IgG-IgM. In type III cryoglobulinemia, the immunoglobulins are polyclonal. Type II and III or mixed cryoglobulinemias are frequently associated with connective tissue disorders, such as lupus erythematosus, rheumatoid arthritis, and Sjögren's syndrome, or may be related to infection—in particular, hepatitis C infection. Idiopathic forms of type II and III cryoglobulinemias are also termed essential mixed cryoglobulinemia.

Clinically, cutaneous lesions in patients with cryoglobulinemia may manifest as chronic palpable purpura, urticaria-like lesions, livedo reticularis, acrocyanosis, digital gangrene, and leg ulcers. Raynaud's phenomenon is common. Systemic manifestations may include arthralgia, hepatosplenomegaly, lymphadenopathy, and glomerulonephritis.

Histopathology. In type I cryoglobulinemia, amorphous material (precipitated cryoglobulins) is deposited subjacent to endothelium and throughout the vessel wall as well as within the vessel lumen, resulting in a thrombus-like appearance. These precipitates stain pink with hematoxylin and eosin and bright red with PAS stain, as opposed to less intense staining of fibrinoid material. Some capillaries are filled with red blood cells, and extensive extravasation of erythrocytes may be present. An inflammatory infiltrate is usually lacking in contrast to mixed cryoglobulinemia, which typically shows an LCV. PAS-positive intramural and intravascular cryoprecipitates may be found also in mixed cryoglobulinemia (Fig. 8-11), although less frequently than in type I cryoglobulinemia.

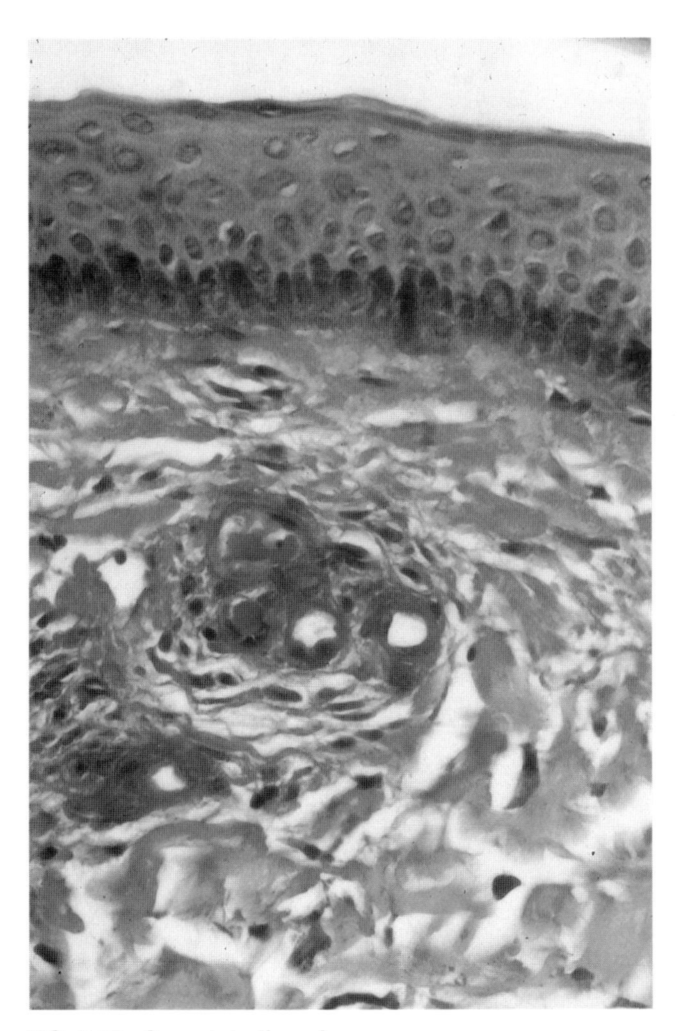

FIG. 8-11. Cryoglobulinemia
PAS-positive bright red cryoprecipitates are visible in small superficial dermal vessels.

Other small-vessel vasculitides with the histologic pattern of an LCV may be found in association with Waldenström's hyperglobulinemia (hyperglobulinemic purpura) and in Schnitzler's syndrome, which manifests as chronic urticaria with macroglobulinemia (usually monoclonal IgM) and other paraproteinemias.

Serum Sickness

This is a syndrome of a morbilliform urticarial eruption, fever, and lymphadenopathy, occuring 7 to 10 days after a primary antigen exposure or 2 to 4 days after a repeat exposure. The antigen may be a drug, from an arthropod sting or from a previous infection, or therapeutic serum globulins.[31] Serum sickness is usually a self-limited condition. There is no distinctive feature in the LCV of serum sickness.

Connective Tissue Disease

Rheumatoid arthritis, lupus erythematosus, and other diseases in the spectrum of connective tissue disease may develop LCV.[32] Clinical and serologic information is critical to the correct interpretation of the cutaneous findings in these clinical settings.

Autoimmune Diseases

Primary Sjögren's syndrome is not associated with connective tissue disease, but may present with purpura in addition to ocular and glandular involvement.[11] The histologic reaction pattern is often an LCV.

Drug-Induced Vasculitis

A hypersensitivity reaction to a drug may result in an LCV.[11,14] Penicillin, thiazides, and sulfonamides are the most common drugs used to induce LCV. Drugs also may induce the pattern of pustular vasculitis.

Paraneoplastic Vasculitis

A wide spectrum of vasculitic processes has been associated with neoplastic disorders.[33] The most common associations include polyarteritis nodosa with hairy cell leukemia and cutaneous small-vessel vasculitis with lymphoproliferative disorders and some carcinomas.

Behçet's Disease

Behçet's disease is a multisystem disease characterized by oral aphthous lesions and at least two of the following criteria: genital aphthae, synovitis, posterior uveitis, cutaneous pustular vasculitis, and meningoencephalitis.[34] It is a disease that is common in the Middle East and Japan, but rare in Northern Europe and the United States. It is associated with HLA-B51. The clinical presentation is extremely variable and so is the vascular involvement. Vascular lesions include not only active inflammatory lesions but also aneurysms, arterial or venous occlusions, and varices.

Histopathology. The histopathologic spectrum of mucocutaneous inflammatory vascular lesions includes, depending on the stage and activity of the lesion, neutrophilic, lymphocytic, and granulomatous vascular reactions. Biopsy specimens of early lesions typically show a neutrophilic vascular reaction. However, fully developed necrotizing leukocytoclastic vasculitis may develop. If the neutrophilic infiltrate is very dense, the pattern of pustular vasculitis may be found (see Fig. 8-8).

Pathogenesis. The etiology of Behçet's disease remains unknown. The vascular injury is presumably immune-mediated, because immune-complex deposition has been demonstrated in vessel walls.[34] Disorders of neutrophils are also being discussed with regard to the etiology of this disease.[34]

Erythema Elevatum Diutinum (EED)

This disease is another rare condition associated with LCV.[35] It is clinically characterized by persistent, initially red to violaceous and later brown to yellow papules, nodules, and plaques. The lesions are typically located on the extensor surfaces of the extremities. The lesions are initially soft, but later they become hard as a result of fibrosis. EED is probably not a distinct disease entity, but rather a clinicopathologic reaction pattern that can be seen in a number of different disease processes, such as inflammatory bowel disease, rheumatoid arthritis, and systemic lupus erythematosus. EED is most often associated with either a monoclonal or polyclonal gammopathy—in particular, IgA hyperglobulinemia.

Histopathology. In its early stages, EED has the histology of an LCV. In later stages, there is formation of granulation tissue and fibrosis. Even though the cellular infiltrate is less pronounced, neutrophils often predominate even then. The capillaries may still show deposits of fibrinoid material or merely fibrous thickening. In the late fibrotic stage, lipid material may also be present as cholesterol clefts.

Microscopic Polyangiitis

MPA, which is discussed in more detail together with classic PAN previously, is again mentioned here because it is an important diagnostic consideration of cutaneous LCV. It falls within the spectrum of pauci-immune vasculitides associated with ANCA. Because there is significant overlap among MPA, WG, and Churg-Strauss syndrome, it is not always possible to categorize patients precisely as to which of these entities is present. In these cases it might be prudent to designate the disease condition as ANCA-positive LCV and not to force it into a particular diagnostic category.

Pathogenesis. The vascular damage in EED is thought to be secondary to immune complexes or immunoglobulin deposition in vessel walls.

Lymphocytic Small-Vessel Vasculitis

A histologic diagnosis of a lymphocytic vasculitis may be made if there is sufficient evidence of vascular damage and the inflammatory infiltrate is predominantly lymphocytic (Fig. 8-12). Often, the vascular damage is subtle and in many cases there may be disagreement among dermatopathologists on whether or not the term "vasculitis" is warranted.[36] Clear-cut evidence of vasculitis is again indisputable if an inflammatory infiltrate is present together with fibrinoid necrosis of the vascular wall. However, these findings are rarely or only focally present in the majority of conditions that have been said to manifest lymphocytic vasculitis.

The disease processes in which lymphocytic vasculitis is commonly observed include arthropod bites, hypersensitivity reactions to drugs, urticarial vasculitis, purpuric dermatitides,

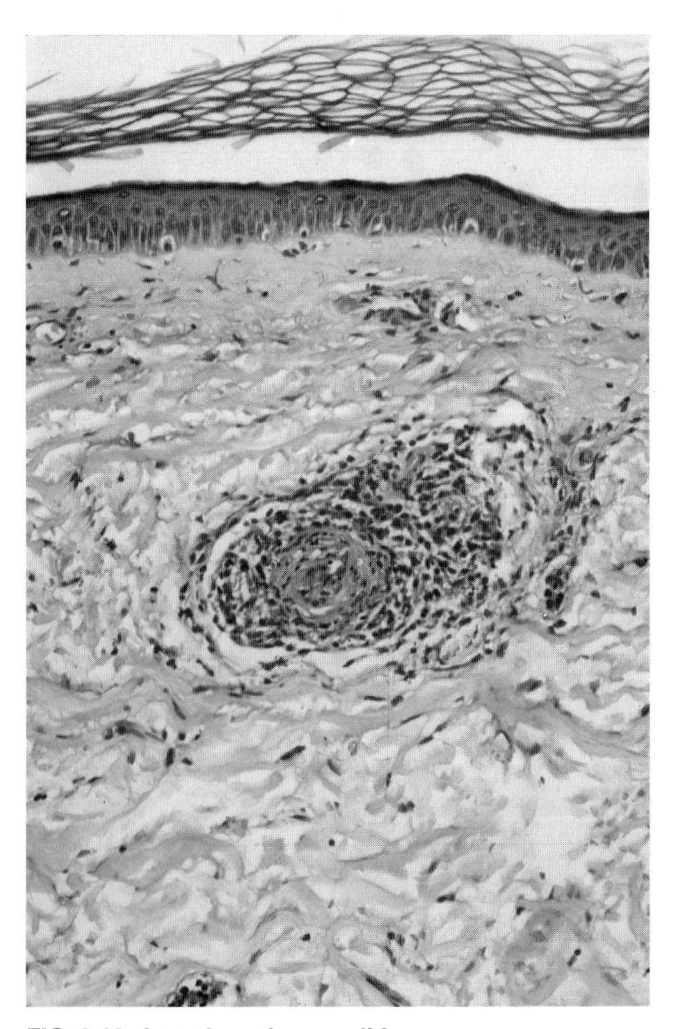

FIG. 8-12. Lymphocytic vasculitis
A dermal vessel is affected by fibroid degeneration and infiltrated by lymphocytes.

TABLE 8-5. *Differential diagnosis of lymphocytic vasculitis and lymphocytic vascular reactions*

Arthropod bites
Drug-induced and other hypersensitivity reactions
Infection-associated reactions (e.g., viral)
Connective tissue diseases
Behçet's disease
Purpuric dermatitides
PLEVA/PLC/LYP
Cutaneous lymphoma
Autoimmune diseases
Pernio
Polymorphous light eruption
Atrophie blanche
Infestations (e.g., scabies)

autoimmune diseases (e.g., Sjögren's syndrome), connective tissue diseases, pernio (chilblains), polymorphous light eruption, atrophie blanche, viral processes, and cutaneous T-cell infiltrates such as pityriasis lichenoides et varioliformis acuta (PLEVA), pityriasis lichenoides chronica (PLC), and lymphomatoid papulosis (LYP) (see Table 8-5). Lymphocytic vasculitis may also be seen in a stage of an otherwise leukocytoclastic or granulomatous vasculitis or in a process that at other times may even be noninflammatory and manifested perhaps as a vasculopathy (e.g., atrophie blanche).

Lymphomatoid Vasculitis and Vascular Reactions

The terms "lymphomatoid vasculitis" and "lymphomatoid vascular reaction" may be used if there is a lymphocytic vasculitis or lymphocytic vascular reaction with significant cytologic atypia of the lymphoid cells (Table 8-6). Although lymphoid nuclear irregularities of some degree may be present in many lymphocytic vascular reactions, probably as a reflection of an activated state of the lymphocytes, lymphoid atypia tends to be particularly well-developed in LYP and some viral processes. The differential diagnosis includes, then, vascular damage in the context of cutaneous lymphoma, such as angiocentric T-cell lymphoma and other lymphomas.[37]

TABLE 8-6. *Differential diagnosis of lymphomatoid vasculitis and vascular reaction*

T-cell lymphoproliferative disorders
Peripheral T-cell lymphoma
Angiocentric T-cell lymphoma
Lymphomatoid papulosis
Lymphomatoid granulomatosis
Angioimmunoblastic lymphadenopathy
Pigmented purpuric dermatitis-like eruptions
Lymphomatoid drug eruptions
Lymphomatoid contact dermatitis
Connective tissue disease
Viral processes
Florid hypersensitivity reactions
Arthropod bites
Scabies infestation

Granulomatous Vasculitis and Granulomatous Vascular Reactions

In the life spans of many inflammatory reactions involving blood vessels, histiocytes may predominate at a certain stage and form granulomas (Fig. 8-13).[11,14] This may occur with no or minimal vascular wall damage or may be associated with fibrinoid degeneration of the vessel wall. In the latter situation, a granulomatous vasculitis is present. The main disease processes that need to be considered in the differential diagnosis of a granulomatous vascular reaction are listed in Table 8-7.

The two main disease processes in which granulomatous vasculitis has been described as prominent and fairly characteristic, although nonspecific, are Wegener's granulomatosis and Churg-Strauss syndrome, which are discussed in more detail here. Other disease processes that enter the differential diagnosis are also mentioned.

Churg-Strauss Syndrome

Churg-Strauss syndrome (CSS) is a systemic disease occurring in asthmatic patients characterized by vasculitis, eosinophilic infiltration of multiple organs, and peripheral eosinophilia. There is considerable overlap of this disease process with other systemic vasculitides, such as PAN and WG, and with other inflammatory disorders exhibiting eosinophils, such as eosinophilic pneumonitis. Hence, there is some confusion surrounding the definition of this syndrome.

Although associations among asthma, eosinophilic and granulomatous tissue reactions, and vasculitis had been previously reported, Churg and Strauss integrated these associations into a syndrome characterized by the clinicopathologic constellation of asthma, fever, hypereosinophilia, eosinophilic tissue infiltrates, necrotizing vasculitis, and extravascular granuloma formation.[38]

The internal organs most commonly involved are the lungs, the gastrointestinal tract, and, less commonly, the peripheral nerves and the heart. In contrast to PAN, renal failure is rare.

Lanham et al.[39] have emphasized that short of autopsy, the classic triad of necrotizing granulomatous vasculitis, eosinophilic tissue infiltration, and extravascular granulomas is extremely difficult to demonstrate because of the focality of the process. They proposed a broader definition of CSS requiring asthma, hypereosinophilia (more than 1.5×10^9 eosinophils per liter), and systemic vasculitis involving two or more extrapulmonary organs.

The incidence of CSS is similar in males and females. It typically presents in the third or fourth decade of life. Patients tend to display several phases of disease development, from nonspecific symptoms of asthma and allergic rhinitis (prodromal phase) to a phase of hypereosinophilia with eosinophilic pneumonitis or gastroenteritis (second phase) and, finally, to systemic vasculitis (third phase). The three disease phases do not always occur sequentially but may on occasion present simultaneously.

Despite multiple reports on CSS, it appears to be rare. Between 1950 and 1974, only 30 cases were identified at the Mayo Clinic.[40] Although Churg and Strauss initially characterized allergic granulomatosis as a "strikingly uniform clinical picture," there is less clarity today about its distinction from other vasculitic processes.

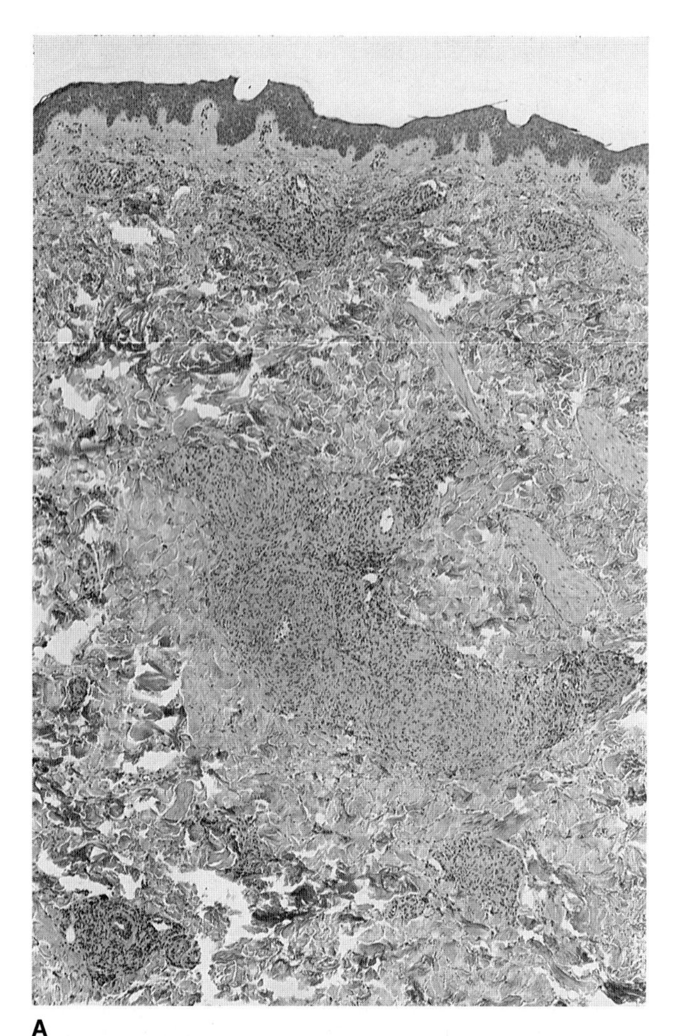

A

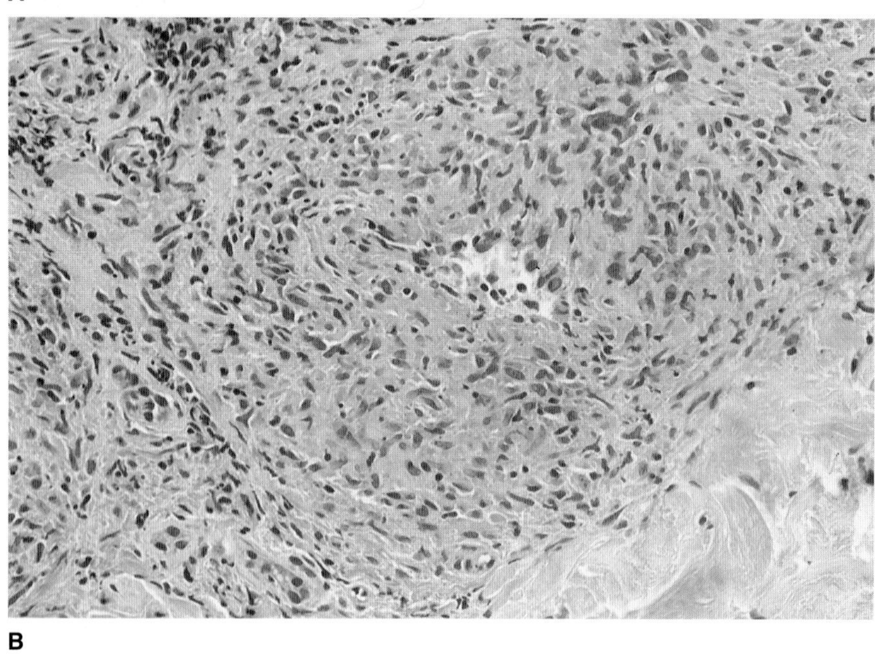

B

FIG. 8-13. Granulomatous vasculitis
Note perivascular histiocytic/granulomatous infiltrate (**A**) and focal vascular damage (**B**).

TABLE 8-7. *Differential diagnosis of granulomatous vascular reactions*

Infection
Wegener's granulomatosis
Churg-Strauss syndrome
Polyarteritis nodosa
Cutaneous Crohn's disease
Drug reaction
Connective tissue disease
Granuloma annulare
Necrobiosis lipoidica
Paraneoplastic phenomena
Angiocentric T-cell lymphoma (lymphomatoid granulomatosis)
Erythema nodosum and erythema nodosum-like reactions

Two types of cutaneous lesions occur in about two-thirds of all patients: (1) hemorrhagic lesions varying from petechiae to extensive ecchymoses, sometimes accompanied by necrotic ulcers and often associated with areas of erythema (similar to Henoch-Schönlein purpura), and (2) cutaneous-subcutaneous nodules. The most common sites of skin lesions are the extremities, but the trunk may also show involvement. In some instances, the petechiae and ecchymoses are generalized. There is also a limited form of allergic granulomatosis, in which, in addition to preexisting asthma, the lesions are confined to the conjunctiva, the skin, and subcutaneous tissue.

Diagnostically helpful laboratory data include peripheral leukocyte counts. CSS is also associated with ANCA. Serum samples from patients with CSS obtained during an active phase of the disease contain anti-MPO (p-ANCA) in the majority of cases (approximately 70%). The levels of anti-MPO have been found to correlate with disease activity. Anti-MPO are found less often in patients with limited forms of the disease. Antiserine proteinase antibodies (c-ANCA) may also be found in patients with CSS, but infrequently so (approximately 7%).

Histopathology. The areas of cutaneous hemorrhage typically show LCV. However, eosinophils may be conspicuous. In some instances, the dermis shows a granulomatous reaction composed predominantly of radially arranged histiocytes and, frequently, multinucleated giant cells centered around degenerated collagen fibers. The central portions of the granulomas contain not only degenerated collagen fibers but also disintegrated cells, particularly eosinophils, in great numbers. These granulomas were initially thought to be characteristic histologic features and were referred to as Churg-Strauss granulomas. However, they are not always present and are not a prerequisite for the diagnosis. Moreover, more recent studies have shown that similar findings can also be observed in other disease processes, such as connective tissue diseases (rheumatoid arthritis and lupus erythematosus), Wegener's granulomatosis, PAN, lymphoproliferative disorders, subacute bacterial endocarditis, chronic active hepatitis, and inflammatory bowel disease (Crohn's disease and ulcerative colitis).[41]

Inflammatory and degenerative changes are found in the subcutaneous tissue. There, the granulomas may attain considerable size through expansion and confluence, thus giving rise to the clinically apparent cutaneous-subcutaneous nodules. The palisading granulomas are embedded in a diffuse inflammatory exudate rich in eosinophils. Strauss suggested that the presence of granulomas in the dermis and in subcutaneous nodules was of significant diagnostic value. However, similar changes have also been observed in other diseases, such as PAN.

Differential Diagnosis. CSS is a clinicopathologic entity. Its diagnosis depends on the clinical picture of respiratory disease, particularly a history of asthma, p-ANCA positivity, and histology compatible and supportive of this diagnosis, especially granulomatous inflammation, necrotizing angiitis, and eosinophilia. The principal differential diagnosis is from PAN, MPA, WG, and the conditions mentioned above that may show extravascular necrotizing granulomas. There appears to be significant overlap with WG and PAN. It is well known that particular patients may shift from one disease category to another over time.

Wegener's Granulomatosis

Wegener's granulomatosis was first recognized as a distinct clinicopathologic disease process in 1936, when Wegener reported three patients with a "peculiar rhinogenic granulomatosis." Goodman and Churg summarized postmortem studies in 1954, from which evolved the classic triad of this clinicopathologic complex characterized by (1) necrotizing and granulomatous inflammation of the upper and lower respiratory tracts, (2) glomerulonephritis, and (3) systemic vasculitis.[42] Liebow and Carrington[43] (1966) and later Deremee et al.[44] (1976) described limited variants of the disease involving the respiratory tract only.

With the recognition of an association between ANCAs and WG, the concept of WG has been modified and the necessity of demonstrating granulomatous inflammation as a prerequisite for the diagnosis of WG has been challenged. A less restrictive definition has been proposed (The Third International Workshop on ANCA, 1991[13]) as *Wegener's vasculitis.* Subsumed under this less restrictive category are ANCA-positive patients with clinical presentations of WG, such as sinusitis, pulmonary infiltrates, and nephritis, and documented necrotizing vasculitis, but without biopsy-proven granulomatous inflammation. Both classic WG and Wegener's vasculitis are considered different manifestations of *Wegener's syndrome,* a more generic term proposed by the Working Classification of ANCA-Associated Vasculitides.

Two-thirds of patients with WG are male, and the mean age of diagnosis is 35 to 54 years. The vast majority of patients are Caucasians. The clinical presentation is extremely variable, ranging from an insidious course with a prolonged period of nonspecific constitutional symptoms and upper respiratory tract findings to abrupt onset of severe pulmonary and renal disease. The most commonly involved anatomic sites include upper respiratory tract, lower respiratory tract, and kidneys. Other organ systems that are commonly affected include joints and skin. Migratory, polyarticular arthralgia of large and small joints is found in up to 85% of patients with WG. Cutaneous involvement is extremely variable in different series, ranging from less than 20% to more than 50% of patients. Skin involvement may manifest as in macular erythematous rash, purpura, papules, papulonecrotic lesions, and nodules with and without ulceration. Occasionally cutaneous lesions are the first manifestation of WG. However, because of their nonspecific appearance, they are frequently recognized as presentations of WG.

The development of assays for ANCA has greatly facilitated the diagnosis of WG and the monitoring of disease activity. In a

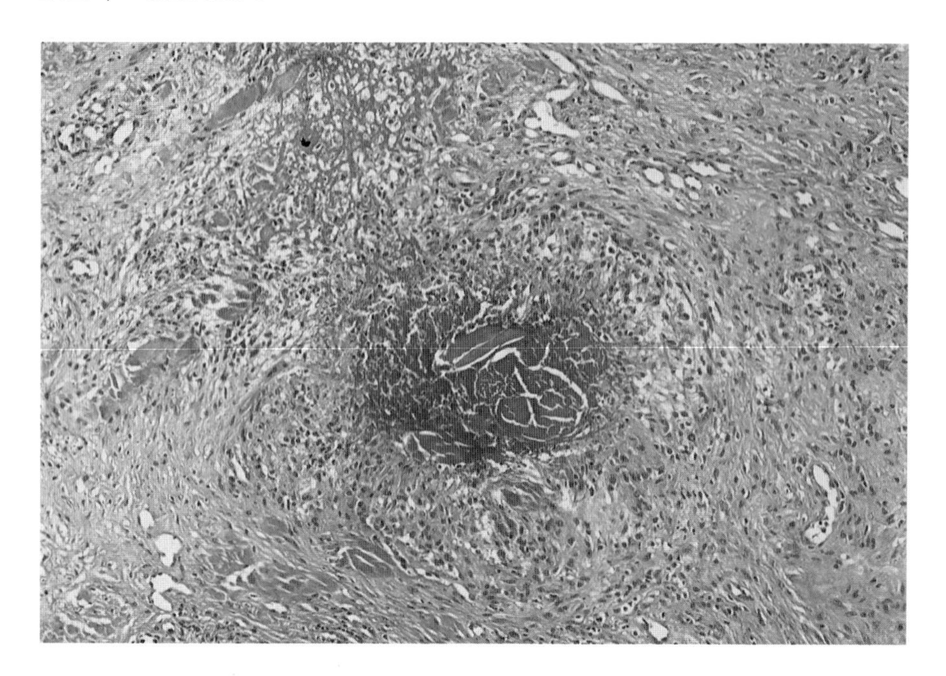

FIG. 8-14. Palisading necrotizing granuloma
An area of fibrinoid dermal necrosis is surrounded by epithelioid histiocytes.

series of 106 patients with WG, sera from 88% of the patients with active disease and 43% of the patients in remission were positive for antiserine proteinase (c-ANCA).

Histopathology. The majority of skin biopsies in patients with WG show nonspecific histopathology, and not all of them are directly related to the pathophysiology of WG.[45] Such nonspecific reaction patterns include perivascular lymphocytic infiltrates. However, in about 25 to 50% of patients, cutaneous lesions have fairly characteristic histopathologic findings. The more frequent distinct reaction patterns include necrotizing/leukocytoclastic small-vessel vasculitis and granulomatous inflammation.[45,46] True granulomatous vasculitis, palisading necrotizing granulomas (Fig. 8-14), or erythema-nodosum-like reaction patterns appear to be rare. In a recent clinicopathologic study of 46 patients with WG, the authors suggested that cutaneous findings characteristic of WG might correlate with disease activity, distribution, and course. The patients with leukocytoclastic vasculitis of the skin tended to have more aggressive courses than patients with cutaneous granulomatous inflammation. LCV commonly presented as palpable purpura or papulonecrotic lesions on the lower extremities. Its presence was often associated with active multiorgan disease. However, patients with cutaneous LCV and limited disease forms also have been reported.

Patients with granulomatous inflammation tended to be younger and to have visceral manifestations of WG less frequently than patients with leukocytoclastic vasculitis, and the disease progressed more slowly in the patients with granulomatous inflammation. However, the presence of granulomatous inflammation does not ensure a benign course, because such findings have also been reported in patients with severe multiorgan WG, thereby giving the inflammatory pattern only limited prognostic value. Both granulomatous inflammation and necrotizing vasculitis may also coexist, particularly in cutaneous ulcers and cutaneous/subcutaneous nodules.

Differential Diagnosis. Both CSS and WG have in common the presence of necrotizing vasculitis and the likelihood of necrotizing granulomatous tissue reactions. The distinction between the two diseases relies primarily on the clinical findings. In contrast to WG, CSS is associated with asthma, lacks lesions in the upper respiratory tract, rarely shows severe renal involvement, and typically is accompanied by eosinophilia or eosinophilic infiltrates and p-ANCA-positivity.

MISCELLANEOUS CONDITIONS WITH USUALLY LIMITED VASCULAR DAMAGE

Pigmented Purpuric Dermatitis

Historically, four variants of purpura pigmentosa chronica have been described: purpura annularis telangiectoides of Majocchi, progressive pigmentary dermatosis of Schamberg, pigmented purpuric dermatitis of Gougerot and Blum, and eczematoid-like purpura of Doucas and Kapentanakis. They are all closely related and often cannot be reliably distinguished on clinical and histologic grounds.[47] Therefore, their classification as distinct entities is not necessary. It is likely that lichen aureus is a closely related variant as well, because the clinical lesion suggests a purpuric component and the histologic findings are similar to those of the other four variants of pigmented purpuric dermatitis (PPD). The general terms "pigmented purpuric dermatitis," "chronic purpuric dermatitis," and "purpura pigmentosa chronica" appear suitable for this disease spectrum.

Clinically, the primary lesion consists of discrete puncta. Gradually, telangiectatic puncta may appear as a result of capillary dilatation, and pigmentation as a result of hemosiderin deposits. In some cases, telangiectasia (Majocchi's disease) predominates; in others, pigmentation (Schamberg's disease) predominates. In Majocchi's disease, the lesions are usually irregular in shape and occur predominantly on the lower legs. In some cases, the findings may mimic those of stasis. Not infrequently, clinical signs of inflammation are present, such as erythema, papules, and scaling (Gougerot-Blum disease) or papules, scaling, and lichenification (eczematoid-like purpura). The disorder is often limited to the lower extremities, but it may be extensive. Mild pruritus may be present. These are no systemic symptoms related to this disease process. Some cases of chronic purpuric dermatitis may be related to a hypersensitivity reaction to drugs. However, in the majority of cases, the etiology of this process is unclear. Eruptions with the clinical and histologic appearance of a pigmented purpuric dermatitis have also been associated with subsequent development of a T-cell lymphoproliferative disorder in some patients. Thus, it is possible that some PPD may be the initial manifestation of T-cell lymphoproliferative disease.[48]

A localized variant of PPD is lichen aureus, in which one or a few patches are present, most commonly on the legs.[49] The patches are composed of closely set, flat papules of a rust, copper, or orange color. In some cases, petechiae are present within the patches. Lichen aureus shows a male predilection and a peak incidence in the fourth decade. The lesions of lichen aureus tend to persist. They typically occur on the lower legs, but may affect many other sites.

Histopathology. The basic process is a lymphocytic perivascular infiltrate limited to the papillary dermis (Fig. 8-15). Epidermal alterations may include slight acanthosis and basal layer vacuolopathy. There is also some variability in the pattern of the dermal infiltrate. In some instances, the infiltrate may assume a bandlike or lichenoid pattern, particularly in the lichenoid variant of Gougerot-Blum disease, and may involve the reticular dermis in a perivascular distribution. Evidence of vascular damage may be present, and the reaction pattern may then be termed lymphocytic vasculopathy, vasculitis, or capillaritis. However, the extent of vascular injury is usually mild and often insufficient to justify the term "vasculitis." Vascular damage commonly consists only of endothelial cell swelling and dermal hemorrhage. Extravasated red blood cells are usually found in the vicinity of the capillaries. However, less commonly one may observe deposition of fibrinoid material in vessel walls. In some instances, the infiltrate involves the epidermis and may be associated with mild spongiosis and patchy parakeratosis. This is observed particularly in some cases of pigmented purpuric lichenoid dermatitis of Gougerot and Blum and eczematoid-like purpura of Doucas and Kapetanakis. The pattern of the infiltrate often is not strictly confined to the perivascular area and may infiltrate the adjacent papillary dermis (between vessels).

In old lesions, the capillaries often show dilatation of their lumen and proliferation of their endothelium. Extravasated red blood cells may no longer be present, but one frequently finds hemosiderin, although in varying amounts. The inflammatory infiltrate is less pronounced than in the early stage.

In lichen aureus, a dense lymphohistiocytic infiltrate is present in the superficial dermis, typically distributed in a bandlike fashion and often associated with an increase in dermal capillaries. Exocytosis of mononuclear cells into the epidermis may be seen. Scattered within the infiltrate are hemosiderin-laden macrophages (Fig. 8-16). The absence or near absence of Civatte bodies or basal layer vasculopathy facilitates the differential diagnosis from lichenoid dermatitides, such as lichen planus.

Differential Diagnosis. PPD may resemble stasis dermatitis because inflammation, dilatation of capillaries, extravasation of erythrocytes, and deposits of hemosiderin occur in both. However, in stasis dermatitis, the process extends much deeper into the dermis, and more pronounced epidermal changes and fibrosis of the dermis are usually present. Changes of intravascular red blood cell sludge and some fibrin deposits also may be seen in stasis, indicating a low flow state. As mentioned earlier, the histologic pattern of PPD may resemble or possibly be an abnormal T-cell process. Careful evaluation of the lesion for epidermotropism and lymphoid atypia, and (of particular importance) good clinicopathologic correlation, are needed to arrive at the correct diagnosis. However, suspicious or equivocal lesions require monitoring and possibly further evaluation for possible progression to cutaneous T-cell lymphoma.

Pathogenesis. The etiology of PPD is essentially unknown, and there are probably several different factors involved. In some instances, PPD is related to drugs and might be interpreted as a hypersensitivity reaction.[50] Some degree of venous insufficiency or stasis is present in many patients with PPD and is likely to be

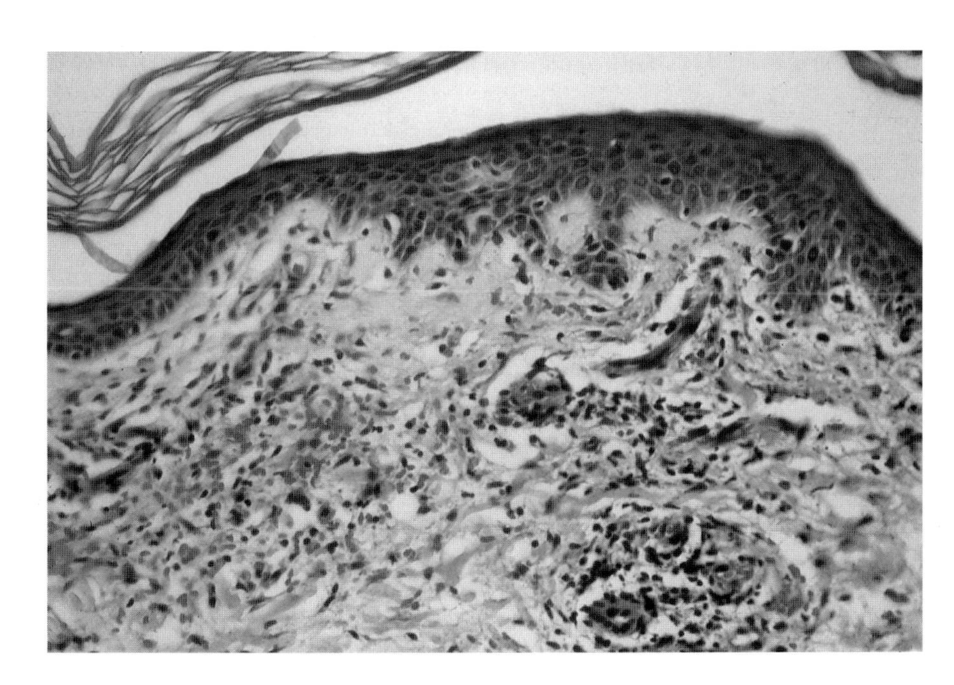

FIG. 8-15. Pigmented purpuric dermatitis
A papillary dermal lymphocytic perivascular infiltrate and extravasation of red blood cells can be seen.

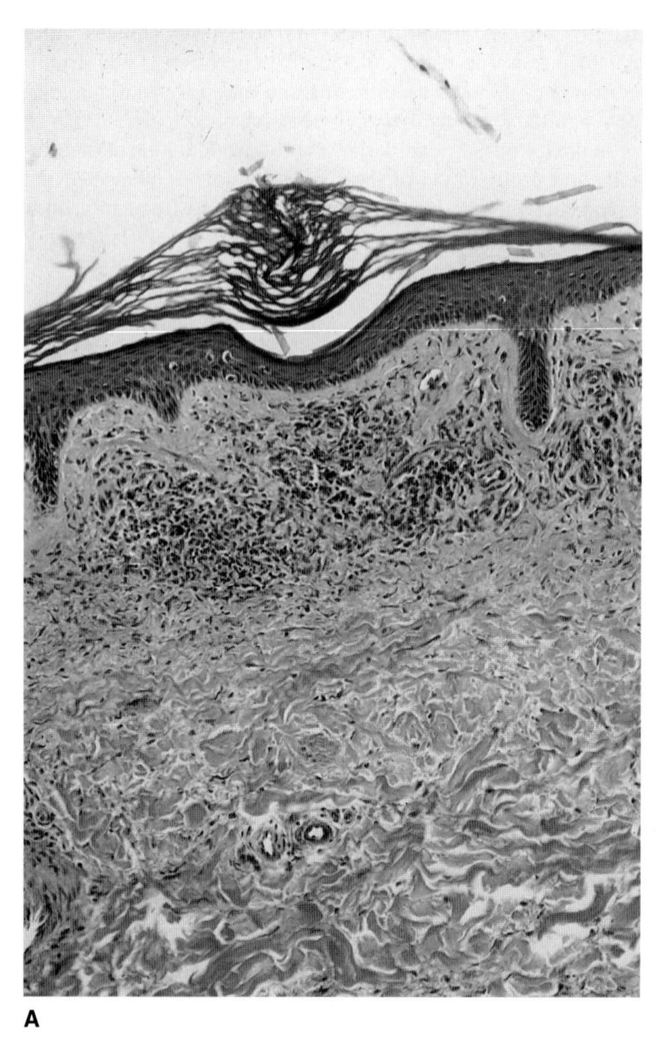

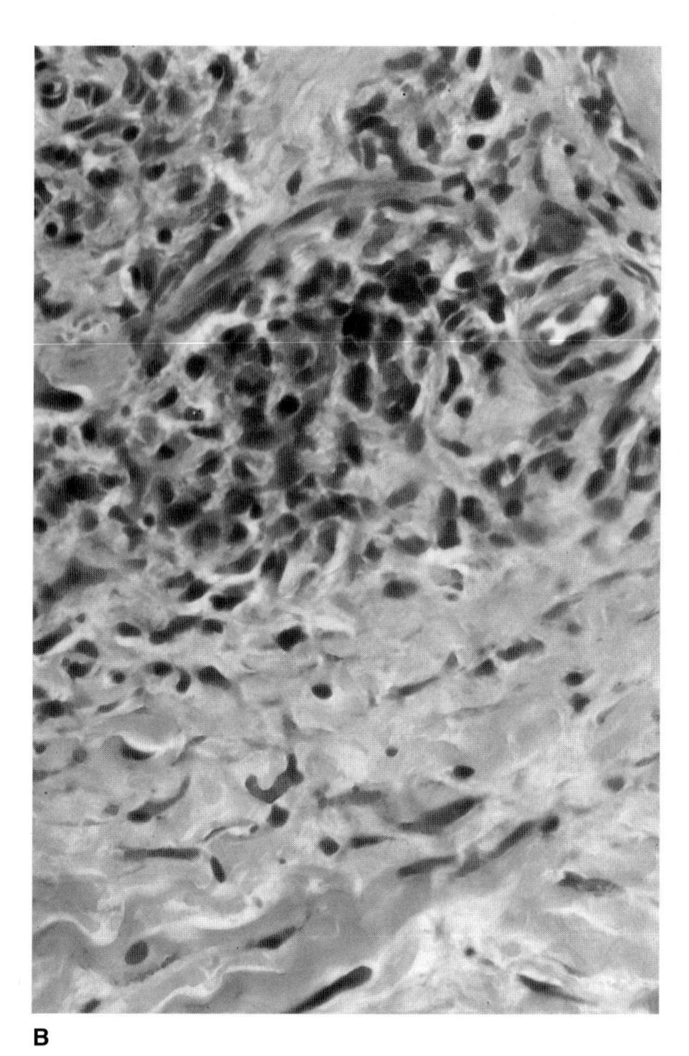

A B

FIG. 8-16. Pigmented purpuric dermatitis
A papillary dermal lymphocytic infiltrate, hemorrhage (**A**), and prominent hemosiderin deposition (**B**) are in evidence.

a factor in the development of PPD in some individuals.[51] As mentioned above, PPD (or a PPD supplement) may represent one of the early presentations of T-cell lymphoproliferative disease.[49] However, this notion requires further study with adequate numbers of patients and long-term follow-up.

Neutrophilic Vascular Reactions

In many clinical conditions, there are reactions characterized by a neutrophilic infiltrate, sometimes even with leukocytoclasis, and some vascular damage (Fig. 8-17).[34] However, the extent of vascular damage is insufficient for necrotizing vasculitis—that is, fibrinoid necrosis is lacking. Such a reaction may need to be distinguished from necrotizing vasculitis, although occasionally it may be seen in a lesion that would eventually manifest or might have manifested fully developed necrotizing vasculitis. It might also be seen in diseases that rarely develop necrotizing vasculitis and may more adequately be categorized within the spectrum of neutrophilic dermatoses or Sweet's-like dermatoses (see later).

Neutrophilic Dermatoses

The term "neutrophilic dermatosis" includes several conditions characterized histologically by (1) a neutrophilic infiltrate, (2) a lack of microorganisms on special stains and cultures, and (3) clinical improvement on systemic steroid treatment.[52] Vascular damage has been observed in these conditions, but it remains unclear whether the vascular injury plays an etiologic role or is merely an epiphenomenon.

Acute Febrile Neutrophilic Dermatosis (Classic Sweet's Syndrome)

Dr. R. D. Sweet described in 1964 a disease process, which he termed "acute febrile neutrophilic dermatosis," that was characterized by acute onset of fever, leukocytosis, and erythematous plaques infiltrated by neutrophils.[52,53] This condition typically occurs in middle-aged women after nonspecific infections of the respiratory or gastrointestinal tract. The lesions tend to be found on the face or extremities and only rarely involve the

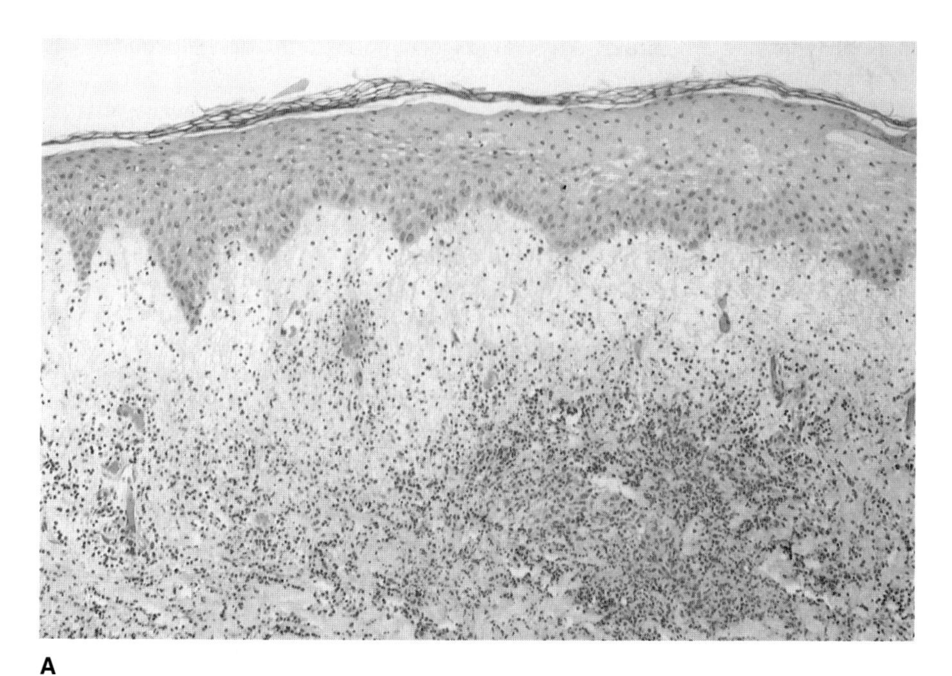

A

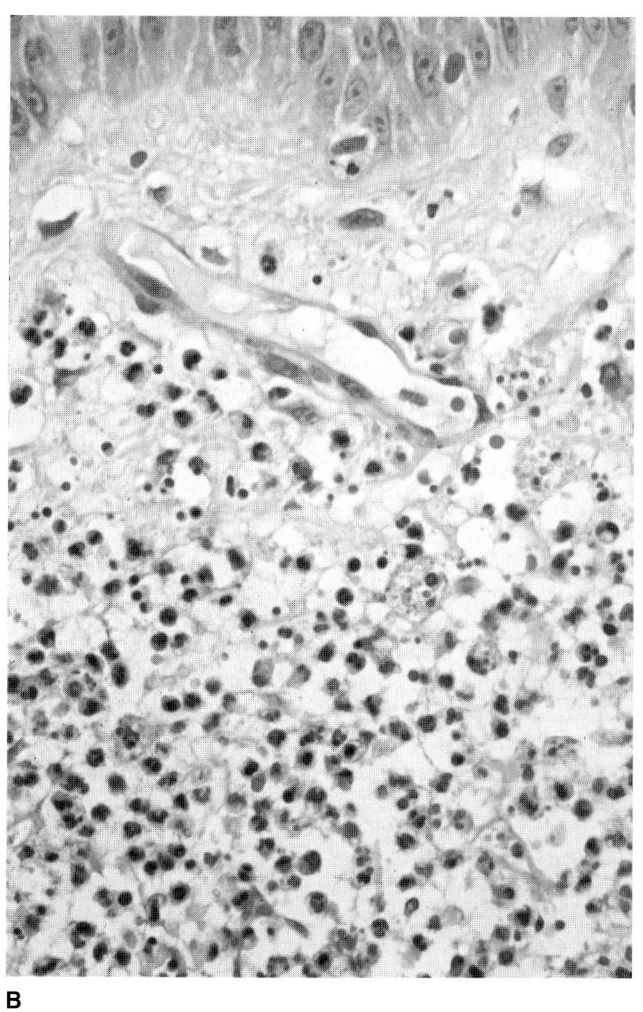

B

FIG. 8-17. Sweet's syndrome
Marked dermal edema (**A**) and a prominent infiltrate primarily composed of neutrophils (**B**) are visible.

trunk. The clinical spectrum of the eruption also may include vesicles and pustules. Involvement of noncutaneous sites, such as eyes, joints, oral mucosa, and visceral sites (lungs, liver, kidneys), has been reported.[53]

Histopathology. There is a dense perivascular infiltrate composed largely of neutrophils (see Fig. 8-17). Some of the neutrophils may show nuclear fragmentation (leukocytoclasis). In addition, there are some mononuclear cells, such as lymphocytes and histiocytes, and occasional eosinophils. The inflammatory cells typically assume a bandlike distribution throughout the papillary dermis. The density of the infiltrate varies and may be limited in a small proportion of cases. There is usually vasodilation and swelling of endothelium with moderate erythrocyte extravasation, and prominent edema of the upper dermis, which in some instances may result in subepidermal blister formation. Extensive vascular damage is not a feature of Sweet's syndrome. The histologic appearance varies depending on the stage of the process. In later stages, lymphocytes and histiocytes may predominate.

Pathogenesis. The disease is thought to be a hypersensitivity reaction, but its etiology is unknown. The three major concepts that have been discussed are immune-complex vasculitis, altered T-cell activation, and altered function of neutrophils.[53] All of them, however, lack sufficient experimental support.

Sweet's-like Neutrophilic Dermatoses

In addition to classic Sweet's syndrome, sterile lesions with neutrophilic infiltrates that improve on steroid treatment can be found in a variety of other clinical conditions (Jorizzo et al; von den Driesch). Such infiltrates can be associated with inflammatory diseases such as autoimmune disorders or with recovery from infection. They may also develop in patients with hemoproliferative disorders or solid tumors, as well as in pregnant women. Many clinicians extend the initial designation of the term "Sweet's syndrome" to include all the different clinical settings in which a Sweet's-like neutrophilic dermatosis may develop.

Clinically, there is typically an abrupt onset of tender or painful erythematous plaques or nodules occasionally with vesicles, pustules, or bullae. Patients tend to have elevated ESR and peripheral leukocytosis generally above 8000 with more than 70% neutrophils. The response to treatment with systemic steroids or potassium iodide is usually excellent.

Histopathology. Histologically, there is a predominantly neutrophilic dermal infiltrate as described for classic Sweet's syndrome. However, depending on the stage of the disease and the adequacy of the sampling, the findings of the biopsy may vary greatly. The reaction pattern may on occasion be quite different from that described for classic Sweet's syndrome. It may, for example, manifest as deep subcutaneous localized suppurative panniculitis. It is important for any pathologist to realize that histologically, the composition and distribution of the infiltrate are not specific enough to rule out an infectious process. Therefore, to arrive at the correct interpretation of a neutrophilic infiltrate, cultures need to be obtained and special stains need to be performed to investigate a potential infectious etiology.

Bowel-Associated Dermatosis-Arthritis Syndrome

This syndrome was initially described in patients after jejunoileal bypass surgery. Subsequently, however, the spectrum of the syndrome has expanded to include other disease processes with typical cutaneous findings and associated bowel disease.[11] Patients may have inflammatory bowel disease or a blind loop after peptic ulcer surgery. The cutaneous lesions are characterized by initial small macules that develop through a papular phase into pustules on a purpuric base. The evolution usually occurs within a 2-day period. The lesions typically reach a size of 0.5 to 1.5 cm. They are typically distributed on the upper part of the body, especially the arms, rather than on the dependent sites of the legs. Cutaneous lesions often occur in crops and are episodical (1 to 2 weeks), with a tendency to recur within months. Fever, myalgias, and arthralgias may accompany the disease process.

Histopathology. The histopathologic changes are usually those of neutrophilic vascular reactions with little or none of the vascular damage observed in Sweet's syndrome and other neutrophilic dermatoses. However, frank necrotizing small-vessel vasculitis may occasionally be noted. In fully developed lesions, the neutrophilic infiltrate and papillary dermal edema may be florid, and subepidermal pustule formation is seen. If vascular damage is observed in such a context, the "term pustular vasculitis" is applied.

Pathogenesis. It has been suggested that antigens derived from intestinal bacteria trigger an immune-complex-mediated reaction with vascular insults.[54]

Pyoderma Gangrenosum

Pyoderma gangrenosum is included in this chapter as well, because in these and other authors' opinions, it represents a clinicopathologic manifestation that falls within the spectrum of neutrophilic dermatoses.[11] As with other neutrophilic dermatoses, it is critical to rule out infection in order to arrive at the correct diagnosis.

Clinically, lesions begin as tender papulopustules or folliculitis that eventually may ulcerate. In the fully developed stage, the lesions are clinically distinct. They have a raised, undermined border, which has a dusky purple hue. Again, as with neutrophilic dermatoses in general, pyoderma gangrenosum may occur as an isolated cutaneous phenomenon or may be a cutaneous manifestation associated with various systemic disease processes, such as inflammatory bowel disease, connective tissue diseases, and lymphoproliferative lesions.

Histopathology. The histologic findings are nonspecific and the diagnosis is primarily clinical. Most authors studying early lesions have reported a primarily neutrophilic infiltrate, which frequently involves follicular structures.[55] Others, however, have stated that the lesions begin with a lymphocytic reaction.[56] Degrees of vessel involvement range from none to fibrinoid necrosis. In the majority of biopsied lesions, a neutrophilic infiltrate is present with some, but limited, vascular damage. Outright vasculitis has been reported and has led to speculations about its possible role in the etiology of pyoderma gangrenosum. Focal vasculitis is often observed in fully developed lesions, but appears secondary to the inflammatory process. The infiltrate tends to be deeper and more extensive than that in classic Sweet's syndrome. The pattern of pustular vasculitis may be present. Fully developed lesions exhibit ulceration, necrosis, and a mixed inflammatory cell infiltrate. Involvement of the deep reticular dermis and subcutis may exhibit primarily mononuclear cell and granulomatous inflammatory reactions.

Granuloma Faciale

Another condition that is often associated with neutrophilic vascular reactions is granuloma faciale (GF).[57] GF presents clinically as one or several asymptomatic, soft, brown-red, slowly enlarging papules or plaques, almost always on the face.

Histopathology. A dense polymorphous infiltrate is present (Fig. 8-18) mainly in the upper half of the dermis, but it may extend into the lower dermis and occasionally even into the subcutaneous tissue. Quite characteristically, the infiltrate does not invade the epidermis or the pilosebaceous appendages but is separated from them by a narrow "grenz" zone of normal collagen. The pilosebaceous structures tend to remain intact. The polymorphous infiltrate consists in large part of neutrophils and eosinophils, but mononuclear cells, plasma cells, and mast cells are also present. Frequently, the nuclei of some of the neutrophils are fragmented, especially in the vicinity of the capillaries, thus forming nuclear dust. Often there is some evidence of vasculitis with deposition of fibrinoid material within and around vessel walls. Occasionally, some hemorrhage is noted. Foam cells are sometimes observed as well as areas of fibrosis in older lesions.

Pathogenesis. Direct immunofluorescence data suggest an immune-complex-mediated event with deposition of mainly IgG in and around vessels.[58]

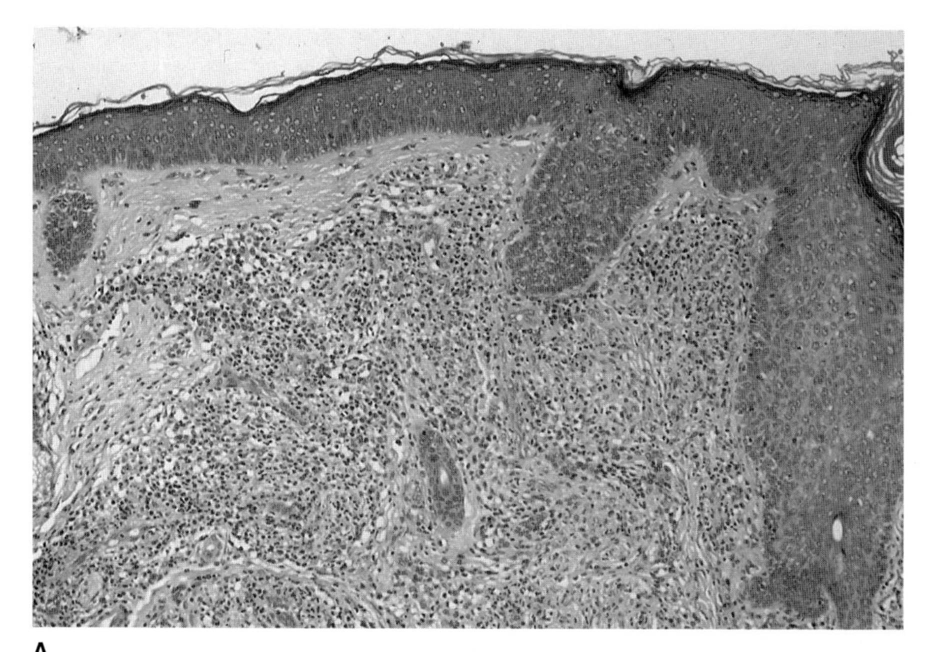

A

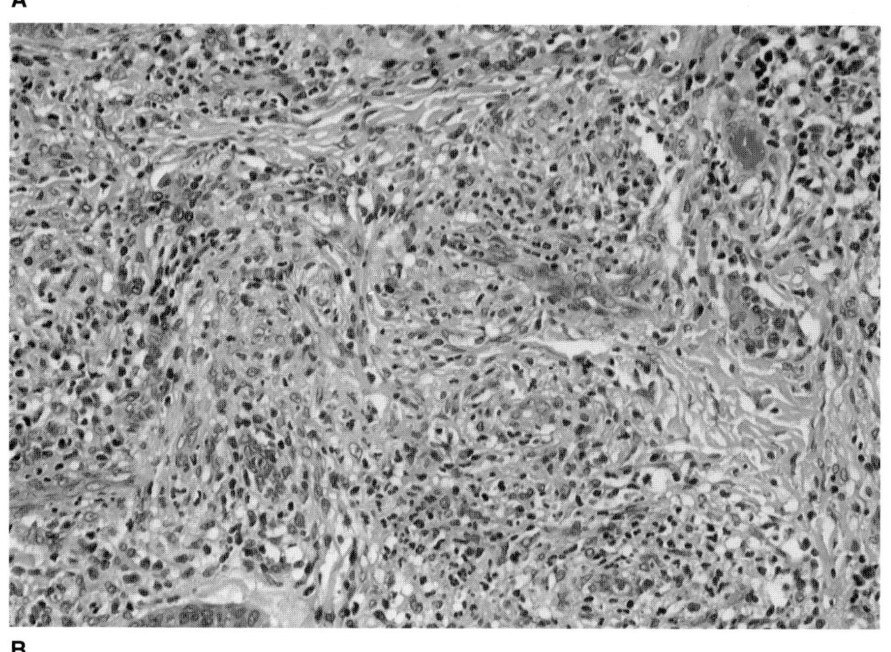

B

FIG. 8-18. Granuloma faciale
Note small grenz zone between epidermis and dermal mixed inflammatory cell infiltrate (**A**), composed of neutrophils, eosinophils, lymphocytes, and histocytes (**B**).

REFERENCES

1. Robboy SJ, Mihm MC, Colman RC et al. The skin in disseminated intravascular coagulation. Br J Dermatol 1973;88:221.
2. Falanga V, Fine MJ, Kapoor WN. The cutaneous manifestations of cholesterol crystal embolization. Arch Dermatol 1986;122:1194.
3. Walker A. Chronic scurvy. Br J Dermatol 1968;80:625.
4. Sneddon IB. Cerebro-vascular lesions and livedos reticularis. Br J Dermatol 1975;77:180.
5. Stiefler RE, Bergfeld WF. Atrophie blanche (review). Int J Dermatol 1982;21:1.
6. Shornick JK, Nichoces BK, Bergstresser PR et al. Idiopathic atrophie blanche. J Am Acad Dermatol 1983;8:792.
7. McCalmont CS, McCalmont TH, Jorizzo JC et al. Livedo vasculitis: Vasculitis or thrombotic vasculopathy? Clin Exp Dermatol 1992;17:4.
8. Degos R, Delort J, Tricot R. Dermatite papulo-squameuse atrophiante. Bull Soc Fr Dermatol Syphiligr 1942;49:148, 281.
9. Doutre MS, Beylot C, Bioulac P et al. Skin lesion resembling malignant atrophic papulosis in lupus erythematosus. Dermatologica 1987;175: 45.
10. Magrinat G, Kerwin KS, Gabriel DA. The clinical manifestations of Degos' syndrome. Arch Pathol Lab Med 1989;113:354.
11. Callen JP. Cutaneous vasculitis: Relationship to systemic disease and therapy. Curr Probl Dermatol 1993;5:45.
12. Fauci AS. The spectrum of vasculitis. Ann Intern Med 1978;89:660.
13. Jennette JC, Falk RJ, Andrassy K et al. Nomenclature of systemic vasculitides: Proposal of an international consensus conference. Arthritis Rheum 1994;37:187.
14. Jennette JC. Vasculitis affecting the skin. Arch Dermatol 1994;130:899.
15. Jennette JC, Falk RJ. Diagnostic classification of antineutrophil cytoplasmic autoantibody-associated vasculitides. Am J Kidney Dis 1991; 16:184.
16. Jennette JC, Falk RJ. Anti-neutrophil cytoplasmic antibodies and associated diseases: A review. Am J Kidney Dis 1990;15:517.
17. Goeken J. Antineutrophil cytoplasmic and anti-endothelial cell antibodies: New mechanisms for vasculitis. Curr Opin Dermatol 1995;19: 75.
18. Diaz-Perez JL, Winkelman RK. Cutaneous periarteritis nodosa. Arch Dermatol 1974;110:407.
19. Baum EW, Sams WM Jr, Payne RR. Giant cell arteritis: A systemic disease with rare cutaneous manifestations. J Am Acad Dermatol 1982; 6:1081.
20. Kussmaul A, Maier K. Ueber eine bisher nicht beschriebene eigenthümliche Arterienerkrankung (Periarteriitis nodosa), die mit Morbus Brightii und rapid fortschreitender allgemeiner Muskellähmung einhergeht. Dtsch Arch Klin Med 1866;1:484.
21. Ferrari E. Veber polylarteritis acuta nodosa (sogerannte periarteritis nodosa) undihre Beziehurgen zur polymyositis and polyneuritis acuta. Beitr Pathol Anat 1903;34:350.
22. Zeek PM. Periarteritis nodosa and other forms of necrotizing angiitis. N Engl J Med 1953;248:764.
23. Davson J, Ball J, Platt R. The kidney in periarteritis nodosa. Q J Med 1948;17:175.
24. deShazo RD, Levinson AI, Lawless OJ, Weisbaum G. Systemic vasculitis with co-existent large and small vessel involvement: A classification dilemma. JAMA 1977;238:1940.
25. Landing BH, Larson EJ. Pathologic features of Kawasaki disease (mucocutaneous lymph node syndrome). Am J Cardiovasc Pathol 1987; 4:75.
26. Johnson WC, Wallrich R, Helwig EB. Superficial thrombophlebitis of the chest wall. JAMA 1962;180:103.
27. Mills JA, Michael BA, Bloch DA et al. The American College of Rheumatology 1990 criteria for the classification of Henoch-Schönlein purpura. Arthritis Rheum 1990;33:1114.
28. Jennette JC, Wieslander J, Tuttle R, Falk RJ. Serum IgA-fibronectin aggregates in patients with IgA nephropathy and Henoch-Schönlein purpura: Diagnostic valve and pathogenic implications. The glomerulor disease collaborative network. Am J Kidney Dis 1991;18:466.
29. Mehregan DR, Hall MJ, Gibson LE. Urticarial vasculitis: A histopathologic and clinical review of 72 cases. J Am Acad Dermatol 1992;26: 441.
30. Cohen SJ, Pittelkow MR, Su WP. Cutaneous manifestations of cryoglobulinemia: Clinical and histopathologic study of 72 patients. J Am Acad Dermatol 1992;26:38.
31. Patel A, Prussick R, Buchanan WW, Sauder DN. Serum sickness-like illness and leukocytoclastic vasculitis after intravenous streptolinase. J Am Acad Dermatol 1991;24:652.
32. Lakhanpal S, Conn DL, Lie JT. Clinical and prognostic significance of vasculitis as early manifestation of connective tissue disease syndromes. Ann Intern Med 1984;101:743.
33. Sanchez-Guerro J, Gutierrez-Urena S, Vidaller A et al. Vasculitis as a paraneoplastic syndrome: Report of 11 cases and review of the literature. J Rheumatol 1990;17:1458.
34. Jorizzo JL, Solomon AR, Zanolli MD et al. Neutrophilic vascular reactions. Arch Dermatol 1988;19:983.
35. LeBoit PE, Yen TSB, Wintroub B. The evolution of lesions in erythema elevatum diutinum. Am J Dermatopathol 1986;8:392.
36. Massa MC, Su WPD. Lymphocytic vasculitis: Is it a specific clinicopathologic entity? J Cutan Pathol 1984;11:132.
37. Thomas R, Vuitch F, Lakhanpl S. Angiocentric T-cell lymphoma masquerading as cutaneous vasculitis. J Rheumatol 1994;21:760.
38. Churg J, Strauss L. Allergic granulomatosis, allergic angiitis, and periarteritis nodosa. Am J Pathol 1951;27:277.
39. Lanham JG, Elkon KB, Pusey CD, Hughes GR. Systemic vasculitis with asthma and eosinophilia: A clinical approach to Churg-Strauss syndrome. Medicine (Baltimore) 1984;63:65.
40. Chumbley LC, Harrison EG Jr, Dereme RA. Allergic granulomatosis and angiitis (Churg-Strauss syndrome): Report and analysis of 30 cases. Mayo Clin Proc 1977;52:477.
41. Finan MC, Winkelman RK. The cutaneous extravascular necrotizing granuloma (Churg-Strauss granuloma) and systemic disease: A review of 27 cases. Medicine (Baltimore) 1983;62:142.
42. Goodman GC, Churg J. Wegener's granulomatosis. Arch Pathol 1954; 58:533.
43. Liebow AA, Carrington CB. Hypersensitivity reactions involving the lung. Trans Stud Coll Physicians Phila 1966;34:47.
44. Deremee RA, McDonald TJ, Harrison EG Jr et al. Wegener's granulomatosis. Mayo Clin Proc 1976;51:777.
45. Barksdale SK, Hallahan CW, Kerr GS et al. Cutaneous pathology in Wegener's granulomatosis. Am J Surg Pathol 1995;19:161.
46. Fauci AS, Wolff SM. Wegener's granulomatosis: Studies in 18 patients and a review of the literature. Medicine (Baltimore) 1973;52:535.
47. Randall SJ, Kierland RR, Montgomery H. Pigmented purpuric eruptions. Arch Dermatol Syphiligr 1951;64:177.
48. Barnhill RL, Braverman IM. Progression of pigmented purpura-like eruptions to mycosis fungoides: Report of three cases. J Am Acad Dermatol 1988;19:25.
49. Waisman M, Waisman M. Lichen aureus. Arch Dermatol 1976;112: 696.
50. Zaun H. Hemorrhagic pigmentary dermatoses. Z Hautkr 1987;62:1485.
51. Shelley WB, Swaminathan R, Shelley ED. Lichen aureus: A hemosiderin tattoo associated with perforator vein incompetence. J Am Acad Dermatol 1984;11:260.
52. Von Den Driesch P. Sweet's syndrome: Acute febrile neutrophilic dermatosis. J Am Acad Dermatol 1994;31:535.
53. Sweet RD. Acute febrile neutrophilic dermatosis. Br J Dermatol 1964; 74:349.
54. Ely PH. The bowel bypass syndrome: A response to bacterial peptidoglycans. J Am Acad Dermatol 1980;2:473.
55. Holt PJA, Davis MG, Saunders KC, Nuki G. Pyoderma gangrenosum. Medicine (Baltimore) 1980;59:114.
56. Su WP, Schroeter AL, Perry HO, Powell FC. Histopathologic and immunopathologic study of pyoderma gangrenosum. J Cutan Pathol 1986; 13:323.
57. Pinkus H. Granuloma faciale. Dermatologica 1952;105:85.
58. Nieboer C, Kalsbeek GL. Immunofluorescence studies in granuloma eosinophilicum faciale. J Cutan Pathol 1977;4:123.

Lever's Histopathology of the Skin, eighth edition, edited by David Elder et al. Lippincott–Raven Publishers, Philadelphia © 1997.

CHAPTER 9

Noninfectious Vesiculobullous and Vesiculopustular Diseases

Lisa M. Cohen, Debra Karp Skopicki, Terence J. Harrist, and Wallace H. Clark Jr.

CLASSIFICATION OF BLISTERS

Definition

A blister is a fluid-filled cavity formed within or beneath the epidermis. The fluid consists of tissue fluid, plasma, and a variable component of inflammatory cells. Blisters may occur in many dermatoses. At first glance, this observation seems to imply that blistering is too general or nonspecific for use in clinical gross evaluation. However, the character of blisters in a given disorder tends to be uniform and to have reproducible characteristics. One useful distinction is the categorization of blisters into *vesicles* (blisters less than 0.5 cm in diameter) and *bullae* (blisters greater than 0.5 cm in diameter). For example, vesicles characteristically occur in dermatitis herpetiformis as opposed to pemphigoid, in which bullae are most commonly observed.

Mechanisms of Blister Formation

The mechanisms for some diseases are shown in Table 9-1. *Spongiosis* is the accumulation of extracellular fluid within the epidermis with resultant separation of the keratinocytes. Pronounced spongiosis leads to disruption of desmosomes and subsequent blister formation. Thus the epidermis has a "spongy" appearance microscopically and the increasing accumulation of fluid leads to a vesicle and, in some instances, to a bulla. Spongiosis is almost always associated with an infiltrate of lymphocytes within the epidermis and around superficial vessels.

Acantholysis results from the loss of appropriate keratinocyte cell-cell contact. Histologic evidence of acantholysis includes the presence of rounded keratinocytes with condensed cytoplasm and large nuclei with peripheral condensation of chromatin and prominent nucleoli.

Reticular degeneration results from ballooning degeneration (intracellular edema) with secondary rupture of the keratinocytes. The remaining desmosomal attachments often connect strands of cytoplasm to intact keratinocytes, giving the epidermis an irregular meshwork appearance.

Cytolysis is the disruption of keratinocytes. It occurs in the normal epidermis when the structural (keratin) matrix of the keratinocyte is overwhelmed by high levels of physical agents such as friction and heat. Friction (mechanical energy applied parallel to the epidermis) leads to the shearing of keratinocytes one from another and of the keratinocytes themselves, giving the characteristic clear, fluid-filled blisters. Minimal friction may lead to cytolysis in subjects whose keratinocytes do not have a normal structural matrix, such as in epidermolysis bullosa simplex and epidermolysis bullosa of the Cockayne-Weber type.

Basement membrane zone disruption or destruction results from primary structural deficiencies as well as from both humoral and cellular immunologically mediated damage. When blisters arise at the epidermal basement membrane zone, any of the specific subanatomic compartments can be affected: (1) the basal keratinocytes, in particular their lower portions; (2) the lamina lucida, an electron lucid area immediately subjacent to the plasma membrane; (3) the lamina densa, composed principally of type IV collagen; and (4) the sublamina densa zone.

L. M. Cohen: Associate Pathologist, Pathology Services, Inc., Cambridge, MA; Associate Pathologist, Beth Israel Hospital, Department of Pathology, Boston, MA; Instructor of Pathology, Harvard Medical School, Boston, MA

D. K. Skopicki: Fellow in Dermatopathology, Beth Israel Hospital/Pathology Services, Inc., Division of Harvard Medical School Dermatopathology Fellowship Program

T. J. Harrist: Medical Director, Pathology Services, Inc., Cambridge, MA; Assistant Professor of Pathology, Harvard Medical School, Boston, MA; Associate Pathologist, Beth Israel Hospital, Department of Pathology, Boston, MA; Director, Beth Israel Hospital/Pathology Services, Inc., Division of Harvard Medical School Dermatopathology Fellowship Program

W. H. Clark Jr.: Consultant in Residence, Pathology Services, Inc., Cambridge, MA; Senior Pathologist, Beth Israel Hospital, Department of Pathology, Boston, MA; Professor of Pathology, Harvard Medical School, Boston, MA

TABLE 9-1. *Some diseases and their mechanisms of blister formation*

Spongiosis	Eczematous dermatitis
	Miliaria
	Pemphigus (early)
	Transient acantholytic dermatosis (one pattern)
Acantholysis	Pemphigus
	Transient acantholytic dermatosis (some patterns)
	Hailey-Hailey disease
	Darier's disease
	Irritant dermatitis (some)
Reticular degeneration	Viral infections
	Eczematous dermatitis (late stage)
Cytolysis	Epidermolysis bullosa simplex
	Epidermolytic hyperkeratosis
	Friction blister
	Erythema multiforme (in part)
	Herpes gestationis (in part)
	Subcorneal pustular dermatosis
	Irritant dermatitis (some)
Basement membrane zone destruction	Bullous pemphigoid
	Cicatricial pemphigoid
	Epidermolysis bullosa acquisita
	Dermatitis herpetiformis
	Linear IgA dermatosis
	Epidermolysis bullosa letalis
	Epidermolysis bullosa dystrophica

Pathologic Evaluation

When blisters are encountered microscopically, systematic analysis can lead to diagnosis in most cases. The critical interpretive assessments to be approached in sequence are as follows: (1) the blister separation plane (Table 9-2), (2) the mechanism(s) of blister formation (see Table 9-1), and (3) the character of the inflammatory infiltrate, including its presence or absence, its pattern, and the specific cell types involved (Table 9-3).

Five principal problems are encountered using this algorithm. The first is that the separation plane may change as blisters age. Second, microscopic slitlike spaces occur within the epidermis in the group of clefting diseases—Darier's disease, Hailey-Hailey disease, and Grover's disease—mimicking true clinical blisters. This group of disorders, however, does not usually present clinically with blisters. Third, evaluation of routine histologic preparations may not allow one to accurately assess the specific mechanism of blister formation. This is particularly true in the subepidermal vesiculobullous disorders. Fourth, the cell types infiltrating the lesions in the vesiculobullous diseases change as the lesions age. Lastly, the histologic descriptions of many of the subepidermal blistering disorders are not accompanied by the rigorous immunological evaluation required today. Many of the subepidermal blistering disorders may strikingly mimic each other clinically, leading to inappropriate diagnosis and making the histologic descriptions in the literature suspect. With these points in mind, the specific disorders and groups of disorders will be discussed.

SPONGIOTIC DERMATITIS

Definition and Evaluation

Spongiotic dermatitis may be acute, subacute, or chronic. The process is dynamic, and each specific type of dermatitis may progress from the acute to the chronic phase. Although the term *spongiotic dermatitis* is occasionally used interchangeably

TABLE 9-2. *Some diseases with their specific separation planes*

Intraepidermal
Subcorneal/granular
Miliaria crystallina
Staphylococcal scalded skin syndrome
Pemphigus foliaceus and variants
Bullous impetigo
IgA pemphigus
Subcorneal pustular dermatosis
Erythema toxicum neonatorum
Transient neonatal pustular melanosis
Acropustulosis of infancy
Spinous
Spongiotic dermatitis
Friction blister (may extend into dermis)
Miliaria rubra
Incontinentia pigmenti
IgA pemphigus
Epidermolytic hyperkeratosis
Hailey-Hailey disease
Suprabasal
Pemphigus vulgaris and variants
Paraneoplastic pemphigus
Darier disease
Subepidermal
Basal keratinocyte necrosis, cytolysis, or damage
Epidermolysis bullosa simplex
Thermal injury (some)
Erythema multiforme
Herpes gestationis
Epidermal basement membrane zone destruction or disruption
Lamina lucida
Bullous pemphigoid
Cicatricial pemphigoid
Herpes gestationis
Dermatitis herpetiformis
Linear IgA dermatosis
Epidermolysis bullosa acquisita
Porphyria cutanea tarda
Epidermolysis bullosa letalis (junctional)
Suction blister
Thermal injury (some)
Sublamina densa
Cicatricial pemphigoid
Linear IgA dermatosis
Epidermolysis bullosa dystrophica
Epidermolysis bullosa acquisita
Bullous systemic lupus erythematosus
Dermal
Penicillamine-induced blisters (iatrogenic)

TABLE 9-3. *Principal infiltrating inflammatory cells in some vesiculobullous dermatoses**

Dermatosis	Principal cell type	Infiltrate
Porphyria		Absent
Variegate		
Cutanea tarda		
Epidermolysis bullosa acquisita (classic)		Absent
Bullous pemphigoid (cell-poor)	Eosinophils	Minimal
Spongiotic dermatitis	Lymphocytes	Present
Erythema multiforme	Lymphocytes	Present
Bullous pemphigoid (cell-rich)	Eosinophils	Present
Herpes gestationis	Eosinophils	Present
Vesiculopustular eruption with hepatobiliary disease	Neutrophils	Present
Dermatitis herpetiformis	Neutrophils	Present
Linear IgA dermatosis	Neutrophils	Present
Epidermolysis bullosa acquisita (inflammatory)	Neutrophils	Present
Bullous SLE	Neutrophils	Present
	Interface dermatitis	
Cicatricial pemphigoid	Mixed neutrophils and eosinophils	Present
	Lymphocytic, bandlike (mucosa only)	
	Eosinophils	
Epidermolysis bullosa acquisita	Mixed neutrophils and eosinophils	Present
Paraneoplastic pemphigus	Lymphocytes—interface dermatitis (lichen planus or erythema multiforme–like)	Present

* These descriptions are accurate in the vast majority of the cases in each dermatosis; however, occasionally the cell types may differ, rendering IF testing mandatory. Other inflammatory cells may be present as a minor component but on occasion are of significant number.

with *eczema*, the word *eczema* lacks specific meaning.[1] *Spongiosis* refers to the accumulation of edema fluid between keratinocytes, in some cases progressing to vesicle formation.

In *acute spongiotic dermatitis*, the stratum corneum is normal and the epidermis is of normal thickness. The degree of spongiosis is variable, extending from slight to marked, with intraepidermal vesiculation in the latter instance. The surrounding keratinocytes may be stellate, surrounded by clear spaces representing the site of fluid collection (Fig. 9-1). Papillary dermal edema is present, correlating with the degree of spongiosis. A lymphohistiocytic infiltrate is present around the superficial plexus, with exocytosis of lymphocytes into spongiotic foci.

In *subacute spongiotic dermatitis*, there is usually mild to moderate spongiosis, occasionally with microvesiculation. The epidermis is moderately acanthotic. The parakeratotic stratum corneum may contain aggregates of coagulated plasma and scattered neutrophils, forming a crust (Fig. 9-2). There is a superficial perivascular lymphohistiocytic infiltrate, which is less prominent than in the acute phase.

In *chronic dermatitis*, there is hyperkeratosis with areas of

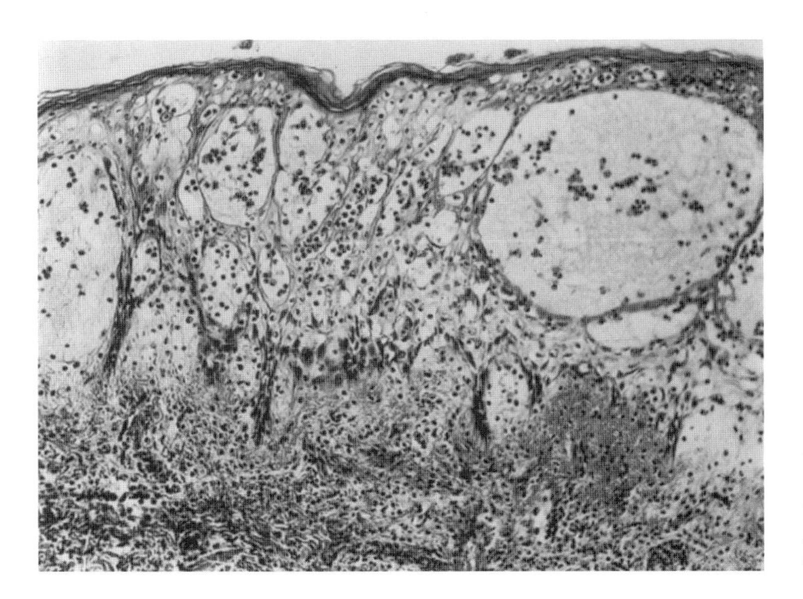

FIG. 9-1. Acute dermatitis: contact dermatitis due to poison ivy
Numerous spongiotic vesicles contain fluid and infiltrating lymphocytes. The stratum corneum is normal, and there is a generous papillary dermal lymphohistiocytic infiltrate.

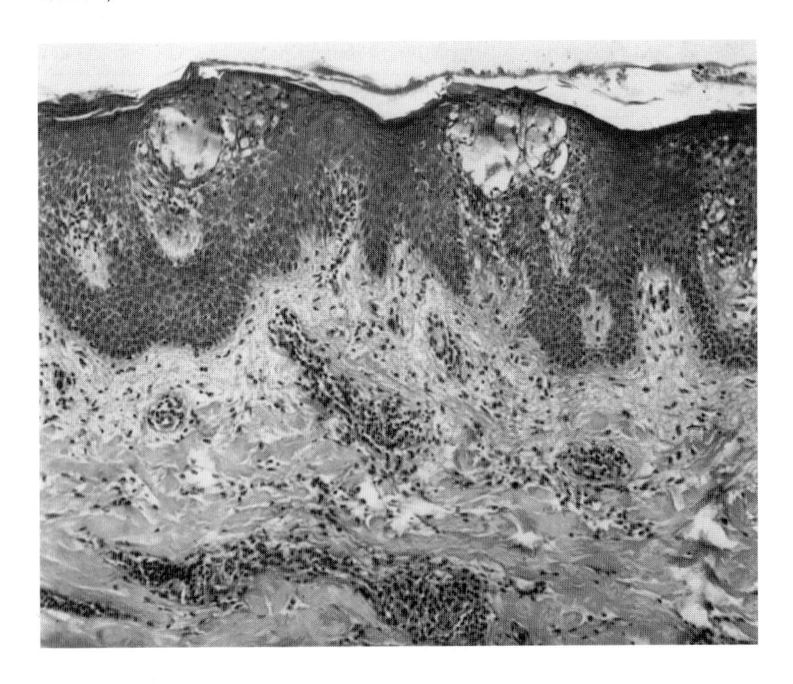

FIG. 9-2. Subacute dermatitis: nummular eczema Spongiotic microvesicles are present in a hyperplastic epidermis with a psoriasiform pattern surmounted by parakeratosis. A moderate perivascular lymphohistiocytic infiltrate is present.

parakeratosis, often hypergranulosis, and moderate to marked acanthosis (Fig. 9-3). Although spongiosis may be present focally, it is minimal. The inflammatory infiltrate is sparse, and papillary dermal fibrosis may be a prominent feature.

Specific Types of Spongiotic Dermatitis

Allergic Contact Dermatitis

The prototype of acute spongiotic dermatitis is allergic contact dermatitis, secondary to exposure to poison ivy. Usually between 24 and 72 hours after exposure to the antigen, the patient develops pruritic, edematous, erythematous papules and plaques and, in some cases, vesicles. Linear papules and vesicles are common in allergic contact dermatitis to poison ivy, reflecting the points of contact between the plant and the skin. Other common causes of allergic contact dermatitis include nickel, paraphenylenediamine, rubber compounds, fragrances, and preservatives in cosmetics. The degree of histologic alterations observed in the reactions to these antigens may be less striking than that secondary to poison ivy.

Histopathology. Early lesions are an acute spongiotic dermatitis. If vesicles develop, they may contain clusters of Langerhans cells. Eosinophils may be present in the dermal infiltrate as well as within areas of spongiosis (see Fig. 9-1). In patients with continued exposure to the antigen, the biopsy may show a subacute or later a chronic spongiotic dermatitis, often lichen simplex chronicus due to rubbing.

Pathogenesis. Allergic contact dermatitis represents a type IV, cell-mediated, delayed hypersensitivity reaction. The reaction is directed against the allergen, often a small hapten com-

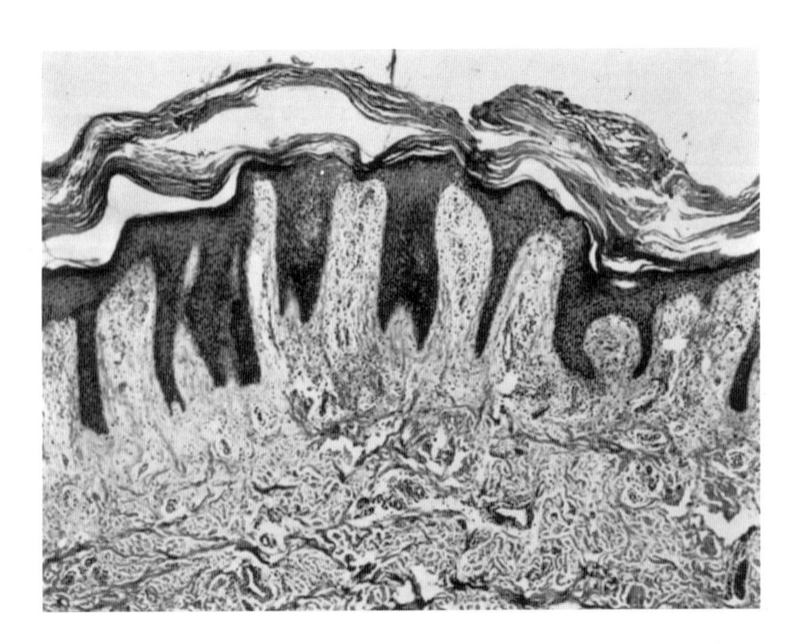

FIG. 9-3. Chronic dermatitis: lichen simplex chronicus There is hyperkeratosis and psoriasiform acanthosis with broadening of the fibrotic papillae. The thick papillary dermal collagen fibers are oriented perpendicular to the overlying epidermis. There is a scant perivascular lymphohistiocytic infiltrate.

plexed with a larger protein in the skin.[2] The immunologic reaction consists of an afferent limb, the sensitization or induction phase, and an efferent limb, the elicitation phase.

Langerhans cells are antigen-presenting cells within the epidermis that bear the receptor for the Fc portion of IgG, the receptor for the third component of complement, and class II major histocompatibility complex (MHC) antigens (HLA-D). Dermal perivascular dendritic cells also express class II MHC antigens and are capable of initiating T cell–mediated contact sensitivity. The perivascular location of these cells is ideal for presentation of antigen to T cells trafficking through the dermis. When the epidermis of mice or hamsters is temporarily deprived of functional Langerhans cells by ultraviolet radiation, contact sensitization to dinitrofluorobenzene (DNFB) does not occur.[3] In allergic contact dermatitis, Langerhans cells carry the antigen through the lymphatics to the regional lymph nodes and present the antigen to CD4+ T lymphocytes in the paracortical region. After 5 to 7 days, some clones of CD4+ T cells become sensitized to the antigen, become activated, multiply, and circulate as memory cells in the bloodstream; some migrate to the skin, ready to react with the antigen if they encounter it. Langerhans cell production of interleukin-1 supports the CD4+ Th1 lymphocyte subset proliferation, which is potentiated by the CD4+ Th1 production of interleukin-2 (IL-2) and autocrine induction of increased IL-2 receptors. The ability to mount a delayed hypersensitivity reaction resides in the Th1 subset.[4]

Upon reexposure to the allergen in the elicitation phase, the efferent limb of the immune reaction, the specifically sensitized T lymphocytes in the circulation, enter the skin. At the site of challenge, Langerhans cells, endothelial cells, perivascular dendritic cells, and monocytes[5,6] process the antigen and present it to the specifically sensitized T cells, which then migrate to the epidermis.[7] The local production of cytokines leads to the arrival of more T cells and amplification of the proinflammatory mechanisms. The important cytokines include those that stimulate lymphocytes (MIP-1β, IL-2, interferon-γ), macrophages (chemotactic factor, MIF, interferon-γ), and/or mast cells and the vasculature (skin reactive factor, interferon-γ).

In 3 to 4 hours after allergen application to the skin of sensitized humans, ultrastructural study reveals noninflammatory epidermal intercellular edema, which is thought to be an extension of the papillary dermal edema.[8] After 6 to 12 hours, a dermal infiltrate composed of lymphocytes and histiocytes is observed with exocytosis into the epidermis. With increasing spongiosis, particularly between 24 and 48 hours, desmosomal attachments are ultimately lost. As a result of separation from the desmosomal attachment plaques, tonofilaments aggregate in the middle of the keratinocyte cytoplasm. After several days, keratinocytes develop intracellular edema, large degenerative cytoplasmic vacuoles, and pyknotic nuclei.[9]

Irritant Contact Dermatitis

This nonallergic inflammatory reaction occurs after exposure to an irritant, a toxic compound that causes a reaction in most individuals who come into contact with it. Common irritants include alkalis, such as soaps, detergents, lye, and ammonia-containing compounds. The irritant response is determined by the type of chemical, its concentration, the mode of exposure, the body site, the barrier function locally, and the age of the patient. Atopy is a predisposing factor. The clinical morphology varies. Chemical burns, usually caused by strong alkalis and acids, lead to immediate painful erythema progressing to vesiculation, necrosis, and, if severe, ulceration. Acute irritant reactions produce a monomorphic picture with scaling, redness, vesicles, pustules, or erosions, and are caused by such mild irritants as detergents and water with additives. Acute irritant contact dermatitis is variable and may be indistinguishable from allergic contact dermatitis. Agents producing this pattern include tretinoin, benzalkonium chloride, dithranol, adhesive tapes, and cosmetics. Chronic irritant contact dermatitis is characterized by dryness, chapping, and absence of vesicles. This reaction pattern in produced by repetitive contact to water, detergent, and solvents.

Histopathology. The histologic picture varies from extensive ulceration, to simply diffuse parakeratosis with congestion and ectasia, to a spongiotic pattern essentially identical to allergic contact dermatitis. The variable features reflect the protean factors discussed above. Some correlations are worthy of note. In some instances, there is significant necrosis with nuclear karyorrhexis and cytoplasmic pallor (Bandmann's achromia).[10] In severe reactions, the necrosis may extend into the dermis. Some irritants such as cantharidin and trichlorethylene produce acantholysis and neutrophilic accumulation in the epidermis.[11] Some reactants, however, may be entirely spongiotic, such as those due to weak irritants, strong irritants in low concentration, and those in the "irritable skin syndrome." Because of these observations and those at positive patch test sites, routine histopathological changes cannot reliably separate irritant from allergic contact reactions, although necrosis, neutrophilic infiltration, and acantholysis are more frequent in the former.

Pathogenesis. First, the irritant chemical must penetrate the cutaneous barrier, the stratum corneum. Detergents, at low concentration, destroy lysosomal enzymes in the stratum corneum, and at higher concentration they dissolve membranes of keratinocytes and lysosomes. Organic solvents may selectively damage blood vessels. Others may be chemotactic for neutrophils.[12] Irritation leads to cytokine expression. In irritant reactions in mice, there was upregulation of IL-1β, IL-6, and IL-10 mRNA.[13] Upregulation of tumor necrosis factor-α (TNF-α) produced by keratinocytes has been shown in vitro and in vivo.[14] Their role in the induction, amplification, and propagation of irritant reactions is poorly understood.

Dyshidrotic Dermatitis

This entity is characterized by recurrent, severely pruritic, deep-seated vesicles that classically involve the lateral aspects of the fingers and, in some cases, the toes. Emotional stress may exacerbate the eruption. In chronic cases, there may be more extensive involvement of the palms and soles. Although the eruption develops acutely, it may become chronic with erythema, lichenification, and fissuring. Secondary impetiginization is common.

Histopathology. Spongiosis and intraepidermal vesiculation occur in acute lesions. There is a superficial perivascular lymphohistiocytic infiltrate with exocytosis of lymphocytes into spongiotic zones. The infiltration is usually mild. In acute lesions, the compact, thickened stratum corneum of acral skin remains intact, and the epidermal thickness is normal. With chronicity, spongiosis diminishes, acanthosis and parakeratosis predominate, and serum may be identified within the stratum corneum. Difficulty in diagnosis may occur because of the formation of vesiculopustules in older lesions.

Autoeczematization or Id Reaction

A sudden generalized or localized vesicular dermatitis developing in association with a defined local dermatitis or infection is known as an "id" reaction. The lesions are pinhead-sized, acuminate or flat-topped, papules. The patient most often has a remote, inflammatory dermatophyte infection, such as bullous tinea pedis or kerion, thus the name *dermatophytid.* In some cases, patients have a severe localized dermatitis, such as stasis dermatitis, with subsequent development of widespread papulovesicular lesions.[15] Other forms of id reactions exist.

Histopathology. The features are those of an acute spongiotic dermatitis, often with micro- or macrovesiculation. Eosinophils may be present.[16] The infiltrating cells are T cells—those within the epidermis are principally CD8+ and those within the dermis are principally CD4+.[17]

Pathogenesis. An id reaction is a secondary vesicular dermatitis that cannot be identified as a common dermatosis, that is of sudden onset, and that is not due to a direct external contactant or infective agent or direct spread of the local infection or dermatosis.[18] It has been postulated to be a hypersensitivity dermatitis to an autoantigen; however, this has never been proven. Several other possibilities exist. First, the reaction may represent a conditioned hyperirritability or responsiveness precipitated by the local infection or dermatitis.[19] Acute local chemical irritation may lower the threshold for an irritant reaction to the same chemical at remote sites. Second, localized dermatitis leads to local production of cytokines by keratinocytes. If the cytokines are hematogenously disseminated, they may lead to distant skin hyperirritability. Lastly, dissemination of antigen (but not of whole infectious agents) from the local site may occur with then a secondary response developing at a site of distant deposition. Recently, microbial antigens have been identified in an id reaction in a patient with tuberculoid leprosy.[20]

Photoallergic Dermatitis

The eruption of photoallergic dermatitis may be due to topical application of, or oral ingestion of, an allergen, resulting in a photocontact dermatitis or photodrug eruption, respectively. Common causes of photodrug eruption include thiazide diuretics, oral hypoglycemics, and phenothiazines. Agents that may elicit a photocontact dermatitis include soaps and cleansers (containing halogenated salicylanilides), perfumes (such as Musk ambrette), topical sulfonamides, sunscreens, benzocaine, and diphenhydramine.[21] The eruption is pruritic and composed of erythematous papules and confluent plaques on sun-exposed skin, usually the face, dorsal aspect of the arms, and the "V" of the neck.

Histopathology. The features are similar to that of an acute allergic contact dermatitis, showing moderate to severe spongiosis, in some cases with vesiculation, and a superficial perivascular lymphohistiocytic infiltrate with exocytosis. A deeper perivascular infiltrate and eosinophils are more common in photoallergic dermatitis induced by systemic ingestion of medications. With chronic exposure to the antigen, there is progression to chronic dermatitis, with diminished spongiosis, less intense inflammation, and more acanthosis. Phototoxic reactions are "sunburn" reactions with epidermal apoptosis and necrosis with intraepidermal to subepidermal blisters—the changes paralleling the degree of damage. Neutrophils are prominent.

Nummular Dermatitis

The eruption is characterized by pruritic, coin-shaped (nummular), erythematous, scaly, crusted plaques. The lesions tend to develop on the extensor surfaces of the extremities.

Histopathology. Nummular dermatitis is the prototype of subacute spongiotic dermatitis (see Fig. 9-2). There is mild to moderate spongiosis, usually without vesiculation, and a superficial perivascular infiltrate composed of lymphocytes, histiocytes, and eosinophils. The epidermis is moderately acanthotic and parakeratotic. The stratum corneum contains aggregates of coagulated plasma and scattered neutrophils, forming a crust. Mild papillary dermal edema and vascular dilatation may be present.

Pathogenesis. The etiology of this entity is unknown. The ultrastructural changes in nummular dermatitis resemble those of contact dermatitis. Intercellular edema is the most conspicuous finding.[22] There is shearing and loss of desmosomes.

Atopic Dermatitis

The eruption is characterized by areas of severe pruritus, erythema, scaling, and excoriation, and with chronicity, lichenification, and lichen simplex chronicus. Many of the cutaneous changes are due to chronic rubbing and scratching. Most patients are diagnosed in childhood, and approximately one third of cases are diagnosed before 1 year of age.[23] There is a female predominance, and many patients have other atopic disorders such as allergic rhinitis or asthma. In infants, the lesions predominate on the face and extensor surfaces of the extremities, but later affect the flexural surfaces. The classically involved sites in older children and adults are the popliteal and antecubital fossae and the sides of the neck. Secondary bacterial infection is common.

Histopathology. In early phases, there is mild spongiosis, exocytosis of lymphocytes, and parakeratosis. Lymphocytes and scattered histiocytes are present around the superficial vascular plexus. In long-standing lesions, the rete ridges are regularly elongated, with less prominent spongiosis and cellular infiltrate. Hyperkeratosis and wedge-shaped hypergranulosis with areas of parakeratosis develop. Vascular endothelial cells may become enlarged.[24] Eosinophils are less conspicuous than in allergic contact or nummular dermatitis. With time, the changes may be those of lichen simplex chronicus.

Pathogenesis. In atopic dermatitis, the absolute number of peripheral blood T lymphocytes may be normal or decreased.[25] In the circulating blood, the number of T cells is decreased, particularly the CD8+ T-lymphocyte subpopulation, leading to an increased CD4 : CD8 ratio.[25] Despite these findings, no known systemic decrease in cell-mediated immunity exists in these patients. Rather, there is a significant localized immunosuppression in the skin, resulting in an increased susceptibility to cutaneous viral and dermatophyte infections, a reduced responsiveness to certain contact allergens, and cutaneous anergy.

Although atopic dermatitis may resemble allergic contact dermatitis clinically and histologically, the former is primarily driven by IL-4 and the latter by IFN-γ.[26] IL-4 induces expression of vascular cell adhesion molecule-1 (VCAM-1) on endothelial cells, which can then selectively recruit eosinophils and basophils to the site of inflammation. It also activates macrophages, induces expression of MHC II antigens on monocytes and B cells, upregulates IgE synthesis by these cells, and induces expression of IgE receptors on Langerhans cells, enhancing their antigen presentation capabilities.

In the lesions of atopic dermatitis, allergen-specific CD4+ T cells accumulate, and facilitated antigen presentation (FAP) occurs. FAP results when IgE-allergen complexes are endocytosed by antigen-presenting cells after binding to the low-affinity FcR type II (CD23). Langerhans cells are then able to process even extremely low allergen protein concentrations bound via these allergen-specific IgE receptors. Upon recognition of processed allergens, the allergen-specific T cells then proliferate, leading to local IL-4 production and further enhancement of allergen-specific immune reactivity.[27]

Two subpopulations of CD4+ T cells, type 1 (Th1) and type 2 (Th2), have a distinct profile of cytokine secretion. Th1 cells are generally recognized for their role in allergic contact dermatitis, allograft rejection, and organ-specific autoimmunity. Th2 cells are believed to contribute to immunoglobulin synthesis (including IgE) and the initiation of allergic disorders.[28] Th1 cells secrete a number of cytokines, including IL-2, interferon-gamma (IFN-γ), and tumor necrosis factor-β. Th2 cells secrete a different cytokine profile, including IL-4, -5, -6, and -10. Both subpopulations are capable of secreting IL-3, TNF-α, and granulocyte-macrophage colony stimulating factor.[28]

In acute lesions of atopic dermatitis, mast cells are normal in quantity but are in various stages of degranulation, indicative of an activated state.[29] In chronic lesions, mast cells are increased in number. They are capable of synthesizing and secreting IL-4, which has many important effects, including its ability to initiate Th2 cell differentiation and proliferation. Although Th2 lymphocytes are a major source of IL-4 in lesions of atopic dermatitis, they require an exogenous source to initiate further IL-4 synthesis, and mast cells likely serve as this exogenous source.[29]

In atopic dermatitis, the correlation of serum IgE and disease activity is controversial. Some patients have high levels of IgE antibodies to the house dust mite *Dermatophagoides pteronyssinus* and to *Pityrosporum orbiculare*, which may play a role in the development of atopic dermatitis.[27,30] IgE assists in antigen capture, as noted above, and probably potentiates allergen-specific responses.[27]

Lichen Simplex Chronicus

Any patient with pruritus who chronically rubs the skin may develop lichen simplex chronicus. It often develops in the setting of atopic dermatitis or allergic contact dermatitis. The lesions are pruritic, thickened plaques often with excoriation, in which the normal skin markings are accentuated, the latter finding known as lichenification.

Histopathology. Lichen simplex chronicus is the prototype for chronic dermatitis (see Fig. 9-3). There is hyperkeratosis interspersed with areas of parakeratosis, acanthosis with irregular elongation of the rete ridges, hypergranulosis, and broadening of the dermal papillae. Slight spongiosis may be observed, but vesiculation is absent. There may be a sparse superficial perivascular infiltrate without exocytosis. In the papillary dermis, there is an increased number of fibroblasts and vertically oriented collagen bundles. As rubbing increases in intensity and chronicity, epidermal hyperplasia becomes more florid, and the fibrosis more marked.

Seborrheic Dermatitis

Clinically, patients develop erythema and greasy scale on the scalp, paranasal areas, eyebrows, nasolabial folds, and central chest. Rarely, patients with seborrheic dermatitis develop generalized lesions. Patients with HIV infection often have severe, recalcitrant disease. In infants, the scalp ("cradle cap"), face, and diaper areas are often involved.

Histopathology. The histopathologic features are a combination of those observed in psoriasis and spongiotic dermatitis. Mild cases may exhibit only a slight subacute spongiotic dermatitis. The stratum corneum contains focal areas of parakeratosis, with a predilection for the follicular ostia, a finding known as "shoulder parakeratosis" (Fig. 9-4). Occasional pyknotic neutrophils are present within parakeratotic foci. There is moderate acanthosis with regular elongation of the rete ridges, mild spongiosis, and focal exocytosis of lymphocytes. The dermis contains a sparse mononuclear cell infiltrate. In HIV-infected patients, the epidermis may contain dyskeratotic keratinocytes, and the dermal infiltrate may contain plasma cells.[31]

Pathogenesis. The pathogenesis is unknown; however, many patients have a good response to oral or topical ketoconazole, suggesting that *Pityrosporum ovale* plays an important role in the pathogenesis of the disease. This postulation is controversial, however, and the organism has not been cultured from lesions.[32]

Stasis Dermatitis

Patients with long-standing venous insufficiency and lower extremity edema may develop pruritic, erythematous, scaly papules and plaques on the lower legs, often in association with brown pigmentation and hair loss.

Histopathology. The epidermis is hyperkeratotic with areas of parakeratosis, acanthosis, and focal spongiosis. There is a superficial, perivascular lymphohistiocytic infiltrate that surrounds plump, thickened capillaries and venules. The superficial dermal vessels may be arranged in lobular aggregates. The proliferation may be florid, mimicking Kaposi's sarcoma (acroangiodermatitis).[33] The reticular dermis is often fibrotic. Hemosiderin is usually present superficially but may be identified about the deep vascular plexus as well.

Differential Diagnosis of Spongiotic Dermatitis

Acute spongiotic dermatitis may be seen histologically in erythema multiforme, pityriasis rosea, guttate parapsoriasis,

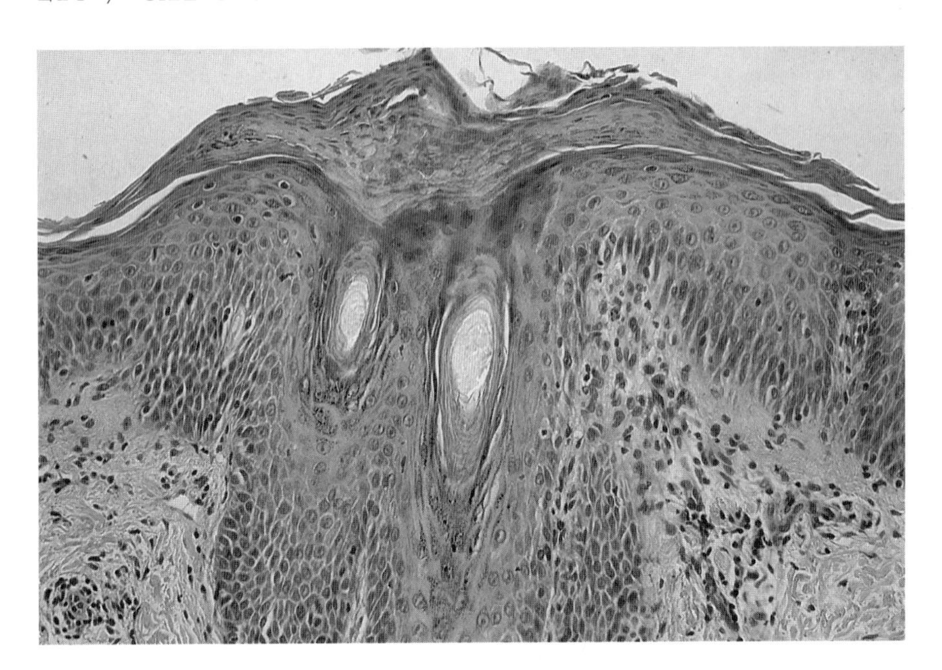

FIG. 9-4. Seborrheic dermatitis There is parakeratotic scale containing a few neutrophils surmounting two vellus follicles. The underlying epidermis is slightly hyperplastic with minimal spongiosis. The dermis contains a scant perivascular infiltrate.

spongiotic drug eruptions, arthropod bite reactions, and dermatophyte infections. In erythema multiforme, dyskeratotic (apoptotic) keratinocytes within and above the basal layer aid in the diagnosis. Lesions of pityriasis rosea contain focal, as opposed to diffuse, areas of spongiosis, exocytosis of lymphocytes, and overlying mounds of parakeratosis. In addition, extravasated erythrocytes may be present within these foci in the epidermis. Guttate parapsoriasis is similar to pityriasis rosea, but it lacks the intraepidermal erythrocytes and has less lymphohistiocytic infiltrate. Spongiotic drug eruptions tend to show a deeper infiltrate and more eosinophils than other forms of acute spongiotic dermatitis. In arthropod bite reactions, the epidermal changes are focal, corresponding to the site of attack, and the infiltrate is wedge-shaped. A periodic acid–Schiff (PAS) stain is necessary to exclude dermatophyte infection.

Pityriasis lichenoides, dermatophyte infection, spongiotic drug eruption, or an arthropod bite reaction may show histopathologic features similar to a *subacute spongiotic dermatitis*. In pityriasis lichenoides et varioliformis acuta, the lesions tend to be circumscribed, and apoptotic keratinocytes, dry neutrophil-rich scale, bandlike interface dermatitis, areas of epidermal necrosis, and a deeper perivascular infiltrate are present. Dermatophyte infections characteristically have neutrophils within the stratum corneum, along with fungal hyphae; however, PAS stain is often necessary to identify the fungal hyphae.

Conditions that reveal a *chronic dermatitis* include pellagra and other nutritional deficiencies, large plaque parapsoriasis, mycosis fungoides, and psoriasis, particularly if altered by therapy. In the nutritional deficiencies, upper epidermal pallor, necrosis, and neutrophilic infiltrate are characteristic. In large plaque parapsoriasis and mycosis fungoides, psoriasiform epidermal hyperplasia is common, but the lymphocytes have nuclear atypia and cerebriform morphology with epidermotropism, in the absence of spongiosis. Lesions of psoriasis may resemble lichen simplex chronicus, but thinning of the suprapapillary plates, confluent parakeratosis, neutrophils within the stratum corneum and upper epidermis, and dilated tortuous capillaries are distinctive.

Other Disorders with Spongiotic Dermatitis

Erythroderma (Generalized Exfoliative Dermatitis)

Erythroderma is characterized by generalized erythema and scale, often in association with fever. The eruption is nonspecific and may be caused by a variety of underlying diseases, such as spongiotic dermatitis, psoriasis, pityriasis rubra pilaris, cutaneous T-cell lymphoma (Sézary syndrome), or a drug eruption. When presenting as erythroderma, the characteristic and specific histopathologic features of these disorders are not well developed, leading to diagnostic confusion.

Histopathology. A careful search for histologic features of any of the above listed etiologies must be undertaken; however, the changes are often those of either a subacute or chronic dermatitis (Fig. 9-5). Thus the histopathologic findings are helpful in establishing the diagnosis in only about 40% of cases.[34] Each case of undetermined origin requires thorough histologic examination through multiple levels, a search for specific histopathologic features, and clinicopathologic correlation. Repeat biopsies and hematologic studies at regular intervals are recommended in patients without definitive diagnosis.

Miliaria

Miliaria develops when sweating is associated with obstruction of the intraepidermal sweat duct. There are three types: miliaria crystallina, miliaria rubra, and miliaria profunda.

Miliaria crystallina develops when the sweat duct is obstructed within the stratum corneum. Asymptomatic, small, superficial, noninflammatory vesicles resembling dewdrops develop, mainly on the trunk, after severe sunburn or with profuse sweating during a febrile illness. The vesicles rapidly subside when sweating ceases or the horny layer overlying the vesicles exfoliates. In some cases, the eruption may be present at birth.[35]

Miliaria rubra (prickly heat) ensues when the sweat duct is obstructed within the deeper layers of the epidermis. It generally

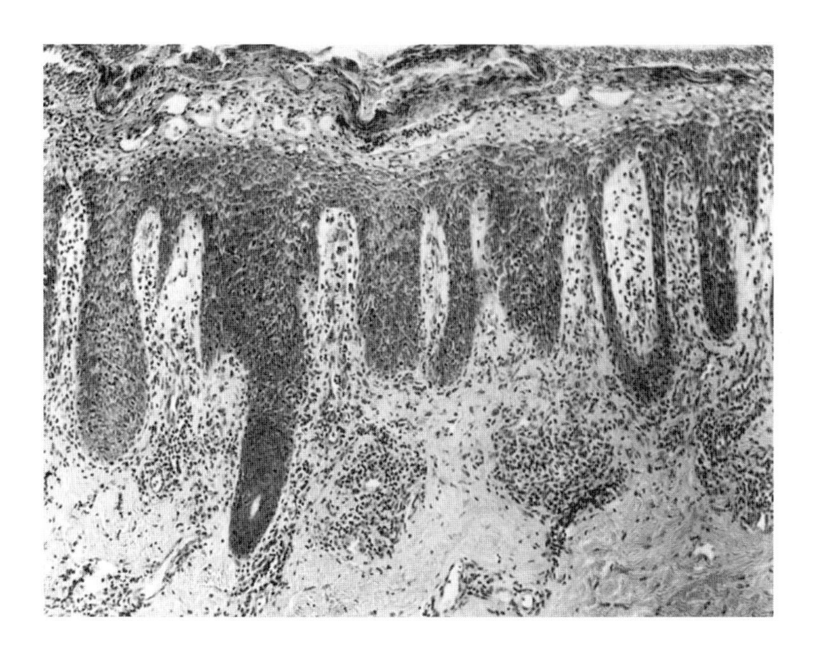

FIG. 9-5. Generalized exfoliative dermatitis due to drug allergy, subacute
There is parakeratosis and marked intercellular and intracellular edema, with psoriasiform acanthosis. Lymphocytes migrate into the epidermis from the perivascular and patchy bandlike infiltrate. A few eosinophils are present.

develops during and after excessive sweating in skin covered by clothing. It may also occur after prolonged covering of the skin by occlusive polyethylene wraps. Anhidrosis and heat intolerance result, particularly when the trunk is occluded.[36,37] The lesions consist of pruritic small papulovesicles surrounded by erythema. Pustules may develop.

Miliaria profunda usually develops after recurrent episodes of miliaria rubra, particularly in tropical climates. The sweat duct is occluded at the dermal-epidermal junction. Lesions are nonpruritic, flesh-colored papules and can result in widespread anhidrosis.

Histopathology. In *miliaria crystallina,* one observes intracorneal or subcorneal vesicles that are in continuity with the underlying sweat duct.[35] A sparse to moderate infiltrate of neutrophils is seen at the periphery of the vesicle. The surrounding epidermis is spongiotic, and there is papillary dermal edema and sparse superficial perivascular inflammation.

In *miliaria rubra,* spongiotic vesicles are found in the stratum malpighii. Serial sectioning shows these vesicles to be in continuity with a sweat duct (Fig. 9-6). Periductal lymphocyte infiltration and spongiosis are seen, as is an infiltrate in the underlying dermis.[38] In many instances, the distal, intraepidermal sweat duct is filled with amorphous "casts" that are PAS-positive and diastase-resistant.[37]

In *miliaria profunda,* the features are similar to those of miliaria rubra but the inflammatory changes involve the lower epidermis and superficial dermis.

Pathogenesis. In *miliaria crystallina,* the obstruction of the sweat duct within the stratum corneum is caused either by mild damage to the epidermis from a preceding sunburn or by exces-

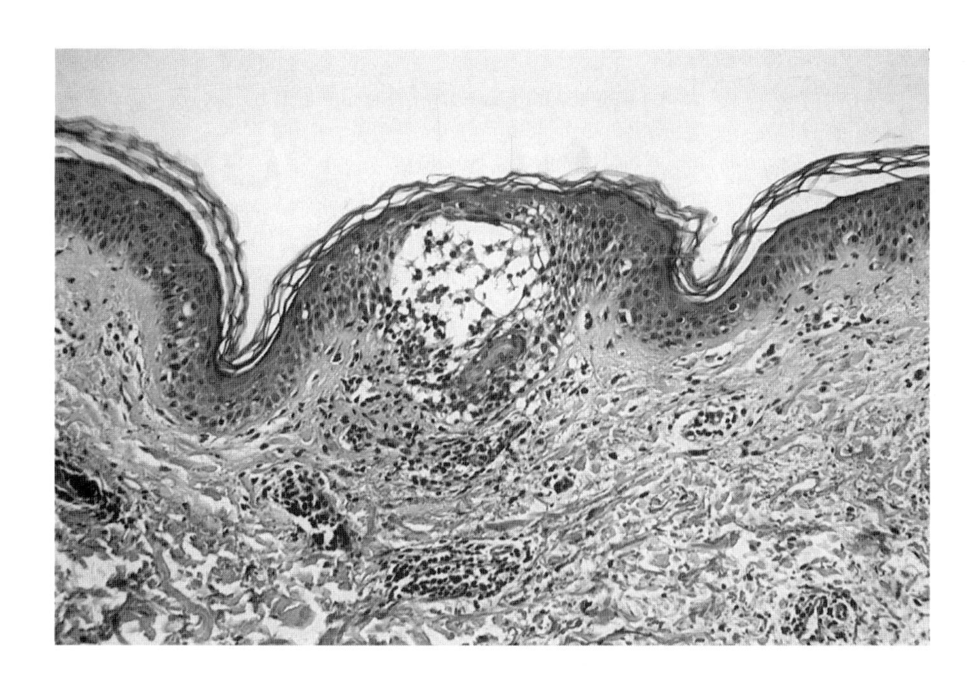

FIG. 9-6. Miliaria rubra
An acrosyringium is surrounded by spongiosis and a spongiotic microvesicle containing fluid, lymphocytes, and a few red blood cells.

sive hydration of the stratum corneum. In neonates, excess hydration of the stratum corneum in utero in combination with immature eccrine ducts may cause swelling of the ductal epithelial cells and occlusion of the duct.[35]

In *miliaria rubra,* increased environmental temperature plays an important role.[39] Aerobic bacteria are thought to contribute to the obstruction of the acrosyringium. In favor of this view are the frequent presence of *Staphylococcus aureus* within the sweat ducts,[40] and the fact that the development of miliaria rubra under an occlusive polyethylene film can be prevented by application of antibacterial solutions.[41]

The PAS-positive, diastase-resistant, amorphous plug within the acrosyringium may occur as a result of injury to the luminal cells, inflammation, and ductal and periductal spongiosis. These changes occur after 48 hours of occlusion and resolve after 14 days, when old, damaged stratum corneum is desquamated. Tape stripping can restore sweating, which supports a reversible, high-level blockage.[37]

Immunological Deficiency Diseases Associated with Spongiotic Dermatitis

Familial Leiner's Disease

In this syndrome, infants develop generalized seborrheic dermatitis, severe diarrhea, recurrent local and systemic infections, and marked wasting. Death is usually due to septicemia. A dysfunction of the fifth component of complement (C5) exists, in addition to other cellular and humoral immune defects.[42]

Hyperimmunoglobulin E Syndrome

In this disease, patients have recurrent pyogenic infections, atopic dermatitis, extreme elevation of serum IgE, and defective neutrophil chemotaxis.[43] The infectious complications include recurrent cold staphylococcal abscesses, furunculosis, otitis, sinusitis, and staphylococcal pneumonia.[44]

Wiscott-Aldrich Syndrome

This X-linked recessive disorder affects males and is characterized by recurrent, systemic bacterial and viral infections, purpura due to thrombocytopenia, and an atopic dermatitis-like eruption. Because of progressive deterioration of cellular immunity, death due to infection or lymphoma ensues in the first decade of life.[45]

Chronic Granulomatous Disease

This X-linked recessive disorder affects males, beginning in infancy with a perioral dermatitis. The dermatitis often progresses to granulomatous lesions accompanied by cervical adenitis.[46] Suppurative and granulomatous infections develop in the skin, lungs, bone, and liver, most commonly due to *Staphylococcus aureus.* Death occurs in most cases in childhood or adolescence. The defect lies in decreased capacity of neutrophils to generate hydrogen peroxide and kill catalase-positive bacteria and fungi.[47] In vitro, neutrophils are unable to reduce nitroblue tetrazolium dye after phagocytosis, a useful screening test for the disease.

PEMPHIGUS GROUP

There are five types of pemphigus: (1) pemphigus vulgaris, with its reactive state, pemphigus vegetans, (2) pemphigus foliaceus, with its lupuslike variant, pemphigus erythematosus, (3) drug-induced pemphigus, (4) IgA pemphigus, and (5) paraneoplastic pemphigus.

As first demonstrated in 1943, acantholysis is the characteristic feature of the bullae of pemphigus.[48] The acantholysis results from in vivo bound antibodies, first discovered in 1964.[49] These antibodies are demonstrable by direct immunofluorescence (DIF) testing of skin and indirect immunofluorescence (IIF) testing of serum. The use of these techniques is now the accepted practice in the diagnosis of all antibody-mediated primary vesiculobullous disorders (see Table 9-4). However, demonstration of the specific antigen against which the antibodies are directed by various techniques (immunoblotting, etc.) is rapidly becoming the gold standard.

Pemphigus Vulgaris

This condition develops primarily in older individuals, presenting with large and flaccid bullae. They break easily and leave denuded areas that tend to increase in size by progressive peripheral detachment of the epidermis (positive Nikolsky sign), leading in some cases to widespread cutaneous involvement. The lesions characteristically involve the oral mucosa, scalp, midface, sternum, and groin. Oral lesions are almost invariably present and are often the first manifestation of the disease.[50] Before corticosteroids became available, the mortality of this disease was high because of fluid loss and superinfection.

Histopathology. It is important that early blisters, preferably small ones, are selected for biopsy. Care should be given to keeping the epidermis attached to the dermis, since the torque applied in punch biopsies may separate the blister roof from the blister base. Therefore, it is advisable to use a refrigerant spray before excising the blister with a punch biopsy, or to excise it with a scalpel. If no recent blister is available, an old one may be moved into the neighboring skin by gentle vertical pressure with a finger (positive Nikolsky sign).[51] The newly created cleavage will reveal early and specific histologic changes.

The earliest recognized change may be either eosinophilic spongiosis, rarely, or more commonly, spongiosis in the lower epidermis (Fig. 9-7A). Acantholysis leads first to the formation of clefts, and then to blisters in a predominantly suprabasal location (see Fig. 9-7B).[48,52,53] The basal keratinocytes, although separated from one another through the loss of attachment, remain firmly attached to the dermis like a "row of tombstones."[52] Thus the blister base is lined by basal keratinocytes clearly separated from one another. Whereas acantholysis usually results in a suprabasal blister, intraepithelial separation may occasionally be higher in the stratum spinosum. Acantholysis may extend into adnexal structures. The blister roof consists of the remaining intact squamous epithelium. Within the blister cavity, there are acantholytic keratinocytes that have rounded, condensed cytoplasm about an enlarged nucleus with peripherally palisaded chromatin and enlarged nucleoli. These may reside singularly or in clusters.

There is little inflammation in the early phase of blister formation. If present, it is usually a sparse, lymphocytic perivascular infiltrate accompanied by dermal edema. If, however, eosinophilic spongiosis is apparent, numerous eosinophils may infiltrate the dermis. The phenomenon of eosinophilic spongiosis occurs occasionally in other bullous diseases, particularly in their early phases, including acute contact dermatitis, pemphigus foliaceus, bullous pemphigoid, herpes gestationis, drug eruptions, spongiotic arthropod bite reactions,[54] and transient acantholytic dermatosis (T. J. Harrist, personal observation).

Several important changes ensue as the lesions age. Firstly, a mixed inflammatory cell reaction consisting of neutrophils, lymphocytes, macrophages, and eosinophils may develop.[52] Because of the instability of the blister roof, erosion and ulceration may occur. Older blisters may also have several layers of keratinocytes at the blister base because of keratinocyte migration and proliferation. Lastly, there may be considerable downward growth of epidermal strands, giving rise to so-called villi (see Fig. 9-7C).

The evaluation of patients with only oral lesions is difficult, because intact blisters are rarely encountered due to the trauma of mastication, and biopsies may show only erosion and ulceration. Patients may be aware of impending blister formation and can be asked to present for a "stat" biopsy at such a time (G. Cohen, personal observation). Indeed, it is best to sample the edge of a denuded area with intact mucosa in an attempt to demonstrate the typical pathologic changes. In patients with only oral lesions, biopsies of intact oral mucosa for DIF testing may be more sensitive than biopsies of lesions for routine light microscopic evaluation.[55]

Cytologic examination using a Tzanck preparation is useful for the rapid demonstration of acantholytic epidermal keratinocytes in the blisters of pemphigus vulgaris. For this purpose, a smear is taken from the underside of the roof and from the base of an early, freshly opened bulla. Giemsa stain is applied with subsequent rinsing and air-drying.[56] Because acantholytic keratinocytes are occasionally seen in various nonacantholytic vesiculobullous or pustular diseases as a result of secondary acantholysis, cytologic examination represents merely a preliminary test and should not supplant histologic examination.[57]

Immunofluorescence (IF) Testing. The edge of a blister with intact surrounding normal skin or uninvolved skin adjacent to a blister should be supplied for biopsy. The tissue may be snap-frozen or transported in Michel's medium. DIF testing is a very reliable and sensitive diagnostic test for pemphigus vulgaris, in that it demonstrates IgG in the squamous intercellular substance in 80% to 95% of cases, including early cases and those with very few lesions, and in up to 100% of cases with active disease (see Fig. 9-7D).[58] It remains positive, often for many years after the disease has subsided.[59] Negative DIF findings when the patient is in remission may be a good prognostic indicator.[60] At this time, DIF testing is thought to be free of false positives. However, on occasion, it may be difficult to distinguish intercellular staining of pemphigus from nonspecific staining that may occur, for example, in spongiotic dermatitis. In recent years, immunoperoxidase methods have achieved roughly the same sensitivity as the IF method, but they have not replaced IF testing as the prime diagnostic tool.[61,62]

Unfixed frozen sections of guinea pig esophagus, monkey esophagus,[59] or normal human skin[63] are used as substrate for IF testing. In general, monkey esophagus is the best substrate for indirect immunofluorescence studies.[58] IgG is demonstrated in the squamous intercellular substance in 80% to 90% of cases,[64] and the titer correlates with disease activity.[65] False positive indirect tests occur. In a series of 1500 patients with circulating pemphigus antibodies, approximately 1% had no evidence of clinical disease.[66] Antibodies that mimic or that may give in vitro deposition in stratified squamous epithelium in the absence of pemphigus have been reported in burns, penicillin allergy, toxic epidermal necrolysis, systemic lupus erythematosus, myasthenia gravis, bullous pemphigoid, cicatricial pemphigoid, lichen planus, and in patients with antibodies directed against blood groups A and B.[66–68] Such antibodies are present in low titer and are thought to be nonpathogenic.

Pathogenesis. There is strong evidence that pemphigus antibodies are pathogenic.

1. In most patients with pemphigus, the antibody titers, as measured by IIF study, correlate with disease activity.[69]
2. Plasmapheresis induces short-term remissions through reduction in pemphigus antibody titers.[70]
3. Pemphigus has developed in neonates born to mothers with active pemphigus secondary to transplacental transfer of maternal IgG.[71]
4. Pemphigus antibody produces positive DIF findings in cutaneous human skin organ cultures with suprabasal acantholysis produced after 24 hours.[72]
5. The partially purified IgG fraction from pooled sera of patients with pemphigus has the same in vitro effect as whole serum.[73]
6. Intraperitoneal injections of the IgG fractions from patients with pemphigus vulgaris into neonatal mice cause blisters with the histological, ultrastructural, and immunofluorescence features of pemphigus vulgaris in 39 of 55 mice.[74]
7. Pemphigus vulgaris IgG F(ab')2 fragments from humans result in acantholysis in neonatal mice.[75]
8. Indeed, the distribution of lesions correlates with the distribution pattern in IF studies of pemphigus vulgaris antigen, whose expression is greatest in buccal mucosa.[76]

The pemphigus vulgaris antigen is a 130kD glycoprotein combined with plakoglobin that is found in desmosomal plaques and cell-cell adhesion junctions.[77] The antigen is desmoglein III, which is a cadherin that mediates cell binding.[78–80] Thus antibody binding with the pemphigus antigen appears to have a profound effect on the integrity of epidermal keratinocyte cell-cell contact. The exact mechanism of acantholysis is unclear. The binding of the antibody to the antigen may directly interfere with desmosomal function. Proteinases, likely induced by pemphigus antigen-antibody union, are thought to play an important role in acantholysis.[81] Plasminogen activator is a possible candidate. It is released by keratinocytes and converts plasminogen to plasmin, which leads to lysis of the intercellular substance and subsequent acantholysis.[82] Although complement fixation by pemphigus antibody may promote acantholysis,[83] acantholysis occurs in experimental systems in the absence of complement.[81]

Ultrastructural Study. The intercellular cement substance, or glycocalyx, is partially or entirely resolved in lesions with early acantholysis.[84] There is widening of the intercellular spaces

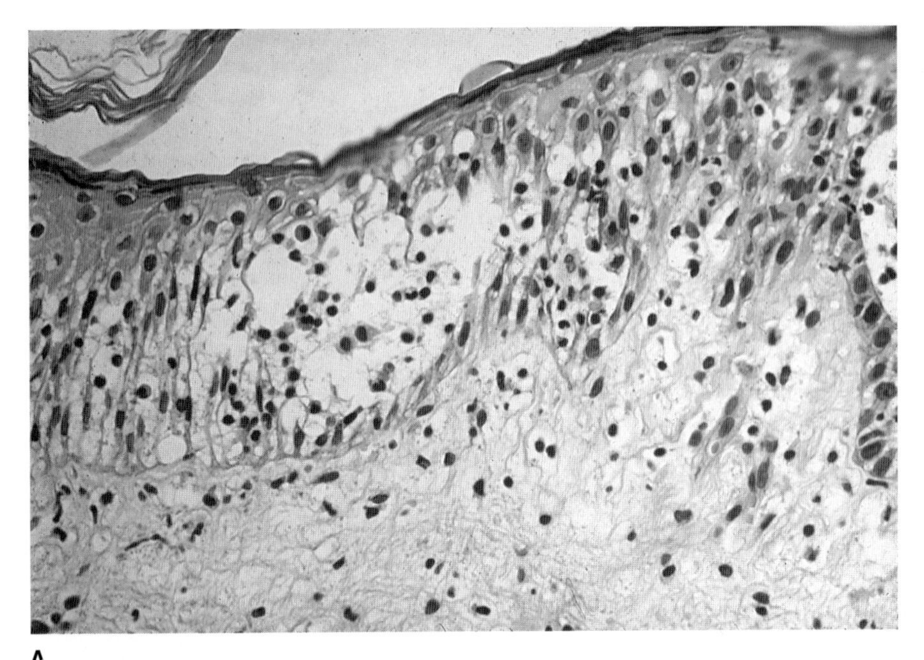

A

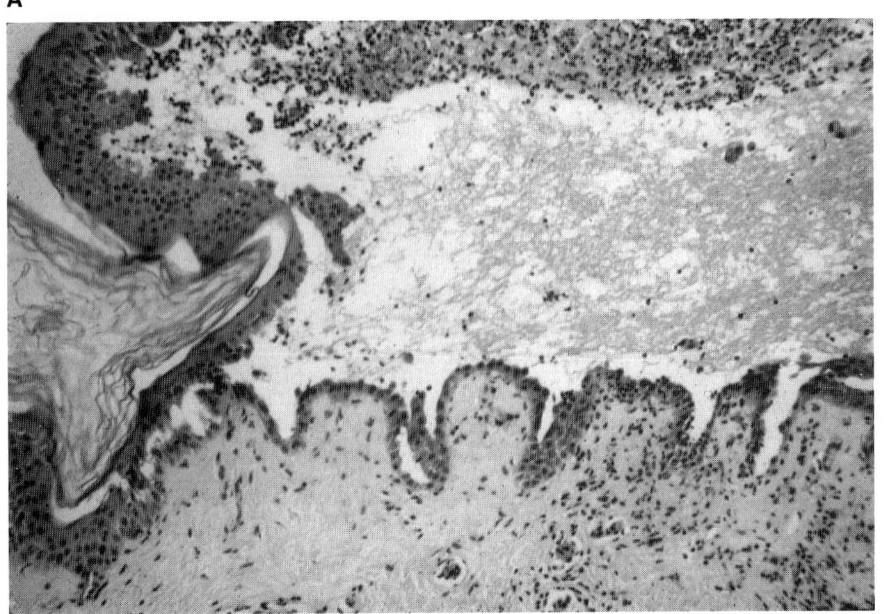

B

FIG. 9-7. Pemphigus vulgaris
(**A**) The earliest changes consist of intercellular edema with eosinophilic spongiosis, leading to loss of intercellular bridges in the lowermost epidermis. (**B**) An intraepidermal acantholytic blister has a suprabasal cleavage plane. Note the initial separation in the surrounding epidermis to the *left*.

with intact desmosomes. As the intercellular space is widened, there is separation of the two opposing attachment plaques of a desmosome, so that single attachment plaques, with adherent tonofilaments, are seen at the periphery of keratinocytes.[85] As acantholysis progresses, the desmosomes gradually disappear and the keratinocytes develop numerous cytoplasmic processes that often interdigitate with one another. All of the early ultrastructural changes in pemphigus vulgaris are extracellular. Only subsequent to the dissolution of the desmosomes does retraction of the tonofilaments to the perinuclear area develop with ultimate degeneration of the acantholytic cells. The cohesion of the basal keratinocytes with the basement membrane zone is not affected in pemphigus vulgaris because of the preservation of structures connecting the basal keratinocytes with the dermis (EM 7). The connection between basal keratinocytes and the dermis contains neither squamous intercellular cement substance nor full desmosomes and remains intact even at stages in which the basal keratinocytes are severely altered.

Differential Diagnosis. In early blisters that are free of secondary changes, such as the degeneration or regeneration of epidermal cells, the histopathology of pemphigus vulgaris is characteristic. Important differential diagnoses include Hailey-Hailey disease and transient acantholytic dermatosis. Hailey-Hailey disease has full-thickness ("dilapidated brick wall") acantholysis, epidermal hyperplasia, and an impetiginized scale crust. The acantholysis does not extend down follicles as it does in pemphigus. Transient acantholytic dermatosis may exhibit small foci of intraepidermal acantholysis, but these are only a few rete wide in contrast to the uniform widespread acantholysis observed in biopsies of pemphigus vulgaris. Disorders that are characterized by focal acantholytic dyskeratosis are readily

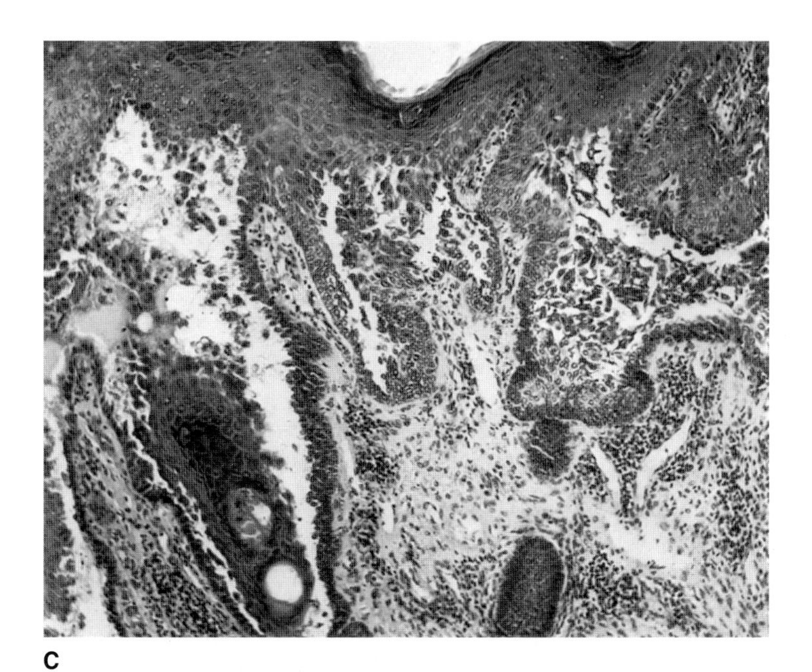

C

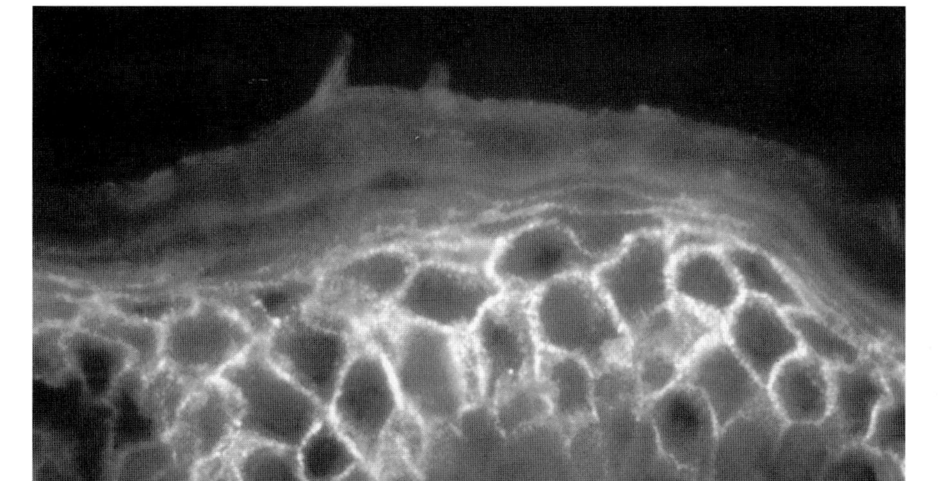

D

FIG. 9-7. ***Continued***
(**C**) An intraepidermal, predominantly suprabasal, blister with numerous acantholytic cells is present. Note the irregular upward growth of papillae lined by a single layer of basal keratinocytes, so-called villi. (**D**) Direct immunofluorescence testing of perilesional skin using fluoresceinated antihuman IgG as test. There is lace-like squamous intercellular substance deposition of IgG, diagnostic and characteristic of pemphigus. In the vast majority of cases, this pattern is shared by both the vulgaris and foliaceus variants.

separated from pemphigus vulgaris by the presence of abnormal granular keratinocytes and parakeratotic cells, so-called corps ronds and corps grains. Although light microscopic examination of pemphigus lesions is important, positive DIF is the gold standard in diagnosis at this time and must be pursued in all cases in which pemphigus vulgaris is considered.

Pemphigus Vegetans

This is an uncommon variant of pemphigus vulgaris, comprising only 1% to 2% of cases.[58,64] Historically, pemphigus vegetans has been divided into the Neumann type and Hallopeau type. In the Neumann type, the disease begins and ends as pemphigus vulgaris, but many of the denuded areas heal with verrucous vegetations that may contain small pustules in early stages. The Hallopeau type is relatively benign, having pustules as the primary lesions instead of bullae. Their development is followed by the formation of gradually enlarging verrucous vegetations, especially in intertriginous areas.[52]

Histopathology. In the Neumann type, the early lesions consist of bullae and denuded areas that have the same histologic picture as that of pemphigus vulgaris. As the lesions age, however, there is formation of villi and verrucous epidermal hyperplasia. Numerous eosinophils are present within the epidermis and dermis, producing both eosinophilic spongiosis and eosinophilic pustules (Fig. 9-8).[52] Acantholysis may not be present in older lesions.

In the Hallopeau type, the early lesions consist of pustules arising on normal skin with acantholysis and formation of small clefts, many in a suprabasal location. The clefts are filled with numerous eosinophils and degenerated acantholytic epidermal

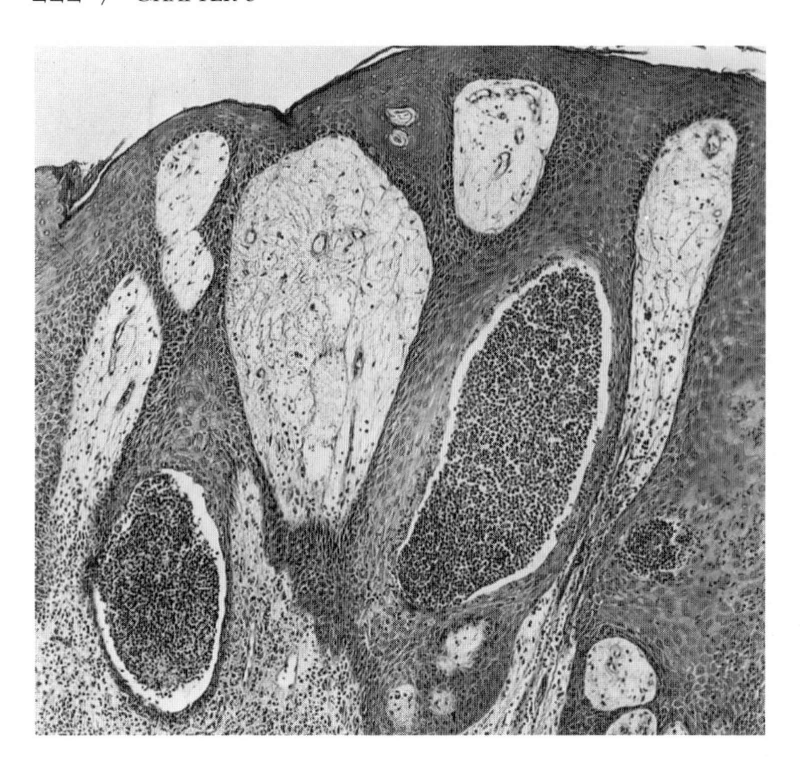

FIG. 9-8. Pemphigus vegetans
Verrucous vegetative epidermal hyperplasia with broad papillae are apparent. Intraepidermal abscesses are composed almost entirely of eosinophils. Zones of acantholysis may be small and difficult to observe.

cells.[86] Early lesions may reveal more eosinophilic abscesses than in the Neumann type.[87] The subsequent verrucous lesions are histologically identical to the Neumann type.

IF Testing. DIF examination reveals squamous intercellular IgG in all recently reported cases.[88,89]

Pathogenesis. Pemphigus vegetans is a variant of pemphigus vulgaris in which verrucous vegetations develop. It is unclear why such vegetations develop in some cases of pemphigus vulgaris and not in others. However, they tend to develop in areas of relative occlusion and maceration with subsequent bacterial infection (T. J. Harrist, personal observation), suggesting a response to superinfection.

Differential Diagnosis. The principal differential diagnosis is pyoderma vegetans, a cutaneous infection caused by either staphylococci or streptococci. The histologic features are similar, but in pyoderma vegetans, neutrophils are more commonly found, and intraepidermal eosinophilic abscesses and acantholysis are rare (Chap. 21). Halogenoderma and blastomycosislike pyoderma must be excluded as well (Chaps. 11 and 23).

Pemphigus Foliaceus

Usually developing in middle-aged individuals, pemphigus foliaceus may have a chronic generalized course or may rarely present as an exfoliative dermatitis. Patients present with flaccid bullae that usually arise on an erythematous base. Erythema, oozing, and crusting are present. Because of their superficial location, the blisters break easily, leaving shallow erosions rather than the denuded areas seen in pemphigus vulgaris. Oral lesions do not occur. The Nikolsky sign is positive, and Tzanck preparation reveals acantholytic granular keratinocytes. Fogo selvagem (endemic pemphigus foliaceus) is clinically, histologically, and immunologically indistinguishable from pemphigus foliaceus.[90,91] It develops in Brazil in people who live close to rivers and streams, the peak incidence being at the end of the rainy season. The cause of fogo selvagem is unknown, but substantial epidemiologic evidence suggests that it is precipitated by an environmental factor. A case control study found that farmers exposed to black fly (*Simulium pruinosum*) bites were much more likely to develop fogo selvagem than farmers who were not bitten.[92]

Histopathology. The earliest change consists of acantholysis in the upper epidermis, within or adjacent to the granular layer, leading to a subcorneal bulla in some instances (Fig. 9-9A). More commonly, enlargement of the cleft leads to detachment of the stratum corneum without bulla formation. The number of acantholytic keratinocytes is usually small, often requiring a careful search to identify them. Secondary clefts may develop, leading to detachment of the epidermis in its midlevel. These clefts may extend to above the basal layer, rarely giving rise to limited areas of suprabasal separation.[93] In the setting of a subcorneal blister, dyskeratotic granular keratinocytes are diagnostic for this disorder. Eosinophilic spongiosis may be prominent with intraepidermal eosinophilic pustules.[94–96] Thus the histologic features of pemphigus foliaceus may have three patterns: (1) eosinophilic spongiosis, (2) a subcorneal blister, often with few acantholytic keratinocytes, and (3) a subcorneal blister with dyskeratotic granular keratinocytes (see Fig. 9-9B), diagnostic for this disorder. The character of the inflammatory infiltrate observed is variable and depends on the age of the lesion, whether a blister is present, whether the superficial portion of the epidermis has been detached, and whether there is impetiginization.

IF Testing. DIF testing of perilesional skin is positive in the vast majority of cases. Two patterns of pemphigus antibody deposition have been described. In most cases, there is full-thickness squamous intercellular substance deposition of IgG. Rarely, IgG may be localized only to the superficial portion of the epidermis.[97] IIF testing of serum reveals squamous intercellular substance deposition of IgG in 80% to 90% of cases.[67]

Pathogenesis. As in pemphigus vulgaris, the antibodies of

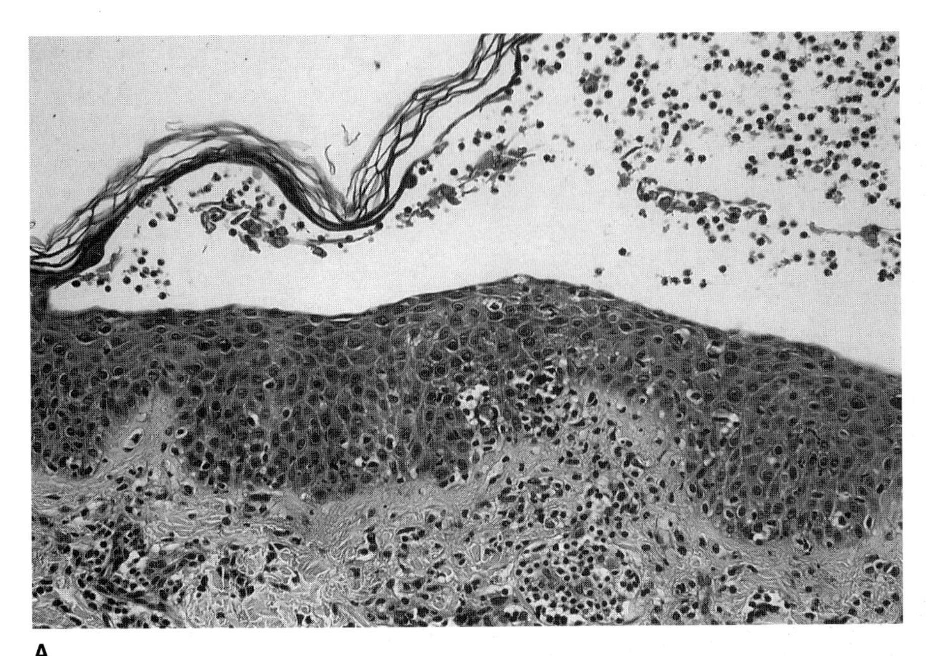

A

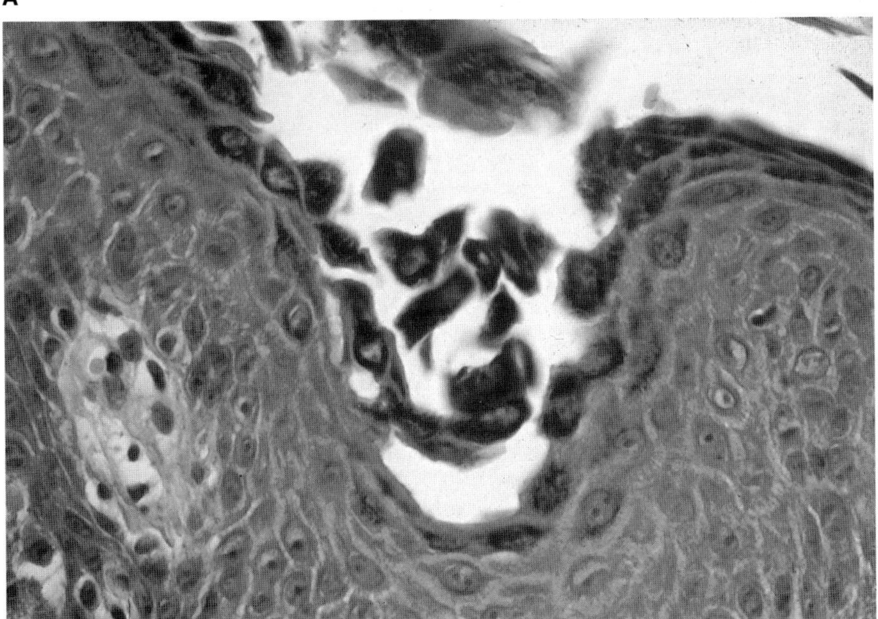

B

FIG. 9-9. Pemphigus foliaceus
(**A**) An intact blister is in a subcorneal location. A few acantholytic cells are present to the *left*, as are numerous neutrophils, the latter a common occurrence in pemphigus foliaceus. (**B**) In the setting of a subcorneal blister, these dyskeratotic acantholytic granular cells are diagnostic of pemphigus foliaceus.

pemphigus foliaceus are pathogenic. The antibodies recognize desmoglein I, which is complexed with plakoglobin.[79,98] Desmoglein I is a 160 kD protein that is an important component of desmosomes. The cleavage plane of pemphigus vulgaris likely differs from pemphigus foliaceus because the differing antibodies have specificity for different adhesion molecules. The pemphigus foliaceus antigen is concentrated in the upper torso and is less prominent in the buccal mucosa, scalp, and lower torso, correlating with lesion distribution.[76]

Ultrastructural Study. There is early loss of intercellular cement substance within the lower epidermis associated with a decrease in the number of desmosomes and formation of tortuous microvilli from the keratinocyte surface. However, acantholysis is most pronounced in the upper layers of the epidermis.[84,85] In the midepidermis, many keratinocytes have perinuclear arrangement of the tonofilaments and homogenization of the perinuclear tonofilament bundles as evidence of dyskeratosis. Marked dyskeratosis distinguishes pemphigus foliaceus from pemphigus vulgaris.[99]

Differential Diagnosis. The differential diagnosis includes staphylococcal scalded skin syndrome (SSSS), impetigo, and subcorneal pustular dermatosis. IF testing may be required to separate SSSS from pemphigus foliaceus, since a small number of acantholytic cells may be observed in SSSS. The lesions of pemphigus foliaceus may become impetiginized and secondarily altered, producing pustules as in impetigo and subcorneal pustular dermatosis. Pemphigus foliaceus contains more acantholytic keratinocytes than do the other two disorders, and pustules are the primary lesions in subcorneal pustular dermatosis. Because the lesions of pemphigus foliaceus may become superinfected, the finding of bacteria does not confirm a diagnosis of bullous impetigo; therefore, IF testing may be critical.

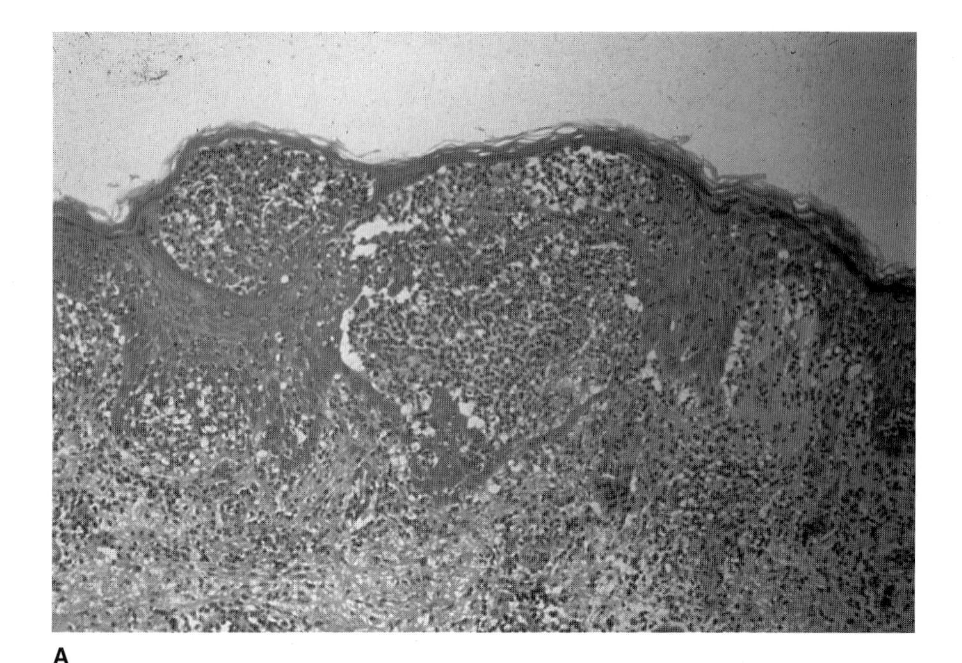

A

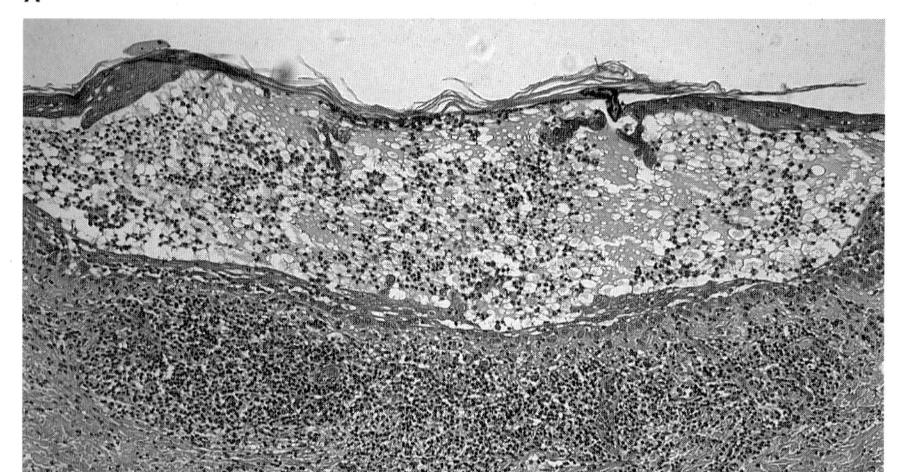

B

FIG. 9-10. IgA pemphigus
(**A**) Intraepidermal pustular variant. Intraepidermal pustules are present in a suprabasal and subcorneal location. Acantholysis is not well developed. (**B**) Subcorneal pustular variant. A subcorneal blister is filled with fluid and numerous neutrophils. A few small clusters of acantholytic cells are apparent.

Pemphigus Erythematosus

Also known as Senear-Usher syndrome, pemphigus erythematosus is a variant of pemphigus foliaceus that gets its name from its lupus erythematosus–like clinical appearance, in which the erythematous plaques and patches are in a butterfly distribution. They may remain localized to this area or may become generalized. No oral lesions are observed.[100]

Histopathology. The light microscopic features are identical to those of pemphigus foliaceus.[52,101] An interface dermatitis may also be apparent in rare cases, making distinction from lupus erythematosus difficult.

IF Testing. DIF testing of perilesional skin reveals squamous intercellular substance deposition of IgG in greater than 75% of cases, and granular deposition of IgM and IgG (i.e., a positive lupus band test) at the dermoepidermal junction. IIF study using monkey esophagus as substrate reveals squamous intercellular substance deposition of IgG in 80% of cases. Antinuclear antibodies are observed in 30% to 80% of cases.[100]

Ultrastructural Study. Pemphigus erythematosus is identical to pemphigus foliaceus in its ultrastructural alterations.

Differential Diagnosis. The differential diagnosis is the same as in pemphigus foliaceus. The presence of an interface dermatitis in some cases leads to confusion with lupus erythematosus and paraneoplastic pemphigus. Subcorneal acantholysis is not a feature of lupus erythematosus.

Drug-Induced Pemphigus

Although immunologic features identical to those of idiopathic pemphigus are reported in most cases of drug-induced pemphigus,[102] evidence now suggests that some drugs may induce acantholysis without production of antibodies.[103] The offending drugs, most frequently penicillamine, captopril, and penicillin derivatives, often contain sulfhydryl groups.[104] The earliest clinical manifestation is that of a nonspecific morbilliform or urticarial eruption. In penicillamine-induced pemphigus, the eruption is characteristic and has been labeled "toxic prepemphigus rash."[103,105] Subsequently, the characteristic lesions of pemphigus develop. Upon cessation of drug therapy, the rash regresses.

Histopathology. The findings in the early eruption are nonspecific, consisting of spongiosis, parakeratosis, and a variable dermal infiltrate. Well-developed lesions are essentially identical to those of pemphigus foliaceus or pemphigus vulgaris. Eosinophilic spongiosis may be prominent.

IF Testing. DIF testing is positive in approximately 90% of patients with drug-induced pemphigus.[103,106] IIF study of serum reveals circulating squamous intercellular substance IgG antibodies in 70% of cases.[106] The antibody titers are usually low and do not appear to correlate with the severity of disease.[105]

Pathogenesis. In those cases in which there is antibody production with subsequent acantholysis, the pathogenesis appears to be identical to that of idiopathic pemphigus. Because the pemphigus antigens have disulfide bonds, sulfhydryl-containing drugs may bind to them.[107,108] Therefore, it is possible that the drug directly affects the keratinocyte adhesion molecules, interferes with their function, and causes subsequent acantholysis, explaining those cases of drug-induced pemphigus that do not have pemphigus antibodies.

IgA Pemphigus

IgA pemphigus is a pruritic vesiculopustular eruption characterized by squamous intercellular IgA deposits and intraepidermal neutrophils. It occurs primarily in middle-aged and elderly individuals, but several cases have been described in children.[109,110] The clinical findings are similar to those in pemphigus foliaceus or subcorneal pustular dermatosis. There are flaccid vesicles, pustules, or bullae that arise on an erythematous base. They often appear in an annular arrangement.[111] Mild leukocytosis, eosinophilia, and IgA kappa paraproteinemia may be noted.[112]

In general, patients may develop one of two types: a subcorneal pustular dermatosislike disorder or an intraepidermal pustular eruption.[109,113,114]

Histopathology. Two patterns are observed that parallel the two clinical presentations. In the first, there are subcorneal vesicopustules or pustules with minimal acantholysis. In the second, intraepidermal vesicopustules or pustules contain small to moderate numbers of neutrophils (Fig. 9-10A and B). One case without neutrophil infiltration has been described.[115]

IF Testing. DIF testing reveals IgA deposition in the squamous intercellular substance throughout the epidermis with increased intensity in the upper layers in some cases of the subcorneal pustular type. Complement and other immunoglobulins are usually not present.[109] However, some cases may have both IgG and IgA present and thus may make a specific diagnosis difficult (i.e., pemphigus vulgaris vs. IgA pemphigus) unless evaluation for antigen specificity is available.[116] IF results are positive in fewer than 50% of reported cases.[117–120] The IgA bound to squamous epithelium is IgA-1. Neither IgA-2, J-chain, nor the secretory component is present.[113] The antibodies are directed against neither the pemphigus vulgaris nor the foliaceus antigen.[114] Rather, the antibodies bind with a 120kD protein (intraepidermal neutrophilic variant) or 115kD and 105kD proteins (subcorneal pustular variant) in desmosomes (desmocollins).

Differential Diagnosis. The subcorneal pustular dermatosis variant is identical to Sneddon-Wilkinson disease. Indeed, many cases reported as Sneddon-Wilkinson disease, in which IF testing was not performed, likely represent the subcorneal pustular dermatosis variant of IgA pemphigus. Pustular psoriasis, bullous impetigo, and pemphigus vulgaris are the principal differential diagnoses. Pustular psoriasis may not be distinguishable on routine light microscopic study, and therefore IF testing may be required.

Paraneoplastic Pemphigus

In this disease, painful oral ulcerations, particularly on the lower lip, have been present in all cases and are associated with a generalized, polymorphous eruption of blisters and lichenoid papules.[121,122] Bronchial and laryngeal erosions may be observed. All patients described, except possibly for one,[123] have had known or occult malignancies, including Hodgkins lymphoma, thymoma, or hematologic malignancy, especially chronic lymphocytic leukemia.[122] Castleman's disease has also been reported in association with paraneoplastic pemphigus. The age of onset is variable, and the course is refractory to treatment. Most patients have died of their skin disease.

A patient with a mixed bullous disease with features of cicatricial pemphigoid and pemphigus has been reported.[124] The patient had a B-cell lymphoma, IgM-paraproteinemia with in vivo bound IgM anti-intercellular substance antibodies, and linearly deposited IgG antiepidermal basement membrane zone antibodies. Histologically, acantholysis similar to pemphigus foliaceus and vulgaris as well as a subepidermal blister were present.

Histopathology. The principal findings are suprabasal acantholysis as seen in pemphigus vulgaris with, in addition, dyskeratosis. Characteristically, there is also a vacuolar interface dermatitis with lichenoid inflammation (Fig. 9-11A and B).[125] Paraneoplastic pemphigus may present exclusively with a lichenoid interface dermatitis in the absence of acantholysis.[126] In addition, some cases may mimic pemphigus vulgaris without a lichenoid interface dermatitis and apoptosis (T. J. Harrist, personal observation).

IF Testing. DIF testing of perilesional skin and mucosa reveals IgG in the squamous intercellular substance in concert with immune reactant deposition at the dermoepidermal junction (see Fig. 9-11C). At the dermoepidermal junction, granular deposition of complement is noted most frequently.[122] Linear deposition of complement, IgG, and IgM, and granular deposition of complement and IgG have been identified in one case each.[121] Whereas circulating paraneoplastic pemphigus antibodies bind to squamous keratinocytes in routine substrates in the majority of cases, the antibodies bind to rat bladder epithelium in all cases. The antibodies are specific for a complex of four polypeptides of molecular weights of 250-, 230-, 210-, and 190kD.[122,127–129] The 250kD and 210kD proteins appear to be

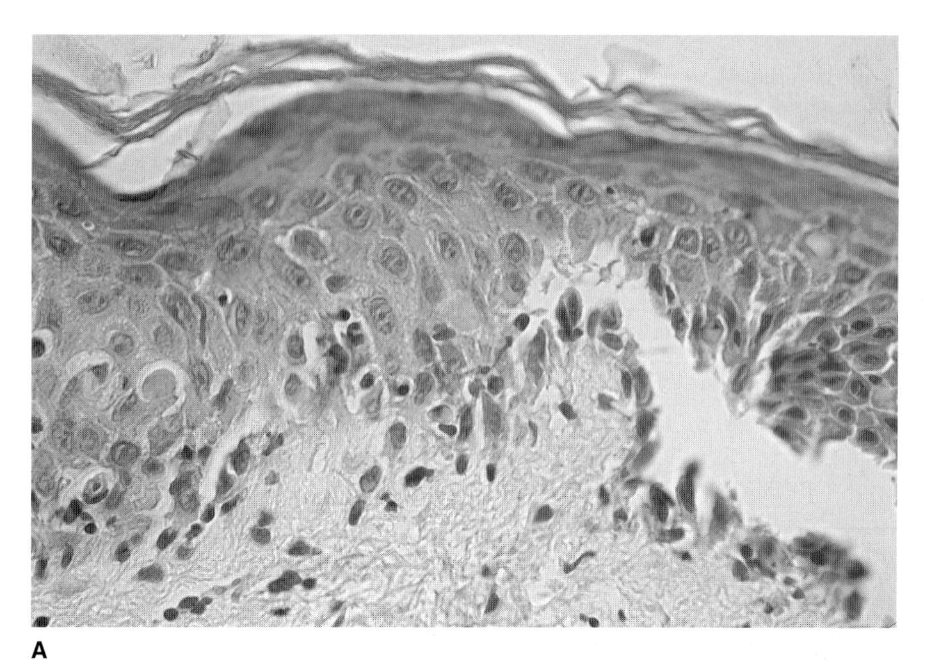

A

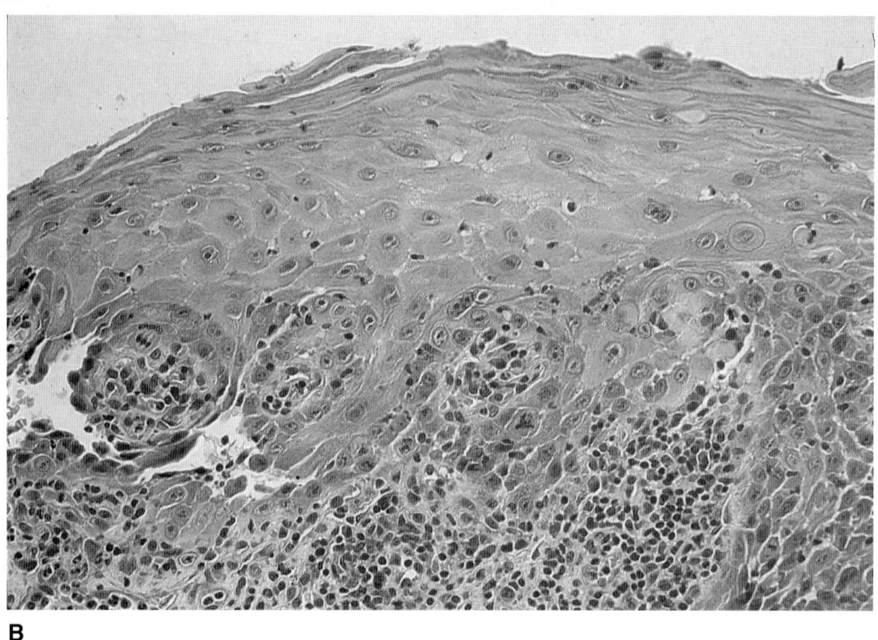

B

FIG. 9-11. Paraneoplastic pemphigus (**A**) Erythema multiforme–like pattern. A cell-poor interface dermatitis is associated with a suprabasal blister. Apoptotic keratinocytes are present. (**B**) Lichen planus–like pattern. There is a cell-rich lichenoid interface dermatitis associated with a suprabasal blister (on the *left*).

desmoplakins I and II. The 230kD antigen corresponds to the BPAg1. The 190kD antigen has not been further characterized.

PEMPHIGOID GROUP

Bullous Pemphigoid

First described in 1953, bullous pemphigoid affects primarily elderly patients with large tense bullae arising on urticarial erythematous bases or on nonerythematous skin.[130] The course is chronic and benign. In contrast to pemphigus, the Nikolsky sign is negative. The lesions involve the trunk, the extremities, and the intertriginous areas, with the oral mucosa involved in about one third of the cases. Bullous pemphigoid may start as a nonspecific eruption suggestive of urticaria or dermatitis, and can persist for weeks or months.[131,132]

Histopathology. In early lesions, papillary dermal edema in combination with a cell-poor or cell-rich perivascular lymphocytic and eosinophilic infiltrate is present. The cell-poor pattern is observed when blisters develop on relatively normal skin (Fig. 9-12) and the cell-rich pattern when the blisters arise on erythematous skin (Fig. 9-13). In the cell-poor pattern, there is usually scant perivascular lymphocytic inflammation with few eosinophils, some scattered throughout the dermis and others near the epidermis.[133,134] In the cell-rich pattern, eosinophilic papillary abscesses may develop with numerous perivascular and interstitial eosinophils intermingled with lymphocytes and neutrophils in the superficial and deep dermis.[135,136] Eosinophilic spongiosis may occur. The blister arises at the dermoepidermal junction.[130,137] Epithelial migration and regeneration may result in an intraepidermal location in older blisters (Fig. 9-14).

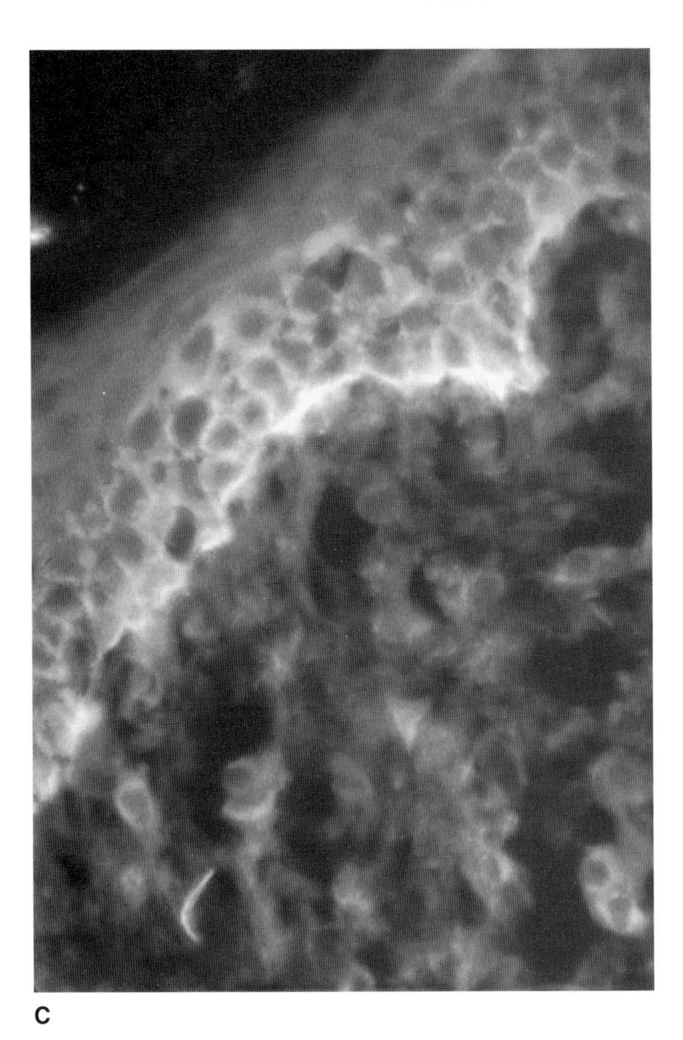

C

FIG. 9-11. *Continued*
(**C**) Direct immunofluorescence testing of perilesional skin using fluoresceinated antihuman IgG as test. There is squamous intercellular substance in lacelike array and linear deposition of IgG at the basement membrane zone. (Courtesy of Drs. Grant Anhalt and Thomas Horn.)

Similar to pemphigus vegetans, a pseudocarcinomatous hyperplasia of the epidermis, subepidermal bullae, and accumulations of eosinophils and lymphocytes may be seen.[138,139]

IF Testing. DIF testing of perilesional skin has shown linear C3 deposition (Fig. 9-15 and Table 9-4) at the dermoepidermal junction in virtually 100% of cases and IgG in 65% to 95%.[67] IIF studies reveal circulating anti–basement membrane zone IgG antibodies in 70% to 80%. Similarly deposited IgA and IgM are observed in about 25% of cases. No correlation exists between the antibody titer and the clinical severity of the disease.[140,141] The IgG is located within the lamina lucida,[142,143] where it appears bound specifically to the hemidesmosomes.[144]

Salt-split skin IF studies are an important diagnostic tool. The technique was first developed in 1984, in which normal human skin was used as a substrate and patient serum as test (indirect salt-split skin technique).[145] The epidermis is reliably split from the underlying dermis through the lamina lucida. Pemphigoid antibodies bind solely to the lower aspect of the basal keratinocytes (the blister roof) in 80% of cases; in about 20% of cases, the antibodies bind to both the lower basal keratinocytes (the roof) and the superior aspect of the base (the blister floor)(Table 9-5). Rarely, it has been reported that pemphigoid antibodies may bind solely to the floor[146,147]; however, these reports have not been substantiated.

Specimens submitted for DIF examination may also be salt-split (direct salt-split skin technique).[148,149] When this technique is used in pemphigoid, IgG is present on the roof or on the roof and the floor (Fig. 9-16A and B). Localization to only the superior aspect of the dermal base has not been reported in bullous pemphigoid using this technique (see Tables 9-4 and 9-5). This pattern is characteristic for epidermolysis bullosa acquisita (see Fig. 9-16C).

Pathogenesis. Pemphigoid antibodies bind to two antigens, a 230kD protein (BPAg1) and a second, 180kD protein (BPAg2).[150,151] The principal antigen, BPAg1, is associated with the cytoplasmic attachment site of hemidesmosomes and is largely within the basal keratinocyte. BPAg2 is a hemidesmosomal antigen now thought to be collagen XVII. The distribution of these antigens within the skin correlates with lesion location.[152] A blistering disorder clinically similar to pemphigoid

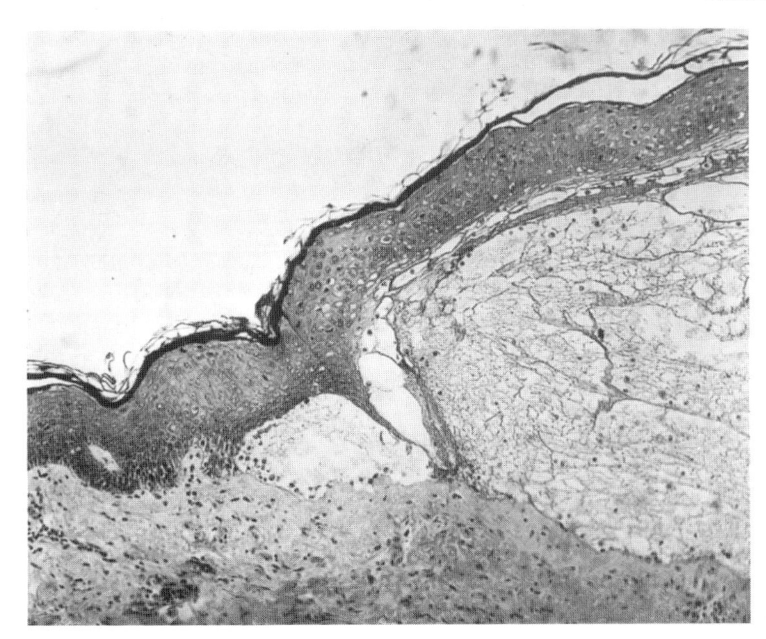

FIG. 9-12. Bullous pemphigoid
A subepidermal bulla contains a net of fibrin but only a few inflammatory cells in this relatively cell-poor variant.

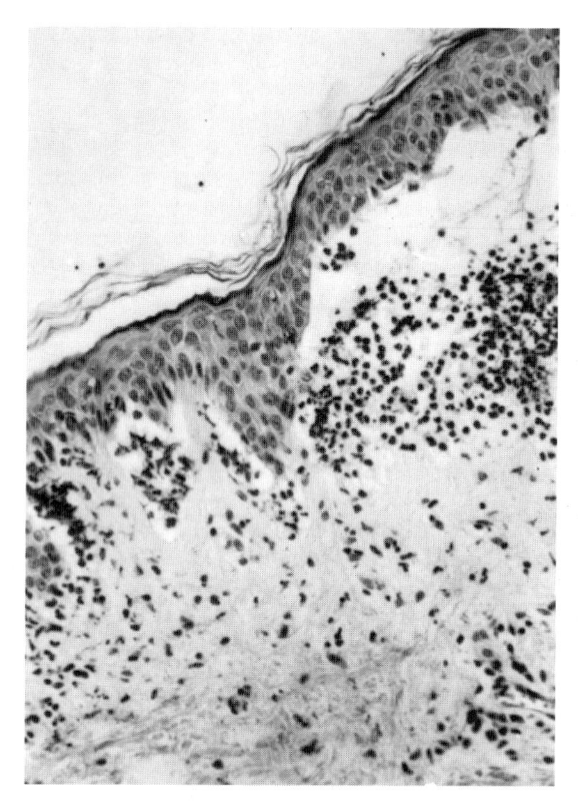

FIG. 9-13. Bullous pemphigoid
A subepidermal bulla arises on erythematous skin. There are microabscesses of eosinophils at the tips of dermal papillae in this cell-rich variant.

has antibodies that recognize a 105kD protein synthesized by both keratinocytes and fibroblasts.[153,154]

Given the known data, a sequence of pathogenetic events may be proposed. Pemphigoid antibodies bind with BPAg1 and BPAg2, activating the complement cascade. The anaphylatoxins, C3a and C4a, are elaborated, activating mast cells. Mast cell activation may be augmented by pemphigoid IgG4, which has homocytotropic properties for mast cells.[155] The mast cells degranulate, releasing a variety of inflammatory mediators, including eosinophil chemotactic factor, neutrophil chemotactic factor, leukotriene B4, proteolytic enzymes, and eosinophil stimulating factor.[156,157] Eosinophil infiltration ensues with subsequent degranulation and release of major basic protein and other proteolytic enzymes. The vessels are hyperpermeable, probably because of the release of vascular permeability factor (VPF) by keratinocytes.[158] Lamina lucida separation develops from injury of basal keratinocytes, disruption of hemidesmosomes, and proteolysis.[159] The role of infiltrating lymphocytes that are predominantly CD4+ is unclear. IL-1 and IL-2, as well as interferon-γ, have been identified in blister fluids.[160]

Ultrastructural Study. Pemphigoid antibodies bind within the lamina lucida, in particular, to the hemidesmosomes.[143,144] The blister arises within the lamina lucida in both the cell-poor and cell-rich lesions. In cell-poor lesions[161] there is disruption of the anchoring filaments without lamina densa fragmentation.[162,163] In contrast, inflammatory lesions of bullous pemphigoid reveal a pronounced infiltrate of eosinophils and mononuclear cells in the dermis with blister formation in the lamina lucida and fragmentation of the lamina densa (EMs 8 and 9).[142,164]

Clinical Variants

Drug-Associated Bullous Pemphigoid

Furosemide, phenacetin, and various penicillins have been associated with bullous pemphigoid.[165–167]

Pemphigoid Localized to the Lower Extremities

Some patients, usually women, present with tense bullae localized to the lower extremities.[168] Histologically, these reveal a cell-poor pattern and have positive IF findings less frequently than routine bullous pemphigoid. At least in one in-

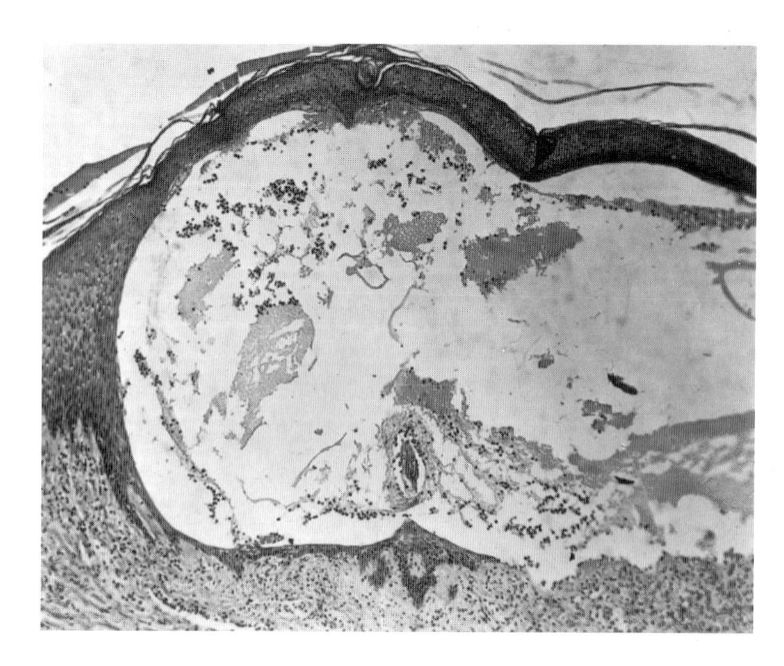

FIG. 9-14. Bullous pemphigoid
A bulla is only partially subepidermal because of regeneration of the epidermis at its floor.

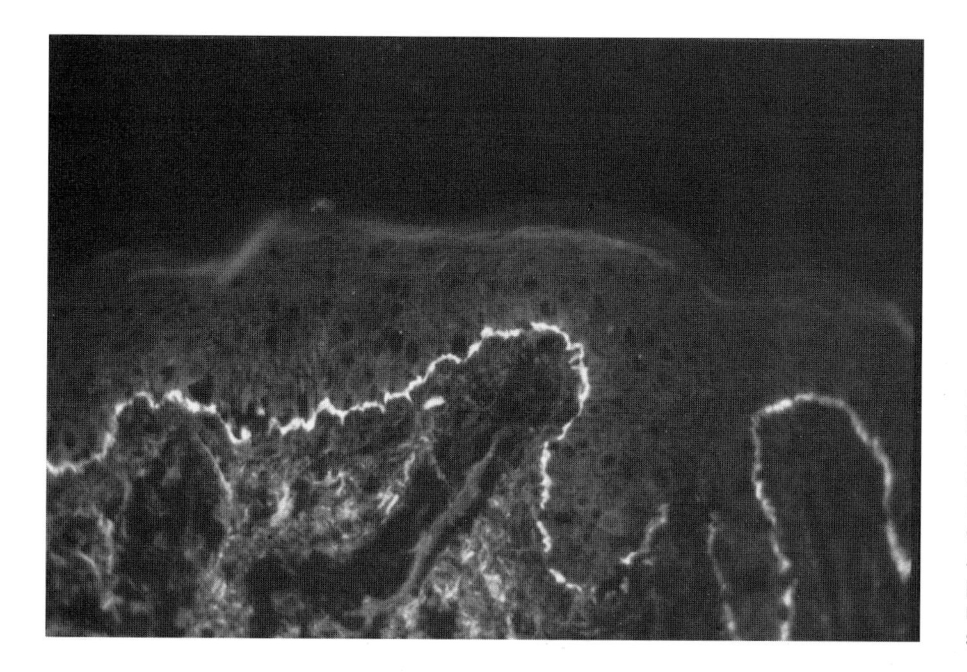

FIG. 9-15. Bullous pemphigoid Direct immunofluorescence testing of perilesional skin using fluoresceinated antihuman C3 as test. There is linearly deposited C3 along the epidermal basement membrane zone. Although characteristic of bullous pemphigoid, this pattern is not diagnostic because it is shared with other subepidermal blistering disorders.

stance, it has been shown that the IgG is directed against BPAg1.[169]

Vesicular Pemphigoid

This variant is worthy of designation only because of its clinical similarity to dermatitis herpetiformis, which may lead to misdiagnosis.

Differential Diagnosis. Histological differentiation of bullous pemphigoid from pemphigus vulgaris is not difficult because of the difference in cleavage planes and the mechanism of blister formation. Bullous pemphigoid is frequently indistinguishable from herpes gestationis; however, herpes gestationis may have greater quantities of infiltrating neutrophils and more basal keratinocyte damage. Epidermolysis bullosa acquisita (inflammatory variant) may have greater numbers of infiltrating neutrophils, but differentiation may be impossible. Dermatitis herpetiformis is characterized by a subepidermal infiltrate of neutrophils with papillary microabscesses. Similarly, linear IgA dermatosis is characterized, in the vast majority of cases, by a neutrophil-rich infiltrate. Erythema multiforme is an interface dermatitis characterized by basal vacuolopathy, dyskeratosis, and a tagging lymphohistiocytic infiltrate along the dermoepidermal junction. Diabetic blisters are noninflammatory, subepithelial in location, and often associated with fibrosis. Some patients with pemphigoid may present only with a superficial perivascular lymphoeosinophilic infiltrate without migration of eosinophils to the dermoepidermal junction. This histologic reaction pattern is most commonly associated with morbilliform

TABLE 9-4. *Direct IF testing in vesiculobullous dermatoses**

Dermatosis	Principal immunoreactant	Site	Pattern
Pemphigus, all variants except:	IgG	ICS	Lacelike
IgA pemphigus	IgA	ICS	Lacelike
Paraneoplastic pemphigus	IgG	ICS	Lacelike
	C3, IgG	BMZ	Linear
	C3, IgG	BMZ	Granular
Bullous pemphigoid	C3, IgG	BMZ	Linear
Cicatricial pemphigoid	C3, IgG	BMZ	Linear
Herpes gestationis	C3	BMZ	Linear
Epidermolysis bullosa acquisita	C3, IgG	BMZ	Linear
Bullous SLE	C3, IgG	BMZ	Linear
	C3, IgG	BMZ	Granular
Dermatitis herpetiformis	IgA	BMZ	Granular
Linear IgA dermatosis	IgA	BMZ	Linear
Erythema multiforme	C3, IgM	BMZ	Granular
	C3, IgM	Vessels	Granular

* Other immunoglobulins may be present, but they are less intense when present and less frequently observed.

ICS: squamous intercellular substance; BMZ: epidermal basement membrane zone.

TABLE 9-5. *Split-skin immunofluorescence results (indirect method)*

Roof only	Roof and base	Base only
Bullous pemphigoid (80%)	Bullous pemphigoid (~15%)	*
Cicatricial pemphigoid	Cicatricial pemphigoid	Cicatricial pemphigoid
		Epidermolysis bullosa acquisita
Linear IgA dermatosis	Linear IgA dermatosis	Linear IgA dermatosis
		Bullous systemic lupus erythematosus
		Porphyria cutanea tarda

* According to some, bullous pemphigoid IgG may localize to the base in the indirect method in 5% of cases. This is not the authors' experience (T. J. Harrist, personal experience), and the status of the cases is uncertain. In the direct methods (see refs. 148 and 149), this finding (bullous pemphigoid antibodies localizing to the base) has not been supported and has not occurred in the experience of T. J. Harrist.

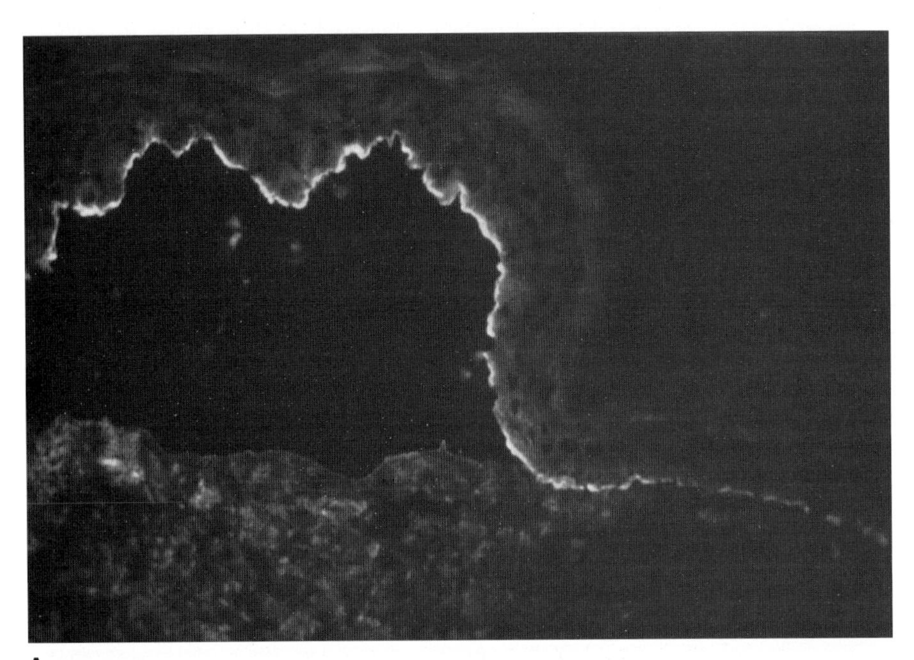

A

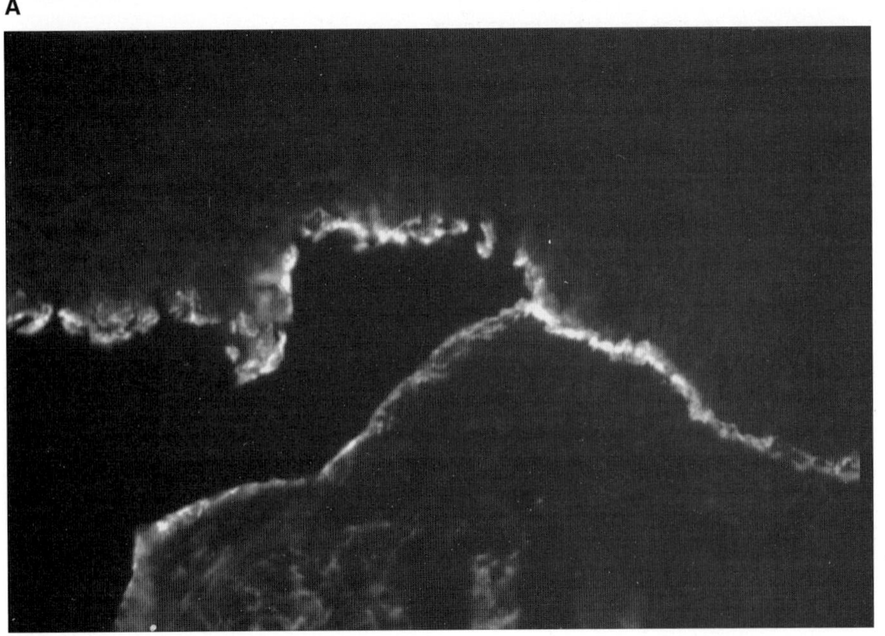

B

FIG. 9-16. Split skin immunofluorescent study using fluoresceinated antihuman IgG as test (**A**) Bullous pemphigoid. IgG is present along the base of the roof and not on the dermal base. (**B**) Bullous pemphigoid. IgG is present on the roof and on the dermal base.

drug eruptions. Rarely, the changes of eosinophilic cellulitis (Well's syndrome) may also herald the presence of pemphigoid. Bullous drug eruptions may present with subepidermal vesicles and eosinophils, and later lesions of dermatitis herpetiformis may contain eosinophils. IF study is necessary to make a specific diagnosis.

Cicatricial Pemphigoid

Historically, a bullous disorder characterized by a chronic course, scarring, and predilection for mucosal surfaces is known as cicatricial pemphigoid. Most patients are elderly, and there is a male predilection. Oral blisters are present in virtually all cases, and ocular involvement is observed in 75% and cutaneous involvement in 33%. The oral lesions are usually small blisters that subsequently erode and ulcerate. Other mucosal surfaces, including the larynx, esophagus, nose, vulva, and anus, may also be involved. Scarring is less evident in these locations than in the conjunctiva, where erythema without blisters and ulceration with subsequent scarring is the rule. Blindness occurs in up to 20% of cases. The cutaneous lesions are of two types: (1) an extensive eruption of bullae that heals without scarring,[130,170,171] and (2) areas of erythema mainly on the face and scalp in which bullae erupt intermittently followed by atrophy and scarring.[172,173] Both types of lesions may be present in the same patient.[174,175] In the Brunsting-Perry variant, there are no mucosal lesions, but rather one to several circumscribed erythematous patches on which recurrent crops of blisters appear with atrophic scarring. The patches are usually confined to the head and neck area.[176,177] Other clinical variants include a widespread nonscarring bullous eruption in which scarring lesions develop only on the head,[178] and widespread bullae that heal with atrophic scars.[179,180]

Histopathology. In cutaneous lesions, a subepidermal blister develops that may extend down adnexae. Neutrophils, histiocytes, and lymphocytes predominate in the inflammatory infiltrate. Eosinophils may or may not be numerous. Lamellar fibrosis beneath the epidermis is a hallmark but may not be present in the initial lesions. Mucosal lesions generally have a lichenoid lymphocytic infiltrate in which neutrophils or eosinophils or both may be present.[181] The changes are often nonspecific in both mucosal and cutaneous lesions, but the above features should lead to consideration of cicatricial pemphigoid.

IF testing. DIF studies reveal linear IgG and C3 in lesional and perilesional skin in approximately 80% of cases. In three series, a total of 35 of 46 patients had linear deposits.[182–184] In most, both IgG and C3 were present, occasionally in association with IgA or IgM. Rarely, only C3 was present.[183] In other cases labeled *cicatricial pemphigoid,* linear IgA was the only immunoglobulin found;[184,185] the best label is therefore *linear IgA bullous dermatosis.* Patients with cicatricial conjunctivitis therefore display only IgA deposits and are best considered a scarring variant of linear IgA dermatosis.[186–188] With respect to the Brunsting-Perry type, 9 of 10 patients had linear IgG at the dermoepidermal junction, 3 of whom had concomitant linear C3.[177,189,190]

IIF testing of serum yields variable results depending on the substrate used (monkey esophagus, guinea pig esophagus, normal human skin, salt-split skin). It appears that circulating antibodies in this disorder may be more readily demonstrated when salt-split human skin is used as substrate, in which IgG may be localized only to the roof or, on occasion, to the base of the induced separation (see Table 9-5).[191,192]

The difference in localization may be explained by differing antigenic specificity of the antibodies. In some cases, the antigen has been the BPAg1,[151] while in others, the BPAg2,[193] a 100kD protein, or epilegrin[194] has been described. All of these antigens occur within the lamina lucida, with epilegrin present in the lower lamina lucida. This may explain the localization of the antibody to the artifactually created blister base in salt-split skin preparations (see Table 9-5). At this point in time, cicatricial pemphigoid is best considered not one disease but several diseases with a similar clinical phenotype of scarring, predilec-

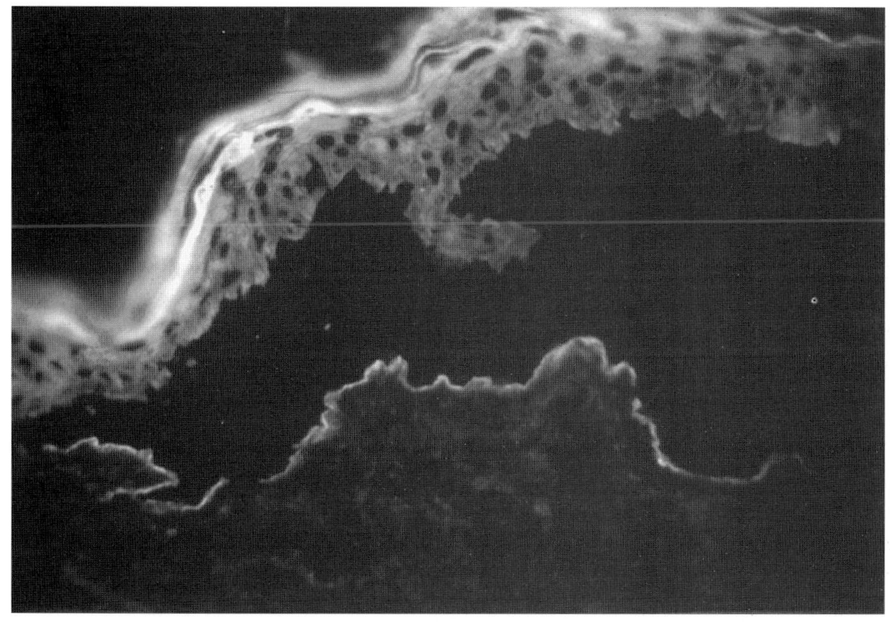
C

FIG. 9-16. *Continued*
(**C**) Epidermolysis bullosa acquisita. IgG is present only on the dermal base.

tion for mucosal and conjunctival surfaces, and subepidermal bullae. Many cases in the literature labeled *cicatricial pemphigoid* without adequate immunological study are best labeled *linear IgA disease* or *epidermolysis bullosa acquisita involving principally mucosal surfaces*.

Ultrastructural Study. Electron microscopic examination revealed in two studies that the oral and cutaneous lesions possess an intact basement membrane zone at the base of the blister.[171,195] In another study of both the oral and cutaneous lesions, the basement membrane zone was destroyed.[196]

Herpes Gestationis

This is a blistering disorder that usually develops during the second to third trimester in pregnant women. It is estimated to occur in 1 in 50,000 pregnancies.[197] Intensely pruritic, urticarial lesions usually develop on the abdomen with subsequent involvement of the extremities, hands, and feet. They usually progress to herpetiform tense vesicles and bullae. The disorder may recur with subsequent pregnancies, menstrual periods, or the use of birth control pills. The course for the mother is benign. There is a debate concerning the possibility of an increased incidence and risk of fetal morbidity and mortality. Recent data indicate that no such risk can be confirmed;[198] however, there has been an association with prematurity and small-for-gestational-age weights.[199] The infant, however, may be born with a mild, transient, vesiculobullous eruption secondary to transplacental transfer of the mediating antibody.[200,201]

Histopathology. In zones of erythema and edema, there is a perivascular infiltrate composed of lymphocytes and many eosinophils. There is marked papillary dermal edema. There may be spongiosis and intracellular edema.[202] Eosinophilic spongiosis may be observed. Focal necrosis of the basal keratinocytes, which has been emphasized by some authors, leads to a subepidermal blister (Fig 9-17).[203]

IF Testing. DIF testing reveals linear deposition of C3 in perilesional skin in virtually all patients.[200] IgG is similarly deposited in 30% to 40%.[201,204] Immunoelectron microscopic study has revealed IgG and C3 to reside within the lamina lucida. Using routine IIF studies of serum, it is uncommon to demonstrate a circulating anti–squamous basement membrane zone antibody. Using in vitro complement fixation, a circulating anti–basement membrane zone IgG is demonstrable in most cases. At this point in time, the use of the label *HG factor* for this antibody is of historical interest only. The BPAg2 is the principal antigen, but the BPAg1 is recognized in some patients as well.[205,206] BPAg2 appears to be a component of type XVII collagen.[207]

Ultrastructural Study. The epidermis at the periphery of bullae shows significant damage, most pronounced in basal keratinocytes, with resultant complete or partial necrosis of epidermal cells.[208] Despite the fact that basal keratinocytes show severe damage, the basal cell plasma membrane and the lamina densa are well preserved and are present at the floor of the blister (EM 11). The hemidesmosomes may be intact in some areas.[209]

VESICULOBULLOUS DERMATOSES WITH AUTOIMMUNITY TO TYPE VII COLLAGEN

Epidermolysis Bullosa Acquisita (EBA)

Classically, EBA is a noninherited disorder of acquired skin fragility.[210,211] This presentation of EBA was the only one recognized until recently. Blisters develop on noninflammatory bases with a predilection for acral areas. Scarring and milia formation ensue. A characteristic nail dystrophy and alopecia are noted. This presentation is associated with malignant lymphoma, amyloidosis, and colitis or enteritis. Histologically, a noninflammatory subepidermal blister is observed along with fibrosis and milia formation. Some patients with EBA may have significant involvement of oral and conjunctival mucosa and therefore may be *cicatricial pemphigoidlike*.[212] However, acral lesions are prominent and nail dystrophy is noted. In this type,

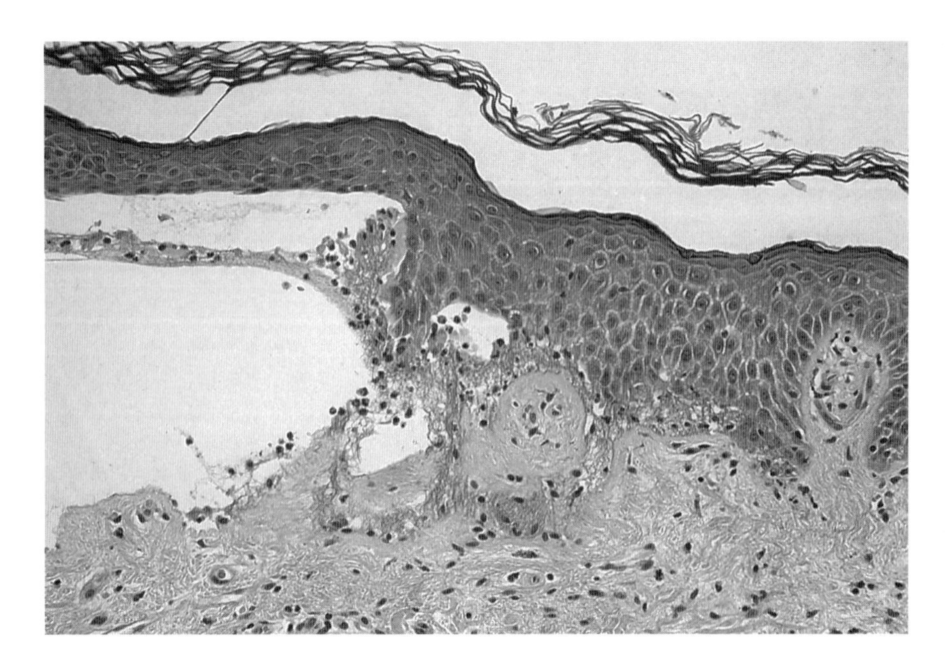

FIG. 9-17. Herpes gestationis A subepidermal blister arises on the basis of basal keratinocyte necrosis in the setting of an eosinophil-rich infiltrate. Note the necrotic keratinocytes on the base of the blister roof.

biopsy from mucosal lesions reveals inflammatory, subepidermal bullae with scarring and milia similar to cicatricial pemphigoid. The histologic changes in cutaneous lesions are identical to those noted in the classic form.

In 1984, five patients with EBA had clinical, histologic, and immunohistologic features characteristic of bullous pemphigoid.[211] They had generalized, pruritic, erythematous macules and papules on which bullae arose. There was less tendency for the lesions to develop acrally and greater involvement of flexural surfaces than in the previously described forms of EBA. At presentation, neither scarring nor milia were discerned; however, delicate scars developed later at the sites of blister formation.

Histopathology. The *bullous pemphigoidlike* presentation described above is the most common form of EBA. The subepidermal blisters are inflammatory. The predominant infiltrating cells are lymphocytes and neutrophils in perivascular and focal interstitial array (Fig. 9-18A and B). Eosinophils are present in small numbers. In the classic form, the subepidermal blisters are noninflammatory.

IF Testing. Examination of perilesional skin using DIF reveals linear deposition of complement at the basement membrane zone in the vast majority of cases. IgG is by far the most common immunoglobulin found, but IgM and IgA may be present as well. Increasing numbers of immunoglobulin subclasses noted at the dermoepidermal junction favor a diagnosis of EBA over bullous pemphigoid. The presence of linear C3 at the dermoepidermal junction alone favors bullous pemphigoid over EBA. However, use of routine DIF cannot reliably distinguish between bullous pemphigoid and EBA. IIF reveals circulating anti–basement membrane zone antibodies in up to 50%.[210,213,214]

Use of the salt-split skin technique leads to the appropriate diagnosis in most cases (see Table 9-5, Fig. 9-16A–C).[215] The

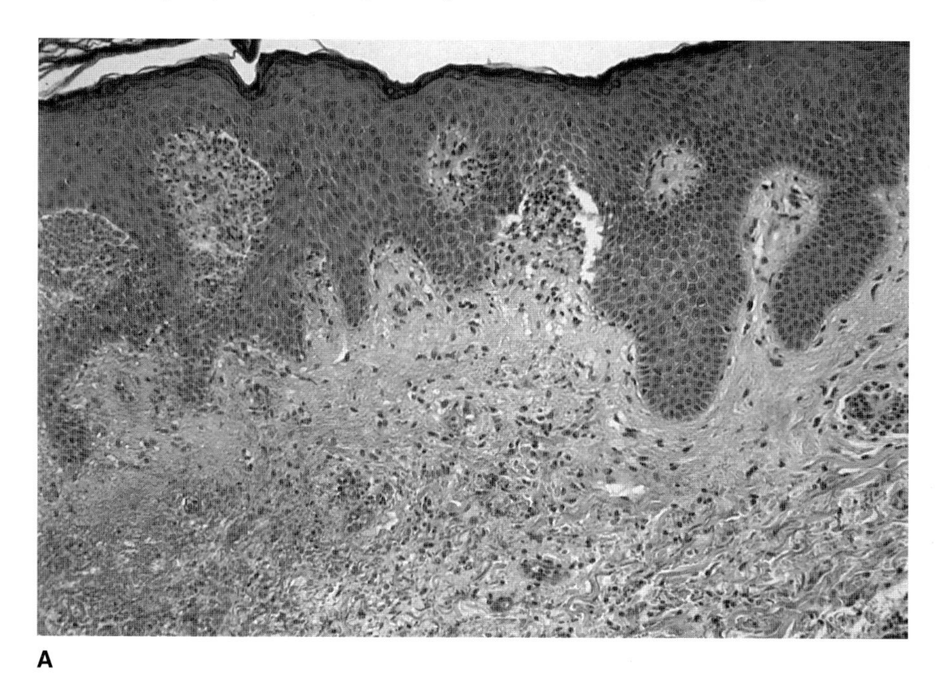

A

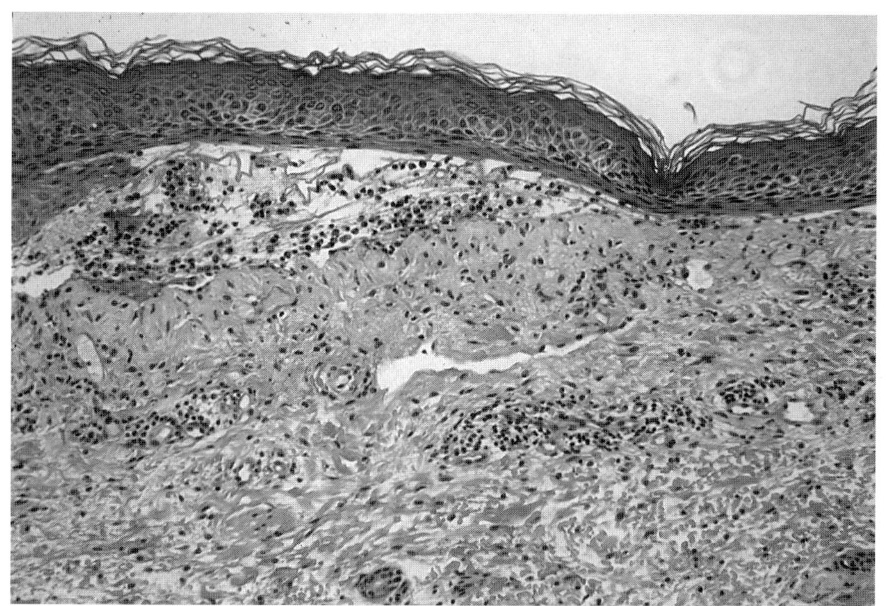

B

FIG. 9-18. Epidermolysis bullosa acquisita, inflammatory variant
(**A**) Early lesion. An infiltrate of eosinophils and neutrophils is present around superficial vessels and in dermal papillae, giving rise focally to separation of the epidermis from the dermis (center). (**B**) Late lesion. A subepidermal blister is apparent, containing principally eosinophils. There is delicate papillary dermal fibroplasia.

antibodies in EBA have specificity for the globular carboxyl terminus of type VII collagen and are deposited beneath the lamina densa.[216,217] Therefore, on salt-split skin studies, IgG is on the floor and not on the roof of the split (see Table 9-5).[215]

Bullous Systemic Lupus Erythematosus (SLE)

Vesicles and bullae may develop in patients with systemic lupus erythematosus. In contrast to dermatitis herpetiformis, they are nonpruritic and may be widespread. In contrast to dermatitis herpetiformis, the lesions are neither symmetrical nor do they have a predilection for extensor surfaces of arms, elbows, or scalp. The lesions may be photodistributed. These patients rarely have classic lesions of discoid, systemic, or subacute cutaneous lupus erythematosus when they develop blisters. In cases from the literature, the vast majority have had a previous history of lupus erythematosus, and most authors have required definitive American Rheumatologic Association (ARA) criteria before making the diagnosis in those patients with bullous lesions. However, at least three patients (who later developed other stigmata of lupus) have presented with a blistering eruption but without previous signs or symptoms of connective tissue disease.[218–221] Bullous lupus erythematosus is most common in women, particularly black women.[222–226] Most of these cases were exquisitely sensitive to dapsone therapy, with rapid involution of the lesions. No correlation with clinical activity of lupus erythematosus was apparent.[225] Some patients with EBA will progress to SLE. (See also Chap. 10.)

Histopathology. Three histologic patterns have been identified in such lesions. The first is striking basal layer vacuolization with subsequent blister formation. The second is vasculitis with subepidermal blister and pustule formation. The third and most common is a dermatitis herpetiformislike histologic pattern. Approximately 25% of cases are said to have a small-vessel, neutrophil-rich leukocytoclastic vasculitis beneath the blister.[225] Histologic features more routinely identified with lupus erythematosus are not present. Another histologic finding that is not emphasized in most case reports is the presence of dermal mucin and hyaluronic acid as defined by alcian blue stain at pH 2.5.[227] The frequency of mucin deposition is unknown.

IF Testing. In all reported cases, IgG and C3 are deposited at the epidermal basement membrane zone. The pattern was linear in more than 50% and was referred to as "granular bandlike" in approximately 25%. IgM and IgA were present in approximately 50% and 60% of cases, respectively. The conflicting pattern of immune reactant deposition is difficult to explain. In these reports, the pattern varies from a "thick band" to a "fine ribbonlike" or "tubular" pattern. The ribbonlike or linear pattern represents antibodies that are bound to rigid, anatomically compartmentalized antigens such as in bullous pemphigoid or epidermolysis bullosa acquisita. In general, granular patterns represent deposition of circulating immune complexes in situ or in situ binding of antigen and antibody in noncompartmentalized zones. Therefore, perhaps some of the cases represent tubular or linear deposition obscured by confluent granular bands (positive lupus band test). IIF study of serum rarely reveals circulating anti–squamous basement membrane zone antibodies that are detected against type VII collagen.[220] It should be noted, however, that salt-split skin preparations may be a more sensitive substrate than whole-skin mounts.

A salt-split skin preparation using patient serum reveals localization to the split floor as in EBA (see Table 9-5). Lastly, Western immunoblots reveal binding to either 290kD or 145kD dermal proteins, components of type VII collagen.[228] However, antibodies to type VII collagen are not present in all cases.

Ultrastructural Study. Immunoelectron microscopic examination reveals electron-dense deposits of IgG at the lower edge of the basal lamina and immediately subjacent dermis in an identical location to the antibody in EBA.[228]

SUBEPIDERMAL IGA-MEDIATED VESICULOBULLOUS DERMATOSES

Dermatitis Herpetiformis

This is an intensely pruritic, chronic recurrent dermatitis that has a slight male predilection. The lesions usually develop in young to middle-aged adults as symmetrical grouped papulovesicles, vesicles, or crusts on erythematous bases. Oral lesions are absent.[229] The elbows, knees, buttocks, scapula, and scalp are commonly involved. There is an increased but rare risk of lymphoma.[230] Dermatitis herpetiformis in association with systemic lupus erythematosus has also been reported.[231]

Histopathology. The typical histologic features are best observed in erythematous skin adjacent to early blisters. In these zones, neutrophils accumulate at the tips of dermal papillae.[232] With an increase in size to microabscesses, a significant admixture of eosinophils may be noted. As microabscesses form, a separation develops between the tips of the dermal papillae and the overlying epidermis, so that early blisters are multiloculated (Fig. 9-19).[233] The presence of fibrin in the papillae may give them a bluish appearance.[234] Within 1 to 2 days, the rete ridges lose their attachment to the dermis, and the blisters then become unilocular (Fig. 9-20) and clinically apparent.[235] At this time, the characteristic papillary microabscesses may be observed at the blister periphery. For this reason, the inclusion of perivesicular skin in the biopsy specimen is of utmost value. The papillary dermis beneath the papillae may have a relatively intense inflammatory infiltrate of neutrophils and some eosinophils. Many neutrophils may exhibit leukocytoclasis. Subjacent to this, a perivascular infiltrate composed of lymphocytes, neutrophils, and eosinophils may be apparent.[134,236] In one study, the diagnostic finding of papillary microabscesses was present in all patients.[237] In another study of 105 biopsy specimens, they were present in only 52%.[238] Apoptotic keratinocytes may be noted above the papillary microabscesses.

IF Testing. In 1967, Cormane described the presence of granular deposits of IgA within the dermal papillae in both lesional and nonlesional skin.[239] IgA is found alone or in combination with other immune reactants in over 95% of cases when uninvolved skin of the forearm or buttock is tested (Fig. 9-21). Fibrillary IgA deposits may also be present. The cutaneous IgA is IgA-1.[240] It is unclear at this time whether J-chain is present, since conflicting data has been reported. Early in the course of the disease, IgA deposits may be absent, and repeat DIF is necessary.[241,242] Some recommend that biopsies be taken from clinically normal skin immediately adjacent to erythema, because false-negative results may occur when blistered or inflamed skin is evaluated.[233,243] Two negative results on DIF testing are a strong indication that the patient does not have der-

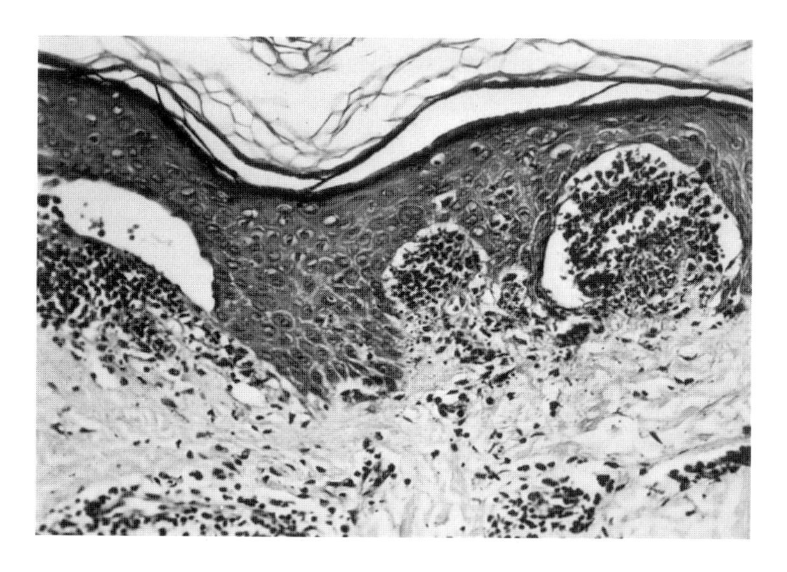

FIG. 9-19. Dermatitis herpetiformis
Dermal papillary microabscesses composed of neutrophils are characteristic. The microabscesses cause separation between the tips of papillae and the epidermis so that the early blisters are multilocular. The presence of fibrin gives them a bluish hue.

matitis herpetiformis. The presence of IgA within the skin is not altered by dapsone therapy. After as long as 2 years, a gluten-free diet results in the disappearance of IgA from the skin.

Circulating IgA antibodies that react against reticulin, smooth muscle endomysium, the dietary antigen gluten, bovine serum albumin, and β-lactoglobin may be present. Using monkey or pig gut as substrate, IIF has been used to detect antiendomysial antibodies, which are present in 52% to 100% of patients.[244,245]

Pathogenesis. Three important findings must be considered in the pathogenesis of dermatitis herpetiformis. First, the disease is associated with a gluten-sensitive enteropathy; second, granular IgA is deposited in the skin; and third, patients have a high frequency of certain HLA antigens. HLA-B8, DR3, and Dqw2 have been identified in high frequency in patients with dermatitis herpetiformis.[246–248] The majority of patients show celiac spruelike changes on jejunal biopsy.[249] This implies that gluten may lead directly to an immunological IgA response or to a defective mucosal barrier that allows entrance of other dietary proteins to which an IgA immunological response may be mounted. The resultant IgA response may lead to deposition of immune complexes, or to in vivo binding of IgA to dietary protein or similar antigens in the skin. At this time, the exact mechanism is unclear.

Ultrastructural Study. The changes in dermatitis herpetiformis resemble those observed in the inflammatory bullae of bullous pemphigoid.[164] Neutrophils are the major inflammatory cell in the former, whereas eosinophils predominate in the latter. Fibrin appears earlier and in greater amount in dermatitis herpetiformis, particularly in dermal papillae (EM 10). While it has been shown immunohistochemically that the early blister forms above the apparently intact lamina lucida,[250] in more advanced lesions the lamina densa has been destroyed, as is noted in the "inflammatory bullae" of bullous pemphigoid.[232,237]

Linear IgA Dermatosis

A group of bullous disorders mediated by IgA antibodies with differing specificities for epidermal basement membrane zone antigens has been labeled *linear IgA dermatosis.* Some patients with linear IgA deposits at the epidermal basement membrane zone are better classified as IgA bullous pemphigoid or IgA epidermolysis bullosa acquisita, since the antibodies have specificity for BPAg1 or type VII collagen, respectively. However, there are two relatively definitive clinical phenotypes that are based on patient age and clinical features—adult linear IgA dermatosis and childhood linear IgA dermatosis (chronic

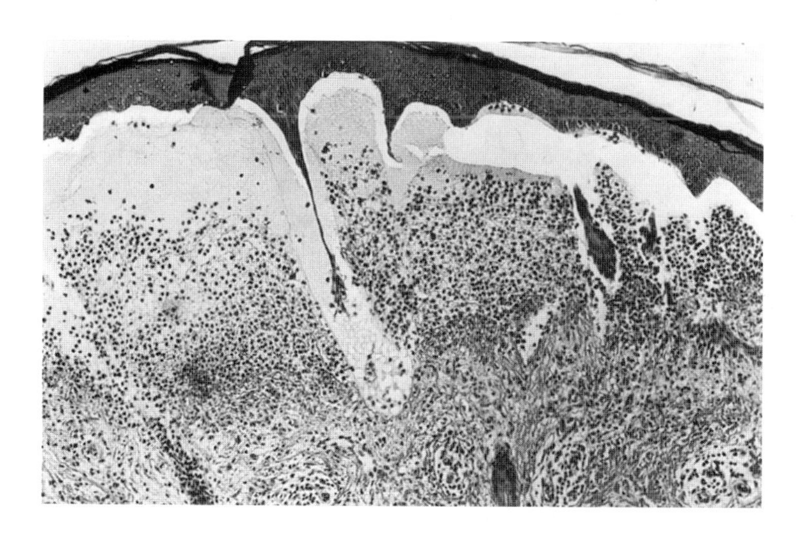

FIG. 9-20. Dermatitis herpetiformis
A fully developed subepidermal blister is no longer multilocular. Most of the infiltrating cells are neutrophils.

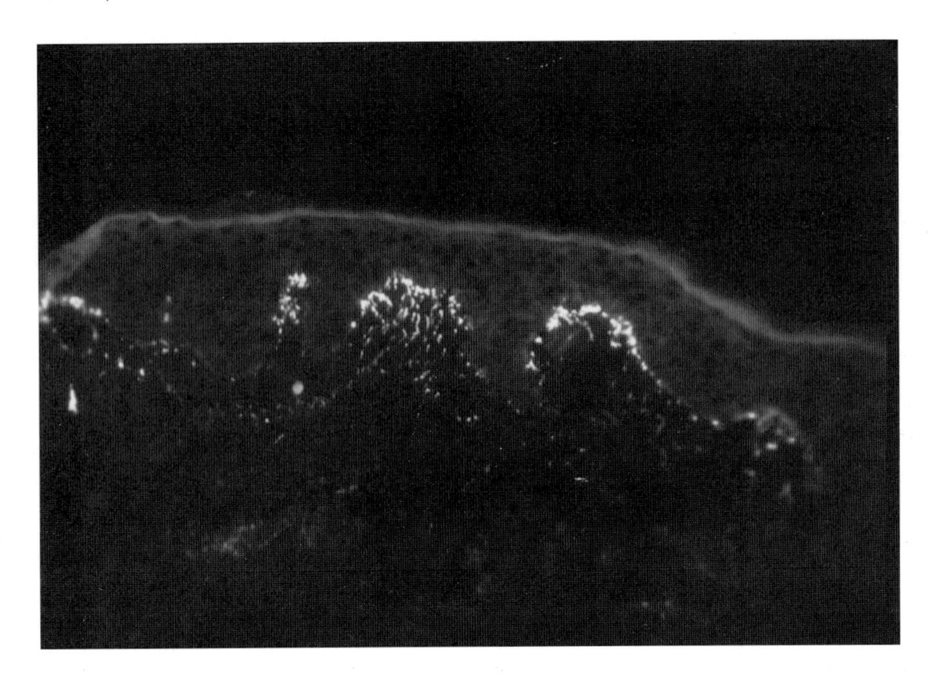

FIG. 9-21. Dermatitis herpetiformis Direct immunofluorescence testing using fluoresceinated antihuman IgA as test. There is granular and thready IgA predominantly at the tips of dermal papillae, at the exact site of the greatest infiltration of neutrophils and the point of earliest subepidermal blister formation.

benign bullous dermatosis of childhood)—and one other is associated with drug therapy.

Adult Type

Vesicles and bullae develop in patients usually over 40 years of age, with a slight female predilection. The lesions are less symmetrical and less pruritic than those in dermatitis herpetiformis but are distributed in similar locations. Ocular and oral lesions may be present in up to 50% of cases. A rare association with systemic lupus erythematosus has been reported.[251] Linear IgA dermatosis has also been associated with lymphoma.[230]

Histopathology. The features are similar if not identical to dermatitis herpetiformis. According to some, there is less tendency for papillary microabscess formation and greater tendency for uniform neutrophil infiltration along the entire dermoepidermal junction and rete in inflamed skin (Fig. 9-22).[252] Rarely, one may observe a principally lymphocytic infiltrate (T. J. Harrist, personal observation), sometimes with numerous neutrophils.[251]

IF Testing. As this test defines the disease, DIF reveals linear IgA along the basement membrane zone in perilesional skin in 100% of cases. One patient presented with linearly deposited IgG initially and only subsequently developed linear IgA deposits.[253] In the vast majority of cases, it is IgA1, but rarely IgA2 is present. When IgG and IgA are present, some detailed immunological study may be needed to allow differential diagnosis with bullous pemphigoid.[254] It has been suggested that, if the IgA deposits are more intense than the IgG deposits and C3

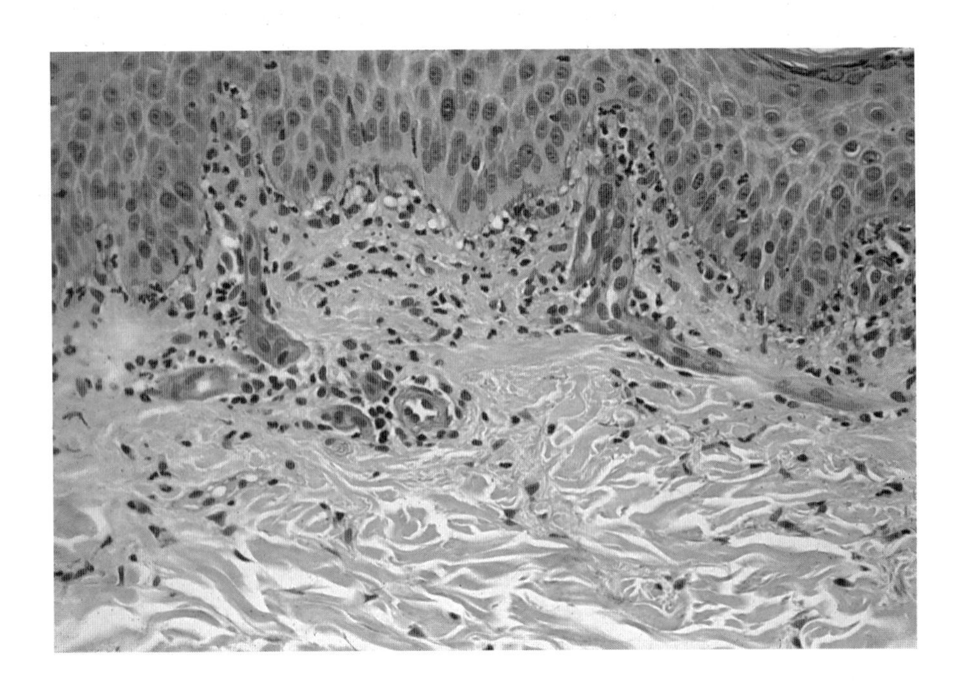

FIG. 9-22. Linear IgA dermatosis Neutrophils infiltrate all along the epidermal basement membrane zone, associated with vacuolopathy (periodic acid–Schiff reagent stain with diastase digestion).

deposition is strong, that linear IgA dermatosis is the best diagnosis.[255] However, it is best considered a distinct disorder labeled *linear IgA/IgG dermatosis* until more data are available. Low titers of circulating anti–squamous basement membrane zone IgA have been identified in only 20% to 30% of cases.[256–259] A recent study, however, has noted such antibodies in up to 75% of patients.[260–261] Split skin results are variable (see Table 9-5).

Pathogenesis. The pathogenesis is unknown.

Ultrastructural Study. The antibodies are deposited principally within the lamina lucida and less commonly beneath the lamina densa.[256,258,262–267]

The antigens against which the IgA is directed include a 97kD protein that may be found in epidermal and dermal extracts.[263] A second antigen is a 285kD protein.[258] These antigens have not been further defined at this time.

Drug-Associated Linear IgA Dermatosis

It is important to note that it is not infrequent for adult-type linear IgA dermatosis to be associated with drug therapy. Vancomycin, lithium, diclofenac, captopril, cifinmandol, and somatostatin have been associated with such presentations.[268–271] Histologically, the changes are identical to idiopathic linear IgA dermatosis in most cases. In some cases, there is an associated lymphoeosinophilic infiltrate in combination with an interface neutrophilic infiltration.

Childhood Type

Originally known as chronic bullous dermatosis of childhood, this disease is unique.[272] The disorder presents in prepubertal, often preschool children, and rarely in infancy. Vesicles or bullae develop on an erythematous or normal base, occasionally giving rise to a so-called string of pearls, a characteristic lesion in which peripheral vesicles develop on a polycyclic plaque.[255,273] They involve the buttocks, lower abdomen, and genitalia, and characteristically have a perioral distribution on the face. Oral lesions may occur.[274] The disorder usually remits by age 6 to 8, but 12% in one series experienced persistent disease.[261,275]

Histopathology. The features are similar to those of the adult-type disease. Some cases, however, resemble bullous pemphigoid because of the presence of eosinophils.[274,276]

IF Testing. DIF testing reveals linearly deposited IgA in virtually 100% of cases.[277] The exact location of the antibody deposition is unclear. At this time, the antigens are thought to be identical to those noted in the adult-type disease.

NONINFECTIOUS VESICULOPUSTULAR DERMATOSES

Erythema Toxicum Neonatorum

A benign, asymptomatic eruption affecting about 40% of term infants usually within 12 to 48 hours after birth, erythema toxicum neonatorum lasts 2 to 3 days and consists of blotchy macular erythema, papules, and pustules that tend to develop at sites of pressure. The eruption is associated with blood eosinophilia.

Histopathology. The macular erythema is characterized by sparse eosinophils in the upper dermis, largely in a perivascular location, and mild papillary dermal edema.

The papules show an accumulation of numerous eosinophils and some neutrophils in the area of the follicle and overlying epidermis (Fig. 9-23). Papillary dermal edema is more intense and eosinophils more numerous.

Mature pustules are subcorneal and are filled with eosinophils and occasional neutrophils. The pustules form as a result of the upward migration of eosinophils to the surface epidermis from within and around the hair follicles.[278]

Pathogenesis. The etiology is unknown. However, two hypotheses have been recently offered. The first is high-viscosity ground substance in the newborn which, because of osmotic changes at birth, causes tissue dilution and inflammation with minor trauma.[279] Second, the eruption has been suggested to be a minor acute graft-versus-host reaction caused by maternal-fetal transfer of lymphocytes during delivery.[280]

Differential Diagnosis. The subcorneal pustules of impetigo and transient neonatal pustular melanosis are not follicular in origin and contain neutrophils rather than eosinophils. A smear of a pustule is helpful to characterize the predominant inflammatory cell. Although many eosinophils are present in the vesicles of incontinentia pigmenti, the vesicle is intraepidermal rather than subcorneal, and spongiosis is present. In addition, necrotic keratinocytes may be prominent in incontinentia pigmenti but are absent in erythema toxicum neonatorum.

Transient Neonatal Pustular Melanosis

Affecting 4.4% of black newborns and 0.6% of white newborns, flaccid vesicopustules with a predilection for the face, trunk, and diaper area develop at birth.[281] These rupture after 1 to 2 days, leaving hyperpigmented macules with collarettes of scale. The development of typical lesions of erythema toxicum neonatorum has been observed days later.[282] Perhaps the two eruptions represent the same disease in different phases, or their coexistence may be on the basis of the frequent occurrence of erythema toxicum neonatorum.

Histopathology. The vesicopustules consist of intracorneal or subcorneal aggregates of neutrophils with an admixture of eosinophils. Fragmented hair shafts may reside within the blister cavity.[282] Within the dermis is an inflammatory infiltrate with some neutrophils and eosinophils. The macules show focal basal hypermelaninosis.[281]

Acropustulosis of Infancy

Recurrent crops of intensely pruritic vesicles or pustules, 1 to 3 mm in diameter, are often mistaken for scabies. They develop primarily in black infants at birth or during the first year of life.[283,284] The lesions occur predominantly on the distal extremities, heal with hyperpigmentation, and resolve in most cases by age 2. Rare cases have been reported in older children.[285]

Histopathology. The intraepidermal or subcorneal vesicopustules contain neutrophils and sparse eosinophils. There is

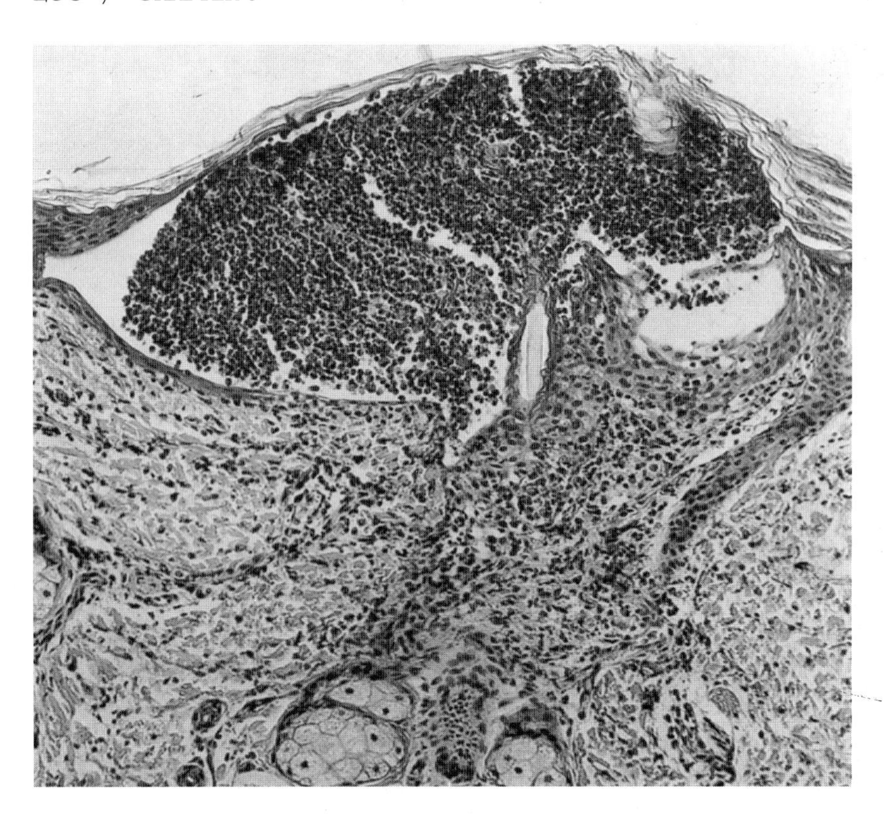

FIG. 9-23. Erythema toxicum neonatrum A subcorneal follicular pustule is filled with eosinophils. There is extensive infiltration of the outer root sheath with eosinophils. (Courtesy of Dieter Luders, MD.)

mild papillary dermal edema and a sparse, mixed, superficial perivascular infiltrate.[286,287]

Pathogenesis. The etiology of infantile acropustulosis is unknown. The disease may be associated with atopic dermatitis and elevated serum IgE levels.[287,288] Direct and indirect immunofluorescence studies have been negative.

Differential Diagnosis. Impetigo, subcorneal pustular dermatosis, candidiasis, and transient neonatal pustular melanosis may be identical to acropustulosis of infancy, so that clinical data are necessary for differentiation. Special stains are necessary to rule out an infectious etiology.

Vesiculopustular Eruption Associated with Hepatobiliary Disease

Recently, seven adults presented with a vesiculopustular eruption, principally on the extremities, in association with hepatobiliary disease.[289] The eruption may herald the hepatobiliary disease. In some instances the lesions evolved from necrotic pustules to atrophic scars. The associated diseases consisted of primary sclerosing cholangitis, hepatitis B infection, and chronic active hepatitis. Cystic fibrosis and Gilbert's syndrome were also observed.

Histopathology. A subepidermal blister developed in association with a subepidermal neutrophilic infiltrate. The subjacent collagen exhibited "fibrinoid degeneration." A suppurative folliculitis was noted in these patients as well.[289] The histologic changes are similar to a previously described diffuse pustular eruption associated with ulcerative colitis.[290]

IF Testing. In two cases, there was no immune reactant deposition. In one case, there was "dermal" and perivascular C3.

Subcorneal Pustular Dermatosis

Also known as Sneddon-Wilkinson disease, subcorneal pustular dermatosis is a chronic disorder first described in 1956, and is characterized by sterile pustules that have a predilection for flexural surfaces and the axillary and inguinal folds.[291] The pustules are seen in an annular or serpiginous arrangement. Pus characteristically accumulates in the lower half of large pustules.[292] Oral lesions do not occur.

Subcorneal pustular dermatosis may be associated with a monoclonal gammopathy, most commonly an IgA paraproteinemia. Some of these cases eventuate in an IgA myeloma.[293]

Histopathology. The pustules are subcorneal and contain neutrophils, with only an occasional eosinophil (Fig. 9-24). The underlying slightly edematous stratum malpighii contains a small number of neutrophils. In some instances, a few acantholytic cells are in the base of the pustule, most likely because of proteolytic enzymes present in the pustular content. They may be partially attached to the epidermis or may lie free in the pustule among the neutrophils.[294] The dermal papillae contain dilated capillaries and a perivascular infiltrate composed of neutrophils and a few eosinophils and mononuclear cells.[295]

IF Testing. In rare reports, DIF study shows IgG and C3 along the basement membrane zone.[296]

Pathogenesis. In some patients, elevated levels of tumor necrosis factor-α in the serum and pustules may be responsible for neutrophil activation.[296]

Ultrastructural Study. The edge of the pustules shows cytolytic changes in the upper epidermis, especially in the granular layer. Dissolution of the plasma membrane and of the cytoplasm of granular cells causes the formation of a subcorneal split. The transepidermal migration of neutrophils and their sub-

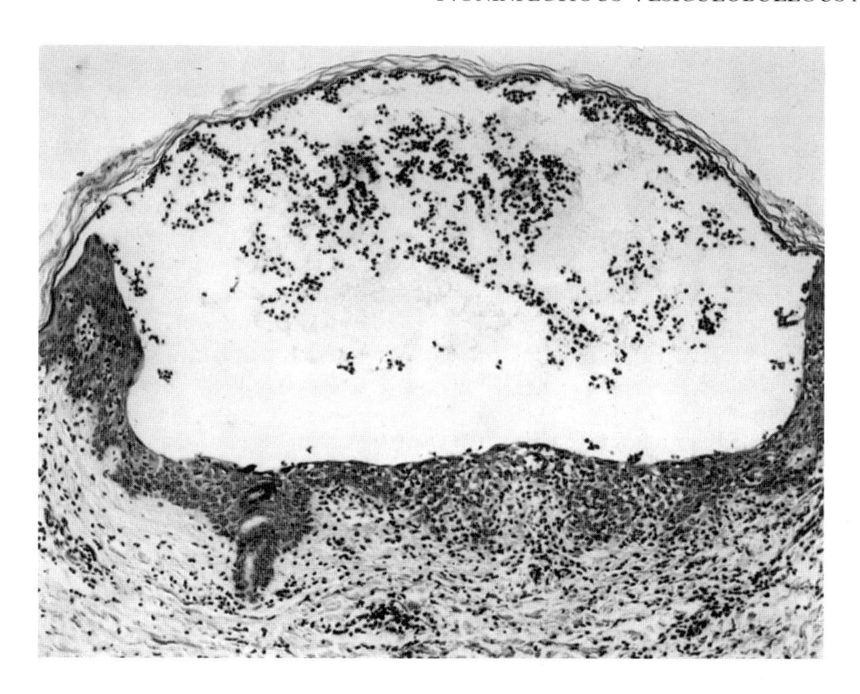

FIG. 9-24. Subcorneal pustular dermatosis A vesiculopustule is present in a subcorneal location. No acantholysis is apparent. Note the similarity to IgA pemphigus.

corneal accumulation are regarded as events secondary to the cellular destruction in the stratum granulosum seen in one study.[297]

Differential Diagnosis. The differential diagnosis includes other entities that show subcorneal pustules. Histologic differentiation from impetigo may be impossible unless bacteria can be demonstrated with a Gram stain. Cultures may be necessary for diagnosis. Histologic differentiation from pemphigus foliaceus or pemphigus erythematosus may also be difficult, since both diseases show subcorneal blisters with acantholysis. Although the acantholysis tends to be more pronounced in pemphigus than in subcorneal pustular dermatosis, clinical information, immunofluorescence testing, and a therapeutic trial of sulfones may be necessary for definitive diagnosis. At least some cases previously diagnosed as subcorneal pustular dermatosis, in which IF studies were not performed, may represent IgA pemphigus.

Although subcorneal pustules occur in both pustular psoriasis and subcorneal pustular dermatosis, spongiform pustules occur only in pustular psoriasis.[292] Some authors regard subcorneal pustular dermatosis as a variant of pustular psoriasis.[298,299]

Erythema Multiforme

Erythema multiforme is an acute, self-limited dermatosis that may be divided into a minor and major form, the latter also known as Stevens-Johnson syndrome. The most frequent etiology in erythema multiforme is infection, *Herpes simplex virus* being the most common agent. In Stevens-Johnson syndrome, medications, in particular sulfonamides, are the offending agents in most patients. Patients with herpes simplex virus–associated erythema multiforme have recurrent lesions, affecting primarily the extremities, with typical target or iris lesions. Those with drug-induced Stevens-Johnson syndrome have truncal involvement, a more purpuric macular eruption, and atypical target lesions.[300] As the name implies, the lesions may be multiform, including macules, papules, vesicles, and bullae. Patients often present with fever. Involvement of the oral, conjunctival, nasal, and genital mucosa is common. In toxic epidermal necrolysis, first described in 1956, a widespread blotchy erythema develops. This is soon followed by the development of large, flaccid bullae and detachment of the epidermis in large sheets, leaving the dermis exposed and giving a moist, eroded appearance.[301] The disease has a high mortality rate because of fluid loss and sepsis. In nearly 90% of cases it is caused by medications, most commonly sulfonamides, β-lactam antibiotics, and nonsteroidal anti-inflammatory drugs.[302] Although once considered necessary treatment, the use of systemic corticosteroids in toxic epidermal necrolysis is controversial. Toxic epidermal necrolysis is widely, but not universally, regarded as a variant of severe erythema multiforme because of its acute course, its frequent occurrence as a drug allergy, and its frequent overlap with Stevens-Johnson disease.[303,304]

Although the presence or absence of mucosal lesions has been used to differentiate the various forms of bullous erythema multiforme, in a recent study no correlation was found, and overall 90% of patients had mucosal lesions.[305] A new classification based on the percentage of body surface area with skin detachment, typical and atypical target lesions, and purpuric macules has subsequently been proposed.

Histopathology. Some authors have previously classified erythema multiforme into a dermal type, epidermal type, and mixed dermal-epidermal type;[306] however, this classification is no longer widely accepted.[307,308] The predominance of epidermal or dermal changes reflects the site of biopsy within an individual lesion and where, in the temporal evolution of the disease, the biopsy is taken. In addition, many cases of primarily "dermal erythema multiforme" may represent hypersensitivity reactions in which interface dermatitis is not the characteristic reaction pattern.

Erythema multiforme is considered the prototype of the vacuolar form of interface dermatitis.[309] Because of its acute nature, there is an orthokeratotic stratum corneum. The earliest changes include vacuolization of the basal cell layer, tagging of lymphocytes along the dermoepidermal junction, and a sparse, superficial, perivascular lymphoid infiltrate (Fig. 9-25). Mild spongiosis and exocytosis are seen. Necrosis of individual keratinocytes in the stratum malpighii occurs, the hallmark of erythema multiforme. Satellite cell necrosis, characterized by intraepidermal lymphocytes in close association with necrotic keratinocytes, is frequently present.

In more papular, edematous lesions, there is papillary dermal edema and more significant spongiosis and inflammation. Intraepidermal vesicles associated with exocytosis may be noted on occasion.[310] Although some authors have noted a significant number of eosinophils in drug-induced erythema multiforme,[311] this has not been noted by others.[307]

In addition to the clinical differences, some histologic differences have been noted between drug-induced and herpes simplex–associated erythema multiforme.[308] In the former, there is more widespread keratinocyte necrosis, microscopic blister formation, and more pigmentary incontinence. In cases associated with herpes simplex virus infection, there is more spongiosis, exocytosis, liquefaction degeneration of the basal layer, and papillary dermal edema. Nuclear dust may be identified in the papillary dermis in the latter.[308]

In toxic epidermal necrolysis, in bullous lesions, and in the central portion of target lesions, there are numerous necrotic keratinocytes, even full-thickness epidermal necrosis, and a subepidermal bulla. The dermal inflammatory infiltrate is more sparse in toxic epidermal necrolysis than in erythema multiforme. Extravasated erythrocytes are commonly found within the blister cavity. Melanophages within the papillary dermis occur in late lesions.

IF Testing. In many patients with erythema multiforme, deposits of IgM and C3 are found in the walls of the superficial dermal vessels.[312,313] Granular deposits of C3, IgM, and fibrinogen may also be present along the dermoepidermal junction.[308,314] In addition, circulating immune complexes have been demonstrated with both a monoclonal rheumatoid factor inhibition assay[313] and a C1q binding radioassay.[315] These findings suggest that immune complex formation or deposition in the cutaneous microvasculature and the dermoepidermal junction play a role in the pathogenesis of erythema multiforme.

In toxic epidermal necrolysis, diffuse epidermal deposition of immunoglobulin and complement in necrotic keratinocytes may be observed.[316] Thus secondary deposition of immune reactants in necrotic keratinocytes may be observed in other forms of erythema multiforme, but the number of dead keratinocytes is usually much less (except in aged blisters).

Pathogenesis. The cellular infiltrate consists largely of CD4+ (helper) lymphocytes, primarily in the dermis, and CD8+ (cytotoxic or suppressor) cells in the epidermis. The mononuclear cells that are associated with necrotic keratinocytes in the process referred to as "satellite cell necrosis" are largely CD8+ cytotoxic lymphocytes similar to those occurring in graft-versus-host disease.[317]

Some authors hypothesize that erythema multiforme represents a type III immune complex–mediated reaction, in which impaired histamine metabolism plays a role in the development of papular lesions and target lesions.[315] An increased number of epidermal Langerhans cells and CD4+ T lymphocytes was noted in the peripheral portion of the target lesions, and a decreased number of Langerhans cells and CD8+ cells were present within the central portion.[315,317] The presence of CD8+ lymphocytes in apposition to necrotic keratinocytes strongly suggests a role for a type IV delayed hypersensitivity reaction. Injury to blood vessels is suggested by the presence of circulating immune complexes and the presence of IgM, C3, fibrinogen, and the herpes antigen in vessel walls and perivascular lymphocytes. This has led some to propose the endothelial cells as a target of injury, that is, a lymphocytic vasculitis,[317] whereas others do not consider erythema multiforme to be a "true vasculitis."[318] Overall, there is evidence to support the theory that the mechanism is a combined type III and IV immune reaction.[317] Susceptibility to erythema multiforme may be related to HLA-DQB1,[319] and recurrent disease to HLA-B62 and -B35.[320]

The association of herpes simplex virus with erythema multiforme has been well documented. Polymerase chain reaction and in situ hybridization have detected herpes simplex virus DNA within lesions of erythema multiforme.[321,322] The virus remains in the skin for up to 3 months after the lesions have healed.[323]

In toxic epidermal necrolysis, the dermal infiltrate is composed of predominantly helper T lymphocytes. Epidermal Langerhans cells are reduced and keratinocyte HLA-DR expression is induced.[324] These changes are similar to those in graft-versus-host disease. The findings suggest a cellular immune reaction, but other mechanisms, such as direct drug cytotoxicity, cannot be excluded.

Ultrastructural Study. The basal lamina is located on the floor or the roof of the blister.[306] The basal cells show marked intracytoplasmic damage with a loss of organelles. Neutrophils and macrophages, rich in lysosomes, are present in the lower epidermis phagocytizing the damaged keratinocytes. In the midepidermis, large, electron-dense, dyskeratotic bodies correspond to the cells with eosinophilic necrosis seen by light microscopy.[306,325] The damaged epidermal cells often contain few or no organelles.[306] Large granular lymphocytes have been identified within the epidermis in close contact with keratinocytes, a finding that supports cell-mediated cytotoxic injury to keratinocytes.[326]

Differential Diagnosis. Necrotic keratinocytes are also a characteristic feature in fixed drug eruptions, pityriasis lichenoides, connective tissue disease, subacute radiation dermatitis, phototoxic dermatitis, acute graft-versus-host disease, viral exanthems, and some drug eruptions. In patients with widespread desquamation or detachment, the differential diagnosis includes toxic epidermal necrolysis and SSSS. Whereas the former involves subepidermal separation, the latter results from separation of the epidermis subcorneally or within the granular layer. Frozen section evaluation of the blister roof is a rapid diagnostic tool to determine the level of the split.

Graft-Versus-Host Disease

Three types of graft-versus-host disease exist. In the two iatrogenic forms, immunodeficient patients receive immunocompetent lymphocytes through bone marrow transplantation (usually allogeneic) or they receive blood products containing immunocompetent lymphocytes from HLA-matched persons.[327]

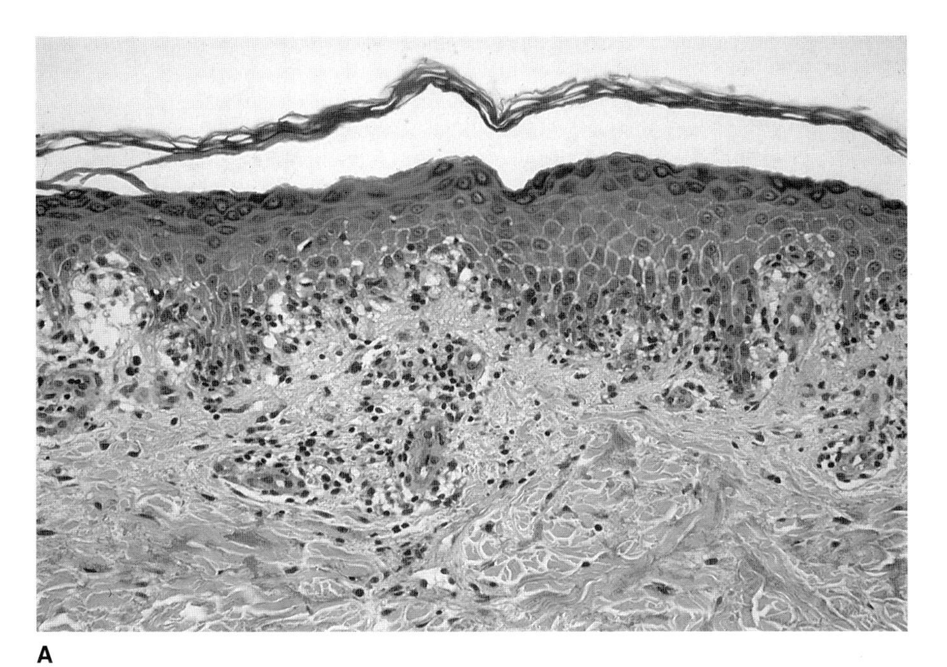

A

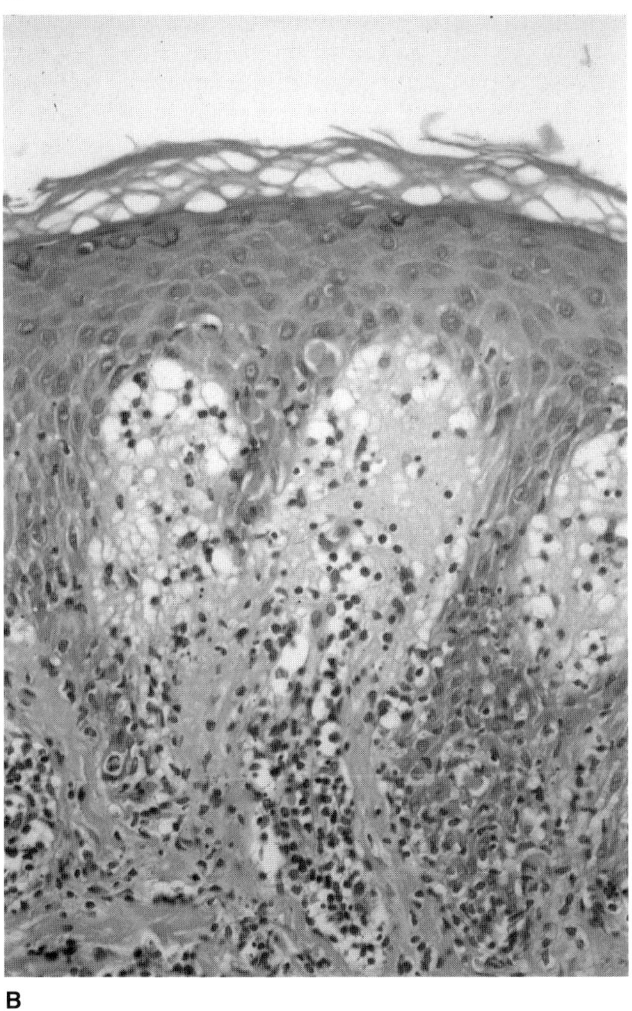

B

FIG. 9-25. Erythema multiforme
There is a superficial perivascular and interface dermatitis with "tagging" of lymphocytes along the dermoepidermal junction with apoptotic keratinocytes. The stratum corneum is normal and there is no acantholysis. Eosinophilic apoptotic keratinocytes are prominent in the epidermis.

In the rare congenital form, maternal lymphocytes normally present in the fetal circulation establish themselves in the fetus and react against their host.[328]

The iatrogenic form of graft-versus-host disease usually follows bone marrow transplantation in patients with aplastic anemia, acute leukemia, or genetic immunodeficiency states. Graft-versus-host reactions occur in approximately 70% of recipients of bone marrow transplantation, and many patients with a graft-versus-host reaction die of infectious complications.[329]

The disease can be divided into an acute and a chronic phase. The acute phase occurs in 75% of patients, and skin lesions develop between 11 and 16 days and peak at 18 days after the transplantation.[330] The chronic phase occurs in about 10% of patients and begins several months (usually after 100 days) to a year after the transplantation.[331] Either phase may occur alone, but many patients have both phases, either merging with one another or separated by an asymptomatic period.[332]

In the *acute phase,* the classic triad includes skin lesions, hepatic dysfunction, and diarrhea. The clinical severity is judged on the extent of the cutaneous eruption, total bilirubin, and stool volume. The eruption is characterized by extensive macular erythema, a morbilliform eruption, purpuric lesions, violaceous scaly papules and plaques, bullae, or in some cases a toxic epidermal necrolysislike epidermal detachment. There is a predilection for the cheeks, ears, neck, upper chest, and palms and soles. Occasionally, follicular papules are seen simulating a folliculitis.[333] Oral lesions may be present. About 30% of patients die from complications of acute graft-versus-host disease. The overall clinical stage, during the first 40 days after transplantation, is useful in identifying patients with progressive and fatal disease.[330] Cutaneous graft-versus-host disease may be due to a synergistic effect from local irradiation.[334]

In the *chronic phase,* an early lichenoid stage and a late sclerotic stage can be distinguished. Each stage can occur without the other.[335] Although usually generalized, the involvement is in rare instances localized to a few areas.[332] In the lichenoid stage, both the cutaneous and oral lesions may be clinically similar to those in lichen planus.[336] In addition, the skin may show extensive erythema and irregular hyperpigmentation. In the late sclerotic stage, dermal sclerosis, atrophy, and poikiloderma may develop. There is cicatricial alopecia, and chronic ulcerations may develop.[332]

Histopathology. The *acute phase* has been divided into four histopathologic grades.[337] In grade 1 disease, there is focal or diffuse vacuolization of the basal cell layer. In grade 2 lesions, spongiosis and dyskeratotic keratinocytes are identified, some in close proximity to epidermal lymphocytes, a phenomenon known as satellite cell necrosis (Fig. 9-26). The necrotic keratinocytes contain a pyknotic nucleus and eosinophilic cytoplasm. Grade 3 lesions are characterized by subepidermal cleft formation, and in grade 4 there is complete loss of the epidermis. There usually is a mononuclear cell infiltrate within the papillary dermis with exocytosis. In fact, some authors require dermal lymphoid inflammation for the diagnosis,[338] since keratinocytic apoptosis and spongiosis may be attributable to the total body irradiation and cytotoxic drugs given prior to bone marrow transplantation. Both the intensity of the lymphoid infiltrate and the earlier appearance of histologic changes correlate with a more severe course.[339] In cases with follicular papules, the involved follicles show degenerate changes in the cells of the follicular epithelium similar to those in the epidermis.[333] In rare cases, basal vacuolization and dyskeratosis of the follicular epithelium may be the only changes.[340]

In the *chronic phase,* the early lichenoid stage may still show evidence of satellite cell necrosis within the epidermis.[341] The overall histologic picture greatly resembles that of lichen planus with hyperkeratosis, hypergranulosis, acanthosis, apoptotic keratinocytes, and a mononuclear cell infiltrate immediately below the epidermis with pigmentary incontinence.[336] As in lichen planus, apoptotic keratinocytes may "drop" into the upper dermis.[341] There may be areas of separation of the basal cell layer from the dermal papillae resembling the clefts seen in severe lichen planus.[332]

In the late sclerotic stage, the epidermis is atrophic, with the keratinocytes being small, flattened, and hyperpigmented. Basal layer vacuolization, inflammation, and colloid body formation are rare or absent.[332] The dermis is thickened, with sclerosis extending into the subcutaneous tissue. The adnexal structures are destroyed.[342,343]

IF Testing. Epithelial basement membrane zone granular IgM deposition is present in 39% of patients with the acute form and in 86% of patients with the chronic form of graft-versus-host disease.[344] In addition, IgM and C3 have been found in the walls of dermal vessels.[342,345] These deposits suggest a possible role for humoral immunity in the pathogenesis of graft-versus-host disease in addition to the well-established role of cellular immunity.

Pathogenesis. Graft-versus-host disease is composed of two distinct clinical entities that each have a different pathogenesis. Acute graft-versus-host disease is produced by the attack of donor immunocompetent T or null lymphocytes against histocompatibility antigens exposed on recipient cells, whereas chronic graft-versus-host disease is produced by immunocompetent lymphocytes that differentiate in the recipient.[346]

The target cell in graft-versus-host disease has been debated. Some authors have shown that rete ridge keratinocytes, where the concentration of stem cells is the greatest, are the preferred target cells because there are more necrotic keratinocytes and inflammatory cells in these zones.[347] Similarly, follicular stem cells in the bulge area may be the target for follicular changes.[348] Induction of an immune reaction against keratinocytes may occur with increased HLA-DR antigen expression on keratinocytes seen in acute and chronic graft-versus-host disease.[349] ICAM-1 expression on keratinocytes correlates with that of HLA-DR antigen as well.[350] Others have found that HLA-DR expression is not necessary for the development of cutaneous disease.[351]

The Langerhans cell may also be a target cell. Although some Langerhans cells may still be present, they are decreased in number and have altered morphology.[349,352,353] Perhaps Langerhans cells are targeted, and keratinocytes are injured as innocent bystanders.[354] Others have found that cutaneous disease is unaffected by anti-Ia antibody in mice, thus suggesting that Langerhans cells are not involved in the pathophysiology of graft-versus-host disease.[355]

In most studies, the cutaneous infiltrate has been found to consist largely of CD8+ suppressor or cytotoxic T lymphocytes; however, both CD4 and CD8 cells may elicit acute graft-versus-host disease.[356,357] It appears that CD3+, CD4−, and CD8+ T cells are present within the epidermis, and CD3+, CD4+, and CD8− T cells are present within the dermal infil-

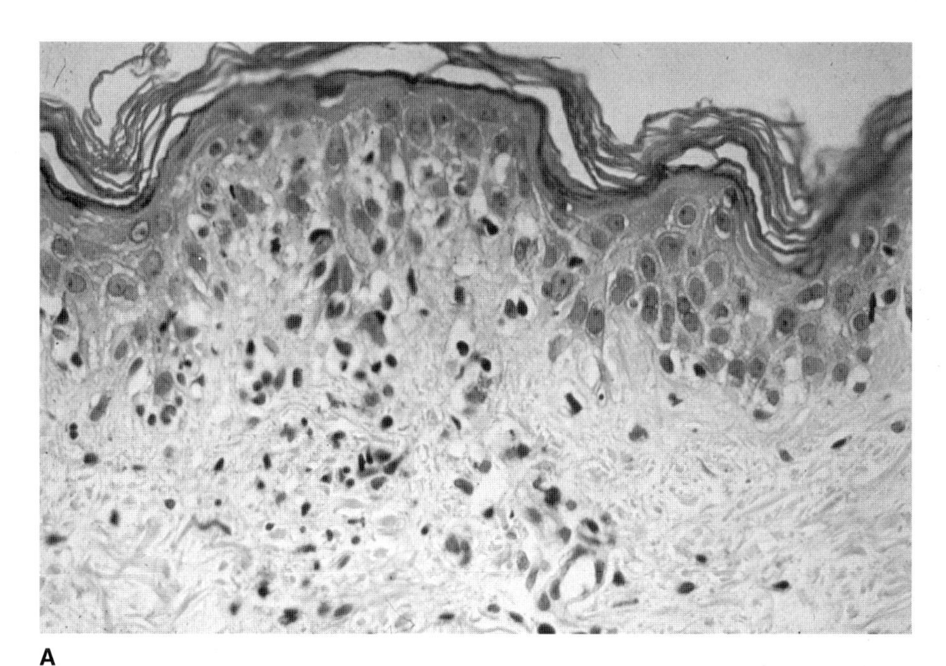

A

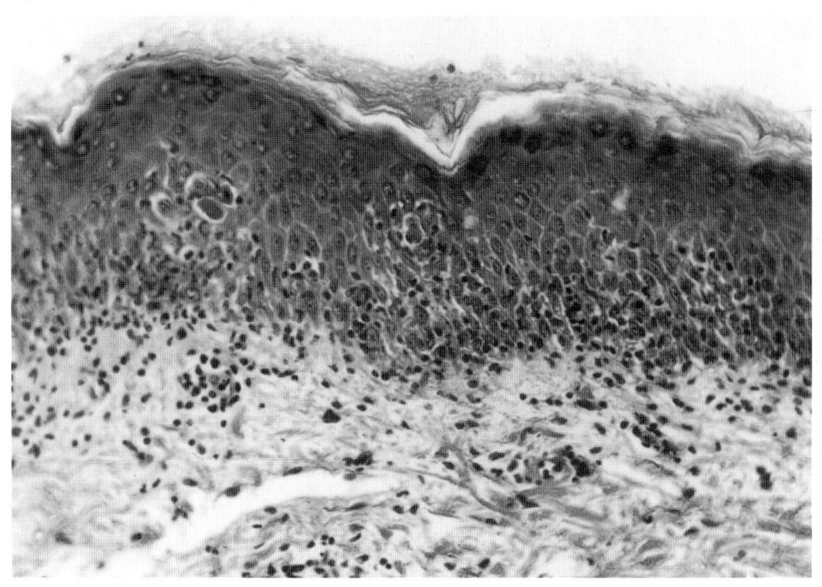

B

FIG. 9-26. Graft-versus-host disease (**A**) There is basal vacuolopathy and a cell-poor interface dermatitis associated with apoptosis (early lesion). (**B**) Necrotic keratinocytes are scattered through the epidermis. Some of them show an associated lymphocyte, a process referred to as a satellite cell necrosis.

trate.[349] Some authors have found that removal of CD8+ cells resulted in an increased severity of disease, thereby suggesting that CD4+ cells cause the greatest degree of graft-versus-host disease.[358] Alternatively, donor CD3−/CD4+/CD8− lymphocytes may be the effector cells.[359]

Finally, the proportion of γ/δ lymphocytes is higher in cutaneous graft-versus-host disease than in controls.[360,361] The surface LFA-1 antigen on T lymphocytes may allow T-cell migration into the epidermis.[355] In addition, endothelial cell marker ELAM-1 may be important in lymphocyte recruitment, whereas CD34 appears to have a negative modulating role.[362] Natural killer cells may participate in the development of skin lesions in concert with T lymphocytes, perhaps by secretion of γ-interferon or tumor necrosis factor-α.[363]

Ultrastructural Study. The necrotic keratinocytic cytoplasm is filled with numerous aggregated tonofilaments.[364] Granule-producing cytotoxic lymphocytes, natural killerlike cells, have been identified in direct cytolytic attack on epithelial cells undergoing apoptosis.[365,366]

Differential Diagnosis. The acute phase of graft-versus-host disease is similar to erythema multiforme, with scattered necrotic keratinocytes and the formation of subepidermal clefts through hydropic degeneration of basal cells. If there is follicular dyskeratosis, the diagnosis is much more likely to be acute graft-versus-host disease.[367] These patients are also at increased risk for drug eruptions, chemotherapy-induced eruptions, and radiation dermatitis, all of which may be indistinguishable from acute graft-versus-host disease.[368,369] Epidermal changes identical to acute graft-versus-host disease may be seen in bone marrow transplant patients without cutaneous lesions.[370]

Vascular injury may be more common in graft-versus-host disease patients than in other bone marrow transplant patients, and thus may serve as a distinguishing feature.[371] A new monoclonal antibody, LN-3, shows increased staining in blood vessels of graft-versus-host disease patients than in controls, and may be a useful diagnostic tool.[372]

The *eruption of lymphocyte recovery* occurs predominantly in patients with acute myelogenous leukemia and bears some resemblance to acute graft-versus-host disease.[373] The eruption is typically morbilliform and develops between 6 and 21 days of chemotherapy, correlating with the earliest recovery of lymphocytes after the nadir. In contrast to patients with graft-versus-host disease, these patients do not develop diarrhea or liver abnormalities. Resolution occurs over several days. Histopathologically, a superficial perivascular mononuclear cell infiltrate, basal vacuolization, spongiosis, and rare dyskeratotic keratinocytes are present. The changes may be indistinguishable from those of early allogeneic or autologous graft-versus-host disease, and clinical information is essential.[374]

Distinguishing between the lichenoid lesions of graft-versus-host disease and lichen planus is often impossible. However, late sclerotic lesions can be differentiated from scleroderma by the marked atrophy of the epidermis. Active synthesis of collagen takes place largely in the upper third of the dermis; in scleroderma, collagen is synthesized mainly in the lower dermis and in the subcutaneous tissue.[341]

Transient Acantholytic Dermatosis

First described in 1970, transient acantholytic dermatosis is characterized by pruritic, discrete papules and papulovesicles on the chest, back, and thighs.[375] In rare instances, vesicles and even bullae are seen.[376]

Most patients are middle-aged or elderly men. Although the disorder is transient in the majority of patients, lasting from 2 weeks to 3 months, it can persist for several years.[377,378] There have been reports of patients with transient acantholytic dermatosis and malignancy, most commonly lymphoproliferative and genitourinary neoplasms.[379,380]

Histopathology. Focal acantholysis and dyskeratosis ("focal acantholytic dyskeratosis") are present. Because these foci are small, they are sometimes found only when step sections are obtained. The acantholysis may occur in four histologic patterns, resembling Darier disease (Fig. 9-27), Hailey-Hailey disease, pemphigus vulgaris, or spongiotic dermatitis. Two or more of these patterns may be found in the same specimen.[377]

IF Testing. In general, IF results are negative.[381] In one study, 5 of 11 patients had C3 deposition in several locations in the epidermis and at the dermoepidermal junction, but there was no consistent pattern.[382] Two other patients were reported to have granular basement membrane zone staining of C3 alone or in combination with IgM on direct IF.[383] IgA and IgM were also noted in colloid bodies, and papillary dermal vascular staining was identified.

Pathogenesis. Although the etiology of transient acantholytic dermatosis remains unknown, there appears to be a relationship to excessive sweating, fever, and bed confinement. Some authors have hypothesized that heat or sweat urea that leaks from the intraepidermal portion of the sweat duct into the surrounding epidermis causes acantholysis.[384] Others dispute this theory and have found the sweat duct to be intact.[385] Finally, interleukin-4 may be responsible for acantholysis, either by induction of plasminogen activator or by stimulation of antibody production.[386]

Ultrastructural Study. In the pemphiguslike zones, there is intradesmosomal separation,[387] fewer desmosomes, and perinuclear aggregation of tonofilament bundles.[388] In the Darier type, features similar to those of Darier disease are present.[389]

Differential Diagnosis. The features that help differentiate transient acantholytic dermatosis from the four diseases that it resembles are the focal nature of the histologic changes and the mixture of patterns. It is important to have clinical information for a definitive diagnosis. IF studies are rarely necessary.

DERMATOPATHIES PRODUCED BY EXTERNAL ENERGY

Friction Blisters

These blisters develop mainly on the soles as a result of prolonged walking, and on the palms and the palmar surfaces of the

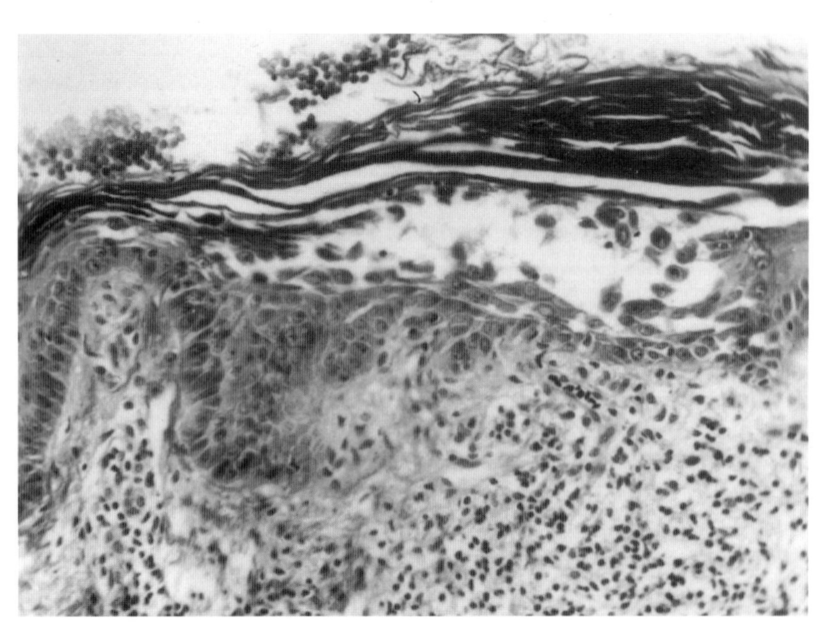

FIG. 9-27. Transient acantholytic dermatosis
There is hypergranulosis, with acantholytic dyskeratotic granular cells. The cleft extends to a suprabasal location.

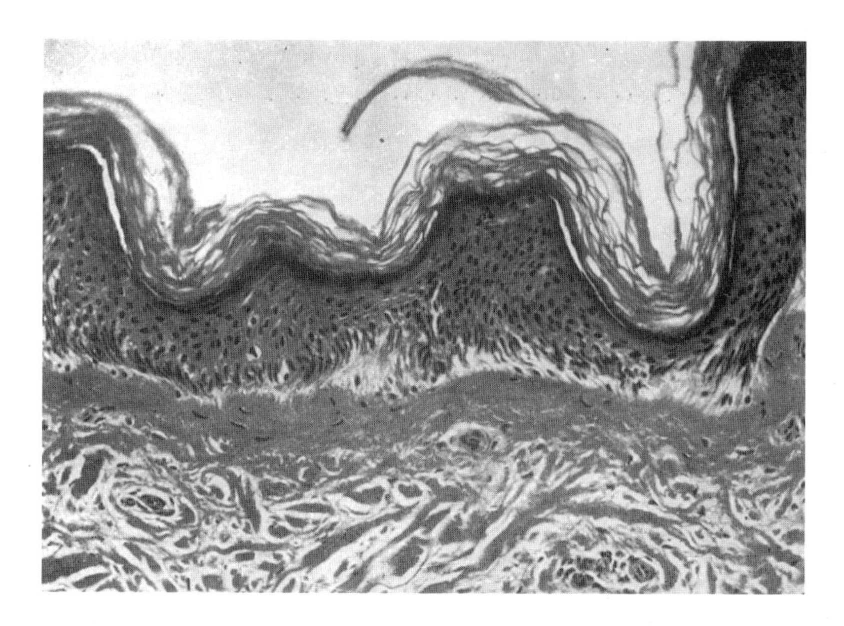

FIG. 9-28. Electrodessication
Both the cytoplasm and nuclei of basal keratinocytes are markedly elongated, with nuclear pyknosis and cytoplasmic hypereosinophilia of the stratum spinosum.

fingers as a result of repetitive actions required in certain occupations or sports. They may occur also as self-inflicted artifacts.[390]

Histopathology. In both naturally occurring and experimentally produced friction blisters, intraepidermal cleavage develops as a result of cytolysis and necrosis of keratinocytes in the upper stratum malpighii.[391] The roof of the blister is composed of the stratum corneum, stratum granulosum, and amorphous cellular debris.[392] Most of the degenerated keratinocytes are pale and are located at the floor of the cleft. The deeper part of the epidermis consists of undamaged cells.[390]

Pathogenesis. Friction blisters are caused by shearing forces within the epidermis. They form only where the epidermis is thick and firmly attached to the underlying tissue.[390]

Ultrastructural Study. Electron microscopy reveals clumped tonofilaments, intracellular edema, small vacuoles at the cell periphery, and areas devoid of organelles.[393]

Electric Burns

It is important that dermatopathologists be familiar with the cutaneous effects of electric current as they are used during electrodesiccation and electrocautery.

Histopathology. Electrodesiccation and electrocautery cause a separation of the epidermis from the dermis. A diagnostic histologic feature is the fringe of elongated, degenerated cytoplasmic processes that protrudes from the lower end of the detached basal cells into the subepidermal space (Fig. 9-28). The nuclei of the basal cells appear stretched vertically. In addition, the upper dermis is homogenized because of coagulation necrosis.[394]

Thermal Burns

In the evaluation of thermal burns, the depth of penetration is of great importance because first- and second-degree burns heal readily, whereas third-degree burns require grafting.

Histopathology. First-degree burns are those in which the lower epidermis, particularly the basal cell layer, remains viable, and only the upper epidermis is affected by heat coagulation. In the affected areas, the nuclei may appear pyknotic and contain perinuclear halos. In a more advanced stage, the nuclei stain faintly eosinophilic or not at all, like "architectural ghosts."[395]

Second-degree burns often show subepidermal blisters and are characterized by partial-thickness dermal necrosis. The lower portion of the cutaneous appendages remains intact, allowing reepithelization to occur. Superficial second-degree burns are associated with necrosis of the surface epidermis and of only a small amount of superficial dermal collagen; in deep second-degree burns, much of the dermal collagen and the cutaneous appendages is injured.[396] In partial-thickness dermal necrosis, the depth of epithelial damage in the cutaneous appendages is a good indicator of the depth of irreversible damage to the collagen. The border between heat-coagulated and normal epithelium is sharp.[395] At a later stage, an inflammatory reaction develops at the junction of the viable and nonviable tissue.

Third-degree burns show full-thickness dermal necrosis with destruction of all cutaneous appendages. The coagulation necrosis may extend to the subcutaneous tissue and to the underlying muscle.[396]

Suction Blisters and Purpura

Negative pressure applied over a circumscribed area may form a subepidermal blister that arises in the lamina lucida. A second reaction, noninflammatory purpura, may also result. The changes may be secondary to overcoming the adhesive forces in the lamina lucida or in vessels.[397]

REFERENCES

1. Ackerman AB, Ragaz A. A plea to expunge the word "eczema" from the lexicon of dermatology and dermatopathology. Am J Dermatopathol 1982;4:315.
2. Eisen HN, Orris L, Belman S. Elicitation of delayed allergic skin reactions with haptens: The dependence of elicitation on hapten combination with protein. J Exp Med 1952;95:473.

3. Streilein JW, Bergstresser PR. Langerhans cell function dictates induction of contact hypersensitivity or unresponsiveness to DNFB in Syrian hamsters. J Invest Dermatol 1981;77:272.
4. Mossman TR, Coffman RL. Th1 and Th2 cells: Different patterns of lymphokine secretion lead to different functional properties. Annu Rev Immunol 1989;7:145.
5. Tse Y, Cooper KD. Cutaneous dermal Ia+ cells are capable of initiating delayed type hypersensitivity responses. J Invest Dermatol 1990; 94:267.
6. Hirshberg H, Braathen LR, Thorsby E. Antigen presentation by vascular endothelial cells and epidermal Langerhans cells: The role of HLA-DR. Immunol Rev 1982;65:57.
7. Epstein EH Jr, Levin DL, Croft JD Jr et al. Mycosis fungoides. Medicine (Baltimore) 1972;15:61.
8. Komura J, Ofuji S. Ultrastructural studies of allergic contact dermatitis in man. Arch Dermatol Res 1980;267:275.
9. Frichot BC III, Zelickson AS. Steroids, lysosomes and dermatitis. Acta Derm Venereol (Stockh) 1972;52:311.
10. Lachapelle JM. Comparative histopathology of allergic and irritant patch test reactions in man. Arch Belg Dermatol 1973;28:83.
11. Willis CM, Stephens SJM, Wilkinson JD. Differential patterns of epidermal leukocyte infiltration in patch test reactions to structurally unrelated chemical irritants. J Invest Dermatol 1993;101:364.
12. Protty C. The molecular basis for skin irritation. In: Brener MM, ed. Cosmetic Surgery Academic. London: 1978;275.
13. Kondo S, Pastore S, Shivji GM et al. Characterization of epidermal cytokine profiles in sensitization and elicitation phases of allergic contact dermatitis as well as irritant contact dermatitis in mouse skin. Lymphokine Cytokine Res 1994;13:367.
14. Lisby S, Muller C, Jongeneel CV et al. Nickel and skin irritants upregulate tumor necrosis factor α mRNA in keratinocytes by different but potentially synergistic mechanisms. Int Immunol 1994;7:343.
15. Kasteler JS, Petersen MJ, Vance JE, Zone JJ. Circulating activated T lymphocytes in autoeczematization. Arch Dermatol 1992;128:795.
16. Ackerman AB. Histologic diagnosis of inflammatory diseases. Philadelphia: Lea and Febiger, 1976;499.
17. Bruynzeel DP, Nieboer C, Boorsma DM et al. Allergic reactions, "spillover" reactions and T cell subsets. Arch Dermatol Res 1983;275: 80.
18. Shelley WB. Id reaction. In: Consultations in dermatology. Philadelphia: Saunders, 1972;262.
19. Roper SS, Jones HE. An animal model for altering the irritability threshold of normal skin. Contact Dermatitis 1985;13:91.
20. Choudri SH, Magro CM, Crowson AN, Nicolle LE. An id reaction to *Mycobacterium leprae*: First documented case. Cutis 1995;54:282.
21. De Leo VA, Harber LC. Contact photodermatitis. In: Fisher AA, ed. Contact Dermatitis. 3rd ed. Philadelphia: Lea and Febiger, 1986;454.
22. Braun-Falco O, Petry G. Feinstruktur der epidermis bei chronischem nummulärem ekzem. Arch Klin Exp Dermatol 1966;224:63.
23. Diepgen TL, Fartasch M. Recent epidemiological and genetic studies in atopic dermatitis. Acta Derm Venereol Suppl (Stockh) 1992;176: 13.
24. Leung DYM, Bhan AK, Schneeberger EE, Geha RS. Characterization of the mononuclear cell infiltrate in atopic dermatitis using monoclonal antibodies. J Allergy Clin Immunol 1983;71:47.
25. Bos JD, Wierenga EA, Smitt JHS et al. Immune dysregulation in atopic eczema. Arch Dermatol 1992;128:1509.
26. Grewe M, Gyufko K, Schöpf E, Krutmann J. Lesional expression of interferon-γ in atopic eczema. Lancet 1994;343:25.
27. Van der Heijden FL, Van Neerven RJJ, Kapsenberg ML. Relationship between facilitated allergen presentation and the presence of allergen-specific IgE in serum of atopic patients. Clin Exp Immunol 1995;99: 289.
28. Del Prete G, Maggi E, Romagnani S. Biology of disease. Human Th1 and Th2 cells: Functional properties, mechanisms of regulation, and role in disease. Lab Invest 1994;70:299.
29. Horsmanheimo L, Harvima IT, Järvikallio A et al. Mast cells are one major source of interleukin-4 in atopic dermatitis. Br J Dermatol 1994; 131:348.
30. Nordvall SL, Lindgren L, Johansson SGO et al. IgE antibodies to *Pityrosporum orbiculare* and *Staphlococcus aureus* in patients with very high serum total IgE. Clin Exp Allergy 1992;22:756.
31. Soeprono FF, Schinella RA, Cockerell CJ, Comite SL. Seborrheic-like dermatitis of acquired immunodeficiency syndrome. J Am Acad Dermatol 1986;14:242.
32. Wikler JR, Nieboer C, Willemze R. Quantitative skin cultures of *Pityrosporum* yeasts in patients seropositive for the human immunodeficiency virus with and without seborrheic dermatitis. J Am Acad Dermatol 1992;27:37.
33. Rao B, Unis M, Poulos E. Acroangiodermatitis: A study of ten cases. Int J Dermatol 1994;33:179.
34. Botella-Estrada R, Sanmartin O, Oliver V et al. Erythroderma: A clinicopathologic study of 56 cases. Arch Dermatol 1994;130:1503.
35. Straka BF, Cooper PH, Greer KE. Congenital miliaria crystallina. Cutis 1991;47:103.
36. Pandolf KB, Griffin TB, Munro EH, Goldman RF. Heat intolerance as a function of percent of body surface involved with miliaria rubra. Am J Physiol 1980;239:R233.
37. Sulzberger MB, Harris DR. Miliaria and anhidrosis III: Multiple small patches and the effects of different periods of occlusion. Arch Dermatol 1972;105:845.
38. Loewenthal LJA. The pathogenesis of miliaria. Arch Dermatol 1961; 84:2.
39. Lillywhite LP. Investigation into the environmental factors associated with the incidence of skin disease following an outbreak of miliaria rubra at a coal mine. Occup Med 1992;42:183.
40. Lyons RE, Levine R, Auld D. Miliaria rubra: A manifestation of staphylococcal disease. Arch Dermatol 1962;86:282.
41. Hölzle E, Kligman AM. The pathogenesis of miliaria rubra: Role of the resident microflora. Br J Dermatol 1978;99:117.
42. Jacobs JC, Miller ME. Fatal familial Leiner's disease. Pediatrics 1972; 49:225.
43. Stanley J, Perez D, Gigli I et al. Hyperimmunoglobulin E syndrome. Arch Dermatol 1978;114:765.
44. Donabedian H, Gallin JI. The hyperimmunoglobulin E recurrent-infection (Job's) syndrome. Medicine (Baltimore) 1983;62:195.
45. Rosen FS. The primary immunodeficiencies: Dermatologic manifestations. J Invest Dermatol 1976;67:402.
46. Weston WL. Disorders of phagocytic function. Arch Dermatol 1976; 112:1589.
47. Dilworth JA, Mandell GL. Adults with chronic granulomatous disease of "childhood." Am J Med 1977;63:233.
48. Civatte A. Diagnostic histopathologique de la dermatite polymorphe douloureuse ou maladie de Duhring-Brocq. Ann Dermatol Syphiligr 1943;3:1.
49. Beutner EH, Jordon RE. Demonstration of skin antibodies in sera of pemphigus vulgaris patients by indirect immunofluorescent staining. Proc Soc Exp Biol Med 1964;117:505.
50. Younus J, Ahmed AR. The relationship of pemphigus to neoplasm. J Am Acad Dermatol 1990;23:482.
51. Asboe-Hansen G. Blister-spread induced by finger pressure, a diagnostic sign of pemphigus. J Invest Dermatol 1960;34:5.
52. Lever WF. Pemphigus and Pemphigoid. Springfield, IL: Charles C. Thomas, 1965.
53. Tappeiner J, Pfleger L. Pemphigus vulgaris: Dermatitis herpetiformis. Arch Klin Exp Dermatol 1962;214:415.
54. Crotty C, Pittelkow M, Muller SA. Eosinophilic spongiosis: A clinicopathologic review of seventy-one cases. J Am Acad Dermatol 1983; 8:337.
55. Arndt K, Harrist TJ. Case records of the Massachusetts General Hospital: Weekly clinicopathological exercises. Case 26-1980. N Engl J Med 1980;303:35.
56. Wheeland RG, Burgdorf WHC, Hoshow RA. A quick Tzanck test. J Am Acad Dermatol 1983;8:258.
57. Graham JH, Bingul O, Burgoon CB. Cytodiagnosis of inflammatory dermatoses. Arch Dermatol 1963;87:118.
58. Korman NJ. Pemphigus. J Am Acad Dermatol 1988;18:1219.
59. Judd KP, Lever WF. Correlation of antibodies in skin and serum with disease severity in pemphigus. Arch Dermatol 1979;115:428.
60. Ratnam KV, Pang BK. Pemphigus in remission: Value of negative direct immunofluorescence in management. J Am Acad Dermatol 1994; 30:547.
61. Kuhn A, Mahrle G, Steigleder GK. Immunohistologische untersuchungen von immundermatosen am rekonstituiertem paraffinschnitt. Hautarzt 1988;39:351.
62. Cerio R, Macdonald DM. Routine diagnostic immunohistochemical labeling of extracellular antigens in formol saline solution-fixed, paraffin-embedded cutaneous tissue. J Am Acad Dermatol 1988;19: 747.

63. Bhogal B, Wojnarowska F, Black MM et al. The distribution of immunoglobulins and the C3 component of complement in multiple biopsies from the uninvolved and perilesional skin in pemphigus. Clin Exp Dermatol 1986;11:49.
64. Korman NJ. Pemphigus. Immunodermatology 1990;8:689.
65. Fitzpatrick RE, Newcomer VD. The correlation of disease activity and antibody titers in pemphigus. Arch Dermatol 1980;116:285.
66. Ahmed AR, Workman S. Anti-intercellular substance antibodies: Presence in serum samples of 14 patients without pemphigus. Arch Dermatol 1983;119:17.
67. Harrist TJ, Mihm MC. Cutaneous immunopathology: The diagnostic use of direct and indirect immunofluorescence techniques in dermatologic disease. Hum Pathol 1979;10:625.
68. Grop PJ, Inderbitzen TM. Pemphigus antigen and blood group substance A and B. J Invest Dermatol 1967;49:285.
69. Anhalt GJ, Patel H, Diaz LA. Mechanisms of immunologic injury (editorial). Arch Dermatol 1983;119:711.
70. Swanson DL, Dahl MV. Pemphigus vulgaris and plasma exchange: Clinical and serologic studies. J Am Acad Dermatol 1981;4:325.
71. Storer JS, Galen WK, Nesbitt LT et al. Neonatal pemphigus vulgaris. J Am Acad Dermatol 1982;6:929.
72. Michel B, Ko CS. Effect of pemphigus or bullous pemphigoid sera and leukocytes on normal skin in organ culture (abstr). J Invest Dermatol 1974;62:541.
73. Schiltz JR, Michel B. Production of epidermal acantholysis in normal human skin in vitro by the IgG fraction from pemphigus serum. J Invest Dermatol 1976;67:254.
74. Anhalt GJ, Labib RS, Vorhees JJ et al. Induction of pemphigus in neonatal mice by passive transfer of IgG from patients with the disease. N Engl J Med 1982;306:1189.
75. Rock B, Labib RS, Diaz LA. Monovalent fab′ immunoglobulin fragments from endemic pemphigus foliaceus autoantibodies reproduce the human disease in neonatal BALB/c mice. J Clin Invest 1990;85: 296.
76. Ioannides D, Hytiroglou P, Phelps RG, Bystryn JC. Regional variation in the expression of pemphigus foliaceus, pemphigus erythematosus, and pemphigus vulgaris antigens in human skin. J Invest Dermatol 1991;96:159.
77. Korman NJ, Eyre RW, Klaus-Kovtun V et al. Demonstration of an adhering-junction molecule (plakoglobin) in the autoantigens of pemphigus foliaceus and pemphigus vulgaris. N Engl J Med 1989; 321:631.
78. Thivolet J. Pemphigus: Past, present, and future. Dermatology 1994; 189(Suppl):26.
79. Stanley JR, Koulu L, Thivolet C. Pemphigus vulgaris and pemphigus foliaceus autoantibodies bind different molecules (abstr). J Invest Dermatol 1984;82:439.
80. Amagai M, Hashimoto T, Shimizu N, Nishikawa T. Absorption of pathogenic autoantibodies by the extracellular domain of pemphigus vulgaris antigen (Dsg3) produced by baculovirus. J Clin Invest 1994; 94:59.
81. Schiltz JR. Pemphigus acantholysis: A unique immunologic injury. J Invest Dermatol 1980;74:359.
82. Hashimoto K, Shafran KM, Webber PS et al. Anti-cell surface pemphigus autoantibodies stimulate plasminogen activated activity of human epidermal cells. J Exp Med 1983;157:259.
83. Hashimoto T, Sugiura M, Kurihara S et al. In vitro complement activation by intercellular antibodies. J Invest Dermatol 1982;78:316.
84. Hashimoto K, Lever WF. An electron microscopic study of pemphigus vulgaris of the mouth with special reference to the intercellular cement. J Invest Dermatol 1967;48:540.
85. Hashimoto K, Lever WF. The intercellular cement in pemphigus vulgaris: An electron microscopic study. Dermatologica 1967;135:27.
86. Rockl H. Uber die pyodermite vegetante von Hallopeau als benigne form des pemphigus vegetans von Neumann nebst einigen bemerkungen zur pyostomatotos vegetans von McCarthy. Arch Klin Exp Dermatol 1964;218:574.
87. Ahmed AR, Blose DA. Pemphigus vegetans, Neumann type and Hallopeau type. Int J Dermatol 1984;23:135.
88. Nelson CG, Apisarnthanarax P, Bean SF, Mullins JF. Pemphigus vegetans of Hallopeau: Immunofluorescence studies. Arch Dermatol 1977;114:627.
89. Lever WF. Pemphigus and pemphigoid: A review of the advances made since 1964. J Am Acad Dermatol 1979;1:2.
90. Beutner EH, Prigenzi LS, Hale LS et al. Immunofluorescent studies of autoantibodies to intracellular areas of epithelia in Brazilian pemphigus foliaceus. Proc Soc Exp Biol Med 1968;127:81.
91. Crosby DL, Diaz LA. Endemic pemphigus foliaceus. In: Bullous Diseases. Dermatologic Clinics. Vol. 11(3). Philadelphia: Saunders, 1993;453.
92. Clovis, Borges, Chaul et al. Environmental risk factors in endemic pemphigus foliaceus (fogo selvagem). J Invest Dermatol 1992;98:A47.
93. Perry HO. Pemphigus foliaceus. Arch Dermatol 1961;83:57.
94. Emerson RW, Wilson Jones E. Eosinophilic spongiosis in pemphigus. Arch Dermatol 1968;97:252.
95. Jablonska S, Chorzelski TP, Beutner EH et al. Herpetiform pemphigus: A variable pattern of pemphigus. Int J Dermatol 1975;14:353.
96. Lagerholm B, Frithz A, Borglund E. Light and electron microscopic aspects of pemphigus herpetiformis (eosinophilic spongiosis) in comparison with other acantholytic disorders. Acta Derm Venereol (Stockh) 1979;59:305.
97. Bystryn JC, Abel E, Defeo C. Pemphigus foliaceus: Subcorneal intercellular antibodies of unique specificity. Arch Dermatol 1974;110: 857.
98. Koulu L, Kusumi A, Steinberg MS et al. Human antibodies against a desmosomal core protein in pemphigus foliaceus. J Exp Med 1984; 160:1509.
99. Wilgram GF, Caulfield JB, Madgic EB. An electron microscopic study of acantholysis and dyskeratosis in pemphigus foliaceus. J Invest Dermatol 1964;43:287.
100. Amerian ML, Ahmed AR. Pemphigus erythematosus: Presentation of four cases and review of the literature. J Am Acad Dermatol 1984;10: 215.
101. Perry HO, Brunsting LA. Pemphigus foliaceus. Arch Dermatol 1965; 91:10.
102. Korman NJ, Eyre RW, Zone J et al. Drug-induced pemphigus: Autoantibodies directed against the pemphigus antigen complexes are present in penicillamine and captopril-induced pemphigus. J Invest Dermatol 1991;96:273.
103. Pisani M, Ruocco V. Drug induced pemphigus. Clin Dermatol 1986; 4:118.
104. Ruocco V, Sacerdoti G. Pemphigus and bullous pemphigoid due to drugs. Int J Dermatol 1991;30:307.
105. Ruocco V, de Luca M, Pisani M et al. Pemphigus provoked by D-penicillamine: An experimental approach using in vitro tissue cultures. Dermatologica 1982;164:236.
106. Yokel BK, Hood AF, Anhalt GJ. Induction of acantholysis in organ explant culture by penicillamine and captopril. Arch Dermatol 1989; 125:1367.
107. Eyre RW, Stanley JR. Human autoantibodies against a desmosomal complex with a calcium-sensitive epitope are characteristic of pemphigus foliaceus patients. J Exp Med 1987;165:1719.
108. Eyre RW, Stanley JR. Identification of pemphigus vulgaris antigen extracted from normal human epidermis and comparison with pemphigus foliaceus antigen. J Clin Invest 1988;81:807.
109. Hodak E, David M, Ingber A et al. The clinical and histopathological spectrum of IgA-pemphigus: A report of two cases. Clin Exp Dermatol 1990;15:433.
110. Saurat JH, Merot Y, Salomon D et al. Pemphigus-like IgA deposits and vesiculopustular dermatosis in a 10-year-old girl. Dermatologica 1987;20:89.
111. Beutner EH, Chorzelski TP, Wilson RM et al. IgA pemphigus foliaceus. J Am Acad Dermatol 1989;20:89.
112. Burrows D, Bingham EA. Subcorneal pustular dermatosis and IgA gammopathy. Br J Dermatol 1984;11:91.
113. Teraki Y, Amagai Z, Hashimoto T et al. Intercellular IgA dermatosis of childhood. Arch Dermatol 1991;127:221.
114. Ebihara T, Hashimoto T, Iwatsuki K et al. Autoantigens for IgA anti-intercellular antibodies of intercellular IgA vesiculopustular dermatosis. J Invest Dermatol 1991;97:742.
115. Neumann E, Dmochowski M, Bowszyc M et al. The occurrence of IgA pemphigus foliaceus without neutrophilic infiltration. Clin Exp Dermatol 1994;19:56.
116. Ohno H, Miyagawa S, Hashimoto T et al. Atypical pemphigus with concomitant IgG and IgA anti-intercellular autoantibodies associated with monoclonal IgA gammopathy. Dermatology 1994;189 (Suppl):115.

117. Hashimoto T, Inamoto N, Nakamura K et al. Intercellular IgA dermatosis with clinical features of subcorneal pustular dermatosis. Arch Dermatol 1987;123:1062.
118. Piette W, Burken RP, Ray TL. Intraepidermal neutrophilic dermatosis: Presence of circulating pemphigus-like IgA antibody specific for monkey epithelium. J Invest Dermatol 1987;88:512.
119. Tagami H, Iwatsuki K, Iwase Y et al. Subcorneal pustular dermatosis with vesiculobullous eruption: Demonstration of subcorneal IgA deposition and a leukocyte chemotactic factor. Br J Dermatol 1983; 109:581.
120. Nishikawa T, Shimizu H, Hashimoto T. Role of IgA intercellular antibodies: Report of clinically and immunologically atypical cases. In: Orfanos CE, Stadler R, Gollnick H, eds. Proceedings of the 17th World Congress of Dermatology. New York: Springer-Verlag, 1987; 383.
121. Mutasim DF, Pelc NJ, Anhalt GJ. Paraneoplastic pemphigus. Dermatologic Clinics 1993;11:473.
122. Anhalt GJ, Kim SC, Stanley JR et al. Paraneoplastic pemphigus: An autoimmune mucocutaneous disease associated with neoplasia. N Engl J Med 1990;323:1729.
123. Ostezan LB, Fabre VC, Caughman W et al. Paraneoplastic pemphigus in the absence of a known neoplasm. J Am Acad Dermatol 1995;33: 312.
124. Bystryn JC, Hodak E, Gao SQ et al. A paraneoplastic mixed bullous skin disease associated with anti-skin antibodies and a B-cell lymphoma. Arch Dermatol 1993;129:870.
125. Horn TD, Anhalt GJ. Histologic features of paraneoplastic pemphigus. Arch Dermatol 1992;128:1091.
126. Stevens SR, Griffiths EM, Anhalt GJ, Cooper KD. Paraneoplastic pemphigus presenting as a lichen planus pemphigoides-like eruption. Arch Dermatol 1993;129:866.
127. Camisa C, Helm TN, Valenzuela R et al. Paraneoplastic pemphigus: Three new cases (abstr). J Invest Dermatol 1992;98:590.
128. Fullerton SH, Woodley DT, Smoller BR et al. Paraneoplastic pemphigus with autoantibody deposition in bronchial epithelium after autologous bone marrow transplantation. JAMA 1992;267:1500.
129. Lam S, Stone MS, Goeken JA et al. Paraneoplastic pemphigus, cicatricial conjunctivitis, and acanthosis nigricans with pachydermatoglyphy in a patient with bronchogenic squamous cell carcinoma. Ophthalmology 1992;99:108.
130. Lever WF. Pemphigus. Medicine (Baltimore) 1953;32:1.
131. Asbrink E, Hovmark A. Clinical variations in bullous pemphigoid with respect to early symptoms. Acta Derm Venereol (Stockh) 1981; 61:417.
132. Amato DA, Silverstein J, Zitelli J. The prodrome of bullous pemphigoid. Int J Dermatol 1988;27:560.
133. Bushkell LL, Jordon RE. Bullous pemphigoid: A cause of peripheral blood eosinophilia. J Am Acad Dermatol 1983;8:648.
134. Eng AM, Moncada B. Bullous pemphigoid and dermatitis herpetiformis: Histologic differentiation. Arch Dermatol 1974;110:51.
135. Jablonska S, Chorzelski T. Kann das histologische bild die grundlage zur differenzierung des morbus duhring mit dem pemphigoid und erythema multiforme darstellen? Dermatol Wochenschr 1963;146:590.
136. Van der Meer JB. Dermatitis herpetiformis: A specific (immunopathological?) entity. Thesis, University of Utrecht, The Netherlands, 1972.
137. Rook AJ, Waddington E. Pemphigus and pemphigoid. Br J Dermatol 1953;65:425.
138. Winkelmann RK, Su WPD. Pemphigoid vegetans. Arch Dermatol 1979;115:446.
139. Kuokkanen K, Helin H. Pemphigoid vegetans. Arch Dermatol 1981; 117:56.
140. Sams WM, Jordon RD. Correlation of pemphigoid and pemphigus antibody with activity of disease. Br J Dermatol 1971;84:7.
141. Person JR, Rogers RS III. Bullous and cicatricial pemphigoid: Clinical, histological, pathogenic, and immunopathological correlations. Mayo Clin Proc 1977;52:54.
142. Schaumburg-Lever G, Rule A, Schmidt-Ullrich B et al. Ultrastructural localization of in vivo bound immunoglobulins in bullous pemphigoid. J Invest Dermatol 1975;64:47.
143. Holubar K, Wolfe K, Konrad K et al. Ultrastructural localization of immunoglobulins in bullous pemphigoid skin. J Invest Dermatol 1975;64:220.
144. Mutasim DF, Anhalt GJ, Diaz LA. Linear immunofluorescence staining of the basement membrane zone produced by pemphigoid antibodies: The result of hemidesmosome staining. J Am Acad Dermatol 1987;16:75.
145. Gammon WR, Briggaman RA, Inman AO et al. Differentiating anti-lamina lucida and anti-sublamina densa anti-BMZ antibodies by indirect immunofluorescence on 1.0 M sodium chloride-separated skin. J Invest Dermatol 1984;82:139.
146. Pang BK, Lee YS, Ratnam KV. Floor-pattern salt-split skin cannot distinguish bullous pemphigoid from epidermolysis bullosa acquisita. Arch Dermatol 1993;129:744.
147. Logan RA, Bhogal B, Das AK et al. Localization of bullous pemphigoid antibody: An indirect immunofluorescence study of 228 cases using a split-skin technique. Br J Dermatol 1987;117:471.
148. Wuepper KD. Repeat direct immunofluorescence to discriminate pemphigoid from epidermolysis bullosa acquisita (correspondence). Arch Dermatol 1990;126:1365.
149. Gammon WR, Kowalewski C, Chorzelski TP et al. Direct immunofluorescence studies of sodium chloride-separated skin in the differential diagnosis of bullous pemphigoid and epidermolysis bullosa acquisita. J Am Acad Dermatol 1990;22:664.
150. Meuller S, Klaus-Kovtun V, Stanley JR. A 230kD basic protein is the major bullous pemphigoid antigen. J Invest Dermatol 1989;92:33.
151. Labib RS, Anhalt GJ, Patel HP et al. Molecular heterogeneity of the bullous pemphigoid antigens as detected by immunoblotting. J Immunol 1986;136:1231.
152. Goldberg DJ, Sablonski M, Bystryn JC. Regional variation in the expression of bullous pemphigoid antigen and location of lesions in bullous pemphigoid. J Invest Dermatol 1984;82:326.
153. Cotell SL, Lapiere JC, Chen JD et al. A novel 105-kDa lamina lucida autoantigen: Association with bullous pemphigoid. J Invest Dermatol 1994;103:78.
154. Chan LS, Cooper KD. A novel immune-mediated subepidermal bullous dermatosis characterized by IgG autoantibodies to a lower lamina lucida component. Arch Dermatol 1994;130:343.
155. Nakagawa T, De Weck AL. Membrane receptors for the IgG4 subclass of human basophils and mast cells. Clin Rev Allergy 1983; 1:197.
156. Varigos GA, Morstyn G, Vadas MA. Bullous pemphigoid blister fluid stimulates eosinophil colony formation and activates eosinophils. Clin Exp Immunol 1982;50:555.
157. Grando SA, Glukhensky BT, Drannik GN et al. Mediators of inflammation in blister fluids from patients with bullous pemphigoid and pemphigus vulgaris. Arch Dermatol 1989;125:925.
158. Brown LF, Harrist TJ, Yeo KT et al. Increased expression of vascular permeability factor (vascular endothelial growth factor) in bullous pemphigoid, dermatitis herpetiformis and erythema multiforme. J Invest Dermatol 1995;104:744.
159. Stahle-Backdahl M, Inoue M, Giudice GJ, Parks WC. 92-kD gelatinase is produced by eosinophils at the site of blister formation in bullous pemphigoid and cleaves the extracellular domain of recombinant 180-kD bullous pemphigoid autoantigen. J Clin Invest 1994;93:2022.
160. Kaneko F, Minagawa T, Takiguchi Y et al. Role of cell-mediated immune reaction in blister formation of bullous pemphigoid. Dermatology 1992;184:34.
161. Braun-Falco O, Rupec M. Elektronenmikroskopische untersuchungen zur dynamik der acantholyse bei pemphigus vulgaris. Arch Klin Exp Dermatol 1967;230:1.
162. Kobayashi T. The dermo-epidermal junction in bullous pemphigoid. Dermatologica 1967;134:157.
163. Lever WF, Hashimoto K. The etiology and treatment of pemphigus and pemphigoid. J Invest Dermatol 1969;53:373.
164. Schaumburg-Lever G, Orfanos CE, Lever WF. Electron microscopic study of bullous pemphigoid. Arch Dermatol 1972;106:662.
165. Fellner MJ, Katz JM. Occurrence of bullous pemphigoid after furosemide therapy. Arch Dermatol 1976;112:75.
166. Kashihara M, Danno K, Miyachi Y et al. Bullous pemphigoid-like lesions induced by phenacetin. Arch Dermatol 1984;120:1196.
167. Hodak E, Ben-Shetrit A, Ingber A, Sandbank M. Bullous pemphigoid: An adverse effect of ampicillin. Clin Exp Dermatol 1990;15:50.
168. Person JR, Rogers RS III, Perry HO. Localized pemphigoid. Br J Dermatol 1976;95:531.
169. Soh H, Hosokawa H, Miyauchi H et al. Localized pemphigoid shares the same target antigen as bullous pemphigoid. Br J Dermatol 1991; 125:73.

170. Behlen CH, Mackay DM. Benign mucous membrane pemphigus with a generalized eruption. Arch Dermatol 1965;92:566.
171. Brauner GJ, Jimbow K. Benign mucous membrane pemphigoid. Arch Dermatol 1972;106:535.
172. Lever WF. Pemphigus conjunctivae with scarring of the skin. Arch Dermatol Syphilol 1942;46:875, and 1944;49:113.
173. Hardy KM, Perry HO, Pingree GC et al. Benign mucous membrane pemphigoid. Arch Dermatol 1971;104:467.
174. Kleine-Natrop HE, Haustein UF. "Benignes Schleimhautpemphigoid" mit rascher Erblindung und generalisierten vernarbenden Hautveränderungen. Hautarzt 1968;19:6.
175. Tagami H, Imamura S. Benign mucous membrane pemphigoid. Arch Dermatol 1974;109:711.
176. Brunsting LA, Perry HO. Benign pemphigoid? A report of seven cases with chronic scarring, herpetiform plaques about the head and neck. Arch Dermatol 1957;75:489.
177. Michel B, Bean SF, Chorzelski T et al. Cicatricial pemphigoid of Brunsting-Perry: Immunofluorescent studies. Arch Dermatol 1977; 113:1403.
178. Hanno R, Foster DR, Bean SF. Brunsting-Perry cicatricial pemphigoid associated with bullous pemphigoid. J Am Acad Dermatol 1980;3:470.
179. Provost TT, Maize JC, Ahmed AR et al. Unusual subepidermal bullous diseases with immunologic features of bullous pemphigoid. Arch Dermatol 1979;115:156.
180. Braun-Falco O, Wolff HH, Ponce E. Disseminiertes vernarbendes pemphigoid. Hautarzt 1981;32:233.
181. Rogers RS III, Seehafer JR, Perry HO. Treatment of cicatricial (benign mucous membrane) pemphigoid with dapsone. J Am Acad Dermatol 1982;6:215.
182. Bean SF. Cicatricial pemphigoid: Immunofluorescent studies. Arch Dermatol 1974;110:552.
183. Griffith MR, Fukuyama K, Tuffanelli D et al. Immunofluorescent studies in mucous membrane pemphigoid. Arch Dermatol 1974;109: 195.
184. Rogers RS III, Perry HO, Bean SF et al. Immunopathology of cicatricial pemphigoid: Studies of complement deposition. J Invest Dermatol 1977;68:39.
185. Reunala T, Rantala J, Histanen J et al. Linear IgA deposition in benign mucous membrane pemphigoid (abstract). J Cutan Pathol 1984;11: 232.
186. Leonard JN, Wright P, Williams DM et al. The relationship between linear IgA disease and benign mucous membrane pemphigoid. Br J Dermatol 1984;110:307.
187. Leonard JN, Hobday CM, Haffenden GP et al. Immunofluorescent studies in ocular cicatricial pemphigoid. Br J Dermatol 1988;118:209.
188. Wojnarowska F, Marsden RA, Bhogal B et al. Childhood cicatricial pemphigoid with linear IgA deposits. Clin Exp Dermatol 1984;9:407.
189. Jacoby WD Jr, Bartholome CW, Ramchand SC et al. Cicatricial pemphigoid (Brunsting-Perry type): Case report and immunofluorescence findings. Arch Dermatol 1978;114:779.
190. Ahmed AR, Salm M, Larson R et al. Localized cicatricial pemphigoid (Brunsting-Perry). Arch Dermatol 1984;120:932.
191. Kelly SE, Wojnarowska F. The use of chemically split tissue in the detection of circulating anti-basement membrane antibodies in bullous pemphigoid and cicatricial pemphigoid. Br J Dermatol 1988;118:31.
192. Fine JD, Neises GR, Katz SI. Immunofluorescence and immunoelectron microscopic studies in cicatricial pemphigoid. J Invest Dermatol 1984;82:39.
193. Bernard P, Prost C, Lecerf V et al. Studies of cicatricial pemphigoid autoantibodies using direct immunoelectron microscopy and immunoblot analysis. J Invest Dermatol 1990;94:630.
194. Domloge-Hultsch N, Anhalt GJ, Gammon WR et al. Antiepilegrin cicatricial pemphigoid: A subepithelial bullous disorder. Arch Dermatol 1994;130:1521.
195. Susi FR, Shklar G. Histochemistry and fine structure of oral lesions of mucous membrane pemphigoid. Arch Dermatol 1971;104:244.
196. Caputo R, Bellone AG, Crosti C. Pathogenesis of the blister in cicatricial pemphigoid and in bullous pemphigoid. Arch Dermatol Forsch 1973;247:181.
197. Shornick JK, Bangert JL, Freeman RG, Gilliam JN. Herpes gestationis: Clinical and histologic features of twenty-eight cases. J Am Acad Dermatol 1983;8:214.
198. Shornick JK. Herpes gestationis. Dermatol Clin 1993;11:527.
199. Shornick JK, Black MM. Fetal risks in herpes gestationis. J Am Acad Dermatol 1992;26:63.
200. Chorzelski TP, Jablonska S, Beutner EH et al. Herpes gestationis with identical lesions in the newborn. Arch Dermatol 1976;112:1129.
201. Katz A, Minta JO, Toole JWP et al. Immunopathologic study of herpes gestationis in mother and infant. Arch Dermatol 1977;113:1069.
202. Piérard J, Thiery M, Kint A. Histologie et ultrastructure de l'herpes gestationis. Arch Belg Dermatol Syphiligr 1969;25:321.
203. Hertz KC, Katz SI, Maize J et al. Herpes gestationis: A clinicopathological study. Arch Dermatol 1976;112:1543.
204. Provost TT, Tomasi TB. Evidence for complement activation via the alternate pathway in skin diseases. J Clin Invest 1973;52:1779.
205. Kelly SE, Bhogal BS, Wojnarowska F et al. Western blot analysis of the antigen in pemphigoid gestationis. Br J Dermatol 1990;122:445.
206. Morrison LH, Labib RS, Zone JJ et al. Herpes gestationis autoantibodies recognize a 180kD human epidermal antigen. J Clin Invest 1988;81:2023.
207. Li K, Tamai K, Tan EM, Uitto J. Cloning of type XVII collagen. J Biochem 1993;268:8825.
208. Schaumburg-Lever G, Saffold OE, Orfanos CE et al. Herpes gestationis: Histology and ultrastructure. Arch Dermatol 1973;107:888.
209. Yaoita H, Gullino M, Katz SI. Herpes gestationis: Ultrastructure and ultrastructural localization on in vivo-bound complement. J Invest Dermatol 1976;66:383.
210. Roenigk HH Jr, Ryan JG, Bergfeld WG. Epidermolysis bullosa acquisita: Report of three cases and review of all published cases. Arch Dermatol 1971;103:1.
211. Gammon WR, Briggaman RA, Woodley DT et al. Epidermolysis bullosa acquisita: A pemphigoid-like disease. J Am Acad Dermatol 1984; 11:820.
212. Dahl MV. Epidermolysis bullosa acquisita: A sign of cicatricial pemphigoid? Br J Dermatol 1979;101:475.
213. Yaoita H, Briggaman RA, Lawly TJ et al. Epidermolysis bullosa acquisita: Ultrastructural and immunologic studies. J Invest Dermatol 1981;76:288.
214. Woodley DT, Gammon WR. Epidermolysis bullosa acquisita. Immunol Ser 1989;46:547.
215. Gammon WR, Fine JD, Briggaman RA. Autoimmunity to type VII collagen: Features and roles in basement membrane zone injury. In: Fine JD, ed. Bullous diseases. New York: Igaku Shoin, 1993;75.
216. Nieboer C, Boorsma DM, Woerdeman MJ, Kalsbeck GL. Epidermolysis bullosa acquisita: Immunofluorescence, electron microscopic and immunoelectron microscopic studies in four patients. Br J Dermatol 1980;102:383.
217. Woodley DT, Burgeson RE, Lunstrum G et al. The epidermolysis bullosa acquisita antigen is the globular carboxy terminus of type VII procollagen. J Clin Invest 1988;81:683.
218. Olansky AJ, Briggaman RA, Gammon WR et al. Bullous systemic lupus erythematosus. J Am Acad Dermatol 1982;7:511.
219. Miller JA, Dowd DM, Dudeney C, Isenberg DA. Vesiculobullous eruption in systemic lupus erythematosus: Demonstration of common anti-DNA antibody idiotype at the dermoepidermal junction. J R Soc Med 1968;79:365.
220. Barton DD, Fine JD, Gammon WR, Sams WM. Bullous systemic lupus erythematosus: An unusual clinical course and detectable circulating antibodies to the epidermolysis bullosa acquisita antigen. J Am Acad Dermatol 1986;15:369.
221. Kettler AH, Bean SF, Duffy JO, Gammon WR. Systemic lupus erythematosus presenting as a bullous eruption in a child. Arch Dermatol 1988;124:1083.
222. Pedro SD, Dahl MV. Direct immunofluorescence of bullous systemic lupus erythematosus. Arch Dermatol 1973;107:118.
223. Jacoby RA, Abraham AA. Bullous dermatosis and systemic lupus erythematosus in a 15-year-old boy. Arch Dermatol 1979;115:1094.
224. Penneys NS, Wiley HS. Herpetiform blisters in lupus erythematosus. Arch Dermatol 1979;115:1427.
225. Hall RP, Lawley TJ, Smith HR, Katz SI. Bullous eruption of systemic lupus erythematosus: Dramatic response to dapsone therapy. Ann Intern Med 1979;97:165.
226. Camisa C, Sharma HM. Vesiculobullous systemic lupus erythematosus: A report of two cases and a review of the literature. J Am Acad Dermatol 1983;9:924.
227. Tsuchida T, Furue M, Kashiwado T, Ishibashi Y. Bullous systemic lupus erythematosus with cutaneous mucinosis and leukocytoclastic vasculitis. J Am Acad Dermatol 1994;31:387.

228. Gammon WR, Woodley DT, Dole KC, Briggaman RA. Evidence that anti-basement membrane zone antibodies in bullous eruption of systemic lupus erythematosus recognized epidermolysis bullosa acquisita autoantigen. J Invest Dermatol 1985;84:472.
229. Tolman MM, Moschella SL, Schneiderman RN. Dermatitis herpetiformis: Specific entity or clinical complex? J Invest Dermatol 1959; 32:557.
230. Leonard JN, Tucker WFG, Fry JS et al. Increased incidence of malignancy in dermatitis herpetiformis. Br Med J 1983;286:16.
231. Aronson AJ, Soltani R, Aronson IK, Ong RT. Systemic lupus erythematosus and dermatitis herpetiformis: Concurrence with Marfan's syndrome. Arch Dermatol 1979;115:68.
232. Piérard J. De l'aspect histologique des plaques érythémateuses de la dermatite herpétiforme de Duhring. Ann Dermatol Syphiligr (Paris) 1963;90:121.
233. Van der Meer JB. Granular deposits of immunoglobulins in the skin of patients with dermatitis herpetiformis: An immunofluorescent study. Br J Dermatol 1969;81:493.
234. Clark WH, Yip SY, Tolman MB. The histiogenesis of dermoepidermal separation in dermatitis herpetiformis (abstr). Clin Res 1968;61: 433.
235. MacVicar DN, Graham JH, Burgoon CF Jr. Dermatitis herpetiformis, erythema multiforme and bullous pemphigoid: A comparative histopathological and histochemical study. J Invest Dermatol 1963; 41:289.
236. Kresbach H, Hartwagner A. Zur differentialdiagnose zwischen dermatitis herpetiformis Duhring und bullösem pemphigoid. Z Hautkr 1968; 43:165.
237. Kint A, Geerts ML, De Brauwere D. Diagnostic criteria in dermatitis herpetiformis. Dermatologica 1976;153:266.
238. Connor BL, Marks R, Wilson Jones E. Dermatitis herpetiformis. Trans St Johns Hosp Dermatol Soc 1972;58:191.
239. Cormane R. Immunofluorescent studies of the skin in lupus erythematosus and other diseases. Pathol Eur 1967;2:170.
240. Olbricht SM, Flotte TJ, Collins AB et al. Dermatitis herpetiformis: Cutaneous deposition of polyclonal IgA1. Arch Dermatol 1986;122: 418.
241. Zone JJ, Carioto LA, LaSalle BA et al. Granular IgA is decreased or absent in never involved skin in dermatitis herpetiformis. Clin Res 1985;33:159.
242. Zone JJ, Sayre, LA, Meyer LJ. Granular IgA is quantitatively greater in perilesional skin than in adjacent uninvolved skin in patients with dermatitis herpetiformis. J Clin Res 1987;35:253.
243. Chorzelski TP, Beutner EH, Jablonska S et al. Immunofluorescence studies in the diagnosis of dermatitis herpetiformis and its differentiation from bullous pemphigoid. J Invest Dermatol 1971;56:373.
244. Kadunce DP, Meyer LJ, Zone JJ. IgA class antibodies in dermatitis herpetiformis: Reaction with tissue antigens. J Invest Dermatol 1989; 93:253.
245. Kumar V, Hemedenger E, Chorzelski T et al. Reticulin and endomysial antibodies in bullous diseases. Comparison of specificity and sensitivity. Arch Dermatol 1987;123:1179.
246. Katz SI, Hertz KC, Rogentine GN et al. HLA-B8 and dermatitis herpetiformis in patients with IgA deposits in skin. Arch Dermatol 1977; 113:155.
247. Strober W. Immunogenic factors. In: Katz SI, moderator. Dermatitis herpetiformis: The skin and the gut. Ann Intern Med 1980;93:857.
248. Hall RP, Sanders ME, Duquesnoy RJ et al. Alterations in HLA-DP and HLA-DQ antigen frequency in patients with dermatitis herpetiformis. J Invest Dermatol 1989;93:501.
249. Marks J, Shuster S, Watson A. Small bowel changes in dermatitis herpetiformis. Lancet 1966;2:1280.
250. Pardo RJ, Penneys NS. Location of basement membrane type IV collagen beneath subepidermal bullous diseases. J Cutan Pathol 1990;17: 336.
251. Lau M, Kaufmann-Grunzinger I, Raghunath M. A case report of a patient with features of systemic lupus erythematosus and linear IgA disease. Br J Dermatol 1991;124:498.
252. Smith SB, Harrist TJ, Murphy GF et al. Linear IgA bullous dermatosis v. dermatitis herpetiformis. Arch Dermatol 1984;120:324.
253. Petersen MJ, Gammon WR, Briggaman RA. A case of linear IgA disease presenting as initially with IgG immune deposits. J Am Acad Dermatol 1986;14;1014.
254. Adachi A, Tani M, Matsubayashi S et al. Immunoelectron microscopic differentiation of linear IgA bullous dermatosis of adults with coexistence of IgA and IgG deposition from bullous pemphigoid. J Am Acad Dermatol 1992;27:394.
255. Chorzelski TP, Jablonska S. IgA linear dermatosis of childhood: Chronic bullous disease of childhood. Br J Dermatol 1979;101:535.
256. Leonard JN, Haffenden GP, Ring NP et al. Linear IgA disease in adults. Br J Dermatol 1982;107:301.
257. Mobacken H, Kastrup W, Ljunghall K et al. Linear IgA dermatosis: A study of ten adult patients. Acta Derm Venereol (Stockh) 1983;63: 123.
258. Wojnarowska F, Whitehead P, Leigh IM et al. Identification of the target antigen in chronic bullous disease of childhood and linear IgA disease of adults. Br J Dermatol 1991;124:157.
259. Peters MS, Rogers RS. Clinical correlations of linear IgA deposition at the cutaneous basement membrane zone. J Am Acad Dermatol 1989;20:761.
260. Wojnarowska F, Marsden RA, Black MM. An updated review of the chronic acquired bullous diseases of childhood. Br J Dermatol 1983; 109:40.
261. Wojnarowska F, Marsden RA, Bhogal B. Chronic bullous disease of childhood, childhood cicatricial pemphigoid, and linear IgA disease of adults. J Am Acad Dermatol 1988;19:792.
262. Prost C, DeLuca C, Combemale P et al. Diagnosis of adult linear IgA dermatosis by immunoelectron microscopy in 16 patients with linear IgA deposits. J Invest Dermatol 1989;92:39.
263. Zone JJ, Taylor TB, Meyer LJ. Identification of the cutaneous basement membrane zone antigen and isolation of antibody in linear immunoglobulin A bullous dermatosis. J Clin Invest 1990;85:812.
264. Meurer M, Schmoeckel C, Braun-Falco O. Dermatitis herpetiformis Duhring miut linearen ablagerungen von IgA (lineare IgA dermatose). Hautarzt 1984;35:230.
265. Yamasaki Y, Hashimoto T, Nishikawa T. Dermatitis herpetiformis with linear-IgA deposition. Acta Derm Venereol (Stockh) 1982;62: 401.
266. Bhogal B, Wojnarowska F, Marsden RA et al. Linear IgA bullous dermatosis of adults and children: An immunoelectron microscopic study. Br J Dermatol 1987;117:289.
267. Pehamberger H, Konrad K, Holubar K. Juvenile dermatitis herpetiformis: An immunoelectron microscopic study. Br J Dermatol 1979; 101:271.
268. Carpenter S, Berg D, Sidhu-Malik N et al. Vancomycin-associated linear IgA dermatosis. J Am Acad Dermatol 1992;26:45.
269. Baden LA, Apovian C, Imber MM et al. Vancomycin-induced linear IgA bullous dermatosis. Arch Dermatol 1988;124:1186.
270. Gabrielsen TO, Staerfelt F, Thune PO. Drug-induced bullous dermatosis with linear IgA deposits along the basement membrane. Acta Derm Venereol (Stockh) 1981;61:439.
271. McWhirter JD, Hashimoto K, Fayne S et al. Linear IgA bullous dermatosis related to lithium carbonate. Arch Dermatol 1987;123:1120.
272. Jordon RE, Bean SF, Trifshauser CT et al. Chronic bullous dermatitis herpetiformis: Negative immunofluorescent tests. Arch Dermatol 1970;101:629.
273. Van der Meer JB, Remme JJ, Nelkins MJJ et al. IgA antibasement membrane antibodies in a boy with pemphigoid. Arch Dermatol 1977; 113:1462.
274. Marsden RA, McKee PH, Bhogal B et al. A study of benign chronic bullous dermatosis of childhood. Clin Exp Dermatol 1980;5:159.
275. Burge S, Wojnarowska F, Marsden A. Chronic bullous dermatosis of childhood persisting into adulthood. Pediatr Dermatol 1988;5:246.
276. Esterly NB, Furey NL, Kirschner BS et al. Chronic bullous dermatosis of childhood. Arch Dermatol 1977;113:42.
277. McGuire J, Nordlund J. Bullous disease of childhood. Arch Dermatol 1973;108:284.
278. Freeman RG, Spiller R, Knox JM. Histopathology of erythema toxicum neonatorum. Arch Dermatol 1960;82:586.
279. Stone OJ. High viscosity of newborn extracellular matrix is the etiology of erythema toxicum neonatorum: Neonatal jaundice? Hyaline membrane disease? Med Hypotheses 1990;33:15.
280. Bassukas ID. Is erythema toxicum neonatorum a mild self-limited acute cutaneous graft-versus-host reaction from maternal-to-fetal lymphocyte transfer? Med Hypothesis 1992;38:334.
281. Ramamurthy RS, Reveri M, Esterly NB et al. Transient neonatal pustular melanosis. J Pediatr 1976;88:831.
282. Ferrandiz C, Coroleu W, Ribera M et al. Sterile transient neonatal pustulosis is a precocious form of erythema toxicum neonatorum. Dermatology 1992;185:18.

283. Jarratt M, Ramsdell W. Infantile acropustulosis. Arch Dermatol 1979; 115:834.
284. Newton JA, Salisbury J, Marsden A, McGibbon DH. Acropustulosis of infancy. Br J Dermatol 1986;115:735.
285. Dromy R, Raz A, Metzker A. Infantile acropustulosis. Pediatr Dermatol 1991;8:284.
286. Bundino S, Zina AM, Ubertalli S. Infantile acropustulosis. Dermatologica 1982;165:615.
287. Palungwachira P. Infantile acropustulosis. Australas J Dermatol 1989; 30:97.
288. McFadden N, Falk ES. Infantile acropustulosis. Cutis 1985;36:49.
289. Magro CM, Crowson AN. A distinctive eruption associated with hepatobiliary disease. Int J Dermatol 1996, in press.
290. O'Loughlin S, Perry HO. A diffuse pustular eruption associated with ulcerative colitis. Arch Dermatol 1978;114:1061.
291. Sneddon IB, Wilkinson DS. Subcorneal pustular dermatosis. Br J Dermatol 1956;68:385.
292. Sneddon IB, Wilkinson DS. Subcorneal pustular dermatosis. Br J Dermatol 1979;100:61.
293. Atukorala DN, Joshi RK, Abanmi A, Jeha MT. Subcorneal pustular dermatosis and IgA myeloma. Dermatology 1993;187:124.
294. Burns RE, Fine G. Subcorneal pustular dermatosis. Arch Dermatol 1959;80:72.
295. Wolff K. Ein beitrag zur nosologie der subcornealen pustulösen dermatose (Sneddon-Wilkinson). Arch Klin Exp Dermatol 1966;224: 248.
296. Grob JJ, Mege JL, Capo C et al. Role of tumor necrosis factor-α in Sneddon-Wilkinson subcorneal pustular dermatosis: A model of neutrophil priming in vivo. J Am Acad Dermatol 1991;25:944.
297. Metz J, Schröpl F. Elktronenmikroskopische untersuchungen bei subcornealer pustulöser dermatose. Arch Klin Exp Dermatol 1970;236: 190.
298. Sanchez N, Ackerman AB. Subcorneal pustular dermatosis: A variant of pustular psoriasis. Acta Derm Venereol Suppl (Stockh) 1979;85: 147.
299. Chimenti S, Ackerman AB. Is subcorneal pustular dermatosis of Sneddon and Wilkinson an entity sui generis? Am J Dermatopathol 1981;3:363.
300. Assier H, Bastuji-Garin S, Revuz J, Roujeau J-C: Erythema multiforme with mucous membrane involvement and Stevens-Johnson syndrome are clinically different disorders with distinct causes. Arch Dermatol 1995;131:539.
301. Lyell A. Toxic epidermal necrolysis: An eruption resembling scalding of the skin. Br J Dermatol 1956;68:355.
302. Schöpf E, Stühmer A, Rzany B et al. Toxic epidermal necrolysis and Stevens-Johnson syndrome. Arch Dermatol 1991;127:839.
303. Lyell A. A review of toxic epidermal necrolysis in Britain. Br J Dermatol 1967;79:662.
304. Ruiz-Maldonado R. Acute disseminated epidermal necroses. J Am Acad Dermatol 1985;13:623.
305. Bastuji-Garin S, Rzany B, Stern RS et al. Clinical classification of cases of toxic epidermal necrolysis, Stevens-Johnson syndrome, and erythema multiforme. Arch Dermatol 1993;129:92.
306. Orfanos CE, Schaumburg-Lever G, Lever WF. Dermal and epidermal types of erythema multiforme. Arch Dermatol 1974;109:682.
307. Ackerman AB, Ragaz A. Erythema multiforme. Am J Dermatopathol 1985;7:133.
308. Howland WW, Golitz LE, Weston WL, Huff JC. Erythema multiforme: Clinical, histopathologic, and immunologic study. J Am Acad Dermatol 1984;10:438.
309. Leboit PE. Interface dermatitis: How specific are its histopathologic features? Arch Dermatol 1993;129:1324.
310. Bedi TR, Pinkus H. Histopathological spectrum of erythema multiforme. Br J Dermatol 1976;95:243.
311. Patterson JW, Parsons JM, Blaylock WK et al. Eosinophils in skin lesions of erythema multiforme. Arch Pathol 1989;113:36.
312. Imamura S, Yanase K, Taniguchi S et al. Erythema multiforme: Demonstration of immune complexes in the sera and skin lesions. Br J Dermatol 1980;102:161.
313. Bushkell LL, Mackel SE, Jordon RE. Erythema multiforme: Direct immunofluorescence studies and detection of circulating immune complexes. J Invest Dermatol 1980;74:372.
314. Finan MC, Schroeter AL. Cutaneous immunofluorescence study of erythema multiforme: Correlation with light microscopic patterns and etiologic agents. J Am Acad Dermatol 1984;10:497.
315. Imamura S, Horio T, Yanase K et al. Erythema multiforme: Pathomechanism of papular erythema and target lesions. J Dermatol 1992; 19:524.
316. King T, Helm TN, Valenzuela R, Bergfeld W. Diffuse intraepidermal deposition of immunoreactants on direct immunofluorescence: A clue to the early diagnosis of epidermal necrolysis. Int J Dermatol 1994;33: 634.
317. Margolis R, Tonnesen MG, Harrist TJ et al. Lymphocyte subsets and Langerhans cells/indeterminate cells in erythema multiforme. J Invest Dermatol 1983;81:403.
318. Huff JC, Weston WL, Tonnesen MG. Erythema multiforme: A critical review of characteristics, diagnostic criteria, and causes. J Am Acad Dermatol 1983;8:763.
319. Khalil I, Lepage V, Douay C et al. HLA DQB1* 0301 allele is involved in the susceptibility to erythema multiforme. J Invest Dermatol 1991;97:697.
320. Schofield JK, Tatnall FM, Brown J et al. Recurrent erythema multiforme: Tissue typing in a large series of patients. Br J Dermatol 1994; 131:532.
321. Aslanzadeh J, Helm KF, Espy MJ et al. Detection of HSV-specific DNA in biopsy tissue of patients with erythema multiforme by polymerase chain reaction. Br J Dermatol 1992;126:19.
322. Brice SL, Krzemien D, Weston WL et al. Detection of herpes simplex virus DNA in cutaneous lesions of erythema multiforme. J Invest Dermatol 1989;93:183.
323. Brice SL, Leahy MA, Ong L et al. Examination of non-involved skin, previously involved skin, and peripheral blood for herpes simplex virus DNA in patients with recurrent herpes-associated erythema multiforme. J Cutan Pathol 1994;21:408.
324. Villada G, Roujeau J-C, Clérici T et al. Immunopathology of toxic epidermal necrolysis. Arch Dermatol 1992;128:50.
325. Prutkin L, Fellner MJ. Erythema multiforme bullosum. Acta Derm Venereol (Stockh) 1971;51:429.
326. Ford MJ, Smith KL, Croker BP et al. Large granular lymphocytes within the epidermis of erythema multiforme lesions. J Am Acad Dermatol 1992;27:460.
327. Anderson KC, Weinstein HJ. Transfusion-associated graft-versus-host disease. N Engl J Med 1990;323:315.
328. Morhenn VB, Maibach HI. Graft vs. host reaction in a newborn. Acta Derm Venereol (Stockh) 1974;54:133.
329. Glucksberg H, Strob R, Fefer A et al. Clinical manifestations of graft-versus-host disease in human recipients of marrow from HLA-matched sibling donors. Transplantation 1975;18:295.
330. Darmstadt GL, Donnenberg AD, Vogelsang GB et al. Clinical, laboratory, and histopathologic indicators of progressive acute graft-versus-host disease. J Invest Dermatol 1992;99:397.
331. Fujii H, Hiketa T, Matsumoto Y et al. Clinical characteristics of chronic cutaneous graft-versus-host disease in Japanese leukemia patients after bone marrow transplantation: Low incidence and mild manifestations. Bone Marrow Transplant 1992;10:331.
332. Shulman HM, Sale GE, Lerner KG et al. Chronic cutaneous graft-versus-host disease in man. Am J Pathol 1978;91:545.
333. Friedman KJ, Leboit PE, Farmer ER. Acute follicular graft-vs-host reaction. Arch Dermatol 1988;124:688.
334. Desbarats J, Seemayer TA, Lapp WS. Irradiation of the skin and systemic graft-versus-host disease synergize to produce cutaneous lesions. Am J Pathol 1994;144:883.
335. James WD, Odom RB. Graft-v.-host disease. Arch Dermatol 1983; 119:683.
336. Saurat JH, Gluckman E, Russel A et al. The lichen planus-like eruption after bone marrow transplantation. Br J Dermatol 1975;93:675.
337. Lerner KG, Kao GF, Storb R et al. Histopathology of graft-versus-host reaction (GvHR) in human recipients of marrow from HLA-matched sibling donors. Transplant Proc 1974;6:367.
338. Horn TD, Bauer DJ, Vogelsang GB, Hess AD. Reappraisal of histologic features of the acute cutaneous graft-versus-host reaction based on an allogeneic rodent model. J Invest Dermatol 1994;103:206.
339. Hymes SR, Farmer ER, Lewis PG et al. Cutaneous graft-versus-host reaction: Prognostic features seen by light microscopy. J Am Acad Dermatol 1985;12:468.
340. Chaudhuri SPR, Smoller BR. Acute cutaneous graft versus host disease: A clinicopathologic and immunophenotypic study. Int J Dermatol 1992;31:270.
341. Janin-Mercier A, Saurat JH, Bourges M et al. The lichen planuslike

and sclerotic phases of the graft versus host disease in man. Acta Derm Venereol (Stockh) 1981;61:187.
342. Spielvogel RL, Goltz RW, Kersey JH. Scleroderma-like changes in chronic graft vs host disease. Arch Dermatol 1977;113:1424.
343. Tanaka K, Sullivan KM, Shulman HM et al. A clinical review: Cutaneous manifestations of acute and chronic graft-versus-host disease following bone marrow transplantation. J Dermatol 1991;18:11.
344. Tsoi MS, Storb R, Jones E et al. Deposition of IgM and C at the dermoepidermal junction in acute and chronic cutaneous graft-vs-host disease in man. J Immunol 1978;120:1485.
345. Ullman S. Immunoglobulins and complement in skin in graft-versus-host disease. Ann Intern Med 1976;85:205.
346. Parkman R, Rappeport J, Rosen F. Human graft versus host disease. J Invest Dermatol 1980;74:276.
347. Sale GE, Shulman HM, Gallucci BB et al. Young rete ridge keratinocytes are preferred targets in cutaneous graft-versus-host disease. Am J Pathol 1985;118:278.
348. Murphy GF, Lavker RM, Whitaker D, Korngold R. Cytotoxic folliculitis in GvHD: Evidence of follicular stem cell injury and recovery. J Cutan Pathol 1990;18:309.
349. Volc-Platzer B, Rappersberger K, Mosberger I et al. Sequential immunohistologic analysis of the skin following allogeneic bone marrow transplantation. J Invest Dermatol 1988;91:162.
350. Norton J, Sloane JP. ICAM-1 expression on epidermal keratinocytes in cutaneous graft-versus-host disease. Transplantation 1991;51:1203.
351. Beschorner WE, Farmer ER, Saral R et al. Epithelial class II antigen expression in cutaneous graft-versus-host disease. Transplantation 1987;44:237.
352. Breathnach SM, Shimada S, Kovac Z, Katz SI. Immunologic aspects of acute cutaneous graft-versus-host disease: Decreased density and antigen-presenting function of Ia+ Langerhans cells and absent antigen-presenting capacity of Ia+ keratinocytes. J Invest Dermatol 1986; 86:226.
353. Lever R, Turbitt M, Mackie R et al. A prospective study of the histological changes in the skin in patients receiving bone marrow transplants. Br J Dermatol 1986;114:161.
354. Breathnach SM, Katz SI. Immunopathology of cutaneous graft-versus-host disease. Am J Dermatopathol 1987;9:343.
355. Shiohara T, Moriya N, Gotoh C et al. Locally administered monoclonal antibodies to lymphocyte function-associated antigen 1 and L3T4 to prevent cutaneous graft-versus-host disease. J Immunol 1988; 141:2261.
356. Murphy GF, Whitaker D, Sprent J, Korngold R. Characterization of target injury of murine acute graft-versus-host disease directed to multiple minor histocompatibility antigens elicited by either CD4+ or CD8+ effector cells. Am J Pathol 1991;138:983.
357. Kawai K, Matsumoto Y, Watanabe H et al. Induction of cutaneous graft-versus-host disease by local injection of unprimed T cells. Clin Exp Immunol 1991;84:359.
358. Dickinson AM, Sviland L, Carey P et al. Skin explant culture as a model for cutaneous graft-versus-host disease in humans. Bone Marrow Transplant 1988;3:323.
359. Sakamoto H, Michaelson J, Jones WK et al. Lymphocytes with a CD4+ CD8-CD3- phenotype are effectors of experimental cutaneous graft-versus-host disease. Proc Natl Acad Sci U S A 1991;88:10890.
360. Horn TD, Farmer ER. Distribution of lymphocytes bearing TCR $\gamma\delta$ in cutaneous lymphocytic infiltrates. J Cutan Pathol 1990;17:165.
361. Norton J, Al-Saffar N, Sloane JP. An immunohistological study of γ/δ lymphocytes in human cutaneous graft-versus-host disease. Bone Marrow Transplant 1991;7:205.
362. Norton J, Sloane JP, Delia D, Greaves MF. Reciprocal expression of CD34 and cell adhesion molecule ELAM-1 on vascular endothelium in acute cutaneous graft-versus-host disease. J Pathol 1993;170:173.
363. Acevedo A, Aramburu J, Lopez J et al. Identification of natural killer (NK) cells in lesions of human cutaneous graft-versus-host disease: Expression of a novel NK-associated surface antigen (Kp43) in mononuclear infiltrates. J Invest Dermatol 1991;97:659.
364. De Dobbeleer GD, Ledoux-Corbusier MH, Achtern GA. Graft versus host reaction: An ultrastructural study. Arch Dermatol 1975;111: 1597.
365. Ferrara JLM, Guillen FJ, Van Dijken PJ et al. Evidence that large granular lymphocytes of donor origin mediate acute graft-versus-host disease. Transplantation 1989;47:50.
366. Sale GE, Gallucci BB, Schubert MM et al. Direct ultrastructural evidence of target-directed polarization by cytotoxic lymphocytes in lesions of human graft-versus-host disease. Arch Pathol Lab Med 1987; 111:333.
367. Davis RE, Smoller BR. T lymphocytes expressing HECA-452 epitope are present in cutaneous acute graft-versus-host disease and erythema multiforme, but not in acute graft-versus-host disease in gut organs. Am J Pathol 1992;141:691.
368. Drijkoningen M, De Wolf-Peeters C, Tricot G et al. Drug-induced skin reactions and acute cutaneous graft-versus-host reaction: A comparative immunohistochemical study. Blut 1988;56:69.
369. Leboit PE. Subacute radiation dermatitis: A histologic imitator of acute cutaneous graft-versus-host disease. J Am Acad Dermatol 1989; 20:236.
370. Elliott CJ, Sloane JP, Sanderson KV et al. The histological diagnosis of cutaneous graft versus host disease: Relationship of skin changes to marrow purging and other clinical variables. Histopathology 1987;11: 145.
371. Dumler JS, Beschorner WE, Farmer ER et al. Endothelial cell injury in cutaneous acute graft-versus-host disease. Am J Pathol 1989;135: 1097.
372. Synovec MS, Braddock SW, Jones J, Linder J. LN-3: A diagnostic adjunct in cutaneous graft-versus-host disease. Mod Pathol 1990;3:643.
373. Horn TD, Redd JV, Karp JE et al. Cutaneous eruptions of lymphocyte recovery. Arch Dermatol 1989;125:1512.
374. Bauer DJ, Hood AF, Horn TD. Histologic comparison of autologous graft-versus-host reaction and cutaneous eruption of lymphocyte recovery. Arch Dermatol 1993;129:855.
375. Grover RW. Transient acantholytic dermatosis. Arch Dermatol 1970; 101:426.
376. Lang I, Lindmaier A, Hönigsman H. Das spektrum der transienten akantholytischen dermatosen. Hautarzt 1986;37:485.
377. Chalet M, Grover R, Ackerman AB. Transient acantholytic dermatosis. Arch Dermatol 1977;113:431.
378. Heenan PJ, Quirk CJ. Transient acantholytic dermatosis. Br J Dermatol 1980;102:515.
379. Guana AL, Cohen PR. Transient acantholytic dermatosis in oncology patients. J Clin Oncol 1994;12:1703.
380. Manteaux AM, Rapini RP. Transient acantholytic dermatosis in patients with cancer. Cutis 1990;46:488.
381. Pehamberger H, Gschnait F, Konrad K et al. Transient acantholytic dermatosis Grover. Z Hautkr 1977;52:841.
382. Bystryn JC. Immunofluorescence studies in transient acantholytic dermatosis (Grover's disease). Am J Dermatopathol 1979;1:325.
383. Millns JL, Doyle JA, Muller SA. Positive cutaneous immunofluorescence in Grover's disease. Arch Dermatol 1980;116:515.
384. Hu C-H, Michel B, Farber EM. Transient acantholytic dermatosis (Grover's disease): A skin disorder related to heat and sweating. Arch Dermatol 1985;121:1439.
385. Gretzula JC, Penneys NS. Transient acantholytic dermatosis: An immunohistochemical study. Arch Dermatol 1986;122:972.
386. Mahler SJ, De Villez RL, Pulitzer DR. Transient acantholytic dermatosis induced by recombinant human interleukin 4. J Am Acad Dermatol 1993;29:206.
387. Kanzaki T, Hashimoto K. Transient acantholytic dermatosis with involvement of oral mucosa. J Cutan Pathol 1978;5:23.
388. Wolff HH, Chalet MD, Ackerman AB. Transitorische akantholytische dermatose (Grover). Hautarzt 1977;28:78.
389. Grover RW, Duffy JL. Transient acantholytic dermatosis. J Cutan Pathol 1975;2:111.
390. Brehmer-Anderson E, Göransson K. Friction blisters as a manifestation of pathomimia. Acta Derm Venereol (Stockh) 1975;55:65.
391. Naylor PFD. Experimental friction blisters. Br J Dermatol 1955;67: 327.
392. Sulzberger MB, Cortese TA Jr, Fishman L et al. Studies on blisters produced by friction. J Invest Dermatol 1966;47:456.
393. Hunter JAA, McVittie E, Comaish JS. Light and electron microscopic studies of physical injury to the skin: II. Friction. Br J Dermatol 1974; 90:491.
394. Winer LH, Levin GH. Changes in the skin as a result of electric current. Arch Dermatol 1958;78:386.
395. Sevitt S. Histological changes in burned skin. In Burns: Pathology and Therapeutic Application. London: Butterworth & Co, 1957;18.
396. Foley FD. Pathology of cutaneous burns. Surg Clin North Am 1970; 50:1200.
397. Metzker A, Merlob P. Suction purpura. Arch Dermatol 1992;128:822.

Lever's Histopathology of the Skin, eighth edition,
edited by David Elder et al. Lippincott–
Raven Publishers, Philadelphia © 1997.

CHAPTER 10

Connective Tissue Diseases

Christine Jaworsky

LUPUS ERYTHEMATOSUS

Lupus erythematosus is a disease that affects multiple organ systems and has a broad range of clinical manifestations. It may take the form of an isolated cutaneous eruption or a fatal systemic illness.

A combination of clinical and laboratory data was used to devise the "Criteria for the Classification of Systemic Lupus Erythematosus" set forth by the American Rheumatism Association (ARA) in 1972, amended in 1982,[1] and later slightly modified.[2] These criteria were developed for classification of patients with systemic lupus erythematosus as opposed to other rheumatic diseases. They are also widely used to diagnose patients with lupus erythematosus. This classification is based on 11 criteria:

1. Malar rash
2. Discoid rash
3. Photosensitivity
4. Oral ulcers, usually painless
5. Arthritis, nonerosive, involving two or more peripheral joints, with tenderness, swelling, or effusion
6. Serositis (pleurisy or pericarditis)
7. Renal disorder (persistent proteinuria exceeding 0.5 g/day or cellular casts)
8. Neurologic disorders (seizures or psychosis)
9. Hematologic disorders (hemolytic anemia; leukopenia of less than 4000/mm^3; lymphopenia of less than 1500/mm^3; or thrombocytopenia of less than 100,000/mm^3)
10. Immunologic disorder (positive LE-cell preparation; anti-DNA in abnormal titer; antibody to Sm nuclear antigen; or false-positive serologic test for syphilis)
11. Antinuclear antibody

A person is judged to have systemic lupus erythematosus (SLE) if any four or more of the 11 criteria are present serially or simultaneously. Furthermore, a diagnosis of SLE is indicated in any patient who has at least three of the following four symptoms: (1) a cutaneous eruption consistent with lupus erythematosus, (2) renal involvement, (3) serositis, or (4) joint involvement.[3] A diagnosis of SLE requires confirmation by laboratory tests. Even though the prognosis of SLE has been greatly improved by early diagnosis and modern methods of treatment, the mortality rate of the disease is between 15% and 25%.[4] Death usually results from infection or severe nephritis.[5]

The importance of adequate laboratory data for evaluation of the seriousness of the illness and its prognosis has long been recognized. Histologic examination of affected tissues in conjunction with serologic and immunofluorescence studies is essential for proper evaluation of a patient with LE.

Cutaneous changes of lupus erythematosus may be subdivided according to the morphology of the clinical lesion and/or its duration (acute, subacute, or chronic). Differentiation between LE subtypes is based upon the constellation of clinical, histological, and immunofluorescence findings.[6] Histologic findings alone may not be sufficient to correctly classify the subtype of the eruption.[7] Not every case of lupus erythematosus can be assigned with certainty to a category because intermediate forms and transitions from one type to another occur.

Chronic Cutaneous Lupus Erythematosus: Discoid LE, Verrucous LE, Tumid LE, LE Panniculitis/Profundus

Discoid Lupus Erythematosus (DLE)

Characteristically, lesions of DLE consist of well-demarcated, erythematous, slightly infiltrated, "discoid" plaques that often show adherent thick scales and follicular plugging. Early and active lesions usually display surrounding erythema. Old lesions often appear atrophic and have hypo- or hyperpigmentation. Occasionally lesions may show verrucous hyperkeratosis, especially at their periphery.[8] Hypopigmentation within previously affected areas is frequent. Rarely, neoplasms have been reported in lesions of lupus erythematosus and have included basal cell carcinoma, squamous cell carcinoma, and atypical fibroxanthoma.[9]

In many instances, the discoid cutaneous lesions are limited to the face, where the malar areas and the nose are predominantly affected. In addition, the scalp, ears, oral mucosa, and vermilion border of the lips may be involved. In patients with involvement of the head and neck unaccompanied initially by

C. Jaworsky: Departments of Dermatology and Pathology, Case Western University and Department of Dermatology, University of Pennsylvania, Philadelphia, PA

systemic lupus erythematosus (SLE), conversion of DLE to SLE is rare (10% risk).

In patients with *disseminated discoid lupus erythematosus,* discoid lesions are seen predominantly on the upper trunk and upper limbs, usually, but not always in association with lesions on the head.[10] SLE may eventually develop in some of these patients.[11] Although discoid cutaneous lesions are typical of DLE, they are also seen in as many as 14% of the patients with SLE.[12]

Histopathology. In most instances of *discoid lesions*, a diagnosis of lupus erythematosus is possible on the basis of a combination of histologic findings. Changes may be apparent at all levels of the skin, but all need not be present in every case. The findings are summarized below:

1. Stratum corneum: hyperkeratosis with follicular plugging
2. Epithelium: thinning and flattening of the stratum malpighii, hydropic degeneration of basal cells, dyskeratosis and squamotization of basilar keratinocytes
3. Basement membrane: thickening and tortuosity
4. Stroma: a predominantly lymphocytic infiltrate arranged along the dermal–epidermal junction, around hair follicles and other appendages, and in an interstitial pattern; interstitial mucin deposition; edema, vasodilatation, slight extravasation of erythrocytes
5. Subcutaneous: slight extension of the inflammatory infiltrate may be present.

The stratum corneum is usually hyperkeratotic. Parakeratosis is not conspicuous, and it may be absent. Keratotic plugs are found mainly in dilated follicular openings (Fig. 10-1A), but they may occur in the openings of eccrine ducts as well. Follicular channels in the dermis may contain concentric layers of keratin instead of hairs.

The most significant histologic change in lupus erythematosus is hydropic degeneration of the basal layer, also referred to as liquefaction degeneration. This change is characterized by vacuolar spaces beneath and between basilar keratinocytes (Fig. 10-1C). In its absence, a histologic diagnosis of lupus erythematosus should be made with caution and only when other histologic findings greatly favor a diagnosis of LE. In addition to liquefaction degeneration, basilar keratinocytes may show individual cell necrosis (apoptosis) and acquire elongate contours like their superficial counterparts, rather than retaining their normal columnar appearance (squamotization). Frequently, the undulating rete ridge pattern is lost and is replaced by a linear array of squamotized keratinocytes (Fig. 10-2A and B).

The epidermal changes vary with the clinical character of lesions; there may be thinning and flattening of the stratum malpighii. A clinically verrucous lesion shows a hyperplastic, papillomatous epidermis with hyperkeratotic scale that simulates a hypertrophic solar keratosis or even a superficially invading squamous cell carcinoma.[13] In lesions of DLE that clinically do not show adherent scaling or keratotic plugging, the epidermis may show few or no changes and, in particular, no hydropic changes in the basal layer.[14]

The basement membrane, normally delicate and inconspicuous, appears thickened and tortuous in long-standing lesions (Fig. 10-1E). This change becomes more apparent with PAS stains (PAS positive, diastase-resistant), and may be found not only at the dermal-epidermal interface but along follicular-dermal junctions as well. These findings correlate with locations of immunoreactant deposits found on direct immunofluorescence testing of affected skin. By contrast, in areas of pronounced hydropic degeneration of the basal cells, the PAS-positive subepidermal basement zone may be fragmented and even absent.[15] Capillary walls may also show thickening, homogenization, and an increase in the intensity of the PAS reaction.

The inflammatory infiltrate in the dermis is usually lymphocytic admixed with plasma cells (Fig. 10-1B and D). Its distribution is a clue to the diagnosis of LE. In active lesions, the infiltrate can be found approximating the dermal-epidermal

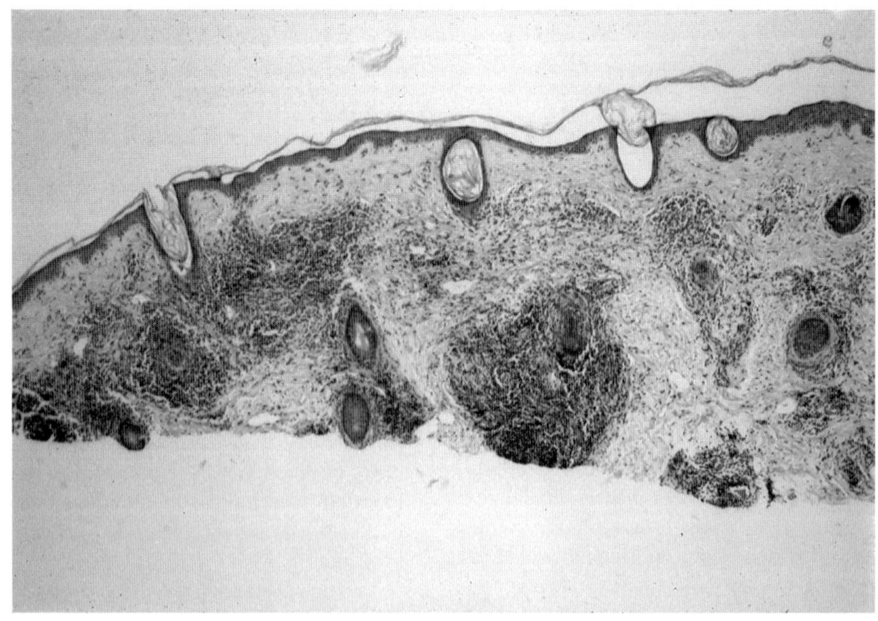

A

FIG. 10-1. Discoid lupus erythematosus
(**A**) The epidermis has lost its rete ridge pattern and shows follicular plugging.

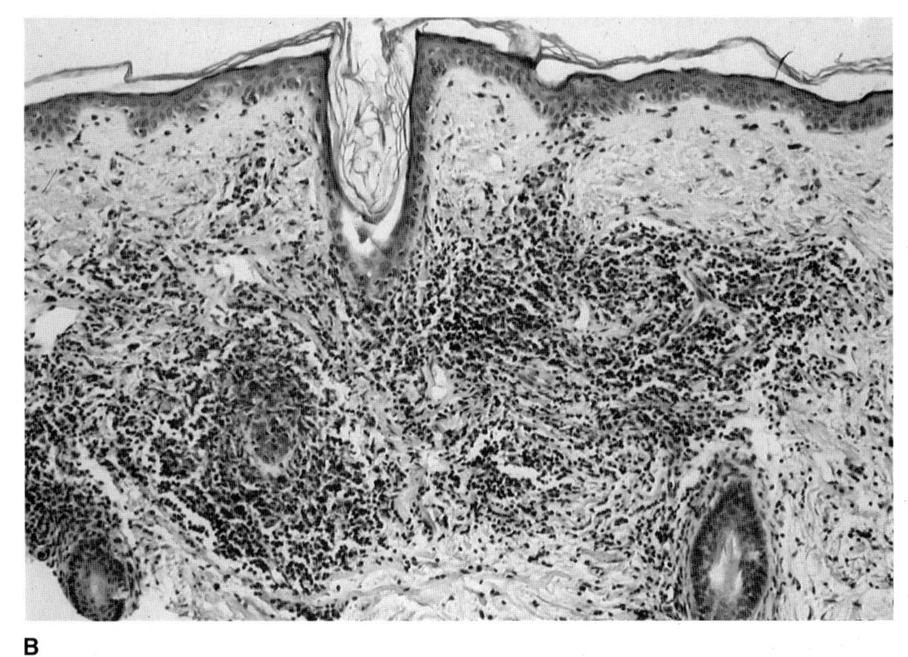

B

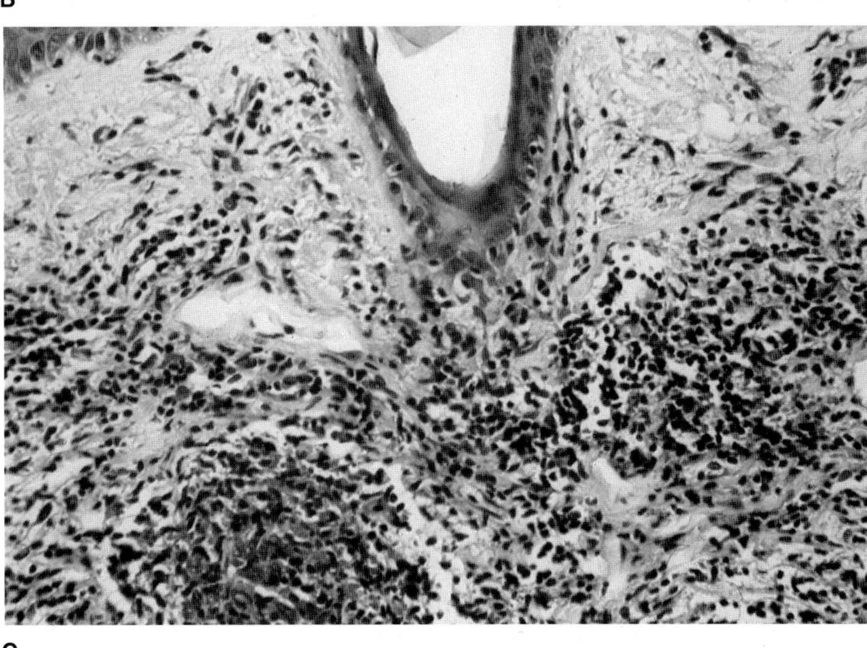

C

FIG. 10-1. *Continued*
(**B**) There is a brisk mononuclear inflammatory infiltrate near the dermal-epidermal junction, which obscures folliculo-dermal junctions. The infiltrate extends in an interstitial pattern into the adjacent stroma. (**C**) Vacuolization of basilar keratinocytes within a follicular ostium. Note the slightly basophilic stromal background indicative of mucin deposition. *(continued on next page)*

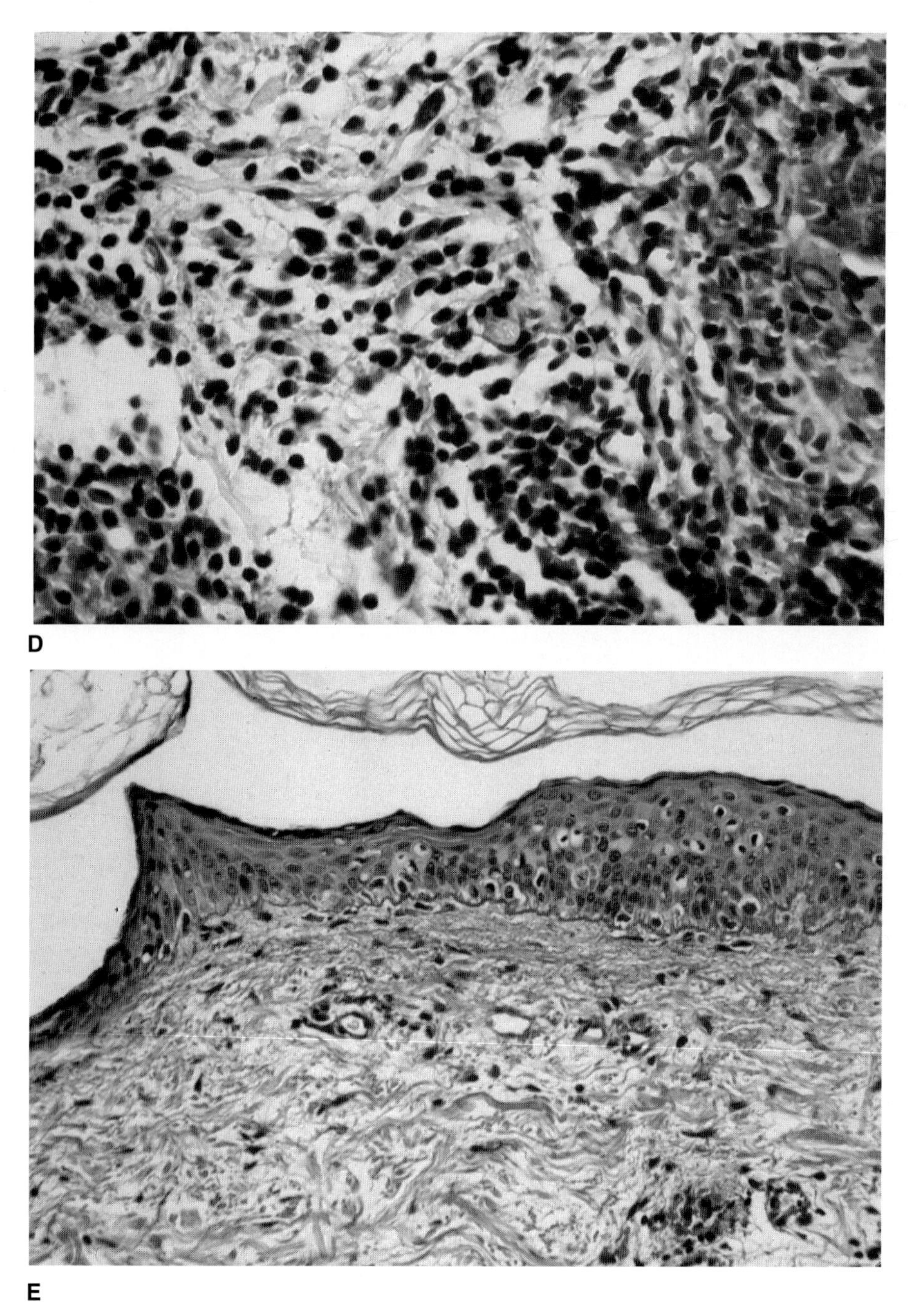

FIG. 10-1. ***Continued***
(**D**) The infiltrate is composed of predominantly lymphocytes admixed with occasional plasma cells. (**E**) PAS stain demonstrating irregularity and tortuosity of the basement membrane zone.

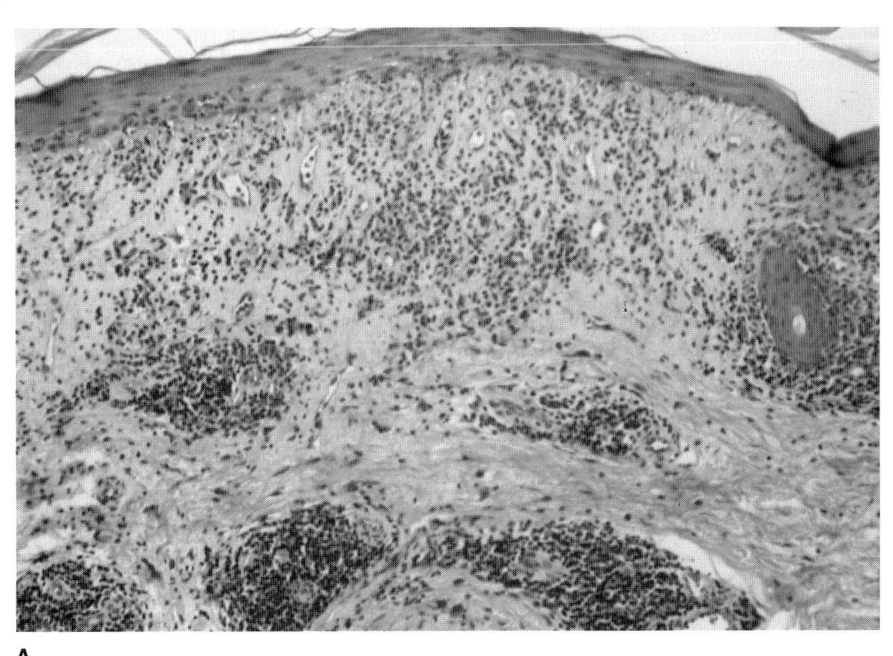

A

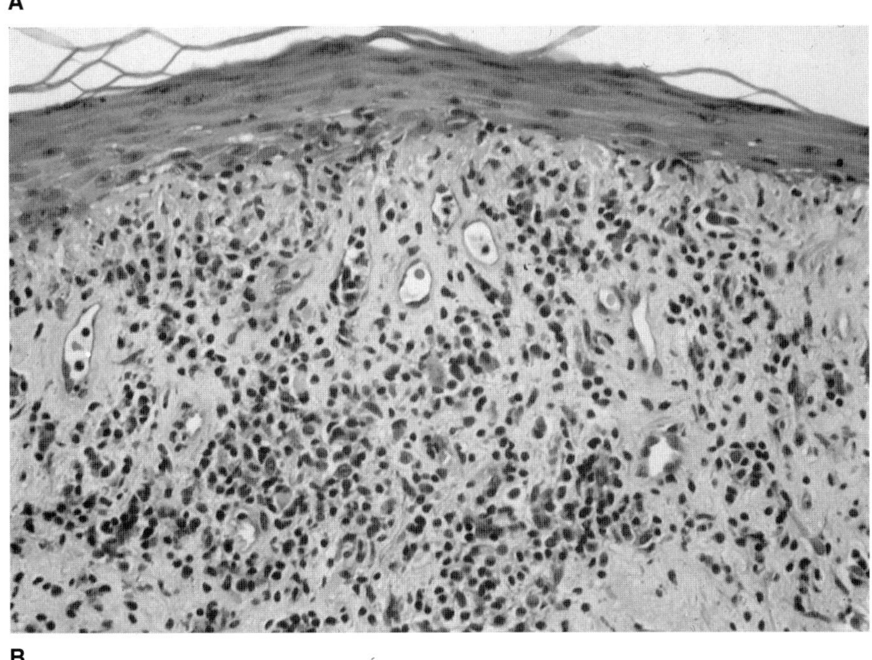

B

FIG. 10-2. Discoid lupus erythematosus
(**A**) Hyperkeratotic stratum corneum overlying an epidermis that has lost its rete ridge pattern. A superficial and deep mononuclear inflammatory infiltrate is also present. (**B**) Squamotization of basilar keratinocytes and formation of colloid bodies.

junction associated with hydropic degeneration. In hair-bearing areas, the infiltrate is located around hair follicles and the sebaceous glands (Fig. 10-1C). Frequently, one can observe hydropic changes in the basal layer of the hair follicles, which may be of diagnostic value in the absence of dermal-epidermal changes. By impinging on pilosebaceous units, the infiltrate causes their gradual atrophy and disappearance. A patchy inflammatory infiltrate also may be present in the upper dermis in an interstitial pattern and around eccrine coils. Occasionally, the infiltrate extends into the subcutaneous fat.

The dermis shows edema and often small foci of extravasated erythrocytes. In dark-skinned persons, melanin is frequently seen within melanophages in the upper dermis because hydropic degeneration in the basal cells causes these cells to lose their melanin (pigmentary incontinence). Vascular channels may be dilated and surrounded by edema. Obliterative and proliferative changes are absent. An increase in the ground substance, hyaluronic acid, is common in the middle and lower dermis and is best demonstrated with colloidal iron or alcian blue stains.[16] Fibrinoid deposits in the dermis are encountered only rarely in discoid lesions, and then only in early discoid lesions.

Colloid bodies, referred to in lichen planus as Civatte bodies, are apoptotic keratinocytes that present as round to ovoid, homogeneous, eosinophilic structures. They may be seen in lesions of DLE, but also in other inflammatory processes where there is damage to basilar keratinocytes (poikiloderma, lichen planus, fixed drug eruptions, lichenoid keratoses). They measure approximately 10 μm in diameter, and are present in the lower epidermis or in the papillary dermis. When located in the dermis, colloid bodies are PAS-positive and diastase-resistant and, on direct immunofluorescence staining, often are found to contain immunoglobulins (IgG, IgM, IgA), complement, and fibrin. This staining does not represent an immunologic phenomenon but is the result of passive absorption.

Differential Diagnosis. The epidermal changes seen in DLE must be differentiated from lichen planus since both diseases may show hydropic degeneration of the basal cell layer. In lichen planus, there is wedge-shaped hypergranulosis and triangular elongation of rete ridges described as "saw-toothing," which are not observed in DLE; in DLE, the epidermis frequently appears flattened. In addition, in lichen planus the infiltrate is superficial (not superficial and deep) and stromal mucin deposition is not seen. (For a discussion of the overlap syndrome lichen planus and lupus erythematosus, see Chap. 7.)

Patchy dermal lymphocytic infiltrates may be seen in five disorders that begin with the letter "L" (called the *five **Ls***). They are **L**upus erythematosus, lymphocytic **L**ymphoma, **L**ymphocytoma cutis, polymorphous **L**ight eruption of the plaque type, and **L**ymphocytic infiltration of the skin of Jessner.

In the absence of significant subepidermal vacuolization, LE must be differentiated from the other four diseases:

- In *lymphocytic lymphoma* atypical lymphocytes are present, are tightly packed, have an interstitial distribution ("Indian filing"), and do not surround pilosebaceous units as in LE.
- In *lymphocytoma cutis* (see Chap. 32), the infiltrate usually is heavier than in lupus erythematosus, may have an interstitial component, shows no tendency to arrange itself around pilosebaceous structures, and often contains an admixture of larger, paler lymphocytes arranged in lymphoid follicles, mimicking germinal center formation.
- In the plaque type of *polymorphous light eruption* there is often a prominent band of papillary dermal edema. The infiltrate is more intense in the superficial than deep dermis and is occasionally admixed with neutrophils. It does not have a folliculocentric arrangement, and is not usually accompanied by stromal mucin deposition (Chap. 12).
- In *Jessner's lymphocytic infiltration of the skin*, the dermal infiltrate may be indistinguishable from that seen in early, nonscarring or purely dermal lesions of lupus erythematosus. The presence of increased numbers of B lymphocytes in the infiltrate may help distinguish this from LE (see later text).[17]

Verrucous Lupus Erythematosus

An exaggerated proliferative epithelial response, which occurs in approximately 2% of patients with chronic cutaneous LE, manifests as verrucous-appearing lesions. Clinically, two types of lesions have been reported in this subset of LE. Lesions may simulate lichen planus or keratoacanthomas. They occur on the face (nose, chin, lips), arms, dorsal aspects of the hands, and occasionally the back. The presence of lesions typical of DLE elsewhere is a helpful clue to the diagnosis.

Histologically, the epidermis is papillomatous, hyperplastic, and surmounted by hyperkeratotic scale. Large numbers of dyskeratotic keratinocytes are usually noted in the lower portion of the epithelium, associated with a band-like mononuclear infiltrate along the dermal-epidermal junction. Older lesions display a thickened basement menbrane zone. A second pattern consists of a cup-shaped keratin-filled crater surrounded by an acanthotic epidermis with elongate rete ridges and a sparse mononuclear infiltrate. These changes, in the presence of a deep dermal perivascular, periappendageal and interstitial infiltrate and mucin deposition, suggest a diagnosis of hypertrophic or verrucous lupus erythematosus.[9]

Tumid Lupus Erythematosus

The dermal form of LE without surface/epithelial changes is known as tumid LE. Clinically, affected patients display indurated papules, plaques, and nodules without erythema, atrophy, or ulceration of the surface. Histologically, superficial and deep dermal perivascular and interstitial lymphocytic infiltrates associated with stromal mucin deposits are observed (Fig. 10-3A–C).[18]

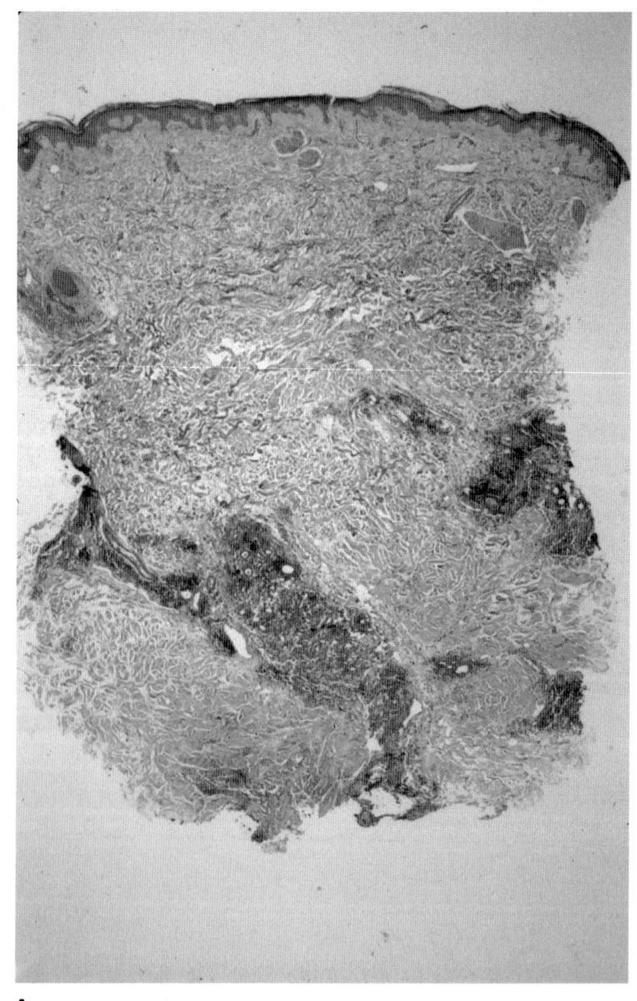

A

FIG. 10-3. Tumid lupus erythematosus
(**A**) There is a deep reticular dermal inflammatory infiltrate surrounding blood vessels and appendages.

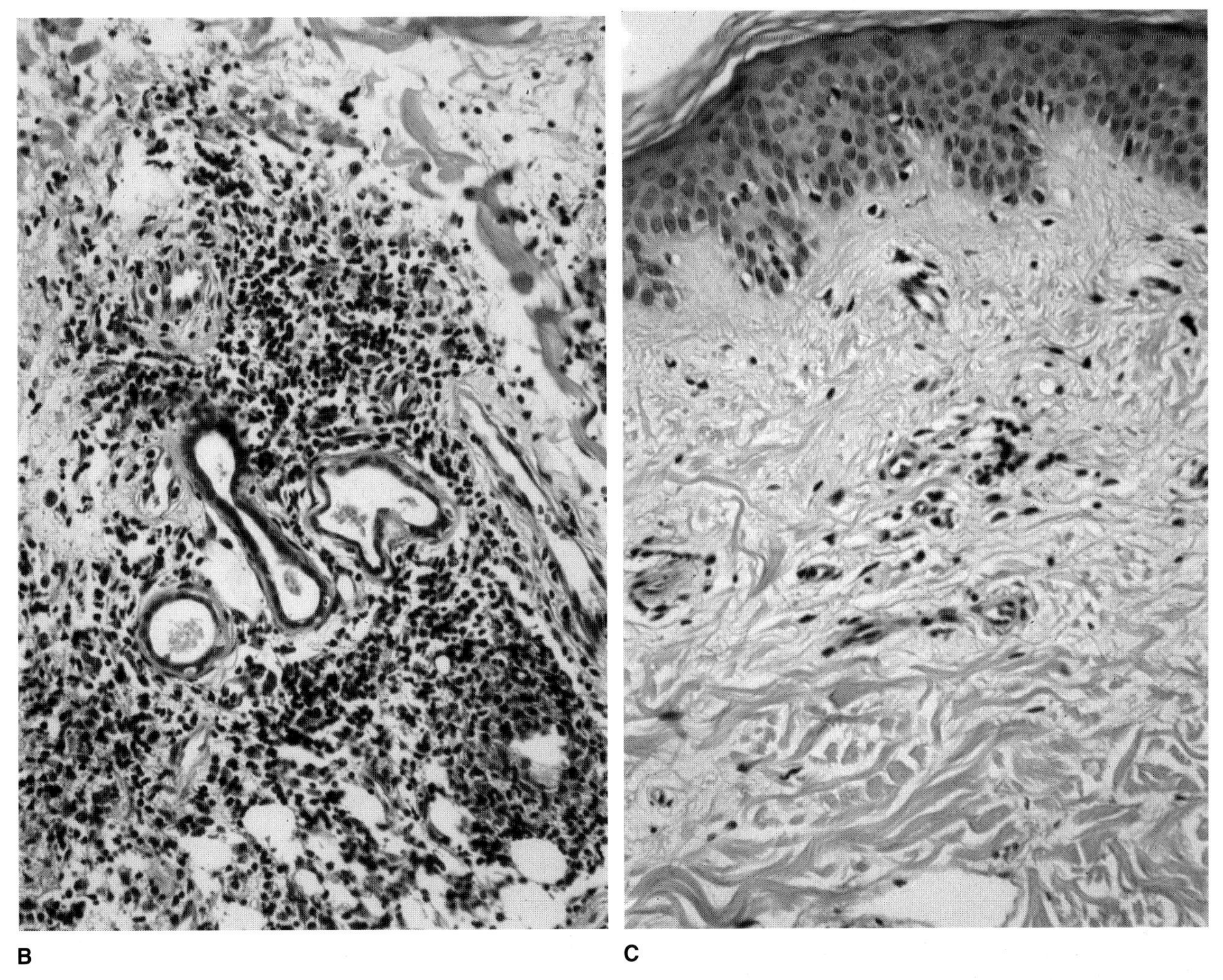

FIG. 10-3. ***Continued***
(**B**) A lymphocytic infiltrate admixed with plasma cells surrounds and separates eccrine ducts and adjacent collagen bundles. The faint bluish hue of the matrix is indicative of mucin deposition. (**C**) The dermal–epidermal junction of this specimen fails to show interface alterations.

Lupus Erythematosus Profundus/Panniculitis

Lupus erythematosus may show changes in adipose tissue associated with the chronic cutaneous or systemic forms. Two-thirds of affected patients have discoid LE lesions. Women are affected three to four times more often than men. Typically, multiple discrete, firm, deep nodules arise on the face, arms (particularly the deltoid area), chest, and/or buttocks. The legs and back may be affected as well. The overlying skin may be normal, erythematous, or atrophic. The panniculitis resolves, leaving depressed atrophic scars.

Subcutaneous adipose tissue may be involved with or without inflammation in the dermis or dermal-epidermal junction. Salient histological findings include a predominantly lobular lymphohistiocytic infiltrate often with plasma cells, occasionally forming germinal centers (Fig. 10-4A–D). Vascular changes include endothelial prominence, thrombosis, calcification, or perivascular fibrosis ("onion-skin" appearance). Fat necrosis with fibrin deposition often eventuates in hyalinization of adipose lobules (see Fig. 10-4C). Stromal mucin deposition may be prominent in well-established lesions.

Subacute Cutaneous Lupus Erythematosus

Subactue cutaneous lupus erythematosus (SCLE) represents about 9% of all cases of lupus erythematosus. It is characterized by extensive erythematous, symmetric nonscarring and nonatrophic lesions that arise abruptly on the upper trunk, extensor surfaces of the arms, and dorsa of the hands and fingers. This eruption has two clinical variants: (1) papulosquamous lesions and (2) annular to polycyclic lesions. Frequently both types of lesions are seen. In some instances, vesicular and discoid lesions with scarring may coexist.

Patients with SCLE may have mild systemic involvement, particularly arthralgias. Approximately 50% fulfill criteria for SLE. Severe SLE, with renal or cerebrovascular disease, develops in only 10% of SCLE.[19] Serologic studies show 70% of

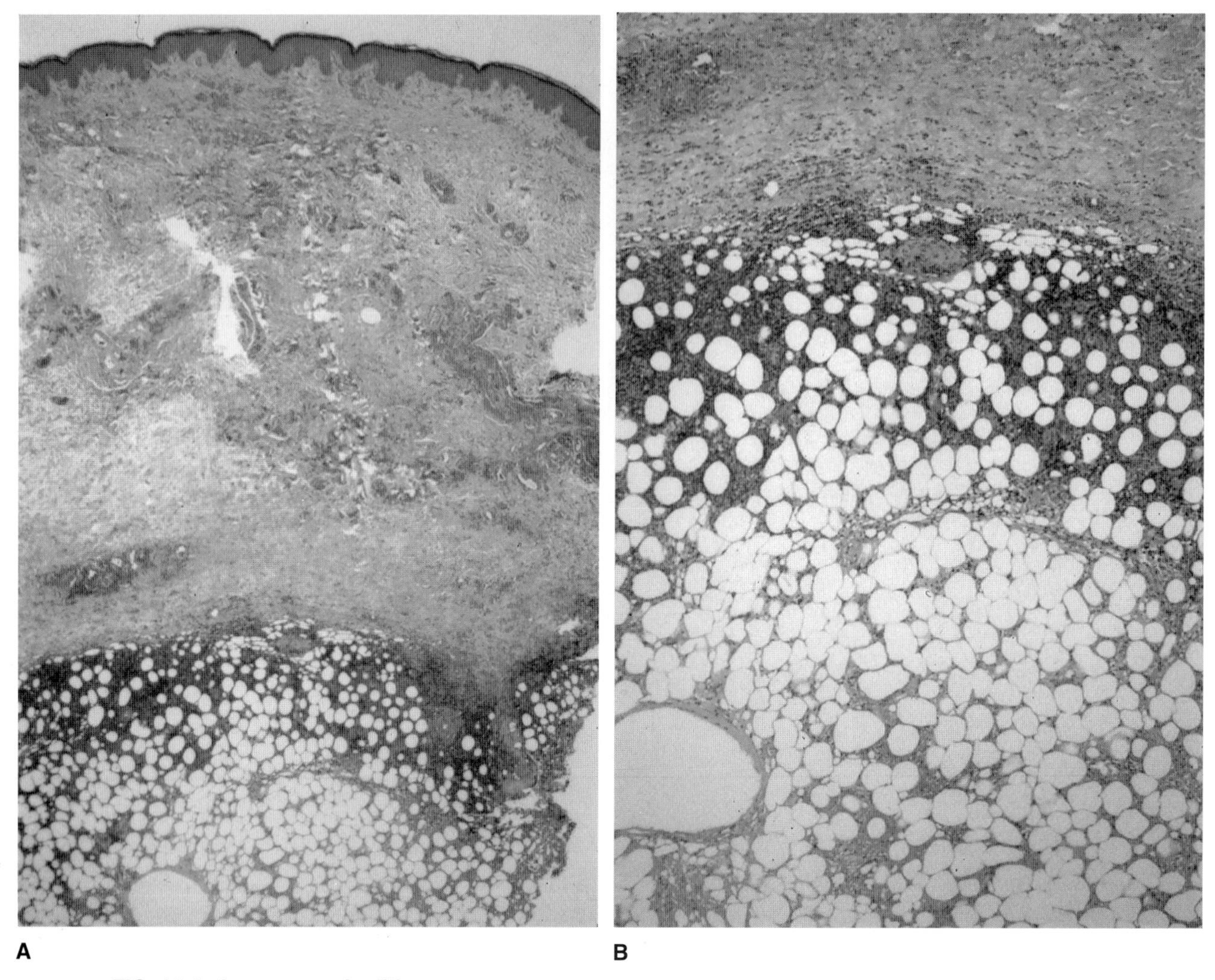

A B

FIG. 10-4. Lupus panniculitis
(**A**) An intense inflammatory infiltrate is present at the dermal-subcutaneous interface and extends into adipose tissue in an interstitial pattern. (**B**) The inflammatory infiltrate outlines individual adipocytes, giving it a lace-like pattern.

affected patients to have the anti-Ro (SS-A) antibody. Patients with SCLE often bear the HLA-DR2 and HLA-DR3 phenotype. SCLE may occur asynchronously with other connective tissue diseases such as Sjögren's syndrome and morphea.

Histopathology. See Histopathology section of Neonatal Lupus Erythematosus.

Neonatal Lupus Erythematosus

Neonatal lupus erythematosus has clinical and histologic skin changes and serologic findings similar to SCLE. Children of mothers with active SLE may develop LE-like symptoms in the neonatal period related to passage of maternal IgG anti-nuclear antibodies (particularly anti-Ro/SSA, anti-La/SSB, or anti-U1RNP autoantibodies) through the placenta. Anti-Ro/SSA are the predominant autoantibodies and are found in approximately 95% of cases. This may result in a transient syndrome characterized by widespread polycyclic, annular, usually nonscarring lesions. There is associated photosensitivity, transient thrombocytopenia, mild hemolytic anemia, leukopenia, and congenital heart block. These changes have their onset at birth to 2 months and usually resolve in the first 6 months of life with decreasing levels of maternal antibodies. The heart block occurs in approximately 50% of affected infants, usually without associated skin lesions, and may be fatal. Of interest, individuals affected with transient neonatal LE may develop SLE as young adults.[20]

Histopathology. Histologic changes in SCLE (and neonatal LE) differ in degree from those in the discoid lesions, and are most intense at the dermal-epidermal interface. They consist of:

1. hydropic degeneration of the basilar epithelial layer, sometimes severe enough to form clefts and subepidermal vesicles
2. colloid bodies in the lower epidermis and papillary dermis (common)
3. edema of the dermis which is more pronounced than in discoid lesions
4. focal extravasation of erythrocytes and dermal fibrinoid deposits (common)
5. less prominent hyperkeratosis and inflammatory infiltrate than in discoid lesions[21]

In comparison with chronic, particularly discoid LE, it is not

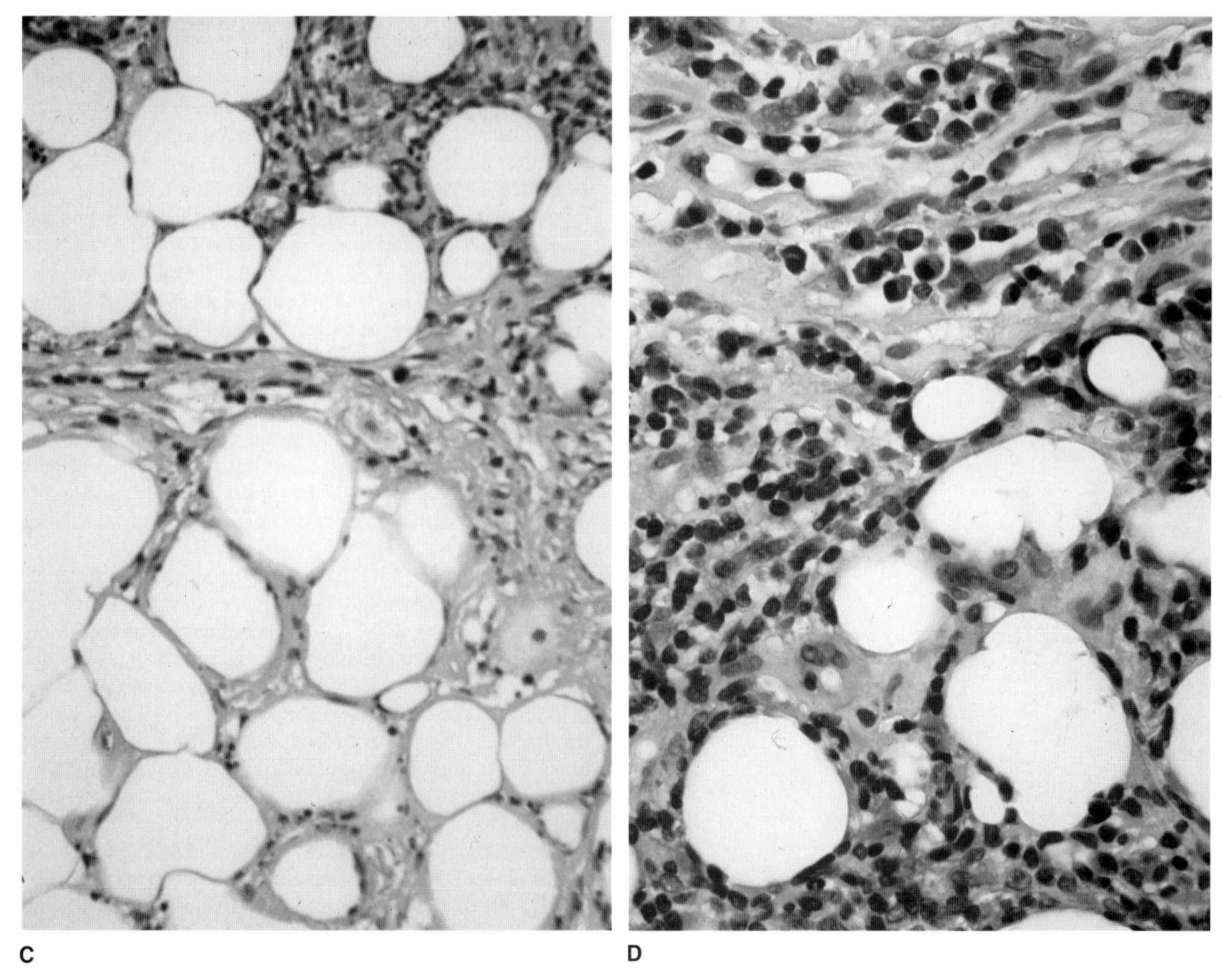

FIG. 10-4. ***Continued***
(**C**) Foam cells indicate adipocyte injury. Note the hyalinized-appearing matrix between adipocytes.
(**D**) A lymphoplasmacytic inflammatory infiltrate splays collagen bundles and adipocytes.

always possible to correctly categorize lesions based on histology alone since there is overlap. Pilosebaceous atrophy is helpful as a discriminating feature and correlates with DLE rather than SCLE.

Systemic Lupus Erythematosus

In SLE the cutaneous manifestations usually appear less suddenly than in SCLE and are less pronounced so that the signs and symptoms of systemic involvement usually overshadow the often subtle form of skin involvement. Usually systemic manifestations, especially joint manifestations, precede the cutaneous lesions. Only approximately 20% of SLE patients demonstrate prominent cutaneous features at the onset of their disease,[21] but approximately 80% will exhibit cutaneous lesions in the course of their disease.[22]

The cutaneous manifestations commonly consist of malar erythema, photosensitivity, palmar erythema, periungual telangiectases, diffuse hair loss as a result of telogen effluvium, and urticarial vasculitis and/or bullous lesions. The erythematous lesions of SLE consist of erythematous, slightly edematous patches without significant scaling and without atrophy. As a rule, the patches are not sharply demarcated. The most common site of involvement is the malar region, but any area of the skin may be involved, particularly the palms and fingers. Occasionally, lesions show a petechial, vesicular, or ulcerative component. Rarely, in the late stage, some of the lesions may assume the appearance of poikiloderma atrophicans vasculare.

Well-defined "discoid" lesions with atrophic scarring, as seen typically in DLE, occur in about 15% of the patients with SLE. They may precede all other clinical manifestations of SLE. A relatively benign course characterizes SLE in most patients with preceding DLE[23]; however, many patients usually have had persistent multiple abnormal laboratory findings from the beginning. This is in contrast to cases of simple DLE, in which most abnormal laboratory findings, if present at all, are transient.

Two variants of SLE, *SLE with genetic deficiency of complement components* and *bullous LE*, bear mention. In the former, the onset of SLE occurs in early childhood and often affects several siblings because of the autosomal recessive mode of transmission.[24] Deficiencies of C2 and C4 result in strikingly similar clinical pictures of extensive lesions similar to DLE with marked scaling, atrophy, and scarring associated with sensitivity to sunlight. In addition, there can be central nervous system involvement and glomerulonephritis, which may be fatal.[25]

In *bullous SLE* subepidermal blisters may arise in previously involved or uninvolved areas. They may form large hemorrhage bullae to herpetiform vesicles, arise suddenly, and show clinical resemblance to lesions of bullous pemphigoid or dermatitis herpetiformis.

The coexistence of SLE and systemic scleroderma or dermatomyositis has been repeatedly described. It is known as overlap syndrome and refers to the coexistence of two related but separate diseases. This is in contrast to *mixed connective tissue disease*, which has become recognized as a disease entity.

For a discussion of the induction of SLE by various drugs, see Drug–Induced Lupus Erythematosus, Chap. 15.

Histopathology. Early lesions of SLE of the erythematous, edematous type may show only slight and nonspecific changes. In well-developed lesions, the histologic changes correspond to those described for subacute cutaneous LE (Fig. 10-5A and B): hydropic degeneration of the basal cell layer occurs in association with edema of the upper dermis and extravasation of erythrocytes.

Fibrinoid deposits in the connective tissue of the skin are often seen in erythematous, edematous lesions, especially in patients with SLE. Such fibrinoid deposits consist of precipitation of fibrin in the ground substance. They appear as granular, strongly eosinophilic, PAS-positive diastase-resistant deposits between collagen bundles, in the walls of dermal vessels, in the papillary dermis or beneath the epidermis in the basement membrane zone. Fibrinoid deposits are not specific for LE. They are seen in association with vascular injury, particularly in leukocytoclastic vasculitis.

The subcutaneous fat is often involved in SLE. Changes similar to those in lupus profundus may be seen, but are usually milder: there may be focal mucin deposition associated with a predominantly lymphocytic infiltrate. Adiopocytes may be separated by edema and fibrinoid deposits. These histologic changes in the subcutaneous fat produce no clinically apparent lesions.

Occasionally, palpable purpuric lesions in SLE patients show

A

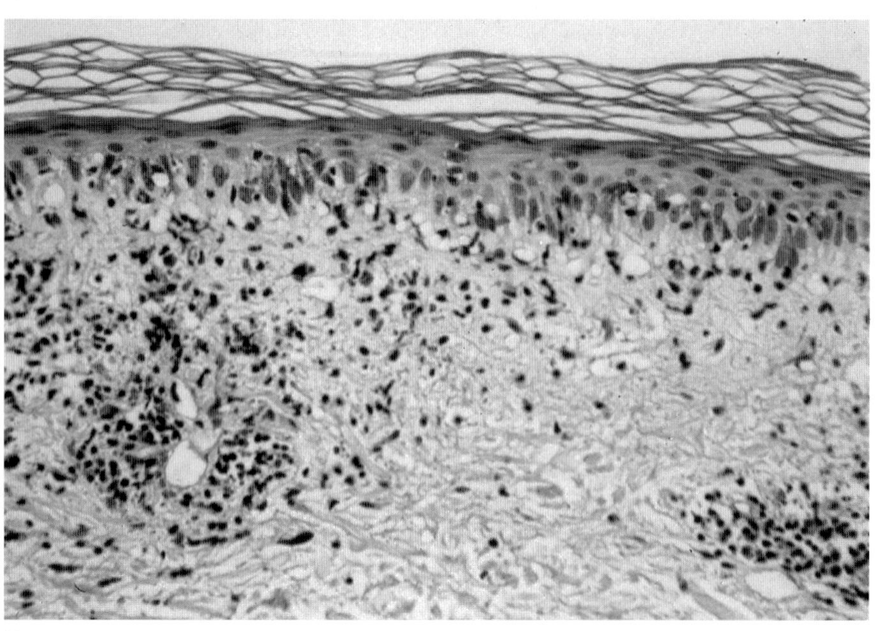

B

FIG. 10-5. Subacute lupus erythematosus
(**A**) A moderate mononuclear inflammatory infiltrate in the upper dermis associated with pronounced dermal edema. (**B**) There is continuous subepidermal vacuolization, pigment incontinence, and focal hemorrhage.

a leukocytoclastic vasculitis histologically indistinguishable from leukocytoclastic vasculitis of other causes: there is endothelial cell swelling, a neutrophilic inflammatory infiltrate, nuclear dust formation, perivenular fibrin deposition, and stromal hemorrhage. Urticaria-like lesions may occur, and show either a leukocytoclastic vasculitis or a perivascular mononuclear infiltrate not diagnostic of lupus erythematosus.[26] Also, white atrophic lesions may occur in SLE that both clinically and histologically resemble those of malignant atrophic papulosis of Degos.[27]

Bullous SLE shows two histologic inflammatory patterns: one is neutrophilic and the other mononuclear. The neutrophilic type simulates dermatitis herpetiformis or linear IgA bullous disease with the formation of papillary microabscesses (Fig. 10-6A–C).[28] Nuclear dust is seen in the papillary microabscesses and in the upper dermis around and within the walls of blood vessels. Direct immunoelectron microscopic studies have localized immunoreactant deposits to beneath the lamina densa, and consist of IgG with or without IgM, and often IgA in a linear or granular pattern. Some patients may also have circulating anti-basement zone antibodies and antibodies directed against type VII collagen. The latter antibodies are similar but not identical to those in epidermolysis bullosa acquisita.[29]

The subepidermal blister associated with a mononuclear inflammatory infiltrate arises in long-standing lesions of cutaneous lupus erythematosus (Fig. 10-7A–C). It likely corresponds to an altered dermal-epidermal interface resulting from inflammation and immunocomplex deposition. This type of change is a part of the spectrum of LE rather than a distinct entity.

Systemic Lesions. Although the etiology of SLE is obscure, it is evident that much of the tissue damage results from deposition of antibody-antigen complexes in affected organ systems.

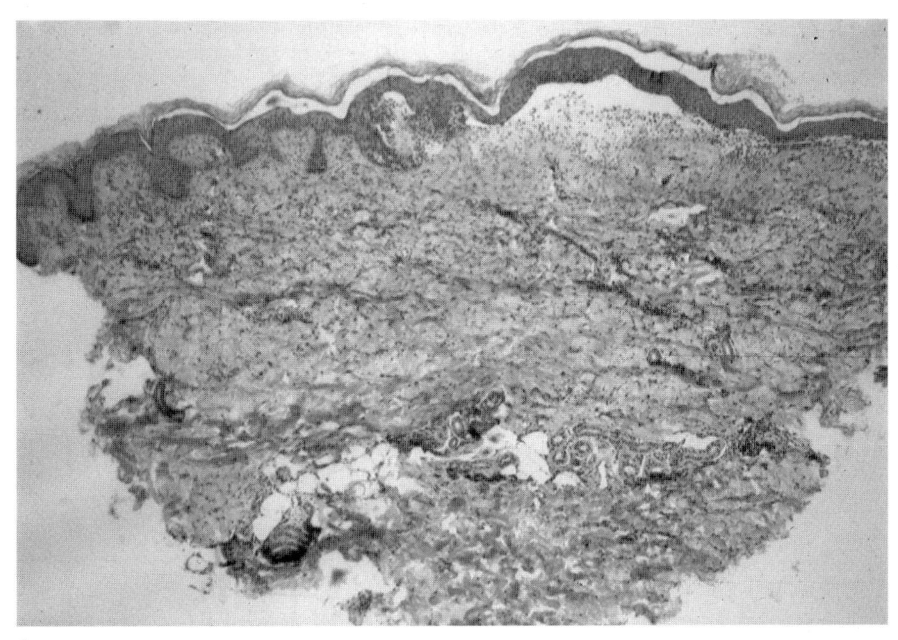

A

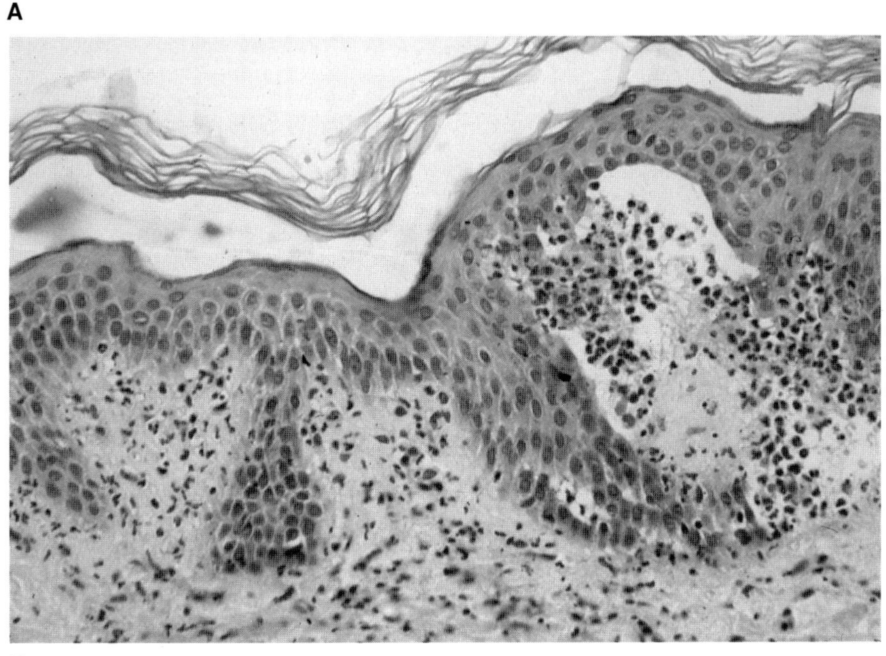

B

FIG. 10-6. Bullous lupus erythematosus, neutrophilic
(**A**) There are several broad-based subepidermal blisters associated with marked papillary dermal edema. (**B**) The papillary dermal abscesses simulate findings of dermatitis herpetiformis; however, neutrophils also invade the epidermis. *(continued on next page)*

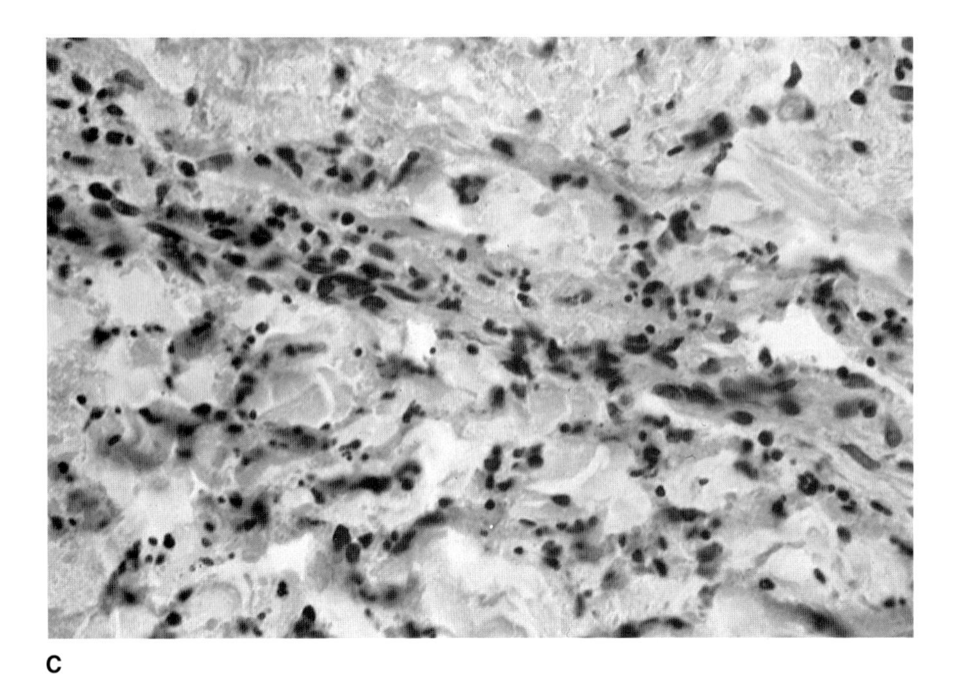

C

FIG. 10-6. ***Continued***
(**C**) Interstitial aggregates of neutrophils in the dermis associated with nuclear dust.

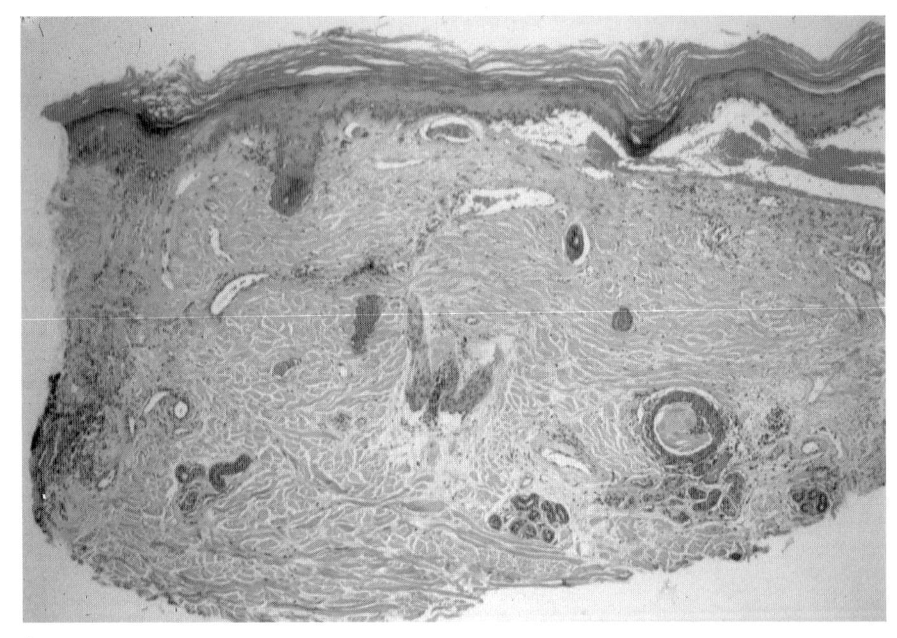

A

FIG. 10-7. Bullous lupus erythematosus, mononuclear
(**A**) A broad subepidermal cleft is present beneath an epidermis that has lost its rete ridge pattern and is surmounted by hyperkeratotic scale. The stroma contains perivascular and periappendageal inflammatory infiltrates.

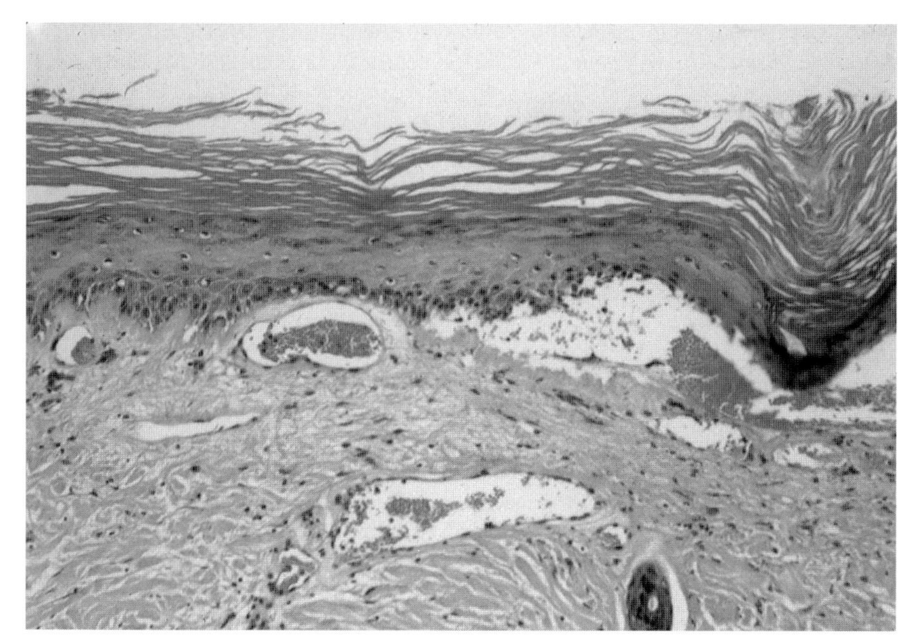

B

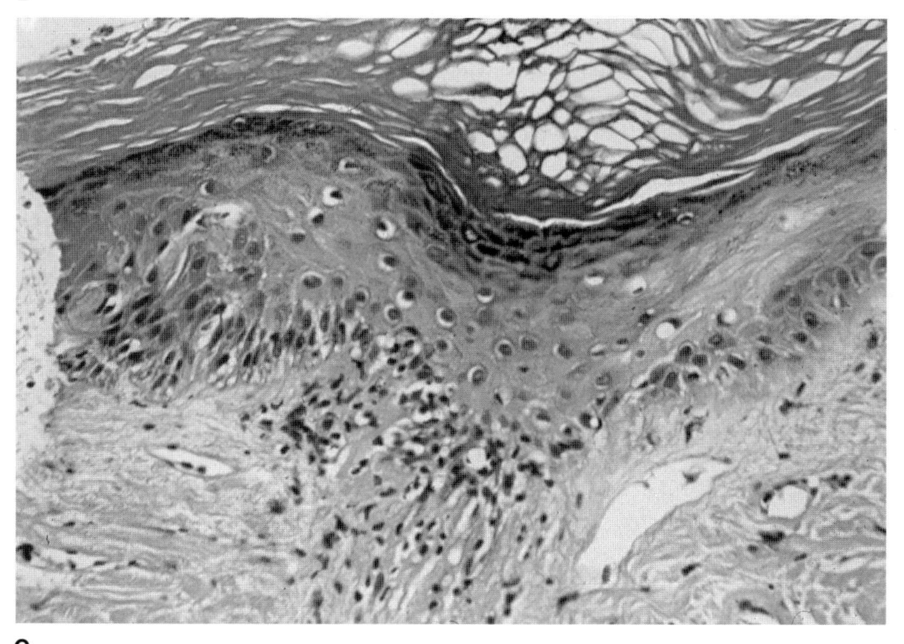

C

FIG. 10-7. *Continued*
(**B**) Along one shoulder the blister cavity contains extravasated erythrocytes. The contralateral edge shows a thickened eosinophilic basement membrane zone. (**C**) Interface alterations are noted along intact dermal-epidermal junction: a mononuclear inflammatory infiltrate tags basilar kerat-inocytes, and is associated with subepidermal vacuolization and a thickened basement membrane.

These immune complexes are demonstrable in renal glomeruli, blood vessels, skin, and the choroid plexus of the brain.

Arthritis occurs most often; however, renal changes are the most important because they are the most common cause of death in SLE. Percutaneous renal biopsy allows determination of the type and degree of histologic changes in the kidneys, which are of prognostic significance regardless of the absence or severity of clinical renal disease.[30] As in skin, immunoglobulin and complement (immunoreactant) deposits are detectable with immunofluorescence and electron microscopic studies.

Four subsets of renal disease have been categorized by the World Health Organization and are summarized later. *Mesangial* immunoglobulin and complement deposits are most frequently seen in SLE. If this process remains stable, there may be no clinical evidence of renal disease or mild proteinuria and/or hematuria. *Focal proliferative glomerulonephritis* (affecting less than 50% of glomerular tufts) shows mesangial changes and segmental deposits of immunoreactants in subendothelial and subepithelial areas and in the basement membranes. This process is associated with proteinuria and often hematuria. *Diffuse proliferative glomerulonephritis* (affecting greater than 50% of glomeruli) shows changes similar to, but more extensive than, those in focal glomerulonephritis. Extensive immunoreactant endothelial and intramembranous deposits correspond to wire loops. Proteinuria and hematuria are common in affected patients; nephrotic syndrome eventually occurs in nearly all patients. If there is disease progression, death may occur within two years from uremia or active SLE. *Membranous glomerulonephritis* is present when there is fairly uniform thickening of the glomerular basement membrane associated with finely granular immunoreactant deposits along the basement membrane in subendothelial locations. This change is nearly always associated with proteinuria and often the nephrotic syndrome. In contrast with diffuse proliferative glomerulonephritis, renal insufficiency is often slowly progressive.

Serositis involving the pleura, epicardium, and peritoneum may show submucosal mononuclear inflammatory infiltrates associated with fibrinoid deposits. In the spleen, periarterial fibrosis around the follicular arteries is common and is highly characteristic of SLE. Thick, concentrically layered rings of sclerotic collagen fibers surround the arteries.

The *verrucous endocarditis of SLE*, the so-called Libman-Sacks endocarditis, occurs mainly on the mitral and tricuspid valves. In the subendothelial connective tissue there are collections of necrotic debris, fibrinoid material, and inflammatory cells forming small vegetations on the valve leaflets.[31]

The *antiphospholipid syndrome* occurs in patients with SLE and other autoimmune diseases who develop immunoglobulins that can prolong phospholipid-dependent coagulation tests. These immunoglobulins occur in association with SLE and other autoimmune diseases, but are found unassociated with them as well. One of these is a lupus anticoagulant and occurs in about 10% of SLE patients. Affected patients are at greater risk for thromboembolic disease including deep venous thrombosis, pulmonary emboli, and other large vessel thrombosis. Other associated findings are recurrent fetal wastage, renal vascular thrombosis, thrombosis of dermal vessels (Fig. 10-8), and thrombocytopenia. Anticardiolipin antibody, a second type of antiphospholipid antibody, occurs five times more often than lupus anticoagulant antibody. It is associated with recurrent arterial and venous thrombosis, valvular abnormalities, cerebrovascular thromboses, and essential hypertension (Sneddon's syndrome).[32] Other cutaneous findings include livedo reticularis, necrotizing purpura, disseminated intravascular coagulation, and stasis ulcers of the ankles.[33]

Pathogenesis and Laboratory Findings. The etiology of lupus erythematosus is considered to be multifactorial at this time and is summarized in Table 10-1. The serologic hallmark of lupus erythematosus is the production of autoantibodies. There is a wide variety of antibodies against different cellular targets. The initial screening test for antinuclear antibodies (ANAs) is indirect immunofluorescence, which provides limited but clinically useful information. Many other assays are available for more specific characterization of ANAs and include immunodiffusion, enzyme-linked immunosorbent assays (ELISA), immunoprecipitation, and immunoblots.

Indirect immunofluorescence detects nuclear, homogenous, rim, speckled, and nucleolar patterns (Table 10-2). The fluorescence ANA test can be regarded as a specific marker for SLE in a rim pattern with a titer of 1:160 or higher and is often indicative of the presence of anti-native or double-stranded DNA antibodies. At a titer of 1:20, about 20% of patients with DLE, most patients with systemic scleroderma, and as many as 5% of normal persons may have a positive reaction. The presence of anti-Sm is indicative of associated lupus nephritis. Antibodies against single-stranded DNA are nonspecific and are found in a variety of diseases. Anti-nRNP antibodies are of diagnostic significance only at high titers because they then indicate mixed connective tissue disease. ANA-negative sera should be examined for the presence of anti-Ro/SSA and La/SSB antibodies, characteristic of subacute and neonatal LE and SLE with genetic deficiency of complement components.

The LE cell test is of historical significance. It consisted of incubating patients' serum with normal white blood cells. In the presence of antibody to whole nucleoprotein (LE factor) damage to nuclei of leukocytes incited phagocytosis of affected nu-

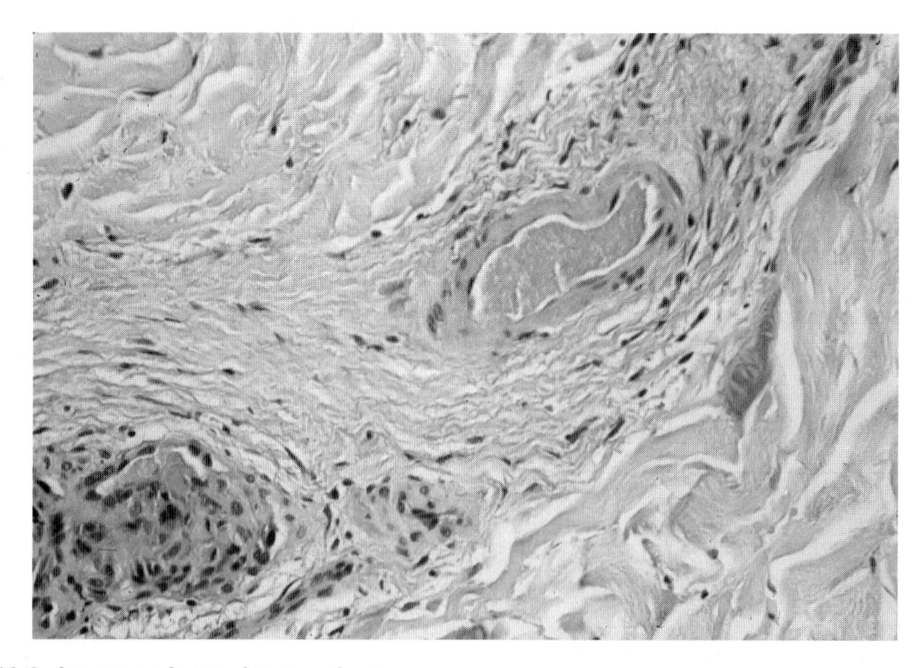

FIG. 10-8. Lupus anticoagulant syndrome
High magnification of pale eosinophilic intravascular thrombi. There is a negligible inflammatory host response.

TABLE 10-1. *Pathogenesis of lupus erythematosus*

Genetic	HLA-DR2	Mothers with newborns with neonatal LE Patients positive for anti–Ro/SSA Older patients with SLE
	HLA-DR3	Younger SLE patients with anti–native DNA antibodies
	HLA-B8 HLA-DR3 HLA-DQ23 HLA-DRw52	Increased frequency in: Mothers with newborns with neonatal LE Females with primary Sjögren's syndrome Female patients with Sjögren's syndrome/LE
Environmental precipitants	Drugs Ultraviolet light Possibly diet	Procainamide, hydralazine
Hormonal influences	Predisposition of females in childbearing years	
Autoimmunity	Every aspect of immune system affected:	
	B cells	Abnormal B lymphocyte maturation and activation Hypergammaglobulinemia
	T cells	Decreased peripheral T lymphocytes T-cell hyperactivity Increased % of CD29+ (memory helper) T cells Preferential loss of CD4, CD45R+ (suppressor inducer) cells in active LE Defective T suppressor function
	Natural killer cell	Normal number of NK cells but decreased NK-cell activity (deficient in active cytotoxicity)
	Antilymphocyte antibody	Lymphocytotoxic antibodies in sera of 80% of SLE patients
	Antinuclear antibodies	Nuclear membrane targets Chromatin targets Ribonucleoprotein targets

clei by unaffected white blood cells. If a smear of the incubated white blood cells is made and stained with Wright's stain, the phagocytized nuclear material may be observed within some of the neutrophils as a large, round, amorphous, smoky, basophilic body of such a large size that it presses the nucleus of the neutrophil against the cell membrane. This represents the LE cell.

Direct immunofluorescence studies detect immunoreactant deposits in affected tissues, particularly the skin and kidneys. A skin biopsy (3 to 4 mm punch) is submitted in saline-impregnated gauze or phosphate-buffered saline, snap frozen, sectioned, and incubated with fluorescein-conjugated antisera to IgA, IgM, IgG, and the third component of complement (C3). In

TABLE 10-2. *Antinuclear antibodies*

Appearance	Pattern	Target site	Associated antibodies	Associated disorder
	Homogenous	Chromatin	Anti-histone Anti-DNA	SLE False + SLE Drug-induced LE
	Rim	Chromatin Nuclear membrane	Anti-DNA Anti-laminin (rare)	SLE
	Fine speckled	Nuclear RNP	Anti-Sm Anti-Ro/SSA Anti-La/SSB Anti-U1RNP	SLE, often with nephritis SLE, Sjögren's syndrome SLE, mixed CTD
		Chromatin	Anti-Ku Anti-topoisomerase 1 (SCL-70)	SLE, scleroderma, myositis Scleroderma
	Discrete speckled	Chromatin	Anti-centromere	CREST
	Nucleolar	Nucleolar RNP Nucleolar components	Anti-U3RNP Anti-RNA polymerase I Anti-Pm-SCl	Scleroderma

TABLE 10-3. *Direct immunofluorescence in lupus erythematosus*

		Result	
Site		Discoid LE	Systemic LE
Sun exposed (e.g., dorsal forearm)	Involved	Positive in >90% of untreated lesions	Positive in 80%–90% of untreated lesions
Sun exposed (e.g., volar forearm)	Uninvolved	Almost always negative	Positive in >80% of untreated SLE
Non sun exposed (e.g., buttock)	Uninvolved	Negative	With active LE: positive in >91% With inactive SLE: positive in 33% Positive result may be indicative of renal involvement

a positive test there is continuous granular deposition of usually two or more immunoreactants (in a band) along the dermal-epidermal junction. Variables that affect test results are the site of the biopsy (sun-exposed vs. sun-protected), duration of the lesion (acute, subacute, chronic), and preceding therapy. The frequency and implications of positive results in DLE and SLE are summarized in Table 10-3.[34,35,36]

Cautious sampling and interpretation of findings are necessary to avoid false-positive and false-negative results. The presence of only one type of immunoreactant, particularly in an intermittent distribution, may be seen in chronically sun-exposed skin or with underlying disorders such as rosacea. False-negative results are often found in acute or subacute lesions and treated lesions. Optimally, an established lesion (present for three months or longer) which has not been treated is submitted for study.[37]

Electron microscopic examination of the cutaneous lesions of both DLE and SLE shows marked changes in the basal cells and the lamina densa. The basal cells show vacuolization of their cytoplasm, which may progress to necrosis and disintegration of the cytoplasm. The colloid or Civatte bodies that may be seen in the epidermis and in the dermis are similar in appearance on electron microscopy to those observed in lichen planus. They are finely filamentous to amorphous granular in appearance and do not possess a delimiting membrane.

The antigen-antibody complexes have been localized with immunoelectron microscopy to beneath the lamina densa. They are seen as irregular aggregates in the uppermost portion of the dermis in the ground substance and occasionally on collagen fibrils. In some instances, small amounts of reaction product are seen also within the lamina densa and the lamina lucida. Localization of immune complexes in lupus erythematosus thus differs from their localization in bullous pemphigoid, in which they are situated entirely within the lamina lucida near the basal cells (see Chap. 9). In bullous SLE, direct immunoelectron microscopy of perilesional skin also shows the reaction product in a continuous band-like distribution below the lamina densa and a separation plane in the dermis below this band, indicating early bulla formation.[38]

The presence of intracytoplasmic tubuloreticular structures has been reported in the cutaneous and renal lesions of SLE and in lesions of DLE. They bear a superficial resemblance to tubuloreticular structures and internal nucleoproteins of paramyxovirus. They are a nonspecific result of cell injury related to increased interferon alpha levels in lupus patients and are not specific for lupus erythematosus.[39]

Jessner's Lymphocytic Infiltration of the Skin

Jessner's lymphocytic infiltration of the skin, first described in 1953,[40] is not a well-understood entity. It is characterized by asymptomatic papules or well-demarcated, slightly infiltrated red plaques, which may develop central clearing. In contrast to lesions of chronic lupus erythematosus, the surface shows no follicular plugging or atrophy. Lesions arise most often on the face, but may also involve the neck and upper trunk.[41] Although this disorder has been reported to occur in childhood,[42] affected patients are usually middle-aged men and women.

Variable numbers of lesions (one to many) often persist for several months or several years. They may disappear without sequelae, or recur at previously involved sites or elsewhere. The eruption may be precipitated or aggravated by sunlight. Antimalarial drugs and/or corticosteroids are useful in controlling this disorder.

Histopathology. The epidermis may be normal but often appears slightly flattened. In the dermis, there are moderately dense perivascular and diffuse infiltrates composed of small, mature lymphocytes admixed with occasional histiocytes and plasma cells (Fig. 10-9A–C). The infiltrate may extend around folliculo-sebaceous units and into subcutaneous adipose tissue.

The histologic differential diagnosis of lymphocytic infiltration of the skin includes the other four of the five "L's": lupus erythematosus, polymorphous light eruption, lymphocytoma cutis, and lymphoma. Lupus erythematosus is compared with lymphocytic infiltrate of the skin in Table 10-4. The latter entity is limited to sun-exposed skin and lacks the hyperkertosis, atrophy, interface changes, and direct immunofluorescence findings noted in lupus. Therefore, lupus should be excluded with serologic and direct immunofluorescence studies.

Approximately 10% of cases of lupus that lack interface alterations and that show negative direct immunofluorescence studies may initially be grouped with lymphocytic infiltration of the skin. Polymorphous light eruptions usually show prominent papillary dermal edema; however, plaque-type polymorphous light eruption may histologically overlap with lymphocytic infiltration of the skin. Clinical features may sometimes separate these two entities.

Immunohistochemical cell marker studies indicate that the predominant component of lymphocytic infiltration of the skin is a mature T lymphocyte. The relative sparsity of B lymphocytes may assist in separation of this entity from lymphocytoma

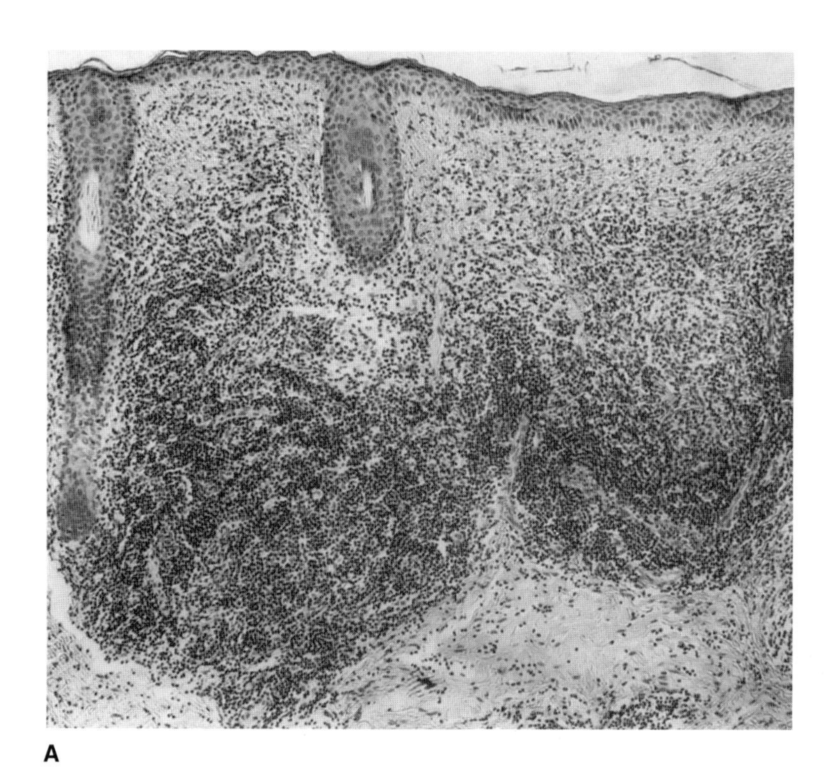

A

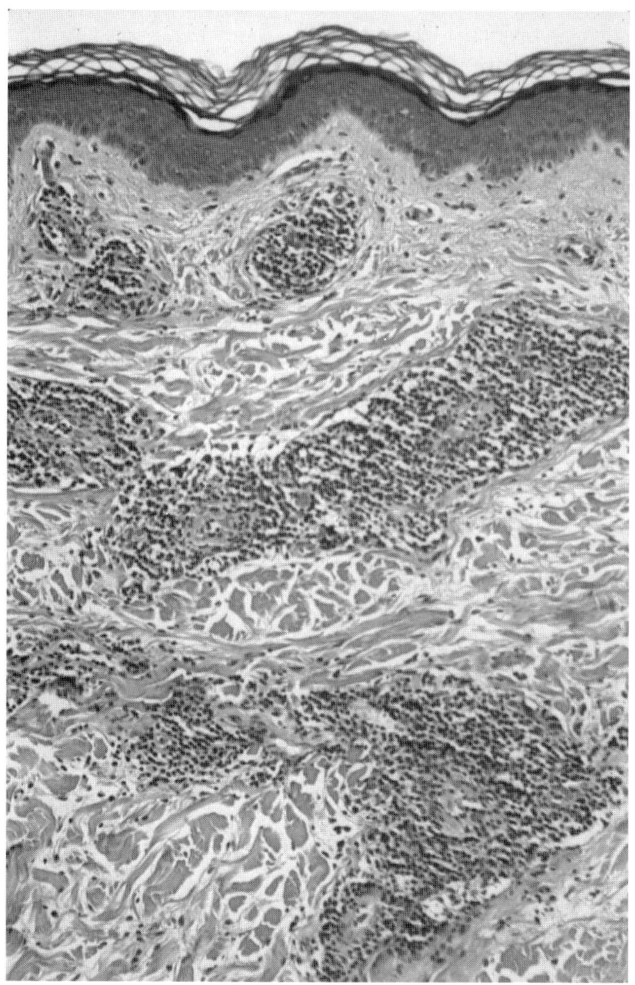

B

FIG. 10-9. Jessner's lymphocytic infiltrate (**A**). The epidermis is normal. The dermis contains large, fairly well demarcated patches of an inflammatory infiltrate composed almost entirely of lymphocytes. (**B**) Another example of Jessner's lymphocytic infiltrate with a less intense mononuclear cell infiltrate. *(continued on next page)*

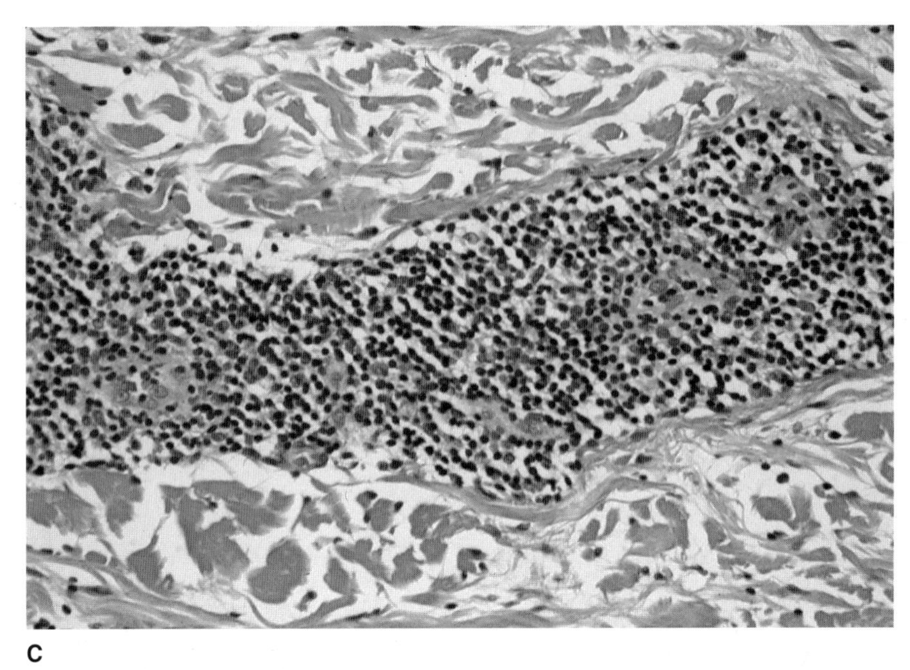

C

FIG. 10-9. ***Continued***
(**C**) A purely lymphocytic infiltrate ensheaths dermal blood vessels.

cutis, which usually displays larger B-cell components with or without associated germinal center formation. Lymphoma cutis may be distinguished with cell-marker analysis, which may show a high proportion of B lymphocytes with a less mature phenotype than expected in skin or cells with aberrant expression of cell-surface antigens.

Pathogenesis. Opinion varies as to whether Jessner's lymphocytic infiltrate of the skin is a distinct entity. The following four views have been expressed: (1) clinical, histological, and immunohistochemical findings warrant its distinction as a separate entity [43]; (2) although some cases represent an entity, others are DLE; (3) all cases are DLE; and (4) it represents an abortive or initial phase of any of the four other diseases with a patchy dermal infiltrate—that is, discoid lupus erythematosus, the plaque type of polymorphous light eruption, lymphocytoma cutis, and lymphocytic lymphoma. The last view appears to be the most likely.[44]

The diagnosis of lymphocytic infiltration of the skin depends upon clinico-pathologic correlation and on longitudinal follow-up. It may be used as a preliminary diagnostic term until a more definitive diagnosis is possible.

TABLE 10-4. *Differences between lymphocytic infiltrates of the skin and discoid lupus erythematosus*

	Lymphocytic infiltrate of the skin	Discoid lupus erythematosus
Distribution	Sun-exposed areas	Sun-exposed areas with or without involvement of non sun-exposed areas
Clinical appearance		
Hyperkeratosis	Absent	Present
Healing with atrophy	Absent	Present
Histopathology		
Interface changes	Absent	Present
Immunofluorescence		
Involved skin	Negative	Positive in 90% of cases

MIXED CONNECTIVE TISSUE DISEASE

Overlapping findings of SLE, scleroderma, and polymyositis associated with the presence of high titers of anti-U1 RNP antibodies have been recognized since 1972 as the syndrome of *mixed connective tissue disease* (MCTD).[45] The first clue to the diagnosis is usually a positive, high-titer speckled ANA. The clinical presentation includes, but is not limited to, edema of the hands, acrosclerosis, Raynaud's phenomenon, synovitis of one or more joints, and myositis that is documented with biopsy or serum elevations of muscle enzymes. Esophageal hypomotility and pulmonary disease may be seen as well. The diagnosis of MCTD may not be made at the outset since symptoms may present in an asynchronous fashion.

Cutaneous lupus erythematosus lesions are found in approximately half of the patients, about as often as "sausage fingers" or sclerodactyly. They cover the entire spectrum of cutaneous lupus erythematosus. Most commonly there are diffuse, nonscarring, poorly demarcated subacute lesions, but some patients show acute malar eruptions as seen in SLE or persistent scarring lesions as seen in DLE.

Patients with high-titer anti-U1 RNP antibodies have a low prevalence of serious renal disease and life-threatening neurologic complications. Although the prognosis of MCTD compares favorably to that of SLE, death may occur from progressive pulmonary hypertension and cardiac complications.[46]

Histopathology. If cutaneous lesions of lupus erythematosus are present, the histologic findings correspond to the type of lesion described in the section on DLE and SLE.

Histogenesis. MCTD, in contrast with most cases of SLE, has no antibodies to DNA. The absence of such antibodies accounts for the rarity of renal disease.

Indirect immunofluorescence studies show the presence of very high titers of serum antibodies directed against extractable ribonuclease-sensitive antigens known as small nuclear ribonucleoproteins (snRNP). They characterize MCTD but are not specific for it. They produce a fine speckled ANA pattern at high dilutions. This speckled pattern corresponds to the widespread distribution of snRNP in the nucleus at sites of active gene transcription, where messenger RNA is being processed.

Direct immunofluorescence staining of normal skin shows deposition of IgG in a speckled (particulate) pattern in epidermal nuclei. Although this finding is typical of MCTD, it is found occasionally also in patients with SLE and other connective-tissue diseases.[47] In addition, patients with MCTD may show a subepidermal lupus band in normal skin. Such a band has been observed in normal sun-exposed skin in about 20% of the cases.

DERMATOMYOSITIS

Dermatomyositis manifests as an inflammatory myopathy with characteristic cutaneous findings. In the absence of cutaneous findings, the diagnosis of polymyositis is applied. Cutaneous findings alone, without muscular involvement, has been termed *amyopathic dermatomyositis* or *dermatomyositis sine myositis*.[48]

Both dermatomyositis and polymyositis are uncommon diseases that have a similar incidence. Both have two peaks of occurrence: one in childhood and one between the ages of 45 and 65.[49] In some instances the cutaneous eruption precedes the development of muscular weakness by many months or even by several years.

Diagnostic criteria for dermatomyositis include proximal symmetric muscle weakness, elevated muscle enzymes, lack of neuropathy on electromyelography, consistent muscle biopsy changes, and cutaneous findings. Involvement of the skeletal muscles causes progressive weakness, vague muscular pain, and later, atrophy of the muscles. The proximal muscles of the extremities and the anterior neck muscles often are the first to be involved. Involvement of the pharynx may result in dysphagia and aspiration of food, and involvement of the diaphragm and of the intercostal muscles may lead to respiratory failure.

Two distinctive cutaneous lesions are found in dermatomyositis. One is violaceous, slightly edematous periorbital patches that primarily involve the eyelids, known as the *heliotrope rash.* The other is discrete red-purple papules over the bony prominences, particularly the knuckles, knees, and elbows, known as *Gottron's papules.* These may evolve into atrophic plaques with pigmentary alterations and telangiectasia and are then known as *Gottron's sign.*

Other cutaneous findings include periungual telangiectasia, hypertrophy of cuticular tissues associated with splinter hemorrhages, photosensitivity, and poikiloderma. Often lesions resembling the erythematous-edematous lesions seen in subacute cutaneous or systemic lupus erythematosus may be found. Subcutaneous and periarticular calcification may be found, particularly in affected children. Calcinosis is usually seen centered in the proximal muscles of the shoulders and pelvic girdle.

Controversy exists over the association of dermatomyositis with malignancy.[50] Interpretation of reports with incidences of 6% to 50% is hampered by the asynchronous development of malignancy in relation to the dermatomyositis. Some series fail to show a significant difference between affected patients and the control population. If malignancy arises with dermatomyositis, it usually occurs in the adult form. Some sources indicate this association is also present in the childhood form, while others view such reports with skepticism. Various tumors have been reported, with ovarian carcinoma perhaps being most frequent.[51]

As with lupus erythematosus, the pathogenesis of the disease is uncertain. Associated antibodies include PM1, Jo1 (correlates with pulmonary fibrosis), Ku (associated with sclerodermatomyositis), and M2. On the whole, the prognosis of dermatomyositis is favorable, especially when treatment with corticosteriods is used. The mortality has been reported to be approximately 14% in some series, with metastatic malignancy a frequent cause of death.[52]

Histopathology. The erythematous-edematous lesions of the skin in dermatomyositis may show only nonspecific inflammation. However, quite frequently the histologic changes are indistinguishable from those seen in SLE. There is epidermal atrophy, basement membrane degeneration, vacuolar alteration of basilar keratinocytes, a sparse lymphocytic inflammatory infiltrate around blood vessels, and interstitial mucin deposition (Fig. 10-10A and B).[53] With severe inflammatory changes, there may be associated subepidermal fibrin deposition. Immune complexes are not detected at the dermal-epidermal junction as in lupus erythematosus.

Old cutaneous lesions with the clinical appearance of poikiloderma atrophicans vasculare usually show a band-like infiltrate under an atrophic epidermis with hydropic degeneration of the basal cell layer (see also the section on poikiloderma atrophicans vasculare). The Gottron's papules overlying the knuckles also show vacuolization of the basal cell layer, but acanthosis rather than epidermal atrophy.[54] Subcutaneous tissue may show focal areas of panniculitis associated with mucoid degeneration of fat cells in early lesions. Extensive areas of calcification may be present in the subcutis at a later stage (see calcinosis cutis, Chap. 17).

Magnetic resonance imaging permits noninvasive assessment of muscle inflammation and may serve as a guide in locating a site for muscle biopsy. Tender proximal muscles of an extremity yield more useful information than atrophic, weak muscles, which show end-stage changes. Three types of changes may be observed in active disease: (1) interstitial inflammatory infiltrates composed of lymphocytes and macrophages; (2) segmental muscle fiber necrosis (loss of skeletal muscle transverse striation, hyalinization of the sarcoplasm, fragmentation and/or phagocytosis of degenerated muscle fragments); or (3) vasculopathy.[55] The latter entity may be seen in the childhood form and shows immunocomplex deposition in vessel walls.[56] Old lesions usually show a rather nonspecific picture of atrophy of the muscle fibers and diffuse interstitial fibrosis with relatively little inflammation.

Systemic Lesions. Changes in organs other than the skin and the striated muscles occur only rarely in dermatomyositis, in contrast to SLE and systemic scleroderma. The myocardium may show changes identical to those in the skeletal muscle but

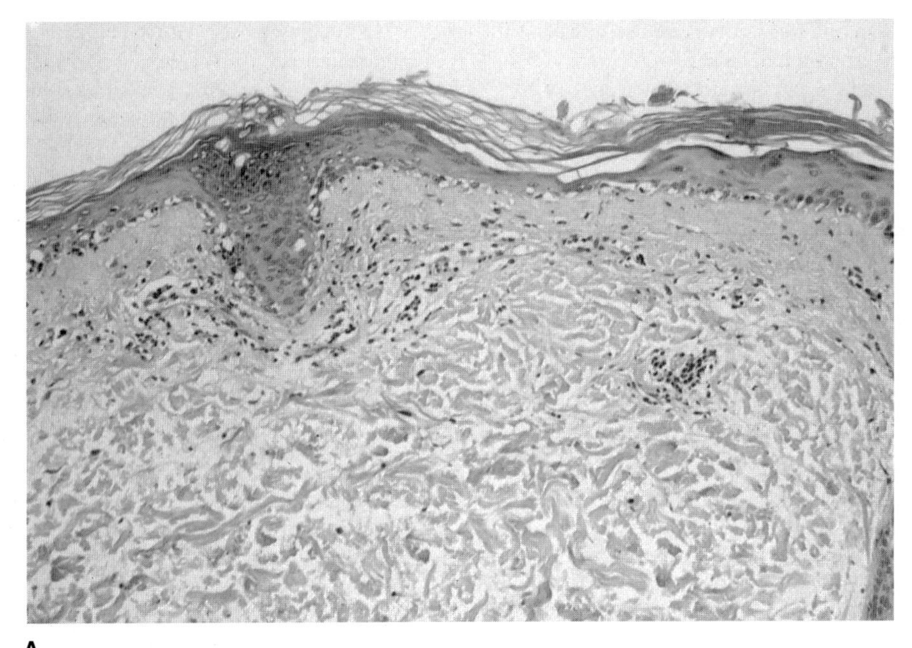

A

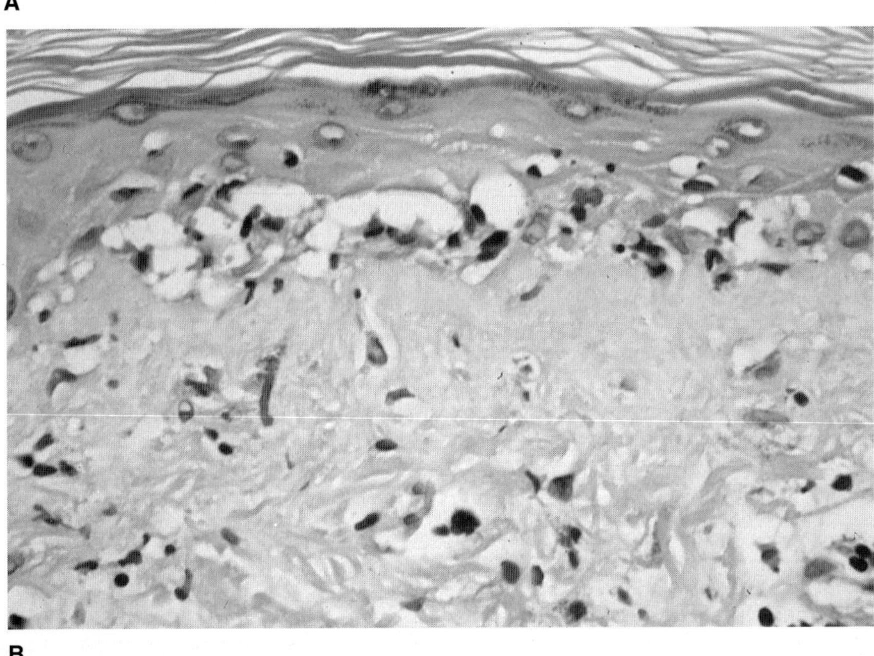

B

FIG. 10-10. Dermatomyositis
(**A**) An atrophic epidermis shows marked vacuolar alteration of basilar keratinocytes associated with a sparse lymphocytic inflammatory infiltrate around superficial dermal vessels. (**B**) Marked vacuolar alteration of basilar keratinocytes associated with sparse lymphocytic infiltrates and papillary dermal melanophages.

less severe. Ulcerative lesions in the gastrointestinal tract, caused by vascular occlusions, have also been described.[57]

Histogenesis. On electron microscopic examination the degenerative changes include focal disintegration of myofilaments and myofibrils, vacuolization, and accumulation of lipid and lysosomes within muscle fibers. As in lupus erythematosus, nonspecific intracytoplasmic tubuloreticular structures may be found in skin and muscles.

Differential Diagnosis. Differentiation of the cutaneous lesions of dermatomyositis from those of subacute cutaneous or systemic lupus erythematosus may be impossible on a histologic basis. It may also be impossible on clinical grounds in cases in which muscular weakness is mild or absent, as it may be in the early stage of dermatomyositis. In such cases, laboratory tests are of great value. The most important is the lupus band test, which is always negative in lesions of dermatomyositis,[58] whereas in lesions of lupus erythematosus it is positive in 90% of the cases. Other tests that are usually negative in dermatomyositis and often positive in lupus erythematosus include urinalysis and renal function tests, as well as tests for antinuclear antibodies, anti-native DNA antibodies, and antibodies to ribonucleoprotein. However, patients with active myositis show an elevation of serum creatine kinase and aldolase.

Poikiloderma Atrophicans Vasculare

Poikiloderma atrophicans vasculare may be seen in three different settings: (1) in association with three genodermatoses; (2) as an early stage of mycosis fungoides; and (3) in association with dermatomyositis and, less commonly, lupus erythematosus.

The three genodermatoses in which the cutaneous lesions have the appearance of poikiloderma atrophicans vasculare are: (1) poikiloderma congenitale of Rothmund–Thomson (Chap. 6), with the lesions of poikiloderma present largely on the face, hands, and feet, and occasionally also on the arms, legs, and buttocks; (2) Bloom's syndrome (Chap. 6), with poikiloderma-like lesions on the face, hands, and forearms; and (3) dyskeratosis congenita (Chap. 6), in which there may be extensive netlike pigmentation of the skin suggestive of poikiloderma atrophicans vasculare.

Poikiloderma-like lesions as features of early mycosis fungoides may be seen in one of two clinical forms: either as the large plaque type of parapsoriasis en plaques, also known as poikilodermatous parapsoriasis (Chap. 7), or as parapsoriasis variegata, also called parakeratosis variegata, which, in its early state, shows papules arranged in a netlike pattern (Chap. 7). Although these two types of parapsoriasis represent an early stage of mycosis fungoides, not all cases progress clinically into fully developed mycosis fungoides.[59] Cases in which no progression toward mycosis fungoides is observed have been described also as *idiopathic poikiloderma atrophicans vasculare*.[60]

The third group of diseases in which lesions of poikiloderma atrophicans vasculare occur is represented by dermatomyositis and SLE. Dermatomyositis is much more commonly seen as the primary disease than lupus erythematosus, and the association with dermatomyositis often is referred to as poikilodermatomyositis. In contrast to mycosis fungoides, in which poikilodermatous lesions are seen in the early stage, the lesions found in dermatomyositis and SLE generally represent a late stage.

Clinically, the term poikiloderma atrophicans vasculare is applied to lesions that, in the early stage, show erythema with slight, superficial scaling, a mottled pigmentation, and telangiectases. In the late stage the skin appears atrophic and the erythema is less pronounced than in the early stage, but the mottled pigmentation and the telangiectases are more pronounced. The clinical picture then resembles chronic radiodermatitis.

Histopathology. In its early stage poikiloderma atrophicans vasculare, without respect to its cause, shows moderate thinning of the stratum malpighii, effacement of the rete ridges, and hydropic degeneration of the basal cells. In the upper dermis there is a band-like infiltrate, which in places invades the epidermis. The infiltrate consists mainly of lymphoid cells but also contains a few histiocytes. Melanophages filled with melanin as a result of pigmentary incontinence are found in varying numbers within the infiltrate. In addition, there is edema in the upper dermis and the superficial capillaries are often dilated. In the late stage the epidermis is apt to be markedly thinned and flattened, but the basal cells still show hydropic degeneration. Melanophages and edema of the upper dermis are still present, and telangiectasia may be pronounced.

The amount and type of dermal infiltrate vary with the underlying cause. In poikiloderma atrophicans vasculare associated with one of the genodermatoses the mononuclear infiltrate is mild and may be absent in the late stage.[61] Similarly, in the late stage of poikiloderma seen in association with dermatomyositis or SLE there is only slight dermal inflammation.[53] In contrast, the amount of inflammatory infiltrate seen in poikiloderma associated with early mycosis fungoides increases rather than decreases with time (Fig. 10-11). In addition, cells with large, hyperchromatic nuclei, so-called mycosis cells, are likely to be present and there is often marked epidermotropism of the infiltrate, which may result in Pautrier microabscesses. Cell-

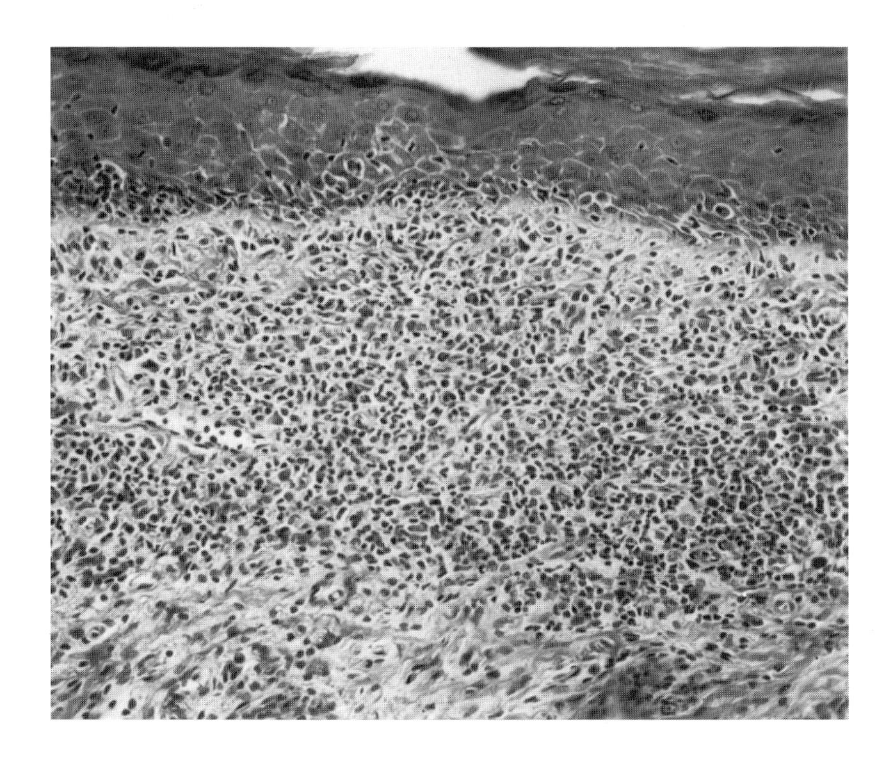

FIG. 10-11. Poikiloderma
The epidermis appears flattened and shows hydropic degeneration of the basal cells. The upper dermis contains a band-like infiltrate, which in places invades the epidermis.

marker analysis of such cases has shown most cells to be T helper/inducer (CD4+) lymphocytes that lack Leu-8 and/or Leu-9 expression, as seen in cutaneous T-cell lymphoma.[62]

SCLERODERMA

Scleroderma (Gr. *skleros*, hard, and *derma*, skin) is a connective tissue disorder characterized by thickening and fibrosis of the skin. Two types of scleroderma exist: circumscribed scleroderma (*morphea*), and systemic scleroderma (*progressive systemic sclerosis*). They are somewhat analogous to the purely cutaneous form of lupus erythematosus (DLE) and the cutaneous plus visceral involvement in systemic lupus erythematosus. Rarely, morphea and systemic scleroderma may coexist. In such instances, the manifestations of morphea arise first and are extensive, whereas those of systemic scleroderma are mild and nonprogressive.[63] Rarely, the manifestations of systemic scleroderma precede those of morphea.[64]

There are also two variants of morphea: atrophoderma of Pasini and Pierini, and eosinophilic fasciitis of Shulman. The latter disease differs sufficiently from morphea so that it will be discussed separately.

Hardening of the skin (sclerodermoid changes) may also arise in association with genetic, metabolic, neurologic, and immunologic disorders, with occupational or chemical exposures, in association with malignancy or as a sequella of infection.[65] Genetic disorders that may show sclerodermatous cutaneous changes include phenylketonuria, progeria, Rothmund–Thomson syndrome and Werner's syndrome. Occupations at risk are jackhammer and chainsaw operators, and those exposed to polyvinyl chloride, silica, and epoxy resins. Patients with metabolic disorders such as porphyria cutanea tarda, primary systemic amyloidosis, Hashimoto's disease, carcinoid syndrome, and childhood diabetes mellitus may show similar cutaneous changes. Chronic graft–versus–host disease frequently shows sclerodermatous changes, while scattered reports in the literature indicate such changes may arise subsequent to silicone and paraffin injections for cosmetic procedures.[66] Chemical agents have been known to induce thickening and hardening of the skin. Specific compounds include polyvinyl chloride, bleomycin, pentazocine, L-5 hydroxytryptophan and carbidopa,[67] Spanish rapeseed oil,[68] and L-tryptophan (eosinophilia-myalgia syndrome).[69]

Morphea

In morphea, or circumscribed scleroderma, the lesions usually are limited to the skin and to the subcutaneous tissue beneath the cutaneous lesions. Occasionally, however, the underlying muscles and rarely the underlying bones are also affected.

Morphea may be divided according to morphology and distribution of lesions into six types: guttate, plaque, linear, segmental, subcutaneous, and generalized. Eosinophilic fasciitis, even though it is the fascial component of subcutaneous morphea, is discussed separately because of its somewhat different clinical and histological appearance.

Guttate lesions occur almost always in association with lesions of the plaque type. Guttate lesions are small and superficial; they resemble the lesions of lichen sclerosus et atrophicus but do not show hyperkeratosis or follicular plugging.

Lesions of the plaque type, the most common manifestation of morphea, are round or oval but through coalescence may assume an irregular configuration. They are indurated, have a smooth surface, and show an ivory color. As long as they are enlarging, they may show a violaceous border, the so-called lilac ring.

Lesions of the linear type occur predominantly on the extremities and on the anterior scalp. When one or several extremities are involved, there is often, in addition to induration of the skin, marked atrophy of the subcutaneous fat and of the muscles, resulting in contractures of muscles and tendons and ankyloses of joints. In children it may result in impaired growth of the affected limb.[70] On the anterior portion of the scalp and on the forehead, linear morphea often has the configuration of the stroke of a saber (*coup de sabre*).[71]

Segmental morphea occurs on one side of the face, resulting in hemiatrophy. Occasionally, morphea en *coup de sabre* and facial hemiatrophy occur together.[71] It is uncertain if Parry-Romberg facial hemiatrophy represents a part of the spectrum of linear scleroderma involving the face.

In subcutaneous morphea (morphea profunda) the involved skin feels thickened and bound to the underlying fascia and muscle. The involved plaques are ill-defined, and the skin of these plaques is smooth and shiny.[72]

Generalized morphea comprises very extensive cases showing a combination of several of the five types just described. It is seen mainly in children, in whom it has been described as disabling pansclerotic morphea[63] but it can also occur in adults. Rarely, bullous lesions are seen in patients with generalized morphea.[73]

The occasional coexistence of lesions of morphea and lichen sclerosus et atrophicus is worthy of note.

There is conflicting data regarding *Borrelia burgdorferi* infection in cases of morphea. Studies indicating that such a relationship exists are primarily from Europe.[74] Studies in North America, and some from Europe, have resulted in negative findings.[75]

Histopathology. The different types of morphea cannot be differentiated histologically. Rather, they differ in regard to severity and to their depth of involvement of the skin. Therefore, it is of great importance that the specimen for biopsy include adequate amounts of subcutaneous tissue, since most of the diagnostic alterations are seen in the lower dermis and in the subcutis.

Although early inflammatory and late sclerotic stages exist, most specimens show an intermediate histologic picture. In the early inflammatory stage, found particularly at the violaceous border of enlarging lesions, the reticular dermis shows thickened collagen bundles and a moderately intense inflammatory infiltrate, predominantly lymphocytic admixed with plasma cells, between the collagen bundles and around the blood vessels (Fig. 10-12A–C). A much more pronounced inflammatory infiltrate than that seen in the dermis often involves the subcutaneous fat and extends upward toward the eccrine glands. Trabeculae subdividing the subcutaneous fat are thickened because of the presence of an inflammatory infiltrate and deposition of new collagen. Large areas of subcutaneous fat are replaced by newly formed collagen, which is composed of fine, wavy fibers, rather than of bundles, and which stains only faintly with hematoxylin-eosin.[76] Vascular changes in the early inflammatory

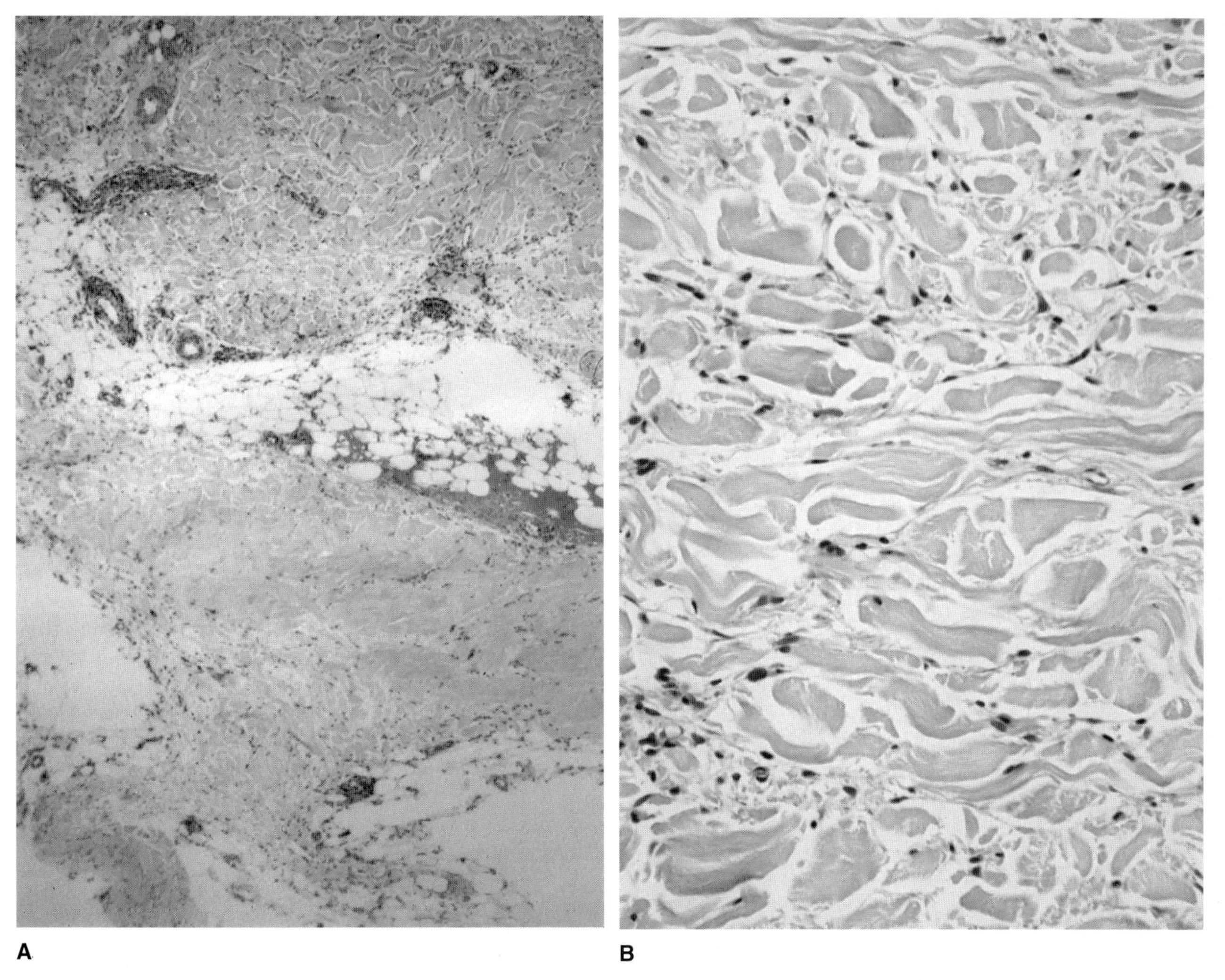

FIG. 10-12. Morphea, early involving the subcutis
(**A**) The trabeculae subdividing the subcutaneous fat are thickened and there is a patchy lymphoplasmacytic infiltrate. Large areas of subcutaneous fat are replaced by newly formed collagen fibers that show only faint staining. (**B**) In the deep reticular dermis, normal collagen bundles contain a subtle interstitial lymphocytic infiltrate. *(continued on next page)*

stage generally are mild both in the dermis and in the subcutaneous tissue. They may consist of endothelial swelling and edema of the walls of the vessels.[77]

In the late sclerotic stage, as seen in the center of old lesions, the inflammatory infiltrate has disappeared almost completely, except in some areas of the subcutis. The epidermis is normal. The collagen bundles in the reticular dermis often appear thickened, closely packed, hypocellular, and stain more deeply eosinophilic than in normal skin (Fig. 10-13A). In the papillary dermis, where the collagen normally consists of loosely arranged fibers, the collagen may appear homogeneous.

The eccrine glands appear markedly atrophic, have few or no adipocytes surrounding them, and appear surrounded by newly formed collagen (Fig. 10-13B). Also, instead of lying near the dermal-subcutaneous junction as in normal skin, they seem to lie higher in the dermis as a result of the replacement of most of the subcutaneous fat by newly formed collagen. This collagen consists of thick, pale, sclerotic, homogeneous or hyalinized bundles with only few fibroblasts (hypocellular). Few blood vessels are seen within the sclerotic collagen; they often have a fibrotic wall and a narrowed lumen.

The fascia and striated muscles underlying lesions of morphea may be affected in the linear, segmental, subcutaneous, and generalized types. The fascia shows fibrosis and sclerosis similar to that seen in subcutaneous tissue. The muscle fibers appear vacuolated and separated from one another by edema and focal collections of inflammatory cells.[78]

Bullae, seen only on rare occasions in generalized and in subcutaneous morphea, arise subepidermally, probably as a result of lymphatic obstruction, causing subepidermal edema.

Differential Diagnosis. Contrasting features of morphea and lichen sclerosus et atrophicus are summarized in Table 10-5. They include relatively little epidermal change in morphea, as compared with thinning of the rete ridges, folllicular plugging, and interface alterations of lichen sclerosus. Reticular dermal changes of fibrosis and inflammation of morphea contrast with edema and loss of elastic tissue in lichen sclerosus. Histologic differentiation of the late stage of morphea from lichen sclero-

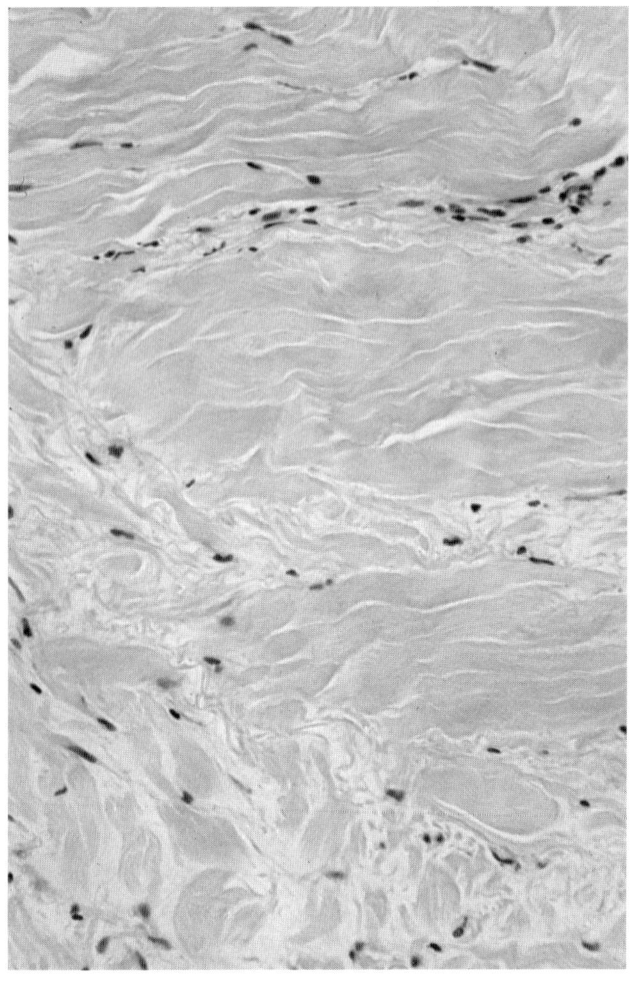

C

FIG. 10-12. *Continued*
(**C**) Contrast with (B): subcutaneous septal collagen is pale, eosinophilic, and hypocellular.

sus et atrophicus may cause difficulties, particularly in view of the fact that the two conditions may coexist.

Systemic Scleroderma

In systemic scleroderma, in addition to involvement of the skin and the subcutaneous tissue visceral lesions are present, leading to death in some patients. The indurated lesions of the skin are not sharply demarcated or "circumscribed," as in morphea, although a few well-demarcated morphea-like patches may occasionally be seen.

Cutaneous involvement usually starts peripherally on the face and hands, gradually extending to the forearms. Facial changes include a mask-like expressionless face, inability to wrinkle the forehead, a beak-like nose, and tightening of the skin around the mouth associated with radial folds. The hands show nonpitting edema involving the dorsa of the fingers, hands, and forearms. Gradually the fingers become tapered, the skin becomes hard, and flexion contractures form. These changes are referred to as acrosclerosis and are associated with Raynaud's phenomenon, which may precede other manifestations by months or even years. Microscopic examination of the nailfold capillary beds shows tortuosity and redundancy of capillary loops with dilatation of the arterioles and venules. Such abnormalities may occasionally be seen in patients with localized scleroderma and herald coexisting or evolving systemic sclerosis.[79]

Systemic sclerosis with limited scleroderma, known as CREST syndrome, is associated with Raynaud's phenomenon in virtually all affected patients. This variant of acrosclerosis, which frequently but not invariably has a favorable prognosis, consists of several or all of the following manifestations: **C**alcinosis cutis, **R**aynaud's phenomenon, involvement of the **E**sophagus with dysphagia, **S**clerodactyly and **T**elangiectases. Death from visceral lesions is rather infrequent in the CREST syndrome.[80]

In about 5% of the cases, the cutaneous lesions first appear on the trunk as so-called *diffuse systemic scleroderma*, often sparing the peripheral portions of the extremities. Raynaud's phenomenon is absent in such patients. There are, however, transitional forms starting out as acrosclerosis with Raynaud's phenomenon but then extending to the proximal portions of the arms and to the trunk. In both forms of systemic scleroderma, the skin in the involved areas is diffusely indurated and, as a result of diffuse fibrosis of the subcutaneous fat, becomes firmly bound to the underlying structures. The skeletal musculature is affected, resulting in weakness and atrophy. Contractures of the muscles and tendons and ankyloses of the joints may develop.

Occasional manifestations pertaining to the skin include diffuse hyperpigmentation, which is seen mainly in diffuse systemic scleroderma. Macular telangiectasias on the face and hands, calcinosis cutis located on the extremities, and ulcerations, especially on the tips of the fingers and over the knuckles, occur predominantly in acrosclerosis. Also vascular ulcers on the lower extremities resembling those seen in atrophie blanche may occur in patients with acrosclerosis.

Histopathology. The histologic appearance of the skin lesions in systemic scleroderma is similar to that of morphea so that histologic differentiation of the two types is not possible. However, in early lesions of systemic scleroderma the inflammatory reaction is less pronounced than in morphea, so that only a mild inflammatory infiltrate is present around the dermal vessels, around the eccrine coils, and in the subcutaneous tissue. The vascular changes in early lesions are slight, as in morphea.[81] In contrast, in the late stage, systemic scleroderma shows more pronounced vascular changes than morphea, particularly in the subcutis. These changes consist of a paucity of blood vessels, thickening and hyalinization of their walls, and narrowing of the lumen. Even in the late stage of systemic scleroderma, the epidermis appears normal, only occasionally showing disappearance of the rete ridges. Aggregates of calcium may also be seen in the late stage within areas of sclerotic, homogeneous collagen of the subcutaneous tissue (see also calcinosis cutis, Chap. 17).

Systemic Lesions. Internal organs are often affected in scleroderma, but their involvement varies greatly in extent and degree. Involvement does not necessarily imply functional compromise, and in many affected patients systemic scleroderma ultimately comes to a standstill. The clinical symptoms produced by reduced pliability, vascular compromise, and subsequent loss of function can be found in the gastrointestinal tract, lungs, heart, and kidneys as well as the skin. In the gastrointestinal tract submucosal fibrosis and replacement of the mus-

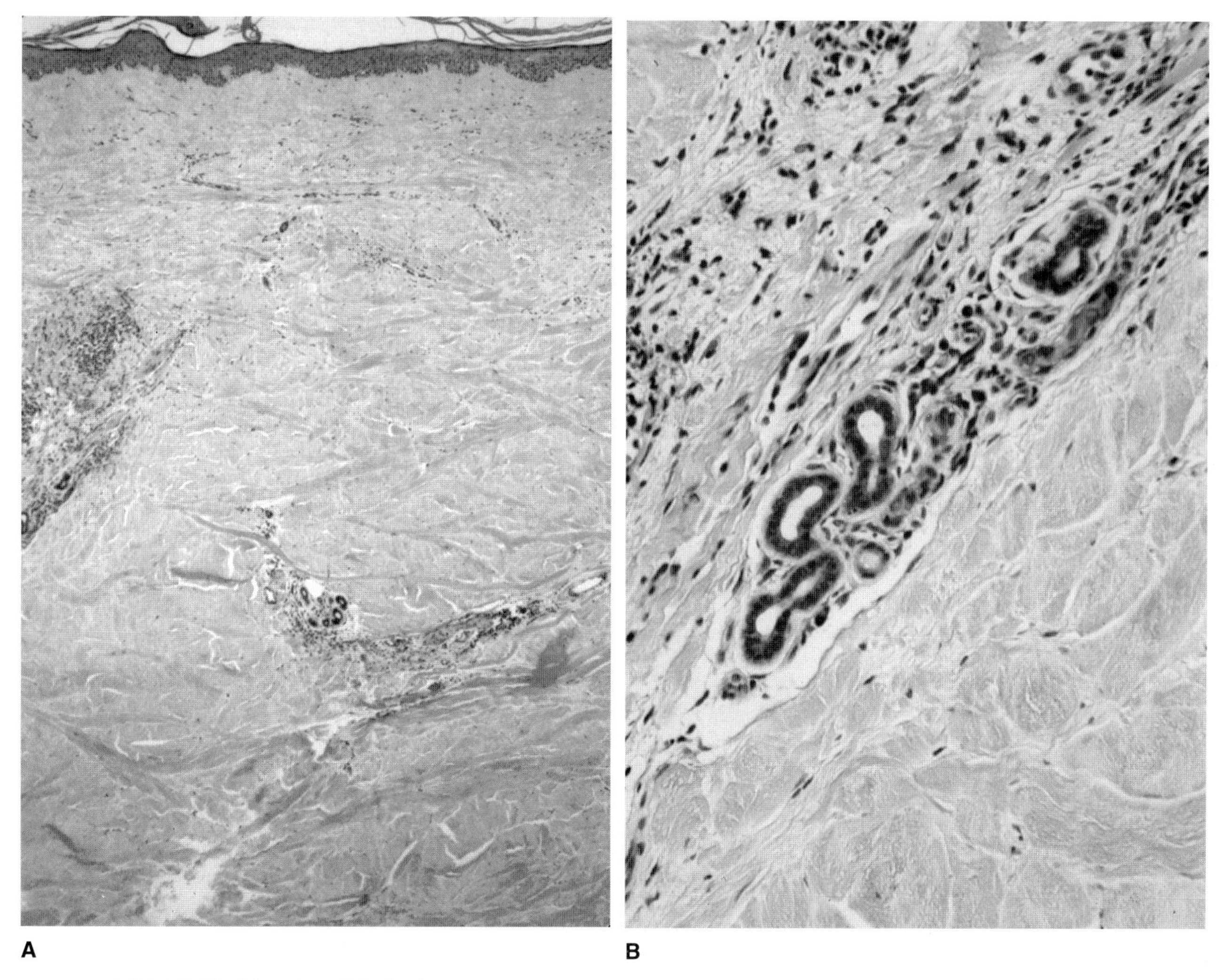

FIG. 10-13. Morphea, late lesion
(**A**) The reticular dermis is hypocellular and shows a paucity of appendageal structures. Eccrine glands are located in the midreticular dermis. (**B**) This eccrine unit has been reduced to a few ducts surrounded by a fibrotic dermis and inflammatory cells, with loss of the adipose tissue that surrounds normal glands.

cularis by fibrosis with intimal thickening of blood vessels give rise to difficulties in swallowing, regurgitation, malabsorption, and eventually ileus. In the lungs interstitial fibrosis, degeneration of alveolar spaces, and intimal thickening of arteries result in dyspnea and cor pulmonale. Cases of pulmonary carcinoma (predominantly bronchoalveolar) have been observed and are associated with the presence of pulmonary fibrosis.[82] The most serious consequences arise in the kidneys. Adventitial fibrosis may affect interlobar, arcuate, and interlobular arteries, while mucoid degeneration affects arcuate and interlobular arteries. Uremia occurs more frequently than rapidly evolving renal failure and hypertension. The latter entity, termed scleroderma renal crisis, is associated with "onion-skin" hyperplasia of arterial walls and may be fatal.[83]

Pathogenesis and Laboratory Findings. The pathogenesis of systemic scleroderma, as with lupus erythematosus, is uncertain

TABLE 10-5. *Contrasting features of morphea and lichen sclerosus et atrophicus*

	Morphea	Lichen sclerosus et atrophicus
Epidermis	Relatively normal No follicular plugging	Thinning of rete Follicular plugging
Dermal-epidermal junction	No hydropic degeneration Subepidermal separation infrequent	Hydropic degeneration of basilar cells Often subepidermal bullae
Dermis	Appears homogenized Papillary dermal collagen elastic fibers present	Marked edema Elastic fibers absent
Subcutis	Inflammation Fibrosis	No inflammation or fibrosis

and may be multifactorial. Histogenetic factors are essentially the same in morphea and systemic scleroderma; they differ only in degree and extent.

The triad of vascular compromise, collagen matrix aberrations, and presence of serologic autoimmune indicators contribute in variable degrees to symptoms and clinical findings in scleroderma and morphea (Table 10-6). Although a relationship to retroviral disease has been suggested, it is speculative and may reflect molecular mimicry of viral antigens.[84]

Microvascular changes. Involved vessels are primarily precapillary arterioles. Changes in the microvasculature have been noted in clinically normal skin. Perivascular edema and functional changes in endothelial cells can be detected early.[85] Precapillary arterioles then show endothelial proliferation and mononuclear inflammatory infiltrates, followed by intimal proliferation and luminal narrowing.[86] Corresponding electron microscopic findings include vacuolization and destruction of endothelial cells, reduplication of the basement membrane, enlargement of the rough endoplasmic reticulum in pericytes and fibroblasts, and perivascular fibrosis. Although widespread arteriolitis may be present in early stages, only rarely does it progress to a necrotizing arteriolitis and eventuate in periarteritis nodosa.[87]

A role for adhesion molecules in the evolution of lesions of scleroderma has been suggested: they are thought to bind mononuclear cells to endothelial cells and facilitate transvascular migration of inflammatory cells into the connective tissue. Interactions with connective-tissue components may lead to the release of cytokines and growth factors, resulting in upregulation of matrix production by fibroblasts and changes in fibroblast phenotype, eventuating in fibrosis.[88]

TABLE 10-6. *Pathogenic factors in scleroderma*

Vascular aberrations	Raynaud's phenomenon
	Intimal hyperplasia of blood vessels
	Adventitial fibrosis
	Vascular abnormalities in other visceral organs
	Microvascular abnormalities
	Enlargement and tortuosity of capillary loops
	Capillary loop dropout
	Thickened and reduplicated basement membrane
	Loss of endothelium
Immunologic factors	T helper cell (CD4+) infiltrates
	Reduction in T-suppressor (CD8+) cells
	Increased soluble interleukin 2 receptors correlate with disease progression and mortality
	Decreased interleukin 1 production by peripheral mononuclear cells
Serologic markers	ANA+ in more than 90% of patients
	Low/absent anti-native (double stranded) DNA, anti-Sm, rare anti-nRNP
	Speckled ANA pattern correlates with anti-centromere antibody on HEp-2 cells and CREST and a relatively favorable prognosis
	Anti-DNA-Topoisomerase 1 (Scl-70)

Collagen matrix aberrations. Analysis of collagen in affected skin has shown excess production of connective-tissue components normally present in the dermis, including types I, III, V, VI, and VII collagen, fibronectin, and proteoglycans.[89,90] Other studies suggest that fibroblasts in localized and systemic scleroderma express some markers of smooth muscle differentiation (myofibroblasts), which may account for their different biologic behavior.[91] Some observers have found loss of CD34+ dendritic cells in affected areas, a finding of uncertain significance.[92]

Serologic/Immunologic markers. Most patients with systemic sclerosis (greater than 90%) and approximately 50% with localized scleroderma (morphea) have a positive ANA. The pattern may be homogenous, speckled, or nucleolar. When using human laryngeal carcinoma cell lines, HEp2, more than 90% of patients with morphea or acrosclerosis have a detectable anticentromere antibody. In patients with systemic sclerosis this antibody is not usually detected. Instead, 20% to 40% of them have antibodies to Scl-70. This antigen has been identified as DNA–topoisomerase I, an intracellular enzyme involved in the uncoiling of DNA before it is transcribed. Antibodies to this enzyme hinder its function. The presence of antibodies to Scl-70 correlates with systemic sclerosis, while the presence of anticentromere antibodies correlates with morphea or CREST and suggests a more favorable prognosis.[93]

In some cases of systemic scleroderma, epidermal nucleolar IgG deposition is seen even in clinically normal skin as a result of high serum concentrations of antibody to nucleolar antigen.[94] Although subepidermal and vascular deposits are regularly absent in the skin in scleroderma, kidney biopsies in patients with renal involvement show diffuse vascular deposits of immunoglobulins, predominantly IgM, or of complement in the intima of the interlobular and arcuate arteries, which by light microscopy often exhibit fibromucinous alterations.[95]

Atrophoderma of Pasini and Pierini

In atrophoderma of Pasini and Pierini there are areas on the trunk, particularly the back, in which the skin appears slightly depressed and has a slate-gray color but shows no other surface changes. The lesions are asymptomatic, bilateral, symmetrical, and sharply but often irregularly demarcated, measuring from 1 to 10 cm in diameter. They often show a "cliff-drop" border, which is largely an optical effect of the slate-gray discoloration. In old lesions, the center of the depressed area may feel slightly indurated.

Histopathology. The histologic changes in early lesions usually are slight and nonspecific, consisting of some thickening of the collagen bundles and a mild, scattered, chronic inflammatory infiltrate.[96] Older lesions show no inflammatory infiltrate, but, in the deeper layers of the dermis, they may show collagen bundles that not only are thickened but also appear tightly packed. In addition, indurated areas may show homogeneous, hyalinized collagen bundles.[97]

Because the collagen bundles in the skin of the back normally are rather thick, it may be difficult to determine whether the collagen shows any changes. It is therefore desirable to take a biopsy specimen not only from the lesion but also from normal skin, either from an area nearby or from the opposite side with subcutaneous fat for comparison.

Pathogenesis. Some authors believe that atrophoderma of Pasini and Pierini is a disease entity, as suggested by the original describers. In favor of this view is that in atrophoderma, the atrophy comes first and the sclerosis possibly appears later, whereas in morphea, the sclerosis comes first and the atrophy appears later.[98]

Most observers view the clinical presentation of atrophoderma to be distinct from morphea: atrophoderma has an earlier onset (second to third decade) and protracted course of 10 to 20 years, and lesions lack a violaceous ring, which characteristically surrounds lesions of morphea. Microscopic findings show similarities to morphea, however, suggesting that atrophoderma of Pasini and Pierini may be a distinct, abortive variant of morphea.[99] To support this view there are instances of coexistent morphea and atrophoderma, as well as reports of transformation of lesions of morphea into atrophoderma.[100] A relationship of this disorder to *Borrelia burgdorferi* infection has been reported but needs more studies to be confirmed.[101]

EOSINOPHILIC FASCIITIS (SHULMAN'S SYNDROME)

First described in 1974,[102] eosinophilic fasciitis is a scleroderma-like disorder characterized by inflammation and thickening of the deep fascia. It has a rapid onset associated with pain, swelling, and progressive induration of the skin leading to exaggerated deep grooving of the skin around superficial veins. This disorder is often accompanied by a peripheral eosinophilia and hypergammaglobulinemia, and has been associated with aplastic anemia. Eosinophilic fasciitis may have its onset with unusual physical exertion; however, more recently it has been reported in association with l-tryptophan ingestion.[103] The latter association is known as eosinophilia-myalgia syndrome, which is clinically and histologically similar to eosinophilic fasciitis.

Eosinophilic fasciitis often involves one or more extremities. The induration may cause a decreased range of motion and, in

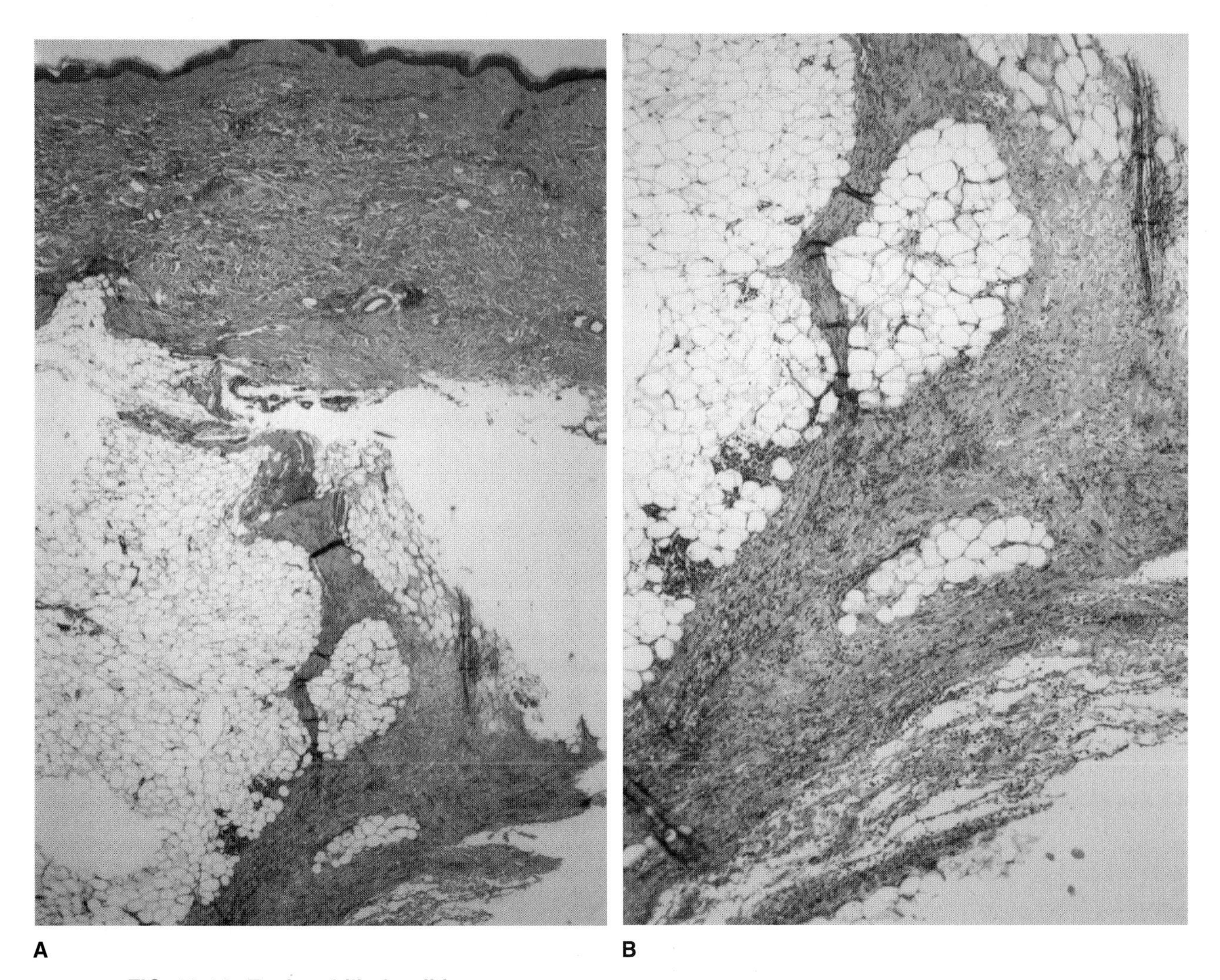

FIG. 10-14. Eosinophilic fasciitis
(**A**) A deep biopsy including fascia. The subcutaneous septum and the fascia appear thickened and contain an inflammatory infiltrate. (**B**) A widened fascia contains an interstitial inflammatory infiltrate that extends to involve adjacent adipose lobules (original magnification ×40). *(continued on next page)*

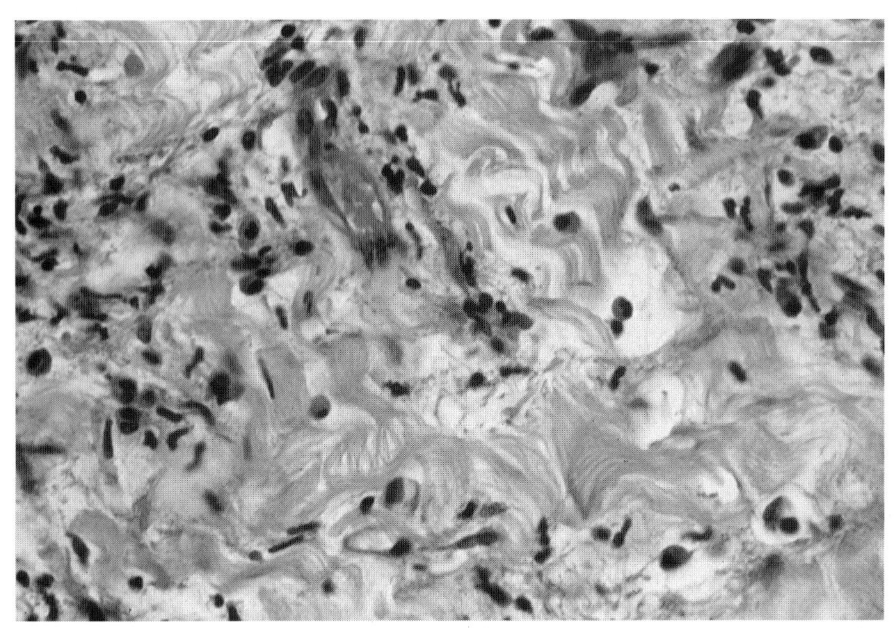

C

FIG. 10-14. *Continued*
(**C**) Among fibrotic bands of collagen is an infiltrate composed of lymphocytes, plasma cells, and occasional eosinophils (original magnification ×400).

severe cases, even joint contractures.[104] In only a few cases are there lesions on the trunk, and the face is almost invariably spared. In nearly all reported cases, Raynaud's phenomenon and visceral lesions of scleroderma have been absent. Only very few instances of incontestable eosinophilic fasciitis have shown evidence of Raynaud's phenomenon [105] or mild pulmonary fibrosis.[106] The disorder has a varied course: some patients improve spontaneously, others improve with corticosteroids, while still others may have relapses and remissions.

Histopathology. A deep wedge biopsy to skeletal muscle including fascia is essential to making the diagnosis of eosinophilic fasciitis. The fascia is markedly thickened, appears homogeneous, and is permeated by a mononuclear inflammatory infiltrate (Fig. 10-14A–C). In some instances the infiltrate in the fascia contains an admixture of eosinophils.[107] The underlying skeletal muscle in some cases shows myofiber degeneration, severe inflammation with a component of eosinophils, and focal scarring; in other cases, however, it is not involved.

In most cases the adipose tissue shows no significant changes, except that the fibrous septa separating deeply located fat lobules are thicker, paler-staining, and more homogeneous and hyaline than normal dermal connective tissue. In other cases, however, the collagen in the lower reticular dermis appears pale and homogeneous, and the entire subcutaneous fat is replaced by horizontally oriented, thick, homogeneous collagen containing only few fibroblasts and merging with the fascia.[108]

Pathogenesis. Whereas at first the impression prevailed that eosinophilic fasciitis was a new syndrome, it soon became apparent that the disorder represents a variant of morphea.[104] Eosinophilic fasciitis shares many features with generalized morphea: they both may show inflammation and fibrosis of the fascia, as well as blood eosinophilia and hypergammaglobulinemia. Also, antinuclear antibodies are present in a significant number of cases.[109] The term morphea profunda, analogous to lupus erythematosus profundus, has been applied to this disorder.[110] Nevertheless, because of its acute onset in most cases, its usual limitation to the structures underlying the skin, and its tendency to resolve, eosinophilic fasciitis deserves recognition as a distinct variant of morphea.[111]

LICHEN SCLEROSUS ET ATROPHICUS

Lichen sclerosus (LS) encompasses the disorders known as *lichen sclerosus et atrophicus*, *balanitis xerotica obliterans* (LS of the male glans and prepuce), and *kraurosis vulvae* (LS of the female labia majora, labia minora, perineum, and perianal region).[112] Lichen sclerosus is an inflammatory disorder of unknown etiology that affects patients 6 months of age to late adulthood. In both males and females genital involvement is the most frequent, and often the only, site of involvement. Extragenital lesions may occur with or without coexisting genital lesions.

Lesions of LS are characterized by white polygonal papules that coalesce to form plaques. Comedo-like plugs on the surface of the plaque correspond to dilated appendageal ostia. The plugs may disappear as the lesion ages, leaving a smooth, porcelain-white plaque. Solitary or generalized lesions may become bullous and hemorrhagic.

In males, involvement of the glans and prepuce often result in phimosis. Although the literature is dominated by reports of LS in incompletely or uncircumcised men,[113] occurrences in circumcised men are reported as well.[114] Neoplasms have been infrequently documented in association with LS; however, a cause and effect relationship has not been established.[112]

In females, contiguous involvement of the labial, perineal, and anal areas has been described clinically as "figure 8" or "keyhole" lesions.[115] Many cases of childhood LS in girls resolve by menarche.[116] If lesions persist, atrophy of the labia and narrowing of the vaginal orifice may ensue. In contrast to lichen sclerosus et atrophicus of the skin, which rarely itches, there is often severe pruritus in the vulvar region. Although neoplasms have been reported in association with LS, the current concensus is that LS is not itself a premalignant condition.[117] Since neoplasms have arisen in areas adjacent to lesions of LS, long-range follow-up of patients with lichen sclerosus et atrophicus of the vulva is advisable.

Of interest, lesions of LS may koebnerize (be provoked by trauma)[118] as well as coexist with morphea.[119,120] In extensive cases of morphea, lichen sclerosus et atrophicus may become superimposed on some of the lesions. It is then best recognized by follicular plugging.[121]

Histopathology. The salient histologic findings in cutaneous lesions of lichen sclerosus et atrophicus are: (1) hyperkeratosis with follicular plugging, (2) atrophy of the stratum malpighii with hydropic degeneration of basal cells, (3) pronounced edema and homogenization of the collagen in the upper dermis, and (4) an inflammatory infiltrate in the mid-dermis.

The hyperkeratosis is so marked that the horny layer is often thicker than the atrophic stratum malpighii, which may be

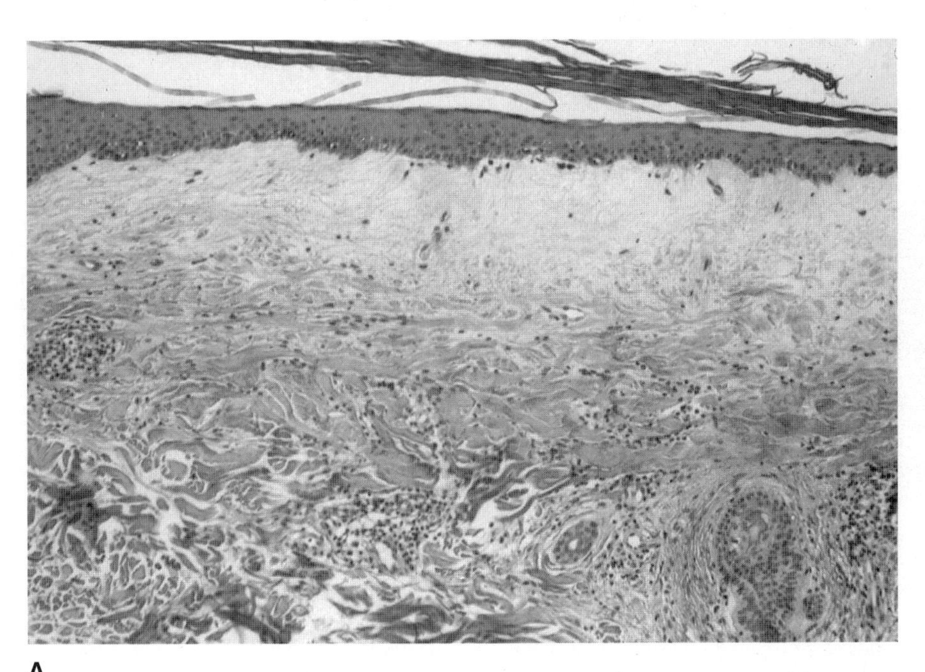

A

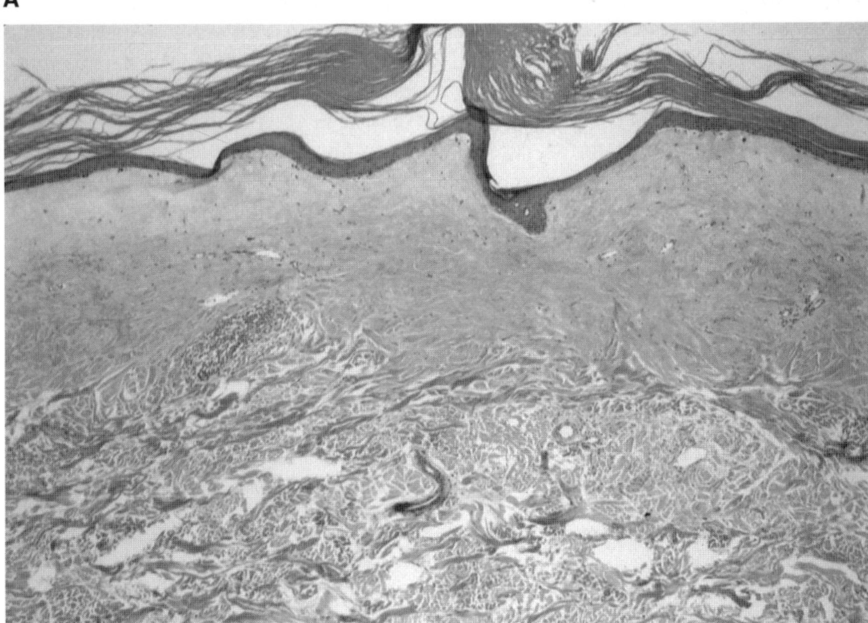

B

FIG. 10-15. Lichen sclerosus
(**A**) An early lesion of lichen sclerosus showing a subepidermal zone of pallor. The compact hyperorthokeratotic scale and atrophic epidermis, zone of pallor, and subjacent, variably dense interstitial lymphocytic inflammatory infiltrate delineating the depth of this process, give the skin a "trilayered" or "striped" appearance (original magnification ×100). (**B**) A well-established lesion, showing a thick hyperkeratotic scale, follicular plugging, an atrophic epidermis, and pale superficial dermal stroma markedly different from normal deep reticular dermis (original magnification ×20). *(continued on next page)*

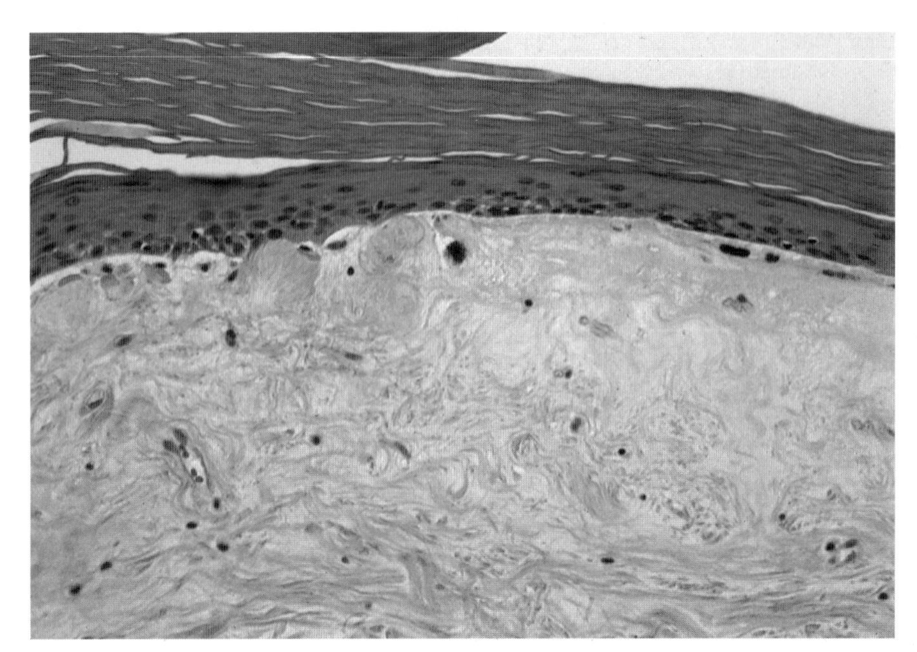

C

FIG. 10-15. *Continued*
(**C**) Intermittent cleft-like spaces separate an atrophic epidermis from a pale dermis, which may contain occasional melanophages (original magnification ×200).

reduced to a few layers of flattened cells (Fig. 10-15A and B). The cells of the basal layer show hydropic degeneration. The rete ridges often are completely absent, although they may persist in a few areas and show some irregular downward proliferation. In such proliferations, hydropic degeneration of the basal cells usually is pronounced.

Plugging of appendageal ostia by keratotic plugs is often associated with atrophy and disappearance of appendageal structures (see Fig. 10-15B). Keratotic plugging is not apparent in mucosal lesions. In the latter areas, particularly the vulva, squamous hyperplasia adjacent to the atrophic epidermis can be found in about one third of patients with LS. There may be varying degrees of "dysplasia" consisting of disorderly arrangement of the cells and enlarged, hyperchromatic nuclei. Transition into carcinoma, however, is said to be rare.[122]

Beneath the epidermis is a broad zone of pronounced lymphedema (Fig. 10-15A and C). Within this zone, the collagenous fibers are swollen and homogeneous and contain only a few nuclei. They stain poorly with eosin and other connective-tissue stains. The blood and lymph vessels are dilated, and there may be areas of hemorrhage. Elastic fibers are sparse and, in old lesions, are absent within the area of lymphedema.[123] In areas of severe lymphedema, clinically visible bullae may form; they are found in subepidermal locations.[124] Shrinkage within the area of lymphedema may occur during the process of dehydration of the specimen, resulting in the formation of pseudobullae, which often are located intradermally.

Except in lesions of long duration, an inflammatory infiltrate is present in the dermis. The younger the lesion, the more superficial is the location of the infiltrate. In very early lesions and at the periphery of somewhat older lesions, the infiltrate may be found in the uppermost dermis, in direct apposition to the basal layer. Soon, however, a narrow zone of edema and homogenization of the collagen displaces the inflammatory infiltrate farther down, so that, in well-developed lesions, the infiltrate is found in the mid-dermis. The infiltrate can be patchy, but it is often band-like and composed of lymphoid cells admixed with plasma cells and histiocytes. In old lesions in which the infiltrate is slight or absent, the collagen bundles in the midportion and lower dermis may appear swollen, homogeneous, and hyperchromatic, thus appearing sclerotic (hence lichen *sclerosus*).

Pathogenesis. Changes in the dermal matrix have been detected in LS. By electron microscopy, collagen fibrils often lack cross striation and in cross sections sometimes have the appearance of empty tubes, suggesting degeneration of collagen fibrils.[125] In some areas new immature collagen of reduced and variable diameter (40–80 nm) is seen.[126] Ultrastructural studies also have shown degeneration of subepidermal elastin and increases in ground substance.[127]

In the epidermis intercellular edema separates epidermal cells that show degenerative changes. There is nearly a complete absence of melanosomes within the keratinocytes. This is the result either of degeneration and disappearance of the melanocytes[126] or of inhibition of the transfer of melanosomes from the melanocytes to the keratinocytes.[128]

Differential Diagnosis. Very early lesions may resemble lichen planus because of the apposition of the inflammatory infiltrate to the basal layer. However, the basal cells are not replaced by flattened squamous cells, as in lichen planus, but appear hydropic, and a subepidermal zone of edema usually has already begun to form in some areas in lichen sclerosus et atrophicus.

Old lesions of lichen sclerosus et atrophicus with thickening and hyperchromasia of the collagen bundles in the midportion and lower dermis and only a slight inflammatory infiltrate may resemble morphea. Nevertheless, the epidermis in morphea, although it may be thin, shows neither hydropic degeneration of the basal cells nor follicular plugging, and the upper dermis in morphea has elastic fibers and shows no zone of edema.[123] Still, in lesions in which lichen sclerosus et atrophicus develops either secondarily to morphea or simultaneously with it, there are, in addition to the epidermal and subepidermal changes of lichen sclerosus et atrophicus, changes indicative of morphea in the lower dermis and in the subcutaneous fat. A definite diagnosis of both lichen sclerosus et atrophicus and morphea in the same lesion can be made only if the newly formed collagen extends into the subcutaneous fat and consists of faintly staining, homogeneous collagen.[129]

REFERENCES

1. Tan EM, Cohen AS, Fries JF et al. The 1982 revised criteria for the classification of systemic lupus erythematosus. Arthritis Rheum 1982; 25:1271.
2. Wechsler HL. Lupus erythematosus (editorial). A clinician's coign of vantage. Arch Dermatol 1983;119:877.
3. Ropes M. Observations on the natural course of disseminated lupus erythematosus. Medicine (Baltimore) 1964:43:387.
4. Hahn BH. Management of systemic lupus erythematosus. In: Kelley WN, Harris ED Jr, Ruddy S, Sledge CB, eds. Textbook of Rheumatology. 4th ed. Philadelphia: Saunders, 1994;1043.
5. Ginzler EM, Schorn K. Outcome and prognosis in systemic lupus erythematosus. Rheum Dis Clin North Am 1988;14:67.
6. David-Bajar KM, Bennion SD, DeSpain JD et al. Clinical, histologic, and immunofluorescent distinctions between subacute cutaneous lupus erythematosus and discoid lupus erythematosus. J Invest Dermatol 1992;99:251.
7. Jerdan MS, Hood AF, Moore GW, Callen JP. Histopathologic comparison of the subsets of lupus erythematosus. Arch Dermatol 1990; 126:52.
8. Uitto J, Santa-Cruz DJ, Eisen AZ, Leone P. Verrucous lesions in patients with discoid lupus erythematosus. Br J Dermatol 1978;98:507.
9. de Berker D, Dissaneyeka M, Burge S. The sequelae of chronic cutaneous lupus erythematosus. Lupus 1992;1:181.
10. O'Loughlin S, Schroeter AL, Jordon RE. A study of lupus erythematosus with particular reference to generalized discoid lupus. Br J Dermatol 1978;99:1.
11. Millard LG, Rowell NR. Abnormal laboratory test results and their relationship to prognosis in discoid lupus erythematosus. Arch Dermatol 1979;115:1055.
12. Estes D, Christian CL. The natural history of systemic lupus erythematosus by prospective analysis. Medicine (Baltimore) 1971;50:85.
13. Vinciullo C. Hypertrophic lupus erythematosus: Differentiation from squamous cell carcinoma. Australas J Dermatol 1986;27:76.
14. Bielicky T, Trapl J. Nichtvernarbender chronischer erythematodes. Arch Klin Exp Dermatol 1963;217:438.
15. Ueki H, Wolff HH, Braun-Falco O. Cutaneous localization of human gamma globulins in lupus erythematosus. Arch Dermatol Forsch 1974;248:297.
16. Panet-Raymond G, Johnson WC. Lupus erythematosus and polymorphous light eruption. Arch Dermatol 1973;108:785.
17. Akasu R, Kahn HJ, From L. Lymphocyte markers on formalin-fixed tissue in Jessner's lymphocytic infiltrate and lupus erythematosus. J Cutan Pathol 1992,19:59.
18. Pandya AG, Sontheimer RD, Cockerell CJ et al. Papulonodular mucinosis associated with systemic lupus erythematosus: Possible mechanisms of increased glycosaminoglycan accumulation. A Am Acad Dermatol 1995;32:199.
19. Sontheimer RD. Subacute cutaneous lupus erythematosus: A decade's perspective. Med Clin North Am 1989;73:1073.
20. Lee LA. Neonatal lupus erythematosus. J Invest Dermatol 1993; 100: 9S.
21. Provost TT. Subsets in systemic lupus erythematosus. J Invest Dermatol 1979;72:110.
22. Gilliam JN. Systemic lupus erythematosus and the skin. In: Lahita RG, ed. Systemic lupus erythematosus. New York: John Wiley & Sons, 1987; 615.
23. Callen JP. Chronic cutaneous lupus erythematosus. Arch Dermatol 1982;118:412.
24. Mascart-Lemone F, Hauptmann G, Goetz J et al. Genetic deficiency of C4 presenting with recurrent infections and a systemic lupus erythematosus-like disease. Am J Med 1983;75:295.
25. Tappeiner G, Hintner H, Scholz S et al. Systemic lupus erythematosus in hereditary deficiency of the fourth component of complement. J Am Acad Dermatol 1982;7:66.
26. Provost TT, Zone JJ, Synkowski D et al. Unusual cutaneous manifestations of systemic lupus erythematosus. Urticaria-like lesions: Correlation with clinical and serologic abnormalities. J Invest Dermatol 1980;75:495.
27. Callen JP. Mucocutaneous changes in patients with lupus erythematosus: The relationship of these lesions to systemic disease. Rhem Dis Clin North Am 1988;14:79.
28. Camisa C. Vesiculobullous systemic lupus erythematosus: A report of four cases. J Am Acad Dermatol 1988;18:93.
29. Gammon WR, Briggaman RA. Bullous SLE: A phenotypically distinctive but immunologically heterogeneous bullous disorder. J Invest Dermatol 1993;100:28S.
30. Schur PH. Clinical features of SLE. In: Kelley WN, Harris ED Jr, Ruddy S, Sledge CB, eds. Textbook of Rheumatology. 4th ed. Philadelphia: Saunders, 1994;1017.
31. Klemperer P, Pollack AD, Baehr G. Pathology of disseminated lupus erythematosus. Arch Pathol 1941;32:569.
32. Asherson RA, Baguley E, Pal C, Hughes GR. Antiphospholipid syndrome: Five year follow up. Ann Rheum Dis 1991;50:805.
33. Bick RL, Baker WF Jr. The antiphospholipid and thrombosis syndromes. Med Clin North Am 1994;78:667.
34. Tuffanelli DL. Cutaneous immunopathology: Recent observations. J Invest Dermatol 1975;65:143.
35. Provost TT, Andres G, Maddison PJ, Reichlin M. Lupus band test in untreated SLE patients. J Invest Dermatol 1980;74:407.
36. Gately LE, Nesbitt LT. Update on immunofluorescent testing in bullous diseases and lupus erythematosus. Dermatol Clin 1994;1:133.
37. Jaworsky C, Murphy GF. Special techniques in dermatology. Arch Dermatol 1989;125:963.
38. Olansky AJ, Briggaman RA, Gammon WR et al. Bullous systemic lupus erythematosus. J Am Acad Dermatol 1982;7:511.
39. Woods VG Jr. Pathogenesis of systemic lupus erythematosus. In: Kelley WN, Harris ED, Ruddy S, Sledge CB, eds. Textbook of Rheumatology. 4th ed. Philadelphia: Saunders, 1994;999.
40. Jessner M, Kanof NB. Lymphocytic infiltration of the skin. Arch Dermatol Syphiligr 1953;68:447.
41. Toonstra J, Wildschut A, Boer J et al. Jessner's lymphocytic infiltration of the skin. Arch Dermatol 1989;125:1525.
42. Higgins CR, Wakeel RA, Cerio R. Childhood Jessner's lymphocytic infiltrate of the skin. Br J Dermatol 1994;131:99.
43. Konttinen YT, Bergroth V, Johansson E et al. A long-term clinicopathologic survey of patients with Jessner's lymphocytic infiltration of the skin. J Invest Dermatol 1987;89:205.
44. Cerio R, Oliver GF, Spaull J et al. The heterogeneity of Jessner's lymphocytic infiltrate (abstr). J Cutan Pathol 1988;15:300.
45. Sharp GC, Irvin WS, Tan EM et al. Mixed connective tissue disease: An apparently distinct rheumatic disease syndrome associated with a specific antibody to an extractable nuclear antigen (ENA). Am J Med 1972;52:148.
46. Ueda N, Mimura K, Meada H et al. Mixed connective tissue disease with fatal pulmonary hypertension and a review of the literature. Virchows Arch A Pathol Anat Histopathol 1984;404:335.
47. Burrows NP, Bhogal BS, Russel Jones R, Black MM. Clinicopathological significance of cutaneous epidermal nuclear staining by direct immunofluorescence. J Cutan Pathol 1993;20:159.
48. Callen JP, Tuffanelli DL, Provost TT. Collagen vascular disease: An update. J Am Acad Dermatol 1994;28:477.
49. Cronin ME, Plotz PH. Idiopathic inflammatory myopathies. Rheum Dis Clin North Am 1990;16:655.
50. Callen JP. Malignancy in polymyositis/dermatomyositis. Clin Dermatol 1988;6:55.
51. Whittmore SE, Rosenshein NB, Provost TT. Ovarian cancer in patients with dermatomyositis. Medicine (Baltimore) 1994;73:153.
52. Bohan A, Peter JB, Bowman RL et al. A computer-assisted analysis of 153 patients with polymyositis and dermatomyositis. Medicine (Baltimore) 1977;56:255.
53. Janis JF, Winkelmann RK. Histopathology of the skin in dermatomyositis. Arch Dermatol 1968;97:640.
54. Hanno R, Callen JP. Histopathology of Gottron's papules. J Cutan Pathol 1985;12:389.
55. DeGirolami UU, Smith TW. Teaching monograph: Pathology of skeletal muscle diseases. Am J Pathol 1982;107:231.
56. Kissel JT, Mendell JR, Rammohan KW. Microvascular deposition of complement membrane attack complex in dermatomyositis. N Engl J Med 1986;314:329.

57. Wainger CK, Lever WF. Dermatomyositis: A report of three cases with postmortem observations. Arch Dermatol Syph 1949;59:196.
58. Harrist TJ, Mihm MC Jr. Cutaneous immunopathology: The diagnostic use of direct and indirect immunofluorescence techniques in dermatologic diseases (review). Hum Pathol 1979;10:625.
59. Samman PD. The natural history of parapsoriasis en plaques (chronic superficial dermatitis) and prereticulotic poikiloderma. Br J Dermatol 1972;87:405.
60. Steigleder GK. Die poikilodermien-genodermien und genodermatosen? Arch Dermatol Syph (Berlin) 1952;194:461.
61. Braun-Falco O, Marghescu S. Kongenitales teleangiektatisches erythem (Bloom-Syndrom) mit diabetes insipidus. Hautarzt 1966;17:155.
62. Lindae ML, Abel EA, Hoppe RT, Wood GS. Poikilodermatous mycosis fungoides and large-plaque parapsoriasis exhibit similar abnormalities of T-cell antigen expression. Arch Dermatol 1988;124:366.
63. Diaz-Perez JL, Connolly SM, Winkelmann RK. Disabling pansclerotic morphea of children. Arch Dermatol 1980;116:169.
64. Ikai K, Tagami H, Imamura S, Hayakawa M. Morphea-like cutaneous changes in a patient with systemic scleroderma. Dermatologica 1979; 158:438.
65. Callen JP, Tuffanelli DL, Provost TT. Collagen-vascular disease: An update. J Am Acad Dermatol 1993;28:477.
66. Sahn EE, Garen PD, Silver RM, Maize JC. Scleroderma following augmentation mammoplasty. Arch Dermatol 1990;126:1198.
67. Joly P, Lampert A, Thomine E, Lauret P. Development of pseudobullous morphea and scleroderma-like illness during therapy with L-5 hydroxytryptophan and carbidopa. J Am Acad Dermatol 1991;25:332.
68. Toxic Epidemic Syndrome Study Group. Toxic epidemic syndrome: Spain, 1981. Lancet 1982;2:697.
69. Oursler JR, Farmer ER, Roubenoff R et al. Cutaneous manifestations of the eosinophilia-myalgia syndrome. Br J Dermatol 1992;127:138.
70. Falanga V, Medsger TA Jr, Reichlin M, Rodnan GP. Linear scleroderma: Clinical spectrum, prognosis, and laboratory abnormalities. Ann Intern Med 1986;104:849.
71. Dilley JJ, Perry HO. Bilateral linear scleroderma en coup de sabre. Arch Dermatol 1968;97:688.
72. Su WPD, Greene SL. Bullous morphea profunda. Am J Dermatopathol 1986;8:144.
73. Synkowski DR, Lobitz WC Jr, Provost TT. Bullous scleroderma. Arch Dermatol 1981;117:135.
74. Buechner SA, Winkelmann RK, Lautenschlager S et al. Localized scleroderma associated with Borrelia burgdorferi infection: Clinical, histologic, and immunohistochemical observations. J Am Acad Dermatol 1993;29:190.
75. Weinecke R, Schlupen EM, Zochling N et al. No evidence for Borrelia burgdorferi-specific DNA in lesions of localized scleroderma. J Invest Dermatol 1995;104:23.
76. Fleischmajer R, Nedwich A. Generalized morphea: I. Histology of the dermis and subcutaneous tissue. Arch Dermatol 1972;106:509.
77. O'Leary PA, Montgomery H, Ragsdale WE. Dermatohistopathology of various types of scleroderma (review). Arch Dermatol 1957;75:78.
78. Hickman JW, Sheils WS. Progressive facial hemiatrophy. Arch Intern Med 1964;113:716.
79. Maricq HR. Capillary abnormalities, Raynaud's phenomenon, and systemic sclerosis in patients with localized scleroderma. Arch Dermatol 1992;128:630.
80. Medsger TA, Masi AT, Rodnan GP et al. Survival with systemic sclerosis (scleroderma). Ann Intern Med 1971;75:369.
81. Fleischmajer R, Nedwich A. Generalized morphea: I. Histology of the dermis and subcutaneous tissue. Arch Dermatol 1972;106:509.
82. Abu-Shakra M, Guillemin F, Lee P. Cancer is systemic sclerosis. Arthritis Rheum 1993;36:460.
83. Tuffanelli DL. Systemic scleroderma. Med Clin North Am 1989;73: 1167.
84. Jablonska S, Blaszczyk M, Chorzelski TP et al. Clinical relevance of immunologic findings in scleroderma. Clin Dermatol 1993;10:407.
85. Prescott RJ, Freemont AJ, Jones CJ et al. Sequential dermal microvascular and perivascular changes in the development of scleroderma. J Pathol 1992;166:255.
86. Haustein UF, Herrmann K, Böhme HJ. Pathogenesis of progressive systemic sclerosis (review). Int J Dermatol 1986;25:286.
87. Toth A, Alpert LI. Progressive systemic sclerosis terminating as periarteritis nodosa. Arch Pathol 1971;92:31.
88. Postlewaithe AE. Connective tissue metabolism including cytokines in scleroderma. Curr Opin Rheumatol 1993;5:766.
89. Rudnicka L, Varga J, Christiano AM et al. Elevated expression of type VII collagen in the skin of patients with systemic sclerosis: Regulation by transforming growth factor-beta. J Clin Invest 1994;93:1709.
90. Varga J, Rudnicka L, Uitto J. Connective tissue alterations in systemic sclerosis (review). Clin Dermatol 1994;12:387.
91. Sappino AP, Masouyé, Saurat JH, Gabbiani G. Smooth muscle differentiation in scleroderma fibroblastic cells. Am J Pathol 1990;137:585.
92. Aiba S, Tabata N, Ohtani H, Tagami H. CD34+ spindle-shaped cells selectively dissapear from the skin lesion of scleroderma. Arch Dermatol 1994;130:593.
93. Aeschlimann A, Meyer O, Bourgeois P et al. Anti-Scl-70 antibodies detected by immunoblotting in progressive systemic sclerosis: Specificity and clinical correlations. Ann Rheum Dis 1989;48:992.
94. Prystowsky SD, Gilliam JN, Tuffanelli D. Epidermal nucleolar IgG deposition in clinically normal skin. Arch Dermatol 1971;114:536.
95. Lapenas D, Rodnan GP, Cavallo T. Immunopathology of the renal vascular lesion of progressive systemic sclerosis (scleroderma). Am J Pathol 1978;91:243.
96. Quiroga ML, Woscoff A. L'atrophodermie idiopathique progressive (Pasini-Pierini) et la sclérodermie atypique lilacée non indurée (Gougerot). Ann Dermatol Syphiligr 1961;88:507.
97. Miller RF. Idiopathic atrophoderma (review). Arch Dermatol 1965; 92:653.
98. Weiner M. In discussion to Eshelman OM: Idiopathic atrophoderma of Pasini and Pierini. Arch Dermatol 1965;92:737.
99. Kencka D, Blaszczyk M, Jablonska S. Atrophoderma Pasini-Pierini is a primary atrophic abortive morphea. Dermatology 1995;190:203.
100. Rupec M. Über die Beziehungen der zirkumskripten sklerodermie zum morbus Pasini-Pierini. Z Hautkr 1962;33:114.
101. Buechner SA, Rufli T. Atrophoderma of Pasini and Pierini: Clinical and histopathologic findings and antibodies to Borrelia burgdorferi in thirty-four patients. J Am Acad Dermatol 1994;30:441.
102. Shulman L. Diffuse fasciitis with hypergammaglobulinemia and eosinophilia: A new syndrome? (abstr). J Rheumatol 1974;1:46.
103. Freundlich B, Werth VP, Rook AH et al. L-Tryptophan ingestion associated with eosinophilic fasciitis but not progressive systemic sclerosis. Ann Int Med 1990;112:758.
104. Golitz LE. Fasciitis with eosinophilia: The Shulman syndrome. Int J Dermatol 1980;19:552.
105. Barriere H, Stalder JF, Berger M et al. Syndrome de Shulman. Ann Dermatol Venereol 1980;107:643.
106. Tamura T, Saito Y, Ishikawa H. Diffuse fasciitis with eosinophilia. Acta Derm Venereol (Stockh) 1979;59:325.
107. Weinstein D, Schwartz RA. Eosinophilic fasciitis. Arch Dermatol 1978;114:1047.
108. Lupton GP, Goette DK. Localized eosinophilic fasciitis. Arch Dermatol 1979;115:85.
109. Jablonska S, Hamm G, Kencka D, Sieminska S. Fasciitis eosinophilica, Übergang in eine eigenartige sklerodermie (sklerodermie-fasciitis). Z Hautkr 1984;59:711.
110. Su WPD, Person JR. Morphea profunda. Am J Dermatopathol 1981; 3:251.
111. Helfman T, Falanga V. Eosinophilic fasciitis. Clin Dermatol 1994;12: 449.
112. Meffert JJ, Davis BM, Grimwood RE. Lichen sclerosus. J Am Acad Dermatol 1995;32:393.
113. Ledwig PA, Weigand DA. Late circumcision and lichen sclerosus et atrophicus of the penis. J Am Acad Dermatol 1989;20:211.
114. Loening-Baucke V. Lichen sclerosus et atrophicus in children. Am J Dis Child 1991;145:1058.
115. Clark JA, Muller SA. Lichen sclerosus et atrophicus in children. Arch Dermatol 1967;95:476.
116. Helm KF, Gibson LE, Muller SA. Lichen sclerosus et atrophicus in children and young adults. Pediatr Dermatol 1991;8:97.
117. Woodruff JD, Baens JS. Interpretation of atrophic and hypertrophic alterations in the vulvar epithelium. Am J Obstet Gynecol 1963;86: 713.
118. Pock L. Koebner phenomenon in lichen sclerosus et atrophicus (letter). Dermatologica 1990;181:76.
119. Shono S, Imura M, Osaku A et al. Lichen sclerosus et atrophicus, morphea and coexistence of both diseases. Histologic studies using lectins. Arch Dermatol 1991;127:1352.
120. Tremaine R, Adam JE, Orizaga M. Morphea coexisting with lichen sclerosus et atrophicus. Int J Dermatol 1990;29:486.

121. Wallace HJ. Lichen sclerosus et atrophicus (review). Trans St Johns Hosp Dermatol Soc 1971;57:9.
122. Hart WR, Norris HJ, Helwig EB. Relation of lichen sclerosus et atrophicus of the vulva to development of carcinoma. Obstet Gynecol 1975;45:369.
123. Steigleder GK, Raab WP. Lichen sclerosus et atrophicus. Arch Dermatol 1961;84:219.
124. Gottschalk HR, Cooper ZK. Lichen sclerosus et atrophicus with bullous lesions and extensive involvement. Arch Dermatol 1947;55:433.
125. Mann PR, Cowan MA. Ultrastructural changes in four cases of lichen sclerosus et atrophicus. Br J Dermatol 1973;89:223.
126. Kint A, Geerts ML. Lichen sclerosus et atrophicus: An electron microscopic study. J Cutan Pathol 1975;2:30.
127. Frances C, Weschler J, Meimon G et al. Investigation of intercellular matrix macromolecules involved in lichen sclerosus. Acta Derm Venereol (Stockh) 1983;63:483.
128. Klug H, Sönnichsen N. Elektronenoptische untersuchungen bei lichen sklerosus et atrophicus. Dermatol Monatsschr 1972;158:641.
129. Uitto J, Santa Cruz DJ, Bauer EA, Eisen AZ. Morphea and lichen sclerosus et atrophicus: Clinical and histopathologic studies in patients with combined features. J Am Acad Dermatol 1980;3:271.

Lever's Histopathology of the Skin, eighth edition,
edited by David Elder et al. Lippincott–
Raven Publishers, Philadelphia © 1997.

CHAPTER 11

Cutaneous Toxicities of Drugs

Thomas Horn

Multiple mechanisms exist by which drugs affect the skin. These mechanisms often relate directly to histologic expression of drug effect. IgE-mediated hypersensitivity to penicillin may manifest as urticaria with dermal edema and a perivascular and interstitial infiltrate of lymphocytes and eosinophils. Necrosis of cutaneous structures may be caused by bleomycin or thio-TEPA independent of preceding inflammation. Human recombinant cytokines given in pharmacologic doses represent a new class of drug. The histopathology of cutaneous eruptions attributable to cytokine therapy varies according to the immunologic effects of the inciting cytokine.

Several medication-related cutaneous eruptions are considered elsewhere in the text, including urticaria (Chap. 7), erythema multiforme (Chap. 9), toxic epidermal necrolysis (Chap. 9), erythema nodosum (Chap. 20), erythroderma (Chap. 9), vasculitis (Chap. 8), and corticosteroid-induced acne (Chap. 18).

EXANTHEMIC DRUG ERUPTIONS

Eruptive and efflorescent cutaneous drug reactions are perhaps the most common adverse effects of medications. Morbilliform and pustular eruptions are considered under this heading. Virtually any drug may be associated with a morbilliform eruption; the nonspecific clinical and histologic changes make definitive implication of a specific agent difficult. The most common class of medications causing morbilliform eruptions is antibacterial antibiotics.[1] The morbilliform rash consists of fine blanching papules, which appear suddenly, are symmetric, and often are brightly erythematous in Caucasian patients.[2]

Various drugs are implicated in acute generalized exanthemic pustulosis.[3] Widespread pustules develop within a period of hours after administration of the offending agent. Although viral infection and mercury exposure are cited as causes, antibacterial antibiotics are most often implicated with a broad range of other medications as well, including acetaminophen. Fever, leukocytosis, purpura, and clinical features suggesting erythema multiforme accompany the pustules.

Histopathology. The typical morbilliform drug eruption displays a variable, often sparse, mainly perivascular infiltrate of lymphocytes and eosinophils. Eosinophils may be absent. Some vacuolization of the dermal-epidermal junction with few apoptotic epidermal cells may be observed, but not to the degree typical of erythema multiforme or toxic epidermal necrolysis.

The largest series describing skin biopsy samples of acute generalized exanthematous pustulosis notes "spongiform superficial pustules (42 of 64 biopsy specimens), papillary edema (39 of 64), polymorphous perivascular infiltrates with eosinophils (22 of 64), and leukocytoclastic vasculitis (13 of 64) with fibrinoid deposition (7 of 13)."[2] (See Figs. 11-1A and B.)

Differential Diagnosis. Distinction of morbilliform drug eruption from viral exanthem in the absence of eosinophils is generally not possible. More than occasional dyskeratotic epidermal cells should prompt consideration of erythema multiforme, toxic epidermal necrolysis, or fixed drug eruption. Currently, the nosology of acute generalized exanthematous pustulosis is unclear. Based strictly on histologic descriptions, distinction from pustular psoriasis, subcorneal pustular dermatosis, and, in some instances, leukocytoclastic vasculitis cannot be made.

DRUG ERUPTIONS PRIMARILY CHARACTERIZED BY INTERFACE DERMATITIS

The histologic features comprising interface dermatitis (see Chap. 9) include vacuolar alteration of the basilar epidermis, necrotic keratinocytes, flattening of basilar keratinocytes, variable infiltration of the upper dermis by lymphocytes and histiocytes, variable exocytosis, and melanophages. These findings may be induced by drugs in several different but reproducible patterns including erythema multiforme, toxic epidermal necrolysis, lichenoid drug eruption, and fixed drug eruption.

ERYTHEMA MULTIFORME AND TOXIC EPIDERMAL NECROLYSIS

Erythema multiforme is characterized by target or "bull's-eye" erythematous edematous macules in varied distribution

T. Horn: Department of Dermatology, Johns Hopkins University, Baltimore, MD

but with predilection for the palms and soles. In contrast, toxic epidermal necrolysis displays diffuse erythema with the patient complaining of tender skin. Blisters may develop in both disorders as well as mucosal and conjunctival involvement. Medications associated with increased risk for these entities include sulfonamides, trimethoprim-sulfamethoxazole, phenobarbital, carbamazipine, phenytoin, oxicam nonsteroidal antiinflammatory agents, allopurinol, chlormezanone, and corticosteroids.[4]

Histopathology. In the spectrum of interface dermatitides, erythema multiforme and toxic epidermal necrolysis display greater keratinocyte necrosis and less inflammation than other disorders. Necrotic keratinocytes are found at all epidermal levels in the fully evolved lesion and may become confluent to form a thoroughly necrotic blister roof. Bullae are subepidermal (see Chap. 9).

LICHENOID DRUG ERUPTION

Lichenoid drug eruption shares clinical similarity to lichen planus. Erythematous to violaceous papules and plaques develop on the trunk and extremities in association with drug ingestion. Implicated agents include gold, antihypertensive medications (especially captopril), penicillamine, and chloroquine.[5]

Histopathology. Lichenoid drug eruption is also similar to lichen planus histologically. In comparison with erythema multiforme and toxic epidermal necrolysis, lichenoid drug eruptions are more heavily inflamed with a more prominent interstitial pattern. Differentiation from lichen planus may not be possible. Numerous eosinophils, parakeratosis, and perivascular inflammation around the mid and deep dermal plexuses are generally absent in lichen planus and should prompt consideration of a lichenoid drug eruption (see also Chap. 7).

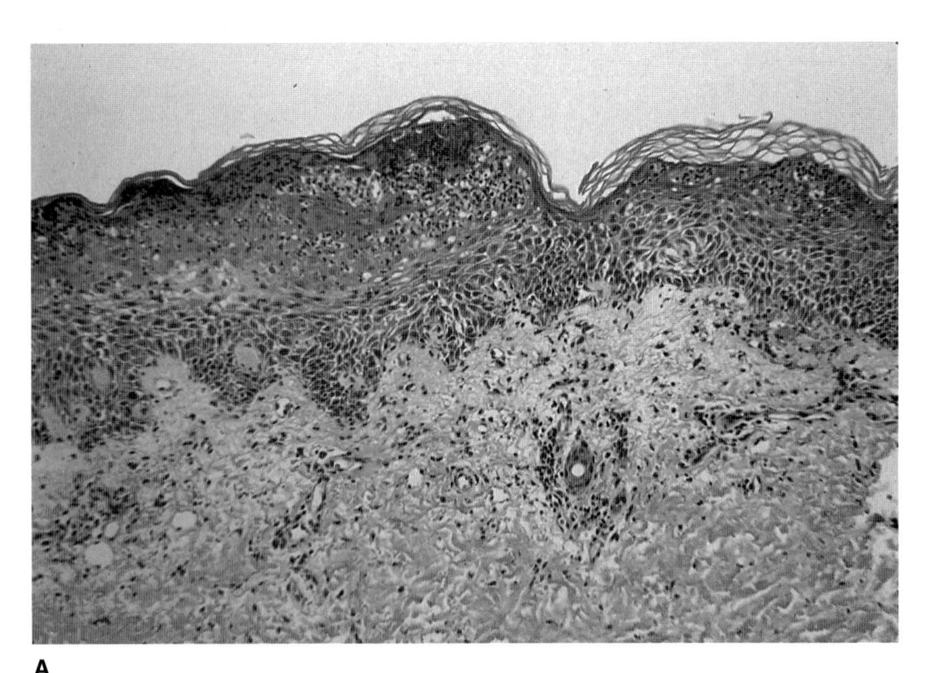

A

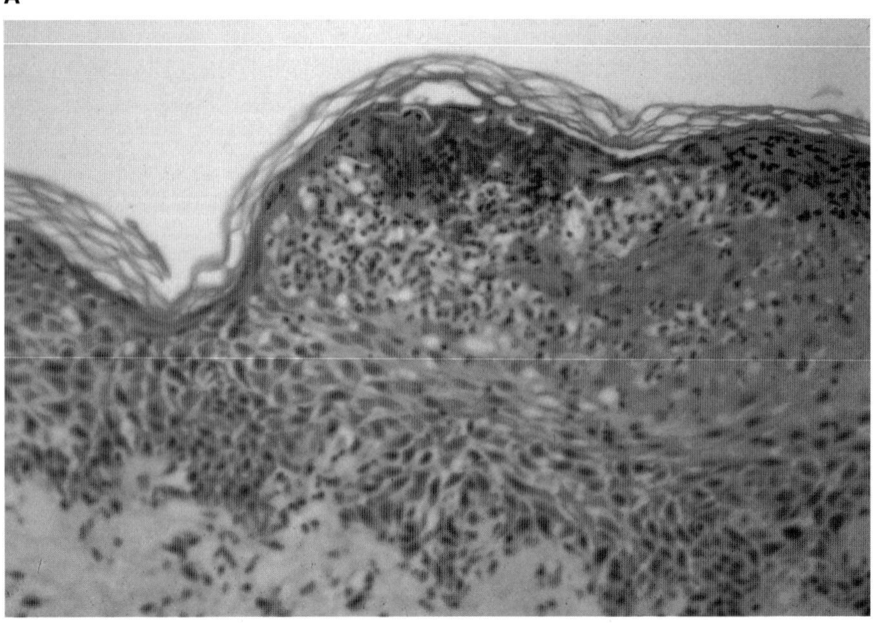

B

FIG. 11-1. Acute generalized exanthematous pustulosis
(**A**) Diffuse spongiosis is present with an upper dermal perivascular infiltrate and upper epidermal pustule. Ampicillin was the inciting drug. (**B**) A subcorneal and intraspinous collection of neutrophils is present.

FIXED DRUG ERUPTION

Fixed drug eruptions show circumscribed lesions that recur persistently at the same site with each administration of the implicated drug. Increasing numbers of lesions may occur with each successive administration. The most common type of fixed drug eruption consists of one or several slightly edematous, erythematous patches that may develop dusky centers, become bullous and, on healing, leave pigmented macules. Fixed drug eruptions occur most commonly after the ingestion of trimethoprim-sulfamethoxazole, acetylsalicylic acid, phenolphthalein, tetracycline, barbiturates, and phenylbutazone, but also occur after ingestion of various other drugs.[6]

Histopathology. The histologic changes observed in fixed drug eruption resemble erythema multiforme and toxic epidermal necrolysis. The frequent presence of hydropic degeneration of the basal cell layer leads to "pigmentary incontinence," which is characterized by the presence of melanin within macrophages in the upper dermis.[7,8] Scattered dyskeratotic keratinocytes with eosinophilic cytoplasm and pyknotic nuclei (often referred to as Civatte bodies, colloid bodies, or dyskeratotic cells) are frequently seen in the epidermis and represent apoptosis. Bullae form by detachment of the epidermis from the underlying dermis.[9] Not infrequently, the epidermis shows extensive confluent necrosis, even in areas in which it has not yet become detached. Confident distinction among fixed drug eruption, erythema multiforme, and toxic epidermal necrolysis, based on examination of a skin biopsy specimen alone, is not always possible.

Pathogenesis. On electron microscopic examination, the dyskeratotic keratinocytes are filled with thick, homogenized keratin tonofilaments and show only sparse remnants of organelles and nuclei. Keratinocytes located in the basal cell layer are often the most severely affected cells. The pigmentary incontinence develops when (1) lymphocytes migrate into the epidermis and cause damage to keratinocytes, which become dyskeratotic; (2) macrophages invade the epidermis and phagocytize the dyskeratotic keratinocytes together with their melanosomes; and (3) the macrophages return to the dermis, where they are able to digest all cellular remnants except for the melanosomes, which are resistant to digestion.[5] The process of pigmentary incontinence in fixed drug eruptions is similar to that occurring in incontinentia pigmenti (see Chap. 6). Expression of keratinocyte intercellular adhesion molecule-1 (ICAM-1, CD54) is sharply limited to lesional epidermis in fixed drug eruption. Localized induction of this adhesion molecule by drugs may explain the sharply circumscribed clinical lesions.[10]

CUTANEOUS REACTIONS TO ANTINEOPLASTIC CHEMOTHERAPEUTIC DRUGS

In general, the cutaneous changes brought about by antineoplastic chemotherapeutic agents are not primarily inflammatory in nature. Rather, the antiproliferative effects common to these drugs disrupt cutaneous cellular metabolism. Clinical manifestations vary. Neutrophilic eccrine hidradenitis presents with erythematous, often acral, plaques several days after cytoreductive chemotherapy. Acral erythema unassociated with primary eccrine changes also occurs after chemotherapy. Hyperpigmentation develops under occluded skin after thio-TEPA administration and in grouped linear streaks after busulfan. Diffuse hyperpigmentation commonly occurs after antineoplastic chemotherapy. Erythema preceding the hyperpigmentation in these settings is minimal or absent.

Histopathology. A common observation after cytoreductive chemotherapy is disruption of the normal pattern of keratinocyte maturation from small cuboidal cells in the basilar epidermis to flattened squames in the stratum corneum. At intervening epidermal levels, keratinocytes are separated by widened intercellular spaces, lose polarity, and display irregular large nuclei, midepidermal mitotic figures, and apoptosis (Figs. 11-2 and 11-3). These changes may be observed in the epidermis after any significant cytoreductive therapy, are not necessarily associated with clinical lesions, and may be termed *epidermal dysmaturation.* Upper dermal melanophages often

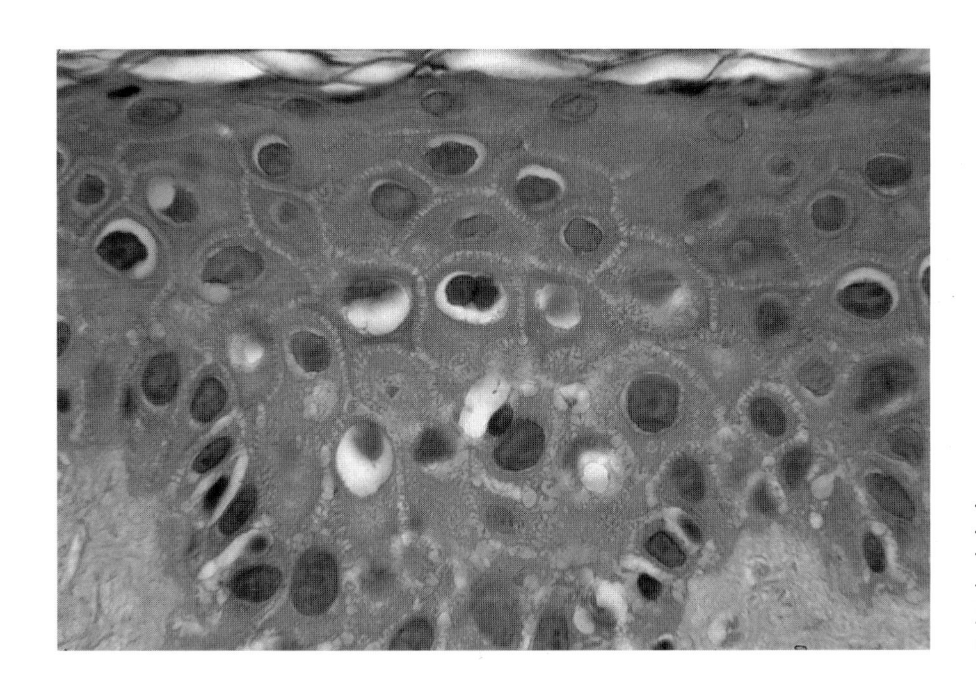

FIG. 11-2. Epidermal dysmaturation due to antineoplastic chemotherapy
This relatively mild example illustrates loss of polarity and disorganization of keratinocytes, including binucleate cells.

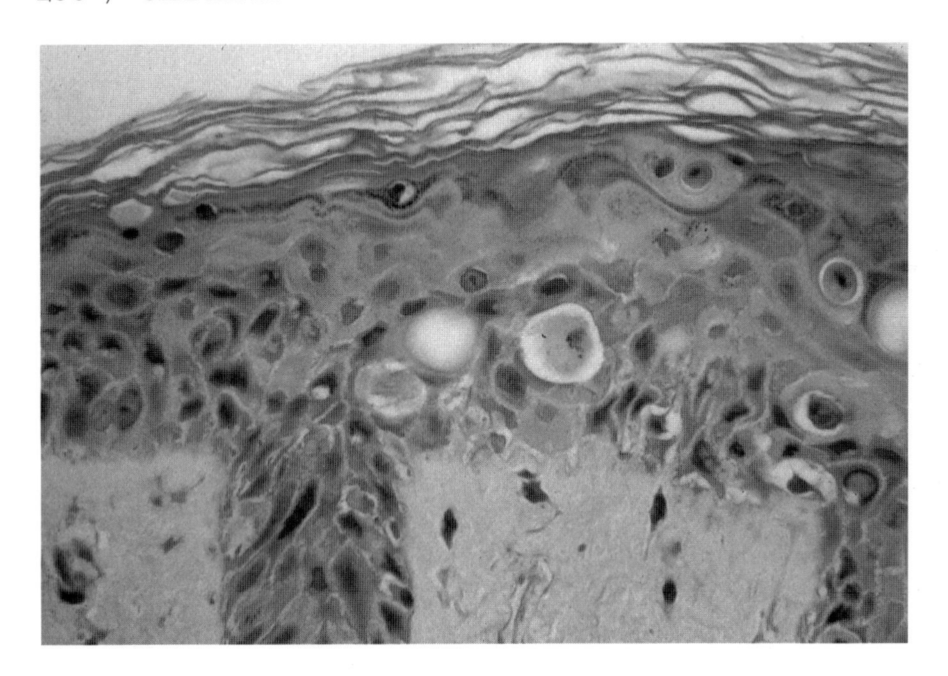

FIG. 11-3. Epidermal dysmaturation due to antineoplastic chemotherapy
Dysmaturation is more advanced in this example, with loss of keratinocyte polarity, highly irregular nuclear contours, multinucleation, and apoptosis.

accompany these changes. In this setting, "starburst" mitotic figures are described after systemic etoposide administration.[11] Numerous mid- and upper-level mitotic figures (so-called "mitotic arrest") are observed after podophyllotoxin application to condyloma. Etoposide and podophyllotoxin are vinca alkaloid derivatives, disrupting mitotic spindle formation by attaching to microtubule proteins.

Several entities in this section are unified by the theory of drug concentration in eccrine sweat. Specimens from patterned *postchemotherapy hyperpigmentation* show vacuolization of basilar epidermis, melanin incontinence, and apoptosis in occluded skin after administration of alkylating agents, specifically thio-TEPA.[12] Inflammation is sparse or absent. Squamous metaplasia of upper eccrine ducts, *syringosquamous metaplasia*, is described after cytoreductive therapies. The normally cuboidal cells lining the duct display irregularly increased amounts of eosinophilic cytoplasm with associated polymorphous inflammation, fibrosis, and necrosis.[13] *Neutrophilic eccrine hidradenitis* consists of variable infiltration of the eccrine coil by neutrophils and lymphocytes with necrosis of secretory epithelium (Figs. 11-4 and 11-5). Individual cells or whole coils show increased cytoplasmic eosinophilia (Fig. 11-6), degeneration of nuclei and loss of integrity of cell walls.[14,15]

Intralesional injection of bleomycin results in epidermal and eccrine necrosis, infiltration of the skin by neutrophils, and expression of HLA-DR and ICAM-1.[16]

Histogenesis. The notion of concentration of antineoplastic chemotherapeutic agents in sweat serves to unify the clinical observation of patterned hyperpigmentation (beneath bandages and electrocardiogram pads in the case of thio-TEPA) and the histologic observations of neutrophilic eccrine hidradenitis and syringosquamous metaplasia. Changes after antineoplastic chemotherapy likely represent a mix of direct toxic effect on the various constituent cells of the skin with secondary inflamma-

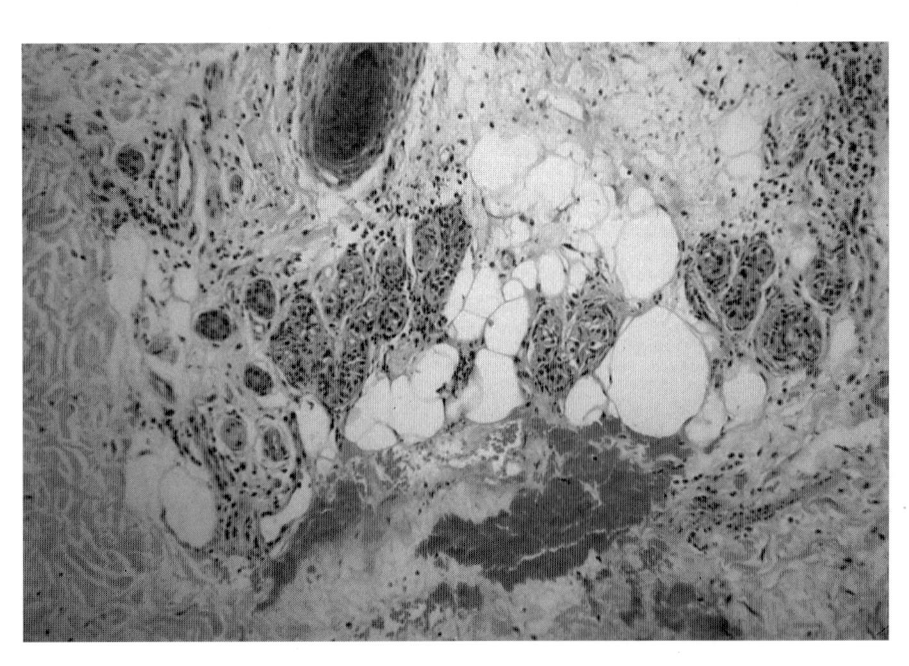

FIG. 11-4. Neutrophilic eccrine hidradenitis
Few inflammatory cells infiltrate and surround the eccrine coil.

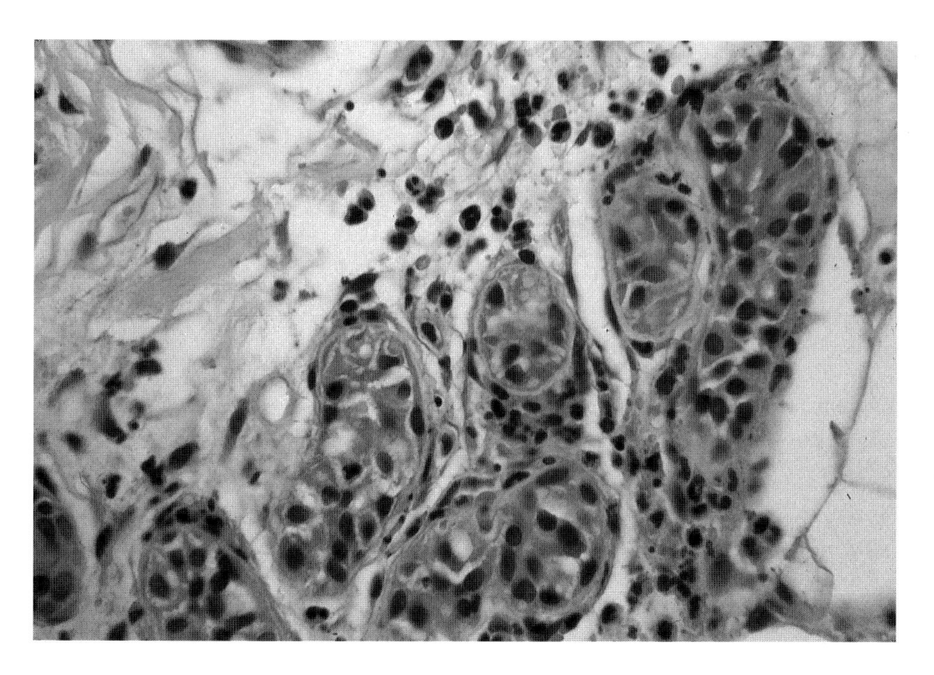

FIG. 11-5. Neutrophilic eccrine hidradenitis
Neutrophils and occasional mononuclear cells are present in the perieccrine adventitia. Some epithelial cells display early necrosis with increased cytoplasmic eosinophilia.

tion incited by cell damage. Other chemotherapy-related cutaneous changes may also involve similar mechanisms—namely, intertriginous erosion/ulceration after isophosphamide[17] and flagellate hyperpigmentation after busulfan.[18] Why specific agents affect specific cell populations in the skin in repeatable fashion is unclear. It is important to note that identification of epidermal dysmaturation assumes considerable importance in establishing the diagnosis of acute graft-versus-host reaction. When possible, the inflammation and apoptosis of a graft-versus-host reaction should be sought in areas unaffected or less affected by dysmaturation.

BULLAE AND SWEAT GLAND NECROSIS IN DRUG-INDUCED COMA

A patient who is in a coma as a result of an accident, illness, or a large dose of a narcotic drug may show, within a few hours, areas of erythema at sites of pressure. Usually within 24 hours, vesicles and bullae develop in the erythematous patches. The incidence of bullae depends on the severity of the coma and is highest in patients who subsequently die. Coma caused by carbon monoxide poisoning can also produce the lesions.[19] The bullae are located at sites subjected to pressure, such as the hands, wrists, scapulae, sacrum, knees, legs, ankles, and heels.

Histopathology. The epidermis shows varying degrees of necrosis. In areas of complete necrosis of the epidermis, the bullae arise subepidermally, but, in areas of only diminished viability showing eosinophilia of the cytoplasm and decreased staining of the nuclei, small intraepidermal vesicles may be seen. Where the epidermis is necrotic in its upper layers but not in its lower layers, even large bullae can form intraepidermally. Blisters may also form in a suprabasal location and may contain some acantholytic cells.[20]

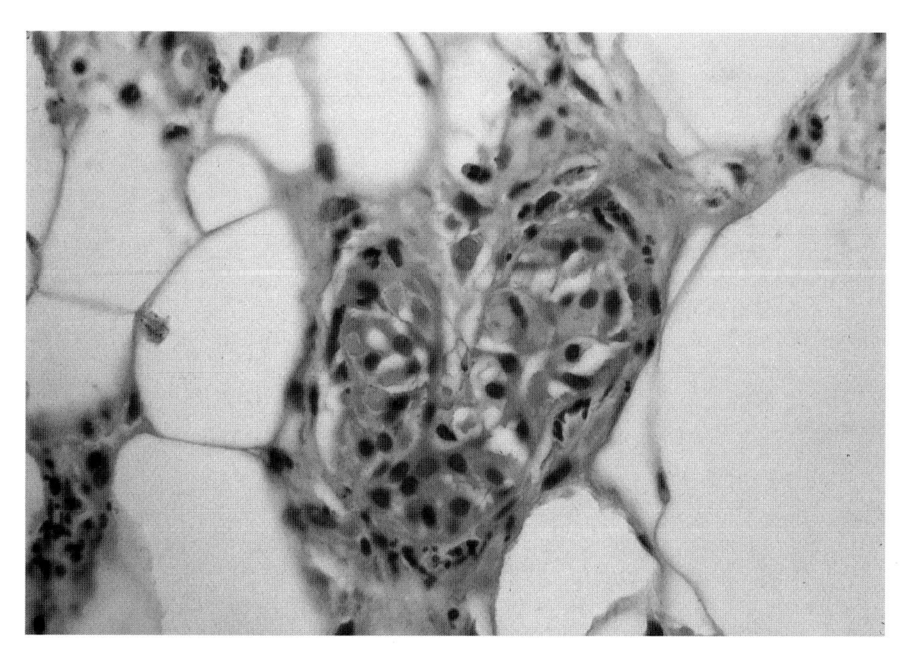

FIG. 11-6. Neutrophilic eccrine hidradenitis
This eccrine coil displays more advanced necrosis.

The secretory cells of the sweat glands show necrosis characterized by eosinophilic homogenization of their cytoplasm and by pyknosis or absence of their nuclei. The sweat ducts usually appear less severely damaged but may also show pale staining or necrosis similar to that of the secretory cells.[21] It is of interest that the sweat gland necrosis is limited to areas in which there are skin lesions. In patients who survive, the necrotic sweat gland epithelium is replaced by normal-appearing epithelial cells within about 2 weeks. In many instances, the pilosebaceous units are also affected with sebaceous gland necrosis and occasional necrosis of the outer and inner root sheaths.

The dermis beneath the bullae, and occasionally also the dermis around the sweat glands, contains a sparse polymorphous infiltrate composed of neutrophils, eosinophils, lymphoid cells, and histiocytes. In addition, some extravasated erythrocytes are often present.

Pathogenesis. The necrosis of the epidermis and sweat glands is a result of both generalized and local hypoxia. The bullae, in turn, are the result of epidermal damage. Coma, whether the result of an accident, an illness, or a drug, causes generalized hypoxia by depressing blood circulation and respiration. In the case of poisoning with carbon monoxide, its binding to hemoglobin acts as an additional factor.[16] Pressure causes further local hypoxia by decreasing blood flow.

CUTANEOUS ERUPTIONS RESULTING FROM ADMINISTRATION OF HUMAN RECOMBINANT CYTOKINES IN PHARMACOLOGIC DOSES

Technologic advances in recombinant DNA research have resulted in the availability of human recombinant cytokines (including colony stimulating factors) for administration to patients in order to effect immunologic manipulation for therapeutic benefit. Based on the actions of human cytokines, specific agents are administered, generally to immunocompromised patients, to enhance the number and/or activity of leukocytes, platelets, or erythrocytes. This action is aimed at hematopoietic cells in the marrow and/or mature leukocytes in the peripheral circulation or tissues.

Mucocutaneous effects of systemic administration of at least 13 cytokines are described (Table 11-1). The findings generally occur (1) at injection sites, (2) as variably distributed eruptions, or (3) as exacerbation or induction of other dermatologic disorders, such as psoriasis.

When asked to examine a skin biopsy specimen from an eruption suspected to be caused by a cytokine, the pathologist should know the temporal relation between administration of the cytokine and appearance of the eruption, white blood cell count, and actions of the cytokine. Ideally, the cutaneous eruption will have begun soon after initiation of cytokine therapy and the histopathology of the eruption will relate in some way to recognized effects of the cytokine.

Histopathology. The morbilliform eruption induced by pharmacologic doses of human recombinant granulocyte-macrophage colony stimulating factor (GM-CSF) illustrates these criteria.[22,23] The upper dermis contains a perivascular and interstitial infiltrate of neutrophils, eosinophils, and lymphocytes (Figs. 11-7 and 11-8). The relative proportion of cell types varies. Macrophages are increased in number and size and may contain melanin when situated in the upper dermis. The epidermis may display intercellular edema with exocytosis of inflammatory cells (Fig. 11-9). Vasculitis is absent.

TABLE 11-1. *Mucocutaneous effects of systemic administration of cytokines*

Cytokine	Reported association
Interleukin-1 alpha and beta	Phlebitis, mucositis[102]
Interleukin-2	Diffuse erythema,[103] exacerbation of psoriasis and autoimmune diseases[104]
Interleukin-3	Flushing[105]
Interleukin-4	Edema[106]
Interleukin-6	Erythematous eruption[107]
GM-CSF	Diffuse eruption (see text)[19]
G-CSF	Neutrophilic dermatosis (see text),[21] vasculitis[108]
Tumor necrosis factor alpha	Erythroderma[109]
Interferon alpha	Alopecia[110]
Interferon beta	Mostly injection site reactions, including vasculitis[111]
Interferon gamma	Exacerbated graft-versus-host reactions[112]

Granulocyte colony stimulating factor (G-CSF) is associated with the development of erythematous plaques that contain numerous neutrophils and upper dermal edema, thus resembling the skin lesions of Sweet's syndrome.[24]

The interested reader is referred to the references for further information.

Pathogenesis. In the case of eruptions associated with GM-CSF and G-CSF, the histologic findings relate to the administration and known actions of the cytokine. In a period of peripheral neutropenia, one finds numerous granulocytes in tissue from these eruptions. Additionally, the effects of GM-CSF on macrophages are demonstrable in the skin by observing their expanded number and size. Immunostains to macrophage/monocyte markers may be useful to highlight this finding.

DRUG-INDUCED PHOTOSENSITIVITY

Drug-induced photosensitivity can be subdivided into photoallergic and phototoxic drug eruptions. Photoallergic drug eruptions represent a T-cell-mediated reaction.

Photoallergic Drug Eruption

In photoallergy, ultraviolet light is required for the allergic reaction to occur. The role of light consists in altering either the hapten itself or the avidity with which the hapten combines with the carrier protein to form a complete photoantigen.[25] Among the photoallergenic drugs are the sulfonamides; the thiazides, such as chlorothiazide and tolbutamide, both of which are aromatic sulfonamides; griseofulvin; the phenothiazines, such as chlorpromazine; quinine; and topical nonsteroidal antiinflammatory medications, including piroxicam.[26] A photoallergic drug eruption causes a photocontact dermatitis in all light-exposed areas. Like any allergic contact dermatitis, it causes itching.

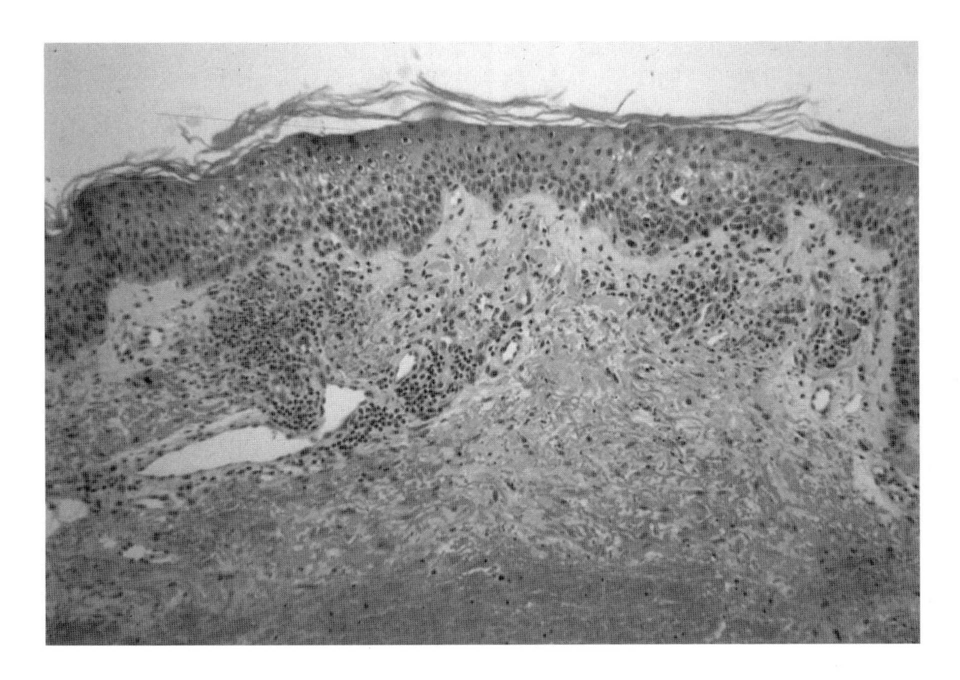

FIG. 11-7. Granulocyte-macrophage colony stimulating factor
A diffuse perivascular and interstitial inflammatory cell infiltrate is present with associated vascular dilatation and epidermal spongiosis.

Histopathology. The histologic appearance of a photocontact dermatitis is that of an allergic contact dermatitis and, as such, shows epidermal spongiosis and microvesiculation, a perivascular lymphocytic infiltrate, and exocytosis, often with eosinophils (see Chap. 9).[27]

Phototoxic Drug Eruption

If given in sufficiently large doses, certain internally administered drugs, in association with exposure to ultraviolet light, may produce a phototoxic dermatitis, which resembles an intensified sunburn. Among the drugs known to elicit a phototoxic response are all drugs capable of producing a photoallergic reaction, provided that they are given in sufficiently high concentrations.[28] Other commonly prescribed phototoxic drugs are certain tetracyclines, such as demeclocycline hydrochloride and doxycycline,[29] quinolones,[30] and psoralens.

Histopathology. A phototoxic drug eruption, like a sunburn reaction, shows both vacuolated keratinocytes (sunburn cells) characterized by an increased volume and pale cytoplasm and apoptotic keratinocytes characterized by a reduced volume and darkly staining cytoplasm.[31] The dermis shows edema and enlargement of endothelial cells.

Chlorpromazine Pigmentation

When chlorpromazine is given in high doses for several years, it may produce in exposed areas of the skin a slate-gray discoloration resembling the discoloration seen in argyria. Exposed parts of the bulbar conjunctivae may show brownish pigmentation.[32]

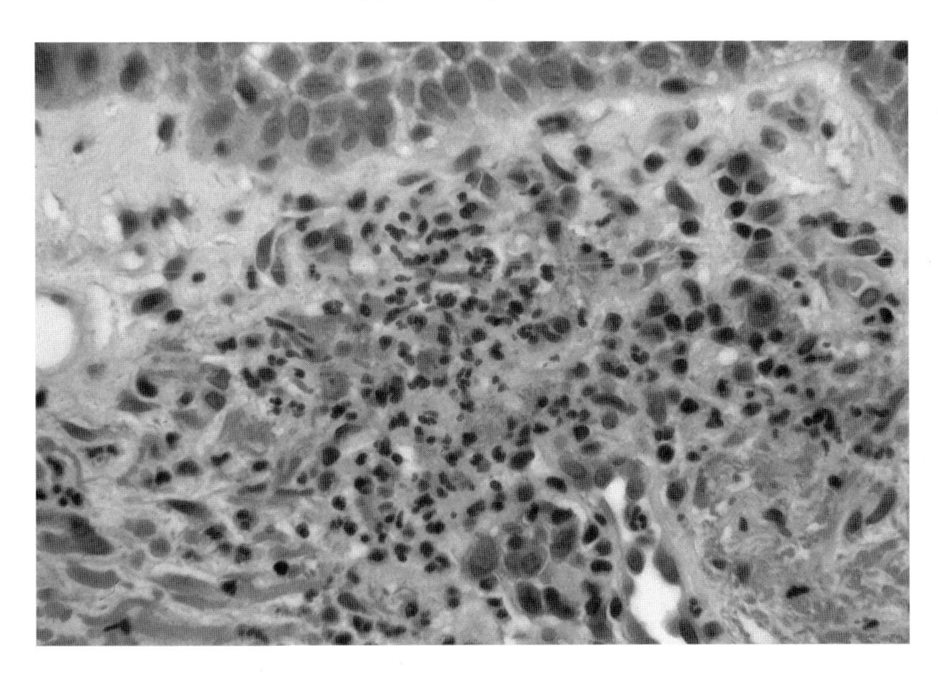

FIG. 11-8. Granulocyte-macrophage colony stimulating factor
The upper dermis contains a collection of neutrophils and eosinophils immediately below the epidermis.

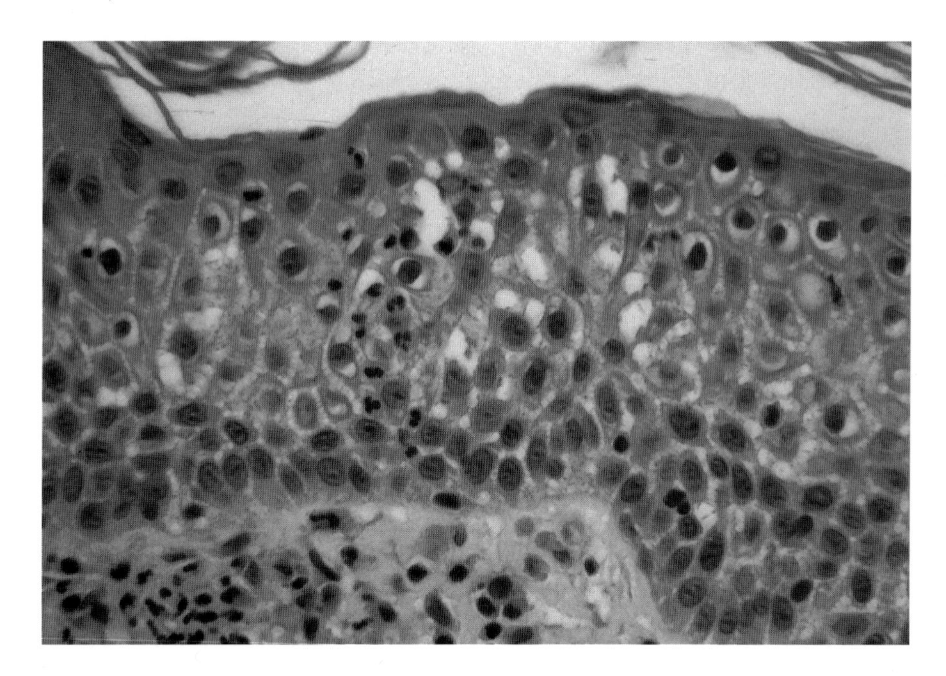

FIG. 11-9. Granulocyte-macrophage colony stimulating factor
Neutrophils extend into the spongiotic epidermis.

Histopathology. The amount of melanin in the basal layer of the epidermis is variable. Considerable accumulation of pigment is found throughout the dermis within macrophages, especially in the vicinity of the capillaries. The pigment has the staining properties of melanin in that it stains black with the Fontana-Masson silver stain and is decolorized by hydrogen peroxide.

In patients who received prolonged treatment with chlorpromazine and who died of unrelated causes, autopsy may reveal in many internal organs melanin-like material that stains black with the Fontana-Masson silver stain and can be decolorized by hydrogen peroxide. This material is found throughout the entire mononuclear-phagocyte system and, to a lesser degree, in the parenchymal cells of the liver, kidneys, and endocrine glands, in myocardial fibers, and in cerebral neurons.[33]

Histogenesis. Electron microscopic examination has confirmed the presence of many melanosome complexes within the lysosomes of dermal macrophages. In addition, round or bizarrely shaped bodies may be seen measuring 0.2 to 3 μm in diameter and possessing such great electron density that no internal structure is recognizable.[34] These bodies are located in macrophages, endothelial cells, pericytes, Schwann cells, and fibroblasts, usually within lysosomes. At times, both electron-dense bodies and melanosome complexes are found within the same lysosome. The electron-dense bodies have been interpreted as a drug metabolite of chlorpromazine or as a lipoprotein complex that is conjugated with chlorpromazine or its metabolites. It has become apparent, however, that the dense bodies histochemically react like melanin.[30] Furthermore, chlorpromazine binds to melanin with a high degree of avidity, with chlorpromazine acting as the electron donor and melanin as the acceptor.[35] It seems likely that the electron-dense bodies represent complexes of melanin with chlorpromazine. These complexes are subsequently carried from the dermis by way of the circulating blood leukocytes to the various internal organs.[36]

Minocycline Pigmentation

The prolonged administration of minocycline, a semisynthetic tetracycline, may result in three distinct types of cutaneous pigmentation[37]: (1) a blue-black pigmentation occurring within areas of inflammation or scarring, usually on the face, especially in active or healed acne lesions[38]; (2) a blue-gray pigmentation of previously normal skin, most commonly seen on the legs but also occurring on the forearms[39]; and (3) a diffuse, muddy brown discoloration, sometimes accentuated in sun-exposed areas.[40] A systemic minocycline-induced hypersensitivity syndrome is reported, predominantly manifested by eosinophilic pneumonitis.[41]

Histopathology. The histologic picture shows differences among the three types. The focal blue-black pigmentation of the face in the first type is associated with macrophages[42] and reacts like hemosiderin. In contrast, the blue-gray pigmentation in the second type, most commonly observed on the legs, shows staining for iron and also reacts with the Fontana-Masson stain; and the muddy brown pigmentation in the third type reveals increased melanization of the basal cell layer and within macrophages in the upper dermis. Overnight immersion of frozen tissue sections in 1 M $MgCl_2$ -ethanol allows the observation of minocycline deposits as yellowish fluorescence by fluorescent microscopy.[43]

Histogenesis. It appears likely that the iron-containing pigment in the first two types of pigmentation represents a drug metabolite-protein complex.[34] The pigment in the second type that reacts with the Fontana-Masson stain does not contain melanin, because it does not bleach with hydrogen peroxide. The pigment in the third type reacts like melanin and represents a phototoxic phenomenon.

Amiodarone Pigmentation

Amiodarone, an iodinated adrenergic blocker used in the treatment of tachyarrhythmias, on long-term (3 to 6 months), high-dose use causes a slate-blue discoloration of sun-exposed skin, especially of the face, in up to 40% of patients.[44] The pigmentation resembles that of argyria.[45] Generally, the hyperpigmentation slowly fades after discontinuation of the drug.

Histopathology. Yellow-brown, slightly refractile pigment granules are seen within macrophages situated principally around blood vessels in the upper reticular dermis. Variable findings are noted using special stains. The granules reportedly stain with the Fontana-Masson stain, indicating the presence of melanin,[46] and with Sudan black, suggesting the presence of lipofuscin.[47] The Perls' iron reaction is negative.[42] In the face of variable staining characteristics, periodic acid-Schiff reliably stains the granules.[41]

Histogenesis. Electron microscopic examination reveals collections of oval or round electron-dense lysosomal granules within macrophages. In addition, myelin-like residual bodies may be seen. Occasionally, there are irregular lipid droplets with the appearance of lipofuscin. Electron-dense granules and myelin-like bodies are found also in peripheral white blood cells and other tissues. The granules contain iodine.[48]

CLOFAZIMINE-INDUCED PIGMENTATION

Clofazimine is administered to patients with leprosy and may cause a pink to pink-brown dyspigmentation soon after initiation of therapy. The pigmentation resolves slowly after discontinuation of clofazimine. The most notably involved areas are the obvious leprosy lesions.[49]

Histopathology. The upper dermis contains numerous foamy macrophages that possess cytoplasm with brown granular pigment. This pigment stains for lipofuscin, but not for melanin or iron.

Pathogenesis. Upon electron microscopy, the macrophages are found to contain phagolysosomes with either lipid or electron-dense granules with a lamellar substructure consistent with lipofuscin or ceroid pigment.[46] The mechanism by which clofazimine causes these changes is unclear.

PENICILLAMINE-INDUCED DERMATOSES

The prolonged administration of penicillamine can cause alterations in collagen and elastic tissue that may result in areas of atrophy of the skin. Anetoderma and elastosis serpiginosa perforans are observed. Damage to epidermal desmosomal elements may induce pemphigus.

Penicillamine-Induced Atrophy of the Skin

Patients on prolonged penicillamine therapy may show atrophy of the skin of the face and neck; light blue, atrophic macules resembling anetoderma; easy bruising resulting in small hemorrhages into the skin followed by milia[50]; or small, white papules at sites of venipuncture in the antecubital fossae.[47]

Histopathology. The anetoderma shows diminution or absence of elastic tissue.[48] The areas of easy bruising of the skin and the papules at sites of venipuncture show either diminution[49] or degeneration and homogenization of collagen.[47]

Histogenesis. The formation of elastic tissue and collagen involves the participation of aldehydes to produce stable cross-links. By reacting with aldehydes to form thiazolidine compounds, penicillamine impairs the formation of such stable cross-links.[51]

Penicillamine-Induced Elastosis Perforans Serpiginosa

Elastosis perforans serpiginosa may occur in patients receiving prolonged treatment with penicillamine. Although the clinical picture does not differ from that of idiopathic elastosis perforans serpiginosa (see Chap. 6), the histologic and electron microscopic features of the altered elastic fibers are unique. Both penicillamine-induced atrophy of the skin and penicillamine-induced elastosis perforans serpiginosa may occur in the same patient.[52]

Histopathology. In comparison with the idiopathic type of elastosis perforans serpiginosa, the penicillamine-induced type, on staining for elastic tissue, shows less hyperplasia of elastic fibers in the papillary dermis, except in areas of active transepidermal elimination. However, in the middle and deep layers of the dermis, a greater number of hyperplastic elastic fibers are present than in idiopathic elastosis perforans serpiginosa. These fibers have an appearance that is specific for penicillamine-induced elastosis perforans serpiginosa. Lateral budding is noted, with the buds arranged perpendicular to the principal fibers. The coarse elastic fibers thus show a serrated, sawtoothlike border and have been aptly compared to the twigs of a bramble bush and have been referred to as "lumpy-bumpy"[49,53] (Fig. 11-10). Similar changes in individual elastic fibers are observed also in nonlesional skin and have been seen in a skeletal artery.[54]

Pathogenesis. On electron microscopic examination, the affected elastic fibers show an inner core that closely resembles a normal elastic fiber with dark microfibrils embedded in electron-lucent elastin. Peripheral to this, a wide, homogeneous, electron-lucent coat is seen that has the appearance of elastin and shows numerous saclike protuberances bulging outward between the adjacent collagen fibers.[49]

DRUG-INDUCED BULLOUS DISORDERS

Several medications are linked to the development of antibody-mediated pemphigus (Table 11-2). Among these, penicillamine is perhaps the most common. The majority of cases of penicillamine-induced pemphigus are pemphigus foliaceus, with rare cases of pemphigus vulgaris and vegetans on record.[55,56] Most cases of pemphigus start between 6 and 12 months after institution of penicillamine therapy. In most instances, the pemphigus subsides shortly after penicillamine is discontinued. In other instances, the disease persists for 1 to 2

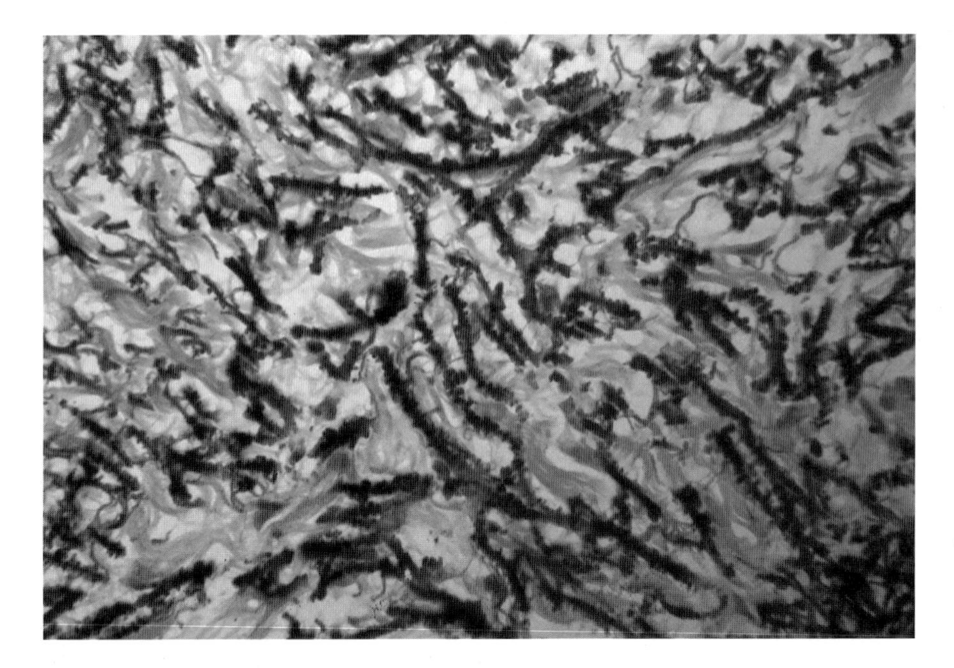

FIG. 11-10. Penicillamine-induced elastosis perforans serpiginosa This elastic tissue stain shows the knobby appearance or lateral budding of the elastic fibers characteristic of penicillamine effect.

years after discontinuation of penicillamine,[56] and in one reported instance it was fatal.[57] Drug induction of subepidermal blisters is also recognized, with vancomycin-induced linear IgA dermatosis as a prime example.[58]

Histopathology. Histologic examination reveals a picture identical with that seen in the blistering disorders not associated with drugs (see Chap. 9).

Pathogenesis. Direct immunofluorescence testing has been positive for intercellular antibodies in most cases of drug-related pemphigus foliaceus and vulgaris.[55] In the rare instances of induced pemphigus erythematosus, subepidermal, in addition to intercellular, deposition of IgG has been noted, just as in the idiopathic type of pemphigus erythematosus.[59] It is not known how penicillamine and captopril induce pemphigus, but it is assumed that the sulfhydryl group common to both drugs alters the intercellular substance into an antigenic structure with subsequent antibody formation. In skin organ culture, both drugs induce acantholysis by addition to the culture medium, presumably by direct action of the drug on a desmosomal structure.[60,61] By immunoprecipitation, it has been shown that autoantibodies in pemphigus foliaceus and vulgaris induced by penicillamine and captopril have the same specificity as in other patients.[62]

DRUG-INDUCED LUPUS ERYTHEMATOSUS

Several drugs may induce a syndrome similar to systemic lupus erythematosus. The drugs that do this most commonly are procainamide, hydralazine, quinidine, chlorpromazine, isoniazid, and propylthiouracil.[63] It is possible that the development of a systemic lupus erythematosus-like syndrome in a patient under medication with these drugs represents the uncovering of latent systemic lupus erythematosus.

Drug-induced systemic lupus erythematosus can be clinically, pathologically, and serologically indistinguishable from spontaneously arising systemic lupus erythematosus. However, cutaneous and renal manifestations are rarer in drug-induced than in spontaneous systemic lupus erythematosus, and pleuropulmonary manifestations are somewhat more common. Usually, but not always, when the medication is discontinued, the clinical and laboratory manifestations subside. Nevertheless, death can occur, especially as a result of renal involvement.[64]

Histopathology. The histologic picture of the cutaneous lesions is the same as in lupus erythematosus (see Chap. 10).

Pathogenesis. Antinuclear antibodies are usually present with anti-single-stranded DNA antibodies. These antibodies bind determinants on histones.[65] Anti-double-stranded DNA antibodies are usually absent. Hypocomplementemia is rare. The occurrence of a lupus band on direct immunofluorescence testing of normal-appearing skin is uncommon.[66] Evidence exists that activated neutrophils convert the implicated drugs to lupus-inducing agents through the action of myeloperoxidase. In an experimental model, absence of extracellular hydrogen peroxide abrogated the cytotoxicity of the drug.[67]

TABLE 11-2. *Drugs causing pemphigus*

Drugs causing pemphigus
Penicillamine
Captopril
Pyritinol
Penicillin
Ampicillin
Rifampin
Pyrazolone derivatives
Cefadroxil
Cephalexin

HALOGEN ERUPTIONS

Ingestion of bromides may cause, besides a pustular eruption, the formation of vegetating, papillomatous plaques called *bromoderma.* The plaques, which usually occur on the lower extremities, often show pustules at their peripheries. Although bromoderma often appears only after prolonged intake of bromides, it may arise soon after administration as well.

Iododerma, usually seen on the face, begins as a rule with multiple pustules that rapidly coalesce into vegetating plaques.[68] Like bromoderma, the plaques of iododerma often show pustules at their peripheries, but they usually show less papillomatous proliferation and a softer consistency than bromoderma, and they often ulcerate. Iododerma is frequently associated with severe systemic signs and symptoms and may be fatal in rare instances.[69] Although the eruption usually arises after prolonged ingestion of iodides, it may start within a few days, especially in patients with chronic renal disease. Iododerma may also start within a few days after a second urography[70] or a second lymphography[68] for which iodine-containing compounds have been used. In one instance, severe iododerma developed 3 days after the first intravenous pyelogram with an iodine-containing compound.[71]

Fluoroderma has been described after the frequent application of a fluoride gel to the teeth for the purpose of preventing caries during ionizing radiation to the face.[72] The lesions consist of scattered papules and nodules on the neck and in the preauricular regions.

Histopathology. The histologic picture in the halogen eruptions is suggestive rather than diagnostic. The difference between bromoderma and iododerma lies largely in the epidermal changes, which usually are much more pronounced in bromoderma, although there is some overlap. The dermal changes are essentially the same and vary with the age of the lesion.

In early lesions, the dermis in both bromoderma and iododerma shows a dense infiltrate of neutrophils, which, in areas of dermal necrosis, show nuclear dust.[73] There may be intradermal abscesses. Eosinophils are present in most cases and may be numerous. Extensive extravasation of erythrocytes may also be seen. At a later stage, the proportion of mononuclear cells increases, and histiocytes may show abundant cytoplasm[68] or large nuclei. The blood vessels are increased in number and dilated, and may show proliferation of endothelium.

The epidermal changes in bromoderma are often pronounced. In addition to papillomatosis, one may observe considerable downward epidermal proliferation, occasionally to such a degree as to produce the picture of pseudocarcinomatous hyperplasia. The acanthosis may center around upper level follicular epithelium. Frequently, intraepidermal abscesses are present (Fig. 11-11). The intraepidermal abscesses are filled with neutrophils, eosinophils, and some desquamated keratinocytes, most of which appear necrotic, although some resemble acantholytic cells. Some epithelial islands in the upper dermis, instead of enclosing an abscess, are filled with keratin.

In iododerma, the epidermis may be eroded or ulcerated. At the margin of the ulcers, one may find intraepidermal abscesses. In old lesions, pseudoepitheliomatous hyperplasia may be encountered.[68]

Fluoroderma has been described only as a mild eruption, but it shares with iododerma and bromoderma the presence of eosinophils, neutrophils, and erythrocytes in the dermis and of microabscesses in the epidermis.[72]

Pathogenesis. Even though there is often a very long interval between the first ingestion of iodides or bromides and the appearance of the cutaneous lesion, halogen eruptions appear to be an allergic phenomenon; once a person has become sensitized, the eruption recurs within a few days upon the readministration of iodides or bromides.

Halogen eruptions probably arise on the basis of delayed hypersensitivity. In one case of iododerma, the patient's lymphocytes underwent blastogenic transformation on exposure to 131I-labeled serum albumin.[73] If an iododerma starts within a few days after the first pyelogram with an iodine-containing compound,[71] previous sensitization to iodine has likely occurred without knowledge of the patient. Also speaking in favor of sensitization is the good response of iododerma to the administration of corticosteroids.[69]

Differential Diagnosis. Intraepidermal abscesses occur in blastomycosis and pemphigus vegetans as well as in the halogen eruptions. However, blastomycosis is easily differentiated by its numerous giant cells and the presence of yeast. In contrast, differentiation from pemphigus vegetans may cause difficulties, especially because eosinophils often are prominent in halogen eruptions as well. Generally, pemphigus vegetans shows a less extensive dermal infiltrate that only rarely contains neutrophils. In pemphigus vegetans, acantholysis usually is pronounced, whereas in halogen eruptions, it is a subtle finding.

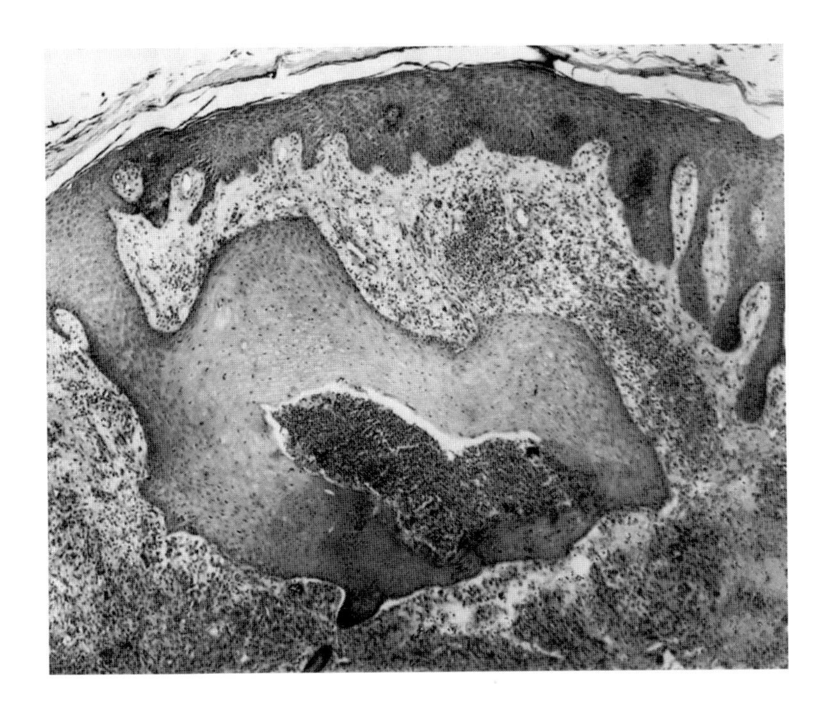

FIG. 11-11. Bromoderma
There is downward proliferation of the epidermis, which encloses a large abscess. The dermis contains a dense inflammatory infiltrate.

ARGYRIA

Argyria is caused by prolonged ingestion of silver salts or their prolonged application to mucous membranes. If the silver salts are ingested, the skin shows a slate-blue discoloration, especially in the exposed areas. Also, the oral mucosa and conjunctivae are often discolored. Even topical application to the oral mucosa or the upper respiratory tract may result in ingestion of sufficient amounts of silver to cause systemic argyria.[74] In some patients with argyria, the nail beds of the fingers (but not of the toes) may show a blue discoloration.[75] On autopsy or during abdominal surgery, internal organs may show a blue discoloration, including the intestines, liver, spleen, and peritoneum.[74,76] Argyria (and chrysiasis) was reported by patients after acupuncture treatment by implantation of the needles.[77] Also, argyria resembling multiple blue nevi was described in a silversmith following multiple cutaneous punctures by a silver filament.[78] Systemic argyria is rare, because patent medications containing silver are no longer available.

Histopathology. Silver is found in the dermis extracellularly as fine, small, round, brown-black granules that appear fairly uniform in size. In contrast, silver is not seen in the epidermis or its appendages. The silver granules measure less than 1 μm in diameter and lie singly and in groups. Although visible in routine stains, they stand out much more clearly when sections are examined with a dark-field microscope. The silver granules then appear as brilliantly refractile, white particles against a dark background. Also, many more granules can be resolved by this method than by direct illumination.

The silver granules are present in the greatest numbers in the basement membrane zone, or membrana propria, surrounding the sweat glands (Fig. 11-12). They are seen in high concentrations in the connective tissue sheaths around the hair follicles and sebaceous glands, in the walls of capillaries, in the arrectores pilorum, and in the nerves.[79] Silver granules are also found in the dermal papillae and scattered diffusely throughout the dermis. Elastic tissue stains reveal a predilection of the granules for elastic fibers, which explains the presence of fingerlike chains of granules projecting into the dermal papillae.[78] The silver has, however, no particular affinity for the epidermal basement membrane zone.

In addition to silver, there is an increase in the amount of melanin, particularly in sun-exposed skin. Increased amounts of melanin are present in some cases only in the epidermis; in other cases, melanin is found also within melanophages scattered throughout the upper dermis.

Comparing the amounts of silver granules in discolored, exposed skin and in nondiscolored, or only slightly discolored, unexposed skin, several investigators have found equal quantities of silver in the same patient. However, exposed skin showing solar elastosis can contain an increased concentration of silver granules in parallel to the increase in elastic tissue. Deposits of silver are also found in internal organs.

Pathogenesis. Electron microscopy reveals that the silver granules lie in most instances almost entirely extracellularly within the dermis.[80] The silver granules consist of aggregates of microgranules, mostly irregularly shaped,[79] and mostly varying in size from 200 and 400 nm in diameter,[81] but ranging up to 1000 nm.

Silver granules are prominently located in the basement membrane (basal lamina) that surrounds sweat glands, endothelial cells, nerve fibers, and smooth muscle cells.[79] Although silver granules may be seen occasionally free in the cytoplasm of macrophages,[82] most authors have only rarely observed silver granules within lysosomes of macrophages[79] or fibroblasts.

The increase in the amount of melanin in the basal cell layer and occasionally also in the upper dermis suggests that the presence of silver in the skin may stimulate melanocytic activity. Increased epidermal melanin is observed also with deposits of other heavy metals, such as iron in hemochromatosis (see Chap. 17) and mercury in mercury pigmentation (see later). The pronounced slate-blue pigmentation in exposed skin is caused by increases in both melanin and silver.

Differential Diagnosis. Histologic differentiation of argyria

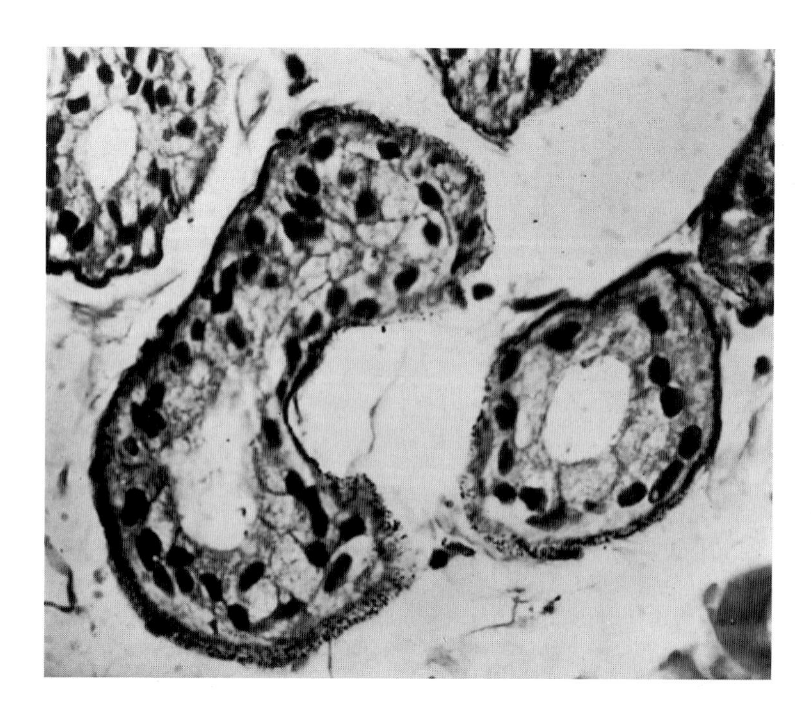

FIG. 11-12. Argyria
Silver granules are present in the membrana propria of the sweat glands. In some places, the granules are so dense that they form a solid black band.

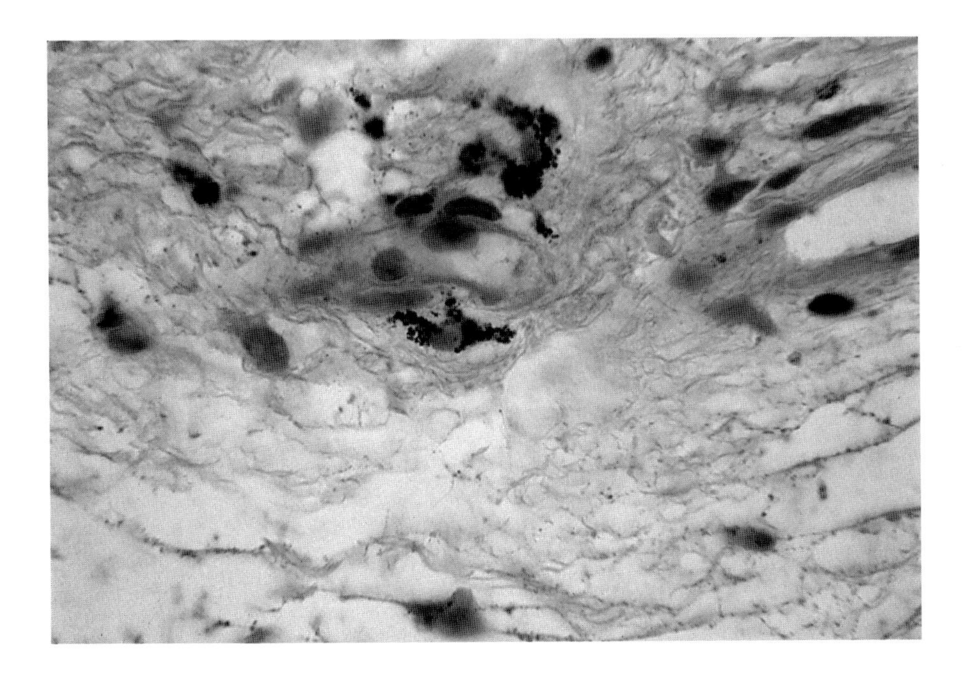

FIG. 11-13. Chrysiasis
Gold granules are noted within upper dermal perivascular macrophages. The gold granules are quite dark and reside within the cytoplasmic processes of macrophages.

from other kinds of pigmentation rarely causes any difficulty because of the uniform size and characteristic distribution of the silver granules. Incubation of sections in a solution consisting of 1% potassium ferricyanide in 20% sodium thiosulfate will result in decolorization of silver. Positive identification of the silver deposits in histologic sections can be accomplished by means of neutron-activation analysis[83] or with an atomic absorption spectrophotometer.[84]

CHRYSIASIS

In chrysiasis, which may follow the prolonged parenteral administration of gold salts as used in the treatment of rheumatoid arthritis, the sun-exposed skin shows a slate-blue discoloration.

Histopathology. Gold granules are larger and more irregularly shaped than silver granules, but they also are light refractile with dark-field examination. The granules are found predominantly within cells, particularly within endothelial cells and within macrophages[85] (Fig. 11-13). Extracellular granules may also be observed (Fig. 11-14). Gold particles are reported to display orange-red birefringence on fluorescence microscopy.[86]

Histogenesis. Electron microscopic examination shows the presence of electron-dense, angulated particles within phagolysosomes of endothelial cells and macrophages.[87] X-ray spectroscopic analysis demonstrates a spectrum consistent with the presence of gold.[87]

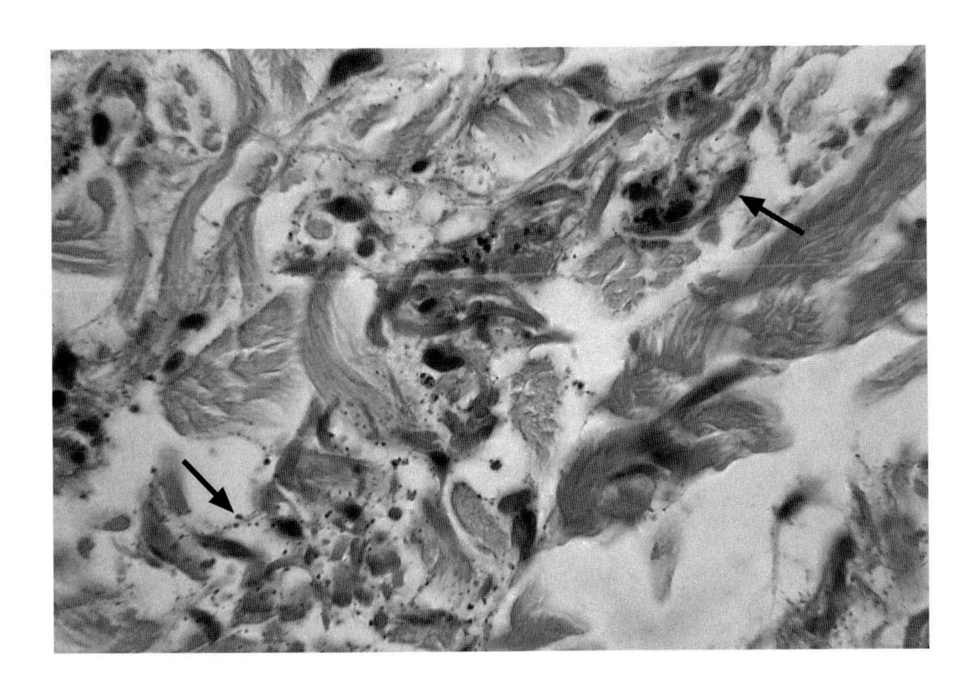

FIG. 11-14. Chrysiasis
Extracellular gold granules are present among the collagen fibers.

MERCURY PIGMENTATION

Regular application of a mercury-containing cream to the face and neck over many years may produce a slate-gray pigmentation of the skin in the areas to which the cream has been applied. Generally, the pigmentation is most pronounced on the eyelids, in the nasolabial folds, and in the folds of the neck.[88] Traumatic implantation of mercury may also occur.

Histopathology. Irregular, brown-black granules are found in the upper dermis, partially free in the dermis and partially within macrophages. In rare instances, granules are seen also in the basal cell layer of the epidermis.[80] Dark-field examination of sections reveals the granules to be brilliantly refractile.[89] On staining with silver nitrate, the amount of melanin in the basal layer of the epidermis may be found to be within normal limits or increased.[89] Traumatic implantation of mercury results in variably sized, often large amorphous deposits of mercury in the dermis and subcutis. Chronic changes include dermal fibrosis and granulomatous inflammation (Fig. 11-15).

Pathogenesis. As seen by electron microscopy, the mercury particles measure approximately 14 nm in diameter and are aggregated into irregular granules with diameters of up to 340 nm. Many granules are associated with elastic fibers, but others are free among the collagen fibers and in macrophages either within lysosomes or free in the cytoplasm.[89] If present in the epidermis, the mercury granules lie in the intercellular spaces of the basal cell layer.[80]

Because the pigmentation is most pronounced in skin folds that are protected from the sun, and there may be no increase in the amount of melanin, it can be concluded that most of the pigmentation is caused by the mercury rather than the melanin.

Differential Diagnosis. Mercury pigmentation differs from a tattoo by the more superficial location of the granules and by refractility of the granules on dark-field examination. Positive identification of the granules as mercury can be made by submission of unstained sections to neutron-activation analysis.[89]

DRUG-INDUCED PSEUDOLYMPHOMA SYNDROME

Phenytoin and carbamazepine[91] may cause a pseudolymphoma syndrome characterized by generalized lymphadenopathy, hepatosplenomegaly, fever, arthralgia, and eosinophilia. Cutaneous findings, occasionally present, may be limited to a few erythematous plaques[92] or nodules or may consist of a generalized macular and papular eruption.[93] Generalized exfoliative dermatitis is reported.[94] In all cases there is improvement and ultimate clearing when the offending agent is discontinued.

Histopathology. On histologic examination of the skin, the infiltrate is often indistinguishable from that of mycosis fungoides (this syndrome is also known as "pseudo-mycosis fungoides") in that there are cerebriform nuclei in the dermal infiltrate and Pautrier microabscesses in the epidermis.[92] In cutaneous nodules, the infiltrate may suggest a cutaneous lymphoma of the non-Hodgkin's type, because large masses of atypical lymphocytes are present in the dermis as well as in the subcutaneous tissue.[95,96]

The enlarged subcutaneous lymph nodes in some cases may show merely reactive hyperplasia[97] but in other cases may suggest lymphoma as a result of the partial loss of normal architecture. In several patients with generalized exfoliative dermatitis, significant numbers of cells in the circulating blood have been Sézary cells.[98] Bone marrow abnormalities are reported.[99]

DRUG-INDUCED PSEUDOPORPHYRIA

Several medications are reported to cause cutaneous lesions that resemble the blisters of porphyria cutanea tarda; however, other cutaneous manifestations are absent. Further, no derangement in porphyrin metabolism is identified. Healing occurs once the medication is discontinued. Implicated drugs include naproxen, furosemide, tetracycline, dapsone, and pyridoxine.[45]

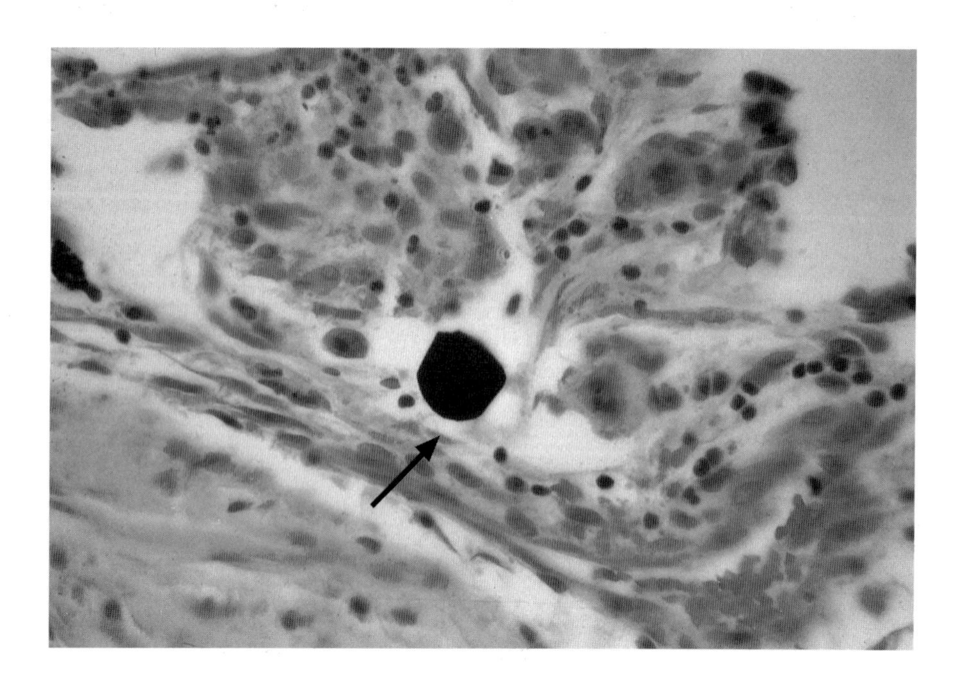

FIG. 11-15. Mercury implantation A mercury droplet is surrounded by lymphocytes and histiocytes.

Histopathology. The blisters resemble the poorly or noninflamed subepidermal bullae of porphyria cutanea tarda (Chap. 17).

Histogenesis. The mechanism by which this reaction occurs is unknown. Unlike porphyria cutanea tarda, no deposits in the skin are revealed by direct immunofluorescence testing (Chap. 10).[100]

PHYTONADIONE-INDUCED PSEUDOSCLERODERMA

Indurated plaques arise at the sites of phytonadione (vitamin K_1) injection after varying lengths of time. Typical sites include the outer thighs, bilaterally. The plaques evolve to resemble scleroderma and are reported to possess an erythematous rim. To date, this complication has been reported only in Europe, raising the possibility of a contaminant in the phytonadione produced regionally.[101]

Histopathology. The histologic features are indistinguishable from those of scleroderma.

REFERENCES

1. Kuokkanen K. Drug eruptions: A series of 464 cases in the Department of Dermatology, University of Turku, Finland, during 1966–70. Acta Allergol 1972;24:407.
2. Cropley TA, Fitzpatrick TBF. Dermatology diagnosis by recognition of clinical, morphologic patterns and syndromes. In: Fitzpatrick TB, Eisen AZ, Wolff K et al. eds. Dermatology in general medicine, New York: McGraw-Hill, 1993;55.
3. Roujeau JC, Bioulac-Sage P, Bourseau C. et al. Acute generalized exanthematous pustulosis. Arch Dermatol 1991;127:1333.
4. Roujeau JC, Kelly JP, Naldi L et al. Medication use and the risk of Stevens-Johnson syndrome or toxic epidermal necrolysis. N Engl J Med 1995;333:1600.
5. Van Hecke E, Kint A, Temmerman L. A lichenoid eruption induced by penicillamine. Arch Dermatol 1981;117:676.
6. Kanwar AJ, Bharija SC, Singh M et al. Ninety-eight fixed drug eruptions with provocation tests. Dermatologica 1988;177:274.
7. Commens C. Fixed drug eruption. Australas J Dermatol 1983;24:1.
8. Masu S, Seiji M. Pigmentary incontinence in fixed drug eruptions. J Am Acad Dermatol 1983;8:520.
9. Korkji W, Soltani K. Fixed drug eruption: A brief review. Arch Dermatol 1984;120:520.
10. Teraki Y, Moriya N, Shiohara T. Drug-induced expression of intercellular adhesion molecule-1 on lesional keratinocytes in fixed drug eruption. Am J Pathol 1995;145:550.
11. Yokel BK, Friedman KJ, Farmer ER et al. Cutaneous pathology following etoposide therapy. J Cutan Pathol 1987;14:326.
12. Horn TD, Beveridge RA, Egorin MJ et al. Observations and proposed mechanism of N,N′,N″-triethylenethiophosphoramide (Thio-TEPA)-induced hyperpigmentation. Arch Dermatol 1989;125:524.
13. Hurt MA, Halvorson RD, Peter FC Jr et al. Eccrine squamous syringometaplasia: A cutaneous sweat gland reaction in the histologic spectrum of "chemotherapy-associated eccrine hidradenitis." Arch Dermatol 1990;126:73.
14. Fitzpatrick JE, Bennion SD, Reed OM et al. Neutrophilic eccrine hidradenitis associated with induction chemotherapy. J Cutan Pathol 1987;14:272.
15. Harrist TJ, Fine JD, Berman RS et al. Neutrophilic hidradenitis: A distinctive type of neutrophilic dermatosis associated with myelogenous leukemia and chemotherapy. Arch Dermatol 1982;118:263.
16. Templeton SF, Solomon AR, Swerlick RA. Intradermal bleomycin infections into normal human skin: A histopathologic and immunopathologic study. Arch Dermatol 1994;130:577.
17. Linassier C, Colombat P, Reisenleiter M et al. Cutaneous toxicity of autologous bone marrow transplantation in nonseminomatous germ cell tumors. Cancer 1990;65:1143.
18. Hymes SR, Simonton SC, Farmer ER et al. Cutaneous busulfan effect in patients receiving bone marrow transplantation. J Cutan Pathol 1985;12:125.
19. Leavell UW, Farley CH, McIntire JS. Cutaneous changes in a patient with carbon monoxide poisoning. Arch Dermatol 1969;99:429.
20. Herschthal D, Robinson MJ. Blisters of the skin in coma induced by amitriptyline and chloracepate dipotassium. Arch Dermatol 1979;115: 499.
21. Brehmer-Andersson E, Pedersen NB. Sweat gland necrosis and bullous skin changes in acute drug intoxication. Acta Dermatol Venereol (Stockh) 1969;49:157.
22. Horn TD, Burke PJ, Karp JE, Hood AF. Intravenous administration of recombinant human granulocyte-macrophage colony-stimulating factor causes a cutaneous eruption. Arch Dermatol 1991;127:49.
23. Mehregan DR, Fransway AF, Edmonson JH, Leiferman KM. Cutaneous reactions to granulocyte-monocyte colony-stimulating factor. Arch Dermatol 1992;128:1055.
24. Park JW, Mehrotra B, Barnett BO et al. The Sweet syndrome during therapy with granulocyte colony-stimulating factor. Ann Int Med 1992;116:996.
25. Harber LC, Baer RL. Pathogenic mechanisms of drug-induced photosensitivity. J Invest Dermatol 1972;58:327.
26. Ophaswongse S, Maibach H. Topical nonsteroidal antiinflammatory drugs: Allergic and photoallergic contact dermatitis and phototoxicity. Contact Dermatitis 1993;29:57.
27. Willis I, Kligman AM. The mechanism of photoallergic contact dermatitis. J Invest Dermatol 1968;51:378.
28. Horio T, Miyauchi H, Asada Y et al. Phototoxicity and photoallergy of quinolones in guinea pigs. J Dermatol Sci 1994;7:130.
29. Frost P, Weinstein GP, Gomez EC. Phototoxic potential of minocycline and doxycycline. Arch Dermatol 1972;105:681.
30. Lasarow RM, Isseroff RR, Gomez EC. Quantitative in vitro assessment of phototoxicity by a fibroblast-neutral assay. J Invest Dermatol 1992;98:725.
31. Gilchrest BA, Soter NA, Stoff JS et al. The human sunburn reaction: Histologic and biochemical studies. J Am Acad Dermatol 1981;5:411.
32. Hays GB, Lyle CB Jr, Wheeler CE Jr. Slate-grey color in patients receiving chlorpromazine. Arch Dermatol 1964;90:471.
33. Greiner AC, Nicolson GA. Pigmentary deposit in viscera associated with prolonged chlorpromazine therapy. Can Med Assoc J 1964;91: 627.
34. Hashimoto K, Wiener W, Albert J et al. An electron microscopic study of chlorpromazine pigmentation. J Invest Dermatol 1966;47:296.
35. Blois MS Jr. On chlorpromazine binding in vivo. J Invest Dermatol 1965;45:475.
36. Sanatove A. Pigmentation due to phenothiazines in high and prolonged doses. JAMA 1965;191:263.
37. Argenyi ZB, Finelli L, Bergfeld WF et al. Minocycline-related cutaneous hyperpigmentation as demonstrated by light microscopy, electron microscopy and x-ray energy spectroscopy. J Cutan Pathol 1987; 14:176.
38. Fenske NA, Millns JL. Cutaneous pigmentation due to minocycline hydrochloride. J Am Acad Dermatol 1980;3:308.
39. Sato S, Murphy GF, Bernard JD et al. Ultrastructural and x-ray microanalytical observations on minocycline-related hyperpigmentation of the skin. J Invest Dermatol 1981;77:264.
40. Pepine M, Flowers DP, Ramos-Caro FA. Extensive cutaneous hyperpigmentation caused by minocycline. J Am Acad Dermatol 1993;28: 292.
41. Kloppenberg M, Dijkmans BA, Breedveld FC. Hypersensitivity pneumonitis during minocycline treatment. Neth J Med 1994;44:210.
42. Altman DA, Fivenson DP, Lee MW. Minocycline hyperpigmentation: A model for in situ phagocytic activity of factor XIIIa positive dermal dendrocytes. J Cutan Pathol 1992;19:340.
43. Okada N, Sato S, Sasou T et al. Characterization of pigmented granules in minocycline-induced cutaneous pigmentation: Observations using fluorescence microscopy and high-performance liquid chromatography. Br J Dermatol 1993;129:403.
44. Waitzer S, Butaney J, From L et al. Cutaneous ultrastructural changes and photosensitivity associated with amiodarone therapy. J Am Acad Dermatol 1987;16:779.
45. Miller AW, McDonald AT. Dermal lipofuscinosis associated with amiodarone therapy. Arch Dermatol 1984;120:646.

46. Rappersberger K, Konrad K, Wieser E et al. Morphological changes in peripheral blood cells and skin in amiodarone-treated patients. Br J Dermatol 1986;114:189.
47. Zachary CB, Slater DN, Holt DW et al. The pathogenesis of amiodarone-induced pigmentation and photosensitivity. Br J Dermatol 1984;110:451.
48. Fitzpatrick JE. New histopathologic findings in drug eruptions. Dermatol Clin 1992;10:19.
49. Job CK, Yoder L, Jacobsen RR et al. Skin pigmentation from clofazimine therapy in leprosy patients: A reappraisal. J Am Acad Dermatol 1990;23:236.
50. Bardach A, Gebhart W, Niebauer G. "Lumpy-bumpy" elastic fibers in the skin and lungs of a patient with penicillamine-induced elastosis perforans serpiginosa. J Cutan Pathol 1979;6:243.
51. Siegel RC. Collagen cross-linking: Effect of D-penicillamine on cross-linking in vitro. J Biol Chem 1977;252:254.
52. Meyrick Thomas RH, Kirby JDT. Elastosis perforans serpiginosa and pseudoxanthoma elasticum-like skin change due to D-penicillamine. Clin Exp Dermatol 1985;10:386.
53. Hashimoto K, McEvoy B, Belcher R. Ultrastructure of penicillamine-induced skin lesions. J Am Acad Dermatol 1981;4:300.
54. Price RG, Prentice RSA. Penicillamine-induced elastosis perforans serpiginosa: Tip of the iceberg? Am J Dermatopathol 1986;8:314.
55. Ruocoo V, Sacrerdoti G. Pemphigus and bullous pemphigoid due to drugs. Int J Dermatol 1991;30:307.
56. Marsden RA, Ryan TJ, Vanhegan RI et al. Pemphigus foliaceus induced by penicillamine. Br Med J 1976;2:1423.
57. Sparrow GP. Penicillamine pemphigus and the nephrotic syndrome occurring simultaneously. Br J Dermatol 1978;98:103.
58. Carpenter S, Berg D, Sidu-Malik N et al. Vancomycin-associated linear IgA dermatosis: A report of three cases. J Am Acad Dermatol 1992;26:45.
59. Yung CW, Hambrick GW Jr. D-penicillamine-induced pemphigus syndrome. J Am Acad Dermatol 1982;6:317.
60. Yokel BK, Hood AF, Anhalt GJ. Induction of acantholysis in organ explant culture by penicillamine and captopril. Arch Dermatol 1989;125:1367.
61. DeDobbeleer G, Godfrine S, Gourdain JM et al. In vitro acantholysis induced by D-penicillamine, captopril, and piroxicam on dead de-epidermized dermis. J Cutan Pathol 1992;19:181.
62. Korman NJ, Eyre RW, Zone J, Stanley JR. Drug-induced pemphigus: Autoantibodies directed against the pemphigus antigen complexes are present in penicillamine and captopril-induced pemphigus. J Invest Dermatol 1991;96:273.
63. Yung RL, Richardson BC. Drug-induced lupus erythematosus. Rheum Dis Clin North Amer 1994;20:61.
64. Whittle TS Jr, Ainsworth SK. Procainamide-induced systemic lupus erythematosus. Arch Pathol 1976;100:469.
65. Pauls JD, Gohill J, Fritzler MJ. Antibodies from patients with systemic lupus erythematosus and drug-induced lupus bind determinants on histone 5(H5). Mol Immunol 1990;27:701.
66. Grossman J, Callerame ML, Condemi JJ. Skin immunofluorescence studies on lupus erythematosus and other antinuclear antibody-positive disease. Ann Intern Med 1974;80:496.
67. Jiang X, Khursigara G, Rubin RL. Transformation of lupus-inducing drugs to cytotoxic products by activated neutrophils. Science 1994;266:810.
68. Perroud H, Delacrétaz J. Iodides végétanes. Ann Dermatol Venereol 1977;104:154.
69. O'Brien TJ. Iodic eruptions. Australas J Dermatol 1987;28:119.
70. Heydenreich G, Larsen PO. Iododerma after high dose urography in an oliguric patient. Br J Dermatol 1997;97:567.
71. Lauret P, Godin M, Bravard P. Vegetating iodides after intravenous pyelogram. Dermatologica 1985;171:463.
72. Blasik LG, Spencer SK. Fluoroderma. Arch Dermatol 1979;115:1334.
73. Rosenberg FR, Einbinder J, Walzer RA et al. Vegetating iododerma. Arch Dermatol 1972;105:900.
74. Marshall JP, Schneider RP. Systemic argyria secondary to topical silver nitrate. Arch Dermatol 1977;113:1077.
75. Plewig G, Lincke H, Wolff HH. Silver-blue nails. Acta Dermatol Venereol (Stockh) 1997;57:413.
76. Gherardi R, Brochard P, Chamek B et al. Human generalized argyria. Arch Pathol 1984;108:181.
77. Suzuki H, Baba S, Uchigasaki S, Murase M. Localized argyria with chrysiasis caused by implanted acupuncture needles. J Am Acad Dermatol 1993;29:833.
78. Rongioletti F, Robert E, Buffa P et al. Blue nevi-like dotted occupational argyria. J Am Acad 1992;27:1015.
79. Pariser RJ. Generalized argyria. Arch Dermatol 1978;114:373.
80. Hönigsman H, Konrad K, Wolfe K. Argyrose: Histologie und Ultrastruktur. Hautarzt 1973;24.
81. Naseman T, Rogge T, Schaeg G. Licht- und elektronenmikroskopische untersuchungen bei der hydrargyrose und der argyrose der haut. Hautarzt 1974;25:534.
82. Johansson EA, Kanerva L, Niemi KM et al. Generalized argyria. Clin Exp Dermatol 1982;7:169.
83. Czitober H, Frischauf H, Leodolter I. Quantitative Untersuchung bei universeller argyrose mittels neutronenaktivierungsanalyse. Virchows Arch A 1970;350:44.
84. Pezzarosa E, Alinovi A, Ferrari C. Generalized argyria. J Cutan Pathol 1983;10:361.
85. Cox AJ, Marich KW. Gold in the dermis following gold therapy for rheumatoid arthritis. Arch Dermatol 1973;108:655.
86. Al-Talib RK, Wright DH, Theaker JM. Orange-red birefringence of gold particles in paraffin wax embedded sections: An aid to the diagnosis of chrysiasis. Histopathology 1994;24:176.
87. Pelachyk JM, Bergfeld WF, McMahon JT. Chrysiasis following gold therapy for rheumatoid arthritis. J Cutan Pathol 1984;11:491.
88. Lamar L, Bliss BO. Localized pigmentation of the skin due to topical mercury. Arch Dermatol 1966;93:450.
89. Burge KM, Winkelmann RK. Mercury pigmentation: An electron microscopic study. Arch Dermatol 1970;102:51.
90. Sigal-Nahum M, Petit A, Gaulier A et al. A nodular cutaneous lymphoproliferative disorder during carbamazepine administration. Br J Dermatol 1992;127:545.
91. Welykyi S, Gradini R, Nakao J et al. Carbamazepine-induced eruption histologically mimicking mycosis fungoides. J Cutan Pathol 1990;17:111.
92. Wolf R, Kahane E, Sandbank M. Mycosis fungoides-like lesions associated with phenytoin therapy. Arch Dermatol 1985;121:1181.
93. Charlesworth EN. Phenytoin-induced pseudolymphoma syndrome. Arch Dermatol 1977;113:477.
94. Harris DW, Ostlere L, Buckley C et al. Phenytoin-induced pseudolymphoma: A report of a case and review of the literature. Br J Dermatol 1992;127:403.
95. Adams JD. Localized cutaneous pseudolymphoma associated with phenytoin therapy: A case report. Australas J Dermatol 1981;22:28.
96. Braddock SW, Harrington D, Vose J. Generalized nodular cutaneous pseudolymphoma associated with phenytoin therapy: Use of T-cell receptor gene rearrangement in diagnosis and clinical review of cutaneous reactions to phenytoin. J Am Acad Dermatol 1992;27:337.
97. Rosenthal CJ, Noguera CA, Coppola A et al. Pseudolymphoma with mycosis fungoides manifestations, hyperresponsiveness to diphenylhydantoin and lymphocyte disregulation. Cancer 1982;49:2305.
98. D'Incan M, Souteyrand P, Bignon YJ et al. Hydantoin-induced cutaneous pseudolymphoma with clinical, pathologic, and immunologic aspects of Sézary syndrome. Arch Dermatol 1992;128:1371.
99. Singer J, Schmid C, Souhami R, Issacson PG. Bone marrow involvement in phenytoin-induced pseudolymphoma. Clin Oncol (R Coll Radiol) 1993;5:397.
100. Howard AM, Dowling J, Varigos G. Pseudoporphyria due to naproxen. Lancet 1985;1:819.
101. Texier L, Gauthier Y, Gauthier O et al. Sclérodermies lombo-fesseères consécutives à des injections intra-musculaires de vitamine K1. Bord Med 1972;7:1571.
102. Brown JM, Grosso MA, Harken AH. Cytokines, sepsis and the skin. Surg Gynecol Obstet, 1989;169:568.
103. Gaspari AA, Lotze MT, Rosenberg SA et al. Dermatologic changes associated with interleukin-2 administration. JAMA 1987;258:1624.
104. Lee RE, Gaspari AA, Lotze MT et al. Interleukin-2 and psoriasis. Arch Dermatol 1988;124:1811.
105. Biesma B, Willemse PHB, Mulder NH et al. Effects of interleukin-3 after chemotherapy for advanced ovarian cancer. Blood 1992;80:1141.
106. Atkins MB, Vachino G, Tilg HJ et al. Phase I evaluation of thrice-

daily intervenous bolus interleukin-4 in patients with refractory malignancy. J Clin Oncol 1992;10:1802.

107. Fleming TE, Mirando WS, Soohoo LF et al. An inflammatory skin eruption associated with recombinant human IL-6. Br J Dermatol 1994;130:534.
108. Glaspy JA, Baldwin GC, Robertson PA et al. Therapy for neutropenia in hairy cell leukemia with recombinant granulocyte colony-stimulating factor. Ann Intern Med 1988;109:789.
109. Yang SC, Grimm EA, Parkinson DR et al. Clinical and immunomodulatory effects of combination immunotherapy with low-dose interleukin-2 and tumor necrosis factor alpha in a patient with advanced non-small cell lung cancer: A phase I trial. Cancer Res 1991;51:3669.
110. Jones GJ, Itri LM. Safety and tolerance of recombinant interferon alpha-2a (Roferon-A) in cancer patients. Cancer 1986;57:1709.
111. Rest EB, Yokel B, Bart B. Local reactions to injection to recombinant human beta interferon. J Cutan Pathol 1995;22:81.
112. Kennedy MJ, Vogelsang GB, Jones RJ et al. Phase I trial of interferon gamma to potentiate cyclosporine-induced graft-versus-host disease in women undergoing autologous bone marrow transplantation for breast cancer. J Clin Oncol 1994;12:249.

Lever's Histopathology of the Skin, eighth edition,
edited by David Elder et al. Lippincott–
Raven Publishers, Philadelphia © 1997.

CHAPTER 12

The Photosensitivity Disorders

John L. M. Hawk, Neil P. Smith,* and Martin M. Black

Cutaneous disorders caused by ultraviolet radiation (UVR), or photodermatoses, consist of drug and chemical photosensitivity, the DNA repair-deficient disorders, the UVR-exacerbated dermatoses, and the largest and commonest group, the idiopathic photodermatoses; these last consist of polymorphic (polymorphous) light eruption, actinic prurigo, hydroa vacciniforme, chronic actinic dermatitis (photosensitivity dermatitis and actinic reticuloid syndrome, persistent light reaction), and solar urticaria.[1,2] Recent careful investigation of the idiopathic group, however, has yielded much circumstantial evidence to suggest that these conditions are all immunologically mediated disorders; the first four perhaps are delayed-type hypersensitivity (DTH) reactions against UVR-induced skin antigen, the exact features of the eruptions very possibly being determined by the cutaneous sites of antigen formation, and the last is probably instead an immediate-type hypersensitivity response against a similarly produced cutaneous or circulating substance.[1] Confirmation of this hypothesis now requires definitive identification of the putative antigens for the conditions.

Drug and chemical photosensitivity, the DNA repair-deficient disorders, and the UVR-exacerbated dermatoses are considered elsewhere in this book; the idiopathic, probably immunologically based photodermatoses are now discussed here.

POLYMORPHIC (POLYMORPHOUS) LIGHT ERUPTION

Polymorphic (polymorphous) light eruption (PMLE) is a commonly occurring, transient, intermittent, UVR-induced eruption of nonscarring, erythematous, itchy papules, plaques, or vesicles of exposed skin, most severe in spring and summer and commonest in young women.[1,2] It is seen mostly at temperate latitudes, affecting up to one in five subjects of any skin coloring; attacks develop during sunny vacations and summer weather, often persisting or recurring, sometimes with gradual reduction in severity, from spring until fall. They follow around 15 minutes to a few hours of sun exposure, or occasionally occur a few days after a period with little exposure, and they begin within hours of irradiation and last for hours, days, or rarely weeks. Some but not necessarily all exposed skin is affected, usually symmetrically; normally uncovered sites are most frequently spared. Diagnosis is made from the history and clinical findings in the presence of normal circulating antinuclear factor and extractable nuclear antigen titers, and of normal urinary, stool, and blood porphyrin concentrations. If there is diagnostic uncertainty, however, histology of a lesion may suggest PMLE, and broad-spectrum or monochromatic irradiation skin tests may induce the typical eruption or else abnormal erythemal or papular responses. Treatment is for the most part prophylactic and often effective. Limitation of UVR exposure, use of appropriate clothing, and regular application of high-protection, broad-spectrum sunscreens during exposure are generally satisfactory for mild disease, and short courses of low-dose psoralen photochemotherapy (PUVA) or UVB phototherapy before summer begins are usually effective in more severe instances. If the eruption should develop despite these measures, a short course of systemic steroid therapy usually rapidly abolishes it. The value of other regularly advocated medications, however, such as antimalarials and beta-carotene, has not been confirmed in controlled trials.

Histopathology. This may vary, but usually there is variable epidermal spongiosis and dermal, perivascular, predominantly mononuclear cell infiltration with edema, which in older lesions may extend into the deeper dermis. The picture may resemble that seen in early lesions of subacute cutaneous lupus erythematosus, except that the infiltrate in PMLE is more commonly around blood vessels than around the pilosebaceous structures, and liquefaction degeneration of the cells of the basal layer is absent (Figs. 12-1 and 12-2); in addition, the degree of papillary dermal edema is usually much greater in PMLE. The cells of the infiltrate are usually T lymphocytes, but occasionally eosinophils and neutrophils are present as well.[1,2]

Pathogenesis. The eruption of PMLE is induced by exposure to UVR, particularly from strong summer sunlight. Artificial reproduction is less easy, and exact action spectra have not been conclusively determined. Nevertheless, the responsible wavelengths appear to be UVB in around a quarter of patients, UVA in half, and both in the remainder. The eruption itself ap-

*Deceased during preparation of manuscript.

J. L. M. Hawk, N. P. Smith, M. M. Black: St. John's Institute of Dermatology, St. Thomas Hospital, London, United Kingdom

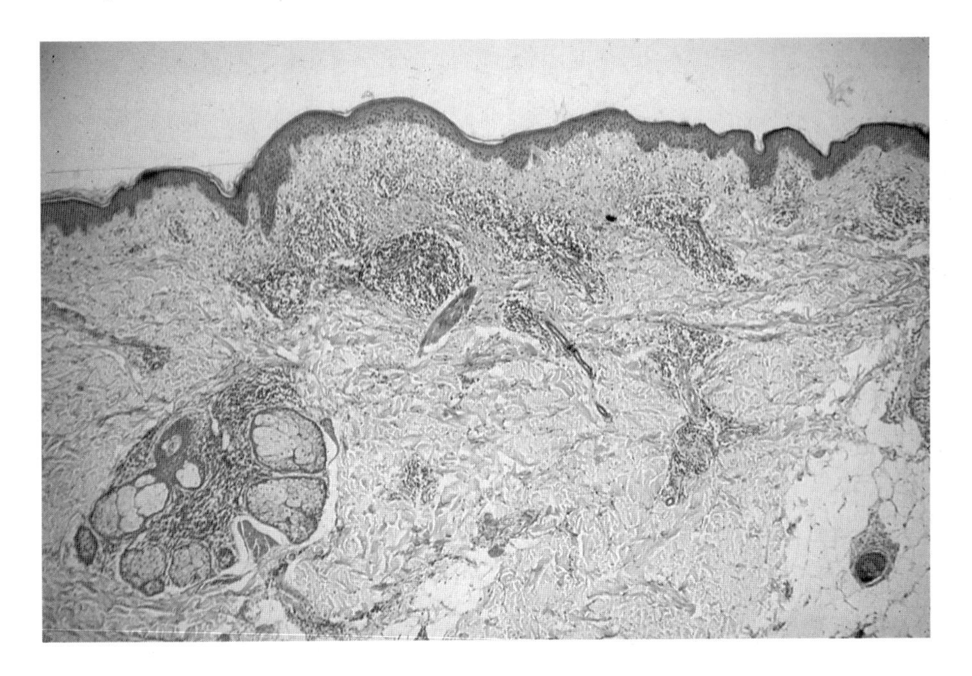

FIG. 12-1. Polymorphic (polymorphous) light eruption
An early plaquelike lesion shows edema of the papillary dermis, with a superficial and deeper perivascular and periappendageal inflammatory infiltrate.

pears very likely to be a DTH response in view of its pattern of dermal cellular infiltration, cytokine production, and adhesion molecule expression, arguably to UVR-induced, endogenous, cutaneous antigen.[1,2]

Differential Diagnosis. PMLE must be differentiated from lupus erythematosus, the porphyrias, other idiopathic photodermatoses, Jessner's lymphocytic infiltrate, cutaneous T-cell lymphoma, rosacea, and rarely other granulomatous infiltrates.[1,2] The diagnosis is generally apparent from the clinical history, in which sun exposure is nearly always clearly incriminated in causing the typical eruption; however, circulating antinuclear antibody and extractable nuclear antigen titers and urinary, stool, and blood porphyrin concentrations must be normal. If doubt persists, the histopathologic findings are usually helpful, although relatively nonspecific.

ACTINIC PRURIGO

Actinic prurigo (AP) is a rare, itchy, papular or nodular, excoriated, chronic summer eruption of the light-exposed and to a lesser extent covered skin of children, usually girls; it generally resolves by early adulthood.[1,2] The face and distal parts of the limbs are most often affected, and the proximal limbs and forehead beneath the hair fringe, being less often exposed, are mostly spared; the buttocks, however, are often involved. Superficial, pitted, or linear scars may be present at the sites of previous lesions; chronic cheilitis and conjunctivitis are also possible. Therapy is often helpful, consisting in mild cases of reduction in sun exposure, use of protective clothing, and application of high-protection, broad-spectrum sunscreens, emollients, and topical steroids. In more severe cases, however, pro-

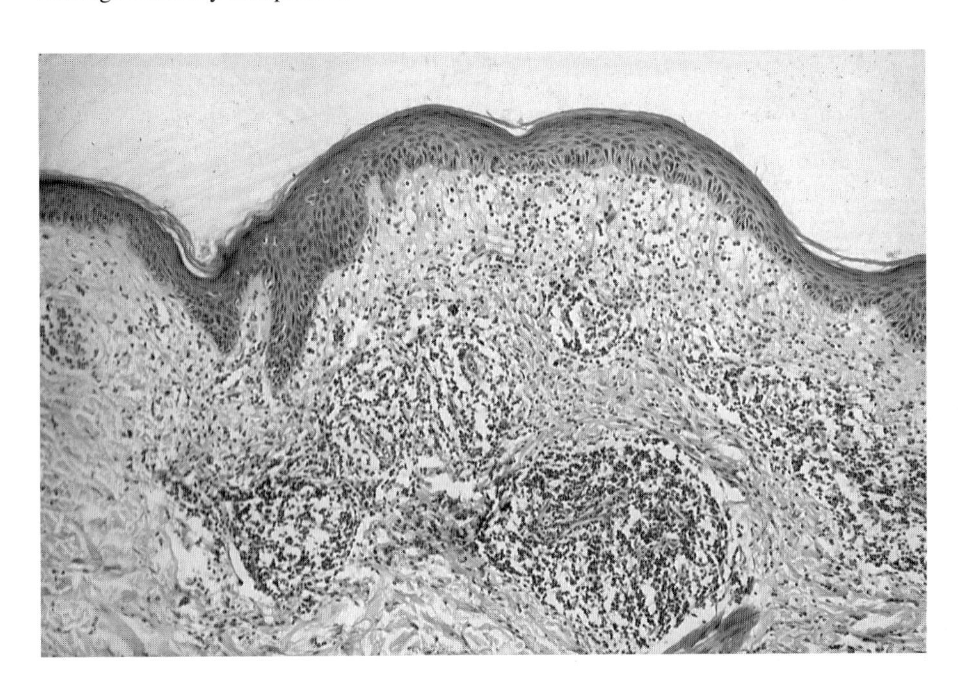

FIG. 12-2. Polymorphic (polymorphous) light eruption
Although there is some epidermal edema, there is no spongiosis or liquefaction degeneration of the basal layer. A prominent degree of edema is apparent in the papillary dermis, and the perivascular inflammatory infiltrate is predominantly lymphocytic.

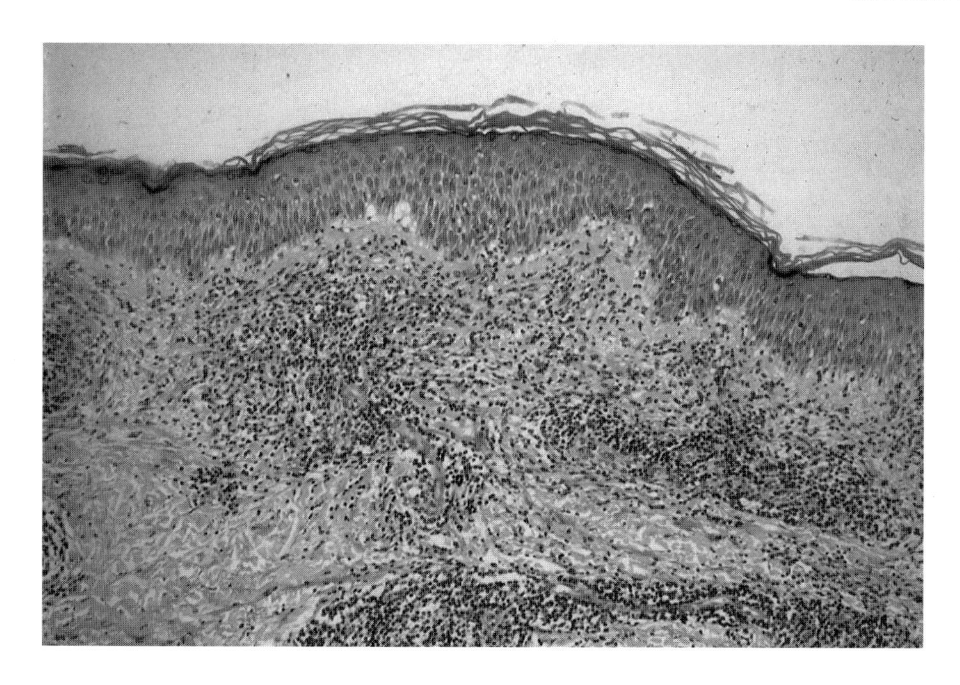

FIG. 12-3. Actinic prurigo
Some overlap with polymorphic light eruption is seen. Edema is present in the papillary dermis along with a heavy upper and middermal perivascular lymphocytic infiltrate.

phylactic low-dose UVB or PUVA irradiation therapy as for PMLE may be useful in appropriate patients; if not, oral thalidomide helps around three quarters of affected subjects, although teratogenicity and moderate peripheral neurotoxicity may preclude its use.[1,2]

Histopathology. The lesions of AP are often excoriated and not diagnostically specific. Early lesions, however, may show variable epidermal spongiosis and dermal perivascular mononuclear cell infiltration similar to that of PMLE (Figs. 12-3 and 12-4); in older lesions there may instead be variable lichenification and a moderately heavy mononuclear cell infiltrate and irregular epithelial hyperplasia similar to those of prurigo nodularis (see Fig. 12-4).[1,2] However, the histology may often be unhelpful, and diagnosis must then be made on other grounds. AP must be differentiated from the same disorders as PMLE, as well as from other causes of prurigo.

Pathogenesis. UVR exposure appears to be of prime importance in the causation of AP, given the greater severity of the disorder in summer and after sun exposure, and the relatively frequent abnormal erythemal or papular skin responses to monochromatic irradiation. Such responses occur in a half to two thirds of patients, often to the UVB wavelengths alone but sometimes also to the UVA.[1] Responses to broad-spectrum irradiation have not been reported. The behavior of AP gives some credence to suggestions that it may be a persistent form of PMLE and thus also a DTH reaction to UVR-induced, endogenous, cutaneous antigen, but this remains highly speculative and no antigen has been identified. The persistence of AP lesions as

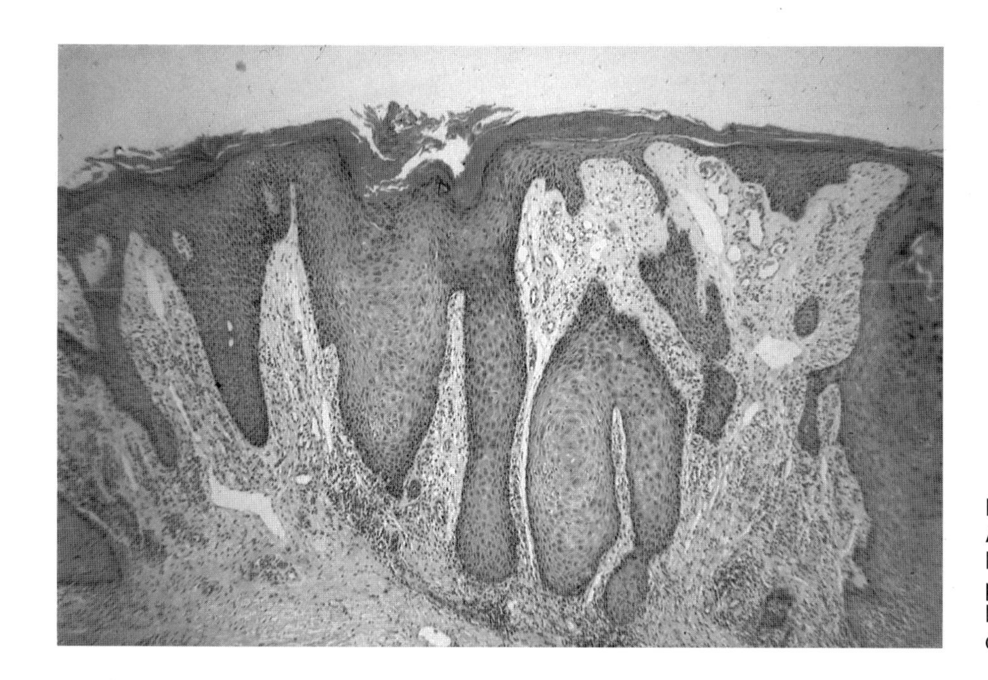

FIG. 12-4. Actinic prurigo
An older lesion shows marked lichenification and epithelial hyperplasia similar to that of prurigo nodularis. A moderately heavy lymphocytic infiltrate is also present.

compared with those of PMLE might well be determined by patient human leukocyte antigen (HLA) type; this appears in almost all cases to be HLA-DR4, found in only 30% of normal subjects, and frequently its rare subtype DRB1*0407, present in only 6% of normal European Caucasoids but relatively common in native Americans, in whom AP is also much more prevalent.[3]

Differential Diagnosis. AP must be differentiated from PMLE, insect bites, scabies, nodular prurigo, and eczema; its seasonal variation, affected sites, and sometimes positive light tests may assist in this differentiation, and the histology may also be helpful, particularly if a lesion is fresh.

HYDROA VACCINIFORME

Hydroa vacciniforme (HV) is a very rare, intermittent, UVR-induced, blistering, scarring eruption of the exposed skin, usually of children.[1,2] The condition generally has onset by age 10 with resolution by early adulthood. Usually sparse, symmetrically scattered, sometimes hemorrhagic vesicles and bullae are characteristic, particularly of the face, ears, and limbs; these may coalesce, umbilicate, and crust over the course of several days, healing thereafter in weeks to leave persistent, disfiguring pock scars. Treatment is difficult. Avoidance of UVR exposure, clothing cover, and application of high-protection, broad-spectrum sunscreens have limited efficacy; in resistant cases, courses of prophylactic low-dose UVB phototherapy or PUVA may sometimes help.

Histology. The principal histologic abnormality is that of intraepidermal vesiculation and reticular degeneration leading to epidermal necrosis. The vesicles are filled with fibrin and acute inflammatory cells, and overlie a dermal cellular infiltrate of predominantly perivascular neutrophils and mononuclear cells (Fig. 12-5).[1,2] The changes are characteristic and essentially diagnostic.

Pathogenesis. The eruption of HV is induced by bright summer sunlight.[1,2] Artificial induction is more difficult and requires repeated broad-spectrum or, less reliably, UVB skin exposure; exact action spectra have not been determined. Blood, urine, and stool porphyrin concentrations, lesional viral studies, and circulating viral, antinuclear factor, and extractable nuclear antigen titers are normal. The dermal perivascular mononuclear cell infiltration of HV and its clinical resemblance to PMLE perhaps suggest similar pathogeneses for the two disorders, arguably therefore both DTH-type immunological responses to UVR-induced, endogenous, cutaneous antigen.

Differential Diagnosis. HV must be differentiated from cutaneous viral disorders, the porphyrias, lupus erythematosus, and other idiopathic photodermatoses by its clinical features and largely diagnostic histopathology, provided always that appropriate viral studies, blood, urine, and stool porphyrin concentrations, and circulating antinuclear factor and extractable nuclear antigen titers are also normal.

CHRONIC ACTINIC DERMATITIS

Chronic actinic dermatitis (CAD) (photosensitivity dermatitis and actinic reticuloid syndrome, persistent light reaction) is a rare, persistent, often disabling, UVR- and occasionally visible light–induced eczema of exposed and sometimes also covered sites.[1,2,4] The condition is most common in elderly men at temperate latitudes, and most severe in summer. It may affect previously normal subjects, or else patients with prior endogenous eczema, photoallergic or allergic contact dermatitis, perhaps oral drug photosensitivity, or even rarely PMLE; allergic contact sensitivity to ubiquitous airborne, sometimes photoactive, agents may coexist. There is usually itchy, scattered or confluent, subacute or chronic eczema of the exposed skin; this may be lichenified or excoriated or, in more severely affected

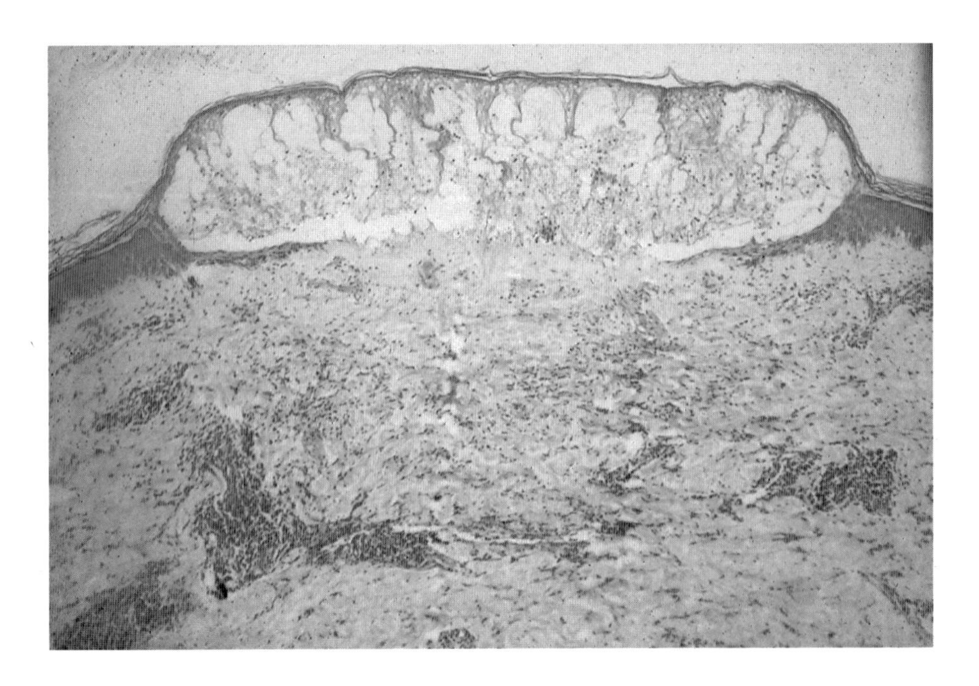

FIG. 12-5. Hydroa vacciniforme Intraepidermal vesiculation is seen leading to epidermal necrosis. The vesicle overlies a dermal perivascular inflammatory infiltrate. (From Sonnex TS, Hawk JLM. British Journal of Dermatology, 1988;118:101–108.)

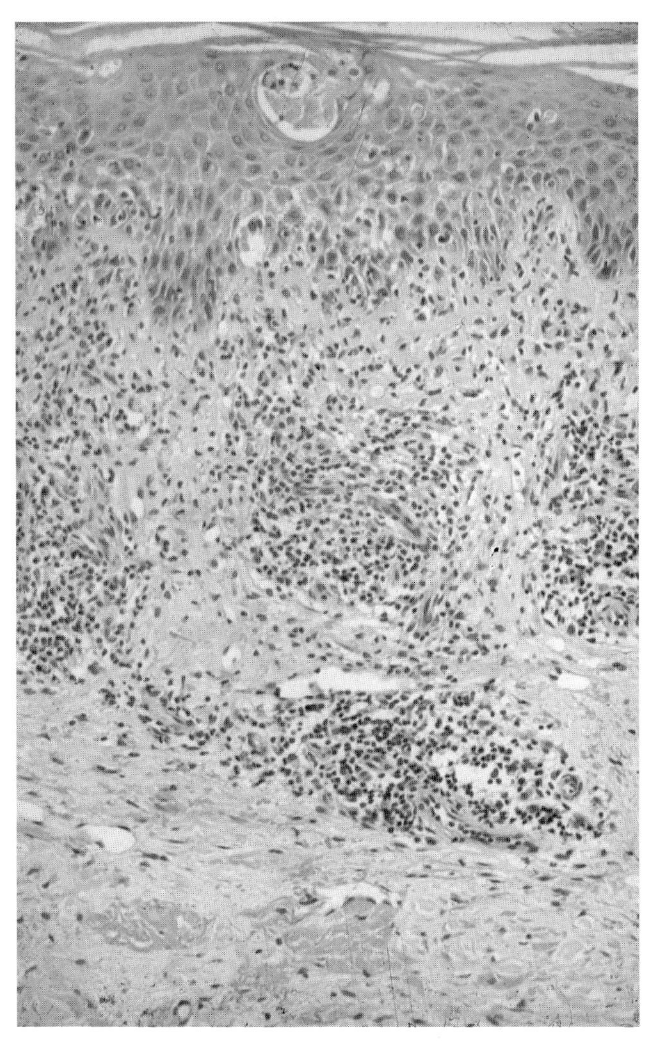

FIG. 12-6. Chronic actinic dermatitis
An early lesion shows epidermal spongiosis with already some lymphoid epidermotropism. A moderately dense lymphoid infiltrate is present in the superficial and mid-dermis.

patients, papular or plaquelike or composed of erythematous, shiny, infiltrated areas on a background of erythema, eczema, or normal skin. Erythroderma is also possible. Malignant transformation has occasionally been claimed but never convincingly demonstrated. Pseudolymphomatous CAD induced by UVB and UVA, and occasionally by visible light, is also known as actinic reticuloid, eczematous CAD induced by UVB is also known as photosensitive eczema or photosensitivity dermatitis, and eczematous CAD evoked by both UVB and UVA is also known as photosensitivity dermatitis; CAD following photoallergic contact dermatitis is also called persistent light reaction. Treatment of CAD is often difficult. Avoidance of UVR exposure, wearing of appropriate protective clothing, and use of high-protection broad-spectrum sunscreens are only rarely effective; if these measures fail, intermittent courses of oral steroids, courses of low-dose PUVA under high-dose oral steroid cover, or immunosuppressive therapy with azathioprine or cyclosporine may be necessary.

Histology. In the early stages of CAD, the histology may resemble that of contact dermatitis, with epidermal spongiosis and a superficial and deeper perivascular inflammatory infiltrate. In older lesions, there is variable acanthosis and the infiltrate is often much heavier. The epidermis, in addition, may contain occasional Pautrier microabscess–like collections of cells, and in the dermis there is often a deep, predominantly perivascular and usually dense mononuclear cell infiltrate containing T lymphocytes, macrophages, eosinophils, and plasma cells; in addition, nuclei may be large, hyperchromatic, and convoluted, and mitotic figures may be present (Figs. 12-6 and 12-7).[1,2,4] If severe, CAD may closely resemble cutaneous T-cell lymphoma. Other features seen in older lesions are the presence of vertically streaked collagen in the papillary dermis and stellate fibroblasts.

Pathogenesis. CAD is clinically and histologically reproducible at all skin sites in the absence of exogenous photosensitizer by UVB alone, by UVB and UVA combined, or rarely by UVB, UVA, and short visible radiation, and the clinical features and pattern of dermal cellular infiltration, cytokine production, and adhesion molecule activation are all very similar to those of allergic contact dermatitis, a known DTH response.[1,2,4] This

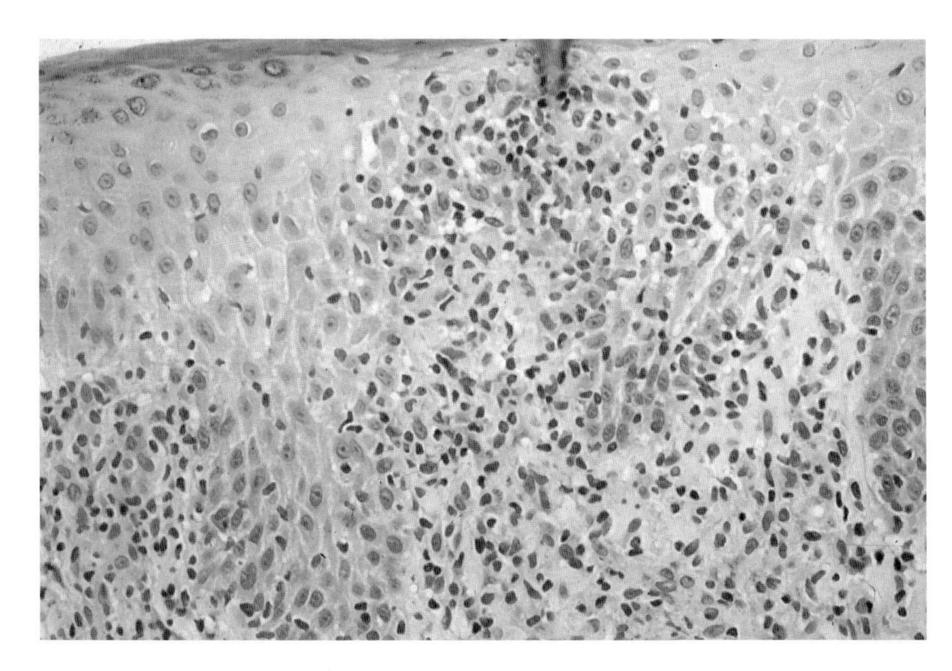

FIG. 12-7. Chronic actinic dermatitis
An older lesion shows epidermal acanthosis and much more prominent lymphoid epidermotropism. Some clusters of lymphocytes resemble early Pautrier microabscesses. A heavy lymphoid dermal infiltrate is seen, without atypia.

strongly suggests that CAD may also be a DTH response, presumably to photo-activated endogenous, cutaneous allergen, and action spectrum studies suggest that the initiating UVR absorber may be DNA or a similar or associated molecule.[5] Concomitant airborne allergic contact dermatitis is very common in CAD, and perhaps increases cutaneous immune responsiveness so as to enable recognition of putative, presumably weak, allergen. Further, CAD is common in elderly men, especially outdoor workers and leisure enthusiasts, and it may well be that simultaneous sunlight and airborne allergen exposure in aged skin leads to relatively easy penetration and slowed clearance of allergens so as to further facilitate development of the condition.

Differential Diagnosis. CAD must be distinguished from other forms of eczema, in particular seborrheic and atopic eczemas and airborne and topical medicament contact dermatitis, as well as from cutaneous T-cell lymphoma, particularly the Sézary syndrome.

SOLAR URTICARIA

Solar urticaria (SU) is a rare UVR- or visible radiation–induced wealing disorder of exposed skin; the more common primary SU occurs spontaneously, and the rare secondary form follows photosensitization to drugs or chemicals.[1,2] Primary SU is slightly more common in women, with onset between ages 10 and 50 years; the eruption develops on exposed skin within 5 to 10 minutes and fades within an hour or two in most instances. Regularly uncovered sites such as the face and the backs of hands are sometimes spared. A tingling sensation and patchy erythema usually precede separate or confluent wealing, the latter sometimes generalized and possibly associated with headache, nausea, bronchospasm, or fainting. Secondary SU generally follows exposure to substances such as tar, pitch, dyes, drugs such as benoxaprofen, or rarely the endogenous metabolite protoporphyrin in erythropoietic protoporphyria. Avoidance of the inducing radiation, use of appropriate sunscreens, or medication with adequate doses of nonsedating antihistamines may help around half of patients. Resistant cases may respond to PUVA or plasmapheresis, but some SU patients fare poorly on all treatment.

Histopathology. There is dermal edema and separation of collagen bundles, along with mild to moderate perivascular neutrophilic and lymphocytic infiltration.[1,2]

Pathogenesis. Any UVR or visible radiation waveband, specific for a given patient, may induce primary SU.[1,2] Wealing is probably mediated through allergic type I hypersensitivity to cutaneous or circulating, irradiation-induced allergen, and presumed circulating antibodies have also been identified, very likely IgE in type. In secondary SU, the eruption probably follows nonimmunological, direct tissue injury. Histamine is probably the major mediator in both forms.

Differential Diagnosis. SU must be differentiated from other light-induced eruptions by its much shorter time course and characteristic wealing, and from other forms of urticaria, particularly physical urticaria induced by heat; the porphyrias, drug and chemical photosensitivity, and lupus erythematosus must also be excluded.

REFERENCES

1. Hawk JLM. Cutaneous photobiology. In: Rook A, Ebling FJG, Champion RH, Burton JL, eds. Textbook of dermatology, 5th ed. Oxford: Blackwell Scientific Publications, 1991;849.
2. Hawk JLM, Norris PG. Abnormal responses to ultraviolet radiation; idiopathic. In: Fitzpatrick TB, Eisen ZA, Wolff K et al., eds. Dermatology in general medicine, 4th ed. New York: McGraw-Hill, 1993;1661.
3. Menagé HduP, Vaughan RW, Baker CS et al. HLA-DR4 may determine expression of actinic prurigo in British patients. J Invest Dermatol 1996;106:362.
4. Ferguson J. Photosensitivity dermatitis and actinic reticuloid syndrome (chronic actinic dermatitis). Semin Dermatol 1990;9:47.
5. Menagé HduP, Harrison GI, Potten CS et al. The action spectrum for induction of chronic actinic dermatitis is similar to that for sunburn inflammation. Photochem Photobiol 1995;62:976.

Lever's Histopathology of the Skin, eighth edition, edited by David Elder et al. Lippincott–Raven Publishers, Philadelphia © 1997.

CHAPTER 13

Disorders Associated with Physical Agents

Heat, Cold, Radiation, or Trauma

David Elder, Rosalie Elenitsas, Bernett Johnson Jr., and Christine Jaworsky

Temperature-dependent skin disorders can be divided into those associated with acute exposure and those associated with chronic exposure to heat or cold. Examples of the former include burns and frostbite. Examples of the latter include erythema ab igne and chilblains, which result from chronic exposure to moderate levels of heat and cold respectively. Unusual or idiosyncratic temperature-dependent skin reactions include Raynaud's phenomenon, cryoglobulinemia, livedo reticularis (see Chap. 8), and cold panniculitis (see Chap. 20) as reactions to cold injury, and physical urticaria, which may be induced by either heat or cold.[1]

BURNS

Burns result from exposure to extremes of heat. The severity of a burn is related to duration of exposure, temperature of the heat source, and skin thickness.[1] The pathogenesis of heat injury involves coagulation necrosis of cellular proteins, enzyme inactivation, and increased capillary permeability, which may in part be due to the release of inflammatory mediators.

Histopathology. In a *first-degree burn* there is no full-thickness necrosis of the epidermis. Depending on the severity of the burn, there may be intraepidermal or subepidermal edema, or there may be evidence of partial-thickness superficial epidermal necrosis. In a *second-degree burn* there is superficial to full-thickness epidermal necrosis, and there is intraepidermal as well as subepidermal edema resulting in a blister that may variously be spongiotic (intraepidermal), subepidermal, or a mixture of the two. Although in a deep second-degree burn there may be necrosis of superficial dermal collagen, for the most part the dermis remains more or less intact and there is potential for epidermal regeneration from the epithelium of skin appendages. In a *third-degree burn* there is full-thickness necrosis of epidermis and dermis with little or no potential for regeneration. Granulation tissue and ultimate scarring are the sequelae of deep second-degree and of third-degree burns. The findings may be complicated by changes due to secondary infection. The scar of a late healed burn is composed of homogeneous or hyalinized collagen. In contrast to a radiation scar, skin appendages are absent from the full-thickness burn scar.[2] After many years, squamous cell carcinoma may develop in the epidermis overlying the burn site (Marjolin's ulcer). Rarely, malignant melanoma has been reported in the same situation.[3]

In acute *sunburn* the epidermis contains scattered eosinophilic keratinocytes that have lost their nuclei. It is likely that these "sunburn cells" are formed by a process of apoptosis, or programmed cell death as a result of irreparable DNA damage. In addition, there is a greater or lesser degree of subepidermal edema, which may result in blister formation. If the sunburn is severe, there may be full-thickness epidermal necrosis but the skin appendages remain viable as a source of regenerated epidermis.

ERYTHEMA AB IGNE

Prolonged exposure to moderate heat emanating from fireplaces, radiators, or heating pads causes a persistent reticular erythema with or without pigmentation. The shins, the lower back, and the buttocks are the most common sites.

Histopathology. The epidermis may show atypical keratinocytes along the basal layer. On staining for elastic tissue, in most cases a great increase in the amount of elastic fibers is seen in the upper dermis and the midportion of the dermis. There is, however, no homogenization with loss of fibrous structure as seen in solar elastosis. In most cases melanin gran-

D. Elder: Department of Pathology, Hospital of the University of Pennsylvania, Philadelphia, PA

R. Elenitsas: Department of Dermatology, University of Pennsylvania, Philadelphia, PA

B. Johnson Jr.: Department of Dermatology, University of Pennsylvania, Philadelphia, PA

C. Jaworsky: Departments of Dermatology and Pathology, Case Western University, Cleveland, OH

ules are found in the upper dermis, and in some cases hemosiderin is also present. The development of "thermal keratoses" and of carcinoma in situ has been reported to occur on the shins.[4–8]

Differential Diagnosis. The absence of basophilic staining in the dermis on staining with hematoxylin and eosin and of homogenization of the elastic fibers differentiates erythema ab igne from solar (actinic) degeneration (Chap. 15).

FROSTBITE

The sequence of events in freezing or nonfreezing cold injury include (1) arterial and arteriolar vasoconstriction, (2) venular and capillary vasodilatation, (3) endothelial leakage, (4) erythrostasis, (5) arteriovenous shunting, (6) segmental vascular necrosis, and (7) massive thrombosis.[9] These processes, with or without actual freezing of tissue, may lead to massive necrosis of tissue. Frostbite occurs when tissue freezes. After rewarming, large blisters form and the necrotic tissue is converted into a hard black eschar. Weeks later, a line of demarcation forms and the tissues distal to the line will undergo autoamputation.[1]

PERNIOSIS

Pernio or chilblain usually consists of tender or painful, raised, violaceous plaques on the fingers or toes referred to as

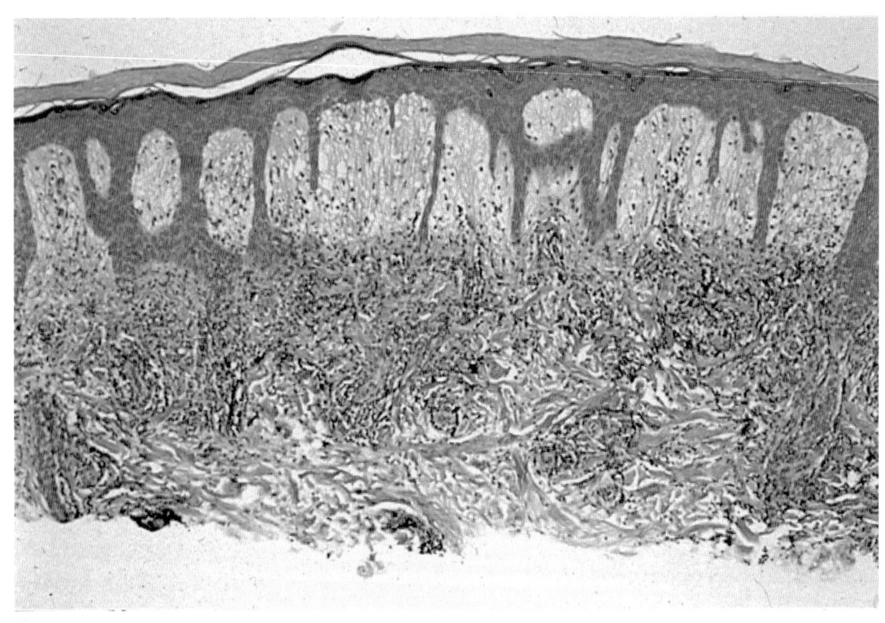

A

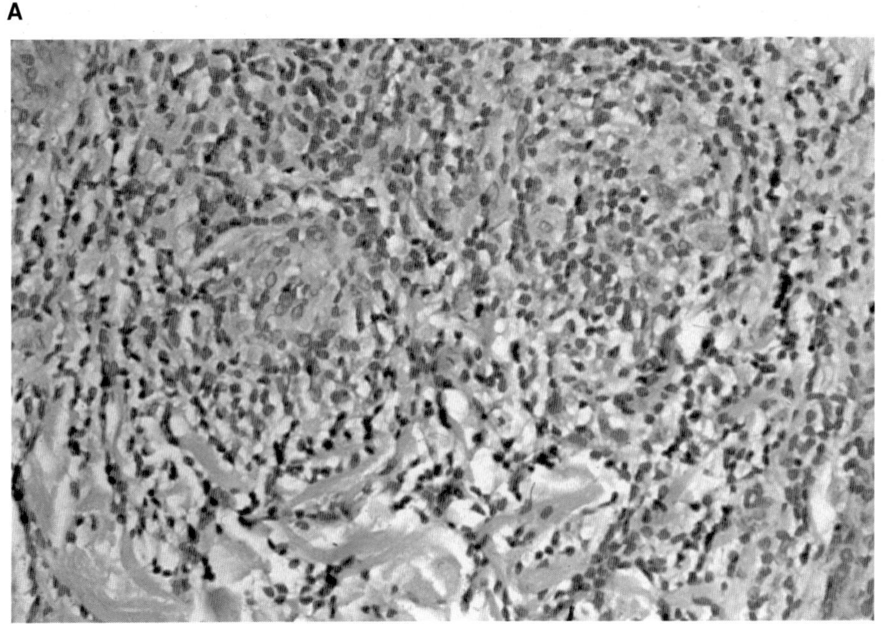

B

FIG. 13-1. Perniosis
(**A**) Intense edema of the papillary dermis and a moderately dense perivascular and interstitial, superficial and deep lymphocytic infiltrate. (**B**) Moderately intense perivascular lymphocytic infiltrate with involvement and some evidence of damage to the vessel wall.

superficial pernio. Occasionally it is found at a more proximal portion of an extremity in a deeper location in the skin or subcutis (see Chap. 20). Pernio is caused in susceptible individuals by prolonged exposure to cold above the freezing point, especially in damp climates.[1]

Histopathology. In superficial pernio, intense edema of the papillary dermis is observed. A marked perivascular mononuclear cell infiltrate is seen in the upper dermis but sparing the edematous papillary dermis. The blood vessels show a diffuse "fluffy" edema of their walls. The mononuclear infiltrate of the vascular walls is suggestive of a lymphocytic vasculitis (Fig. 13-1).

In deep pernio an intense mononuclear cell perivascular infiltrate extends throughout the dermis into the subcutaneous fat. The blood vessels show a similar edema as the superficial form of pernio.[10,11]

RADIATION DERMATITIS

An early (acute) stage and a late (chronic) stage of radiation dermatitis are recognized. Early radiation dermatitis develops after large doses of x-rays or radium. Erythema develops within about a week. This may heal with desquamation and pigmentation. If the dose was high enough, painful blisters may develop at the site of erythema. In that case, healing usually takes place with atrophy, telangiectasia, and irregular hyperpigmentation. Subsequent to very large doses ulceration occurs, generally within two months. Such an ulcer may heal ultimately with severe atrophic scarring, or it may not heal.

Late (chronic) radiation dermatitis occurs from a few months to many years after the administration of fractional doses of x-rays or radium. The skin shows atrophy, telangiectasia, and irregular hyper- and hypopigmentation. Ulceration, as well as foci of hyperkeratosis, may be seen within the areas of atrophy. Squamous cell carcinomas or basal cell epitheliomas may develop. The former tend to arise in areas of severe radiation damage, and the latter in areas in which the radiation damage is rather mild.[12]

Histopathology. In early radiation dermatitis, there is intracellular edema of the epidermis with pyknosis of the nuclei. The cells of the hair follicles, sebaceous glands, and sweat glands also show acute degenerative changes. An inflammatory infiltrate is seen throughout the dermis and may permeate the epidermis. Some of the blood vessels are dilated, whereas others, especially large ones in the deep portions of the dermis, show edema of their walls, endothelial proliferation, and even thrombosis. The collagen bundles show edema. In cases with blisters, the degenerated epidermis is detached from the dermis, and, if ulceration is present, not only the epidermis but also the upper dermis undergo necrosis. The area of necrosis is then surrounded by neutrophils.[13]

In late radiation dermatitis, the epidermis is irregular, showing atrophy in some areas and variable hyperplasia in others. Hyperkeratosis is common. The cells of the stratum malpighii show degenerative changes, such as edema and homogenization. In addition, they may show a disorderly arrangement and individual cell keratinization. Some of the nuclei may be atypical. The epidermis may also show irregular downward growth and may even grow around telangiectatic vessels, which may become nearly enclosed in the epidermis (Fig. 13-2).

In the dermis, the collagen bundles are swollen and often show hyalinization. They may stain irregularly and appear faintly eosinophilic in some areas and deeply eosinophilic in others. In response to the degeneration of collagen, new collagen may form throughout the dermis. Large, bizarre, stellate "radiation fibroblasts" may be found.[14] The nuclei of these cells may be enlarged, irregular, and hyperchromatic. This "radiation atypia" differs from that seen in neoplasms because the cellularity is low and the atypical nuclei are scattered among other, less atypical cells. Thus, the atypia is "random" rather than "uniform," as is characteristic of malignant neoplasms. Striking and rather characteristic changes may be observed in the blood vessels. Those located in the deep dermis often show fibrous thickening of their walls, so that the lumen may be nearly or entirely occluded. Some of the vessels show thrombosis and recanaliza-

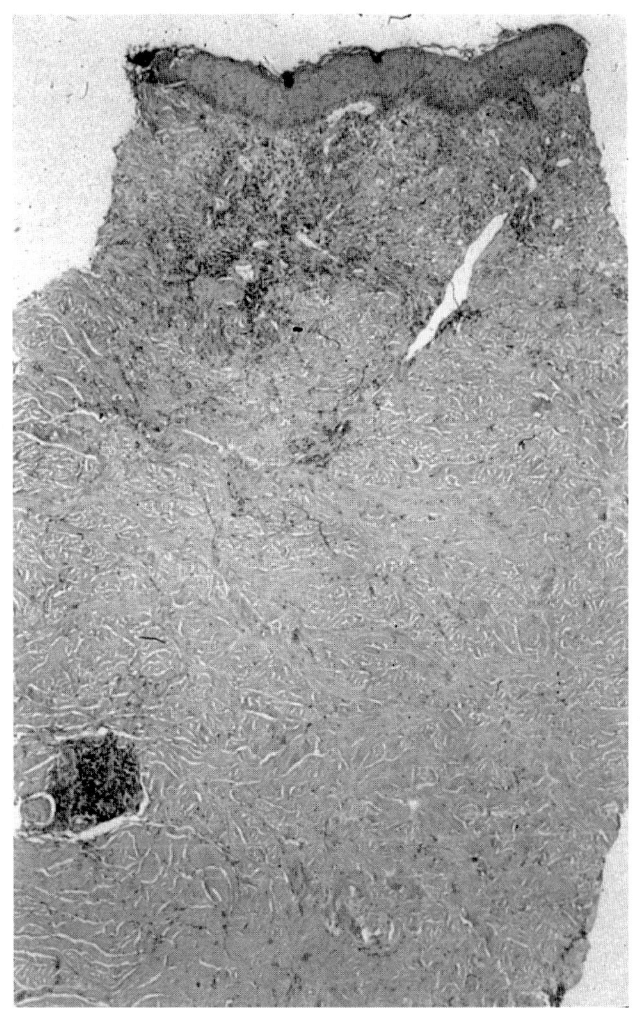

A

FIG. 13-2. Radiation dermatitis
(**A**) Radiation fibrosis. The normal architecture of the reticular dermis collagen is replaced by homogenized collagen. There are inflammation and telangiectasia of superficial vessels. In contrast to a burn scar, skin appendages are present in the scar. *(continued on next page)*

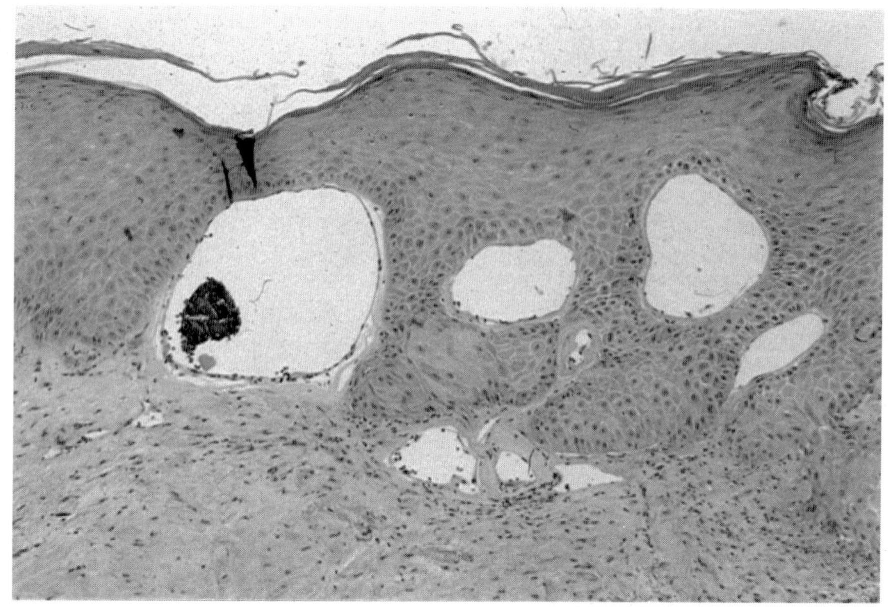

B

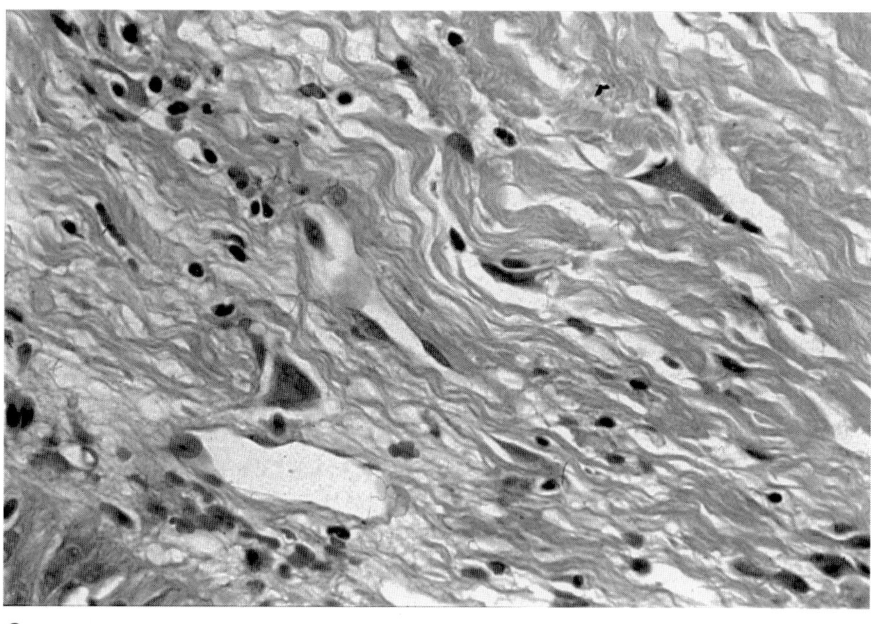

C

FIG. 13-2. *Continued*
(**B**) Telangiectatic vessels in a radiation scar. The epidermis tends to grow around and enclose the dilated vessels. (**C**) Radiation atypia. Scattered fibroblasts contain enlarged, irregular, and hyperchromatic nuclei. Other cells are not atypical, and the cellularity is low. This "random" atypia and the low cellularity tend to distinguish radiation atypia from neoplastic atypia, in which the cellularity is usually high, the atypia is uniform, and mitoses are usually present.

tion. In contrast, the vessels of the upper dermis may be telangiectatic. Also, there may be lymphedema in the subepidermal region. Hair structures and sebaceous glands are absent, but the sweat glands usually are preserved at least in part, except in areas of severe injury.

In severe cases of late radiation dermatitis, ulceration occurs. The deep-lying, large blood vessels in the regions of such ulcers often are completely occluded.

Squamous cell carcinomas arising in late radiation dermatitis often show a high degree of malignancy with a tendency to metastasize. Frequently, they are of the spindle cell type (see Chap. 30).[15] Basal cell epitheliomas tend to be less invasive and destructive.[16,17] The occurrence of a sarcoma is rare. A few fairly convincing cases have been published, most of them diagnosed as malignant fibrous histiocytoma (see Chap. 33).[18,19] Many of these tumors are quite undifferentiated so that a spin-

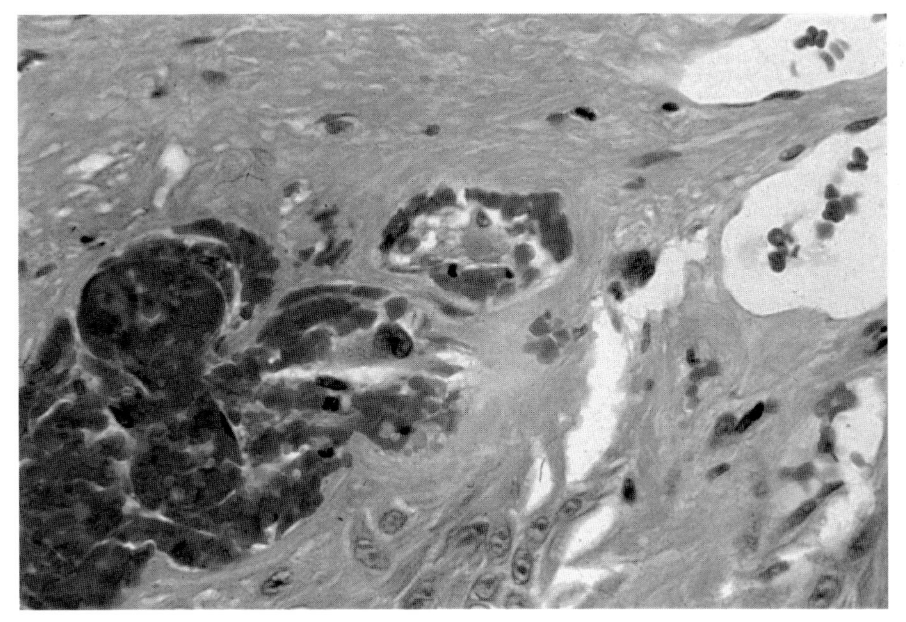

D

FIG. 13-2. *Continued*
(**D**) Radiation atypia. Scattered endothelial cells contain atypical nuclei similar to those of the fibroblasts depicted above. These appearances must be differentiated from angiosarcoma, in which atypia is more uniform and channels lined by a single layer of cells infiltrate among dermal collagen bundles.

dle-cell squamous cell carcinoma can be ruled out only by means of electron microscopy or through the use of monoclonal antibodies (see Chaps. 29, 33).

Differential Diagnosis. The epidermal changes of late radiation dermatitis may be similar to those of either an atrophic or a hyperplastic solar keratosis. However, the dermal changes differ. In solar keratosis there is basophilic degeneration limited to the upper dermis, whereas in late radiation dermatitis degenerative changes of the collagen extend deep into the dermis.

SUBCUTANEOUS FIBROSIS AFTER RADIATION THERAPY

Radiation therapy for cancer may concentrate the dose of radiation well below the skin surface at the site of deep tumors. It may lead, however, to the development of subcutaneous fibrosis several months after radiotherapy. In order for recurrent tumor to be ruled out, a deep biopsy, including muscle, is needed.

Histopathology. Histologic examination shows a band of fibrosis overlying degenerated skeletal muscle. The blood vessels show thickening of the walls and endothelial proliferation.[20] Random atypia of fibroblasts and endothelial cells is usually evident.

CALCANEAL PETECHIAE (BLACK HEEL)

An asymptomatic, pigmented, macular lesion is found on one or both heels immediately above the hyperkeratotic border of the foot. The margin of the lesion is ill defined and speckled. The lesion is traumatic in origin and is caused by any sport, such as basketball, tennis, or football, that leads to slamming of the foot against the shoe. The importance of the lesion lies in its clinical resemblance to a malignant melanoma.

Histopathology. Extravasated erythrocytes may be found in the dermal papillae. Often, however, the histologic changes are limited to the stratum corneum, where one observes rounded collections of amorphous, yellow-brown material representing lysed red blood cells. The amorphous material does not stain blue with Perls' stain, as hemosiderin would. However, positive peroxidase and benzidine reactions prove that the material is derived from hemoglobin.[21,22]

Pathogenesis. Small foci of hemorrhages move from the tips of the dermal papillae into the epidermis and are found in the thick keratin layer of the heel. The Perls' stain for iron is negative because of the absence of phagocytosis of the lysed red blood cells in the stratum corneum.[23,24]

REFERENCES

1. Page EH, Shear NH. Temperature-dependent skin disorders. J Am Acad Dermatol 1988;18:1003.
2. Weedon D. Reactions to physical agents. In: Weedon D, ed. The skin. Edinburgh: Churchill Livingstone, 1992;571.
3. Fleming MD, Hunt JL, Purdue GF et al. Marjolin's ulcer: A review and reevaluation of a difficult problem. J Burn Care Rehabil 1990;11: 460.
4. Finlayson GR, Sams WM Jr, Smith JG Jr. Erythema ab igne: A histopathological study. J Invest Dermatol 1966;46:104.
5. Hurwitz RM, Tisserand ME. Erythema ab igne. Arch Dermatol 1987; 123:21.
6. Shahrad P, Marks R. The wages of warmth: Changes in erythema ab igne. Br J Dermatol 1977;97:179.
7. Johnson WC, Butterworth T. Erythema abligne. Arch Dermatol 1971; 104:128.
8. Arrington JH III, Lockman DS. Thermal keratoses and squamous cell

carcinoma in situ associated with erythema ab igne. Arch Dermatol 1979;115:1226.
9. Kulka JP. Cold injury of the skin. Arch Environ Health 1965;11:484.
10. Wall LM, Smith NP. Perniosis: A histopathological review. Clin Exp Dermatol 1981;6:263.
11. Herman EW, Kezis JS, Silvers DN. A distinctive variant of pernio. Arch Dermatol 1981;117:26.
12. Lazar P, Cullen SI. Basal cell epithelioma and chronic radiodermatitis. Arch Dermatol 1963;88:172.
13. Epstein E. Radiodermatitis. Springfield, IL: Charles C. Thomas, 1962.
14. Young EM Jr, Barr RJ. Sclerosing dermatosis. J Cutan Pathol 1985;12: 426.
15. Sims CF, Kirsch N. Spindle-cell epidermoid epithelioma simulating sarcoma in chronic radiodermatitis. Arch Dermatol Syph 1948;57:63.
16. Totten RS, Antypes PG, Dupertuis SM et al. Pre-existing roentgen-ray dermatitis in patients with skin cancer. Cancer 1957;10:1024.
17. Anderson NP, Anderson HE. Development of basal cell epithelioma as a consequence of radiodermatitis. Arch Dermatol Syph 1951;63:586.
18. Seo IS, Warner TFCS, Warren JS et al. Cutaneous postirradiation sarcoma: Ultrastructural evidence of pluripotential mesenchymal cell derivation. Cancer 1985;56:761.
19. Souba WW, McKenna RJ Jr, Meis J et al. Radiation-induced sarcomas of the chest wall. Cancer 1986;57:610.
20. James WD, Odom RB. Late subcutaneous fibrosis following megavoltage radiotherapy. J Am Acad Dermatol 1980;3:616.
21. Kirton V, Price MW. "Black heel." Trans St Johns Hosp Dermatol Soc 1965;51:80.
22. Crissey JT, Peachey JC. Calcaneal petechiae. Arch Dermatol 1961;83: 501.
23. Rufli T. Hyperkeratosis haemorrhagica. Hautarzt 1980;31:606.
24. Mehregan AH. Perforating dermatoses: A clinicopathologic review. Int J Dermatol 1977;16:19.

Lever's Histopathology of the Skin, eighth edition,
edited by David Elder et al. Lippincott–
Raven Publishers, Philadelphia © 1997.

CHAPTER 14

Noninfectious Granulomas

Philip E. Shapiro

FOREIGN-BODY REACTIONS

Foreign substances, when injected or implanted accidentally into the skin, can produce a focal, nonallergic foreign-body reaction, or in persons specifically sensitized to them, a focal allergic response.[1] In addition, certain substances formed within the body may produce a nonallergic foreign-body reaction when deposited in the dermis or the subcutaneous tissue. Such endogenous foreign-body reactions are produced, for instance, by urates in gout and by keratinous material in pilomatricoma, as well as in ruptured epidermoid and trichilemmal cysts.

Histopathology. A *nonallergic* foreign-body reaction typically shows a granulomatous response with histiocytes and giant cells around the foreign material. Often, some of the giant cells are of the foreign-body type, in which the nuclei are in haphazard array. In addition, lymphocytes are usually present, as may be plasma cells and neutrophils. Frequently, some of the foreign material is seen within macrophages and giant cells, a finding that of course is of great diagnostic value. The most common cause of a foreign-body granuloma is rupture of a hair follicle or follicular cyst, and sometimes only the cyst contents, rather than residual cyst wall, is identifiable (Fig. 14-1). Exogenous substances producing nonallergic foreign-body reactions are, for instance, silk and nylon sutures (Fig. 14-2), wood, paraffin and other oily substances, silicone gel, talc, surgical glove starch powder, and cactus spines. Some of these substances—nylon sutures, wood, talc, surgical glove starch powder, and sea-urchin spines—are doubly refractile on polarizing examination. Double refraction often is very helpful in localizing foreign substances.

An *allergic* granulomatous reaction to a foreign body typically shows a sarcoidal or tuberculoid pattern consisting of epithelioid cells with or without giant cells. Phagocytosis of the foreign substance is slight or absent. Substances that in sensitized persons produce an allergic granulomatous reaction are, for instance, zirconium, beryllium, and certain dyes used in tattoos. Some substances that at first act as foreign material may later on, after sensitization has occurred, act as allergens, as in the case of sea-urchin spines and silica.

P. E. Shapiro: Dermatopathology Laboratory of New England, Hartford, CT

A histologic decision as to whether a granuloma is of the foreign-body type or of the allergic type is not always possible. A granuloma of the allergic type is more likely to have roundish, well-circumscribed collections of epithelioid histiocytes and less likely to have multinucleated histiocytes of the foreign-body type.

Nonallergic Foreign-Body Reactions

Paraffinoma

Foreign-body reactions following injections of oily substances such as mineral oil (paraffin) occur as irregular, plaque-like indurations of the skin and subcutaneous tissue.[2] Ulceration or abscesses may develop. The interval between the time of injection and the development of induration or ulceration may be many years.

The misleading term *sclerosing lipogranuloma* was given to paraffinoma of the male genitalia because of the disproved assumption that it was a local reactive process following injury to adipose tissue.[3,4]

Histopathology. Paraffinomas have a "Swiss cheese" appearance because of the presence of numerous ovoid or round cavities that show great variation in size (Fig. 14-3). These cavities represent spaces occupied by the oily substance.[5] The spaces between the cavities are taken up in part by fibrotic connective tissue and in part by a cellular infiltrate of macrophages and lymphocytes. Some of the macrophages have the appearance of foam cells. Variable numbers of multinucleated foreign-body giant cells are present.

In frozen sections of paraffinoma, the foreign material stains orange with Sudan IV or oil red O, although less so than neutral fat.[5]

Silicone Granuloma

Reactions to medical-grade silicone have occurred after injection of its liquid form for cosmetic purposes, or from leakage or rupture of silicone gel from breast implants. In the United

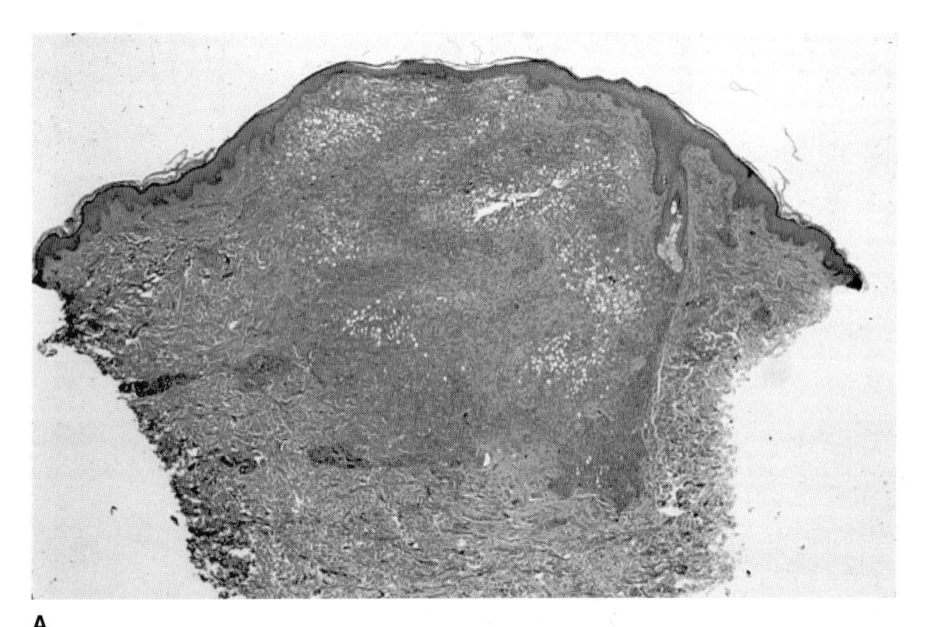

A

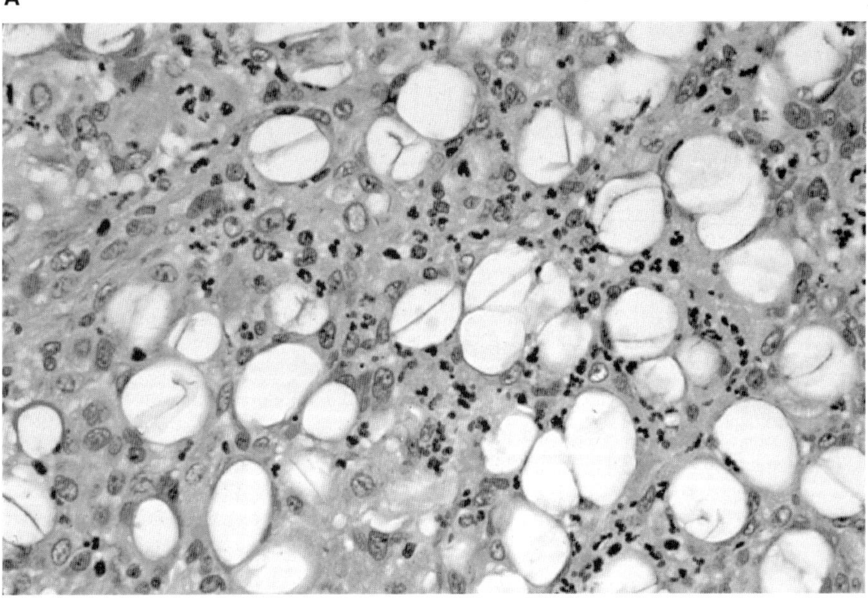

B

FIG. 14-1. Ruptured epidermoid cyst
(**A**) There is a nodular infiltrate with histiocytes and neutrophils, without an obvious cyst wall. (**B**) Cornified cells (squames), representing cyst contents, are within spaces that are surrounded by neutrophils and histiocytes.

States, the injection of liquid silicone is now banned, and it is no longer used as the gel in breast implants, in part because of controversy surrounding the unproven hypothesis that silicone leads to autoimmune disease in some individuals. Leakage from silicone breast implants, which are still in use in Europe, can cause development of subcutaneous nodules and plaques.[6]

Histopathology. As in paraffinoma, numerous ovoid or round cavities of varying sizes are seen, resulting in a "Swiss cheese" appearance. These spaces are what remain after the silicone has been removed during processing, although occasionally scant residual silicone is seen as colorless, irregularly shaped, refractile, nonpolarizable material within the spaces. Histiocytes may be present between the cavities; they can be foamy or multinucleated and accompanied by lymphocytes and eosinophils.[6,7] In addition, varying degrees of fibrosis are present.

Talc Granuloma

Talc (magnesium silicate) may produce granulomous inflammation when introduced into open wounds. Historically, talc was used as powder on gloves, but this use has been abandoned for many years, with starch being the currently used surgical dusting powder.[8] However, talc may still be introduced into wounds, either because of accidental contamination by a surgeon who uses talcum powder[8] or because talcum may be incorporated into the actual rubber glove during manufacturing.[9]

Histopathology. Histologic examination reveals histiocytes and multinucleated giant cells, some of which may contain visible particles of talc. Talc crystals can be needle-shaped with a yellow-brown or blue-green hue, and appear as white birefringent particles with polarized light.[9] Their presence can be con-

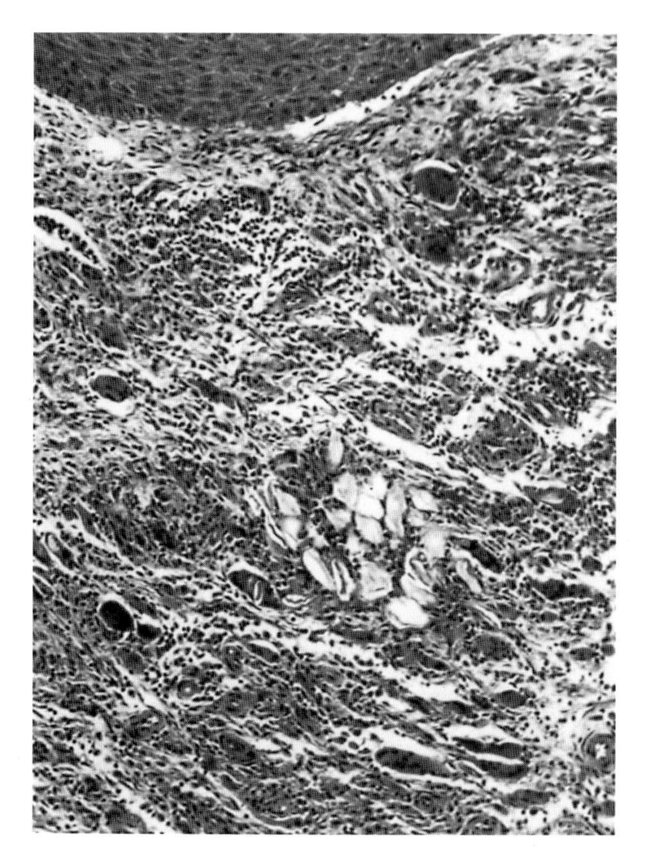

FIG. 14-2. Foreign-body granuloma caused by a nylon suture
The nylon suture is in the center of the field. Around it is a dense inflammatory infiltrate containing numerous foreign-body giant cells.

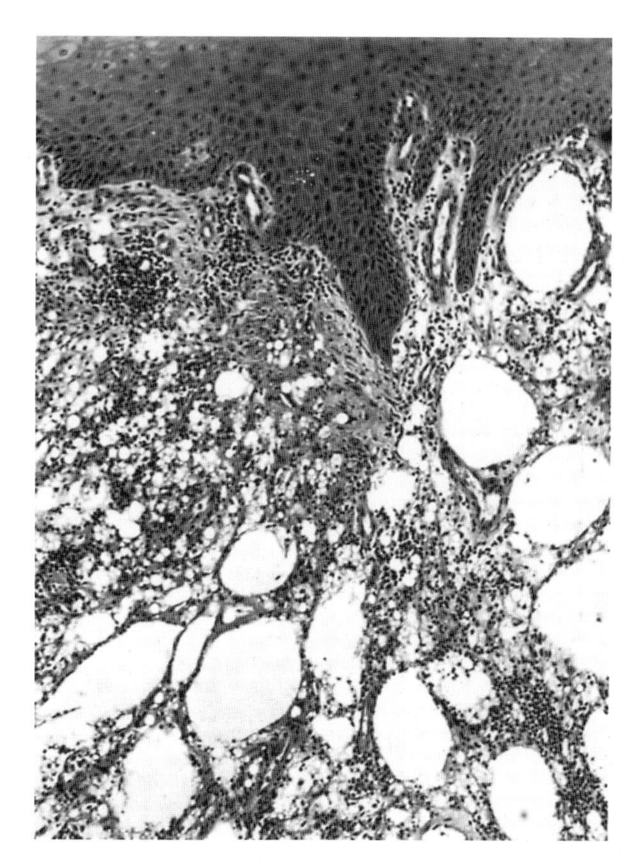

FIG. 14-3. Lipid granuloma caused by the injection of mineral oil (paraffinoma)
The many large and small oval or round cavities that give the section a "Swiss cheese" appearance represent spaces that were filled with mineral oil (paraffin).

firmed by x-ray diffraction studies[10] or energy dispersive x-ray analysis.[9]

Starch Granuloma

Granulomas may result from the contamination of wounds with surgical gloves powdered with corn starch.[8]

Histopathology. A foreign-body reaction with multinucleated giant cells is present. Scattered through the infiltrate, one observes starch granules as ill-defined ovoid basophilic structures measuring 10 to 20 μm in diameter. Most of the granules are seen within the foreign-body giant cells. They react with periodic acid–Schiff (PAS) and methenamine silver and, on examination in polarized light, are birefringent, showing a Maltese cross configuration.[11]

Cactus Granuloma

Cactus granulomas show within days or weeks after the injury tender papules from which cactus spines may still protrude. They may be extruded spontaneously within a few months.

Histopathology. Early papules, a few days after the injury, show in the dermis fragments of cactus spicules that are associated with an intense, perivascular lymphohistiocytic infiltrate containing many eosinophils. After a few weeks, the infiltrate consists of lymphocytes, macrophages, and giant cells.[12,13] Sharply marginated spicules are seen both within giant cells and lying free in the dermis. The spicules are PAS-positive.[14]

Interdigital Pilonidal Sinus

In barbers, the implantation of human hair in the interdigital web spaces may cause small, asymptomatic, or slightly tender openings.[15] Similar lesions have been observed in dog groomers.[16]

Histopathology. Histologic examination reveals a sinus tract lined by epidermis and containing one or several hairs, thus resembling a hair follicle. Either the sinus tract encases the hair completely, or, if the hair extends deeper than the sinus tract, one finds at the lower end of the hair a foreign-body giant cell reaction intermingled with inflammatory cells.[15,17]

Allergic Foreign-Body Reactions

Sea-Urchin Granuloma

Injuries from the spines of sea urchins occur most commonly on the hands and feet. Even if the friable spines have been only incompletely removed, the wounds tend to heal after spontaneous extrusion of most of the foreign material.[18,19] However, in some persons, violaceous nodules appear at the sites of injury after a latent period of 2 to 12 months.[20]

Histopathology. The nodules are composed largely of epithelioid cells and giant cells.[18] Doubly refractile material may be present in the granulomas.[19] If remnants of a spine are still present, they are surrounded by a wall of leukocytes and many large foreign-body giant cells.[19]

Pathogenesis. The appearance of sarcoidlike granulomas after a latent interval of months in only a small proportion of the injured patients suggests a delayed hypersensitivity reaction.[20] The spines of sea urchins, in addition to the calcified material, contain remnants of epithelial cells.[20] The double refraction that may be found in the granulomas may be due to the presence of a small amount of silica in the calcified spines.[19]

Silica Granuloma

Silica (silicon dioxide) is contained in rocks, soil, sand, and glass. It frequently contaminates accidental wounds, in which it sets up a foreign-body reaction of limited duration followed by fibrosis.[21] In the vast majority of cases, silica causes no further trouble. In exceptional cases, a delayed hypersensitivity granulomatous reaction occurs at the site of the old scar.[22] The mean interval for this delayed hypersensitivity reaction is approximately 10 years, but it may be less than a year or more than 50 years after the original injury.[23] When this reaction occurs, indurated papules or nodules develop at the site of injury.

Histopathology. In silica granuloma, there are groups of epithelioid histiocytes with a lymphocytic infiltrate that tends to be sparse.[22–26] Foreign-body giant cells may be abundant or absent, and Langhans' giant cells also may be present. If multinucleated histiocytes are not numerous, a picture resembling sarcoid is produced (Fig. 14-4). However, the diagnosis of sarcoidosis is easily excluded by the presence, especially within giant cells, of crystalline particles varying in size from barely visible to 100 μm in length; they represent silica crystals. When examined with polarized light, these particles are doubly refractile. The presence of silicon can be confirmed by x-ray spectrometric or energy dispersive x-ray analysis.[23,26]

Pathogenesis. Evidence suggests that the sarcoidlike granulomatous response to silica that occurs long after initial injury represents a delayed-type hypersensitivity reaction.[22–24,27]

Zirconium Granuloma

Deodorant sticks containing zirconium lactate and creams containing zirconium oxide may cause a persistent eruption composed of soft, red-brown papules in the areas to which they have been applied. Zirconium lactate is no longer present in antiperspirants sold in the United States. However, a granulomatous reaction has also been described in response to roll-on antiperspirant containing aluminum-zirconium complex.[28]

Histopathology. Histologic examination shows large aggregates of epithelioid cells with a few giant cells and a sparse or moderately dense lymphocytic infiltrate, producing a picture that may be indistinguishable from sarcoidosis.[29–31] Because of the small size of the zirconium particles, they cannot be detected on examination with polarized light.[29] Their presence, however, can be demonstrated by spectrographic analysis[30] or energy dispersive x-ray analysis.[28]

Pathogenesis. Evidence that zirconium granulomas develop on the basis of an allergic sensitization to zirconium includes the following: (1) they occur only in persons sensitized to zirconium;[32] (2) the pattern of granulomous inflammation is like that of other granulomatous dermatitides that have been attributed to delayed-type hypersensitivity reactions; and (3) autoradiographic analysis of experimentally induced lesions in sensitized individuals reveals no zirconium within epithelioid cells.[33]

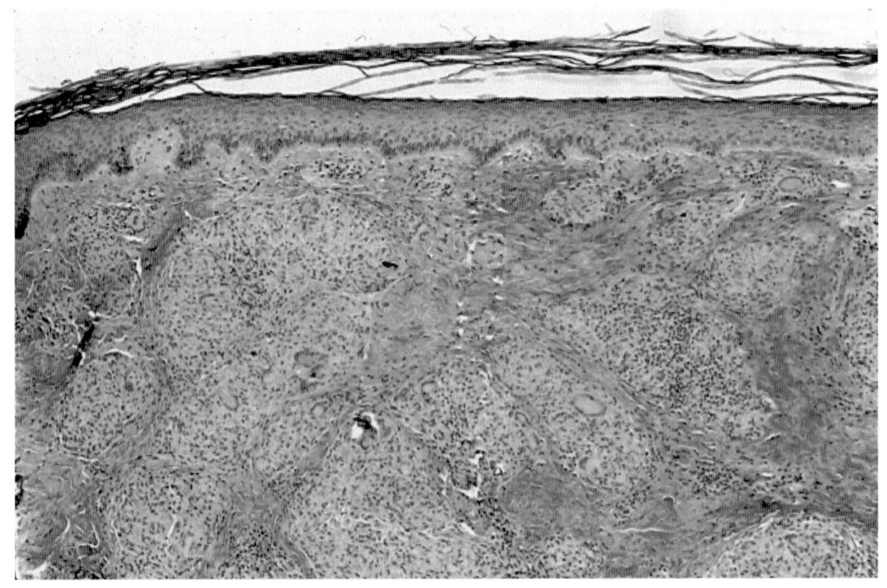

FIG. 14-4. Silica granuloma
(**A**) There are well-circumscribed collections of epithelioid histiocytes with a sparse infiltrate of lymphocytes. Note the vertical knife mark caused by the foreign body.

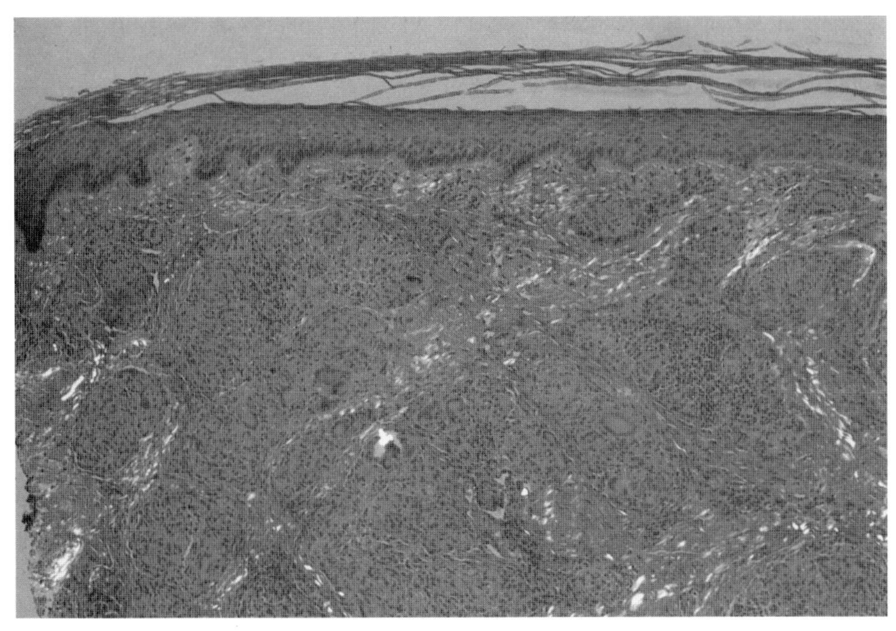

B

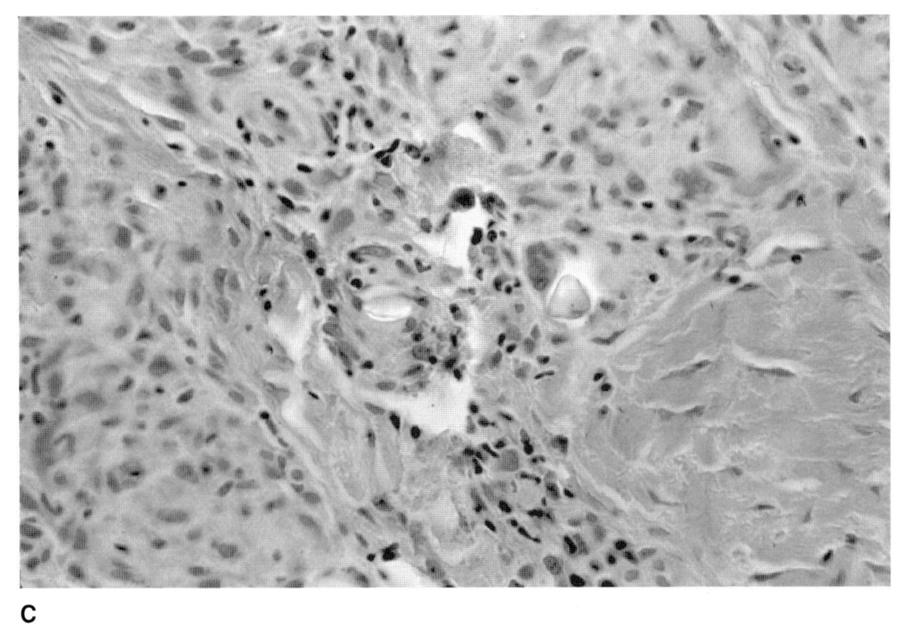

C

FIG. 14-4. ***Continued***
(**B**) Sections from *A* viewed under polarized light revealing doubly refractile foreign material. (**C**) Foreign material containing silica is present in spaces surrounded by epithelioid histiocytes.

Aluminum Granuloma

Single or multiple subcutaneous persistent nodules may appear several months after the subcutaneous injection of diphtheria, tetanus, or pertussis vaccine that are aluminum-adsorbed. The aluminum adjuvant is thought to prolong the period of activity of the vaccine, thus increasing the immunologic response.

Histopathology. The most striking finding is the presence of nodular aggregations of lymphocytes with lymphoid follicles and germinal centers in the dermis and subcutis. There is fibrosis, which may occur in bands that separate the lymphocytic nodules. Eosinophils may be prominent.[34,35] The granulomatous component consists of histiocytes with ample cytoplasm and, in some cases, a few giant cells or large areas of eosinophilic necrosis surrounded by histiocytes in a palisade.[35] PAS staining, with or without diastase digestion, gives the impression of a granular cytoplasm in the macrophages.[34]

Pathogenesis. Electron microscopic examination reveals irregular membrane-bound electron-dense material within macrophages. X-ray microanalysis has shown that the electron-dense material contains aluminum.[34]

Zinc-Induced Granuloma

Local allergic reactions to insulin are not uncommon. However, the granulomatous response, which may occur with zinc-containing insulin preparations, is rare. It may begin with sterile furunculoid lesions.[36]

Histopathology. The early furunculoid lesions show a dense neutrophilic infiltrate and many birefringent rhomboidal crystals of zinc insulin. Later, fibrosis and granulomatous inflammation develop.[36,37]

Berylliosis

Beryllium granulomas are mostly of historical interest. Up to 1949, beryllium-containing compounds were widely used in the manufacture of fluorescent light tubes. Two diseases resulted from this: systemic berylliosis and local beryllium granulomas. Systemic berylliosis developed in some workers in plants manufacturing fluorescent tubes through inhalation of these compounds. Systemic berylliosis primarily shows pulmonary involvement, which results in death in about one third of the patients.[38] Beryllium may reach the skin through the blood circulation and cause cutaneous granulomas. However, this was a rare event, having been observed in one series in only 4 instances among 535 patients with systemic berylliosis.[38] The granulomas consist of only a few papular lesions over which the skin remains intact.

Purely local beryllium granulomas occurred in persons who cut themselves on broken fluorescent tubes that were coated with a mixture containing zinc-beryllium silicate.[39] The cutaneous granulomas after laceration show as their first sign incomplete healing of the laceration, followed by swelling, induration and tenderness, and, finally, central ulceration.[40]

Histopathology. The cutaneous granulomas of systemic berylliosis are like those of sarcoidosis, showing very slight or no caseation.[38] The cutaneous granulomas following laceration, in contrast to the cutaneous granulomas of systemic berylliosis, show central necrosis, which may be pronounced.[39] A moderately dense infiltrate of lymphocytes may be present, resembling the granulomas of tuberculosis. The epidermis shows acanthosis and possibly ulceration. No particles of beryllium are seen in histologic sections, but its presence in the lesions can be demonstrated by spectrographic analysis.[40]

Pathogenesis. Systemic berylliosis develops on the basis of a delayed hypersensitivity reaction.[41,42]

Tattoo Reactions

Clinically apparent inflammatory reactions to tattoos are quite rare. They have been observed most commonly with red dyes containing mercuric sulfide, such as cinnabar (Chinese red). More recently, there has been a move away from using mercury-containing dyes toward the use of dyes containing other red pigments, such as ferric hydrate (sienna or red ochre), cadmium selenide (cadmium red), and organic dyes, but such mercury-free red dyes may also produce adverse reactions.[43,44] Reactions have also been reported with chrome green,[45] cobalt blue,[46] purple manganese salts,[47] yellow cadmium sulfide,[48] and iron oxide.[49] In some instances, an allergic response to the pigment has been suggested by a positive patch test.

Histopathology. Tattoos that are not clinically inflamed ordinarily show irregularly shaped granules of dye that are located within macrophages and extracellularly in the dermis, without any inflammatory reaction (Fig. 14-5).[50]

Inflammatory reactions in clinically inflamed tattoos may or may not be granulomatous. Photoexacerbation has been described with reactions to red pigments[43,44] and yellow pigments.[48] Nongranulomatous reactions include a perivascular lymphocytic infiltrate with pigment-containing macrophages,[43,50] a lichenoid response, which in some instances may resemble lichen planus or hypertrophic lichen planus[43,44,51,52] and a pseudolymphomatous picture with a dense, nodular or diffuse, predominantly lymphocytic infiltrate that also contains histiocytes and coarse tattoo pigment granules.[53,54]

Granulomatous reactions may be either of the sarcoidal type[45,55,56] or the foreign-body type[45,49] A tuberculoid pattern has also been described in response to cobalt blue, but this may have been due to a mycobacterial infection.[57] The granulomatous responses show tattoo granules scattered throughout the infiltrate. In the sarcoidal type, the infiltrate contains nodules of epitheloid histiocytes, and in the foreign-body type, there are obvious multinucleated histiocytes of the foreign-body type. A sparse or dense lymphocytic infiltrate may be present. In the sarcoidal type of reaction, the regional lymph nodes may also participate, with tattoo granules in the lymph nodes.[58] There are a few reports of patients with sarcoidal granulomas in their tattoos who also had pulmonary disease,[55,56,59,60] uveitis,[46,61] or erythema nodosum,[55] suggesting a systemic hypersensitivity response to the tattoo, or true sarcoidosis.

Pathogenesis. Electron microscopic examination of tattoo marks without an allergic reaction shows that most tattoo granules are located within macrophages, where they often lie within membrane-bound lysosomes. In addition, some tattoo granules are found free in the dermis.[62]

Bovine Collagen Implant

Injectable bovine collagen is used for cosmetic purposes, principally on the face to diminish "wrinkles," such as glabellar creases and prominent nasolabial folds. A small minority of patients will develop an allergic granulomatous response at the site of injection. This response usually develops within one month of injection, is manifested by induration and erythema, and usually resolves spontaneously in less than a year.[7]

Histopathology. The bovine collagen differs from native collagen by staining paler and being less fibrillar, and by its nonbirefringence when examined with polarized light. It may lie within the center of a palisaded granuloma containing many foreign-body giant cells, or it may be associated with a more diffuse granulomatous reaction. There is a variable associated infiltrate of lymphocytes, eosinophils, plasma cells, and neutrophils that tends to spare the implanted collagen.[7]

SARCOIDOSIS

Sarcoidosis is a systemic granulomatous disease of undetermined etiology. A distinction is made between the rare subacute, transient type of sarcoidosis and the usual chronic, persistent type.

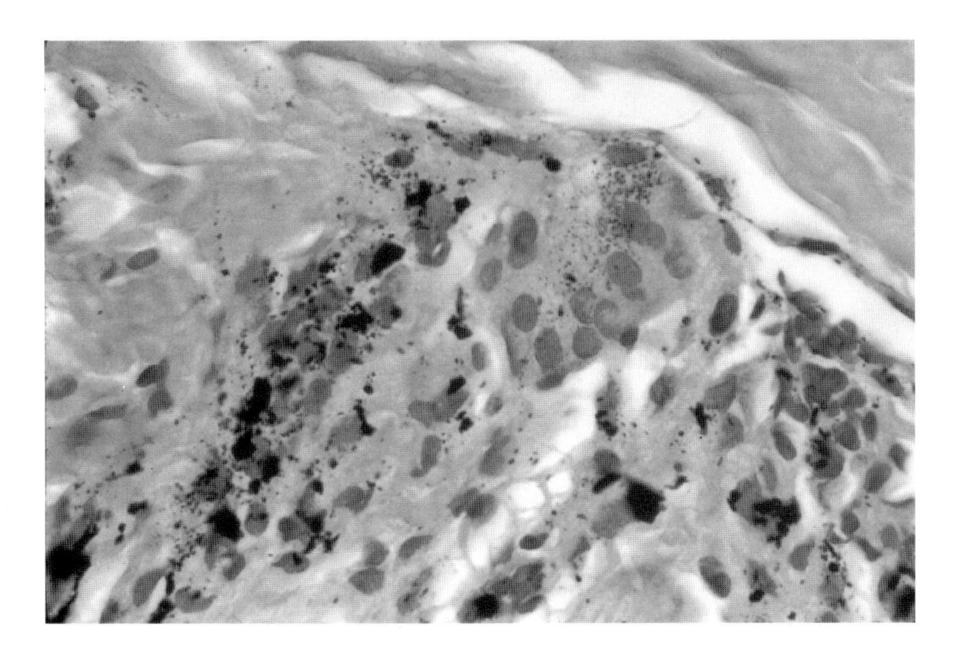

FIG. 14-5. Tattoo
A traumatic tattoo (graphite) showing black particles with irregular outlines and varied sizes, both intracellularly within macrophages and extracellularly.

In subacute, transient sarcoidosis, erythema nodosum is associated with hilar adenopathy and fever and, in some cases, also with migrating polyarthritis and acute iritis. The disease subsides in almost all patients within a few months without sequelae. Cutaneous manifestations other than erythema nodosum do not occur.[63,64] Occasionally, there is enlargement of some of the subcutaneous lymph nodes, such as the submental or cervical lymph nodes.[65]

In chronic, persistent sarcoidosis, cutaneous lesions are encountered in about one fourth of the patients who are seen in medical departments.[66] In contrast, cutaneous lesions are the only manifestation of sarcoidosis in about one-fourth of the patients with sarcoidosis seen in dermatologic departments, since in three combined series 25 of 104 patients had lesions limited to the skin.[67–69] The most common type of cutaneous lesion consists of brown-red or purple papules and plaques. Through central clearing, annual or circinate lesions may result. When the papules or plaques are situated on the nose, cheeks, and ears, the term *lupus pernio* is applied.[70]

A rather rare form of sarcoidosis is the lichenoid form, in which small, papular lesions are found.[71] Very rare manifestations of sarcoidosis are erythrodermic, ichthyosiform, atrophic, ulcerating, verrucous, angiolupoid, hypopigmented, and alopecic. In erythrodermic sarcoidosis, the erythroderma may be generalized[72] or may consist of extensive, sharply demarcated, brown-red, slightly scaling patches with little or no palpable infiltration.[73] In ichthyosiform sarcoidosis, areas of ichthyosis are found on the lower extremities[74] but at times also elsewhere on the skin.[75] Rarely, there are extensive atrophic lesions.[76] They may undergo ulceration.[77] Multiple ulcers have been described also in plaquelike lesions.[78] Angiolupoid sarcoid is characterized by a prominent telangiectatic component.[79] Lesions of hypopigmented sarcoid appear as macules with or without an associated papular or nodular compent.[80]

Subcutaneous nodules of sarcoidosis are quite rare. Originally described by Darier and Roussy,[81] they may occur in association with other cutaneous lesions[73] or alone.[82]

Systemic sarcoidosis occasionally coexists with granuloma annulare.[67] Cutaneous lesions of sarcoidosis may localize in areas of scarring, as in herpes zoster scars.[83] Tattoos[59] or other causes of exogenous material in the skin[84] may be the site of lesions of sarcoidosis.

Histopathology. The lesions of erythema nodosum occurring in subacute, transient sarcoidosis have the same histologic appearance as "idiopathic" erythema nodosum.[65]

Like lesions in other organs, the cutaneous lesions of chronic, persistent sarcoidosis are characterized by the presence of circumscribed granulomas of epithelioid cells, so-called epithelioid cell tubercles showing little or no necrosis.

The papules, plaques, and lupus pernio–type lesions show variously sized aggregates of epithelioid cells scattered irregularly through the dermis with occasional extension into the subcutaneous tissue.[85] In the erythrodermic form, the infiltrate shows rather small granulomas of epithelioid cells in the upper dermis intermingled with numerous lymphocytes,[73,86] and, rarely, also giant cells.[87] Typical epithelioid cell tubercles are found in the ichthyosiform lesions,[75] in ulcerated areas,[78] and in areas of atrophy.[88] Verrucous sarcoid shows prominent acanthosis and hyperkeratosis.[89] Biopsies of hypopigmented sarcoid may reveal granulomas, which may have a perineural component, or no granulomatous component at all.[90] In subcutaneous nodules, epithelioid cell tubercles lie in the subcutaneous fat.[82]

In typical lesions of sarcoidosis of the skin, the well-demarcated islands of epithelioid cells contain only few, if any, giant cells (Fig. 14-6), usually of the Langhans' type. A moderate number of giant cells can be found in old lesions. These giant cells may be quite large and irregular in shape. Giant cells may contain asteroid bodies or Schaumann bodies. Asteroid bodies, which are more common, are star-shaped eosinophilic structures that, when stained with phosphotungstic acid–hematoxylin, produce a center that is brown-red and spikes that are blue.[73] Schaumann bodies are round or oval, laminated, and calcified, especially at their periphery. They stain dark blue because of the presence of calcium. Neither of the two bodies is specific for sarcoidosis; they have been observed in other granulomas, such as tuberculosis, leprosy, and berylliosis.

Classically, sarcoid has been associated with only a sparse lymphocytic infiltrate, particularly at the margins of the epithelioid cell granulomas (see Fig. 14-6). Because of this sparse infiltrate of lymphocytes, the granulomas have been referred to as "naked" tubercles. However, lymphocytic infiltrates in sarcoid may occasionally be dense, as in tuberculosis (Fig. 14-7). Occasionally, a slight degree of necrosis showing eosinophilic staining is found in the center of some of the granulomas (Fig. 14-8).[85] A reticulum stain of sarcoid reveals a network of reticulum fibers surrounding and permeating the epithelioid cell granulomas. If the granulomas of sarcoidosis involute, fibrosis extends from the periphery toward the center, with gradual disappearance of the epithelioid cells.[85]

Systemic Lesions. The lungs are the most common organ to produce clinical manifestations in the chronic, persistent type of sarcoidosis, doing so in about 50% of the cases.[64] The lesions may be either nodular or disseminated with extensive parenchymal fibrosis of the lungs. In the latter type of involvement, cavities form not infrequently, and aspergillosis with pulmonary hemorrhage may ensue.[90a]

In about 25% of the patients, ocular manifestations, consisting most commonly of a chronic iridocyclitis, occur. Splenomegaly exists in about 17%. In about 12%, osseous granulomas are present, most commonly in the phalanges of the fingers and toes. Involved phalanges appear swollen and deformed, often sausage-shaped.[91] Also, the skull may show lesions,[92] appearing in roentgenograms as circumscribed lytic lesions. About 8% of the patients have involvement of large salivary glands, usually of the parotid gland.[64] In about 5%, one encounters paresis of a cranial nerve, most commonly of the facial nerve.[64] Asymptomatic enlargement of the hilar lymph nodes is present in 70%, of peripheral lymph nodes in 30%, and of the liver in 20% of the patients.[64,93]

Sarcodosis, although usually a benign disease, may lead to death. The mortality rate of sarcoidosis lies between 5% and 6%.[64,93] The most common cause of death from sarcoidosis is insufficiency of the right side of the heart resulting from massive involvement of the lungs with parenchymal fibrosis. Rather

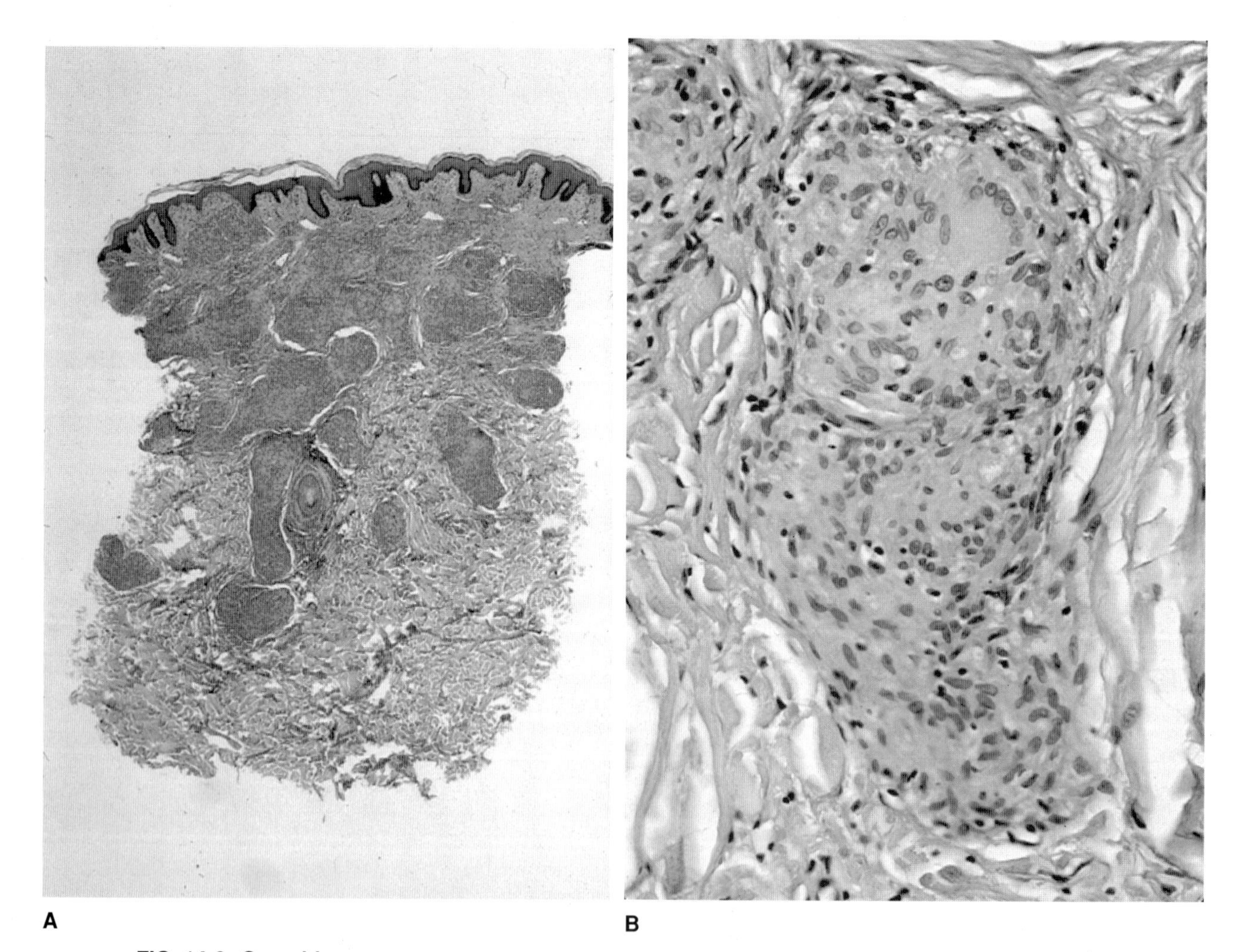

FIG. 14-6. Sarcoid
(**A**) Well-circumscribed collections of epithelioid histiocytes. (**B**) A well-circumscribed collection of epithelioid histiocytes with a sparse infiltrate of lymphocytes.

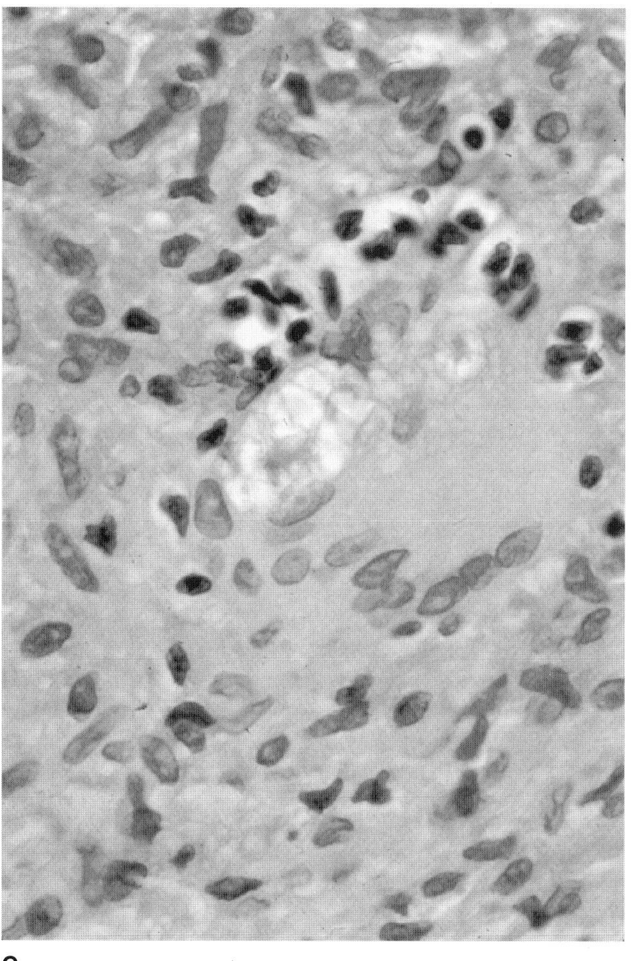

C

FIG. 14-6. ***Continued***
(**C**) In the center of the photograph are two star-shaped, eosinophilic asteroid bodies.

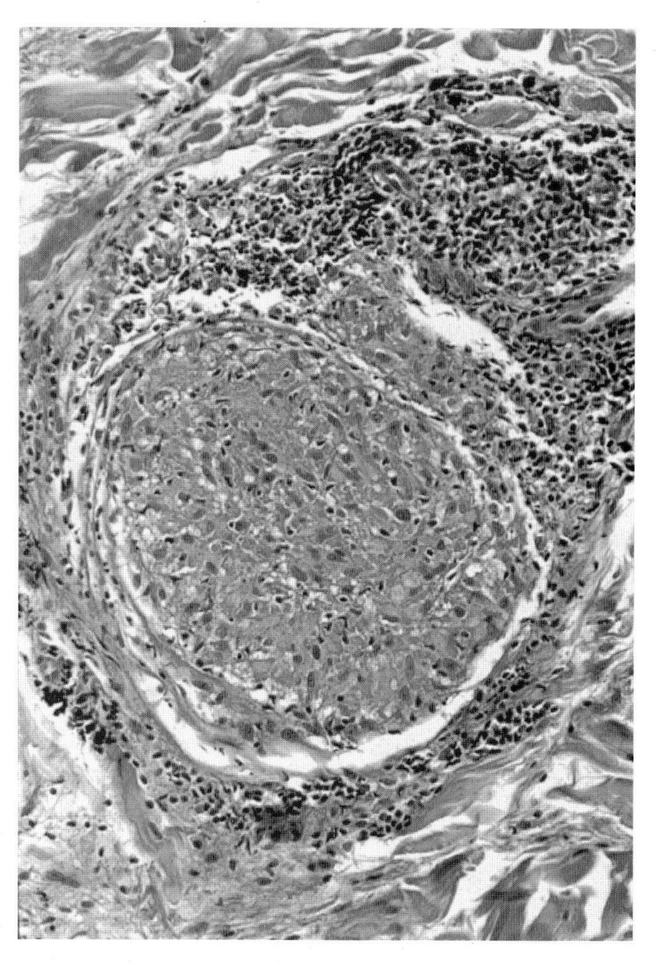

FIG. 14-7. Sarcoid
An unusually dense lymphocytic infiltrate surrounding the epithelioid histiocytes.

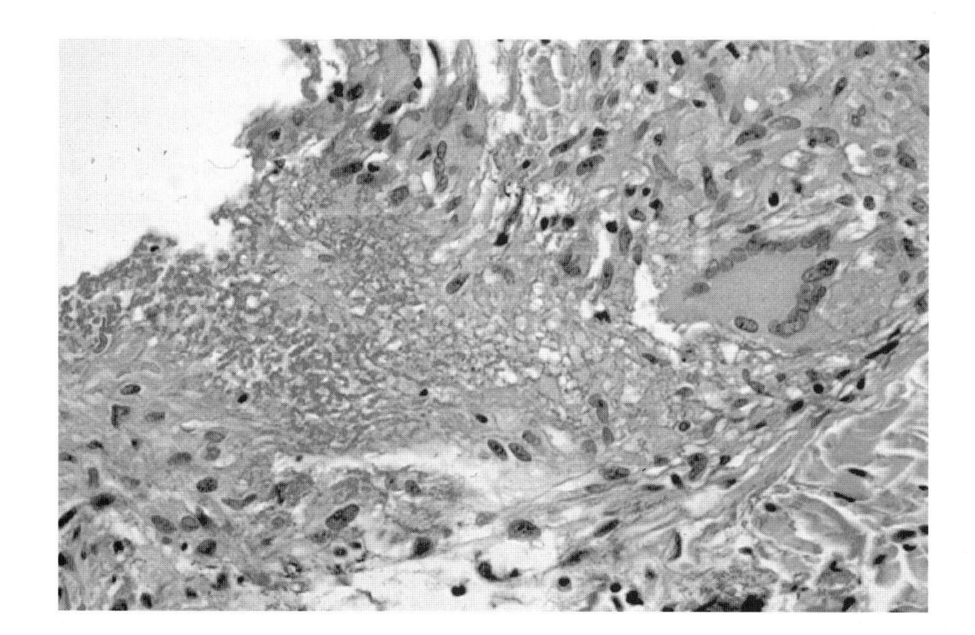

FIG. 14-8. Sarcoid
Fibrinoid material within the granulomatous component.

rare is death from pulmonary hemorrhage or from tuberculosis superimposed on sarcoidosis of the lungs. Another possible fatal complication is renal insufficiency resulting from hypercalcemia and hypercalciuria[94] or from sarcoidal glomerulonephritis.[95] In very rare instances only, death results from massive involvement of the myocardium[96] or of the liver.[97] Hypopituitarism from involvement of either the pituitary gland or the hypothalamus is also a rare fatal complication.[98]

Definitive diagnosis of chronic systemic sarcoidosis should be based on biopsy, since it may be mimicked by other diseases, such as tuberculosis. If skin lesions are present, they are the obvious choice for biopsy. If no skin lesions are present, a Kveim test may be useful. Kveim test involves intradermal injection of antigen derived from heat-sterilized suspension of sarcoidal tissue, particularly spleen or lymph node. The site is sampled 6 weeks later, with a positive result being the formation of a sarcoid-like granuloma.[99,100] The test has a sensitivity of about 80%, with false-positive reactions occurring in less than 2%.[101] However, Kveim antigen is not widely available. The most accepted alternative approach for confirming a presumptive diagnosis of systemic sarcoidosis is fiberoptic bronchoscopy with transbronchial lung biopsy.[102]

Pathogenesis. The cause of sarcoidosis is unknown, and the disease may not have the same pathogenesis in all individuals. Alterations in immunologic status have long been recognized, including impaired delayed-type hypersensitivity reactions to cutaneous antigens (anergy), a shift of helper T lymphocytes from peripheral blood to sites of disease activity, and hypergammaglobulinemia.[103] However, current thinking suggests that these immunologic phenomena represent a response to an as yet unidentified antigen.[104] Mycobacteria especially have been postulated to represent the antigen source, but conflicting data, including some using PCR-based technology, have left the issue unresolved for the present.[104]

Electron microscopic examination of epitheloid cells fails to show any evidence of bacterial fragments, unlike the macrophages seen in granulomas caused by mycobacteria, although the cells contain primary lysosomes, some autophagic vacuoles, and complex, laminated residual bodies.[105] The giant cells form through the coalescence of epitheloid cells with partial fusion of their plasma membranes. The Schaumann bodies probably form from laminated residual bodies of lysosomes. The asteroid bodies consist of collagen showing the typical 64-nm to 70-nm periodicity. It seems likely that the collagen is trapped between epithelioid cells during the stage of giant-cell formation.[105]

Differential Diagnosis. The histologic differentiation of lesions of sarcoidosis from lupus vulgaris may be very difficult, and it is occasionally impossible. There is no absolute histologic criterion by which the two diseases can be differentiated with certainty. However, as a rule, the infiltrate in sarcoidosis lies scattered throughout the dermis, whereas the infiltrate in lupus vulgaris is located close to the epidermis. Furthermore, sarcoidosis usually shows only few lymphoid cells at the periphery of the granulomas, giving them the appearance of "naked" epithelioid cell tubercles, whereas lupus vulgaris often shows a marked inflammatory reaction around and between the granulomas. The granulomas of sarcoidosis usually show much less central necrosis than the granulomas of lupus vulgaris[106]; however, not all biopsies of tuberculosis show necrosis, and some biopsies of sarcoid do. The epidermis in sarcoidosis is usually normal or atrophic, whereas in lupus vulgaris, in addition to atrophy, areas of ulceration, acanthosis, and pseudocarcinomatous hyperplasia are not uncommon. The absence of identifiable mycobacteria with acid-fast stain cannot be used to exclude tuberculosis, because in lupus vulgaris the organisms are scarce and may be difficult or impossible to find.

Occasionally, foreign-body granulomas can resemble sarcoidosis. Polariscopic examination in search of doubly refractile material, such as silica, should be performed on biopsies suspected of being sarcoidosis. The papular type of acne rosacea occasionally shows "naked" tubercles indistinguishable from those of sarcoidosis, but unlike sarcoid, they are usually perifollicular.

Tuberculoid leprosy, which may show just a sparse lymphocytic infiltrate, may also be difficult to distinguish from sarcoidosis; only 7% of cases of tuberculoid leprosy show acid-fast bacilli, and then only a few, so that they may easily be overlooked.[107] The most likely place to find bacilli is within degenerated dermal nerves, because the epithelioid cell granulomas of tuberculoid leprosy form around dermal nerves that are undergoing necrosis. Thus, the epithelioid cell granulomas of tuberculoid leprosy show small areas of central necrosis more often than those of sarcoidosis. Also, the granulomas of tuberculoid leprosy, in contrast with those of sarcoidosis, follow nerves and therefore often appear elongated.[108] Clinical correlation may be required to distinguish between these two diseases. For example, in the United States, leprosy virtually can be excluded if a patient has not been in an endemic area (either in a foreign country or where it is carried in armadillos domestically, e.g., Texas and Louisiana) or has not had prolonged close contact with another individual with the disease.

CHEILITIS GRANULOMATOSA (MIESCHER-MELKERSSON-ROSENTHAL SYNDROME)

The classic triad of Miescher-Melkersson-Rosenthal syndrome consists of recurrent labial edema, relapsing facial paralysis, and fissured tongue.[109] However, not all patients have the classic triad. In a review of 220 patients, labial swelling was seen in 84%, facial palsy in 23%, and fissured tongue in 60%.[109] Whereas monosymptomatic labial edema is recognized as part of the syndrome, lingua plicata by itself is not, since this is not uncommon in the general population. One occasionally observes, either in addition to or in place of swelling of the lips, swelling of the forehead, the chin, the cheeks, the eyelids, or the tongue.[110] The submandibular or submental lymph nodes may be enlarged.[111] Swelling of the buccal mucosa, gingiva, and pallet also can occur.[109] Chronic swelling of the vulva or of the foreskin has been described as a genital counterpart of chelitis granulomatosa.[112,113]

Histopathology. Granulomatous inflammation is not present in all biopsies of clinically involved lips.[114] There may be just edema and a predominately perivascular but also interstitial lymphoplasmacytic infiltrate that may be sparse or quite dense, producing a nodular appearance. If granulomas are present, they are noncaseating and tend to be small and scattered (Fig. 14-9). The collections of epithelioid histiocytes may be poorly circumscribed and are often associated with lymphocytes, but occasionally larger and/or "naked" tubercles are present, producing a picture like that of sarcoid.[111,114–118] The lymph nodes may also show granulomatous inflammation.[119]

Pathogenesis. The cause of the disorder is unknown. Idiosyncratic reactions to exogenous factors, such as food additives, have been postulated to be causal in some cases.[120] A relationship to sarcoidosis, originally assumed by some authors,[119] does not exist. Likewise, this syndrome appears to be distinct from Crohn's disease, which may also produce granulomatous inflammation of the lip.[120,121]

CHEILITIS GLANDULARIS

Cheilitis glandularis is a rare condition. It has been described mostly in adults but also in children. Diagnosis is based primarily on clinical features.[122] The characteristic picture consists of persistent enlargement and eversion of the lower lip. Ducts appear to be enlarged and exude mucoid material or clear fluid that may be accentuated by gentle squeezing.[122,123] A papular component may be present.[124]

Histopathology. Various histologic findings have been reported, none consistently, probably because the condition may

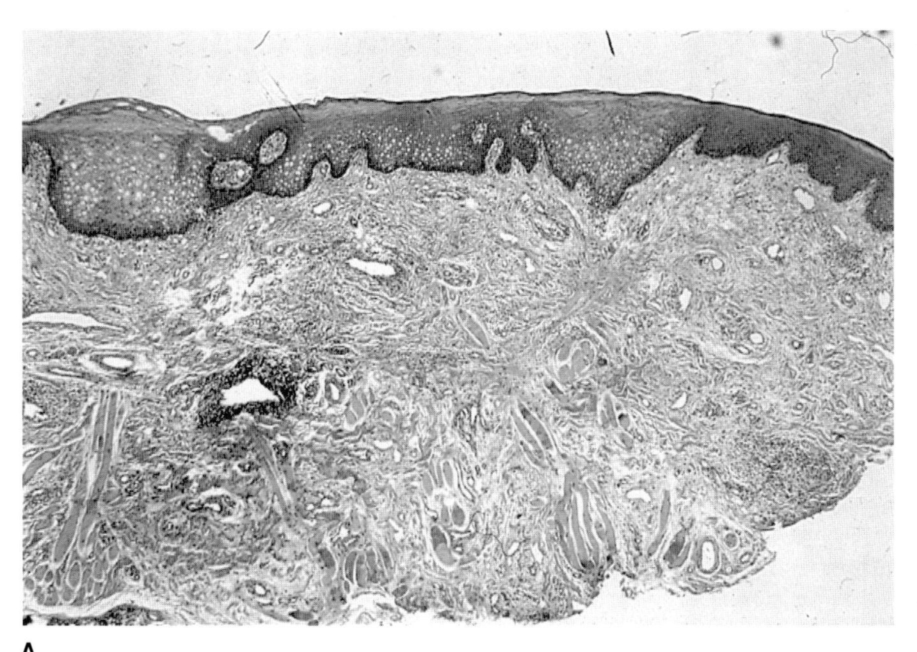

A

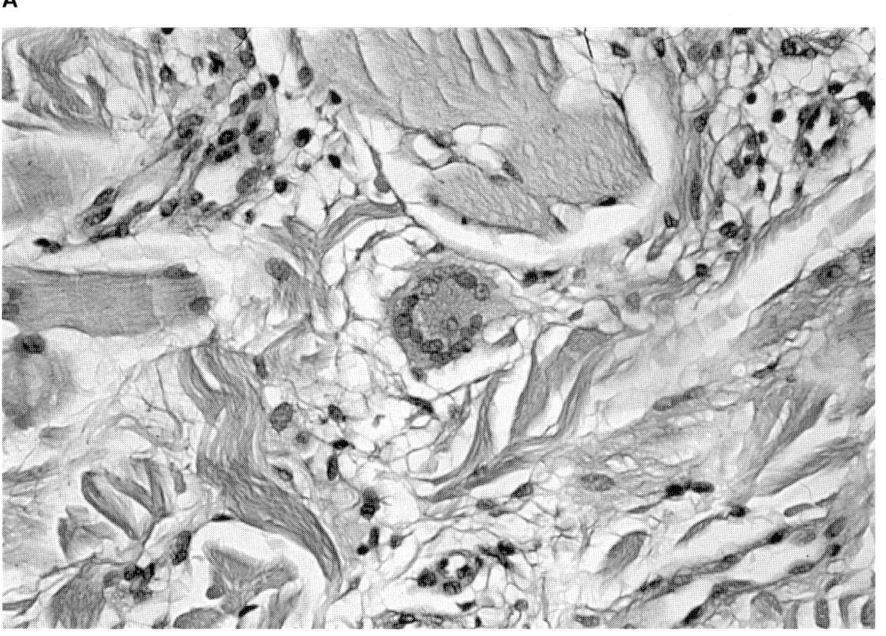

B

FIG. 14-9. Miescher-Melkersson-Rosenthal syndrome
(**A**) Biopsy of lip mucosa showing slight vascular ectasia, edema, and a sparse inflammatory infiltrate. (**B**) A sparse granulomatous component. (Courtesy of Carolyn Carroll, MD.)

not represent a specific disease (see section on Pathogenesis). Salivary gland hyperplasia, duct ectasia, fibrosis, and inflammation with lymphocytes, plasma cells, and histiocytes have been described.[123,124] However, any or all of these features may be absent.[122] Hyperkeratosis can also occur.[122]

Pathogenesis. Cheilitis glandularis is probably caused by several different factors. Marked, chronic sun and wind exposure has been implicated as a common cause, and it has been suggested that this is not truly a disorder of salivary glands, since they may appear histologically normal.[122] An atopic diathesis, factitious cheilitis, and hereditary factors have also been implicated.[122,124] There are older reports in the literature that describe an increased incidence of squamous cell carcinoma in association with cheilitis glandularis.[125] This is probably a consequence of actinic damage, which tends to be associated with this condition and which may be exacerbated by the eversion of the lip.[125]

GRANULOMA ANNULARE

Granuloma annulare occurs most commonly in children and young adults but occurs in all age groups. The lesions of granuloma annulare consist of small, firm, asymptomatic papules that are flesh-colored or pale red and are often grouped in a ringlike or circinate fashion. There usually are several lesions, but there may be just one, or there may be many. The lesions are found most commonly on the hands and feet. Though chronic, they subside after a number of years. Unusual variants of granuloma annulare include (1) a generalized form, consisting of hundreds of papules that are either discrete or confluent but only rarely show an annular arrangement[126,127]; (2) perforating granuloma annulare, with umbilicated lesions occurring usually in a localized distribution,[128,129] and rarely in a generalized distribution[130,131]; (3) erythematous granuloma annulare, showing large, slightly infiltrated erythematous patches, with a palpable border, on which scattered papules may subsequently arise;[132] and (4) subcutaneous granuloma annulare, in which subcutaneous nodules occur, especially in children, either alone or in association with intradermal lesions.[133–135] The subcutaneous nodules have a clinical appearance similar to rheumatoid nodules, although there is a greater tendency to occur on the legs and feet,[136,137] and there is no history of arthritis. A very rare, deep, destructive form of granuloma annulare has also been described.[138]

A correlation between generalized papular granuloma annulare and diabetes mellitus has been observed by several authors.[127,139,140] Granuloma annulare has also been reported to develop at the site of resolved herpes zoster[141,142] and occasionally in association with necrobiosis lipoidica,[143] sarcoid,[144] and AIDS.[145]

Histopathology. Histologically, granuloma annulare shows an infiltrate of histiocytes and a sparse perivascular infiltrate of lymphocytes. The histiocytes may be present in just an interstitial pattern without apparent organization, or in a well-developed palisade completely surrounding areas with prominent mucin (Figs. 14-10 and 14-11). Patterns between these two extremes occur, and typically a single biopsy will show histiocytes that are not palisaded, slightly palisaded, and well palisaded. Although degenerated collagen is present, as is small quantities of fibrin,[144] it is the increased mucin that is the hallmark of granuloma annulare. The increased mucin is almost always apparent on routinely stained sections as faint blue material with a stringy and finely granular appearance. Stains such as colloidal iron and alcian blue can be used to highlight mucin if it is not clearly apparent. Occasionally, sections will not reveal increased mucin, particularly those lacking a palisaded arrangement of histiocytes. In biopsies with well-developed palisades, the central mucinous area is commonly accompanied by a few nuclear fragments or neutrophils. Plasma cells are present rarely, and a sparse to moderately dense infiltrate of eosinophils occurs in a small percentage of biopsies. Multinucleated histiocytes are present more often than not, but they are usually few and often subtle. They can occasionally be seen to have engulfed short, thick, blue-gray elastic fibers.[146] The histiocytic infiltrate is usually present throughout the full thickness of the dermis or the middle and upper dermis, but occasionally just the superficial or deep dermis is involved.[147]

On rare occasions in granuloma annulare, there are aggregations of epithelioid histiocytes, usually with some giant cells

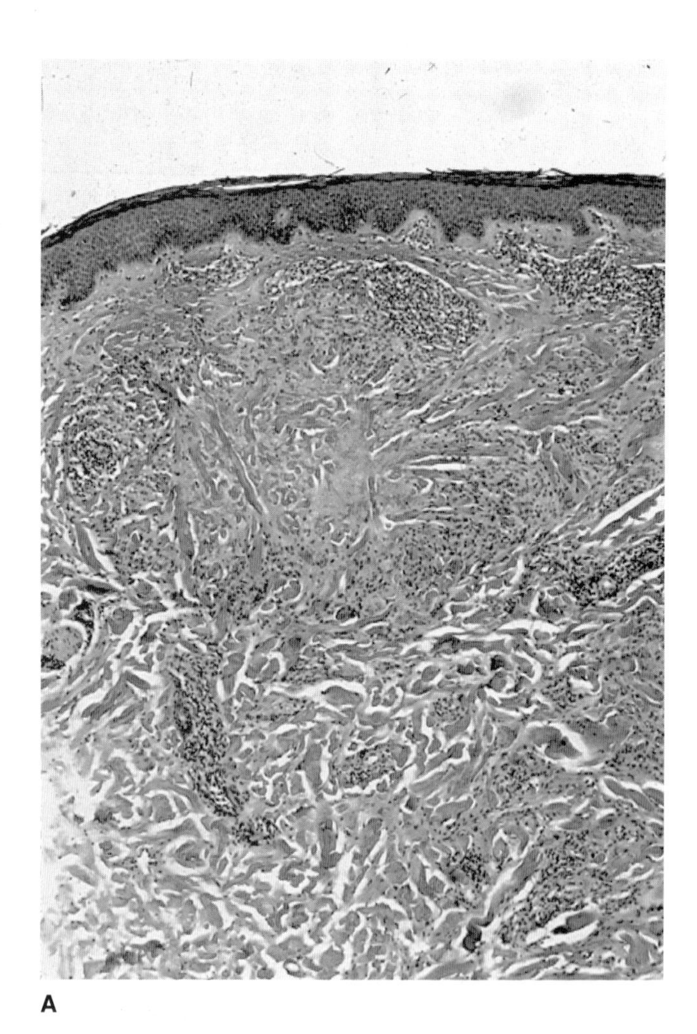

A

FIG. 14-10. Granuloma annulare
(**A**) Granuloma annulare showing a palisade of histiocytes in the upper dermis with a perivascular lymphocytic infiltrate.

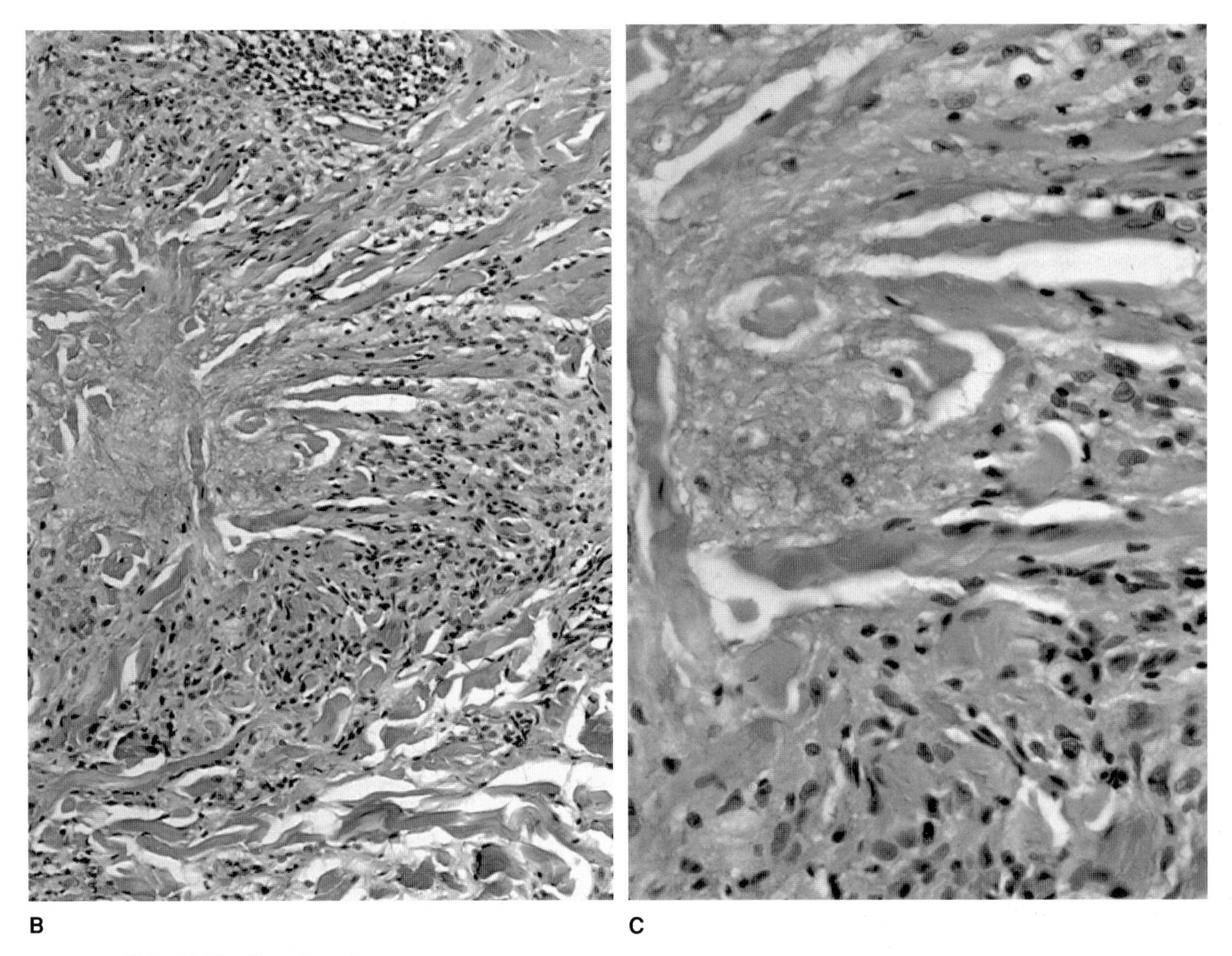

FIG. 14-10. ***Continued***
(**B**) A palisade of histiocytes surrounding mucin. (**C**) Higher magnification showing mucin that has a faint feathery blue appearance in routinely stained sections.

and a rim of lymphoid cells, that resemble the epithelioid cell nodules of sarcoidosis.[144,147] These usually differ from the nodular aggregations of sarcoid, however, by being less well circumscribed and lacking asteroid bodies.

Vascular changes in granuloma annulare are variable but generally are not regarded as conspicuous.[148] In some instances, however, there are fibrinoid deposits in vessel walls and occlusion of vascular lumina.[149]

Among the variants of granuloma annulare mentioned, the usual histologic picture is found in the generalized form[126] and the erythematous form.[132] In perforating granuloma annulare, at least part of the palisading granulomatous process is located very superficially and is associated with disruption of the epidermis.[128–131]

The subcutaneous nodules of granuloma annulare usually show large foci of palisaded histiocytes surrounding areas of degenerated collagen and prominent mucin with a pale appearance[150]; however, biopsies in which mucin was not apparent or the central area appeared more fibrinoid have also been reported (Fig. 14-12).[136,137]

Pathogenesis. Electron microscopic examination reveals degeneration of both collagen and elastic fibers in granuloma annulare.[144] The macrophages (histiocytes) show a high content of primary lysosomes and considerable cytoplasmic activity with release of lysosomal enzymes into the extracellular space.[151] Synthesis of types I and III collagen also occurs, probably as a reparative response.[152] A cell-mediated immune response also appears to be involved, with a prominent presence of activated helper T cells.[153,154] An immunoperoxidase study of the histiocytic population showed staining for lysozyme, but not for the other macrophage markers HAM 56 or KP1.[155]

Blood vessel deposits of IgM and the third component of complement (C3) have been observed by some investigators,[154] but others have found them only rarely[156] or not at all.[157] Thus the existence of an immune complex vasculitis in granuloma annulare[154] appears unlikely.

Differential Diagnosis. Granuloma annulare and necrobiosis lipoidica may resemble one another histologically. Although much has been written about the difficulty of separating these disorders histologically,[148] it should be pointed out that the distinction can be easily accomplished clinically in most circumstances.[158] Furthermore, although it is true that histologic dis-

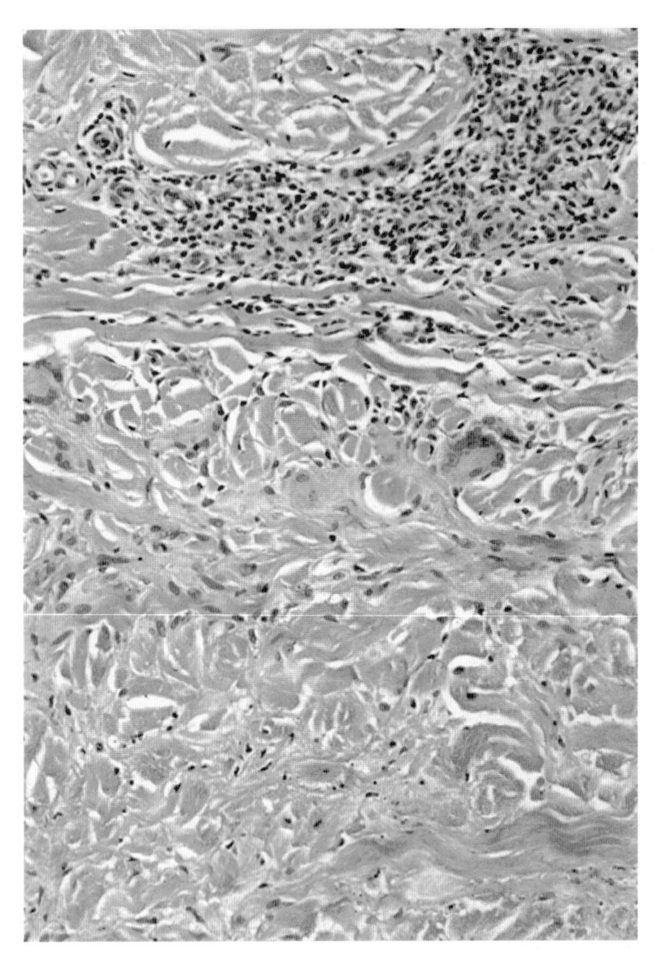

FIG. 14-11. Granuloma annulare
The interstitial type of granuloma annulare, with histiocytes between collagen bundles, including rare multinucleated histiocytes, and a perivascular infiltrate of lymphocytes.

tinction may be impossible, usually it can be accomplished by using the following criteria: (1) Although either disease may involve the dermis diffusely, necrobiosis lipoidica rarely involves just one focus of the dermis or predominantly the upper half of the dermis, whereas granuloma annulare commonly does. (2) Histiocytes in palisades that completely encircle altered connective tissue are more common in granuloma annulare, whereas histiocytes in linear array that are horizontally oriented in a somewhat tiered fashion are more typical of necrobiosis lipoidica. (3) Abundant mucin is typical of granuloma annulare and distinctly uncommon in necrobiosis lipoidica. (4) Necrobiosis lipoidica often shows dermal sclerosis and thickened subcutaneous septa, whereas granuloma annulare does not (the sclerosis often produces a straight edge to the sides of a punch biopsy, in contrast to the inward retraction and/or more irregular edge seen in biopsies without sclerosis). Other features that are more characteristic of necrobiosis lipoidica include the presence of a larger number of giant cells, more pronounced vascular changes such as thickened blood vessel walls, and prominent plasma cells in the deep dermis. Furthermore, necrobiosis lipoidica is more likely to show extensive deposits of lipids or nodular lymphocytic infiltrates in the deep dermis or subcutis,[159] although these features are not commonly seen.

The interstitial type of granuloma annulare, in which palisades of histiocytes are not well developed, is less likely to be confused with necrobiosis lipoidica and more likely to be confused with a process that can also show a superficial and deep lymphocytic infiltrate, such as the inflammatory stage of morphea, but the subtle presence of histiocytes in an interstitial pattern usually allows a definitive diagnosis. This pattern can also be simulated by cutaneous T-cell lymphoma, which can have a granulomatous infiltrate with a granuloma annulare–like pattern.[160] Such examples of cutaneous T-cell lymphoma can usually be recognized for what they are by the presence of at least some epidermotropism, a dermal lymphocytic infiltrate that is more dense around the superficial plexus than the deep one, and/or a somewhat lichenoid component to the infiltrate. The interstitial type of granuloma annulare may also resemble a xanthoma; distinction is usually possible because in granuloma annulare a foamy appearance to the histiocytes is either completely lacking or very subtle, whereas in xanthoma at least some of the histiocytes are obviously foamy. Another distinguishing feature is that granuloma annulare tends to show an obvious perivascular lymphocytic infiltrate, whereas xanthomas do not.[161]

Differentiation of subcutaneous granuloma annulare from a rheumatoid nodule is not always possible on histologic grounds, but subcutaneous granuloma annulare is more likely than rheumatoid nodule to show abundant mucin and less likely to show foreign-body giant cells and prominent stromal fibrosis.[150]

Finally, it should be remembered that granuloma annulare and other palisading granulomas may be simulated by epithelioid sarcoma, which may also contain mucin. Clues that a biopsy is epithelioid sarcoma include ulceration or recurrence, areas of necrosis that include necrotic epithelioid cells, and cytologic atypia. Although atypia tends not to be striking, the epithelioid cells in epithelioid sarcoma usually show more nuclear hyperchromasia and pleomorphism, more mitotic figures, larger size, and redder cytoplasm than do the histiocytes of granuloma annulare.[162]

NECROBIOSIS LIPOIDICA

Two thirds of patient with necrobiosis lipoidica have overt diabetes at the time of diagnosis. Of the rest, all but 10% will develop diabetes within 5 years, have abnormal glucose tolerance, or have a history of diabetes in at least one parent. Of all patients with diabetes, less than 1% develop necrobiosis lipoidica.[140]

In well-developed necrobiosis lipoidica, one observes clinically one or several sharply but irregularly demarcated patches or plaques, usually on the shins.[163] They appear yellow-brown in the center and purplish at the periphery. Whereas the periphery of the lesions may show slight induration, the center of the lesions gradually becomes atrophic and shows telangiectases, and it may break down to form an ulcer. When lesions first begin, red-brown papules can be observed. In addition to the shins, lesions may be present elsewhere on the lower extremities, including the ankles, calves, thighs, popliteal areas, and feet. In about 15% of the cases, lesions are present also in areas other

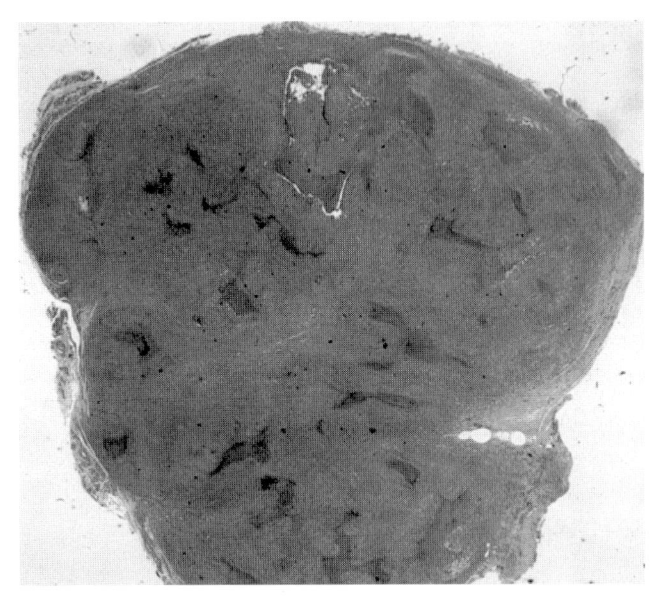

A

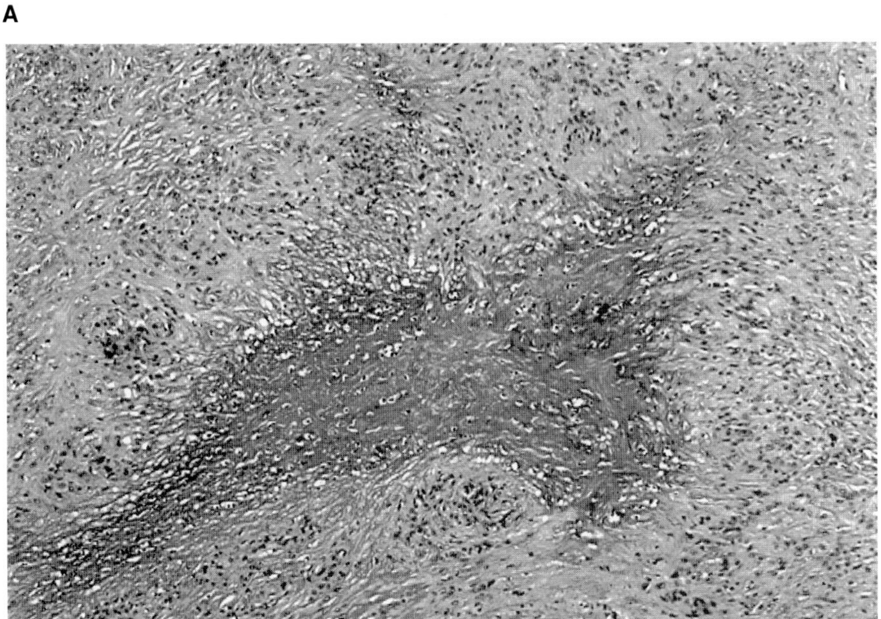

B

FIG. 14-12. Subcutaneous granuloma annulare (pseudorheumatoid nodule)
(**A**) A well-circumscribed subcutaneous nodule with many areas of histiocytes in a palisade surrounding fibrinoid material. (**B**) Histiocytes in a palisade around fibrinoid material.

than the legs, especially on the dorsa of the hands, fingers, and forearms. Rarely, the head and abdomen are affected. Necrobiosis lipoidica with lesions exclusively outside the legs is extremely rare; it was reported to occur in 1% of patients with necrobiosis lipoidica.[164]

Lesions located in areas other than the legs may appear raised and firm and may have a papular, nodular, or plaquelike appearance without atrophy; they may clinically resemble granuloma annulare.[164] Involvement of the scalp with large, atrophic patches occurs occasionally; it has been reported not only in association with lesions on the shins and elsewhere[165,166] but also, rarely, as the only lesion present.[167,168]

In rare instances, transfollicular elimination of necrotic material takes place in necrobiosis lipoidica, producing small hyperkeratic plugs within a plaque.[169] Necrobiosis lipoidica occasionally coexists with sarcoid[170] or granuloma annulare.[143]

Histopathology. On histologic examination, the epidermis may be normal, atrophic, or hyperkeratotic. In some instances, the surface of the biopsy shows ulceration. Usually the entire thickness of the dermis or its lower two thirds is affected by a process that can show a variable degree of granulomous inflammation, degeneration of collagen, and sclerosis (Fig. 14-13), but occasionally only the upper dermis is affected.[147,148,158,171] The granulomous component is usually conspicuous, and the histiocytes may or may not be arranged in a palisade. Occasionally there are just a few scattered epithelioid histiocytes and giant cells. The latter picture is more likely to occur in sections in which sclerosis is extensive, and occasionally in such biopsies several sections must be examined before the granulomatous component becomes apparent. Giant cells are usually of the Langhans' or foreign-body type; occasionally, Touton cells or asteroid bodies[172] are seen. If the histiocytes are arranged in a palisade, the palisades tend to be somewhat horizontally oriented and/or in a vaguely tiered fashion. Occasionally, histiocytes may be seen to completely encircle altered connective tissue, particularly degenerated collagen, but more commonly, altered connective tissue is not completely surrounded by histiocytes. This alteration of connective tissue has also been referred to as "necrobiosis." The altered collagen appears different from normal collagen tinctorially by having a paler grayer hue and structurally by appearing more fragmented and more haphazardly arranged; it may also appear more compact. Areas of sclerosis with a decreased number of fibroblasts can be seen. A clue to the presence of sclerosis can be found by looking at the sides of the biopsy specimen, which tend to be straight with less of the inward retraction of the dermis ordinarily associated with punch biopsies. Increased mucin is usually inapparent or just subtle, in contrast to granuloma annulare. Other findings include a sparse to moderately dense, primarily perivascular lymphocytic infiltrate, plasma cells in the deep dermis in some biopsies, involvement of the upper subcutis with thickened fibrous septa, and lipids (which may be present in foamy histiocytes,[173] which may be inferred from the presence of cholesterol clefts, or which can be detected extracellularly with special stains on fresh tissue). Older lesions show telangiectases superficially. Blood vessels, particularly in the middle and lower dermis, often exhibit thickening of their walls with proliferation of their endothelial cells. The process may lead to partial and rarely to complete occlusion of the lumen. The thickened walls appear heavily infiltrated with PAS-positive, diastase-resistant material.[148] Vascular changes of this type are seen particularly near areas in which the collagen bundles appear thickened and

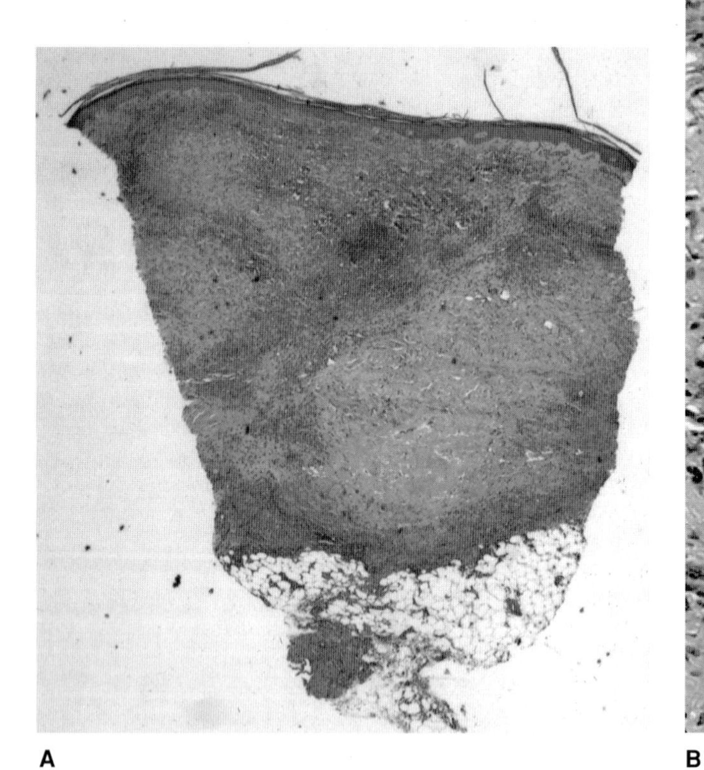
A

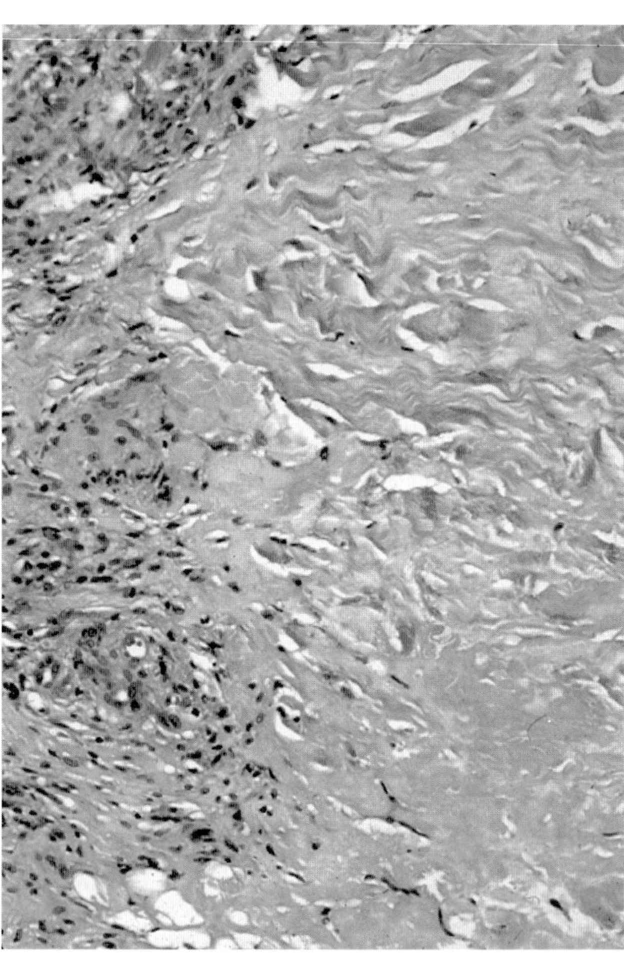
B

FIG. 14-13. Necrobiosis lipoidica
(**A**) The presence of sclerosis can be identified by the relatively straight edges of the punch biopsy. The infiltrate involves the full thickness of the dermis and upper subcutis and is arranged in a tierlike fashion. (**B**) Histiocytes and lymphocytes on the left surrounding degenerated collagen in the lower right corner. Compared to the normal collagen above it, the degenerated collagen has a more compact appearance and appears more gray-blue than pink.

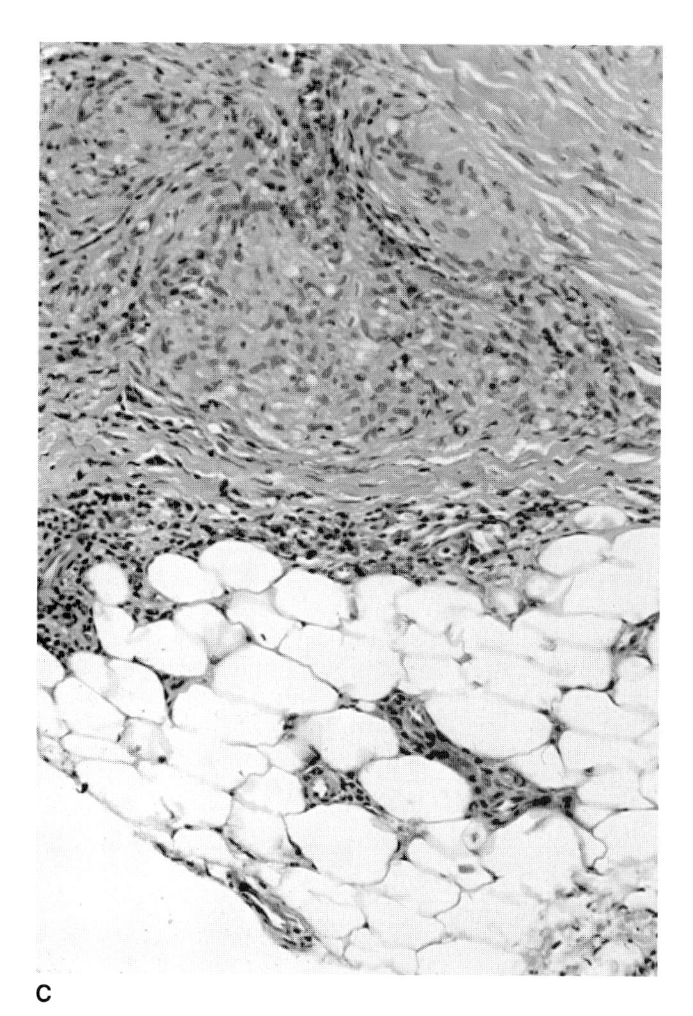

C

FIG. 14-13. *Continued*
(**C**) Epithelioid histiocytes in the deep dermis and lymphocytes and plasma cells at the dermal-subcutaneous junction.

hyalinized. Whereas the vascular changes often are conspicuous in lesions of the lower legs, they usually are mild or absent elsewhere.[168]

One cannot reliably determine on the basis of histologic findings if a patient has diabetes, although the presence of a pattern with more obvious palisading and degeneration of collagen has been correlated with such.[171]

Pathogenesis. The cause of necrobiosis lipoidica is unknown, and it is unclear whether the degeneration of collagen is a primary or secondary event.[163] Some authors have expressed their belief that the degeneration of collagen is due to vascular changes and that, in cases in which clinical or latent diabetes exists, the diabetes is the cause of the vascular changes.[174] However, evidence against a vascular cause is the absence of vascular abnormality in about one-third of biopsies examined,[171] and the fact that vessels that are affected are often situated in the lower layers of the dermis and are of a larger caliber than the type of vessel affected by diabetic microangiopathy.

Electron microscopic examination shows degenerative changes in collagen and elastin with loss of cross-striation in collagen fibrils. Collagen synthesis by fibroblasts is decreased.[175]

Direct immunofluorescence studies have shown that necrobiotic areas contain fibrinogen, and deposits of immunoglobulin and C3 have been found in the vessel walls,[176,177] but this is not a consistent finding.[178]

Differential Diagnosis. Differentiation of necrobiosis lipoidica from granuloma annulare was discussed in the section on granuloma annulare.

Occasionally, necrobiosis lipoidica shows discrete collections of epithelioid cells that may resemble those seen in sarcoidosis.[165,171] However, alteration of the collagen aids in the differential diagnosis.[165]

Necrobiotic xanthogranuloma with paraproteinemia can simulate necrobiosis lipoidica but differs by showing a more dense, diffuse infiltrate with a greater proportion of foamy histiocytes, and by showing more extensive inflammation of the subcutis with greater disruption of the normal subcutaneous architecture.

For a discussion of differentiation of necrobiosis lipoidica from annular elastolytic granuloma, see the section on annular elastolytic granuloma later in this chapter.

RHEUMATOID NODULES

Rheumatoid nodules occur in patients with rheumatoid arthritis, particularly over extensor surfaces, such as the proximal ulna, the olecranon process, and the metacarpophalangeal and proximal interphalangeal joints.[179] They may occur elsewhere, such as the back of the hands, over amputation stumps,[180] and rarely in extracutaneous sites, such as the lung and heart.[181,182] The nodules vary in size from a few millimeters to 5 cm and may be solitary or numerous.[181] Rarely, rheumatoid nodules show a central draining perforation.[183] Rheumatoid factor is almost always found in high titer; rarely, nodules may precede apparent joint disease.[179] There are also a few reports of patients with systemic lupus erythematosus and rheumatoid nodules.[184–186]

Pseudorheumatoid nodule is a term that has been applied to nodules in the subcutis that mimic rheumatoid nodules histologically but that develop in the absence of rheumatoid arthritis (or systemic lupus erythematosus).[134,135,137] These occur in children or adults. The subsequent development of rheumatoid arthritis occurs infrequently in adults and rarely, if ever, in children. Because some of these nodules occur in patients with other lesions that are typical of intradermal granuloma annulare,[134,135] the nodules have been considered to represent a subcutaneous variant of granuloma annulare.

Histopathology. Rheumatoid nodules occur in the subcutis and lower dermis and show one or several areas of fibrinoid degeneration of collagen that stain homogeneously red (Figs. 14-14 and 14-15). Nuclear fragments and basophilic material may be present, but mucin is almost always minimal or absent.[150] These areas are surrounded by histiocytes in a palisaded arrangement. Foreign-body giant cells are present in about 50% of biopsies.[150] In the surrounding stroma, there is a proliferation of blood vessels and fibrosis. A fairly sparse infiltrate of other inflammatory cells is associated with the histiocytes and surrounding stroma. Lymphocytes and neutrophils are most common, but mast cells, plasma cells, and eosinophils may be present. Occasionally, lipid is seen.[134,150] Vasculitis has been described[187] but is not usually encountered.[150] In perforating

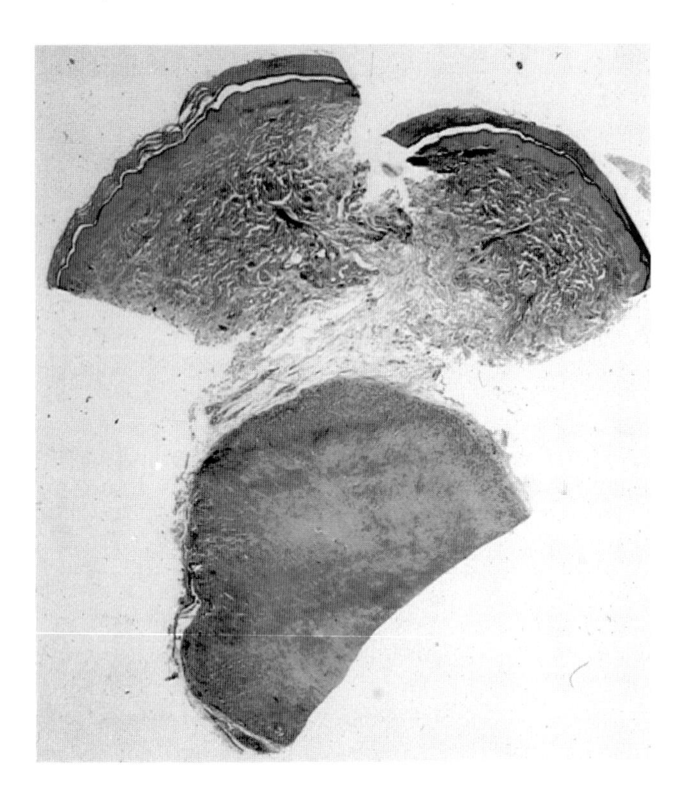

FIG. 14-14. Rheumatoid nodule
A palisaded granuloma in the subcutis, a typical location for a rheumatoid nodule.

rheumatoid nodules, the central fibrinoid material connects to the overlying skin surface.[183]

Pathogenesis. Factors that have been implicated in the formation of rheumatoid nodules include trauma and a specific T-cell–mediated immune reaction.[179]

Differential Diagnosis. The principal differential diagnosis is subcutaneous granuloma annulare, which was discussed in the section on granuloma annulare. A distinction should be made from epithelioid sarcoma, which was also covered in that section. Nonabsorbable sutures may produce periarticular palisaded granulomas like those of rheumatoid nodule[188]; in such instances, there should be a history of previous surgery, and birefringent suture material should be visible under polarized light. Rheumatic fever produces nodules (rheumatic nodules), especially over the elbows, knees, scalp, knuckles, ankles, and spine,[189] which were confused with rheumatoid nodules in the early part of the century. Histologically, a rheumatic fever nodule is less likely to show central, homogeneous fibrinoid necrosis, a palisade of histiocytes is usually not as well developed, and fibrosis is minimal or absent.[181,190] Rarely, an infectious process, such as cryptococcosis, can produce a deep palisaded granuloma. It can be differentiated from rheumatoid nodule because the palisade surrounds primarily necrotic debris and organisms, rather than fibrinoid material.

ANNULAR ELASTOLYTIC GIANT-CELL GRANULOMA

Annular elastolytic giant-cell granuloma is the name that is currently in vogue for a condition with unclear nosologic status,

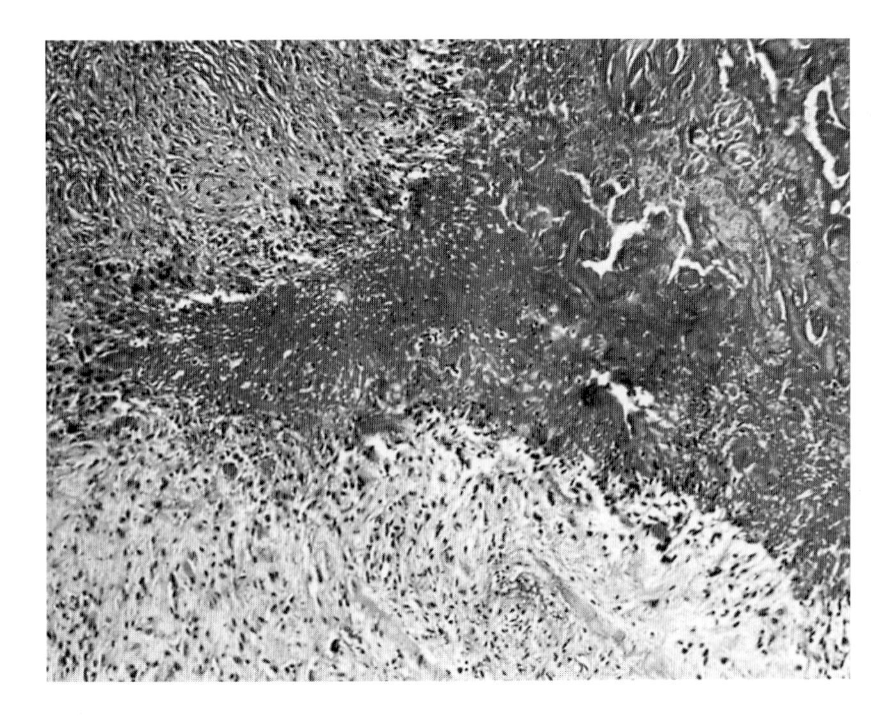

FIG. 14-15. Rheumatoid nodule
There is a large, central zone of fibrinoid degeneration surrounded by histiocytes in a palisaded arrangement.

especially whether or not it truly distinct from granuloma annulare.[191–193] It almost always occurs on sun-exposed skin, such as the face, neck, dorsum of hand, forearm, and arm, and hence the previous name *actinic granuloma*[194]; however, there are a few reports of similar lesions involving sun-protected sites.[195–197] The lesions clinically resemble granuloma annulare. They are typically large, somewhat annular plaques. The border may be serpiginous and is slightly raised, approximately 3 mm wide, and pearly or slightly red or brown. The central zone may show depigmentation and/or atrophy. Smaller papules may also occur, and lesions may be solitary, few, or numerous.[194,198,199] Other names under which these lesions have been described include *atypical necrobiosis lipoidica of the face and scalp*,[200] *Miescher's granuloma of the face*,[199] and *granuloma multiforme*.[198] A possibly related process occurs on the conjunctiva.[201]

Histopathology. The histologic features are best appreciated in a radial biopsy that contains the central zone, the elevated border, and the skin peripheral to the ring.[194,198,199] The central zone shows the hallmark of the disease, that is, near or total absence of elastic fibers, best appreciated with an elastic tissue stain (e.g., Verhoeff–van Gieson) (Fig. 14-16). The collagen in this zone may show horizontally oriented fibers producing a slight scarlike appearance. By contrast, the zone peripheral to the annulus shows an increased amount of thick elastotic material with the staining properties of elastic tissue. The transitional zone at the raised border shows a granulomatous infiltrate with either of the patterns seen in granuloma annulare, that is, histiocytes arranged interstitially between collagen bundles or, less commonly, in a palisade. Occasionally, there are contiguous epithelioid histiocytes in small clusters. Multinucleated histiocytes are conspicuous, usually being large and containing as many as a dozen nuclei, mostly in haphazard arrangement, but sometimes in ringed array. Elastotic fibers are present adjacent to and within the giant cells. Asteroid bodies that stain like elastic fibers may be found in the giant cells.[199] The infiltrate also contains lymphocytes and often some plasma cells. Mucin is not present.

Differential Diagnosis. The principal differential diagnosis is granuloma annulare, which may in fact be an artificial distinction. Since engulfment of abnormal elastic fibers can also occur in granuloma annulare[146] as well as in other granulomatous processes, it has been argued that the elastophagocytosis of annular elastolytic giant-cell granuloma does not qualify it as a distinct entity different from granuloma annulare on sun-damaged skin.[192] Although some elastolysis has also been described in granuloma annulare,[198] it is the complete loss of elastic tissue in the central zone that has been used as the primary basis for separating the diseases. Other features that have been evoked for distinguishing them is the presence of larger and more numerous giant cells, and the absence of mucin in annular elastolytic giant-cell granuloma.

Necrobiosis lipoidica differs by the lack of a central zone of elastolysis and the presence of degenerated collagen, sclerosis, and, in some circumstances, lipids and vascular changes. Furthermore, annular elastolytic giant-cell granuloma involves mostly the upper and middle dermis, whereas necrobiosis lipoidica tends to affect the deep dermis and sometimes the subcutis at least as much as the upper dermis.

GRANULOMA GLUTEALE INFANTUM

Granuloma gluteale infantum, first described in 1971,[202] shows asymptomatic, round to oval, smooth, raised nodules, reddish blue in color, from a few millimeters to a few centimeters in diameter, and irregularly distributed over the region of the skin that is covered by diapers.[202–204] Although usually seen in infants, it has also been described in incontinent adults.[205,206]

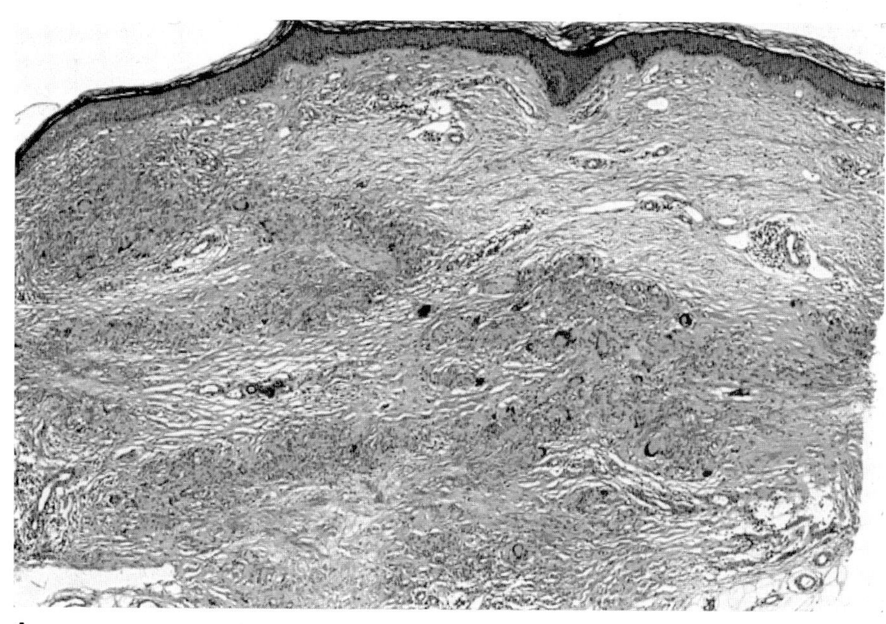
A

FIG. 14-16. Annular elastolytic granuloma
(**A**) Several areas of histiocytes arranged in a palisade with obvious multinucleated histiocytes and fibrosis. (*continued on next page*)

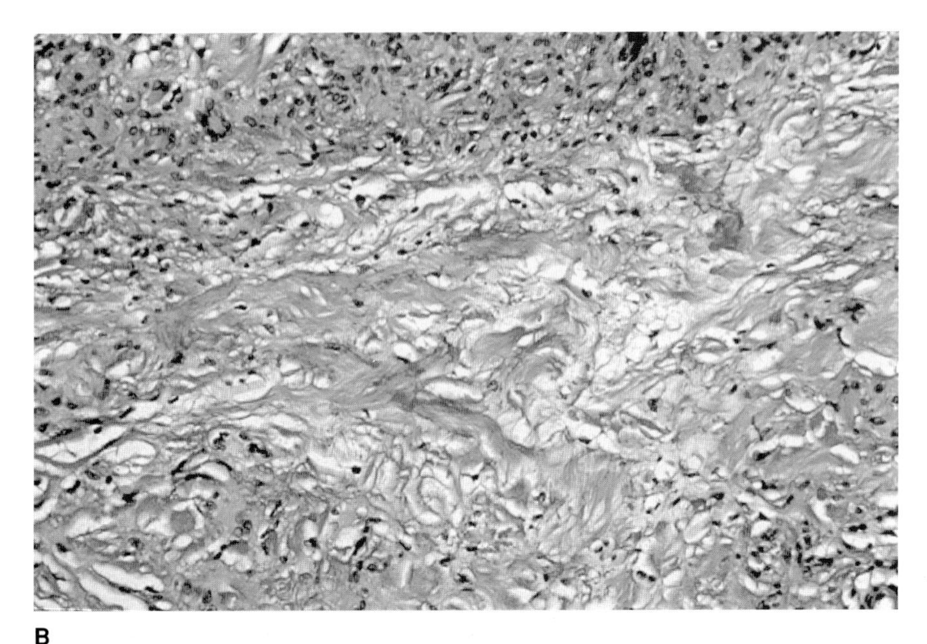

B

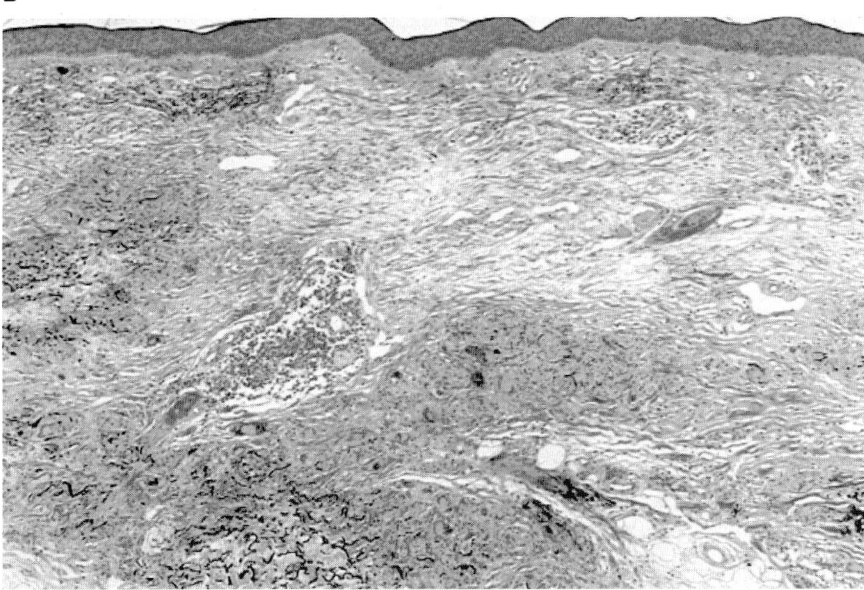

C

FIG. 14-16. *Continued*
(**B**) Histiocytes arranged in a palisade around connective tissue that is slightly fibrotic, without obvious mucin. (**C**) Elastic tissue stain shows absence of elastic tissue in the center of the lesion.

Histopathology. Acanthosis is usually present. A dense mixed infiltrate is seen throughout the dermis. Lymphocytes, histiocytes, plasma cells, neutrophils, and eosinophils may all be seen.[204] In addition, there may be microabscesses composed of neutrophils and eosinophils, as well as extravasation of erythrocytes together with a proliferation of capillaries.[202] Multinucleated histiocytes or well-developed granulomas are not a feature of the infiltrate. In a few instances, staining with the PAS reaction has revealed spores and pseudohyphae consistent with the presence of *Candida albicans* in the stratum corneum,[207] but fungi are often not detected.

Pathogenesis. In nearly all patients described in the literature, the development of granuloma gluteale infantum has been preceded by a diaper dermatitis, which only in some instances has been associated with a *C albicans* infection.[203] It appears very likely that exogenous factors are the cause of the eruption.[202] Topical applications of fluorinated corticosteroid preparations for a prolonged period of time and prolonged wearing of plastic diapers have been implicated, but a consistent cause has not been identified.[208]

REFERENCES

1. Epstein WL, Shahen JR, Krasnobrod H. The organized epithelioid cell granuloma: Differentiation of allergic (zirconium) from colloidal (silica) types. Am J Pathol 1963;43:391.
2. Behar TA, Anderson EE, Barwick WJ. Sclerosing lipogranulomatosis: A case report of scrotal injection of automobile transmission fluid and literature review of subcutaneous injection of oils. Plastic Reconstr Surg 1993;91:352.
3. Smetana HF, Bernhard W. Sclerosing lipogranuloma. Arch Pathol 1950;50:296.

4. Newcomer VD, Graham JH, Schaffert RR et al. Sclerosing lipogranuloma resulting from exogenous lipids. Arch Dermatol 1956;73:361.
5. Oertel VC, Johnson FB. Sclerosing lipogranuloma of male genitalia. Arch Pathol 1977;101:321.
6. Mason J, Apisarnthanarax P. Migratory silicone granuloma. Arch Dermatol 1981;117:366.
7. Morgan AW. Localized reactions to injected therapeutic materials: Part 2. J Cutan Pathol 1995;22:289.
8. Ellis H. Pathological changes produced by surgical dusting powders. Ann R Coll Surg Engl 1994;76:5.
9. Kasper CS, Chandler PJ. Talc deposition in skin and tissues surrounding silicone gel-containing prosthetic devices. Arch Dermatol 1994; 130:48.
10. Tye MJ, Hashimoto K, Fox F. Talc granulomas of the skin. JAMA 1966;198:1370.
11. Leonard DD. Starch granulomas. Arch Dermatol 1973;107:101.
12. Snyder RA, Schwartz RA. Cactus bristle implantation. Arch Dermatol 1983;119:152.
13. Suzuki H, Baba S. Cactus granuloma of the skin. J Dermatol 1993;20: 424.
14. Winer LH, Zeilenga RH. Cactus granuloma of the skin. Arch Dermatol 1955;72:566.
15. Joseph HL, Gifford H. Barber's interdigital pilonidal sinus. Arch Dermatol 1954;70:616.
16. Price SM, Popkin GL. Barber's interdigital hair sinus: A case report in a dog groomer. Arch Dermatol 1976;112:523.
17. Goebel M, Rupec M. Interdigitaler pilonidaler sinus. Dermatol Wochenschr 1967;153:341.
18. Rocha G, Fraga S. Sea urchin granuloma of the skin. Arch Dermatol 1962;85:406.
19. Haneke E, Kolsch I. Seeigelgranulome. Hautarzt 1980;31:159.
20. Kinmont PDC. Sea-urchin sarcoidal granuloma. Br J Dermatol 1965; 77:335.
21. Epstein E, Gerstl B, Berk M et al. Silica pregranuloma. Arch Dermatol 1955;71:645.
22. Eskeland G, Langmark F, Husby G. Silicon granuloma of the skin and subcutaneous tissue. Acta Pathol Microbiol Scand Suppl 1974;248: 69.
23. Mowry RG, Sams WM Jr, Caulfield JB. Cutaneous silica granuloma. Arch Dermatol 1991;127:692.
24. Rank BK, Hicks JD. Pseudotobercoloma granulosum silicoticum. Br J Plast Surg 1972;25:42.
25. Arzt L. Foreign body granulomas and Boeck's sarcoid. J Invest Dermatol 1955;24:155.
26. Schwechat-Millet M, Ziv R, Trau H et al. Sarcoidosis versus foreign-body granuloma. Int J Dermatol 1987;26:582.
27. Epstein WL. Granulomatous hypersensitivity. Prog Allergy 1967;11: 38.
28. Skelton HG III, Smith KJ, Johnson FB et al. Zirconium granuloma resulting from an aluminum zirconium complex: A previously unrecognized agent in the development of hypersensitivity granulomas. J Am Acad Dermatol 1993;28:874.
29. Williams RM, Skipworth GB. Zirconium granulomas of the glabrous skin following treatment of Rhus dermatitis. Arch Dermatol 1959;80: 273.
30. Baler GR. Granulomas from topical zirconium in poison ivy dermatitis. Arch Dermatol 1965;91:145.
31. Lopresti PJ, Hambrick GW. Zirconium granuloma following treatment of Rhus dermatitis. Arch Dermatol 1965;92:188.
32. Shelley WB, Hurley HJ. The allergic origin of zirconium deodorant granulomas. Br J Dermatol 1958;70:75.
33. Epstein WL, Skahen JR, Krasnobrod H. Granulomatous hypersensitivity to zirconium: Localization of allergin in tissue and its role in formation of epithelioid cells. J Invest Dermatol 1962;38:223.
34. Slater DN, Underwood JCE, Durrant TE et al. Aluminum hydroxide granulomas: Light and electron microscopic studies and x-ray microanalysis. Br J Dermatol 1982;107:103.
35. Fawcett HA, Smith NP. Injection-site granuloma due to aluminum. Arch Dermatol 1984;120:1318.
36. Morgan AW. Localized reactions to injected therapeutic materials: Part I. J Cutan Pathol 1995;22:193.
37. Jordaan HF, Sandler M. Zinc-induced granuloma: A unique complication of insulin therapy. Clin Exp Dermatol 1989;14:227.
38. Stoeckle JD, Hardy HL, Weber AL. Chronic beryllium disease. Am J Med 1967;46:545.
39. Neave HJ, Frank SB, Tolmach J. Cutaneous granulomas following laceration by fluorescent light bulbs. Arch Dermatol Syph 1950;61: 401.
40. Dutra FR. Beryllium granulomas of the skin. Arch Dermatol Syph 1949;60:1140.
41. Hanifin JM, Epstein WL, Cline MJ. In vitro studies of granulomatous hypersensitivity to beryllium. J Invest Dermatol 1970;55:284.
42. Henderson WR, Fukuyama K, Epstein WL et al. In vitro demonstration of delayed hypersensitivity in patients with berylliosis. J Invest Dermatol 1972;58:5.
43. Bendsoe N, Hansson C, Sterner O. Inflammatory reactions from organic pigments in red tattoos. Acta Derm Venereol (Stockh) 1991;71: 70.
44. Sowden JM, Byrne JPH, Smith AG et al. Red tattoo reactions: X-ray microanalysis and patch test studies. Br J Dermatol 1991;124:576.
45. Loewenthal LJA. Reactions in green tattoos. Arch Dermatol 1960;82: 237.
46. Rorsman H, Dahlquist I, Jacobsson S et al. Tattoo granuloma and uveitis. Lancet 1969;2:27.
47. Schwartz RA, Mathias CG, Miller CH et al. Granulomatous reaction to purple tattoo pigment. Contact Dermatitis 1987;16:198.
48. Bjornberg A. Reactions to light yellow tattoos from cadmium sulfide. Arch Dermatol 1963;88:267.
49. Rubinanes EI, Sanchez JL. Granulomatous dermatitis to iron oxide after permanent pigmentation of the eyebrows. J Dermatol Surg Oncol 1993;19:14.
50. Goldstein AP. Histologic reactions in tattoos. J Dermatol Surg Oncol 1979;5:896.
51. Winkelmann RK, Harris RB. Lichenoid delayed hypersensitivity reactions in tattoos. J Cutan Pathol 1979;6:59.
52. Clarke J, Black MM. Lichenoid tattoo reactions. Br J Dermatol 1979; 100:451.
53. Blumental G, Okun MR, Ponitch JA. Pseudolymphomatous reaction to tattoos. J Am Acad Dermatol 1982;6:485.
54. Zinberg M, Heilman E, Glickman F. Cutaneous pseudolymphoma rusulting from a tattoo. J Dermatol Surg Oncol 1982;8:955.
55. Sowden JM, Cartwright PH, Smith AG et al. Sarcoidosis presenting with a granulomatous reaction confined to red tattoos. Clin Exp Dermatol 1992;17:446.
56. Weidman AI, Andrade R, Franks AG. Sarcoidosis. Arch Dermatol 1966;94:320.
57. Bjornberg A. Allergic reaction to cobalt in light blue tattoo markings. Acta Derm Venereol (Stockh) 1961;41:259.
58. Hanada K, Chiyoya S, Katebira Y. Systemic sarcoidal reaction in tattoo. Clin Exp Dermatol 1985;10:479.
59. Collins P, Evans AT, Gray W, Levison DA. Pulmonary sarcoidosis presenting as a granulomatous tattoo reaction. Br J Dermatol 1994; 130:658.
60. Dickinson JA. Sarcoidal reactions in tattoos. Arch Dermatol 1969; 100:315.
61. Mansour AM, Chan CC. Recurrent uveitis preceded by swelling of skin tattoos. Am J Ophthalmol 1991;111:515.
62. Abel EA, Silberberg I, Queen D. Studies of chronic inflammation in a red tattoo by electron microscopy and histochemistry. Acta Derm Venereol (Stockh) 1972;52:453.
63. Putkonen T. Symptomenkomplex der beginnenden Sarkoidose. Dermatol Wochenschr 1966;152:1455.
64. James DG, Siltzbach LE, Sharma OP et al. A tale of two cities: A comparison of sarcoidosis in London and New York. Arch Intern Med 1969;123:187.
65. Wood BT, Behlen CH II, Weary PE. The association of sarcoidosis, erythema nodosum and arthritis. Arch Dermatol 1966;94:406.
66. Olive KE, Kataria YP. Cutaneous manifestations of sarcoidosis. Arch Int Med 1985;145:1811.
67. Umbert P, Winkelmann RK. Granuloma annulare and sarcoidosis. Br J Dermatol 1977;97:481.
68. Veien NK. Cutaneous sarcoidosis treated with levamisole. Dermatologica 1977;154:185.
69. Hanno R, Needelman A, Eiferman RA et al. Cutaneous sarcoidal granulomas and the development of systemic sarcoidosis. Arch Dermatol 1981;117:203.
70. Spiteri MA, Matthey F, Gordon T et al. Lupus pernio: A clinical-radiological study of thirty-five cases. Br J Dermatol 1985;112:315.

71. Okamoto H, Horio T, Izumi T. Micropapular sarcoidosis simulating lichen nitidus. Dermatologica 1985;170:253.
72. Morrison JGL. Sarcoidosis in a child, presenting as an erythroderma with keratotic spines and palmar pits. Br J Dermatol 1976;95:93.
73. Lever WF, Freiman DG. Sarcoidosis: A report of a case with erythrodermic lesions, subcutaneous nodes and asteroid inclusion bodies in giant cells. Arch Dermatol Syph 1948;57:639.
74. Kelly AP, Ichthyosiform sarcoid. Arch Dermatol 1978;114:1551.
75. Kauh YC, Goody HE, Luscombe HA. Ichthyosiform sarcoidosis. Arch Dermatol 1978;114:100.
76. Bazex J, Dupin P, Giordano F. Sarcoidose cutanée et viscérale. Ann Dermatol Venereol 1987;114:685.
77. Hruza GJ, Kerdel FA. Generalized atrophic sarcoidosis with ulcerations. Arch Dermatol 1986;122:320.
78. Schwartz RA, Robertson DB, Tierney LM et al. Generalized ulcerative sarcoidosis. Arch Dermatol 1982;118:931.
79. Rongioletti F, Bellisomi A, Rebora A. Disseminated angiolupoid sarcoidosis. Cutis 1987;40:341.
80. Cornelius CE, Stein KM, Hanshaw WJ, Spott DA. Hypopigmentation and sarcoidosis. Arch Dermatol 1973;198:249.
81. Darier J, Roussy G. Un cas de tumeurs benignes multiples: Sarcoides sous-cutanees ou tuberculides nodulaires hypodermiques. Ann Dermatol Syph 1904;2:144.
82. Vainsencher D, Winkelmann RK. Subcutaneous sarcoidosis. Arch Dermatol 1984;120:1028.
83. Bisaccia E, Scarborough A, Carr RD. Cutaneous sarcoid granuloma formation in herpes zoster scars. Arch Dermatol 1983;119:788.
84. Walsh NMG, Hanly JG, Tremaine R, Murray S. Cutaneous sarcoidosis and foreign bodies. Am J Dermatopathol 1993;15:203.
85. Barrier HJ, Bogoch A. The natural history of the sarcoid granuloma. Am J Pathol 1953;29:451.
86. Wigley JEM, Musso LA. A case of sarcoidosis with erythrodemic lesions. Br J Dermatol 1951;63:398.
87. Mittag H, Rupec M, Kalbfleisch H et al. Zur frage der erythrodermischen sarkoidose. Z Hautkr 1986;61:673.
88. Chevrant-Breton J, Revillon L, Pony JC et al. Sarcoidose à manifestations cutanées extensives ulcéreuses et atrophiantes. Ann Dermatol Venereol 1977;104:805.
89. Glass LA, Apisarnthanarax P. Verrucous sarcoidosis simulating hypertrophic lichen planus. Int J Dermatol 1989;28:539.
90. Alexis JB. Sarcoidosis presenting as cutaneous hypopigmentation with repeatedly negative skin biopsies. Int J Dermatol 1994;32:44.
90a. Israel HL, Ostrow A. Sarcoidosis and aspergilloma. Am J Med 1969; 47:243.
91. Van-Landuyt H, Zultak M, Blanc D et al. Sarcoidose ostéocutanée chronique multilante. Ann Dermatol Venereol 1988;115:587.
92. Bodie BF, Kheir SM, Omura EF. Calvarial sarcoid mimicking metastatic disease. J Am Acad Dermatol 1980;3:401.
93. Maycock RL, Bertrand P, Morison CE et al. Manifestations of sarcoidosis. Am J Med 1963;35:67.
94. Longcope WT, Freiman DG. A study of sarcoidosis. Medicine (Baltimore) 1952;31:1.
95. McCoy RC, Fisher CC. Glomerulonephritis associated with sarcoidosis. Am J Pathol 1972;68:339.
96. Roberts WC, McAllister HA Jr, Ferrans VJ. Sarcoidosis of the heart. Am J Med 1977;63:86.
97. Mistilis SP, Green JR, Schiff L. Hepatic sarcoidosis with portal hypertension. Am J Med 1964;36:470.
98. Selenkow HA, Tyler HR, Matson DD et al. Hypopituitarism due to hypothalamic sarcoidosis. Am J Med Sci 1959;238:456.
99. Rupec M, Korb G, Behrend H. Feingewebliche untersuchungen zur entwicklung des positiven Kveim-tests. Arch Klin Exp Dermatol 1970;237:811.
100. Steigleder GK, Silva A Jr, Nelson CT. Histopathology of the Kveim test. Arch Dermatol 1961;84:828.
101. Siltzbach LE, James DG, Neville E et al. Course and prognosis of sarcoidosis around the world. Am J Med 1974;57:847.
102. Koerner SK, Sakowitz AJ, Appelman RI et al. Transbronchial lung biopsy for the diagnosis of sarcoidosis. N Engl J Med 1975;293:268.
103. James DG, Williams WJ. Immunology of sarcoidosis. Am J Med 1982;72:5.
104. Weissler JC. Southwestern Internal Medicine Conference. Sarcoidosis: Immunology and clinical management. Am J Med Sci 1994;307:233.
105. Azar HA, Lunardelli C. Collagen nature of asteroid bodies of giant cells in sarcoidosis. Am J Pathol 1969;57:81.
106. Civatte J. Sarcoidose et infiltrats tuberculoides. Ann Dermatol Syphiligr 1963;90:5.
107. Azulay RD. Histopathology of skin lesions in leprosy. Int J Lepr 1971; 39:244.
108. Wiersema JP, Binford CH. The identification of leprosy among epithelioid cell granulomas of the skin. Int J Lepr 1972;40:10.
109. Zimmer WM, Rogers RS III, Reeve CM, Sheridan PJ. Orofacial manifestations of Melkersson-Rosenthal syndrome. Oral Surg Oral Med Oral Pathol 1992;74:610.
110. Wagner G, Oberste-Lehn H. Zur kenntnis der symptomatologie der granulomatosis idiopathica. Z Hautkr 1963;32:166.
111. Hornstein OP. Melkersson-Rosenthal Syndrome. Curr Probl Dermatol 1975;5:117.
112. Westemark P, Henriksson TG. Granulomatous inflammation of the vulva and penis: A genital counterpart to cheilitis granulomatosa. Dermatologica 1979;158:269.
113. Hoede N, Heidbückel U, Korting GW. Vulvitis granulomatosa chronica: Melkersson-Rosenthal vulvitis. Hautarzt 1982;33:218.
114. Greene RM, Rogers RS III. Melkersson-Rosenthal syndrome: A review of 36 patients. J Am Acad Dermatol 1989;21:1263.
115. Miescher G. Über essentielle granulomatöse makrocheilie (cheilitis granulomatosa). Dermatologica 1945;91:57.
116. Hornstein O. Uber die pathogenese des sogenannten Melkersson-Rosenthal syndroms (einschliesslich der "cheilitis granulomatosa" Miescher). Arch Klin Exp Dermatol 1961;212:570.
117. Allen CM, Camisa C, Hamzeh S, Stephens L. Cheilitis granulomatosa: Report of six cases and review of the literature. J Am Acad Dermatol 1990;23:444.
118. Cohen HA, Cohen Z, Ashkenasi A et al. Melkersson-Rosenthal syndrome. Cutis 1994;54:327.
119. Hering H, Scheid P. Kritische bemerkungen zum Melkersson-Rosenthal syndrom als teilbild des Morbus Besnier-Boeck-Schaumann. Arch Dermatol Syph (Berlin) 1954;197;344.
120. Editorial. Orofacial granulomatosis. Lancet 1991;338:20.
121. Kano Y, Shiohara T, Yasita A, Nagashima M. Granulomatous cheilitis and Crohn's disease. Br J Dermatol 1990;123:409.
122. Swerlick RA, Cooper PH. Cheilitis glandularis: A re-evaluation. J Am Acad Dermatol 1984;10:466.
123. Rada DC, Koranda FC, Katz FS. Cheilitis glandularis: A disorder of ductal ectasia. J Dermatol Surg Oncol 1985;11:372.
124. Weir TW, Johnson WC. Cheilitis glandularis. Arch Dermatol 1971; 103:433.
125. Michalowski R. Cheilitis glandularis, heterotopic salivary glands and squamous cell carcinoma of the lips. Br J Dermatol 1962;74:445.
126. Dicken CH, Carrington SG, Winkelmann RK. Generalized granuloma annulare. Arch Dermatol 1969;99:556.
127. Haim S, Friedman-Birnbaum R, Shafrir A. Generalized granuloma annulare: Relationship to diabetes mellitus as revealed in 8 cases. Br J Dermatol 1970;83:302.
128. Owens DW, Freeman RG. Perforating granuloma annulare. Arch Dermatol 1971;103:64.
129. Lucky AW, Prose ND, Bove K et al. Papular umbilicated granuloma annulare. Arch Dermatol 1992;128:1375.
130. Duncan WC, Smith JD, Knox JM. Generalized perforating granuloma annulare. Arch Dermatol 1973;108:570.
131. Samlaska CP, Sandberg GD, Maggio KL, Sakas EL. Generalized perforating granuloma annulare. J Am Acad Dermatol 1992;27:319.
132. Ogino A, Tamaki E. Atypical granuloma annulare. Dermatologica 1978;156:97.
133. Rubin M, Lynch FW. Subcutaneous granuloma annulare. Arch Dermatol Syphiligr 1966;93:416.
134. Kerl H. Knotige rheumatische hautmanifestationen und ihre differentialdiagnose. Z Hautkr 1972;47:193.
135. Lowney ED, Simons HM. "Rheumatoid" nodules of the skin. Arch Dermatol 1963;88:853.
136. Salomon RJ, Gardepe SF, Woodley DT. Deep granuloma annulare in adults. Int J Dermatol 1986;25:109.

137. Evans MJ, Blessing K, Gray ES. Pseudorheumatoid nodule (deep granuloma annulare) of childhood: Clinicopathologic features of twenty patients. Pediatr Dermatol 1994;11:6.
138. Dabski K, Winkelmann K. Destructive granuloma annulare of the skin and underlying soft tissues: Report of two cases. Clin Exp Dermatol 1991;16:218.
139. Romaine R, Rudner EJ, Altman J. Papular granuloma annulare and diabetes mellitus. Arch Dermatol 1968;98:152.
140. Jelinek JE. Cutaneous manifestations of diabetes mellitus. Int J Dermatol 1994;33:605.
141. Zanolli MD, Powell BL, McCalmont T et al. Granuloma annulare and disseminated herpes zoster. Int J Dermatol 1992;31:55.
142. Friedman JJ, Fox BJ, Albert HL. Granuloma annulare arising in herpes zoster scars. J Am Acad Dermatol 1986;14:764.
143. Crosby DL, Woodley DT, Leonard DD. Concomitant granuloma annulare and necrobiosis lipodica. Dermatologica 1991;183:225.
144. Umbert P, Winkelmann RK. Histologic, ultrastructural, and histochemical studies of granuloma annulare. Arch Dermatol 1977;113: 1681.
145. Calista D, Landi G. Disseminated granuloma annulare in acquired immunodeficiency syndrome: Case report and review of the literature. Cutis 1995;55:158.
146. Burket JM, Zelickson AS. Intracellular elastin in generalized granuloma annulare. J Am Acad Dermatol 1986;14:975.
147. Gray HR, Graham JH, Johnson WC. Necrobiosis lipoidica: A histopathological and histochemical study. J Invest Dermatol 1965; 44:369.
148. Wood MG, Beerman H. Necrobiosis lipoidica, granuloma annulare, and rheumatoid nodule. J Invest Dermatol 1960;34:139.
149. Dahl MV, Ullman S, Goltz RW. Vasculitis in granuloma annulare. Arch Dermatol 1977;113:463.
150. Patterson JW. Rheumatoid nodule and subcutaneous granuloma annulare: A comparative histologic study. Am J Dermatopathol 1988;10:1.
151. Wolff HH, Maciejewski W. The ultrastructure of granuloma annulare. Arch Dermatol Res 1977;259:225.
152. Kallioinen M, Sandberg M, Kinnunen T, Oikarinen A. Collagen synthesis in granuloma annulare. J Invest Dermatol 1992;98:463.
153. Buechner SA, Winkelmann RK, Banks PM. Identification of T-cell subpopulations in granuloma annulare. Arch Dermatol 1983;119: 125.
154. Modlin RL, Vaccaro SA, Gottlieb B et al. Granuloma annulare: Identification of cells in the cutaneous infiltrate by immunoperoxidase techniques. Arch Pathol 1984;108:379.
155. Mullans E, Helm KF. Granuloma annulare: An immunohistochemical study. J Cutan Pathol 1994;21:135.
156. Thyresson HN, Doyle JA, Winkelmann RK. Granuloma annulare: Histopathologic and direct immunofluorescence study. Acta Derm Venereol (Stockh) 1980;60:261.
157. Nieboer C, Kalsbeek GL. Direct immunofluorescence studies in granuloma annulare, necrobiosis lipoidica and granulomatosis disciformis Mieschner. Dermatologica 1979;158:427.
158. Laymon CW, Fischer I. Necrobiosis lipoidica (diabeticorum?). Arch Dermatol Syph 1949;59:150.
159. Alegre VA, Winkelmann RK. A new histopathologic feature of necrobiosis lipoidica diabeticorum: Lymphoid nodules. J Cutan Pathol 1988;15:75.
160. Shapiro PE, Pinto FJ. The histologic spectrum of mycosis fungoides/Sezary syndrome (cutaneous T-cell lymphoma). Am J Surg Pathol 1994;18:645.
161. Cooper PH. Eruptive xanthoma: A microscopic simulant of granuloma annulare. J Cutan Pathol 1986;13:207.
162. Chase DR, Enzinger FM. Epithelioid sarcoma: Diagnosis, prognostic indicators, and treatment. Am J Surg Pathol 1985;9:241.
163. Lowitt MH, Dover JS. Necrobiosis lipoidica. J Am Acad Dermatol 1991;25:735.
164. Muller SA, Winkelmann RK. Necrobiosis lipoidica diabeticorum. Arch Dermatol 1966;93:272.
165. Mehregan AH, Pinkus H. Necrobiosis lipoidica with sarcoid reaction. Arch Dermatol 1961;83:143.
166. Mackey JP. Necrobiosis lipoidica diabeticorum involving scalp and face. Br J Dermatol 1975;93:729.
167. Gaethe G. Necrobiosis lipoidica diabeticorum of the scalp. Arch Dermatol 1964;89:865.
168. Metz G, Metz J. Extracrurale manifestion der necrobiosis lipoidica: Isolierter befall des kopfes. Hautarzt 1977;28:359.
169. Parra CA. Transepithelial elimination in necrobiosis lipoidica. Br J Dermatol 1977;96:83.
170. Gudmundson K, Smith O, Dervan P, Powell FC. Necrobiosis lipoidica and sarcoidosis. Clin Exp Dermatol 1991;16:287.
171. Muller SA, Winkelmann RK. Necrobiosis lipoidica diabeticorum. Arch Dermatol 1966;94:1.
172. Smith JG Jr, Wansker BA. Asteroid bodies in necrobiosis lipoidica. Arch Dermatol 1956;74:276.
173. Nicholas L. Necrobiosis lipoidica diabeticorum with xanthoma cells. Arch Dermatol 1943;48:606.
174. Bauer MF, Hirsch P, Bullock WK et al. Necrobiosis lipoidica diabeticorum: A cutaneous manifestation of diabetic microangiopathy. Arch Dermatol 1964;90:558.
175. Oikarinen A, Mörtenhumer M, Kallioinen M et al. Necrobiosis lipoidica: Ultrastructural and biochemical demonstration of a collagen defect. J Invest Dermatol 1987;88:227.
176. Ullman S, Dahl MV. Necrobiosis lipoidica. Arch Dermatol 1977;113: 1671.
177. Quimby SR, Muller SA, Schroeter AL. The cutaneous immunopathology of necrobiosis lipoidica diabeticorum. Arch Dermatol 1988;124:1364.
178. Laukkanen A, Fraki JA, Vaatainen N et al. Necrobiosis lipoidica: Clinical and immunofluorescent study. Dermatologica 1986;172:89.
179. Veys EM, De Keyser F. Rheumatoid nodules: Differential diagnosis and immunohistological findings. Ann Rheum Dis 1993;52:625.
180. Chalmers IM, Arneja AS. Rheumatoid nodules on amputation stumps: Report of three cases. Arch Phys Med Rehabil 1994;75:1151.
181. Moore CP, Willkens RF. The subcutaneous nodule: Its significance in the diagnosis of rheumatic disease. Semin Arthritis Rheum 1977;7:63.
182. Suliani RJ, Lansman S, Konstadt S. Intracardiac rheumatoid nodule presenting as a left atrial mass. Am Heart J 1994;127:463.
183. Horn RT Jr, Goette DK. Perforating rheumatoid nodule. Arch Dermatol 1982;118:696.
184. Dubois EL, Friou GJ, Chandor S. Rheumatoid nodules and rheumatoid granulomas in systemic lupus erythematosus. JAMA 1972;220; 515.
185. Schofield JK, Cerio R, Grice K. Systemic lupus erythematosus presenting with "rheumatoid nodules." Clin Exp Dermatol 1992;17:53.
186. Hahn BH, Yardley HH, Stevens MD. Rheumatoid "nodules" in systemic lupus erythematosus. Ann Intern Med 1970;72:49.
187. Sokoloff L, McCluskey RT, Bunim JJ. Vascularity of the early subcutaneous nodule of rheumatoid arthritis. Arch Pathol 1953;55:475.
188. Alguacil-Garcia A. Necrobiotic palisading suture granulomas simulating rheumatoid nodule. Am J Surg Pathol 1993;17:920.
189. Hayes RM, Gibson S. An evaluation of rheumatic nodules in children. JAMA 1942;119:554.
190. Kiel H. The rheumatic subcutaneous nodules and simulating lesions. Medicine (Baltimore) 1938;17:261.
191. Dahl MV. Is actinic granuloma really granuloma annulare? Arch Dermatol 1986;122:39.
192. Ragaz A, Ackerman AB. Is actinic granuloma a specific condition? Am J Dermatopathol 1979;1:43.
193. Hanke CW, Bailin PL, Roenigk HH Jr. Annular elastolytic giant cell granuloma. J Am Acad Dermatol 1979;1:413.
194. O'Brien JP. Actinic granuloma. Arch Dermatol 1975;111:460.
195. Yanagihara M, Kato F, Mori S. Extra- and intra-cellular digestion of elastic fibers by macrophages in annular elastolytic giant cell granuloma. J Cutan Pathol 1987;14:303.
196. Sina B, Wood C, Rudo K. Generalized elastophagocytic granuloma. Cutis 1992;49:355.
197. Boneschi V, Brambilla L, Fossati S et al. Annular elastolytic giant cell granuloma. Am J Dermatopathol 1988;10:224.
198. Steffen C. Actinic granuloma (O'Brien). J Cutan Pathol 1988;15:66.
199. Mehregan AH, Altman J. Miescher's granuloma of the face. Arch Dermatol 1973;107:62.
200. Dowling GB, Wilson Jones E. Atypical (annular) necrobiosis lipoidica of the face and scalp. Dermatologica 1967;135:11.

201. Steffen C. Actinic granuloma of the conjunctiva. Am J Dermatopathol 1992;14:253.
202. Tappeiner J, Pfleger L. Granuloma glutaeale infantum. Hautarzt 1971; 22:383.
203. Uyeda K, Nakayasu K, Takaishi Y. Kaposi sarcoma-like granuloma on diaper dermatitis. Arch Dermatol 1973;107:605.
204. Simmons IJ. Granuloma gluteale infantum. Australas J Dermatol 1977;18:20.
205. Maekawa Y, Sakazaki Y, Hayashibara T. Diaper area granuloma of the aged. Arch Dermatol 1978;114:382.
206. Fujita M, Ohno S, Danno K, Miyachi Y. Two cases of diaper area granuloma of the adult. J Dermatol 1991;18:671.
207. Delarétaz J, Grigoriu D, De Crousaz H et al. Candidose nodulaire de la région inguino-génitale et des fesses (granuloma glutaeale infantum). Dermatologica 1972;144:144.
208. Sweidan NA, Salman SM, Kibbi AG, Zaynoun ST. Skin nodules over the diaper area. Arch Dermatol 1989;125:1703.

Lever's Histopathology of the Skin, eighth edition,
edited by David Elder et al. Lippincott–
Raven Publishers, Philadelphia © 1997.

CHAPTER 15

Degenerative Diseases and Perforating Disorders

Edward R. Heilman and Robert J. Friedman

SOLAR (ACTINIC) ELASTOSIS

Senile changes in areas of the skin not regularly exposed to sunlight manifest themselves clinically only in thinning of the skin and a decrease in the amount of subcutaneous fat. In contrast, there are often pronounced changes in the appearance of the exposed skin of elderly persons, especially those with fair complexions. These changes, however, are the result of chronic sun exposure rather than of age. In exposed areas, especially on the face, the skin shows wrinkling, furrowing, and thinning. In addition, there may be an irregular distribution of pigment. In the nuchal region, the skin, after many years of exposure to the sun, may appear thickened and furrowed. This is referred to as cutis rhomboidalis nuchae.

Two variants of circumscribed solar elastosis occur on the arms rather than on the face: *actinic comedonal plaques,*[1] consisting of solitary nodular plaques with a cribriform appearance and comedone-like structures, and *solar elastotic bands of the forearm,*[2] consisting of cordlike plaques across the flexor surfaces of the forearms.

Histopathology. In skin not regularly exposed to sunlight, there is a progressive disappearance of elastic tissue in the papillary dermis with age. It involves the oxytalan fibers, which in young age form a thin, superficial network perpendicular to the dermal-epidermal junction. Electron microscopically, the oxytalan fibers consist solely of microfibrils (Chap. 3). In middle age, the oxytalan fibers in the papillary dermis are split and fewer than at a young age, and in old age they may be absent.[3]

In the skin of the face exposed to the sun, especially in persons with fair complexions, hyperplasia of the elastic tissue is usually evident on histologic examination by the age of 30, even though clinically the skin may appear normal. No white person past 40 years of age has normal elastic tissue in the skin of the face.[4] The elastic fibers have increased in number, and they are thicker, curled, and tangled.

E. R. Heilman: Departments of Dermatology and Pathology, SUNY Health Sciences Center, Brooklyn, NY; Dermpath, Scarsdale, NY

R. J. Friedman: Department of Dermatology, NYU School of Medicine, New York, NY; Dermpath, Scarsdale, NY

In patients with clinically evident solar elastosis of the exposed skin, staining with hematoxylin-eosin reveals, in the upper dermis, basophilic degeneration of the collagen separated from a somewhat atrophic epidermis by a narrow band of normal collagen. In the areas of basophilic degeneration, the bundles of eosinophilic collagen have been replaced by amorphous basophilic granular material.

With elastic tissue stains, the areas of basophilic degeneration stain like elastic tissue and therefore are referred to as elastotic material (Fig. 15-1). The elastotic material usually consists of aggregates of thick, interwoven bands in the upper dermis[2]; but in areas of severe solar degeneration, the elastotic material may have an amorphous rather than a fibrous appearance and may extend into the lower portions of the dermis rather than being confined to the upper dermis.[5]

On staining with silver nitrate, the distribution of melanin in the basal cell layer may appear irregular in that areas of hyperpigmentation alternate with areas of hypopigmentation.[5]

In the actinic comedonal plaques described as occurring on the arms, dilated, corneocyte-filled follicles may be present within areas of elastotic, amorphous material.[1] Similarly, the elastotic bands on the forearms consist of nodular collections of amorphous material.[2]

Histogenesis. Electron microscopic examination of areas of solar elastosis shows elastotic material as the main component. Even though this elastotic material resembles elastic tissue in its chemical composition, it differs significantly in appearance from aged elastic fibers in unexposed, aged skin. Instead of showing amorphous electron-lucent elastin and aggregates of electron-dense microfibrils (Chap. 3), the thick fibers of elastotic material show two structural components: a fine granular matrix of medium electron density and, within this matrix, homogeneous, electron-dense, irregularly shaped inclusions.[6] The electron-dense inclusions seem to develop by means of a condensation process in the granular matrix.[2] The respective proportion for each of the two components can vary between 30% and 70% of the volume.[7] Microfibrils such as those observed in normal or aged elastic fibers are absent. Accordingly, immunoelectron microscopy shows that the elastotic material has retained its antigenicity for elastin but not for microfibrils.[8]

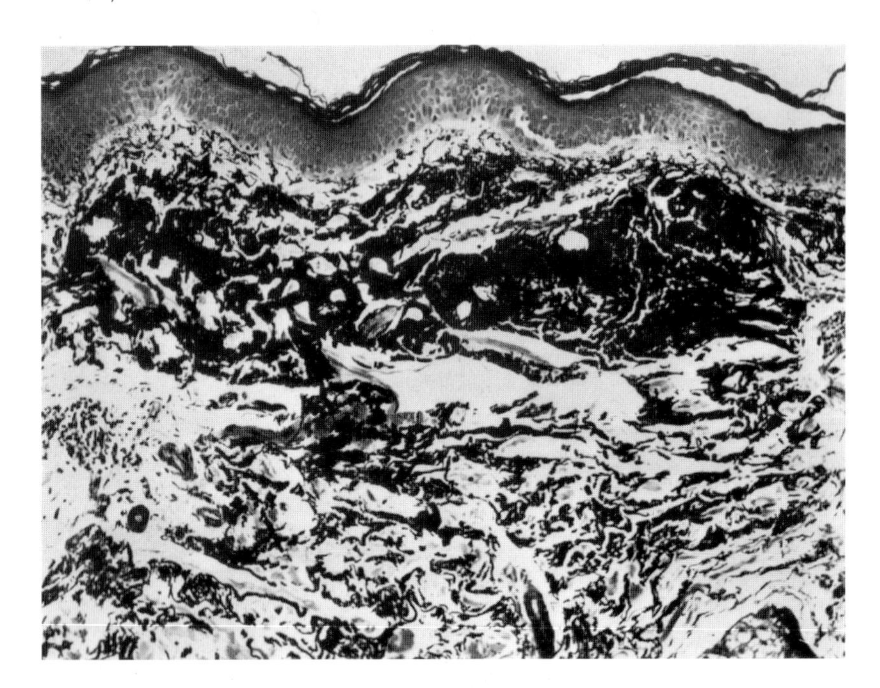

FIG. 15-1. Solar (actinic) degeneration In the upper dermis, separated from the epidermis by a narrow band of normal collagen, there are aggregates of thick, interwoven bands of elastotic material staining like elastic tissue.

The number and size of elastotic fibers are greatly increased over the number and size of elastic fibers found in normal or aged skin. Extensive amorphous material can be seen around the elastotic fibers and also among the collagen fibrils. Collagen fibrils are diminished in number, with those present often showing a diminished electron density, a diminished contrast in cross striation, and a splitting up into filaments at their ends.[9] The fibroblasts show the characteristics of actively synthesizing cells in that they possess an extensive, dilated, rough endoplasmic reticulum containing amorphous or fine granular material that is excreted into the extracellular space.[2,10] Often, strands of fine granular material are discernible between the surfaces of active fibroblasts and masses of elastotic material.[6]

It can be concluded that the elastotic material is newly formed as the result of an altered function of fibroblasts, which are no longer capable of producing normal elastic fibers or collagen. The elastotic material is not regarded as a degeneration product of preexisting elastic fibers.

The elastotic material that histochemically stains like elastic tissue resembles elastic tissue in its chemical composition and its physical and enzymatic reactions. Thus, the amino acid composition of the elastotic tissue resembles that of elastin and differs significantly from that of collagen. In particular, the elastotic material, like elastic tissue, has a much lower content of hydroxyproline than collagen.[11] Moreover, the elastotic material in unfixed sections shows the same brilliant autofluorescence as do elastic fibers on examination with the fluorescence microscope,[12] and both the elastotic material and elastic tissue are susceptible to elastase digestion.[13]

The elastotic material contains a large amount of acid mucopolysaccharides, as indicated by staining with alcian blue. A significant portion of these acid mucopolysaccharides may be sulfated because prior incubation with hyaluronidase removes only 50% to 75% of the alcian-blue-positive staining. The basophilia of the elastotic material, however, is not affected by incubation with hyaluronidase.[14]

The irregular distribution of melanin in the epidermis observed in some patients with solar degeneration, when studied by electron microscopy, is found to be caused largely by an impairment of pigment transfer from melanocytes to keratinocytes. Although some keratinocytes contain many melanosomes, others contain few or no melanosomes. The latter are surrounded by dendrites laden with melanosomes.[15]

Differential Diagnosis. For a discussion of differentiation of solar elastosis from pseudoxanthoma elasticum, see Chap. 3.

FAVRE-RACOUCHOT SYNDROME (NODULAR ELASTOSIS WITH CYSTS AND COMEDONES)

In Favre-Racouchot syndrome, the facial skin shows, especially lateral to the eyes, multiple open and cystically dilated comedones.

Histopathology. Dilated pilosebaceous openings and large, round, cystlike spaces are lined by a flattened epithelium and represent greatly distended hair follicles.[16,17] Both the dilated pilosebaceous openings and the cystlike spaces are filled with layered horny material. The sebaceous glands are atrophic. Solar elastosis often is pronounced,[16] but it may be slight or absent.[18] Because the comedones are open, they do not tend to become inflamed[19] (see section on Acne Vulgaris).

PERFORATING DISORDERS

The perforating disorders comprise a group of unrelated pathologic abnormalities sharing the common characteristic of transepidermal elimination. This phenomenon is characterized by the elimination or extrusion of altered dermal substances and, in some cases, by such material behaving as foreign material.

Traditionally, four diseases have been included in this group: *Kyrle's disease* (hyperkeratosis follicularis et parafollicularis in cutem penetrans), *perforating folliculitis, elastosis perforans serpiginosum,* and *reactive perforating collagenosis.* In addition, an important fifth condition known as *perforating disorder of renal failure and/or diabetes* has been added to this group.[20]

Although transepidermal elimination is a prominent feature in all these conditions, it has also been described as a secondary phenomenon in other entities, including such inflammatory disorders as granuloma annulare, one variant of pseudoxanthoma elasticum, and chondrodermatitis nodularis helicis. Needless to say, there is a long list of other conditions that can exhibit transepidermal elimination as an associated reaction pattern.

Kyrle's Disease

Kyrle's disease is a rare disorder, described by Kyrle in 1916,[21] that may actually comprise a group of disorders with similar epidermal-dermal reaction patterns associated with chronic renal failure, diabetes, prurigo nodularis, and even keratosis pilaris. Therefore, the discussion of Kyrle's disease and perforating disorders of chronic renal disease and/or diabetes has a very broad overlap in terms of their clinical and pathologic features.

Clinical Features. This eruption presents with a large number of papules, some coalescing into plaques, numbering in the hundreds and often distributed on the extremities. Although some may appear to involve the follicular units, these lesions are more likely to be extrafollicular. The typical patient is young to middle aged and often has a history of diabetes mellitus. The papules are dome shaped, 2 to 8 mm in diameter, with a central keratotic plug. Excoriations often are found in the vicinity of these lesions. Linear lesions related to possible "Koebnerization" have been described.

Histopathology. The essential histopathologic findings include (1) a follicular or extrafollicular cornified plug with focal parakeratosis embedded in an epidermal invagination, (2) basophilic degenerated material identified in small collections throughout the plug with absence of demonstrable collagen and elastin, (3) abnormal vacuolated and/or dyskeratotic keratinization of the epithelial cells extending to the basal cell zone, (4) irregular epithelial hyperplasia, and (5) an inflammatory component that is typically granulomatous with small foci of suppuration (Fig. 15-2). In most instances it is important to perform elastic tissue stains and even trichrome stains to exclude perforating elastic fibers as in elastosis perforans serpiginosum or collagen fibers as in reactive perforating collagenosis.[22]

Histogenesis. The primary event is claimed to be a disturbance of epidermal keratinization characterized by the formation of dyskeratotic foci and acceleration of the process of keratinization. This leads to the formation of keratotic plugs with areas of parakeratosis.[23–25] Because the rapid rate of differentiation and keratinization exceeds the rate of cell proliferation, the parakeratotic column gradually extends deeper into the abnormal epidermis, leading in most cases to perforation of the parakeratotic column into the dermis. Perforation is not the cause of Kyrle's disease, as originally thought,[21] but rather represents the consequence or final event of the abnormally sped-up keratinization. This rapid production of abnormal keratin forms a plug which acts as a foreign body, penetrating the epidermis and inciting a granulomatous inflammatory reaction. A certain similarity exists between the parakeratotic column in Kyrle's disease and that observed in porokeratosis Mibelli.[24] In both conditions, a parakeratotic column forms as the result of rapid and faulty keratinization of dyskeratotic cells, but, whereas in Kyrle's disease the dyskeratotic cells are often used up so that disruption of the epithelium occurs, the clone of dyskeratotic cells can maintain itself in porokeratosis Mibelli by extending peripherally.

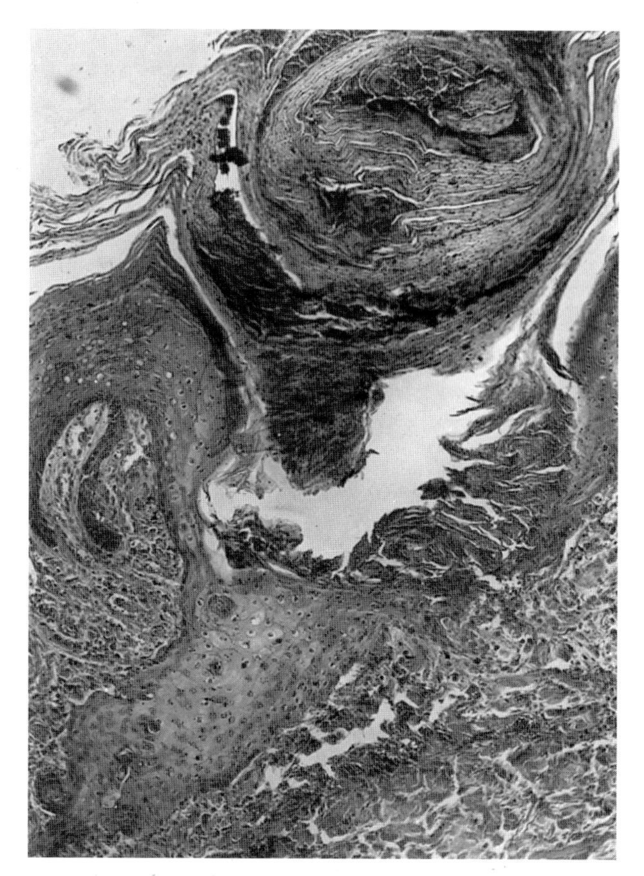

FIG. 15-2. Kyrle's disease
A heavy keratotic, partly parakeratotic plug containing basophilic debris lies in an invagination of the epidermis. On the left side of the invagination, where there are no granular cells, a parakeratotic column arises from epidermal cells that appear vacuolated and dyskeratotic. On the right side of the invagination, there is a disruption of the epidermal cells. Thus, the plug is in direct contact with the dermis, which, in this area, shows degeneration with inflammatory and foreign-body giant cells. (Courtesy of Joseph M. Hitch, MD.)

Differential Diagnosis. See Table 15-1.

Perforating Folliculitis

Perforating folliculitis is a perforating disorder that has many features overlapping with Kyrle's disease and perforating disorders of renal disease/diabetes. As described by Mehregan and Coskey[26] this is a relatively uncommon disorder usually observed in the second to fourth decades and is characterized by erythematous follicular papules with central keratotic plugs.

TABLE 15-1. *Differential diagnoses of perforating disorders*

Disease	Primary defect	Distinctive features	Histogenesis
Kyrle's disease	Focus of dyskeratotic rapidly proliferating cells in the epidermis	Follicular or extrafollicular cornified plug embedded in an epidermal invagination associated with epithelial hyperplasia and absence of demonstrable collagen and elastin	Disturbance of keratinization, forming a plug that acts as a foreign body penetrating the epidermis and inciting a granulomatous inflammatory reaction
Perforating folliculitis	Hyperkeratotic plug in follicular unit containing a retained hair	Compact ortho and parakeratotic plug with degenerated collagen, altered elastin, and mixed inflammatory cell infiltrate including neutrophils	A primary irritant causing follicular hyperkeratosis resulting in a mechanical breakdown of the follicle wall by the hair shaft
Elastosis perforans serpiginosum	Formation of numerous thickened coarse elastic fibers in the superficial dermis	Formation of narrow channel through an acanthotic epidermis with elimination of eosinophilic elastic fibers	Thickened elastic fibers act as mechanical irritants or "foreign bodies"
Reactive perforating collagenosis	Subepidermal focus of altered collagen caused by trauma	Formation of cup-shaped vertically oriented channel with transepidermal elimination of degenerated collagen	Histochemically altered collagen acts as "foreign body"
Perforating disorder secondary to chronic renal disease and/or diabetes mellitus	Chronic rubbing due to pruritis, resulting in follicular hyperkeratosis and perforation	A combination of features similar to that seen in perforating folliculitis, reactive perforating collagenosis, and prurigo nodularis	Exogenously altered skin in pruritic diabetics and patients with chronic renal disease

The lesions are 2 to 8 mm in diameter and tend to be localized to the extensor surfaces of the extremities and the buttocks. The key to making this diagnosis is the clinical and histologic identification of a follicular unit as the primary site for the inflammatory process.

Histopathology. The main pathologic abnormalities consist of (1) a dilated follicular infundibulum filled with compact ortho and parakeratotic cornified cells; (2) degenerated basophilic staining material, comprised of granular nuclear debris from nuclear neutrophils, other inflammatory cells, and degenerated collagen bundles; (3) one or more perforations through the follicular epithelium; and (4) an associated perifollicular inflammatory cell infiltrate composed of lymphocytes, histiocytes, and neutrophils (Fig. 15-3). Additionally, altered collagen and refractile eosinophilically altered elastic fibers are found adjacent to the sites of perforation. When serial sections through the specimen are examined, a remnant of the hair shaft can sometimes be found.

Histogenesis. Perforating folliculitis is the end result of abnormal follicular keratinization most likely caused by irritation, either chemical or physical, and even chronic rubbing. A portion of a curled-up hair is often seen close to or within the area of perforation or even in the dermis, surrounded by a foreign-body granuloma.[26]

Differential Diagnosis. In Kyrle's disease, the keratinous plug may be extrafollicular, the perforation usually is present deep in the invagination at the bottom of the keratinous plug, and no eosinophilic degeneration of elastic fibers is found. In addition, in Kyrle's disease, epithelial hyperplasia is a significant feature. For a discussion of the differential diagnosis of perforating folliculitis from elastosis perforans serpiginosum, see the following section on Differential Diagnosis for Elastosis Perforans Serpiginosum.

Elastosis Perforans Serpiginosum

Elastosis perforans serpiginosum (EPS) is the most distinctive of the perforating disorders because it demonstrates the best example of transepidermal elimination. In EPS, increased numbers of thickened elastic fibers are present in the upper dermis and altered elastic fibers are extruded through the epidermis. It is a rare disorder that affects young individuals with a peak incidence in the second decade. Men are affected more often than women. EPS is primarily a papular eruption localized to one anatomic site and most commonly affecting the nape of the neck, the face, or the upper extremities. The papules are typically 2 to 5 mm in diameter. These papules are arranged in arcuate or serpiginous groups and may coalesce.

Of particular importance is the association of EPS with systemic diseases. The important associations include Down's syndrome, Ehlers-Danlos syndrome, osteogenesis imperfecta, pseudoxanthoma elasticum, and Marfan's syndrome. In addition, on rare occasions EPS is observed in association with Rothmund-Thompson syndrome or other connective tissue disorders, and as a secondary complication of penicillamine administration.

Histopathology. The essential findings include a narrow transepidermal channel that may be straight, wavy, or of corkscrew shape and thick, coarse elastic fibers in the channel admixed with granular basophilic staining debris (Fig. 15-4). A mixed inflammatory cell infiltrate accompanies the fibers in the channel. Also observed are abnormal elastic fibers in the upper dermis in the vicinity of the channel. In this zone the elastic fibers are increased in size and number. As these fibers enter the lower portion of the channel, they maintain their normal staining characteristics, but as they approach the epidermal surface they may not stain as expected with elastic stains (Fig. 15-5).[27]

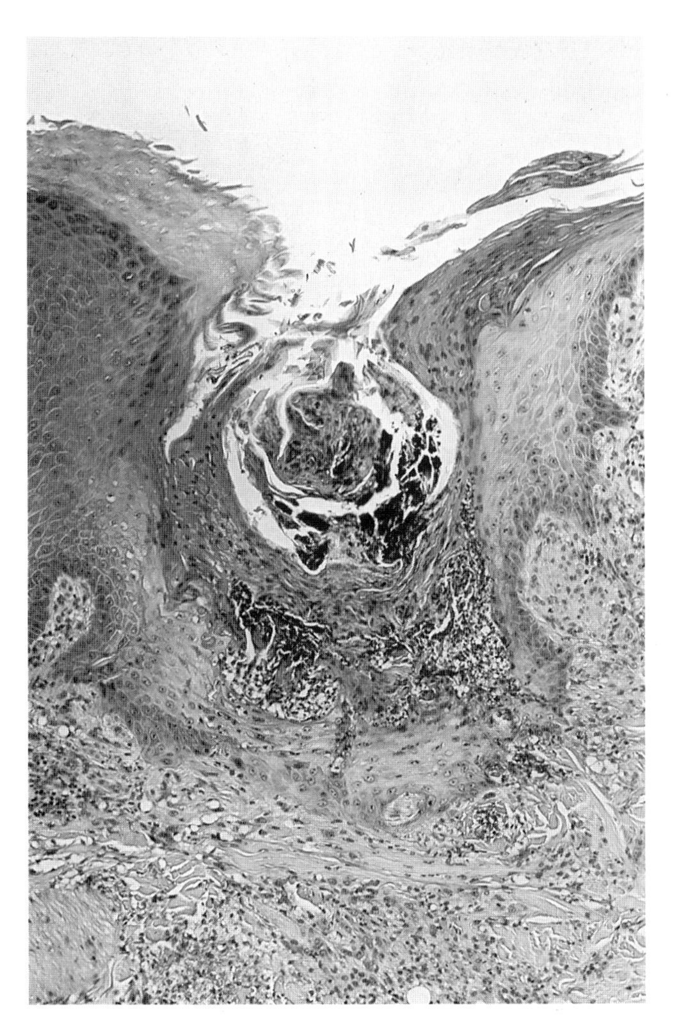

FIG. 15-3. Perforating folliculitis
A dilated follicular unit contains a keratotic plug with an admixture of basophilic staining debris. The follicular epithelium is perforated, and there are degenerated collagen fibers in the surrounding dermis.

Histogenesis. The cause of EPS is not known. Because the elastic fibers show no obvious abnormality within the dermis except hyperplasia, it is conceivable that the thickened elastic fibers act as mechanical irritants or "foreign bodies" and provoke an epidermal response in the form of hyperplasia. The epidermis then envelops the irritating material and eliminates it through transepidermal channels. The degeneration of the elastic fibers within the channels probably is caused by proteolytic enzymes set free by degenerating inflammatory cells.[27] The channel is formed as a reactive phenomenon through which the "foreign bodies" are extruded. Because copper metabolism is essential to the formation of elastin and because the administration of penicillamine, a copper chelating agent, has been found to induce EPS, several authors have concluded that the primary abnormality begins with a defect in the metabolism of this essential element.[28]

Differential Diagnosis. Both Kyrle's disease and perforating folliculitis have in common with elastosis perforans serpiginosum a central keratotic plug and a perforation through which degenerated material is eliminated. In addition, perforating folliculitis, like elastosis perforans serpiginosum, shows the elimination of degenerated eosinophilic elastic fibers. However, neither of the two diseases shows the great increase in elastic tissue that is observed in elastosis perforans serpiginosum in the uppermost dermis and particularly in the dermal papillae on staining with elastic tissue stains.

Reactive Perforating Collagenosis

Reactive perforating collagenosis (RPC) is a rare perforating disorder in which altered collagen is extruded by means of transepidermal elimination. True, classic RPC is a genodermatosis that is inherited as an autosomal dominant or recessive trait.[29,30] The lesions are precipitated by trauma, arthropod assaults, folliculitis, and even exposure to cold. RPC occurs early in life, and both genders are equally affected.

The primary clinical lesion is a small papule that enlarges to the size of 5 to 10 mm with a hyperkeratotic central umbilication. Often the lesion appears eroded. These lesions spontaneously regress, leaving superficial scars with postinflammatory pigmentary alteration.

An adult, acquired type of RPC has been described in association with diabetes mellitus and chronic renal failure[31–33] but may in fact represent a variant of perforating disorder secondary to chronic renal disease and/or diabetes (see text following).

Histopathology. The classic lesion shows a vertically oriented, shallow, cup-shaped invagination of the epidermis, forming a short channel (Fig. 15-6A). The channel is lined by acanthotic epithelium along the sides. At the base of the invagination there is an attenuated layer of keratinocytes that in some foci appear eroded. Within the channel there is densely packed degenerated basophilic staining material and basophilically altered collagen bundles. Vertically oriented perforating bundles of collagen are present interposed between the keratinocytes of the attenuated bases of the invagination (see Fig. 15-6B). It is important that a Masson-trichrome stain be done to confirm that the fibers are collagen.

Histogenesis. The basic process in reactive perforating collagenosis consists of the transepidermal elimination of histochemically altered collagen. Nevertheless, as delineated by electron microscopy, the collagen fibrils appear intact, with regular periodicity.[34]

Perforating Disorder Secondary to Chronic Renal Failure and/or Diabetes Mellitus

This newly established dermatosis,[35] which combines clinical features of Kyrle's disease and histologic features of perforating folliculitis, occurs quite commonly in patients with chronic renal failure.[20] In most instances, the lesions arise within a few months after renal dialysis has been started.[36,37] The lesions are usually located mainly on the extensor surfaces of the lower extremities but are often extensive. They consist of follicular papules and often have a central keratotic plug.[38] They may coalesce to form verrucous plaques.

Histopathology. Small lesions tend to have the histologic picture of perforating folliculitis, with the perforation, if it occurs, in the infundibular portion of the hair follicle.[36,37] In larger lesions, perforations are apt to be at the base of the follicular

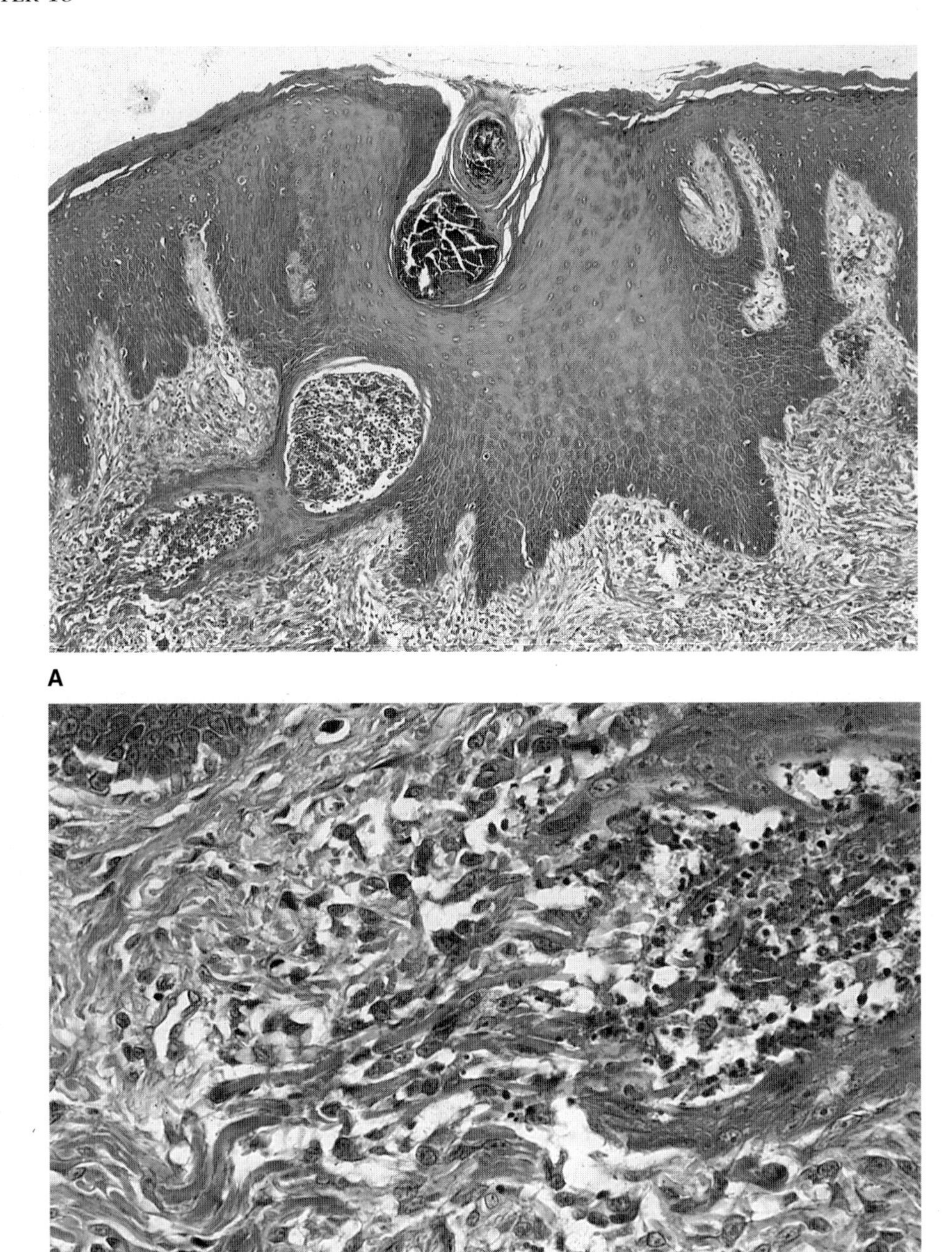

FIG. 15-4. Elastosis perforans serpiginosum
(A) A narrow, curved channel through an acanthotic epidermis is shown. The upper portion of the channel contains basophilic necrotic material. The lower portion of the channel contains, in addition to necrotic material, degenerated elastic fibers. **(B)** There are thickened degenerated elastic fibers at the origination of the transepidermal channel.

invagination.[39,40] Both types of perforations may be observed in a single biopsy specimen.[35] In some instances, no follicular structure can be identified, and in these cases the lesions can be indistinguishable from reactive perforating collagenosis with superimposed features of prurigo nodularis.

Histogenesis. The usual occurrence of a papular eruption with features of a perforating disorder in association with renal dialysis has led to speculations that this disease may be caused by the accumulation of a poorly dialyzable "uremic" substance.[36] In a few instances, however, the disorder has occurred without dialysis.[35,38,40] This condition may have appeared only recently because hemodialysis has been prolonging the lives of chronic renal failure patients,[35] which raises the possibility that this disorder is simply a manifestation of chronically rubbed skin as a result of pruritis with a prominent follicular component.

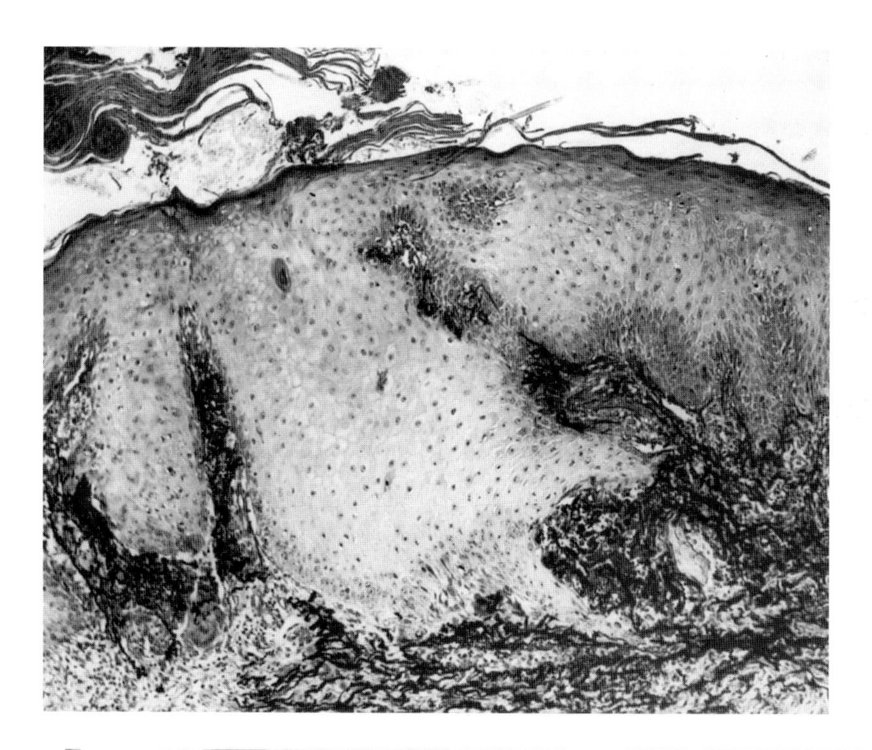

FIG. 15-5. Elastosis perforans serpiginosum
The great increase in both the amount and the size of the elastic fibers in the uppermost dermis and particularly in the dermal papillae is pathognomonic for elastosis perforans serpiginosum.

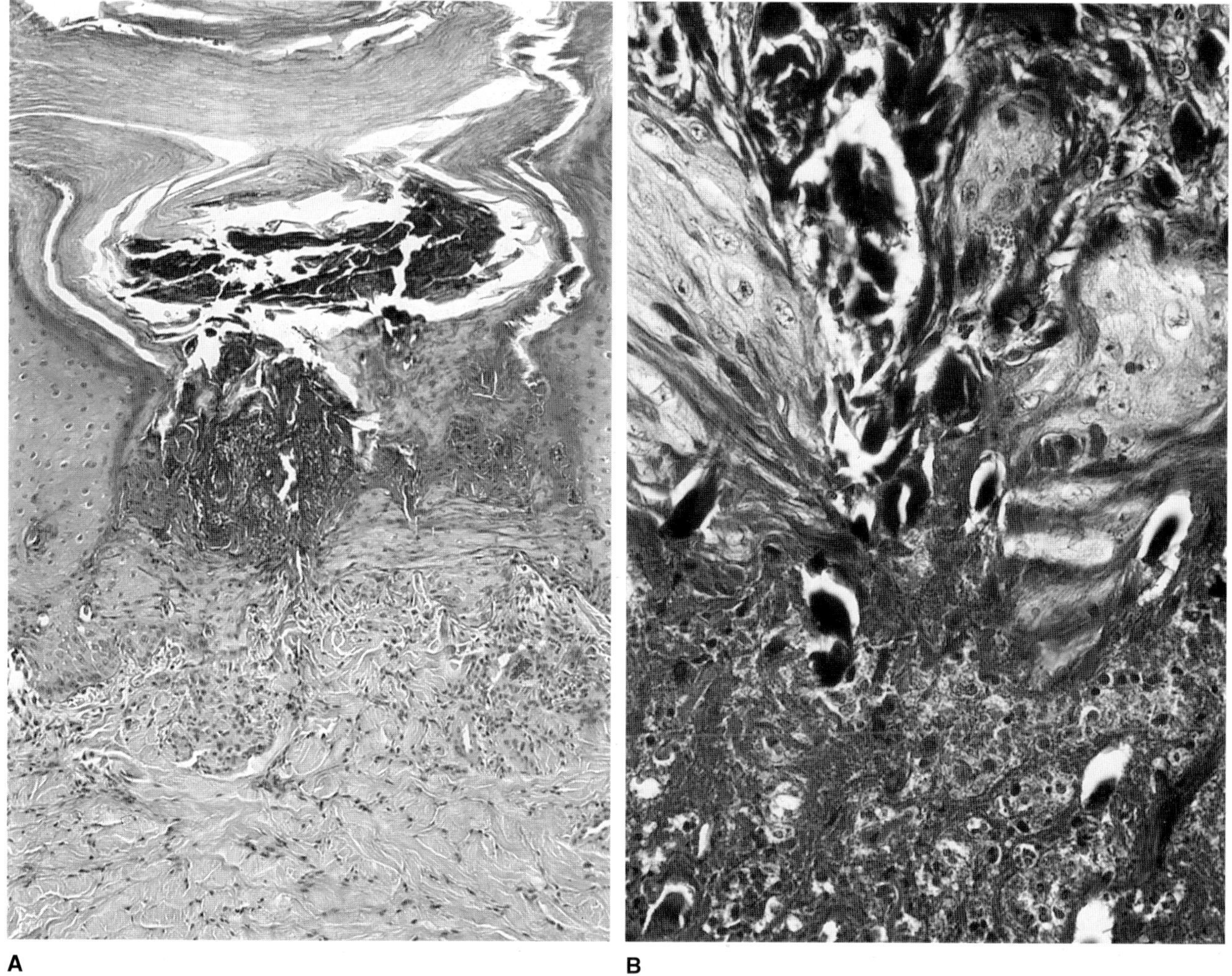

FIG. 15-6. Reactive perforating collagenosis
(A) Cup-shaped, vertically oriented channel containing degenerated collagen bundles and basophilic staining material. (**B**) Darkly stained degenerated collagen fibers perforating an attenuated epithelium and extending into the base of the channel.

PERFORATING CALCIFIC ELASTOSIS (PERIUMBILICAL PERFORATING PSEUDOXANTHOMA ELASTICUM)

In perforating calcific elastosis, also referred to as periumbilical perforating pseudoxanthoma elasticum, a gradually enlarging, well-demarcated, hyperpigmented patch or plaque may be seen in the periumbilical region in middle-aged, multiparous women.[41] The patch or plaque is in some instances atrophic with discrete keratotic papules[42]; in other instances, it has a verrucous border,[43] and in still others it has a fissured, verrucous surface throughout.[44] The size of the lesion varies from 2 to 14 cm.

In one elderly patient with chronic renal failure undergoing hemodialysis, lesions of "perforating pseudoxanthoma elasticum" have been reported on each breast.[45]

Histopathology. Numerous altered elastic fibers are observed in the reticular dermis. They are short, thick, and curled, and are encrusted with calcium salts, as shown by a positive von Kossa stain. They are thus indistinguishable from the elastic fibers seen in pseudoxanthoma elasticum (Fig. 15-7).[41] As in pseudoxanthoma elasticum, the elastic fibers are visible even in

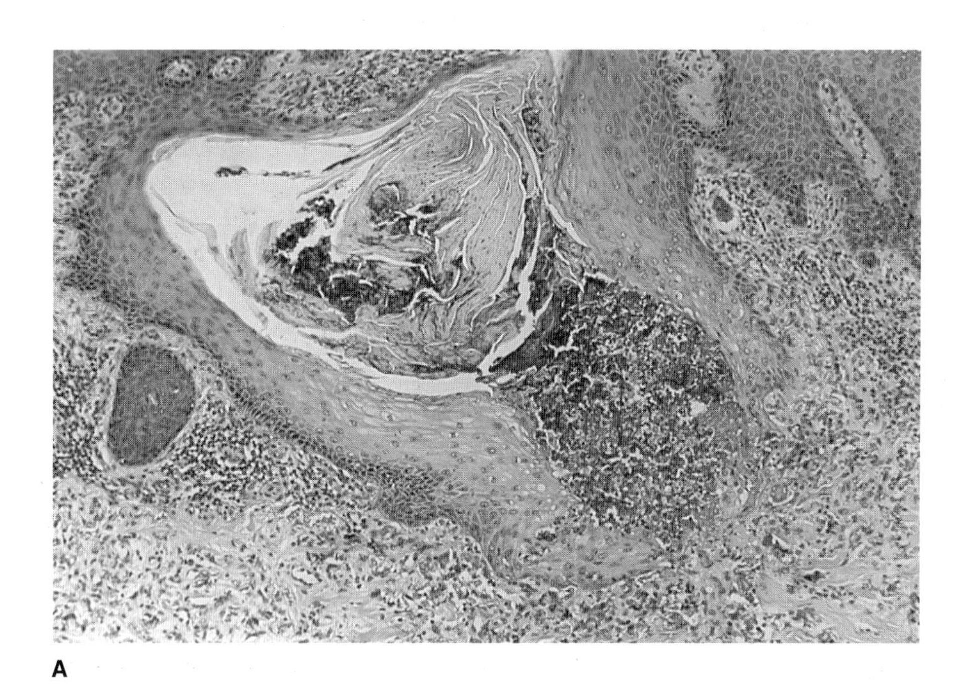

A

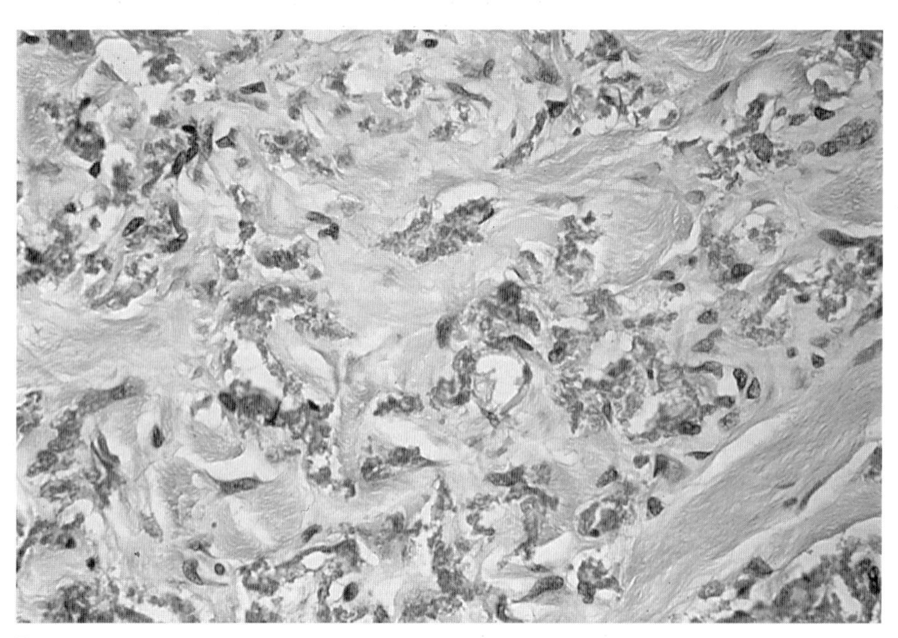

B

FIG. 15-7. Perforating calcific elastosis
(**A**) Irregular transepidermal channel containing degenerated elastic fibers encrusted by calcium salts. (**B**) Increased number of curled elastic fibers encrusted by calcium salts in the upper dermis, a finding indistinguishable from pseudoxanthoma elasticum.

sections stained with hematoxylin-eosin, owing to their basophilia.[42] In contrast to pseudoxanthoma elasticum, however, the altered elastic fibers in perforating calcific elastosis are extruded to the surface either through the epidermis in a wide channel[43] or through a tunnel in the hyperplastic epidermis that ends in a keratin-filled crater.[42]

HYPERKERATOSIS LENTICULARIS PERSTANS (FLEGEL'S DISEASE)

A rare dermatosis first described in 1958,[46] hyperkeratosis lenticularis perstans consists of asymptomatic, flat, hyperkeratotic papules from 1 to 5 mm in diameter, located predominantly on the dorsa of the feet and on the lower legs. Removal of the adherent, horny scale causes slight bleeding. In addition to the central horny scale, larger papules often have a peripherally attached collarette of fine scaling. In two reported instances, extensive papular lesions were present on the oral mucosa.[47]

The disorder starts in late life and persists indefinitely. An autosomal dominant transmission has been noted in several instances.[48–50]

Histopathology. In some instances, the histologic picture is nonspecific, showing hyperkeratosis with occasional areas of parakeratosis, irregular acanthosis intermingled with areas of flattening of the stratum malpighii, and vascular dilation with a moderate amount of perivascular round cell infiltration.[51] It seems, however, that if the specimen is obtained from a well-developed, markedly hyperkeratotic lesion, a characteristic, although not necessarily diagnostic, histologic picture may be revealed. The lesion shows a greatly thickened, compact, strongly eosinophilic horny layer standing out in sharp contrast to the less heavily stained basket-weave keratin of the uninvolved epidermis.[52] The underlying stratum malpighii appears flattened, with thinning or even absence of the granular layer.

Acanthosis is observed at the periphery. In some instances, bordering on the central depression, the epidermis at the periphery forms a papillomatous elevation resembling a church spire.[46,53,54] The dermal infiltrate is composed largely of lymphoid cells and is located as a narrow band fairly close to the epidermis with a rather sharp demarcation at its lower border.

Histogenesis. Under electron microscopic examination, the absence of membrane-coating granules was noted in some cases and regarded as the primary lesion of hyperkeratosis lenticularis perstans.[47,50]

A defect in the membrane-coating granules seems indeed to play a role in Flegel's disease, because in other cases in which membrane-coating granules were present, the granules lacked a lamellar internal structure and appeared vesicular.[55,56] In one case, both lamellar and vesicular bodies were observed, with lamellar bodies greatly predominating in uninvolved epidermis and vesicular bodies in lesional epidermis.[57]

STRIAE DISTENSAE

Striae distensae occur most commonly on the abdomen, on the thighs, and in the inguinal region. They consist of bands of thin, wrinkled skin that at first are red, then purple, and finally white.

Histopathology. The epidermis is thin and flattened. There is a decrease in the thickness of the dermis. The upper portion of the dermis shows straight, thin collagen bundles arranged parallel to the skin surface and transverse to the direction of the striae. The elastic fibers are arranged similarly. Fine elastic fibers predominate in early lesions, whereas in older lesions they are thick.[58] Within the striae, nuclei are scarce and sweat glands and hair follicles are absent.[59]

Histogenesis. The histologic findings support the view that striae distensae are scars.[59] They occur in conditions associated with increased production of glucocorticoids by the adrenal glands. Among these conditions are pregnancy, obesity, adolescence, and especially Cushing's disease.[60] In obesity, the increased adrenocortical activity is a consequence of the obesity, and the production of glucocorticoids returns to normal when the body weight is reduced.[61] Similarly, the occurrence of striae in nonobese adolescents, as noted in 35% of the girls and 15% of the boys examined, is associated with an increase in 17-kerosteroid excretion.[62] Striae may also form in response to prolonged intake of corticosteroids or following the prolonged local application of corticosteroid creams to the skin.[60] The action of the glucocorticoids consists of an antianabolic effect suppressing both fibroblastic and epidermal activity, as tissue culture studies have shown.[63]

WRINKLING DUE TO MIDDERMAL ELASTOLYSIS

Wrinkling due to middermal elastosis is a rare disorder first described in 1977.[64] It occurs in middle-aged women and consists of widespread, large areas of fine wrinkling. The wrinkling may be associated with small, soft, papular lesions consisting of tiny perifollicular protrusions, leaving the hair follicle itself as an indented center.[65] Some of the lesions may be preceded by urticaria[64] or erythematous patches.[66]

Histopathology. In this condition there is a selective absence of elastic tissue strictly limited to the middermis of involved areas.[64] The perifollicular protrusions around indented hair follicles result from preservation of a thin layer of elastic tissue in the immediate vicinity of the follicles. This causes the hair follicles to appear retracted while the perifollicular skin protrudes.[65]

Histogenesis. Electron microscopic examination reveals fragments of normal-appearing elastic fibers within macrophages.[67]

MACULAR ATROPHY (ANETODERMA)

Macular atrophy, or anetoderma, is characterized by atrophic patches located mainly on the upper trunk. The skin of the patches is thin and blue-white and bulges slightly. The lesions may give the palpating finger the same sensation as a hernial orifice. Two types of macular atrophy are generally distinguished: the Jadassohn type, in which the atrophic lesions initially appear red and, on histologic examination, show an inflammatory infiltrate; and the Schweninger-Buzzi type, which clinically is noninflammatory from the beginning. However, not every case can be clearly assigned to one or the other of these two types; many clinically noninflammatory cases show an inflammatory infiltrate when examined histologically.[68] The justification for distinguishing between the inflammatory and noninflammatory types has therefore been questioned.[69] In many patients, new lesions continue to appear over a period of several years.

It appears dubious that a secondary form of macular atrophy occurs in the courses of various diseases, such as syphilis, lupus erythematosus, and leprosy.[70] The macular atrophy then represents the atrophic stage of the preceding disease.[71] One instance of macular atrophy has been observed after prolonged treatment with penicillamine.[72]

Histopathology. Early, erythematous lesions usually show a moderately pronounced perivascular infiltrate of mononuclear cells.[73] In a few instances, however, the early inflammatory lesions show a perivascular infiltrate in which neutrophils and eosinophils predominate and nuclear dust is present, resulting in a histologic picture of leukocytoclastic vasculitis.[74,75]

The elastic tissue may still appear normal in the early stage of an erythematous lesion.[76] Usually, however, it is already decreased or even absent within the lesion. In cases in which there is a decrease in the amount of elastic tissue, mononuclear cells may be seen adhering to elastic fibers.[73]

Longstanding, noninflammatory lesions generally show a more or less complete loss of elastic tissue, either in the papillary and upper reticular dermis or in the upper reticular dermis only. A perivascular and periadnexal round-cell infiltrate of varying intensity is invariably present, so that a distinction of an inflammatory and a noninflammatory type is not justified. In some instances, the involved areas show small, normal elastic fibers, which are probably the result of resynthesis, or abnormal, irregular, granular, twisted, fine fibers.[68]

Histogenesis. Electron microscopic examination of lesions reveals a few thin, irregular elastic fibers, with more or less complete loss of the amorphous substance elastin but with relative conservation of the microfibrils. Macrophages, lymphocytes, and some plasma cells are observed. It appears possible that partial destruction by elastases originating in the macrophages occurs, because it is known that the elastases preferentially destroy the amorphous substance of the elastic fibers.[77]

ACRO-OSTEOLYSIS

The term *acro-osteolysis* refers to lytic changes on the distal phalanges. Three types are recognized: familial; idiopathic, nonfamilial; and occupational, which is associated with exposure to vinyl chloride gas.

The *familial type* affects mainly the phalanges of the feet and is associated with recurrent ulcers on the soles.[78]

The *idiopathic type* affects the hands more severely than the feet. Involvement of the distal phalanges of the fingers causes shortening of the fingers. This variant may be associated with Raynaud's phenomenon. Only one case has been described, with cutaneous lesions consisting of numerous yellow papules 2 to 4 mm in diameter and showing a linear distribution and coalescence into plaques, mainly on the arms.[78]

Occupational acro-osteolysis, like the idiopathic type, causes shortening of the fingers due to osteolysis. This variant is often associated with Raynaud's phenomenon and progressive thickening of the skin of the hands and forearms simulating scleroderma. There may be erythema of the hands, and the thickening may consist of papules and plaques.[79] The skin of the face may show diffuse induration.[80] In addition, there may be thrombocytopenia, portal fibrosis, and impaired hepatic and pulmonary function.[81]

Histopathology. The histologic changes in the papules and plaques of idiopathic and occupational acro-osteolysis consist of thickening of the dermis, with swelling and homogenization of the collagen bundles, indistinguishable from scleroderma. Staining for elastic tissue shows disorganization of the elastic fibers, which appear thin and fragmented.[78–80]

Histogenesis. Vinyl chloride disease is an immune-complex disorder associated with hyperimmunoglobulinemia, cryoglobulinemia, and evidence of in vivo activation of complement.[81] The immunologic nature of the disease explains why it is developed by fewer than 3% of the workers exposed to vinyl chloride gas.[79]

REFERENCES

1. Eastern JS, Martin S. Actinic comedonal plaque. J Am Acad Dermatol 1980;3:633.
2. Raimer SS, Sanchez RL, Hubler WR et al. Solar elastic bands of the forearm: An unusual chronic presentation of actinic elastosis. J Am Acad Dermatol 1986;15:650.
3. Frances C, Robert L. Elastin and elastic fibers in normal and pathologic skin. Int J Dermatol 1984;23:166.
4. Kligman AM. Early destructive effect of sunlight on human skin. JAMA 1969;210:2377.
5. Mitchell RE. Chronic solar dermatosis: A light and electron microscopic study of the dermis. J Invest Dermatol 1967;48:203.
6. Nürnberger F, Schober E, Marsch WC et al. Actinic elastosis in black skin. Arch Dermatol Res 1978;262:7.
7. Marsch WC, Schober E, Nürnberger F. Zur ultrastruktur und morphogenese der elastischen faser und der aktinischen elastose. Z Hautkr 1979;54:43.
8. Matsuta M, Izaki S, Ide C et al. Light and electron microscopic immunohistochemistry of solar elastosis. J Dermatol 1987;14:364.
9. Braun-Falco O. Die morphogenese der senil-aktinischen elastose. Arch Klin Exp Dermatol 1969;235:138.
10. Ebner H. Über die entstehung des elastotischen materials. Z Hautkr 1969;44:889.
11. Smith JG Jr, Davidson E, Sams WM Jr et al. Alterations in human dermal connective tissue with age and chronic sun damage. J Invest Dermatol 1962;39:347.
12. Niebauer G, Stockinger L. Über die senile elastose. Arch Klin Exp Dermatol 1965;221:122.
13. Findley GH. On elastase and the elastic dystrophies of the skin. Br J Dermatol 1954;66:16.
14. Sams WM Jr, Smith JG Jr. The histochemistry of chronically sun-damaged skin. J Invest Dermatol 1961;37:447.
15. Olsen RL, Nordquist J, Everett MA. The role of epidermal lysosomes in melanin physiology. Br J Dermatol 1970;83:189.
16. Favre M, Racouchot J. L'élastéidose cutanée nodulaire à kystes et à comédons. Ann Dermatol Syphiligr 1951;78:681.
17. Helm F. Nodular cutaneous elastosis with cysts and comedones: Favre-Racouchot syndrome. Arch Dermatol 1961;84:666.
18. Hassounah A, Piérard EG. Keratosis and comedos without prominent elastosis in Favre-Racouchot disease. Am J Dermatopathol 1987;9:15.
19. Fanta D, Niebauer G. Aktinische (senile) komedonen. Z Hautkr 1976; 51:791.
20. Sehgal VN, Jain S, Thappa DM et al. Perforating dermatoses: A review and report of four cases. J Dermatol 1993; 20:329.
21. Kyrle J. Hyperkeratosis follicularis et parafollicularis in cutem penetrans. Arch Dermatol Syphilol 1916;123:466.
22. Carter VH, Constantine VS. Kyrle's disease: I. Clinical findings in five cases and review of literature. Arch Dermatol 1968;97:624.
23. Constantine VS, Carter VH. Kyrle's disease: II. Histopathologic findings in five cases and review of the literature. Arch Dermatol 1968;97: 633.

24. Tappeiner J, Wolff K, Schreiner E. Morbus kyrle. Hautarzt 1969;20: 296.
25. Bardach H. Dermatosen mit transepithelialer perforation. Arch Dermatol Res 1976;257:213.
26. Mehregan AH, Coskey RJ. Perforating folliculitis. Arch Dermatol 1968;97:394.
27. Mehregan AH. Elastosis perforans serpiginosa: A review of the literature and report of 11 cases. Arch Dermatol 1968;97:381.
28. Neilson, Christensen, Hentzer et al.
29. Weiner AL. Reactive perforating collagenosis. Arch Dermatol 1970; 102:540.
30. Kanan MW. Familial reactive perforating collagenosis and intolerance to cold. Br J Dermatol 1974;91:405.
31. Poliak SC, Lebwohl MG, Parris A et al. Reactive perforating collagenosis associated with diabetes mellitus. N Engl J Med 1982;306:81.
32. Cochran RJ, Tucker SB, Wilkin JK. Reactive perforating collagenosis of diabetes mellitus and renal failure. Cutis 1983;31:55.
33. Beck HI, Brandrup F, Hagdrup HK et al. Adult, acquired reactive perforating collagenosis. J Cutan Pathol 1988;15:124.
34. Fretzin DF, Beal DW, Jao W. Light and ultrastructural study of reactive perforating collagenosis. Arch Dermatol 1980;116:1054.
35. Garcia-Bravo B, Rodriguez-Pichardo A, Camacho F. Uraemic follicular hyperkeratosis. Clin Exp Dermatol 1985;10:448.
36. Hurwitz RM, Weiss J, Melton ME et al. Perforating folliculitis in association with hemodialysis. Am J Dermatopathol 1982;4:101.
37. White CR Jr, Heskel NS, Pokorny DJ. Perforating folliculitis of hemodialysis. Am J Dermatopathol 1982;4:109.
38. Noble JP, Guillemette J, Eisenmann D et al. Hyperkératose à type de bouchons kératosiques au cours de l'insuffisance rénale chronique et des maladies métaboliques. Ann Dermatol Venereol 1982;109:471.
39. Stone RA. Kyrle-like lesions in two patients with renal failure undergoing dialysis. J Am Acad Dermatol 1981;5:707.
40. Hood AF, Hardegen GL, Zarate AR et al. Kyrle's disease in patients with chronic renal failure. Arch Dermatol 1982;118:85.
41. Pruzan D, Rabbin PE, Heilman ER. Periumbilical perforating pseudoxanthoma elasticum. J Am Acad Derm 1992;26:642.
42. Hicks J, Carpenter CL Jr, Reed PJ. Periumbilical perforating pseudoxanthoma elasticum. Arch Dermatol 1979;115:300.
43. Lund HZ, Gilbert CF. Perforating pseudoxanthoma elasticum. Arch Pathol 1976;100:544.
44. Schwartz RA, Richfield DF. Pseudoxanthoma elasticum with transepidermal elimination. Arch Dermatol 1978;114:279.
45. Nickoloff BJ, Noodleman R, Abel EA. Perforating pseudoxanthoma elasticum associated with chronic renal failure and hemodialysis. Arch Dermatol 1985;121:1321.
46. Flegel H. Hyperkeratosis lenticularis perstans. Hautarzt 1958;9:362.
47. Van de Staak WJBM, Bergers AMG, Bougaarts P. Hyperkeratosis lenticularis perstans: Flegel. Dermatologica 1980;161:340.
48. Bean SF. The genetics of hyperkeratosis lenticularis perstans. Arch Dermatol 1972;106:72.
49. Beveridge GW, Langlands AO. Familial hyperkeratosis lenticularis perstans associated with tumours of the skin. Br J Dermatol 1973;88: 453.
50. Frenk E, Tapernoux B. Hyperkeratosis lenticularis perstans: Flegel. Dermatologica 1976;153:253.
51. Bean SF. Hyperkeratosis lenticularis perstans. Arch Dermatol 1969;99: 705.
52. Price ML, Wilson Jones E, MacDonald DM. A clinicopathological study of Flegel's disease: Hyperkeratosis lenticularis perstans. Br J Dermatol 1987;116:681.
53. Raffle EJ, Rogers J. Hyperkeratosis lenticularis perstans. Arch Dermatol 1969;100:423.
54. Krinitz K, Schafer I. Hyperkeratosis lenticularis perstans. Dermatol Monatsschr 1971;157:438.
55. Squier CA, Eady RAJ, Hopps RM. The permeability of epidermis lacking normal membrane-coating granules: An ultrastructural tracer study of Kyrle-Flegel disease. J Invest Dermatol 1978;70:361.
56. Tezuka T. Dyskeratotic process of hyperkeratosis lenticularis perstans: Flegel. Dermatologica 1982;164:379.
57. Kanitakis J, Hermier C, Hokayem D et al. Hyperkeratosis lenticularis: Flegel's disease. Dermatologica 1987;174:96.
58. Tsuji T, Sawabe M. Elastic fibers in striae distensae. J Cutan Pathol 1988;15:215.
59. Zheng P, Lavker RM, Kligman AM. Anatomy of striae. Br J Dermatol 1985;112:185.
60. Epstein NW, Epstein WL, Epstein JH. Atrophic striae in patients with inguinal intertrigo. Arch Dermatol 1963;87:450.
61. Simkin B, Arce R. Steroid excretion in obese patients with colored abdominal striae. N Engl J Med 1962;266:1031.
62. Sisson WR. Colored striae in adolescent children. J Pediatr 1954;45:520.
63. Klehr N. Striae cutis atrophicae: Morphokinetic examinations in vitro. Acta Derm Venereol Suppl (Stockh) 1979;85:105.
64. Shelley WB, Wood MC. Wrinkles due to idiopathic loss of middermal elastic tissue. Br J Dermatol 1977;97:441.
65. Brenner W, Gschnait F, Konrad K et al. Non-inflammatory dermal elastolysis. Br J Dermatol 1979;99:335.
66. Delacrétaz J, Perroud H, Vulliemin JF. Cutis laxa acquise. Dermatologica 1977;155:233.
67. Heudes AM, Boullie MC, Thomine E et al. Élastolyse acquise en nappe du derme moyen. Ann Dermatol Venereol 1988;115:1041.
68. Venencie PY, Winkelmann RK. Histopathologic findings in anetoderma. Arch Dermatol 1984a; 120:1040.
69. Venencie PY, Winkelmann RK, Moore BA. Anetoderma: Clinical findings, association, and long-term follow-up evaluation. Arch Dermatol 1984;120:1032.
70. Deluzenne R. Les anétodermies maculeuses. Ann Dermatol Syphililigr (Paris) 1956;83:618.
71. Edelson Y, Grupper C. Anétodermie maculeuse et lupus érythémateux. Bull Soc Fr Dermatol Syphiligr 1970;77:753.
72. Davis W. Wilson's disease and penicillamine-induced anetoderma. Arch Dermatol 1977;113:976.
73. Kossard S, Kronman KR, Dicken CH et al. Inflammatory macular atrophy: Immunofluorescent and ultrastructural findings. J Am Acad Dermatol 1979;1:325.
74. Cramer HJ. Zur Histopathogenese der dermatitis atrophicans maculosa. Dermatol Wochenschr 1963;147:230.
75. Hellwich M, Nickolay-Kiesthardt J. Kasuistischer beitrag zur anetodermia jadassohn. Z Hautkr 1986;61:1638.
76. Miller WM, Ruggles CW, Rist TE. Anetoderma. Int J Dermatol 1979; 18:43.
77. Venencie PY, Winkelmann RK. Ultrastructural findings in the skin lesions of patients with anetoderma (abstr). Arch Dermatol 1984b;120: 1084.
78. Meyerson LB, Meier GC. Cutaneous lesions in acroosteolysis. Arch Dermatol 1972;106:224.
79. Markowitz SS, McDonald CJ, Fethiere W et al. Occupational acroosteolysis. Arch Dermatol 1972;106:219.
80. Veltmann, G, Lange CE, Stein G. Die Vinyl krankheit Mautarzt 1978;29:177.
81. Fine RM. Acro-osteolysis: Vinyl chloride induced "scleroderma." Int J Dermatol 1976;15:676.

Lever's Histopathology of the Skin, eighth edition,
edited by David Elder et al. Lippincott–
Raven Publishers, Philadelphia © 1997.

CHAPTER 16

Cutaneous Manifestations of Nutritional Deficiency States and Gastrointestinal Disease

Cynthia Magro, A. Neil Crowson, and Martin Mihm Jr.

DEFICIENCIES OF VITAMINS, OTHER AMINO ACIDS, AND MINERALS

Scurvy

The manifestations of scurvy, due to vitamin C (ascorbic acid) deficiency, have been known for 3000 years. In 1753, Sir James Lynd demonstrated the efficacy of citrus fruits in the prevention of this condition,[1] which is characterized by follicular purpuric macules with or without follicular hyperkeratosis and cork screw hairs, ecchymoses, particularly in the pretibial areas, and conjunctival and gingival hemorrhages, the latter associated with gingival hyperplasia (Color Fig. 16-1).[2] Subcutaneous hemorrhage with woody edema of the lower extremities and hemarthrosis may occur. Nonspecific aches and pains and impaired wound healing are frequent. Anemia, possibly related to decreased amounts of active folate and blood loss, is present in approximately 75% of individuals.[3] For humans, the principal source of vitamin C, a substance which cannot be synthesized from glucose derivatives, is fruits and vegetables. Scurvy occurs in those who avoid these foods; especially predisposed are the elderly, chronic alcoholics, and renal dialysis patients, in whom a diet lacking vitamin C is not infrequent.

Histopathology. Follicular hyperkeratosis and perifollicular erythrocyte extravasation without an accompanying vasculopathy are characteristic. Extensive extravasations are usually associated with deposits of hemosiderin within and outside of macrophages. A coiled hair may emanate from the dilated follicular orifice.[4]

Differential Diagnosis. Other pauci-inflammatory hyperkeratotic dermatoses that should be considered in the differential diagnosis include keratosis pilaris, vitamin A deficiency, pityriasis rubra pilaris, ichthyosis vulgaris, and a resolving lichenoid follicular hyperkeratotic process such as lichen planopilaris, lichen spinulosus, or lupus erythematosus. Coiled or "corkscrew" hairs are not pathognomonic of scurvy and may be seen in certain ectodermal dysplasia syndromes.

Pathogenesis. Most manifestations of scurvy can be attributed to defective collagen synthesis. Lysine and proline hydroxylase enzymes require vitamin C to reduce Fe^{+3} during the reaction. In vitamin C deficiency, the end product, hydroxyproline, which stabilizes the collagenous domain of procollagen, is deficient.[2] Ultrastructurally, the dermal fibroblasts appear shrunken and show a decreased amount of rough endoplasmic reticulum.[6] Around these fibroblasts, one observes increased amounts of extracellular filamentous or amorphous material that has failed to polymerize into normal collagen fibrils. The extravasation of red cells is caused by vacuolar degeneration of endothelial cells, junctional separation of adjoining endothelial cells, and detachment of the basement membrane from the endothelium in capillaries and small venules.[6]

Vitamin A Deficiency (Phrynoderma)

Seen mainly in Asia and Africa, vitamin A deficiency is rare in the United States but may occur following intestinal bypass surgery for obesity.[7] Dryness and roughness of the skin along with conical follicular keratotic plugs characterize the cutaneous changes. Night blindness, xerophthalmia, and keratomalacia also occur.

Histopathology. The skin shows moderate hyperkeratosis with distension of the upper part of the follicle by large, horny plugs.[7] Sebaceous glands are greatly reduced in size and may exhibit epithelial atrophy.[8] In severe cases both eccrine and sebaceous glands may exhibit squamous metaplasia.[9]

Differential Diagnosis. Other causes of a pauci-inflammatory interfollicular and follicular hyperkeratotic process include pityriasis rubra pilaris, ichthyosis vulgaris, and resolved lesions of lupus erythematosus and lichen planopilaris. Spotty parakeratosis, hyperplasia of the epidermis, and a superficial dermal infiltrate with basilar vacuolar change are additional histologic

C. Magro: Pathology Services, Inc., Cambridge, MA; Beth Israel Hospital and Harvard Medical School, Boston, MA

A. N. Crowson: Misericordia General Hospital and Central Medical Laboratories, Winnipeg, Manitoba, Canada

M. Mihm Jr.: Chief of Dermatology and Dermatopathology, Albany Medical College, Albany, NY

features that distinguish pityriasis rubra pilaris from phrynoderma. Superficial dermal fibroplasia with melanophage accumulation is the hallmark of resolved lichen planopilaris and lupus erythematosus. Sebaceous gland atrophy has been described in pellagra. Squamous metaplasia of the eccrine apparatus has been seen with methotrexate therapy and graft-versus-host disease.

Acquired Vitamin B_3 Deficiency (Pellagra)

The word "pellagra" is derived from two Italian words, "pelle" meaning "skin" and "agra" meaning "sharp burning" or "rough". Although primarily ascribed to niacin (vitamin B_3) deficiency, other vitamin deficiencies or protein malnutrition[10] appear integral to the development of the pellagra symptom complex. Presenting as cutaneous lesions, gastrointestinal symptoms, and mental changes, pellagra has been given the acronym of the three Ds: dermatitis, diarrhea, and dementia. In the United States, the enrichment of whole wheat flour with niacin has almost eliminated pellagra; however, it is still prevalent in other countries such as Mexico and in some nations in Africa where cornmeal is the main constituent of the diet. Occurrence in the United States is mainly in chronic alcoholics and in patients with anorexia nervosa, malignant gastrointestinal tumors, and intestinal parasitosis.[10] Its appearance in carcinoid syndrome is believed to reflect a depression of endogenous niacin production by tumor cell diversion of tryptophan toward serotonin.[11] Pellagra has also been reported in patients receiving isoniazid, pyrazinamide, hydantoin, ethionamide, phenobarbital, azathioprine, and chloramphenicol. Isoniazid, a structural analogue of niacin, can cause suppression of endogenous niacin production.

Three basic skin eruptions occur in pellagrins.[12] The first is a photo-induced eruption that is intensely erythematous and subsequently exfoliates to yield a hyperpigmented residuum. The second type of eruption is characterized by painful erythematous erosions in genital and perineal areas possibly induced by pressure, heat, and trauma.[10] The increased skin fragility may reflect aberrations in the collagen and elastic fiber content of the skin. Pellagrins may develop a seborrheic dermatitis-like rash involving the face, scalp, and neck. Oral manifestations include beefy, red, cracked lips, and a fissured or smooth, red, sore tongue. Among the neurological symptoms are dementia, psychosis, anxiety, defective memory, burning sensations, sudden attacks of falling, dizziness, and headaches. A cause of sudden death is central pontine myelinolysis.[10]

Histopathology. Psoriasiform epidermal hyperplasia with hyperkeratosis, parakeratosis, and a lymphocytic perivascular inflammatory cell infiltrate characterize initial lesions. Additional features include scattered necrotic keratinocytes, granular cell layer loss, and architectural disarray with dysmaturation (a personal observation). Depigmentation of the basal layer with accumulation of fat droplets is described, as is vacuolation of cells within the granular and spinous layers.[13] Epidermal atrophy, hypermelanosis, vascular ectasia, and sebaceous atrophy characterize end-stage lesions.[13] Seborrheic dermatitis-like lesions may show sebaceous gland hyperplasia with follicular dilatation. Fragmentation, swelling, and thickening of elastic fibers, swelling of collagen fibers, and merging of elastic tissue with collagen have been described. A morphology indistinguishable from necrolytic migratory erythema and acrodermatitis enteropathica has been reported, comprising intracellular edema with vacuolar change of the upper stratum Malpighii and keratinocyte necrosis, sometimes accompanied by neutrophilic infiltration of the degenerating upper stratum Malpighii, subcorneal pustulation localized to or in isolation from these areas, and folliculitis.[10,14]

Pathogenesis. A deficiency in urocanic acid caused by a reduction in histidine and histidase activity has been postulated as a possible mechanism of photosensitivity in pellagra; urocanic acid protects the skin from ultraviolet (UV) wavelengths by absorbing light in the UVB range.[10] Kynurenic acid, a metabolic byproduct of the tryptophan-kynurenine-nicotinic pathway, accumulates in pellagra as a result of a deficiency of nicotinamide which blocks the formation of kynurenic acid. Kynurenic acid induces a phytotoxic reaction in skin subjected to long-way UV radiation ranging from 350 to 380 mm.[10] Some of the gastrointestinal symptoms may relate to degenerative changes of the dorsal vagal nuclei. The neurological symptoms may be due to chromatolysis of various cortical and brain stem nuclei.[10]

Differential Diagnosis. The histopathology is similar to the nutritional dermatoses acrodermatitis enteropathica and necrolytic migratory erythema. In addition, those dermatitides associated with hyperkeratosis, a maturation disarray, and/or scattered degenerating keratinocytes need to be considered as discussed in the differential diagnosis section of necrolytic migratory erythema.

Congenital Vitamin B_3 Deficiency (Hartnup Disease)

Named after the family in which it was first described in 1956, Hartnup disease is a distinctive autosomal recessive syndrome comprising pellagrinous skin[15,16] neurological abnormalities including mental deterioration and cerebellar ataxia, and abnormal aminoaciduria.[17] The intermittent skin eruption is seen primarily in the summer at times of maximal sun exposure and at times resembles either poikiloderma vascular atrophicans[18] or, when vesicles are prominent, hydroa vacciniforme.[19] Hartnup disease, in contrast to pellagra, does not respond to treatment with niacin.[19]

Histopathology. The histopathology usually resembles pellagra. Poikilodermatous lesions manifest flattening of the epidermis and prominent dermal melanophage accumulation.[18]

Pathogenesis. An intestinal and renal tubular defect of tryptophan absorption leads to a deficiency in endogenous niacin, accounting for the pellagra-like symptomatology. Chromatographic studies of urine show persistent aminoaciduria, particularly of tryptophan and of indolic substances derived from tryptophan.[16,18]

OTHER FORMS OF NUTRITIONAL DERMATOSES

Necrolytic Migratory Erythema (Glucagonoma Syndrome)

First described in 1942 in a patient with a pancreatic islet cell carcinoma,[20] this distinctive dermatosis, which precedes all other symptoms of pancreatic carcinoma by several years,[21] is most commonly seen in association with a glucagon-secreting

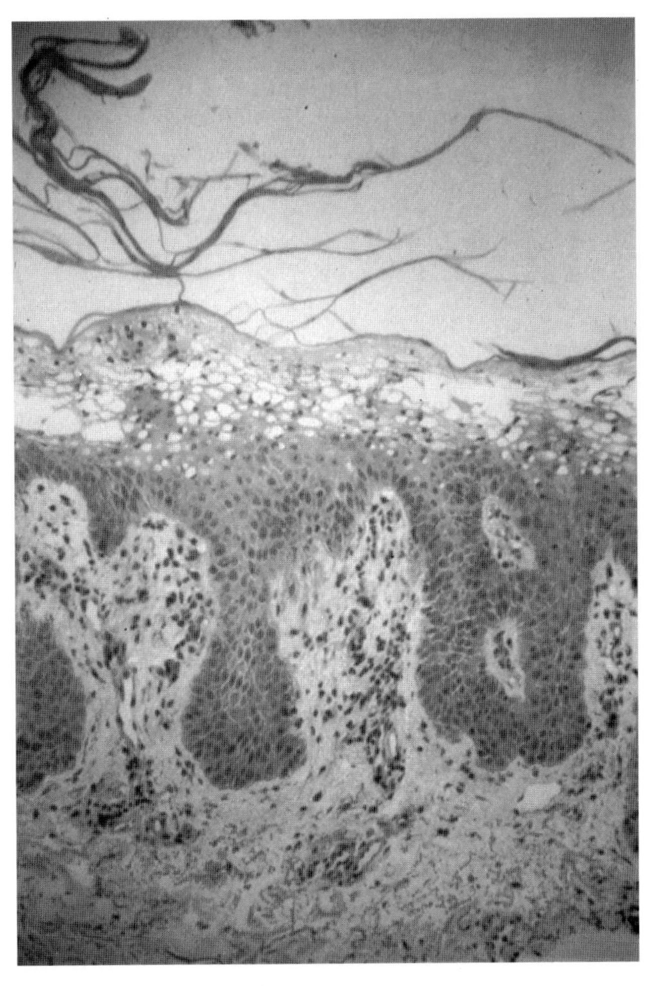

FIG. 16-1. Necrolytic migratory erythema (glucagonoma syndrome)
Subacute lesion showing psoriasiform hyperplasia of the epidermis and striking hydropic change within the superficial half of the stratum malpighii. Scattered dyskeratotic cells are also noted within the hydropic epithelium. There is an overlying loosely adherent parakeratotic scale.

alpha cell tumor of the pancreas. Surgical extirpation of the neoplasm may result in resolution of the eruption.[22]

The manifestations of glucagonoma syndrome include cutaneous and mucosal lesions, weight loss, anemia, adult-onset diabetes, glucose intolerance, and elevation of serum glucagon level. Skin lesions are situated mainly on the face in perioral and perinasal distribution, the perineum, genitals, shins, ankles, and feet and include erythema, erosions, and flaccid vesicular-pustular lesions that rupture easily and often have a circinate appearance due to peripheral spreading. Rapid healing together with the continuous development of new lesions result in daily fluctuations of the eruption. Cheilitis and glossitis also exist.

Histopathology. The characteristic acute lesion shows abrupt necrosis of the upper layers of the stratum spinosum, which may detach from the subjacent viable epidermis. Keratinocyte degeneration varies from marked hydropic swelling to cytoplasmic eosinophilic with nuclear pyknosis (Fig. 16-1). Neutrophilic chemotaxis to the necrotic epithelium may eventuate in a subcorneal pustule. Chronic lesions have as their hallmark a psoriasiform dermatitis. In both acute and chronic lesions there is architectural disarray, reflecting a maturation defect; it manifests as basal layer hyperplasia, vacuolar change, and a deficient granular layer.[14] The epidermis is surmounted by a broad parakeratotic scale (Fig. 16-2). Candida may be noted.[23]

Pathogenesis. Patients with glucagonoma have sustained gluconeogenesis resulting in a negative nitrogen balance, with protein amino acid degradation, even of epidermal proteins.[24] In addition to glucagonoma, necrolytic migratory erythema has been reported with hepatic cirrhosis,[25] a jejunal adenocarcinoma with hepatic dysfunction, and malabsorption with villous atrophy;[26] glucagon levels may be normal. A comparable syndrome in dogs develops in the setting of diabetes mellitus and hepatic cirrhosis.[23] In all of these conditions malabsorption and diarrhea lead to isolated deficiencies of certain essential fatty acids, zinc, and amino acids. The pathophysiology may reflect in part a phospholipid fatty acid abnormality in cells due to defective delta-6-desaturase enzyme, which is known to be inhibited by zinc deficiency and excess alcohol. In patients with un-

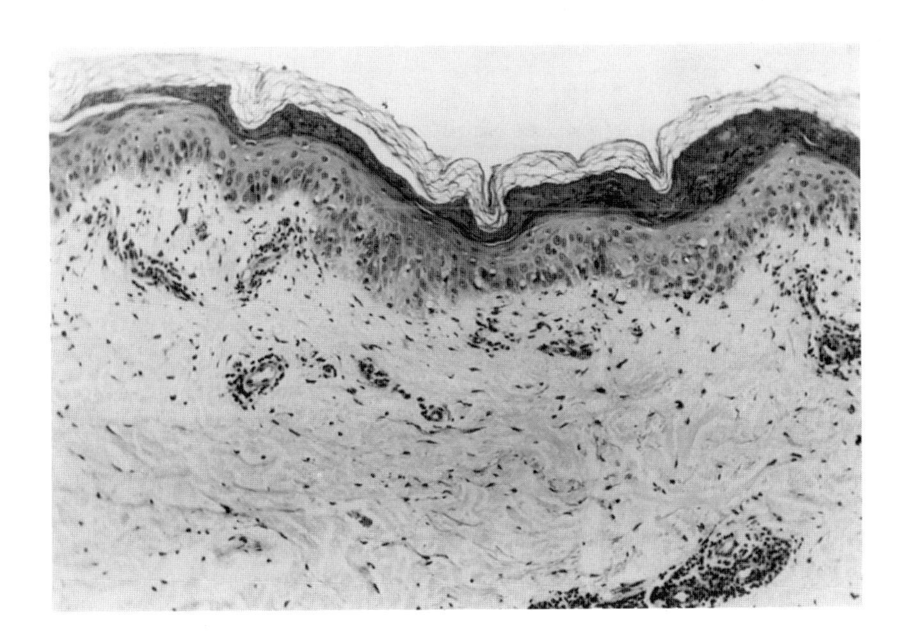

FIG. 16-2. Necrolytic migratory erythema (glucagonoma syndrome)
The lower portion of the stratum malpighii appears viable, whereas the upper portion shows necrolysis or "sudden death." The necrolytic portion manifests cytoplasmic eosinophilic homogenization with pyknotic nuclei.

resectable glucagonoma who manifest necrolytic migratory erythema, infusion of amino acids has resulted in rapid clearing of the cutaneous lesions.[27]

Differential Diagnosis. The histopathology is similar to other nutritional dermatoses, namely acrodermatitis enteropathica and pellagra. Those dermatitides associated with hyperkeratosis, a maturation disarray, and/or scattered degenerating keratinocytes such as graft-versus-host disease, subacute cutaneous lupus erythematosus, dermatomyositis, pityriasis rubra pilaris, and toxic drug eruptions, particularly those that are photo-induced, also should be considered.

Acrodermatitis Enteropathica

Acrodermatitis enteropathica, first described in 1942,[28] is transmitted as an autosomal recessive trait. Caused by defective intestinal absorption of zinc,[29] it usually manifests in the first 4–10 weeks of life in bottle–fed infants as an acral and periorificial cutaneous eruption accompanied by intractable diarrhea and diffuse partial alopecia. Cutaneous lesions manifest as areas of moist erythema, occasionally associated with vesiculobullous and/or pustular lesions.[30] Untreated cases eventuate in death from malnutrition and infection because of immunologic defects caused by zinc deficiency, the latter including decreased natural killer cell activity, impaired delayed-type hypersensitivity, and thymic atrophy.[31] Paronychia, stomatitis, photophobia, blepharitis, conjunctivitis, corneal opacities, and hoarseness are additional manifestations. An acquired form occurs in patients receiving intravenous hyperalimentation with low zinc content,[32] in infants who are fed breast milk low in zinc,[33] in patients with Crohn's disease, and in the setting of AIDS nephropathy when proteinuria eventuates in excessive loss of protein-bound zinc.[31]

Histopathology. The upper part of the epidermis shows pallor due to intracellular edema and is surmounted by a confluent, thick, parakeratotic scale that may contain neutrophils. There is granular cell layer diminution and focal dyskeratosis. As with necrolytic migratory erythema, there may be architectural disarray and maturation delay. Subcorneal vesicles may be present. The epidermis is of variable thickness, manifesting both psoriasiform hyperplasia and atrophy. In a few instances acantholysis is seen.[30,33] Superinfection with Candida may occur (Fig. 16-3).

Pathogenesis. Defective intestinal absorption of zinc has been demonstrated in children with acrodermatitis enteropathica,[34] resulting in plasma zinc levels well below the normal range of 68 to 112 μg/dl. Oral administration of zinc sulfate eventuates in rapid and complete resolution of the disease. Electron microscopy shows evidence of abnormal keratinization with decreased keratohyalin granules and increased numbers of keratinosome-derived lamellae within intercellular spaces. Keratinosomes[35] contain several zinc-dependant enzyme systems, the metabolism of which may be affected.

Differential Diagnosis. Pellagra, necrolytic migratory erythema, and acrodermatitis enteropathica are histologically very similar, sharing a constellation of histologic features that should suggest a diagnosis of nutritional dermatosis. They all have in common confluent parakeratosis, granular layer diminution, epidermal pallor and focal dyskeratosis, psoriasiform hyperplasia, architectural disorder, and maturation delay.[14] Other considerations raised in the differential diagnosis section of necrolytic migratory erythema should also be entertained.

Kwashiorkor

Kwashiorkor is a form of protein malnutrition coupled by carbohydrate excess resulting in reduction of a patient's weight by 20% to 40%. Primary manifestations include generalized hypopigmentation that begins circumorally and in the pretibial

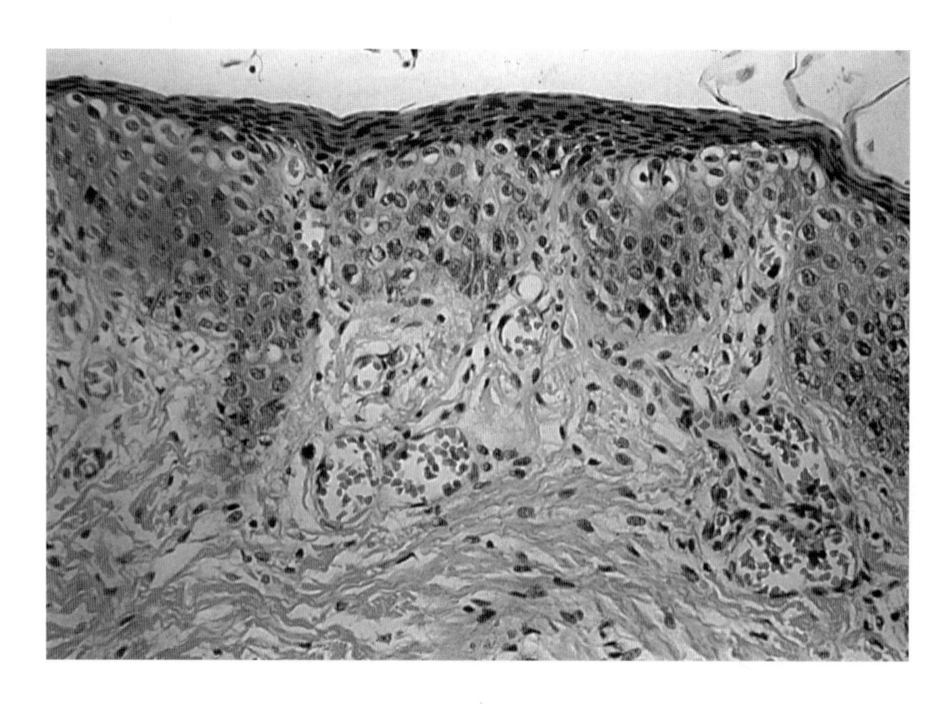

FIG. 16-3. Acrodermatitis enteropathica
The epidermis demonstrates psoriasiform hyperplasia, dysmaturation, granular cell layer diminution, and vacuolar change. The epidermis is surmounted by a compact parakeratotic scale. Vascular ectasia is also present.

regions. With disease progression, hyperpigmented plaques with a waxy texture develop over the elbows, ankles, and in the intertriginous areas. Dryness, desquamation, and decreased skin elasticity occur. "Crazy pavement" or "flaky-paint dermatosis" describes the extensive desquamation with erosions and fissuring that may be seen in severe cases.[36] Hair abnormalities include a diffuse alopecia, alternating bands of normal and hypopigmented hair referred to as the "flag" sign, and an unusual reddish brown discoloration called hypochromotrichia.[36] Extracutaneous manifestations include cerebral atrophy secondary to loss of myelin lipid,[37] diarrhea, hepatic steatosis, and mucosal abnormalities such as a smooth tongue, angular stomatitis, and perianal and nasal erosions.

Histopathology. The histologic picture of skin lesions is not diagnostic but is said to resemble pellagra.[38] The changes include psoriasiform hyperplasia with hyperkeratosis and increased pigmentation throughout the epidermis or atrophy with irregular shortening and flattening of the rete.[38]

Pathogenesis. The etiology of the edema includes reduced capillary blood flow, hypoalbuminemia, and increased peripheral vasoconstriction.[39]

CUTANEOUS MANIFESTATIONS OF GASTROINTESTINAL DISEASE

Pyoderma Gangrenosum

First described in 1930,[40] pyoderma gangrenosum was once considered pathognomonic of idiopathic ulcerative colitis, but has since been described in association with a wide variety of disorders including roughly 5% of patients with Crohn's disease. Beginning as folliculocentric pustules or fluctuant nodules, the lesions ulcerate and have sharply circumscribed violaceous, raised edges in which necrotic pustules may be seen. The disease most commonly occurs in adults who are 30 to 50 years old, on the lower extremities and trunk. Occasionally it occurs in childhood, affecting the buttocks, perineal region, and head and neck area.[41] Koebnerization occurs at sites of trauma including intravenous puncture sites, surgical wounds, and peristomal sites.[42] Roughly 70% of cases are associated with four main categories of systemic diseases.[43] In addition to inflammatory bowel disease, pyoderma gangrenosum has been associated with hematological disorders including acute lymphoid and myeloid leukemias and myeloma, rheumatological conditions including rheumatoid arthritis and lupus erythematosus, and hepatopathies[44] namely chronic active hepatitis, primary biliary cirrhosis, and sclerosing cholangitis.[45] Both a superficial granulomatous variant[46] and a vesiculopustular variant, comprising disseminated vesicles and necrotizing pustules, some follicular-based, have been observed without accompanying systemic disease. The vesiculopustular variant has also been used in association with ulcerative colitis and in association with underlying liver disease.[45,47]

Histopathology. Pyoderma gangrenosum has a dichotomous tissue reaction, showing central necrotizing suppurative inflammation usually with ulceration, and, peripherally, a lymphocytic vascular reaction comprising perivascular and intramural lymphocytic infiltrates, usually without fibrin deposition or mural necrosis (Fig. 16-4). Transitional areas show neutrophils in a loose cuff around the angiocentric lymphocytic infiltrates, defining a mixed lymphocytic and neutrophilic vascular reaction compatible with a Sweet's-like vascular reaction. Bullous lesions may also demonstrate a Sweet's-like vascular reaction with perivascular disintegrating neutrophilic infiltrates hemorrhage and without accompanying mural necrosis or luminal fibrin deposition. There is marked edema and a more superficially disposed pattern of dermal neutrophilia pathergy.[49,50] Although a neutrophil-predominant leukocytoclastic vasculitis may be observed in areas of maximal tissue pathology, pyoderma gangrenosum does not reflect a primary vasculitis. In some cases a necrotizing pustular follicular reaction may be the central nidus of the lesion, particularly in the vesicular pustular

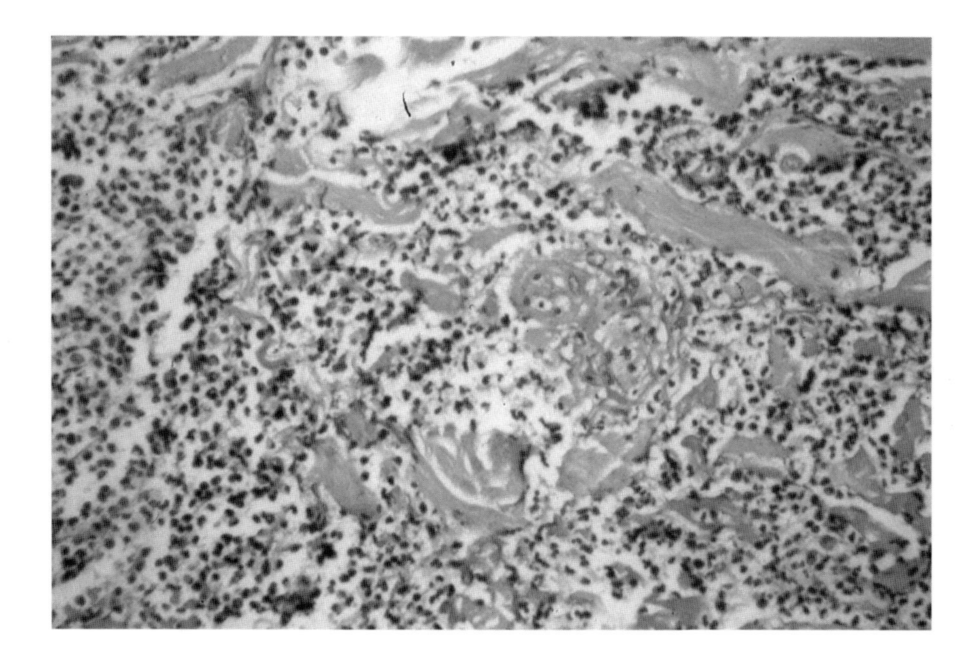

FIG. 16-4. Pyoderma gangrenosum
The center of the lesion shows a neutrophilic infiltrate with leukocytoclasia and dermolysis.

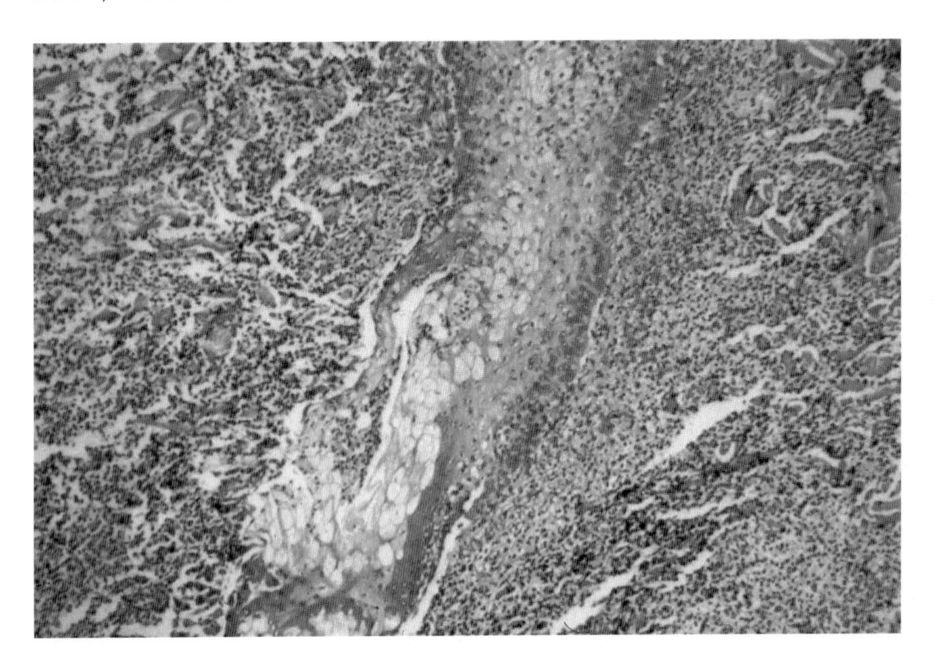

FIG. 16-5. Pyoderma gangrenosum The central nidus of tissue pathergy may be a necrotizing pustular follicular reaction.

variant associated with ulcerative colitis or hepatobiliary disease (Fig. 16-5). In the superficial granulomatous variant, florid pseudoepitheliomatous hyperplasia along with the intraepithelial and superficial dermal suppurative granulomatous inflammation with admixed plasma cells and eosinophils may be observed.[46] Cases of pyoderma gangrenosum associated with Crohn's disease may have areas of granulomatous inflammation.

Differential Diagnosis. An incipient lesion of pyoderma gangrenosum may be indistinguishable from Sweet's syndrome; the latter is rarely folliculocentric and does not show lysis of dermal collagen or vessel wall necrosis in areas of maximum dermal neutrophilic infiltration. In addition, clinical features usually make the distinction possible. Because of prominent follicular involvement, the differential diagnosis should also include other causes of necrotizing pustular follicular reactions with an accompanying vasculopathy such as mixed cryoglobulinemia, Behçet's disease, rheumatoid vasculitis, herpetic folliculitis, acute pustular bacterid, and pustular drug reactions.[51] These other conditions frequently have a necrotizing mononuclear cell or neutrophil predominant vasculitis in contrast to the non-necrotizing vascular reaction of pyoderma gangrenosum. Other causes of a Sweet's-like vascular reaction should be considered, such as the bowel arthritis dermatosis syndrome, Behçet's disease, idiopathic pustular vasculitis, rheumatoid arthritis, acute pustular bacterid, and Sweet's syndrome.[48]

Pathogenesis. Direct immunofluorescence testing supports a vasculopathy by virtue of perivascular deposition of immunoreactants, mainly IgM and C3,[52] in more than half of patients. This change occurs in nonspecific vessel injury and does not support a humoral-based pathogenesis. Defective cell immunity without humoral abnormalities has been implicated in some patients.[53] Immunoelectrophoresis has revealed monoclonal gammopathy, most commonly of the IgA type, in 10% of patients with pyoderma gangrenosum.[54] The good response of systemic corticosteroid administration suggests an immunogenic cause.[53]

Bowel-Associated Dermatosis–Arthritic Syndrome (Bowel Bypass Syndrome)

An intermittent eruption, mainly on the extremities, may appear after intestinal bypass surgery for morbid obesity and following extensive small bowel resection. Purpuric macules and papules that may evolve into necrotizing vesiculo-pustular lesions are characteristic. Polyarthritis, malaise, and fever are often associated with and may precede the eruption.[55] Although originally called the bowel bypass syndrome, it now bears the more appropriate appellation, bowel arthritis dermatosis syndrome, as a similar picture may develop in patients with diverticulosis, peptic ulcer disease, and idiopathic inflammatory bowel disease.[56,57,58,59]

Histopathology. Characteristically, there is a perivascular lymphocytic infiltrate with a peripheral cuff of disintegrating neutrophils, erythrocyte extravasation, and absent or minimal fibrin deposition consistent with a Sweet's-like vascular reaction; a leukocytoclastic vasculitis occurs less often.[59] Papillary dermal edema may be striking and may lead to subepidermal vesiculation.[55] Epidermal pustulation, variable epithelial necrosis, and massive superficial dermal neutrophilia complete the picture (Fig. 16-6) and define pustular vasculitis.[55]

Pathogenesis. Circulating immune complexes, including those containing cryoproteins, are demonstrable in most patients. The antigenic trigger may be peptidoglycans from intestinal bacteria,[56] which are structurally and antigenically similar to the peptidoglycan of *Streptococcus*. The latter exacerbate symptoms in patients with this condition and also produce a similar syndrome in animals.[56] Direct immunofluorescence testing has shown linear and granular deposits of immunoglobulins and complement along the dermal-epidermal junction and within vessels.[56] One study showed *Escherichia coli* antigens in a granular array along the dermal-epidermal junction. Via an indirect methodology, a pemphigus-like pattern of intercellular staining has been reported,[56] the significance of which is unclear.

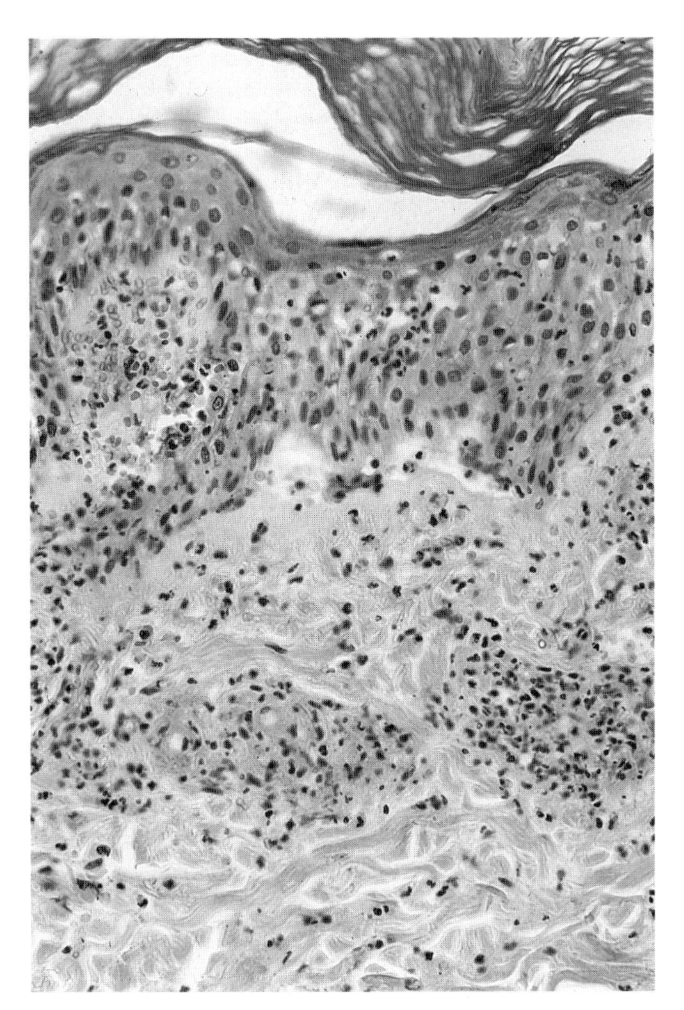

FIG. 16-6. Bowel arthritis dermatosis syndrome
Pustular vasculitis characterized by dermal papillae microabscess formation along with a leukocytoclastic vasculitis involving dermal papillae capillaries.

Differential Diagnosis. The differential diagnosis of bowel arthritis dermatosis syndrome includes Sweet's syndrome, incipient pyoderma gangrenosum, and certain of the pustular vasculitides such as acute pustular bacterid related to antecedent streptococcal infection, septic vasculitis due to *Meningococcus* and *Gonococcus*, Behçet's syndrome, leukocytoclastic vasculitis in patients with a pustular psoriasiform diatheses,[60] idiopathic pustular vasculitis, and acute generalized exanthemous pustulosis.[60] The distinction may be impossible in those conditions that manifest a Sweet's-like vascular reaction—namely, Behçet's disease, Sweet's syndrome, pyoderma gangrenosum, acute pustular bacterid, and idiopathic pustular vasculitis.

SPECIFIC DISEASES

Aphthosis (Behçet's Disease)

Behçet's disease is a symptom complex of oral and genital ulceration and iritis that has a world-wide distribution but is most common in the Pacific rim and eastern Mediterranean.[61,62] The presence of oral ulceration plus any two signs of genital ulceration, skin lesions (e.g., pustules or nodules), or eye lesions (e.g., uveitis or retinal vasculitis) is held to be diagnostic.

The cutaneous lesions include erythema nodosum–like nodules, vesicles, pustules, pyoderma gangrenosum, Sweet's syndrome, a pustular reaction to needle trauma, superficial migratory thrombophlebitis, ulceration, infiltrative erythema, acral purpuric papulonodular lesions, and acneiform folliculitis.[63,64]

The extracutaneous manifestations are categorized as oral and/or genital aphthae, vasculo-, ocular-, entero- or neuro-Behçet's disease, renal disease, and arthritis. Oral apthosis recurring at least three times over a 12-month period is essential to the diagnosis.[62] In vasculo-Behçet's disease, aneurysms and occlusive venous and arterial main vessel lesions occur. The ocular manifestations include uveitis, hypopyon iritis, optic neuritis, and choroiditis. Entero-Behçet's disease manifests as diarrhea, constipation, abdominal pain, vomiting, and melena. Neuro-Behçet's disease presents as brain stem dysfunction, meningoencephalitis, organic psychiatric symptoms, and mononeuritis multiplex.[63] Asymptomatic microhematuria and/or proteinuria are among the renal manifestations. An oligoarthritis may involve the wrist, elbow, knee, or ankle joints.

Histopathology. The cutaneous lesions can be categorized histopathologically into three main groups: vascular, extravascular with or without vasculopathy, and acneiform.

The pathologic spectrum of the cutaneous vasculopathy encompasses a mononuclear cell vasculitis with variable mural and luminal fibrin deposition; a paucicellular thrombogenic vasculopathy (Fig. 16-7); and a neutrophilic vascular reaction involving capillaries and veins of all calibers. The mononuclear cell reaction may be frankly granulomatous or it may be lymphocytic predominant to define a lymphocytic vasculitis. The neutrophilic vascular reaction may resemble that of Sweet's syndrome (Fig. 16-8)[65] or a leukocytoclastic vasculitis. Diffuse extravascular mononuclear cell– and/or neutrophil–predominant inflammation of the dermis and/or panniculus may occur with or without the aforementioned vascular changes. The histiocytes infiltrating the panniculus may manifest phagocytosis of cellular debris. Suppurative or mixed suppurative and granulomatous folliculitis with or without vasculitis characterizes the acneiform lesions. Acral purpuric papulonodular lesions show a lymphocytic interface dermatitis with lymphocytic exocytosis, dyskeratosis, and a perivascular lymphocytic infiltrate, recapitulating the mucosal histopathology.[64]

Extracutaneous lesions histopathologically mirror the skin changes. Oral aphthous ulcers demonstrate a central diffuse neutrophilic infiltrate with necrosis of the epithelium and connective tissue pathergy of the corium, and peripherally, a border showing dense lymphocytic infiltration of the corium associated with lymphocytic exocytosis and degenerative epithelial changes. In our experience, genital aphthae have the same appearance (Fig. 16-9).[63] The large vessel arteriopathy represents an ischemic sequelum of a mononuclear cell vasculitis of the vasa vasorum, while venous thrombosis may be due in part to an underlying hypercoagulable state as discussed later. A lymphocytic vascular reaction with or without mural and intraluminal fibrin deposition is the histopathology of neuro-, entero-, ocular-, and arthritic Behçet's disease, with other organ changes such as demyelination and intestinal ulceration reflecting resultant ische-

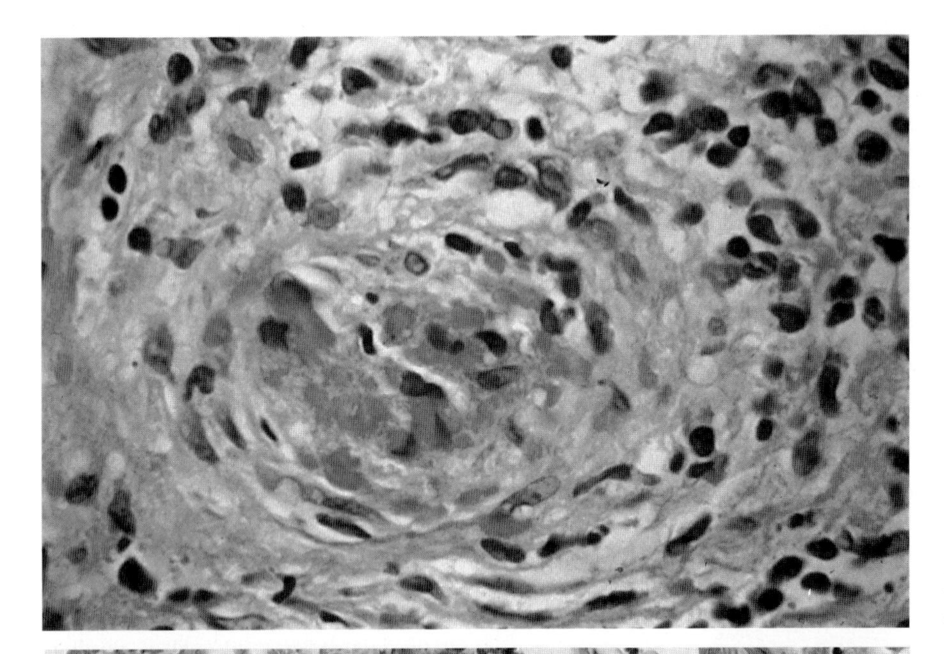

FIG. 16-7. Behçet's disease
Another characteristic vascular reaction pattern is a pauci-inflammatory thrombogenic vasculopathy.

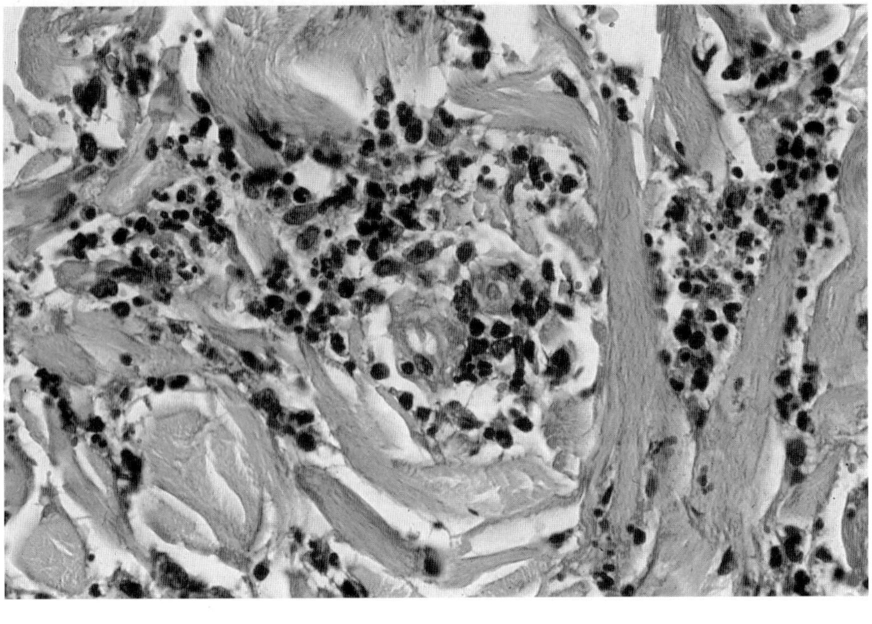

FIG. 16-8. Behçet's disease
There is a Sweet's-like vascular reaction manifested by angiocentric mononuclear cell and neutrophilic infiltrates with erythrocyte extravasation and leukocytoclasia but without accompanying mural and intraluminal fibrin deposition.

mia.[64] The renal histopathology includes IgA nephropathy, focal and diffuse proliferative glomerulonephritis, and amyloidosis.[67]

Differential Diagnosis. The lymphocytic vasculitis observed in Behçet's disease may mimic that seen in association with systemic lupus erythematosus, rheumatoid arthritis,[68] Sjögren's syndrome, relapsing polychondritis, Degos' disease, and paraneoplastic vasculitis in the setting of lymphoproliferative disease. Granulomatous vasculitis may also be observed in Wegener's granulomatosis, allergic granulomatosis of Churg-Strauss, Crohn's disease, sarcoidosis, acquired hypogammaglobulinemia, a post-herpetic eruption,[69] paraneoplastic syndrome (related to underlying hematological malignancy), rheumatoid arthritis, hypersensitivity reactions to certain infections including syphilis and tuberculosis,[70] scleroderma, and late-stage lesions of microscopic polyarteritis nodosa. Other causes of a Sweet's-like vasculopathy include Sweet's syndrome, bowel arthritis dermatosis, pyoderma gangrenosum, and idiopathic pustular vasculitis.[48] Conditions that combine a vasculitis with a folliculitis include pyoderma gangrenosum, mixed cryoglobulinemia, rheumatoid vasculitis, and bacterid.[51]

Pathogenesis. An immunogenetic basis is likely in view of the association with certain HLA types, namely HLA-B5, HLA-B12, HLA-B27, and HLA-B51.[71] Patients have shown a heightened immune response to antigenic components of certain streptococcal species[72,73] and *Mycobacterium tuberculosis.*[74] Other implicated organisms include herpes simplex,[75] Epstein-

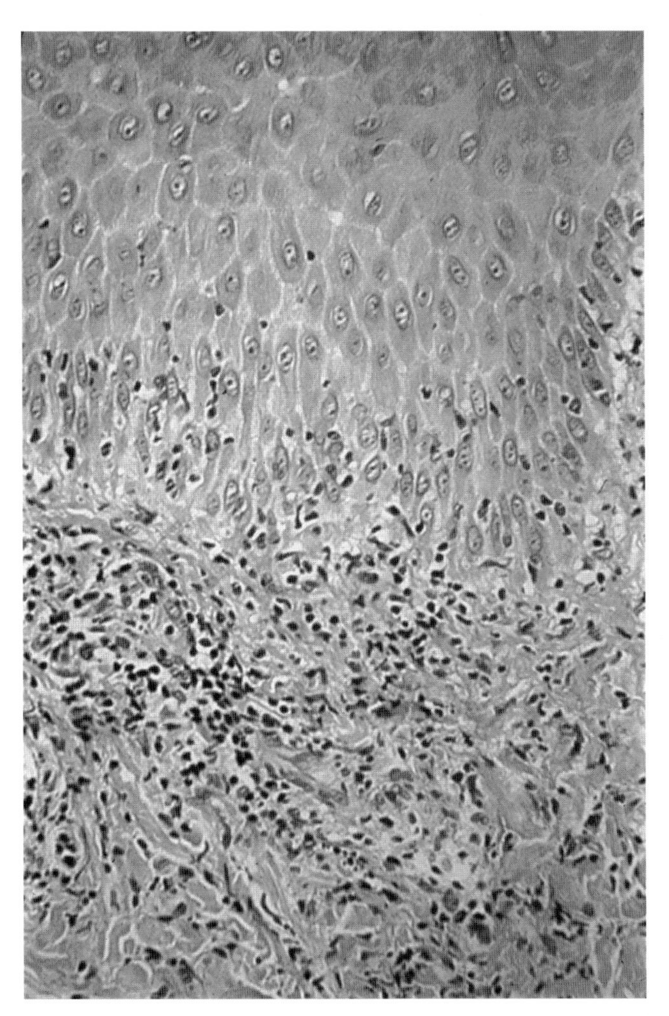

FIG. 16-9. Behçet's disease
Although the center of an oral or vulvar aphthous ulcer is predominated by a neutrophilic response, biopsies of the periphery typically show a lymphocyte predominate infiltrate both in an extravascular and angiocentric disposition with variable lymphocytic exocytosis.

Barr virus,[76] and human immunodeficiency virus (HIV).[77] Underlying abnormalities in T-lymphocyte function may be integral to this aberrant response related to the synthesis by microorganisms and mammalian tissue of a family of polypeptides termed heat shock proteins (HSP).[78,79] These proteins are produced by cells exposed to stresses such as increased temperature. Sensitized T cells and T-cell clones specific to the 65-kD mycobacterial HSP have been reported in rheumatoid arthritis.[80] T lymphocytes from patients with Behçet's disease in one study exhibit a greater stimulation by this HSP compared to normal controls or patients with unrelated disease.[81] The gamma-delta T-cell subset is the principal populace that responds to the mycobacterial 65-kD HSP, an observation that may account for the increase in circulating gamma-delta T cells in patients with Behçet's disease or with antecedent streptococcal or mycobacterial infections.[82]

Tissue neutrophilia may relate to the presence of HLA-B51, which has been associated with neutrophil hyperreactivity;[83] neutrophil functions are also increased in Behçet's disease.[84]

Vascular thrombosis has been attributed to antibody mediated endothelial injury,[85] protein C or S deficiency,[86] factor XII deficiency, inhibition of plasminogen activator, and circulating lupus anticoagulant.[87–89]

INFLAMMATORY BOWEL DISEASE

Crohn's Disease (Regional Enteritis)

First described in 1932, Crohn's disease is an idiopathic disorder of the gastrointestinal tract. The diagnosis is based on a constellation of radiologic, pathologic, and endoscopic data, namely deep mucosal fissures, fistula formation, transmural inflammation, discontinuous colonic and small bowel disease with preferential right-sided involvement, and sarcoidal granulomatous and fibrosing inflammation of the mucosa and submucosa.[90] Concomitant extraintestinal manifestations include fever, anemia, lupus anticoagulant, ophthalmic disease such as uveitis and episcleritis, colitic monoarticular large-joint arthritis, polyarthritis, spondylitis, amyloidosis,[91] renal lithiasis with resultant hydronephrosis,[92] cerebral vascular occlusions, and a spectrum of cutaneous eruptions.

Skin manifestations, principally restricted to patients with colonic disease, occur in 14% to 44% of patients with Crohn's disease depending upon whether or not perianal disease is considered a cutaneous manifestation.[90] Ulcers, fissures, sinus tracts, abscesses, and vegetant plaques may extend in continuity from sites of intra-abdominal involvement to the perineum, buttocks, or abdominal wall, ostomy sites, or incisional scars. When sterile granulomatous skin lesions arise at sites discontinuous from the gastrointestinal tract, the appellation "metastatic Crohn's disease" is applied.[93] Clinically, metastatic Crohn's disease presents as solitary or multiple nodules, plaques, ulcers, lichenoid lesions, or violaceous perifollicular papules involving extremities, intertriginous areas, abdominal skin folds, or genitalia.[94] Erythema nodosum,[95] the most common cutaneous manifestation of Crohn's disease,[90] and pyoderma gangrenosum develop in 15% and 1.5% of patients, respectively. Palmar erythema, a pustular response to trauma,[95] erythema multiforme usually with mucosal involvement,[95,96] epidermolysis bullosa acquisita, hidradenitis suppurative, rosacea, secondary cutaneous oxalosis, malabsorption-related acrodermatitis enteropathica,[95] and vasculitic lesions including benign cutaneous polyarteritis nodosa have also been described. Digitate hyperkeratosis reminiscent of punctate porokeratosis is also described.[97] Cutaneous necrosis as a complication of circulating lupus anticoagulant may also occur.

Oral lesions, manifesting as "cobblestone" lesions, aphthous ulcers, lip swelling, and pyostomatitis vegetans, occur in roughly 5% of patients with Crohn's disease.[95]

Histopathology. The perianal mucosal lesions and oral lesions of pyostomatitis vegetans show pseudoepitheliomatous hyperplasia in conjunction with suppurative granulomatous inflammation within the epithelium and subjacent corium

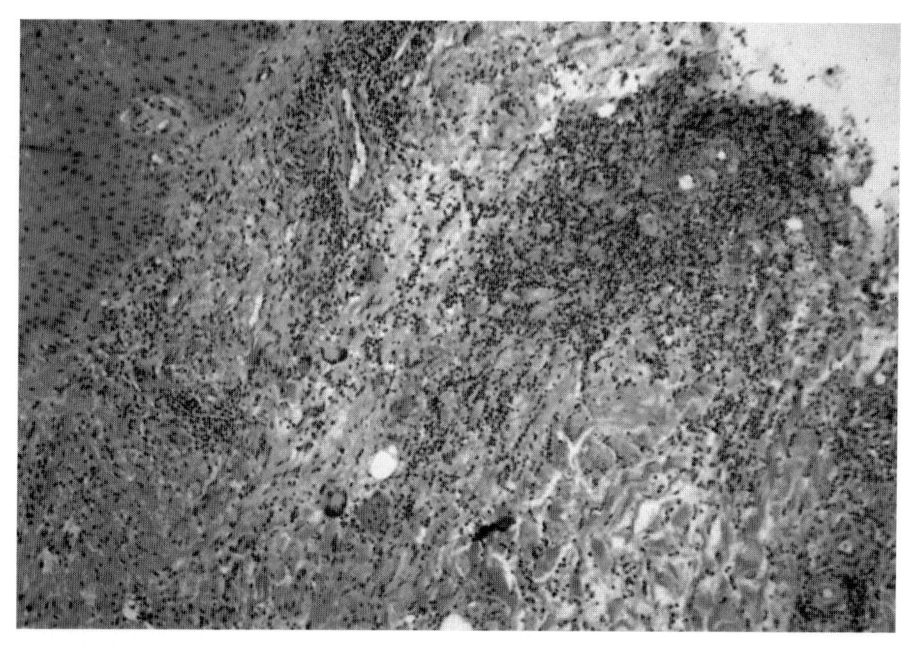

FIG. 16-10. Crohn's disease
Biopsy shows suppurative granulomatous inflammation accompanied by a severe necrotizing leukocytoclastic and granulomatous vasculitis; morphology is indistinguishable from cutaneous Wegener's granulomatosis and reminiscent of pyostomatitis vegetans, a prototypic oral lesion of Crohn's disease.

(Fig. 16-10). The most frequent histologic patterns seen in metastatic Crohn's disease are nonsuppurative granulomata which may assume a sarcoidal or diffuse pattern, frequently in close apposition to the epidermis and granulomatous vasculitis. Histological examination of the erythema nodosum–like lesion may show one of four patterns: (1) septal panniculitis consistent with classic erythema nodosum, (2) dermal-based sarcoidal granulomata,[98] (3) a dermal-based small-vessel granulomatous[99] or leukocytoclastic vasculitis, or (4) benign cutaneous polyarteritis nodosa. The latter shows mural infiltration by histiocytes and neutrophils with variable mural fibrinoid necrosis confined to the muscular arteries of the subcutaneous fat (see Fig. 16-12); occasional vessel involvement of the peripheral nerves and skeletal muscle of the affected extremity to produce mononeuritis and myositis respectively may occur.[100] A pauci-inflammatory thrombogenic vasculopathy characterizes the cutaneous infarcts associated with lupus anticoagulant. Necrobiosis lipoidica–like or granuloma annulare–like foci[101] may also be seen defined by areas of collagen necrobiosis with concomitant mucin or fibrin deposition and a palisading histiocytic infiltrate. Unlike idiopathic granuloma annulare or necrobiosis lipoidica, there usually is an accompanying leukocytoclastic vasculitis, thrombogenic or a granulomatous vasculopathy, and foci of extravascular neutrophilia.[101] Dense neutrophilic infiltration of the dermis accompanied by scattered giant cells has been reported as a unique histologic pattern.[102] We have also seen this pattern of suppurative granulomatous inflammation in concert with the aforementioned necrobiosis lipoidica or granuloma annulare tissue reaction. Cases of lip swelling show non-necrotizing granulomatous inflammation.[95]

The histology of pyoderma gangrenosum has been previously discussed.

Differential Diagnosis. The differential diagnosis of sarcoidal granulomatous inflammation in the skin includes sarcoidosis, id reactions to antecedent streptococcal or mycobacterial infections,[103] acquired hypogammaglobulinemia, rosacea, paraneoplastic histiocytopathies such as those associated with low-grade lymphoproliferative disease, rheumatoid arthritis, and granulomatous inflammatory reactions to ingested or inoculated inorganic compounds such as silica, zirconium, and beryllium. The lesions resembling benign cutaneous polyarteritis nodosa differ from systemic polyarteritis nodosa by virtue of confinement of the vasculitis to the subcutaneous fat without dermal involvement.[100] The changes of pyostomatitis vegetans also should raise the possibility of Wegener's granulomatosis, mycobacterial infection, blastomycosis, and histoplasmosis. The histopathology of the lip swelling may mimic that of Melkersson-Rosenthal syndrome.[95]

Pathogenesis. A common morphology shared by the intestinal and cutaneous disease is one of sarcoidal granulomatous inflammation, suggesting an integral role for cell mediated immunity in the pathogenesis of the lesions. Circulating immune complexes have been detected in some patients[95] and likely are the pathogenetic basis of the necrotizing vasculitis. Lastly, a subset of patients with Crohn's disease has antineutrophil cytoplasmic antibodies.

Ulcerative Colitis

Ulcerative colitis is an idiopathic inflammatory bowel disease involving the large intestine with rectal involvement being

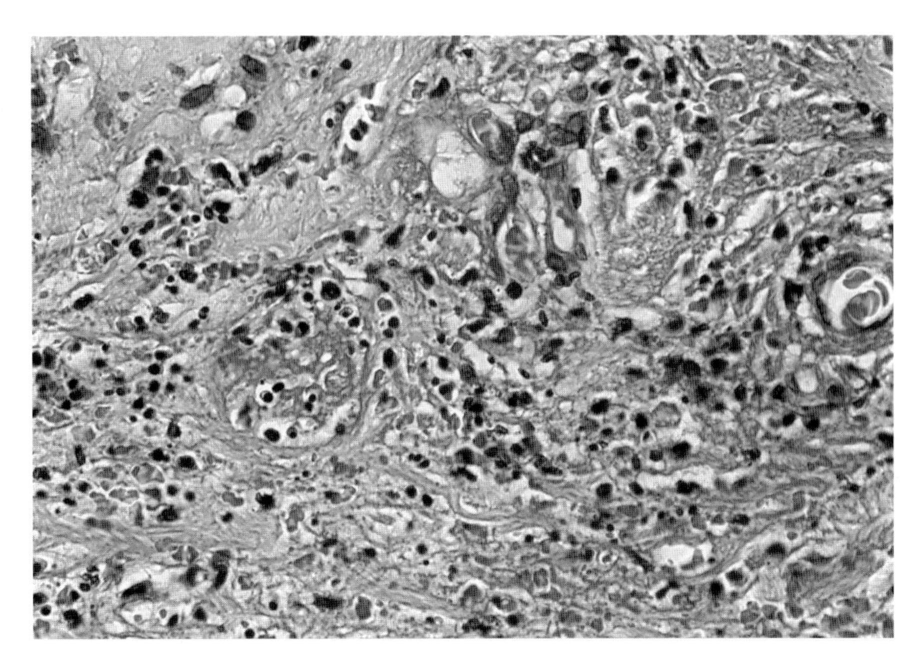

FIG. 16-11. Ulcerative colitis
Biopsy of the lesion illustrated in Color Fig. 16-3 revealed an angiocentric disintegrating neutrophilic infiltrate with accompanying mural and fibrin deposition with leukocytoclastic vasculitis. Immunofluorescent studies demonstrated vascular IgA deposition.

almost ubiquitous. It is characterized by glandular destruction and inflammation of variable intensity. Glandular dysplasia eventuating in carcinoma complicates the clinical course, particularly in patients with disease of pediatric onset. Extramucosal associations include chronic active hepatitis, primary sclerosing cholangitis, pulmonary vasculitis,[104] chronic fibrosing alveolitis, limited Wegener's granulomatosis of the lung,[105] pulmonary apical fibrosis, large-joint monoarticular arthritis, polyarthritis, and ankylosing spondylitis. Cutaneous manifestations may occur, the spectrum of which encompasses vasculitis, erythema nodosum, pyoderma gangrenosum, superficial migratory thrombophlebitis, and cutaneous thrombosis with resultant gangrene,[106] the latter two manifestations possibly related to underlying lupus anticoagulant or cryofibrinogenemia.[107] Pyoderma gangrenosum is more frequently associated with ulcerative colitis than with Crohn's disease and erythema nodosum more frequently with Crohn's disease. The lesions of pyoderma gangrenosum also include an unusual disseminated vesiculopustular variant.[108]

Histopathology. Pyoderma gangrenosum and erythema nodosum, the most common cutaneous manifestations of ulcerative colitis, are discussed elsewhere. Cutaneous vasculitis in association with ulcerative colitis includes IgA associated leukocytoclastic vasculitis[109] and benign cutaneous polyarteritis nodosa (Figs. 16-11 and 16-12). We have seen a patient with ulcerative colitis who developed a necrotizing suppurative granulomatous tissue reaction reminiscent of cutaneous Wegener's granulomatosis. A pauci-inflammatory thrombogenic vasculopathy involving vessels throughout the dermis and subcutis characterizes the histomorphology of associated lupus anticoagulant and/or cryofibrinogenemia.[107]

Celiac Disease

Celiac disease, a malabsorption syndrome due to small-intestine damage caused by a humoral immune response to ingested gluten, is prototypically associated with dermatitis herpetiformis.[110,111] A leukocytoclastic vasculitis has also been described in patients with celiac disease.[112] The proposed etiologic basis is an Arthus type III immune reaction with antigen penetration of the abnormal mucosa as the immunogenic trigger. Underlying mixed cryoglobulinemia[113] may occur, as may mesangial nephritis, the latter a sequela of circulating immune complexes.[111] The clinical presentation and histopathology is similar to other forms of leukocytoclastic vasculitis.

HEPATOBILIARY DISEASE

Sclerosing Cholangitis and Primary Biliary Cirrhosis

Pyoderma gangrenosum, particularly a disseminated superficial vesiculopustular variant,[114] and dermatitis herpetiformis have been described in association with sclerosing cholangitis.[45] Also, diffuse superficial pyoderma gangrenosum has been described in patients with ulcerative colitis, an associated finding in 70% of patients with sclerosing cholangitis. Isolated case reports of elastosis perforans serpiginosa with coexisting Down's syndrome[115] and disseminated warts along with primary combined immune deficiency and progressive multifocal leukoencephalopathy have been described in association with

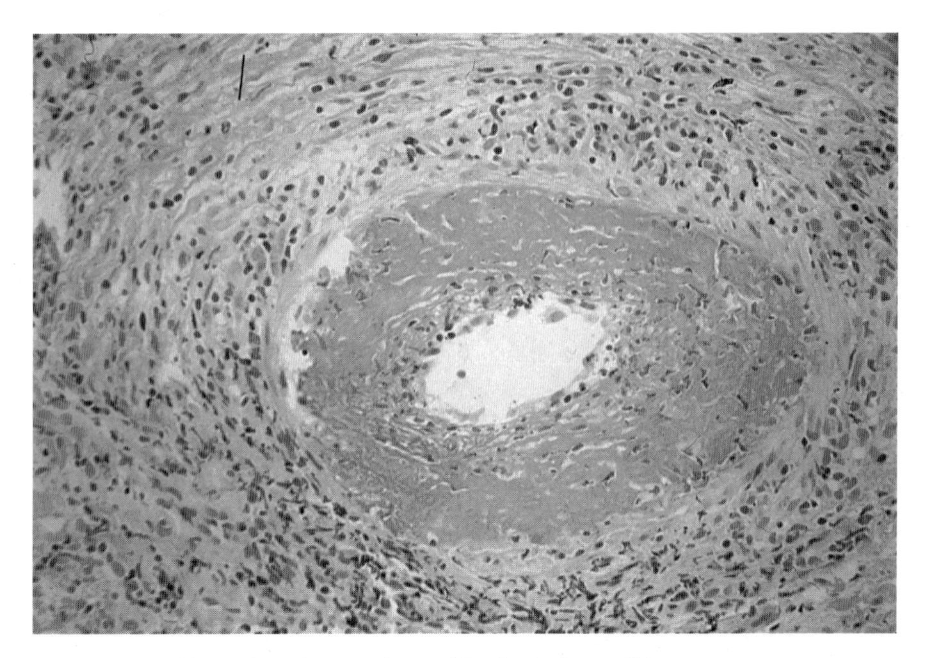

FIG. 16-12. Polyarteritis nodosa in a patient with ulcerative colitis
Within the subcutaneous fat, the wall of a subcutaneous artery demonstrates striking fibrinoid necrosis and is surrounded and permeated by disintegrating neutrophilic infiltrates unaccompanied by small-vessel involvement. The findings are typical for benign cutaneous polyarteritis nodosa.

sclerosing cholangitis. Cutaneous manifestations seen with primary biliary cirrhosis include lichen planus,[116] CREST, sarcoidal granulomata,[117] and vitiligo.[118]

Histopathology. Vesiculopustular pyoderma gangrenosum is characterized by a necrolytic subepithelial blister in which massive papillary edema is accompanied by sheets of neutrophils within the blister cavity, and prominent leukocytoclasia often centered around follicles. Peripheral to the areas of neutrophilia, angiocentric mononuclear-cell infiltrates with minimal accompanying vascular injury are observed (Fig. 16-13).

Pathogenesis. Although of unclear pathogenetic significance, antineutrophil cytoplasmic antibodies (ANCA) in a perinuclear pattern have been detected in 72% of patients with primary sclerosing cholangitis and ulcerative colitis.[119,120] ANCA have also been described in Wegener's granulomatosis, microscopic polyarteritis nodosa, and idiopathic crescentic glomerulonephritis. Patients with primary sclerosing cholangitis and concomitant ulcerative colitis[121] have circulating antibodies to colonic epithelial cells.[122] An immunogenic basis has also been proposed for primary sclerosing cholangitis in view of the association with HLA-B8 and/or HLA-DR3 antigens.

Hepatitis

Hepatitis can be broadly categorized into infectious and noninfectious causes. Most of the former are viral and are mediated by hepatitis A, B, C, and delta, cytomegalovirus, Epstein-Barr virus, and, rarely, varicella, measles, and herpes simplex. Of the latter, only chronic active hepatitis of autoimmune etiology will be considered, which is a necro-inflammatory disorder of unknown etiology with a predilection for young women.[123] Both the clinical presentation and liver chemistry profile may resemble infectious hepatitis. Hepatitis C antibodies have been demonstrated in patients with classic autoimmune hepatitis, a finding reputed to represent a nonspecific response that disappears during remission. Conversely, an autoantibody profile mimicking chronic active hepatitis may be seen in hepatitis C.[123] Other laboratory abnormalities include anemia, hypergammaglobulinemia, positive lupus erythematosus cell preparations, and positive antibodies to non–organ-specific antibodies, such as antinuclear antibodies, antineutrophil cytoplasmic antibodies, and antibodies to smooth muscle and liver/kidney microsomes.[123]

The principal cutaneous manifestations of viral and autoimmune hepatitis are lichen planus, leukocytoclastic vasculitis,[124] porphyria cutanea tarda,[125] erythema multiforme,[126] pyoderma gangrenosum,[127] and Gianotti-Crosti syndrome.[128] Lichen planus has been reported in patients with hepatitis C, chronic active hepatitis of unknown etiology, and primary biliary cirrhosis (Fig. 16-14).[129] The vasculitis may be on the basis of mixed cryoglobulinemia in the setting of hepatitis C infection.[124] The porphyria and erythema multiforme eruptions also have been described in association with hepatitis C.

Papular acrodermatitis[128] (Gianotti-Crosti syndrome) represents a primary infection with hepatitis B virus, acquired through the skin or mucous membranes, which is characterized by a nonpruritic, erythematous, papular eruption on the face, extremities, and buttocks. The eruption usually lasts about three weeks and is associated with lymphadenopathy and an acute, usually anicteric hepatitis of at least two-months duration that only rarely progresses to chronic liver disease. Hepatitis B surface antigenemia is present.[128] A similar eruption may be produced by several other viruses, such as Epstein-Barr virus, coxsackie B virus, and cytomegalovirus,[130] in which case there is often no hepatitis or lymphadenopathy.

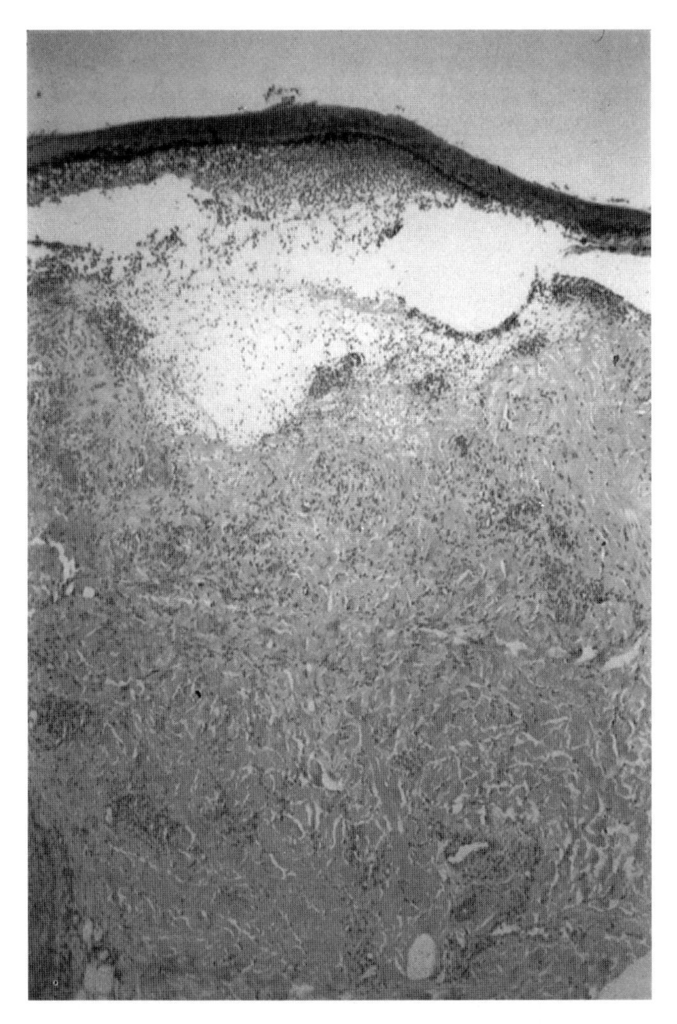

FIG. 16-13. Vesicular pustular pyoderma gangrenosum A biopsy of the lesion demonstrated marked subepidermal edema and a subjacent intense neutrophilic and lymphocytic infiltrate with tissue pathergy confined to the superficial dermis.

Histopathology. The histologic appearance of the papules in Gianotti-Crosti syndrome includes a moderately dense infiltrate of lymphocytes and histiocytes in the upper and mid-dermis that are found mainly around capillaries that exhibit endothelial swelling, accompanied by erythrocyte extravasation.[128] Focal spongiosis, parakeratosis with mild acanthosis, and a focal interface dermatitis complete the picture.[130] The histopathology of lichen planus, pyoderma gangrenosum, erythema multiforme, leukocytoclastic vasculitis, and porphyria cutanea tarda is described in other sections of the book. Mixed cryoglobulinemia differs from conventional leukocytoclastic vasculitis by the presence of intraluminal eosinophilic deposits that are strongly PAS positive.

Pathogenesis. The sera of all patients with hepatitis B–induced papular acrodermatitis exhibit hepatitis B surface antigens by radioimmunoassay. Antibodies to hepatitis B surface antigens are not detected during the eruptive phase, but only six to twelve months after the eruption; patients with antibodies become hepatitis B surface antigen–negative, suggesting a role for humoral immunity in their recovery.

Acrokeratosis Neoplastica (Bazex Syndrome)

First described in 1965,[131] this rare but clinically distinctive dermatosis is associated with either a primary malignant neoplasm of the upper aerodigestive tract or metastatic cancer to the lymph nodes of the neck. Thickening of the periungual and subungual skin and of the palms and soles occurs initially when the neoplasm is silent. Subsequently, the skin of the ears, nose, face, and the trunk and extremities becomes involved and shows a violaceous color, peeling, and fissuring.[132,133] The palmar lesions may resemble Reiter's disease.

Histopathology. Ill-defined perivascular lymphocytic infiltrates containing a few pyknotic neutrophils in the upper dermis along with mild acanthosis, hyperkeratosis, and scattered parakeratotic foci are described. Eosinophilic and vacuolar degeneration of the spinous layer may be noted.[133]

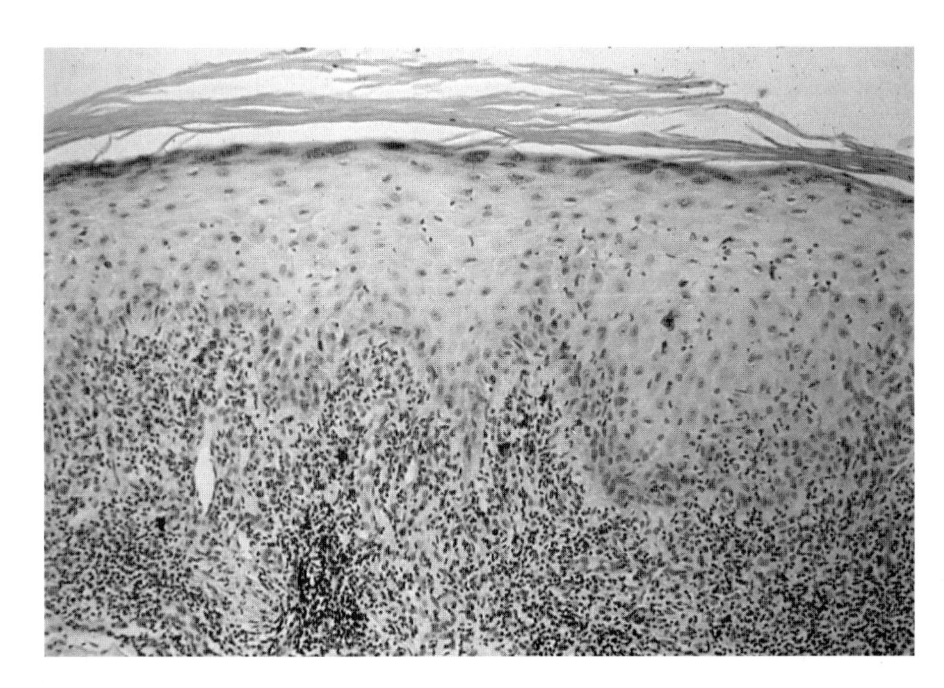

FIG. 16-14. Lichen planus arising in the setting of hepatitis C infection This patient with hepatitis C developed an eruption clinically compatible with lichen planus. The histomorphology confirms the diagnosis by virtue of a dense band-like lymphocytic infiltrate in apposition to an epidermis showing hypergranulosis and surmounted by a hyperkeratotic scale.

REFERENCES

1. Statters DJ, Asokan VS, Littlewood SM, Snape J. Carcinoma of the caecum in a scorbutic patient. Br J Clin Pract 1990;44:738.
2. Levine M. New concepts in the biology and biochemistry of ascorbic acid. N Eng J Med 1986;314:892.
3. Stokes PL, Melikiah V, Leeming RL et al. Folate metabolism in scurvy. Am J Clin Nutr 1975;28:126.
4. Ellis CN, Vanderveen EE, Rasmussen JE. Scurvy: A case caused by peculiar dietary habits. Arch Dermatol 1984;120:1212.
5. Abramovits–Ackerman W, Bustos T, Simosa–Leon V et al. Cutaneous findings in a new syndrome of autosomal recessive ectodermal dysplasia with corkscrew hairs. J Am Acad Derm 1992;27:917.
6. Hashimoto K, Kitabchi AE, Duckworth WC et al. Ultrastructure of scorbutic human skin. Acta Derm Venereol (Stockh) 1970;50:9.
7. Wechsler HL. Vitamin A deficiency following small-bowel bypass surgery for obesity. Arch Dermatol 1979;115: 73.
8. Frazier CN, Hu C. Nature and distribution according to age of cutaneous manifestations of vitamin A deficiency. Arch Dermatol Syph 1936;33: 825.
9. Bessey OA, Wolbach SB. Vitamin A, physiology and pathology. JAMA 1938;110:2072.
10. Hendricks, WM. Pellagra and pellagralike dermatoses: Etiology, differential diagnosis, dermatopathology, and treatment. Semin Dermatol 1991;10(Review):282.
11. Castiello RJ, Lynch PJ. Pellagra and the carcinoid syndrome. Arch Dermatol 1972;105:574.
12. Spivak JL, Jackson DL. Pellagra: An analysis of 18 patients and a review of the literature. Johns Hopkins Med J 1977;140:295.
13. Montgomery H. Nutritional and vitamin deficiency. In: Dermatopathology. Vol. 1. New York: Harper and Row, 1967;260.
14. Ackerman AB. Histologic diagnosis of inflammatory skin diseases: A method by pattern analysis. Philadelphia: Lea and Febiger, 1978; 269:512.
15. Dent CE. Hartnup disease: An inborn error of metabolism. Arch Dis Child 1957;32:363.
16. Halvorsen L, Halvorsen S. Hartnup disease. Pediatrics 1963;31:29.
17. Baron DN, Dent CE, Harris H et al. Hereditary pellagralike skin rash with temporary cerebellar ataxia, constant renal aminoaciduria and other bizarre chemical features. Lancet 1956;2:421.
18. Clodi PH, Deutsch E, Niebauer G. Krankheitsbild mit poikilodermieartigen hautveranderungen, aminoacidurie und Indolaceturie. Arch Klin Exp Dermatol 1964;218:165.
19. Ashurst PJ. Hydroa vacciniforme occurring in association with Hartnup disease. Br J Dermatol 1969;81:486.
20. Becker SW, Kahn D, Rothman S. Cutaneous manifestations of internal malignant tumors. Arch Dermatol Syph 1942;45:1069.
21. Domen RE, Shaffer MB Jr, Finke J, et al. The glucagonoma syndrome. Arch Intern Med 1980;140:262.
22. Binnick AN, Spencer SK, Dennison WL Jr et al. Glucagonoma syndrome. Arch Dermatol 1977;113:749.
23. Kasper CS, McMurray K. Necrolytic migratory erythema without glucagonoma versus canine superficial necrolytic dermatitis: Is hepatic impairment a clue to pathogenesis? J Am Acad Dermatol 1991; 25:534.
24. Kaspar CS. Necrolytic migratory erythema: Unresolved problems in diagnosis and pathogenesis. A case report and literature review. Cutis 1992;49:120.
25. Blackford S, Wright S, Roberts DL. Necrolytic migratory erythema without glucagonoma: The role of dietary essential fatty acids. Br J Dermatol 1991;125:460.
26. Goodenberger DM, Lawley TJ, Strober W, et al. Necrolytic migratory erythema without glucagonoma. Arch Dermatol 1977; 115:1429.
27. Fujita J, Seino Y, Isida H, et al. A functional study of a case of glucagonoma exhibiting typical glucagonoma syndrome. Cancer 1986;57:860.
28. Danbolt N, Closs K. Akrodermatitis enteropathica. Acta Derm Venereol (Stockh) 1942;23:127.
29. Moynahan EJ. Acrodermatitis enteropathica: A lethal inherited zinc-deficiency disorder. Lancet 1974;2:399.
30. Gonzalez JR, Botet MV, Sanchez JL. The histopathology of acrodermatitis enteropathica. Am J Dermatopathol 1982;4:303.
31. Reichel M, Mauro TM, Ziboh VA, et al. Acrodermatitis enteropathica in a patient with the acquired immunodeficiency syndrome. Arch Dermatol 1992;128:415.
32. Bernstein B, Leyden JL. Zinc deficiency and acrodermatitis enteropathica after intravenous hyperalimentation. Arch Dermatol 1978; 114:1070.
33. Niemi KM, Anttila PH, Kanerva L, Johansson E. Histopathological study of transient acrodermatitis enteropathica due to decreased zinc in breast milk. J Cutan Pathol 1989;16:382.
34. Weissman K, Hoe S, Knudsen L, et al. Zinc absorption in patients suffering from acrodermatitis enteropathica and in normal adults assessed by whole-body counting technique. Br J Dermatol 1979;101: 573.
35. Ortega SS, Cachaza JA, Tovar IV, Feijboo MF. Zinc deficiency dermatitis in parenteral nutrition: An electron-microscopic study. Dermatologica 1985;171:163.
36. Albers SE, Brozena SJ, Fenske NA. A case of kwashiorkor. Cutis 1993;51:445.
37. Househam KC. Computed tomography of the brain in kwashiorkor: A follow up study. Arch Dis Child 1991;66:623.
38. Montgomery H. Nutritional and vitamin deficiency. In: Dermatopathology. Vol. 1. New York: Harper and Row, 1967;264.
39. Richardson D, Iputo J. Effects of kwashiorkor malnutrition on measured capillary filtration rate in forearm. Am J Physiol 1992; 262:H496.
40. Brunsting LA, Goeckerman WE, O'Leary PA. Pyoderma (ecthyma) gangrenosum. Arch Dermatol 1930;22:655.
41. Graham JA, Hansen KK, Rabinowitz LG, Esterly NB. Pyoderma gangrenosum in infants and children. Pediatr Dermatol 1994;11:10.
42. Cairns BA, Herbst CA, Sartor BR et al. Peristomal pyoderma gangrenosum and inflammatory bowel disease. Arch Surg 1994;129:769.
43. Schwaegerle SM, Bergfeld WF, Senitzer D et al. Pyoderma gangrenosum: A review. J Am Acad Dermatol 1988;18:559.
44. Callen JP. Pyoderma gangrenosum and related disorders. Med Clin North Am 1989;73:1247.
45. Magro CM, Crowson AN. Vesiculopustular eruption of hepatobiliary disease. Int J Dermatol (in press).
46. Wilson-Jones E, Winkelmann RK. Superficial granulomatous pyoderma: A localized vegetative form of pyoderma gangrenosum. J Am Acad Dermatol 1988;18:511.
47. Ayres G. Pyoderma gangrenosum: An unusual syndrome of ulcerative vesicles in arthritis. Arch Dermatol 77:269.
48. Jorizzo JL, Solomon AR, Zanolli M, Lehin B. Neutrophilic vascular reactions. J Am Acad Dermatol 1988;19:983.
49. Pye RJ, Choudhury C. Bullous pyoderma as a presentation of acute leukemia. Clin Exp Dermatol 1977;2:33.
50. Koester G, Tarnower A, Levisohn D, Burgdorf W. Bullous pyoderma gangrenosum. J Am Acad Dermatol 1993;29:875.
51. Magro CM, Crowson AN, Harrist TJ. Inflammatory folliculocentric vasculopathy syndromes: A distinctive manifestation of systemic disease. Lab Invest 74(Abstract):43A.
52. Powell FC, Schroeter AL, Perry HO, Su WPD. Direct immunofluorescence in pyoderma gangrenosum. Br J Dermatol 1983;108:287.
53. Holt PJA, Davies MG, Saunders KC, et al. Pyoderma gangrenosum: Clinical and laboratory findings in 15 patients with special reference to polyarthritis. Medicine 1980;59:114.
54. Powell FC, Schroeter AL, Su D, Perry HO. Pyoderma gangrenosum and monoclonal gammopathy. Arch Dermatol 1983;119:468.
55. Morrison JGL, Fourie ED. A distinctive skin eruption following small-bowel bypass surgery. Br J Dermatol 1980;102:467.
56. Ely PH. The bowel bypass syndrome: A response to bacterial peptidoglycans. J Am Acad Dermatol 1980;2:473.
57. Jorizzo JL, Apisarnthanarax P, Subrt P, et al. Bowel-bypass syndrome without bowel bypass: Bowel-associated dermatosis-arthritis syndrome. Arch Intern Med 1983;143:457.
58. Dicken CH. Bowel-associated dermatosis-arthritis syndrome: Bowel bypass syndrome without bowel bypass. J Am Acad Dermatol 1986; 14:792.
59. Goldman JA, Casey HL, Davidson ED et al. Vasculitis associated with intestinal bypass surgery. Arch Dermatol 1979;115:725.
60. Magro CM, Crowson AN, Peeling R. Vasculitis as the pathogenetic basis of Reiter's disease. Hum Pathol 1995;26:633.
61. O'Duffy JD. Behçet's syndrome. New Eng J Med 1990;322:326.

62. Main DM, Chamberlain MA. Clinical differentiation of oral ulceration in Behçet's disease. Br J Rheumatol 1992;31:767.
63. Magro CM, Crowson AN. Cutaneous manifestations of Behçet's disease. Int J Dermatol 1995; 34(Review):159.
64. King R, Crowson AN, Murray E, Magro CM. Acral purpuric papulonodular lesions as a manifestation of Behçet's disease. Int J Dermatol 1995;34:190.
65. Oguz O, Serdaroglu S, Turzin Y et al. Acute febrile neutrophilic dermatosis (Sweet's syndrome) associated with Behçet's disease. Int J Dermatol 1992;31:645.
66. Koc Y, Gullu I, Akpek G et al. Vascular involvement in Behçet's Disease. J Rheumatol 1992;19:402.
67. Akutsu Y, Itami N, Tanaka M et al. IgA nephritis in Behçet's disease: Case report and review of the literature. Clin Nephrol 1990;34:52.
68. Sokoloff L, Bunin JJ. Vascular lesions in rheumatoid arthritis. J Chronic Dis 1957;5:668.
69. Langenberg A, Yen TS, LeBoit PE. Granulomatous vasculitis occurring after cutaneous herpes zoster despite absence of viral genome. J Am Acad Dermatol 1991;24:429.
70. Choudhri S, Magro CM, Nicolle L, Crowson AN. A unique id reaction to *Mycobacterium leprae*: First documented case. Cutis 1994;54:282.
71. Lehner T, Batchelor JR, Challacombe SJ, Kennedy L. An immunogenetic basis for the tissue involvement in Behçet's syndrome. Immunology 1979;37:895.
72. Namba K, Ueno T, Okita M. Behçet's disease and streptococcal infection. Jpn J Ophthalmol 1986;30:385.
73. Yokota K, Hayashi S, Fujii N et al. Antibody response to oral streptococci in Behçet's disease. Microbiol Immunol 1992;36:815.
74. Efthimiou J, Hay PE, Spiro SG, Lane DJ. Pulmonary tuberculosis in Behçet's syndrome. Br J Dis Chest 1988; 82:300.
75. Studd M, McCance DJ, Lehner T. Detection of HSV-1 DNA in patients with Behçet's syndrome and in patients with recurrent oral ulcers by the polymerase chain reaction. J Med Microbiol 1991;34:39.
76. Hamzaoui K, Kahan A, Ayed K, Hamza M. Cytotoxic T cells against herpes simplex virus in Behçet's disease. Clin Exp Rheumatol 1991; 9:131.
77. Stein CM, Thomas JE. Behçet's disease associated with HIV infection. J Rheumatol 1991;18:1427.
78. Lamb JR, Young DB. T cell recognition of stress proteins: A link between infectious and autoimmune disease. Mol Biol Med 1990;7:311.
79. Lehner T, Lavery E, Smith R et al. Association between the 65 kilodalton heat shock protein, *Streptococcus sangui* and the corresponding antibodies in Behçet's syndrome. Infect Immun 1991;59:1424.
80. Holoshitz J, Koning JE, Coligan JE et al. Isolation of CD4- CD8-mycobacterial reaction T lymphocyte clones from rheumatoid arthritis synovial fluid. Nature 1989;39:226.
81. Pervin K, Childerstone A, Shinnick T et al. T cell epitope expression of mycobacterial and homologous human 65-kilodalton heat shock protein peptide in short term cell line from patient with Behçet's disease. J Immunol 1993;151:2273.
82. Suzuki Y, Hoshi K, Matsuda T, Mizushima Y. Increased peripheral blood gamma delta+ T cells and natural killer cells in Behçet's disease. J Rheumatol 1992;19:588.
83. Sensi A, Gavioli R, Spisani S et al. HLA B51 antigen associated with neutrophil hyperactivity. Dis Markers 1991;9:327.
84. Pronai L, Ichikawa Y, Nakazawa H, Arimori S. Enhanced superoxide generation and the decreased superoxide scavenging activity of peripheral blood leukocytes in Behçet's disease: Effects of colchicine. Clin Exp Rheumatol 1991;9:227.
85. Aydintung AO, Tokgoz G, D'Cruz DP et al. Antibodies to endothelial cells in patients with Behçet's disease. Clin Immunol Immunopathol 1993;67:157.
86. Disdier P, Harle JR, Mouly A et al. Case report: Behçet's syndrome and factor XII deficiency. Clin Rheumatol 1992;11:422.
87. Chafa O, Fischer AM, Meriane F et al. Behçet's syndrome associated with protein S deficiency. Thromb Haemost 1992;67:1.
88. Hampton KK, Chamberlain MA, Menon DK, Davies JA. Coagulation and fibrinolytic activity in Behçet's disease. Thromb Haemost 1991; 66:292.
89. Al-Dalaan A, Al-Ballaa SR, Al-Janadi S et al. Association of anti-cardiolipin antibodies with vascular thrombosis and neurological manifestation of Behçet's disease. Clin Rheumatol 1993;12:28.
90. Greenstein AJ, Janowitz HD, Sachar DB. The extra-intestinal complications of Crohn's disease and ulcerative colitis: A study of 700 patients. Medicine (Baltimore) 1976;55:401.
91. Werther JL, Schapira A, Rubenstein O, Janowitz HD. Amyloidosis in regional enteritis: A report of 5 cases. Am J Med 1960;29:416.
92. Present DH, Rabinowitz JC, Bank PA, Janowitz HD. Obstructive hydronephropathy. N Eng J Med 1969;280:523.
93. Shum D, Guenther L. Metastatic Crohn's disease: Case report and review of the literature. Arch Dermatol 1990;126:645.
94. Buckley C, Bayoumi A-HM, Sarkany I. Metastatic Crohn's disease. Clin Exp Dermatol 1990;15:131.
95. Burgdorf W. Cutaneous manifestations of Crohn's disease. J Am Acad Dermatol 1981;5:689.
96. Lebwohl M, Fleischmajer R, Janowitz H et al. Metastatic Crohn's disease. J Am Acad Dermatol 1984;10:33.
97. Aloi FG, Molinero A, Pippione M. Parakeratotic horns in a patient with Crohn's disease. Clin Exp Dermatol 1989;14:79.
98. Witkowski JA, Parish LC, Lewis JE. Crohn's disease, non-caseating granulomas on the legs. Acta Derm Venereol (Stockh) 1977;57:181.
99. Burgdorf W, Orken M. Granulomatous perivasculitis in Crohn's disease. Arch Dermatol 1981;117:674.
100. Diaz-Perez JL, Winkelmann RK. Cutaneous polyarteritis nodosa. Arch Dermatol 1974;110:407.
101. Magro CM, Crowson AN, Regauer S. Granuloma annulare and necrobiosis lipoidica as a manifestation of systemic disease. Hum Pathol 1996;27:50.
102. Smoller BR, Weishar M, Gray MH. An unusual cutaneous manifestation of Crohn's disease. Arch Pathol Lab Med 1990;114:609.
103. Choudrhi SM, Magro CM, Nicolle LM, Crowson AN. An id reaction to *Mycobacterium leprae*: First documented case. Cutis 1994;54:282.
104. Collins WJ, Bendig DW, Taylor WF. Pulmonary vasculitis complicating childhood ulcerative colitis. Gastroenterology 1979;77:1091.
105. Kedziora JA, Wolff M, Chang J. Limited forms of Wegener's granulomatosis in ulcerative colitis. Am J Roentgenol Radium Ther Nucl Med 1975;125:127.
106. Stapleton SR, Curley RK, Simpson WA. Cutaneous gangrene secondary to focal thrombosis: An important cutaneous manifestation of ulcerative colitis. Clin Exp Dermatol 1989;14:387.
107. Ball GV, Goldman LN. Chronic ulcerative colitis, skin necrosis, and cryofibrinogenemia. Ann Int Med 1976;85:464.
108. Barnes L, Lucky AW, Bucuvales JC et al. Pustular pyoderma gangrenosum associated with ulcerative colitis in childhood. J Am Acad Dermatol 1986;15:608.
109. Peters AJ, van de Waal Bake AW, Daha MR, Breeveld FC. Inflammatory bowel disease and ankylosing spondylitis with cutaneous vasculitis, glomerulonephritis and circulating IgA immune complexes. Ann Rheum Dis 1990;49:638.
110. Scott BB, Young S, Raja SM et al. Celiac disease and dermatitis herpetiformis: Further studies of their relationship. Gut 1976;17:759.
111. Moothy AV, Zimmerman SW, Maxim PE. Dermatitis herpetiformis and celiac disease: Association with glomerulonephritis, hypocomplementemia and circulating immune complexes. JAMA 1978;239:2019.
112. Meyers S, Dikman S, Spiera H et al. Cutaneous vasculitis complicating celiac disease. Gut 1981;22:61.
113. Doe WF, Evans D, Hobb JR, Booth CC. Celiac disease, vasculitis and cryoglobulinemia. Gut 1972;13:112.
114. Laajam MA, al-Mofarreh MA, al-Zayyani NR. Primary sclerosing cholangitis in chronic ulcerative colitis: Report of cases in Arabs and review. Trop Gastroenterol 1992;13(Review):106.
115. O'Donnell, Kelly P, Dervan P et al. Generalized elastosis perforans serpinginosa in Downe's syndrome. Clin and Exp Dermatol 1992;17:31.
116. Graham-Brown RAC, Sarkany I, Sherlock S. Lichen planus and primary biliary cirrhosis. Br J Dermatol 1982;106:699.
117. Harrington AC, Fitzpatrick JE. Cutaneous sarcoidal granulomas in a patient with primary biliary cirrhosis. Cutis 1992;49:271.
118. Zauli D, Crespi C, Miserocchi F et al. Primary biliary cirrhosis and vitiligo. J Am Acad Dermatol 1986;15:105.
119. Snook JA, Chapman RW, Fleming K, Jewell DP. Anti-neutrophil nuclear antibody in ulcerative colitis, Crohn's disease and primary sclerosing cholangitis. Clin Exp Immunol 1989;76:30.
120. Hardarson S, LaBrecque DR, Mitros FA et al. Antineutrophil cytoplasmic antibody in inflammatory bowel and hepatobiliary diseases: High prevalence in ulcerative colitis, primary sclerosing cholangitis, and autoimmune hepatitis. Am J Clin Pathol 1993;99:277.

121. Olsson R, Danielsson A, Jarnerot G et al. Prevalence of primary sclerosing cholangitis in patients with ulcerative colitis. Gastroenterology 1991;100:1319.
122. Chapman RW, Cottone M, Selby WS et al. Serum autoantibodies, ulcerative colitis and primary sclerosing cholangitis. Gut 1990;27: 86.
123. Krawitt EL. Autoimmune hepatitis: Classification, heterogeneity and treatment. Am J Med 1994;96:23S.
124. Durand JM, Lefevre P, Harle JR et al. Cutaneous vasculitis and cryoglobulinemia type II associated with hepatitis C virus infection. Lancet 1991;337:499.
125. Fargion S, Piperno A, Cappellini MD et al. Hepatitis C virus and porphyria cutanea tarda: Evidence of a strong association. Hepatology 1995;21:1754.
126. Antinori S, Esposito R, Aliprandi C, Tadini G. Erythema multiforme and hepatitis C. Lancet 1991;337:428.
127. Byrne JP, Hewitt M, Summerly R. Pyoderma gangrenosum associated with active chronic hepatitis. Arch Dermatol 1976;112:1297.
128. Gianotti F. Papular acrodermatitis of childhood and other papulovesicular acro-located syndromes (review). Br J Dermatol 1979;100:49.
129. Jubert C, Pawlotsky JM, Pouget F et al. Lichen planus and hepatitis C virus-related chronic active hepatitis. Arch Dermatol 1994;130:73.
130. Spear RL, Winkelman RK. Gianotti-Crosti syndrome: A review of 10 cases not associated with hepatitis B infection. Arch Dermatol 1984; 120:891.
131. Bazex A, Salvador R, Dupre A et al. Syndrome paraneoplastique a type d'hyperkeratose des extremities. Bull Soc Fr Dermatol Syphiligr 1965;72:182.
132. Pecora AL, Landsman L, Imgrund SP et al. Acrokeratosis neoplastica (Basex syndrome). Arch dermatol 1983;119:820.
133. Bazex A, Griffith A. Acrokeratosis paraneoplastica: a new cutaneous marker of malignancy. Br J Dermatol 1980;103:301.

Lever's Histopathology of the Skin, eighth edition,
edited by David Elder et al. Lippincott–
Raven Publishers, Philadelphia © 1997.

CHAPTER 17

Metabolic Diseases of the Skin

John Maize and John Metcalf

AMYLOIDOSIS

Amyloid

The term "amyloid" is applied to extracellular proteinaceous deposits that are resistant to proteolytic digestion and have distinctive physical properties. Deposits can be localized to a body site or can be "systemic," involving several organs and tissues.

By light microscopy, amyloid appears amorphous, eosinophilic, and hyaline. Characteristic staining qualities distinguish it from other glassy, pink substances. The Congo-red stain results in a brick red staining reaction and apple-green birefringence, and amyloid stains metachromatically with crystal violet and methyl violet stains. These staining characteristics result from the cross-beta-pleated sheet conformation of the polypeptide backbones of the amyloid fibrils. These fibrils, which ultrastructurally are 7.5 nm in width and of indeterminate length, are formed by the polymerization of small, soluble polyanionic proteins, ranging from 3 to 30 kDa. Amyloid-P component, GAGS, fibronectins, and other connective tissue components are also incorporated into the deposit of aggregated fibrils.[1]

Chemically, there are more than 16 different amyloids, which, although sharing the physical properties outlined above, are distinguished by having different protein constituents and diverse origins. It has been recommended that classification of amyloidoses be based on the fibril protein whenever possible.[2]

Cutaneous deposition of amyloid can result from any one of several systemic disease processes. However, cutaneous amyloid deposits can also result from local processes limited to the skin.

Systemic Amyloidoses That Involve the Skin: AL (Immunoglobulin Light Chains)

In its systemic form, this disease is also known as primary systemic amyloidosis. This uncommon disease results from a plasma cell dyscrasia with production of monoclonal light chains.[3] The heart, smooth and skeletal muscle, and other soft tissues, as well as the kidneys, liver, and spleen, are frequently involved. However, deposits can be localized to the skin (and lungs).[1] When they are restricted to the skin, the terms "amyloidosis cutis nodularis atrophicans" and "nodular amyloidosis" have been applied. Heart failure, gastrointestinal bleeding, and renal failure can be fatal complications of the systemic form.[4,5] Among cutaneous lesions, petechiae and ecchymoses are most common.[5] They are the result of involvement of cutaneous blood vessels and are observed mainly on the face, especially on the eyelids and in the periorbital region. Minor trauma may precipitate these lesions, referred to by some as "pinch purpura." In addition, there may be discrete or coalescing papules or plaques. They usually have a waxy color but may be blue-red as the result of hemorrhage into them.[6,7] In rare instances, one observes firm cutaneous or subcutaneous nodules or plaques or areas of induration of the skin resembling morphea.[8] Bullae that may be induced by minor trauma and may be hemorrhagic occur occasionally.[7,9,10] Among oral lesions, macroglossia is common, occurring in 17% of the patients.[4]

Histopathology. Examination of cutaneous lesions in the systemic form of the disease reveals faintly eosinophilic amorphous, often fissured masses of amyloid deposited in the dermis and in the subcutaneous tissues. Quite frequently, accumulations of amyloid are deposited close to the epidermis. They may or may not be separated from the overlying epidermis by a narrow zone of collagen (Fig. 17-1). They are rarely deposited around individual elastic fibers.[11] The involvement of the walls of blood vessels is responsible for the frequent presence of extravasated erythrocytes. Inflammatory cells are lacking or scarce.[10] Bullae arise by cleavage in extensive dermal amyloid deposits and form intradermally, rather than at the dermal-epidermal junction.[9,10]

In the subcutaneous tissue, there may be large aggregates of amyloid with infiltration of the walls of blood vessels and so-called amyloid rings, which are formed by the deposition of amyloid around individual fat cells.[10] The fat cells may then appear as if cemented together by the amyloid.

Even if there are no skin lesions, fine-needle aspirates of the abdominal fat often are of use in documenting the diagnosis[12,13] (Fig. 17-2). Tissue biopsies of normal-appearing skin yield positive results in about 40% of all patients.[8,14] These biopsies show small deposits in the walls of small blood vessels in the dermis

J. Maize: Department of Dermatology, Medical University of South Carolina, Charleston, SC
J. Metcalf: Pathology and Laboratory Medicine, Medical University of South Carolina, Charleston, SC

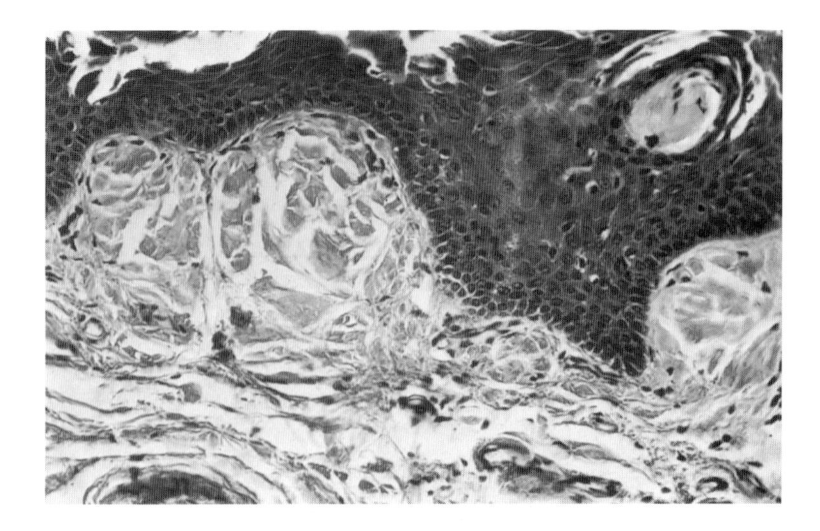

FIG. 17-1. Primary systemic amyloidosis
Amorphous, fissured masses of amyloid are present in the upper dermis. The amyloid material greatly resembles that observed in colloid milium (see Fig. 17-4).

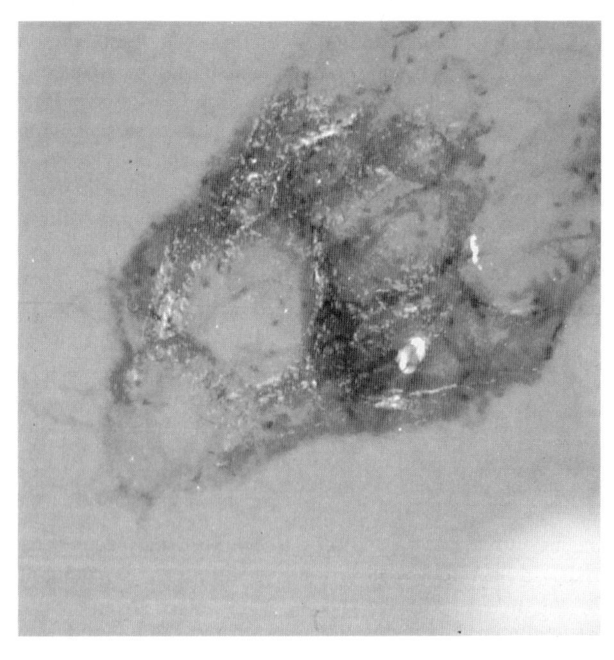

FIG. 17-2. Primary systemic amyloidosis
Amyloid deposited in subcutaneous fat exhibits green birefringence when stained with Congo red in this aspirate from the abdominal fat pad.

or the subcutaneous tissue but occasionally also around eccrine glands and lipocytes. The forearm is the recommended area for biopsy.[14]

When localized to the skin, the nodular amyloid deposits are surrounded by a dense plasmacytic infiltrate and production of the immunoglobulin light chains is thought to occur locally.[15]

Relationship with Multiple Myeloma. AL amyloidosis results from the production of monoclonal immunoglobulins and/or free light chains, usually λ light chains, by an abnormal population of B-cells. The vast majority of the patients (90%) have monoclonal protein in urine or serum (Bence-Jones protein).[16] If there is overtly malignant plasma cell neoplasia it is referred to as multiple myeloma. Systemic amyloidosis is found in 5 to 15% of multiple myeloma patients. The majority of patients with AL amyloidosis do not have overt multiple myeloma, however. These patients have an underlying B-cell dyscrasia and, despite having no tumor masses, show an increased plasma cell population on bone marrow examination. It is uncertain whether or not this patient population will inevitably develop multiple myeloma.

Pathogenesis. In the systemic form of AL amyloidosis, the amyloid originates from monoclonal immunoglobulin light chains produced by plasma cells in the bone marrow. In the localized form, the amyloid is thought to be produced by the local plasma cell infiltrate, and, as in the systemic form, the amyloid protein has immunocytochemical characteristics of AL amyloid.[15]

Ultrastructurally, amyloid deposits consist of irregularly arranged straight, nonbranching filaments that often appear hollow because their peripheries appear electron-dense in comparison with their centers. These filaments are 6 to 7 nm in diameter but are of indeterminate length.[17–19]

AA (Serum Amyloid A) Amyloidosis

Also known as secondary systemic amyloidosis, AA amyloidosis can result from chronic inflammatory disease or recurring bouts of acute inflammation such as tuberculosis, complications of bronchiectasis, and chronic osteomyelitis. It is now relatively rare in industrialized countries since the development of modern antibiotic therapy, and most cases in the United States and Western Europe are associated with chronic rheumatoid arthritis or related disorders.[20] At time of diagnosis, the vast majority of patients have renal insufficiency or the nephrotic syndrome. There are no cutaneous lesions.

Histopathology. AA amyloid is deposited in parenchymatous organs such as the kidneys, liver, spleen, and adrenal. These deposits are found first in the interstitium and blood vessel walls; with progression, the deposits gradually replace the parenchyma. Deposits within the glomeruli and peritubular tissues result in renal failure.

Fine-needle aspiration biopsy of the subcutaneous fat and staining of the aspirated material by the Congo-red method is the most sensitive method of diagnosis.[12,13,21,22] Tissue biopsy of skin with underlying subcutaneous fat demonstrates deposits of AA amyloid around lipocytes, in blood vessel walls, around eccrine glands, and sometimes free in the dermis.[14]

Pathogenesis. AA amyloid is thought to be derived from serum amyloid A (SAA), an apoprotein complex of high-density lipoprotein (HDL3) that is synthesized by hepatocytes and is normally present in the serum in barely detectable concentrations. Production is stimulated by inflammation via IL-1 and other cytokines. AA protein is then formed when SAA undergoes carboxy terminal cleavage.[23–25] This process takes place within lysosomes of macrophages that are receiving antigenic stimulation by a variety of chronic diseases.[26] The amyloid is then deposited extracellularly.

Primary Localized Cutaneous Amyloidosis

Lichen Amyloidosis and Macular Amyloidosis

Lichen amyloidosis and macular amyloidosis are best considered as different manifestations of the same disease process. Lichen amyloidosis is characterized by closely set, discrete, brown-red papules that often show some scaling and that are most commonly located on the legs, especially the shins, although they may occur elsewhere. Through the coalescence of papules, plaques may form on the legs. These plaques often have verrucous surfaces and then resemble hypertrophic lichen planus or lichen simplex chronicus. Usually the lesions of lichen amyloidosis itch severely. It is assumed by some authors that the pruritis leads to damage of keratinocytes by scratching and to subsequent production of amyloid.[27,28]

Macular amyloidosis is characterized by pruritic macules showing pigmentation with a reticulated or rippled pattern. Although macular amyloidosis may occur anywhere on the trunk or extremities, the upper back is a fairly common site.[29] In Southeast Asia, where macular amyloidosis is common, prolonged friction from a rough nylon towel or a back scratcher is thought to be its cause.[30] The eruption can be easily passed off as postinflammatory hyperpigmentation by physicians unfamiliar with the condition.[31]

Macular amyloidosis and lichen amyloidosis sometimes occur together in the same patient, and lichenoid amyloidosis can arise in a setting of macular amyloidosis, presumably due to scratching.[32,33] When treated by intralesional injection of steroids, the lichenoid lesions can become macular.

Histopathology. Lichen and macular amyloidosis show deposits of amyloid that are limited to the papillary dermis. Most of the amyloid is situated within the dermal papillae. Although the deposits usually are smaller in macular amyloidosis than in lichen amyloidosis, differentiation of the two on the basis of the amount of amyloid is not possible.[31] The two conditions actually differ only in the appearance of the epidermis, which is hyperplastic and hyperkeratotic in lichen amyloidosis. Occasionally, the amount of amyloid in macular amyloidosis is so small that it is missed, even when special stains are used on frozen sections. In such instances, more than one biopsy may be necessary to confirm the diagnosis.[34]

In areas in which the entire dermal papilla is filled with amyloid, the amyloid appears homogeneous in both lichen and macular forms. In lesions in which the dermal papillae are only partially filled, as seen more often in macular amyloidosis, the amyloid has a globular appearance and resembles the colloid bodies found in lichen planus (Fig. 17-3A, B, and C). These amyloid bodies in some areas lie in direct contact with the overlying basal cells of the epidermis. Similar colloid bodies are also found in some sections within the epidermis, but, in contrast with those located at the epidermal-dermal junction, they do not stain as amyloid. In addition, there often is a striking degree of pigmentary incontinence.

Histogenesis. The light microscopic findings in lichen and macular amyloidosis suggest that degenerating epidermal cells are discharged into the dermis, where they are converted into amyloid. The epidermal origin of the amyloid in lichen and macular amyloidosis is supported by electron microscopy.[35,36] Also on electron microscopy, the degenerating epidermal cells resemble the colloid bodies observed in lichen planus. They contain the following components: (1) tonofilaments; (2) degenerated, wavy tonofilaments that are thicker but less electron-dense than normal tonofilaments; (3) lysosomes; and (4) typical filaments of amyloid, 6 to 10 nm thick, that are straight and nonbranching.[36] It is postulated that the degenerated, wavy tonofilaments are recognized as foreign and are digested by the cell's own lysosomes. Such digestion produces amyloid filaments. A conversion of tonofilaments into amyloid filaments requires that the alpha-pleated sheet configuration of the tonofilaments change into the beta configuration of amyloid.[37] However, immunohistochemical studies suggest that components of the lamina densa and anchoring fibrils are also associated with amyloid deposits. Further ultrastructural examination shows disruption of the lamina densa overlying these deposits.[38]

On direct immunofluorescence, all specimens of lichen or macular amyloidosis fluoresce positively for immunoglobulins or complement, particularly immunoglobulin M (IgM) and the third component of complement (C3). Staining for kappa and lambda light chains is positive. The immunofluorescent pattern is globular and thus is similar to that of lichen planus, except for the absence of fibrin. It suggests that the globular aggregates of lichenoid or macular amyloidosis, like the colloid bodies of lichen planus, act as a filamentous sponge into which immunoglobulins and complement are absorbed.[39]

The epidermal derivation of the amyloid in lichen and macular amyloidosis is supported by histochemical and immunologic findings. In contrast to the amyloid of systemic amyloidosis, the amyloid of lichenoid and macular amyloidosis shows fluorescence for disulfide bonds as normally seen in the stratum corneum, suggesting that cross-linking of sulfhydryl groups occurs in amyloidogenesis.[40] Furthermore, immunofluorescence studies with an antikeratin antiserum have shown intense staining of the amyloid for the antikeratin antibody.[41]

After full agreement apparently had been reached about the keratogenic origin of the amyloid in lichen and macular amyloidosis, some dissenting opinions were expressed. In one study, amyloid stained negatively for keratin determinants and the positive reactions obtained by previous investigators were regarded as nonimmunologic, because amyloid deposits can easily absorb immunoglobulins.[42] Degenerating collagen was regarded as the site of formation of amyloid.[43] Other authors found direct amyloid fibril formation at the basal surfaces of living basal cells in lichen amyloidosis.[44]

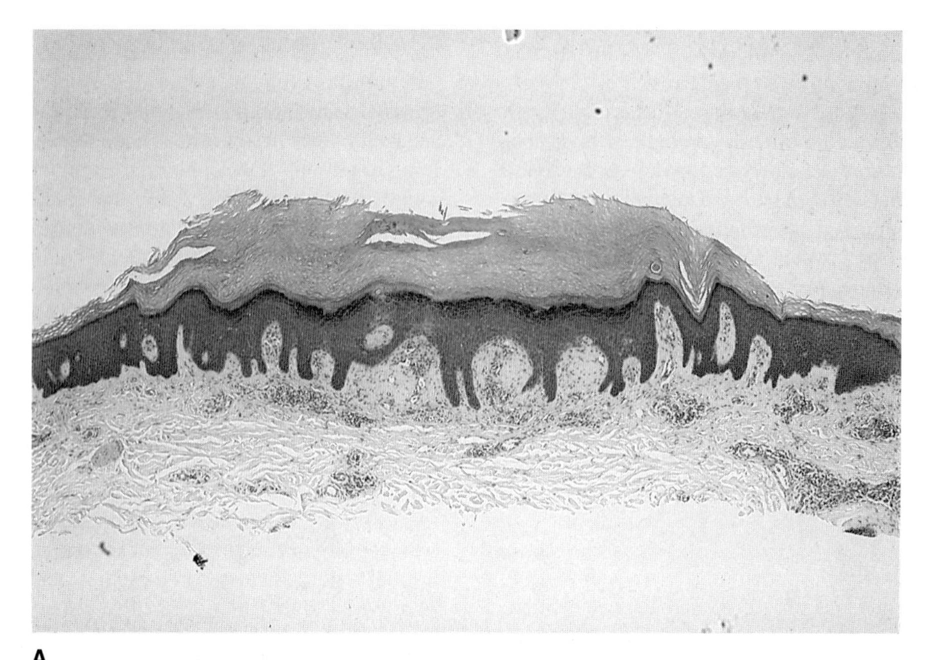

A

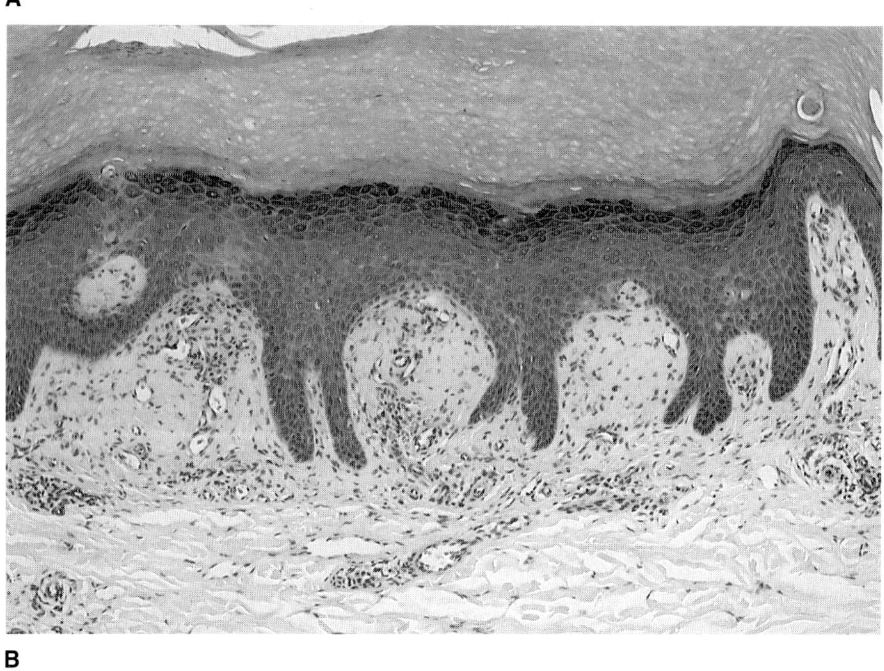

B

FIG. 17-3. Lichen amyloidosis
There is hyperkeratosis and epidermal hyperplasia. Dermal papillae are rounded and contain globular deposits of amyloid. (**A**: H&E, original magnification ×40; **B**: H&E, original magnification ×100; **C**: H&E, original magnification ×200).

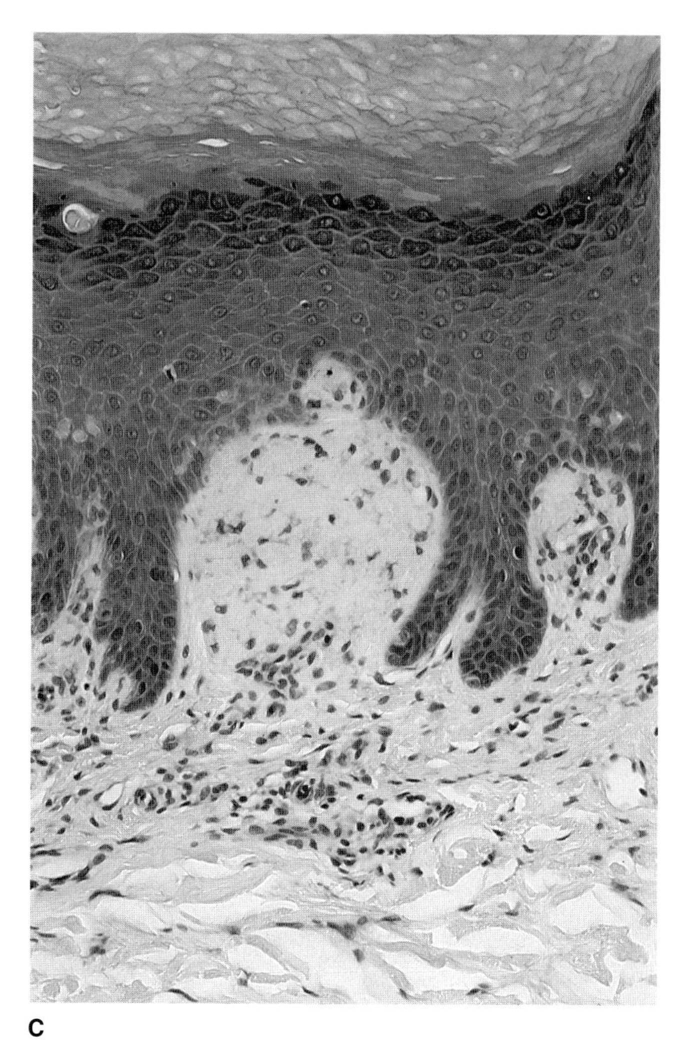

FIG. 17-3. *Continued*

The amyloid that may be found in the stroma or in the adjacent connective tissue of basal cell carcinoma and other epithelial tumors has an appearance on electron microscopy and direct immunofluorescence similar to that of lichen and macular amyloidosis, suggesting that it too is derived from tonofilaments.[45] This amyloid also shows positive staining with antikeratin antiserum.[41]

Nodular Amyloidosis

Nodular amyloidosis is a rare condition in which nodular deposits of AL amyloid are deposited in the skin, but in which there is no apparent systemic involvement. One or several nodules are encountered, usually on the legs[46] or face[47] but occasionally elsewhere. The nodules commonly measure from 1 to 3 cm in diameter. In their centers, the skin may appear atrophic.[48] In exceptional instances, plaques are observed.[49]

Histopathology. Beneath an atrophic epidermis are large masses of amyloid, which extend through the entire dermis into the subcutaneous fat. Amyloid deposits are also found within the walls of blood vessels, in the membrana propria of the sweat glands, and around fat cells.[49] A lymphoplasmacytic infiltrate is scattered through the masses of amyloid and at the periphery.[15,47,48,50] In addition to clusters of plasma cells, Russell bodies and amyloid-containing foreign-body giant cells may be seen.[51]

Differential Diagnosis. On a histologic basis, differentiation of nodular amyloidosis from primary systemic amyloidosis is not possible.

COLLOID MILIUM AND NODULAR COLLOID DEGENERATION

There are three types of colloid degeneration of the skin: (1) juvenile colloid milium, (2) adult colloid milium, and (3) nodular colloid degeneration. Types 1 and 3 are very rare.

Juvenile colloid milium has its onset before puberty and shows numerous round or angular, brownish, waxy papules located mainly on sun-exposed areas, particularly the face.[52,53] In nearly half of the reported cases there is a family history, and the possibility of a hereditary defect has been postulated.[53]

Adult colloid milium, which starts in adult life, is clinically indistinguishable from the juvenile type, except that in some instances it involves the dorsa of the hands in addition to the face and neck.[54,55] Sun exposure often seems to be a precipitating factor.[52]

Nodular colloid degeneration shows either a single large nodule on the face[56] or multiple nodules on the face[57] or the chin and scalp.[58] Sun exposure does not seem to play a role, because in some instances, the lesions are limited to the trunk.[59]

Histopathology. The histologic findings differ in the three types of colloid degeneration, because the colloid in the juvenile form is of epidermal origin, and that in the other two forms is of dermal origin.[52,60]

In juvenile colloid milium, fissured colloid masses fill the papillary dermis. The overlying epidermis is flattened, and basal cells show transformation into colloid bodies.[61] Ultrastructurally, the colloid material is found within individual basal keratinocytes above an intact basement membrane and in extracellular aggregates in the dermis. These deposits contain remnants of nuclear membrane material, degenerating cell organelles, and desmosomes. The fibrillary structure is similar to that of amyloid ultrastructurally, although staining with Congo red failed to result in birefringence, and other stains for amyloid were negative in the case reported by Handfield-Jones et al.[53]

In adult colloid milium, a narrow zone of connective tissue usually separates the homogeneous masses of colloid located in the papillary dermis from the overlying epidermis (Fig. 17-4). Elastic tissue staining shows some elastic fibers in this narrow zone of connective tissue.[52] In addition, solar elastotic fibers are usually seen at the base of the colloid deposits.[62]

In nodular colloid degeneration, the epidermis is flattened. The upper three fourths of the dermis are filled with pale pink, homogeneous material; in some lesions, even the entire dermis is filled with this material[58] (Fig. 17-5). Scattered nuclei of fibroblasts are present within the colloid.[56] There are scattered clefts or fissures, and some dilated capillaries. The hair follicles and sebaceous glands appear well-preserved.[57]

Pathogenesis. The colloid in all three types shows considerable resemblance to amyloid—not only in its histologic appearance but also in its histochemical reactions.[62]

Histochemical staining shows that colloid, like amyloid, is PAS-positive and diastase-resistant. Staining with Congo red

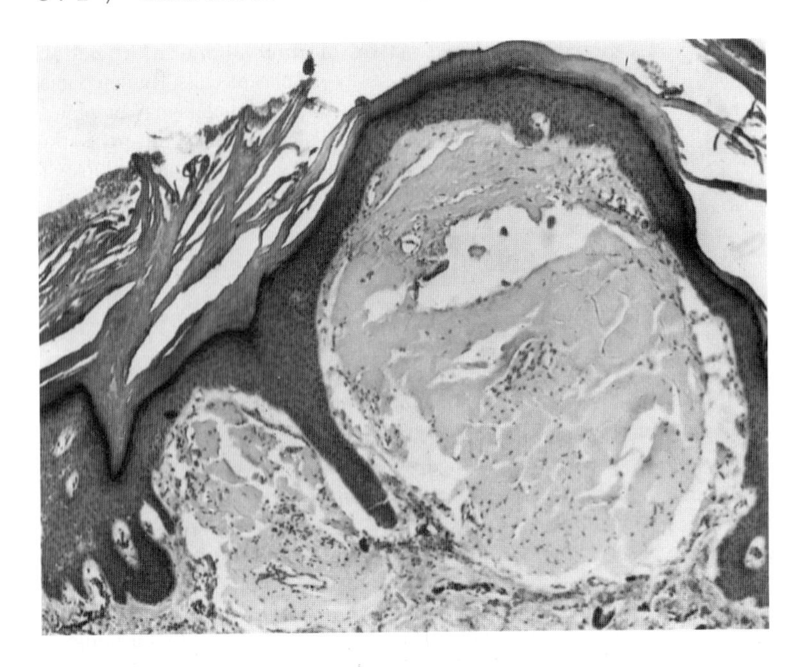

FIG. 17-4. Colloid milium, adult type
Two round, homogeneous, fissured masses of colloid are present in the uppermost dermis. The colloid material greatly resembles the amyloid material observed in primary systemic amyloidosis (see Fig. 17-1).

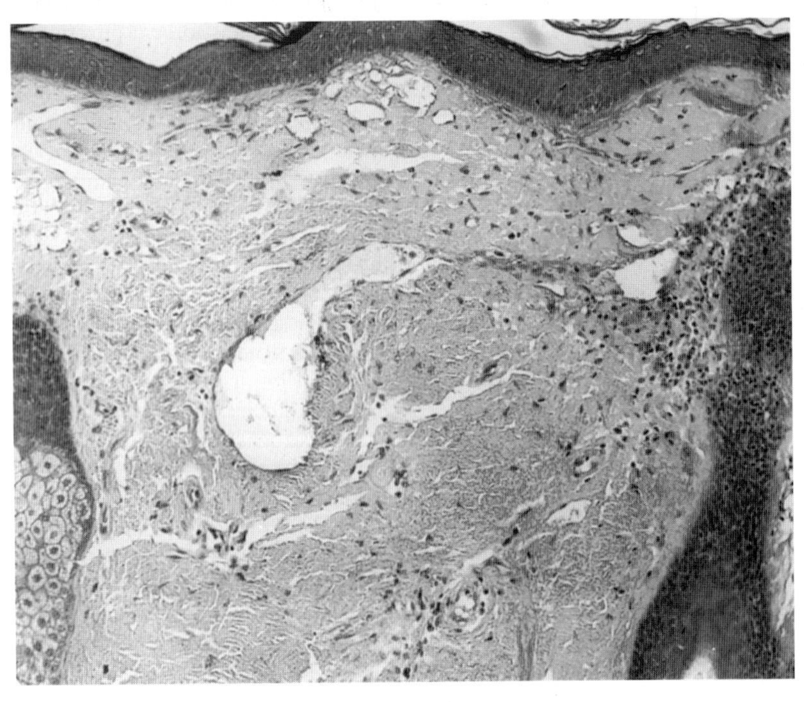

FIG. 17-5. Nodular colloid degeneration
Large masses of colloid are present throughout the dermis. Scattered nuclei of fibroblasts are present within the colloid. The cutaneous appendages are well-preserved.

results in green birefringence (sometimes weak), and the colloid fluoresces after staining with thioflavin T.[62] However, it does not react with pagoda red and other cotton dyes.[63] Serum amyloid P not only is a component of normal and abnormal dermal elastic fibers, but reportedly can be stained immunocytochemically in colloid milium.[64] Juvenile colloid milium exhibits a positive immunostaining reaction to polyclonal antikeratin antibody. This suggests that the histogenesis of this process may differ from that of the adult form in that the colloid in juvenile colloid milium is more likely derived from keratinocytes.[65]

Electron microscopy in a case of juvenile colloid milium has shown that the colloid consists of tightly packed bundles of filaments, 8 to 10 nm thick, in a wavy or whorled arrangement.[60] The colloid, which forms by filamentous degeneration of tonofilaments, maintains a cytoid configuration in the dermis and may contain nuclear remnants.[65,66]

In adult colloid milium, the colloid masses are seen on electron microscopic examination to consist primarily of a granulofibrillar, amorphous substance. On high magnification, very fine filaments, only 2 nm wide, may be seen embedded in the amorphous substance.[52,64] There is rather conclusive evidence that colloid is derived from elastic fibers through sequential degenerative changes. This can be observed at the periphery of the lesion, where colloid is being produced, and within the colloid, where one sees fibrils with a tubular structure and a diameter of 10 nm that are strikingly similar to the microfibrils of elastic fibers.[54] The colloid in adult colloid milium thus represents a final product of severe solar degeneration.[64]

The colloid in nodular colloid degeneration, similar to that in adult colloid milium, consists of an amorphous substance and short, wavy, irregularly arranged filaments.[58] The diameter of these filaments is 3 to 4 nm.[56] These electron microscopic findings exclude nodular amyloidosis as the diagnosis, because in this condition the filaments have a diameter of about 6 to 7 nm and are long and straight.

LIPOID PROTEINOSIS (HYALINOSIS CUTIS ET MUCOSAE; URBACH-WIETHE DISEASE)

This rare disorder is inherited as an autosomal recessive trait. First described by Siebenmann[67] in 1908, it was established as a distinct clinical and histologic entity by Urbach and Wiethe[68] in 1929. In 1932, Urbach coined the term "lipoid proteinosis."[69]

Clinically, there are papular and nodular lesions on the face. Areas of diffuse infiltration associated with hyperkeratosis are observed on the elbows, knees, hands, and occasionally elsewhere. The papules and nodules on the face cause pitted scars, giving the skin a pigskin-leather appearance. Verrucous plaques can form in areas of friction.[70] Beads of small nodules may be present along the free margins of the eyelids. The tongue is firm because of diffuse infiltration. Extension of the infiltration to the frenulum of the tongue restricts normal movement of the tongue, and infiltration of the vocal cords causes hoarseness, which may be present at birth. Convulsive seizures are not uncommon.[71,72]

Histopathology. There is extensive cutaneous deposition of amorphous eosinophilic material surrounding capillaries, sweat coils and in the thickened papillary dermis (Fig. 17-6). Focal deposits are found in the deeper dermis. In verrucous lesions, the homogeneous bundles often are oriented perpendicular to the skin surface. This hyaline material is PAS-positive and resistant to diastase digestion. Staining with alcian blue at pH 2.9 is slightly positive and is sensitive to hyaluronidase digestion.[73] The presence of lipids is variable and likely results from adherence of lipids to glycoproteins, rather than from abnormal lipid production.[74]

Systemic Lesions. Intracranial calcification has been noted quite frequently in x-ray examination of patients with lipoid proteinosis and has been held responsible for convulsive seizures in these patients.[71,75] Autopsy findings have established that the calcium is deposited within the walls of capillaries located in the hippocampal gyri of the temporal lobes.[76] The fact that, after decalcification, a mantle of PAS-positive material is observed around the endothelium of these vessels indicates that hyalinization precedes calcification of the capillary walls.

The widespread distribution of the pericapillary hyalin deposits has been established by biopsies and autopsies. Deposits have been found in the submucosae of the upper respiratory and digestive tracts and in the submucosae of the stomach, jejunum, rectum, and vagina; in the retina between the vitreous membrane and the pigment epithelium; and in the testes, pancreas, lungs, kidneys, and elsewhere.[72,76]

Pathogenesis. Two different substances present in lesions of lipoid proteinosis have the light microscopic appearance of hyalin because they consist of homogeneous eosinophilic material and are PAS-positive and diastase-resistant.[73,77] Their different appearances and origins, however, become evident on electron microscopy.[78,79] One is true hyalin, produced by fibroblasts, and the other represents hyalin-like material consisting of multiplications of basal laminae and is produced by a variety of cells (see later), but not by fibroblasts.

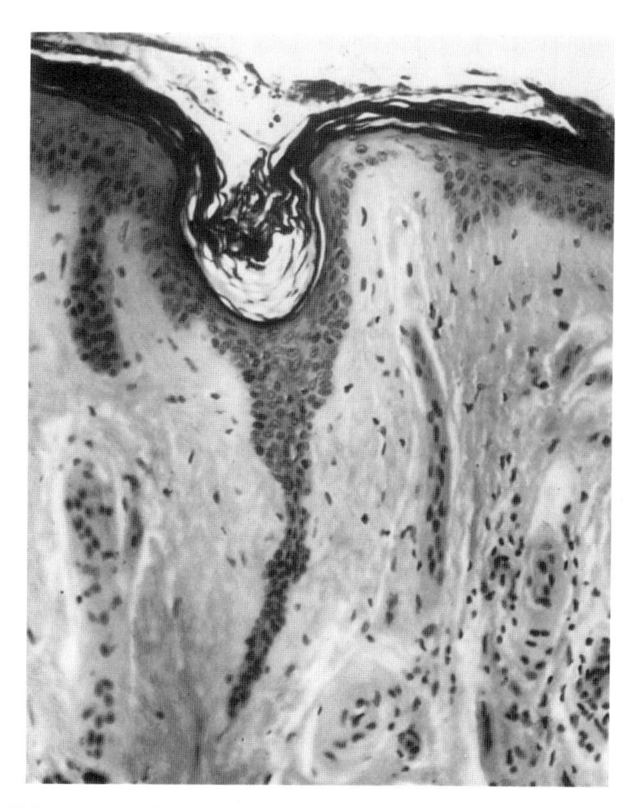

FIG. 17-6. Lipoid proteinosis
The hyaline material consists of thick, homogeneous bundles that extend perpendicular to the skin surface. In addition, thick hyaline mantles surround the blood vessels.

Lipids are not an essential feature of the disease. They can be removed with lipid solvents without damage to the protein-carbohydrate complex of the true hyalin. This suggests that the lipids are either free or loosely bound to the hyaline.[80]

Although the pathogenesis of LP is not well understood, it may result from one or several enzyme defects leading to abnormal accumulation of glycoproteins.[81]

There is also evidence to support altered distribution of genetically distinct collagen types.[82]

On electron microscopic examination, three major alterations are noted in the dermis: (1) a considerable thickening of basal laminae; (2) massive depositions of amorphous material (hyalin), predominantly in the upper dermis and around blood vessels;[83] and (3) a marked reduction in the number and size of collagen fibrils.[79,82]

The thickening of the basal laminae in multiple layers is evident around small blood vessels, skin appendages, smooth muscle cells, perineuria, and Schwann cells.[84] In contrast, there is almost no multiplication of the basal lamina of the epidermis.[84] Around capillaries, basal laminae consist of as many as 20 layers, and occasionally even more, arranged in a concentric "onion-skin" arrangement.[83] Interspersed between these layers are fine collagen fibrils in an amorphous matrix. The thickened basement membranes stain intensively for laminin and collagen type IV.[79]

A unique feature of hyalinosis cutis et mucosae consists of large depositions of amorphous material in the dermis. The exact chemical nature of this hyaline material is not known, but it is a noncollagenous glycoprotein that contains neither laminin nor fibronectin.[79]

The collagen within the areas of hyalin deposits appears as fine but otherwise normal fibrils arranged in bundles or in random fashion. Most fibrils have a diameter less than 50 nm, compared with the usual size of 70 to 140 nm. Involved skin shows a fivefold reduction in collagen type I, the major collagen species of normal skin, and to a lesser extent in collagen type III, as indicated by cell culture studies. As judged by the contents of glycine and hydroxyproline, normal skin contains about 80% collagen, but involved skin in hyalinosis cutis et mucosae contains only 20% collagen as the result of a large accumulation of noncollagenous glycoproteins.

Cultured fibroblasts from lesions of hyalinosis cutis et mucosae have shown an increased synthesis of noncollagenous proteins at the expense of newly synthesized collagens. The hyaline material in hyalinosis cutis et mucosae originates from the overproduction of noncollagenous proteins, most of which are normal constituents of human skin.[79]

Differential Diagnosis. Porphyria shows deposits of hyalin-like material around the superficial dermal capillaries indistinguishable from the perivascular deposits of hyalin-like material seen in lipoid proteinosis. However, involvement of the membrana propria of the sweat glands is rare, and no true dermal hyaline is present. In addition, the cutaneous lesions in porphyria are limited to sun-exposed areas.

PORPHYRIA

Seven types of porphyria are recognized (Table 17-1). The light sensitivity in the six types with cutaneous lesions is caused by wavelengths that are absorbed by the porphyrin molecule. These wavelengths lie in the 400-nm range, respresenting long-wave ultraviolet light (UVA) and visible light.[85]

In *erythropoietic porphyria*, a very rare disease which typically develops during infancy or childhood, recurrent vesiculobullous eruptions in sun-exposed areas of the skin gradually result in mutilating ulcerations and scarring. It is inherited in an autosomal recessive pattern.[86] Hypertrichosis and brown-stained teeth that fluoresce are additional features.[87,88]

In *erythropoietic protoporphyria*, the usual reaction to light is erythema and edema followed by thickening and superficial scarring of the skin.[89] In rare instances, vesicles are present that may resemble those seen in hydroa vacciniforme.[90–92] The protoporphyrin is formed in reticulocytes in the bone marrow and is then carried in circulating erythrocytes and in the plasma. When a smear of blood from a patient is examined under a fluorescence microscope, large numbers of red-fluorescing ery-

TABLE 17-1. *Classification of the porphyrias*

Porphyrias	Type; heredity; onset	Cutaneous manifestations	Extra-cutaneous manifestations	Urine	Feces	Erythrocytes	Enzymatic defect
Erythropoietic porphyria	Ery; Rec; Infancy	Blisters, severe scarring	Red teeth; hemolytic anemia	Uro I	Copro I	Uro I, stable fluorescence	Uroporphyrinogen III cosynthase
Erythropoietic protoporphyria	Ery; Dom; Childhood	Burning, edema, thickening, rarely blisters	Rarely fatal liver disease	Negative	Protoporphyrin continuously	Protoporphyrin, transient fluoresence	Ferrochelatase (Heme synthase)
Acute intermittent porphyria (AIP)	Hep; Dom; Young adulthood	Negative	Abdominal pain, neuropathy, psychoses	ALA, PBG continuously	Negative	Negative	Uroporphyrinogen I synthase
Porphyria variegata	Hep; Dom; Young adulthood	Same as PCT	Same as AIP	ALA, PBG during attacks	Protoporphyrin continuously	Negative	Protoporphyrinogen oxidase
Porphyria cutanea tarda (PCT)	Hep; Dom; Middle age	Blisters, scarring, thickening	Decreased liver function, siderosis	Uro III, continuous fluorescence		Negative	Uroporphyrinogen decarboxylase
Hepatoerythrocytic porphyria (homozygous form of PCT)	Ery and Hep; Dom; Childhood	Blisters, severe scarring, thickening	Decreased liver function	Uro I, Uro III	Copro I, Copro III	Protoporphyrin	Uroporphyrinogen decarboxylase
Hereditary coproporphyria	Hep; Dom; Young adulthood	Same as PCT	Same as AIP	Copro, ALA, PBG during attacks	Copro continuously	Negative	Coproporphyrinogen oxidase

AIP = acute intermittent porphyria; ALA = delta-aminolevulinic acid; Copro = coproporphyrin; Dom = autosomal dominant; Ery = erythropoietic; Hep = hepatic; PBG = porphobilinogen; PCT = porphyria cutanea tarda; Rec = autosomal recessive; Uro = uroporphyrin.

throcytes are observed. The protoporphyrin is cleared from the plasma by the liver and excreted into the bile and feces.[93] It is not found in the urine. In rare instances, fatal liver disease develops quite suddenly, usually in persons of middle age[94] but occasionally in patients only in the second decade of life.[95,96] (See also Histogenesis.)

In *porphyria variegata*, different members of the same family may have either cutaneous manifestations identical to those of porphyria cutanea tarda or systemic involvement analogous to acute intermittent porphyria, or both, or the condition may remain latent.[92,97] The presence of protoporphyrin in the feces distinguishes porphyria variegata from porphyria cutanea tarda (see Table 17-1).[98] Also, a sharp fluorescence emission peak at 626 nm is specific for the plasma of porphyria variegata.[99,100]

In *porphyria cutanea tarda*, a dominantly inherited disorder, three forms can be distinguished: sporadic, familial, and hepatoerythropoietic.[101] In the *sporadic form*, only the hepatic activity of uroporphyrinogen decarboxylase is decreased. Almost all patients are adults, and no clinical evidence of porphyria cutanea tarda is found in other members of the patient's family. Although the sporadic form can occur without any precipitating factor,[102] in most instances, in addition to the inherited enzymatic defect, an acquired damaging factor to liver function is needed. The damaging agent most commonly is ethanol but may also be estrogens.[103]

In the *familial form*, in addition to the hepatic activity, the extrahepatic activity of uroporphyrinogen decarboxylase is decreased to about 50% of normal. The enzymatic activity usually is determined on the erythrocytes. The familial form may occur at any age, including childhood, and often, but not always, there is a family history of overt porphyria cutanea tarda.

In the very rare *hepatoerythropoietic form*, the skin lesions appear in childhood and the activity of uroporphyrinogen decarboxylase in all organs is decreased to less than 10% of normal. Family studies suggest that these patients are homozygous for the gene that causes porphyria cutanea tarda.[101]

Clinically, the sporadic form of porphyria cutanea tarda, by far the most common type of porphyria, shows blisters that arise through a combination of sun exposure and minor trauma, mainly on the dorsa of the hands but sometimes also on the face. Mild scarring may result. The skin of the face and the dorsa of the hands often are thickened and sclerotic. Hypertrichosis of the face is common. Evidence of hepatic cirrhosis with siderosis is regularly present but generally is mild.[104] In rare instances, a malignant hepatoma or a carcinoma metastatic to the liver induces porphyria cutanea tarda.[105] In the familial form of porphyria cutanea tarda, the clinical picture is similar to that of the sporadic form, but the changes are more pronounced. In the hepatoerythropoietic form, the manifestations are even more severe. On clinical grounds, the symptoms of most patients resemble those of erythropoietic porphyria, but when symptoms are milder they resemble those of erythropoietic protoporphyria.[106] Vesicular eruptions lead to ulceration, severe scarring, partial alopecia, and sclerosis.[107] Erythrocytes and teeth may show fluorescence.[108] Liver damage develops with increasing age.[109]

In *hereditary coproporphyria*, a very rare disorder, there are episodic attacks of abdominal pain and a variety of neurologic and psychiatric disturbances analogous to those observed in acute intermittent porphyria and porphyria variegata.[110] In some cases, there are also cutaneous manifestations indistinguishable from those of porphyria cutanea tarda and porphyria variegata.[110,111]

Histopathology. The histologic changes in the skin lesions are the same in all six types of porphyria with cutaneous lesions. Differences are based on the severity rather than on the type of porphyria. Homogeneous, eosinophilic material is regularly observed, and bullae are present in some instances. In addition, sclerosis of the collagen is present in old lesions.[112,113]

In mild cases, homogeneous, pale, eosinophilic deposits are limited to the immediate vicinity of the blood vessels in the papillary dermis.[113] These deposits are best visualized with a PAS stain, because they are PAS-positive and diastase-resistant.

In severely involved areas, which are most common in erythropoietic protoporphyria, the perivascular mantles of homogeneous material are wide enough in the papillary dermis to coalesce with those of adjoining capillaries. In addition, deeper blood vessels may show homogeneous material around them, and similar homogeneous material may be found occasionally around eccrine glands.[114] PAS staining demonstrates this material particularly well. In some instances, it also contains acid mucopolysaccharides, shown with alcian blue or the colloidal iron stain,[113] or lipids, demonstrable with Sudan IV or Sudan black B.[90,114] In addition, the PAS-positive epidermal-dermal basement membrane zone may be thickened.[113]

In areas of sclerosis, which occur especially in porphyria cutanea tarda, the collagen bundles are thickened. In contrast to scleroderma, PAS-positive, diastase-resistant material is often present in the dermis in perivascular locations.[113]

The bullae, which are most common in porphyria cutanea tarda and least common in erythropoietic protoporphyria, arise subepidermally (Fig. 17-7A and B). Some blisters are dermolytic and arise beneath the PAS-positive basement membrane zone;[115] others form in the lamina lucida and are situated above the PAS-positive basement membrane zone[116] (Fig. 17-8). It has been suggested that the blisters in porphyria cutanea tarda in mild cases arise within the junctional zone, but that in severe cases they form beneath the PAS-positive basement membrane zone and thus heal with scarring.[117] It is quite characteristic of the bullae of porphyria cutanea tarda that the dermal papillae often extend irregularly from the floor of the bulla into the bulla cavity.[100,118] This phenomenon, referred to as "festooning," is explained by the rigidity of the upper dermis induced by the presence of eosinophilic material within and around the capillary walls in the papillae and the papillary dermis.

The epidermis forming the roof of the blister often contains eosinophilic bodies that are elongate and sometimes segmented.[119] These "caterpillar bodies" are PAS-positive and diastase-resistant. Ultrastructurally, they have been found to contain three components: (1) cellular organelles, including melanosomes, desmosomes, and mitochondria; (2) colloid that may be located intracellularly or extracellularly; and (3) electron-dense material thought to be of basement membrane origin.[120]

Pathogenesis. The substance around dermal vessels has the appearance of hyalin because it consists of homogeneous, eosinophilic material and is PAS-positive and diastase-resistant. However, just as the perivascular material in lipoid proteinosis, it is only hyalin-like and consists of multiplications of basal laminae.[121] True hyalin, which is present in large amounts in the dermis of lipoid proteinosis, and is produced by fibroblasts as amorphous material, is absent.

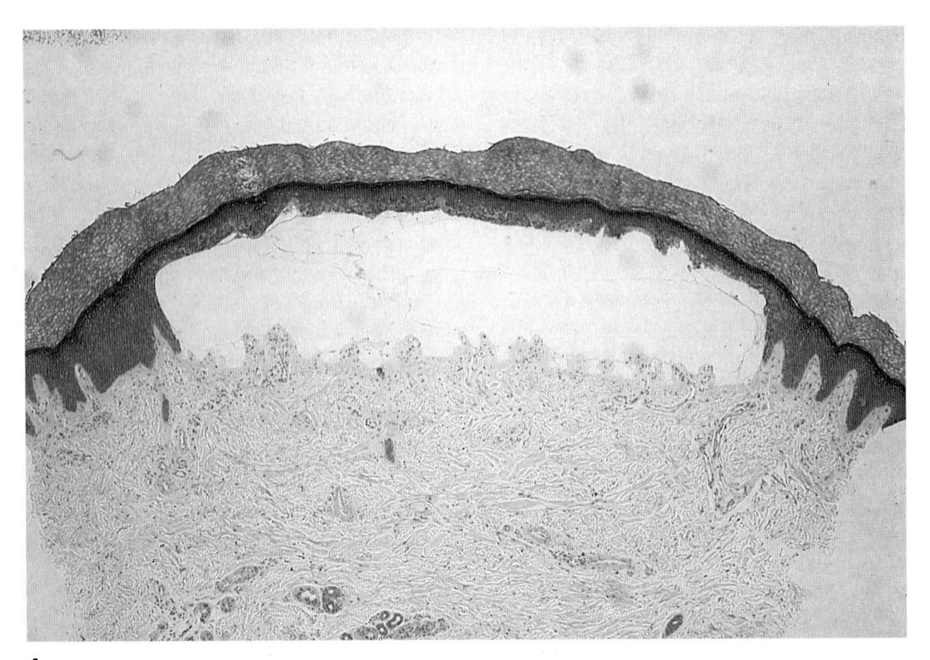

A

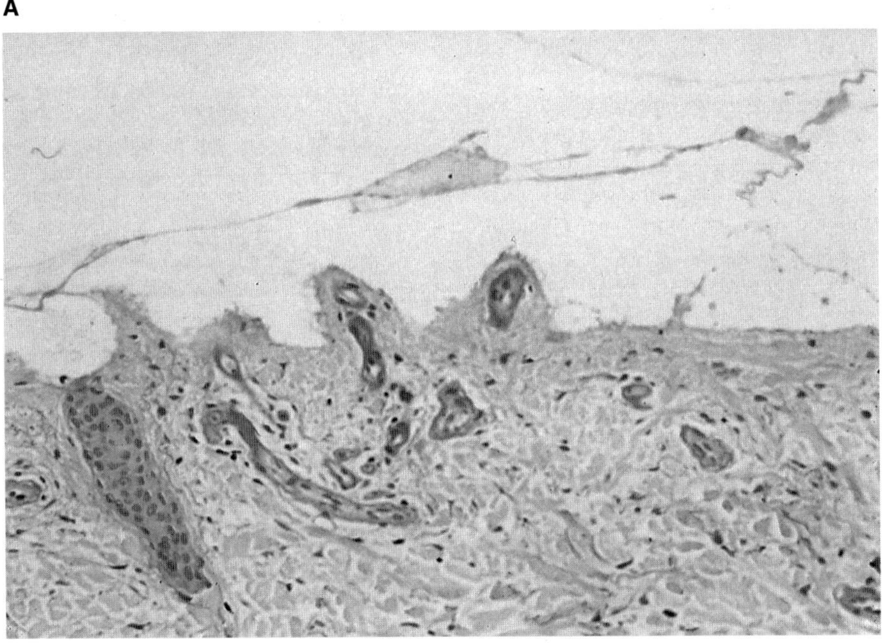

B

FIG. 17-7. Porphyria cutanea tarda
(**A**) There is a subepidermal blister. The architecture of the dermal papillae remains intact. The dermis contains no significant inflammatory infiltrate (H&E). (**B**) Vessels within preserved dermal papillae at the blister base are surrounded by PAS-positive diastase-resistant deposits (D-PAS).

On electron microscopic examination, one observes concentric multiplications of the basement membrane around the dermal blood vessels. Peripheral to this multilayered basement membrane, one observes a thick mantle of unlayered material with the same filamentous and amorphous composition as that of the basement membrane. Often, a gradual transition from the layered to the unlayered zone can be observed.[121,122] Scattered through the thick, unlayered zone are solitary collagen fibrils with an average diameter of only 35 nm, in contrast to the 100 nm of mature collagen.[112,121] In cases with severe involvement, intermingled filamentous and amorphous material is seen throughout the upper dermis and even in the middermis.

Proof that the perivascular material in porphyria represents excessively synthesized basement membrane material and as such contains type IV collagen is provided by positive immunofluorescence staining with anti-type IV collagen monospecific antibody.[123] The presence of small collagen fibrils analogous to reticulum fibrils suggests the presence also of type III collagen.

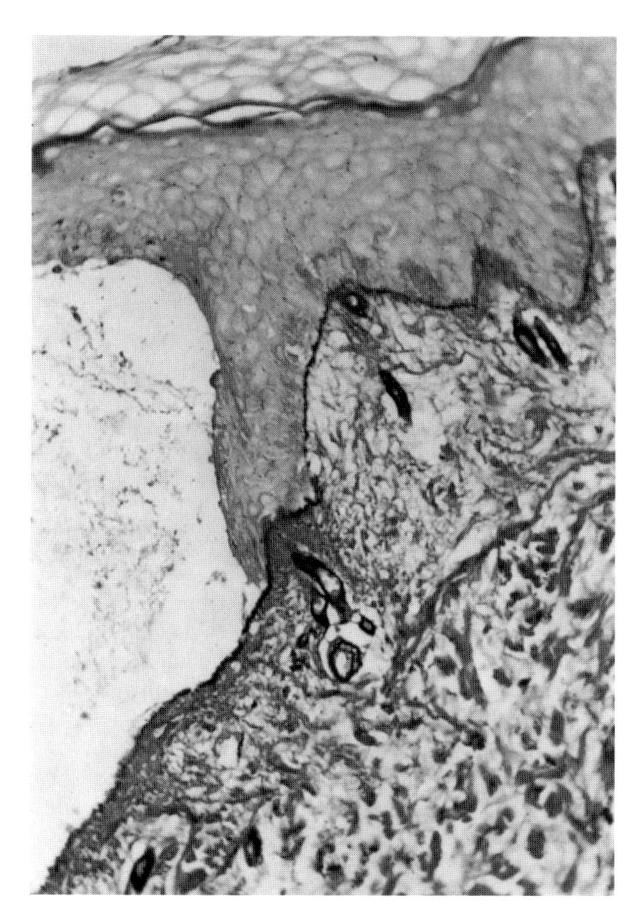

FIG. 17-8. Porphyria cutanea tarda
On staining with the PAS reaction after diastase digestion, the PAS-positive basement membrane zone is observed at the floor of the blister. PAS-positive hyalin is present in the walls of capillaries in the upper dermis.

Direct immunofluorescence testing has revealed in the majority of patients the presence of immunoglobulins, particularly IgG,[113] and occasionally also of complement,[124] in the walls of blood vessels and at the epidermal-dermal junction of light-exposed skin. It is unlikely that these deposits indicate an immunologic phenomenon; rather, they are the result of "trapping" of immunoglobulins and complement in the filamentous material.

The *enzymatic defect* that causes each form of prophyria is known (see Table 17-1). Enzyme determinations may be carried out on cultured skin fibroblasts, erythrocytes, or liver tissue.

Liver damage is generally mild and chronic in porphyria cutanea tarda. In erythropoietic protoporphyria, however, liver function tests are usually normal, even though microscopic deposits of protoporphyrin in the liver are frequently found.[91] Yet, in rare instances, death occurs from liver failure developing swiftly after the initial detection of hepatic dysfunction.[94] Patients with liver failure have very high levels of protoporphyrin in the erythrocytes and, at the time of death, show extensive deposits of protoporphyrin in a cirrhotic liver. The protoporphyrin in hepatocytes and Kupffer cells appears as dark brown granules.[96] This pigment exhibits birefringence on polariscopic examination and, in unstained sections viewed with ultraviolet light, shows red autofluorescence.[94] In patients with normal liver function tests, biopsy of the liver may or may not show portal and periportal fibrosis.[95]

Pseudoporphyria Cutanea Tarda

In patients with chronic renal failure who are receiving maintenance hemodialysis, an eruption indistinguishable from that of porphyria cutanea tarda may develop on the dorsa of the hands and fingers during the summer months.[125] Rarely, blisters are seen also on the face, and atrophic scarring develops.[126] In a series of 180 patients receiving hemodialysis, 28 (16%) showed this type of eruption.[127] Normal porphyrin levels in urine, stool, and plasma are the rule in hemodialyzed patients developing clinical signs of porphyria cutanea tarda. However, in a few patients receiving hemodialysis for chronic renal failure, a true porphyria cutanea tarda coexists.[128,129] In such patients, if a certain degree of diuresis persists, urinalysis may not be representative of the porphyria metabolism, and the plasma and fecal porphyrins should always be measured.[130]

Porphyria cutanea tarda may also occur following the ingestion of certain drugs, such as furosemide, nalidixic acid, tetracycline hydrochloride, and naproxen.[131] Because many patients on hemodialysis for renal failure also are receiving furosemide, withdrawal of the drug can determine whether the dialysis or the medication is the cause of the pseudoporphyria, because in drug-induced cases, withdrawal of the drug is curative.[131]

Histopathology. In patients with pseudoporphyria, the histologic picture is indistinguishable from that seen in mild cases of porphyria. The superficial blood vessels show thickened walls, and the PAS-positive basement membrane zone is often thickened as well. Blisters are subepidermal, with festooned dermal papillae. The blisters usually are situated above the PAS-positive basement membrane zone.[126,131]

Pathogenesis. Electron microscopic findings are identical to those of porphyria.[127] As in porphyria, immunoglobulins are often observed in vessel walls and at the epidermal-dermal junction. Complement is also occasionally present.[125,127]

CALCINOSIS CUTIS

There are four forms of calcinosis cutis: metastatic calcinosis cutis, dystrophic calcinosis cutis, idiopathic calcinosis cutis, and subepidermal calcified nodule.

Metastatic Calcinosis Cutis

Metastatic calcification develops as the result of hypercalcemia or hyperphosphatemia. Hypercalcemia may result from (1) primary hyperparathyroidism, (2) excessive intake of vitamin D,[132] (3) excessive intake of milk and alkali,[133] or (4) extensive destruction of bone through osteomyelitis or metastases of a carcinoma.[134] Hyperphosphatemia occurs in chronic renal failure as the result of a decrease in renal clearance of phosphorus and is associated with a compensatory drop in the serum calcium level. The low level of ionized calcium in the serum stimulates parathyroid secretion, leading to secondary hyperparathyroidism and to resorption of calcium and phosphorus from bone. The demineralization of bone causes both osteodystrophy and metastatic calcification.[135,136]

Metastatic calcification most commonly affects the media of the arteries and the kidneys. In addition, other visceral organs, such as the myocardium, the stomach, and the lungs,[135,137] may be involved.

Metastatic calcification in the subcutaneous tissue is occasionally observed in association with renal hyperparathyroidism,[135] in uremia,[138] in hypervitaminosis D,[132] and as the result of excessive intake of milk and alkali,[133] but rarely in primary hyperparathyroidism.[134] Palpable, hard nodules, occasionally of considerable size, are located mainly in the vicinity of the large joints.[135] With an increase in size, the nodules may become fluctuant.[139]

Calciphylaxis is a life-threatening condition in which there is progressive calcification of small and medium-sized vessels of the subcutis with subsequent vascular compromise resulting in ischemia and necrosis. It most frequently arises in the setting of hyperparathyroidism associated with chronic renal failure.[140] Calciphylaxis is often, but not always, associated with an elevated serum calcium/phosphate product.[141]

Clinically, the lesions present as a panniculitis or vasculitis. Bullae, ulcerations, or a lividoreticulosis-like eruption can be present.[140,141]

Instances of *cutaneous metastatic calcinosis* are rare. Most reports have concerned patients with renal hyperparathyroidism and osteodystrophy. The cutaneous lesions may consist of firm, white papules,[142] papules in a linear arrangement,[139] symmetric, nodular plaques,[136] or papules and nodules from which a granular, white substance can be expressed.[143]

Mural calcification of arteries and arterioles in the deep dermis or in the subcutaneous tissue occurs rarely in primary hyperparathyroidism[144] but somewhat more frequently in secondary hyperparathyroidism subsequent to renal disease and particularly if subsequent to dialysis for chronic renal disease or to renal allograft.[145,146] This may lead to occlusion of these vessels and to infarctive ulcerations, especially on the legs.

Histopathology. Calcium deposits are recognized easily in histologic sections, because they stain deep blue with hematoxylin-eosin. They stain black with the von Kossa stain for calcium. As a rule, the calcium occurs as massive deposits when located in the subcutaneous fat (Fig. 17-9) and usually as granules and small deposits when located in the dermis. Large deposits of calcium often evoke a foreign-body reaction, so that giant cells, an inflammatory infiltrate, and fibrosis may be present around them.[136]

In areas of infarctive necrosis, as a result of calcification of dermal or subcutaneous arteries or arterioles, the involved vessels show calcification of their walls and intravascular fibrosis with attempts at recanalization of the obstructed lumina.[144] Mural calcification often is most pronounced in the internal elastic membranes of arteries or arterioles.[145]

The histologic changes in calciphylaxis include calcium deposits in the subcutis, chiefly within the walls of small and medium-sized vessels. These deposits can be associated with endovascular fibrosis, thrombosis, or global calcific obliteration.[147] Calcification can also be identified within the soft tissues (Fig. 17-10). The vascular lesions result in ischemic and/or gangrenous necrosis of the subcutaneous fat and overlying skin.

It is particularly important that these findings be recognized in order that appropriate therapy, which often includes parathyroidectomy, might be instituted immediately.

Dystrophic Calcinosis Cutis

In dystrophic calcinosis cutis, the calcium is deposited in previously damaged tissue. The values for serum calcium and phosphorus are normal, and the internal organs are spared. There may be numerous large deposits of calcium

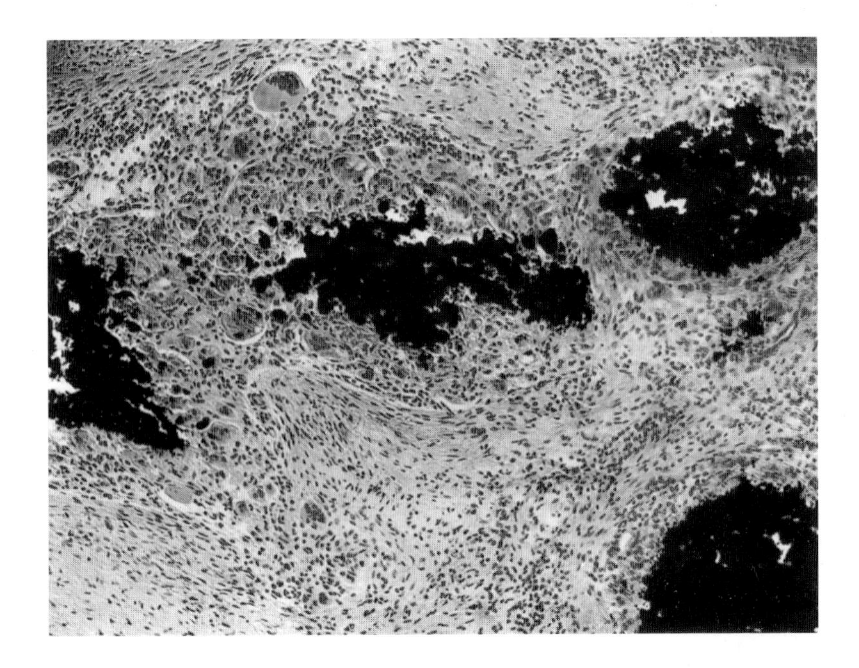

FIG. 17-9. Metastatic calcinosis cutis
The condition was caused by hypercalcemia produced by prolonged and excessive intake of vitamin D. The von Kossa stain for calcium demonstrates irregular masses of calcium surrounded by a foreign-body giant-cell reaction in the subcutaneous fat.

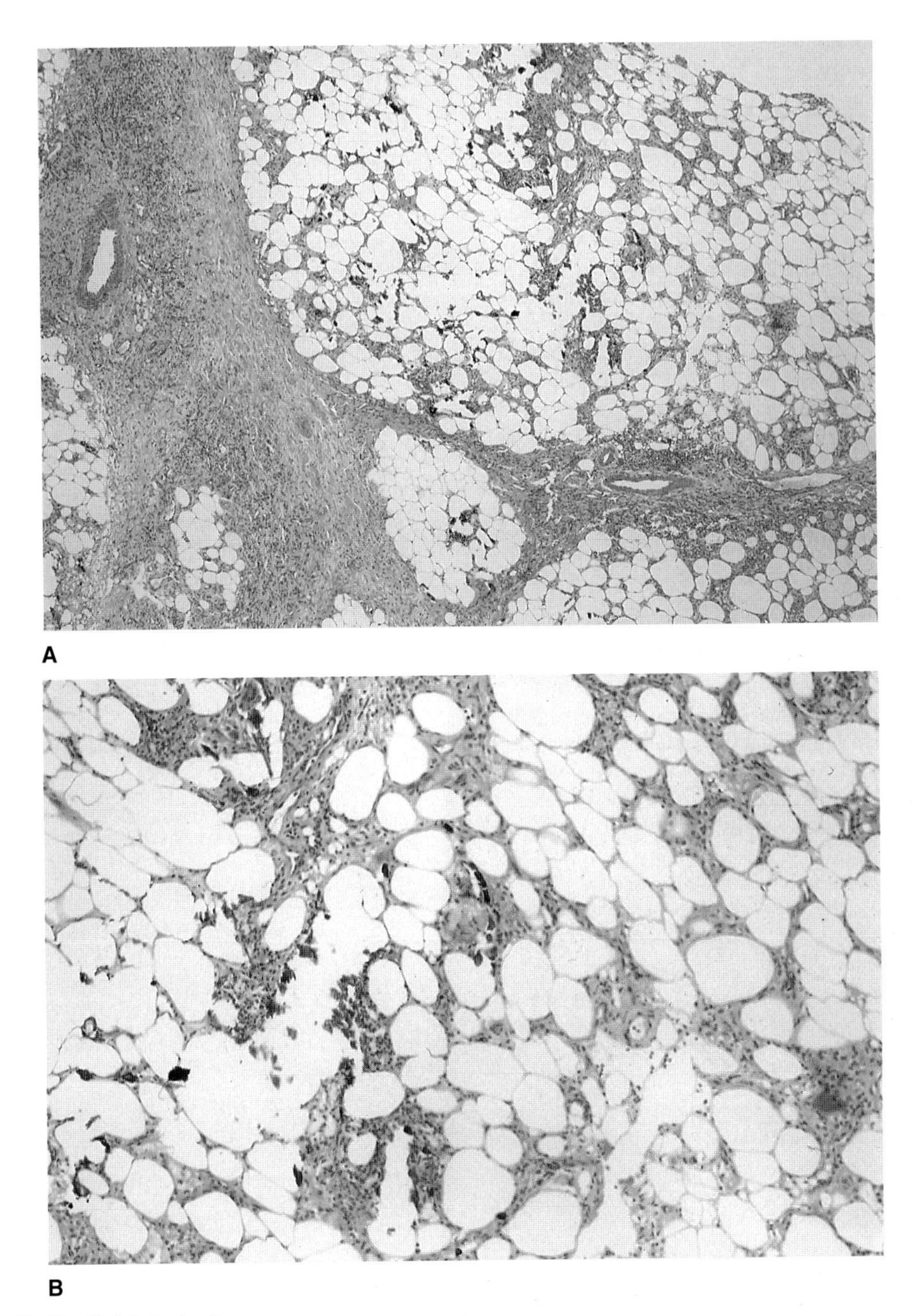

FIG. 17-10. Calciphylaxis
There is a panniculitis with associated calcification of soft tissues in the walls of small vessels (**A**: H&E, original magnification ×20; **B**: H&E, original magnification ×100).

(calcinosis universalis) or only a few deposits (calcinosis circumscripta).

Calcinosis universalis occurs as a rule in patients with dermatomyositis, but, exceptionally, it has also been observed in patients with systemic scleroderma.[148] Large deposits of calcium are found in the skin and subcutaneous tissue and often in muscles and tendons.[149] In dermatomyositis, if the patient survives, the nodules of dystrophic calcinosis gradually resolve.

Calcinosis circumscripta occurs as a rule in patients with systemic scleroderma; rarely, however, it may be observed in patients with widespread morphea.[150,151] Generally, in the presence of calcinosis, systemic scleroderma manifests itself as acrosclerosis. The association of acrosclerosis and calcinosis is often referred to as the Thibierge-Weissenbach syndrome or as the CREST syndrome, because the manifestations usually consist of calcinosis cutis, Raynaud's phenomenon, esophageal dysfunction, sclerodactyly, and telangiectasia.[148,150,152] Patients with this syndrome often have a better prognosis than those with generalized scleroderma or systemic sclerosis. Clinically, calcinosis circumscripta shows successively appearing areas of induration that often break down and extrude white, chalky material.

Lupus erythematosus is only rarely associated with dystrophic calcinosis cutis.[153]

In addition to occurring in the connective tissue diseases, dystrophic calcinosis is often seen in subcutaneous fat necrosis of the newborn and, rarely, in the subcutaneous nodules occurring in Ehlers-Danlos disease.

Histopathology. As in metastatic calcinosis cutis, the calcium in dystrophic calcinosis cutis usually is present as granules or small deposits in the dermis and as massive deposits in the subcutaneous tissue.[151] A foreign-body giant-cell reaction is often found around large deposits of calcium.[154] The calcium deposits usually are located in areas in which the collagen or fatty tissue appears degenerated as a result of the disease preceding the calcinosis.

Idiopathic Calcinosis Cutis

Even though the underlying connective tissue disease in some instances of dystrophic calcinosis cutis may be mild and can be overlooked unless specifically searched for, there remain cases of idiopathic calcinosis cutis that resemble dystrophic calcinosis cutis but show no underlying disease.[155–157]

One entity is regarded as a special manifestation of idiopathic calcinosis cutis: tumoral calcinosis. It consists of numerous large, subcutaneous, calcified masses that may be associated with papular and nodular skin lesions of calcinosis.[158,159] The disease usually is familial and is associated with hyperphosphatemia.[159,160] Otherwise, the resemblance of tumoral calcinosis to the dystrophic calcinosis universalis observed with dermatomyositis is great.

Histopathology. Tumoral calcinosis shows in the subcutaneous tissue large masses of calcium surrounded by a foreign-body reaction.[154] Intradermal aggregates are present in some cases. Discharge of calcium may take place through areas of ulceration or by means of transepidermal elimination.[159]

Pathogenesis. Two authors have studied lesions of idiopathic calcinosis cutis by electron microscopy.[155,156] They agree that the deposits consist of pleomorphic calcium phosphate (apatite) crystals. However, according to one opinion the earliest deposits of calcium are situated in the ground substance,[155] whereas according to the other the earliest calcium deposits lie within collagen fibrils and subsequently extend into the ground substance as the apatite crystals grow.[156]

Idiopathic Calcinosis of the Scrotum

Idiopathic calcinosis of the scrotum consists of multiple asymptomatic nodules of the scrotal skin. The nodules begin to appear in childhood or in early adult life, increase in size and number, and sometimes break down to discharge their chalky contents.[161]

Histopathology. At one time the accepted view was that some of the calcific masses in calcinosis of the scrotum were surrounded by a granulomatous foreign-body reaction and others were not.[161,162] However, in recent publications in which numerous scrotal nodules were examined, some of the lesions were epidermal cysts, whereas other cystic lesions showed calcification of their keratin contents, and still others showed ruptures of their epithelial walls. The cyst wall was eventually destroyed, leaving only dermal collections of calcium. Thus, according to this view, calcinosis of the scrotum represents the end stage of dystrophic calcification of scrotal epidermal cysts.[163,164] Other authors who also had examined either several patients or multiple nodules agreed that the lesions originated from cysts. One author favored eccrine duct milia as the origin because of a positive reaction for carcinoembryonic antigen, a marker of eccrine sweat glands.[165] Another author found various types of cysts: epidermal, pilar, and indeterminate cysts showing various degrees of calcification.[166] One can assume that early lesions start out as cysts but, as they age and calcify, lose their cyst walls. It is likely that authors who found no cyst walls were examining old lesions.

Subepidermal Calcified Nodule

In subepidermal calcified nodule, also referred to as cutaneous calculi, usually a single small, raised, hard nodule is present. Occasionally, however, there are two or three nodules,[167,168] and in some instances there are numerous[169] or even innumerable[170] nodules. Most patients are children, but in some patients a nodule is present at birth[171] or does not appear until adulthood.[172] In most instances, the surface of the nodule is verrucous, but it may be smooth. The most common location of the nodule is the face.

Histopathology. The calcified material is located predominantly in the uppermost dermis, although in large nodules it may extend into the deep layers of the dermis. The calcium is present largely as closely aggregated globules (Fig. 17-11). In some instances, however, there is also one or several large, homogeneous masses of calcified material[167,168] (Fig. 17-12). Both the globules and the homogeneous masses occasionally contain well-preserved nuclei.[167] Macrophages and foreign-body giant cells may be arranged around the large, homogeneous masses.[167] The epidermis is often hypertrophic. Calcium granules may be observed within the epidermis, indicative of transepidermal elimination.[170,173]

Pathogenesis. The primary event seems to be the formation of large, homogeneous masses that undergo calcification and break up into numerous calcified globules.[168] The origin of the homogeneous masses is obscure. It is not likely that they originate from a specific preexisting structure, such as sweat ducts[171] or nevus cells,[172] as has been assumed.

GOUT

In the early stage of gout, there usually are irregularly recurring attacks of acute arthritis. In the late stage, deposits of monosodium urate form within and around various joints, leading to chronic arthritis with destruction in the joints and the adjoining bone. During this late stage, urate deposits, called tophi, may occur in the dermis and subcutaneous tissue. The incidence of tophaceous lesions in gout has significantly decreased since 1950, from 14% to 3%, even though the incidence of gout has

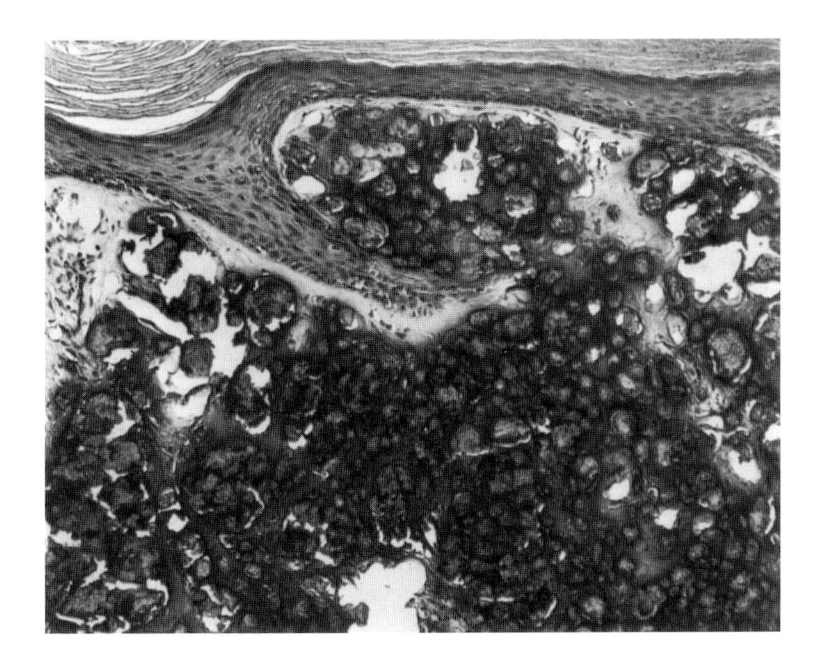

FIG. 17-11. Subepidermal calcified nodule
Granules and globules of calcium are located beneath the epidermis.

remained unchanged. Improved methods of treatment account for this decrease.[174]

Tophi are observed most commonly on the helix of the ears, over the bursae of the elbows, and on the fingers and toes.[175] They may attain a diameter of several centimeters. When large, tophi may discharge a chalky material. In rare instances, gout may present as tophi on the fingertips or as panniculitis on the legs without the coexistence of a gouty arthritis.[176,177]

Histopathology. For the histologic examination of tophi, fixation in absolute ethanol or an ethanol-based fixative, such as Carnoy's fluid, is preferable to fixation in formalin; aqueous fixatives such as formalin dissolve the characteristic urate crystals, leaving only amorphous material.[178] Anhydrous tissue processing is also important to preserve the urate crystals.

On fixation in alcohol, tophi can be seen to consist of variously sized, sharply demarcated aggregates of needle-shaped urate crystals lying closely packed in the form of bundles or sheaves. The crystals often have a brownish color and are doubly refractile on polariscopic examination (Fig. 17-13). The aggregates of urate crystals are often surrounded by a palisaded granulomatous infiltrate containing many foreign-body giant cells[179] (Fig. 17-14). The urate crystals appear black and the surrounding tissue yellow when the sections are stained with 20% silver nitrate solution.[180]

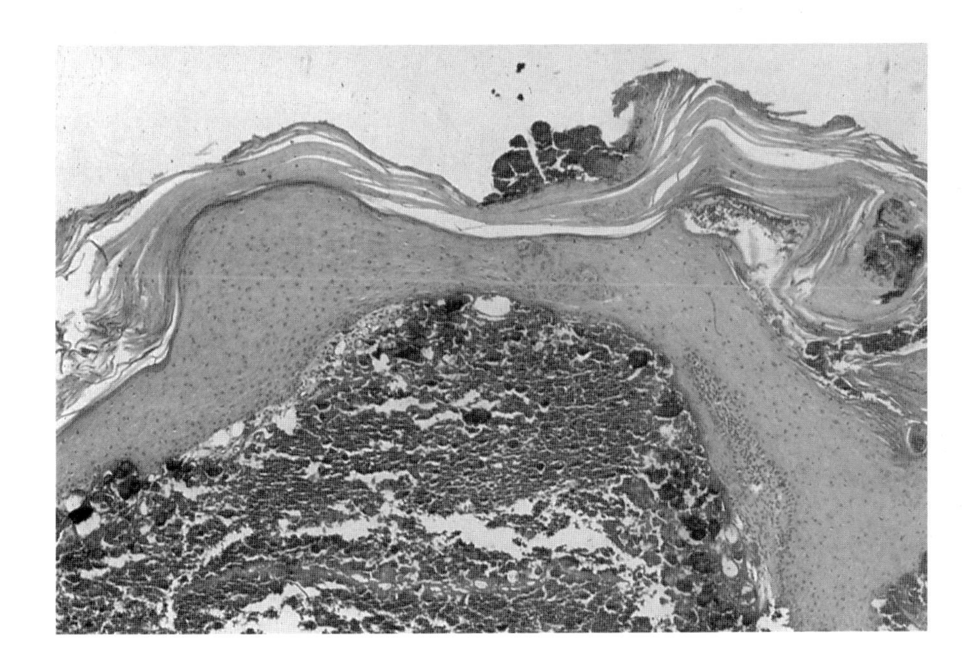

FIG. 17-12. Subepidermal calcified nodule
A large deposit of calcium in the dermis distorts the overlying epidermis (H&E).

Even when the specimen has been fixed in formalin, the diagnosis of gout can be made without difficulty because of the characteristic rim of foreign-body giant cells and macrophages surrounding the aggregates of amorphous material. As a secondary phenomenon, calcification, and occasionally ossification, may take place in the sodium urate aggregates.

Histogenesis. Gout, a dominantly inherited disorder, is characterized by hyperuricemia. An asymptomatic stage of hyperuricemia precedes the development of gouty arthritis by many years. Patients with gout are a heterogeneous group. In some patients, diminished renal excretion of uric acid accounts for the hyperuricemia; in others, an excessive production of uric acid from increased purine biosynthesis is found. In still other patients with gout, both excessive synthesis of uric acid and decreased renal excretion of uric acid are found.[181]

OCHRONOSIS

There are two types of ochronosis: endogenous ochronosis (alkaptonuria), which is inherited as an autosomal recessive trait, and localized exogenous ochronosis, which is caused by

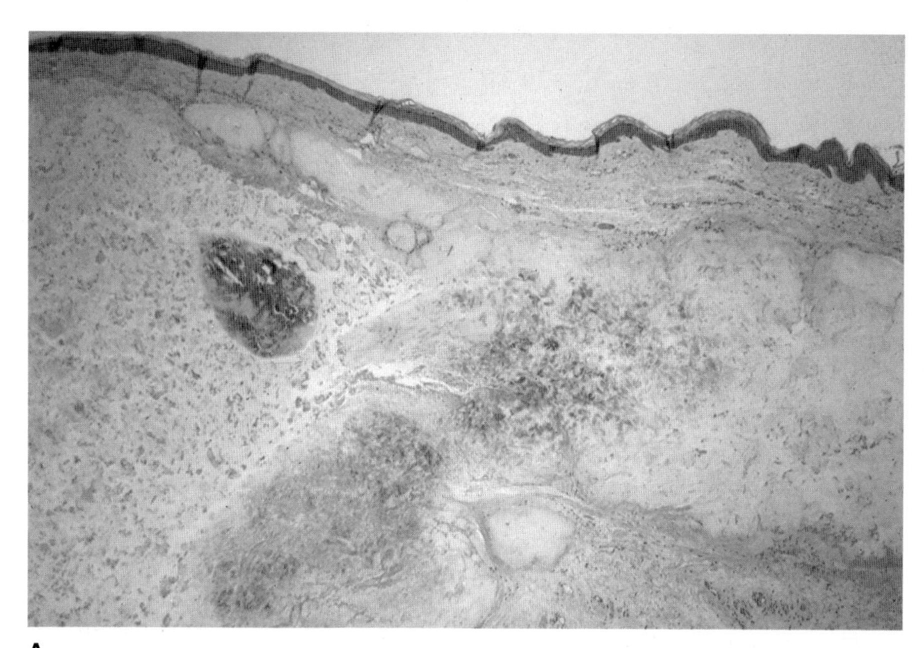

A

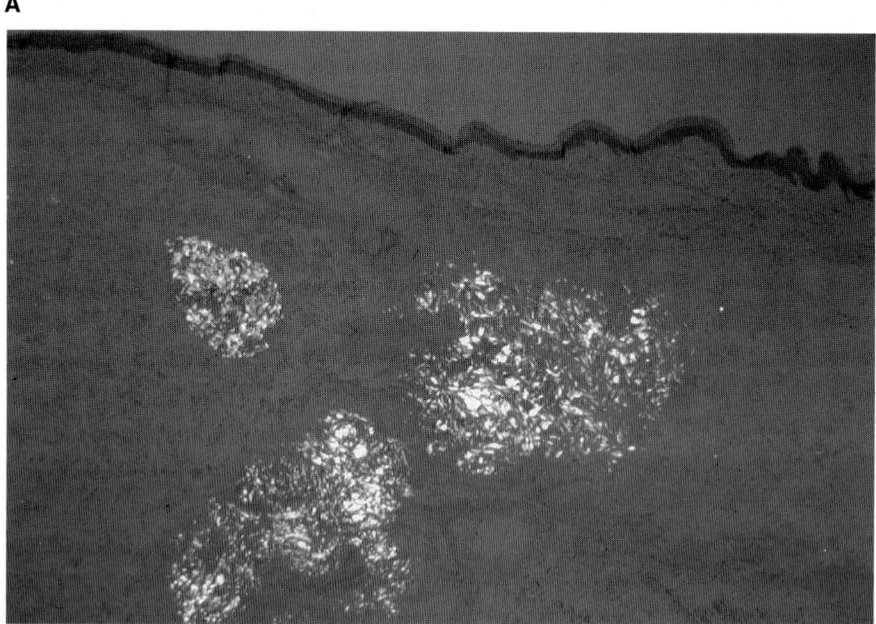

B

FIG. 17-13. Gouty tophus
(**A**) There are deposits of urate crystals in the reticular dermis that have a brownish color. The lucent areas show where some urate crystals were removed during processing of the tissue (H&E). (**B**) Polarization with a red filter reveals birefringent urate crystals representing the brownish material in the H&E-stained section.

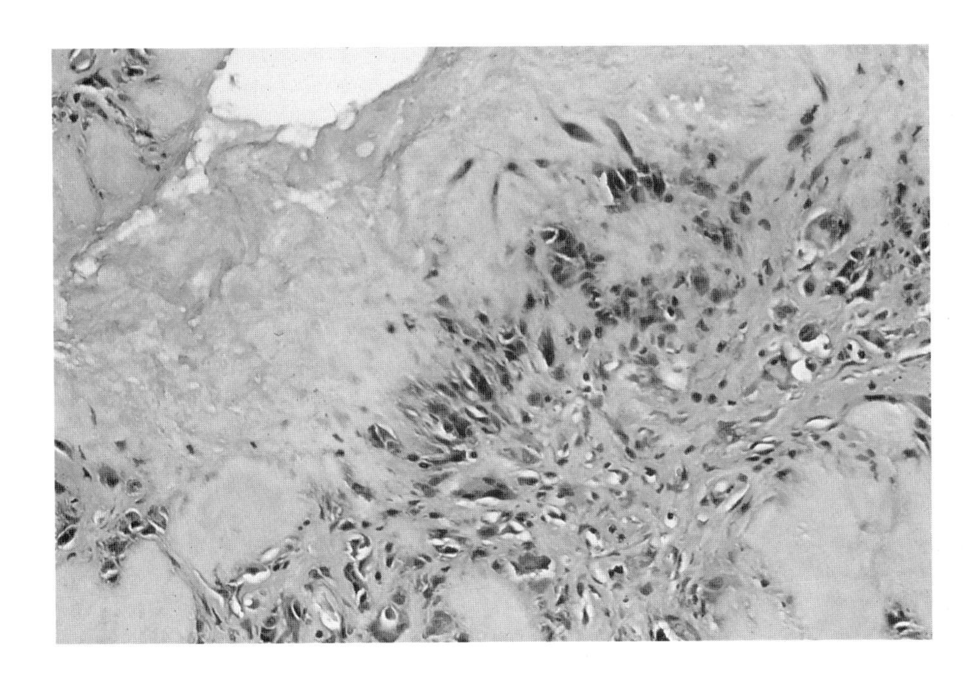

FIG. 17-14. Gouty tophus
There are macrophages and multinucleated giant cells surrounding the urate deposits in the dermis (H&E).

the topical application of a hydroquinone cream to exposed parts of the skin in order to lighten the color of dark skin.

As the result of the lack of homogentisic acid oxidase in endogenous ochronosis, homogentisic acid accumulates over the course of years in many tissues—especially in the cartilages of the joints, the ears, and the nose; in ligaments and tendons; and in the sclerae. This results in osteoarthritis; in blackening of cartilages, ligaments, and tendons; and in patchy pigmentation of the sclerae. In the course of time, homogentisic acid accumulates in the dermis in sufficient amounts to cause patchy brown pigmentation of the skin. The gene for homogentisic acid oxidase maps to chromosome 3q.[182]

In localized exogenous ochronosis, there is a macular blue-black hyperpigmentation of portions of the face to which the hydroquinone cream was applied.[183] In more severely involved areas, blue-black papules, milia, and nodules can occur.

Histopathology. Involvement of the skin is essentially identical in endogenous and exogenous ochronosis, although it is often more pronounced in exogenous ochronosis.[184] The ochronotic pigment, as seen in sections of the dermis stained with hematoxylin-eosin, has a yellow-brown or ochre color; thus, the name ochronosis.

The skin shows ochronotic pigment as fine granules free in the tissue and in the endothelial cells of blood vessels, in the basement membrane and the secretory cells of sweat glands, and within scattered macrophages.[185] The most striking finding, however, is the ochronotic pigment within collagen bundles, causing homogenization and swelling of the bundles. Some collagen bundles assume a bizarre shape; they appear rigid and tend to fracture transversely with jagged or pointed ends[186] (Fig. 17-15). As the result of the breaking up of degenerated collagen bundles, irregular, homogeneous, light brown clumps lie free in the tissue. The altered dermal connective tissue does not stain with silver nitrate as melanin does but becomes black when stained with cresyl violet or methylene blue.[187] In addition, ochronotic pigment can be found within elastic fibers.[188] In nodular ochronosis, a granulomatous response surrounds this material.[189] Transfollicular elimination of ochronotic fibers may occur in patients with severe disease.[190]

Pathogenesis. In *endogenous ochronosis*, because of an inborn lack of homogentisic acid oxidase, the two amino acids tyrosine and phenylalanine cannot be catabolized beyond homogentisic acid. Most of the homogentisic acid is excreted in the urine. The urine, on standing or after the addition of sodium hydroxide, turns black (alkaptonuria) because, through oxidation and polymerization, homogentisic acid is converted into a dark-colored insoluble product. However, some of the homogentisic acid gradually accumulates in certain tissues. It is bound irreversibly to collagen fibers as a polymer after oxidation to benzoquinone-acetic acid.[191]

In *exogenous ochronosis*, the topically applied hydroquinone inhibits the activity of homogentisic acid oxidase in the skin, resulting in the local accumulation of homogentisic acid, which polymerizes to form ochronotic pigment. In effect, this process mimics the cutaneous manifestation of endogenous ochronosis.[184]

On electron microscopic examination of early lesions, one observes deposition of amorphous, electron-dense ochronotic pigment around individual collagen fibrils within collagen fibers.[192] This causes the collagen fibrils to lose their periodicity and to degenerate. Gradually, the collagen fibrils disappear as they are replaced by ochronotic pigment. Ultimately, the ochronotic pigment occupies entire collagen fibers and, by fusion, entire collagen bundles.[192] Cross sections of the bundles then reveal a large, homogeneous, electron-dense aggregate that in some instances shows remnants of collagen fibrils at its periphery, as well as macrophages containing particles of chronotic pigment.[188,193] Particles of ochronotic pigment can also be found in elastic fibers.[188]

MUCINOSES

There are six types of cutaneous mucinosis: (1) generalized myxedema; (2) pretibial myxedema; (3) lichen myxedematosus or papular mucinosis; (4) reticular erythematous mucinosis or

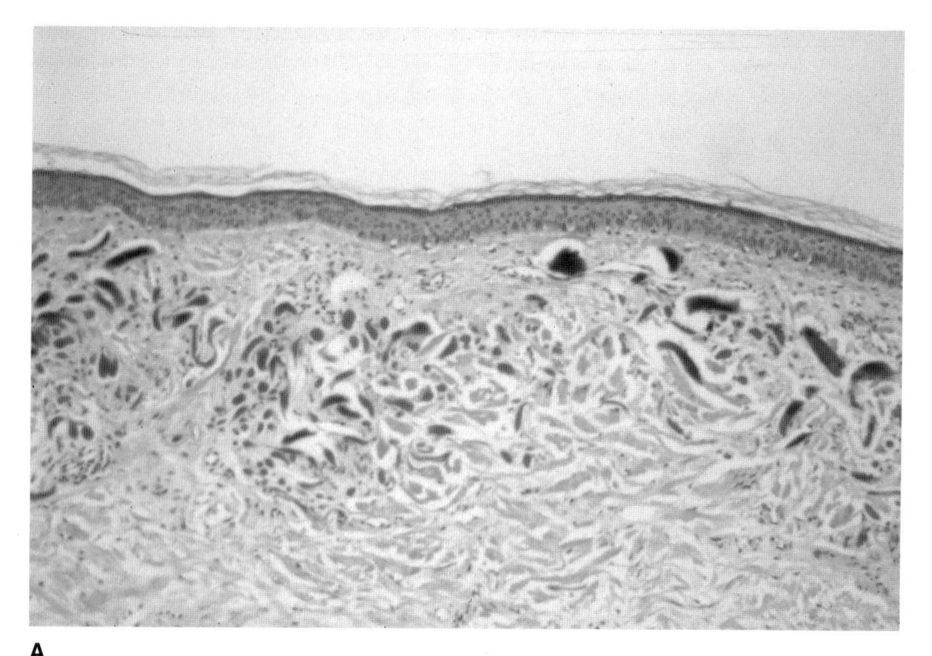

A

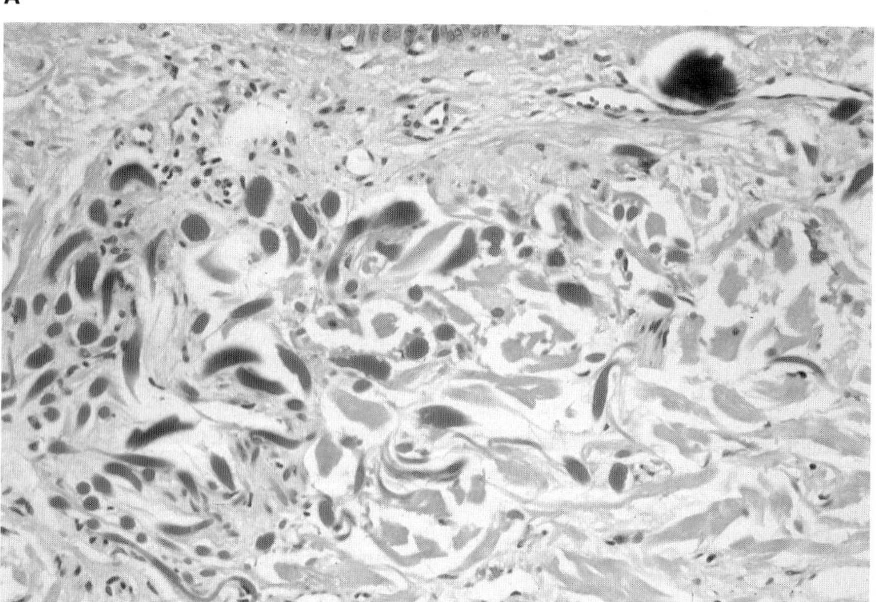

B

FIG. 17-15. Exogenous ochronosis
Yellowish orange-colored collagen bundles are present in the superficial reticular dermis. Some are abnormally thickened (**A**: H&E, original magnification ×100; **B**: H&E, original magnification ×200).

plaquelike mucinosis; (5) self-healing juvenile cutaneous mucinosis; and (6) scleredema.

Regular demonstration of the presence of mucin in the dermis is possible only in pretibial myxedema, in self-healing juvenile cutaneous mucinosis, and in lichen myxedematosus. In reticular erythematous mucinosis, it is possible in most cases. In generalized myxedema, the amount of mucin usually is too small to be demonstrable, and in scleredema, mucin may be present only in the early stage.

The mucin found in these six diseases represents an increase in the mucin that is normally present in the ground substance of the dermis. It consists of proteins bound to hyaluronic acid, an acid mucopolysaccharide or glycosaminoglycan. As a result of the great water-binding capacity of hyaluronic acid, dermal mucin contains a considerable amount of water. This water is largely removed during the process of dehydration of the specimen; consequently, in routine sections, the mucin, because of its marked shrinkage, appears largely as threads and granules.

The mucin present in the six types of mucinosis stains a light blue in sections stained with hematoxylin-eosin. It also stains with colloidal iron. It is alcian-blue-positive at pH 2.5 but negative at pH 0.5 and shows metachromasia with toluidine blue at pH 7.0 and 4.0 but no metachromasia below pH 2.0.[194] It is PAS-negative (indicating the absence of neutral mucopolysaccharides) and aldehyde-fuchsin-negative (indicating the absence of sulfated acid mucopolysaccharides). The mucin is completely removed on incubation of histologic sections with testicular hyaluronidase for 1 hr at 37° C.[195]

Generalized Myxedema

In generalized myxedema, caused by hypothyroidism, the entire skin appears swollen, dry, pale, and waxy. It is firm to the touch. In spite of its edematous appearance, the skin does not pit on pressure. There is often a characteristic facial appearance: the nose is broad, the lips are swollen, and the eyelids are puffy.

Histopathology. The epidermis may show slight orthohyperkeratosis and follicular plugging. Usually, routinely stained sections show no abnormality in the dermis, except in severe cases, in which one may observe swelling of the collagen bundles with splitting up of the bundles into individual fibers with some blue threads and granules of mucin interspersed.[196] However, with histochemical stains, such as colloidal iron, alcian blue, or toluidine blue, it is possible, at least in severe cases, to demonstrate small amounts of mucin, mainly in the vicinity of the blood vessels and hair follicles.

Pretibial Myxedema

Usually, the lesions are limited to the anterior aspects of the legs, but they may extend to the dorsa of the feet. They consist of raised, nodular, yellow, waxy plaques with prominent follicular openings that give a peau d'orange appearance. Similar lesions rarely occur on the radial aspect of the forearms.[197]

Pretibial myxedema usually occurs in association with thyrotoxicosis and not infrequently becomes more pronounced after treatment of the thyrotoxicosis. It nearly always occurs in association with exophthalmos. Rarely, pretibial myxedema, with or without exophthalmos, occurs in nonthyrotoxic thyroid disease such as chronic lymphocytic thyroiditis; the patient is then either euthyroid or hypothyroid.[198]

Histopathology. The epidermis and papillary dermis are usually normal. Mucin in large amounts is present in the dermis, particularly in the upper half (Fig. 17-16). As a result, the dermis is greatly thickened. The mucin occurs not only as individual threads and granules but also as extensive deposits resulting in the splitting up of collagen bundles into fibers and wide separation of the fibers. As a result of shrinkage of the mucin during the process of fixation and dehydration, there are empty spaces within the mucin deposits. The number of fibroblasts is not increased as a rule, but in areas in which there is much mucin, some fibroblasts have a stellate shape and are then referred to as mucoblasts.[196,199]

Pathogenesis. On electron microscopic examination, the collagen bundles and fibers are separated by wide, electron-lucent, empty spaces. The fibroblasts that produce the mucin are stellate-shaped with long, thin cytoplasmic processes and exhibit dilated cisternae of the rough endoplastic reticulum. An amorphous, moderately electron-dense material coats the surface of the fibroblasts. This material is also present in small, irregular clumps within the otherwise empty-appearing spaces.[199] At high magnification, the amorphous material appears as a complex of microfibrils and granules, forming a network.[200]

Of interest is the almost invariable presence of long-acting thyroid stimulator (LATS) in the serum of patients with pretibial myxedema. There is, however, a rather poor correlation between the severity of the skin lesions and the level of serum LATS; furthermore, LATS is detected in 40% to 60% of patients with an active exophthalmic goiter but without pretibial myxedema. Thus, LATS cannot be regarded as the cause of pretibial myxedema.[201] It is likely that the IgG LATS represents an autoantibody that is produced by lymphocytes in thyroid disease, especially in thyrotoxicosis, and is a reflection, rather than a cause, of the underlying disease.[198]

The restriction of the myxedema largely to the pretibial area may be explained by the finding that fibroblasts from the pretibial area synthesize two to three times more hyaluronic acid than do fibroblasts from other areas when incubated with serum from patients with pretibial myxedema.[202]

Differential Diagnosis. Pretibial myxedema must be differentiated from pretibial mucinosis associated with venous stasis.

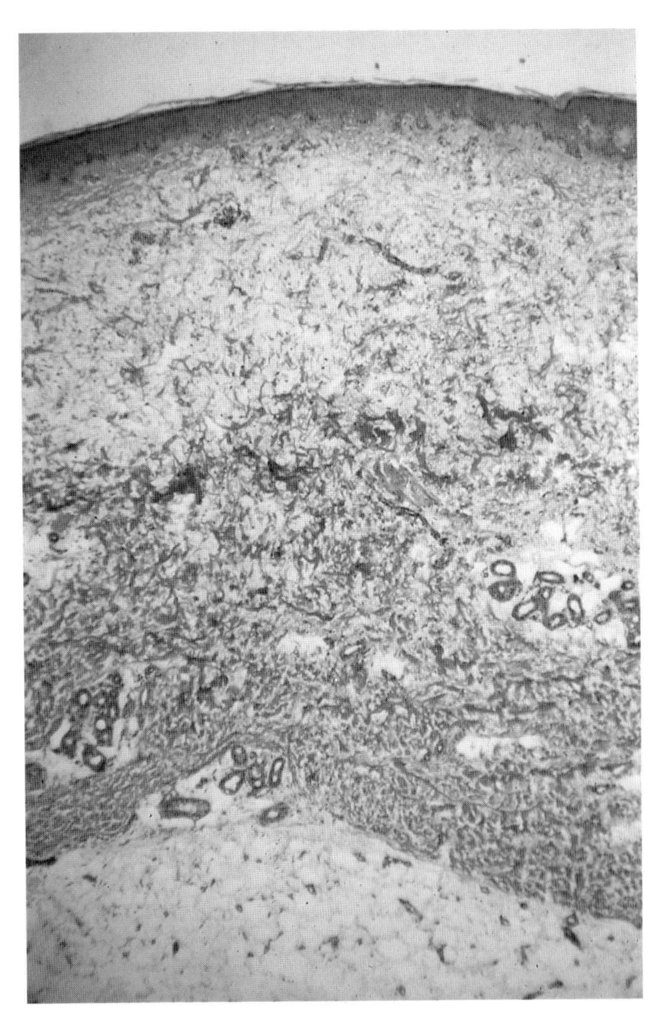

A

FIG. 17-16. Pretibial myxedema
(A) At scanning magnification, the epidermis and papillary dermis are normal. The collagen fibers in the reticular dermis are widely separated by deposits of mucin (H&E). *(continued on next page)*

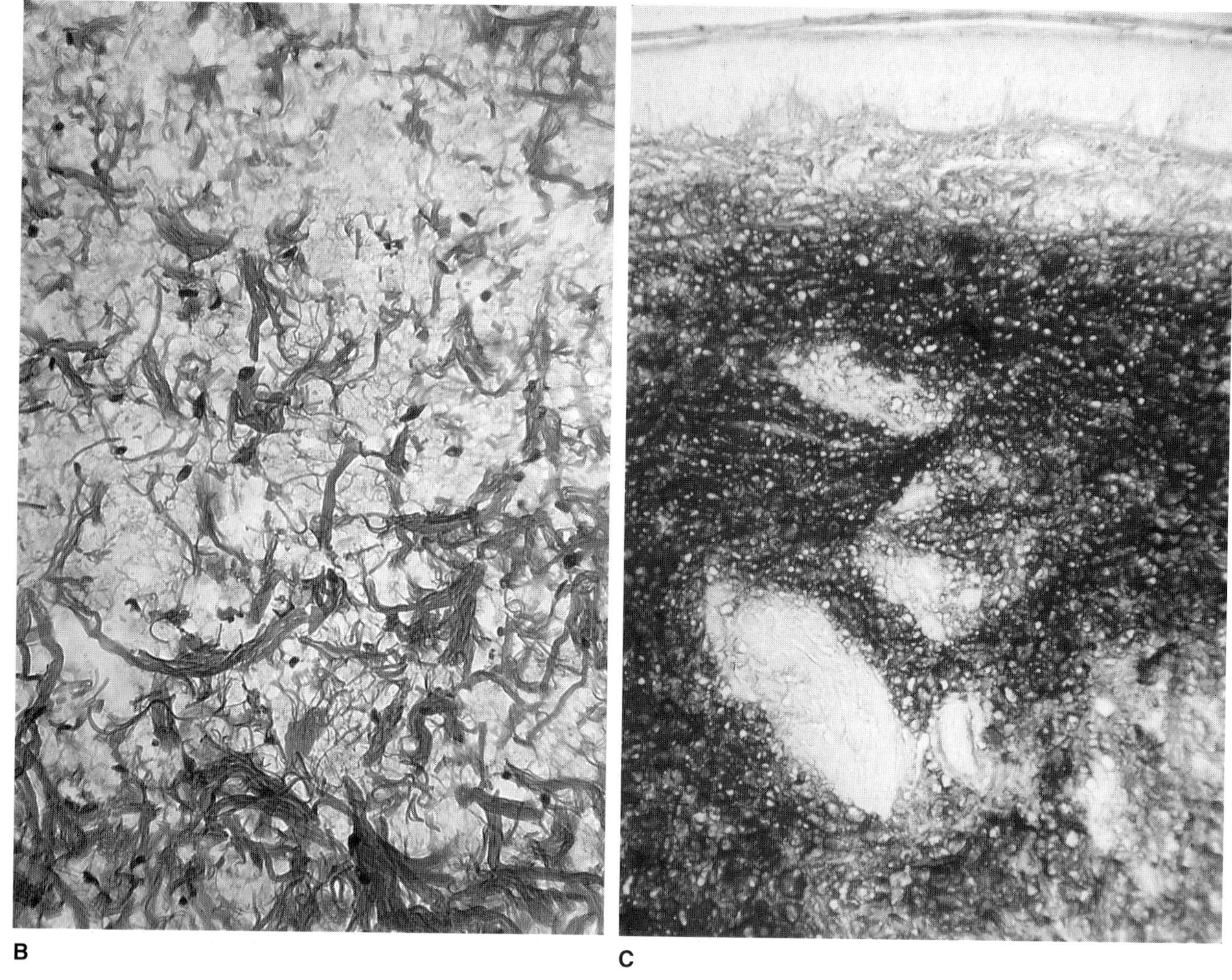

FIG. 17-16. *Continued*
(**B**) At higher magnification, stellate fibroblasts are evident among the separated collagen fibers (H&E). (**C**) The colloidal iron stain confirms the presence of abundant mucin in the reticular dermis.

In pretibial mucinosis, the excess mucin is localized to the thickened papillary dermis and is accompanied by angioplasia and siderophages.[203]

Lichen Myxedematosus

Lichen myxedematosus, or papular mucinosis, is characterized by a more or less extensive eruption of asymptomatic, soft papules generally 2 to 3 mm in diameter. Although densely grouped, they usually do not coalesce. The face and arms are the most commonly affected areas. In some instances, in addition to papules, large nodules may be present, especially on the face.[204] Although the disease is very chronic, spontaneous resolution has been reported.[205]

In a variant of lichen myxedematosus called *scleromyxedema*, one finds a generalized eruption of papules as in lichen myxedematosus and, in addition, diffuse thickening of the skin associated with erythema. There is marked accentuation of the skin folds, particularly on the face. Scleromyxedema can be differentiated from scleroderma clinically by the papular component and the absence of telangiectasias. Transitions of lichen myxedematosus to scleromyxedema do occur. Acral persistent papular mucinosis presents multiple small papular lesions on the hands and forearms.[206] The clinical and histopathologic features resemble the discrete papular form of lichen myxedematosus.[207] The detection of IgA monoclonal gammopathy in one case also suggests that it is a localized variant of lichen myxedematosus.[208] Cutaneous mucinosis of infancy may also represent a localized form of papular mucinosis on the upper extremities unassociated with monoclonal gammopathy.[209]

Histopathology. In lichen myxedematosus, fairly large amounts of mucin are present. In contrast with pretibial myxedema, however, the mucinous infiltration is found only in circumscribed areas, is most pronounced in the upper dermis, and is associated with an increase in fibroblasts and collagen[210,211] (Fig. 17-17). The collagen bundles may show a rather irregular arrangement.

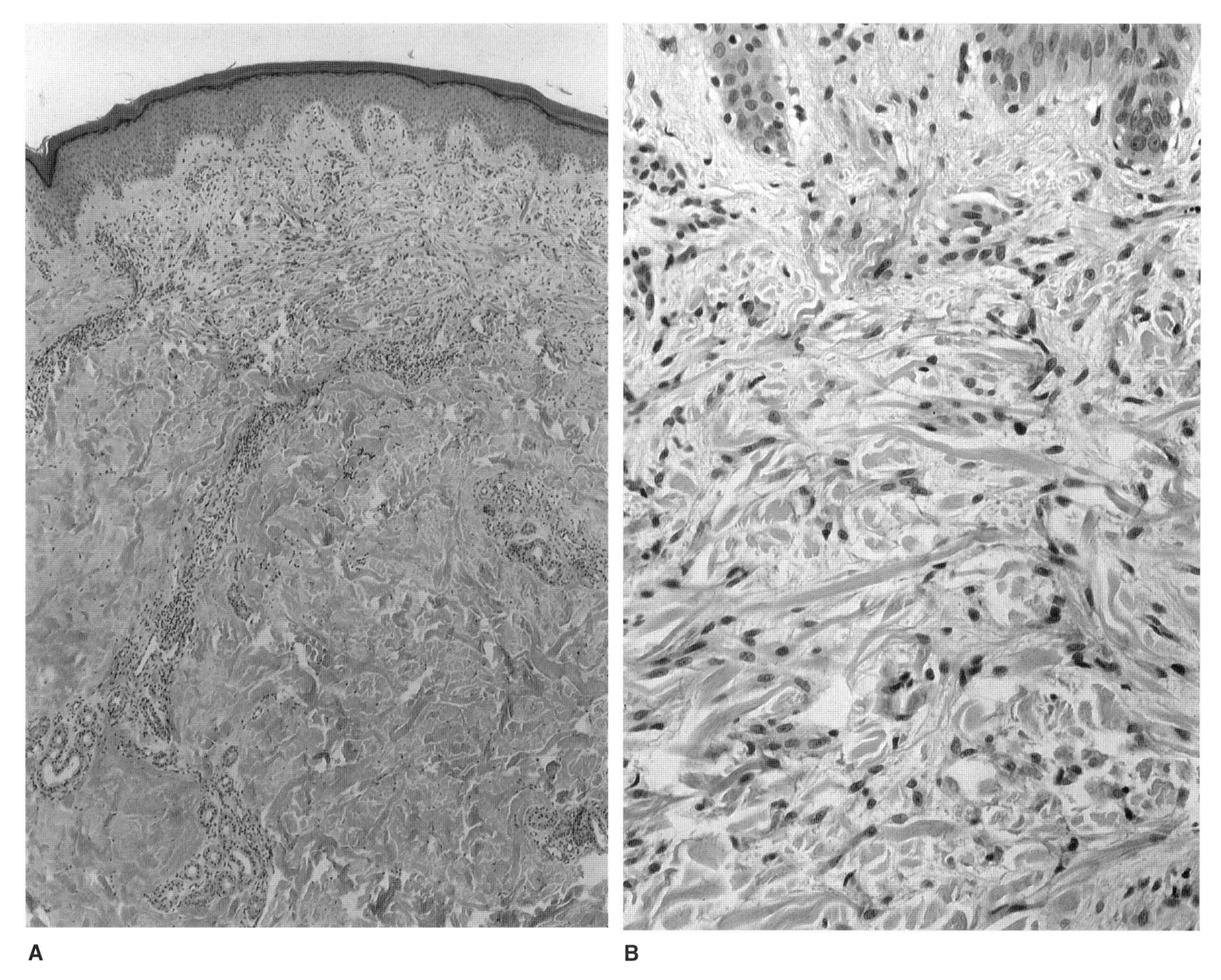

FIG. 17-17. Lichen myxedematosus
(**A**) At scanning power, a dome-shaped papule is evident. The papillary and superficial reticular dermis contain abundant mucin (H&E). (**B**) In addition to mucin, there is an increased number of plump fibroblasts in the upper dermis (H&E).

Scleromyxedema

The histologic picture found in the papules in scleromyxedema resembles that observed in lichen myxedematosus. In the diffusely thickened skin, there is extensive proliferation of fibroblasts, throughout the dermis, associated with irregularly arranged bundles of collagen. In many areas, the collagen bundles are split into individual fibers by mucin. As a rule, the amount of mucin is greater in the upper half than in the lower half of the dermis.[212]

Autopsy examination of patients with scleromyxedema usually has not shown mucinous deposits in any internal organs.[211–213] However, in one case, mucin was detected in renal papillae, and in another it was found in the adventitia and media of blood vessels in several organs.[214,215]

Pathogenesis. Electron microscopic examination of scleromyxedema reveals an increase in the number of fibroblasts. They show considerable activity, as indicated by the presence of a markedly dilated rough endoplasmic reticulum and long cytoplasmic processes. These fibroblasts produce both collagen and ground substance. The presence of many collagen fibrils with reduced diameter, similar to those in scleroderma, indicates that it is young collagen. In many areas, there are small bundles of young collagen fibrils, with each fibril richly coated with ground substance.[216]

The presence of a *monoclonal component* (M component) or paraprotein in the sera of patients with lichen myxedematosus and scleromyxedema has been noted in nearly all cases that have been adequately tested. Its absence has been noted in a few cases[217]; in another case, it was absent at first but present later on.[218]

In nearly all instances, the paraprotein is an IgG, although other immunoglobulin classes occur on rare occasions.[213,219] The IgG paraprotein is a very basic protein because of an increased lysine content in its light chains.[220] Thus, in most instances, it migrates more slowly than gamma globulin on serum electrophoresis and may even migrate toward the cathode rather than toward the anode.[221] In instances in which it migrates with the same speed as gamma-globulin, immunoelectrophoresis is required for its recognition.[222] The IgG of lichen myxedematosus differs from the IgG of multiple myeloma not only by usually showing slower electrophoretic migration but also by the fact that its IgG molecules nearly always possess light chains of the lambda type, although light chains of the kappa type have occasionally been found.[223,224] In contrast, in multiple myeloma with elevated values for IgG, only about one-third of the reported cases with IgG molecules have lambda light chains, and two-thirds have kappa light chains.[225] In addition to showing a monoclonal IgG, many cases of lichen myxedematosus show hyperplasia of plasma cells in the bone marrow.[213,214,222,226] These plasma cells have been shown to synthesize the monoclonal IgG.[224] In some cases, the plasma cells in the bone marrow have been regarded as atypical in appearance.[227] However, only one case fulfilling the criteria for coexisting multiple myeloma has been documented.[228]

The role of the monoclonal IgG in lichen myxedematosus is not clear. Its presence in the dermal mucin has been demonstrated by direct immunofluorescence.[227,229,230] Furthermore, the serum containing the paraprotein stimulates the production of hyaluronic acid and prostaglandin E by fibroblasts in vitro.[231] However, although the serum from patients with lichen myxedematosus stimulates fibroblast proliferation in vitro, the purified IgG paraprotein itself has no direct effect on fibroblast proliferation.[232]

Reticular Erythematous Mucinosis

Erythematous, reticulated areas with irregular but well-defined margins are present, usually in the center of the chest and of the upper back. This disorder was first described in 1960 as being composed of confluent papules and was called plaquelike mucinosis, but similar cases showing coalescent macules, rather than papules, were designated reticular erythematous mucinosis in 1974.[233,234] It has since become apparent that macular and papular lesions can coexist.[235] In rare instances, lesions spare the trunk and are present on the arms and face.[236] The eruption is asymptomatic. It is chronic but usually responds well to small doses of antimalarial drugs of the 4-aminoquinoline group, such as chloroquin.

Histopathology. Two histologic features are usually present: small amounts of dermal mucin and a mild or moderately pronounced mononuclear infiltrate situated predominantly around blood vessels and hair follicles.[233,234] The infiltrate is composed of helper T cells.[237]

In papular lesions, the mucin usually is fairly conspicuous. As a rule, mucin can be recognized even in routinely stained sections (Fig. 17-18). The mucin stains with alcian blue and usually also with mucicarmine. In addition, there often is metachromasia on staining with toluidine blue or with the Giemsa stain.[233,234] Fibroblasts with bipolar processes are located in the mucinous deposits.[238]

In macular lesions, the mucin may be missed in routinely stained sections and become apparent only on staining with alcian blue. In some instances, no mucin is found, even on staining with alcian blue,[239] but if an alcian-blue stain is negative in paraffin-embedded sections, it may be positive in unfixed, frozen sections.[240] If this is negative, too, the diagnosis depends on the presence of the mononuclear infiltrate, the clinical appearance, and the response of the patient to treatment with antimalarial drugs.

Differential Diagnosis. Reticular erythematous mucinosis, Jessner's lymphocytic infiltrate of skin, and lupus erythematosus share in common a perivascular and perifollicular lymphocytic infiltrate and increased mucin among collagen bundles. In Jessner's lymphocytic infiltrate, the lymphocytic infiltrate is usually much more dense than that in reticular erythematous mucinosis. Lupus erythematosus almost always shows vacuolar changes in the basal layer of the epidermis and follicular units, but in the rare tumid lesions, vacuolar changes may be inconspicuous. Thus it may not be possible to distinguish between the tumid lesions of lupus erythematosus and reticular erythematous mucinosis by conventional microscopy.

Self-Healing Juvenile Cutaneous Mucinosis

This rare dermatosis has been described only in children. It has a sudden onset and undergoes spontaneous resolution within a few months. Infiltrated plaques with a corrugated surface are observed on the torso, and nodules occur on the face and in the periarticular region. There may be associated fever, arthralgias, muscle tenderness, and weakness.[241]

Histopathology. Abundant mucinous material, alcian-blue-positive at pH 2.5, is present mainly in the upper reticular dermis.[242] There may be a superficial perivascular lymphocytic infiltrate and a slight increase in the number of mast cells and fibroblasts in the zone of mucin deposition.

Scleredema

Scleredema, occasionally called scleredema adultorum even though it may occur in children and infants, is characterized by diffuse, nonpitting swelling and induration of the skin.[243,244] Three groups can be recognized:[245] one with abrupt onset, one with insidious onset, and one preceded by diabetes. In the first group, the scleredema starts abruptly during or within a few weeks after an upper respiratory tract infection. The skin lesions may clear within a few months or the disease may take a prolonged course. In the second group, the scleredema starts insidiously, for no apparent reason, spreads gradually, and takes a chronic course. The disease in the third group is preceded by diabetes for years, starts insidiously, and persists indefinitely. Usually, the scleredema starts on the face and extends to the neck and upper trunk. Unlike scleroderma, the hands and feet are always spared. In about 75% of the patients, complete resolution takes place within a few months; in the remaining 25%, the disease may persist for as long as 40 years.[246] Although visceral lesions may occur, death from scleredema is rare.

Diabetes is commonly associated with persistent scleredema and, in most of these instances, is quite resistant to antidiabetic therapy.[246] It has been suggested that the association of persistent scleredema with maturity-onset diabetes be recognized as a special form of scleredema.[247]

Histopathology. The dermis in scleredema is about three times thicker than normal (Fig. 17-19). The collagen bundles are thickened and separated by clear spaces, causing "fenestration" of the collagen. The secretory coils of the sweat glands, surrounded by fat tissue, are located in the upper dermis or mid-

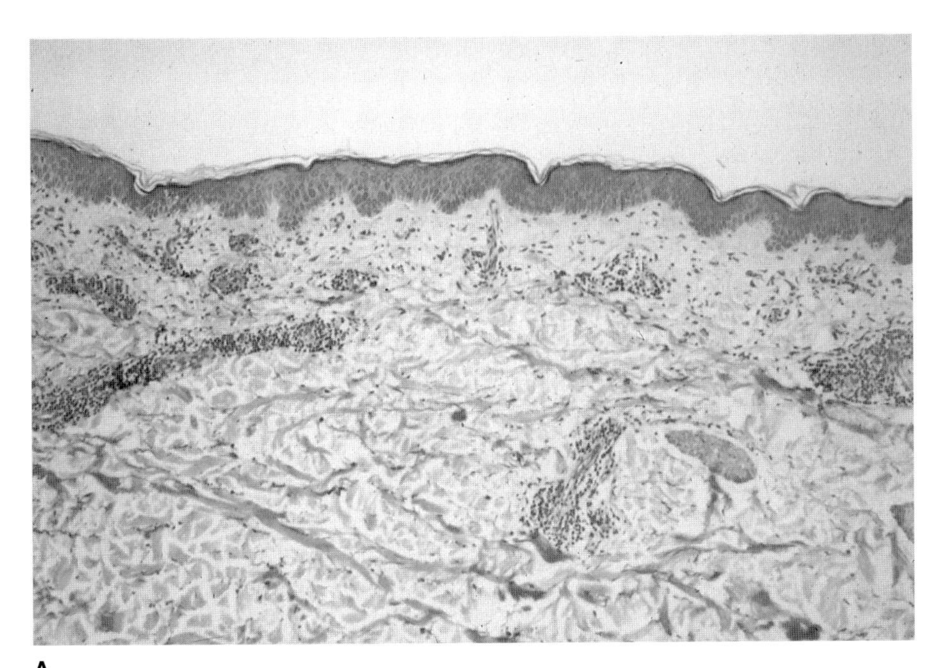

A

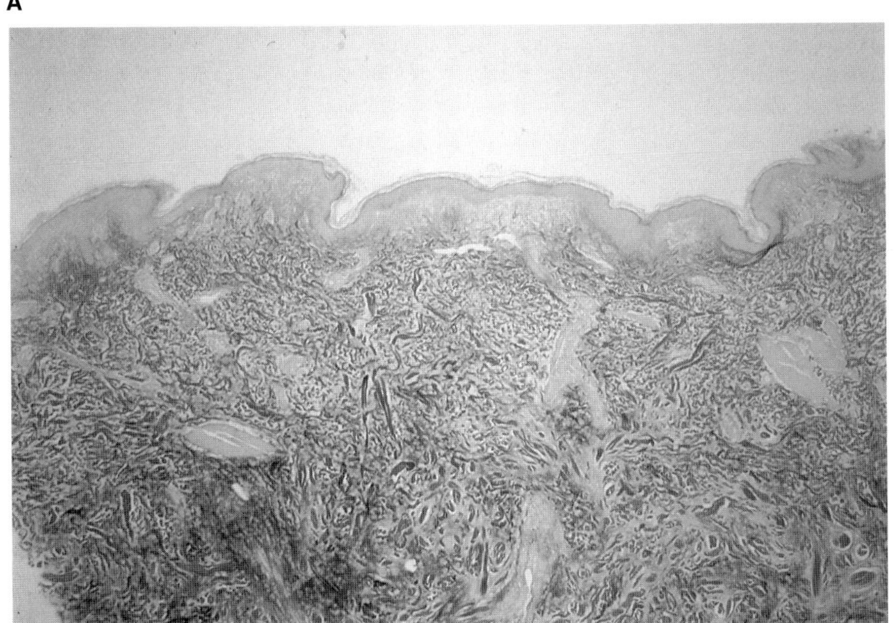

B

FIG. 17-18. Reticular erythematous mucinosis
(**A**) There is a moderate perivascular infiltrate of lymphocytes around blood vessels in the dermis (H&E). (**B**) Colloidal iron staining reveals abundant mucin among collagen fibers.

dermis rather than, as normally, in the lower dermis or at the junction of the dermis and the subcutaneous fat. Because the distance between the epidermis and the sweat glands is unchanged, it can be concluded that much of the subcutaneous fat in scleredema has been replaced by dense collagenous bundles.[248] No increase in the number of fibroblasts is noted in association with the hyperplasia of the collagen; in fact, their number may be strikingly decreased.[249]

In many instances, especially in early cases, histochemical staining reveals the presence of hyaluronic acid between the bundles of collagen, particularly in the areas of fenestration. Staining with toluidine blue usually reveals metachromasia, which is most evident at pH 7.0, weaker at pH 5.0, and absent at pH 1.5, indicating the presence of only nonsulfated acid mucopolysaccharides.[194] Although the hyaluronic acid is usually present throughout the dermis, it may be present only in the deeper portion of the dermis[250] (Fig. 17-20).

In some instances, staining with toluidine blue at pH 7.0 is more intense if unfixed cryostat sections are used in place of formalin-fixed material.[251] In some cases, even frozen sections have failed to stain with alcian blue or toluidine blue.[252] It may be postulated that, in cases of long standing in which the disease has reached a steady stage of collagen turnover, staining for hyaluronic acid may give negative results.[248] In cases of scleredema in which formaldehyde-fixed specimens fail to show acid mucopolysaccharides, they may show them on fixation in 0.05% cetylpyridinium chloride solution and staining with alcian blue at pH 2.5.[244] It has been stated that fixation with 1%

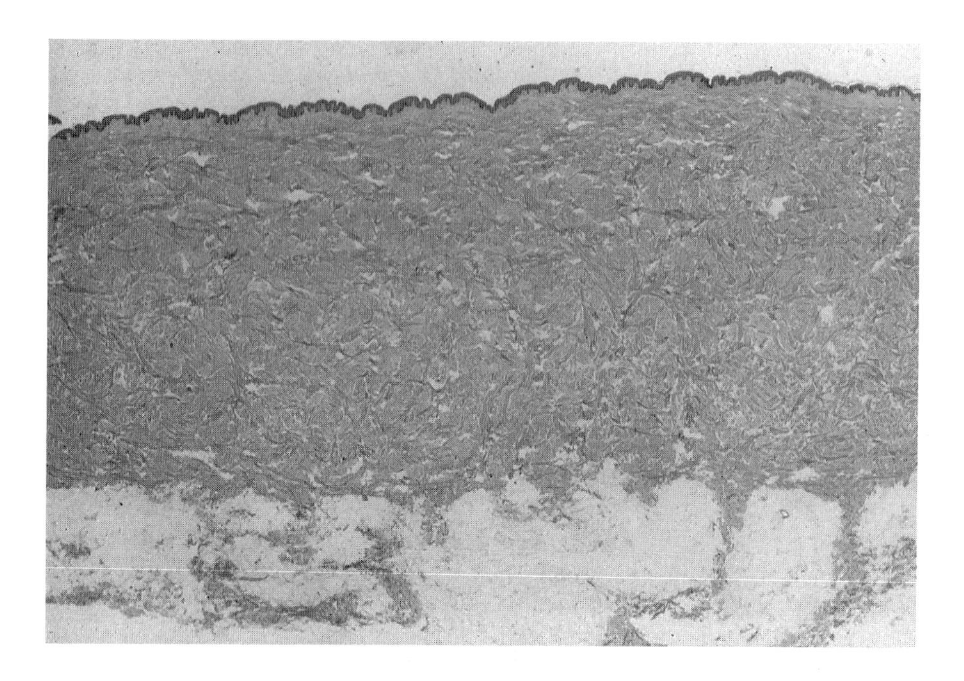

FIG. 17-19. Scleredema
Panoramic view showing only a greatly thickened reticular dermis. The subcutis is not involved as in scleroderma (H&E).

cetylpyridinium chloride solution in standard formalin fixative combined with colloidal iron staining gives the best results.[253]

Systemic Lesions. Occasionally, the tongue and some skeletal muscles are involved, and, on histologic examination, the muscle bundles show edema and loss of striation.[252,254] In a few reported cases, pleural and pericardial effusions were present.[252,255] In one case, the disease terminated in death, and autopsy revealed, in addition to pleural and pericardial effusions, diffuse edema of the heart, the liver, and the spleen.[256]

Pathogenesis. In many patients with longstanding scleredema, a monoclonal gammopathy is found in the serum. Usually the paraprotein is either IgG-kappa or IgG-lambda.[249] In other cases, it has been IgA-kappa, IgA-lambda, or IgM-lambda.[257] There can be coexistence of scleredema with multiple myeloma.[258] No immunoglobulin deposits have been found in involved skin sites.[249]

Differential Diagnosis. It can be difficult to differentiate between end-stage scleroderma in which inflammation is no longer present and scleredema. As a rule, however, in scleroderma, the collagen in the reticular dermis and subcutaneous tissue appears homogenized and hyalinized and stains only lightly with eosin and with the Masson trichrome stain, but in scleredema, the collagen bundles are thickened without being hyalinized and stain normally with eosin and the trichrome stain.[248]

MUCOPOLYSACCHARIDOSES

The mucopolysaccharidoses (MPS) comprise a group of storage diseases in which, as the result of a deficiency of specific lysosomal enzymes, there is inadequate degradation of mucopolysaccharides, or glycosaminoglycans. Consequently, this material accumulates within lysosomes of various cells in many organs, including the skin. Greatly elevated levels of mucopolysaccharides are present in the blood serum and in the urine. Ten enzymatically distinct types of mucopolysaccharidosis have been identified, and most appear to have allelic variants.[259]

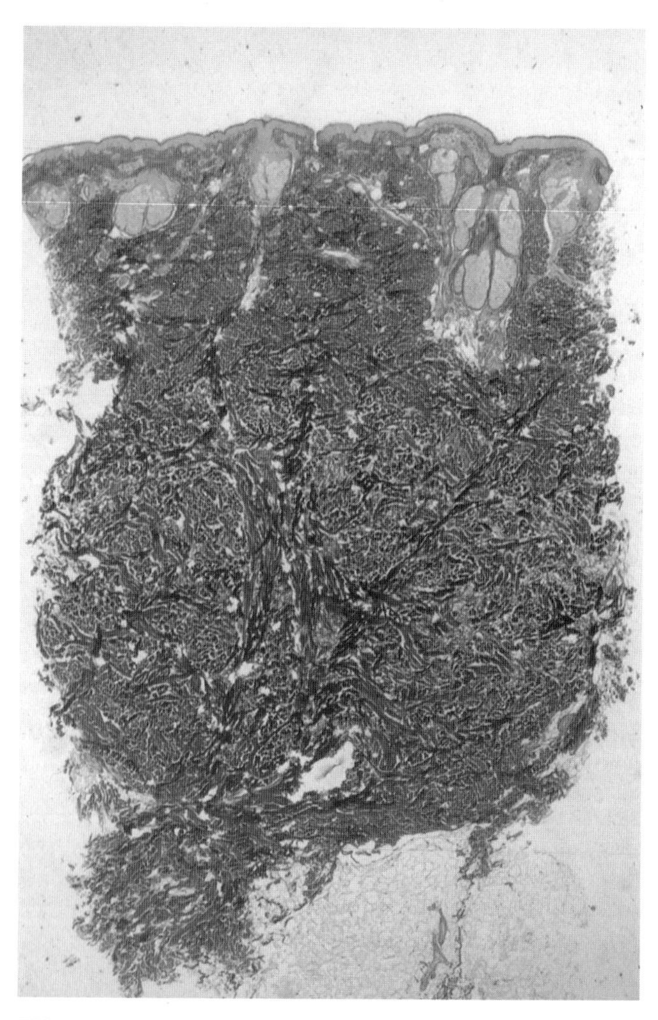

FIG. 17-20. Scleredema
Colloidal iron staining of an early case reveals increased mucin in the middle and lower dermis.

Thus, there is marked variation in the manifestations not only from type to type, but also within the same type. The most common features, any or all of which may be present or absent, include dwarfism, skeletal deformities, hepatosplenomegaly, corneal clouding, and progressive mental deterioration with premature death from cardiorespiratory complications. In many instances, there is a characteristic facial appearance—thick lips, flattened nose, and hirsutism—referred to as gargoylism. The mode of transmission is autosomal recessive in all types of MPS except type II, the Hunter syndrome, which is X-linked recessive.

Of the 10 types of MPS, only types I to III will be discussed here. MPS I presents as three distinctive variants, even though they are all caused by a deficiency of the same enzyme. MPS I H, Hurler's syndrome, causes severe mental retardation and death, usually within the first decade of life.[260] In contrast, persons with MPS I S, Scheie's syndrome, have normal intelligence, no dwarfism, and a normal life expectancy.[261] MPS I H/S, the Hurler-Scheie syndrome, is intermediate between MPS I H and MPS I S. MPS II, Hunter's syndrome, occurs in a severe form, with mental retardation and early death, and in a mild form, in which mental function is normal and survival to adult life is the rule.[262] MPS III, Sanfilippo's syndrome, has mild somatic changes but severe mental retardation.[263]

The skin in all 10 types of MPS usually appears thickened and inelastic. However, the only type in which distinctive cutaneous lesions are found frequently, although not invariably, is MPS II, Hunter's syndrome. These lesions consist of ivory white papules or small nodules, usually 3 to 4 mm in diameter, that may coalesce to form ridges in a reticular pattern on the upper trunk, especially in the scapular region.[262,264] This condition has been referred to as "pebbling" of the skin.

Histopathology. In all 10 types of MPS, the normal-appearing or slightly thickened skin, on staining with the Giemsa stain or toluidine blue, shows metachromatic granules within fibroblasts, so that the fibroblasts resemble mast cells.[260] The granules also stain with alcian blue and with colloidal iron.[261] Fixation in absolute alcohol in some instances demonstrates the metachromasia better than fixation in formalin.[265] In addition, metachromatic granules are occasionally present in some epidermal cells and in the secretory and ductal cells of eccrine glands.[260,266,267]

The cutaneous papules observed only in Hunter's syndrome show not only metachromatic granules within dermal fibroblasts but also extracellular deposits of metachromatic material between collagen bundles and fibers.[264,265]

In all types of mucopolysaccharidosis, metachromatic granules are visible also in the cytoplasm of circulating lymphocytes when smears of them are stained with toluidine blue after fixation in absolute methanol, a finding that aids in the rapid diagnosis of mucopolysaccharidosis.[268]

Histogenesis. Biochemical studies have shown that, in MPS I, as a result of a deficiency in alpha-l-iduronidase, there is an increased urinary excretion of heparan sulfate and dermatan sulfate (chondroitin sulfate).[259] In MPS II, the same two substances are excessively excreted owing to a deficiency in iduronate sulfatase. In MPS III, there is excessive excretion of heparan sulfate. Successful bone marrow transplantation in children with Hurler's syndrome can restore the previously deficient alpha-1-iduronidase level.[269]

By staining for acid phosphatase and by electron microscopy, the metachromatic granules in the skin and in the lymphocytes have been identified as lysosomes that contain acid mucopolysaccharides, which they are incapable of degrading.[267,268]

Electron microscopic examination of the skin reveals in most fibroblasts numerous electron-lucent, greatly dilated, membrane-bound vacuoles representing lysosomes. Some of the vacuoles contain granular material or, less commonly, myelin-like structures representing residual bodies.[261,270] Lysosomes are present also in macrophages, showing the same characteristics as in fibroblasts.[263] In addition, from 5% to 20% of the epidermal cells contain lysosomal vacuoles, with acid phosphatase activity, varying from a solitary vacuole to 20 or 30 vacuoles per cell.[266]

The dermal Schwann cells also contain electron-lucent lysosomes. In addition, some Schwann cells occasionally show laminated membranous structures ("zebra bodies"). These structures resemble those found in the brains of some patients with mucopolysaccharidosis. In the brain, they contain gangliosides as the result of a deficiency in the lysosomal hydrolase beta-d-galactosidase.[266] The deposition of gangliosides in the brain leads to mental deterioration through the degeneration and loss of neurons.[269]

ACANTHOSIS NIGRICANS

There are eight types of acanthosis nigricans: malignant, benign inherited, obesity-associated, syndromic, acral, unilateral, drug-induced, and mixed.[271] The malignant type differs from the benign types by showing more extensive and more pronounced lesions, by its progressiveness, and by its onset usually after the age of 40. The histologic picture is essentially the same in all types.

The *malignant* type is associated with a malignant tumor—most commonly an abdominal, and particularly a gastric, carcinoma.[272] However, it may also occur with squamous cell carcinoma, with sarcomas, and with Hodgkin's and non-Hodgkin's lymphomas.[271] In some cases, the skin lesions precede the symptoms of malignancy. The sign of Leser-Trélat, which is characterized by the sudden appearance of numerous seborrheic keratoses in association with a malignant tumor, may be an early stage or incomplete form of the malignant type of acanthosis nigricans. The seborrheic keratoses observed in this sign may be accompanied or followed by lesions of acanthosis nigricans.[271]

The *benign inherited* type usually has its onset during infancy or early childhood. It is an autosomal dominant trait.[273]

Syndromic acanthosis nigricans is especially linked to syndromes associated with insulin resistance.[274] In the HAIR-AN syndrome, which affects younger women, there is hyperandrogenemia (HA), insulin resistance (IR), and acanthosis nigricans (AN).[271] Another subset links autoimmune states such as lupus erythematosus with uncontrolled diabetes mellitus, acanthosis nigricans, and ovarian hyperandrogenism. These patients have antibodies to the insulin receptor. Acanthosis nigricans has also been associated with insulin resistance in obesity, hypothyroidism, and congenital generalized lipodystrophy.[275–277]

Acanthosis nigricans-like lesions have been induced by high dosages of nicotinic acid.[278] Acanthosis nigricans has also oc-

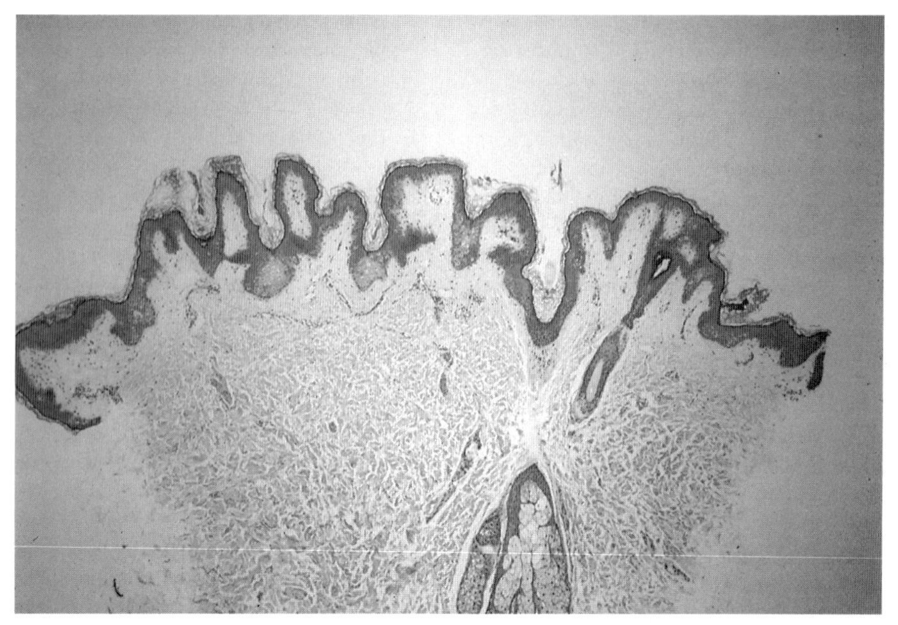

A

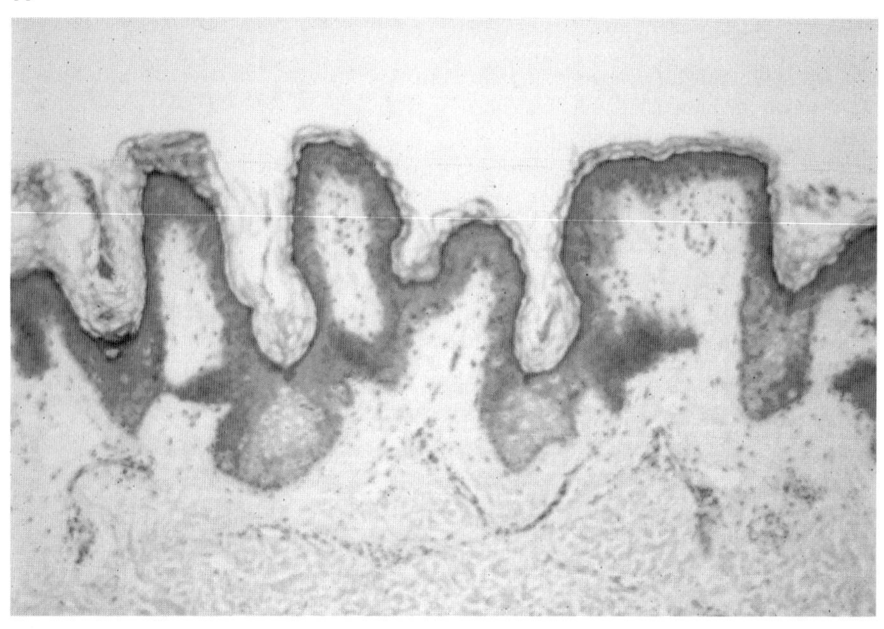

B

FIG. 17-21. Acanthosis nigricans
(**A**) There are papillomatous projections of the dermis (H&E). (**B**) The epidermis is not increased in thickness above the papillomatous projections. The stratum corneum shows loose, basket-weave orthokeratosis (H&E).

curred following use of oral contraceptives, following use of the folic acid antagonist triazinate, and as a localized reaction to insulin.[273,279,280]

Clinically, acanthosis nigricans presents papillomatous brown patches, predominantly in the intertriginous areas such as the axillae, the neck, and the genital and submammary regions. In extensive cases of acanthosis nigricans of the malignant type, mucosal surfaces, such as the mouth, the vulva, and the palpebral conjunctivae, may be involved.[272] In the acral type, there is velvety hyperpigmentation of the dorsa of the hands and feet.

Histopathology. Histologic examination reveals hyperkeratosis and papillomatosis but only slight, irregular acanthosis and usually no hyperpigmentation. Thus, the term *acanthosis nigricans* has little histologic justification.

In a typical lesion, the dermal papillae project upward as fingerlike projections. The valleys between the papillae show mild to moderate acanthosis and are filled with keratotic material (Fig. 17-21). Horn pseudocysts can occur in some cases.[281] The epidermis at the tips of the papillae and often also on the sides of the protruding papillae appears thinned.

Slight hyperpigmentation of the basal layer is demonstrable with silver nitrate staining in some cases but not in others.[282] The brown color of the lesions is caused more by hyperkeratosis than by melanin.

In the acanthosis nigricans lesions of the polycystic ovary syndrome, there are prominent deposits of glycosaminoglycan consisting mostly of hyaluronic acid in the papillary dermis.[283]

Histogenesis. The inherited type of acanthosis nigricans can be classified as a type of epidermal nevus. In persons who have acanthosis associated with insulin resistance, high levels of insulin may activate insulin-like growth factor-1 receptors and thereby mediate epidermal proliferation.[284] Malignant acanthosis nigricans most likely is mediated by growth factors that are secreted by the associated neoplasm such as transforming growth factor-alpha.[285] The basal cells from one patient with syndromic acanthosis nigricans demonstrated unusually high expression of the rare keratins 18 and 19.[281]

Differential Diagnosis. Differentiation of acanthosis nigricans from other benign papillomas, particularly from linear epidermal nevi and from the hyperkeratotic type of seborrheic keratosis, may be difficult. As a rule, however, linear epidermal nevi show more marked acanthosis than acanthosis nigricans and have a more compact orthokeratotic stratum corneum. Furthermore, the pilosebaceous units in linear epidermal nevi are rudimentary. Acanthosis nigricans cannot be distinguished histologically from confluent and reticulated papillomatosis.

Confluent and Reticulated Papillomatosis

Confluent and reticulated papillomatosis shows slightly hyperkeratotic and papillomatous pigmented papules that are confluent in the center and reticulated at the periphery.[286] The site of predilection is the sternal region. In the view of some authors, this disorder represents a variant of acanthosis nigricans.[287] However, its location and reticulated pattern are distinctive.

Histopathology. Mild hyperkeratosis and papillomatosis are present, as is focal acanthosis, limited largely to the valleys between elongated papillae.[287] Thus, the histologic changes are similar to but milder than those of acanthosis nigricans.

Histogenesis. Heavy colonization with *Pityrosporum orbiculare* has been observed in patients with confluent and reticulated papillomatosis, so that this disorder has been regarded as a peculiar host reaction to *P orbiculare*.[288,289] However, in a review of the literature, it was found that, even though potassium hydroxide preparations had yielded positive findings for yeast in 10 cases, there were positive findings for yeast and hyphae in only one case and negative results in 20 cases.[290] Considering the common presence of the yeast phase as a nonpathogen, the role of *Malassezia* (*Pityrosporum*) as the cause of confluent and reticulated papillomatosis can be discounted.

IDIOPATHIC HEMOCHROMATOSIS

In idiopathic hemochromatosis, large amounts of iron are deposited in various organs of the body, especially in the parenchymal cells of the liver and pancreas and in the myocardial fibers. The classic tetrad of idiopathic hemochromatosis consists of hepatic cirrhosis, diabetes, hyperpigmentation of the skin, and cardiac failure.

Unless there is early recognition and adequate treatment by phlebotomy, hemochromatosis is a fatal disorder as the result of liver failure, heart disease, or hepatocellular carcinoma, which occurs in about one-third of the patients with advanced hemochromatosis.[291]

Pigmentation of the skin is present in more than 90% of the patients with idiopathic hemochromatosis at the time the diagnosis is made, but it is often so mild as to attract little attention.[292,293] The pigmentation is most pronounced in exposed areas, especially on the face. Its color usually is brown or bronze but may be blue-gray. The pigmentation is caused largely by melanin and not by iron. In addition to pigmentation, ichthyosis-like changes, koilonychia, and hair loss are common.

Histopathology. Histologic examination of pigmented skin, especially from exposed areas, shows melanin to be present in increased amounts in the basal layer of the epidermis.[292,294] Hemosiderin can be demonstrated in the skin of most patients with the aid of an iron stain, such as Perls' stain. It is found as blue-staining granules, mainly around blood vessels, both extracellularly and within macrophages, and in the basement membrane zone of the sweat glands and within cells of the connective tissue surrounding these glands.[294] Siderosis around eccrine glands appears specific for idiopathic hemochromatosis.[292] In rare instances, some iron is present in the epidermis, particularly in the basal cell layer, and in the epithelial cells of the sweat glands.[295]

In selecting a site for biopsy, it is not necessary to choose a pigmented area, because if deposits of iron are present in the skin, they are not limited to the areas of pigmentation. It is important, however, not to take a specimen from the legs, where deposits of iron are frequently found in association with even minor venous stasis or as a consequence of a preceding inflammation that may no longer be evident.

A skin biopsy no longer represents an important test for establishing the diagnosis of idiopathic hemochromatosis; it is merely of confirmatory value. Determinations in the serum of the level of iron, of the iron-binding capacity, as measured by the degree of saturation of transferrin with iron, of the plasma ferritin concentration, and, above all, biopsy of the liver, have replaced the skin biopsy in importance.[293]

Histogenesis. Idiopathic hemochromatosis is an autosomal recessive disorder. It is one of the most common abnormal genes in the United States: about 10% of the U.S. population are carriers of the disease.[296] This figure implies a homozygote frequency of two or three persons per 1000. The gene for hemochromatosis is linked to HLA-A and D65105 on chromosome 6p.[297]

The exact nature of the defect leading to excessive iron storage is not known. Although iron absorption through duodenal mucosa is excessive, it is not known if this is the primary event. The degree of saturation of transferrin with iron is very high. Consequently, not all of the iron passing from the intestinal tract can be bound to transferrin, and it is therefore deposited in a variety of organs. Iron accumulates particularly in the parenchyma of the liver and pancreas and in the myocardium, and by damaging the cells in which it accumulates, it causes hepatic cirrhosis, diabetes, and cardiac insufficiency.

Two observations indicate that the cutaneous pigmentation in idiopathic hemochromatosis is caused by melanin and not by hemosiderin. The first observation concerns a patient who, in addition to having idiopathic hemochromatosis, had vitiligo. The areas of vitiligo were fully depigmented despite the finding on histologic examination that they contained just as much iron as deeply pigmented areas.[294] The second observation was made in a black patient with idiopathic hemochromatosis who had three epidermal cysts. Although the patient had noticed no change in his skin color, he had observed progressive darkening of the cysts, and histologic examination revealed considerable amounts of melanin both in the walls of the cysts and in their keratinous contents.[298]

The increase in the amount of melanin found in the skin of patients with hemochromatosis is brought about by iron in the skin. The iron stimulates melanocytic activity either by increasing oxidative processes or by reacting with epidermal sulfhydryl groups and reducing their inhibitory effect on the enzyme system governing melanin synthesis.[299,300]

VITAMIN A DEFICIENCY (PHRYNODERMA)

Deficiency of vitamin A is very rare in the United States, occurring mainly in Asia and Africa. It has been recently described, however, as occurring after small bowel bypass surgery for obesity.[301,302] Vitamin A deficiency results in cutaneous changes to which the name *phrynoderma* has been given. These changes consist of dryness and roughness of the skin and the presence of conical, follicular keratotic lesions. In addition to causing cutaneous changes, deficiency of vitamin A may cause night blindness, xerophthalmia, and keratomalacia.

Histopathology. The skin shows moderate hyperkeratosis with marked distention of the upper parts of the hair follicles by large, horny plugs.[301,303] The horny plugs may perforate the follicular epithelium.[302] The sebaceous gland lobules are greatly reduced in size. There may also be atrophy of the sweat glands, such as flattening of the secretory cells.[304] In severe cases, the sweat glands and sebaceous glands may undergo keratinizing metaplasia.[305]

Differential Diagnosis. Histologic differentiation of phrynoderma from ichthyosis vulgaris and keratosis pilaris is impossible, except in very severe cases of phrynoderma, in which the sweat glands and the sebaceous glands show keratinizing metaplasia. Pityriasis rubra pilaris differs from phrynoderma by showing, in addition to hyperkeratosis and follicular plugging, stuttering parakeratosis, irregular epidermal hyperplasia, and an inflammatory infiltrate in the upper dermis.

PELLAGRA

Pellagra is caused by a deficiency of nicotinic acid (niacin) or its precursor, the essential amino acid tryptophan. As a dietary deficiency disease, it may occur in chronic alcoholics and patients with anorexia nervosa.[306] It may also occur in patients with the carcinoid syndrome; the tumor cells divert tryptophan toward serotonin, thus depressing endogenous niacin production.[307] In addition, pellagra is a well-recognized complication of isoniazid therapy for tuberculosis. Because isoniazid is a structural analog of niacin, it can cause the suppression of endogenous niacin production.[308] Because 5-fluorouracil inhibits the conversion of tryptophan to nicotinic acid, it also may precipitate pellagra.[309]

Pellagra presents cutaneous lesions, gastrointestinal symptoms, and mental changes, resulting in the triad of the three Ds: dermatitis, diarrhea, and dementia.

The cutaneous lesions are precipitated by sunlight. A symmetrical photosensitive dermatitis predominantly involves the dorsa of the hands, wrists, and forearms, the face, and the nape of the neck. In the early stage, there is erythema, which usually is sharply demarcated; in severe cases, it may be accompanied by vesicles or bullae. Later, the skin becomes thickened, scaly, and pigmented.

Histopathology. The histologic changes of the skin are nonspecific. Early lesions present a superficial perivascular lymphocytic inflammatory infiltrate in the upper dermis. Vesicles, if present, arise as in erythema multiforme either subepidermally, owing to vacuolar degeneration of the basal layer and edema in the papillary dermis, or intraepidermally, owing to degenerative changes in the epidermis.[310]

In older lesions, one observes hyperkeratosis with areas of parakeratosis and prominent but irregular epidermal hyperplasia. The amount of melanin in the basal layer of the epidermis often is increased. Late lesions may show epidermal atrophy, and the dermis may show fibrosis in addition to chronic inflammation.[310]

Hartnup Disease

First described in 1956 and named in 1957 after the family in which it was first observed, Hartnup disease is transmitted as an autosomal recessive trait.[311,312] It first manifests itself in early childhood and often improves with advancing age. A photosensitivity eruption is present that usually is indistinguishable from pellagra.[313] However, in some cases, the cutaneous reaction to sun exposure resembles poikiloderma atrophicans vasculare or, because of the prominence of vesicles, hydroa vacciniforme.[314,315] In addition, there may be cerebellar ataxia and mental retardation. Niacin is used to treat Hartnup disease.[313]

Histopathology. The cutaneous eruption in Hartnup disease usually shows the same histologic changes observed in pellagra (see earlier). In patients with poikiloderma-like changes, one observes atrophy of the epidermis and the presence of a chronic inflammatory infiltrate and of melanophages in the upper dermis.[314]

Histogenesis. The sun-sensitivity eruption with its resemblance to pellagra is caused by an enzymatic defect in the transport of tryptophan and a resultant decrease in the endogenous production of niacin. The defect in tryptophan transport consists of both an intestinal defect in tryptophan absorption and a renal tubular defect causing inadequate reabsorption of amino acids, including tryptophan. Chromatographic study of the urine shows a constant aminoaciduria, particularly the presence of tryptophan and of indolic substances derived from tryptophan—a finding that establishes the diagnosis.[314]

OCULOCUTANEOUS TYROSINOSIS

Oculocutaneous tyrosinosis, also referred to as the Richner-Hanhart syndrome and tyrosinemia type II, is transmitted as an autosomal recessive trait. It is characterized by very tender hyperkeratotic papules and plaques on the palms and soles arising in infancy or childhood; bilateral keratitis, which may lead to corneal opacities; and mental retardation. In some families, however, ocular changes are absent.[316] A diet low in tyrosine and phenylalanine improves the disease manifestations.

Histopathology. In most instances, the histologic findings in the keratotic lesions are not diagnostic, showing merely orthokeratotic hyperkeratosis with hypergranulosis and acanthosis.[317] In one reported case, vertical parakeratotic columns were present over the openings of the acrosyringia. Multinucleated keratinocytes and dyskeratotic cells were noted in the spinous layer.[318] A large intraepidermal bulla seen in another patient probably was also the result of irritation.[319]

Histogenesis. Tyrosinemia maps to chromosome 16q 22.1 to 16q 22.2.[313] As a result of a genetic deficiency in hepatic tyrosine aminotransferase, excessive amounts of tyrosine are found in the blood, urine, and tissues. It can be assumed that excessive amounts of intracellular tyrosine enhance cross-links between aggregated tonofilaments. On electron microscopic examination, aggregations of tonofilaments and needle-shaped tyrosine crystalline inclusions are found in keratinocytes.[318]

REFERENCES

1. Sipe JD. Amyloidosis. Crit Rev Clin Lab Sci 1994;31:325.
2. Husby G. Nomenclature and classification of amyloid and amyloidosis. J Intern Med 1992;232:511.
3. Glenner GG, Harbaugh J, Ohms JI et al. An amyloid protein: The amino-terminal variable fragment of an immunoglobulin light chain. Biochem Biophys Res Commun 1970;41:1287.
4. Kyle RA, Bayrd ED. Amyloidosis: Review of 236 cases. Medicine (Baltimore) 1975;54:171.
5. Kyle RA. Amyloidosis. Int J Dermatol 1980;19:537 and 1981;20:20.
6. Natelson EA, Duncan EC, Macossay CR et al. Amyloidosis palpebrarum. Arch Intern Med 1979;125:304.
7. Beacham BE, Greer KE, Andrews BS et al. Bullous amyloidosis. J Am Acad Dermatol 1980;3:506.
8. Brownstein MH, Helwig EB. The cutaneous amyloidosis. II. Systemic forms. Arch Dermatol 1970;102:20.
9. Bluhm JF III, Johnson SC, Norback DH. Bullous amyloidosis. Arch Dermatol 1980;116:1164.
10. Westermark P. Amyloidosis of the skin: A comparison between localized and systemic amyloidosis. Acta Derm Venereol (Stockh) 1979; 59:341.
11. Sepp N, Pichler E, Breathnach SM et al. Amyloid elastosis: Analysis of the role of amyloid P component. J Am Acad Dermatol 1990; 22:27.
12. Blumenfeld W, Hildebrandt RH. Fine needle aspiration of abdominal fat for the diagnosis of amyloidosis. Acta Cytol 1993;37:170.
13. Libbey CA, Skinner M, Cohen AS. Use of abdominal fat tissue aspirate in the diagnosis of systemic amyloidosis. Arch Intern Med 1983; 143:1549.
14. Rubinow A, Cohen AS. Skin involvement in generalized amyloidosis. Ann Intern Med 1978;88:781.
15. Masuda C, Mohri S, Nakajima H. Histopathological and immunohistochemical study of amyloidosis cutis nodularis atrophicans: Comparison with systemic amyloidosis. Br J Dermatol 1988;119:33.
16. Kyle RA. Amyloidosis: Introduction and overview. J Intern Med 1992;232:507.
17. Hashimoto K, Kumakiri M. Colloid: Amyloid bodies in PUVA-treated human psoriatic patients. J Invest Dermatol 1979;72:70.
18. Glenner GG, Page DL. Amyloid, amyloidosis and amyloidogenesis. Int Rev Exp Pathol 1976;15:2.
19. Goettler E, Anton-Lamprecht I, Kotzur B. Amyloidosis cutis nodularis. Hautarzt 1976;27:16.
20. Gertz MA. Secondary amyloidosis (AA). J Intern Med 1992;232:517.
21. Westermark P. Occurrence of amyloid deposits in the skin in secondary systemic amyloidosis. Acta Pathol Microbiol Scand [A] 1972; 80:718.
22. Orifila C, Giraud P, Modesto A et al. Abdominal fat tissue aspirate in human amyloidosis: Light, electron, and immunofluorescence studies. Hum Pathol 1986;17:366.
23. Levin M, Granklin EC, Frangione B, Pras M. The amino acid sequence of a major nonimmunoglobulin component of some amyloid fibrils. J Clin Invest 1972;51:2773.
24. Benditt EP, Eriksen N. Amyloid protein SAA is associated with high density lipoprotein from human serum. Proc Natl Acad Sci USA 1977; 74:4025.
25. Skinner M. Protein AA/SAA. J Intern Med 1992;232:513.
26. Breathnach SM, Black MM. Systemic amyloidosis and the skin. Clin Exp Dermatol 1979;4:517.
27. Jambrosic J, From L, Hanna W. Lichen amyloidosus. Am J Dermatopathol 1984;6:151.
28. Leonforte JF. Sur l'origine de l'amyloidose maculeuse. Ann Dermatol Venereol 1987;114:801.
29. Shanon J, Sagher F. Interscapular cutaneous amyloidosis. Arch Dermatol 1970;102:195.
30. Wong CK, Lin CS. Friction amyloidosis. Int J Dermatol 1988;27:302.
31. Brownstein MH, Hashimoto K. Macular amyloidosis. Arch Dermatol 1972;106:50.
32. Brownstein MH, Hashimoto K, Greenwald G. Biphasic amyloidosis: Link between macular and lichenoid forms. Br J Dermatol 1973;88: 25.
33. Bedi TR, Datta BN. Diffuse biphasic cutaneous amyloidosis. Dermatologica 1979;158:433.
34. Black MM, Wilson Jones E. Macular amyloidosis. Br J Dermatol 1971;84:199.
35. Kumakiri M, Hashimoto K. Histogenesis of primary localized cutaneous amyloidosis: Sequential change of epidermal keratinocytes to amyloid via filamentous degeneration. J Invest Dermatol 1979;73: 150.
36. Hashimoto K, Kobayashi H. Histogenesis of amyloid in the skin. Am J Dermatopathol 1980;2:165.
37. Glenner GG. Amyloid deposits and amyloidosis: The betafibrilloses. N Engl J Med 1980;302:1283.
38. Horiguchi Y, Fine JD, Leigh IM et al. Lamina densa malformation involved in histogenesis of primary localized amyloidosis. J Invest Dermatol 1992;99:12.
39. MacDonald DM, Black MM, Ramnarain N. Immunofluorescence studies in primary localized cutaneous amyloidosis. Br J Dermatol 1977;96:635.
40. Danno K, Horis T. Sulphhydryl and disulphide stainings of amyloid: A comparison with hyaline body. Acta Derm Venereol (Stockh) 1981; 61:285.
41. Masu S, Hosokawa M, Seiji M. Amyloid in localized cutaneous amyloidosis: Immunofluorescence studies with anti-keratin antiserum. Acta Derm Venereol (Stockh) 1981;61:381.
42. Ishii M, Asai Y, Hamada T. Evaluation of cutaneous amyloid employing auto-keratin antibodies and the immunoperoxidase technique (PAP method). Acta Derm Venereol (Stockh) 1984;64:281.
43. Ishii M, Terao Y, Hamada T. Formation of amyloid from degenerating collagen islands in primary cutaneous amyloidosis (abstr). Clin Exp Dermatol 1987;12:302.
44. Westermark P, Norén P. Two differenent pathogenetic pathways in lichen amyloidosus and macular amyloidosis. Arch Dermatol Res 1986;278:206.
45. Weedon D, Shand E. Amyloid deposits in the skin in secondary systemic amyloidosis. Br J Dermatol 1979;101:141.
46. Potter BA, Johnson WC. Primary localized amyloidosis cutis. Arch Dermatol 1971;103:448.
47. Goerttler E, Anton-Lamprecht I, Kotzur B. Amyloidosis cutis nodularis. Hautarzt 1976;27:16.
48. Rodermund OE. Zur amyloidosis cutis nodularis atrophicans (Gottron 1950). Arch Klin Exp Dermatol 1967;230:153.
49. Lindemayr W, Partsch H. Plattenartig infiltrierte lokalisierte hautamyloidose. Hautarzt 1970;21:104.
50. Brownstein MH, Helwig EB. The cutaneous amyloidoses: I. Localized forms. Arch Dermatol 1970;102:8.
51. Northcutt AD, Vanover MJ. Nodular cutaneous amyloidosis involving the vulva. Arch Dermatol 1985;121:518.

52. Ebner H, Gebhart W. Vergleichende untersuchungen bei juvenilem und adultem Colloid Milium. Arch Dermatol Res 1978;261:231.
53. Handfield-Jones SE, Atherton DJ, Black MM et al. Juvenile colloid milium: Clinical, histological and ultrastructural features. J Cutan Pathol 1992;19:434.
54. Kobayashi A, Hashimoto K. Colloid and elastic fibre: Ultrastructural study on the histogenesis of colloid milium. J Cutan Pathol 1983;10:111.
55. Stone MS, Tschen JA. Colloid milium. Arch Dermatol 1986;122:711.
56. Dupre A, Bonafe JF, Pieraggi MT et al. Paracolloid of the skin. J Cutan Pathol 1979;6:304.
57. Sullivan M, Ellis FA. Facial colloid degeneration in plaques. Arch Dermatol 1961;84:816.
58. Kawashima Y, Matsubara T, Kinbara T et al. Colloid degeneration of the skin. J Dermatol 1977;4:115.
59. Reuter MJ, Becker SW. Colloid degeneration (collagen degeneration) of the skin. Arch Dermatol Syph 1942;46:695.
60. Ebner H, Gebhart W. Colloid milium: Light and electron microscopic investigations. Clin Exp Dermatol 1977;2:217.
61. Percival BH, Duthie DA. Notes on a case of colloid pseudomilium. Br J Dermatol 1948;60:399.
62. Graham JH, Marques AS. Colloid milium: A histochemical study. J Invest Dermatol 1967;49:497.
63. Yanagihara M, Mehregan AM, Mehregan DR. Staining of amyloid with cotton dyes. Arch Dermatol 1984;120:1184.
64. Hashimoto K, Black M. Colloid milium: A final degeneration product of actinic elastoid. J Cutan Pathol 1985;12:147.
65. Hashimoto K, Nakayama H, Chimenti S et al. Juvenile colloid milium: Immunohistochemical and ultrastructural studies. J Cutan Pathol 1989;16:164.
66. Kumakiri M, Hashimoto K. Histogenesis of primary localized cutaneous amyloidosis: Sequential change of epidermal keratinocytes to amyloid via filamentous degeneration. J Invest Dermatol 1979;73: 150.
67. Siebenmann F. Über mitbeteiligung der schleimhaut bei allgemeiner hyperkeratose der haut. Arch Laryng Rhin 1908;20:101.
68. Urbach E, Wiethe C. Lipoidosis cutis et mucosae. Virchows Arch A 1929;273:285.
69. Konstantinov K, Kabakchiev P, Karchev T et al. Lipoid proteinosis. J Am Acad Dermatol 1992;27:293.
70. Paller AS. Histology of lipoid proteinosis. JAMA 1994;272:564.
71. Holtz KH, Schulze W. Beitrag zur klinik und pathogenese der hyalinosis cutis et mucosae (Lipoid-proteinose Urbach-Wiethe). Arch Dermatol Syph (Berlin) 1950;192:206.
72. Caplan RM. Visceral involvement in lipoid proteinosis. Arch Dermatol 1967;95:149.
73. Fleischmajer R, Nedwich A, Ramos E, Silva J. Hyalinosis cutis et mucosae. J Invest Dermatol 1969;52:495.
74. Shore RN, Howard BV, Howard WJ, Shelley WB. Lipoid proteinosis: Demonstration of normal lipid metabolism in cultured cells. Arch Dermatol 1974;110:591.
75. Laymon CW, Hill EM. An appraisal of hyalinosis cutis et mucosae. Arch Dermatol 1957;75:55.
76. Holtz KH. Über gehirn-und augenveränderungen bei hyalinosis cutis et mucosae (lipoid-proteinose) mit autopsiebefund. Arch Klin Exp Dermatol 1962;214:289.
77. Van der Walt IJ, Heyl T. Lipoid proteinosis and erythropoietic protoporphyria. Arch Dermatol 1971;104:501.
78. Kint A. A comparative electron microscopic study of the perivascular hyaline from porphyria cutanea tarda and from lipoid proteinosis. Arch Klin Exp Dermatol 1970;239:203.
79. Fleischmajer R, Krieg T, Dziadek M et al. Ultrastructure and composition of connective tissue in hyalinosis cutis et mucosae skin. J Invest Dermatol 1984;82:252.
80. McCusker JJ, Caplan RM. Lipoid proteinosis (lipoglycoproteinosis). Am J Pathol 1962;40:599.
81. Bauer EA, Santa-Cruz DJ, Aisen AL. Lipoid proteinosis: In vivo and in vitro evidence for a lysosomal storage disease. J Invest Dermatol 1981;76:119.
82. Harper JI, Duance VC, Sims TJ, Light ND. Lipoid proteinosis: An inherited disorder of collagen metabolism? Br J Dermatol 1985;113: 145.
83. Moy LS, Moy RL, Matsuoka LY et al. Lipoid proteinosis: Ultrastructural and biochemical studies. J Am Acad Dermatol 1987;16:1193.
84. Ishibashi A. Hyalinosis cutis et mucosae. Defective digestion and storage of basal lamina glycoprotein synthesized by smooth muscle cells. Dermatologica 1982;165:7.
85. Konrad K, Hönigsmann H, Gschnait F et al. Mouse model for protoporphyria: II. Cellular and subcellular events in the photosensitivity flare of the skin. J Invest Dermatol 1975;65:300.
86. Meola T, Lim HW. The porphyrias. Dermatol Clin 1993;11:583.
87. Stretcher GS. Erythropoietic porphyria. Arch Dermatol 1977;113: 1553.
88. Murphy GM, Hawk JLM, Nicholson DC et al. Congenital erythropoietic porphyria. Clin Exp Dermatol 1987;12:61.
89. Gschnait F, Wolff K, Konrad K. Erythropoietic protoporphyria: Submicroscopic events during the acute photosensitivity flare. Br J Dermatol 1975;92:545.
90. Ryan EA. Histochemistry of the skin in erythropoietic protoporphyria. Br J Dermatol 1966;78:501.
91. De Leo VA, Mathews-Roth M, Poh-Fitzpatrick M et al. Erythropoietic protoporphyria: Ten years experience. Am J Med 1976;60:8.
92. Harber LC, Poh-Fitzpatrick MB, Walther RR. Cutaneous aspects of the porphyrias. Acta Derm Venereol Suppl (Stockh) 1982;100:9.
93. Mathews-Roth MM. Erythropoietic protoporphyria: Diagnosis and treatment. N Engl J Med 1977;297:98.
94. MacDonald DM, Germain D, Perrot H. The histopathology and ultrastructure of liver disease in erythropoietic protoporphyria. Br J Dermatol 1981;104:7.
95. Cripps DJ, Goldfarb SS. Erythropoietic protoporphyria: Hepatic cirrhosis. Br J Dermatol 1978;98:349.
96. Wells MM, Golitz LE, Bender BJ. Erythropoietic protoporphyria with hepatic cirrhosis. Arch Dermatol 1980;116:429.
97. Fromke VL, Bossenmair I, Cardinal R et al. Porphyria variegata: Study of a large kindred in the United States. Am J Med 1978;65:80.
98. Mustajoki P. Variegate porphyria. Ann Intern Med 1978;89:238.
99. Poh-Fitzpatrick MB. A plasma porphyrin fluorescence marker for variegate porphyria. Arch Dermatol 1980;116:543.
100. Corey TJ, De Leo VA, Christianson H et al. Variegate porphyria: Clinical and laboratory features. J Am Acad Dermatol 1980;2:36.
101. Elder GH. Recent advances in the identification of enzyme deficiencies in the porphyrias (comment). Br J Dermatol 1983;108:729.
102. Köstler E, Seebacher C, Riedel H et al. Therapeutische und pathogenetische aspekte der porphyria cutanea tarda. Hautarzt 1986;37: 210.
103. Roenigk HH, Gottlob ME. Estrogen-induced porphyria cutanea tarda. Arch Dermatol 1970;102:260.
104. Elder GH, Lee GB, Tovey JA. Decreased activity of hepatic uroporphyrinogen decarboxylase in sporadic porphyria cutanea tarda. N Engl J Med 1978;299:274.
105. Keczkes K, Barker DJ. Malignant hepatoma associated with acquired cutaneous porphyria. Arch Dermatol 1976;112:78.
106. Czarnecki DB. Hepatoerythropoietic porphyria. Arch Dermatol 1980; 116:307.
107. Simon N, Berkó G, Schneider I. Hepato-erythropoietic porphyria presenting as scleroderma and acrosclerosis in a sibling pair. Br J Dermatol 1977;663.
108. Lim HW, Poh-Fitzpatrick MB. Hepatoerythropoietic porphyria: A variant of childhood-onset porphyria cutanea tarda. J Am Acad Dermatol 1984;11:1103.
109. Hönigsmann H, Reichel K. Hepatoerythrozytäre Porphyrie. Hautarzt 1979;30:95.
110. Roberts DT, Brodie MJ, Moore MR et al. Hereditary coproporphyria presenting with photosensitivity induced by the contraceptive pill. Br J Dermatol 1977;96:549.
111. Hunter GA. Clinical manifestations of the porphyrias: A review. Australas J Dermatol 1979;20:120.
112. Kint A. A comparative electron microscopic study of the perivascular hyaline from porphyria cutanea tarda and from lipoid proteinosis. Arch Klin Exp Dermatol 1970;239:203.
113. Epstein JH, Tuffanelli DL, Epstein WL. Cutaneous changes in the porphyrias. Arch Dermatol 1973;107:689.
114. Ozasa S, Yamamoto S, Maeda M et al. Erythropoietic protoporphyria. J Dermatol 1977;4:85.
115. Wolff K, Hönigsmann H, Rauschmeier W et al. Microscopic and fine structural aspects of porphyrias. Acta Derm Venereol Suppl (Stockh) 1982;100:17.

116. Klein GF, Hintner H, Schuler G et al. Junctional blisters in acquired bullous disorders of the dermal-epidermal junction zone. Br J Dermatol 1983;109:499.
117. Nagato N, Nonaka S, Ohgami T et al. Mechanism of blister formation in porphyria cutanea tarda. J Dermatol Tokyo 1987;14:551.
118. Feldaker M, Montgomery H, Brunsting LA. Histopathology of porphyria cutanea tarda. J Invest Dermatol 1955;24:131.
119. Egbert BM, LeBoit PE, McCalmont T et al. Caterpillar bodies: Distinctive, basement membrane-containing structures in blisters of porphyria. Am J Dermatopathol 1993;15:199.
120. Raso DS, Greene WB, Maize JC et al. Caterpillar bodies of porphyria cutanea tarda ultrastructurally represent a unique arrangement of colloid and basement membrane bodies. Am J Dermatopathol 1996; 18:24.
121. Anton-Lamprecht I, Meyer B. Zur ultrastruktur der haut bei protoporphyrinämie. Dermatologica 1970;141:76.
122. Ryan EA, Madill GT. Electron microscopy of the skin in erythropoietic protoporphyria. Br J Dermatol 1968;80:561.
123. Murphy GM, Hawk JLM, Magnus JA. Late-onset erythropoietic protoporphyria with unusual cutaneous features. Arch Dermatol 1985; 121:1309.
124. Cormane RH, Szabo E, Tio TY. Histopathology of the skin in acquired and hereditary porphyria cutanea tarda. Br J Dermatol 1971;85:531.
125. Gilchrest B, Rowe JW, Mihm MC Jr. Bullous dermatosis in hemodialysis. Ann Intern Med 1975;83:480.
126. Thivolet J, Euvrard S, Perrot H et al. La pseudo-porphyrie cutanée tardive des hémodialyses. Ann Dermatol Venereol 1977;104:12.
127. Perrot H, Germain D, Euvrard S et al. Porphyria cutanea tardalike dermatosis by hemodialysis. Arch Dermatol Res 1977;259:177.
128. Poh-Fitzpatrick MB, Bellet N, De Leo VA et al. Porphyria cutanea tarda in two patients treated with hemodialysis for chronic renal failure. N Engl J Med 1978;299:292.
129. Poh-Fitzpatrick MB, Masullo AS, Grossman ME. Porphyria cutanea tarda associated with chronic renal failure and hemodialysis. Arch Dermatol 1980;116:191.
130. Harlan SL, Winkelmann RK. Porphyria cutanea tarda and chronic renal failure. Mayo Clin Proc 1983;58:467.
131. Judd LE, Henderson DW, Hill DC. Naproxen-induced pseudoporphyria. Arch Dermatol 1986;122:451.
132. Wilson CW, Wingfield WL, Toone EC Jr. Vitamin D poisoning with metastatic calcification. Am J Med 1953;14:116.
133. Wermer P, Kuschner M, Riley EA. Reversible metastatic calcification associated with excessive milk and alkali intake. Am J Med 1953;14: 108.
134. Mulligan RM. Metastatic calcification. Arch Pathol 1947;43:177.
135. Katz AI, Hampers CL, Merrill JP. Secondary hyperparathyroidism and renal osteodystrophy in chronic renal failure (review). Medicine (Baltimore) 1969;48:333.
136. Kolton B, Pedersen J. Calcinosis cutis and renal failure. Arch Dermatol 1974;110:256.
137. Kuzela DC, Huffer WE, Conger JD et al. Soft tissue calcification in chronic dialysis patients. Am J Pathol 1977;86:403.
138. Parfitt AM. Soft tissue calcification in uremia. Arch Intern Med 1969; 124:544.
139. Putkonen T, Wangel GA. Renal hyperparathyroidism with metastatic calcification of the skin. Dermatologica 1959;118:127.
140. Ivker RA, Woosley J, Briggaman RA. Calciphylaxis in three patients with end-stage renal disease. Arch Dermatol 1995;131:63.
141. Cockerell CJ, Dolan ET. Widespread cutaneous and systemic calcification (calciphylaxis) in patients with the acquired immuno-deficiency syndrome and renal disease. J Am Acad Dermatol 1992;26:559.
142. Posey RE, Ritchie EB. Metastatic calcinosis cutis with renal hyperparathyroidism. Arch Dermatol 1967;95:505.
143. Eisenberg E, Bartholow PV Jr. Reversible calcinosis cutis. N Engl J Med 1963;268:1216.
144. Winkelmann RK, Keating FR Jr. Cutaneous vascular calcification, gangrene and hyperparathyroidism. Br J Dermatol 1970;83:263.
145. Chan YL, Mahoney JF, Turner JJ et al. The vascular lesions associated with skin necrosis in renal disease. Br J Dermatol 1983;109:85.
146. Leroy D, Barrellier MT, Zanello D. Purpura réticulé et nécrotique (à type d'angiodermite nécrotique) dû à des calcifications artérielles au cours d'une insufficiance rénale chronique. Ann Dermatol Venereol 1984;111:461.
147. Fischer AH, Morris DJ. Pathogenesis of calciphylaxis: Study of three cases with literature review. Hum Pathol 1995;26:1055.
148. Velayos EE, Masi AT, Stevens MB et al. The "CREST" syndrome: Comparison with systemic sclerosis (scleroderma). Arch Intern Med 1979;139:1240.
149. Muller SA, Winkelmann RK, Brunsting LA. Calcinosis in dermatomyositis. Arch Dermatol 1959;79:669.
150. Muller SA, Brunsting LA, Winkelmann RK. Calcinosis cutis: Its relationship to scleroderma. Arch Dermatol 1959;80:15.
151. Holmes R. Morphoea with calcinosis. Clin Exp Dermatol 1979;4:125.
152. Carr RD, Heisel EB, Stevenson TD. CREST syndrome. Arch Dermatol 1965;92:519.
153. Kabir DJ, Malkinson FD. Lupus erythematosus and calcinosis cutis. Arch Dermatol 1969;100:17.
154. Reich H. Das Teutschlaender-Syndrom. Hautarzt 1963;14:462.
155. Paegle RD. Ultrastructure of mineral deposits in calcinosis cutis. Arch Pathol 1966;2:474.
156. Cornelius CE III, Tenenhouse A, Weber JC. Calcinosis cutis. Arch Dermatol 1968;98:219.
157. Haim S, Friedman-Birnbaum R. Two cases of circumscribed calcinosis. Dermatologica 1971;143:111.
158. Whiting DA, Simson IW, Kallmeyer JC et al. Unusual cutaneous lesions in tumoral calcinosis. Arch Dermatol 1970;102:465.
159. Pursley TV, Prince MJ, Chausmer AB et al. Cutaneous manifestations of tumoral calcinosis. Arch Dermatol 1979;115:1100.
160. Mozaffarian G, Lafferty FW, Pearson OH. Treatment of tumoral calcinosis with phosphorus deprivation. Ann Intern Med 1972;77: 741.
161. Shapiro L, Platt N, Torres-Rodriquez VM. Idiopathic calcinosis of the scrotum. Arch Dermatol 1970;102:199.
162. Fisher BK, Dvoretzky I. Idiopathic calcinosis of the scrotum. Arch Dermatol 1978;114:957.
163. Bode U, Plewig G. Klassifikation follikulärer zysten. Hautarzt 1980; 31:1.
164. Swinehart JM, Golitz LE. Scrotal calcinosis: Dystrophic calcification of epidermoid cysts. Arch Dermatol 1982;118:985.
165. Dare AJ, Axelsen RA. Scrotal calcinosis: Origin from dystrophic calcification of eccrine duct milia. J Cutan Pathol 1988;15:142.
166. Song DH, Lee KH, Kang WH. Idiopathic calcinosis of the scrotum. J Am Acad Dermatol 1988;19:1095.
167. Woods B, Kellaway TD. Cutaneous calculi. Br J Dermatol 1963;75:1.
168. Tezuka T. Cutaneous calculus: Its pathogenesis. Dermatologica 1980; 161:191.
169. Shmunes E, Wood MG. Subepidermal calcified nodules. Arch Dermatol 1972;105:593.
170. Eng AM, Mandrea E. Perforating calcinosis cutis presenting as milia. J Cutan Pathol 1981;8:247.
171. Winer LH. Solitary congenital nodular calcification of the skin. Arch Dermatol Syph 1952;66:204.
172. Steigleder GK, Elschner H. Lokalisierte calcinosis. Hautarzt 1957; 8:127.
173. Duperrat B, Goetschel G. Calcification nodulaire solitaire congénitale de la peau (Winer, 1952). Ann Dermatol Syphiligr 1963;90:283.
174. O'Duffy JD, Hunder GG, Kelly PJ. Decreasing prevalence of tophaceous gout. Mayo Clin Proc 1975;50:227.
175. Lichtenstein L, Scott HW, Levin MH. Pathologic changes in gout. Am J Pathol 1956;32:871.
176. Lopez Redondo MJ, Requena L, Macia M et al. Fingertip tophi without gouty arthritis. Dermatology 1993;187:140.
177. LeBoit PE, Schneider S. Gout presenting as lobular panniculitis. Am J Dermatopathol 1987;9:334.
178. King DF, King LA. The appropriate processing of tophi for microscopy. Am J Dermatopathol 1982;4:239.
179. Gottron HA, Korting GW. Chronische hautgicht. Arch Klin Exp Dermatol 1957;204:483.
180. Cohen PR, Schmidt WA, Rapini RP. Chronic tophaceous gout with severely deforming arthritis: A case report with emphasis on histopathologic considerations. Cutis 1991;48:445.
181. Seegmiller JE. Skin manifestations of gout. In: Eisen AZ, Wolff K et al., eds. Dermatology in general medicine. 4th ed. New York: McGraw-Hill, 1993;1894.
182. Janocha S, Wolz W, Srsen S et al. The human gene for alkaptonuria (AKU) maps to chromosome 3q. Genomics 1994;19:5.

183. Snider RL, Thiers BT. Exogenous ochronosis. J Am Acad Dermatol 1993;28:662.
184. Penneys NS. Ochronosislike pigmentation from hydroquinone bleaching creams. Arch Dermatol 1985;121:1239.
185. Lichtenstein L, Kaplan L. Hereditary ochronosis. Am J Pathol 1954; 30:99.
186. Findlay GH, Morrison JGL, Simson IW. Exogeneous ochronosis and pigmented colloid milium from hydroquinone bleaching creams. Br J Dermatol 1975;93:613.
187. Laymon CW. Ochronosis. Arch Dermatol 1953;67:553.
188. Teller H, Winkler K. Zur klinik und histopathologie der endogenen ochronose. Moutarzt 1973;24:537.
189. Dogliotti M, Leibowitz M. Granulomatous ochronosis: A cosmetic-induced skin disorder in blacks. Afr Med J 1979;56:757.
190. Jordaan HF, Van Niekerk DJT. Transepidermal elimination in exogenous ochronosis. Am J Dermatopathol 1991;13:418.
191. Zannoni VG, Malawista SE, La Du BN. Studies on ochronosis: II. Studies on benzoquinone-acetic acid, a probable intermediate in the connective tissue pigmentation of alcaptonuria. Arthritis Rheum 1962;5:547.
192. Atwood HD, Clifton S, Mitchell RE. A histological, histochemical and ultrastructural study of dermal ochronosis. Pathology 1971;3:115.
193. Tidman MJ, Horton JJ, Macdonald DM. Hydroquinone-induced ochronosis: Light and electron-microscopic features. Clin Exp Dermatol 1986;11:224.
194. Holubar K, Mach KW. Scleredema (Buschke). Acta Derm Venereol (Stockh) 1967;47:102.
195. Johnson WC, Helwig EB. Cutaneous focal mucinosis. Arch Dermatol 1966;93:13.
196. Cawley EP, Lupton CH Jr, Wheeler CE et al. Examination of normal and myxedematous skin. Arch Dermatol 1957;76:537.
197. Wortsman JD, Traycoff RB, Stone S. Preradial myxedema in thyroid disease. Arch Dermatol 1981;117:635.
198. Lynch PJ, Maize JC, Lisson JC. Pretibial myxedema and nonthyrotoxic thyroid disease. Arch Dermatol 1973;107:107.
199. Konrad K, Brenner W, Pehamberger H. Ultrastructural and immunological findings in Graves' disease with pretibial myxedema. J Cutan Pathol 1980;7:99.
200. Ishii M, Nakagawa M, Hamada T. An ultrastructural study of pretibial myxedema utilizing improved ruthenium red stain. J Cutan Pathol 1984;11:125.
201. Schermer DR, Roenigk HH Jr, Schumacher OP et al. Relationship of long-acting thyroid stimulator to pretibial myxedema. Arch Dermatol 1970;102:62.
202. Cheung HS, Nicoloff JT, Kamiel MB et al. Stimulation of fibroblast biosynthetic activity by serum of patients with pretibial myxedema. J Invest Dermatol 1978;71:12.
203. Somach SC, Helm TN, Lawlor KB et al. Pretibial mucin: Histologic patterns and clinical correlation. Arch Dermatol 1993;129:1152.
204. Hill TG, Crawford JN, Rogers CC. Successful management of lichen myxedematosus. Arch Dermatol 1976;112:67.
205. Hardie RA, Hunter JAA, Urbaniak S et al. Spontaneous resolution of lichen myxedematosus. Br J Dermatol 1979;100:727.
206. Flowers SL, Cooper PM, Landes HB. Acral persistent papular mucinosis. J Am Acad Dermatol 1989;21:293.
207. Stephens CJM, McKee PH, Black MM. The dermal mucinoses: Advances in dermatology 1993;8:201.
208. Borradori L, Aractingi S, Blanc F et al. Acral persistent papular mucinosis and IgA monoclonal gammopathy. Dermatology 1992;185:134.
209. Lum D. Cutaneous mucinosis of infancy. Arch Dermatol 1980;116:198.
210. Dalton JE, Seidell MA. Studies on lichen myxedematosus (papular mucinosis). Arch Dermatol 1954;67:194.
211. Montgomery H, Underwood LJ. Lichen myxedematosus: differentiation from cutaneous myxedemas or mucoid states. J Invest Dermatol 1953;20:213.
212. Rudner EJ, Mehregan A, Pinkus H. Scleromyxedema. Arch Dermatol 1966;93:3.
213. Braun-Falco O, Weidner F. Skleromyxödem Arndt-Gottron mit knochenmarks-plasmocytose und myositis. Arch Belg Dermatol Syphiligr 1970;26:193.
214. Perry HO, Montgomery H, Stickney JM. Further observations on lichen myxedematosus. Ann Intern Med 1960;53:955.
215. McGuiston CH, Schoch EP Jr. Autopsy findings in lichen myxedematosus. Arch Dermatol 1956;74:259.
216. Hardemeier T, Vogel A. Elektronenmikroskopische befunde beim sklerömyxodem Arndt-Gottron. Arch Klin Exp Dermatol 1970;237: 722.
217. Howsden SM, Herndon JH Jr, Freeman RG. Lichen myxedematosus. Arch Dermatol 1975;111:1325.
218. Carli-Basset C, Lorette G, Alison Y et al. Apparition retardée d'une mucinose papuleuse. Ann Dermatol Venereol 1979;106:175.
219. Harris RB, Perry HO, Kyle RA et al. Treatment of scleromyxedema with melphalan. Arch Dermatol 1979;115:295.
220. Lawrence DA, Tye MJ, Liss M. Immunochemical analysis of the basic immunoglobulin in papular mucinosis. Immunochemistry 1972; 9:41.
221. Shapiro CM, Fretzin D, Norris S. Papular mucinosis. JAMA 1970; 214:2052.
222. Piper W, Hardmeier T, Schäfer E. Das skleromyxödem Arndt-Gottron: Eine paraproteinämische ekrankung. Schweiz Med Wochenschr 1967;97:829.
223. Archibald GC, Calvert HT. Hypothyroidism and lichen myxoedematosus. Arch Dermatol 1977;113:684.
224. Lai A, Fat RFM, Suurmond D, Radl J et al. Scleromyxedema (lichen myxedematosus) associated with a paraprotein, IgG_1 of the type kappa. Br J Dermatol 1973;88:107.
225. James K, Fudenberg H, Epstein WL et al. Studies on a unique diagnostic serum globulin in papular mucinosis (lichen myxedematosus). Clin Exp Immunol 1967;2:153.
226. Feldman P, Shapiro L, Pick AI et al. Scleromyxedema. Arch Dermatol 1969;99:51.
227. McCarthy JT, Osserman E, Lombardo PC et al. An abnormal serum globulin in lichen myxedematosus. Arch Dermatol 1964;89:446.
228. Muldrow ML, Bailin PH. Scleromyxedema associated with IgG lambda multiple myeloma. Clev Clin Q 1983;50:189.
229. Rowell NR, Waite A, Scott DG. Multiple serum protein abnormalities in lichen myxedematosus. Br J Dermatol 1969;81:753.
230. Sawada Y, Ohashi M. Scleromyxedema. J Dermatol (Tokyo) 1980; 7:207.
231. Yaron M, Yaron I, Yust I et al. Lichen myxedematosus (scleromyxedema) serum stimulates hyaluronic acid and prostaglandin E production by human fibroblasts. J Rheumatol 1985;12:171.
232. Harper RA, Rispler J. Lichen myxedematosus serum stimulates human skin fibroblast proliferation. Science 1978;199:545.
233. Perry HO, Kierland RR, Montgomery H. Plaque-like form of cutaneous mucinosis. Arch Dermatol 1960;82:980.
234. Steigleder GK, Gartmann H, Linker U. REM-syndrome: Reticular erythematous mucinosis (round-cell erythematosis): A new entity? Br J Dermatol 1974;91:191.
235. Quimby SR, Perry HO. Plaque-like cutaneous mucinosis: Its relationship to reticular erythematous mucinosis. J Am Acad Dermatol 1982; 6:856.
236. Morison WL, Shea CR, Parrish JA. Reticular erythematous mucinosis syndrome. Arch Dermatol 1979;115:1340.
237. Braddock SW, Kay HD, Maennle D et al. Clinical and immunologic studies in reticular erthematous mucinosis and Jessner's lymphocytic infiltrate of skin. J Am Acad Dermatol 1993;28:691.
238. Herzberg J. Das REM-Syndrom. Z Hautkr 1981;56:1317.
239. Stephens CJM, Das AK, Black MM et al. The dermal mucinoses: A clinicopathologic and ultrastructural study. J Cutan Pathol 1990;17:319.
240. Balogh E, Nagy-Vezekényi K, Fórizs E. REM syndrome. Acta Derm Venereol (Stockh) 1980;60:173.
241. Caputo R, Grima HR, Gelmetti C. Self-healing juvenile cutaneous mucinosis. Arch Dermatol 1995;131:459.
242. Pucevich MV, Latour DL, Bale GF et al. Self-healing juvenile cutaneous mucinosis. J Am Acad Dermatol 1984;11:327.
243. Cron RQ, Swetter SM. Scleredema revisited: A post-streptococcal complication. Clin Pediatr (Phila) 1994;33:606.
244. Heilbron B, Saxe N. Scleredema in an infant. Arch Dermatol 1986; 122:1417.
245. Venencie PY, Powell FC, Su WPD et al. Scleredema: A review of thirty-three cases. J Am Acad Dermatol 1984;11:128.
246. Fleischmajer R, Raludi G, Krol S. Scleredema and diabetes mellitus. Arch Dermatol 1970;101:21.
247. Krakowski A, Covo J, Berlin C. Diabetic scleredema. Dermatologica 1973;146:193.
248. Fleischmajer R, Perlish JS. Glycosaminoglycans in scleroderma and scleredema. J Invest Dermatol 1972;58:129.

249. Kövary PM, Vakilzadeh F, Macher E et al. Monoclonal gammopathy in scleredema. Arch Dermatol 1981;117:536.
250. Roupe G, Laurent TC, Malmström A et al. Biochemical characterization and tissue distribution of the scleredema in a case of Buschke's disease. Acta Derm Venereol (Stockh) 1987;67:193.
251. Niebauer G, Ebner H. Skleroedema (Buschke). Dermatol Monatsschr 1970;156:940.
252. Curtis AC, Shulak BM. Scleredema adultorum. Arch Dermatol 1965; 92:526.
253. Matsuoka LY, Wortsman J, Dietrich JG et al. Glycosaminoglycans in histologic sections. Arch Dermatol 1987;123:862.
254. Reichenberger M. Betrachtungen zum Skleroedema adultorum Buschke. Hautarzt 1964; 15:339.
255. Vallee BL. Scleredema: A systemic disease. N Engl J Med 1946;235: 207.
256. Leinwand I. Generalized scleredema: Report with autopsy findings. Ann Intern Med 1951;34:226.
257. Ohta A, Uitto J, Oikarinen AI et al. Paraproteinemia in patients with scleredema. J Am Acad Dermatol 1987;16:96.
258. Sansom JE, Sheehan AL, Kennedy CT, Delaney TJ. A fatal case of scleredema of Buschke. Br J Dermatol 1994;130:669.
259. Wenstrup RJ, Pinnell SR. The genetic mucopolysaccharides. In: Fitzpatrick TB, Eisen AZ, Wolff K et al., eds. Dermatology in general practice. 4th ed. New York: McGraw-Hill, 1993;1971.
260. Hambrick GW Jr, Scheie HG. Studies of the skin in Hurler's syndrome. Arch Dermatol 1962;85:455.
261. Horiuchi R, Ishikawa H, Ishii Y et al. Mucopolysaccharidosis with special reference to Scheie syndrome. J Dermatol 1976;3:171.
262. Prystowsky SD, Maumenee IH, Freeman RG et al. A cutaneous marker in the Hunter syndrome. Arch Dermatol 1977;113:602.
263. Lasser A, Carter DM, Mahoney MJ. Ultrastructure of the skin in mucopolysaccharidoses. Arch Pathol 1975;99:173.
264. Zivony DI, Spencer DM, Qualman SJ, Bechtel M. Ivory colored papules in a young boy. Arch Dermatol 1995;131:81.
265. Freeman RG. A pathological basis for the cutaneous papules of mucopolysaccharidosis: II. The Hunter syndrome. J Cutan Pathol 1977;4:318.
266. Belcher RW. Ultrastructure of the skin in the genetic mucopolysaccharidoses. Arch Pathol 1972;94:511.
267. Belcher RW. Ultrastructure and function of eccrine glands in the mucopolysaccharidoses. Arch Pathol 1973;96:339.
268. Belcher RW. Ultrastructure and cytochemistry of lymphocytes in the genetic mucopolysaccharidoses. Arch Pathol 1972;93:1.
269. Whitley CB, Belani KG, Change PN et al. Long-term outcome of Hurler syndrome following bone marrow transplantation. Am J Med Genet 1993;46:209.
270. De Cloux RJ, Friederici HHR. Ultrastructural studies of the skin in Hurler's syndrome. Arch Pathol 1969;88:350.
271. Schwartz RA. Acanthosis nigricans. J Am Acad Dermatol 1994; 31:1.
272. Mikhail GR, Fachnie DM, Drukker BH et al. Generalized malignant acanthosis nigricans. Arch Dermatol 1979;115:201.
273. Curth HO. Classification of acanthosis nigricans. Int J Dermatol 1976;15:592.
274. Rendon MI, Cruz PD, Sontheimer RD et al. Acanthosis nigricans: A cutaneous marker of tissue resistance to insulin. J Am Acad Dermatol 1989;21:461.
275. Hud JA Jr, Cohen JB, Wagner JM, Cruz PD. Prevalence and significance of acanthosis nigricans in an adult obese population. Arch Dermatol 1992;128:941.
276. Ober KP. Acanthosis nigricans and insulin resistance associated with hypothyroidism. Arch Dermatol 1985;121:229.
277. Oseid S, Beck-Nielsen H, Pedersen O. Decreased binding of insulin to its receptor in patients with congenital generalized lipodystrophy. New Engl J Med 1977;296:245.
278. Stals H, Vercammen C, Peters C, Morren MA. Acanthosis nigricans caused by nicotinic acid. Dermatology 1994;189:203.
279. Greenspan AH, Shupack JL, Foo SH et al. Acanthosis nigricans hyperpigmentation secondary to triazinate therapy. Arch Dermatol 1985; 121:232.
280. Fleming MG, Simon SI. Cutaneous insulin reaction resembling acanthosis nigricans. Arch Dermatol 1986;122:1054.
281. Bonnekuh B, Wevers A, Spangenberger H et al. Keratin patterns of acanthosis nigricans in syndrome-like association with polythelia, polycystic kidneys, and syndactyly. Arch Dermatol 1993;129:1177.
282. Brown J, Winkelmann RK. Acanthosis nigricans: A study of 90 cases (review). Medicine (Baltimore) 1968;47:33.
283. Wortsman J, Matsuoka LY, Kupchella CE et al. Glycosaminoglycan deposition in the acanthosis nigricans lesions of the polycystic ovary syndrome. Arch Intern Med 1983;143:1145.
284. Cruz PD, Hud JA. Excess insulin binding to insulin-like growth factor receptors: Proposed mechanism for acanthosis nigricans. J Invest Dermatol 1992;98:82S.
285. Wilgenbus K, Lentner A, Kuckelkorn R et al. Further evidence that acanthosis nigricans maligna is linked to enhanced secretion by the tumour of transforming growth factor alpha. Arch Dermatol Res 1992; 284:266.
286. Gougerot H, Carteaud A. Papillomatose pigmentée innominée. Bull Soc Fr Dermatol Syphiligr 1927;34:719.
287. Kesten BM, James HD. Pseudoatrophoderma colli, acanthosis nigricans, and confluent and reticular papillomatosis. Arch Dermatol 1957; 75:525.
288. Roberts SDB, Lachapelle JM. Confluent and reticulate papillomatosis (Gougerot-Carteaud) and Pityrosporon orbiculare. Br J Dermatol 1969;81:841.
289. Yesudian P, Kamalam S, Razack A. Confluent and reticulated papillomatosis (Gougerot-Carteaud). Acta Derm Venereol (Stockh) 1973; 53:381.
290. Nordby CA, Mitchell AJ. Confluent and reticulated papillomatosis responsive to selenium sulfide. Int J Dermatol 1986;25:194.
291. Fairbanks VF, Baldus WP. Hemochromatosis: The neglected diagnosis. Mayo Clin Proc 1986;61:296.
292. Chevrant-Breton J, Simon M, Bourel M et al. Cutaneous manifestations of idiopathic hemo-chromatosis: Study of 100 cases. Arch Dermatol 1977;113:161.
293. Milder MS, Cook JD, Stray S et al. Idiopathic hemochromatosis: An interim report. Medicine (Baltimore) 1980;59:34.
294. Perdrup A, Poulsen H. Hemochromatosis and vitiligo. Arch Dermatol 1964;90:34.
295. Weintraub LR, Demis DJ, Conrad ME et al. Iron excretion by the skin: Selective localization of iron^{59} in epithelial cells. Am J Pathol 1965; 46:121.
296. Crosby WH. Hemochromatosis: The missed diagnosis. Arch Intern Med 1986;146:1209.
297. Stone C, Pointon JJ, Halliday JW et al. Isolation of CA dinucleotide repeats close to D6S105: Linkage disequilibrium with hemochromatosis. Hum Mol Genet 1994;3:2043.
298. Leyden JL, Lockshin NA, Kriebel S. The black keratinous cyst: A sign of hemochromatosis. Arch Dermatol 1972;106:379.
299. Robert P, Zürcher H. Pigmentstudien: I. Mitteilung: Über den einfluss von schwermetallverbindungen, hämin, vitaminen, mikrobiellen toxinen, hormonen und weiteren stoffen auf die dopamelaninbildung in vitro und die pigmentbildung in vivo. Dermatologica 1950;100:217.
300. Buckley WR. Localized argyria. Arch Dermatol 1963;88:531.
301. Wechsler HL. Vitamin A deficiency following small-bowel bypass surgery for obesity. Arch Dermatol 1979;115:73.
302. Barr DJ, Riley RJ, Green DJ. Bypass phrynoderma: Vitamin A deficiency associated with bowel-bypass surgery. Arch Dermatol 1984; 120:919.
303. Fasal P. Clinical manifestations of vitamin deficiencies as observed in the Federated Malay States. Arch Dermatol Syph 1944;50:160.
304. Frazier CN, Hu C. Nature and distribution according to age of cutaneous manifestations of vitamin A deficiency. Arch Dermatol Syph 1936;33:825.
305. Bessey OA, Wolbach SB. Vitamin A: Physiology and pathology. JAMA 1938;110:2072.
306. Rapaport MJ: Pellagra in a patient with anorexia nervosa. Arch Dermatol 1985;121:255.
307. Castiello RJ, Lynch PJ. Pellagra and the carcinoid syndrome. Arch Dermatol 1972;105:574.
308. Cohen LK, George W, Smith R. Isoniazid-induced acne and pellagra. Arch Dermatol 1974;109:377.
309. Stevens HP, Ostlere LS, Begent RHJ et al. Pellagra secondary to 5-fluorouracil. Br J Dermatol 1993;128:578.
310. Moore RA, Spies TD, Cooper ZK. Histopathology of the skin in pellagra. Arch Dermatol Syph 1942;46:106.
311. Baron DN, Dent CE, Harris H et al. Hereditary pellagralike skin rash with temporary cerebellar ataxia, constant renal aminoaciduria and other bizarre chemical features. Lancet 1956;2:421.

312. Dent CE. Hartnup disease: An inborn error of metabolism. Arch Dis Child 1957;32:363.
313. Goldsmith LA. Biochemical diseases. In: Alper JA. Genetic disorders of the skin. St. Louis: Mosby-Yearbook, 1991;64.
314. Clodi PH, Deutsch E, Niebauer G. Krankheitsbild mit poikilodermieartigen hautveränderungen, aminoacidurie und indolaceturie. Arch Klin Exp Dermatol 1964;218:165.
315. Ashurst PJ. Hydroa vacciniforme occurring in association with Hartnup disease. Br J Dermatol 1969;81:486.
316. Rehák A, Selim MM, Yadav G. Richner-Hanhart syndrome (tyrosinaemia-II): Report of four cases without ocular involvement. Br J Dermatol 1981;104:469.
317. Larrègue M, De Giacomoni P, Odièvre P et al. Modification des kératinocytes au cours de la tyrosinose oculo-cutanée: Syndrome de Richner-Hanhart. Ann Dermatol Venereol 1980;107:1023.
318. Shimizu N, Ito M, Ito K et al. Richner-Hanhart's syndrome: Electron microscopic study of the skin lesions. Arch Dermatol 1990;126:1342.
319. Zaleski WA, Hill A, Kushniruk W. Skin lesions in tyrosinosis: Response to dietary treatment. Br J Dermatol 1973;88:335.

Lever's Histopathology of the Skin, eighth edition,
edited by David Elder et al. Lippincott–
Raven Publishers, Philadelphia © 1997.

CHAPTER 18

Inflammatory Diseases of the Epidermal Appendages and of Cartilage

Edward Abell

ACNE VULGARIS

Acne vulgaris is a disease of adolescence and early adulthood that only occasionally persists later into adult life—more often in women. Chiefly affecting the face, upper back, and chest, it produces two types of lesions: comedones and inflammatory lesions. Comedones may be closed "whiteheads" or open "blackheads." Closed comedones much more frequently evolve into inflammatory lesions. Inflammatory lesions may also arise from diminutive follicular lesions or microcomedones, which are not clinically observed. Once developed, inflammatory follicular papules may evolve into pustulation or inflammatory nodules, the latter of which may be the origin of subsequent cysts. Cystic acne may result in severe scarring. Acne fulminans, a rare inflammatory variant of acne, occurs mainly in young male patients, evolving rapidly into tender, ulcerated, crusted lesions that scar. It can be associated with fever and polyarthralgia.[1]

Histopathology. The development of a comedone involves a complex but incompletely understood process that results in dilatation and thinning of the infundibular epithelial wall. The follicular lumen acquires a plug of loosely arranged keratinized cells and a substantial sebaceous column (arising from the associated sebaceous glands) that contains sebaceous material and microorganisms. The lipid materials of the sebaceous column are substantially removed by the use of fat solvents in histologic processing. In closed comedones, the follicular orifice remains more or less normal in size, but when the process leads to dilatation of the follicular ostia, this then characterizes an open comedone. In both types of comedones, only mild mononuclear cell infiltrates are present around the vessels in the adjacent papillary dermis. Attenuation of the follicular wall may be extreme and result in wall rupture.[2] Release of follicular contents into the dermis generates great increases in the inflammatory reaction with initial accumulation of neutrophils. When follicular rupture is superficial, it tends to lead to the development of a clinical pustule (Fig. 18-1), but when it occurs in the deeper dermis, an inflammatory nodule is formed. Foreign-body granulomatous inflammation develops in response to retention of comedonal material in the dermis, and if the follicular damage is severe, extensive scarring can result. In severe forms of acne (cystic acne and acne fulminans), cellular infiltrates become very extensive, and connective tissue necrosis and large dermal abscesses develop.[3] Epithelial outgrowth of the damaged follicle may tend to encapsulate and exteriorize the inflammatory debris, simulating the process of a perforating collagenosis.[2]

Pathogenesis. Acne is a multifactorial condition, initially requiring sex hormone release and activation of the sebaceous glands.

Three major factors are concerned with the development of this condition: androgens, sebum, and *Propionibacterium acnes.*

Substantial evidence indicates the role of androgens in activating sebum production.[4–6] Testosterone and dihydrotestosterone (DHT) appear to be the hormones that activate sebum production. DHT is enzymatically produced in the tissues by the enzyme 5A-reductase. Increased levels of serum androgens have been related to severe cystic acne,[7] but the majority of acne patients—particularly male patients—do not show abnormal hormone levels. Elevated androgen levels in women occur more frequently[8] but may also be elevated in similar proportion in women with hirsutism without acne. It has been suggested that this may reflect differences in the breakdown products of DHT in the target tissue.[9] Androgens, therefore, are derived from two sources: precursor androgens of glandular original (gonadal and adrenal), and target tissue androgens derived from the peripheral conversion of plasma precursors to more potent androgens. The precise roles of these androgenic hormones in the production of acne lesions remain controversial. It has been suggested that in patients with mild acne the serum levels of precursor androgens are normal and that in these circumstances only tissue androgen levels are elevated.[10]

Sebum production in acne is elevated and appears to correlate with the severity of the condition.[11] The beneficial effect of Isotretinonin (13-cis-retinoic acid) appears to result largely from reduction in sebum production: "Remove sebum and you remove acne."[12] After two months of treatment with oral Isotretinonin, a 70% reduction in sebum excretion is obtained,[13]

E. Abell: The Dermatopathology Laboratory, St. Francis Medical Center, Pittsburgh, PA

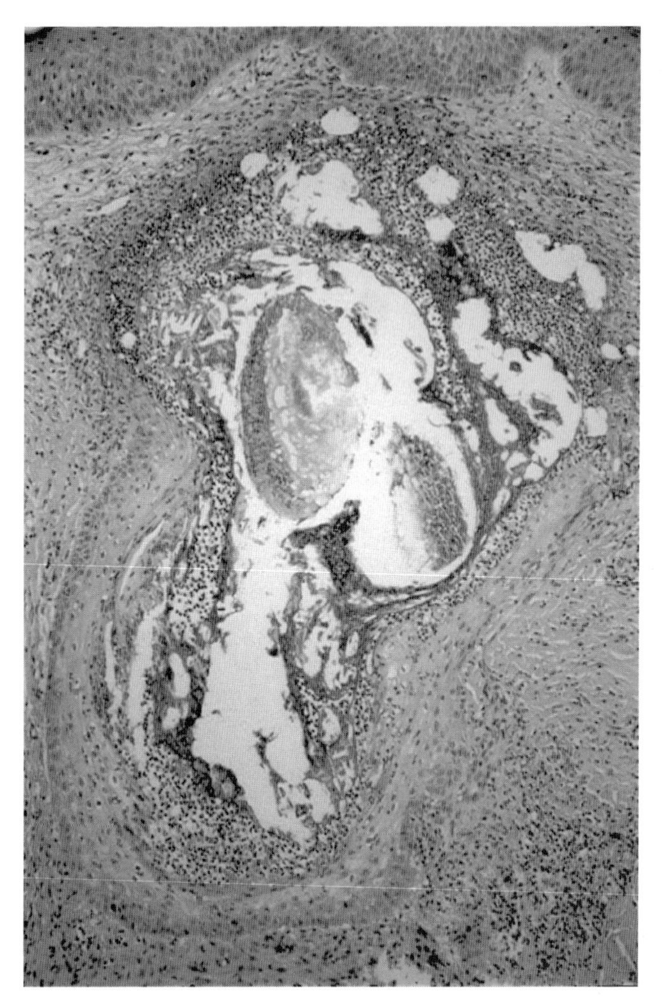

FIG. 18-1. Acne
A closed comedone has ruptured the thinned infundibular wall, and a superficial pustule has developed. Note large sebaceous column in center.

and after four months a reduction of 88% may be obtained.[14] These changes are associated histologically with a marked reduction in sebaceous gland size.[14] Substantial reduction in *P acnes* levels has also been detected in acne patients taking oral Isotretinonin,[13] and follicular hyperkeratinization may also be reduced.[15]

Of all the microorganisms identified in the follicular infundibulum, only *P acnes* appears to be consistently involved in the pathogenesis of acne lesions, even though the population levels of this organism in lesional skin may not be consistently greater than those in normal skin.[16,17] Immunologic reactivity to this organism may contribute to the inflammatory response in acne lesions. Acne patients may demonstrate elevated serum antibody levels and increased immediate hypersensitivity to *P acnes* and may exhibit cell-mediated immunity to this organism as well, as can be shown by an increase in lymphocyte transformation as a result of exposure to *P acnes* antigen.[18] A good correlation has been detected between delayed skin test reactivity to this organism and the severity of inflammatory lesions in acne vulgaris.[19]

The beneficial effects of both systemic and topical antibiotics on acne patients are generally attributed to their suppressive effects on *P acnes*.[20] However, some studies suggest that this may not be so. Oral tetracycline may improve acne without reducing the population of *P acnes*,[17] and topical erythromycin may also produce a beneficial effect without depressing bacterial levels in open comedones.[21]

Comedone development is associated with increased epithelial cell proliferation in the lower portion of the infundibulum, as can be measured by tritium labeling techniques.[22] This leads to overproduction of keratin materials, which appear to bind more avidly as a result of increased levels of intercellular adhesion materials.[23] If accumulation of keratin and sebaceous material is associated with dilatation of the follicular orifice, a blackhead develops. This structure has a reasonable expectation of ultimate discharge of materials to the surface. If this dilatation is not achieved, continued thinning and ultimate rupture of the infundibular wall becomes more probable. The black color of open comedones appears to be related to the densely packed keratinocytes and to the bacteria and bacterial breakdown products located at the surface.[24] Generation of inflammation in acne lesions is in itself a complex problem. Potential instigators of inflammation may be derived from the breakdown products of the sebaceous lipids, from byproducts derived from the *P acnes* organism, and by various immunologic mechanisms produced against this organism.[25]

ROSACEA

Rosacea is an inflammatory condition of the face that is more common after the age of 30. It is usually bilateral but occasionally is unilateral or focal, producing diffuse erythema within which scattered telangiectasia, papules, and occasional pustules develop. It characteristically affects the nose, cheeks, glabella, and chin, and if it is severe, lesions may spread to the neck and exceptionally disseminated lesions may be observed.[26] Rhinophyma, a late complication that occurs almost exclusively in men, is a result of bullous swelling of the soft tissue. Eye changes—especially blepharitis and conjunctivitis—are quite common in rosacea, and in 5% of the cases a painful keratitis can develop.[27] Rosacea can precipitate persistent facial lymphedema.

Histopathology. Pathologic changes may vary considerably from case to case, reflecting the clinical presentation.[28] Vascular dilatation of upper and middermal vessels, with perivascular and perifollicular lymphohistiocytic inflammation and occasional plasma cells, is generally present in all cases. Lymphatic dilatation is usual and often prominent (Fig. 18-2). Dermal infiltrates may accumulate into small nodular aggregates and develop a granulomatous organization. Epithelioid histiocytes in a tuberculoid pattern may accumulate, and there can be occasional multinucleate giant cells[29] (Fig. 18-3). Foreign-body granuloma may develop around the debris and organisms released following follicular damage and rupture.[30] Follicular involvement can also be quite variable: when this is a minor feature, there may be infundibular spongiosis and exocytosis, but more severe involvement demonstrates accumulation of neutrophils into a superficial pustular folliculitis.

Granulomatous infiltrates are said to occur in about 10% of all cases of rosacea.[29,31] Caseous degeneration has been said to be absent,[32,33] but caseation necrosis has been recently identi-

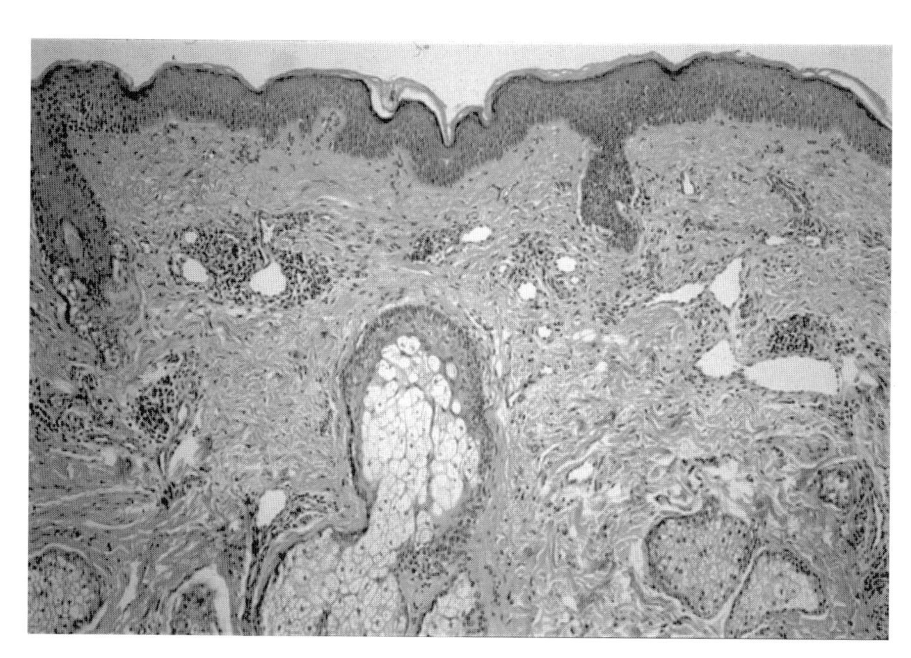

FIG. 18-2. Rosacea
Perivascular dermal infiltrates are associated with pronounced dilatation of small vessels and lymphatics: "telangiectatic rosacea."

fied in about 10% of patients showing granulomatous inflammation.[34] In rhinophyma, sebaceous gland hyperplasia becomes very prominent, and the sebaceous ducts are dilated and filled with keratin material and sebum. There may be dermal fibroplasia and an increase in connective tissue.

Pathogenesis. Rosacea is not associated with an increase in sebum excretion.[35] Sun damage appears to be an almost constant associated feature of rosacea.[36] The role of demodex organisms in this condition has been debated for decades. Reports have claimed significant association of mites in biopsied tissue,[30,37] but other studies have not identified any association that would support this claim.[33,38] A definitive view cannot therefore be stated, but it seems probable that rosacea may have a multifactorial etiology.[39]

Immunoglobulins and complement components have been identified at the dermal-epidermal junction in patients with rosacea,[40,41] but these findings have been disputed.[42] The apparent presence of immune deposits in the skin may be a reflection of changes associated with chronic actinic injury.

The concept of rosacea-like tuberculids appears to have evolved because of the granulomatous pathology exhibited in more severe papular forms of this disorder. A direct relationship with active tuberculosis is now largely discounted.

Differential Diagnosis. Subacute cutaneous lupus erythematous and telangiectatic forms of rosacea can clinically look very much alike. The pathologic changes in the incomplete or tumid form of lupus erythematosus (LE) can also closely mimic the minor perivascular inflammatory change observed in telan-

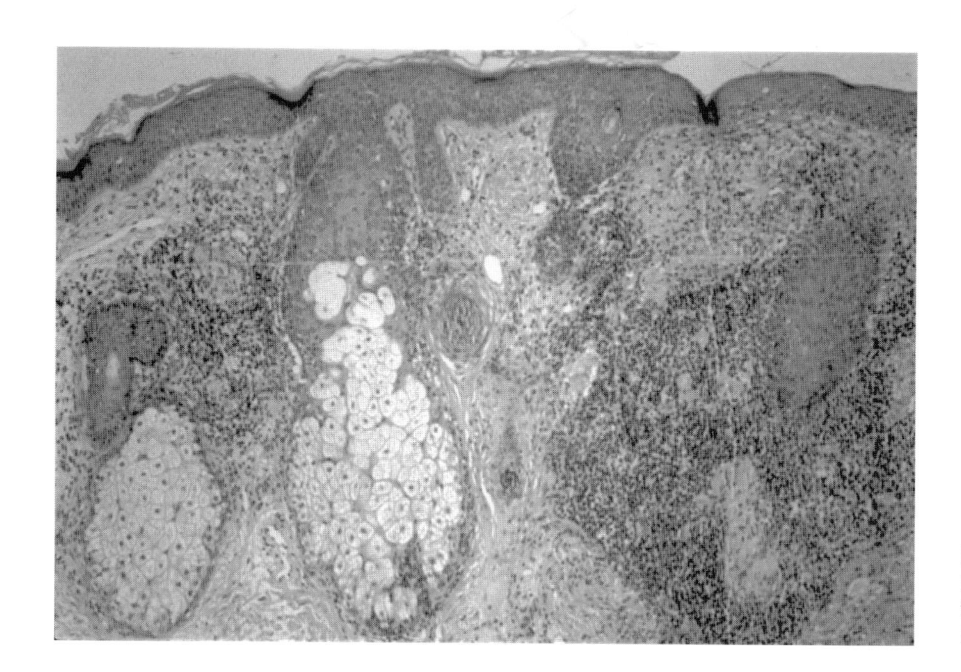

FIG. 18-3. Rosacea
Perivascular and perifollicular infiltrates are denser, and focal epithelioid granulomata have developed.

giectatic forms of rosacea. However, rosacea consistently lacks the epidermal injury that is characteristic of LE.

Granulomatous rosacea can certainly mimic the histopathology of atypical mycobacterial infections, but much less frequently can organized granulomatous change mimic lupus vulgaris and cutaneous sarcoidosis. Other investigative procedures and tissue cultures may be necessary to define these diagnoses more precisely.

LUPUS MILIARIS DISSEMINATUS FACIEI

Although now considered a variant of rosacea, lupus miliaris disseminatus faciei has its own distinct clinical presentation. Characteristic lesions are discrete papules—single papules or small groups of flesh-colored or mildly erythematous papules—involving the face but specifically involving the eyelids and upper lip, which are areas where rosacea lesions are uncommon.[43] This condition lacks the erythema and telangiectasia of rosacea. Papules often persist for 12 to 24 months but can heal spontaneously.[44] This condition is often very resistant to standard rosacea therapy.

Histopathology. Biopsy specimens sectioned through the central portion of a papular lesion demonstrate one of the most highly characteristic patterns of cutaneous histopathology. Surrounding a usually large area of caseous necrosis, aggregates of epithelioid histiocytes and occasional multinucleate giant cells form a substantial "tubercle" (Fig. 18-4). Sparse lymphoid infiltrates are observed peripherally.[44–46]

Pathogenesis. Despite the histologic picture, no direct relationship with tuberculosis has been documented for this condition. Although it is considered to belong to the rosacea group of disorders, its etiology is entirely unknown. It has been suggested that the histopathology suggests a mechanism associated with cell-mediated immunity because of the strong lysozyme staining of the epithelioid and giant cells.[47]

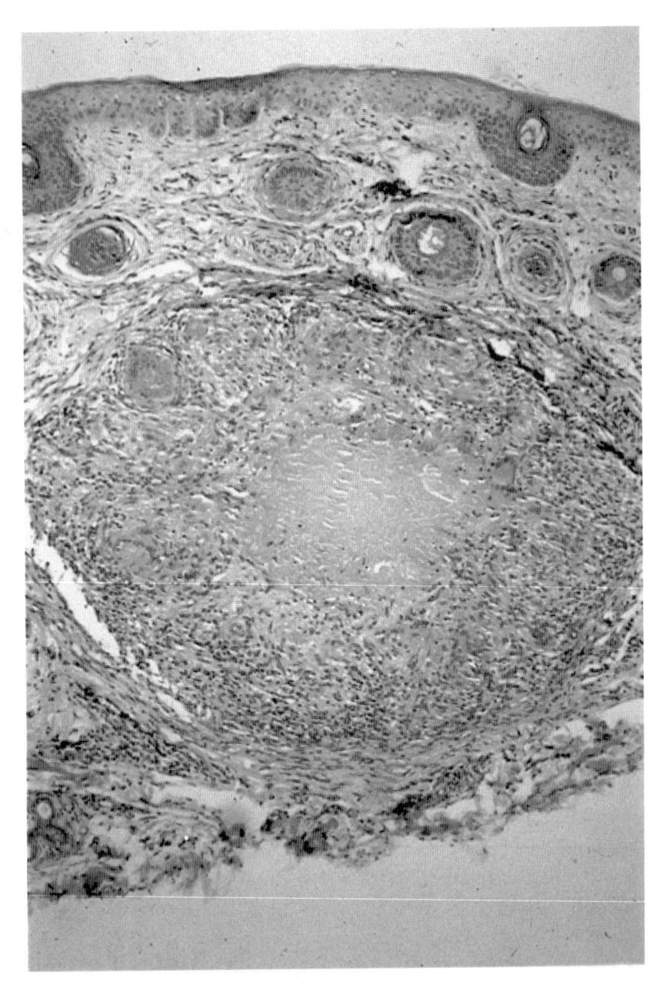

FIG. 18-4. Lupus miliaris disseminatus faciei
Focal "tuberculoid" granuloma with central caseation. Several multinucleate giant cells are present.

PERIORAL DERMATITIS

Recognition of this relatively common facial eruption gains importance because of its resemblance to rosacea, seborrheic dermatitis, and occasionally lupus erythematosus.[48] Predominantly affecting white women of European extraction from the mid teens into middle age, it produces fine papules—singly, grouped, or confluent—with minimal scaling in the perioral area and more rarely in periocular distribution. Pinhead-size pustules may occur in more severe cases, but the condition lacks significant telangiectasia and appears to be unassociated with solar elastosis.

Histopathology. Fully developed lesions show a spongiotic edema of follicular infundibulum with mild mononuclear cell exocytosis (Fig. 18-5). Similar changes may be observed in the epidermis overlying the involved follicles. The adjacent dermis shows perivascular lymphohistiocytic infiltrates, and in rare cases plasma cells may be prominent. Minor lesions may exhibit only dermal inflammation, elastosis is usually absent, and lesions tend to lack the dermal edema and telangiectasia characteristic of rosacea.[49]

An alternative histopathologic assessment has been offered[50] in which biopsies obtained from this condition show pathologic changes more consistent with those of rosacea, with granulomatous lesions being found also.

Pathogenesis. Perioral dermatitis was first described as a light-sensitive seborrheid,[51] but subsequent investigation has suggested a very large number of possible etiologies for this condition, including candida organisms; bacteria, particularly of fusiform type; demodex mites; a wide range of contactants, whether irritant or allergic (including cosmetics and fluoride-containing toothpaste); hormones (including the birth control pill and topical corticosteroids, particularly of potent type); as well as emotional and systemic conditions. A comprehensive review of this information is recommended.[52]

KERATOSIS PILARIS

This common persistent condition characteristically affects the lateral aspect of the arms, thighs, and buttocks. Keratotic follicular papules sometimes immediately surrounded by erythema are present. The condition is usually asymptomatic and is

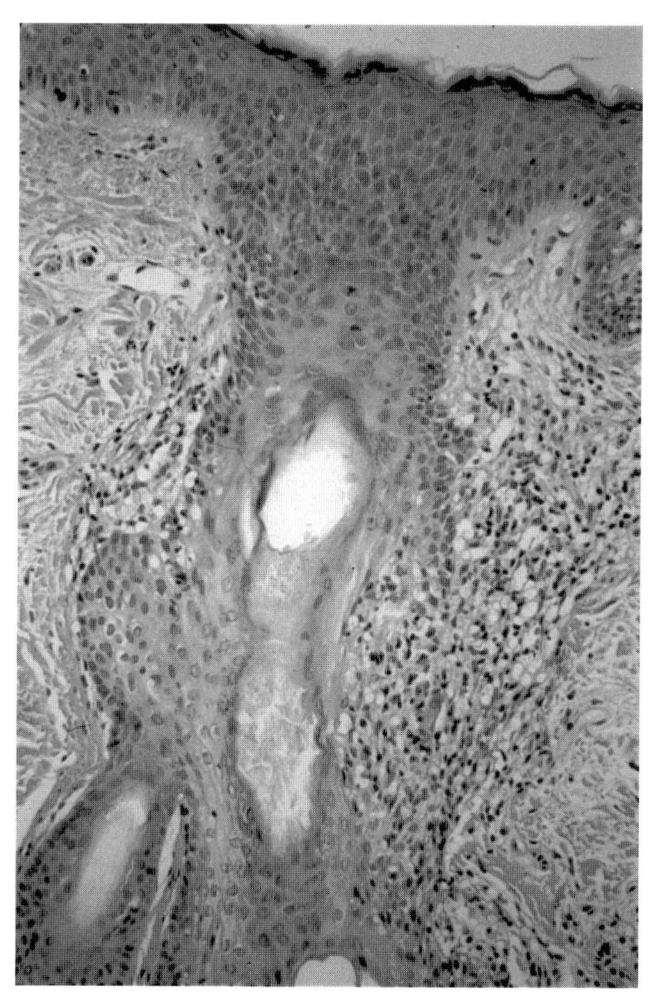

FIG. 18-5. Perioral dermatitis
An early lesion showing infundibular spongiosis and exocytosis, and adjacent dermal infiltrates.

only occasionally more generalized. Keratosis pilaris may be seen in association with ichthyosis vulgaris,[53] and it appears to be more common in patients with atopic dermatitis as well. Similar lesions may form a part of the presentation of a variety of more extensive erythematous keratinizing disorders.

Histopathology. An orthokeratotic keratin plug blocks and dilates the orifice and upper portion of the follicular infundibulum (Fig. 18-6). A twisted hair shaft may be trapped within this keratin material, and mild perivascular mononuclear cell infiltrates are usually present in the adjacent dermis.

Pathogenesis. The cause of this condition is unknown, but genetic factors may be involved. A similar condition, lichen spinulosus,[54] shows a very similar pathology except that the keratin material extends rather more substantially beyond the follicular orifice and the mass may contain one or more hair shafts.[55] Lesions similar to those of keratosis pilaris may arise in phrynoderma (see Chap. 16), but the follicular keratin plug is said to be of parakeratotic type.[56] Keratosis pilaris atrophicans[57] represents a spectrum of clinical conditions in which the follicle involved undergoes atrophy and scarring destruction. Scarring alopecia of the scalp may also occur in this condition.

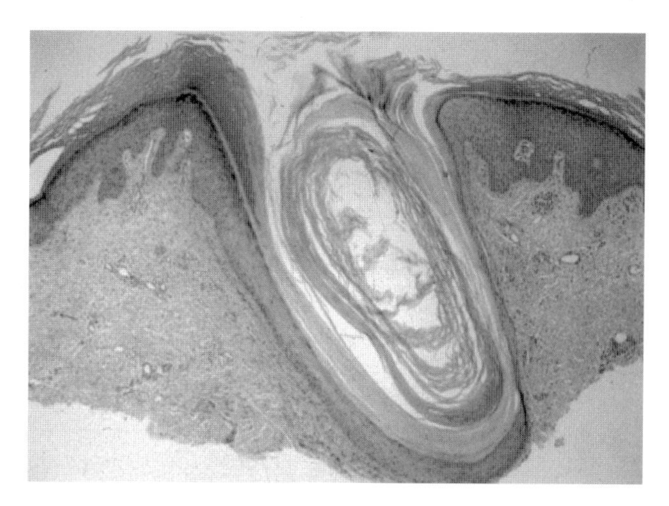

FIG. 18-6. Keratosis pilaris
An orthokeratotic plug dilates a follicular ostia. Minimal perivascular infiltrates are present in adjacent dermis.

DISSEMINATE AND RECURRENT INFUNDIBULAR FOLLICULITIS

This condition, described initially in 1968, demonstrates sheeted, itchy, skin-colored follicular papules resembling goose flesh.[58] It affects the trunk and upper extremities predominantly, may last for several months or even for years,[58,59] and occurs almost exclusively in black patients.

Histopathology. Affected follicles show infundibular spongiosis with mononuclear cell exocytosis (Fig. 18-7). The follicle may show keratin retention, and parakeratosis may develop at the orifice.[58,59] The adjacent dermis may exhibit some edema and mild perivascular lymphocytic infiltrates. Although this is not diagnostically specific pathology, it can be characteristic in the appropriate clinical setting.

Pathogenesis. No cause has been found for this odd, itchy condition. Contact allergy has not been documented. An inflammatory response to endogenous components of the follicle may be involved.

EOSINOPHILIC PUSTULAR FOLLICULITIS

Described originally in adult Japanese patients in 1970 by Ofuji,[60] this condition demonstrates broad patches of itchy follicular papules and pustules involving particularly the face, trunk, and arms. The involved areas may take on various configurations; there may be central healing and peripheral spread. The condition is now known to be geographically more widespread and may be seen in children.[61,62] It occurs also in patients with HIV infection,[63] and extrafollicular lesions with involvement of both palms and soles are documented.[64] Scarring alopecia through scalp involvement has also been reported.[65] Moderate leukocytosis and eosinophilia in the peripheral blood are also present.

Histopathology. Involved follicles may show spongiotic change with exocytosis extending from the sebaceous gland and its duct throughout the infundibular zone. Lymphocytes with

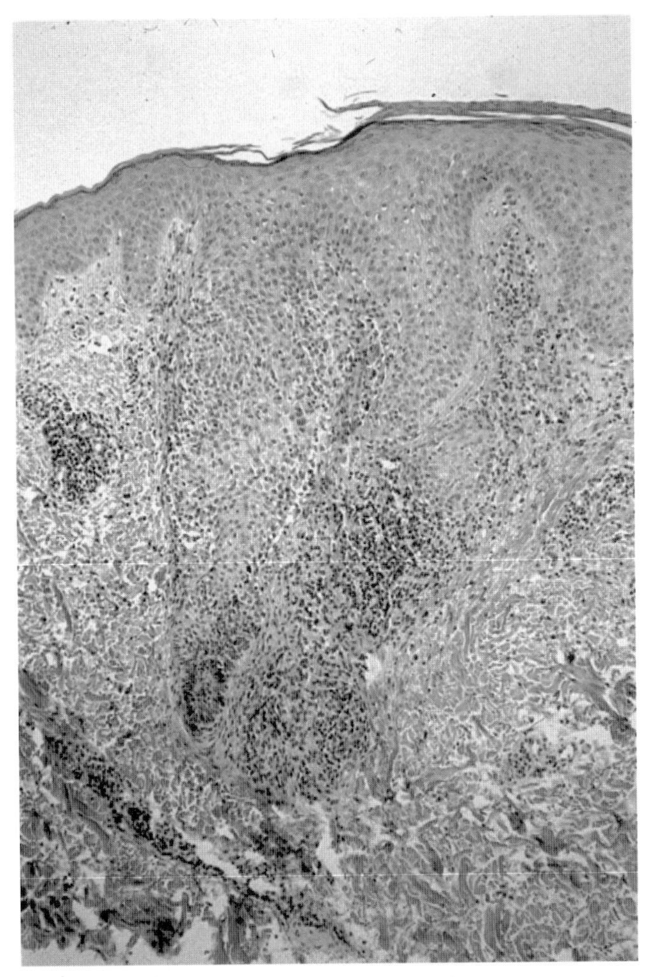

FIG. 18-7. Disseminated and recurrent infundibular folliculitis
Spongiosis and mononuclear cell exocytosis with dermal infiltrates are present. Note parakeratosis and mild spongiotic changes at surface.

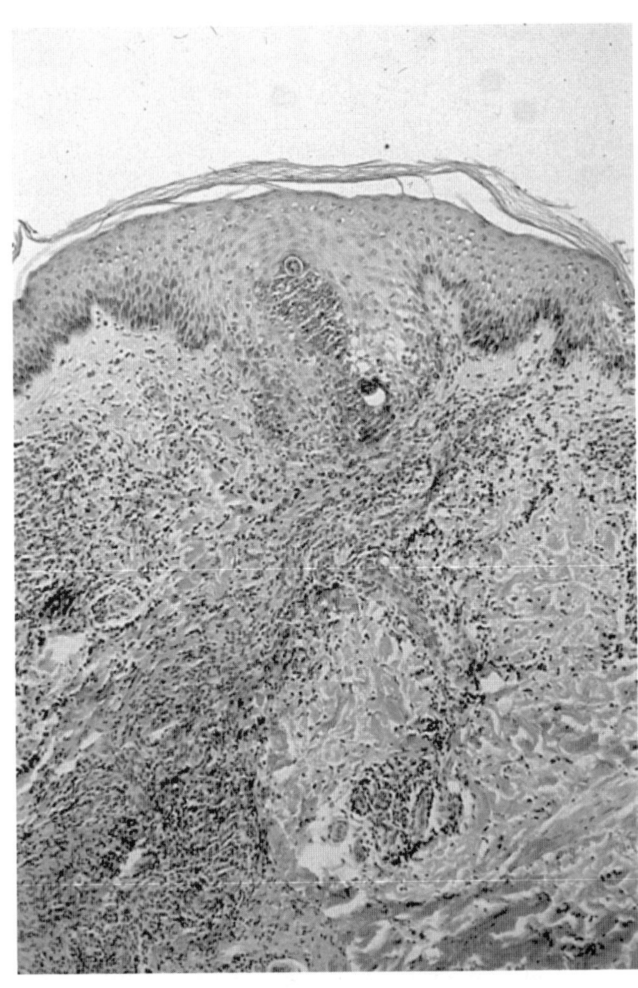

FIG. 18-8. Eosinophilic pustular folliculitis
An early lesion with micropustule developing within the epidermal portion of the follicular infundibulum. Note dense adjacent infiltrate of lymphocytes and eosinophils.

some eosinophils migrate into the epidermis initially in a somewhat diffuse pattern, but micropustular aggregation develops (Fig. 18-8) and the ultimate lesion is an infundibular eosinophilic pustule.[65,66] The epidermis adjacent to the follicle may be involved and demonstrate eosinophilic microabscess formation.[67] The adjacent dermis shows perivascular infiltrates of lymphocytes and numerous eosinophils.[68] In HIV-related lesions, the inflammatory process appears to be focused at the level of the follicular isthmus and sebaceous duct.[69]

Pathogenesis. The cause of this condition is not known. Pemphigus-like antibody involving the lower portion of the epidermis has been demonstrated,[70] and antibody directed against the cytoplasm of the basal cells of the outer root sheath of follicles has also been reported.[71] Neutrophil and eosinophil chemotactic factors in stratum corneum extracts from lesions have also been demonstrated.[72] Cell adhesion molecule expression activation may be involved in the selective migration of eosinophils and lymphocytes into the involved hair follicle epithelium.[73]

Differential Diagnosis. Erythema toxicum neonatorum produces eosinophilic follicular pustules, and intraepidermal vesicles with eosinophils can be seen in acropustulosis and in the vesicular phase of incontinentia pigmenti, and these might be diagnostic considerations for follicular and extrafollicular lesions of eosinophilic pustular folliculitis. The clinical presentation of these conditions would generally be substantially different. However, identical eosinophilic pustular eruptions have been described in association with *Pseudomonas* infection[74] and also in dermatophyte fungal infection.[75]

EOSINOPHILIC CELLULITIS (WELLS' SYNDROME)

This rare dermatosis was fully characterized in 1979[76] as a sudden eruption of a variable number of bright erythematous patches, which over a period of a few days expand into indurated erythematous plaques that may be painful or sore. The overlying epidermis may produce vesicles or small blisters. The disease, if untreated, may persist for a few weeks or months and may be recurrent. Associated or provoking stimuli may include insect bites and cutaneous parasitosis, cutaneous viral infections and drug reactions, leukemic and myeloproliferative disorders,

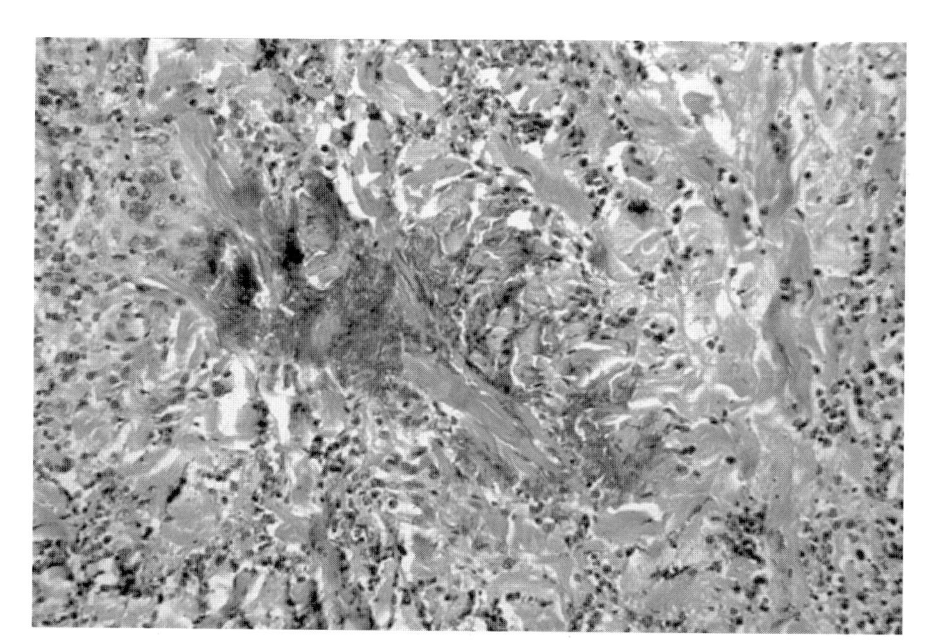

FIG. 18-9. Eosinophilic cellulitis A "flame figure" set in a diffuse dermal infiltrate of mixed mononuclear cells and eosinophils.

and atopic dermatitis and fungal infections. Although patients are usually adults, the condition has also been described in children.[77] Peripheral blood eosinophilia is usually present.

Histopathology. Early lesions demonstrate diffuse but dense dermal infiltrates of eosinophils; eosinophil degranulation is prominent.[76] Infiltrates generally extend throughout the dermis and may involve the subcutaneous tissue or occasionally the underlying muscle.[78] Where the epidermis is substantially involved, multilocular spongiotic intraepidermal vesicles develop,[79] but blistering is usually of subepidermal type. Eosinophils are found in the epidermis.

Older lesions show more extensive eosinophil degranulation; the granular material aggregates focally around collagen fibers, forming the characteristic "flame figures"[76] (Fig. 18-9). These foci may develop a palisade of macrophages and sometimes giant cells.[79,80] In florid lesions, necrobiosis may develop within the palisading histiocytic reaction.[81]

Pathogenesis. Immunofluorescence staining identifies eosinophil major basic protein deposition in the granules of the flame figures.[82] However, electron microscopic examination reveals that collagen fibers remain intact, suggesting that a primary degeneration of collagen is not a factor in initiating flame figure formation.[83]

TRICHORRHEXIS INVAGINATA (NETHERTON'S SYNDROME OR BAMBOO HAIR)

Scalp hair of individuals with trichorrhexis invaginata, almost always of autosomal recessive inheritance pattern, is short, sparse, and brittle. This condition is usually found in association with ichthyosis linearis circumflexa, which is characterized by migratory polycyclic scaly lesions.[84] In a few instances, as described in the original case,[85] trichorrhexis invaginata is found in association with lamellar icthyosis.

Histopathology. Involved hair shafts show a bamboo deformity. A portion of the distal hair shaft ("ball") invaginates into an expanded proximal portion ("cup").[86]

Pathogenesis. Invagination occurs at the site of an intermittent keratinizing defect of the hair cortex resulting from incomplete conversion of -SH groups into S-S linkages in the protein of the cortical fibers. This defect leads to cortical cell softness and the bamboo deformity.[87]

TRICHOSTASIS SPINULOSA

This follicular condition, which is not uncommon in middle-aged and older individuals, occurs predominantly on the face and middle back. It may be clinically inapparent or present as raised follicular spicules.

Histopathology. Affected hair follicles demonstrate retention of small hair shafts enveloped in a keratinous sheath within the dilated infundibulum, this mass often projecting substantially from the skin surface.[88] As many as 20 or more hair shafts may be trapped in this way.

Pathogenesis. The retained hairs demonstrate normal telogen club structures, which suggest a normally functioning follicle. It seems likely that the entrapment is a result of hyperkeratosis in the follicular infundibulum, producing an obstruction to normal hair shedding.[89]

ALOPECIA AREATA

Alopecia areata is characterized by complete or nearly complete absence of hair in one or more circumscribed areas of the scalp. Inflammatory change is not clinically obvious, and the follicular openings are preserved. Complete scalp involvement (alopecia totalis) may occur suddenly or through prolonged progressive disease, and complete or nearly complete loss of the entire body hair (alopecia universalis) can occur also. Involvement of the eyebrows and eyelashes and a pitted defect in the nail plates are additional features of this condition. Although the majority of patients undergo spontaneous resolution, others show grumbling persistent disease, and fewer patients have permanent hair loss. In the areas of active hair shedding, a short,

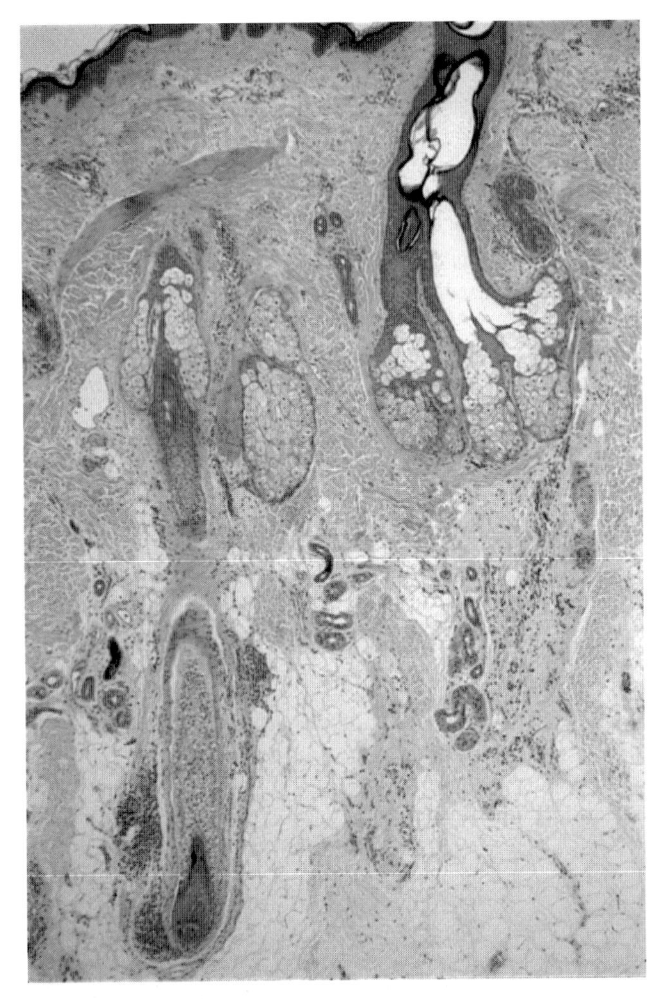

FIG. 18-10. Alopecia areata
Lymphocytic infiltrates are present around inferior portion and bulb of a regenerating anagen follicle, but note other diminutive follicles, one with peribulbar lymphocytes, and also lymphocytes along course of follicular sheaths in deeper dermis.

fractured hair shaft may be identified—the characteristic "exclamation point" hair.

Histopathology. Headington[90] has suggested that the pathology of alopecia areata reflects four distinct stages into which this disorder can be divided: (1) acute hair loss, (2) persistent (chronic) baldness, (3) partial telogen-to-anagen conversion (incomplete recovery), and (4) normal recovery.

In all phases, the critically diagnostic pathologic sign is lymphocytic infiltrates in the peribulbar area of anagen follicles (Fig. 18-10), or follicles in early catagen. The lymphocytic infiltrates are present around the receding epithelial remnant but also in the area of the collapsing follicular sheaths. While still in anagen, lymphocytes may be seen sparsely infiltrating the matrix epithelium (Fig. 18-11). Follicular structures diminish in size rapidly and become miniaturized, and as a result are identified more superficially in the dermis. In the early active hair loss phase, diminutive follicles are observed predominantly in early or late catagen, and this persists into the chronic active baldness phase. In incomplete recovery, diminutive anagen follicles may be quite numerous, many showing some peribulbar lymphocytic infiltrates. If such follicles are able to elaborate hair shafts, these shafts tend to be without melanin pigment. In longstanding cases, the inflammatory infiltrates appear to diminish.[91] Lymphocytes may invade both the bulbs and the outer root sheaths of early recovering anagen hairs. In severe alopecia universalis and totalis of long duration (a decade or more), functional follicular structures may be diminished in number and some scarring of the follicular sheaths may be identified.[92]

When biopsy specimens are sectioned transversely early in the disease, it can be demonstrated that the number of follicles is not diminished but that follicles enter a persistent phase of telogen (telogen germinal units) and that there is a diminution of normal club telogen follicles.[93] These findings suggest that the inflammatory damage to the follicular bulb precipitates abnormal catagen, which, without the elaboration of the "club" structure, allows immediate shedding of the hair shaft.

Pathogenesis. The lymphocytic infiltrates in the peribulbar area consist substantially of T helper lymphocytes.[94,95] In normal subjects, Langerhans' cells are found only in the upper portions of hair follicles, but they can be found in the bulbar area in patients with alopecia areata in the persistent stage.[96] The presence of bulbar Langerhans' cells and of activated T-lymphocytic infiltrates favor an immune mechanism for the cause of this condition.

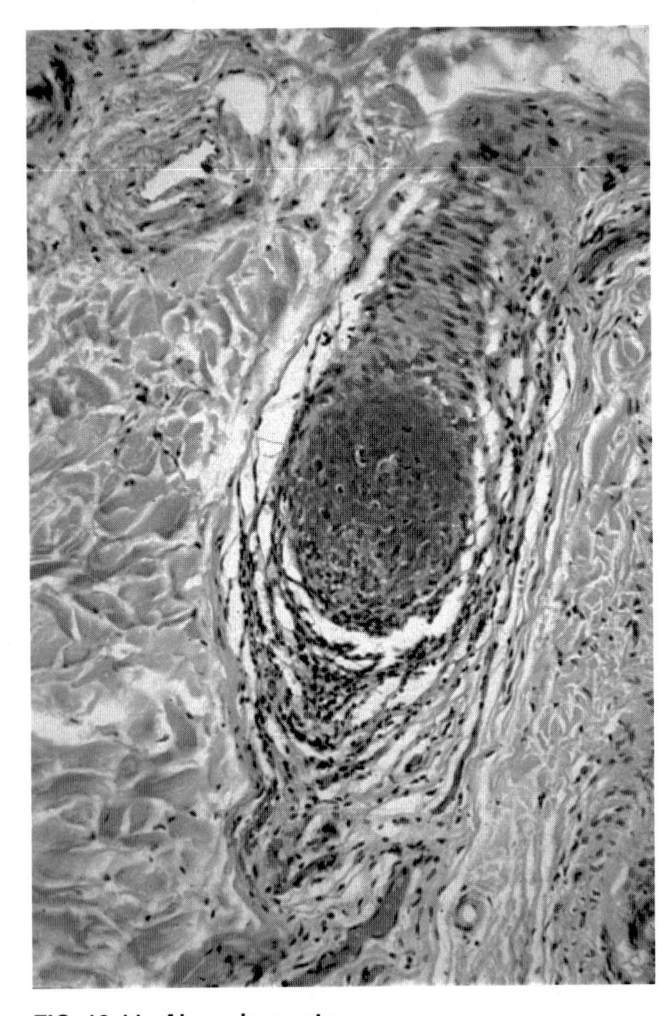

FIG. 18-11. Alopecia areata
A small anagen recovery follicle shows developing peribulbar lymphocytic infiltrate. Note sparse lymphocytes in matrix epithelium.

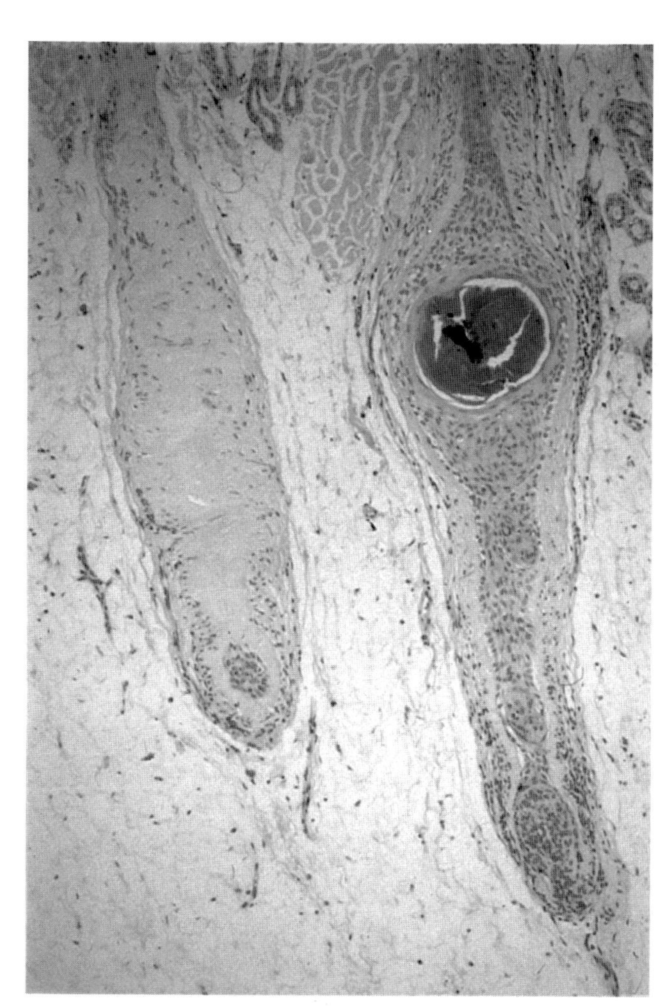

FIG. 18-12. Trichotillomania
Two adjacent catagen follicles, one with focal hemorrhage and pigment cast in collapsing outer root sheath.

Familial cases of alopecia areata are well recognized, suggesting a possible genetic predisposition. HLA class II antigen associations have recently been recognized in defining at least two types of alopecia areata.[97] Expression of cell adhesion molecules in the matrix epithelium, dermal papilla, and adjacent vessels has been demonstrated, suggesting a mechanism for leukocyte infiltration.[98,99]

Differential Diagnosis. Although the follicles may diminish in size in androgenetic alopecia, dermal infiltrates, when present in this condition, remain superficial, perivascular, and peri-infundibular, and biopsy specimens from active alopecia areata are rarely, if ever, a diagnostic problem when the peribulbar infiltrates are identified. Alopecia syphilitica, however, may produce follicular infiltrates that can very closely mimic those of active alopecia areata.[100]

TRICHOTILLOMANIA

Compulsive avulsion of hair shafts leads to zones of thin, ragged, broken stubble on the affected scalp. If the damage is done in localized fashion it can occasionally mimic alopecia areata. Follicular breakage and loss may occasionally be associated with evidence of damage to the scalp by erosions or crusts.

Histopathology. The most important findings in biopsy specimens are an increase in catagen hairs (up to 75%), pigmentary defects and casts, evidence of traumatized hair bulbs, and trichomalacia.[101] Occasionally, follicles may be identified still in anagen but empty because of hair shaft avulsion. Follicles can show considerable distortion of the bulbar epithelium and sometimes conspicuous hemorrhage (Fig. 18-12).[101,102] Hair shaft avulsion may deposit melanin pigment in the hair papilla and peribulbar connective tissue (Fig. 18-13). Pigment casts are also frequently identified in the isthmus or infundibulum (Fig. 18-14). Trichomalacia, described as a complete but distorted, fully developed terminal hair in its bulb (Fig. 18-15), is relatively uncommon but is specific for trichotillomania. These various injuries to the bulbar portions of follicles are not accompanied by significant inflammatory infiltrates.

Differential Diagnosis. Trichotillomania is not associated with miniaturization of follicles. This feature and the lack of deep perifollicular infiltrates usually serve to differentiate trichotillomania from alopecia areata. Histologic findings in early traction alopecia are said to be identical with those of trichotillomania, but fewer follicles are involved, the changes are less dramatic, and vellus hairs are preserved.[103]

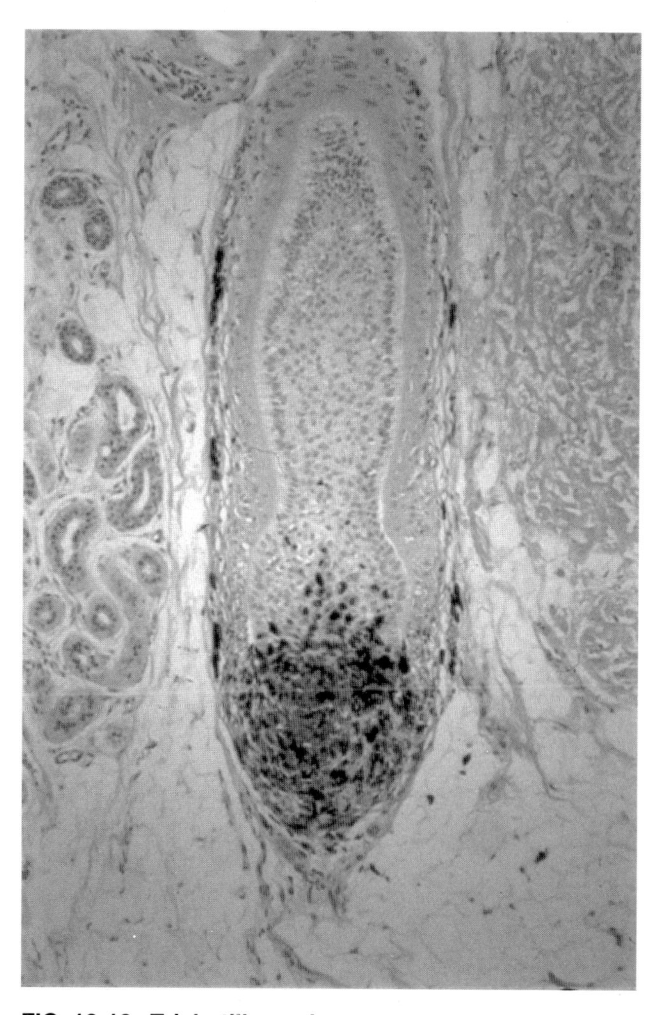

FIG. 18-13. Trichotillomania
Damaged catagen follicle showing melanin pigment release from matrix into dermal papilla and sheath.

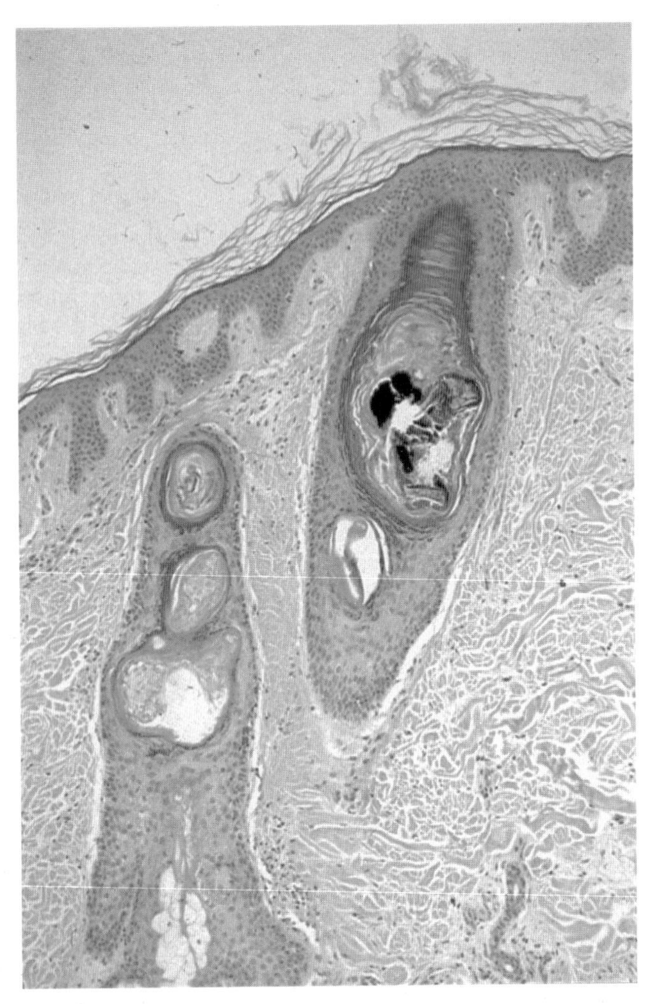

FIG. 18-14. Trichotillomania
Pigment cast in follicular infundibulum.

TELOGEN EFFLUVIUM

Telogen effluvium represents the increased or excessive shedding of hair in the telogen phase of the growth cycle. Shed hair shafts are recognizable because of the telogen club structure formed in this phase of the growth cycle, and this structure also makes normal telogen readily recognizable in histologic sections. This condition has several precipitating causes or associated conditions, but shedding tends to occur in a diffuse pattern throughout the scalp. The original clinical concept was identified initially by Kligman,[104] but this clinical concept has been substantially elaborated more recently by Headington,[105] who has described five different processes by which this excessive telogen shedding may occur. Briefly, these processes depend on changes that occur in the length of the anagen period of growth, and on the active process of release of hair shafts in telogen.

Histopathology. Using routine biopsy specimens and conventional sectioning, only a subjective assessment of the proportion of follicles in telogen can be obtained. More objective specimens can be obtained only by using horizontal sections of punch biopsy scalp material.[106] Telogen effluvium does not show significant dermal inflammatory infiltrates, nor should there be evidence of diminution of follicular and hair shaft size, unless telogen effluvium occurs in patients with established androgenetic or another form of involutional alopecia. Proportions of normal telogen follicles in excess of 15% are considered to be abnormal and suggest the likely presence of telogen effluvium.[105,107] However, others have suggested that a level of 25% is necessary for definitive diagnosis.[103,104] Timing of the biopsy clearly affects the pathologic changes observed. Should a biopsy be obtained in the very early stages of recovery, early anagen regeneration follicles will also be present (Fig. 18-16), but if recovery is substantial, the histopathologic assessment may be entirely normal.

Pathogenesis. Telogen effluvium may be associated with a variety of hormonal disturbances and is perhaps most commonly associated with the postpartum period of pregnancy. Hormone medication and a wide variety of drugs may also be involved. Fever, systemic conditions, nutritional deficiency states, and psychological stress are also situations in which hair loss of this type may occur to a greater or lesser extent.[105,108]

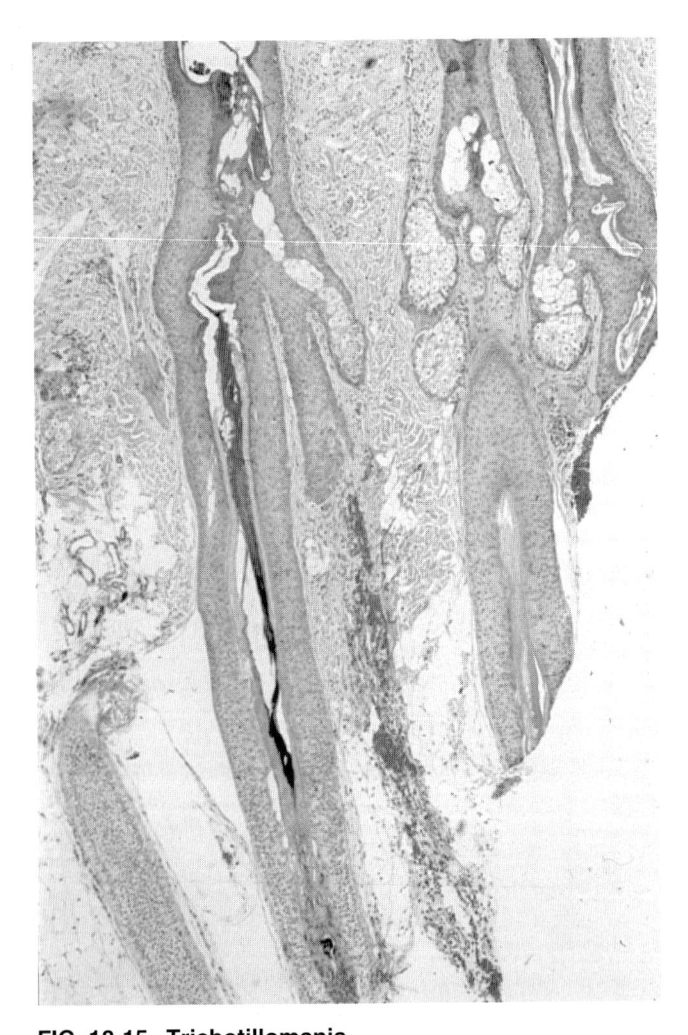

FIG. 18-15. Trichotillomania
Trichomalacia, a fully developed and pigmented but distorted hair shaft, is demonstrated in center follicle.

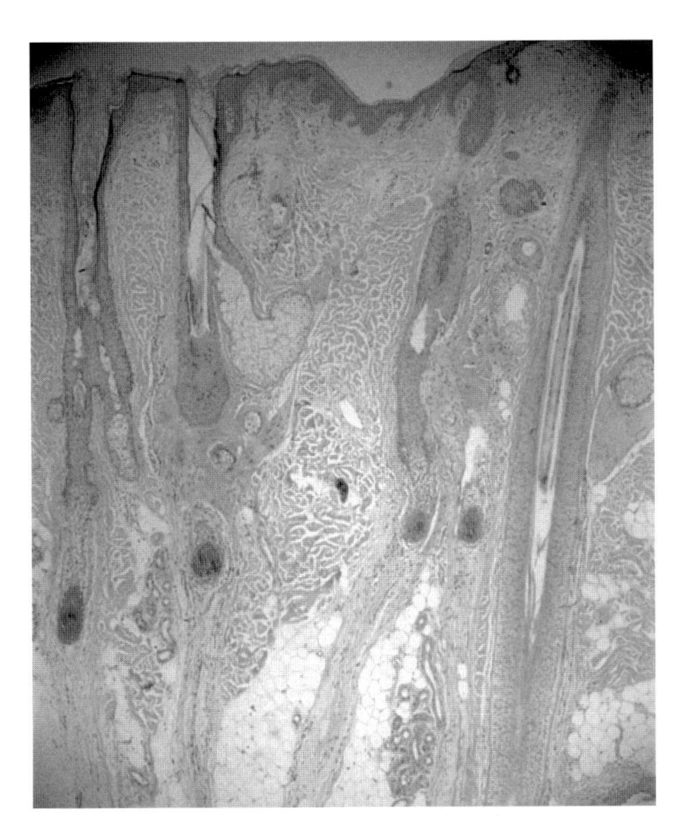

FIG. 18-16. Telogen effluvium, early recovery phase Note the "club" telogen follicle and four follicles in early anagen regeneration.

ANDROGENETIC ALOPECIA

The expression of androgenetic alopecia requires an exaggerated androgenic influence on hair follicles in certain areas of the scalp; this frequently shows a familial and probably genetic inheritance pattern. Hair shafts become progressively finer and shorter, with true alopecia occurring only as a later event. This involutional process slowly evolves to become so severe that the scalp skin becomes exposed to a greater or lesser extent. Initially in male patients, bifrontal thinning occurs, often with similar changes over the vertex, but in the full expression of the condition, there may be almost total baldness of the entire frontovertical area of the scalp. This process can also occur in women, although much less frequently and with lesser severity so that significant balding is quite unusual.

Histopathology. Satisfactory evaluation of this condition can be achieved only from transverse sectioning of punch biopsy material.[106] Diminution of follicular size, most effectively measured by assessment of mean hair shaft diameter, can be obtained with relative simplicity using an optical micrometer. Because this approach allows assessment of all follicles in the specimen, direct counting of anagen, telogen, and catagen follicles can be undertaken and the percentages of each obtained. Samples smaller than 4 mm in diameter show insufficient numbers of follicles for meaningful results.

Reduction of follicular size appears to be randomized, so that, initially, normal-size follicles coexist with an increased number of smaller ones, whereas, ultimately, follicular reduction becomes more persistent and obvious (Fig. 18-17).[109,110] These changes are associated with this reduction in follicular size and there is a progressive increase in the percentage of telogen follicles, both of normal club pattern and with increasing severity of this condition, diminutive or persistent telogen epithelial remnants (telogen germinal units).[106] These structures appear to represent epithelial remnants of telogen follicles that no longer respond to the stimulus to return to anagen growth.

Ultimately, there may be a reduction in the density of follicles in the affected areas of the scalp.[107] Superficial perivascular and peri-infundibular mononuclear cell infiltrates have been described with some consistency in this condition.[111,112] Peri-infundibular fibroplasia ultimately leading to focal follicular scarring has been reported,[111] and this may be the explanation for the reduced follicular density. The diminution of follicles leads to a substantial increase in the number of empty follicular sheaths in the deeper dermis and subcutaneous tissue.

Pathogenesis. The pattern of balding indicates that only certain follicles are susceptible to the involution effect produced by androgens. It has been suggested that androgens effect this in-

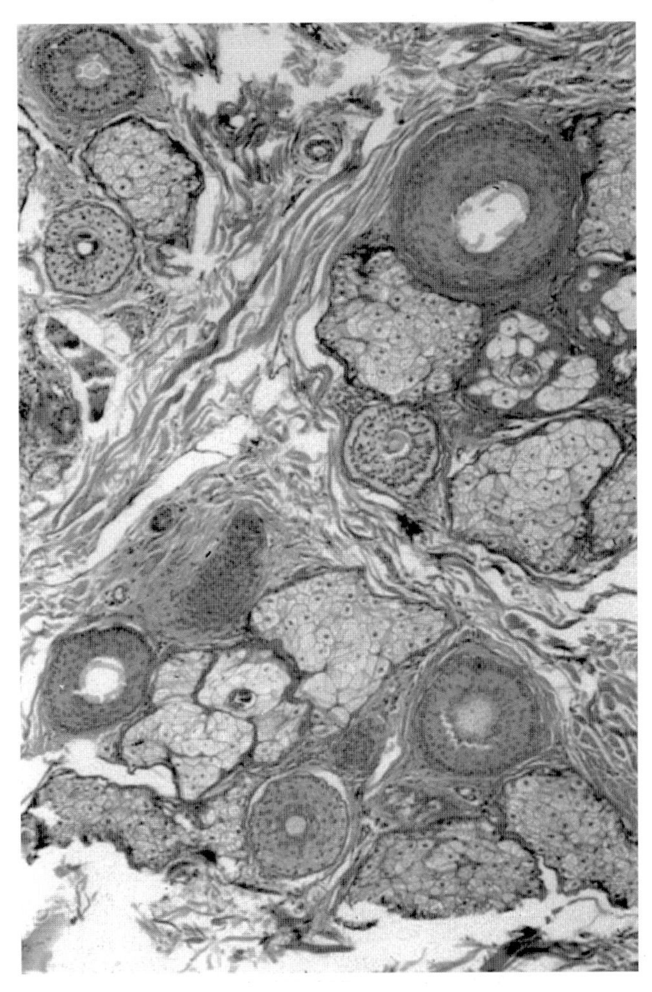

FIG. 18-17. Androgenetic alopecia, horizontal section Sectioned follicles show great variation of size with many small follicles. Note two "club" telogen follicles in lower portion of figure and more central undifferentiated epithelial tissue (telogen germinal unit).

fluence by way of receptors in the hair papillae,[113] and more recent studies have shown that papillae from balding scalp follicles contain higher levels of androgen receptor.[114] Androgen receptor expression may be genetically controlled. Investigations bearing on the genetic and hormonal aspects of androgenetic alopecia have been recently reviewed.[115,116]

SCARRING ALOPECIA

A very large number of dermatologic conditions may lead to follicular damage sufficient to produce destruction and replacement of the pilosebaceous structures by scar tissue.[117] Localized infections and inflammatory conditions—including lupus erythematosus and lichen planopilaris, which are common causes of scarring alopecia, as well as diffuse scarring alopecia associated with cutaneous scleroderma—will be discussed in the relevant sections of this text under which they are more appropriately classified.

The condition of pseudopelade will be described here.

PSEUDOPELADE (BROCQ)

In this uncommon condition, scattered, irregularly outlined patches of noninflammatory alopecia progressively develop. Islands of normal skin may be left within these scarred zones. The condition is more common in women and occasionally develops in childhood. After a lengthy period of activity the condition ultimately burns out completely, leaving permanent but variably severe scarring alopecia. This clinical pattern may arise in association with inflammatory conditions, and larger series of these cases have included some that on biopsy ultimately show underlying lichen planopilaris, lupus erythematosus, and scleroderma.[118] Brocq is the eponym of pseudopelade most appropriately applied to those cases that appear to be of idiopathic origin.

Histopathology. In the truly idiopathic cases of pseudopelade, variable lymphocytic infiltrates may be seen in the superficial dermis in perivascular or loosely peri-infundibular arrangement.[119] Massive lymphocytic infiltration associated with apoptosis has been reported also.[120] The inflammatory phase may be short, and biopsies may show no significant inflammatory infiltrates.[117] Infiltrates may extend into the follicular epithelium and occasionally into the sebaceous glands. Deep perifollicular inflammation is not detected.[121]

Most biopsies are obtained when scarring is established. Scar tissue replaces the entire site of the pilosebaceous apparatus (Fig. 18-18). Exceptional sebaceous glands may be preserved, but the arrector pili muscle remains behind, isolated in the middermis. The scar tract of the follicle may extend into the subcutaneous tissue,[122] and the remnant of the elastic fiber sheath of the damaged follicle may be retained at this site.[123] Although elastic tissue staining of specimens in this condition generally shows substantial preservation of the elastic fiber network in the reticular dermis, it is customary to identify loss of the fiber network in the upper dermis, in the site of the preexisting upper infundibular epithelium.[123] The surface epidermis retains its normal architecture.

Differential Diagnosis. In active cases of lichen planopilaris and discoid lupus erythematosus, the characteristic distribution of inflammatory infiltrates and the involvement of the basal epidermis of the follicular infundibulum and the surface epidermis usually allow rapid discrimination between these two conditions. When lichen planopilaris and discoid lupus erythematosus are in inflammatory remission or have burned out, the resultant damage from these conditions may prove to be a diagnostic problem.[124] Elastic tissue stains may help to discriminate between them and direct immunofluorescence testing may be helpful by demonstrating immunoglobulin and complement deposits in the dermal-epidermal junctional zone in lupus erythematosus.[125]

The scarring alopecia resulting from destructive inflammatory folliculitis (including folliculitis decalvans), as well as that following chronic tractional alopecia, hot comb alopecia, and the follicular degeneration syndrome, may create very similar patterns of predominantly focal follicular scarring alopecia, and clinical correlation is always necessary for accurate assessment of biopsy specimens.

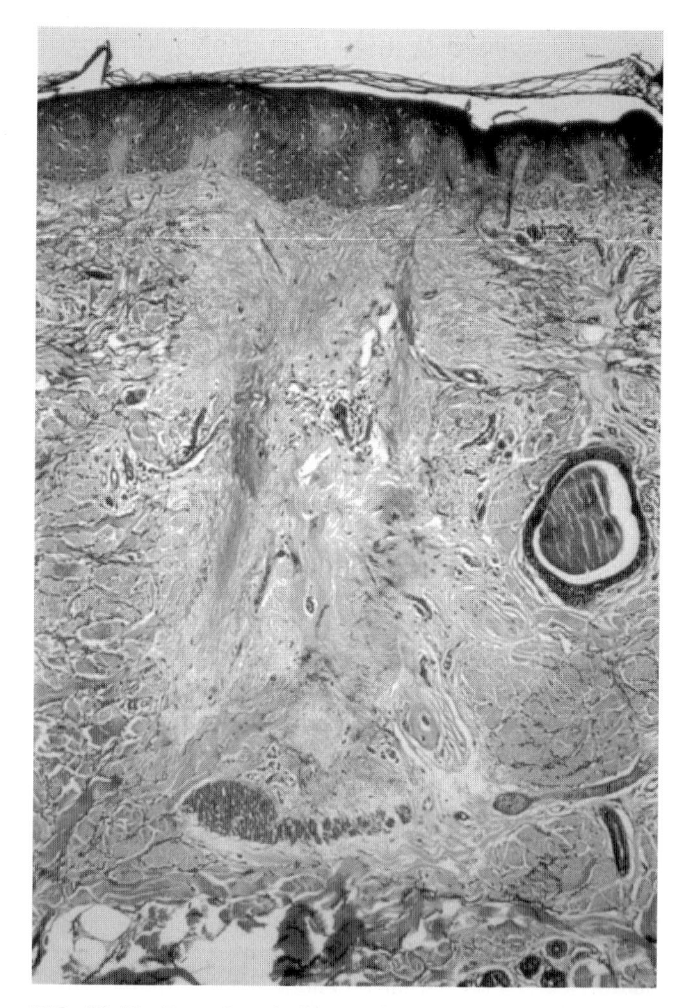

FIG. 18-18. Pseudopelade
Elastic stain. A vertically oriented scar replaces previous pilosebaceous structure. Note preserved fiber network in adjacent reticular dermis.

The diffuse dermal thickening and homogenization of collagen fiber that occur in localized scleroderma usually make it easy to differentiate this condition from pseudopelade.

ALOPECIA MUCINOSA (FOLLICULAR MUCINOSIS)

Described in 1957 by Pinkus,[126] this condition is now classified into two types: a primary (idiopathic) type and a secondary (symptomatic) variety. When these types can be distinguished, the primary form, which may lead to permanent alopecia, tends to have a shorter but benign course. On the other hand, the secondary type is often associated with lymphomas of which the majority are of cutaneous T-cell type (mycosis fungoides), and this condition may evolve over many years, with a fatal outcome.

The skin lesions consist of grouped erythematous papules and/or plaques that may be markedly indurated or even nodular. Alopecia is conspicuous only when it affects terminal hair-bearing areas.

The benign (primary) form, which tends to affect children and young adults more frequently, is often confined to the head and neck but may be disseminated. The lymphoma-related (secondary) form tends to develop more uniformly widespread plaques and is almost always an adult disorder. These patterns are not consistently diagnostically predictive, however, and the adult plaque form can run a long, benign course.[127]

There has been controversy as to the ability of histopathologists to distinguish between the primary and secondary forms. Initially it was considered that the histopathology could be predictive.[127] Later, some researchers concluded that transition from the benign form to the lymphomatous type could occur,[128,129] but others disputed this finding.[130,131] More recently, a large study of 59 cases concluded that there was no clinical or pathologic pattern by which the ultimate outcome of the condition could be predicted.[132] Complicating the situation is the finding of follicular mucinosis in association with other lymphomas (Hodgkin's disease,[132–134] cutaneous B-cell lymphoma,[135] and chronic lymphatic leukemia[134]), together with a substantial number of inflammatory cutaneous disease disorders (chronic discoid lupus erythematosus,[136] angiolymphoid hyperplasia,[137] verruca,[131] alopecia areata,[138] leprosy,[139] and melanocytic nevus[140]). These numerous processes associated with production of follicular epithelial mucins certainly suggest that this is a relatively nonspecific reaction pattern.

Histopathology. Vacuolar change, resembling reticular degeneration but sometimes evolving into more extensive cavitation of the outer root sheath and sebaceous gland epithelium within which mucin is deposited, characterizes this condition[141] (Fig. 18-19). Occasionally, little mucin can be detected, perhaps because of removal of this water-soluble material in the processing procedure.[142]

Mucin deposits consist of acid mucopolysaccharide, which stains metrochromatically with Giemsa stain or toluidine blue as well as with alcian blue in acid pH. Mucin consists predominantly of hyaluronic acid, because the material can be substantially removed by prior digestion with hyaluronidase. The periodic acid–Schiff (PAS) reaction also demonstrates a moderate amount of positive material throughout the involved pilosebaceous apparatus, and, because this can be digested by diastase, this material represents glycogen.[141]

The inflammatory infiltrates are lymphocytes and histiocytes, but there also may be eosinophils. Exocytosis into the outer root sheath epithelium, the sebaceous gland epithelium, and occasionally the lower portion of the infundibular epithelium occurs. Atypical lymphocytic infiltrate in both the adventitia and the epithelial component substantially indicates a lymphoma-associated lesion (Fig. 18-20). Although individual pathologic criteria are not in themselves diagnostic of either type of follicular mucinosis, increased density of the perifollicular infiltrate and more substantial epidermotropism have been considered to favor a follicular lesion of cutaneous T-cell lymphoma type.[143] This study suggested that prominent eosinophilia of the infiltrate and more substantial mucin deposition tended to favor a benign process. These findings were not substantiated, however, in a more recent study.[132]

Pathogenesis. Electron microscopic studies have demonstrated that the mucin is a product of the outer root sheath ep-

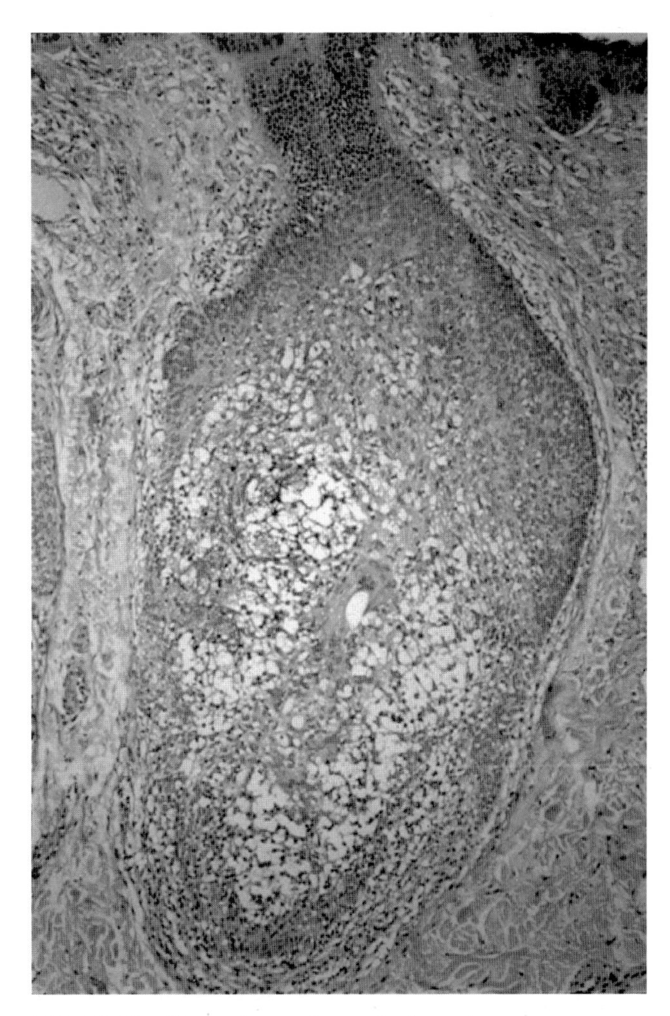

FIG. 18-19. Alopecia mucinosa (primary)
A follicular infundibulum shows reticular degeneration with exocytosis and mucin deposition, but note sparse dermal infiltrates.

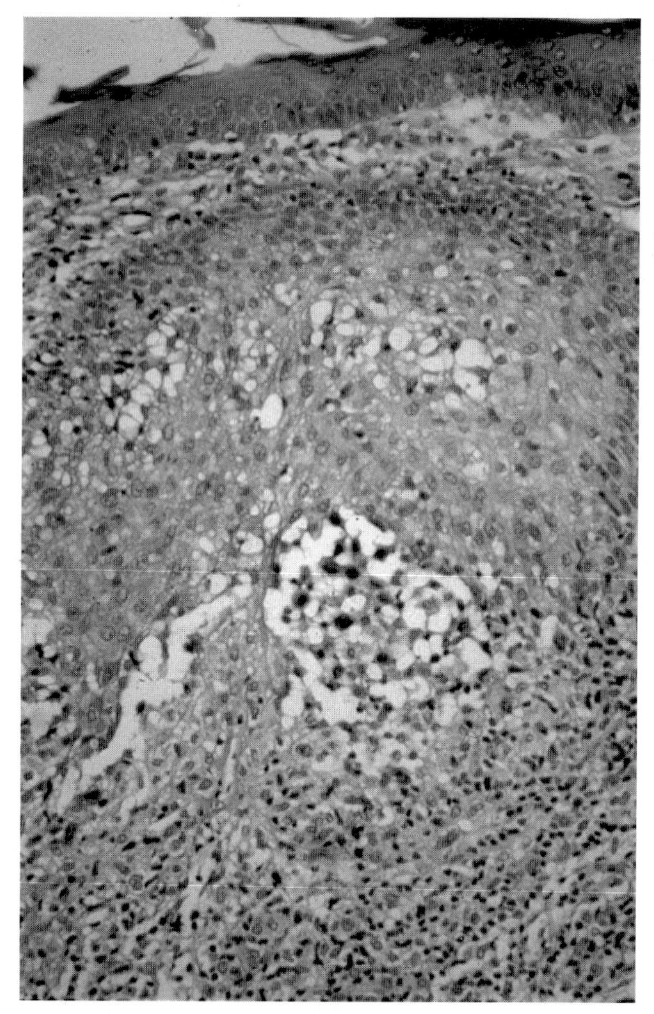

FIG. 18-20. Alopecia mucinosa (secondary) Atypical lymphocytes aggregate in an infundibular structure showing mucinous vacuolar degeneration.

ithelial cells. The cytoplasm shows prominent, dilated, rough-surfaced endoplasmic reticulum containing fine, granular, filamentous material that is secreted into the intercellular spaces.[144] Clonal proliferation of T lymphocytes has been documented in cutaneous T-cell lymphoma presenting with follicular mucinosis, as shown by T-cell receptor gene rearrangement analysis.[145]

SYRINGOLYMPHOID HYPERPLASIA WITH ALOPECIA

This rare, chronic dermatosis, first described in 1969,[146] occurs only in adult males who present with patchy, often hyperpigmented, fine keratin-plugged follicular papules. The condition produces both alopecia and anhidrosis. There may be diminished sensation.

Histopathology. Dense lymphocytic infiltrates are present in the adventitial dermis of sweat ducts and glands, which show epithelial hyperplasia. Exocytosis accompanies these changes, and the lumina of the ducts may be obliterated.[147,148]

Pathogenesis. Of the few cases reported to date, two have been associated with follicular mucinosis. In one of these, the follicular condition was considered to be of idiopathic or benign type.[149] In the other case, the infiltrates were considered to represent cutaneous T-cell lymphoma, and clonal proliferation of T lymphocytes was demonstrated by T-cell receptor gene rearrangement analysis.[148]

FOX-FORDYCE DISEASE

Fox-Fordyce disease, which occurs almost exclusively in women, demonstrates firm, itchy follicular papules in those areas where apocrine glands occur (axillae, areolae, and genital areas). This condition represents apocrine miliaria.[150]

Histopathology. Obstruction of the intraepidermal apocrine duct occurs through formation of a keratin plug in the follicular infundibulum at its insertion site. A spongiotic vesicle occurs behind or below this obstructing plug and may represent an apocrine sweat-retention vesicle, which may rupture. Infundibular acanthosis may then follow, and inflammatory cells may be present in the adjacent dermis in a perivascular pattern. Vesicles may show exocytosis. Step sections of biopsy material are usually needed to show this lesion adequately.[151,152]

Pathogenesis. Complete apocrine anhidrosis occurs in this condition, as demonstrated by the lack of secretion following intradermal injections of 1:1000 solution of epinephrine into the affected area.[150]

CHONDRODERMATITIS NODULARIS HELICIS

This condition presents as a single (rarely multiple), exquisitely tender, small, dull erythematous nodule on the superior rim of the helix (less frequently on the antihelix). The lesions develop crust and ulceration in the center, producing elevated margins that may mimic basal cell carcinoma. Lesions tend to persist indefinitely.

Histopathology. Epidermal ulceration is usually present, and the intact epidermal margin is edematous and acanthotic. A crust of exudate, parakeratosis, and dermal debris covers the surface of the ulceration.[153] The dermis directly below the ulcerated zone shows homogeneous acellular collagen degeneration and necrosis, which may reach the perichondrial tissue below (Fig. 18-21). The viable connective tissue adjacent to the zone of degeneration shows vascular proliferation with inflammatory cells of lymphohistiocytic type, and there may be some fibroplasia and occasional plasma cells.[154,155] Glomus cell aggregates have been described in these vascularized granulation tissue–like areas.[156] The perichondrial tissue may be thickened and may seem to migrate into the base of the dermal necrosis.[157] Cartilaginous degeneration can occur, although it is usually minimal, with diminution of cell nuclei. If cartilaginous degeneration is severe, there may be focal calcification and ossification.[158]

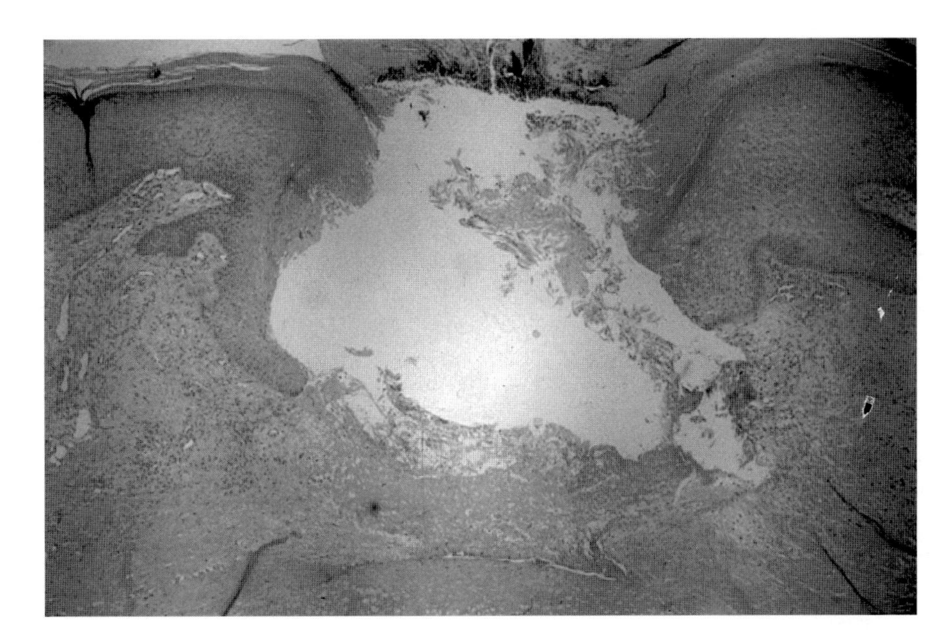

FIG. 18-21. Chondrodermatitis nodularis helicis
A sharply defined crusted ulcer extends to the perichondrium of ear cartilage. Note degenerate dermal tissue in the base and granulation tissue–like reaction adjacent.

Pathogenesis. As the name indicates, it was initially thought that this condition resulted from cartilaginous degeneration. Doubt about this origin was sustained by cases occurring in the absence of cartilaginous involvement. The condition is now more commonly attributed to dermal degeneration most likely resulting from vascular insufficiency, whether induced by trauma, pressure, cold, or the complication of solar elastotic degenerative change. The limited vasculature and lack of subcutaneous tissue insulation may both contribute to this situation. The condition has also been considered to represent a perforating disorder in which the epithelium attempts to eliminate actinically damaged connective tissue.[153,157,159] The severe tenderness of the lesion may be related to the glomoid capillary proliferation.[159]

RELAPSING POLYCHONDRITIS

This condition, although often episodic, generally runs a progressively destructive course. The onset usually consists of auricular chondritis and arthritis, but involvement of the cartilage of the nose and respiratory tract is frequently observed, as is ocular inflammation. Mortality is about 25%, most commonly from respiratory tract involvement or cardiac valvular damage.[160]

Ear and nose involvement consists of intermittent attacks of painful erythema and swelling. Rarely, only one ear is involved.[161] Ultimately, the ears become soft and flabby as a result of cartilaginous degeneration, and the nose assumes a saddle nose deformity.[162] Cutaneous lesions occur occasionally, consisting of purpuric or erythema nodosum–like lesions.[160,163]

About one-third of the patients have other manifestations of rheumatic or autoimmune diseases, and there may be associated leukocytoclastic vasculitis.[160,163,164] Indeed, it has been suggested that the cartilaginous damage may be secondary to the primary vasculitis.[165] A condition that combines features of Behçet's disease with relapsing polychondritis has been described,[166] and a case of relapsing polychondritis with coexisting pseudocyst of the auricle has been documented.[167]

Histopathology. In early lesions, only the marginal chondrocytes appear degenerate, showing vacuolization, nuclear pyknosis, and loss of basophilia as a result of the release of chondroitin sulfate from the matrix with resulting faint eosinophilia.[168] An elastic tissue stain shows clumping and destruction of the cartilaginous elastic fibers.[169] A dense, inflammatory infiltrate develops in the perichondrium, encroaching on the cartilage. Neutrophils, lymphocytes, and plasma cells, together with macrophages, may be present. With succeeding episodes and more extensive destruction of chondrocytes and their phagocytosis, the involved areas are infiltrated by fibrous tissue.[170]

Cutaneous lesions in this condition may show a vasculitis with occlusion of vessels and lymphocytic infiltrates with eosinophils.[163] There may be an associated systemic vasculitis or arteritis of the aorta or large arteries.[160] Erythema elevatum diutinum has also been reported in cutaneous lesions of patients with relapsing polychondritis.[171]

Pathogenesis. Circulating antibodies to type II collagen have been detected in patients with relapsing polychondritis.[172,173] Type II collagen is found exclusively in cartilage. The antibodies are generally found only in patients with active disease.[174] Circulating immune complexes can often be demonstrated.[172] The antibodies are directed against native and undenatured collagen, suggesting a primary role for these antibodies rather than a secondary one in response to cartilaginous injury.[172] Deposition of immunoglobulin and complement components in the inflamed cartilage of patients has also been detected.[167,168]

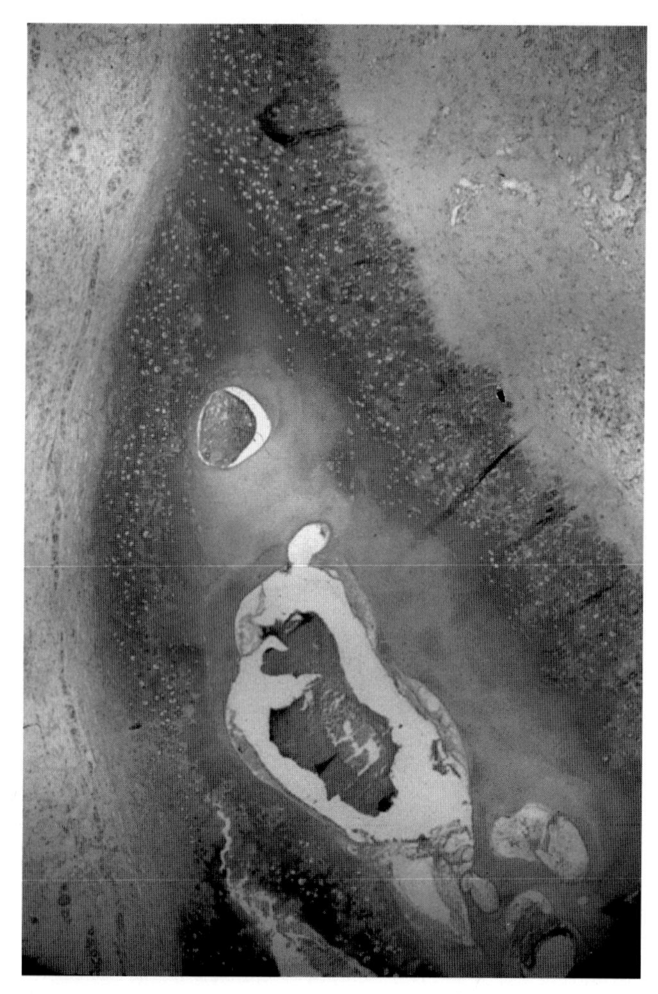

FIG. 18-22. Pseudocyst of the auricle
Mucicarmine stain. A mucin containing cystic cavity is present within the ear cartilage. Note the surrounding amorphous degenerate cartilage.

PSEUDOCYST OF THE AURICLE

In pseudocyst of the auricle, an asymptomatic, fluctuant swelling is observed on the upper portion of the anterior aspect of the ear, measuring about 1 cm in diameter. The cyst arises spontaneously, and only rarely are both ears involved.[175] When the cyst is punctured, a clear, deep yellow, viscous fluid is obtained.

Histopathology. An intracartilaginous cavity without an epithelial lining is found on histologic examination. The cyst wall consists of auricular cartilage, which is partially degenerated, appearing as eosinophilic amorphous material (Fig. 18-22).[176]

Pathogenesis. Pseudocyst of the auricle has been described in association with relapsing polychondritis.[167] It has been suggested that the degenerative change and intracartilaginous cavitation occur following the release of lysosomal enzymes.[177]

REFERENCES

1. Goldschmidt H, Leyden JJ, Stein KH. Acne fulminans. Arch Dermatol 1977;113:444.
2. Strauss JS, Kligman AM. The pathologic dynamics of acne vulgaris. Arch Dermatol 1960;82:779.
3. Massa MC, Su WPD. Pyoderma faciale: A clinical study of twenty-nine patients. J Am Acad Dermatol 1982;6:84.
4. Pochi PE, Strauss JS. Endocrinologic control of the development and activity of the human sebaceous gland. J Invest Dermatol 1974;62:191.
5. Thody AJ, Shuster S. Control and function of sebaceous glands. Physiol Rev 1989;69:383.
6. Imperato-McGinley J, Gautier T, Cal LQ et al. The androgen control of sebum production: Studies of subjects with dihydrotestosterone deficiency and complete androgen insensitivity. J Clin Endocrinol Metab 1993;76:524.
7. Marynick SP, Chakmakjian ZH, McCaffree DL, Herndon JH. Androgen excess in cystic acne. N Engl J Med 1983;308:981.
8. Lucky AW, McGuire J, Rosenfield RL et al. Plasma androgens in women with acne vulgaris. J Invest Dermatol 1983;81:70.
9. Toscano V, Balducci R, Blanchi P et al. Two different pathogenetic mechanisms may play a role in acne and in hirsutism. Clin Endocrinol 1993;39:551.
10. Lookingbill DP, Horton R, Demens LM et al. Tissue production of androgen in women with acne. J Am Acad Dermatol 1985;12:481.
11. Strauss JS, Pochi PE, Downing DT. Acne perspectives. J Invest Dermatol 1974;62:321.
12. Shuster S. Acne: The ashes of a burnt out controversy. Acta Derm Venereol Suppl (Stockh) 1985;120:34.
13. Leyden JJ, McGinley KJ. Effect of 13-cis-retinoic acid on sebum production and *Propionibacterium acnes* in severe nodulocystic acne. Arch Dermatol Res 1982;272:331.
14. Goldstein JA, Comite H, Mescon H, Pochi PE. Isotretinoin in the treatment of acne, histologic changes, sebum production, and clinical observations. Arch Dermatol 1982;118:555.
15. Melnik B, Kinner T, Plewig G. Influence of oral isotretinoin treatment on the composition of comedonal lipids. Arch Dermatol Res 1988;280:97.
16. Leyden JJ, McGinley KJ, Mills OH, Kligman AM. *Propionibacterium* levels in patients with and without acne vulgaris. J Invest Dermatol 1975;65:382.
17. Cove JH, Cunliffe WJ, Holland KT. Acne vulgaris: Is the bacterial population size significant? Br J Dermatol 1980;102:277.
18. Puhvel SM, Amirian D, Weintraub J, Reisner RM. Lymphocyte transformation in subjects with nodulo-cystic acne. Br J Dermatol 1977;97:205.
19. Kersey P, Sussman M, Dahl M. Delayed skin test reactivity to *Propionibacterium acnes* correlates with severity of inflammation in acne vulgaris. Br J Dermatol 1980;103:651.
20. Akers WA, Allen AM, Burnett JW et al. Systemic antibiotics for treatment of acne vulgaris. Arch Dermatol 1975;111:1630.
21. Resh W, Stoughton RB. Topically applied antibiotics in acne vulgaris. Arch Dermatol 1976;112:182.
22. Plewig G. Morphologic dynamics of acne vulgaris. Acta Derm Venereol Suppl (Stockh) 1980;89:9.
23. Lavker RM, Leyden JJ. Lamellar inclusions in follicular horny cells: A new aspect of abnormal keratinization. J Ultrastruct Res 1979;69:362.
24. Zelickson AS, Mottaz JH. Pigmentation of open comedones. Arch Dermatol 1983;119:567.
25. Leyden JJ. New understandings of the pathogenesis of acne. J Am Acad Dermatol 1995;32:15S.
26. Marks R, Wilson-Jones E. Disseminated rosacea. Br J Dermatol 1969;81:16.
27. Meschig R. Ophthalmological complications of rosacea. In: Marks R, Plewig G, eds. Acne and related disorders. London: Dunitz, 1989;321.
28. Ramelet AA. Rosacée: Étude histopathologique de 75 cas. Ann Dermatol Venereol 1988;115:801.
29. Marks R, Harcourt-Webster JN. Histopathology of rosacea. Arch Dermatol 1969;100:683.
30. Grosshans EM, Kremer M, Maleville J. *Demodex folliculorum* und die histogenese der granulomatösen rosacea. Hautartz 1974;25:166.

31. Rufli T, Cajacob A, Schuppli R. Rosacea granulomatosa, Demodex-Granulomatose. Dermatologica 1982;165:310.
32. Mullanax MG, Kierland RR. Granulomatous rosacea. Arch Dermatol 1970;101:206.
33. Erlach E, Gerbart W, Niebauer G. Zur pathogenese der granulomatösen rosacea. Z Hautkr 1976;51:459.
34. Helm KF, Menz J, Gibson LE, Dicken CH. A clinical and histopathologic study of granulomatous rosacea. J Am Acad Dermatol 1991;25: 1038.
35. Burton JL, Pye RJ, Meyrick G, Shuster S. The sebum excretion rate in rosacea. Br J Dermatol 1975;92:541.
36. Logan RA, Griffiths WAD. Climatic factors and rosacea. In: Marks R, Plewig G, eds. Acne and related disorders. London: Dunitz, 1989;311.
37. Forton F, Seys B. Density of *Demodex folliculorum* in rosacea: A case-control study using standardized skin surface biopsy. Br J Dermatol 1993;128:650.
38. Ecker RI, Winkelmann RK. Demodex granuloma. Arch Dermatol 1979;115:343.
39. Wilkin JK. Rosacea, pathophysiology and treatment. Arch Dermatol 1994;130:359.
40. Jablonska S, Chorzelski T, Maciejowska E. The scope and limitations of the immunofluorescence method in the diagnosis of lupus erythematosus. Br J Dermatol 1970;83:242.
41. Gajewska M. Rosacea in common male baldness. Br J Dermatol 1975; 93:63.
42. Abell E, Black MM, Marks R. Immunoglobulin and complement deposits in the skin in inflammatory facial dermatoses. Br J Dermatol 1974;91:281.
43. Ukei H, Masuda T. Lupus miliaris disseminatus faciei. Hautarzt 1979; 30:553.
44. Kumano K, Tani M, Murata Y. Dapsone in the treatment of miliary lupus of the face. Br J Dermatol 1983;109:57.
45. Scott KW, Calnan CD. Acne agminata. Trans St Johns Hosp Dermatol Soc 1967;53:60.
46. Simon N. Ist der Lupus miliaris disseminatus tuberkulöser ätiologie? Hautarzt 1975;26:625.
47. Mihara K, Isoda M. Immunohistochemical study of lysozyme in lupus miliaris disseminatus faciei. Br J Dermatol 1986;115:187.
48. Mihan R, Ayres S. Perioral dermatitis. Arch Dermatol 1964;89:803.
49. Marks R, Black MM. Perioral dermatitis: A histopathological study of 26 cases. Br J Dermatol 1971;84:242.
50. Ramelet AA, Delacretaz J. Étude histo-pathologique de la dermatite périorale. Dermatologica 1981;163:361.
51. Furmess GM, Lewis HM. Light sensitive seborrheid. Arch Dermatol 1957;75:245.
52. Kerr REI, Thomson J. Perioral dermatitis. In: Fitzpatrick TB, Eisen AZ, Wolff K et al., eds. Dermatology in general medicine. New York: McGraw-Hill, 1993;735.
53. Mevorah B, Marazzi A, Frenk E. The prevalence of accentuated palmoplantar markings and keratosis pilaris in atopic dermatitis, autosomal dominant ichthyosis vulgaris and control dermatological patients. Br J Dermatol 1985;112:679.
54. Friedman SJ. Lichen spinulosus. A clinicopathologic review of thirty five cases. J Am Acad Dermatol 1990;22:261.
55. Boyd AS. Lichen spinulosus: Case report and overview. Cutis 1989; 43:557.
56. Nakjang Y, Yuttanavivat T. Phrynoderma: A review of 105 cases. J Dermatol (Tokyo) 1988;15:531.
57. Arndt KA, Rand RE. Follicular syndromes with inflammation and atrophy. In: Fitzpatrick TB, Eisen AZ, Wolff K et al., eds. Dermatology in general medicine. New York: McGraw-Hill, 1993:766.
58. Hitch JM, Lund HZ. Disseminate and recurrent infundibulofolliculitis. Arch Dermatol 1972;105:580.
59. Owen WR, Wood C. Disseminate and recurrent infundibulofolliculitis. Arch Dermatol 1979;115:174.
60. Ofuji S, Ogino A, Horio T et al. Eosinophilic pustular folliculitis. Acta Derm Venereol (Stockh) 1970;50:195.
61. Lucky AW, Esterly NS, Heskel N et al. Eosinophilic pustular folliculitis in infancy. Pediatr Dermatol 1984;1:202.
62. Duarte AM, Kramer J, Yusk JW et al. Eosinophilic pustular folliculitis in infancy and childhood. Am J Dis Child 1993;147:197.
63. Rosenthal D, LeBoit PE, Klumpp L, Berger TG. Human immunodeficiency virus associated eosinophilic folliculitis. Arch Dermatol 1991; 127:206.
64. Ishibashi A, Nishiyama Y, Miyata C, Chujo T. Eosinophilic pustular folliculitis (Ofuji). Dermatologica 1974;149:240.
65. Orfanos CE, Sterry W. Sterile eosinophile pustulose. Dermatologica 1978;157:193.
66. Ofuji S. Eosinophilic pustular folliculitis. Dermatologica 1987;174: 53.
67. Holst R. Eosinophilic pustular folliculitis. Br J Dermatol 1976;95:661.
68. Guillaume JC, Dubertret L, Cosnes A et al. Folliculite à éosinophiles (maladie d'Ofuji). Ann Dermatol Venereol 1979;106:347.
69. McCalmont TH, Altemus O, Maurer T, Berger TG. Eosinophilic folliculitis. Am J Dermatopathol 1995;17:439.
70. Vakilzadeh F, Suter L, Knop J, Macher E. Eosinophilic pustulosis with pemphigus-like antibody. Dermatologica 1981;162:265.
71. Nunzi E, Parodi A, Rebora A. Ofuji's disease. J Am Acad Dermatol 1985;12:268.
72. Takematsu H, Tagami H. Eosinophilic pustular folliculitis: Studies on possible chemotactic factors involved in the formation of pustules. Br J Dermatol 1986;114:209.
73. Teraki Y, Konohana I, Shiohara T et al. Eosinophilic pustular folliculitis (Ofuji's disease) immunohistochemical analysis. Arch Dermatol 1993;129:1015.
74. Brenner S, Wolf R, Ophir J. Eosinophilic pustular folliculitis of unknown cause? J Am Acad Dermatol 1994;31:210.
75. Haupt HM, Stern JB, Weber CB. Eosinophilic pustular folliculitis: Fungal folliculitis? J Am Acad Dermatol 1990;23:1012.
76. Wells GC, Smith NP. Eosinophilic cellulitis. Br J Dermatol 1979;100: 101.
77. Anderson CR, Jenkins D, Tron V, Prendiville JS. Wells' syndrome in childhood: Case report and review of literature. J Am Acad Dermatol 1995;33:857.
78. Spigel GT, Winkelmann RK. Wells' syndrome. Arch Dermatol 1979; 115:611.
79. Fisher GB, Greer KE, Copper PH. Eosinophilic cellulitis (Wells' syndrome). Int J Dermatol 1985;24:101.
80. Brehmer-Andersson E, Kaaman T, Skog E, Frithz A. The histopathogenesis of the flame figure in Wells' syndrome based on five cases. Acta Derm Venereol (Stockh) 1986;66:213.
81. Newton JA, Greaves MW. Eosinophilic cellulitis (Wells' syndrome) with florid histological changes. Clin Exp Dermatol 1988;13:318.
82. Peters MS, Schroeter AL, Gleich GJ. Immunofluorescence identification of eosinophil granule major basic protein in the flame figures of Wells' syndrome. Br J Dermatol 1983;109:141.
83. Stern JB, Sobel HJ, Rotchford JP. Wells' syndrome: Is there collagen damage in the flame figures? J Cutan Pathol 1984;11:501.
84. Hurwitz S, Kirsch N, McGuire I. Reevaluation of ichthyosis and hair shaft abnormalities. Arch Dermatol 1971;103:266.
85. Netherton EW. A unique case of trichorrhexis nodosa: "Bamboo hairs". Arch Dermatol 1958;78:483.
86. Greene SL, Muller SA. Netherton's syndrome. J Am Acad Dermatol 1985;13:329.
87. Ito M, Ito K, Hashimoto K. Pathogenesis in trichorrhexis invaginata (bamboo hair). J Invest Dermatol 1984;83:1.
88. Sarkany J, Gaylarde PM. Trichostasis spinulosa and its management. Br J Dermatol 1971;84:311.
89. Goldschmidt H, Hojyo-Tomoka MT, Kligman AM. Trichostasis spinulosa. Hautarzt 1975;26:299.
90. Headington JT. The histopathology of alopecia areata. J Invest Dermatol 1991;96:69S.
91. Messenger AG, Slater DN, Bleehen SS. Alopecia areata: Alterations in the hair growth cycle and correlation with the follicular pathology. Br J Dermatol 1986;114:337.
92. Abell E, Gruber HM. A histopathologic reappraisal of alopecia areata. J Cutan Pathol 1987;14:347.
93. Headington JT, Mitchell A, Swanson N. New histopathologic findings in alopecia areata studied in transverse section. J Invest Dermatol 1981;76:325.
94. Todes-Taylor N, Turner R, Wood GS et al. T cell subpopulations in alopecia areata. J Am Acad Dermatol 1984;11:216.
95. Khoury EL, Price VH, Abdel-Salam MM et al. Topical minoxidil in alopecia areata: No effect on the perifollicular lymphoid infiltration. J Invest Dermatol 1992;99:40.
96. Kochiyama A, Hatamochi A, Ueki H. Increased number of OKT6-positive dendritic cells in the hair follicles of patients with alopecia areata. Dermatologica 1985;171:327.

97. Colombe BW, Price VH, Khoury EL et al. HLA class II antigen associations help to define two types of alopecia areata. J Am Acad Dermatol 1995;33:757.
98. Nickoloff BJ, Griffiths CEM. Aberrant intercellular adhesion molecule-1 (ICAM-1) expression by hair follicle epithelial cells and endothelial leukocyte adhesion molecule-1 (ELAM-1) by vascular cells are important adhesion molecule alterations in alopecia areata. J Invest Dermatol 1991;96:91S.
99. McDonagh AJG, Snowden JA, Stierle C et al. HLA and ICAM-1 expression in alopecia areata in vivo and in vitro: The role of cytokines. Br J Dermatol 1993;129:250.
100. Lee JYY, Hsu ML. Alopecia syphilitica, a simulator of alopecia areata: Histopathology and differential diagnosis. J Cutan Pathol 1991;18:87.
101. Muller SA. Trichotillomania: A histopathologic study in sixty-six patients. J Am Acad Dermatol 1990;23:56.
102. Mehregan AH. Trichotillomania. Arch Dermatol 1970;102:129.
103. Sperling LL, Lupton GP. Histopathology of non-scarring alopecia. J Cutan Pathol 1995;22:97.
104. Kligman AM. Pathologic dynamics of human hair loss: I. Telogen effluvium. Arch Dermatol 1961;83:175.
105. Headington JT. Telogen effluvium. Arch Dermatol 1993;129:356.
106. Headington JT. Transverse microscopic anatomy of the human scalp. Arch Dermatol 1984;120:449.
107. Whiting DA. Diagnostic and predictive value of horizontal sections of scalp biopsy specimens in male pattern androgenetic alopecia. J Am Acad Dermatol 1993;28:755.
108. Fiedler VC, Hafeez A. Diffuse alopecia: Telogen hair loss. In: Olsen E, ed. Disorders of hair growth. New York: McGraw-Hill, 1994;241.
109. Headington JT, Novak E. Clinical and histologic studies of male pattern baldness treated with topical minoxidil. Curr Ther Res 1984;36:1098.
110. Abell E. Histologic response to topically applied minoxidil in male-pattern alopecia. Clin Dermatol 1988;6:191.
111. Abell E. Pathology of male pattern alopecia. Arch Dermatol 1984; 120:1607.
112. Kligman AM. The comparative histopathology of male-pattern baldness and senescent baldness. Clin Dermatol 1988;6:108.
113. Randall VA, Thornton MJ, Hamada K, Messenger AG. Mechanism of androgen action in cultured dermal papilla cells derived from human hair follicles with varying responses to androgens in vivo. J Invest Dermatol 1992;98:86S.
114. Hibberts NA, Randall VA. Balding scalp dermal papilla cells contain higher levels of androgen receptors than those of non-balding scalp ones. Br J Dermatol 1993;129:478.
115. Olsen EA. Androgenetic alopecia. In: Olsen EA, ed. Disorders of hair growth. New York: McGraw-Hill, 1994;257.
116. Sawya ME, Hordinsky MK. Advances in alopecia areata and androgenetic alopecia. In: Callen JP, Dahl MV, Golitz LE et al., eds. Advances in dermatology. St. Louis: Mosby–Year Book 1992;211.
117. Elston DM, Bergfeld WF. Cicatricial alopecia (and other causes of permanent alopecia). In: Olsen EA, ed. Disorder of hair growth. New York: McGraw-Hill, 1994;285.
118. Braun-Falco O, Bergner T, Heilgemeir GP. Pseudopelade Brocq-krankheitsbild oder krankheitsentität. Hautarzt 1989;40:77.
119. Templeton SF, Solomon AR. Scarring alopecia: A classification based upon microscopic criteria. J Cutan Pathol 1994;21:97.
120. Pierard-Franchimont C, Pierard GE. Massive lymphocyte-mediated apoptosis during the early stage of pseudopelade. Dermatologica 1986;172:254.
121. Ioannides G. Alopecia: A pathologist's view. Int J Dermatol 1982;21: 316.
122. Braun-Falco O, Imai S, Schmoeckel C et al. Pseudopelade of Brocq. Dermatologica 1986;172:18.
123. Pinkus H. Differential patterns of elastic fibers in scarring and non-scarring alopecias. J Cutan Pathol 1978;5:93.
124. Nayar M, Schomberg K, Dawber RPR, Millard PR. A clinicopathological study of scarring alopecia. Br J Dermatol 1993;128:533.
125. Jordon RE. Subtle clues to diagnosis by immunopathology: Scarring alopecia. Am J Dermatopathol 1980;2:157.
126. Pinkus H. Alopecia mucinosa: Inflammatory plaques with alopecia characterized by root sheath mucinosis. Arch Dermatol 1957;76:419.
127. Emmerson RW. Follicular mucinosis: A study of forty-seven patients. Br J Dermatol 1969;81:395.
128. Pinkus H. Commentary: Alopecia mucinosa. Arch Dermatol 1983; 119:698.
129. Sentis HJ, Willemze R, Scheffer E. Alopecia mucinosa progressing into mycosis fungoides: A long-term follow-up of two patients. Am J Dermatopathol 1988;10:478.
130. Kim R, Winkelmann RK. Follicular mucinosis (alopecia mucinosa). Arch Dermatol 1962;85:490.
131. Hempstead RW, Ackerman AB. Follicular mucinosis: A reaction pattern in follicular epithelium. Am J Dermatopathol 1985;7:245.
132. Gibson LE, Muller SA, Leiferman KM, Peters MS. Follicular mucinosis: Clinical and histopathologic study. J Am Acad Dermatol 1989; 20:441.
133. Stewart M, Smoller BR. Follicular mucinosis in Hodgkin's disease: A poor prognostic sign? J Am Acad Dermatol 1991;24:784.
134. Mehregan AD, Gibson EL, Muller AS. Follicular mucinosis: Histopathologic review in 33 cases. Mayo Clin Proc 1991;66:387.
135. Benchikhi H, Wechsler J, Rethers L et al. Cutaneous B-cell lymphoma associated with follicular mucinosis. J Am Acad Dermatol 1995;33: 673.
136. Cabré J, Korting GW. Zum symptomatischen charakter der "Mucinosis follicularis": Ihr Vorkommen beim Lupus erythematodes chronicus. Dermatol Wochenschr 1964;149:513.
137. Wolff HH, Kinney J, Ackerman AB. Angiolymphoid hyperplasia with follicular mucinosis. Arch Dermatol 1978;114:229.
138. Fanti PA, Tosti A, Morelli R et al. Follicular mucinosis in alopecia areata. Am J Dermatopathol 1992;14:542.
139. Lazaro-Medina A, Tianco EA, Avila JM. Additional markers for the type I reactional states in borderline leprosy. Am J Dermatol 1990;12: 417.
140. Jordaan HF. Follicular mucinosis in association with a melanocytic nevus: A report of two cases. J Cutan Pathol 1987;14:122.
141. Johnson WC, Higdon RS, Helwig EB. Alopecia mucinosa. Arch Dermatol 1969;79:395.
142. Braun-Falco O. In the discussion of Zambal Z: Ablagerungen in der Haut bei Alopecia mucinosa. Arch Klin Exp Dermatol 1970;237:155.
143. Logan RA, Headington JT. Follicular mucinosis: A histologic review of 80 cases. J Cutan Pathol 1988;15(abstr):324.
144. Ishibashi A. Histogenesis of mucin in follicular mucinosis: An electron microscopic study. Acta Derm Venereol (Stockh) 1976;56:163.
145. Zelickson BD, Peters MS, Muller SA et al. T-cell receptor gene rearrangement analysis: Cutaneous T-cell lymphoma, peripheral T-cell lymphoma, and premalignant and benign cutaneous lymphoproliferative disorders. J Am Acad Dermatol 1991;25:787.
146. Sarkany I. Patchy alopecia, anhidrosis, eccrine gland wall hypertrophy and vasculitis. Proc R Soc Med 1969;62:157.
147. Vaklizadeh F, Brocker EB. Syringolymphoid hyperplasia with alopecia. Br J Dermatol 1984;110:95.
148. Tomaszewski MM, Lupton GP, Krishnan J et al. Syringolymphoid hyperplasia with alopecia. J Cutan Pathol 1994;21:520.
149. Berger TG, Goette DK. Eccrine proliferation with follicular mucinosis. J Cutan Pathol 1987;14:188.
150. Shelley WB, Levy EJ. Apocrine sweat retention in man: II. Fox-Fordyce disease (apocrine miliaria). Arch Dermatol 1956;73:38.
151. MacMillan DC, Vickers HR. Fox-Fordyce disease. Br J Dermatol 1971;84:181.
152. Mevorah B, Duboff GS, Wass RW. Fox-Fordyce disease in prepubescent girls. Dermatologica 1968;136:43.
153. Goette DK. Chondrodermatitis nodularis chronica helicis: A perforating necrobiotic granuloma. J Am Acad Dermatol 1980;2:148.
154. Newcomer VD, Steffen CG, Sternberg TH, Lichtenstein L. Chondrodermatitis nodularis chronica helicis. Arch Dermatol 1953;68:241.
155. Shuman R, Helwig EB. Chrondrodermatitis helicis. Am J Clin Pathol 1954;24:126.
156. Haber H. Chondrodermatitis nodularis chronica helicis. Hautarzt 1960;11:122.
157. Leonforte JE. Le nodule douloureux de l'oreille: Hyperplasie épidermique avec élimination transépithéliale. Ann Dermatol Venereol 1979;106:577.
158. Garcia E, Silva L, Martins O, Da Silva Picoto A. Bone formation in chondrodermatitis nodularis helicis. J Dermatol Surg Oncol 1980;6: 582.
159. Santa Cruz DJ. Chondrodermatitis nodularis helicis: A transepidermal perforating disorder. J Cutan Pathol 1980;7:70.
160. McAdam LP, O'Hanlan MA, Bluestone R, Pearson CM. Relapsing polychondritis: Prospective study of 23 patients and a review of the literature. Medicine (Baltimore) 1976;55:193.

161. Case records of the Massachusetts General Hospital: Relapsing polychondritis. New Engl J Med 1982;307:1631.
162. Thurston CS, Curtis AC. Relapsing polychondritis. Arch Dermatol 1966;93:664.
163. Weinberger A, Myers AR. Relapsing polychondritis associated with cutaneous vasculitis. Arch Dermatol 1979;115:980.
164. Michet CJ, McKenna CH, Luthra HS, O'Fallon WM. Relapsing polychondritis: Survival and predictive role of early disease manifestations. Ann Intern Med 1986;104:74.
165. Handrock K, Gross W. Relapsing polychondritis as a secondary phenomenon of primary systemic vasculitis. Ann Rheum Dis 1993;52:895.
166. Orme RL, Norlund JJ, Barich L, Brown T. The magic syndrome: Mouth and genital ulcers with inflamed cartilage. Arch Dermatol 1990;126:940.
167. Helm TN, Valenzuela R, Glanz S et al. Relapsing polychondritis: A case diagnosed by direct immunofluorescence and coexisting with pseudocyst of the auricle. J Am Acad Dermatol 1992;26:315.
168. Valenzuela R, Cooperrider PA, Gogate P et al. Relapsing polychondritis. Hum Pathol 1980;11:19.
169. Feinerman LK, Johnson WC, Weiner J, Graham JH. Relapsing polychondritis. Dermatologica 1970;140:369.
170. Barranco VP, Minor DP, Solomon H. Treatment of polychondritis with dapsone. Arch Dermatol 1976;112:1286.
171. Bernard P, Bedane C, Delrous JL et al. Erythema elevatum diutinum in a patient with relapsing polychondritis. J Am Acad Dermatol 1992;26:312.
172. Foidart JM, Abe S, Martin GR et al. Antibodies to type II collagen in relapsing polychondritis. N Engl J Med 1978;299:1203.
173. Terato K, Shimozuru Y, Katayama K et al. Specificity of antibodies to type II collagen in rheumatoid arthritis. Arthritis Rheum 1990;33:1493.
174. Foidart JM, Katz SI. Relapsing polychondritis. Am J Dermatopathol 1979;1:257.
175. Fukamizu H, Imaizumi S. Bilateral pseudocysts of the auricles. Arch Dermatol 1984;120:1238.
176. Glamb R, Kim R. Pseudocyst of the auricle. J Am Acad Dermatol 1984;11:58.
177. Cohen PR, Grossman ME. Pseudocyst of the auricle: Case report and world literature review. Arch Otolaryngol Head Neck Surg 1990;116:1202.

Lever's Histopathology of the Skin, eighth edition,
edited by David Elder et al. Lippincott–
Raven Publishers, Philadelphia © 1997.

CHAPTER 19

Inflammatory Diseases of the Nail

Thomas D. Griffin

An understanding of the normal anatomy and histology of the nail unit precedes understanding the pathology that may occur there (see Chap. 3, Histology of the Skin: Nails). Inflammatory pathologic processes in the nail unit affect mainly the matrix, nail bed, hyponychium, and nail folds. Changes in the nail plate occur secondarily. A basic understanding of where pathologic processes affect the nail unit will guide the practitioner in choosing a site of biopsy. As in other clinical situations, understanding the location and type of pathology leads to more effective diagnosis and treatment of the disease process.

Because of the unique anatomy of the nail unit, there is a limited number of possible reaction patterns to inflammatory processes. These reaction patterns may have different features from those seen in the skin. Because the nail unit produces a product, the nail plate, some inflammatory processes of the nail matrix may lead to irreversible damage resulting in an abnormal or absent plate, much akin to processes affecting the hair unit that lead to scarring alopecia. On the other hand, processes affecting the nail bed and hyponychium that do not affect the formation of the plate may affect its shape or adhesiveness. The nail bed responds to injury by becoming metaplastic, that is, by switching from onycholemmal keratinization (without keratohyalin granules) to epidermoid keratinization. It becomes hyperplastic, showing hyperkeratosis, parakeratosis, hypergranulosis, marked spongiosis, and exudative scale crust formation. The products of this reaction build up between the nail bed and plate. This process leads to the altered shape and shedding patterns of the nail plate that are common to several diseases affecting the nail bed, such as psoriasis and onychomycosis.

Inflammatory diseases may also affect the nail folds. When the ventral surface of the proximal nail fold is affected, one may see inflammation of the cuticle and alterations of the dorsal surface of the nail plate. Eczema and contact dermatitis of the fingers may affect both the proximal and lateral nail folds.

Inflammatory processes affecting the nail may have many overlapping features. Although a specific diagnosis may be made in many cases, such as in lichen planus affecting the matrix, often it may be difficult to distinguish between, for example, psoriasis and eczema affecting the nail bed.

T. D. Griffin: Department of Dermatology, University of Pennsylvania, Glenside, PA

BIOPSY OF THE NAIL UNIT

Biopsy of the nail unit is recommended in many cases when the diagnosis is in doubt or when definitive histopathologic diagnosis is needed before beginning therapy.

Nail matrix biopsy is best performed after reflecting back the proximal nail fold.[1] The nail plate may remain intact or may be avulsed before the biopsy. It is of utmost importance to avoid bisecting the matrix. One should obtain a 2- to 3-mm punch biopsy from the center of the matrix so that the excision is entirely within and surrounded by matrix. It is also important to avoid both the curvilinear portion of the lunula and the most proximal portion of the matrix, since interruption of these areas may lead to defects in the nail plate.

The nail bed may be sampled using a punch biopsy through the nail plate down to the periosteum.[2] Longitudinal incisional biopsies may also be done. In this procedure, en bloc removal of the lateral nail fold, matrix, bed, and hyponychium is done. This procedure is excellent for defining disease processes of the nail unit. It is probably too extensive for routine nail biopsies and is not necessary for making a histopathologic diagnosis in most cases.

The proximal nail fold region may be sampled by a punch biopsy or a transverse excisional biopsy.[2] Care must be taken to avoid going so deep in this area as to transect the tendon of the extensor digitorum communis, which inserts into the proximal dorsal portion of the terminal phalanx. Transection of this tendon will result in a drop deformity of the distal phalanx. One must also avoid the distal free margin of the proximal nail fold to prevent notching.

ECZEMATOUS DERMATITIS

Most forms of eczematous dermatitis affect the nail unit, with atopic dermatitis being most common. Contact dermatitis due to nail cosmetics or occupational exposure may affect all areas of the nail unit. Nail plate changes usually result from matrix or proximal nail fold involvement. Onycholysis may be due to nail bed involvement that begins distally at the hyponychium and spreads inward to involve the nail bed. Secondary chronic paronychial infection may occur. The biopsy should be focused on the site of involvement, usually the nail bed or nail matrix. The histologic changes include spongiosis and exocytosis of mononuclear cells, and an acanthotic epidermis. Stains for fungal organisms should be performed to rule out onychomycosis.

PSORIASIS

Nail involvement in psoriasis may occur in up to 50% of patients. Nail changes may occur in up to 80% of patients with psoriatic arthritis. In 10 percent of patients with psoriasis, nail involvement may be the only manifestation.

Psoriasis may involve any part of the nail unit, including the matrix, nail bed, hyponychium, and nail folds. Biopsy through the nail plate and nail bed is preferred for diagnosis of psoriasis involving the nail. Sections should be stained with hematoxylin-eosin and also with periodic acid–Schiff (PAS) stain or silver methenamine stain to rule out fungal infection. Because psoriasis and onychomycosis share many clinical and histologic features, a positive fungal stain is the only reliable way of distinguishing histologically between psoriasis and onychomycosis.[3]

Psoriatic involvement of the proximal nail matrix causes clinical pitting and roughening of the surface of the nail plate. Histologically, one sees foci of parakeratosis on the surface of the plate, which, when shed, leave pits in the plate. Involvement of the mid- and distal matrix leads to clinical leukonychia. Once again, the histology is that of foci of parakeratosis in the nail plate; however, in leukonychia, the parakeratotic cells are located in the deeper portions of the plate.

The "oil drop sign" of psoriatic nails is a reddish-brown discoloration of the nail bed and hyponychium.[4] It represents an early, acute focus of psoriasis involving the nail bed. One sees hyperkeratosis and parakeratosis with collections of neutrophils in the stratum corneum representing a Munro microabscess. The nail bed epidermis may show hypergranulosis with focal hypogranulosis. There is elongation of the dermal papillae with dilatation and proliferation of capillaries surrounded by lymphocytes, histiocytes, and occasional neutrophils (Fig. 19-1). Distal nail onycholysis shows a similar histology and therefore has a similar histogenesis. The split in psoriatic onycholysis occurs between where neutrophils and parakeratotic foci are located within the plate and the underlying hyponychium.[5] The yellow leading edge of onycholytic nail correlates with the presence of neutrophils in the nail plate keratin.

Ultimately, well-developed psoriasis of the nail bed leads to subungual hyperkeratosis and exudate, which lift the nail plate off the bed. The nail bed epithelium shows psoriasiform acanthosis with elongated rete ridges and capillary proliferation. Neutrophils may be present in the superficial epidermis and within the keratin. Late or chronically traumatized psoriatic nails may develop features of lichen simplex chronicus,[6] including marked compact orthokeratosis, hypergranulosis, and fibrosis of the papillary dermis, characterized by vertical streaks of coarse collagen fibers.

LICHEN PLANUS

The incidence of nail involvement occurring in association with lichen planus ranges from 1% to 10%.[7] Lichen planus may involve the nail alone, though isolated nail involvement is rare in children. Lichen planus may involve the nail matrix, nail bed, and hyponychium. Examination and understanding of the pathogenesis of clinical changes will aid the clinician in determining where to sample the nail unit.

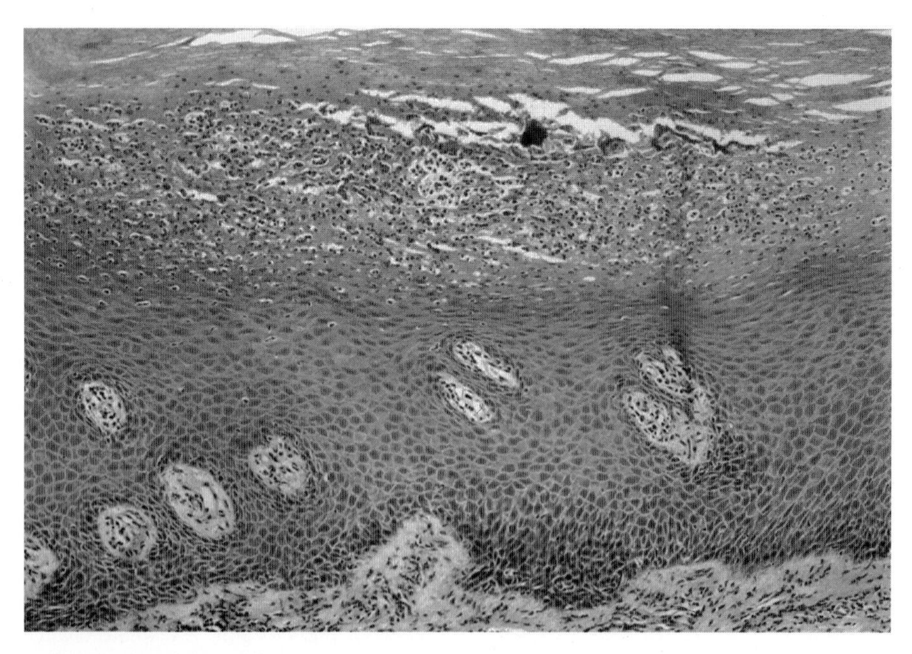

FIG. 19-1. Psoriasis of the nail bed
A Munro microabscess is seen in the lower portion of the nail plate. There is absence of the granular layer, acanthosis of the nail bed epidermis, with spongiosis and exocytosis of mononuclear cells and vascular ectasia of vessels in the underlying papillary dermis.

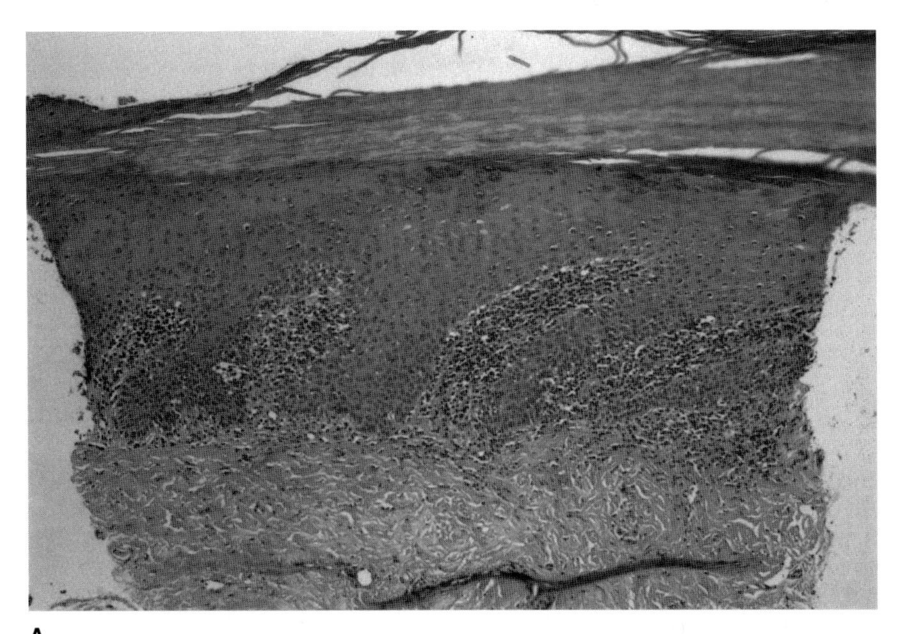

A

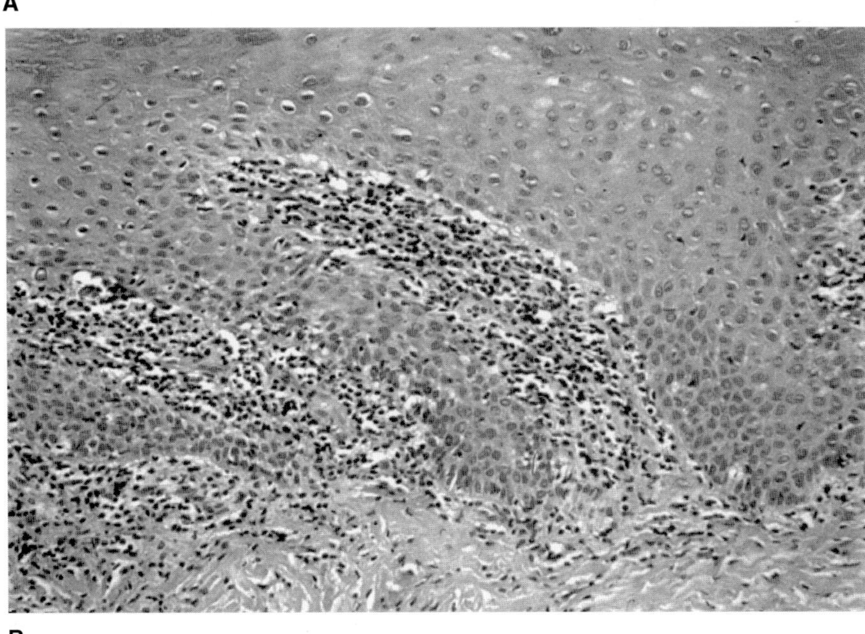

B

FIG. 19-2. Lichen planus of the nail matrix
(**A**) One sees hyperkeratosis, hypergranulosis, acanthosis of the epidermis, and vacuolar degeneration at the dermoepidermal junction with disruption of the rete pattern. (**B**) A bandlike infiltrate of lymphocytes and histiocytes obscures the dermoepidermal junction.

Involvement of the proximal nail matrix leads to longitudinal grooves and ridges (onychorrhexis) of the nail plate. As in lichen planus of the skin, one sees hyperkeratosis, hypergranulosis, vacuolar degeneration, necrotic keratinocytes, Civatte bodies, and a bandlike infiltrate of lymphocytes and histiocytes accompanied by melanophages (Fig. 19-2). If lichen planus of the proximal nail matrix is treated early in its course, onychorrhexis may be reversible. As with other skin appendages, such as hair, if the process progresses, fibrosis and scarring may result, leading to permanent deformity.

If the nail matrix is involved diffusely, onychoschizia (lamellar changes with fragility and brittleness) results. Once again, if treated before scarring occurs, the changes are reversible. When severe, unchecked lichen planus of the matrix occurs in the pterygia form. The matrix is replaced by scar connecting the proximal nail fold to the nail bed. As a result, the two epithelia adhere and grow distally together, constituting a pterygium.

Occasionally, lichen planus of the nail bed alone may occur. Proximal onycholysis, to be differentiated from distal onycholysis in psoriasis, occurs because of involvement of the proximal nail bed. The nail plate is otherwise normal. Papular lesions of lichen planus may occur in various locations of the nail bed and lead to focal atrophy. As a result, the overlying nail plate will be focally dimpled or spooned (koilonychia).

BULLOUS DISEASES

Several vesiculobullous diseases may affect the nail unit. In Darier-White disease, nail changes usually occur in association with other clinical findings. Rarely, involvement may be limited to the nail alone. Nail changes may occur in the proximal nail fold, matrix, nail bed, and hyponychium. The proximal nail fold may show keratotic papules that are histologically similar to those of acrokeratosis verruciformis of Hopf. However, in addition to papillary epidermal hyperplasia, focal areas of suprabasilar acantholysis may be seen.[8]

Involvement of the nail matrix in Darier-White disease is usually located in the distal lunula and manifests clinically as a white longitudinal streak. Histologically, this leukonychia is due to foci of persistent parakeratosis in the lower nail plate related to the usual histology of Darier-White disease of the distal matrix.

The nail bed and hyponychium are commonly involved in Darier-White disease. Involvement may be mild, leading to red and white longitudinal streaks. More severe involvement leads to wedge-shaped, distal, subungual keratosis, accompanied by nail fragility. In time, the nail plate may become markedly thickened. The nail bed epithelium becomes hyperplastic with parakeratosis between the nail bed and nail plate. Suprabasilar clefts are absent in the nail bed.[8] An interesting finding is the presence of atypical keratinocytes in the nail bed epidermis, many of which may be multinucleated.[8]

Nail involvement in pemphigus vulgaris is uncommon but may affect the proximal and lateral nail folds, leading to chronic paronychia and superficial nail plate changes.[9] Biopsy of the involved nail fold reveals suprabasilar acantholysis and positive direct immunofluorescence with IgG and C3 in the intercellular spaces of the epidermis. Involvement of the matrix causes onychomadesis (proximal separation of the nail plate).[10] Pemphigus foliaceus may also affect the nail unit.

Bullous and cicatricial pemphigoid have been reported to involve the nail unit, with clinical effects implicating involvement of both matrix and nail bed, including longitudinal splits and pterygium formation.[11]

Erythema multiforme and toxic epidermolysis may affect the nail matrix, resulting in either sloughing of the nail or, in some cases, scarring, leading to anonychia or pterygium formation.[12] Epidermolysis bullosa in many of its manifestations affects the nail unit. Epidermolysis bullosa simplex may cause onycholysis or onychogryphosis. In epidermolysis bullosa simplex–herpetiformis, nail dystrophy or anonychia may result from subungual blister formation. Junctional epidermolysis bullosa may lead to dystrophy and anonychia in all of its forms. Nail changes have been described for the Cochayne-Touraine, Albopapuloid, and Hallopeau-Siemens varieties of dystrophic epidermolysis bullosa.[13]

CONNECTIVE TISSUE DISEASE

The nail unit is affected by most types of connective tissue disease, primarily in the microvasculature of the proximal nail fold.[14] In vivo capillary microscopy reveals dilated capillary loops with adjacent hemorrhage and avascularity. This pattern is present in 80% to 95% of patients with progressive systemic sclerosis. However, an identical clinical pattern may be seen in patients with dermatomyositis, other connective tissue disease, and idiopathic Raynaud phenomenon. A crescent-shaped biopsy of the proximal nail fold reveals deposits of eosinophilic PAS-positive material in the keratin of the cuticle.[14] These deposits tend to be more extensive in patients with connective tissue disease and in patients with more severe in vivo capillary microscopy abnormalities. More data are needed to determine if a proximal nail fold biopsy to evaluate for the presence and degree of PAS-positive deposits is of value in predicting the development of connective tissue disease in patients with idiopathic Raynaud phenomenon.

INFECTION

Fungal infection of the nails may be the most common nail disorder.[15] There are four main types: distal subungual onychomycosis, proximal subungual onychomycosis, white superficial onychomycosis, and candidal onychomycosis. Distal subungual onychomycosis is the most common form and is usually caused by *Trichophyton rubrum*. The fungus initially invades the hyponychium and lateral nail folds, causing yellowing, onycholysis, and eventual subungual hyperkeratosis. Biopsy of the nail bed shows hyperkeratosis. A PAS stain should be performed on all nail biopsies. This stain reveals fungal organisms that are usually located in the lower stratum corneum near the nail bed epidermis (Fig. 19-3). The nail bed epidermis shows acanthosis, spongiosis, and exocytosis of lymphocytes and histiocytes. In proximal subungual onychomycosis, infection initially involves the area of the proximal nail fold. Proximal white subungual onychomycosis is rare in the general population but common in patients affected with the human immunodeficiency virus (HIV).[16] In these patients, proximal white subungual onychomycosis is caused by *T rubrum*. On the other hand, superficial white onychomycosis is caused by *T mentagrophytes*, located on the superficial nail plate only.[15] In HIV-infected persons, superficial white onychomycosis is usually caused by *T rubrum*.[16] *Candida* species are a common cause of chronic paronychia. *Candida* may involve the nail plate and nail bed in patients with chronic mucocutaneous candidiasis and in HIV-infected patients. *Candida albicans* is the major fungus affecting the nail in pediatric patients with AIDS and may cause hypertrophic nail bed infection.[16]

Bacterial infections caused by *Staphylococcus aureus* and *Pseudomonas aeruginosa* occur mainly in the nail folds and lead to acute paronychia. Bacteria may also be involved along with *Candida* in chronic paronychia. *Pseudomonas* may colonize onycholytic nail plates, leading to green discoloration.[15]

Sarcoptes scabiei may involve the nail unit. Organisms are often present in distal subungual hyperkeratotic debris found in the hyponychium and may be a cause of persistent epidemics of scabies. Norwegian scabies may cause severe involvement of the nail folds.[17]

Herpes simplex type I or II may cause herpetic whitlow or herpetic paronychia involving the nail folds.

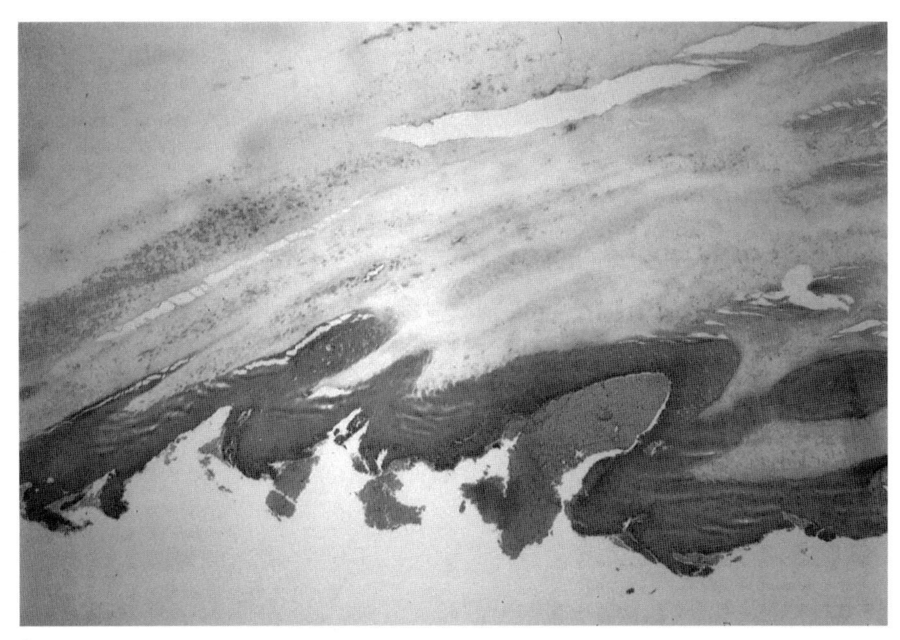

A

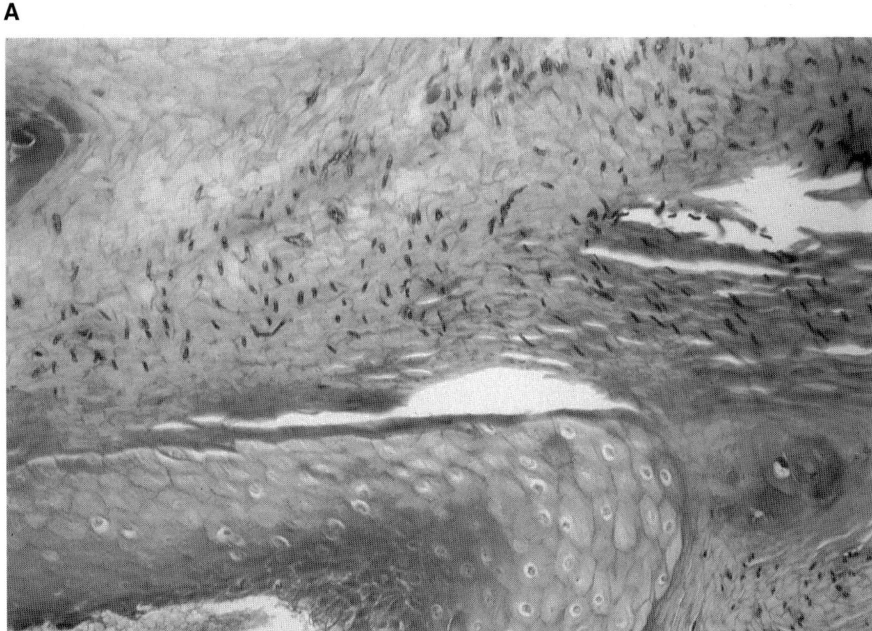

B

FIG. 19-3. Onychomycosis
(**A**) The features seen are hyperkeratosis with alternating columns of parakeratosis. There is papillomatous acanthosis of the epidermis, which at high power shows spongiosis with exocytosis of mononuclear cells. (**B**) Staining with PAS and diastase shows septate hyphal elements located in the lower stratum corneum and concentrated in areas of parakeratosis (H&E, original magnification ×2; PAS with diastase, original magnification ×20).

REFERENCES

1. Scher RK. Surgical gems: Biopsy of the matrix of nail. J Dermatol Surg Oncol 1980;6:19.
2. Scher RK. Punch biopsies of the nails: A simple, valuable procedure. J Dermatol Surg Oncol 1978;4:528.
3. Kouskoukis CE, Scher RK, Ackerman AB. What histologic finding distinguishes onychomycosis and psoriasis? Am J Dermatopathol 1983;5:501.
4. Kouskoukis CE, Scher RK, Ackerman AB. The "oil drop" sign of psoriatic nails: A clinical finding specific for psoriasis. Am J Dermatopathol 1983;5:259.
5. Robbins TO, Kouskoukis CE, Ackerman AB. Onycholysis in psoriatic nails. Am J Dermatopathol 1983;5:39.
6. Kouskoukis CE, Scher RK, Ackerman AB. The problem of features of

lichen simplex chronicus complicating the histology of diseases of the nail. Am J Dermatopathol 1984;6:45.
7. Scher RK, Ackerman AB. Lichen planus. Am J Dermatopathol 1983; 5:375.
8. Zaias N, Ackerman AB. The nail in Darier-White disease. Arch Dermatol 1973;107:193.
9. Dhawan SS, Zaias N, Pena J. The nail fold in pemphigus vulgaris (letter). Arch Dermatol 1990;126:1374.
10. Parameswara VR, Chinnappaiah Naik RP. Onychomedesis associated with pemphigus vulgaris. Arch Dermatol 1981;117:759.
11. Burge SM, Powell SM, Ryan TJ. Cicatricial pemphigoid with nail dystrophy. Clin Exp Dermatol 1985;10:472.
12. Wancher B, Thornmann J. Permanent anonychia after Stevens-Johnson syndrome. Arch Dermatol 1977;113:970.
13. Pearson RW. Clinical pathologic types of epidermolysis bullosa in non-dermatological complications. Arch Dermatol 1988;124:718.
14. Scher RK, Tom DWK, Lally EV, Bogaars HA. The clinical significance of periodic acid-Schiff-positive deposits in cuticle-proximal nail fold biopsy specimens. Arch Dermatol 1985;121:1406.
15. Cowen PR, Scher RK. Geriatric nail disorders: Diagnosis and treatment. J Am Acad Dermatol 1992;26:521.
16. Daniel CR, Norton LA, Scher RK. The spectrum of nail disease in patients with human immunodeficiency virus infection. J Am Acad Dermatol 1992;27:93.
17. Scher RK. Subungual scabies. Am J Dermatopathol 1983;5:187.

Lever's Histopathology of the Skin, eighth edition,
edited by David Elder et al. Lippincott–
Raven Publishers, Philadelphia © 1997.

CHAPTER 20

Inflammatory Diseases of the Subcutaneous Fat

N. Scott McNutt, Abelardo Moreno, and Félix Contreras

A histopathologic classification of *panniculitis* is based on the microscopic and macroscopic changes in the subcutaneous fat. The diseases presented in this chapter are divided into groups based on their patterns of involvement of the anatomic structures in the subcutis (Table 20-1). However, for definite diagnoses, it is important to consider whether or not there are associated changes, for example in the overlying dermis and epidermis, as well as what types of inflammatory cells are involved. The subcutaneous fat can be divided into the following anatomic regions: the septa between fat lobules, the fat lobules themselves, the blood vessels, and the nerves. When the septa are involved by inflammation the histologic changes include septal widening due to edema, hemorrhage, fibrosis, or inflammatory infiltration by neutrophils, eosinophils, and macrophages, with or without granuloma formation. Involvement of the fat lobules includes necrosis, cellular infiltration, and fibrosis. Necrosis of fat is common and the different types of necrosis have been classified by etiology as ischemic, traumatic, enzymatic, metabolic, and infectious. The cellular infiltrate associated with necrosis can be composed predominantly of polymorphonuclear leukocytes (neutrophils and eosinophils), lymphocytes (occasionally with germinal centers), and macrophages (with or without granulomas). Fibrosis of the fat lobules is a late event, which is the end result of multiple causes of lobular panniculitis ranging from that due to simple trauma to that due to complex connective-tissue diseases. By analysis of the anatomic patterns of involvement of these regions, it is possible to make a specific diagnosis in a patient with panniculitis even when the interactions between inflammatory cells and target cells in panniculitis show considerable overlap in their basic mechanisms at the cellular and molecular levels.

Although the classification of panniculitis stresses the differences between the lobules of fat and the interlobular septa, there is an intimate relationship between the two. The septa contain the major blood vessels and nerves that supply the delicate plexus of vessels within the fat lobules and also contain the major vessels that pass on to the overlying dermis. When blood vessels are the target of inflammation, the different sizes of the involved blood vessels are important in the classification of panniculitis. The relative sizes of the blood vessels and their wall structures can cause certain diseases to be localized in the fat. Inflammation of the walls of large vessels often involves only the fat lobules immediately adjacent to the vessel. The medium-sized vessels are in the septa and inflammation of their walls leads to septal inflammation and secondary ischemic destruction of the fat lobules. Inflammation of small vessels can affect the septa, lobules, or both. The relatively sluggish blood flow through the small vessels in the fat facilitates the exudation of substances and the emigration of inflammatory cells into the panniculus. For example, immune complexes or medications can be deposited in the walls of these vessels. Moreover, the subcutaneous fat cells, or adipocytes, form a closely regulated metabolic reserve, on which certain chemical compounds interact preferentially; for example, pancreatic lipases that have been released into the circulating blood or fat-soluble chemicals and medications can localize in the fat and cause metabolic or inflammatory changes.

In the upper portion of the panniculus are the secretory coils of eccrine and apocrine glands and the lower portion of hair follicles. Consequently, diseases of the skin appendages can involve the panniculus secondarily. The subcutis also has a lower border on the fascia and inflammatory diseases that affect the fascia can penetrate upward into the septa and lobules.

Unfortunately, a significant problem is that the clinical appearance of the lesions of panniculitis is not very specific since most patients have deep erythematous nodules. A consideration of the clinical distribution, number of lesions, and whether or not they are ulcerated help in the formulation of a clinical differential diagnosis. Some early clinical studies led to the description of clinical "entities," such as Weber-Christian disease or panniculitis of Rothmann and Makai, which unfortunately exhibit nonspecific histopathologic changes that occur in a variety of actual diseases that cause panniculitis.

Another major problem in the classification of panniculitis is often that the size of the biopsy is inadequate. The individual lobules of fat may be more than 1 mm in diameter and several

N. S. McNutt: Department of Dermatopathology, New York Hospital—Cornell University Medical Center, New York, NY

A. Moreno: Departarmento de Anatomia Patoligica, Hospital de Bellvitge, Barcelona, Spain

F. Contreras: Department of Pathology, Hospital "La Paz," Madrid, Spain

TABLE 20-1. *Classification of panniculitis*

I. With prominent vasculitis (septal or lobular)	II. Without prominent vasculitis	III. Mixed patterns
A. Neutrophilic 1. Leukocytoclastic immune-complex vasculitis 2. Subcutaneous polyarteritis nodosa 3. Thrombophlebitis 4. Type 2 leprosy reaction (erythema nodosum leprosum) B. Lymphocytic 1. Nodular vasculitis 2. Perniosis 3. Angiocentric lymphomas C. Granulomatous 1. Nodular vasculitis/erythema induratum 2. Type 2 leprosy reaction 3. Wegener's granulomatosis 4. Churg-Strauss allergic granulomatosis	A. Septal inflammation 1. Lymphocytic and mixed a. Erythema nodosum and variants 2. Granulomatous a. Palisaded granulomatous diseases b. Sarcoidosis c. Subcutaneous infection; tuberculosis, syphilis 3. Sclerotic a. Scleroderma b. Eosinophilic fasciitis c. Ischemic liposclerosis d. Toxins B. Lobular inflammation 1. Neutrophilic a. Infection b. Ruptured folliculitis and cysts c. Pancreatic fat necrosis 2. Lymphocytic a. Lupus panniculitis b. Post-steroid panniculitis c. Lymphoma/leukemia 3. Macrophagic a. Rosai-Dorfman disease b. Histiocytic cytophagic panniculitis 4. Granulomatous a. Erythema induratum/nodular vasculitis b. Palisaded granulomatous diseases c. Sarcoidosis, Crohn's disease 5. Mixed inflammation, with many foam cells a. α_1-antitrypsin deficiency b. Weber-Christian disease c. Traumatic fat necrosis 6. Eosinophilic a. Eosinophilic panniculitis b. Arthropod bites, parasites 7. Enzymatic fat necrosis a. Pancreatic enzyme panniculitis 8. Crystal deposits a. Sclerema neonatorum b. Subcutaneous fat necrosis of the newborn c. Gout d. Oxalosis 9. Embryonic fat pattern a. Lipoatrophy b. Lipodystrophy	In the natural progression of lesions of vasculopathic panniculitis, as well as in septal or lobular panniculitis, a complex mixture of patterns can result depending on the stage of the evolution of the disease. For example, factitial panniculitis can exhibit a mixed pattern with microscopic features (hematoma, foreign bodies, dermal lesions, fibrosis) that fit into more than one category.

lobules and septa are needed to discern accurately a pattern of involvement. Consequently, an adequate biopsy should be an elliptical, excisional, or incisional one that gives at least a specimen of fat 6 mm in greatest dimension, and should include deep subcutis as well as the overlying skin. Only a few diagnoses can be made on a specimen of aspirated fat or a needle or punch biopsy of a nodule in the subcutis; the use of these biopsy modalities is to be discouraged for purposes of histologic classification of panniculitis.

A third problem is that most of the lesions have a time course in which there occurs an early form of inflammation with varying degrees of vascular changes, followed by a stage of phagocytosis of fat and a more or less pronounced granulomatous reaction, and by a final stage of fibrosis. Such a time course is evident in the overall lesion and may also be different in various areas of the lesion. With small biopsies or with a nonspecific pattern of inflammation, a simple categorical diagnosis of "panniculitis" may be necessary until further studies and clinical follow-up information allows the placement of the disease into a more exact category.[1–3]

Table 20-1 presents a summary of the classification of panniculitis. Not all of the disease entities listed are discussed in this chapter; some can be found elsewhere in greater detail: *cutaneous polyarteritis nodosa* (Chap. 8), *sarcoidosis*, *granuloma annulare*, *rheumatoid nodule* (Chap. 14), and *gummatous tertiary syphilis* (Chap. 22).

ERYTHEMA NODOSUM

Clinical Presentation. An acute form and a chronic form of erythema nodosum exist, which differ in their clinical manifestations but do not have recognized differences in their histologic characteristics.

In the *acute form* of erythema nodosum, there is a sudden appearance of tender, bright red or dusky red-purple nodules that only slightly elevate the level of the skin surface (Color Fig. 20-1). The nodules vary from 1 to 5 cm in diameter and have a strong predilection for the anterior surfaces of the lower legs, although they also may occur elsewhere, especially on the calves, thighs, and, in severe cases, on the forearms, hands, and even the face. They occur mostly on the dependent regions of the body. The lesions do not ulcerate and generally involute within a few weeks. As a result of the intermittent appearance of new lesions, the disease may persist for several months. The acute disease often is accompanied by fever, malaise, leukocytosis, and arthropathy.[4] The lesions are tender and warm. Lesions near a joint can mimic an arthritis. Focal hemorrhages are common and can cause the lesions to resemble bruises (*erythema contusiforme*). Bilateral hilar adenopathy can be present in patients with acute erythema nodosum without sarcoidosis since a number of pulmonary infections can produce both hilar adenopathy and erythema nodosum.[4] Erythema nodosum occurs in 10% to 20% of patients with sarcoidosis and is thought to portend a good prognosis.[4]

The *chronic form* of erythema nodosum is also known as *erythema nodosum migrans*[5] or subacute nodular migratory panniculitis of Vilanova and Piñol.[6] There are one or several red, subcutaneous nodules that are found, usually unilaterally, on the lower leg. Vilanova observed that almost all the patients were women (16 to 65 years of age) with a solitary lesion and a recent history of sore throat and arthralgia. Tenderness is slight or absent. The nodules enlarge by peripheral extension into plaques, often with central clearing. The duration may be from a few months to a few years.

Histopathology. The histologic changes are present mainly in the subcutaneous tissue. The overlying dermis often has only a minimal to moderate perivascular lymphocytic infiltrate.

In the *early lesions* of *acute erythema nodosum* there is edema of the septa with a lymphohistiocytic infiltrate, having a slight admixture of neutrophils and eosinophils (Fig. 20-1).[7] Focal fibrin deposition and extravasation of erythrocytes occur frequently.[1] Often the inflammation is most intense at the periphery of the edematous septa and extends into the periphery of the fat lobules between individual fat cells in a lace-like fashion. Necrosis of the fat is not prominent. Rarely, clusters of neutrophils are present or the infiltrate is predominantly neutrophilic (Fig. 20-2).[8] Clusters of macrophages around small blood vessels, or a slit-like space, occur in early lesions and are known as Miescher's radial nodules (Fig. 20-3).[9,10] The degree of vascular involvement is variable.[1,11] There is usually edema of the walls of veins with separation of the muscular layers. Infiltration by lymphocytes is common, but neutrophils and eosinophils can also be present. Necrosis of the vessel walls is very rare but has been observed in a few patients with lesions clinically indistinguishable from erythema nodosum.[12] Focally, vasculitis may be found in a few patients with recurrent erythema nodosum that is secondary to medications or estrogenic oral contraceptives.

Later lesions of acute erythema nodosum show widening of the septa, often with fibrosis and with inflammation at the edges of the septa and involving the periphery of the fat lobules (Figs. 20-4 and 20-5). Neutrophils usually are absent and the vascular changes are less prominent than in early lesions. There are more

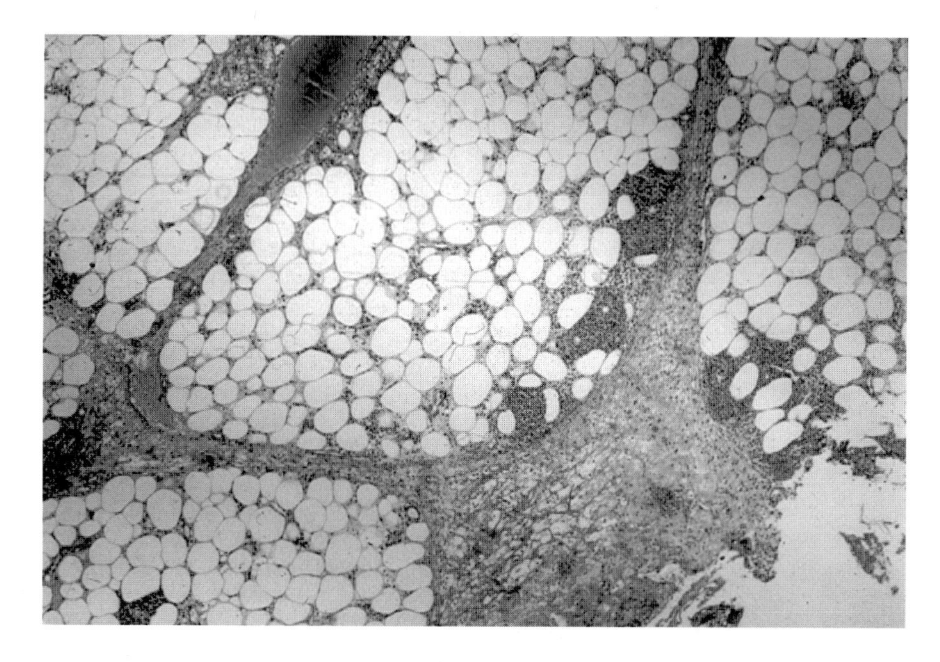

FIG. 20-1. Erythema nodosum, acute The septa are edematous and a mixed inflammatory infiltrate is in the septa with extension into the periphery of the fat lobules.

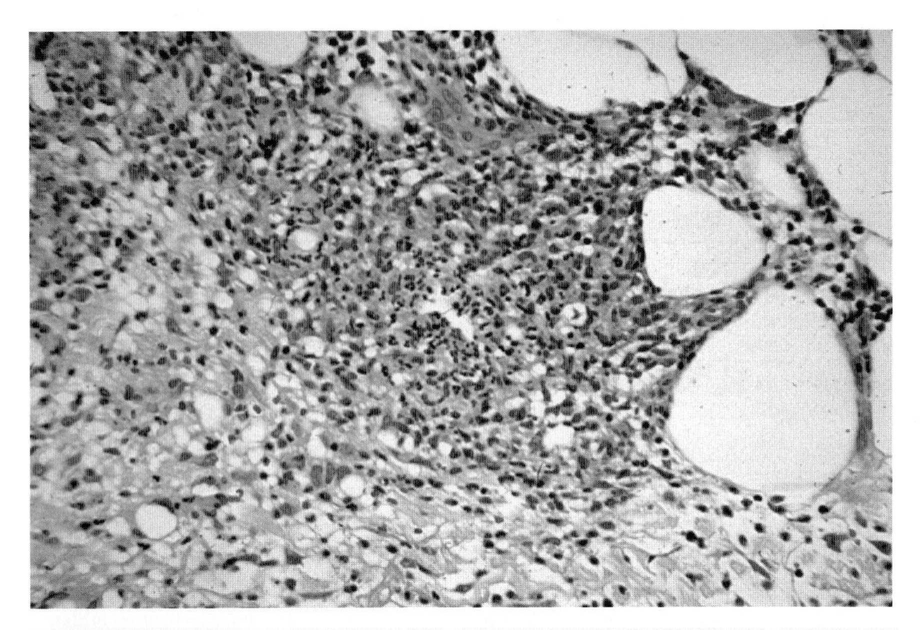

FIG. 20-2. Erythema nodosum, acute
In early lesions, neutrophils can be abundant and tend to cluster at the interface between septa and lobules.

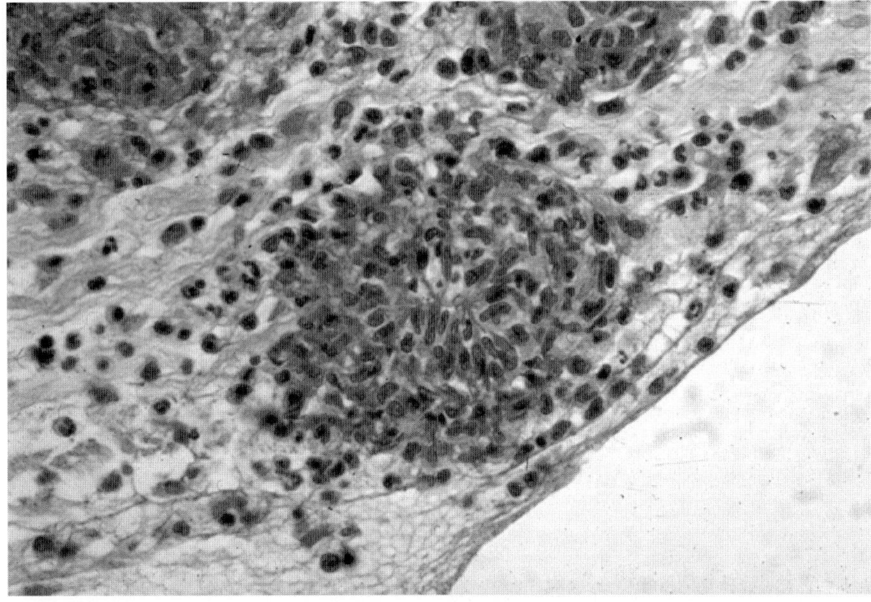

FIG. 20-3. Erythema nodosum, acute
Clusters of macrophages in radial arrays form Miescher's nodules.

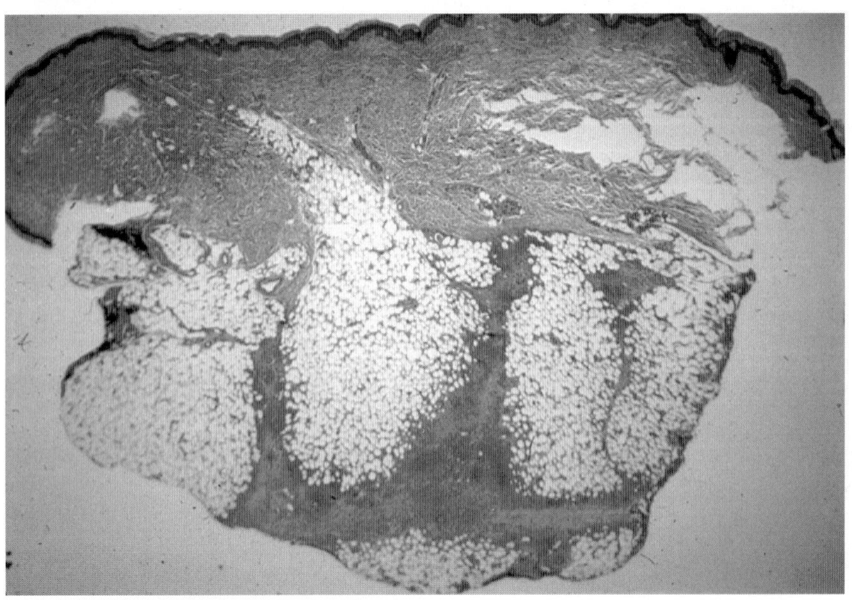

FIG. 20-4. Erythema nodosum
At low magnification, portions of two septa and three fat lobules can be seen. The inflammation has produced widening of the septa and inflammation extending into the periphery of the fat lobules.

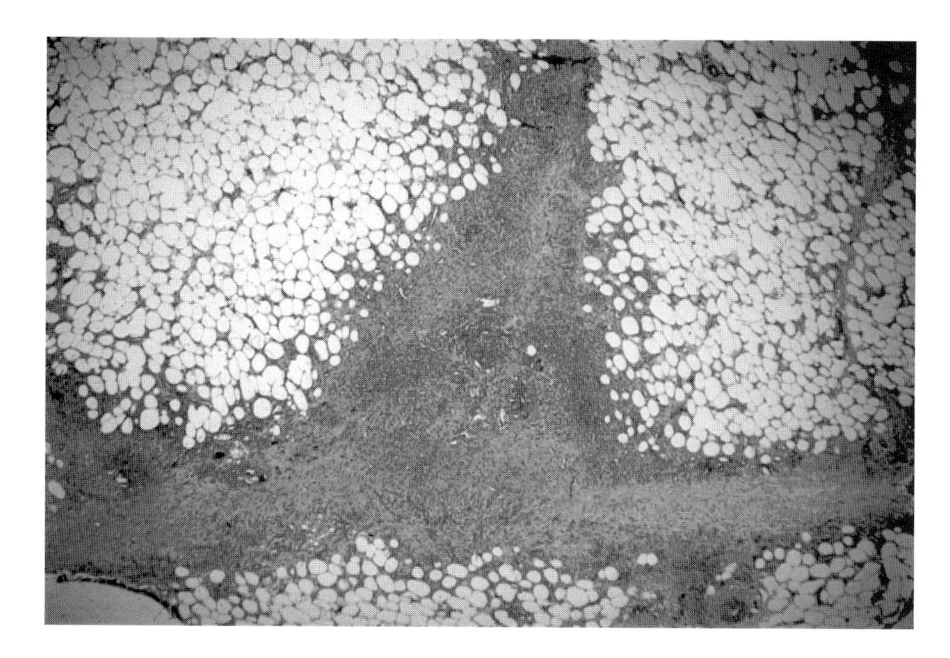

FIG. 20-5. Erythema nodosum There is inflammation not only in the septa but also concentrated at the margins of septa and fat lobules.

macrophages in the infiltrate. Macrophages at the edges of the fat lobules phagocytize lipid from damaged adipocytes and the small droplets of lipid in their cytoplasm give them a "foam-cell" appearance. Granulomas formed by macrophages, without lipid deposition, are more frequent when late lesions are compared to the early ones (Fig. 20-6). The granulomas are often loosely formed with macrophages predominating in a focus with multinucleated giant cells. Occasionally, well-formed, discrete sarcoidal granulomas occur in small numbers in the septa. The multinucleated giant cells usually have an irregular distribution of nuclei in the cytoplasm. The oldest lesions have septal widening and fibrosis with a decrease in all of the inflammatory cells, except for a few persisting at the periphery of the fat lobules.

In *chronic erythema nodosum*, the histologic findings are generally the same as those of the late stages of acute erythema nodosum. However, granuloma and lipogranuloma formation often is more pronounced. There is vascular proliferation and thickening of the endothelium with extravasation of erythrocytes.[13] In some instances numerous well-formed granulomas can be found and consist of epithelioid macrophages and giant cells without caseous necrosis.[1] Although significant degrees of vasculitis have been observed by some authors,[6,14] others have found vascular changes to be slight or absent.[15,16] The presence of thickened fibrotic septa with marked capillary proliferation and massive granulomatous reactions have lead several authors to consider erythema nodosum migrans as an entity separate from the late lesions of acute erythema nodosum.[17]

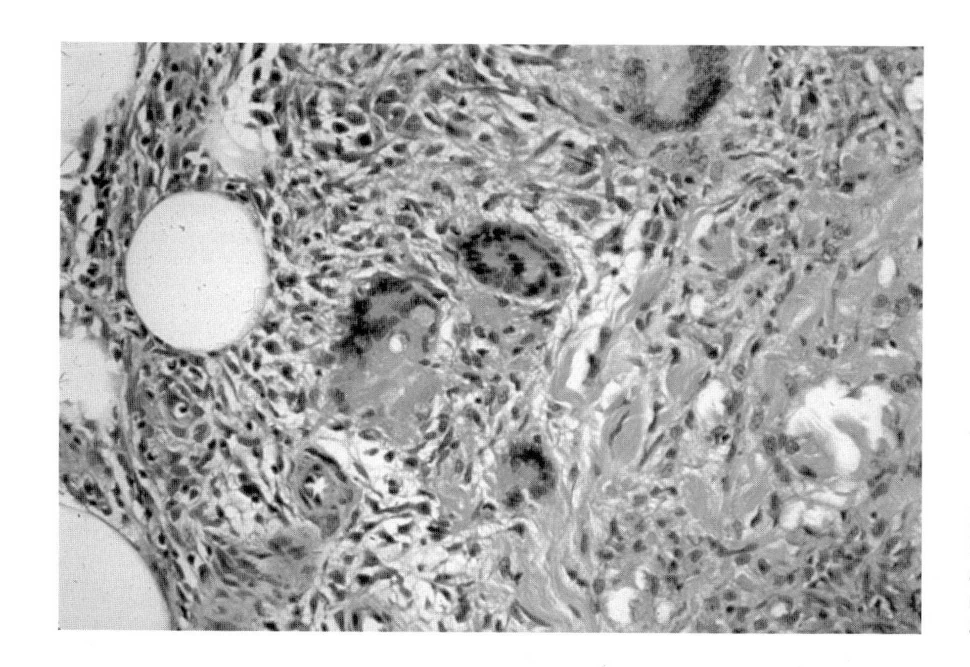

FIG. 20-6. Erythema nodosum Fibrosis, lymphocytic infiltration, and accumulations of macrophages and multinucleated cells in the septa characterize the mid-phase lesions.

Pathogenesis. Although the cause of erythema nodosum cannot always be determined in an individual patient, streptococcal infection is the most common among the known causes, as evidenced by elevation of antistreptolysin O titers. The diseases that can be associated with erythema nodosum are numerous and have been reviewed.[18] They may be divided into: infections with bacteria, fungi, or protozoa; viral diseases; malignancies; and miscellaneous conditions. The most frequent bacterial infections are streptococcal infection, tuberculosis, *Yersinia enterocolitica* infection,[19] brucellosis, leptospirosis, tularemia, and clamydial infection. The most frequently associated fungal infections are coccidioidomycosis, histoplasmosis,[20] dermatophytosis, and blastomycosis. Protozoal infections such as toxoplasmosis can cause erythema nodosum. Among the associated viral and rickettsial infections are herpes simplex, infectious mononucleosis, lymphogranuloma venereum, ornithosis, and psittacosis. Erythema nodosum occurs with some cases of leukemia and Hodgkin's disease as well as with other cancers, particularly after irradiation or other treatment. Among the miscellaneous associations several diseases can cause considerable difficulty in diagnosis, particularly sarcoidosis, which can have erythema nodosum as part of a symptom complex in acute sarcoidosis along with slight hilar adenopathy, fever, arthralgias, and occasionally acute iritis. The sarcoidal granulomas that can occur in erythema nodosum are less frequent and are associated with edema, in contrast to the abundant granulomas that occur in subcutaneous sarcoidosis. Likewise, Crohn's disease can be associated with erythema nodosum[4] and the two diseases can be difficult to distinguish from each other histologically in the skin involvement unless there is ulceration.[21] Other conditions are Behçet's disease[22] and ulcerative colitis. Erythema nodosum and Sweet's syndrome have been reported in the same patient.[23] Among the many medications that can cause erythema nodosum, estrogens and oral contraceptives[24] and sulfonamides are common ones, and rare ones include: aminopyrine, antimony compounds, arsphenamine, bromides, iodides, phenacetin, salicylates, immunizations, and vaccinations. Such a great diversity in inciting agents and circumstances suggests that several mechanisms may be capable of triggering the clinical and histopathologic changes that are classified as erythema nodosum.

Direct immunofluorescence studies have shown deposits of immunoglobulins only very rarely in the blood vessel walls in erythema nodosum.[2] Small amounts of complement in the vessel walls and abundant fibrin around the vessels are frequent but nonspecific findings. On electron microscopic examination, nonspecific vascular changes consisting of damage to endothelial cells and lymphocytic infiltration have been described.[25]

The occurrence of erythema nodosum in response to medications and to tuberculin skin testing in patients with a positive reaction suggests that a type IV delayed hypersensitivity reaction may play an important role, given the paucity of reports of immunoglobulin deposition and failure to demonstrate circulating immune complexes.[26] However, in some patients a type III immune-complex reaction could be responsible. Circulating immune complexes and rheumatoid factors have been detected in some patients with sarcoidosis and erythema nodosum.[27] The predilection for the anterior shins and for dependent parts of the body suggests that trauma or sluggish blood flow play a role in the localization of the lesions.

Differential Diagnosis. Erythema nodosum needs to be distinguished from *erythema induratum* and *nodular vasculitis.* Vasculitis and zones of fat necrosis are absent in erythema nodosum and frequent in erythema induratum. In patients suspected to have erythema nodosum but with necrotizing vasculitis, the possibility of cutaneous polyarteritis nodosa must be considered. In the latter disease, medium-sized arteries rather than veins or small-caliber blood vessels are affected, and there is necrosis of the walls of the affected arteries. Instead, nodular vasculitis has mainly lymphocytic infiltration with fibrous thickening and obliteration of vascular lumens. *Superficial migratory thrombophlebitis,* unlike erythema nodosum, has a large vein containing thrombus in the center of the lesion. Syphilitic gummas are ulcerative irregular lesions with depressed scars. *Subcutaneous tuberculosis* can mimic erythema nodosum in lesions that are extending from underlying organs or bone. Stains for acid-fast organisms and cultures are needed. Subcutaneous tuberculosis can spare the upper portion of the panniculus whereas erythema nodosum does not. Erythema nodosum does not have granulomas or sclerosis in the overlying dermis, and in this way can be distinguished from most cases of sarcoidosis, scleroderma, necrobiosis lipoidica diabeticorum, ruptured follicular cysts, and factitial traumatic panniculitis.

EOSINOPHILIC PANNICULITIS

Clinical Features. The diagnosis of eosinophilic panniculitis is based on the histological appearance of numerous eosinophils in the fat, which can be found as a reaction pattern in the following clinical diseases: erythema nodosum, vasculitis, arthropod bites, parasitic infection, drug injections, Well's syndrome, hypereosinophilic syndrome, and eosinophilic leukemia.[28–32]

Histopathology. Usually there is a mixed inflammatory infiltrate of lymphocytes, macrophages, and numerous eosinophils involving both septa and lobules of the subcutis (Fig. 20-7). A pure infiltrate of normal eosinophils indicates hypereosinophilic syndrome, in contrast to eosinophilic leukemia, in which the eosinophils are cytologically atypical. The eosinophils aggregate on collagen and degranulate to form flame figures in Well's syndrome. The histologic sections should be searched for parasites, but they may be in the gastrointestinal tract or other sites, in which case the panniculitis is a reaction to circulating antigens.

Differential Diagnosis. The differential diagnosis includes reactions to foreign bodies (polarize the sections), reactions to parasites, deep arthropod bite reactions, or drug injections. Peripheral blood studies will rule out eosinophilic leukemia, which also has eosinophilic precursor cells in the infiltrate in the fat. Macrophages can ingest eosinophil granules from degranulated eosinophils in a variety of hypersensitivity reactions and should be distinguished from true eosinophilic myelocytes and metamyelocytes. A hypereosinophilic syndrome has been reported in several patients with lymphoid abnormalities that are clonal T-cell proliferations.[33,34]

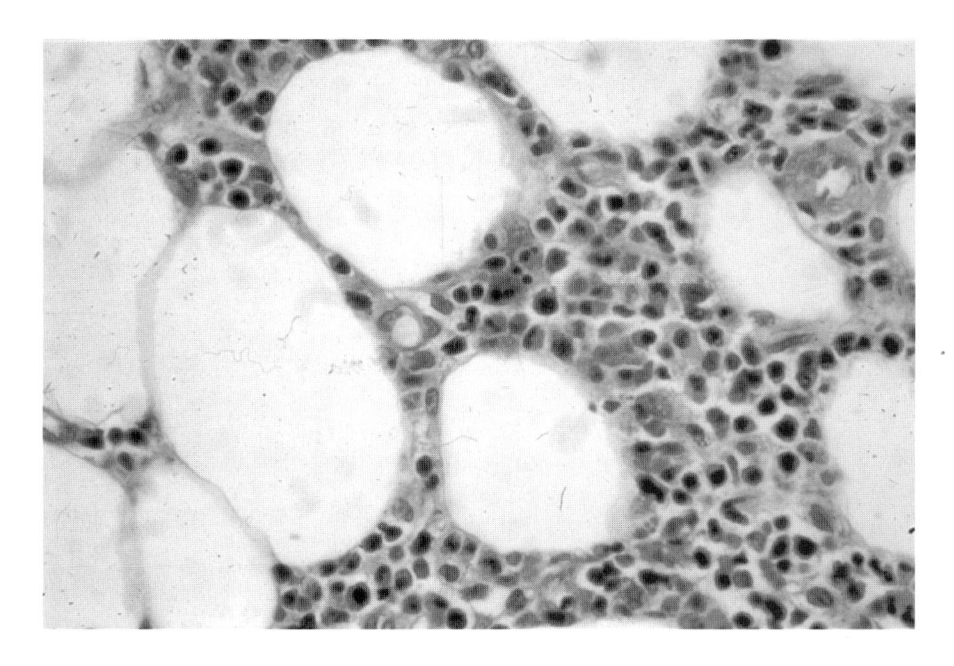

FIG. 20-7. Eosinophilic panniculitis
Eosinophils are very abundant in the mixed inflammatory infiltrate that affects both septa and lobules.

PANNICULITIS ASSOCIATED WITH SEVERE α_1-ANTITRYPSIN DEFICIENCY

Clinical Features. Patients born with a severe deficiency of α_1-antitrypsin (AAT) have exaggerated damage due to inflammation in the skin, for example after trauma to the subcutis. AAT deficiency is estimated to be present in one out of every 3500 live births in the white population.[35] The enzyme is the major component of the α-1 peak on serum electrophoresis and is an inhibitor of the serine proteases trypsin, chymotrypsin, plasmin, thrombin, and neutrophil-produced elastase. The antitrypsin proenzyme is produced in the liver but is not secreted in most of the affected individuals. Liver disease is often the presenting problem, including hepatomegaly, neonatal cholestatic jaundice, and cirrhosis in children.[36,37] Large PAS-positive, diastase-resistant globules of proenzyme can be seen in hepatocytes, especially near the fibrous septa. Inflammation in the lung leads to unopposed release of neutrophil elastase that produces panacinar emphysema, involving destruction from respiratory bronchioles to alveolar ducts and alveoli. The pulmonary disease usually becomes evident in young to middle-aged adults. Skin lesions present after trauma as recurrent nodules that can drain a yellow fluid derived from the enzymatic breakdown of the fibrous tissue and fat (Fig. 20-8).[38–40]

Histopathology. Biopsies of well-developed lesions show a mixed pattern of septal and lobular inflammation characterized by many neutrophils and destruction of the fat and the fibrous septa (Fig. 20-9). Sterile abscesses surround and isolate fat lobules (Fig. 20-10).[41] Late lesions have a macrophage and lymphocytic infiltrate with many foam cells and fibrosis.[40,42] The macrophages can exhibit cytophagic activity and particularly can ingest neutrophil fragments and extravasated erythrocytes.

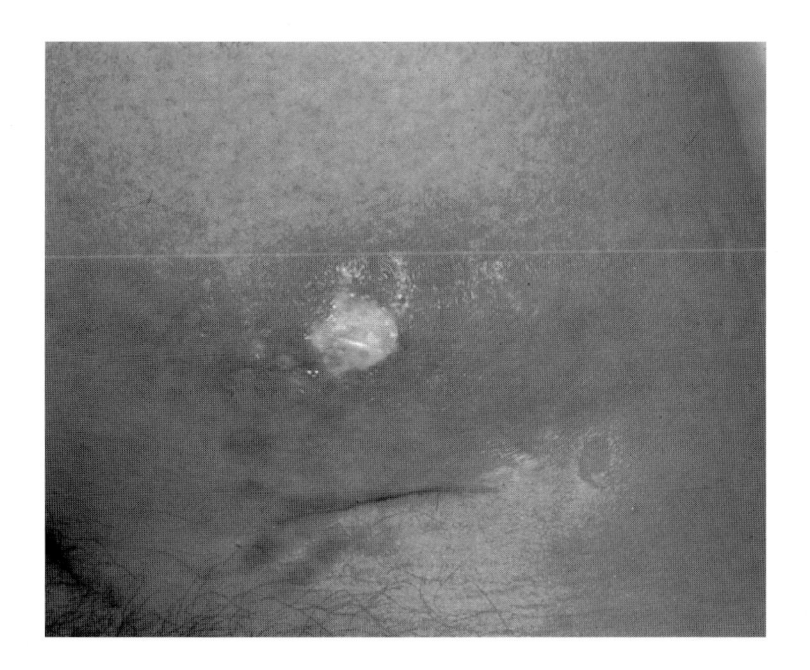

FIG. 20-8. α_1-Antitrypsin deficiency panniculitis
The gross lesions vary from subtle erythematous deep nodules to ulcerated lesions, often at sites of trauma. This advanced lesion is ulcerated and has a discharge of necrotic fat and fluid. (Courtesy of Dr. J. T. Headington.)

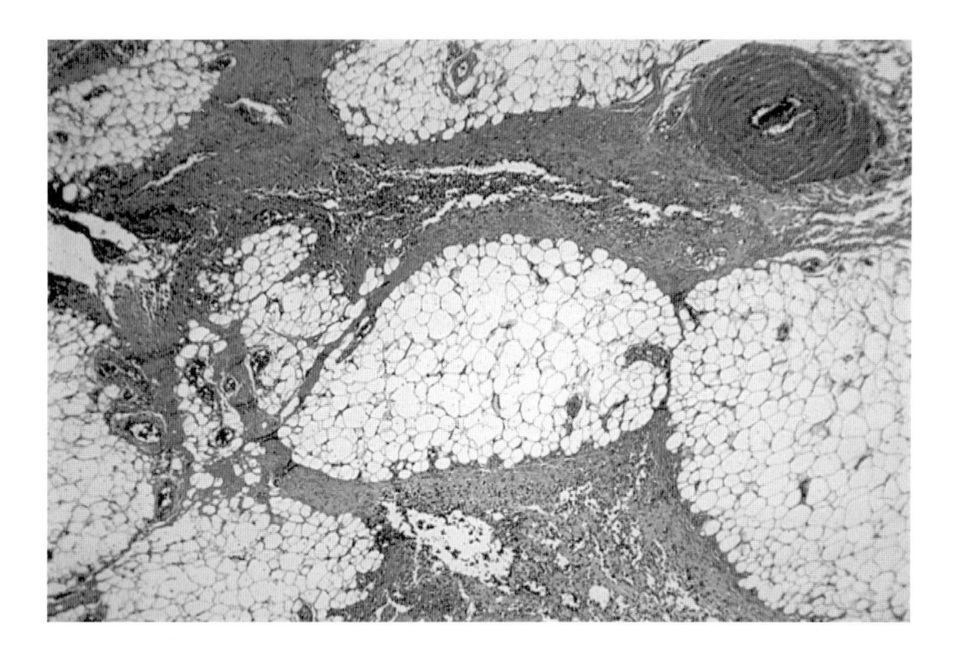

FIG. 20-9. α_1-Antitrypsin deficiency panniculitis
There are neutrophilic abscesses in the septa surrounding the fat lobules. Vasculitis is absent.

Biopsies of early lesions have not been studied in a series of cases, but in some patients, the early manifestations are neutrophilic infiltrates between collagen bundles in the dermis, with scattered solitary neutrophils and small collections of neutrophils in the septa and lobules of the subcutaneous fat.[43] Depending on the size of the lesion, the subcutaneous involvement can be patchy with necrotic foci contrasting with normal fat lobules in the vicinity.[40,42]

Differential Diagnosis. The histopathologic changes are not specific for AAT deficiency but rather are shared by a number of diseases that can be responsible for *necrotizing panniculitis*. A biopsy of a subcutaneous nodule occasionally shows a nonspecific pattern of necrotizing acute inflammation characterized by fat necrosis and a massive neutrophilic infiltrate, often accompanied by karyorrhexis, fibrin deposition, focal vasculitis, and histiocytic reparative reaction. These changes can represent a very acute form of ischemic necrosis (liquefaction necrosis) in cases of nodular vasculitis, but also can be associated with AAT deficiency, pyoderma gangrenosum, inflammatory reaction near ulcers from a variety of causes, as well as can represent changes due to infection by pyogenic bacteria including mycobacteria.[44] If a meticulous study, including cultures and enzymatic studies, fails to reveal a satisfactory final diagnosis, then the term "necrotizing panniculitis" can be a suitable histologic diagnosis until other methods or information become available.

The clinical features of AAT deficiency overlap with those of Weber-Christian disease to the extent that a determination of serum levels of the enzyme should be performed on all cases clinically suspected of having Weber-Christian disease or any patient with ulcerating and necrotizing panniculitis. Weber-Christian disease is more restricted to the fat lobules than AAT

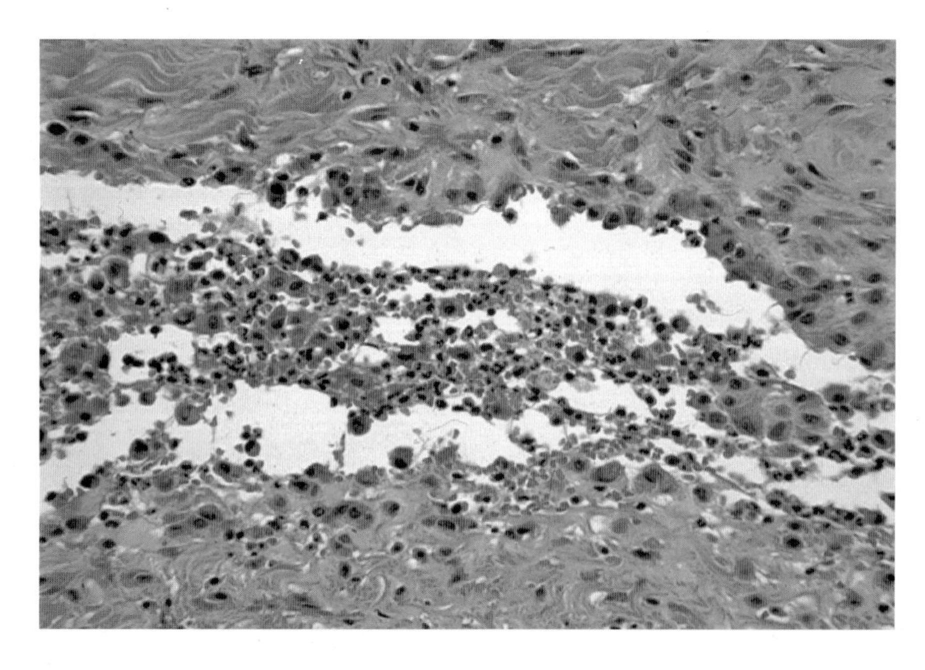

FIG. 20-10. α_1-Antitrypsin deficiency panniculitis
Neutrophils, macrophages, and extravasated erythrocytes are in the sterile abscesses in the septa.

deficiency panniculitis, which involves septa, lobules, and overlying dermis.[43] Histiocytic cytophagic panniculitis (often a form of subcutaneous T-cell lymphoma with reactive histiocytosis) is in the differential diagnosis due to the fact that cytophagic activity also occurs in AAT deficiency. The prominence of neutrophils in AAT deficiency is in contrast to the lymphocytes in histiocytic cytophagic panniculitis. In the early lesions, infection needs to be ruled out since erysipelas can have similar histology. Serum electrophoresis is important in detecting affected and carrier individuals with AAT deficiency.

SUPERFICIAL MIGRATORY THROMBOPHLEBITIS

Clinical Presentation. Multiple, tender, erythematous nodules are found usually on the lower legs but occasionally on the arms or trunk.[45,46] After several days a cord-like induration a few centimeters long can be felt.[47] As the old lesions resolve, usually within a few weeks, new nodules may erupt. Recurrent migratory thrombophlebitis can occur as a manifestation of Behçet's disease; it is also part of Trousseau's syndrome, in which there is an associated visceral carcinoma.

Histopathology. The lesion is centered around a large vein in the subcutis, usually in a septal location and occasionally in the deep vascular plexus at the junction of deep dermis and subcutis (Fig. 20-11). The affected vein has a thick wall with the smooth muscle distributed in fascicles in the wall. The lumen often is completely occluded by thrombus. An inflammatory infiltrate extends between the muscle bundles and only a short distance into the tissue surrounding the vein.[48] In early lesions, the infiltrate is composed of many neutrophils, but later it consists mainly of lymphocytes, macrophages, and a few giant cells.[45,46] If recanalization of the lumen of the vein takes place, granulomas with giant cells can be found within the wall and the lumen of the affected vessel. These granulomas participate in the resorption of the thrombus.[47]

Differential Diagnosis. Owing to the elevated hydrostatic pressure in the veins of the lower legs in ambulatory patients, the walls of the veins have an increased amount of elastic fibers and smooth muscle in their walls. They can be distinguished from arteries when there is minimal inflammation and when elastic tissue stains show an absence of an internal elastic lamina. Thrombus usually occludes the lumen of veins in superficial migratory thrombophlebitis. Polyarteritis nodosa affects arteries and is recognized if the affected vessels can be identified as arteries based on lumen diameter, wall thickness, internal elastic lamina, and location.

ERYTHEMA INDURATUM (NODULAR VASCULITIS)

Clinical Presentation. The lesions of erythema induratum, also known as "nodular vasculitis," consist of painless but somewhat tender, deep-seated, circumscribed, nodular, subcutaneous infiltrations of the lower legs, especially on the calves. Gradually, the infiltrations extend toward the surface, forming blue-red plaques that can ulcerate before healing with atrophy and scarring (Color Fig. 20-2). Recurrences are common and often are precipitated by the onset of cold weather. Women are more commonly affected than men. "Nodular vasculitis" was proposed by Montgomery as a term for those cases with erythema induratum-like lesions that were not associated with tuberculosis.[13,48]

Histopathology. In contrast to erythema nodosum that is mainly a septal panniculitis, erythema induratum (nodular vasculitis) initially is mainly a lobular panniculitis due to vasculitis that produces ischemic necrosis of the fat lobule with relatively less involvement of the structures of the septa (Fig. 20-12). The fat necrosis can be extensive, caseous as well as coagulative, and elicits granulomatous inflammation (Figs. 20-13 and 20-14).

Epithelioid cells and giant cells form broad zones of inflammation surrounding the necrosis but also can form well-delimited granulomas of the tuberculoid type (Fig. 20-15). Ziehl-Neelsen stains are negative for intact mycobacteria.[49] In approximately one third of cases, granulomas are sparse or

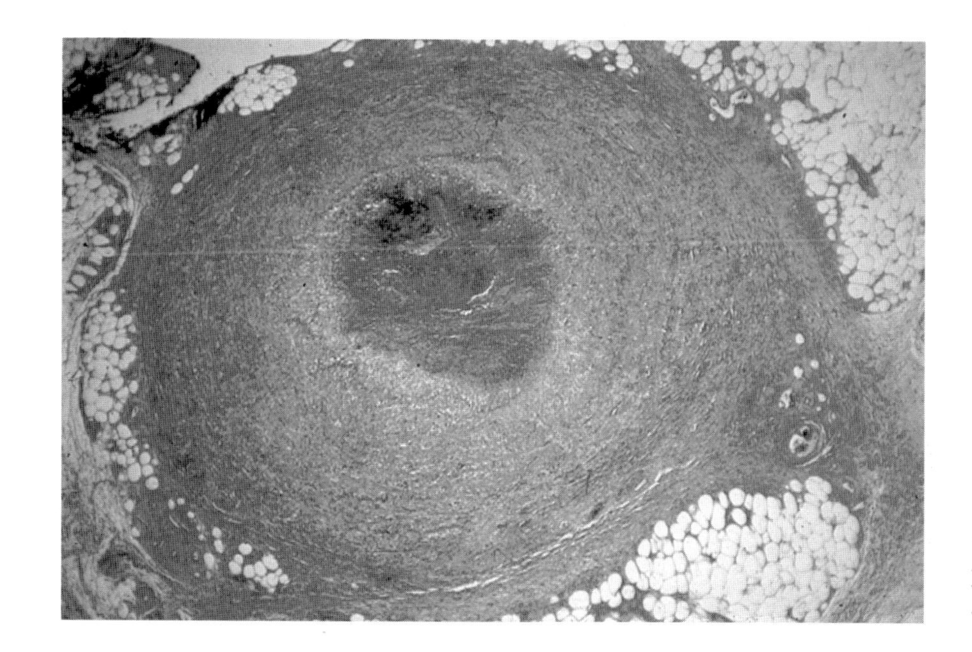

FIG. 20-11. Thrombophlebitis A thrombus occludes the lumen of the vein, which has an edematous wall with an inflammatory infiltrate.

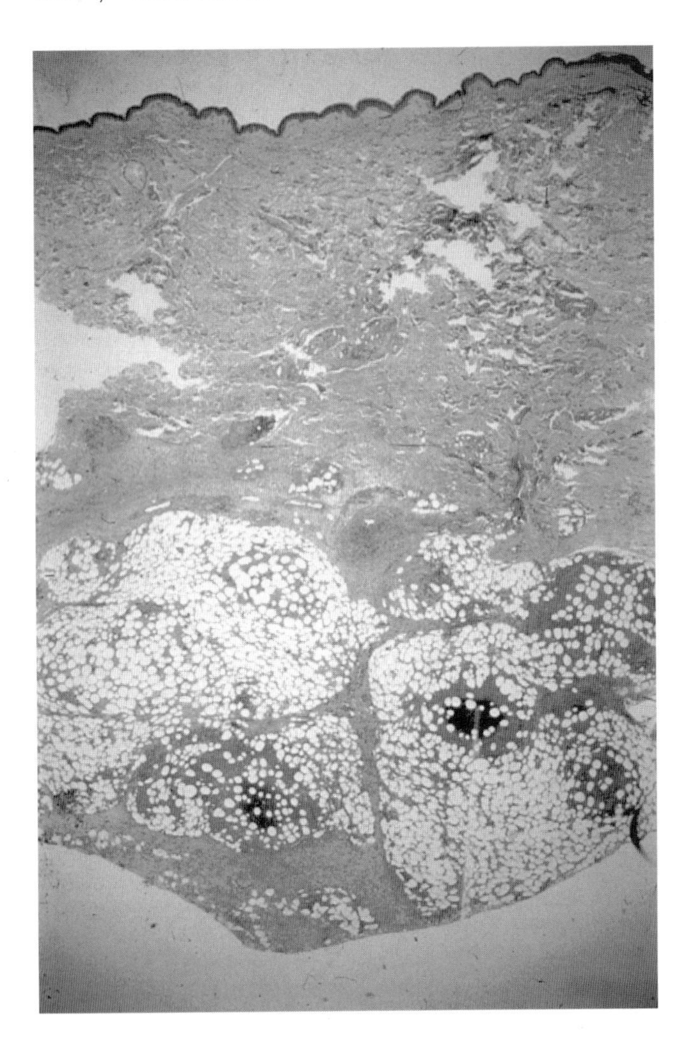

FIG. 20-12. Nodular vasculitis/erythema induratum, early lesion
Vasculitis in the deep plexus is associated predominantly with lobular panniculitis but septa are also involved to a lesser extent.

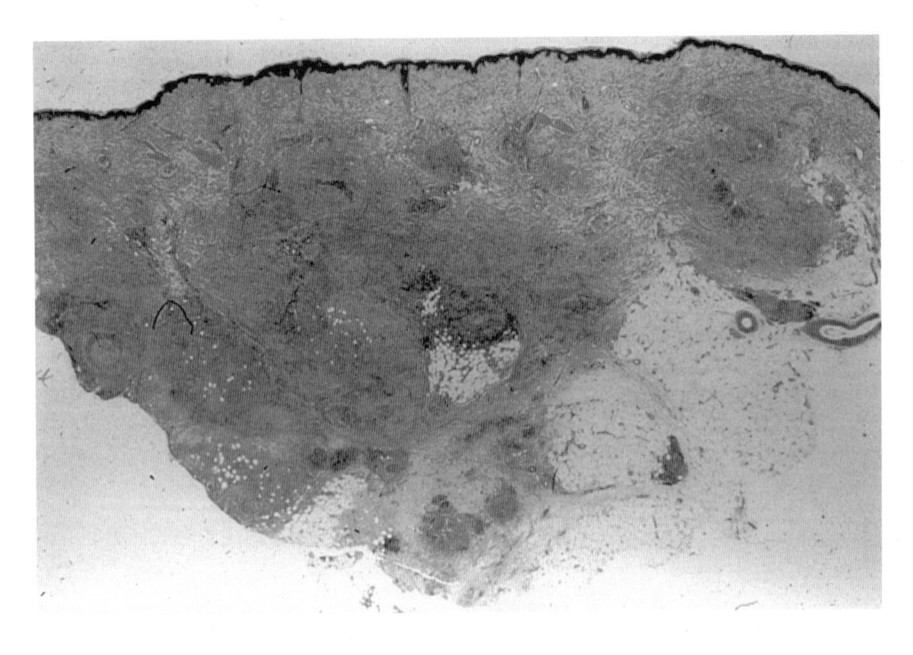

FIG. 20-13. Nodular vasculitis/erythema induratum, late lesion
Vasculitis and granulomatous inflammation involve the deep dermal and subcutaneous vessels, producing both lobular and septal panniculitis.

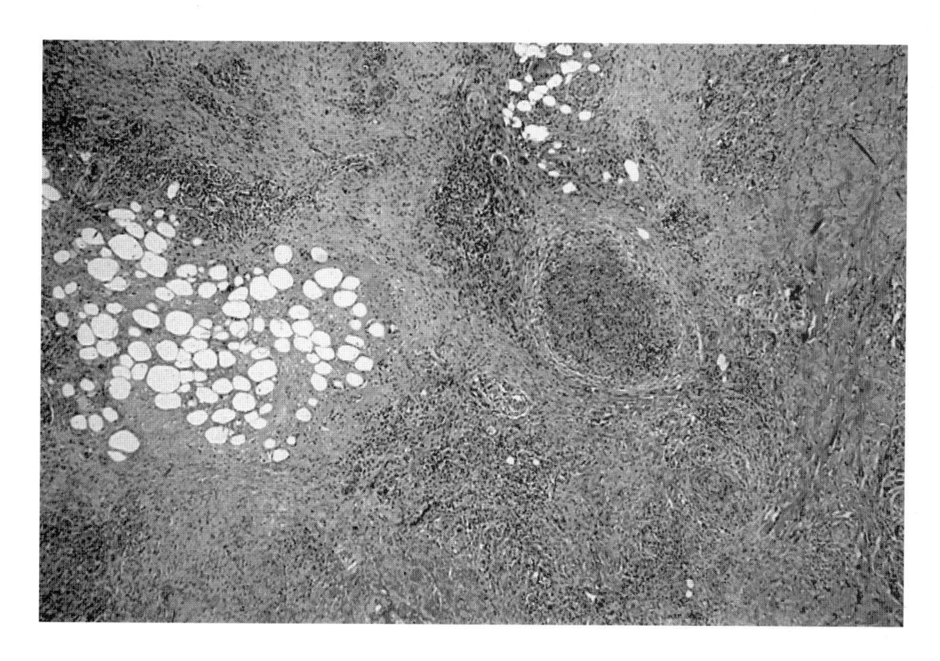

FIG. 20-14. Nodular vasculitis/erythema induratum
Adjacent to regions of lobular fat necrosis, there are infiltrates of lymphocytes and macrophages that can be arranged in well-formed granulomas.

absent and lymphocytes and plasma cells predominate.[49] Both the tuberculoid granulomas and the lymphoid infiltrate extend between the fat cells, largely replacing them.

Vascular changes are extensive and severe. Arteries and veins of small and medium size show infiltration of their walls by a dense lymphoid or granulomatous inflammatory infiltrate (See Fig. 20-15), associated with endothelial swelling and edema of the vessel walls and fibrous thickening of the intima.[48] Thrombosis and occlusion, or just compromise, of the lumen can produce extensive ischemic and caseous necrosis of the fat in about half of the cases. Extensive necrosis leads to involvement of the overlying dermis and subsequent ulceration. The necrotic fat has fat cysts, with surrounding amorphous, finely granular, eosinophilic material containing some pyknotic nuclei. Later lesions contain many foamy histiocytes surrounding the areas of fat necrosis.

Those cases that have been associated with tuberculosis have been designated "erythema induratum," whereas those not associated with tuberculosis have been called "nodular vasculitis."[13,48]

Pathogenesis. Erythema induratum in the past has been caused by a hypersensitivity reaction to tuberculosis, which is a "tuberculid." However neither inoculation of lesional tissue into guinea pigs nor cultures of such tissue have yielded isolates of tubercle bacilli. Also, erythema induratum responds to treatment with corticosteroids.[50] In contrast, evidence against erythema induratum being a tuberculid consists of the finding that active tuberculosis is no more frequent in patients with erythema induratum than in the general population. Also, patients with tuberculosis can develop erythema nodosum.[51] A delayed hypersensitivity reaction seems likely to be the basis of nodular vasculitis in nontuberculous patients since S100-positive, dendritic cells are increased in number within granulomas near the vessels in nodular vasculitis and not in polyarteritis nodosa.[52] These dendritic cells could present antigens to T cells.

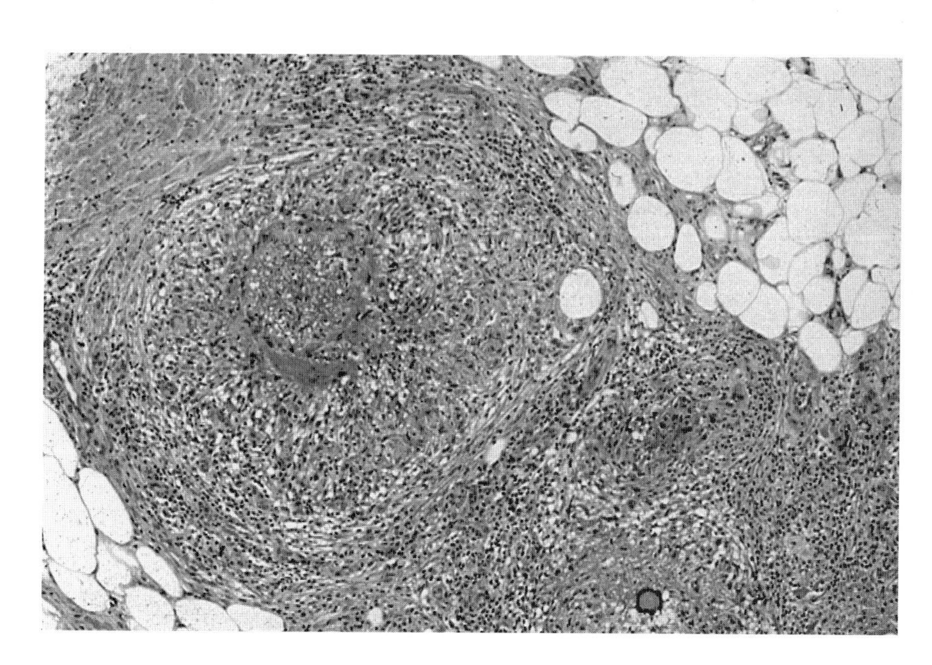

FIG. 20-15. Nodular vasculitis/erythema induratum
The infiltration of vessel walls by lymphoid cells can be granulomatous.

The primary event in erythema induratum is a vasculitis of the subcutaneous arteries and veins. If fat necrosis develops it is the result of ischemia following vascular damage.

Differential Diagnosis. Erythema induratum can be distinguished from erythema nodosum by the prominent lymphohistiocytic vasculitis in erythema induratum, which is only found very rarely in erythema nodosum. When caseation necrosis is present it clearly separates erythema induratum from erythema nodosum but not from direct cutaneous mycobacterial infection, which lacks the vasculitis of erythema induratum. Mycobacteria can be difficult to find in subcutaneous lesions of tuberculosis and are absent from erythema induratum on the Ziehl-Neelsen method for acid-fast staining. Detection of DNA from *M tuberculosis* in lesions of erythema induratum by polymerase chain reaction[53] but with negative cultures suggests a hypersensitivity reaction to fragments of tubercle bacilli.[54]

The difficult distinctions are between *erythema induratum*, *thrombophlebitis*, and subcutaneous *polyarteritis nodosa*, all of which can produce the clinical picture of nodules on the legs with vasculitis. Polyarteritis nodosa has neutrophilic infiltrates and fibrinoid necrosis of arterial vessel walls, whereas erythema induratum and nodular vasculitis have lymphohistiocytic infiltrates of the vessel walls with intimal proliferation and thrombosis. Elastic tissue stains are helpful in some lesions for distinguishing small arteries affected by polyarteritis from small veins affected by thrombophlebitis. However, the anatomic distinction between arteries and veins can be difficult when the inflammation in polyarteritis destroys the elastic fibers and when the elastic tissue is increased in the walls of veins due to stasis and venous hypertension commonly present in the lower legs. Deep biopsies and step sections in the tissue blocks may be necessary to demonstrate the focal necrotizing vasculitis in polyarteritis nodosa since thrombosis and reactive changes near these foci can closely resemble nodular vasculitis in routine sections. At times only a general diagnosis of "panniculitis with vasculitis" can be given until other biopsies or additional clinical information clarify the nature of the disorder.

LUPUS ERYTHEMATOSUS PANNICULITIS

Clinical Features. In patients with chronic cutaneous lupus erythematosus, the lesions can be deep and can involve the panniculus either alone or accompanied by dermal lesions.[55–57] The patients can have either chronic discoid lupus erythematosus or systemic lupus erythematosus. Most commonly, the skin lesions are firm, indurated subcutaneous nodules, and the overlying skin shows no specific changes.

The lesions are deep nodules and plaques that tend to involve the skin of the trunk and proximal extremities, particularly the lateral aspects of the upper arms, thighs, and buttocks. Symmetrical lesions on the anterior chest or upper arms can suggest a traumatic or factitial dermatitis, and indeed trauma may play a role in the localization of the lupus lesions to these sites. Approximately 70% of these patients also have other lesions that are typical of discoid lupus erythematosus and approximately 50% have evidence of mild systemic lupus erythematosus.[57] The lesions are painful and have a tendency to ulcerate and to heal leaving depressed scars. When the overlying skin is involved there is a loss of hair, erythema, poikiloderma, and epidermal atrophy. The patients may present with localized depressions of lipoatrophy alone.[58] The term "lupus profundus" has been used both for lupus panniculitis and also for discoid lupus erythematosus lesions that involve the dermis and extend deeply into the subcutis. Lesions that begin as a pure panniculitis over time can develop dermal sclerosis and deep depressions in the skin surface.

Histopathology. The histologic sections show a deep lymphocytic infiltration in the fat lobules and in the septa.[55] Lymphoid aggregates, nodules, and germinal centers, also known as follicular centers, are common.[55,59] Usually there is mucinous edema of the septa and of the overlying dermis. The dermis can have a superficial and deep perivascular lymphocytic infiltrate with plasma cells or can have all of the changes of lesions of discoid lupus erythematosus. A distinctive feature is the so-called "hyaline necrosis" of the fat, in which portions of the fat lobule

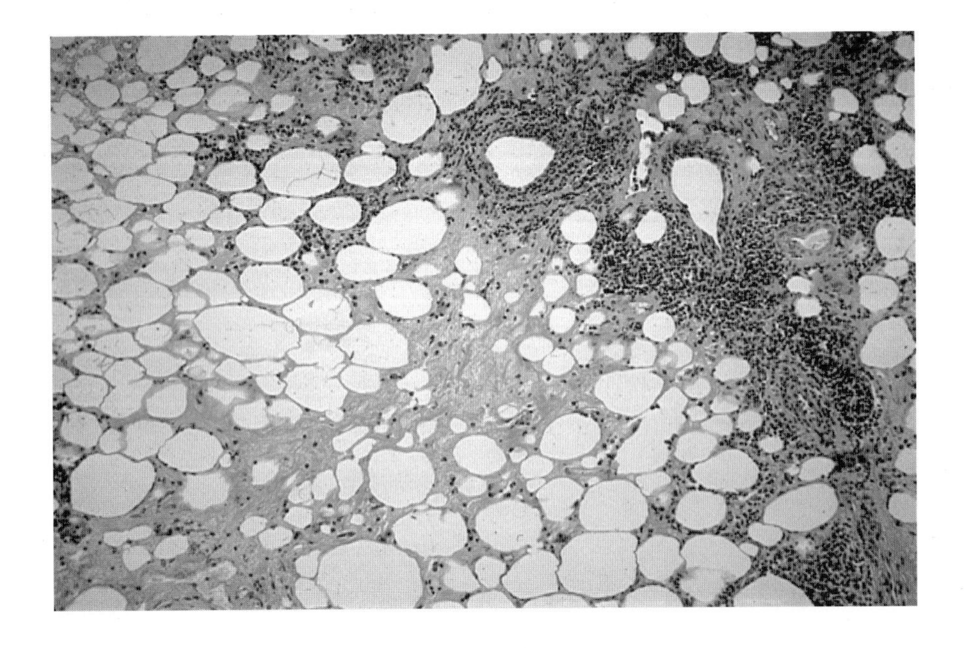

FIG. 20-16. Lupus panniculitis Necrotic fat lobules contain hyalinized interstitial fibrin deposits and a dense lymphocytic infiltrate adjacent to the necrotic zones.

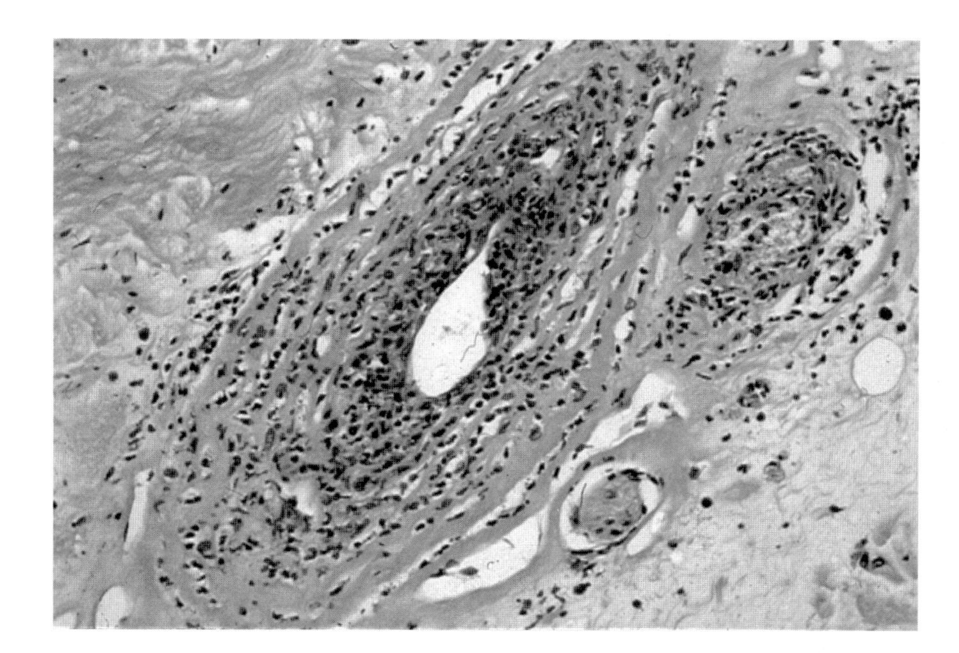

FIG. 20-17. Lupus panniculitis Blood vessels have lymphocytic infiltration of their walls with concentric fibrosis.

have lost nuclear staining of the fat cells and there is an accumulation of fibrin and other proteins in a homogeneous eosinophilic matrix between residual fat cells and extracellular fat globules (Fig. 20-16).[55] Blood vessels are infiltrated by lymphoid cells and can have restriction of their lumen diameter (Fig. 20-17). Calcification may be present in older lesions.

Pathogenesis. Approximately 50% of patients with lupus profundus have positive immunofluorescence at the dermal-epidermal junction and hair follicle basement membrane, especially with granular deposition of IgM and C3 and linear fibrin deposits. Many cases also have granular IgM and C3 as well as fibrin associated with deep dermal and subcutaneous blood vessel walls. Fibrin is distributed diffusely in the panniculus, both in the lobules and in the septa in areas of hyaline necrosis. It seems likely that trauma may be involved in the localization of lesions, perhaps through increased vascular permeability and leakage of circulating antinuclear antibodies or immune complexes into the fat lobules. A few patients have had lupus panniculitis in the presence of a genetic partial deficiency of C2 and C4[60] and a lupus-like syndrome has been reported in approximately one-third of patients with C2 deficiency.[61,62] In patients with complement at the dermal-epidermal junction, deposition of the so-called membrane-attack complex, composed of C5b–9, can also be demonstrated.

Differential Diagnosis. Cases of lupus panniculitis have been given the diagnosis of Weber-Christian disease in the past, and the overlap in histologic appearances may prevent any distinction between these two diseases. However, Weber-Christian disease can be sharply localized just to the fat lobules; in contrast, lupus panniculitis tends to cause mucinous edema (detectable on alcian blue stains) and inflammation around the blood vessels of the dermis. Immunofluorescence and serologic studies allow a positive diagnosis of lupus erythematosus in many instances.

A particularly troublesome differential diagnosis is between lupus panniculitis and subcutaneous T-cell lymphoma or B-cell lymphoma. Each may have dense lymphoid infiltrates in the fat, and usually the lymphoma cells have cytologically atypical lymphocytes. However, a significant proportion of subcutaneous T-cell lymphomas are composed of small cells that lack obvious cytologic atypia. Immunohistochemical studies can show a pure T-helper or T-suppressor population, but T-cell receptor gene rearrangements often are necessary for showing clonality in the lymphoid infiltrate.

Erythema induratum, like lupus panniculitis, also shows hyaline necrosis and vasculitis. There is more granulomatous inflammation than in most cases of lupus panniculitis. Erythema induratum lacks the mucinous edema of the dermis.

RELAPSING FEBRILE NODULAR NONSUPPURATIVE PANNICULITIS (WEBER-CHRISTIAN DISEASE)

Clinical Presentation. The diagnosis of Weber-Christian disease is a diagnosis of exclusion. It is made much less frequently now than it was in the 1950 to 1970 period, probably due to the greater power of current laboratory testing to reveal lupus erythematosus panniculitis, AAT deficiency panniculitis, or histiocytic cytophagic panniculitis in cases that might have been classified as Weber-Christian disease in the past. The classical clinical description is a disease characterized by the appearance of crops of tender nodules and plaques in the subcutaneous fat, usually in association with mild fever. The lower extremities are favored sites, but lesions can occur also on the trunk, the upper extremities, and rarely on the face. The lesions may ulcerate (Color Fig. 20-3); as they involute, they leave depressions in the skin surface. The overlying skin usually shows no involvement other than mild erythema.

The disease occurs most frequently in middle-aged women, although it has been seen in both sexes and at all ages including the neonatal period.[63] In general, the prognosis is good, with the attacks gradually becoming less severe and ultimately ceasing.[64] However, if systemic panniculitis is present, the disease may be fatal.[65]

This clinical description has significant overlap with that of lupus erythematosus panniculitis or histiocytic cytophagic panniculitis, which must be ruled in or out. The name Weber-Christian disease has been used in such a general fashion by some authors that the term loses meaning beyond being a clinical syndrome with nodular panniculitis for which the etiology has not yet been determined.[66]

Histopathology. The histopathologic appearance itself is not sufficiently specific to exclude the other diseases mentioned in the differential diagnosis. The classical description of the disease is that of a lobular panniculitis that evolves through three phases.

The first phase occurs when there is only erythema and induration clinically. There is acute inflammation of the fat lobules with degeneration of fat cells accompanied by an infiltrate of neutrophils, lymphocytes, and macrophages (Fig. 20-18 and 20-19). Neutrophils may predominate, but abscesses do not occur.[67]

The second phase is recognized histologically after the lesions have been present for several days. The infiltrate is discretely localized to the fat lobules (see Fig. 20-18) and consists mainly of macrophages but usually also with a few lymphocytes and plasma cells. Many of the macrophages near the fat cells have ingested fat particles and have developed vacuolated cytoplasm that gives them the name "foam cells" (Fig. 20-20). These foam cells can be large and often some of them are multinucleated. A few multinucleated cells without foamy cytoplasm also may be found. Foamy macrophages replace the fat lobules and extracellular lipid masses (misnamed "microcysts") result from lysis of the adipose cells or from breakdown of the foamy macrophages. In some cases, the lesions perforate the skin surface and discharge a sterile, oily liquid.

The third phase is found in the clinical lesions that are depressed and indurated. The histologic preparations show many fibroblasts and scattered lymphocytes and a few plasma cells that have replaced the fat and the foam cells. Collagen deposition results in dense fibrosis. Usually the epidermis and dermis are spared unless there is perforation and drainage through the skin. Vascular changes usually are mild, with only endothelial proliferation and edema and thickening of the vessel walls.[68,69]

Systemic Lesions. The occurrence of systemic lesions separates Weber-Christian disease from most other causes of panniculitis, except for histiocytic cytophagic panniculitis and AAT deficiency panniculitis. Four types of lesions have been described in autopsy material[69]: (1) involvement of the perivisceral adipose tissue, including mesenteric and omental fat; (2) involvement of intravisceral adipose tissue, which causes focal necroses in liver or spleen and may be followed by macrophage infiltration and enlargement of these organs,[69] occasionally even with jaundice[65,70]; (3) involvement of the bone marrow, resulting in interference in hematopoiesis and anemia[69]; and (4) accumulation of large amounts of oily fluid in either the peritoneal or pleural cavity.[69]

Among the nonfatal extracutaneous manifestations painful osteolytic lesions have been described. On histologic examination, the bone lesions have fat necrosis, lymphocytic infiltration, fat-laden macrophages, and multinucleated giant cells.[71]

Pathogenesis. If Weber-Christian disease exists as a distinct disease,[8,72] the cause is unknown. An immune mechanism is suspected because high levels of circulating immune complexes have been reported.[65]

Differential Diagnosis. The histologic appearance of Weber-Christian disease is most distinctive during the second phase, since there is such a preponderance of foam cells discretely localized to the subcutaneous fat lobules. In rare instances, erythema nodosum can have a predominance of neutrophils and can resemble the first phase of Weber-Christian disease.[8] The neutrophilic phase of Weber-Christian disease is so short that biopsies of several lesions, including a well-developed older lesion, should exclude erythema nodosum, which is mainly a septal panniculitis, whereas Weber-Christian is mainly a lobular panniculitis.

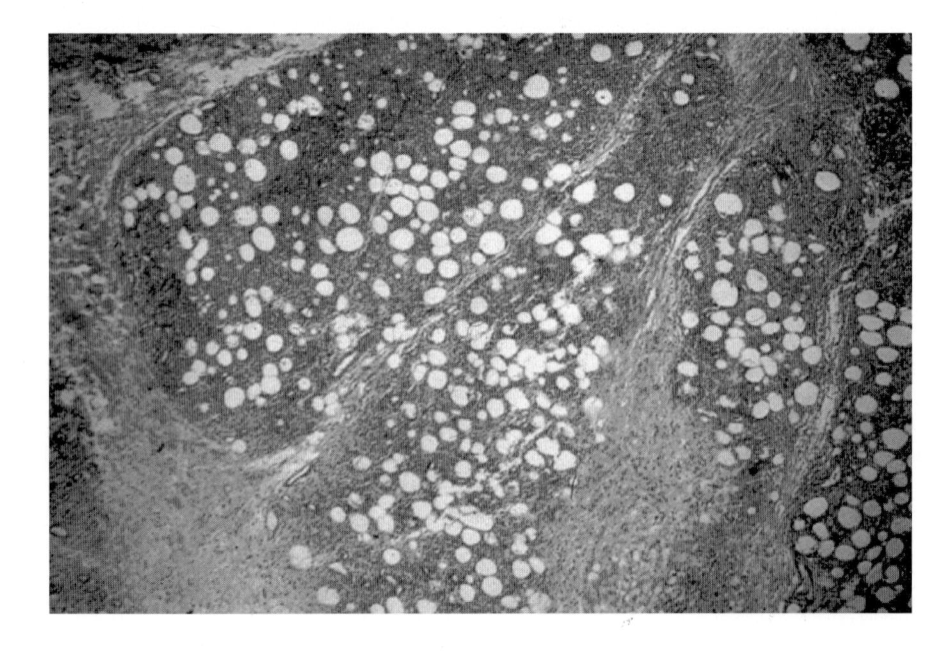

FIG. 20-18. Weber-Christian disease, early lesion
A dense lymphoid infiltrate is sharply localized to the fat lobules without vasculitis.

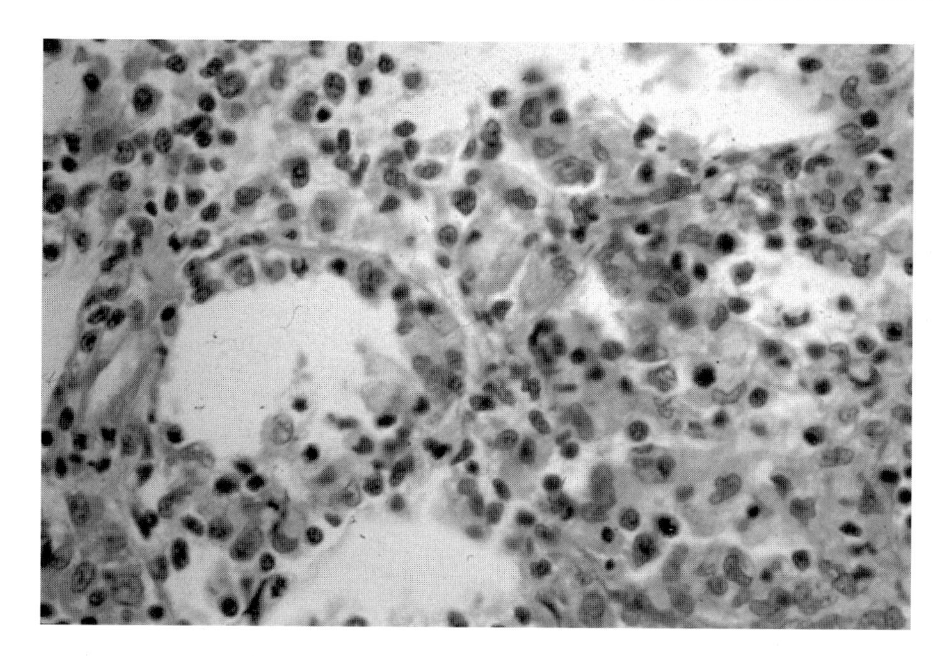

FIG. 20-19. Weber-Christian disease, early lesion
The infiltrate is composed mainly of lymphocytes and macrophages with variable numbers of neutrophils.

Subcutaneous fat necrosis in pancreatic disease can produce lesions that clinically resemble those in Weber-Christian disease, but the histology is very different in the extensive necrosis of fat cells and the presence of bluish precipitates of calcium with fatty acids in the fat lobules after pancreatic enzyme digestion.

Histiocytic cytophagic panniculitis can mimic the clinical appearance of Weber-Christian disease but is histologically different in the presence of macrophages and multinucleated cells with phagocytosis of erythrocytes, lymphocytes, and neutrophils to produce so-called "bean bag cells," rather than the phagocytosis of fat to produce mainly foam cells.[73]

PANNICULITIS ROTHMANN-MAKAI

The term "panniculitis Rothmann-Makai" was proposed in 1945 as the designation for a "heterogeneous group of cases of idiopathic panniculitis that do not fit into any of the distinctly defined syndromes, such as Weber-Christian syndrome, erythe-

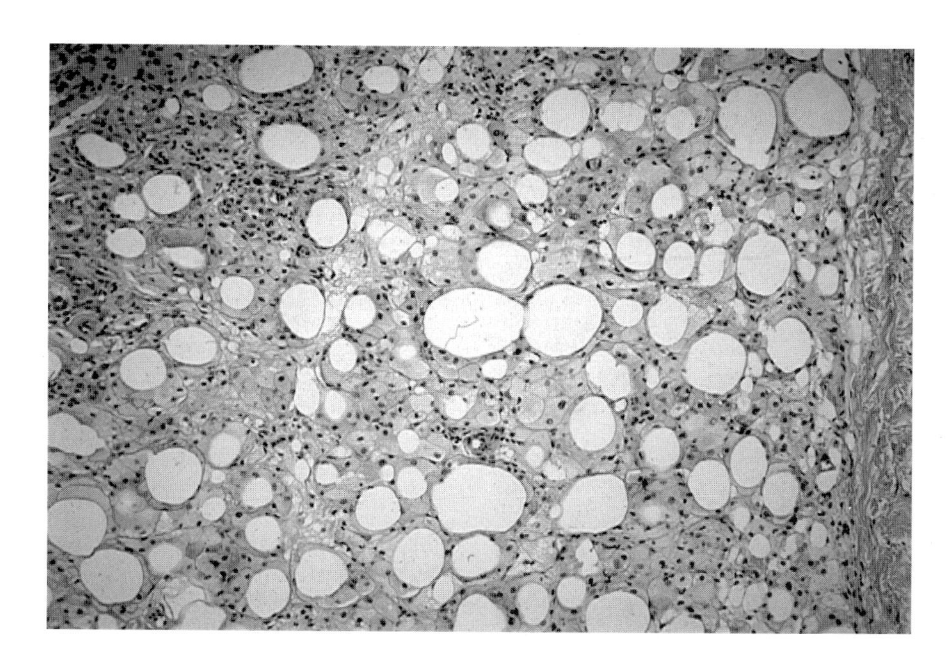

FIG. 20-20. Weber-Christian disease, later lesion
The fat is necrotic and has been extensively replaced by lipid-laden macrophages or "foam cells."

ma nodosum, or erythema induratum."[74] This diagnostic term is based entirely on negative criteria[75] and consequently should be avoided. It seems preferable to refer to such cases as "unclassified panniculitis" until more definitive studies are available.

PANNICULITIS DUE TO PHYSICAL OR CHEMICAL AGENTS

Clinical Features. Trauma may be due to physical injury or chemical injury, such as that produced by injection of noxious substances. Physical injury can be produced by blunt pressure or impact, cold or excessive heat, or electrical injury. All of these factors can produce firm nodules in the subcutaneous fat. In many instances, these various inciting agents can be distinguished best by the clinical history and distribution of the lesions. Surreptitious injections of noxious substances can produce bizarre clinical and histological patterns of lesions but are suspected clinically by their distribution only in areas easily reached by the patient (*factitial panniculitis*). Drug injections by nurses usually are located in the deltoid region or on the buttocks. Insulin injections, often on the thigh and lower abdomen, can result in subcutaneous lesions. Meperidine hydrochloride or Demerol[76] and pentazocine or Talwin[77] injections are known to produce traumatic panniculitis. The injection of oily substances such as paraffin or silicone has been common for cosmetic effects, but reactions to these substances or to contaminants in them produce a panniculitis.[78,79] Mentally ill persons and drug addicts may purposely or inadvertently inject themselves with foreign substances, such as feces or milk, sometimes used to dilute or cut narcotics. These various physical or chemical traumas lead to indurated subcutaneous nodules that may undergo liquefaction, ulcerate, and discharge pus or a thick oily fluid. Healing leaves depressed scars.[80] Lesions produced by extreme cold usually do not ulcerate unless associated with pernio or vasculitis with cryoglobulinemia. Cold injury may occur in children after eating an iced food such as a popsicle.[81–83] The cold injury produces nodules or plaques that appear from one to three days after exposure and subside spontaneously within two weeks. Excessive heat and electrical injury usually are accompanied by ulceration and eschar formation.

Histopathology. The injection of the various toxic agents will produce a variable histologic picture of acute inflammation, with aggregation of neutrophils and focal fat necrosis with hemorrhage.[80] Older lesions have infiltrates of lymphocytes and macrophages with fibrosis (Fig. 20-21).[77] Vasculitis usually is absent. Polarized light may reveal foreign material in injection sites.[76] The injection of oily liquids leads to the formation of many pockets of fatty material "fat cysts," often with a surrounding fibrous reaction containing foamy macrophages, that produces a "Swiss-cheese appearance" after the fat is extracted during routine histologic processing.[78,79] Fixation of the tissue in osmium tetroxide may be useful since endogenous lipids (but not most exogenous lipids) contain many unsaturated double bonds that react readily with osmium tetroxide to produce a black deposit of reduced osmium oxides.[84,85]

Trauma due to cold injury initially has an infiltrate of lymphocytes and macrophages near the blood vessels of the deep plexus at the junction of dermis and subcutis. Such changes have also been described in perniosis. Biopsies at the third day, the height of the reaction, show rupture of the fat cells with fat pockets in the tissue surrounded by an infiltrate of lymphocytes, macrophages, neutrophils, and occasional eosinophils.[82,86]

Pathogenesis. The subcutaneous fat of children is more sensitive to cold injury than that of older children and adults. In all newborn infants and in 40% of infants 6 months of age, the application of an ice cube to the skin produces nodules of cold panniculitis. By 9 months of age only occasional infants have such cold reactivity.[83] The greater degree of saturation of the lipids in newborns raises the crystallization temperature of the fats and produces greater susceptibility to cold injury.[87] This mechanism of injury also is involved in *sclerema neonatorum.*

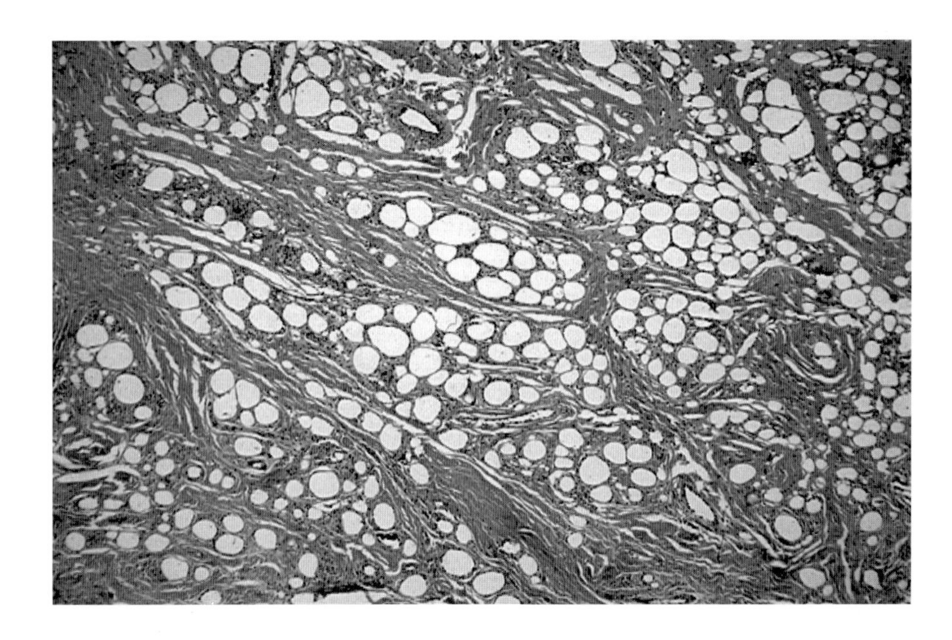

FIG. 20-21. Traumatic panniculitis Pressure necrosis has caused extensive necrosis of the fat followed by fibrosis around the distorted lobules.

LOCALIZED LIPOATROPHY AND LIPODYSTROPHY

Clinical Features. Both localized lipoatrophy and lipodystrophy can have lesions with a similar clinical appearance; however, lipoatrophy usually involves one or several circumscribed, round, depressed areas, from one to several centimeters in diameter. In contrast, lipodystrophy produces the loss of large areas of subcutaneous fat. Most cases of lipodystrophy are of the cephalothoracic type and involve the face, neck, upper extremities, and upper trunk. Some cases have been noted that extend downward from the iliac crest. Lipodystrophy has been reported with diabetes[88] and with glomerulonephritis.[89] Lipoatrophic panniculitis also occurs in *connective tissue panniculitis.*[90]

Histopathology. Lesions of lipodystrophy are described with total loss of the subcutaneous fat producing dermis adjacent to fascia.[88] However, localized lipoatrophy has been described as having two types: inflammatory and noninflammatory or "involutional" types. In the inflammatory type, multiple lesions are common and have a lymphocytic infiltrate around the blood vessels and scattered diffusely in the fat lobules.[58] Areas of fat necrosis can be present with infiltration by macrophages.

In the involutional type, usually there is only a solitary lesion that exhibits a decrease in size of the individual adipocytes. They are separated from each other by abundant eosinophilic, hyaline material, or in some instances by mucoid material.[91]

SUBCUTANEOUS NODULAR FAT NECROSIS IN PANCREATIC DISEASE

Clinical Features. In patients with pancreatitis or pancreatic neoplasms, the release of lipase enzymes into the blood can lead to nodules of fat necrosis in the subcutis. The pretibial region is the most common site of the nodules, but they may occur on the thighs, buttocks, and elsewhere (Color Fig. 20-4). The nodules usually are tender and red and may be fluctuant,[92] but they only rarely discharge oily fluid through fistulae.[93] Abdominal pain is present in most cases of pancreatitis but absent in pancreatic carcinoma when the nodules appear. Arthralgia in the ankles is a common early symptom.[94] The carcinomas of the pancreas are usually of the acinar cell type.[93]

Histopathology. The histologic appearance of the subcutaneous nodules in pancreatic disease is characteristic in most instances.[94] In the foci of fat necrosis, there are ghost-like fat cells having thick, faintly stained cell peripheries and no nuclear staining (Fig. 20-22). Calcification forms basophilic granules in the cytoplasm of the necrotic fat cells, and sometimes lamellar deposits around individual fat cells or patchy basophilic deposits at the periphery of the fat necrosis (Fig. 20-23).[92] A polymorphous infiltrate surrounds the foci of fat necrosis and consists of neutrophils, lymphoid cells, macrophages, foam cells, and foreign-body giant cells.[95] There can be extensive hemorrhage into the lesions. Old lesions have macrophages, foam cells, lymphocytes, and fibroblasts, with fibrosis and hemosiderin deposition.[92] In some cases with pancreatic enzyme panniculitis, possibly with early lesions, biopsies of subcutaneous nodules show only a nonspecific pattern of a necrotizing panniculitis with a neutrophilic inflammatory response. Multiple biopsies and deep biopsies may allow a definitive diagnosis.

Systemic Lesions. Fat necrosis also occurs in internal organs. The symptoms of arthralgia are due to periarticular fat necrosis.[95] Fat necrosis is common also in the pancreas and surrounding fat tissue and in the fat of the omentum, mesentery, pericardial, and perirenal regions, as well as in the mediastinum and bone marrow.[92] Calcium precipitation can be extensive enough to produce life-threatening hypocalcemia.

Pathogenesis. The damaged or tumorous pancreatic acinar cells release lipase, phospholipase, trypsin, and amylase into the surrounding tissues and blood. The serum values for amylase and lipase usually are elevated transiently and may not be de-

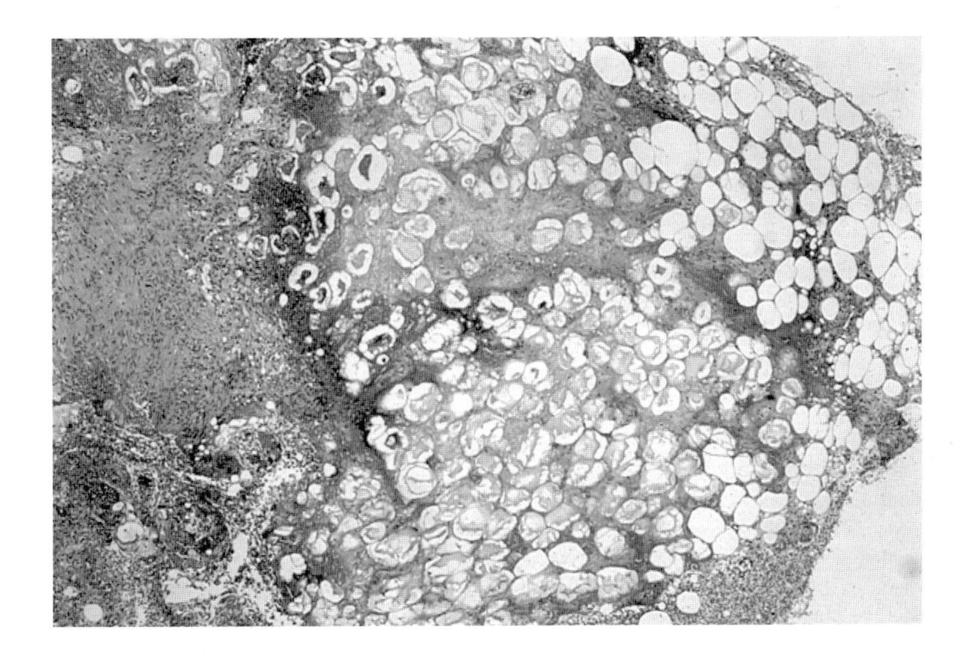

FIG. 20-22. Pancreatic enzyme panniculitis
Necrotic fat cells contain eosinophilic deposits of partially hydrolyzed fat. Calcification forms granular basophilic material. Focal hemorrhage is frequent.

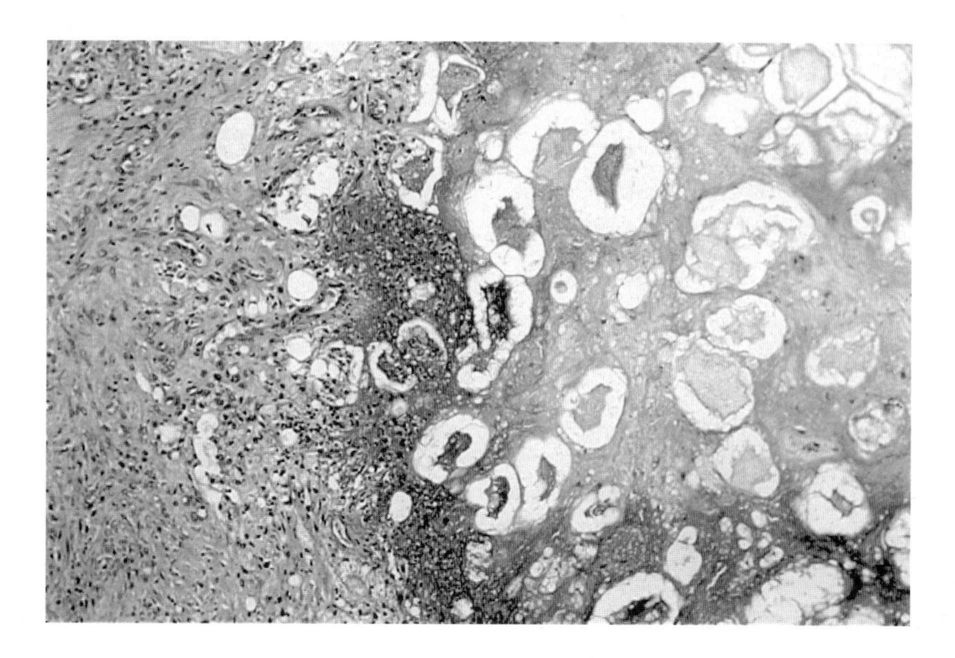

FIG. 20-23. Pancreatic enzyme panniculitis
Many neutrophils are present at the margin of the zone of calcification and fat necrosis.

tected in all cases. Amylase levels often peak two to three days after the appearance of the subcutaneous nodules.[94] Lipase can be detected in the regions of fat necrosis and in ascitic fluid.[96] It is not clear how the pancreatic proenzymes become activated in producing fat necrosis. Local changes in vascular permeability due to trauma or other circulating enzymes, such as trypsin or phospholipase A2, may allow the pancreatic lipase to enter the interstitial compartment of the fat lobules and produce fat necrosis. Free fatty acids released by the lipolysis combine with calcium to form the soapy basophilic deposits in the tissue.[97] Enzymatic damage to the integrity of the vascular wall can produce extensive hemorrhage.

Differential Diagnosis. The usual diagnostic distinction is between fat necrosis due to pancreatic disease and to physical trauma, but clinically may include also erythema nodosum, erythema induratum, nodular vasculitis, α_1-antitrypsin deficiency panniculitis, disseminated infection, or Weber-Christian disease. Only pancreatic fat necrosis produces the basophilic deposits of calcium precipitated with an abundance of free fatty acids. The other entities all can have neutrophils in the fat. Basophilic debris from neutrophil nuclei must be distinguished from calcium deposits. Septic foci of bacterial or fungal infection require special stains for organisms. Despite vascular damage and hemorrhage, neutrophilic vasculitis usually is absent in fat necrosis due to pancreatic disease. Old lesions that have resorbed the calcium soaps cannot be distinguished easily from the other entities.

SCLEREMA NEONATORUM

Clinical Features. Sclerema neonatorum is a very rare disorder, usually in premature infants, that is characterized by a diffuse, rapidly spreading, nonpitting, hardening of the subcutaneous fat of neonates in the first few days of life. The skin seems wax-like, tight, cold, and indurated. Death usually supervenes in a few weeks, if untreated. On autopsy, the subcutis is greatly thickened, hardened, and lard-like. Most infants with sclerema neonatorum are cyanotic at birth, have difficulty maintaining their body temperature, and have a major debilitating illness.[87]

Histopathology. The subcutaneous tissue owes its thickening to the increase in size of the fat cells and to the presence of wide, intersecting fibrous bands.[87] The lipid crystals inside the fat cells produce rosettes of fine needle-like clefts. In frozen sections, the crystals are not extracted and are visible in polarized light.[98] In most instances there is very little evidence of any inflammatory reaction to the fat necrosis, but very rarely there is an inflammatory reaction containing giant cells.[98,99] Characteristically, the changes develop rapidly, are extensive, and elicit less inflammatory reaction than those of subcutaneous fat necrosis of the newborn or of localized cold panniculitis in young children.

Systemic Lesions. In most cases of sclerema neonatorum, the changes are limited to the subcutaneous fat.[87] However, in two cases autopsy revealed lesions in the visceral fat that were identical to those in the subcutis. In one case the lesions were widespread,[98] while in the other the systemic lesions were limited to the perirenal and retroperitoneal fat.[99]

Pathogenesis. Compared to the fat of the adult, the subcutaneous fat of the newborn has a greater ratio of saturated to unsaturated fatty acids, which produces solidification of the fat at higher temperatures. In sclerema neonatorum these changes are exaggerated so that the neutral fat (triglyceride) crystallizes at room temperature. The increased ratio of saturated (palmitic or stearic acid) to unsaturated fatty acids (such as oleic acid) may be produced by defective enzyme pathways that lead to an excess of saturated fatty acids.[87] X-ray diffraction studies have shown that the crystals in the fat cells are due to triglycerides.[100] It is likely that the use of thermally controlled incubators for premature infants has caused this disease to be extremely rare. This same mechanism of injury is operative in localized cold panniculitis in infants.

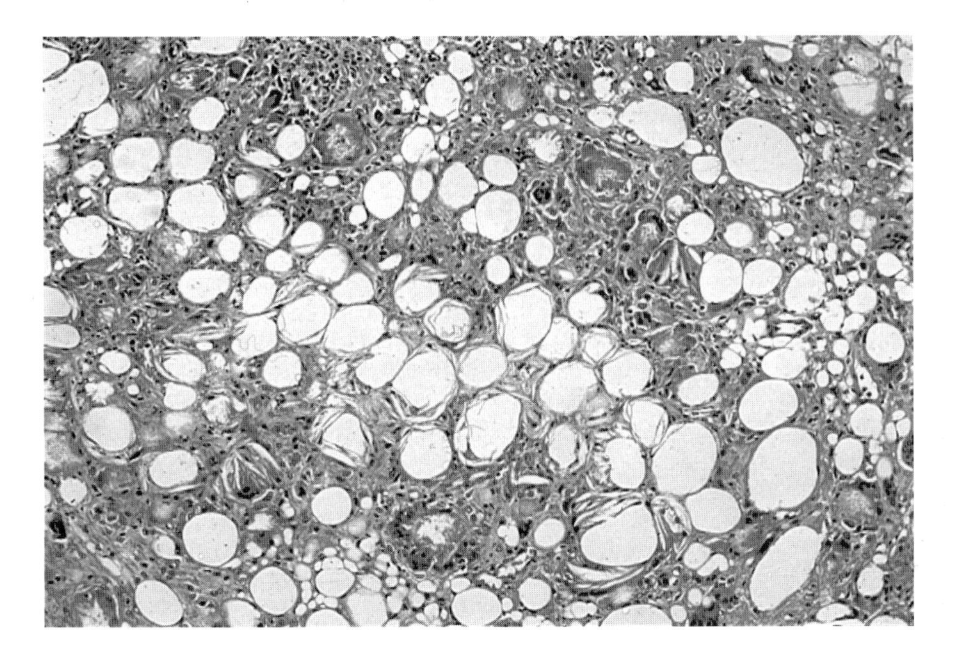

FIG. 20-24. Subcutaneous fat necrosis of the newborn
There is a lobular infiltrate of macrophages and lymphocytes with many slender clefts in the fat cells where crystals of fat were located.

Differential Diagnosis. Generalized edema due to an immature renal system can mimic some aspects of sclerema neonatorum but the generalized edema is pitting, while sclerema is not. Lymphedema (Milroy's disease) can produce nonpitting lymphedema, particularly of the legs, in an otherwise healthy infant. Biopsies are not advised but show dilation of lymphatics. Erysipelas is more demarcated, warm, and tender than sclerema.

SUBCUTANEOUS FAT NECROSIS OF THE NEWBORN

Clinical Features. Subcutaneous fat necrosis of the newborn usually occurs in premature or full-term infants, often after delivery with forceps. Indurated nodules and plaques appear in the subcutis a few days after birth. Rarely, in cases with numerous nodules, the lesions may discharge a caseous material.[101] The patient's health generally is good and the nodules resolve spontaneously after a few weeks or months. Rarely, some infants are severely ill and die.[101] In 16 reported cases, the subcutaneous fat necrosis was associated with hypercalcemia, and three patients died.[102] The development of extensive subcutaneous fat necrosis has been reported in infants following induced hypothermia used in cardiac surgery.[103] An underlying defect in composition and metabolism of fat has been assumed to exist in such cases.

Histopathology. Focal areas of fat necrosis are present in the fat lobules and are infiltrated by macrophages and foreign-body giant cells (Fig. 20-24). The fat deposits in the macrophages and giant cells contain crystalline fat, which forms needle-shaped clefts in a radial arrangement (Fig. 20-25).[104] In frozen sections, the radial clefts contain doubly refractile crystals. Calcium deposits usually are small and are scattered in the necrotic fat. If the necrosis is extensive, calcium deposits may be large and require several years to be resorbed.

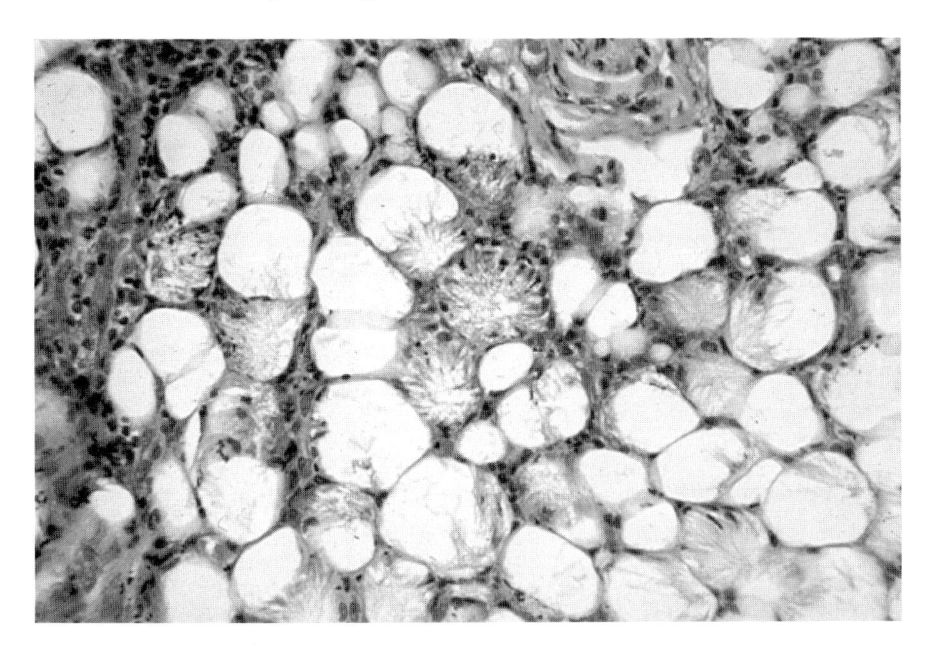

FIG. 20-25. Subcutaneous fat necrosis of the newborn
Macrophages and multinucleated giant cells contain radial crystalline arrays of fat.

Pathogenesis. Electron microscopic examination shows that the phagocytosis of fat crystals starts with the invasion of fat cells by cytoplasmic projections of macrophages. Subsequently, fat crystals are seen within the cytoplasm of macrophages and of foreign-body giant cells, which result from the fusion of macrophages.[104]

The cause of subcutaneous fat necrosis of the newborn is not known. There is debate about the role of trauma since many of the patients have been premature infants who were born by forceps delivery or who otherwise endured a difficult delivery. However, lesions were reported in a child delivered by cesarean section.[104]

Differential Diagnosis. Both subcutaneous fat necrosis of the newborn and sclerema neonatorum have crystalline arrays of needle-like clefts in the fat. Sclerema is a catastrophic diffuse illness that gives little time for extensive inflammation so that in sclerema there is an absence of focal areas of fat necrosis with macrophages and giant cells. In sclerema, there is also an absence of calcifications and the presence of wide bands of fibrous tissue in the subcutis.[87] Treatment of children with high doses of steroids—for example, as was done for rheumatic fever—can produce *post-steroid panniculitis* with subcutaneous lesions very similar histologically to those of subcutaneous fat necrosis of the newborn.[105] The deep nodules usually occur within one to thirty days after the cessation of high-dose steroid treatment. Traumatic fat necrosis has focal areas of necrosis and inflammation but lacks the crystals of fat. Localized infection can be difficult to exclude but the infants with subcutaneous fat necrosis are generally rather healthy and are not septic.

CALCIFYING PANNICULITIS

Clinical Features. Patients with end-stage renal disease or hyperparathyroidism may develop indurated, erythematous, cold, subcutaneous and dermal nodules, and plaques (Color Fig. 20-5). The lesions can progress to extensive dry gangrenous necrosis of the skin and subcutis. The lesions can be related to the prior administration of medications containing calcium or phosphates, so that the balance of calcium to phosphate is so disturbed as to favor precipitation of calcium phosphate salts in the tissue. Plaques often are localized at usual sites of subcutaneous injection such as the thighs and abdomen.

Histopathology. The early or minimal lesions of patients with this disorder often have calcification of the media of the blood vessels in the subcutis (Fig. 20-26). In calciphylaxis associated with chronic renal failure, fibrointimal hyperplasia occludes the lumen of small arteries.[106] In severe cases, calcium phosphate crystals form in the interspaces between fat cells in the lobules of subcutaneous fat. The affected vessels can undergo thrombosis with ischemic necrosis of the subcutaneous fat and the overlying dermis and epidermis.

Pathogenesis. Calciphylaxis is a condition in which the balance of calcium and phosphate favors precipitation of calcium phosphate at the sites of trauma, injection of medications containing calcium or phosphate compounds, or in vessel walls. The patients usually have end-stage renal disease and less commonly hyperparathyroidism. Case reports indicate that the phenomenon of calcium precipitation can be induced locally by injections of an anticoagulant drug such as calcium heparinate,[107] by infusions containing excess phosphate, or for unknown reasons during hemodialysis.[108] In young children extensive subcutaneous calcifications can result from subcutaneous fat necrosis of the newborn. In adults the differential diagnosis also includes a prior episode of pancreatic fat necrosis. The extensive calcification of the media of small arterioles is distinctive for calciphylaxis.

LIPOMEMBRANOUS CHANGE OR LIPOMEMBRANOUS PANNICULITIS

Clinical Features. Patients with severe stasis, diabetes, and other causes of arterial vascular insufficiency to the lower legs can develop indurated plaques in the subcutis. They are depressed and painful, but rarely ulcerate.[109,110] The lesions are defined microscopically by the presence of lipomembranes around fat deposits or "cysts." Lipomembranous change has

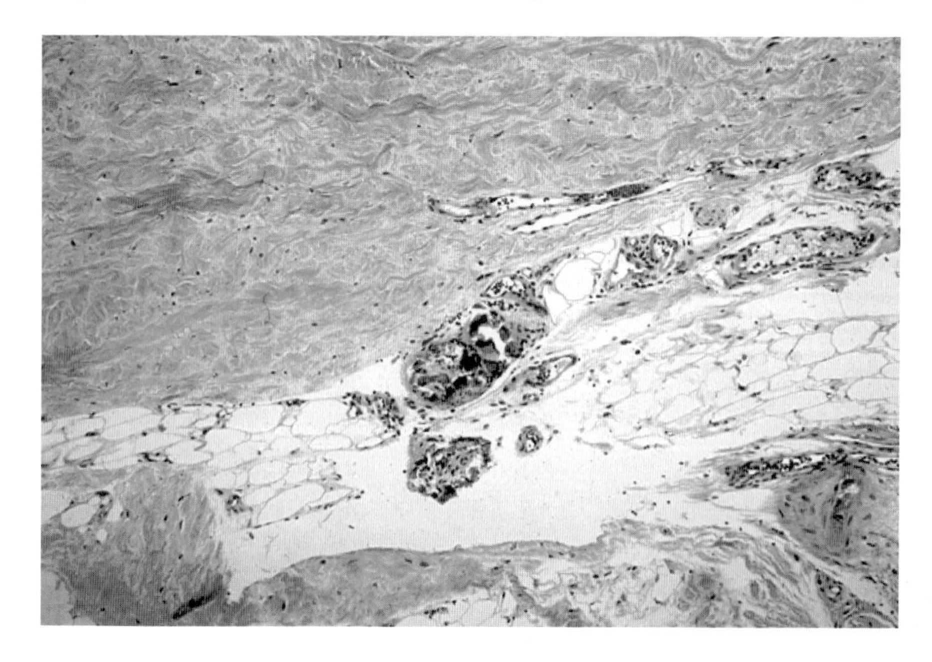

FIG. 20-26. Calcifying panniculitis Precipitation of calcium phosphate salts in the blood vessel walls produces a blue deposit. These deposits lead to thrombosis and ischemic necrosis of the adjacent fat and overlying skin.

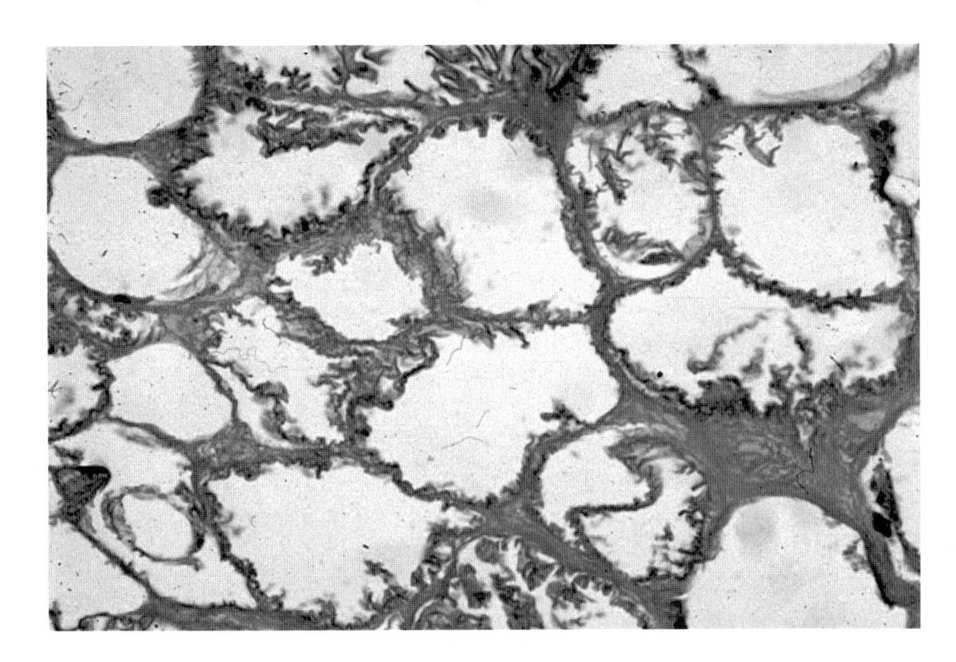

FIG. 20-27. Lipomembranous panniculitis
Necrosis of the fat has produced a layer of pale eosinophilic material, a "lipomembrane," around the periphery of the fat globules.

been found also in lupus erythematosus panniculitis and in morphea.[111]

Histopathology. Biopsies deep into the fat show a lobular panniculitis with focal macrophage infiltration and fibrosis around the shrunken lobules. At the border of the lobules with the septa there are fat cysts that are lined by a thin eosinophilic layer of protein that has fine, feathery projections into the fat cavity (Fig. 20-27). This layer is called a lipomembrane and is positive on PAS (Fig. 20-28) and elastic-tissue stains. Early lesions have focal areas of fat necrosis, such as those produced by partial ischemia.

Differential Diagnosis. This is not a very specific entity and probably reflects the tendency of necrotic fat to accumulate fibrin and other material at the surface of the exposed fat. However, extensive lipomembranous change is rare in simple traumatic fat necrosis in comparison to ischemic panniculitis.

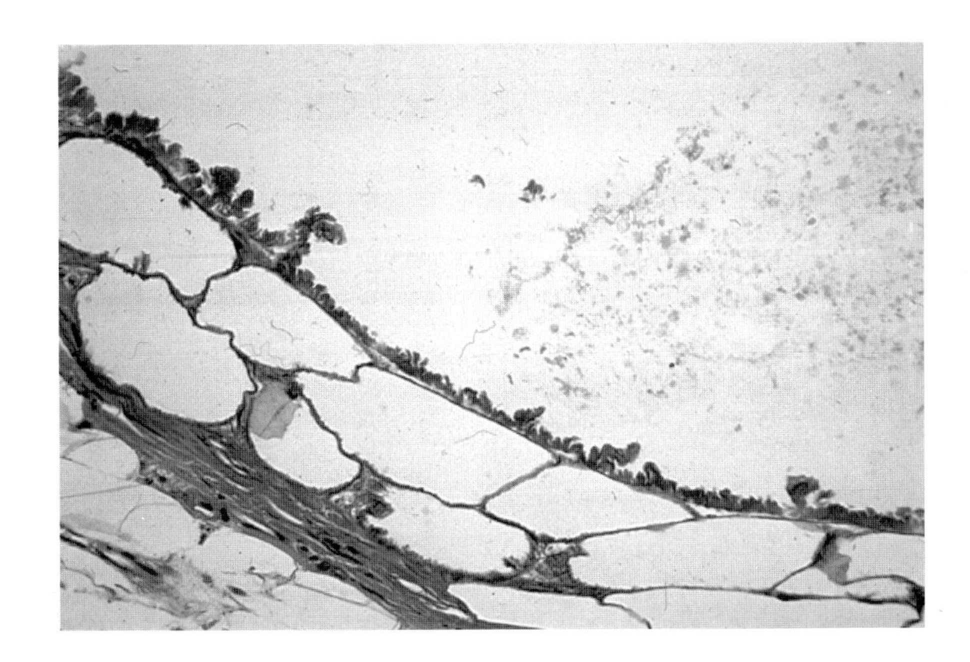

FIG. 20-28. Lipomembranous panniculitis
Lipomembranes have feathery projections into the fat globules and are PAS positive (PAS stain).

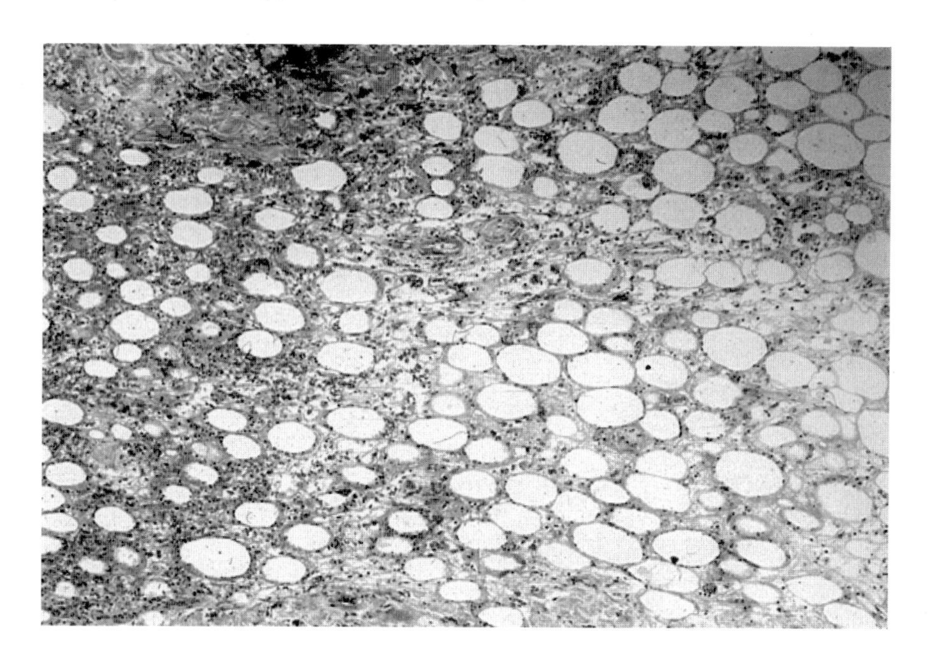

FIG. 20-29. Histiocytic cytophagic panniculitis
There is hemorrhagic necrosis of the fat with an infiltrate of lymphocytes and macrophages.

HISTIOCYTIC CYTOPHAGIC PANNICULITIS (SUBCUTANEOUS T-CELL LYMPHOMA WITH HEMOPHAGOCYTIC SYNDROME)

Clinical Features. Histiocytic cytophagic panniculitis is a frequently fatal systemic disease that is characterized by recurrent, widely distributed, painful subcutaneous nodules associated with malaise and fever.[73,112–114] The nodules can be hemorrhagic (Color Fig. 20-6). Ulcers can be present.[115] Hepatosplenomegaly, pancytopenia, and progressive liver dysfunction develop in most cases.[116] The patients may follow a long chronic course or the disease can be fulminant. The patients usually die a hemorrhagic death due to depletion of blood coagulation factors. Aggressive chemotherapeutic intervention, analogous to that used for malignant histiocytosis, has resulted in remission in one patient.[117] In some patients, the disease seems limited to the skin and subcutaneous tissue and follows a more benign course.[112]

Histopathology. A deep biopsy usually shows both subcutaneous and dermal nodules composed of macrophages and a

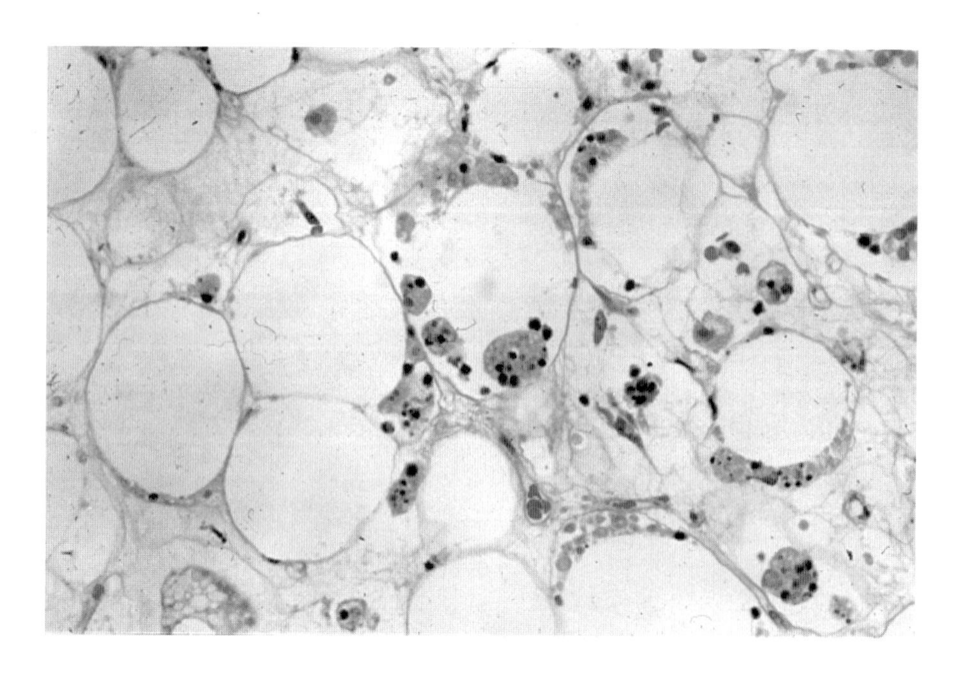

FIG. 20-30. Histiocytic cytophagic panniculitis
Macrophages and multinucleated cells ingest lymphocytes and erythrocytes to form so-called "bean bag cells."

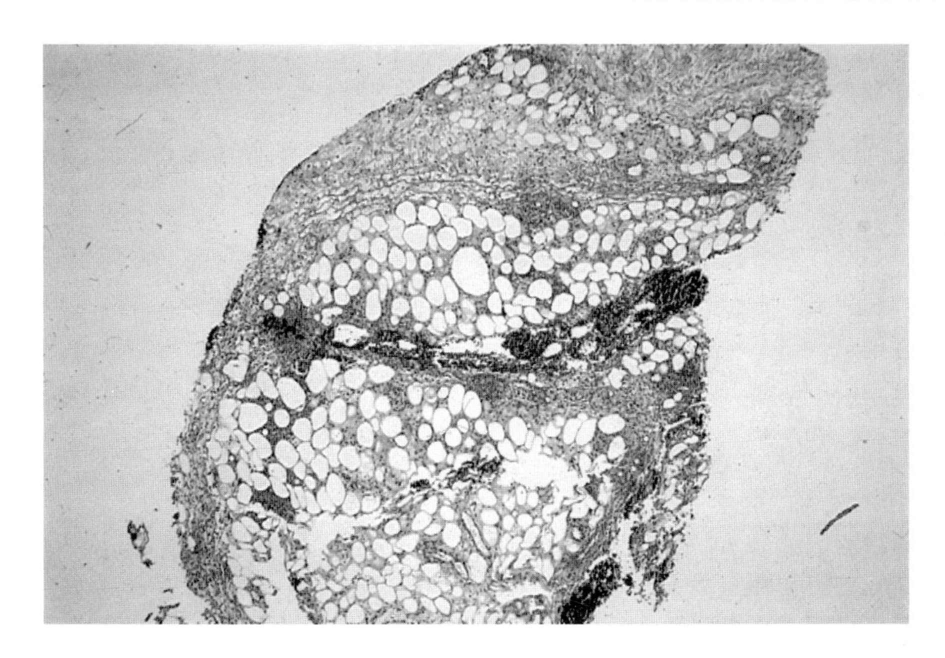

FIG. 20-31. Mycobacterial panniculitis
Direct mycobacterial infection of the panniculus has produced both a septal and lobular panniculitis.

mixed inflammatory infiltrate. In the subcutis the inflammation is both septal and lobular (see Color Fig. 20-6). Often there is necrosis and hemorrhage (Fig. 20-29). The nuclei of the macrophages are within the range of sizes and shapes seen in benign inflammatory disorders. In some areas the macrophages become so engorged by phagocytosis of erythrocytes, lymphocytes, and cell fragments that they have been named "bean bag cells" (Fig. 20-30).[73] In some patients early lesions contain a rather dense infiltrate of small lymphocytes and only focal areas with cytophagic histiocytes.

The involvement of other organs by similar cytophagic macrophages leads to diffuse infiltration of liver, bone marrow, spleen, lymph nodes, myocardium, lungs, and gastrointestinal tract.[118] The cytophagic macrophages can deplete almost all of the bone marrow elements.

Pathogenesis. When originally described, the disease was differentiated from malignant histiocytosis by the fact that the nuclei of the macrophages in the cytophagic panniculitis were not cytologically atypical. Due to the fulminant course in some patients, the disease is considered by some to be a variant form of malignant histiocytosis that can remain confined to the skin and subcutis for a protracted period.[119] However, more recently the similarity to terminal hemophagocytic syndromes associated with lymphomas[120,121] has led to consideration that the cytophagic panniculitis is the result of an abnormal lymphocyte population that has stimulated benign macrophages to engage in fulminant hemophagocytosis.[122–126] Viral infections that are associated with hemophagocytic syndromes, without lymphoma, usually do not have panniculitis.

MISCELLANEOUS PANNICULITIS

The administration of bromide and iodide compounds can produce a panniculitis, usually in association with changes in the overlying epidermis and dermis. Due to the decrease in therapeutic use of bromide and iodide compounds, the number of patients with this disorder has decreased dramatically. In reactions to bromide or iodide administration there is epidermal hyperplasia that can develop pseudoepitheliomatous features and intraepidermal abscesses of neutrophils and eosinophils. Allergy to potassium bromide has been demonstrated in some patients by a lymphocyte-transformation test.[127]

Painful lipomatous masses can develop in severely obese patients with histological evidence of inflammation of nerves and endocrine abnormalities. This disease, called adiposis dolorosa or Dercum's disease, is rare, occurs in middle age, and affects females more than males.[128,129]

Mycobacterial infection of the fat can produce a *mycobacterial panniculitis* that can mimic erythema nodosum (Figs. 20-31 and 20-32) as well as erythema induratum.[130] Special stains for acid-fast bacteria and cultures are important for the identification of the mycobacteria that are responsible. Often nontuberculous mycobacteria are involved in countries with a low incidence of tuberculosis.

Morphea or scleroderma can produce a panniculitis that has dense infiltrates of lymphocytes and plasma cells at the periphery of the fat lobules, particularly at the junction of deep reticular dermis and the subcutis. Characteristically the septa are widened and have hyalinized sclerotic collagen. Similar changes in the collagen are noted in the overlying dermis in most cases. Some of the changes are similar to those of lupus panniculitis so that immunofluorescence and serologic tests are needed to distinguish them.[131–133] Discoid lupus erythematosus with panniculitis has more fibrinoid necrosis of the dermis, which stains more brightly eosinophilic than the staining of the pale sclerotic collagen bundles of morphea or scleroderma panniculitis.

Pyoderma gangrenosum can produce ulcers that are difficult to distinguish from those of an ulcerating panniculitis.[21,134]

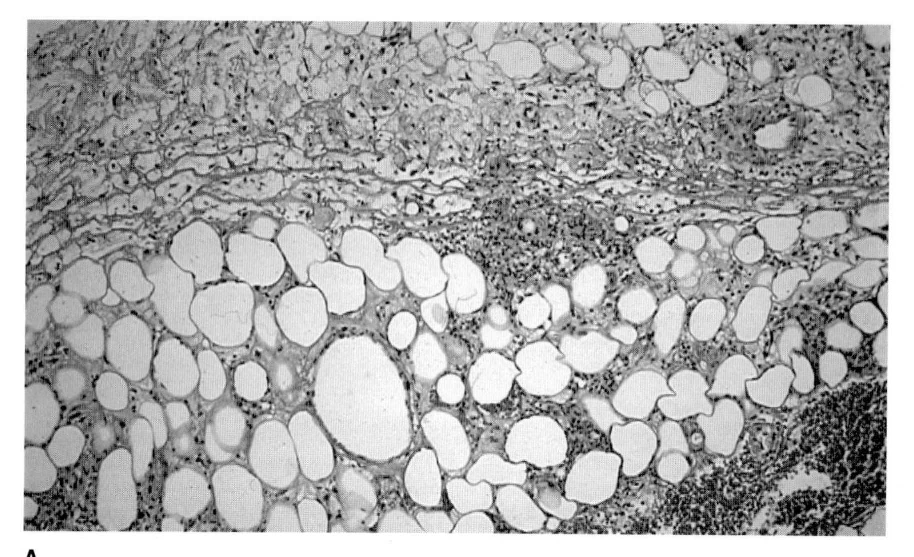

A

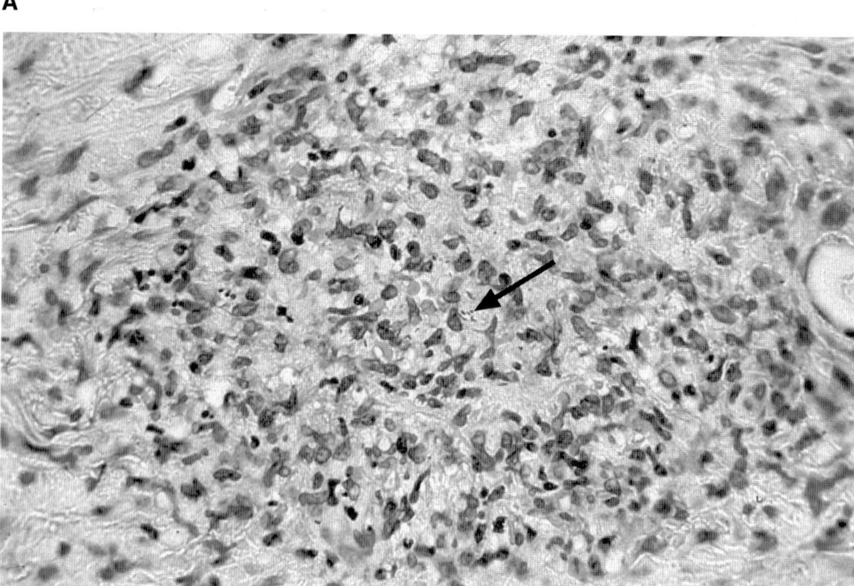

B

FIG. 20-32. Mycobacterial panniculitis
(**A**) Collections of neutrophils, edema and small granulomas can closely mimic the histology of erythema nodosum. (**B**) Staining for mycobacteria shows that numerous red, acid-fast bacilli (arrow) are present in this example (AFB stain).

However, the gross appearance of pyoderma gangrenosum is characteristic in the irregularity of the ulcers, their shallowness, and the undermined violaceous borders. Biopsies taken at the edges of the ulceration may show pustules and lymphocytic inflammation in the dermis with extension of the lymphoid cells into the septa and lobules of the panniculus. The lesions do not have the extensive necrosis of the fat that is present in erythema induratum or the macrophage infiltration into the lobules of Weber-Christian disease. The sterile abscesses of α_1-antitrypsin deficiency panniculitis resemble those of pyoderma gangrenosum, but extend deeper than pyoderma gangrenosum, which lacks abscesses in the fat.

REFERENCES

1. Winkelmann RK, Forstrom L. New observations in the histopathology of erythema nodosum. J Invest Dermatol 1975;65:441.
2. Niemi KM, Forstrom L, Hannuksela M et al. Nodules on the legs. Acta Derm Venereol (Stockh) 1977;57:145.
3. Pierini LE, Abulafia J, Wainfeld S. Idiopathic lipogranulomatous hypodermitis. Arch Dermatol 1969;98:290.

4. Braverman IM. Skin signs of systemic disease. Philadelphia: Saunders, 1981;476.
5. Bafverstedt B. Erythema nodosum migrans. Acta Derm Venereol (Stockh) 1968;48:381.
6. Vilanova X, Pinol Aguadé J. Subacute nodular migratory panniculitis. Br J Dermatol 1959;71:45.
7. Ackerman AB, Ragaz A. The Lives of Lesions: Chronology in Dermatopathology. New York: Masson Publishing USA, Inc., 1984;65.
8. Forstrom L, Winkelmann RK. Acute panniculitis. Arch Dermatol 1977;113:909.
9. Miescher G. Zur histologie des erythema nodosum. Acta Derm Venereol (Stockh) 1947;27:447.
10. Sanchez Yus E, Sanz Vico MD, de Diego V. Miescher's radial granuloma: A characteristic marker of erythema nodosum. Am J Dermatopathol 1989;11:434.
11. Zabel M. Zur histopathologie des erythema nodosum. Z Hautkr 1977; 52:1253.
12. Ackerman AB. In answer to "Questions to the editorial board." Am J Dermatopathol 1983;5:409.
13. Montgomery H. Dermatopathology. New York: Hoeber Medical Division, Harper & Row, 1967;1.
14. Fine RM, Meltzer HD. Chronic erythema nodosum. Arch Dermatol 1969;100:33.
15. Hannuksela M. Erythema nodosum migrans. Acta Derm Venereol (Stockh) 1973;53:313.
16. Forstrom L, Winkelmann RK. Granulomatous panniculitis in erythema nodosum. Arch Dermatol 1975;111:335.
17. Prestes C, Winkelmann RK, Su WPD. Septal granulomatous panniculitis: Comparison of the pathology of erythema nodosum migrans (migratory panniculitis) and chronic erythema nodosum. J Am Acad Dermatol 1990;22:477.
18. Weedon D. Systemic pathology. Vol. 9. New York: Churchill Livingstone 1992;1.
19. DeBois J, van de Pitte J, de Greef H. Yersinia enterocolitica as a cause of erythema nodosum. Dermatologica 1978;156:65.
20. Medeiros AA, Marty SD, Tosh FE et al. Erythema nodosum and erythema multiforme as clinical manifestations of histoplasmosis in a community outbreak. N Engl J Med 1966;274:415.
21. Gellert A, Green ES, Beck ER, Ridley CM. Erythema nodosum progressing to pyoderma gangrenosum as a complication of Crohn's disease. Postgrad Med J 1983;59:791.
22. Chun SI, Su WPD, Lee S, Rogers RS. Erythema nodosum-like lesions in Behçet's syndrome. J Cutan Pathol 1989;16:259.
23. Blaustein A, Moreno A, Noguera J, de Moragas JM. Septal granulomatous panniculitis in Sweet's syndrome. Arch Dermatol 1985;121: 785.
24. Salvatore MA, Lynch PJ. Erythema nodosum, estrogens, and pregnancy. Arch Dermatol 1980;116:557.
25. Haustein UF, Klug H. Ultrastrukturelle untersuchungen der blutgefasse beim erythema nodosum. Dermatol Monatsschr 1977;163:13.
26. Nunnery E, Persellin RH, Pope RM. Lack of circulating immune complexes in uncomplicated erythema nodosum. J Rheumatol 1983;10: 991.
27. Verrier Jones J, Cummings RH, Asplin CM et al. Evidence of circulating immune complexes in erythema nodosum and early sarcoidosis. Ann N Y Acad Sci 1976;278:212.
28. Winkelmann RK, Frigas E. Eosinophilic panniculitis: A clinicopathologic study. J Cutan Pathol 1986;13:1.
29. Burket JM, Burket BJ. Eosinophilic panniculitis. J Am Acad Dermatol 1985;12:161.
30. Glass LA, Zaghloul AB, Solomon AR. Eosinophilic panniculitis associated with recurrent parotitis. Am J Dermatopathol 1989;11:555.
31. Ollague W, Ollague J, Guevara de Veliz A, Penaherrera S. Human gnathostomiasis in Ecuador: Nodular migratory eosinophilic panniculitis. Int J Dermatol 1984;23:647.
32. Kato N. Eosinophilic panniculitis. J Dermatol 1993;20:185.
33. Whittaker SJ, Jones RR, Spry CJF. Lymphomatoid papulosis and its relationship to "idiopathic" hypereosinophilic syndrome. J Am Acad Dermatol 1988;18:339.
34. Cogan E, Schandene L, Crusiaux A et al. Clonal proliferation of type 2 helper T cells in a man with the hypereosinophilic syndrome. N Engl J Med 1994;330:535.
35. Fagerhol MK, Cox DW. The Pi polymorphism: Genetic, biochemical and clinical aspects of human alpha-1-antitrypsin. Adv Hum Genet 1981;11:1.
36. Eriksson S, Carlson J, Velez R. Risk of cirrhosis and primary liver cancer in alpha-1-antitrypsin deficiency. N Engl J Med 1986;314:736.
37. Sveger T. Alpha-1-antitrypsin deficiency in early childhood. Pediatrics 1978;62:22.
38. Breit SN, Clark P, Robinson JP et al. Familial occurrence of alpha-1-antitrypsin deficiency and Weber-Christian disease. Arch Dermatol 1983;119:198.
39. Bleumink E, Klokke HA. Protease-inhibitor deficiencies in a patient with Weber-Christian panniculitis. Arch Dermatol 1984;120:936.
40. Smith KC, Su WP, Pittelkow MR, Winkelmann RK. Clinical and pathologic correlations in 96 patients with panniculitis, including 15 patients with deficient levels of alpha-1-antitrypsin. J Am Acad Dermatol 1989;21:1192.
41. Hendrick SJ, Silverman AK, Solomon AR, Headington JT. Alpha-1-antitrypsin deficiency associated with panniculitis. J Am Acad Dermatol 1988;18:684.
42. Smith KC, Pittelkow MR, Su WPD. Panniculitis associated with severe alpha-1-antitrypsin deficiency: Treatment and review of the literature. Arch Dermatol 1987;123:1655.
43. Geller JD, Su WPD. A subtle clue to the histopathologic diagnosis of early alpha-1-antitrypsin deficiency panniculitis. J Am Acad Dermatol 1994;31:241.
44. Langenberg A, Egbert B. Neutrophilic tuberculous panniculitis in a patient with polymyositis. J Cutan Pathol 1993;20:177.
45. Samlaska CP, James WD. Superficial thrombophlebitis: I. Primary hypercoagulable states. J Am Acad Dermatol 1990;22:975.
46. Samlaska CP, James WD. Superficial thrombophlebitis: II. Secondary hypercoagulable states. J Am Acad Dermatol 1990;23:1.
47. Schuppli R. Zur atiologie der phlebitis saltans. Hautarzt 1959;10:466.
48. Montgomery H, O'Leary PA, Barker NW. Nodular vascular diseases of the legs: Erythema induratum and allied conditions. JAMA 1945; 128:335.
49. Rademaker M, Lowe DG, Munro DD. Erythema induratum (Bazin's disease). J Am Acad Dermatol 1989;21:740.
50. van der Lugt L. Some remarks about tuberculosis of the skin and tuberculids. Dermatologica 1965;131:26.
51. Thompson R, Urbach F. Erythema induratum. Int J Dermatol 1987;26: 402.
52. Cribier B. Étude immunohistochimique de la vasculite nodulaire: Role possible d'une hypersensibilite retardée cellulaire. Ann Dermatol Venereol 1992;119:958.
53. Penneys NS, Leonardi CL, Cook S et al. Identification of *Mycobacterium tuberculosis* DNA in five different types of cutaneous lesions by the polymerase chain reaction. Arch Dermatol 1993;129:1594.
54. Ollert MW, Thomas P, Korting HC et al. Erythema induratum of Bazin: Evidence of T-lymphocyte hyperresponsiveness to purified protein derivative of tuberculin. Report of two cases and treatment. Arch Dermatol 1993;129:469.
55. Sanchez NP, Peters MS, Winkelmann RK. The histopathology of lupus erythematosus panniculitis. J Am Acad Dermatol 1981;5:673.
56. Izumi AK, Takiguchi P. Lupus erythematosus panniculitis. Arch Dermatol 1983;119:61.
57. Tuffanelli DL. Lupus panniculitis. Sem Dermatol 1985;4:79.
58. Peters MS, Winkelmann RK. Localized lipoatrophy: Atrophic connective tissue disease panniculitis. Arch Dermatol 1980;116:1363.
59. Harris RB, Duncan SC, Ecker RI, Winkelmann RK. Lymphoid follicles in subcutaneous inflammatory disease. Arch Dermatol 1979;115: 442.
60. Taieb A, Hehunstre JP, Goetz J et al. Lupus erythematosus panniculitis with partial genetic deficiency of C2 and C4 in a child. Arch Dermatol 1986;122:576.
61. Meyer O, Hauptmann G, Tappeiner G et al. Genetic deficiency of C4, C2 or C1q and lupus syndromes: Association with anti-Ro(SS-A) antibodies. Clin Exp Immunol 1985;62:678.
62. Provost TT, Arnett FC, Reichlin M. C2 deficiency, lupus erythematosus and anticytoplasmic Ro(SS-A) antibodies. Arthritis Rheum 1983; 26:1533.
63. Hendricks WM, Ahmad M, Gratz E. Weber-Christian syndrome in infancy. Br J Dermatol 1978;98:175.
64. Albrectsen B. The Weber-Christian syndrome, with particular reference to etiology. Acta Derm Venereol (Stockh) 1960;40:474.

65. Ciclitira PJ, Wight DGD, Dick AP. Systemic Weber-Christian disease. Br J Dermatol 1980;103:685.
66. Thiers BH. Relapsing febrile nonsuppurative nodular panniculitis (Weber-Christian disease). In: Demis DJ, McGuire J, eds. Clinical dermatology. Philadelphia: Harper & Row, 1984;1.
67. Lever WF. Nodular nonsuppurative panniculitis (Weber-Christian disease). Arch Dermatol 1949;59:31.
68. Cummins LJ, Lever WF. Relapsing febrile nodular nonsuppurative panniculitis (Weber-Christian disease). Arch Dermatol Syphilol 1938; 38:415.
69. Steinberg B. Systemic nodular panniculitis. Am J Pathol 1953;29: 1059.
70. Miller JL, Kritzler RA. Nodular nonsuppurative panniculitis. Arch Dermatol Syphilol 1943;47:82.
71. Pinals RS. Nodular panniculitis associated with an inflammatory bone lesion. Arch Dermatol 1970;101:359.
72. MacDonald A, Feiwel M. A review of the concept of Weber-Christian panniculitis with a report of five cases. Br J Dermatol 1968;80:355.
73. Winkelmann RK, Bowie EJW. Hemorrhagic diathesis associated with benign histiocytic, cytophagic panniculitis and systemic histiocytosis. Arch Intern Med 1980;140:1460.
74. Baumgartner W, Riva G. Panniculitis, die herdformige fettgewebsentzundung. Helv Med Acta (Suppl)1945;12:3.
75. Schuppli R. Die panniculitis typus Rothmann-Makai. In: Marchionini A, ed. Handbuch der haut- und geschlectskrankheiten. Vol. II. Berlin: Springer-Verlag, 1965;2.
76. Forstrom L, Winkelmann RK. Factitial panniculitis. Arch Dermatol 1974;110:747.
77. Parks DL, Perry HO, Muller SA. Cutaneous complications of pentazocine injections. Arch Dermatol 1971;104:231.
78. Oertel YC, Johnson FB. Sclerosing lipogranuloma of the male genitalia. Arch Pathol 1977;101:321.
79. Winer LH, Steinberg TH, Lehman R et al. Tissue reactions to injected silicone liquids. Arch Dermatol 1964;90:588.
80. Ackerman AB, Mosher DT, Schwamm HA. Factitial Weber-Christian syndrome. JAMA 1966;198:731.
81. Rotman H. Cold panniculitis in children. Arch Dermatol 1966;94:720.
82. Duncan WC, Freeman RG, Heaton CL. Cold panniculitis. Arch Dermatol 1966;94:722.
83. Epstein EH Jr, Oren ME. Popsicle panniculitis. N Engl J Med 1970; 282:966.
84. Best EW, Mason HL, Deweerd JW et al. Sclerosing lipogranuloma of the male genitalia produced by mineral oil. Mayo Clin Proc 1953;28: 623.
85. Newcomer VD, Graham JH, Schaffert RR et al. Sclerosing lipogranuloma resulting from exogenous lipids. Arch Dermatol 1956;73:361.
86. Beacham BE, Cooper PH, Buchanan S et al. Equestrian cold panniculitis in women. Arch Dermatol 1980;116:1025.
87. Kellum RE, Ray TL, Brown GR. Sclerema neonatorum. Arch Dermatol 1968;97:372.
88. Taylor WB, Honeycutt WM. Progressive lipodystrophy and lipoatrophic diabetes. Arch Dermatol 1961;84:31.
89. Chartier S, Buzzanga JB, Paquin F. Partial lipodystrophy associated with a type 3 form of membranoproliferative glomerulonephritis. J Am Acad Dermatol 1987;16:201.
90. Handfield-Jones SE, Stephens CJ, Mayou BJ, Black MM. The clinical spectrum of lipoatrophic panniculitis encompasses connective tissue panniculitis. Br J Dermatol 1993;129:619.
91. Peters MS, Winkelmann RK. The histopathology of localized lipoatrophy. Br J Dermatol 1986;114:27.
92. Cannon JR, Pitha JV, Everett MA. Subcutaneous fat necrosis in pancreatitis. J Cutan Pathol 1979;6:501.
93. De Graciansky P. Weber-Christian syndrome of pancreatic origin. Br J Dermatol 1967;79:278.
94. Hughes PSH, Apisarnthanarax P, Mullins JF. Subcutaneous fat necrosis associated with pancreatic disease. Arch Dermatol 1975;111:506.
95. Mullin GT, Caperton EM Jr, Crespin SR et al. Arthritis and skin lesions resembling erythema nodosum in pancreatic disease. Ann Intern Med 1968;68:75.
96. Millns JL, Evans HL, Winkelmann RK. Association of islet cell carcinoma of the pancreas with subcutaneous fat necrosis. Am J Dermatopathol 1979;1:273.
97. Levine N, Lazarus GS. Subcutaneous fat necrosis after paracentesis: Report of a case in a patient with acute pancreatitis. Arch Dermatol 1976;112:993.
98. Zeek P, Madden EM. Sclerema adiposum neonatorum of both internal and external adipose tissue. Arch Pathol 1946;41:166.
99. Flory CM. Fat necrosis of the newborn. Arch Pathol 1948;45:278.
100. Horsfield GI, Yardley HJ. Sclerema neonatorum. J Invest Dermatol 1965;44:326.
101. Oswalt GC Jr, Montes LF, Cassady G. Subcutaneous fat necrosis of the newborn. J Cutan Pathol 1978;5:193.
102. Norwood-Galloway A, Lebwohl M, Phelps RG et al. Subcutaneous fat necrosis of the newborn with hypercalcemia. J Am Acad Dermatol 1987;16:435.
103. Silverman AK, Michels EH, Rasmussen JE. Subcutaneous fat necrosis in an infant, occurring after hypothermic cardiac surgery. J Am Acad Dermatol 1986;15:331.
104. Tsuji T. Subcutaneous fat necrosis of the newborn: Light and electron microscopic studies. Br J Dermatol 1976;95:407.
105. Roenigk HH Jr, Haserick JR, Arundell FD. Poststeroid panniculitis. Arch Dermatol 1964;90:387.
106. Fischer AH, Morris DJ. Pathogenesis of calciphylaxis: Study of three cases with literature review. Hum Pathol 1995;26:1055.
107. Buchet S, Blanc D, Humbert P et al. La panniculite calcifiante. Ann Dermatol Venereol 1992;119:659.
108. Lowry LR, Tschen JA, Wolf JE, Yen A. Calcifying panniculitis and systemic calciphylaxis in an end-stage renal patient. Cutis 1993;51: 245.
109. Alegre VA, Winkelmann RK, Aliaga A. Lipomembranous changes in chronic panniculitis. J Am Acad Dermatol 1988;19:39.
110. Jorizzo JL, White WL, Zanolli MD et al. Sclerosing panniculitis. Arch Dermatol 1991;127:554.
111. Snow JL, Su WPD, Gibson LE. Lipomembranous (membranocystic) changes associated with morphea: A clinicopathologic review of three cases. J Am Acad Dermatol 1994;31:246.
112. White JW Jr, Winkelmann RK. Cytophagic histiocytic panniculitis is not always fatal. J Cutan Pathol 1989;16:137.
113. Garcia Consuegra J, Barrio MI, Fonseca E et al. Histiocytic cytophagic panniculitis: Report of a case in a 12-year-old girl. Eur J Pediatr 1991;150:468.
114. Peters MS, Su WPD. Panniculitis. Dermatol Clin 1992;10:37.
115. Willis SM, Opal SM, Fitzpatrick JE. Cytophagic histiocytic panniculitis: Systemic histiocytosis presenting as chronic, nonhealing, ulcerative skin lesions. Arch Dermatol 1985;121:910.
116. Alegre VA, Winkelmann RK. Histiocytic cytophagic panniculitis. J Am Acad Dermatol 1989;20:177.
117. Alegre VA, Fortea JM, Camps C, Aliaga A. Cytophagic histiocytic panniculitis: Case report with resolution after treatment. J Am Acad Dermatol 1989;20:875.
118. Crotty CP, Winkelmann RK. Cytophagic histiocytic panniculitis with fever, cytopenia, liver failure, and terminal hemorrhagic diathesis. J Am Acad Dermatol 1981;4:181.
119. Ducatman BS, Wick MR, Morgan TW et al. Malignant histiocytosis: A clinical, histologic, and immunohistochemical study of 20 cases. Hum Pathol 1984;15:368.
120. Jaffe ES, Costa J, Fauci AS et al. Malignant lymphoma and erythrophagocytosis simulating malignant histiocytosis. Am J Med 1983;75: 741.
121. Avinoach I, Halevy S, Argov S, Sacks M. Gamma/delta T-cell lymphoma involving the subcutaneous tissue and associated with a hemophagocytic syndrome. Am J Dermatopathol 1994;16:426.
122. Gonzalez CL, Medeiros LJ, Braziel RM, Jaffe ES. T-cell lymphoma involving subcutaneous tissue: A clinicopathologic entity commonly associated with hemophagocytic syndrome. Am J Surg Path 1991; 15:17.
123. Peters MS, Winkelmann RK. Cytophagic panniculitis and B cell lymphoma. J Am Acad Dermatol 1985;13:882.
124. Aronson IK, West DP, Variakojis D et al. Panniculitis associated with cutaneous T-cell lymphoma and cytophagic histiocytosis. Br J Dermatol 1985;112:87.
125. Perniciaro C, Zalla MJ, White JW Jr, Menke DM. Subcutaneous T-cell lymphoma: Report of two additional cases and further observations. Arch Dermatol 1993;129:1171.

126. Hytiroglou P, Phelps RG, Wattenberg DJ, Strauchen JA. Histiocytic cytophagic panniculitis: Molecular evidence for a clonal T-cell disorder. J Am Acad Dermatol 1992;27:333.
127. Diener W, Kruse R, Berg P. Halogenpannikulitis auf kaliumbromid. Monatsschr Kinderheilkd 1993;141:705.
128. Dercum FX. Adiposis dolorosa. Am J Med Sci 1982;104:521.
129. Winkelman NW, Eckel JL. Adiposis dolorosa (Dercum's disease): A clinicopathologic study. JAMA 1925;85:1935.
130. Santa Cruz DJ, Strayer DS. The histologic spectrum of the cutaneous mycobacterioses. Hum Pathol 1982;13:485.
131. Su WPD, Person JR. Morphea profunda: A new concept and a histopathologic study of 23 cases. Am J Dermatopathol 1981;3:251.
132. Winkelmann RK. Panniculitis in connective tissue disease. Arch Dermatol 1983;119:336.
133. Winkelmann RK, Padilha-Goncalves A. Connective tissue panniculitis. Arch Dermatol 1980;116:291.
134. Powell FC, Schroeter AL, Su WPD, Perry HO. Pyoderma gangrenosum and monoclonal gammopathy. Arch Dermatol 1983;119:468.

Lever's Histopathology of the Skin, eighth edition, edited by David Elder et al. Lippincott–Raven Publishers, Philadelphia © 1997.

CHAPTER 21

Bacterial Disease

Sebastian Lucas

IMPETIGO

Two types of impetigo occur: impetigo contagiosa, or nonbullous impetigo, usually caused by group A streptococci; and bullous impetigo, including the staphylococcal scalded-skin syndrome, which is caused by *Staphylococcus aureus.*[1]

Impetigo Contagiosa

Impetigo contagiosa is primarily an endemic disease of preschool-age children that may occur in epidemics. Very early lesions consist of vesicopustules that rupture quickly and are followed by heavy, yellow crusts. Most of the lesions are located in exposed areas. An occasional sequela is acute glomerulonephritis. As a rule, however, the nephritis following impetigo contagiosa has a favorable long-term prognosis.[2]

Histopathology. The vesicopustule arises in the upper layers of the epidermis above, within, or below the granular layer (see Classification of Bullae, Chap. 9). It contains numerous neutrophils (Fig. 21-1). Not infrequently, a few acantholytic cells can be observed at the floor of the vesicopustule.[3] Occasionally, Gram-positive cocci can also be found within the vesicopustule, both within neutrophils and extracellularly.[4]

The stratum malpighii underlying the bulla is spongiotic, and neutrophils often can be seen migrating through it. The upper dermis contains a moderately severe inflammatory infiltrate of neutrophils and lymphoid cells.

At a later stage, when the bulla has ruptured, the horny layer is absent, and a crust composed of serous exudate and the nuclear debris of neutrophils may be seen covering the stratum malpighii.

Pathogenesis. In the United States, group A streptococci used to be the most frequently recovered organisms in patients with impetigo contagiosa, either alone or in association with *S aureus.*[5] However, the predominant pathogen responsible for impetigo has been changing. In recent years, cultures of specimens from patients with impetigo in nearly all instances have grown coagulase-positive *S aureus* that has proved resistant to penicillin and ampicillin but has responded to antibiotics such as cloxacillin.[6,7] More recently, topical mupirocin, which has excellent activity against methicillin-resistant *S aureus* (MSRA), has been used.[1] Group A streptococci may be found in combination with staphylococci.[1] In Great Britain, *S aureus* has been the most commonly recovered organism for a long time.[8]

Differential Diagnosis. Histologic differentiation of impetigo contagiosa from subcorneal pustular dermatosis and from pemphigus foliaceus can be difficult. However, only impetigo shows Gram-positive cocci in the bulla cavity. In addition, pemphigus foliaceus usually shows fewer neutrophils, more acantholytic cells, and occasionally some dyskeratotic granular cells (Chap. 9).

Bullous Impetigo and Staphylococcal Scalded-Skin Syndrome

Phage group II staphylococci may produce bullous impetigo and the staphylococcal scalded-skin syndrome.

Bullous impetigo occurs mainly in newborns, infants, and young children. Occasionally, it is observed in adults, particularly in those with deficiencies in cell-mediated immunity.[9,10] It is characterized by vesicles that rapidly progress to flaccid bullae with little or no surrounding erythema. The contents of the bullae are clear at first; later on, they may be turbid. Bullous impetigo may spread and become generalized, so that clinical distinction from staphylococcal scalded-skin syndrome may be impossible.[11] An important difference, however, is that cultures from intact bullae of bullous impetigo, unlike those of the staphylococcal scalded-skin syndrome, grow phage group II *S aureus.*

Staphylococcal scalded-skin syndrome, first described more than 100 years ago[12] and also known as Ritter's disease, occurs largely in the newborn and in children younger than 5 years. It rarely occurs in adults[13–15] or in older children[16] except in the presence of a severe underlying disease.[17]

The disease begins abruptly with diffuse erythema and fever. Large, flaccid bullae filled with clear fluid form and rupture almost immediately. Large sheets of superficial epidermis separate and exfoliate. The disease runs an acute course and is fatal

S. Lucas: UMDS Department of Histopathology, St. Thomas' Hospital, London, United Kingdom

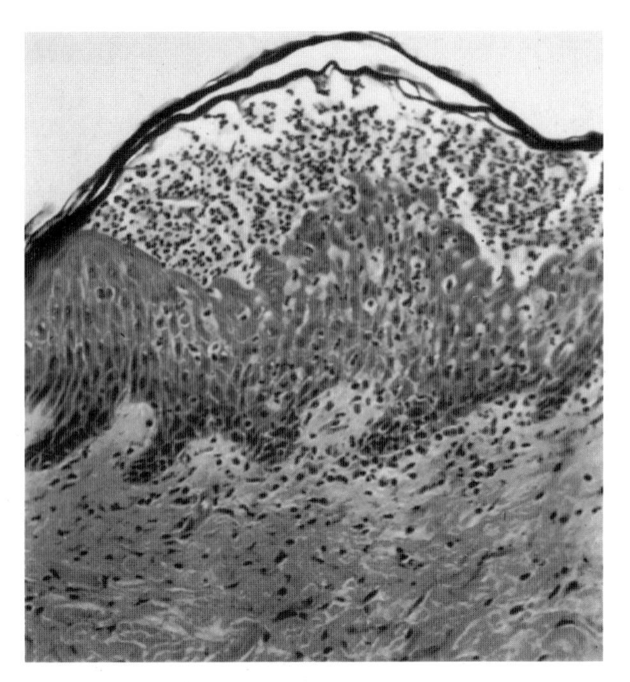

FIG. 21-1. Impetigo contagiosa
A subcorneal pustule containing numerous neutrophils is present. The underlying stratum malpighii shows spongiosis, and neutrophils are seen migrating through it (original magnification ×200).

in less than 4% of all cases in children.[18] Most fatalities occur in neonates with generalized lesions. In contrast, in the rare cases of staphylococcal scalded-skin syndrome occurring in adults, the prognosis is much worse, with a mortality rate exceeding 50%. Death is usually related to the coexistent disease or to immunosuppressive therapy given for it.[13] Both bullous impetigo and staphylococcal scalded-skin syndrome are transmissible and can cause epidemics in nurseries, where they may occur together.[19]

An important difference between the two diseases is that no phage group II staphylococci can be grown from the bullae of the staphylococcal scalded-skin syndrome, in contrast to the bullae of bullous impetigo. The absence of phage group II staphylococci from the bullae of staphylococcal scalded-skin syndrome results from the fact that these staphylococci are present at a distant focus. Usually, the distant focus is extracutaneous and consists of a purulent conjunctivitis, rhinitis, or pharyngitis.[18] Rarely, the distant focus consists of a cutaneous infection[14] or a septicemia.[13] The bullae are caused by a staphylococcal toxin referred to as exfoliatin (see section on Pathogenesis).

Histopathology. In both bullous impetigo and staphylococcal scalded-skin syndrome, the cleavage plane of the bulla, like that in impetigo contagiosa, lies in the uppermost epidermis either below or, less commonly, within the granular layer. A few acantholytic cells are often seen adjoining the cleavage plane.[18] In contrast to impetigo contagiosa, however, there are few or no inflammatory cells within the bulla cavity. In bullous impetigo, the upper dermis may show a polymorphous infiltrate, whereas in the staphylococcal scalded-skin syndrome the dermis is usually free of inflammation.[11]

Pathogenesis. The causative factor is the exfoliative toxin (ET, or exfoliatin) produced by group II *S aureus* strains. The mechanism of the separation through the stratum granulosum is not known, but binding to filaggrin may be involved.[17,20] The toxins may have serine protease activity.[22] When cultures of phage group II staphylococci obtained either from the bullae of bullous impetigo or from the distant sites of infection in staphylococcal scalded-skin syndrome, or the exotoxin exfoliatin isolated from such cultures, are injected subcutaneously into newborn mice, they produce generalized exfoliation with intraepidermal cleavage, largely at the level of the stratum granulosum.[19,20] The reason that only neonatal mice develop generalized exfoliation is that adult mice excrete test doses of exfoliatin rapidly, within a few hours, but newborn mice excrete exfoliatin slowly. This probably results from the fact that the newborn kidney is not fully developed.[23] In humans, the ability of adult kidneys to excrete exfoliatin produced by phage group II staphylococci explains the rarity of staphylococcal scalded-skin syndrome in adults, and the increased susceptibility to the disease in adult patients with chronic renal failure.[17] In addition, most adults are protected by antibodies to the toxin, which are less prevalent in young children.[17]

Electron microscopy shows that the cleavage plane of lesions in humans as well as in mice is at the interface between the spinous and granular layers, with some upward extension into the lower granular layer. Splitting occurs without damage to adjacent acantholytic keratinocytes.[18] Exfoliatin appears to act primarily on the intercellular substance, because, in studies carried out on newborn mice, the intercellular spaces widen and microvilli form before the desmosomes separate within their interdesmosomal contact zone.[24,25]

Differential Diagnosis. Both staphylococcal scalded-skin syndrome and severe erythema multiforme of the toxic epidermal necrolysis or Lyell type show clinically extensive detachment of the epidermis and thus may clinically resemble one another. This has resulted in confusion in the past, so that at one time both diseases were referred to as Lyell's disease or toxic epidermal necrolysis. However, the two diseases can be easily differentiated histologically; in severe erythema multiforme, the entire, or nearly the entire, epidermis detaches itself, with considerable necrosis of the epidermal cells (Chap. 9), whereas in staphylococcal scalded-skin syndrome only the uppermost portion of the epidermis becomes detached, with relatively slight damage to the underlying epidermal cells.[26]

In fulminating cases in which rapid differentiation between the two diseases is required, one may obtain a freshly made peel of skin by eliciting the Nikolsky phenomenon. The peel is placed in normal saline solution and frozen in it to form a block. Sections cut with a cryostat and stained with hematoxylin-eosin then show the histologic differences just described.[27] In addition, a Tzanck smear may be obtained from the denuded base, fixed with 95% methyl alcohol for 1 minute, and then stained with the Giemsa or Wright stain for 5 minutes. In the staphylococcal scalded-skin syndrome, the smear shows elongated epithelial cells with relatively small nuclei, as seen in the upper epidermis, and no inflammatory cells. In severe erythema multiforme of the toxic epidermal necrolysis type, the smear shows either cuboidal cells with relatively large nuclei, as seen in the lower epidermis, or inflammatory cells, or both.[26,27]

ECTHYMA

Ecthyma is essentially ulcerated impetigo contagiosa. It occurs chiefly below the knees as multiple crusted ulcers. It is clearly streptococcal in origin, because skin cultures are nearly always positive for group A streptococci. In addition, coagulase-positive staphylococci as secondary invaders can frequently be cultured from lesions.[28]

Histopathology. A nonspecific ulcer is observed with numerous neutrophils both in the dermis and in the serous exudate at the floor of the ulcer.

ERYSIPELAS

Erysipelas is an acute superficial cellulitis of the skin caused by group A streptococci. It is characterized by the presence of a well-demarcated, slightly indurated, dusky red area with an advancing, palpable border. In some patients, erysipelas has a tendency to recur periodically in the same areas. In the early antibiotic era, the incidence of erysipelas appeared to be on the decline and most cases occurred on the face. More recently, however, there appears to have been an increase in the incidence, and facial sites are now less common whereas erysipelas of the legs is predominant.[29] Potential complications in patients with poor resistance or after inadequate therapy may include abscess formation, spreading necrosis of the soft tissue, infrequently necrotizing fasciitis, and septicemia.[29] Nephritic and cardiac complications are rare because erysipelas is usually produced by nonnephritogenic and nonrheumatogenic strains of streptococci.[29]

Histopathology. The dermis shows marked edema and dilatation of the lymphatics and capillaries. There is a diffuse infiltrate, composed chiefly of neutrophils, that extends throughout the dermis and occasionally into the subcutaneous fat. It shows a loose arrangement around dilated blood and lymph vessels. If sections are stained with the Giemsa or Gram stain, streptococci are found in the tissue and within lymphatics.[30]

In cases of recurring erysipelas, the lymph vessels of the dermis and subcutaneous tissue show fibrotic thickening of their walls with partial or complete occlusion of the lumen.[31]

NECROTIZING FASCIITIS

Necrotizing fasciitis, like erysipelas, is caused by group A beta-hemolytic streptococci and it shows rapidly spreading erythema. However, the erythema is ill-defined and progresses to painless ulceration and necrosis along fascial planes. Whereas erysipelas involves the more superficial layers of the skin, cellulitis extends more deeply into the subcutaneous tissues.[32] Although virtually all cases of erysipelas are caused by beta-hemolytic streptococci, primarily group A, the differential diagnosis of cellulitis is much more extensive. In addition to group A streptococci, possible etiologic agents include *Staphylococcus aureus* and, less frequently, *Streptococcus pneumoniae, Haemophilus influenzae,* and (rarely) a laundry list of other organisms including vibrios, Gram-negative bacteria such as pseudomonas, areromonas, clostridia and other anaerobes, legionella, *Erysipelothrix rhusiopathiae,* and *Helicobacter cinaedi.*[32] Minor trauma is frequently a predisposing factor. There has been a recent increase in reports of necrotizing fasciitis due to group A streptococci, and these infections are commonly associated with the onset of shock and organ failure, which are manifestations of the streptococcal toxic shock syndrome.[32] Unless treated by wide surgical debridement, necrotizing fasciitis is often fatal.[33] Probing of the subcutaneous tissue discloses extensive undermining and a serosanguineous exudate.[34]

Histopathology. The histologic picture is characterized by acute and chronic inflammation with necrosis (Figs. 21-2, 21-3, and 21-4). Often there is thrombosis of blood vessels as the

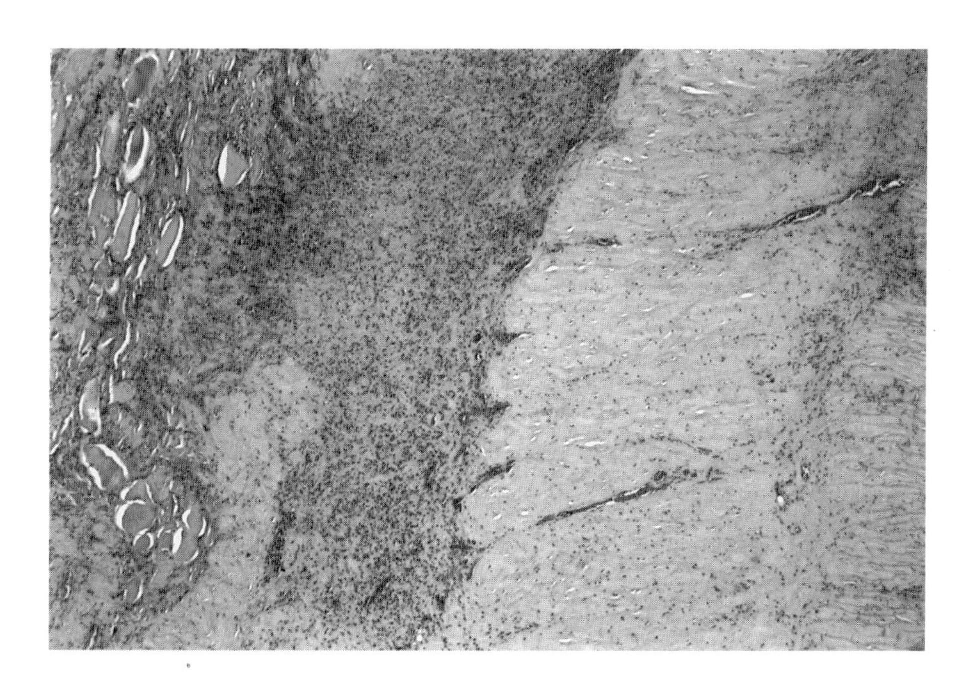

FIG. 21-2. Necrotizing fasciitis Necrosis of muscle (left) and fascia in a patient with a staphylococcal infection complicating a hysterectomy.

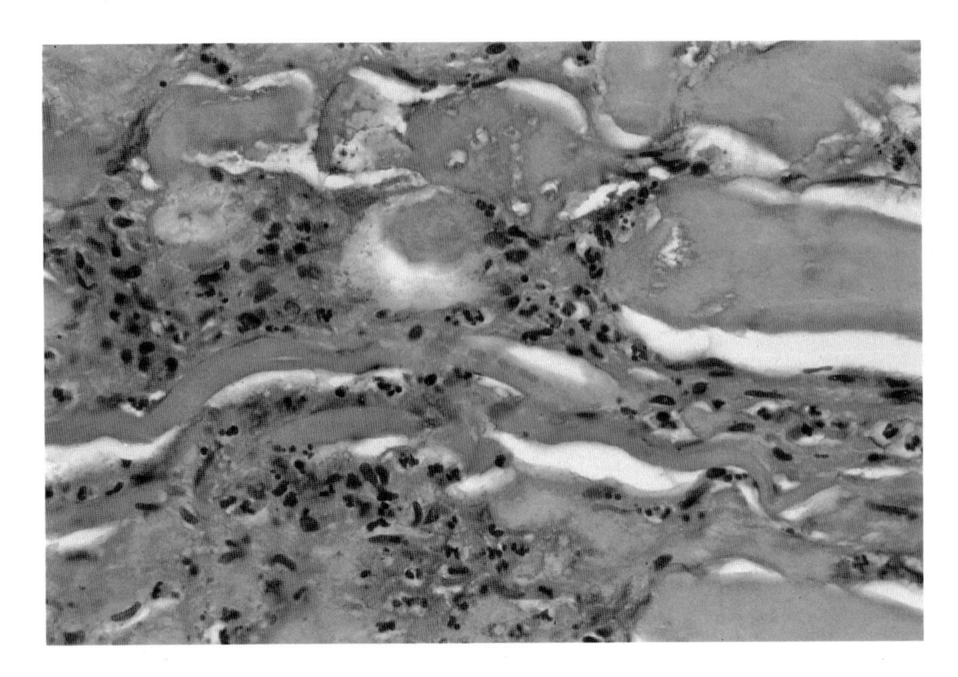

FIG. 21-3. Necrotizing fasciitis
Necrotic muscle surrounded by degenerating neutrophils.

result of damage to vessel walls from the inflammatory process.[33] The key feature in distinguishing necrotizing fasciitis from a less threatening superficial cellulitis is the location of the inflammation. In the former, the inflammation involves the subcutaneous fat, fascia, and muscle in addition to the dermis. A biopsy may be submitted at the time of surgical debridement for frozen section examination. In an appropriate setting, the presence of edema and neutrophils in these deep locations supports the diagnosis.[32,35] Frank necrosis may not be demonstrable, and bacteria are frequently not evident in an initial biopsy.

ACUTE SUPERFICIAL FOLLICULITIS

Impetigo Bockhart

Impetigo Bockhart, caused by staphylococci, is characterized by an eruption of small pustules, many of which are pierced by hairs.

Histopathology. Impetigo Bockhart presents a subcorneal pustule situated in the opening of a hair follicle. The upper por-

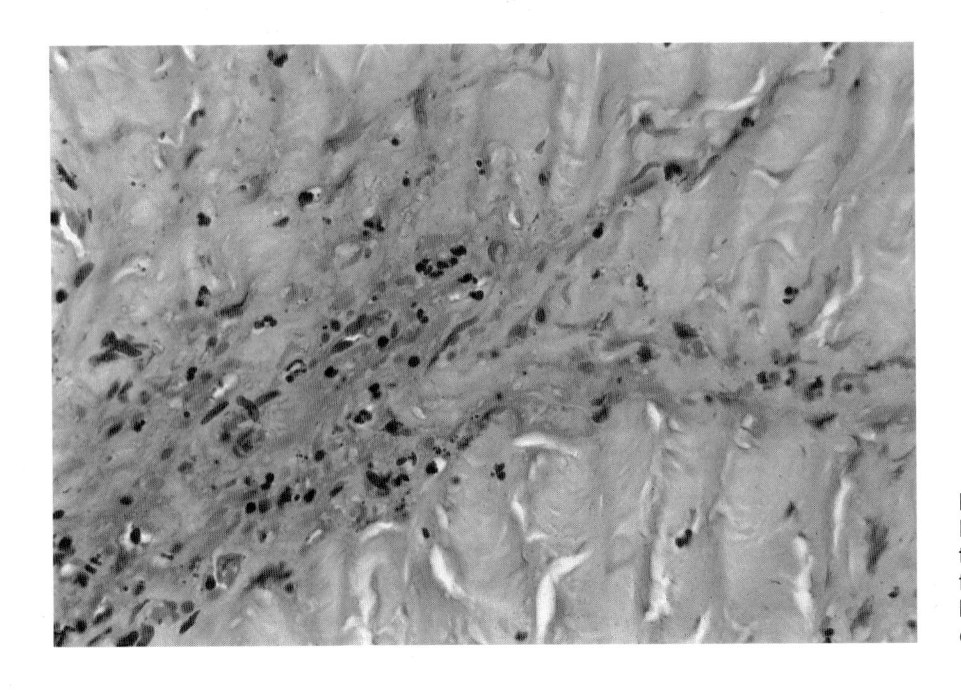

FIG. 21-4. Necrotizing fasciitis
Fascia with focal edema and neutrophils. Presence of neutrophils in the fascia is compatible with fasciitis in a biopsy specimen, even in the absence of demonstrable necrosis.

tion of the hair follicle is surrounded by a considerable inflammatory infiltrate composed predominantly of neutrophils.

Pseudomonas Folliculitis

In recent years, patients have exhibited outbreaks of pruritic macules, papules, and follicular pustules after using heated swimming pools, whirlpools, or "hot tubs." The eruption usually starts 8 to 48 hours after exposure in a contaminated facility and usually resolves spontaneously within 7 to 10 days.[36]

Histopathology. There is distension and disruption of a hair follicle, the pilar canal of which is filled with a dense infiltrate of neutrophils. There also is a perifolliculitis, and the epithelium of the hair follicle may be disrupted.[36,37]

Pathogenesis. The causative organism is *Pseudomonas aeruginosa,* which is ubiquitous in nature and may be found in soil, in fresh water, and on human skin. Proper chlorination and maintenance of pools decrease the population of *Pseudomonas.*

ACUTE DEEP FOLLICULITIS (FURUNCLE)

A furuncle is caused by staphylococci and consists of a tender, red, perifollicular swelling terminating in the discharge of pus and of a necrotic plug.

Histopathology. A furuncle shows an area of perifollicular necrosis containing fibrinoid material and many neutrophils. At the deep end of the necrotic plug, in the subcutaneous tissue, is a large abscess. A Gram stain shows small clusters of staphylococci in the center of the abscess.[38]

CHRONIC SUPERFICIAL FOLLICULITIS

Acne varioliformis, or acne necrotica, is characterized by recurrent, small, indolent, follicular papules on the forehead and scalp. The lesions undergo central necrosis and usually heal with small, pitted scars.[39]

Histopathology. Early lesions show a marked perifollicular lymphocytic infiltrate with exocytosis of lymphocytes into the external root sheath. This is followed by necrosis of the hair follicle and of the perifollicular epidermis. Late lesions have central cores of necrotic tissue.[39]

CHRONIC DEEP FOLLICULITIS

Folliculitis barbae is a deep-seated infection of the bearded region in men. There are follicular papules and pustules followed by erythema, crusting, and boggy infiltration of the skin. Abscesses may or may not be present. Scarring and permanent hair loss usually ensue.

Folliculitis decalvans occurs predominantly in men. Scattered through the scalp are bald, atrophic areas showing follicular pustules at their peripheries. In some instances, other hairy areas, such as the bearded and pubic regions and the axillae[40] and the eyebrows and eyelashes,[41] are also involved. Through peripheral spreading, the atrophic areas gradually increase in size.[42]

Folliculitis keloidalis nuchae represents a chronic folliculitis on the nape of the neck in men that causes hypertrophic scarring. In early cases, there are follicular papules, pustules, and occasionally abscesses. The lesions are replaced gradually by indurated fibrous nodules.

Histopathology. In early lesions of all three forms of chronic deep folliculitis, one observes a perifollicular infiltrate composed largely of neutrophils but also containing lymphoid cells, histiocytes, and plasma cells. The infiltrate develops into a perifollicular abscess leading to destruction of the hair and hair follicles. Older lesions show chronic granulation tissue containing numerous plasma cells, as well as lymphoid cells and fibroblasts.[43] Often, foreign-body giant cells are present around remnants of hair follicles, and particles of keratin may be located near the giant cells.[44] As healing takes place, fibrosis is observed. If there is hypertrophic scar formation, as in folliculitis keloidalis nuchae, numerous thick bundles of sclerotic collagen are present.

PSEUDOFOLLICULITIS OF THE BEARD

Pseudofolliculitis of the beard represents a foreign-body inflammatory reaction surrounding an ingrown beard hair. It occurs in men with curly hair, especially blacks, who shave closely. Clinically, one observes follicular papules and pustules resembling those of a bacterial folliculitis.

Histopathology. As a result of its curvature, the advancing sharp free end of the hair, as it approaches the skin, causes an invagination of the epidermis accompanied by inflammation and, often, an intraepidermal microabscess. As the hair enters the dermis, a more severe inflammatory reaction develops with downgrowth of the epidermis in an attempt to ensheath the hair. This is accompanied by abscess formation within the pseudofollicle and a foreign-body giant cell reaction at the tip of the invading hair.[45]

FOLLICULAR OCCLUSION TRIAD (HIDRADENITIS SUPPURATIVA, ACNE CONGLOBATA, AND PERIFOLLICULITIS CAPITIS ABSCEDENS ET SUFFODIENS)

The three diseases included in the follicular occlusion triad have similar pathogeneses and similar histopathologic findings.[46] Quite frequently, two of the three diseases, and occasionally all three diseases, are encountered in the same patient.[47–49] All three diseases represent a chronic, recurrent, deep-seated folliculitis resulting in abscesses and followed by the formation of sinus tracts and scarring. Although the primary etiology of these conditions is not bacterial, they are discussed in this chapter because the differential diagnosis includes the deep bacterial folliculitides.

In *hidradenitis suppurativa,* the axillary and anogenital regions are affected. Acute and chronic forms can be distinguished.[50] The acute form exhibits red, tender nodules that become fluctuant and heal after discharging pus. In the chronic form, deep-seated abscesses lead to the discharge of pus through sinus tracts. Severe scarring results.[51]

Acne conglobata, an entity different from acne vulgaris, occurs mainly on the back, buttocks, and chest and only rarely on the face or the extremities. In addition to comedones, fluctuant

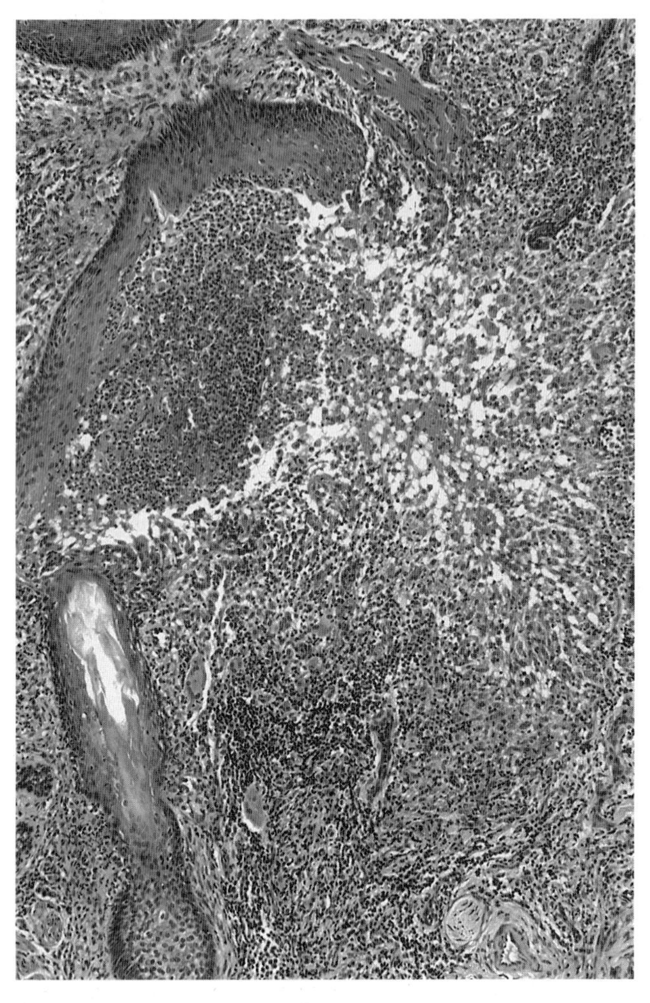

FIG. 21-5. Acute folliculitis
Hair shaft disrupted by acute inflammation that spreads into the dermis (H&E, medium power).

nodules discharging pus or a mucoid material occur, as well as deep-seated abscesses that discharge through interconnecting sinus tracts.[52]

In *perifolliculitis capitis abscedens et suffodiens,* nodules and abscesses as described for acne conglobata occur in the scalp.[53]

Pilonidal sinus is often considered to be a part of this group of disorders ("follicular occlusion tetrad"). Its pathogenesis appears to be similar, and it is often present in patients with one or more of the other members of the group.

Histopathology. Early lesions in all three diseases of the follicular occlusion triad show follicular hyperkeratosis with plugging and dilatation of the follicle. The follicular epithelium may proliferate or may be destroyed (Figs. 21-5 to 21-9). At first there is little inflammation, but eventually a perifolliculitis develops with an extensive infiltrate composed of neutrophils, lymphocytes, and histiocytes. Abscess formation results and leads to the destruction first of the pilosebaceous structures and later also of the other cutaneous appendages. Apocrine glands in hidradenitis suppurativa of the axillae or groin regions may be secondarily involved by the inflammatory process. In response to this destruction, granulation tissue containing lymphoid and plasma cells, and foreign-body giant cells related to fragments of keratin and to embedded hairs, infiltrates the area near the remnants of hair follicles (see Fig. 21-7). As the abscesses extend deeper into the subcutaneous tissue, draining sinus tracts develop that are lined with epidermis. In areas of healing, extensive fibrosis may be observed (see Fig. 21-6).[49]

Pathogenesis. The common initiating event in the three diseases of the follicular occlusion triad appears to be follicular hyperkeratosis leading to retention of follicular products.[54] Thus, the designation *hidradenitis suppurativa* is a misnomer, because involvement of apocrine as well as of eccrine glands represents a secondary phenomenon and is the result of extension of the inflammatory process into deep structures.

It appears doubtful that the diseases comprising the follicular occlusion triad are caused primarily by bacterial infection, because cultures from unopened abscesses often are negative.[55]

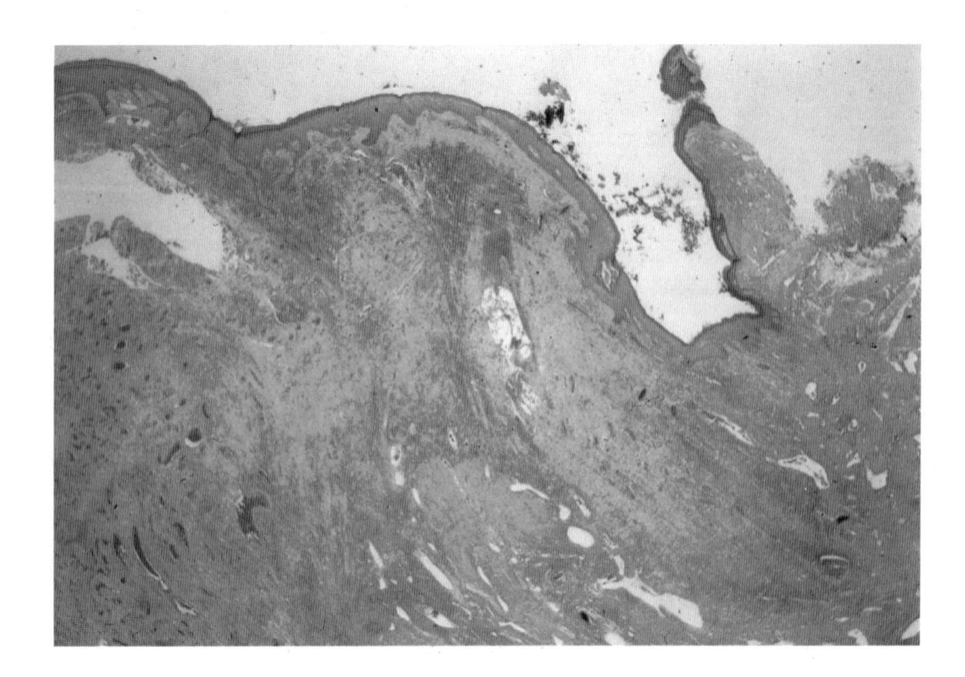

FIG. 21-6. Follicular occlusion disorder (perifolliculitis capitis abscedens et suffodiens)
In this lesion from the scalp, there are sinuses lined by granulation tissue and containing hairs, extending through the dermis and into the panniculus.

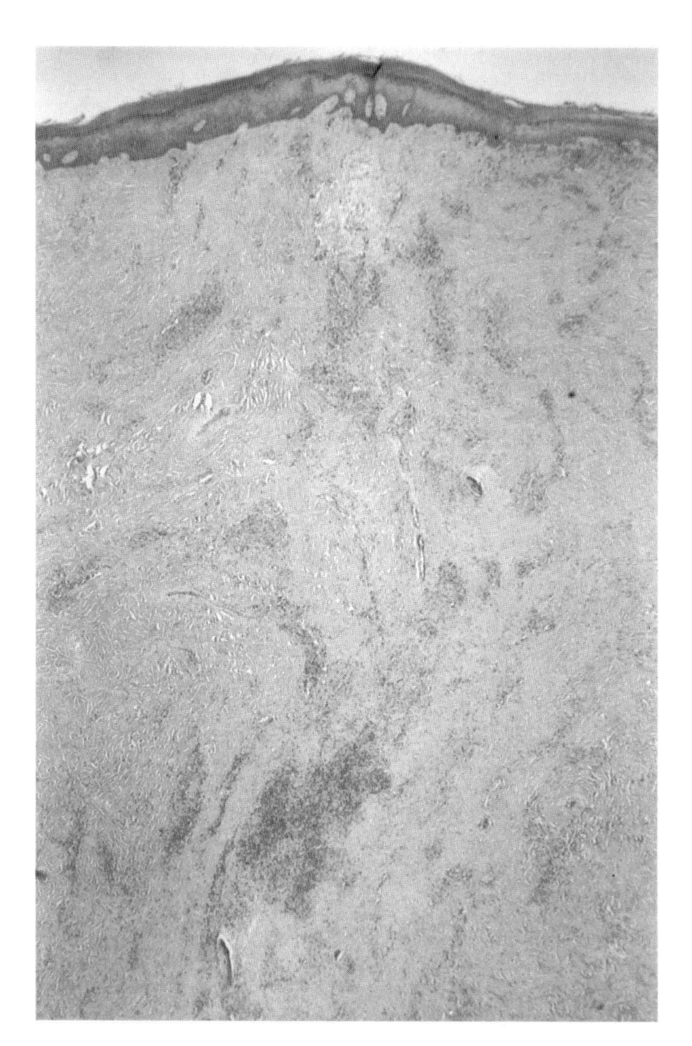

FIG. 21-7. Follicular occlusion disorder
In an end-stage region, there is scarring with patchy inflammation, which tracks down a healed sinus at the site of a destroyed hair follicle.

The beneficial effect of the internal administration of corticosteroid suggests that the three diseases represent antigen-antibody reactions resulting in tissue breakdown. Defects in cell-mediated immunity exist in some patients with hidradenitis suppurativa[55] but not in others.[50]

BLASTOMYCOSIS-LIKE PYODERMA (PYODERMA VEGETANS)

Two entirely different diseases have been described under the term *pyoderma vegetans* or *pyodermite végétante of Hallopeau*. One disease, now referred to as pemphigus vegetans of Hallopeau, shows the typical intercellular immunofluorescence of the pemphigus group on direct immunofluorescence testing (see Chap. 9). The other disease represents a vegetating tissue reaction, possibly secondary to bacterial infection.[56] In order to emphasize the difference between it and pemphigus vegetans of Hallopeau, it is preferable to refer to this disease as blastomycosis-like pyoderma rather than as pyoderma vegetans.[57]

Blastomycosis-like pyoderma shows one or multiple large, verrucous, vegetating plaques with scattered pustules and elevated borders.[56] The plaques show considerable resemblance to those observed in blastomycosis (see Chap. 23). The location of the plaques varies considerably from case to case. In some instances, the face and legs are affected[56,57]; in others it is the intertriginous areas.[58] Some authors have observed an association with ulcerative colitis.[58,59]

Histopathology. The two major features of blastomycosis-like pyoderma are pseudocarcinomatous hyperplasia and multiple abscesses in the dermis as well as in the hyperplastic epidermis. The abscesses are composed of neutrophils in some cases[56,57] and of eosinophils in others.[58,59]

Pathogenesis. Bacteria, most commonly *Staphylococcus aureus,* can be regularly found in blastomycosis-like pyoderma; however, the presence of several different strains and the variable response of patients to antibiotic therapy suggest that the bacteria are secondary invaders,[57] although they may be responsible for the vegetating tissue reaction.[56] A deficiency in cellular immunity[60] and a decrease in the chemotactic activity of the neutrophils[61] have also been observed.

Differential Diagnosis. In cases with largely eosinophils in

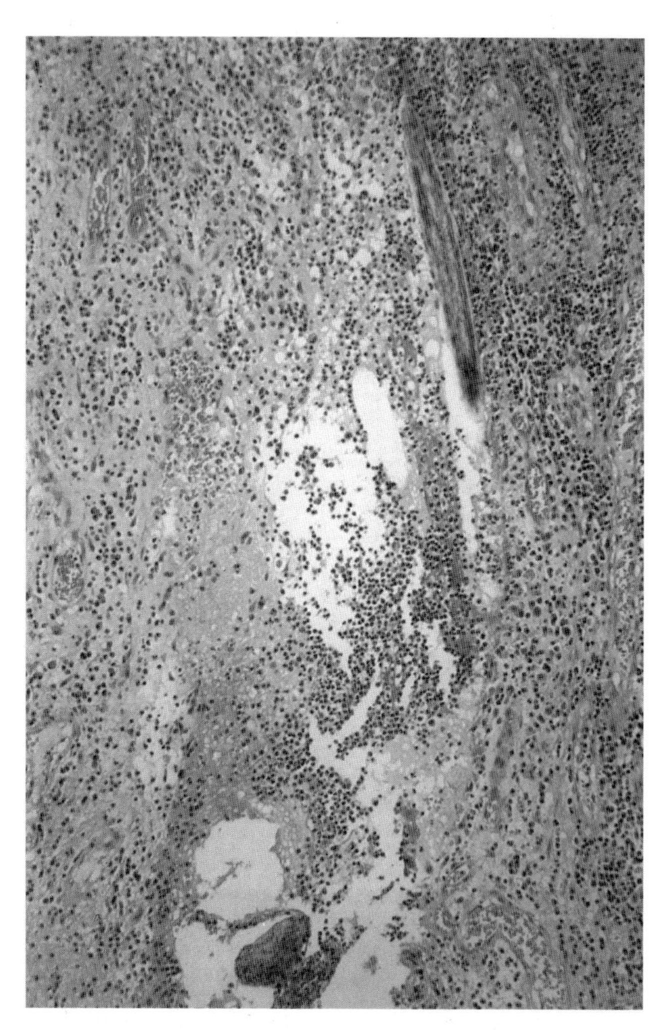

FIG. 21-8. Follicular occlusion disorder
An actively inflamed sinus contains hairs surrounded by neutrophils, granulation tissue, and scar tissue.

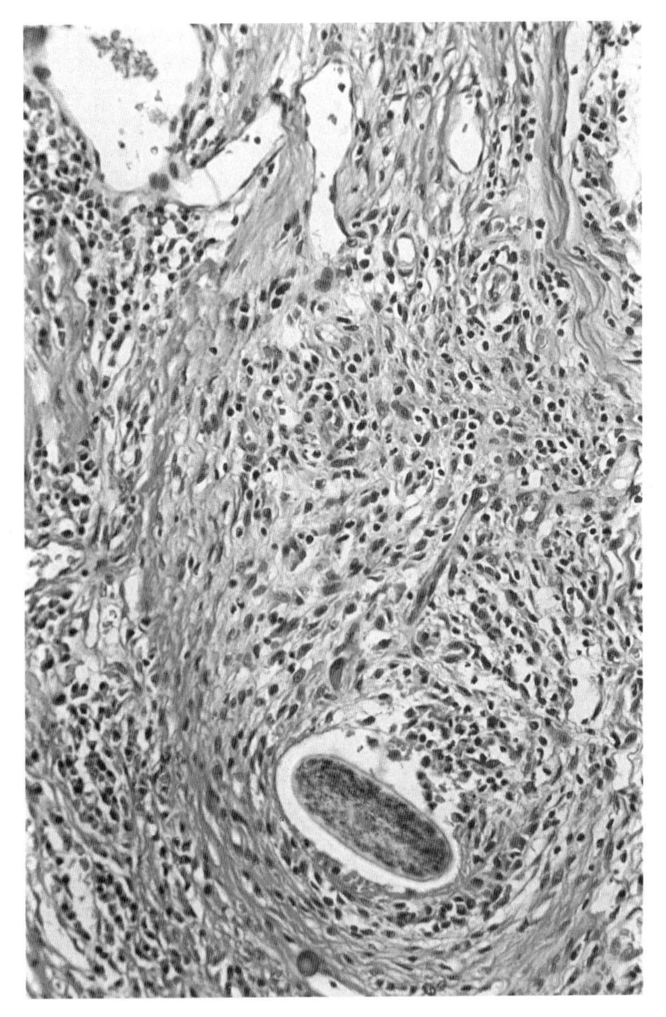

FIG. 21-9. Follicular occlusion disorder
In an apparent early lesion, granulation tissue and inflammation surround a hair at the base of a largely destroyed hair follicle.

the abscesses, pemphigus vegetans must be excluded by direct immunofluorescence.[62] If there is marked pseudocarcinomatous hyperplasia, multiple biopsies may be necessary for differentiation from true squamous cell carcinoma.

TOXIC SHOCK SYNDROME

The toxic shock syndrome (TSS) is an acute febrile illness usually caused by certain toxin-producing strains of *Staphylococcus aureus*. Occasionally, however, group A beta-hemolytic *Streptococcus* can cause this illness.[63] In the initial report in 1978, the disease was described in a series of seven children.[64] Although many cases have been associated in recent years with the use of superabsorbent vaginal tampons by menstruating women, additional reported settings for TSS have included surgical wound infections of the skin,[65] empyema, fasciitis, osteomyelitis, peritonsillar abscesses, and other infections.[66] Fever, hypotension or shock, an extensive rash resembling scarlet fever or sunburn, and involvement of three or more organ systems are the initial defining manifestations, whereas desquamation occurs 1 to 2 weeks after the onset.[67] In rare instances, bullae are also present.[68,69] In addition, there may be a conjunctivitis and an oropharyngitis. Internal organs may be affected by a toxic encephalopathy, thrombocytopenia, renal failure, or hepatic damage. Mortality has been estimated at 5% to 10%.[70]

Histopathology. Although in some cases the findings in the skin are not specific,[71] in most instances the histologic findings are quite characteristic, consisting of a superficial perivascular and interstitial mixed-cell infiltrate containing neutrophils and sometimes eosinophils, foci of spongiosis containing neutrophils, and scattered necrotic keratinocytes that sometimes are arranged in clusters within the epidermis.[72] If bullae are present, they are subepidermal in location.[68,69]

Pathogenesis. Even though in rare cases *Staphylococcus aureus* bacteremia occurs, the cause of the toxic shock syndrome is a toxin that is produced locally at the site of a toxigenic staphylococcal infection. Several toxins have been implicated in toxic shock syndrome, including toxic shock syndrome toxin-1 (TSST-1) and the staphylococcal enterotoxins B, C, and F.[67,73] Susceptibility to disease correlates with absence of protective antibodies to the toxin, and cytokine activation may be involved in some aspects of its pathogenesis.[67] Streptococcal TSS has been associated with bacteriemia and extensive necrotizing fasciitis, unlike the staphyloccocal syndrome usually associated with occult or minor focal infections.[67] Streptococcal TSS appears to be caused also by toxins produced by the bacteria, including pyrogenic exotoxin A, which shares some homologies with TSST-1.[74]

ACUTE SEPTICEMIA

Three types of acute fulminating septicemia have cutaneous manifestations that are diagnostically significant. They are those caused by *Neisseria meningitidis*, *Pseudomonas*, and *Vibrio vulnificus*.

Acute Meningococcemia

Fulminating septicemic infections with *N meningitidis* exhibit extensive purpura consisting of both petechiae and ecchymoses. The centers of the petechiae may show small pustules. In addition, shock, cyanosis, and severe consumption coagulopathy occur.[75] Without treatment, death may result within 12 to 24 hours. On autopsy, extensive hemorrhaging is found in many internal organs, especially the lungs, kidneys, and adrenals.

On rare occasions, acute septicemia with purpura can be produced by other organisms, such as *Diplococcus pneumoniae*, *Streptococcus*, or *Staphylococcus aureus*.[76]

Histopathology. The cutaneous petechiae and ecchymoses show, in many dermal vessels, thrombi composed of neutrophils, platelets, and fibrin. In addition, there is an acute vasculitis with considerable damage to the vascular walls resulting in large and small areas of hemorrhaging into the tissue. Neutrophils and nuclear dust are present within and around the damaged vessels.[77] In most instances, many meningococci can be demonstrated in the luminal thrombi, within vessel walls, and around vessels as Gram-negative diplococci. They are present in the cytoplasm of endothelial cells and neutrophils and also extracellularly.[77,78] Intraepidermal and subepidermal pustules filled with neutrophils may also be observed.[78]

Pathogenesis. In the past, vascular collapse and death were attributed to massive bilateral hemorrhaging into the adrenal glands and were known as the Waterhouse-Friderichsen syndrome. However, it was then learned that death can occur without significant damage to the adrenals.[79] Therefore, it was assumed that the generalized hemorrhagic diathesis was caused by the consumptive depletion of plasma clotting factors and the resulting disseminated intravascular coagulation.[80] It seems likely, however, that there are two distinct pathogenic mechanisms operating in acute meningococcemia.[75] First, a shocklike terminal phase is associated with the development of widespread thrombosis of the pulmonary microcirculation. These thrombi, which are caused by meningococcal toxins, are composed of leukocytes and fibrin and often also contain meningococci. They produce severe cor pulmonale, which cannot be prevented by treatment with heparin. Similar microthrombi are found also in the skin, spleen, heart, and liver. Second, a meningococcal endotoxin produces disseminated intravascular coagulation resulting in thrombi composed of fibrin only. These thrombi are found in the capillaries of the adrenal cortex and the kidneys and may cause hemorrhagic infarction of the adrenal glands and renal cortical necrosis. This secondary phase of the disease can be modified with heparin therapy, but its control does not improve survival, because the adrenal and renal lesions are not immediately life-threatening, in contrast to the pulmonary lesions, which result in shock and death.

Pseudomonas Septicemia

The classic and diagnostic cutaneous lesions of *Pseudomonas aeruginosa* or *Pseudomonas cepacia* septicemia are referred to as *ecthyma gangrenosum*. *Pseudomonas* septicemia usually occurs in debilitated, leukemic, or severely burned patients, particularly after they have received treatment with several antibiotics. The cutaneous lesions may be single but usually are multiple. They consist of punched-out ulcers about 1 cm in diameter that have hemorrhagic borders. They usually are preceded by hemorrhagic bullae.[81] In Tzanck smears prepared from the bases of the lesions, Gram-negative rods can be identified, confirming the diagnosis. Because of the rapid fatality of *Pseudomonas* septicemia, early institution of intravenous treatment with gentamicin sulfate is indicated.

In rare instances of *Pseudomonas* septicemia, multiple large, indurated, subcutaneous nodules are observed in addition to the cutaneous ulcers.[82,83]

Occasionally, lesions of ecthyma gangrenosum have been observed in immunocompromised patients without bacteremia; these cases have better prognoses.[84]

Histopathology. The ulcers show at their bases a necrotizing vasculitis with only scant neutrophilic infiltration and little nuclear dust. There is, however, extensive bacillary infiltration of the perivascular region and of the adventitia and media of blood vessels. Nevertheless, the intima and the lumen usually are spared.[85] *Pseudomonas* bacilli first invade the walls of the deep subcutaneous vessels and then spread along the surfaces of the vessels to the dermis.[86] By causing perivascular and vascular necrosis, the bacilli cause extravasation of erythrocytes and the formation of ulcers (Figs. 21-10 and 21-11).

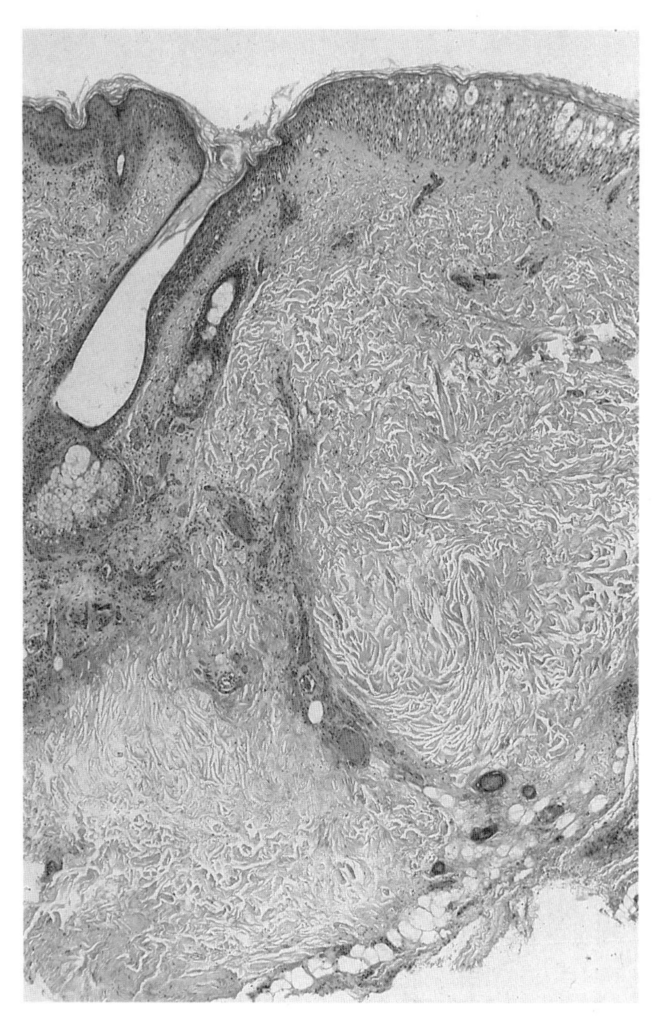

FIG. 21-10. Pseudomonas septicemia
Skin showing superficial infarction (right), basophilic material (near the middle), and deep vessels in the dermis (H&E, low power).

The subcutaneous nodules are the result of cellulitis caused by the presence of large numbers of *Pseudomonas* bacilli.[82]

Vibrio Vulnificus Septicemia

Vibrio vulnificus infections occur in coastal regions of the United States. Raw seafood consumption, particularly raw oysters, or wounds acquired in marine environments can cause the infection. *V vulnificus* is a virulent pathogen, producing significant morbidity and, unless treated, mortality, especially in patients with cirrhosis of the liver.

Striking skin lesions are an early sign of septicemic infection. Indurated plaques show blue discoloration, vesicles, and bullae. Large ulcers may develop.[87]

Histopathology. Noninflammatory bullae form as the result of dermal necrosis, which is caused by the extracellular toxin

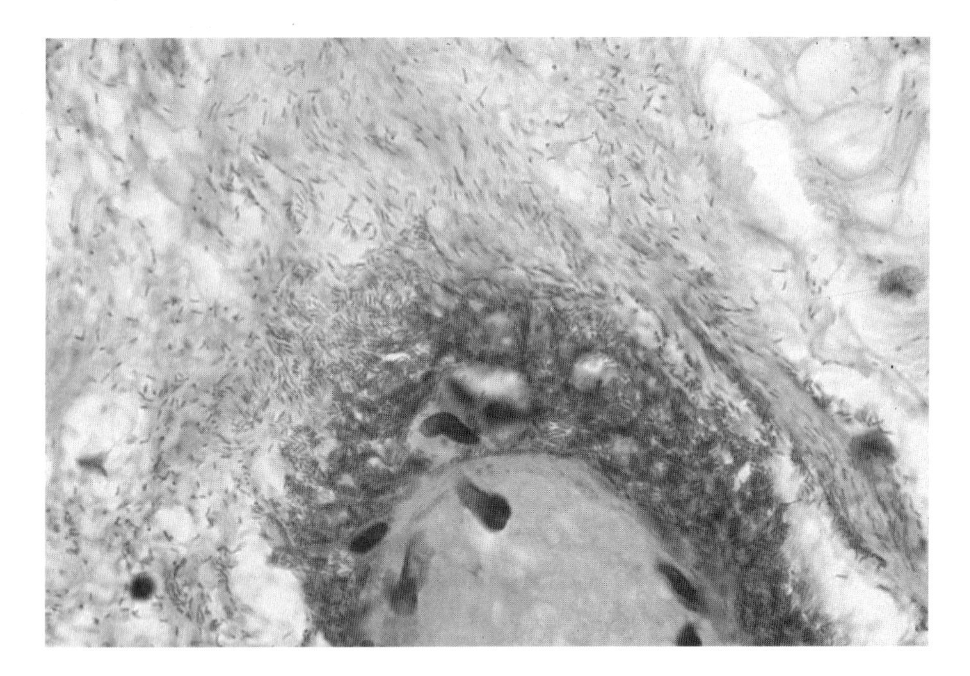

FIG. 21-11. Pseudomonas septicemia
Bacilli infiltrating the deep vessel wall and into the surrounding dermis. The lumen is thrombosed. There is no inflammation (H&E, high power).

produced by the bacterium. Clusters of bacteria may be seen in dermal vessels without associated dermal infiltrate.[88]

Pathogenesis. V vulnificus is a Gram-negative rod that is motile by means of a single polar flagellum. It can be isolated from the blood and bullae of patients with this infection.

CHRONIC SEPTICEMIA

Meningococcemia and gonococcemia can occur in association with a chronic intermittent, benign eruption.

Chronic Meningococcemia

In patients with partial immunity to *Neisseria meningitidis*, an infection with this organism produces chronic meningococcemia. This disease is characterized by recurrent attacks of fever, each lasting about 12 hours, associated with migratory joint pains and a papular and petechial eruption. Positive blood cultures are obtained during the febrile attacks.

Histopathology. The cutaneous lesions of chronic meningococcemia, in contrast to those of acute meningococcemia, show no bacteria and no vascular thrombosis or necrosis. Instead, one observes in papular lesions a perivascular infiltrate composed largely of lymphoid cells and only a few neutrophils.[89,90] In petechial lesions, one may find, in addition to a limited area of perivascular hemorrhage, a fairly high percentage of neutrophils and fibrinoid material in the walls of the vessels, so that the histologic picture resembles that of a leukocytoclastic vasculitis.[90] The presence of meningococci cannot be demonstrated, not even through direct immunofluorescence testing.[89]

Chronic Gonococcemia

Patients with chronic gonococcemia, also referred to as disseminated gonococcal infection,[91] like those with chronic meningococcemia, have intermittent attacks of fever and polyarthralgia. The cutaneous lesions of the two diseases are also similar, except that those of chronic gonococcemia are few in number and have a predominantly acral distribution. In contrast to chronic meningococcemia, there are often, in addition to papules and petechiae, vesicopustules with hemorrhagic halos and, rarely, hemorrhagic bullae. Blood cultures often are positive for *Neisseria gonorrhoeae*, but only during attacks of fever. A search for gonococci should also be made in possible sites of primary infection.

Histopathology. The capillaries in the upper dermis and middermis are surrounded by an infiltrate of neutrophils and a variable admixture of mononuclear cells and red cells. There often is nuclear dust, as in leukocytoclastic vasculitis. Fibrinoid material may be present in the walls of some vessels, and fibrin thrombi in some lumina.[92] Pustular lesions are usually observed in intraepidermal locations with neutrophils both within them and in the underlying dermis.[93] Bullae are subepidermal in location.[94]

Gram-negative diplococci are observed in tissue sections only on rare occasions in the walls of blood vessels.[95] They are found more readily in direct smears of pus from freshly opened pustules. It is of interest that direct smears reveal gonococci more commonly than cultures.[96] However, *N gonorrhoeae* can frequently be identified in tissue sections by use of fluorescent-antibody techniques.[97] For this purpose, fluorescein-labeled antigonococcus globulin is used. Diplococci, as well as single cocci and disintegrated antigenic material, are then observed, largely in perivascular locations. The reason that direct smears are more apt to show diplococci than cultures and that the fluorescent-antibody technique is particularly effective in demonstrating gonococci lies in the fact that smears and the fluorescent-antibody technique are not dependent on living organisms, as are cultures.

Pathogenesis. Whereas most strains of gonococci are susceptible to the bactericidal action of normal serum, those causing disseminated gonococcal infection are resistant.[91]

MALAKOPLAKIA

Malakoplakia may affect various organs, most commonly the urinary tract and the gastrointestinal tract.[97a] In rare instances, it involves the skin.[98,99] The lesions are the result of an inability of macrophages to phagocytose bacteria adequately. The most common organism grown in cultures of tissue material is *Escherichia coli,*[98,100] but in some instances other bacteria such as *Staphylococcus aureus, Rhodococcus equi,* and nontuberculosis mycobacteria[101] are cultured. Some patients with lesions of malakoplakia have altered immune responsiveness as a result of carcinoma, autoimmune systemic diseases such as systemic lupus erythematosus, or immunosuppressive therapy for lymphoma or for renal transplantation.[102]

Cutaneous malakoplakia lesions are chronic, and may be associated with internal lesions. The appearance of the cutaneous lesions is nonspecific and variable. Most commonly, one observes a fluctuant area,[101] a draining abscess,[100] draining sinuses,[102] or an ulcer; however, in some patients, a solitary, tender nodule or a cluster of tender papules is observed. The cutaneous disease is benign and self-limited.

Histopathology. There are sheets of large histiocytes containing fine, eosinophilic granules in their cytoplasm. Many of them contain, in addition to the granules, ovoid or round basophilic inclusions, referred to as Michaelis-Gutmann bodies, that vary in size from 5 to 15 μm (Fig. 21-12).[99] These bodies either are homogeneous or have a "target" appearance by showing concentric laminations. The infiltrate may also contain lymphocytes, plasma cells, and polymorphs.

The Michaelis-Gutmann inclusion bodies and the cytoplasmic granules are PAS-positive, diastase-resistant, and alcian-blue-positive. In addition, the Michaelis-Gutmann bodies stain with the von Kossa stain for calcium and contain small amounts of iron that may be demonstrated by Perls' stain. With the Gram stain, Gram-negative bacteria may be seen in some of the histiocytes, and, in the rare case caused by mycobacteria, Ziehl-Neelsen stain reveals the organisms. The bodies may be observed in skin scrapings of lesions.[103]

Pathogenesis. Electron microscopic examination reveals that the cytoplasm of the granular cells contains numerous phagolysosomes corresponding to the PAS-positive granules. Some phagolysosomes contain lamellae in a concentric arrangement.[99] The Michaelis-Gutmann bodies develop within phagolysosomes by the progressive deposition of electron-dense calcific material on the whorled or concentric lamellae until they are ultimately completely calcified. Bacteria may be observed in the cytoplasm of the granular cells and in various stages of digestion within phagolysosomes.[101]

Malakoplakia represents an acquired defect in the lysosomal killing and digestion of phagocytized bacteria. Deficiencies of β-glucuronidase and of $3',5'$ guanosine monophosphate dehydrongenase have been documented.[100,104]

MYCOBACTERIAL INFECTIONS

Taxonomically, the mycobacteria are divided into two major groups, the rapid growers and the slow growers in culture. *Mycobacterium leprae* lies outside this scheme because it cannot be cultured in vitro. Within each group the species are organized in subgroups according to certain culture (growth requirement) and biochemical characteristics. Among the infections to be considered in this chapter, the important slow growers are *M tuberculosis* complex, including BCG; the *M avium* complex, including *M avium* and *M intracellulare*; the *M kansasii* complex; the complex that includes *M marinum* and *M ulcerans*; and mycobacteria with special growth requirements, such as *M haemophilum*. Rapid growers that affect the skin include *M fortuitum* complex, which also includes *M chelonei.*[105] Many other mycobacteria can occasionally cause skin lesions.[106–108]

Tuberculosis and leprosy bacilli are intracellular parasites that are found in the tissues of humans (and occasionally animals). Transmission requires exposure to infected people. The other mycobacteria are abundant in nature in both soil and water, and exposure to infection occurs throughout life, although usually without significant clinical disease.

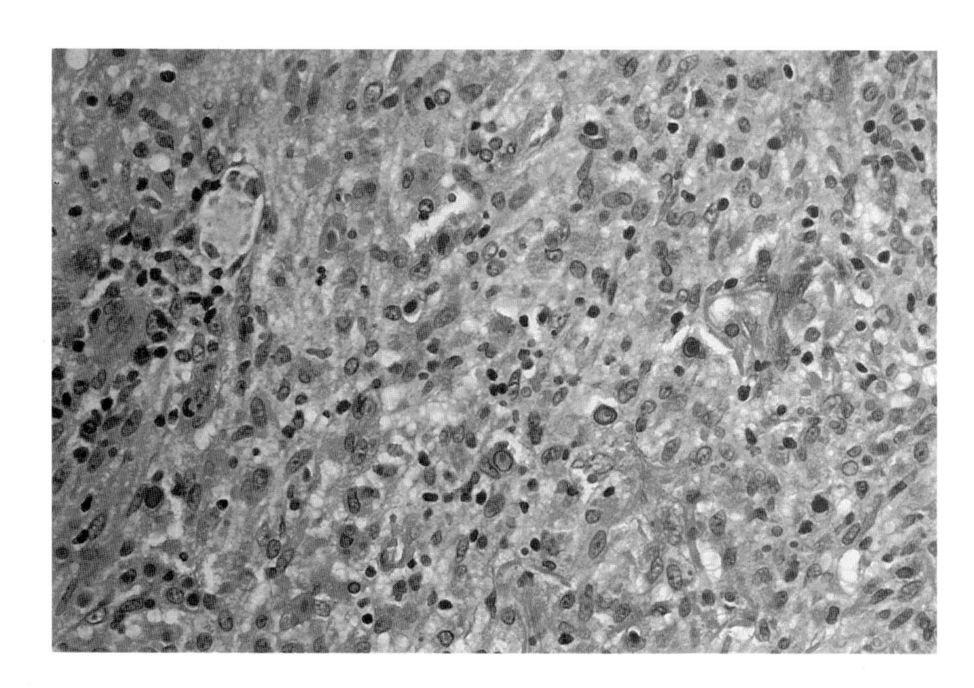

FIG. 21-12. Malakoplakia
Sheets of macrophages with eosinophilic cytoplasm; several in the center contain Michaelis-Gutmann inclusion bodies (H&E, high power).

Mycobacteria are bacilli that are weakly Gram-positive and are classically identified in histologic sections by stains that exploit their resistance to decoloration by acid—i.e., acid-fast bacilli.[109] All mycobacteria apart from the leprosy bacillus (see later) are well stained by the standard Ziehl-Neelsen technique.

TUBERCULOSIS

Tuberculosis was until recently considered to be a diminishing clinical problem in industrialized nations while remaining a dominant public health problem in resource-poor countries. However, there is a resurgence of tuberculosis everywhere because of a combination of factors, including immigration from endemic countries (particularly in Asia and Africa), increased movement of refugees, the HIV pandemic, and poverty.[110] As a result, cutaneous tuberculosis remains a clinical and diagnostic problem.[111,112]

Infection of the skin and subcutis by *Mycobacterium tuberculosis* occurs by three routes: (1) by direct inoculation into the skin (causing a primary chancre, or tuberculosis verrucosa cutis, or tuberculosis cutis orificialis lesions); (2) by hematogenous spread from an internal lesion (causing lupus vulgaris, miliary tuberculosis, and tuberculous gumma lesions); and (3) from an underlying tuberculous lymph node by direct extension (causing scrofuloderma). For descriptive purposes, these different tuberculous dermatitides are delineated (a modified "Beyt classification" is used).[107] But in clinical practice, many cases do not readily fit into these clinical and histologic categories.[108,113,114]

The basic reaction of human tissues to tuberculous bacilli is a sequence, first of acute nonspecific inflammation during which the bacilli multiply and cannot be phagocytosed and killed by neutrophil polymorphs. Macrophages then phagocytose the organisms, but their efficacy in killing them depends crucially on enhanced activation. T-cell allergy to tuberculous antigens induces secretion of cytokines that recruit and activate macrophages, which become epithelioid cells. Some will fuse to form giant cells, the typical form of which in tuberculosis is the Langhans' giant cell with the nuclei arranged around the periphery of the cytoplasm. As delayed hypersensitivity increases, there is caseation necrosis within the granuloma, caseation being a homogeneous eosinophilic infarctlike necrotic process whereby the macrophages die. It is probably mediated by cytokines (such as tumor necrosis factor) and the macrophage proteases. This necrotic process inactivates or kills many of the mycobacteria in the lesion, but it does not eliminate them.[115,116]

The necrotic granuloma is thus typical of tuberculosis and other mycobacterial infections, but it is not specific, being seen in numerous other infections that involve this type of cell-mediated immunity (e.g., histoplasmosis, syphilis, and leishmaniasis).

The determinants of what happens in tuberculosis infection therefore include the virulence of the organism (tuberculosis is more virulent than most of the nontuberculosis mycobacteria), the size of the inoculum, the route of infection, and the immune status of the patient. It is evident that if cell-mediated immunity is impaired, the T-cell/macrophage system will not operate to contain the infection. The resulting pathology is generally less granulomatous (fewer activated macrophages) and has a higher density of mycobacteria. Such conditions are HIV infection with its sequel of AIDS (acquired immunodeficiency syndrome), steroid therapy, and cytotoxic drugs.

Primary Tuberculosis

Primary infection with tuberculosis occurs only rarely on the skin. Children or adults may acquire it following minor trauma or contact with infected material—as a result, for instance, of mouth-to-mouth artificial respiration,[117] inoculation during an autopsy,[118] needle-stick injury,[119] or inoculation during tattooing.[120] Usually, the cutaneous lesion arises within 2 to 4 weeks after the inoculation. It consists of an asymptomatic crust-covered ulcer referred to as tuberculous chancre. The regional lymph nodes become enlarged and tender and may suppurate and produce draining sinuses.

Histopathology. The histologic development of the lesion is very much like that observed in experimental cutaneous inoculation of the guinea pig. In the earliest phase, the histologic picture is that of an acute neutrophilic reaction, with areas of necrosis resulting in ulceration. Numerous tubercle bacilli are present, particularly in the areas of necrosis.[118] After 2 weeks, monocytes and macrophages predominate. Three to 6 weeks after onset, epithelioid cells and giant-cell granulomas develop, followed by caseation necrosis within the granuloma mass (Fig. 21-13). In time, the necrosis lessens, and the number of tubercle bacilli decreases until it is so greatly reduced that the bacilli may be impossible to demonstrate in histologic sections. Simultaneous with the decrease in the number of tubercle bacilli in the lesion, the tuberculin test with purified protein derivative (PPD), previously negative, becomes positive. The draining lymph nodes receive tubercle bacilli and enlarge through developing caseating granulomas, parallel to a primary infection in the lung.

Tuberculosis Verrucosa Cutis

Tuberculosis verrucosa cutis represents an inoculated exogenous infection of the skin in persons with a degree of immunity—i.e., previous exposure to tuberculosis. In tuberculosis verrucosa cutis, one usually observes a single lesion presenting as a verrucous plaque with an inflammatory border and showing gradual peripheral extension. The verrucous surface exhibits fissures from which pus often can be expressed. The most common sites are the hands and, in children, the knees, buttocks, and thighs.

Histopathology. The histologic picture includes hyperkeratosis and acanthosis. Beneath the epidermis, there is an acute inflammatory infiltrate. Abscess formation may be observed in the upper dermis or within downward extensions of the epidermis. In the middermis, tuberculoid granulomas with a moderate amount of necrosis are usually present. Tubercle bacilli are more numerous in this disease than in lupus vulgaris and occasionally can be demonstrated histologically (Fig. 21-14).

Miliary Tuberculosis of the Skin

Involvement of the skin with miliary tuberculosis is rare in the immunocompetent, occurring mostly in infants and only oc-

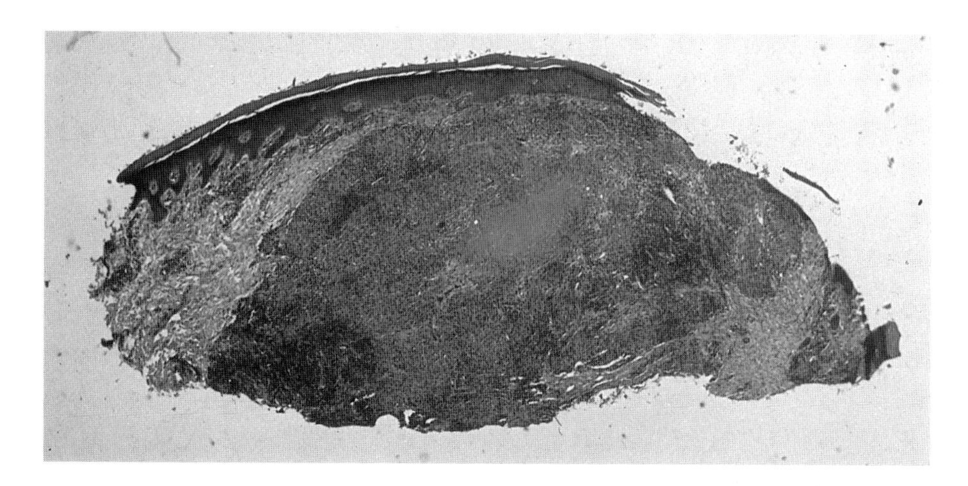

FIG. 21-13. Tuberculosis
A prosector's wart from inoculation of the finger from a tuberculous cadaver. There is central caseation necrosis with dense macrophage and lymphocyte surround (H&E, low power).

casionally in adults. Usually, internal involvement is widespread as a result of hematogenous dissemination, and the cutaneous eruption is generalized, consisting of erythematous papules and pustules 2 to 5 mm in diameter.[121] The tuberculin test generally is negative. The disease has a high fatality rate.

There exists, however, a milder form of hematogenous dissemination of tubercle bacilli in neonates born of tuberculous mothers. This form shows limited visceral involvement and only a few scattered erythematous papules with central crusts.[122]

Histopathology. In severe cases, the center of the papule shows a microabscess containing neutrophils, cellular debris, and numerous tubercle bacilli. This is surrounded by a zone of macrophages with occasional giant cells. In the milder form, the histologic picture in the skin is similar, except that the Ziehl-Neelsen stain is negative for acid-fast organisms.

Lupus Vulgaris

The lesions of lupus vulgaris are usually found on the head or neck. The skin of and around the nose is frequently involved.[123] The lesions consist of one or a few well-demarcated, reddish brown patches containing deep-seated nodules, each about 1 mm in diameter. If the blood is pressed out of the skin with a glass slide, these nodules stand out clearly as yellow-brown macules, referred to, because of their color, as apple-jelly nodules. The disease is very chronic, with slow, peripheral extension of the lesions. In the course of time, the affected areas become atrophic, with contraction of the tissue. It is a characteristic feature of lupus vulgaris that new lesions may appear in areas of atrophy. Superficial ulceration or verrucous thickening of the skin occurs occasionally. Squamous cell carcinoma develops at the margins of ulcers in rare instances.

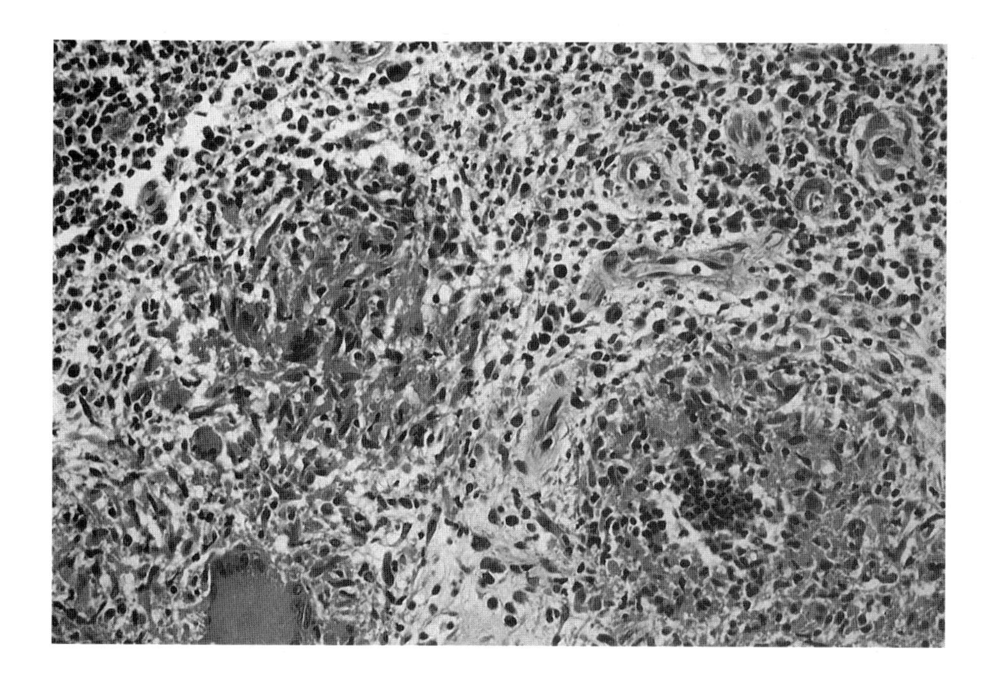

FIG. 21-14. Tuberculosis
An epithelioid cell granuloma, an adjacent giant cell, and a granuloma with central acute inflammation. Occasional acid-fast bacilli were observed in this case (H&E, high power).

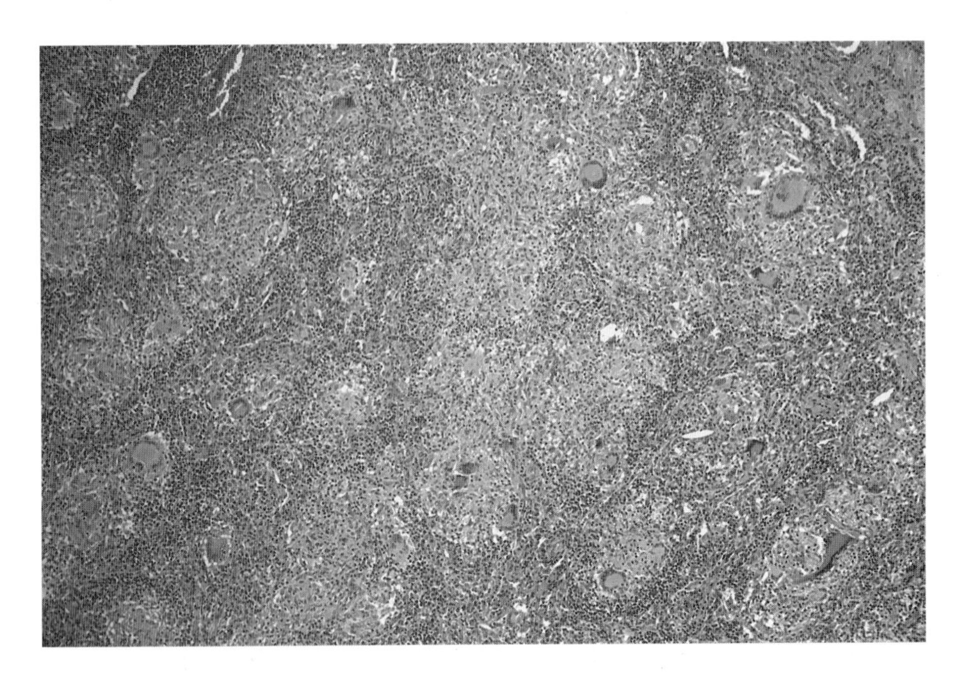

FIG. 21-15. Lupus vulgaris
Near-confluent nonnecrotizing epithelioid cell granulomas in the dermis (H&E, medium power).

Histopathology. Tuberculoid granulomas composed of epithelioid cells and giant cells are present. Caseation necrosis within the tubercles is slight or absent.[124] Although the giant cells usually are of the Langhans' type, with peripheral arrangement of the nuclei, some can be of the foreign-body type, with irregular arrangement of the nuclei. There is an associated infiltrate of lymphocytes (Figs. 21-15 and 21-16). Sometimes this may be more prominent that the granulomatous component. The inflammation is most pronounced in the upper dermis, but in some areas it may extend into the subcutaneous layer. Tuberculoid granulomas cause destruction of the cutaneous appendages. In areas of healing, extensive fibrosis may be present.

Secondary changes in the epidermis are common. The epidermis may undergo atrophy and subsequent destruction, causing ulceration, or it may become hyperplastic, showing acanthosis, hyperkeratosis, and papillomatosis. At the margins of ulcers, pseudoepitheliomatous hyperplasia often exists. Unless a deep biopsy is done in such cases, one may see only the epithelial hyperplasia and a nonspecific inflammation, and the diagnosis may be missed.[123] In rare instances, squamous cell carcinoma supervenes.[125]

Tubercle bacilli are present in such small numbers that they can very rarely be demonstrated by staining methods. Polymerase chain reaction (PCR) detection of mycobacterial DNA is more often positive.[126] In some instances of lupus vulgaris when an old focus of primary infection cannot be detected, a positive tuberculin test and the response to antituberculous therapy must suffice as proof of a tuberculous etiology.

Pathogenesis. Lupus vulgaris is a form of secondary or reactivation tuberculosis developing in previously infected and

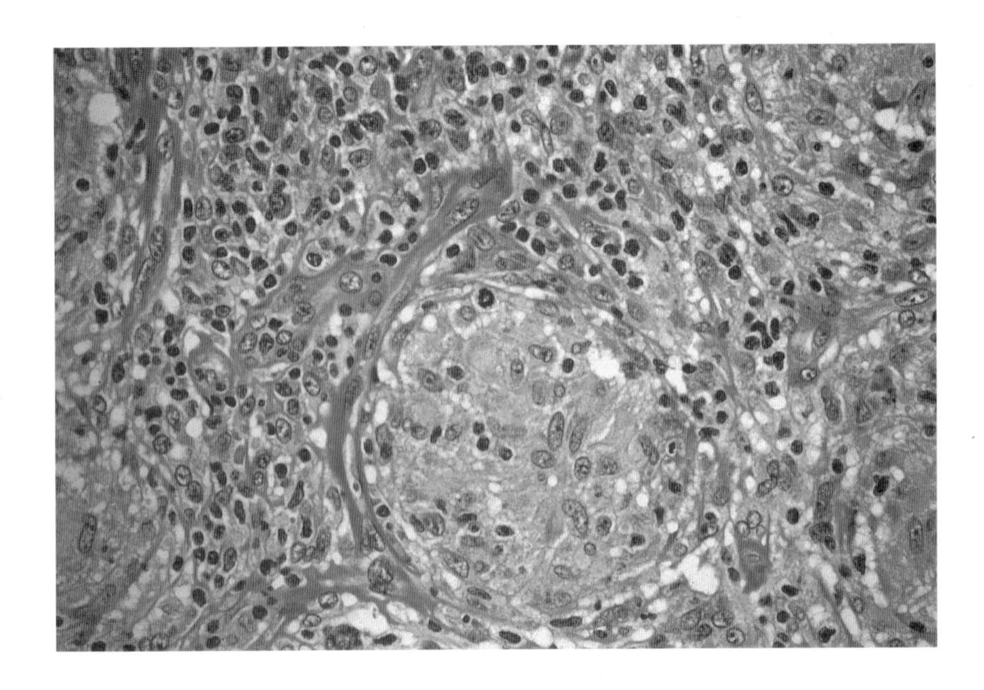

FIG. 21-16. Lupus vulgaris
Same lesion as in Fig. 21-9, showing an epithelioid cell granuloma (H&E, high power).

sensitized persons. Hypersensitivity to PPD tuberculin is high. Although the mode of infection is often not apparent, the disease rarely seems to be the result of an exogenous reinfection of the skin; usually it results from hematogenous spread from an old, reactivated focus in the lung or from lymphatic extension from a tuberculous cervical lymphadenitis.[107]

Scrofuloderma

Scrofuloderma represents a direct extension to the skin of an underlying tuberculous infection present most commonly in a lymph node or a bone. The lesion first manifests itself as a blue-red, painless swelling that breaks open and then forms an ulcer with irregular, undermined, blue borders.

Histopathology. The center of the lesion usually exhibits nonspecific changes, such as abscess formation or ulceration. In the deeper portions and at the periphery of the lesion, if the biopsy specimen is adequate, one usually sees tuberculoid granulomas with a considerable amount of necrosis and a pronounced inflammatory reaction. Usually, the number of tubercle bacilli is sufficient for them to be found in histologic sections.

Tuberculous Gumma

Hematogenous infection of the skin from an internal lesion may result in a large dermal or subcutaneous nodule that is necrotic and ultimately ulcerates the epidermis.

Histopathology. Most of the lesion is caseation necrosis with a rim of epithelioid cells and giant cells (Figs. 21-17 and 21-18). Acid-fast bacilli are scanty.

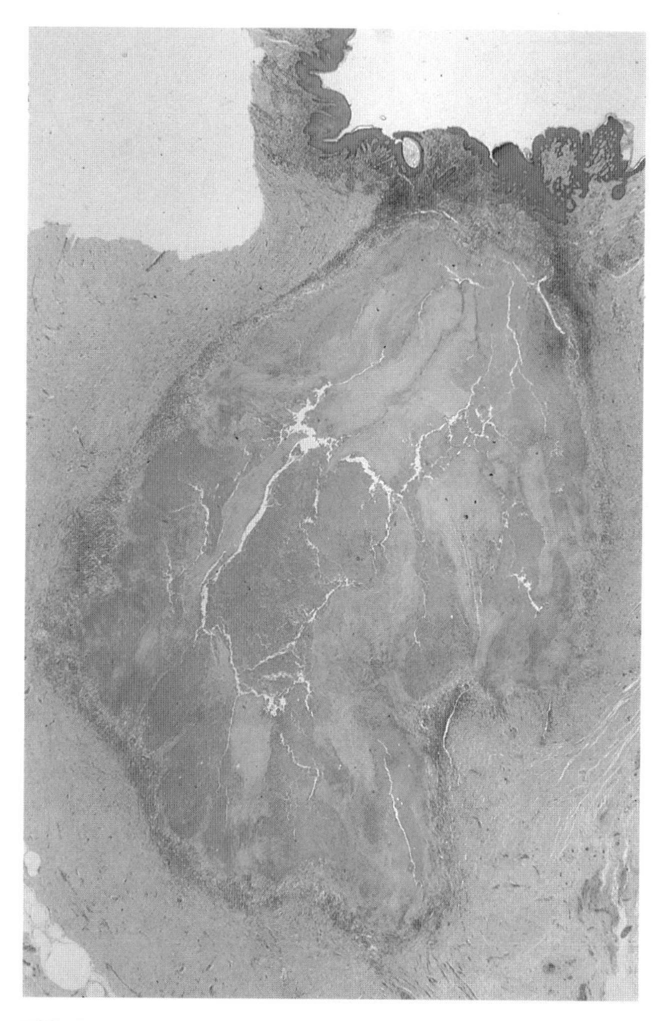

FIG. 21-17. Tuberculosis
A tuberculoma-like appearance with much caseation necrosis in the dermis (H&E, low power).

Tuberculosis Cutis Orificialis

The lesions of tuberculosis cutis orificialis are shallow ulcers with a granulating base occurring singly or in small numbers on or near the mucosal orifices of patients with advanced internal tuberculosis. The infection has spread by direct contamination from an internal lesion that is excreting bacilli. Most patients have a low degree of immunity. The ulcers, which are often very tender, may occur inside the mouth, on the lips, around the anus, or on the perineum.[127] In the case of genitourinary tuberculosis, ulcers may occur on the vulva.

Histopathology. The histologic picture may show merely an ulcer surrounded by a nonspecific inflammatory infiltrate. In most instances, tuberculoid granulomas with pronounced necrosis are found deep in the dermis.[127] Tubercle bacilli are usually readily demonstrated in the sections, even when the histologic appearance is nonspecific.

Differential Diagnosis of Cutaneous Tuberculosis

Because tuberculosis can produce such a wide variety of inflammatory reactions—nonnecrotic granulomas, necrotic granulomas, nonspecific acute inflammation, and epithelial hyperplasia[113]—it is not surprising that many other lesions have similar histologic appearances. These other lesions include sarcoidosis, mycoses, leishmaniasis, nontuberculosis mycobacterioses and leprosy, syphilis, foreign-body implantation reactions, Wegener's granulomatosis, and rosacea.

Sarcoidosis usually has little lymphocytic reaction around the granulomas, unlike most forms of granulomatous tuberculosis. When necrosis occurs in a sarcoid, it is usually fibrinoid in type rather than caseating. A thorough search for acid-fast bacilli, a search for fungal infection with PAS and Grocott stains, and the use of polarizing light to exclude foreign material are obviously important in arriving at a diagnosis. Clinical data and the result of a tuberculin test are also significant. Culture of a lesion should establish the diagnosis in most cases. Recently, the use of PCR technology on paraffin sections to detect specific mycobacterial DNA has proved useful in confirming tuberculosis in the absence of evident organisms in sections.[128]

Tuberculids

The *tuberculids,* a term first proposed in 1896,[129] according to some authors comprise two types of dermatoses: papulonecrotic tuberculids and lichen scrofulosorum.[130,131] Cases of

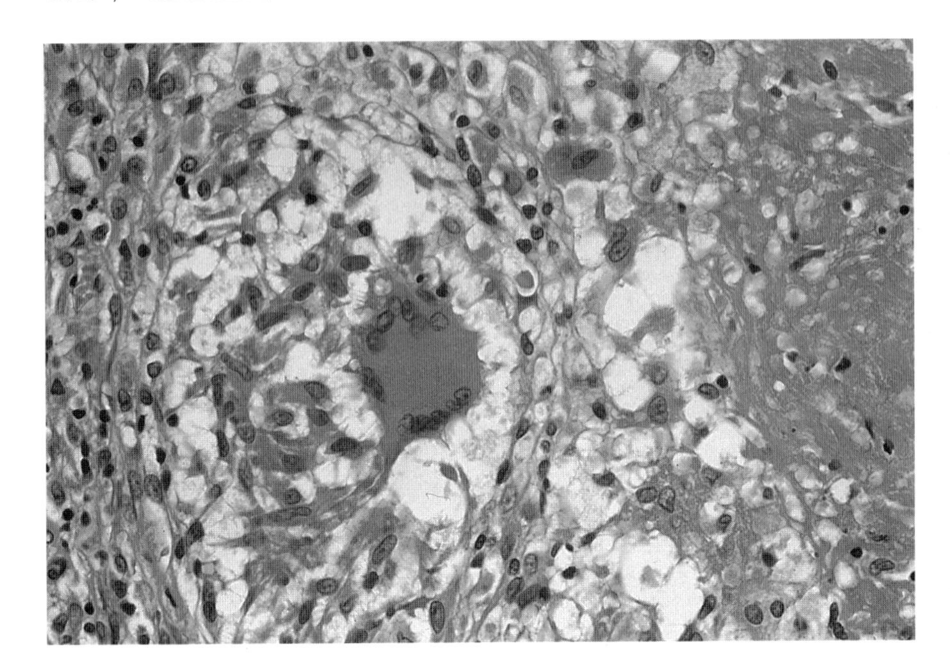

FIG. 21-18. Tuberculosis
Same lesion as in Fig. 21-7, showing the edge of the necrosis with epithelioid cells and giant cells (H&E, high power).

nodular vasculitis, when associated with tuberculosis, are included within the group of tuberculids and are called erythema induratum (Bazin's disease; see Chap. 8).

Tuberculids are skin lesions in patients with tuberculosis, often occult, elsewhere in the body. The most common sites of infection are lymph nodes.[132] By definition, stains for acid-fast bacilli and culture for mycobacteria are negative; delayed hypersensitivity skin tests for tuberculosis are positive, and the lesions heal on antituberculous therapy. Recently, using the PCR technique, mycobacterial DNA has been identified in some lesions.[133] This supports the concept of tuberculids as immunologic reactions to degenerate dead bacilli or antigenic fragments thereof that have been deposited in the skin and subcutis.

Papulonecrotic Tuberculids

Papulonecrotic lesions are erythematous papules that usually develop on the limbs in a symmetrical distribution.[134] They ulcerate and heal, leaving depressed scars. These tuberculids often recur until treated. Occasionally they may develop into lupus vulgaris.

Histopathology. Vascular involvement is observed in early lesions. It may consist of a leukocytoclastic vasculitis[130] or a lymphocytic vasculitis.[135] In either case, it is associated with fibrinoid necrosis and thrombotic occlusion of individual vessels.[135] Subsequently, a wedge-shaped area of necrosis forms, with its broad base toward the epidermis[134] (Figs. 21-19 and 21-20). As this wedge is gradually cast off, epithelioid and

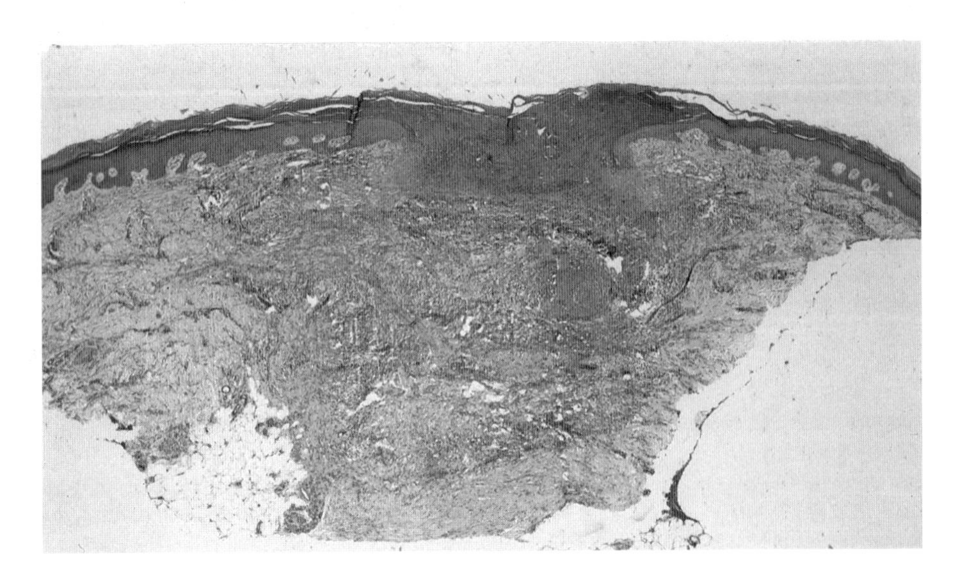

FIG. 21-19. Papulonecrotic tuberculid
Wedge-shaped infarction of the dermis and epidermis, caused by vasculitis (H&E, low power).

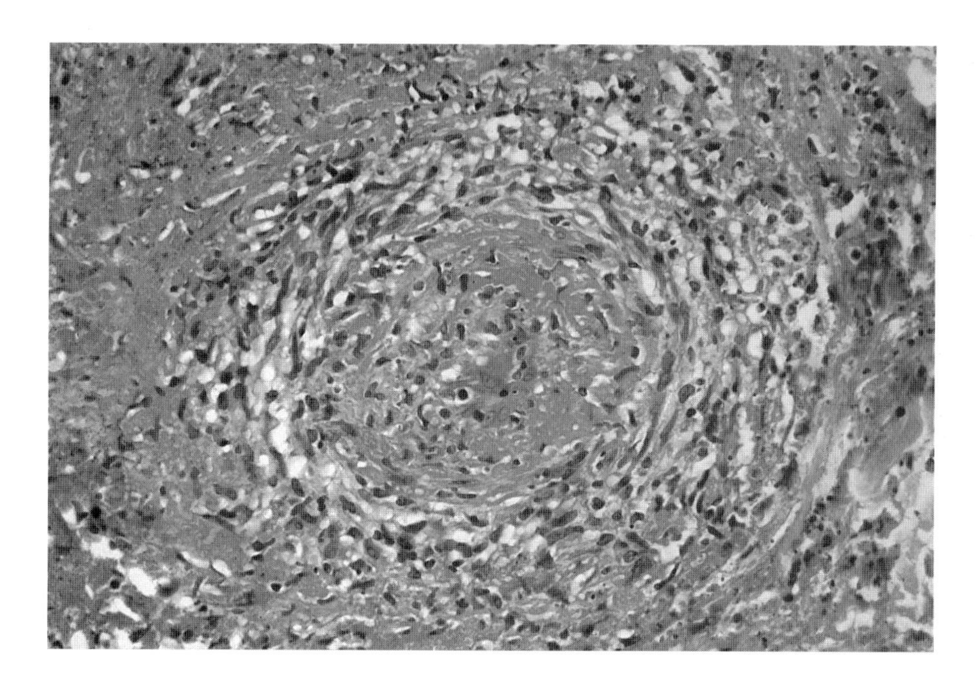

FIG. 21-20. Papulonecrotic tuberculid
Necrotizing vasculitis of a dermal artery, with granulomatous surround (H&E, high power).

giant cells gather around its periphery, although focal granuloma formation is poor. Follicular necrosis or suppuration may occur, although diffuse acute inflammatory cells are infrequent. Ziehl-Neelsen stains are, of course, negative.

Differential Diagnosis. Numerous conditions may be confused clinically or histopathologically with papulonecrotic tuberculids. They include pityriasis lichenoides acuta, syphilides, miliary tuberculosis, perforating granuloma annulare, and suppurative folliculitis.[134]

Lichen Scrofulosorum

This lesion consists of yellow or brown follicular papules, 0.5 to 3.0 mm in diameter, on the trunk. They heal without scarring.

Histopathology. Superficial dermal granulomas are observed, usually in the vicinity of hair follicles or sweat ducts. The granulomas are composed of epithelioid cells, with some Langhans' giant cells and a narrow margin of lymphoid cells at the periphery (Fig. 21-21). Generally, caseation necrosis is absent.[131]

Differential Diagnosis. Distinction of lichen scrofulosorum from sarcoidosis may be impossible on histologic grounds alone.

Pathogenesis. The histogenesis of tuberculids is still unclear. Tubercle bacilli are absent in tuberculids, either because they have arrived hematogenously in fragmented form or because they have been destroyed at the sites of the tuberculids by immunologic mechanisms. Mycobacterial DNA is, however, demonstrable in many cases.[133,136] The reaction in the papulonecrotic tuberculid consists of an Arthus reaction with vasculitis followed by a delayed hypersensitivity response with granuloma formation.[130] In the case of lichen scrofulosorum, there is only a delayed hypersensitivity reaction resulting in granuloma formation.[131]

Tuberculid-type reactions are also described with nontuberculosis mycobacteria (*Mycobacterium bovis* and *M avium*).[137,138]

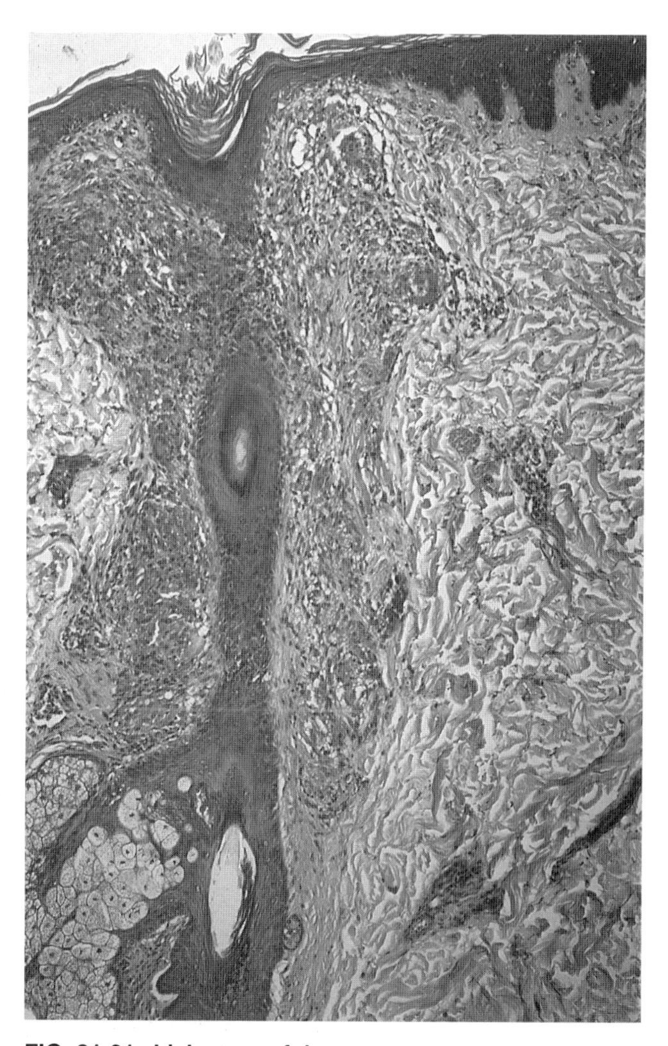

FIG. 21-21. Lichen scrofulosorum
Nonnecrotizing epithelioid cell granulomas alongside a hair shaft (H&E, low power).

INFECTIONS WITH NONTUBERCULOSIS MYCOBACTERIA

Among the nontuberculosis, nonleprosy mycobacterial infections of the skin, those caused by *Mycobacterium marinum* are the most common among nonimmunosuppressed people.[139] Unlike *M tuberculosis,* which is transmitted from person to person, nontuberculosis mycobacteria are abundant in nature, in soil and water, and contact is frequent in most zones of the world.[106,140]

These skin infections may be acquired by direct inoculation into the skin or by hematogenous spread from a visceral focus. Increased use of immunosuppression in medicine (e.g., for transplantation and cancer chemotherapy) and the pandemic of HIV/AIDS have resulted in many more mycobacterial skin infections. The cell-mediated immune system is a major defense against such organisms and is affected or destroyed during the course of these immunosuppressive conditions. The clinical and histopathologic patterns are also altered, with organisms being found in greater density than in immunocompetent persons.

The histopathologic picture in nontuberculosis mycobacterioses is just as variable as the clinical picture and may present nonspecific acute and chronic inflammation, suppuration and abscess formation, or tuberculoid granulomas with or without caseation.[113,141] In some instances, both tissue reactions occur concurrently. The presence or absence of acid-fast bacilli depends on the tissue reaction. In suppurative lesions, numerous acid-fast bacilli often can be found.

Infection with *Mycobacterium kansasii*

M kansasii is usually a lymph node and pulmonary infection,[142] and skin lesions are unusual. Implantation causes a chronic cutaneous nodule and sometimes ulceration.[143] The lesions are often crusted. There may be sporotrichoid spread up the extremity.[139,144] In immunocompromised patients such as those with HIV infection, there may be multiple visceral lesions (lung and bone) with hematogenous dissemination to skin. The skin lesions are acute abscesses with large numbers of acid-fast bacilli (Fig. 21-22).

Infection with *Mycobacterium avium-intracellulare*

M avium complex infection is a common cause of cervical lymph node mycobacteriosis in normal children, and of pulmonary disease in previously damaged lungs.[106] Prior to the HIV pandemic, skin infections were rare, with hematogenously borne lesions in skin and subcutis observed in patients usually with immunosuppressing diseases.[108]

Severely immunocompromised patients such as those with HIV infection have a very high prevalence of *M avium-intracellulare* bacteremia,[145] and many show one or more cutaneous papules and nodules.[146,147] Steroid therapy also predisposes to skin lesions. The histology may be granulomatous or mixed acute and chronic inflammatory, as with tuberculosis.[106] Sometimes there is a histology resembling that of lepromatous leprosy (Figs. 21-23). Macrophages contain large numbers of bacilli without necrosis, and a spindle cell transformation of macrophages, forming a histoidlike lesion (as in leprosy), can occur (see Figs. 21-23 and 21-24).[148,149]

Infection with *Mycobacterium marinum*

Infections with *M marinum* can be contracted through minor abrasions incurred while bathing in swimming pools or in ocean or lake water or while cleaning home aquariums.[150] Infected swimming pools have caused epidemics, the largest of which affected 290 persons.[151] The period of incubation usually is about 3 weeks, but may be longer.[139]

Clinically, most of the lesions caused by *M marinum* are solitary and consist of indolent, dusky red, hyperkeratotic, papillomatous papules, nodules, or plaques. Superficial ulceration is occasionally observed. The fingers, knees, elbows, and feet are

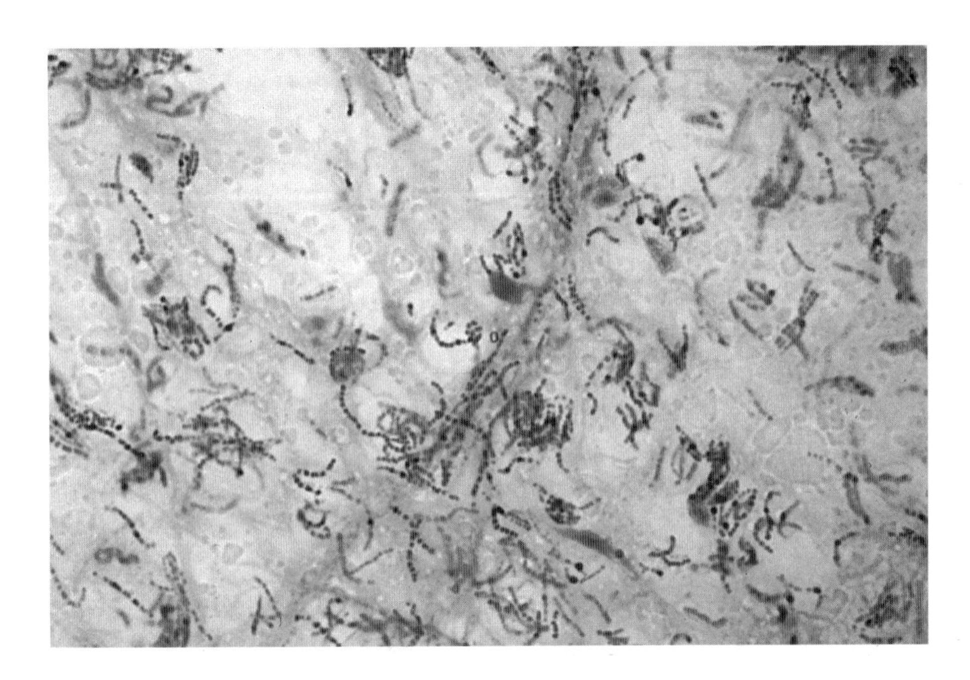

FIG. 21-22. *Mycobacterium kansasii* infection
Needle aspirate of a skin lesion on an immunocompromised patient. Abundant elongated and beaded acid-fast bacilli typical of *M kansasii* (Ziehl-Neelsen, high power).

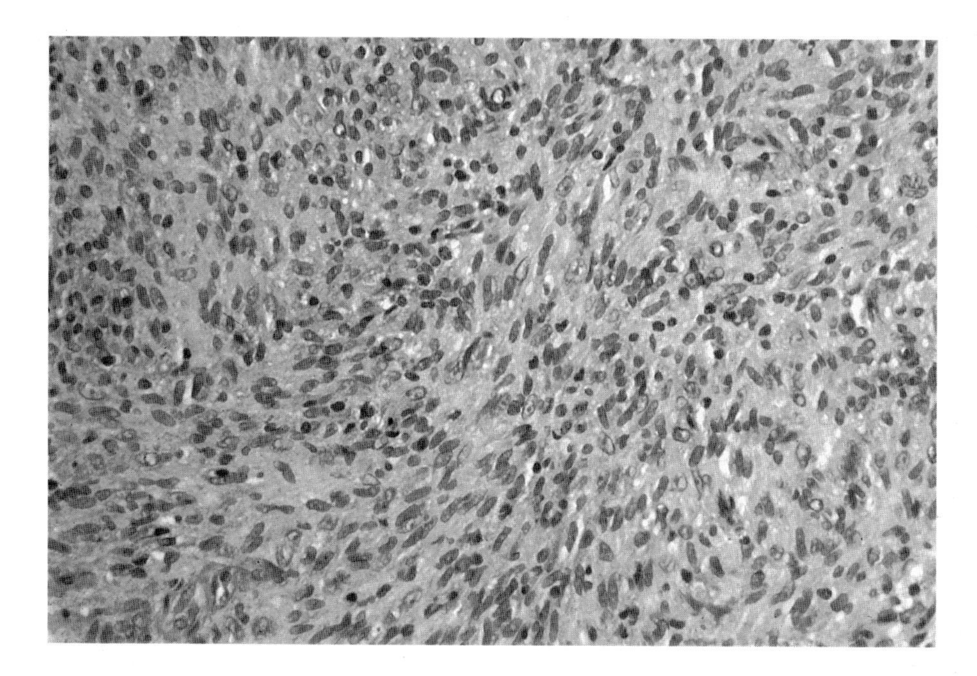

FIG. 21-23. *Mycobacterium avium-intracellulare* infection
Spindle cell proliferation of macrophages (pattern similar to that observed in histoid leprosy) (H&E, high power).

most commonly affected. In some instances, satellite papules arise and ascending sporotrichoid spread occurs.[152] Lesions may form at different sites in the case of multiple injuries. Although spontaneous healing usually takes place within a year, the lesions persist in some patients for many years. A few HIV-associated cases have been reported.[153] Fatal disseminated *M marinum* infection is rare.[154]

Histopathology. Early lesions no more than 2 or 3 months old show a nonspecific inflammatory infiltrate composed of neutrophils, monocytes, and macrophages. In lesions about 4 months old, a few multinucleated giant cells and a few small epithelioid cell granulomas usually are present, and in lesions 6 months old or older, typical tubercles or tuberculoid structures may be seen.[155] Areas of necrosis are only occasionally present in the centers of the granulomas. The epidermis often shows papillomatosis and hyperkeratosis with an acute inflammatory infiltrate, and ulceration (Fig. 21-25).

Acid-fast bacilli usually can be identified in histologic sections of early lesions that show a nonspecific inflammatory infiltrate. In contrast, tuberculoid granulomas generally no longer show acid-fast organisms unless areas of central necrosis are present. Although primary lesions usually require a few months for the formation of tuberculoid granulomas, the sporotrichoid nodules that arise later show tuberculoid granulomas and a lack of acid-fast bacilli even when they have been present for only a few weeks.

Differential Diagnosis. The granulomatous reaction produced by *M marinum* is similar to that observed in tuberculosis verrucosa cutis or lupus vulgaris. The pattern of pseudoepitheliomatous hyperplasia with granulomas and polymorphonuclear

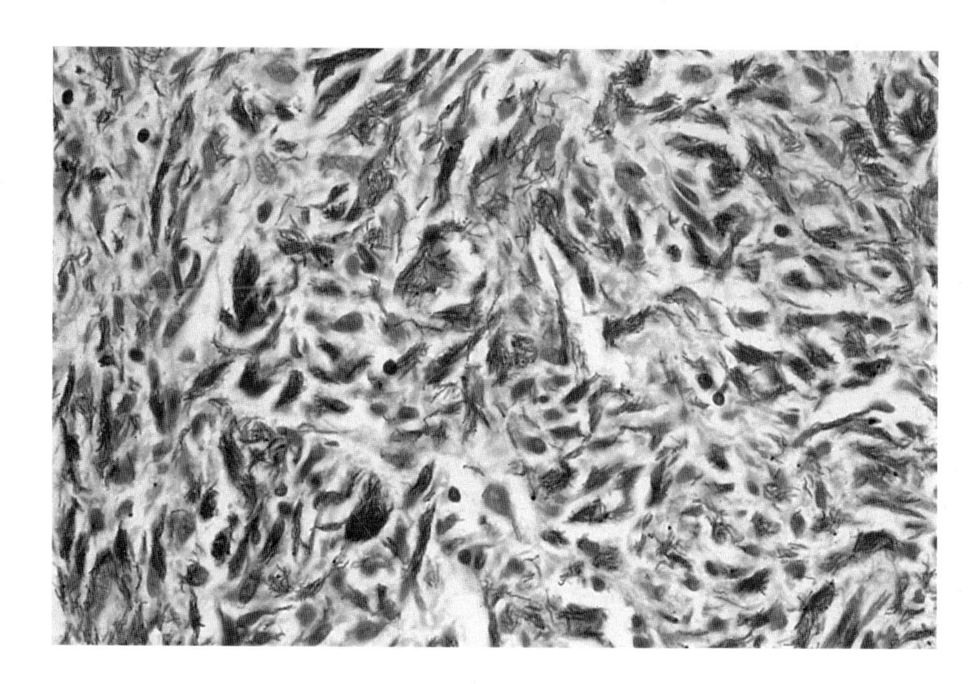

FIG. 21-24. *Mycobacterium avium-intracellulare* infection
Same lesion as in Fig. 21-15, showing abundant acid-fast bacilli, similar to histoid leprosy (Ziehl-Neelsen, high power).

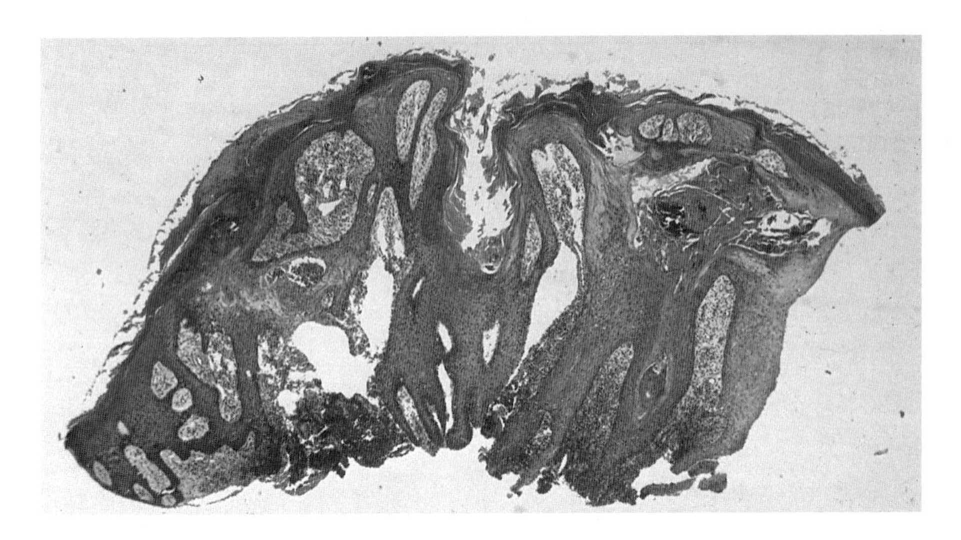

FIG. 21-25. *Mycobacterium marinum* infection
A marked pseudoepitheliomatous epidermal hyperplasia, with acute inflammatory foci within the epidermis (H&E, low power).

neutrophil infiltrate is also seen in several cutaneous mycoses (e.g., sporotrichosis and chromoblastomycosis), so fungal stains need to be examined alongside Ziehl-Neelsen stains. For definitive identification, culture may be necessary.

Buruli Ulcer (*M ulcerans*)

Buruli ulceration, an infection caused by a nontuberculosis mycobacterium, *M ulcerans,* is endemic in West and Central Africa, Central America, and South Australia.[156–158] The infection commences as a cutaneous nodule that ulcerates down to fat and bone with extensive undermining of the epidermis.[159] These painless ulcers are usually located on extremities. Penetrating trauma is a recognized antecedent factor, but the organism has yet to be isolated in nature.[158]

Histopathology. The infection begins as a subcutaneous nodule exhibiting "ghost" ischemic-type fat necrosis with deposition of fibrin (Fig. 21-26), and hematoxyphilic clumps of mycobacteria. Ulceration proceeds as the epidermis loses its vascular supply. Ziehl-Neelsen stains reveal vast numbers of acid-fast bacilli in the necrotic fat (Figs. 21-27 and 21-28). Thrombosed vessels are observed. In time, a granulomatous reaction commences from the depth and sides of the ulcer; healing and reepithelialization take place with considerable scarring. Acid-fast bacilli decline in number during healing.[156,157,160]

Pathogenesis. The widespread necrosis of subcutaneous tissue is caused by an exotoxin elaborated by *M ulcerans.* This toxin causes necrosis when inoculated into guinea pig skin.[161,162] Like *M marinum, M ulcerans* shows optimal cultural growth at 30° to 33° C. Healing coincides with development of delayed hypersensitivity to the mycobacterium.

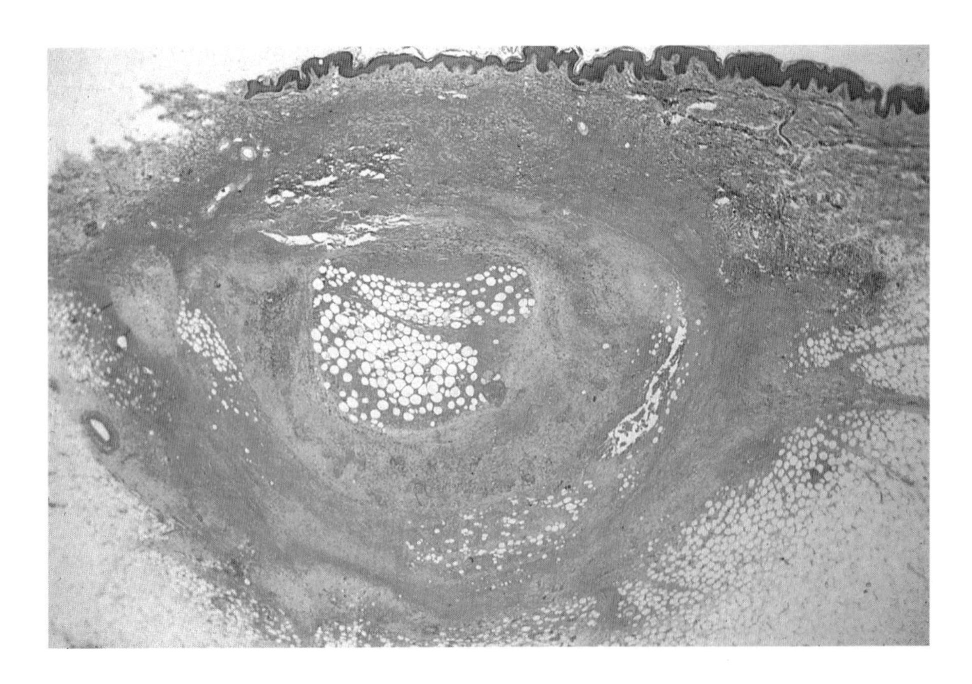

FIG. 21-26. Buruli ulcer (*Mycobacterium ulcerans* infection)
Early, preulcerating lesion, with pandermal and subcutaneous fat necrosis (H&E, low power).

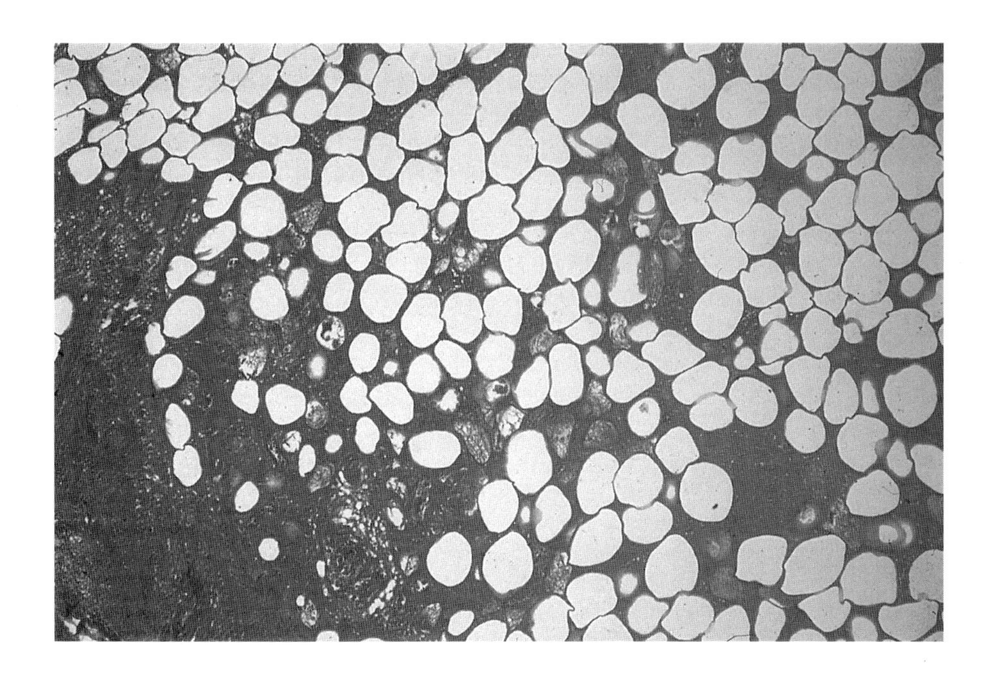

FIG. 21-27. Buruli ulcer
The ischemic-type fat necrosis, without cellular reaction (H&E, medium power).

Other Nontuberculosis Mycobacterioses

Infections in the skin and subcutis caused by the rapid growers, *M chelonei* and *M fortuitum,* are associated with medical injections through unsterile contaminated needles and cannulae.[106,163] Sporotrichoid spread can occur with *M chelonei*.[164] The inflammatory reaction is usually a mixed acute (neutrophilic) and chronic (granulomatous) response, with acid-fast bacilli visible on sections.[106] Localized and disseminated *M haemophilum* infection is reported in patients with HIV and other causes of immunosuppression.[136,165–167]

Bacille Calmette-Gúerin (BCG) is the most commonly used vaccine, yet it rarely results in significant cutaneous lesions. Persisting ulcerating lesions may be observed. Histologically, these lesions are caseating granulomas in the dermis, as seen in tuberculosis, but acid-fast bacilli are rarely observed. In immunocompromised patients, there may be generalized cutaneous nodules, and histology shows abundant bacilli, poorly formed bacilli, and variable or no necrosis.[168]

LEPROSY

Leprosy is caused by *M leprae* and predominantly affects the skin and peripheral nerves. The disease is endemic in many tropical and subtropical countries but is declining in incidence. The Indian subcontinent, Southeast Asia, sub-Saharan countries in Africa, and Brazil comprise the areas most affected at present.[169]

The mode of transmission of leprosy is unknown, but it is probably inhalation of bacilli,[106] which may be excreted from the nasal passages of a multibacillary patient or possibly im-

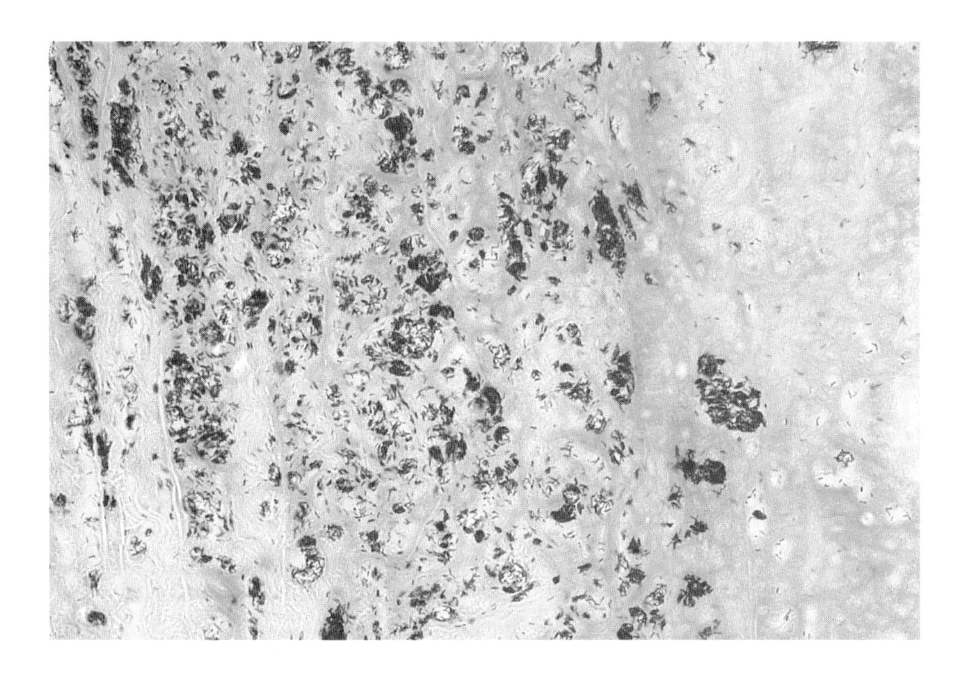

FIG. 21-28. Buruli ulcer
Clumps of acid-fast bacilli within the fat necrosis (Ziehl-Neelsen, high power).

planted from organisms in the soil. Direct person-to-person infection by means of the skin occurs rarely if at all. After inhalation, it is likely that bacilli pass through the blood to peripheral and cutaneous nerves, where infection and host reaction commence.

Immunopathologic Spectrum of Leprosy

The sequence of disease pathogenesis is complex, is very chronic, and depends on host-parasite immunologic responses. The leprosy bacillus is nontoxic, and clinicopathologic manifestations are the result of immunopathology and/or the progressive accumulation of infected cells. Leprosy is the best example of a disease showing an immunopathologic spectrum whereby the host immune reaction to the infective agent ranges from apparently none to marked, with a consequent range of clinicopathologic manifestations.[170,171] Tuberculoid leprosy indicates a high cellular immune response (i.e., T cells and macrophage activation) and few bacilli in tissues; at the opposite pole, lepromatous leprosy indicates an absent cellular immune response to *M leprae* antigens, with no macrophage activation and abundant bacilli in tissues. The spectrum of leprosy is a continuum, and patients may move in either direction according to host response and treatment. The standard delineation follows that of Ridley and Jopling,[170] with categories defined along the spectrum by a combination of clinical, microbiological, histopathologic, and immunologic indices: TT (tuberculoid), BT (borderline tuberculoid), BB (midborderline), BL (borderline lepromatous), and LL (lepromatous). The term "borderline" is used to denote patterns that share some features of both tuberculoid and lepromatous leprosy.[170,172]

TT and LL patients are stable, the former often self-healing and the latter remaining heavily infected unless given appropriate chemotherapy. Patients presenting at the BT point will often downgrade toward BL leprosy in the absence of treatment. The central point of the spectrum (BB) is the most unstable, with most patients downgrading to LL if not treated. The term "indeterminate leprosy" is used to describe patients presenting with very early leprosy lesions that cannot be categorized definitely along the immunopathologic spectrum (cannot be determined as BT or LL, for example).

It is likely that in endemic zones, a high proportion of people are infected by *M leprae* but either have full immunity and no disease, or have developed one or a few lesions that have self-healed without significant morbidity. The progression of infection and disease is summarized in Fig. 21-29. Patients with determined leprosy are most numerous at the BT and LL points of the spectrum.

Staining of *M leprae* Bacilli

The classical method for demonstrating leprosy bacilli in lesions is a modified Ziehl-Neelsen stain, where the degree of acid and alcohol removal of carbol fuchsin is less than in the methods used for identifying other mycobacteria. The Fite methods are the most commonly used.[173] Recently, a periodic acid-carbol pararosanilin has been advocated.[174] Methanamine silver stains are also useful in detecting fragmented acid-fast bacilli. The sensitivity of detection of acid-fast bacilli by histologic means remains poor, because about 1000 bacilli per cubic centimeter of tissue must be present in order to detect one bacillus in a section. For lesions where bacilli are scanty, it is recommended that at least six sections be examined before declaring them negative. The standard enumeration of leprosy bacilli in lesions—the bacterial index (BI)—follows Ridley's logarithmic scale (which applies to both skin biopsies and slit skin smears)[172]:

BI = 0: no bacilli observed
BI = 1: 1 to 10 bacilli in 10 to 100 high-power fields (hpf, oil immersion)
BI = 2: 1 to 10 bacilli in 1 to 10 hpf
BI = 3: 1 to 10 bacilli per hpf
BI = 4: 10 to 100 bacilli per hpf
BI = 5: 100 to 1000 bacilli per hpf
BI = 6: >1000 bacilli per hpf

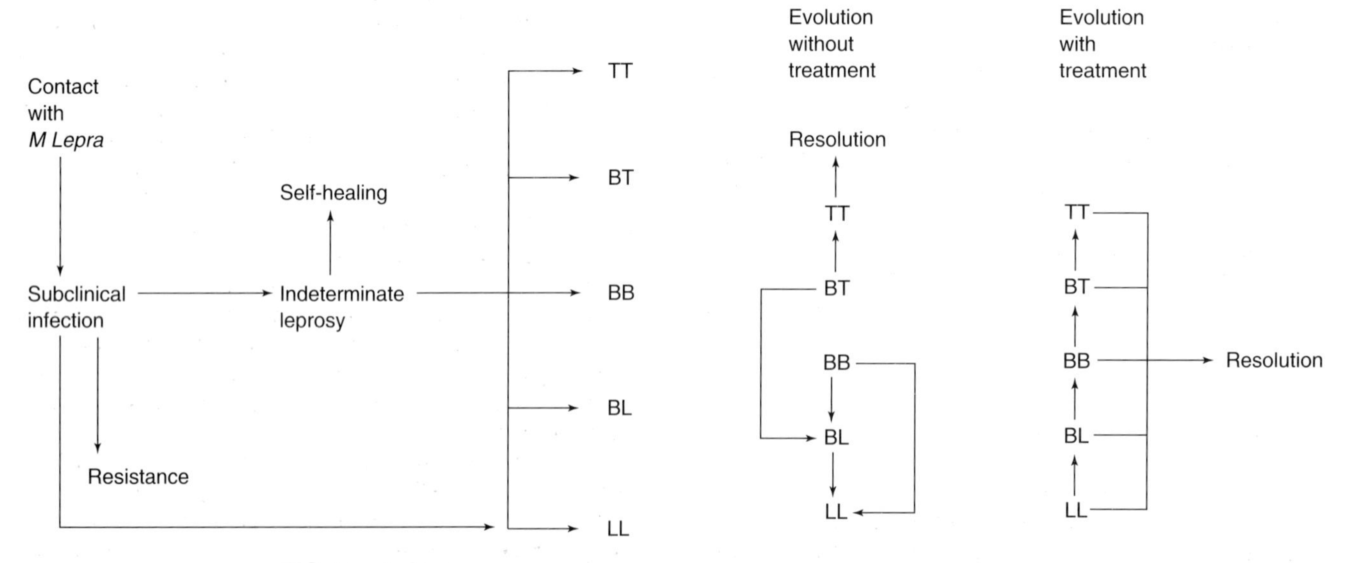

FIG. 21-29. Leprosy
The sequence of events that may follow infection with *Mycobacterium leprae*.

Solid-staining bacilli indicate that the organisms are capable of multiplication. Fragmented (beaded) and granular acid-fast bacilli indicate that they are dead. Patients with no bacilli detectable in lesions are termed paucibacillary; those with some or many bacilli are multibacillary (this distinction is important in determing the duration of chemotherapy).[175]

Immunocytochemical methods for demonstrating mycobacterial antigens have a limited role. The most frequently used is a polyclonal anti-BCG antibody.[176] In untreated lesions, it will not detect small numbers of bacilli if ordinary histochemical methods have proved negative. However, immunocytochemistry does have a role in demonstrating the presence of leprosy antigen after the bacilli have fragmented, been partly digested by macrophage enzymes, and lost their acid-fast staining quality (see later).

Clinical Pathology of Leprosy

For general discussions of clinical leprosy and leprosy pathology, the reader is referred to Pfaltzgraff and Ramu[177] and Job.[178]

Early, Indeterminate Leprosy

Many patients present with obvious or advanced skin and peripheral nerve lesions (the latter are primarily nerve enlargement and the consequences of anaesthesia): these patients have "determined leprosy." However, the earliest detectable skin lesion comprises one or a few hypopigmented macules with variable loss of sensation. Any part of the body may be affected.

Histopathology. There is mild lymphocytic and macrophage accumulation around neurovascular bundles, the superficial and deep dermal vessels, sweat glands, and erector pili muscle; focal lymphocytic invasion into the lower epidermis and into the dermal nerves may be observed. No formed epithelioid cell granulomas are present (if they were, it would not be indeterminate leprosy but a tuberculoid leprosy). Schwann cell hyperplasia is a feature, but it is highly subjective. Not all these features are present in every case. The diagnosis hinges on finding one or more acid-fast bacilli in the sites of predilection: in nerve, in erector pili muscle, just under the epidermis, or in a macrophage about a vessel. Without demonstrating bacilli, the diagnosis can only be presumptive (Figs. 21-30 and 21-31).

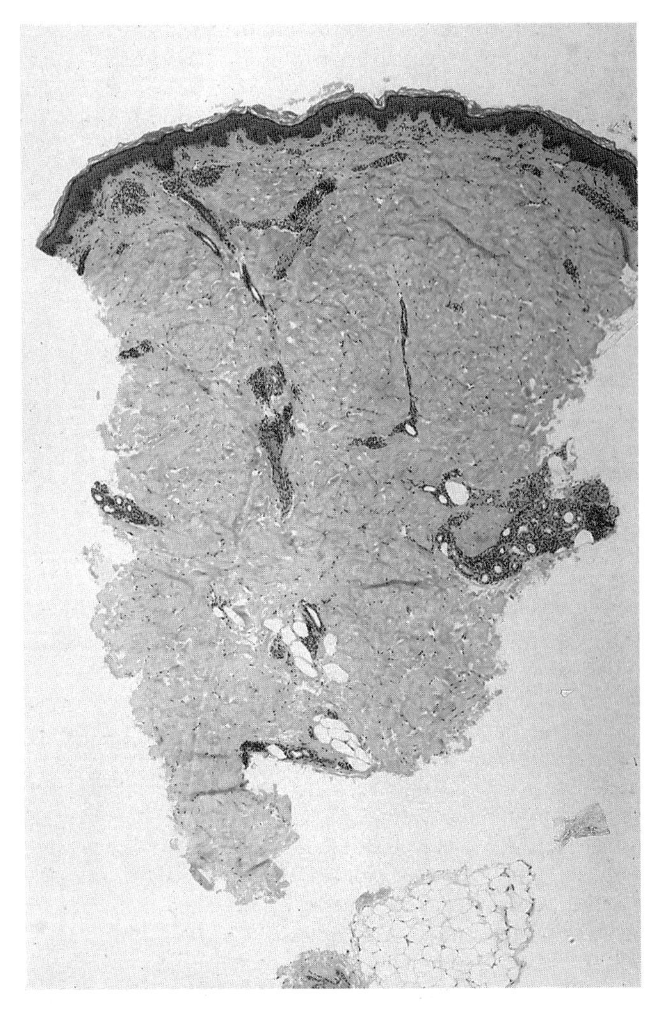

FIG. 21-30. Indeterminate leprosy
Slight pandermal perineurovascular and periappendageal chronic inflammation (H&E, low power).

The leprosy delayed hypersensitivity skin test, the Mitsuda reaction, may be of use in predicting the outcome of indeterminate leprosy (should it not be treated properly). Mitsuda-negative patients with indeterminate leprosy are more likely to become lepromatous, whereas Mitsuda-positive patients are likely to become tuberculoid or to self-heal without developing tuberculoid lesions.

Lepromatous (LL) Leprosy

Lepromatous leprosy initially has cutaneous and mucosal lesions, with neural changes occurring later. The lesions usually are numerous and are symmetrically arranged. There are three clinical types: macular, infiltrative-nodular, and diffuse. In the macular type, numerous ill-defined, confluent, either hypopigmented or erythematous macules are observed. They are frequently slightly infiltrated. The infiltrative-nodular type, the classical and most common variety, may develop from the macular type or arise as such. It is characterized by papules, nodules, and diffuse infiltrates that are often dull red. Involvement of the eyebrows and forehead often results in a leonine facies, with a loss of eyebrows and eyelashes. The lesions themselves are not notably hypoesthetic, although, through involvement of the large peripheral nerves, disturbances of sensation and nerve paralyses develop. The nerves that are most commonly involved are the ulnar, radial, and common peroneal nerves.

The diffuse type of leprosy, called Lucio leprosy, which is most common in Mexico and also in Central America, shows diffuse infiltration of the skin without nodules. This infiltration may be quite inconspicuous except for the alopecia of the eyebrows and eyelashes it produces. Acral, symmetric anesthesia is generally present.[179]

A distinctive variant of lepromatous leprosy, the histoid type, first described in 1963,[180] is characterized by the occurrence of well-demarcated cutaneous and subcutaneous nodules resembling dermatofibromas. It frequently follows incomplete chemotherapy or acquired drug resistance, leading to bacterial relapse.

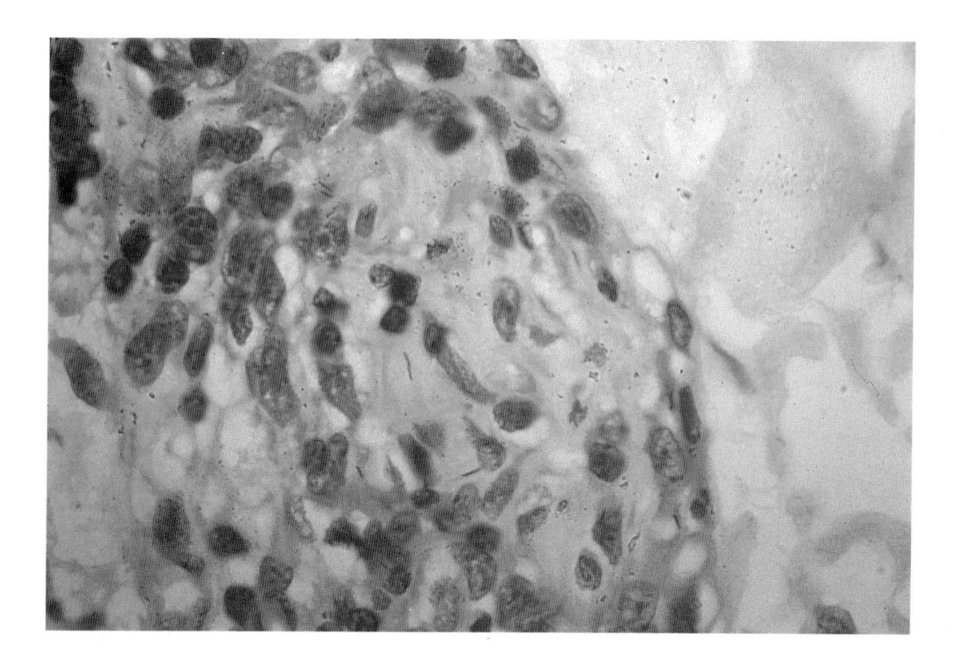

FIG. 21-31. Indeterminate leprosy High-power view of a nerve with surrounding lymphocytes and a few intraneural acid-fast bacilli (Wade-Fite, high power).

Rarely, lepromatous leprosy can present as a single lesion, rather than as multiple lesions.[181]

Histopathology. Lepromatous leprosy, in the usual macular or infiltrative-nodular lesions, exhibits an extensive cellular infiltrate that is almost invariably separated from the flattened epidermis by a narrow grenz zone of normal collagen (Fig. 21-32). The infiltrate causes the destruction of the cutaneous appendages and extends into the subcutaneous fat. In florid early lesions, the macrophages have abundant eosinophilic cytoplasm and contain a mixed population of solid and fragmented bacilli (BI = 4 or 5) (Fig. 21-33). The bacilli, on Wade-Fite staining, can be seen to measure about 5.0 by 0.5 μm, and if solid may be packed like cigars. Bacilli are commonly observed in endothelial cells also. There is no macrophage activation to form epithelioid cell granulomas. Lymphocyte infiltration is not prominent, but there may be many plasma cells.

In time, and with antimycobacterial chemotherapy, degenerate bacilli accumulate in the macrophages—the so-called lepra cells or Virchow cells—which then have foamy or vacuolated cytoplasm (Figs. 21-34 and 21-35). They resemble xanthoma cells and, on staining with fat stains, are shown to contain lipid—largely neutral fat and phospholipids—rather than cholesterol. The Wade-Fite stain reveals that the bacilli are fragmented or granular and, especially in very chronic lesions, disposed in large basophilic clumps called globi (Fig. 21-36). In lepromatous leprosy, in contrast to tuberculoid leprosy, the nerves in the skin may contain considerable numbers of leprosy bacilli, but remain well-preserved for a long time and slowly become fibrotic.

The histopathology of Lucio (diffuse) leprosy is similar, but with a characteristic heavy bacillation of the small blood vessels in the skin.[179]

Histoid Leprosy

Histoid leprosy shows the highest loads of bacilli (the BI is frequently 6), and the majority are solid-staining, arranged in clumps like sheaves of wheat. The macrophage reaction is un-

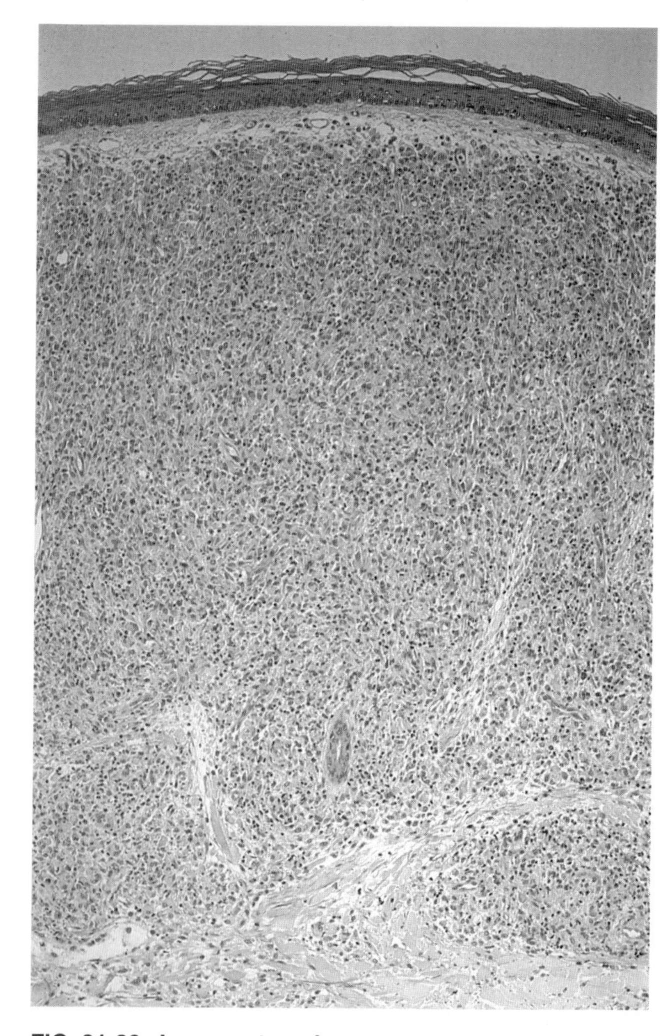

FIG. 21-32. Lepromatous leprosy Skin in a florid case of multibacillary leprosy with a mass of macrophages in the dermis (no granuloma formation), leaving a clear grenz zone under the epidermis (H&E, low power).

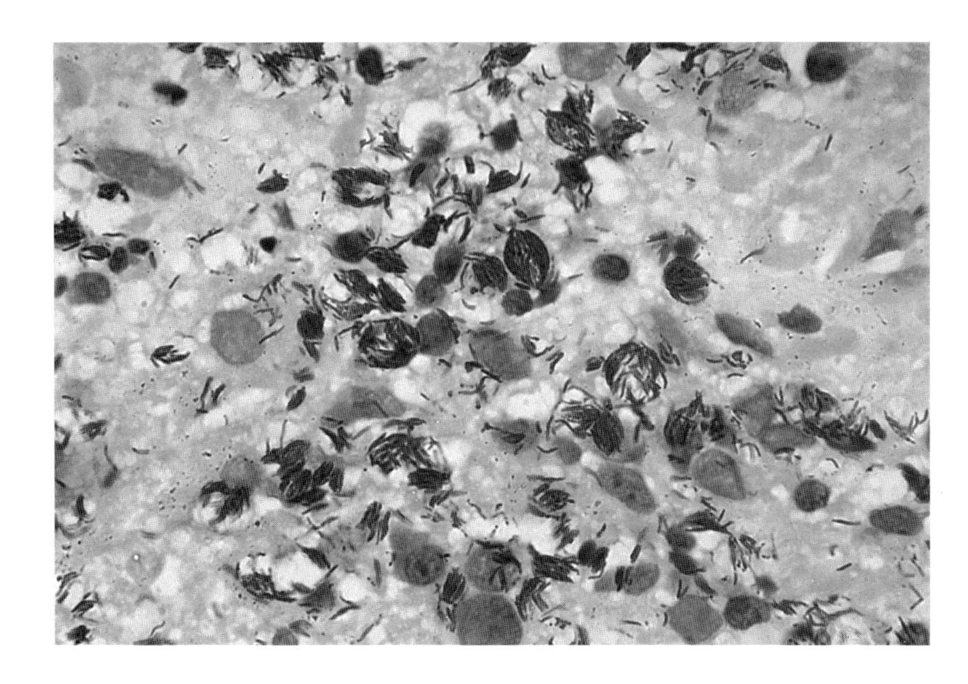

FIG. 21-33. Lepromatous leprosy Acid-fast bacilli, mostly solid, in large numbers (Wade-Fite, high power).

usual in that the cells frequently become spindle-shaped and oriented in a storiform pattern, similar to those of a fibrohistiocytoma (Fig. 21-37). The epidermis may be stretched over such dermal expansile nodules.

When lepromatous leprosy is treated, the bacilli die rapidly and become fragmented within weeks or months. However, it can take several years for the bacterial debris to be cleared by host macrophages. The *M leprae* antigen may persist even longer, and can be demonstrated by immunocytochemical stains (Wade-Fite or silver) even when no bacilli are evident (Fig. 21-38).

Borderline Lepromatous (BL) Leprosy

The lesions of BL leprosy are less numerous and less symmetrical than LL lesions and often display some central dimples.

Histopathology. The important difference between LL and BL leprosy histology is that in BL the lymphocytes are more prominent and there is a tendency for some activation of macrophages to form poorly to moderately defined granulomas. Perineural fibroblast proliferation, forming an "onion skin" in cross section, is typical. Foamy cells are not prominent, and globi do not usually accumulate; the BI ranges from 4 to 5.

Midborderline (BB) Leprosy

The skin lesions are irregularly dispersed and shaped erythematous plaques with punched-out centers. There may be small satellite lesions. Edema is prominent in the lesions.

Histopathology. In BB leprosy, the macrophages are uniformly activated to epithelioid cells but are not focalized into distinct granulomas, and lymphocytes are scanty. There are no

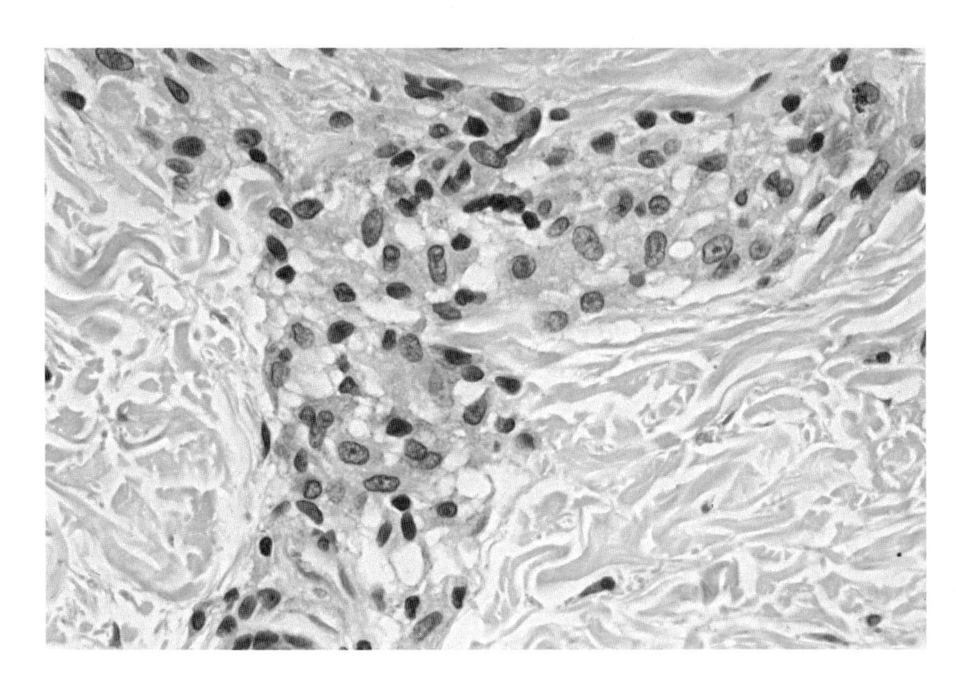

FIG. 21-34. Lepromatous leprosy More common type than that in Fig. 21-23, with smaller foci of perivascular and foamy macrophages (H&E, medium power).

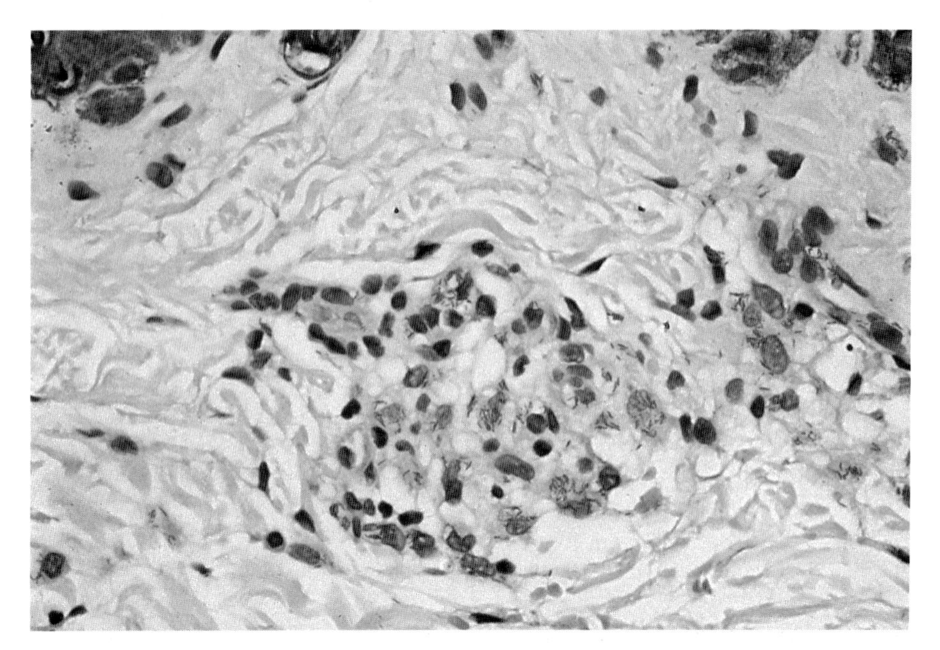

FIG. 21-35. Lepromatous leprosy
Same case as in Fig. 21-26, with numerous acid-fast bacilli, many degenerate, in macrophages (Wade-Fite, high power).

Langhans' giant cells. The BI ranges from 3 to 4. Dermal edema is prominent between the inflammatory cells.

Borderline Tuberculoid (BT) Leprosy

The lesions are asymmetrical and may be scanty. They are dry, hairless plaques with central hypopigmentation. Nerve enlargement is usually found, and the lesions are usually anesthetic.

Histopathology. Granulomas with peripheral lymphocytes follow the neurovascular bundles and infiltrate sweat glands and erector pili muscles. Langhans' giant cells are variable in number and are not large in size. Granulomas along the superficial vascular plexus are frequent, but they do not infiltrate up into the epidermis. Nerve erosion and obliteration are typical (Figs. 21-39 and 21-40). Acid-fast bacilli are scanty (BI ranges from 0 to 2) and are most readily found in the Schwann cells of nerves. Immunocytochemical staining for S-100 protein often

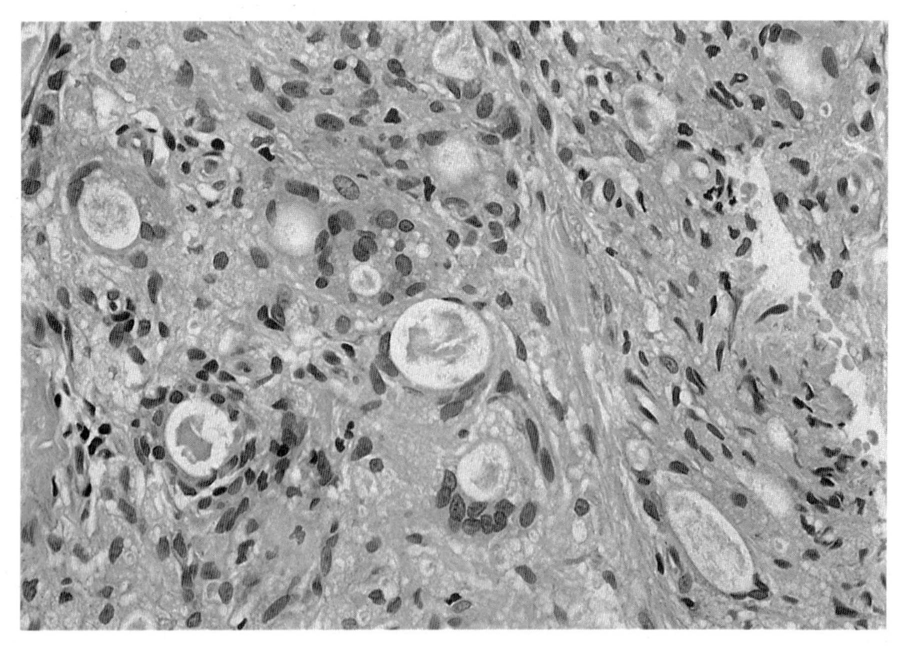

FIG. 21-36. Lepromatous leprosy
Old treated lesion, with large masses (globi) of agglomerated basophilic dead mycobacteria within macrophages (H&E, high power).

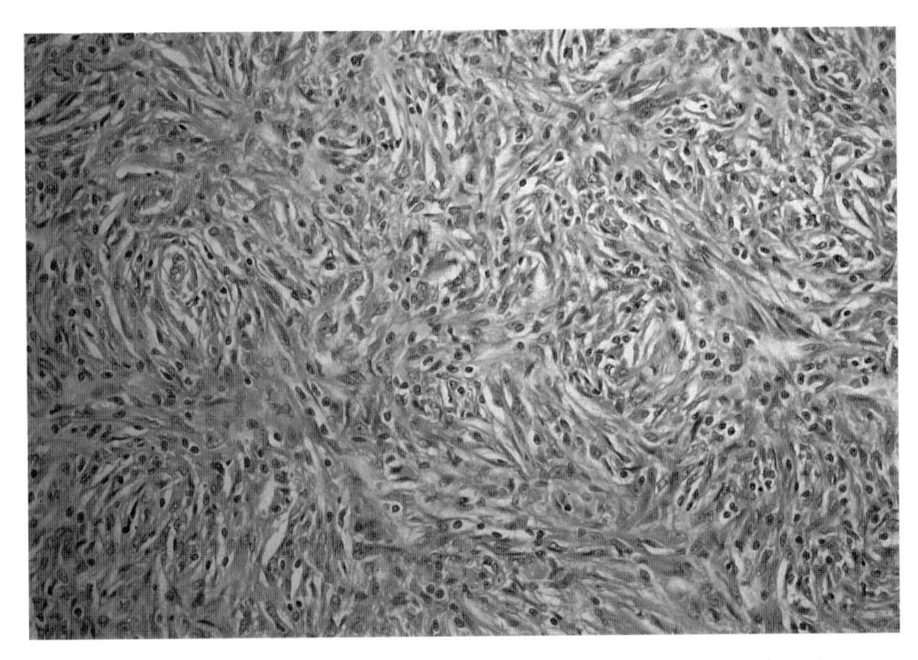

FIG. 21-37. Lepromatous leprosy
A histoid lesion, with spindle cell proliferation of macrophages, resembling a fibrohistiocytoma. The acid-fast bacillus stain showed vast numbers of organisms (similar to the *M avium-intracellulare* lesion, Fig. 21-16) (H&E, high power).

demonstrates the perineural and intraneural granuloma well (Fig. 21-41).

Tuberculoid (TT) Leprosy

The skin lesions of TT leprosy are scanty, dry, erythematous, hypopigmented papules or plaques with sharply defined edges. Anaesthesia is prominent (except on the face). The number of lesions ranges from one to five. Thickened local peripheral nerves may be found. The lesions heal rapidly on chemotherapy.

Histopathology. Primary TT leprosy has large epithelioid cells arranged in compact granulomas along with neurovascular bundles, with dense peripheral lymphocyte accumulation. Langhans' giant cells are typically absent. Dermal nerves may

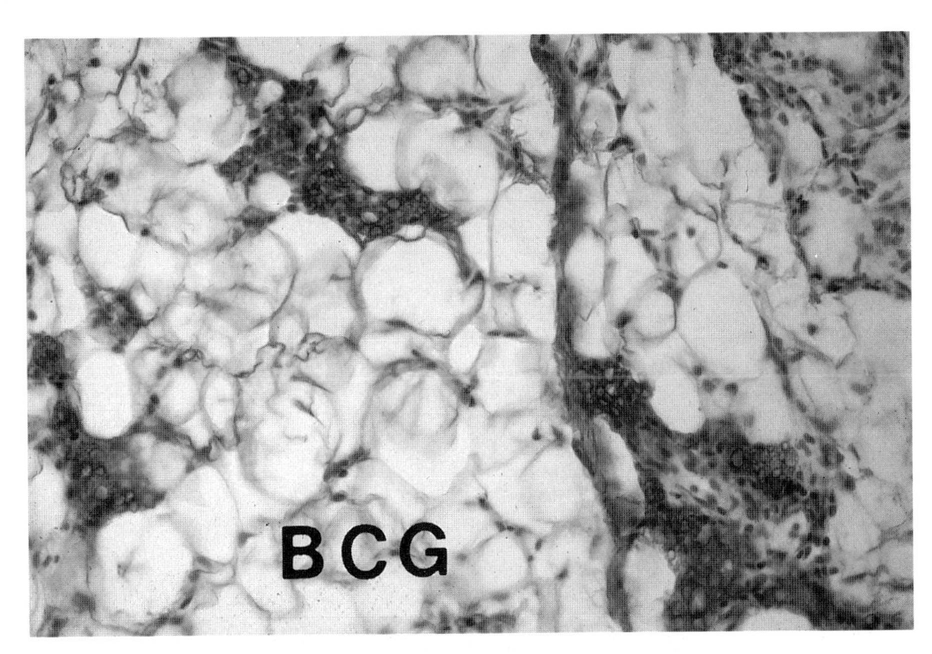

FIG. 21-38. Lepromatous leprosy
Old treated lesion; foamy macrophages remain, but no acid-fast bacilli were visible. However, an antimycobacterial immunocytochemical stain reveals persistent leprosy antigen (Anti-BCG, medium power).

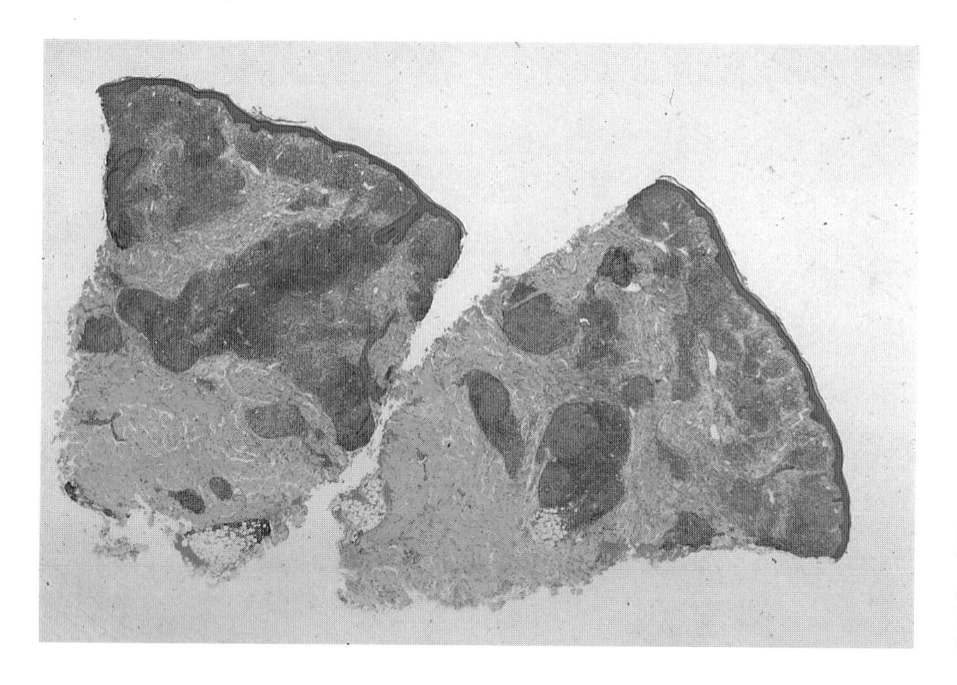

FIG. 21-39. Tuberculoid leprosy Two sections of a typical lesion, showing pandermal perineurovascular granulomas and lymphocytes (H&E, low power).

be absent (obliterated) or surrounded and eroded by dense lymphocyte cuffs (Fig. 21-42). Acid-fast bacilli are rarely found, even in nerves. A second pattern of TT leprosy is found in certain reactional states (see later).

Peripheral Nerves

In all these patterns of leprosy, the major peripheral nerves are often undergoing parallel pathologies. The inflammation is similar, and the same classification system is applied. However, the density of acid-fast bacilli is often a logrithm higher than in the nearby skin.[182]

Leprosy Reactions

Leprosy reactions are classified into two main types (1 and 2). A third reaction is specific to Lucio multibacillary leprosy.[177,183]

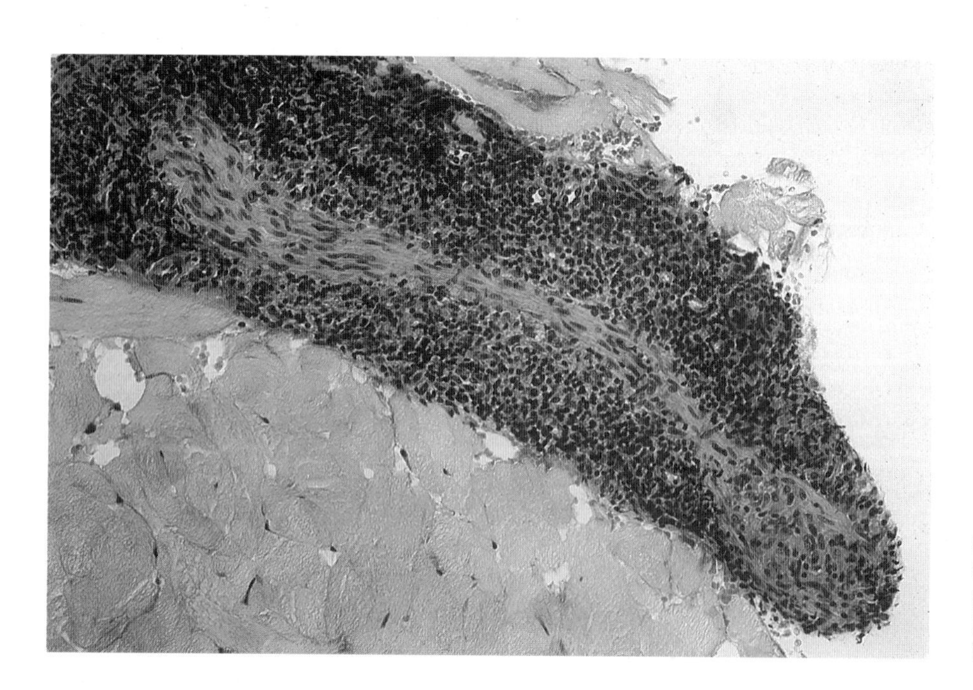

FIG. 21-40. Tuberculoid leprosy One pattern of neuritis; dense lymphocytosis surrounding and eroding into the deep dermal nerve (H&E, high power).

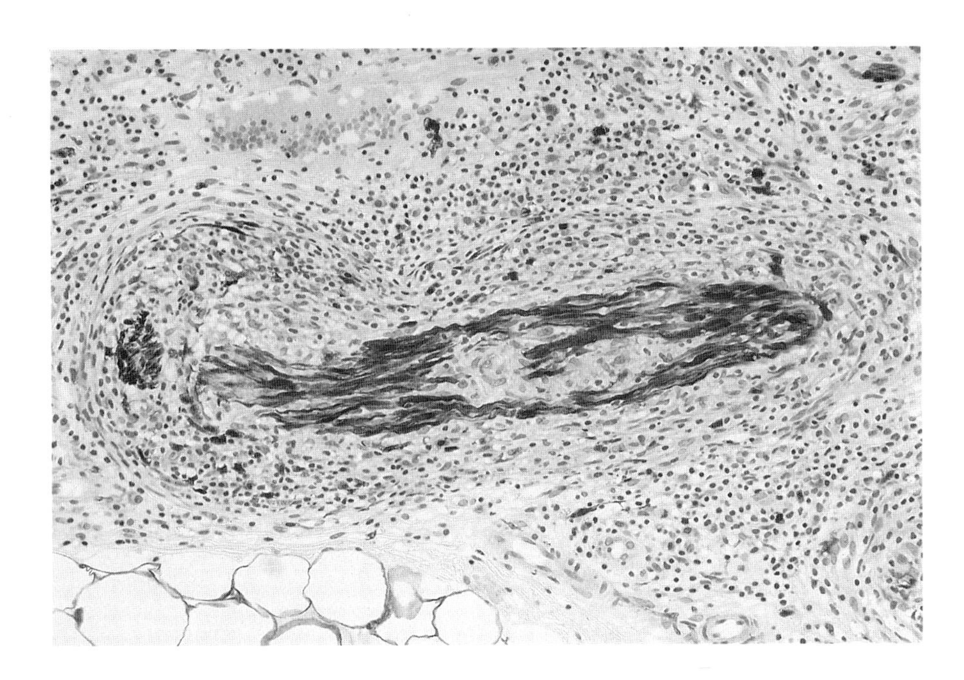

FIG. 21-41. Tuberculoid leprosy Typical endoneuritis demonstrated by immunocytochemical staining of Schwann cells. There is an intraneural granuloma disrupting the Schwann cells (Anti-S-100 protein, medium power).

Type 1 Reactions

Because the immunopathologic spectrum of leprosy is a continuum, patients may move along it in both directions. Should such shifts be rapid, they induce an inflammatory reaction with edema that results in enlargement of lesions with more erythema. Shifts toward the tuberculoid pole are called upgrading or reversal reactions; shifts toward the lepromatous pole are termed downgrading reactions. Both are aspects of delayed hypersensitivity, or type 1, leprosy reactions. TT patients are stable. BT patients may downgrade without treatment. Multibacillary patients, particularly those at the BL point, frequently upgrade on chemotherapy, and about one quarter of them will exhibit significant reactions. BB patients are most unstable and will move either way depending on therapy, often with reactions. The most important aspect of type 1 reactions is not the skin but the condition of the peripheral nerves, in which a similar inflammatory process is going on; reaction induces increased intraneural inflammation and edema, which is damaging. At worst, there is caseous necrosis of large peripheral nerves resulting from upgrading reactions.

Histopathology. The histopathology of type 1 reactions has still not been well evaluated.[184] The distinction between upgrading and downgrading reactions is difficult to make and may require serial examinations. Typically, there is edema within and about the granulomas, and proliferation of fibrocytes in the dermis. In upgrading reactions, the granuloma becomes more epithelioid and activated, and Langhans' giant cells are larger (Fig. 21-43); there may be erosion of granulomas into the lower epidermis, and there may be fibrinoid necrosis within granulomas and even within dermal nerves. In downgrading reactions, necrosis is much less common, and over time the density of bacilli increases. Multibacillary leprosy patients who upgrade on therapy show old foamy macrophages and degenerate bacilli admixed with new epithelioid cell granulomas.

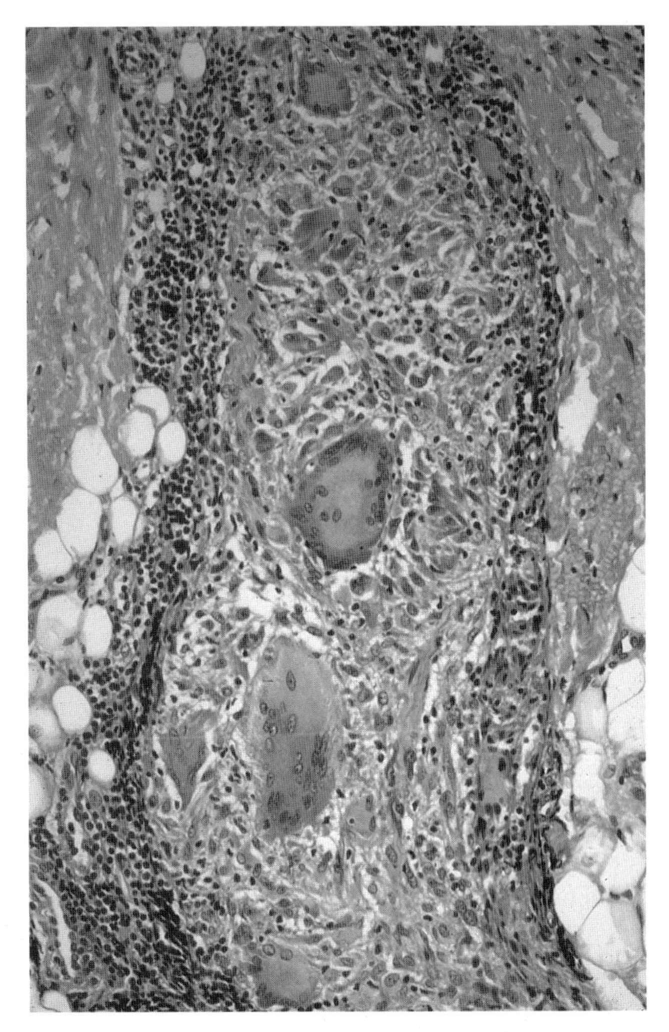

FIG. 21-42. Tuberculoid leprosy Another pattern of neuritis; giant-cell granulomas within the dermal nerve disrupting the Schwann cells and axons (H&E, high power).

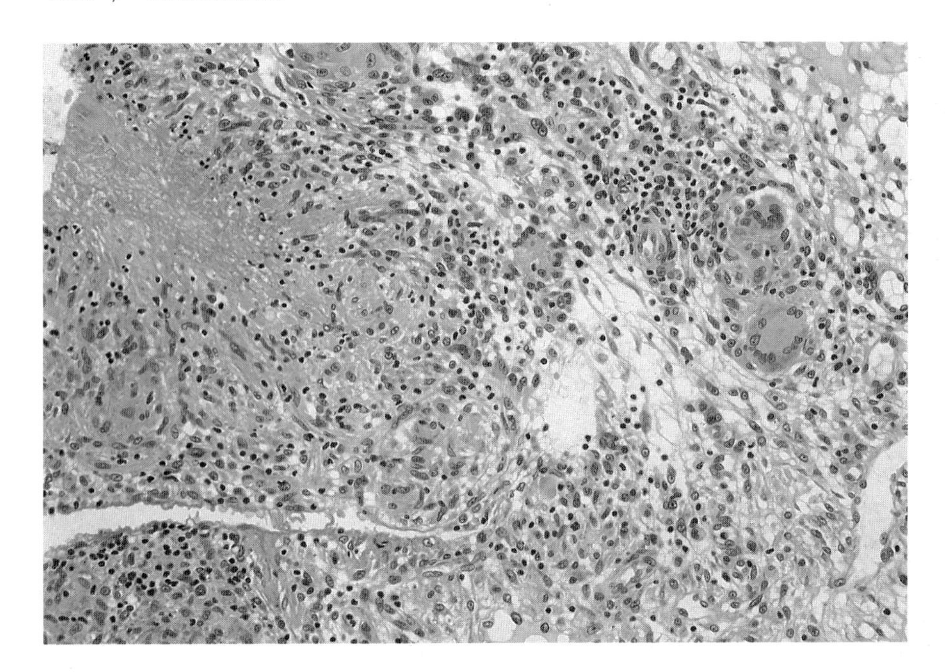

FIG. 21-43. Leprosy: type 1 reaction (delayed hypersensitivity) Within the granuloma there are edema, fibrinoid necrosis, and Langhans' giant cells (H&E, high power).

Type 2 Reaction: Erythema Nodosum Leprosum (ENL)

Erythema nodosum leprosum, or ENL, occurs most commonly in LL leprosy and less frequently in borderline lepromatous (BL) leprosy.[177] It may be observed not only in patients under treatment but also in untreated patients. Clinically, the reaction has a greater resemblance to erythema multiforme than to erythema nodosum. On the skin one observes tender, red plaques and nodules together with areas of erythema and occasionally also purpura and vesicles. Ulceration, however, is rare. The eruption is widespread and is accompanied by fever, malaise, arthralgia, and leukocytosis. New lesions appear for only a few days in some cases but for weeks and even years in others. This is the only type of reactional leprosy that responds to treatment with thalidomide.

Histopathology. In erythema nodosum leprosum, the lesions are foci of acute inflammation superimposed on chronic multibacillary leprosy (Fig. 21-44). Polymorph neutrophils may be scanty or so abundant as to form a dermal abscess with ulceration.[185] Whereas foamy macrophages containing fragmented bacilli are usual, in some patients no bacilli remain and macrophages have a granular pink hue on Wade-Fite staining, indicating mycobacterial debris. An antimycobacterial immunocytochemical stain (e.g., anti-BCG) will indicate abundant antigen. A necrotizing vasculitis affecting arterioles, venules, and capillaries occurs in some cases of ENL; these patients may have superficial ulceration.

Lucio Reaction

The Lucio reaction occurs exclusively in diffuse lepromatous leprosy, in which it is a fairly common complication. It usually occurs in patients who have received either no treatment or inadequate treatment. In contrast to erythema nodosum leprosum, fever, tenderness, and leukocytosis are absent. The lesions consist of barely palpable, hemorrhagic, sharply marginated, irregular plaques. They develop into crusted lesions and, particularly on the legs, into ulcers. There may be repeated attacks or continuous appearance of new lesions for years.

Histopathology. In the Lucio reaction, vascular changes are critical.[179] Endothelial proliferation leading to luminal obliteration is observed in association with thrombosis in the medium-sized vessels of the dermis and subcutis. There is a sparse, largely mononuclear infiltrate. Dense aggregates of acid-fast bacilli are found in the walls and the endothelium of normal-appearing vessels, as well as in vessels with proliferative changes. Ischemic necrosis, brought on by the vascular occlusion, leads to hemorrhagic infarcts and results in crusted erosions or frank ulcers.

Electron Microscopy of Leprosy

Under electron microscopy, *M leprae* can be seen to consist of an electron-dense cytoplasm lined by a trilaminal plasma membrane. Outside of this membrane lies the bacterial cell wall surrounded by a radiolucent area, the waxy coating typical of mycobacteria.[109] Lepra bacilli are found in the skin, predominantly in macrophages and in Schwann cells.

Pathogenesis of Leprosy

With respect to immunologic reactivity, patients with lepromatous leprosy have a defect in cell-mediated immune responses to the lepra bacilli, which therefore cannot be eradicated from the body spontaneously.[186,187] The primary defect lies in the T lymphocytes, which can be stimulated only slightly or not at all to react against the lepra bacilli and thus do not adequately activate macrophages to destroy phagocytosed bacilli. This defect is specific for *M leprae* because patients with lepromatous leprosy show normal immunologic responses to antigens other than lepromin in both in vivo and in vitro testing.

The specific inability of T lymphocytes obtained from patients with lepromatous leprosy to react against lepromin is

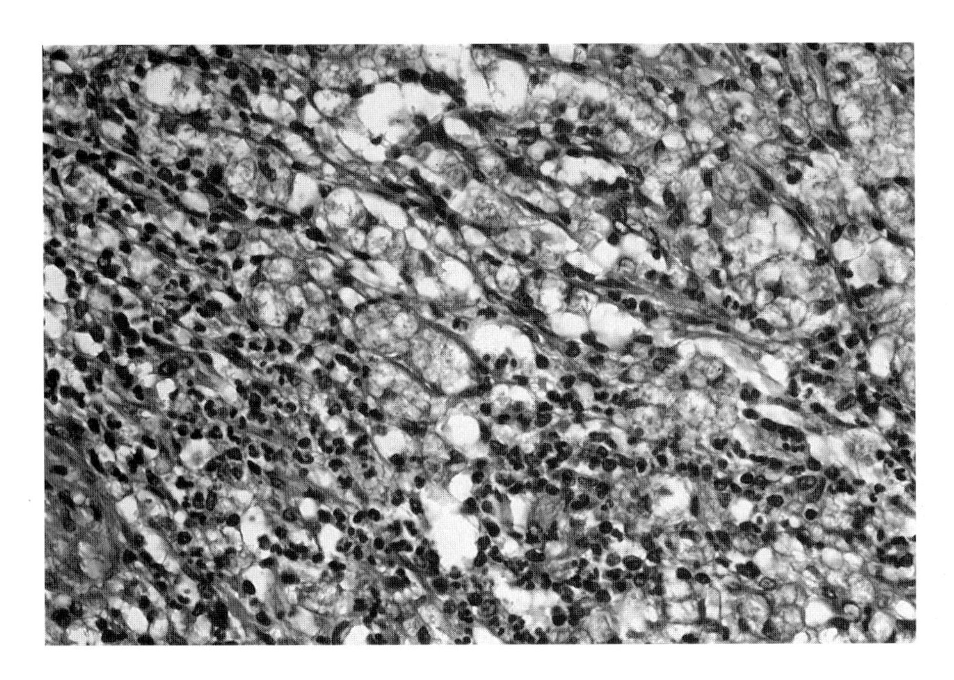

FIG. 21-44. Leprosy: erythema nodosum leprosum (ENL; type 2 reaction)
Foamy macrophages and a polymorphonuclear cell infiltrate (H&E, high power).

shown by the fact that, when these lymphocytes are incubated with lepromin, they show little or no production of macrophage migration inhibiting factor (MIF). In contrast, the lymphocytes of patients with tuberculoid leprosy produce significant amounts of MIF on exposure to lepromin. One modern view is that in tuberculoid patients, exposure to leprosy antigens results in a predominant T helper 1 (Th-1) cytokine secretion profile, which results in macrophage activation. Conversely, in lepromatous patients, the cytokine profile (Th-2) inhibits cell-mediated immunity and promotes humoral immunity, which does not contribute to host defense.[186,188] In reversal reactions, there is an increase in the lymphocyte response to lepromin during the reaction and a decrease during the postreaction phase.

Analysis of T-cell subsets in lesions have shown that in tuberculoid leprosy, with its high degree of resistance to the leprosy bacilli, the T helper lymphocytes are distributed evenly throughout the epithelioid cell aggregates, and the suppressor T lymphocytes are restricted to the peripheries of the granulomas. In lepromatous leprosy, both helper and suppressor T lymphocytes are distributed diffusely throughout the lesions.[189,190] It is noteworthy that the distribution of helper and suppressor T cells in tuberculoid leprosy is similar to that observed in sarcoidosis.

In patients with either erythema nodosum leprosum or the Lucio reaction, deposits of IgG and the third component of complement (C3), as well as circulating immune complexes, have been found in the vessel walls of the dermal lesions. This suggests that both reactions are mediated by immune complexes (Gell and Coombes type III reaction).[176]

The lepromin skin test, or Mitsuda test, consists of the intradermal injection of a preparation of *M leprae* derived from autoclaved infected human tissue. A positive reaction consists of the formation of a nodule measuring 5 mm or more in diameter after 2 to 4 weeks. On histologic examination, the nodule shows an epithelioid cell granuloma. The reaction is positive only in the high-resistance (tuberculoid and borderline tuberculoid) forms of the disease. In indeterminate leprosy, it may be positive or negative. The test reveals the inability of patients at the lepromatous end of the spectrum to react to the injection of *M leprae* with an epithelioid cell granuloma, and its main value is therefore as a marker of specific cell-mediated immunity to this organism, which varies continuously along the immunopathologic spectrum.

HIV Infection and Leprosy

Because HIV induces a generalized immunosuppressive state, and because a wide range of intracellular infectious agents normally controlled by the T-cell/macrophage system may proliferate to cause significant disease, it was expected that leprosy might also be affected. Specifically, the disease might become more prevalent in HIV and leprosy coendemic areas, and individual patients might downgrade toward lepromatous disease as their HIV disease progresses. However, epidemiologic studies have shown no effect of HIV infection on the incidence of leprosy in properly controlled studies,[191,192] nor has a change in the proportions of tuberculoid versus lepromatous patients been noted.[193] At present, the only clinicopathologic difference between HIV-infected and noninfected leprosy patients that is suggested is an increased likelihood of HIV-positive patients undergoing type 1 upgrading reactions.[193,194] This rather paradoxical phenomenon awaits further evaluation.

Histopathologic Differential Diagnosis

The leprosy bacillus cannot yet be grown in vitro. Tuberculoid (granulomatous) leprosy needs to be distinguished from the many other granulomatous dermatitides. The presence of acid-fast bacilli in nerves is conclusive proof of leprosy, as is the demonstration of an intraneural granuloma. The S-100 stain may highlight this phenomenon,[195] although in practice, if the diagnosis is in doubt after investigation with ordinary stains, this immunocytochemical method is not usually diagnostic either. In leprosy, naked granulomas are found only in BB leprosy, and acid-fast bacilli will be found in the lesions. Sarcoidosis may rarely cause granulomas to form within peripheral nerves[196] but does not appear to do so in dermal nerves. The general vertical perineurovascular distribution of granulomatous inflammation and involvement of sweat glands in tuberculoid leprosy are helpful. The presence or absence of plasma cells or of intraepidermal lymphocytes is not helpful. Unlike other mycobacterial skin infections such as tuberculosis, and unlike granulomatous leishmaniasis, the epidermis in tuberculoid leprosy is usually flat and nonhyperplastic. Intragranuloma necrosis (fibrinoid or caseating) occurs in leprosy in type 1 reactions—sometimes spontaneously; this can be confused with necrobiotic lesions such as granuloma annulare. Necrosis within a nerve that is granulomatous is diagnostic of leprosy.

Early, indeterminate leprosy overlaps with many specific and nonspecific dermatitides manifesting perineurovascular lymphocytic infiltrates. Finding bacilli in critical sites (in nerve, under the epidermis, in erector pili muscle, or in macrophages) is critical. In the absence of bacilli and the presence of a pandermal infiltrate, leprosy can only be suspected. Problems may arise from contaminant mycobacteria in staining solutions and in the water baths used for floating out sections. Such organisms are usually above the plane of the section, overlap the cell nuclei, and usually stain darker than *M leprae*. The use of PCR for identifying paucibacillary leprosy in skin sections and tissues has not been as successful as it once was thought to be.[197]

Ultimately, there is a proportion of suspect paucibacillary leprosy lesions for which the histopathologist cannot make a firm diagnosis either way; and intra- and interobserver variation may be considerable.[198] Clinical diagnosis of single-lesion leprosy is also imperfect.[181]

Lepromatous leprosy infiltrates can resemble xanthoma, although the cytoplasmic granularity is more coarse in the latter disease. The presence of acid-fast bacilli is obviously important, and in long-treated lesions that may cause confusion, antimycobacterial immunocytochemistry is helpful. Erythema nodosum leprosum may be overlooked because it is a combined chronic and acute inflammatory infiltrate, but once thought of, the presence of bacilli or antigen is diagnostic. Certain other mycobacterioses in immunosuppressed patients, such as *M avium-intracellulare*, may produce histoidlike multibacillary lesions[148] (see Figs. 21-23 and 21-24); however, nerves are not involved in this infection.

ANTHRAX

Anthrax, caused by *Bacillus anthracis*, is enzootic in many countries.[199] It occurs occasionally among workers in tanneries and wool-scouring mills through the handling of infected hides, wool, or hair imported from Asia. The lesion starts as a papule. The papule enlarges, and a hemorrhagic pustule forms.[200] After the pustule has ruptured, a thick, black eschar covers the area. Marked erythema and edema surround the lesion. Characteristically, pain is slight or absent.

Histopathology. At the site of the eschar, the epidermis is destroyed, and the ulcerated surface is covered with necrotic tissue. There is marked edema of the dermis. Vasculitis, hemorrhage, and variable acute and chronic inflammatory infiltrate are observed (Figs. 21-45 and 21-46).

Anthrax bacilli are present in large numbers and can be recognized in sections stained with the Gram stain. The bacillus is large, rod-shaped, encapsulated, Gram-positive, 6 to 10 μm long, and 1 to 2 μm thick. Anthrax bacilli are found particularly in the necrotic tissue toward the surface of the ulcer but also in the dermis (Fig. 21-47). Phagocytosis of the bacilli by either neutrophils or histiocytes is absent.

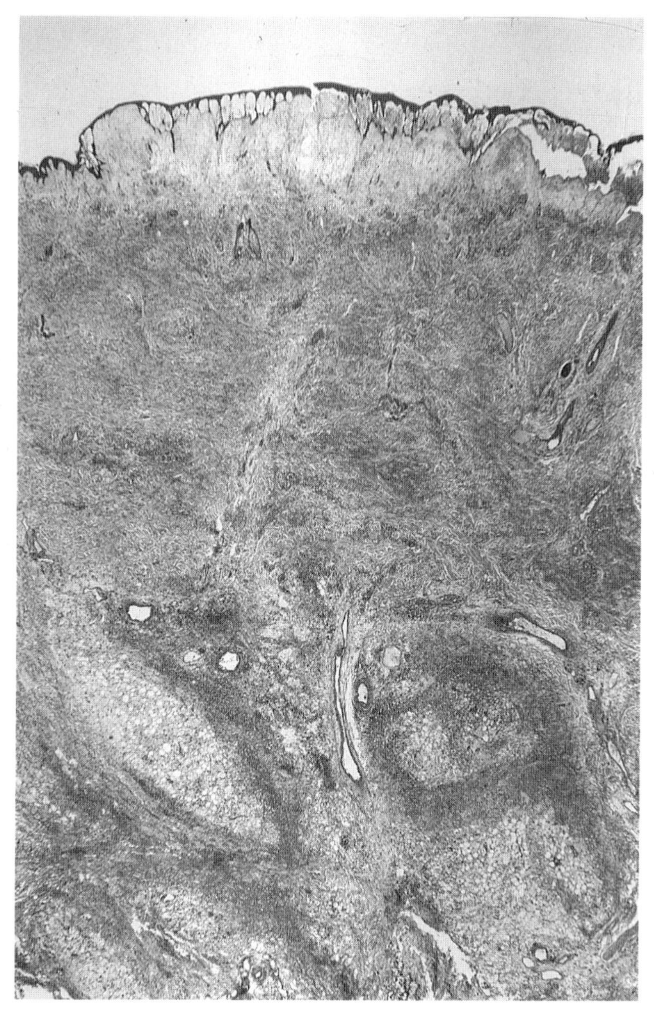

FIG. 21-45. Anthrax
Acute lesion with epidermal necrosis and pandermal inflammation (H&E, low power).

TULAREMIA

Tularemia is caused by *Francisella tularensis*, a small, Gram-negative, pleomorphic coccobacillus. It is usually acquired by humans through direct contact with rodents, but it may be transmitted from rodents to humans by insects, such as mosquitoes, ticks, or deer flies.[201] The disease often occurs in small epidemics. There are two types: ulceroglandular, the more common type, and typhoidal. These types reflect differences in host response. In ulceroglandular tularemia, there is a vigorous inflammatory reaction, pneumonia is less common, and the patient's prognosis is good. In the typhoidal form, there are few localizing signs, pneumonia is more common, and the mortality without therapy is much higher.

In the ulceroglandular type, one or several painful ulcers occur as primary lesions at the site of infection, usually on the hands. Tender subcutaneous nodes may form along the lymph vessels that drain the primary lesion or lesions. There is consid-

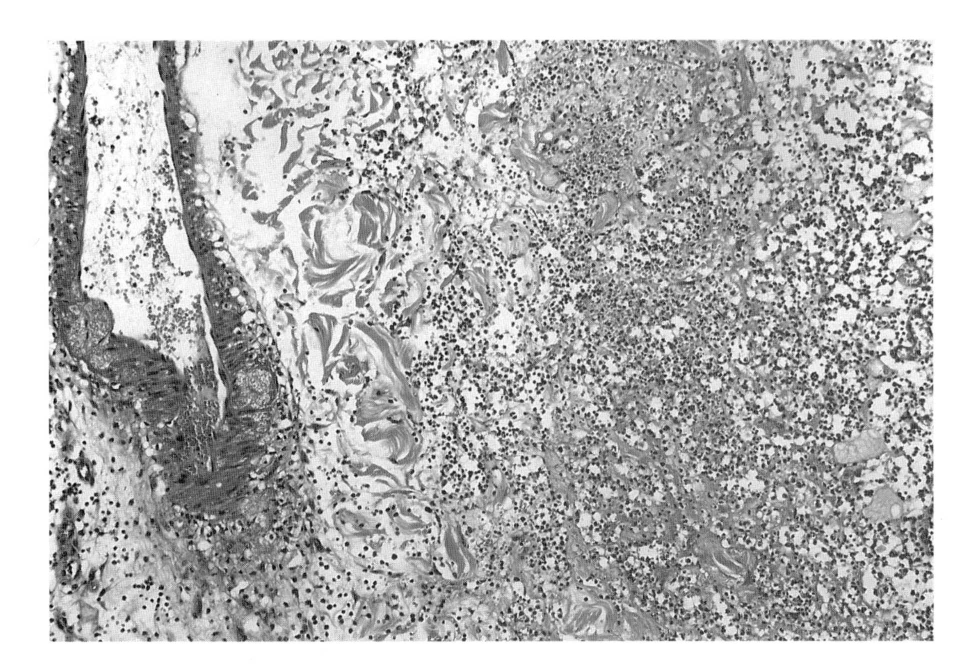

FIG. 21-46. Anthrax
Acute inflammation and a necrotizing vasculitis (H&E, medium power).

erable swelling of the regional lymph nodes, and the infection is associated with marked constitutional symptoms. Healing of the lesions takes place in 2 to 5 weeks.[202,203]

Histopathology. The primary ulcer shows at its base a nonspecific inflammatory infiltrate associated with a granulomatous reaction. In some cases, only a moderate number of epithelioid cells and a few giant cells are observed.[202] In others, however, large, well-developed tuberculoid granulomas are apparent. These granulomas may show central necrosis with the presence of nuclear dust. Late lesions may show epithelioid cell tubercles that have no central necrosis and are surrounded by only a slightly inflammatory reaction, and they may thus have an appearance resembling that of sarcoidosis.[204]

The tender nodes that may be found along lymph vessels show multiple granulomas deep in the dermis and extending into the subcutaneous tissue. The central zones of necrosis in the granulomas may attain a much greater size than in the primary ulcer. Similarly, the regional lymph nodes show multiple granulomas with centrally located abscess necrosis or caseous necrosis.[202,205]

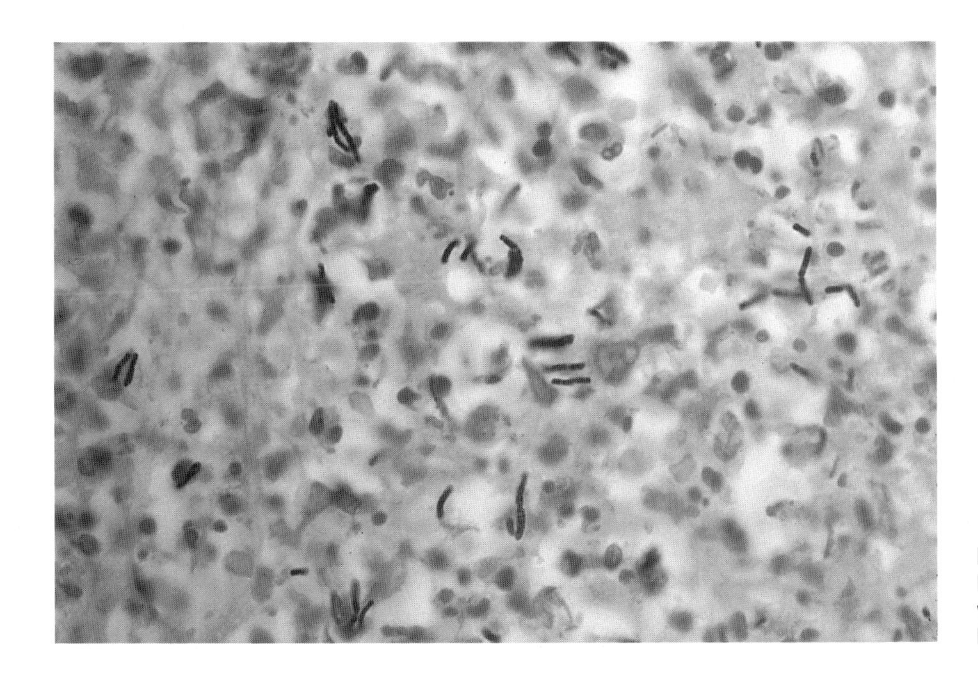

FIG. 21-47. Anthrax
Numerous Gram-positive thick bacilli within the acute inflammation (Gram, high power).

ROCKY MOUNTAIN SPOTTED FEVER

Rocky Mountain spotted fever is caused by *Rickettsia rickettsii*, a small, pleomorphic coccobacillus that is an obligate intracellular parasite. It is transmitted by ticks from infected animals. Contrary to its name, the disease is encountered most commonly in the Southeast of the United States and has been acquired even within New York City.[206,207]

After an incubation period of 1 to 2 weeks, chills and fever develop, and a few days later, a rash appears that begins on the extremities and spreads to the trunk. The lesions at first are macular to papular but become purpuric within 2 to 3 days. There may be only petechiae, but in fatal cases widespread ecchymoses are common. Gangrene may result from small vessel occlusion.[208] Because the diagnosis may not be made in the beginning and the course may be rapid, mortality exceeds 10%, despite the effectiveness of antibiotics such as tetracycline and chloramphenicol if given in time. Whenever a diagnosis of Rocky Mountain spotted fever is suspected, a search should be made for an eschar indicating the site of a tick bite. One may find a hemorrhagic crust 8 to 10 mm in diameter surrounded by an erythematous ring. In some severe systemic cases, there are no obvious skin lesions.[208,209]

Histopathology. The small vessels of the dermis and of the subcutaneous fat exhibit a necrotizing vasculitis with a perivascular infiltrate consisting mostly of lymphocytes and macrophages. There is extravasation of erythrocytes. As a result of injury to the endothelial cells, luminal thrombosis and microinfarcts occur. The causative organism, which measures 0.3 by 1 μm, is too small to be visible by light microscopy using ordinary stains. However *R rickettsii* can be identified in sections of skin lesions by immunocytochemistry.[210] Coccal and bacillary forms are observed in endothelial cells in association with perivascular lymphocytic infiltration. Electron microscopic examination of the tick bite site demonstrates rickettsial organisms within the cytoplasm and the nuclei of endothelial cells. These organisms appear as electron-dense, round or oval structures surrounded by an electron-lucent halo. The entire organism is bounded by a limiting cell wall. The organisms range in size from 0.3 to 0.5 μm in greatest diameter.

CHANCROID

Chancroid, caused by *Haemophilus ducreyi*, is a sexually transmitted disease leading to one or several ulcers, chiefly in the genital region.[211,212] The ulcers exhibit little if any induration and often have undermined borders. They are usually tender. Inguinal lymphadenitis, either unilateral or bilateral, is common and, unless treated, often results in an inguinal abscess.

Histopathology. The histologic changes observed beneath the ulcer are sufficiently distinct to permit a presumptive diagnosis of chancroid in many instances. The lesion consists of three zones overlying each other and shows characteristic vascular changes[212,213] (Fig. 21-48). The surface zone at the floor of the ulcer is rather narrow and consists of neutrophils, fibrin, erythrocytes, and necrotic tissue. The next zone is fairly wide and contains many newly formed blood vessels showing marked proliferation of their endothelial cells. As a result of the endothelial proliferation, the lumina of the vessels are often occluded, leading to thrombosis. In addition, there are degenerative changes in the walls of the vessels. The deep zone is composed of a dense infiltrate of plasma cells and lymphoid cells (Fig. 21-49).

FIG. 21-48. Chancroid
Skin ulcer with the three-zone pattern of inflammation (H&E, low power).

Demonstration of bacilli in tissue sections stained with Giemsa stain or Gram stain is occasionally possible (Fig. 21-50). The bacilli are most apt to be found between the cells of the surface zone.[213] However, in smears of serous exudate obtained from the undermined edge of the ulcer, the bacilli usually can be seen on staining with the Giemsa or Gram stain. *H ducreyi* is a fine, short, Gram-negative coccobacillus, measuring about 1.5 by 0.2 μm, often arranged in parallel chains. In situ hybridization may also specify chancroid organisms.[214] Electron microscopy reveals that the bacilli are extracellular and thus rarely visible in phagosomes of macrophages.[215]

The diagnosis of chancroid is confirmed by culture on selective blood-enriched agar.[216]

Chancroid may clinically resemble donovanosis by showing nontender or only slightly tender, indurated ulcers without undermined margins.[217] On the other hand, particularly in the presence of several lesions, herpes simplex has to be excluded,

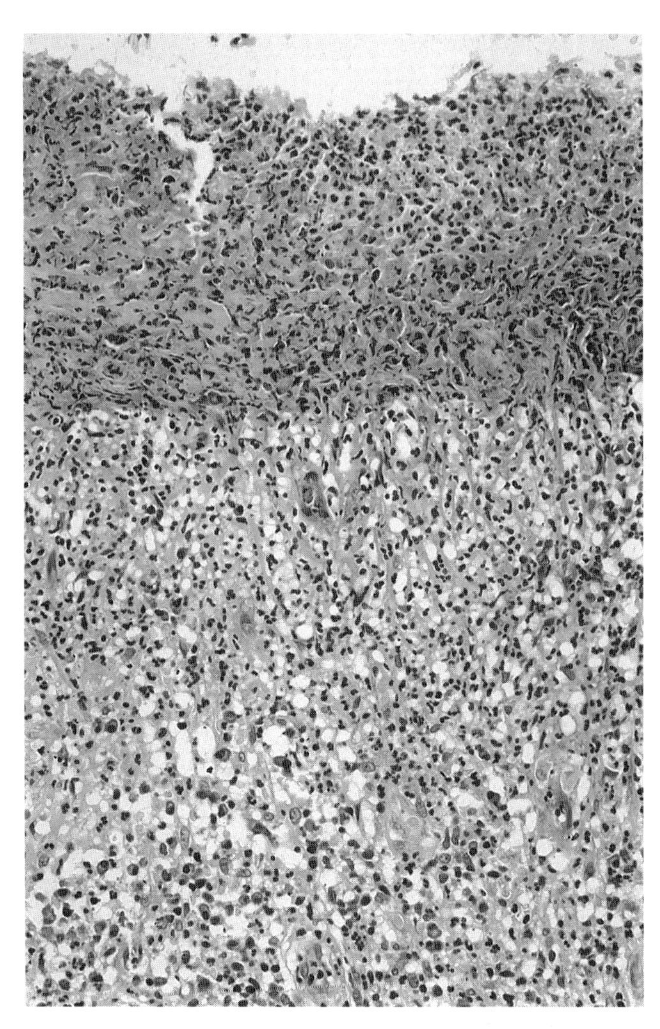

FIG. 21-49. Chancroid
Superficial necrotic zone, underlying granulation tissue, and deeper fibrosis with plasma cells (H&E, medium power).

although in herpes simplex the ulcerations usually are not as deep as those in chancroid.

GRANULOMA INGUINALE (DONOVANOSIS)

Granuloma inguinale, also called donovanosis, is a sexually transmitted disease caused by *Calymmatobacterium granulomatis*.[218] The organism is a Gram-negative short bacillus, about 2 to 3 μm long, with bipolar staining. The disease is endemic, but relatively uncommon, in the tropics.[219]

Granuloma inguinale occurs in the genital or perianal region either as a single lesion or as several lesions.[220] The lesions consist of ulcers filled with exuberant granulation tissue that bleeds easily (the characteristic beefy appearance). The borders of the ulcers are elevated and often have serpiginous outlines. Because the lesions spread by peripheral extension, they may attain a large size. In some instances, ulceration leads to mutilation resulting from destruction of tissue.[221] In others, excessive granulation tissue causes vegetating lesions. Occasionally, squamous cell carcinoma supervenes.[222] Local lymphadenopathy occurs through secondary infection of ulcerated skin.

Histopathology. At the edge of the ulcer, the epidermis exhibits acanthosis that may reach the proportions of pseudocarcinomatous hyperplasia. Present in the dermis is a dense infiltrate that is composed predominantly of histiocytes and plasma cells (Fig. 21-51). Scattered throughout this infiltrate are small abscesses composed of neutrophils. The number of lymphoid cells is conspicuously small.[213]

The macrophages, which may be large, have a typical vacuolated appearance; these vacuoles contain bacilli and comprise the so-called "Donovan bodies." *C granulomatis* does not stain with hematoxylin-eosin stains but is well delineated by the Warthin-Starry method as short bacilli, either singly or in clumps[213,223] (Fig. 21-52). Giemsa stain shows bipolar condensations of stain. Electron microscopy reveals that the bacteria reside in phagosomes.[224]

Differential Diagnosis. Overdiagnosis of carcinoma is pos-

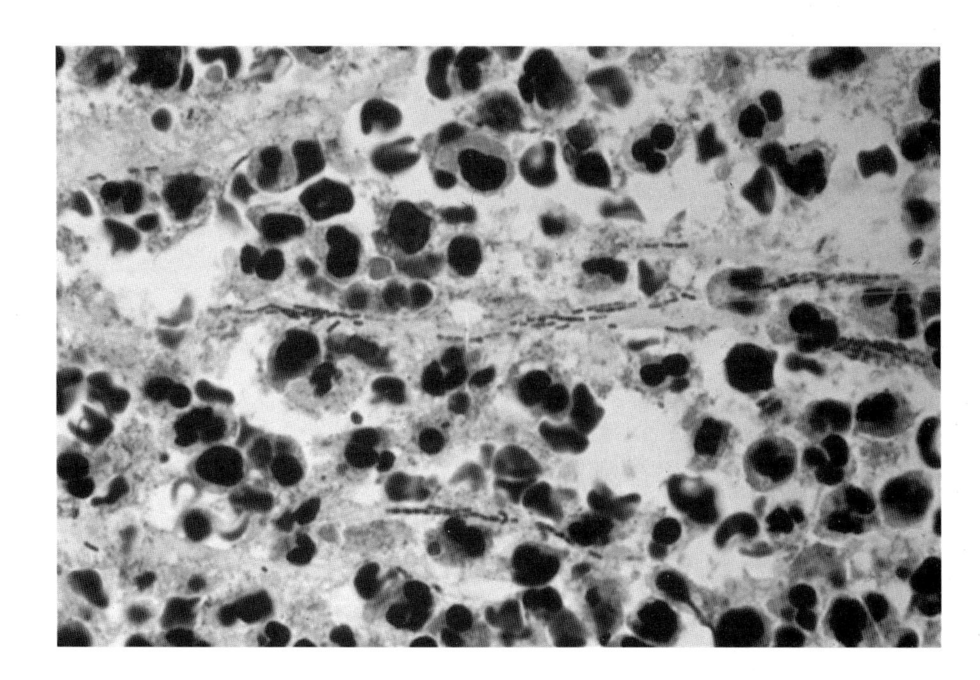

FIG. 21-50. Chancroid
Bacilli (in the superficial zone) lying in parallel chains (Giemsa, high power). (Courtesy of Dr. A. Freinkel, South Africa.)

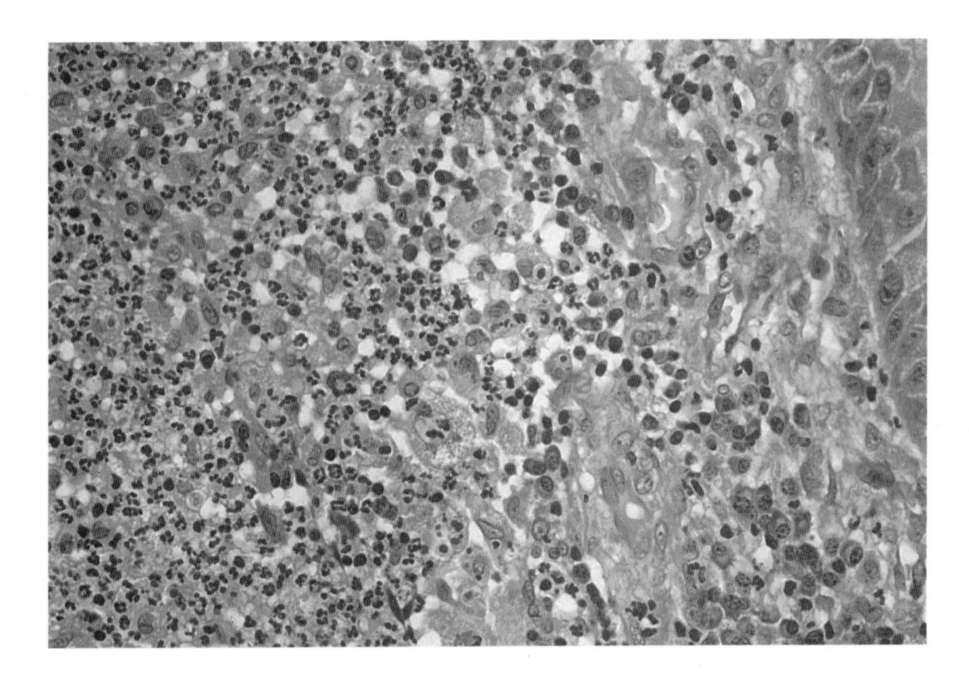

FIG. 21-51. Donovanosis
Acute inflammation intermixed with basophilic foamy macrophages (H&E, high power).

sible because of the epithelial hyperplasia. The inflammatory pattern is similar to that observed in rhinoscleroma.

RHINOSCLEROMA

Rhinoscleroma is a chronic infectious but only mildly contagious disease caused by *Klebsiella rhinoscleromatis*, a Gram-negative bacillus. The nose, pharynx, larynx, trachea, and occasionally also the skin of the upper lip are distorted and infiltrated with hard, granulomatous masses. The disorder always begins in the nose. Although formerly endemic in Central Europe, it is now encountered mainly in Central America and Africa.[225–227]

Histopathology. The cellular infiltrate is a chronic granulation tissue with abundant plasma cells and Mikulicz cells. Polymorphs may be present (but they cannot kill the bacteria). Russell bodies (plasma cells with retained globules of immunoglobulins) are frequently observed. The characteristic cell is the Mikulicz cell, a large histiocyte measuring from 10 to 100 μm in diameter (Fig. 21-53). It has a pale, vacuolated cytoplasm. Within the cytoplasm of the Mikulicz cells, one finds many bacilli (Fig. 21-54). They can be seen faintly in sections stained with hematoxylin and eosin but are better visualized with the Giemsa stain or a Warthin-Starry silver stain.[228] They are also stained red by the PAS technique. They are Gram-negative rods that measure 2 to 3 μm in length and appear round or ovoid in cross section. Immunocytochemistry can also be used to confirm rhinoscleroma.[226,229]

In longstanding lesions, marked fibrosis is present. The mucosal epithelium overlying the cellular infiltrate often exhibits

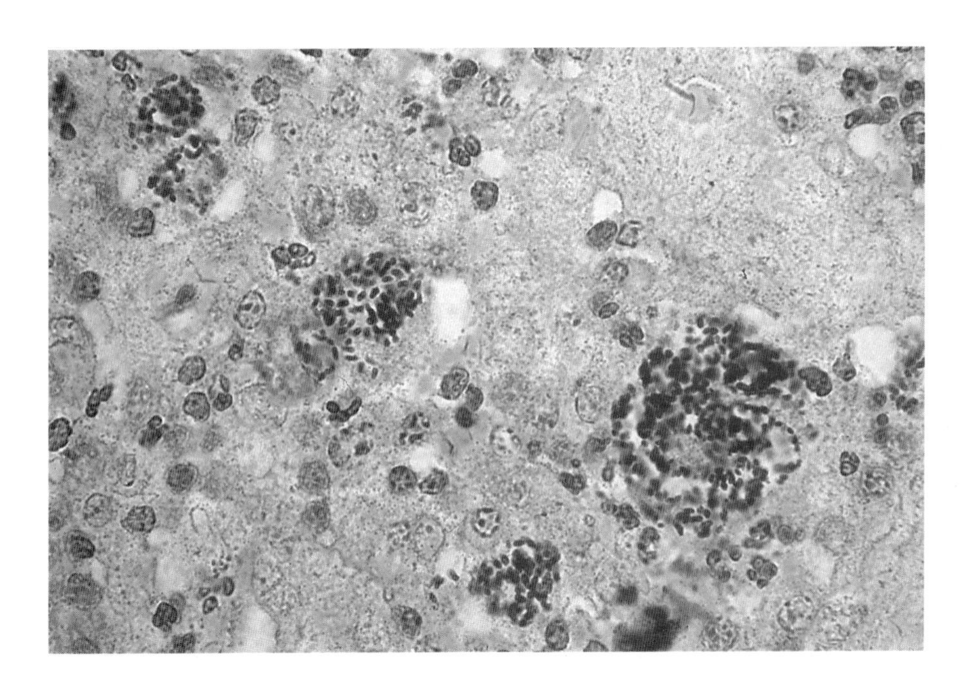

FIG. 21-52. Donovanosis
Bacilli within macrophages (Warthin-Starry, high power).

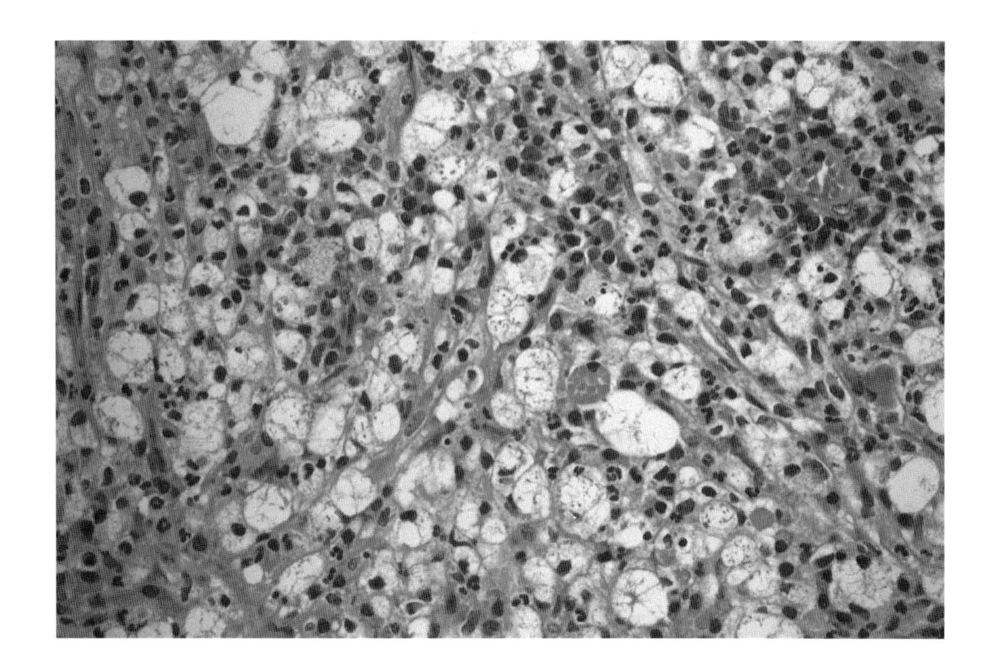

FIG. 21-53. Rhinoscleroma
Foamy macrophages (Mikulicz cells) and plasma cells (H&E, high power).

hyperplasia, which may be so pronounced as to give rise to a mistaken diagnosis of squamous cell carcinoma.

Electron microscopy reveals numerous phagosome vacuoles of varying size within the Mikulicz cells. Some vacuoles contain one or a few bacilli up to 4 μm in length. They are surrounded by a characteristic coat of finely granular, filamentous material arranged in a radial fashion. This coating material contains mucopolysaccharides and is responsible for the positive PAS reaction of the bacteria.[227]

Differential Diagnosis. The histopathology of rhinoscleroma is essentially similar to that of donovanosis (granuloma inguinale). Foamy, vacuolated macrophages are also observed in many other chronic inflammatory conditions (e.g., leprosy, chronic staphyloccocal abscess, mycoses, and leishmaniasis), but special stains and associated clinicopathologic features usually enable their distinction. (See Table 24-1 for a differential diagnosis of parasitized histiocytes.) Plasma cells and Russell bodies, similarly, correlate with chronicity in many diverse infections, such as treponematoses, amoebiasis, leishmaniasis, and tuberculosis.

LYMPHOGRANULOMA VENEREUM

Lymphogranuloma venereum is a sexually transmitted disease caused by *Chlamydiae trachomatis*. Chlamydiae are obligate intracellular parasites with a unique biphasic life cycle.[230]

The incubation period of lymphogranuloma venereum varies from 3 to 30 days but averages 7 days. The primary lesion is a small erosion or papule 5 to 8 mm in size. This lesion heals

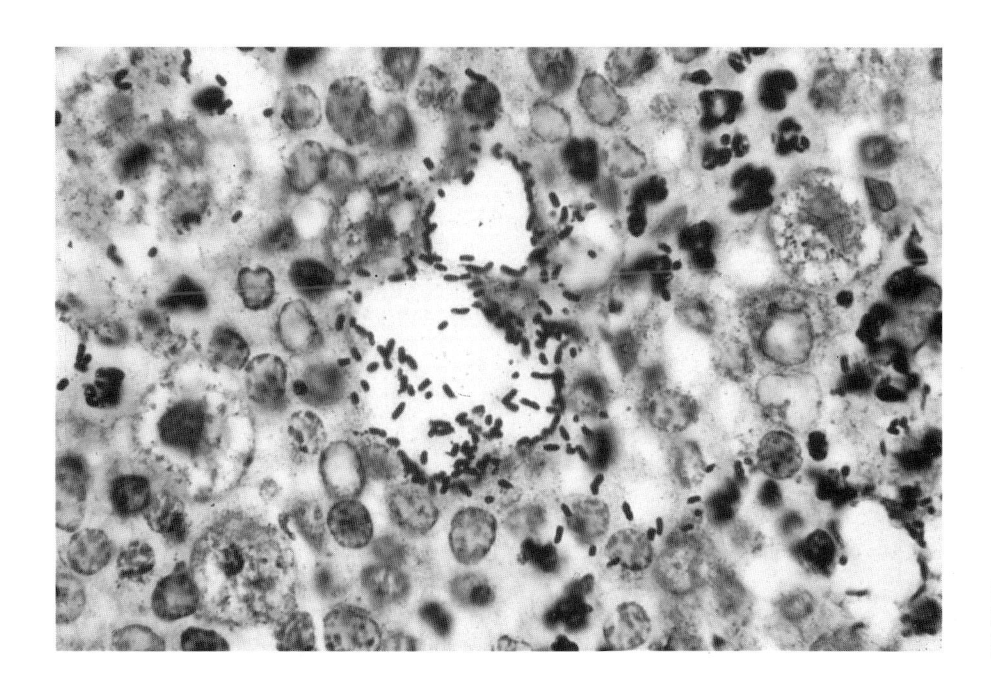

FIG. 21-54. Rhinoscleroma
Bacilli within the macrophages (Warthin-Starry, high power).

within a few days and may pass unnoticed. Within 1 to 2 weeks after the appearance of the primary lesion, enlargement of the inguinal lymph nodes begins. Inguinal lymphadenopathy occurs in most men infected with this disease but in only some women. The involved inguinal lymph nodes at first are firm but subsequently develop multiple areas of suppuration, resulting in draining sinuses. The lymphadenopathy usually subsides within 2 to 3 months. Rarely, elephantiasis of the penis and scrotum or chronic penile ulcerations arise as a late complication.[231]

In women in whom the infection begins in the lower portion of the vagina, drainage is to the iliac and anorectal lymph nodes rather than to the inguinal lymph nodes, and may result in proctitis.[220] Rectal stricture and perineal ulcerations are fairly common late complications in these women. Lymph stasis may lead to marked vulvar edema, referred to as esthiomene.[106] Proctitis and rectal stricture also occur in homosexual men.[232]

Histopathology. The changes in the initial papule are nonspecific. There is ulceration and a nonspecific granulation tissue.[213] In the lymph nodes, stellate abscesses with surrounding epithelioid cells and macrophage giant cells represent the characteristic lesion. A similar pathology is seen in cat-scratch disease nodes. Ordinary histologic stains do not demonstrate the infecting organisms in skin or node. The diagnosis may be confirmed by culture of a skin lesion or lymph node, and serology is useful.[233]

Chlamydiae undergo a developmental cycle and, as can be seen by electron microscopy, occur in two forms: elementary body and initial body.[230] The elementary body is adapted to an extracellular environment and is infective for other cells. It measures about 0.3 μm in diameter and consists of a round, electron-dense inner body surrounded by an electron-lucid halo and a membrane. After entering a host cell by means of phagocytosis, it develops into a metabolically active initial body 0.5 to 1 μm in diameter. Multiplication takes place by division of the nucleus. This division results in two elementary bodies, which on leaving the host cell can infect other cells.[230]

CAT-SCRATCH DISEASE

The skin lesion develops 2 to 4 days after a scratch or bite from a cat. It may be macular, papular, or a nodule, usually on the arm or hand. Two to 3 weeks later, a large, tender swelling of a group of lymph nodes develops in the drainage area of the scratch. The cat scratch heals in a normal fashion, but the affected lymph nodes become fluctuant as a result of suppuration. The average duration of lymph node enlargement is 2 months.[234,235]

Histopathology. The primary papules at the site of the scratch show one or several acellular areas of necrobiosis in the dermis. These areas are of various shapes, including round, triangular, and stellate. Surrounding them are several layers of histiocytic and epithelioid cells, with the innermost layer exhibiting a palisading arrangement. A few giant cells may be present. The periphery of the epithelioid cell reaction is surrounded by a zone of lymphoid cells.

The reaction in the lymph nodes is similar to that observed in the skin, except that the central areas of necrosis in the epithelioid cell granulomas undergo abscess formation through the accumulation of numerous neutrophils. Macrophage giant cells are also present. As the abscesses enlarge, they become confluent.

Delicate, pleomorphic, Gram-negative bacilli can be demonstrated with the Warthin-Starry silver impregnation stain peripheral to the necrosis of involved lymph nodes[236] and in the skin at the primary site of inoculation.[237] Immunocytochemistry also reveals the bacilli,[238,239] and serodiagnostic tests are available.[240] For specific identification (see later), PCR techniques and in vitro culture may be used.[241]

Electron microscopic examination reveals that the bacteria are invariably extracellular and form small clusters. They are 0.8 to 1.5 μm long and 0.3 to 0.5 μm wide, with homogeneous bacterial walls.[242]

Taxonomically, two bacterial species, both members of the alpha-2 subgroup of proteobacteria but not closely related, are associated with cat-scratch disease. *Afipia felis* is the cause of a minority of cases,[238,243] and *Bartonella henselae* (previously *Rochalimaea henselae*) causes the majority.[240] *B henselae* is carried in the blood and oral cavities of cats.[244]

BACILLARY ANGIOMATOSIS

Bacillary angiomatosis is a new disease, first described in 1983[245] as a skin or disseminated infection in patients immunosuppressed by HIV infection.[240] It is also rarely encountered in patients with other immunocompromising conditions and even in immunocompetent people.[246,247] The agents are two Gram-negative bacilli of the alpha-2 subgroup of proteobacteria, originally termed *Rochalimaea spp* but now grouped with *Bartonella*: *B quintana* and *B henselae*.[240] The pathology is similar to that of the late cutaneous stage of bartonellosis, caused by *B bacilliformis*.[248] As with cat-scratch disease, exposure to cats is a major risk factor for acquiring this infection.[249]

The skin lesions are reddish or brown papules on any part of the body, usually in large numbers, that resemble Kaposi's sarcoma. They may also present as subcutaneous lumps without skin involvement.[240,250,251]

Histopathology. The epidermis may be flat or hyperplastic. In the dermis there are single or multinodular proliferations of capillaries accompanied by an inflammatory infiltrate that includes variable numbers of neutrophil polymorphs and mononuclear cells, as well as edema. Leukocytoclasia is frequently observed.[250,252] Characteristic of bacillary angiomatosis are extracellular deposits of palely hematoxyphilic granular material (Fig. 21-55). Warthin-Starry staining reveals these deposits to be dense masses of short bacilli (Fig. 21-56). The Grocott-Gomori methenamine silver method also demonstrates the argyrophilic bacilli.[246] These bacilli may also be delineated by modified Gram stains such as the Brown-Hopps stain.

Differential Diagnosis. The major differential diagnoses are Kaposi's sarcoma, pyogenic granuloma, and epithelioid hemangioma.[252] The presence of clumps of bacilli is obviously important. The capillary proliferation does not have the organized arborizing quality of that in pyogenic granuloma. Spindle cell proliferation and intracellular hyaline globules as seen in Kaposi's sarcoma are not features of bacillary angiomatosis, and Kaposi's sarcoma does not include polymorphs; however, the two conditions may be difficult to distinguish, and many pathologists have learned about bacillary angiomatosis from being informed that the lesions of "Kaposi's sarcoma" disappeared on treatment with antibiotics. Epithelioid hemangioma has plumper (histiocytoid) endothelial cell proliferation and no acute inflammation.

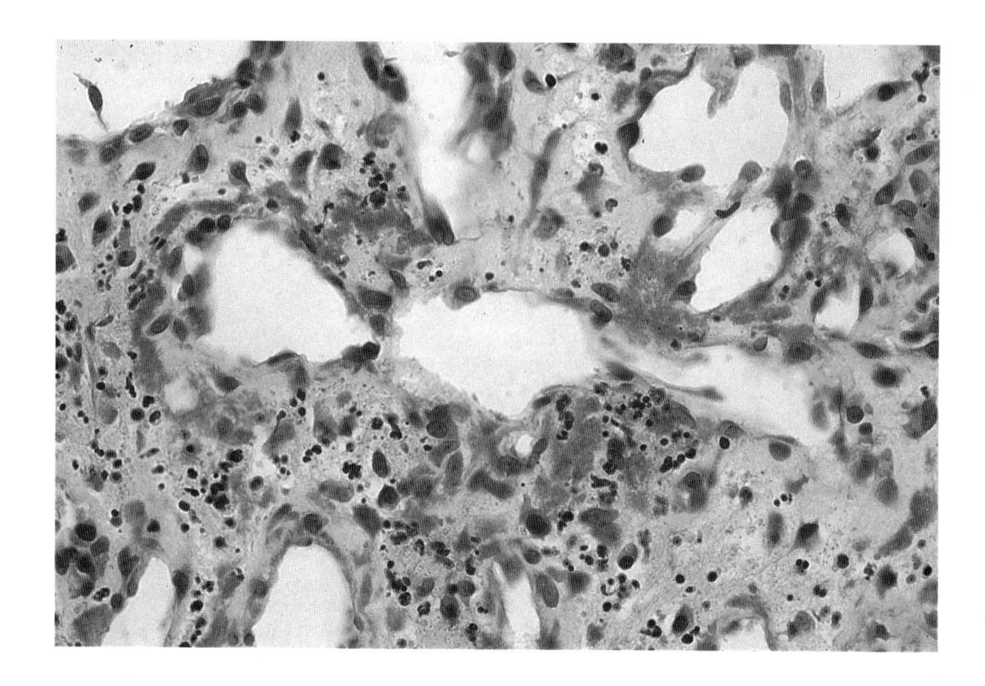

FIG. 21-55. Bacillary angiomatosis Dermis shows vascular proliferation, leukocytoclasia, and smudges of basophilic extracellular material (the bacteria) (H&E, high power). (Courtesy of Dr. N. Francis, London.)

BOTRYOMYCOSIS

Botryomycosis is not a fungal infection but a chronic suppurative infection of skin (and other organs such as lungs and meninges) in which pyogenic bacteria form granules similar to those seen in mycetoma.[253] Although immunosuppressed patients, including those with HIV infection, may acquire botryomycosis,[254] most patients have no known immune defect. Occasionally the lesion is associated with another dermatosis such as follicular mucinosis.[255]

The skin lesions are local nodules, ulcers, or sinuses communicating with deep abscesses. They occur mainly on the extremities.

Histopathology. The dermal inflammation is predominantly that of neutrophil polymorph abscesses with surrounding granulation tissue and fibrosis. Within the abscesses are granules (grains) shaped like a bunch of grapes, hence the name of the disease (Figs. 21-57 and 21-58). The grains may vary from 20 μm to 2 mm in diameter. They are composed of closely aggregated nonfilamentous bacteria with a peripheral, radial deposition of intensely eosinophilic material—a Hoeppli-Splendore (HS) reaction. The bacteria are usually *Staphylococcus aureus*, but streptococci and certain Gram-negative bacilli such as *Proteus, Pseudomonas,* and *E coli* are sometimes found. Gram stains delineate these broad categories of infection, although sometimes the organisms in Gram-positive infections are degenerate and lose their Gram-positive staining reaction (Fig. 21-59). The HS reaction material comprises antibody and fibrin.

The overlying epithelium often exhibits pseudoepitheliomatous hyperplasia. Transepithelial elimination of grains may be observed (as with mycetoma).[256]

Pathogenesis. Local implantation of infection may be a

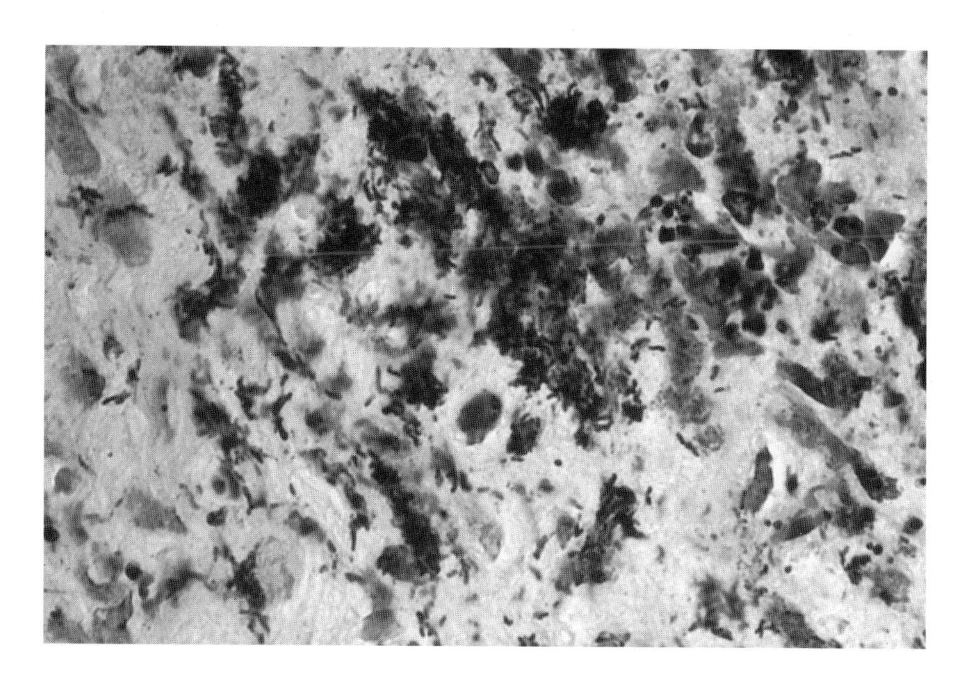

FIG. 21-56. Bacillary angiomatosis Clumps of extracellular bacilli (Warthin-Starry, high power).

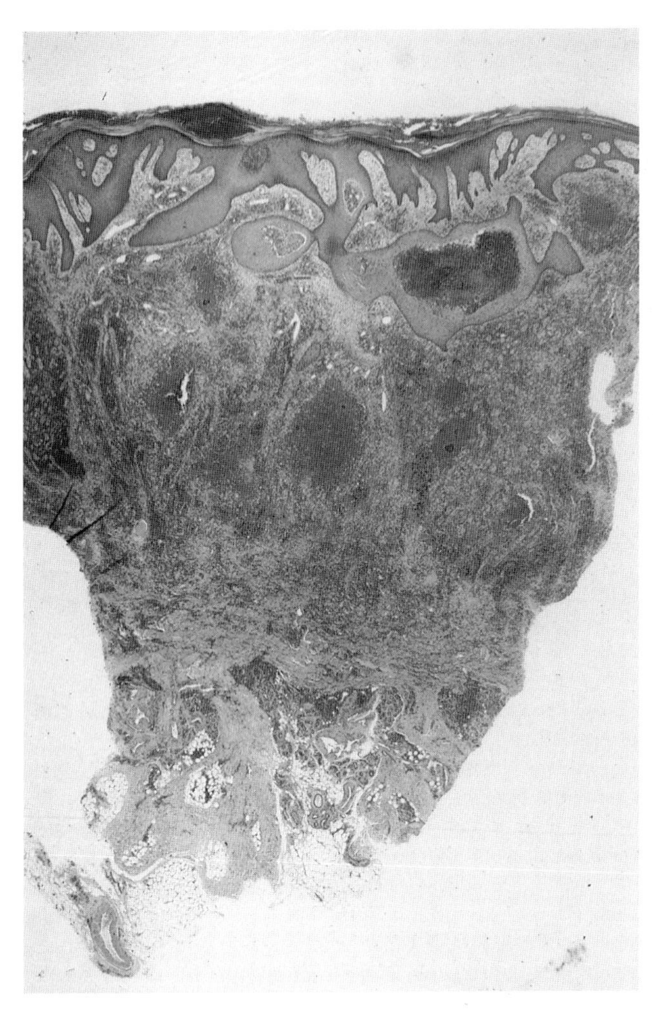

FIG. 21-57. Botryomycosis
There is pseudoepitheliomatous hyperplasia, and small abscesses in the dermis containing clumps of bacteria (H&E, low power).

factor in some cases, with persistence of a foreign body. Bacteremia is documented in many patients, but in others the lesions appear de novo. The characteristic formation of the peribacterial HS reaction probably prevents phagocytosis and intracellular killing of the bacteria, leading to chronicity.

NOCARDIOSIS

Nocardia species are Gram-positive, weakly acid-fast, filamentous, branching bacilli that are ubiquitous in the soil. The main species are *N asteroides,* which is global in distribution, and *N brasiliensis,* which is found mainly in the Americas.[257,258]

N asteroides is an opportunist agent, and immunocompromised patients, such as those with HIV infection[259,260] and organ transplant recipients, are liable to nocardiosis. Infection of the skin follows direct implantation from the environment, hematogenous spread from pulmonary infection, or direct spread through the chest wall from a lung lesion. The skin lesions include erythematous nodules, pustular ulcers, and sinuses. They may be single or multiple.

N brasiliensis affects immunocompetent as well as immunosuppressed people. The primary and secondary skin lesions are similar to those of *N asteroides*. Sporotrichoid spread up a limb, with lymphatic involvement, may occur.[261] Both species may produce a chronic mycetoma-like lesion with much fibrosis and tissue destruction.

Histopathology. The bacteria induce a mixed acute abscess and granulomatous response in the skin, with fibrosis. Occasionally the bacteria are clumped together with a surrounding Hoeppli-Splendore reaction (see sections on Botryomycosis and Mycetoma). More often they are more loosely dispersed and resemble *Actinomycosis* species. Hematoxylin-eosin stains demonstrate the bacilli poorly. They are 1 μm in diameter, filamentous, branching, beaded, Gram-positive, Grocott-silver-positive, and usually weakly acid-fast so that a modified Ziehl-Neelsen stain appropriate for leprosy bacilli stains them. This

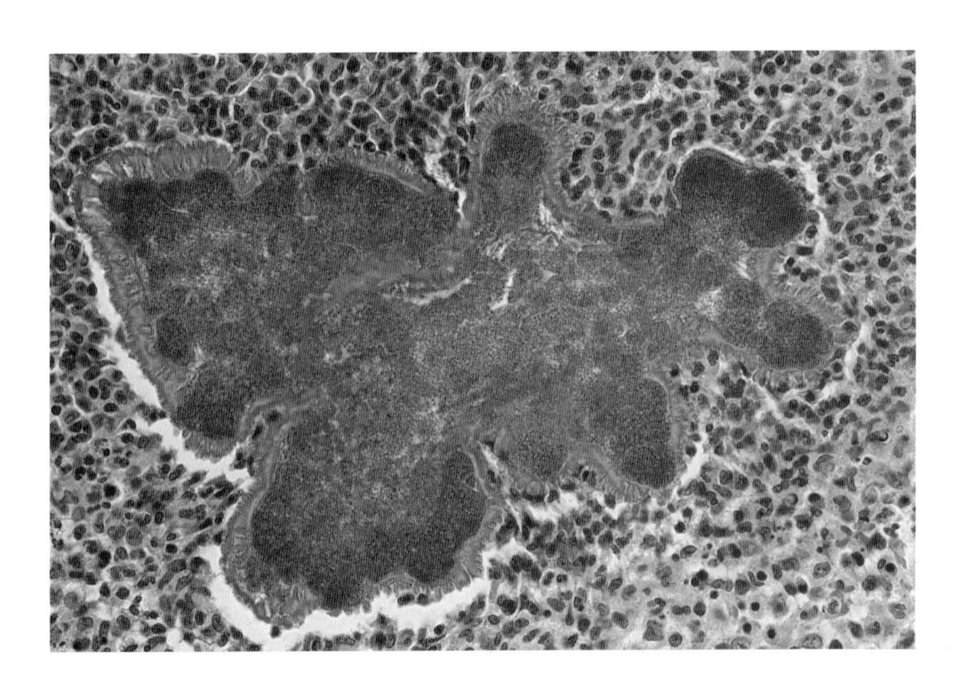

FIG. 21-58. Botryomycosis
An abscess within which is a basophilic bacterial clump with an eosinophilic surrounding Hoeppli-Splendore reaction (H&E, high power).

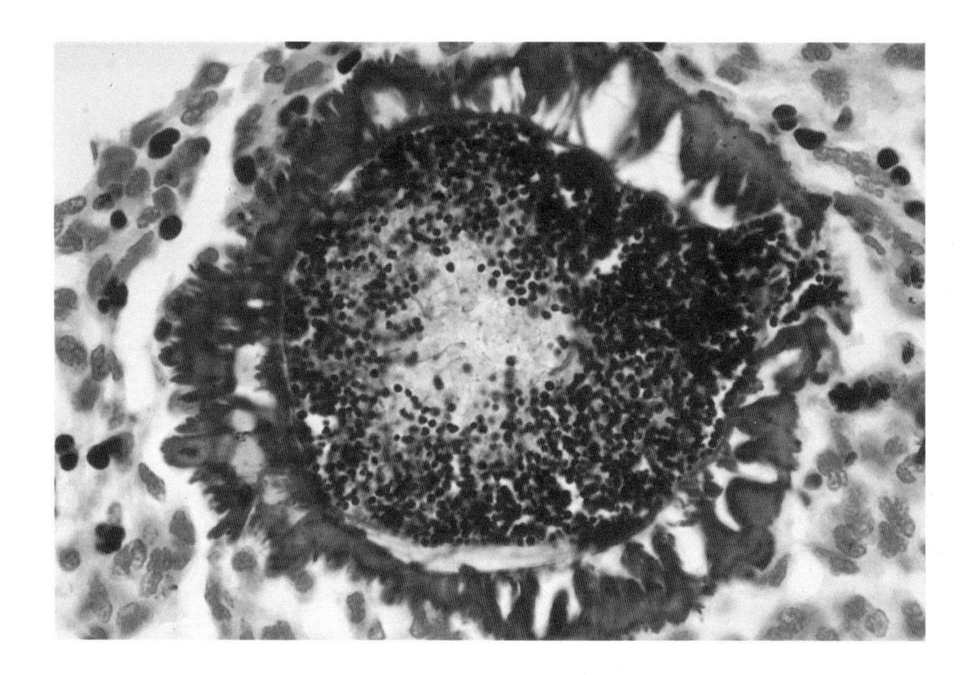

FIG. 21-59. Botryomycosis
A staphylococcal lesion showing Gram-positive cocci (centrally they are degenerate and nonstaining) (Gram, high power).

latter feature assists in the distinction of *Nocardia* from *Actinomyces* and related bacilli; specific antisera with immunocytochemistry are also helpful,[259] and culture is definitive. The shape of the organisms distinguishes them from mycobacteria. The Grocott silver method is the most sensitive screening stain for nocardiosis.

ACTINOMYCOSIS

Actinomyces israelii is a Gram-positive, branching, filamentous bacterium. It resides as a commensal organism in the oral cavity and tonsillar crypts. The main clinicopathologic manifestations are cervicofacial, thoracic, and intestinal actinomycosis.[262] In the first of these, skin lesions result from extension of suppuration from the oral mucosa through to the facial skin, with sinus formation and discharge of pus and sulfur granules (see later). Thoracic and intestinal infections may produce discharging sinuses onto the skin from infection tracking outward from lung and gut.[263] On rare occasions, purely cutaneous actinomycotic infection occurs, and hematogenous dissemination can produce multiple skin sinuses. An infected pilonidal sinus of the penis has been reported.[264]

Histopathology. The inflammatory reaction to actinomycotic infection is typically a chronic abscess with polymorphs, surrounding granulation tissue, and fibrosis.[265] The organisms are usually tangled together in a matted colony, forming a granule or grain (like botryomycosis and mycetoma). These grains, commonly termed "sulfur granules," may be 20 μm to 4 mm in diameter. The bacilli within are 1-μm-diameter filaments that are hematoxyphilic and Gram-positive (Fig. 21-60). They stain with the Grocott silver method. Often only the peripheral fila-

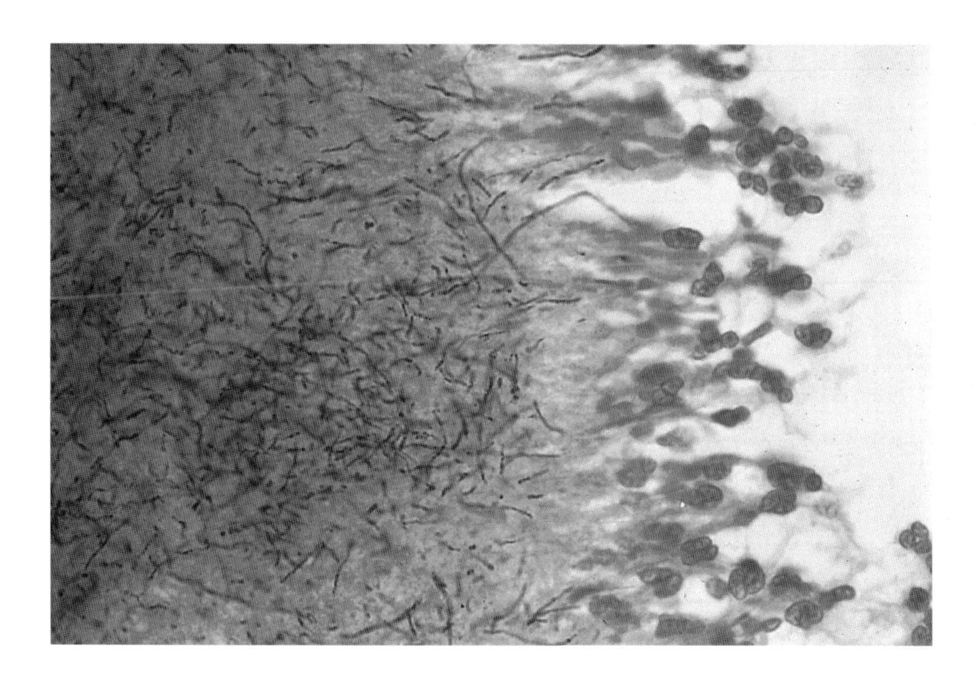

FIG. 21-60. Actinomycosis
The edge of a grain, showing Gram-positive filaments (Gram, high power).

ments stain with the Gram method, because of degeneration of the inner bacteria. The peripheral filaments often terminate in a club. A Hoeppli-Splendore reaction may be found peripheral to the bacteria in the grain. The histologic differentiation from nocardiosis is discussed previously.

REFERENCES

1. Dagan R. Impetigo in childhood: Changing epidemiology and new treatments. Pediatr Ann 1993;22:235.
2. Kaplan EL, Anthony BF, Chapmann SS et al. Epidemic acute glomerulonephritis associated with type 49 streptococcal pyoderma. Am J Med 1970;48:9.
3. Steigleder GK. Zur differentialdiagnose des pemphigus vulgaris aus dem blasengrundausstrich. Arch Klin Exp Dermatol 1955;202:1.
4. Kouskoukis CE, Ackerman AB. What histologic finding distinguishes superficial pemphigus and bullous impetigo? Am J Dermatopathol 1984;66:179.
5. Peter G, Smith AL. Group A streptococcal infections of the skin and pharynx. N Engl J Med 1977;297:311.
6. Schachner L, Taplin D, Scott G et al. A therapeutic update of superficial skin infections. Pediatr Clin North Am 1983;30:397.
7. Coskey RJ, Coskey LA. Diagnosis and treatment of impetigo. J Am Acad Dermatol 1987;17:62.
8. Noble WC, Presbury D, Connor BL. Prevalence of streptococci and staphylococci in lesions of impetigo. Br J Dermatol 1974;91:115.
9. Levine J, Norden CW. Staphylococcal scalded-skin syndrome in an adult. N Engl J Med 1972;287:1339.
10. Reid LH, Weston WL, Humbert JR. Staphylococcal scalded skin syndrome. Arch Dermatol 1974;109:239.
11. Elias PM, Levy SW. Bullous impetigo: Occurrence of localized scalded skin syndrome in an adult. Arch Dermatol 1976;112:856.
12. Ritter von Rittershain G. Die exfoliative dermatitis jüngerer säuglinge. Centralzeitschrift für Kinderheilkunde 1878;2:3.
13. Ridgway HB, Lowe NJ. Staphylococcal syndrome in an adult with Hodgkin's disease. Arch Dermatol 1979;115:589.
14. Pachinger W. Staphylogenes Lyell-syndrome bei einer erwachsenen mit agranulocytose. Z Hautkr 1980;55:57.
15. Diem E, Konrad K, Graninger W. Staphylococcal scalded-skin syndrome in an adult with fatal disseminated staphylococcal sepsis. Acta Derm Venereol (Stockh) 1982;62:295.
16. Borchers SL, Gomez EC, Isseroff RR. Generalized staphylococcal scalded skin syndrome in an anephric boy undergoing hemodialysis. Arch Dermatol 1984;120:912.
17. Hardwick N, Parry CM, Sharpe GR. Staphylococcal scalded skin syndrome in an adult: Influence of immune and renal factors. Brit J Dermatol 1995;132:468.
18. Elias PM, Fritsch P, Epstein EH Jr. Staphylococcal scalded skin syndrome (review). Arch Dermatol 1977;113:207.
19. Melish ME, Glasgow LA. The staphylococcal scalded-skin syndrome. N Engl J Med 1970;282:1114.
20. Melish ME, Glasgow LA, Turner MD. The staphylococcal scalded-skin syndrome: Isolation and partial characterization of the exfoliative toxin. J Infect Dis 1972;125:129
21. Smith TP, Bailey CJ. Epidermolytic toxin from *Staphylococcus aureus* binds to filaggrins. FEBS Lett 1986;194:309.
22. Bailey CJ, Smith TP. The reactive serine residue of epidermolytic toxin A. Biochem J 1990;269:535.
23. Fritsch P, Elias P, Varga J. The fate of staphylococcal exfoliation in newborn and adult mice. Br J Dermatol 1976;95:275.
24. Wuepper KD, Dimond RL, Knutson DD. Studies of the mechanism of epidermal injury by a staphylococcal epidermolytic toxin. J Invest Dermatol 1975;65:191.
25. Dimond RL, Wolff HH, Braun-Falco O. The staphylococcal scalded skin syndrome. Br J Dermatol 1977;96:483.
26. Dimond RL, Wuepper KD. Das staphylogene Lyell-syndrom. Hautarzt 1977;28:447.
27. Amon RB, Dimond RL: Toxic epidermal necrolysis: Rapid differentiation between staphylococcal- and drug-induced disease. Arch Dermatol 1975;111:1433.
28. Kelly C, Taplin D, Allen AM. Streptococcal ecthyma. Arch Dermatol 1971;103:306.
29. Grosshans E. The red face: Erysipelas. Clin Dermatol 1993;11:307.
30. Swartz MN, Weinberg AN. Erysipelas. In: Fitzpatrick TB, Eisen AZ, Wolff K et al, eds. Dermatology in general medicine. 3rd ed. New York: McGraw-Hill, 1987;2104.
31. Tappeiner J, Pfleger L: Zur histopathologie cutaner lymphgefässe beim chronisch-rezidivierenden erysipel der unteren extremitäten. Hautarzt 1964;15:218.
32. Bisno AL, Stevens DL. Streptococcal infections of skin and soft tissues. New Engl J Med 1996;334:240.
33. Buchanan CS, Haserick JR. Necrotizing fasciitis due to group A beta-hemolytic streptococci. Arch Dermatol 1970;101:664.
34. Koehn GS. Necrotizing fasciitis. Arch Dermatol 1978;114:581.
35. Stamenkovic I, Lew PD. Early recognition of potentially fatal necrotizing fasciitis: The use of frozen section biopsy. N Engl J Med 1984; 310:1689.
36. Silverman AR, Nieland ML. Hot tub dermatitis: A familial outbreak of *Pseudomonas* folliculitis. J Am Acad Dermatol 1983;8:153.
37. Fox AB, Hambrick GW JR. Recreationally associated *Pseudomonas aeruginosa* folliculitis. Arch Dermatol 1984;120:1304.
38. Pinkus H. Furuncle. J Cutan Pathol 1979;6:517.
39. Kossard S, Collins A, McCrossin J. Necrotizing lymphocytic folliculitis. J Am Acad Dermatol 1987;16:1007.
40. Bogg A. Folliculitis decalvans. Acta Derm Venereol (Stockh) 1963; 43:14.
41. Suter L: Folliculitis decalvans. Hautarzt 1981;32:429.
42. Laymon CW, Murphy RJ. The cicatricial alopecias. J Invest Dermatol 1947;8:99.
43. Meinhof W, Braun-Falco O. Über die folliculitis sycosiformis atrophicans barbae Hoffman: Sycosis lupoides Milton-Brocq, ulerythema sycosiforme unna. Dermatol Wochenschr 1966;152:153.
44. Moyer DG, Williams RM. Perifolliculitis capitis abscedens et suffodiens. Arch Dermatol 1962;85:378.
45. Strauss JS, Kligman AM. Pseudofolliculitis of the beard. Arch Dermatol 1956;74:533.
46. Pillsbury DM, Shelley WB, Kligman AM. Dermatology. Philadelphia: Saunders, 1956;481.
47. McMullan FH, Zeligman I. Perifolliculitis capitis abscedens et suffodiens. Arch Dermatol 1956;73:256.
48. Moyer DG, Williams RM. Perifolliculitis capitis abscedens et suffodiens. Arch Dermatol 1962;85:378.
49. Hyland CH, Kheir SM. Follicular occlusion disease with elimination of abnormal elastic tissue. Arch Dermatol 1980;116:925.
50. Dvorak VC, Root RK, MacGregor RR. Host-defensive mechanisms in hidradenitis suppurative. Arch Dermatol 1977;113:450.
51. Brunsting HA. Hidradenitis suppurativa: Abscess of the apocrine sweat glands. Arch Dermatol Syphiligr 1939;39:108.
52. Strauss JS. Acne conglobata. In: Fitzpatrick TB, Eisen AZ, Wolff K et al., eds. Dermatology in general medicine. 2nd ed. New York, McGraw-Hill, 1979;452.
53. Moschella SL, Klein MH, Miller RJ. Perifolliculitis capitis abscedens et suffodiens. Arch Dermatol 1967;96:195.
54. Curry SS, Gaither DH, King LE Jr. Squamous cell carcinoma arising in dissecting perifolliculitis of the scalp. J Am Acad Dermatol 1981; 4:673.
55. Djawari D, Hornstein OP. Recurrent chronic pyoderma with cellular immunodeficiency. Dermatologica 1980;116:116.
56. Su WPD, Duncan SC, Perry HO. Blastomycosis-like pyoderma. Arch Dermatol 1979;115:170.
57. Williams HM Jr, Stone OJ. Blastomycosis-like pyoderma. Arch Dermatol 1966;93:226.
58. Brunsting LA, Underwood LJ. Pyoderma vegetans in association with chronic ulcerative colitis. Arch Dermatol Syphilol 1949;60:161.
59. Forman L. Pemphigus vegetans of Hallopeau. Arch Dermatol 1978; 114:627.
60. Getlik A, Farkas J, Palenikova O et al. Pyoderma vegetans bei zellulärer immunitätsdefizienz. Dermatol Monatsschr 1980;166:645.
61. Djawari D, Hornstein OP. In vitro studies on microphage functions in chronic pyoderma vegetans. Arch Dermatol Res 1978;263:97.
62. Ruzicka T, Goerz G. Beobachtungen bei der pyodermite végétante Hallopeau. Z Hautkr 1979;54:24.
63. Bartter T, Dascal A, Carrol K et al. Toxic strep syndrome. Arch Intern Med 1988;148:1421.
64. Todd J, Fishaut M, Kapral F et al. Toxic shock syndrome caused by phage group I *Staphylococci*. Lancet 1978;2:1116.

65. Huntley AC, Tanabe JL. Toxic shock syndrome as a complication of dermatologic surgery. J Am Acad Dermatol 1987;16:227.
66. Rheingold AL, Hargrett NT, Dan BB et al. Non-menstrual toxic shock syndrome: A review of 130 cases. Ann Intern Med 1992;96:871.
67. Resnick SD. Staphylococcal toxin-mediated syndromes in childhood. Semin Dermatol 1992;11:11.
68. Abdul-Karim FW, Lederman MM, Carter JR et al. Toxic shock syndrome. Hum Pathol 1981;12:16.
69. Elbaum DJ, Wood C, Abuabara F et al. Bullae in a patient with toxic shock syndrome. J Am Acad Dermatol 1984;10:267.
70. Findley RF, Odom RB. Toxic shock syndrome (review). Int J Dermatol 1982;21:117.
71. Weston WL, Todd JK. Toxic shock syndrome. J Am Acad Dermatol 1981;4:478.
72. Hurwitz RM, Ackerman AB. Cutaneous pathology of the toxic shock syndrome. Am J Dermatopathol 1985;7:563.
73. Smith JH, Krull F, Cohen GH et al. A variant of toxic shock syndrome: Clinical, microbiologic, and autopsy findings. Arch Pathol 1983;107:351.
74. Stevens DL, Tanner MH, Winship J et al. Severe group A streptococcal infections associated with a toxic shock-like syndrome and scarlet fever toxin A. N Engl J Med 1989;321:1.
75. Dalldorf FG, Jennette JC. Fatal meningococcal septicemia. Arch Pathol 1977;101:6.
76. Plaut ME. Staphylococcal septicemia and pustular purpura. Arch Dermatol 1969;99:82.
77. Hill WR, Kinney TD. The cutaneous lesions in acute meningococcemia. JAMA 1947;134:513.
78. Shapiro L, Teisch JA, Brownstein MH. Dermatohistopathology of chronic gonococcal sepsis. Arch Dermatol 1973;107:403.
79. Ferguson JH, Chapman OD. Fulminating meningococcic infections and the so-called Waterhouse-Friderichsen syndrome. Am J Pathol 1948;24:763.
80. Winkelstein A, Songster CL, Caras TS et al. Fulminant meningococcemia and disseminated intravascular coagulation. Arch Intern Med 1969;124:55.
81. Hall JH, Callaway JL, Tindall JP et al. *Pseudomonas aeruginosa* in dermatology. Arch Dermatol 1968;97:312.
82. Schlossberg D. Multiple erythematous nodules as a manifestation of *Pseudomonas aeruginosa* septicemia. Arch Dermatol 1980;116:446.
83. Bazel J, Grossman ME. Subcutaneous nodules in pseudomonas sepsis. Am J Med 1986;80:528.
84. Huminer D, Siegman-Igra Y, Morduchowicz G et al. Ecthyma gangrenosum without bacteremia: Report of six cases and review of the literature. Arch Intern Med 1987;147:299.
85. Mandell JN, Feiner HP, Price NM et al. *Pseudomonas cepacia* endocarditis and ecthyma gangrenosum. Arch Dermatol 1977;113:199.
86. Dorff GI, Geimer NF, Rosenthal DR et al. Pseudomonas septicemia: Illustrated evolution of its skin lesion. Arch Intern Med 1971;128:591.
87. Wickboldt LG, Sanders CV. *Vibrio vulnificus* infection: Case report and update since 1970. J Am Acad Dermatol 1983;9:243.
88. Tyring SK, Lee PC. Hemorrhagic bullae associated with *Vibrio vulnificus* septicemia. Arch Dermatol 1986;122:818.
89. Ognibene AJ, Ditto MR. Chronic meningococcemia. Arch Intern Med 1964;114:29.
90. Nielsen LT. Chronic meningococcemia. Arch Dermatol 1970;102:97.
91. Schoolnik GK, Buchanan TM, Holmes KK et al. Gonococci causing disseminated gonococcal infection are resistant to the bactericidal action of normal human sera. J Clin Invest 1976;58:163.
92. Shapiro L, Teisch JA, Brownstein MR. Dermatohistopathology of chronic gonococcal sepsis. Arch Dermatol 1973;107:403.
93. Björnberg A. Benign gonococcal sepsis. Acta Derm Venereol (Stockh) 1970;50:313.
94. Ackerman AB. Hemorrhagic bullae in gonococcemia. N Engl J Med 1970;282:793.
95. Ackerman AB, Miller RC, Shapiro L. Gonococcemia and its cutaneous manifestations. Arch Dermatol 1965;91:227.
96. Abu-Nassar H, Fred HL, Yow EM. Cutaneous manifestations of gonococcemia. Arch Intern Med 1963;112:731.
97. Kahn G, Danielson D. Septic gonococcal dermatitis. Arch Dermatol 1969;99:421.
97a. Stanton MJ, Maxted W. Malakoplakia: A study of the literature and current concepts of pathogenesis, diagnosis and treatment. J Urol 1981;125:139.
98. McClure J. Malakoplakia. J Pathol 1983;140:275.
99. Palou J, Torras H, Baradad M et al. Cutaneous malakoplakia. Dermatologica 1988;176:288.
100. Abou NI, Pombejara C, Sagawa A et al. Malakoplakia: Evidence for monocyte lysosomal abnormality correctable by cholinergic agonist in vitro and in vivo. N Engl J Med 1973;297:1413.
101. Sencer O, Sencer H, Uluoglu O et al. Malakoplakia of the skin. Arch Pathol 1979;103:446.
102. Sian CS, McCabe RE, Lattes CG. Malakoplakia of skin and subcutaneous tissue in a renal transplant recipient. Arch Dermatol 1981;117:654.
103. Kumar PV, Tabbei SZ. Cutaneous malakoplakia diagnosed by scraping cytology. Acta Cytol 1988;32:125.
104. Schwartz DA, Ogden PO, Blumberg HM, Honig E. Pulmonary malakoplakia in a patient with the acquired immunodeficiency syndrome: Differential diagnostic considerations. Arch Pathol Lab Med 1990;114:1267.
105. Goodfellow M, Wayne LG. Taxonomy and nomenclature. In: Ratledge C, Stanford J, eds. The biology of the mycobacteria. London: Academic Press, 1982;470.
106. Lucas SB. Mycobacteria and the tissues of man. In: Ratledge C, Stanford J, eds. The biology of the mycobacteria. Vol 3. London: Academic Press, 1988;107.
107. Beyt BE, Ortbals DW, Santa Cruz DJ et al. Cutaneous mycobacteriosis: Analysis of 34 cases with a new classification of disease. Medicine (Baltimore) 1980;60:95.
108. Saxe N. Mycobacterial skin infections. J Cutan Pathol 1985;12:300.
109. Draper P. The anatomy of mycobacteria. In: Ratledge C, Stanford J, eds. The biology of the mycobacteria. London: Academic Press, 1982; 9.
110. Raviglione MC, Snider DE, Kochi A. Global epidemiology of tuberculosis: Morbidity and mortality of a worldwide epidemic. JAMA 1995;273:220.
111. Farina MC, Gegundez MI, Pique E et al. Cutaneous tuberculosis: A clinical, histopathologic, and bacteriologic study. J Am Acad Dermatol 1995;33:433.
112. Sehgal VN, Jain MK, Srivastava G. Changing pattern of cutaneous tuberculosis: A prospective study. Int J Dermatol 1989;28:231.
113. Santa Cruz DJ, Strayer DS. The histopathologic spectrum of the cutaneous mycobacteriosis. Hum Pathol 1982;13:485.
114. Kakakhel K, Fritsch P. Cutaneous tuberculosis. Int J Dermatol 1989; 28:355.
115. Dannenberg AM. Immune mechanisms in the pathogenesis of pulmonary tuberculosis. Rev Infect Dis 1989;11:S369.
116. Rook GAW, Bloom BR. Mechanisms of pathogenesis of tuberculosis. In: Bloom BR, ed. Tuberculosis: Pathogenesis, protection and control. Washington, DC: American Society for Microbiology Press, 1994;485.
117. Helman KM, Muschenheim C. Primary cutaneous tuberculosis resulting from mouth-to-mouth respiration. N Engl J Med 1965;273:1035.
118. Goette DK, Jacobson KW, Doty RD. Primary inoculation tuberculosis of the skin. Arch Dermatol 1978;114:567.
119. Kramer F, Sasse SA, Simms JC, Leedom JM. Primary cutaneous tuberculosis after a needle-stick injury from a patient with AIDS and undiagnosed tuberculosis. Ann Intern Med 1993;119:594.
120. Horney DA, Gaither JM, Lauer R et al. Cutaneous inoculation tuberculosis secondary to "jailhouse tattooing." Arch Dermatol 1985; 121:648.
121. Rietbroek RC, Dahlmans RPM, Smedts F et al. Tuberculosis cutis miliaris disseminata as a manifestation of miliary tuberculosis: Literature review and report of a case of recurrent skin lesions. Rev Infect Dis 1991;13:265.
122. McCray MK, Esterly NB. Cutaneous eruption in congenital tuberculosis. Arch Dermatol 1981;117:460.
123. Warin AP, Wilson-Jones E. Cutaneous tuberculosis of the nose with unusual clinical and histologic features leading to a delay in diagnosis. Clin Exp Dermatol 1977;2:235.
124. Marcoral J, Servitje O, Moreno A et al. Lupus vulgaris: Clinical, histologic, and bacteriologic study of 10 cases. J Am Acad Dermatol 1992;26:404.
125. Haim S, Friedman-Birnbaum R. Cutaneous tuberculosis and malignancy. Cutis 1978;21:643.
126. Serfling U, Penneys NS, Loenardi CL. Identification of *Mycobacterium tuberculosis* DNA in a case of lupus vulgaris. J Am Acad Dermatol 1993;28:318.

127. Regan W, Harley W. Orificial and pulmonary tuberculosis. Australas J Dermatol 1979;20:88.
128. Penneys NS, Leonardi CL, Cook S et al. Identification of *Mycobacterium tuberculosis* DNA in five different types of cutaneous lesions by PCR. Arch Dermatol 1993;129:1594.
129. Darier MJ. Des "tuberculides" cutanees. Arch Dermatol Syph 1896; 7:1431.
130. Morrison JGL, Furie ED. The papulonecrotic tuberculide. Br J Dermatol 1974;91:263.
131. Smith NP, Ryan TJ, Sanderson RV et al. Lichen scrofulosorum: A report of four cases. Br J Dermatol 1976;94:319.
132. Breathnach SM, Black MM. Atypical tuberculide (acne scrofulosorum) secondary to tuberculous lymphadenitis. Clin Exp Dermatol 1981;6:339.
133. Victor T, Jordaan HF, van Niekerk DJ et al. Papulonecrotic tuberculid. Identification of *Mycobacterium tuberculosis* DNA by polymerase chain reaction. Am J Dermatopathol 1992;14:491.
134. Jordaan HF, van Niekerk DJ, Louw M. Papulonecrotic tuberculid: A clinical, histopathololgical and immunohistochemical study of 15 patients. Am J Dermatopathol 1994;16:474.
135. Wilson-Jones E, Winkelmann RK. Papulonecrotic tuberculid: A neglected disease in Western countries. J Am Acad Dermatol 1986; 14:815.
136. Degitz K, Steidl M, Thomas P et al. Aetiology of tuberculids. Lancet 1993;341:239.
137. Iden DL, Rogers RS, Schroeter AL. Papulonecrotic tuberculid secondary to *Mycobacterium bovis*. Arch Dermatol 1978;114:564.
138. Williams JT, Pulitzer DR, DeVillez RL. Papulonecrotic tuberculid secondary to disseminated *Mycobacterium avium* complex. Int J Dermatol 1994;33:109.
139. Horowitz EA, Sanders WE. Other mycobacterial species. In: Mandell GL, Bennett JE, Dolin R, eds. Principles and practice of infectious diseases. New York: Churchill Livingstone, 1995;2264.
140. von Reyn CF, Barber TW, Arbeit RD et al. Evidence of previous infection with *Mycobacterium avium-Mycobacterium intracellulare* complex among healthy subjects: An international study of dominant mycobacterial skin test reactions. J Infect Dis 1993;168:1553.
141. Inwald D, Nelson M, Cramp M et al. Cutaneous manifestations of mycobacterial infection in patients with AIDS. Br J Dermatol 1994; 130:111.
142. Kennedy C, Chin A, Lien RAM et al. Leprosy and human immunodeficiency virus infection: A closer look at the lesions. Int J Dermatol 1990;29:130.
143. Hanke CW, Temofeew RK, Slama SL. *Mycobacterium kansasii* infection with multiple cutaneous lesions. J Am Acad Dermatol 1987; 16:1122.
144. Owens DW, McBride ME. Sporotrichoid cutaneous infection with *Mycobacterium kansasii*. Arch Dermatol 1969;100:54.
145. Nightingale SD, Byrd LT, Southern PM et al. Incidence of *Mycobacterium avium-intracellulare* complex bacteremia in human immunodeficiency virus-positive patients. J Infect Dis 1992;165:1082.
146. Havlir DV, Ellner JJ. *Mycobacterium avium* complex. In: Mandell GL, Bennett JE, Dolin R, eds. Principles and practice of infectious diseases. New York: Churchill Livingstone, 1995;2250.
147. Barbaro DJ, Orcutt VL, Coldiron BM. *Mycobacterium avium-Mycobacterium intracellulare* infection limited to the skin and lymph nodes in patients with AIDS. Rev Infect Dis 1989;11:625.
148. Wood C, Nickoloff BJ, Todes-Taylor NR. Pseudotumour resulting from atypical mycobacterial infection: A "histoid" variety of *Mycobacterium avium-intracellulare* complex infection. Am J Clin Pathol 1985;83:524.
149. Cole GW, Gebhard J. *Mycobacterium avium* infection of the skin resembling lepromatous leprosy. Br J Dermatol 1979;101:71.
150. Huminer D, Pitlik SD, Block C et al. Aquarium-borne *Mycobacterium marinum* skin infection. Arch Dermatol 1986;122:698.
151. Philpott JA, Woodburne AR, Philpott OS et al. Swimming pool granuloma. Arch Dermatol 1963;88:158.
152. Dickey RF. Sprotrichoid mycobacteriosis caused by *M marinum* (balnei). Arch Dermatol 1969;98:385.
153. Debat-Zoguereh D, Bonnet E, Mars ME et al. Mycobactériose cutanée à *Mycobacterium marinum* au cours de l'infection par le VIH. Méd Mal Infect 1993;23:37.
154. Tchornobay AM, Claudy AL, Perrot JL et al. Fatal disseminated *Mycobacterium* infection. Int J Dermatol 1992;31:286.
155. Travis WD, Travis LB, Roberts GD et al. The histopathologic spectrum in *Mycobacterium marinum* infection. Arch Pathol Lab Med 1985;109:1109.
156. Heyman J. Out of Africa: Observations on the histopathology of *Mycobacterium ulcerans*. J Clin Pathol 1993;46:5.
157. Connor DE, Lunn HF. Buruli ulceration. Arch Pathol 1966;81:183.
158. Marston BJ, Diallo MO, Horsburgh CR et al. Emergence of Buruli ulcer disease in the Daloa region of Côte d'Ivoire. Am J Trop Med Hyg 1995;52:219.
159. Uganda Buruli Group. Clinical features and treatment of pre-ulcerative Buruli lesions: *Myucobacterium ulcerans* infection. Br Med J 1970;2:390.
160. Hayman J, McQueen A. The pathology of *Mycobacterium ulcerans* infection. Pathol 1983;17:594.
161. Pimsler M, Sponsler TA, Meyers WM. Immunosuppressive properties of the soluble toxin from *Mycobacterium ulcerans*. J Infect Dis 1988; 157:577.
162. Hockmeyer WT, Krieg RE, Reich M, Johnson RD. Further characterization of *Mycobacterium ulcerans* toxin. Infect Immun 1978;21:124.
163. Wallace RJ, Swenson JM, Silcox VA et al. Spectrum of disease due to rapidly growing mycobacteria. Rev Infect Dis 1983;5:657.
164. Murdoch ME, Leigh IM. Spirotrichoid spread of cutaneous *Mycobacterium chelonei* infection. Clin Exp Dermatol 1989;14:309.
165. McGovern J, Bix BC, Webster G. *Mycobacterium haemophilium* skin disease successfully treated with excision. J Am Acad Dermatol 1994; 30:269.
166. Rogers PL, Walker RE, Lane HC et al. Disseminated *Mycobacterium haemophilum* infection in two patients with the acquired immunodeficiency syndrome. Am J Med 1988;84:640.
167. Kristjansson M, Bieluch VM, Byeff PD. *Mycobacterium haemophilum* infection in immunocompromised patients: Case report and review of the literature. Rev Infect Dis 1991;13:906.
168. Abramowsky C, Gonzalez B, Sorensen RU. Disseminated BCG infections with primary immunodeficiencies. Am J Clin Pathol 1993; 100:52.
169. Noordeen SK. Eliminating leprosy as a public health problem. Int J Lepr 1995;63:559.
170. Ridley DS, Jopling WH. Classification of leprosy according to immunity: A five-group system. Int J Lepr 1966;34:255.
171. Ridley DS. Histological classification and the immunological spectrum of leprosy. Bull World Health Organization 1974;51:451.
172. Ridley DS. Skin biopsy in leprosy. Basel: Ciba Geigy, 1990.
173. Lowy L. Processing of biopsies for leprosy bacilli. J Med Lab Technol 1956;13:558.
174. Harada K. A modified allochrome procedure for demonstrating mycobacteria in tissue sections. Int J Lepr 1977;45:49.
175. van Brakel WH, de Soldenhoff R, McDougall AC. The allocation of leprosy patients into paucibacillary and multibacillary groups for multidrug therapy, taking into account the number of body areas affected by skin, or skin and nerve lesions. Lepr Rev 1992;63:231.
176. Ridley MJ, Ridley DS. The immunopathology of erythema nodosum leprosum: The role of extravascular complexes. Lepr Rev 1983; 54:95.
177. Pfaltzgraff RE, Ramu G. Clinical leprosy. In: Hastings RC, ed. Leprosy. Edinburgh: Churchill Livingstone, 1994;237.
178. Job CK. Pathology of leprosy. In: Hastings RC, ed. Leprosy. Edinburgh: Churchill Livingstone, 1994;193.
179. Rea TH, Ridley DS. Lucio's pheonomenon: A comparative histological study. Int J Lepr 1979;47:161.
180. Wade HW. The histoid variety of lepromatous leprosy. Int J Lepr 1963;31:129.
181. Pönnighaus JM. Diagnosis and management of single lesions in leprosy. Lepr Rev 1996;67:89.
182. Ridley DS, Ridley MJ. The classification of nerves is modified by delayed recognition of *M leprae*. Int J Lepr 1986;54:596.
183. Ridley DS. Pathogenesis of leprosy and related diseases. London: Wright, 1988.
184. Ridley DS, Radia KB. The histological course of reactions in borderline leprosy and their outcome. Int J Lepr 1981;49:383.
185. Hussain R, Lucas SB, Kifayet A et al. Clinical and histological discrepancies in diagnosis of ENL reactions classified by assessment of acute phase proteins SAA and CRP. Int J Lepr 1995;63:222.
186. Ottenhoff THM. Immunology of leprosy: Lessons from and for leprosy. Int J Lepr 1994;62:108.

187. Choudhuri K. The immunology of leprosy: Unravelling an enigma. Int J Lepr 1995;63:430.
188. Salgame P, Abrams JS, Clayberger C et al. Differing lymphokine profiles of functional subsets of human CD4 and CD8 T cell clones. Science 1991;254:279.
189. Modlin RL, Hofman FM, Meyer PR et al. In situ demonstration of T lymphocyte subsets in granulomatous inflammation: Leprosy, rhinoscleroma and sarcoidosis. Clin Exp Immunol 1983;51:430.
190. Modlin RL, Rea TH. Immunopathology of leprosy. In: Hastings RC, ed. Leprosy. Edinburgh: Churchill Livingstone, 1994;225.
191. Orege PA, Fine PEM, Lucas SB et al. A case control study of human immunodeficiency virus-1 (HIV-1) infection as a risk factor for tuberculosis and leprosy in western Kenya. Tubercle Lung Dis 1993;74:377.
192. Pönnighaus JM, Mwanjasi LJ, Fine PEM et al. Is HIV infection a risk factor for leprosy? Int J Lepr 1991;59:221.
193. Lucas SB. HIV and leprosy (editorial). Lepr Rev 1993;64:97.
194. Blum L, Flageul B, Sow S et al. Leprosy reversal reaction in HIV-positive patients. Int J Lepr 1993;61:214.
195. Fleury RN, Bacchi CE. S-100 protein and immunoperoxidase technique as an aid in the histopathologic diagnosis of leprosy. Int J Lepr 1987;55:338.
196. Gainsborough N, Hall SM, Hughes RAC, Leibowitz S. Sarcoid neuropathy. J Neurol 1991;238:177.
197. De Wit MYL, Faber WR, Krieg SR et al. Application of a polymerase chain reaction for the detection of *Mycobacterium leprae* in skin tissues. J Clin Microbiol 1991;29:906.
198. Fine PEM, Job CK, Lucas SB et al. The extent, origin and implications of observer variation in the histopathological diagnosis of leprosy. Int J Lepr 1993;61:270.
199. Lew D. *Bacillus anthracis:* Anthrax. In: Mandell GL, Bennett JE, Dolin R, eds. Principles and practice of infectious disease. New York: Churchill Livingstone, 1995;1885.
200. Breathnach AF, Turnbull PCB, Eykyn SJ, Twort CHC. A labourer with a spot on his chest. Lancet 1996;347:96.
201. Penn RL. Francisella tularensis: Tularemia. In: Mandell GL, Bennett JE, Dolin R, eds. Principles and practice of infectious disease. New York: Churchill Livingstone, 1995;2060.
202. Kodama BF, Fitzpatrick JE, Gentry RH. Tularemia. Cutis 1994; 54:279.
203. Myers SA, Sexton DJ. Dermatologic manifestations of arthropod-borne diseases. Infect Dis Clin North Am 1994;8:689.
204. Cerny Z. Skin manifestations of tularaemia. Int J Dermatol 1994; 33:468.
205. von Schroeder HP, McDougall EP. Ulceroglandular and pulmonary tularemia: A case resulting from a cat bite to the hand. J Hand Surg 1993;18:132.
206. Salgo MP, Telzak EE, Carrie B et al. A focus of Rocky Mountain spotted fever within New York City. N Engl J Med 1985;318:1345.
207. Raoult D, Walker DH. *Rickettsia rickettsii.* In: Mandell GL, Bennett JE, Dolin R, eds. Principles and practice of infectious disease. New York: Churchill Livingstone, 1995;1721.
208. Kirkland KB, Marcom P, Sexton DJ et al. Rocky mountain spotted fever complicated by gangrene: Report of six cases and review. Clin Infect Dis 1993;16:629.
209. Sexton DJ, Corey GR. Rocky mountain "spotless" and "almost spotless" fever: A wolf in sheep's clothing. Clin Infect Dis 1992;15:439.
210. White WL, Patrick JD, Miller LR. Evaluation of immunoperoxidase techniques to detect *Rickettsia rickettsii* in fixed tissue sections. Am J Clin Pathol 1994;101:747.
211. Morse SA. Chancroid and *Haemophilus ducreyi.* Clin Microbiol Rev 1989;2:137.
212. Moxon ER. *Haemophilus ducreyi:* Chancroid. In: Mandell GL, Bennett JE, Dolin R, eds. Principles and practice of infectious disease. New York: Churchill Livingstone, 1995;2047.
213. Freinkel AL. Histological aspects of sexually transmitted genital lesions. Histopathology 1987;11:819.
214. Parsons LM, Shayegani M, Waring AL, Bopp LH. DNA probe for the identification of *Haemophilus ducreyi.* J Clin Microbiol 1989; 27:1441.
215. Marsch WC, Haas N, Stuttgen G. Ultrastructural detection of *Haemophilus ducreyi* in biopsies of chancroid. Arch Dermatol Res 1978;263:153.
216. Fiumara NJ, Rothman K, Tang S. The diagnosis and treatment of chancroid. J Am Acad Dermatol 1986;15:939.
217. Werman BS, Herskowitz LJ, Olansky S et al. A clinical variant of chancroid resembling granuloma inguinale. Arch Dermatol 1983; 119:890.
218. Ballard RC. Calymmatobacterium granulomatis: Donovanosis. In: Mandell GL, Bennett JE, Dolin R, eds. Principles and practice of infectious disease. New York: Churchill Livingstone, 1995, in 2210.
219. Sehgal VN, Shyam Prasad AL. Donovanosis: Current concepts. Int J Dermatol 1986;25:8.
220. Lucas SB. Tropical pathology of the female genital tract and ovaries. In: Fox H, ed. Haines and Taylor obstetrical and gynaecological pathology. Edinburgh: Churchill Livingstone, 1995; in press.
221. Spagnolo DV, Coburn PR, Cream JJ, Azadian BS. Extrangenital granuloma inguinale (donovanosis) diagnosed in the United Kingdom: A clinical, histological, and electron microscopical study. J Clin Pathol 1984;37:945.
222. McKay CR, Binch WI. Carcinoma of the vulva following granuloma inguinale. Am J Syph 1952;36:511.
223. Hirsch BC, Johnson WC. Pathology of granulomatous disease: Mixed inflammatory granulomas. Int J Dermatol 1984;23:585.
224. Davis CM, Collins C. Granuloma inguinale: An ultrastructural study of Calymmatobacterium granulomatis. J Invest Dermatol 1969; 53:315.
225. Okoth-Olende CA, Bjerregaard B. Scleroma in Africa: A review of cases from Kenya. East Afr Med J 1990;67:231.
226. Meyer PR, Shum TK, Becker TS, Taylor CR. Scleroma (rhinoscleroma): A histologic immunohistochemical study with bacteriologic correlates. Arch Pathol Lab Med 1983;107:377.
227. Shum TK, Whitaker CW, Meyer PR. Clinical update on rhinoscleroma. Laryngoscope 1982;92:1149.
228. Hoffman E, Loose LD, Harkin JC. The Mikulicz cell in rhinoscleroma. Am J Pathol 1973;73:47.
229. Gumprecht TF, Nichols PW, Meyer PR. Identification of rhinoscleroma by immunoperoxidase technique. Laryngoscope 1983;93:627.
230. Jones RE. Chlamydia trachomatis. In: Mandell GL, Bennett JE, Dolin R, eds. Principles and practice of infectious disease. New York: Churchill Livingstone, 1995;1679.
231. Hopsu-Havu VK, Sonck CE. Infiltrative, ulcerative and fistular lesions of the penis due to lymphogranuloma venereum. Br J Vener Dis 1973;49:193.
232. Bolan RK, Sands M, Schachter J et al. Lymphogranuloma venereum and acute ulcerative proctitis. Am J Med 1982;72:703.
233. Barnes RC. Laboratory diagnosis of human chlamydial infections. Clin Microbiol Rev 1989;2:119.
234. Carithers HA. Cat scratch disease: An overview based on a study of 1,200 patients. Am J Dis Child 1985;139:1124.
235. Lucas SB. Cat scratch disease (editorial). J Pathol 1991;163:93.
236. Wear DJ, Margileth AM, Hadfield TL et al. Cat scratch disease: A bacterial infection. Science 1983;221:1403.
237. Margileth AM. Dermatologic manifestations and update of cat scratch disease. Pediatr Dermatol 1988;5:1.
238. Yu X, Raoult D. Monoclonal antibodies to *Afipia felis:* A putative agent of cat scratch disease. Am J Clin Pathol 1994;101:603.
239. Min K-W, Reed JA, Welch DF, Slater LN. Morphologically variable bacilli of cat scratch disease are identified by immunocytochemical labelling with antibodies to *Rochlimaea henselae.* Am J Clin Pathol 1994;101:607.
240. Adal KA, Cockerell CJ, Petri WA. Cat scratch disease, bacillary angiomatosis, and other infections due to *Rochalimea.* N Engl J Med 1994;330:1509.
241. Clarridge JE, Raich TJ, Pirwani D et al. Strategy to detect and identify *Bartonella* species in routine clinical laboratory yields *Bartonella henselae* from HIV-positive patients and unique *Bartonella* strain from his cat. J Clin Microbiol 1995;33:2107.
242. Kudo E, Sakaki A, Sumitomo M et al. An epidemiological and ultrastructural study of lymphadenitis caused by Warthin-Starry positive bacteria. Virchows Arch [A] 1988;412:563.
243. Brenner DJ, Hollis DG, Moss CW et al. Proposal of *Afipia* gen. nov. with *Afipia felis* sp. nov. (formerly the cat scratch bacillus), *Afipia clevelandensis* sp. nov. (formerly the Cleveland Clinic Foundation strain), *Afipia broomeae* sp. nov., and three unnamed genospecies. J Clin Microbiol 1991;29:2450.
244. Koehler JE, Glaser CA, Tappero JW. *Rochalimaea henselae* infection: A new zoonosis with the domestic cat as reservoir. JAMA 1994; 271:531.

245. Stoler MH, Bonfiglio TA, Steigbigel RT, Pereira M. An atypical subcutaneous infection associated with AIDS. Am J Clin Pathol 1983; 80:714.
246. Milde P, Brunner M, Borchard F et al. Cutaneous bacillary angiomatosis in a patient with chronic lymphocytic leukaemia. Arch Dermatol 1995;131:933.
247. Itin PH, Fluckiger R, Zbinden R, Frei R. Recurrent pyogenic granuloma with satellitosis: A localised variant of bacillary angiomatosis? Dermatol 1994;189:409.
248. Cottell SL, Noskin GA. Bacillary angiomatosis: Clinical and histologic features, diagnosis and treatment. Arch Intern Med 1994; 154:524.
249. Tappero JW, Mohle-Boetani J, Koehler JE et al. The epidemiology of bacillary angiomatosis and bacillary peliosis. JAMA 1993;269:770.
250. Cockerell CJ. The clinico-pathologic spectrum of bacillary (epithelioid) angiomatosis. In: Rotterdam H, Racz P, Greco MA, Cockerell CJ, eds. Progress in AIDS Pathology. Vol II. New York: Field & Wood, 1990;111.
251. Schinella RA, Greco MA. Bacillary angiomatosis presenting as a soft-tissue tumour without skin involvement. Hum Pathol 1990;21:567.
252. LeBoit PE, Berger TG, Egbert BM, Beckstead JA et al. Bacillary angiomatosis: The histopathology and differential diagnosis of a pseudoneoplastic infection in patients with HIV disease. Am J Surg Pathol 1989;13:909.
253. Hacker P. Botryomycosis. Int J Dermatol 1983;22:455.
254. Toth IR, Kazal HL. Botryomycosis in acquired immunodeficiency syndrome. Arch Pathol Lab Med 1987;111:246.
255. Harman RR, English MP, Halford M et al. Botryomycosis: A complication of extensive follicular mucinosis. Br J Dermatol 1980;102:215.
256. Goette DK. Transepithelial elimination in botryomycosis. Int J Dermatol 1981;20:198.
257. Curry WA. Human nocardiosis: A clinical review with selected case reports. Arch Intern Med 1980;140:818.
258. Berd D. *Nocardia brasiliensis* infection in the United States: A report of nine cases and a review of the literature. Am J Clin Pathol 1973; 59:254.
259. Lucas SB, Hounnou A, Peacock CS et al. Nocardiosis in HIV-positive patients: An autopsy study in West Africa. Tubercle Lung Dis 1994; 75:301.
260. Uttamchandari RB, Daikos GL, Reyes RR et al. Nocardiosis in 30 patients with advanced human immunodeficiency virus infection: clinical features and outcome. Clin Infect Dis 1994;18:348.
261. Tsuboi R, Takamori K, Ogawa H et al. Lymphocutaneous nocardiosis caused by *Nocardia asteriodes:* Case report and review of the literature. Arch Dermatol 1986;122:1183.
262. Russo TA. Agents of actinomycosis. In: Mandell GL, Bennett JE, Dolin R, eds. Principles and practice of infectious diseases. New York: Churchill Livingstone, 1995;2280.
263. Brown JR. Human actinomycosis: A study of 181 subjects. Hum Pathol 1973;4:319.
264. Rashid AM, Williams RM, Parry D, Malone PR. Actinomycosis associated with a pilonidal sinus of the penis. J Urol 1992;148:405.
265. Behberhani MJ, Heeley JD, Jordan HV. Comparative histopathology of lesions produced by *Actinomyces israelii, A.naeslundii,* and *A. viscosus* in mice. Am J Pathol 1983;110:267.

Lever's Histopathology of the Skin, eighth edition,
edited by David Elder et al. Lippincott–
Raven Publishers, Philadelphia © 1997.

CHAPTER 22

Treponemal Diseases

A. Neil Crowson, Cynthia Magro, and Martin Mihm Jr.

The treponemal diseases, broadly classified as venereal and nonvenereal, are caused by motile bacteria of the family *Spirochetacea*, which also includes the genera *borrelia* and *leptospira*. The pathogenic treponemes resemble each other morphologically, being characterized in dark-field and biopsy preparations as coiled, silver-staining organisms measuring 6 to 20 μm by 0.10 to 0.18 μm, and show a high degree of DNA homology.[1] The nonvenereal treponematoses include yaws, pinta, and endemic syphilis.

VENEREAL SYPHILIS

Acquired syphilis, caused by *Treponema pallidum*, has afflicted humanity since at least the fifteenth century.[2] Although it was a major cause of morbidity and mortality in the early twentieth century, public health programs and the advent of penicillin so reduced its incidence in First World countries that, by the mid-1980s, most physicians were unfamiliar with its signs and symptoms.[1] However, the incidence of acquired syphilis is increasing; in 1990, the incidence was 20 per 100,000 in the United States and 360 per 100,000 in parts of Africa. This may relate to the outbreak of human immunodeficiency virus infection, with which acquired syphilis is linked epidemiologically. *T pallidum* is generally spread through contact between infectious lesions and disrupted epithelium at sites of minor trauma incurred during sexual intercourse. The transmission rate is between 10% and 60%.

Primary syphilis is defined by a skin lesion, or chancre, in which organisms are identified; it typically arises 21 days after exposure at the inoculation site, and is classically a painless, brown-red, indurated, round papule, nodule, or plaque 1 to 2 cm in diameter. Lesions may be multiple or ulcerative, and the regional lymph nodes may be enlarged.

Secondary syphilis results from the hematogenous dissemination of organisms, resulting in more widespread clinical signs accompanied by constitutional symptoms inclusive of fever, malaise, and generalized lymphadenopathy. A generalized eruption occurs, comprising brown-red macules and papules, papulosquamous lesions resembling guttate psoriasis, and, rarely, pustules.[3] Lesions may be follicular-based, annular, or serpiginous, particularly in recurrent attacks of secondary syphilis. Other skin signs include alopecia and condylomata lata, the latter comprising broad, raised, gray, confluent papular lesions arising in anogenital areas, pitted hyperkeratotic palmoplantar papules termed "syphilis cornee," and, in rare severe cases, ulcerating lesions that define "lues maligna." Some patients develop mucous patches composed of multiple shallow, painless ulcers.

Meningovascular syphilis is usually observed in tertiary syphilis after 7 to 12 years of disease[4] but can occur in the secondary stage and be symptomatic; usually, it manifests as basilar meningitis and can be associated with cranial nerve palsies.[5] Acute transverse myelitis occurs in rare cases[6] as is glomerulonephritis, and an occasional patient suffers from self-limited hepatitis.

Primary- and secondary-stage lesions may resolve without therapy or go unnoticed by the patient, who then passes into a latent phase. The latter may be subdivided into early and late stages, an arbitrary distinction that may be helpful in guiding the therapeutic approach. The Center for Disease Control bases its distinction of the early (infectious) latent stage from the late (noninfectious) latent stage on whether the duration of the infection is less or more than 1 year, respectively. The World Health Organization uses a 2-year period to make this distinction. After a variable latent period, the patient enters the *tertiary stage*.

Tertiary syphilis comprises gummatous skin and mucosal lesions ("benign tertiary syphilis"), cardiovascular manifestations, and neurological manifestations. The skin lesions may be solitary or multiple, and can be divided into superficial nodular and deep gummatous types. The nodular type has a smooth, atrophic center with a raised, serpiginous border. The gummatous lesions present as subcutaneous swellings that ulcerate.[7]

Congenital syphilis, on the rise since the mid-1980s,[8] is a diagnosis rendered when organisms are observed by dark-field, fluorescent antibody, or conventional histochemical techniques in lesion, placenta, or umbilical cord.[9] A case is deemed to be

A. N. Crowson: Central Medica Laboratories and Misericordia General Hospital, Winnipeg, Manitoba, Canada
C. Magro: Pathology Services, Inc.; Department of Pathology, Beth Israel Hospital/Harvard University, Cambridge, MA
M. Mihm Jr.: Chief, Dermatology and Dermatopathology, Albany Medical College, Albany, NY

presumptive when an infant is born to a mother who had inadequately treated or untreated syphilis at the time of delivery, or when an infant or child with a reactive treponemal test for syphilis exhibits evidence of congenital syphilis by virtue of physical or long-bone radiological examination, a reactive cerebrospinal fluid (CSF) VDRL, an elevated CSF protein or white blood cell count of unknown cause, or quantitative treponemal titres four times higher than the mother's at the time of birth.[9] Clinical signs include rhinitis, chancres, or a maculopapular desquamative rash.[8] Infection occurs by a transplacental route, affecting more than 50% of infants born to mothers with primary or secondary syphilis, roughly 40% of those born to mothers in the early latent stage, and only 10% of those born to mothers with late latent infections.[9]

Histopathology of Syphilis. The two fundamental pathologic changes in syphilis are (1) swelling and proliferation of endothelial cells and (2) a predominantly perivascular infiltrate composed of lymphoid cells and often plasma cells. In late secondary and tertiary syphilis, there are also granulomatous infiltrates of epithelioid histiocytes and giant cells.

Primary Syphilis

The epidermis at the periphery of the syphilitic chancre reveals changes comparable to those observed in lesions of secondary syphilis—namely, acanthosis, spongiosis, and exocytosis of lymphocytes and neutrophils. Toward the center, the epidermis gradually becomes thinner and appears edematous and permeated by inflammatory cells. In the center, the epidermis may be absent. The papillary dermis appears edematous. A dense perivascular and interstitial lymphohistiocytic and plasmacellular infiltrate spans the entire thickness of the dermis (Fig. 22-1); the lymphocytes are principally of T helper/inducer subset. Neutrophils are often admixed. An obliterative endarteritis characterized by endothelial swelling and mural edema is observed (Fig. 22-2).

By silver staining with the Levaditi stain or the Warthin-Starry stain and by immunofluorescent techniques, spirochetes are usually identified along the dermal-epidermal junction and within and around blood vessels. If seen in their full length, which is rare, spirochetes generally show 8 to 12 spiral convolutions, each measuring from 1 to 1.2 μm in length (Fig. 22-3). If spirochetes are stained with silver, it should be remembered that silver also stains melanin and reticulum fibers. Differentiation may cause some difficulties but should be possible based on the fact that the melanin in the dendritic processes of melanocytes has a granular appearance, the granules being thicker and more heavily stained than *T pallidum.*[10] Reticulin fibers, although wavy, do not exhibit a spiral appearance.

Histologic examination of enlarged regional lymph nodes in primary syphilis most commonly reveals a chronic inflammatory cell infiltrate containing many plasma cells. In addition, there are endothelial hyperplasia and follicular hyperplasia. Spirochetes are numerous and can nearly always be identified with the Warthin-Starry stain. In some cases, noncaseating granulomas resembling those of sarcoidosis are found in the lymph nodes.[11]

Histogenesis. T pallidum can be demonstrated by histochemistry or by immunohistochemistry. The latter comprises immunofluorescent methods in frozen[12] or fresh specimens and immunoperoxidase methods employable in fixed tissues.[13] By electron microscopy, the organism can be seen in both intra- and extracellular dispositions in the epidermis and dermis[14]—within keratinocyte nuclei,[15] fibroblasts,[15,16] nerve fibers,[17] blood vessel endothelia, and the lumina of lymphatic channels.[15] Phagocytic vacuoles of macrophages and neutrophils may contain organisms,[18] as may the cytoplasm of plasma cells. Ultrastructurally, the organism is 8 to 16 μm in length with regular spirals, a wavelength of 0.9 μm, and an amplitude of 0.2 μm, and a cytoplasmic body 0.13 μm in diameter with tapering ends, all enveloped by a 7-nm trilaminar cytoplasmic membrane.[19] The organisms attach to host cells by

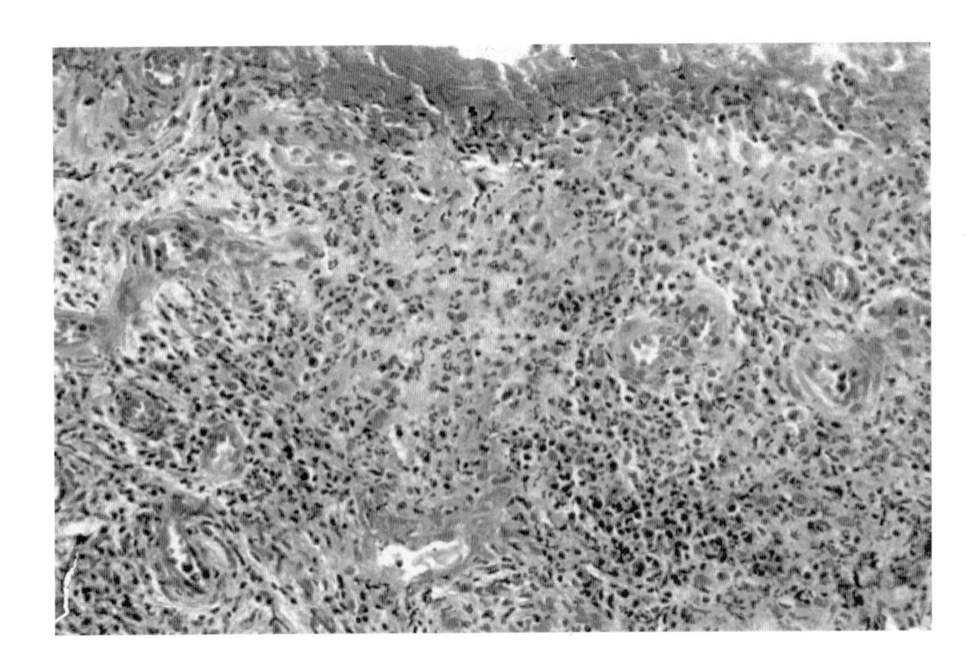

FIG. 22-1. Primary syphilitic chancre
The epithelium is eroded and the corium contains a dense plasma-cell-rich infiltrate. There is neovascularization with secondary necrotizing vasculitic changes manifested by mural fibrin deposition.

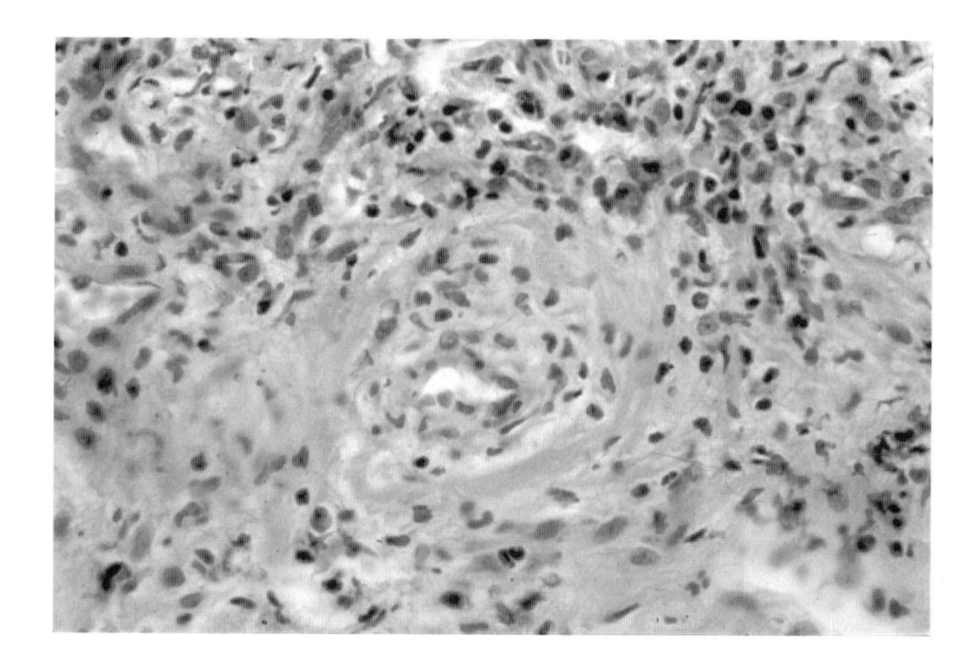

FIG. 22-2. Primary syphilitic chancre
There is endarteritis obliterans manifested by endothelial cell swelling, endothelial hyperplasia, and expansion of vessel walls by edema and a lymphohistiocytic infiltrate with resultant lumenal attenuation. A diffuse extravascular plasma-cell-rich infiltrate is present.

means of acorn-shaped nosepieces. The contractile motility of the spirochete is mediated by three or four axial filaments that course the length of the cytoplasmic body.[20] A paraplastic membrane surrounds these axial filaments in young organisms, but is replaced by an electron-dense amorphous substance produced by the host cell as an immunological response in older spirochetes.[17]

Differential Diagnosis. Lesions of chancroid are the most difficult to differentiate clinically from a syphilitic chancre. The characteristic histopathology of chancroid is one of dense lymphohistiocytic infiltrates with a paucity of plasma cells and a granulomatous vasculitis. An epidermal reaction pattern similar to the syphilitic chancre is observed—namely, psoriasiform epidermal hyperplasia and spongiform pustulation. A Giemsa or alcian blue stain reveals coccobacillary forms between keratinocytes and along the dermal-epidermal junction. The infiltrate is composed mainly of T helper lymphocytes and histiocytes including Langerhans' cells.[21]

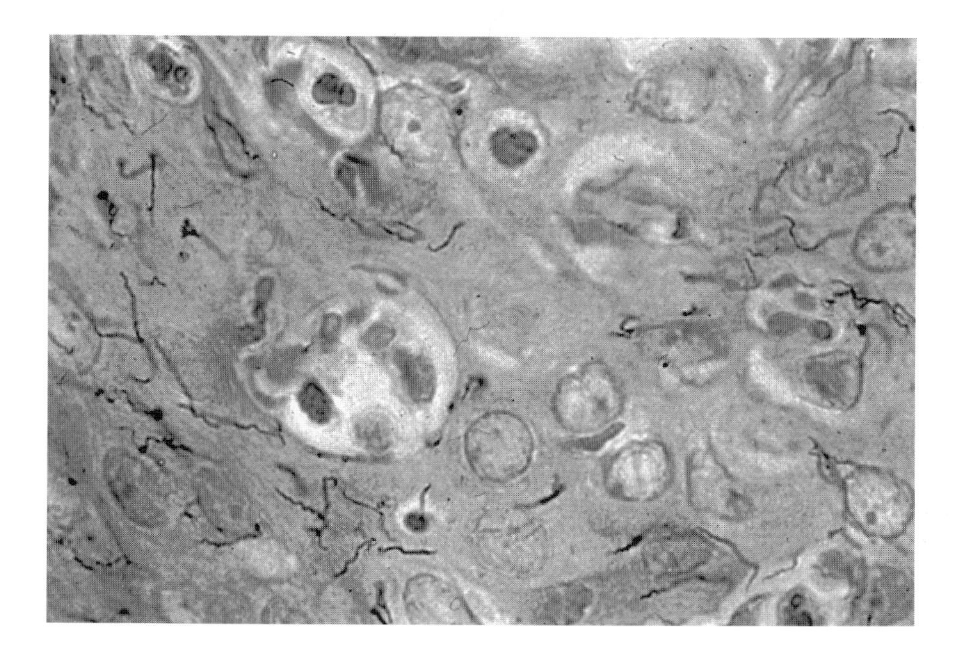

FIG. 22-3. Primary syphilitic chancre
A silver stain reveals numerous elongate coiled spirochetes ranging in length from 8 to 12 μm in a perivascular disposition.

Secondary Syphilis

There is considerable histologic overlap among the various clinical forms of secondary syphilis, such as the macular, papular, and papulosquamous types.[22,23] Nevertheless, epidermal changes are least pronounced in the macular type and most pronounced in the papulosquamous type of lesion.

Biopsies generally reveal psoriasiform hyperplasia of the epidermis with spongiosis and basilar vacuolar alteration. Exocytosis of lymphocytes, spongiform pustulation, and parakeratosis also may be observed (Fig. 22-4).[10,22] The parakeratosis may be patchy or broad, with or without intracorneal neutrophilic abscesses. Although lesions may mimic psoriasis, attenuation of the suprapapillary plate is uncommon. Scattered necrotic keratinocytes may be observed. Ulceration is not a feature of macular, papular, or papulosquamous lesions of secondary syphilis.

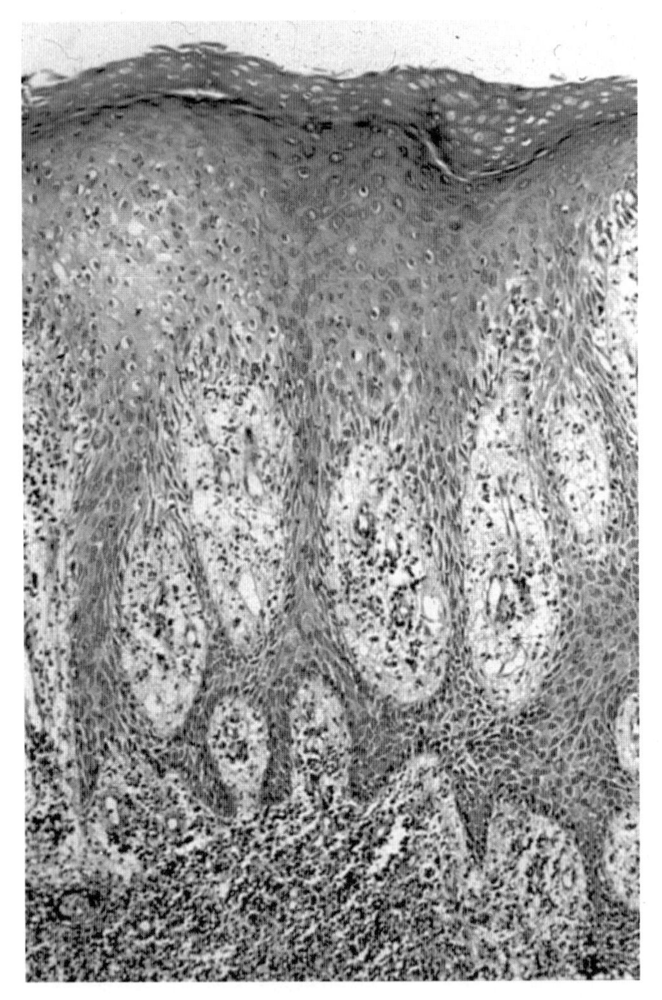

FIG. 22-4. Secondary syphilis
There is psoriasiform hyperplasia of the epidermis with concomitant intracellular edema and exocytosis of lymphocytes; the epidermis is surmounted by an orthohyperkeratotic and parakeratotic scale. There is prominent papillary dermal edema with resultant basilar vacuolar alteration. A dense, bandlike lymphocytic infiltrate with admixed plasma cells hugs the dermal-epidermal junction, defining a concomitant lichenoid tissue reaction.

The dermal changes include marked papillary dermal edema and a perivascular and/or periadnexal infiltrate that may be lymphocyte predominant, lymphohistiocytic, histiocytic predominant, or frankly granulomatous and that is of greatest intensity in the papillary dermis and extends as loose perivascular aggregates into the reticular dermis. Obscuration of the superficial vasculature and a lichenoid morphology observed in some cases (see Fig. 22-4), and a cell-poor infiltrate is seen in others (Fig. 22-5). In a few cases, when the infiltrate is heavy, atypical-appearing nuclei may be present and may then suggest the possibility of mycosis fungoides[24] or non-Hodgkin's lymphoma. Neutrophils are not infrequent and may permeate the eccrine coil to produce a neutrophilic eccrine hidradenitis.[10] Granulomatous inflammation is almost invariable in lesions of greater than 4 months duration[23] and may be present in some cases of early syphilis.[25] A plasma cell component is inconspicuous or absent in 25% of the cases (Fig. 22-6).[22] Eosinophils are not usually observed. Vascular changes such as endothelial swelling and mural edema may accompany the angiocentric infiltrates and are present in only about half of the cases.[22] Frank necrotizing injurious vascular alterations are distinctly unusual. A silver stain is recommended in all cases that are suspected of being secondary syphilis; it shows the presence of spirochetes in about a third of the cases of secondary syphilis, mainly within the epidermis and less commonly around the blood vessels of the superficial plexus. In some instances, the silver stain is positive even when dark-field examination of the patient's lesions is negative.[10] By the immunofluorescent technique, all cases are positive. Phenotypic analysis of the infiltrate reveals a lymphoid populace composed mainly of T cells with an equal proportion of cytotoxic and T helper cells.

There are several histologic variants of secondary syphilis—namely, condylomata lata, syphilitic alopecia, pustular lesions, syphilis cornee, and lues maligna. Lesions of condylomata lata show all of the aforementioned changes observed in macular, papular, and papulosquamous lesions, but more florid epithelial hyperplasia and intraepithelial microabscess formation are observed.[10,26] A Warthin-Starry stain shows numerous treponemes.[17]

Biopsies of syphilitic alopecia may demonstrate a superficial and deep perivascular and perifollicular lymphocytic and plasmacellular infiltrate that permeates the outer root sheath epithelium with a concomitant perifollicular fibrosing reaction.[10] An involutional tendency characterized by increased numbers of telogen hairs is observed. A concomitant necrotizing pustular follicular reaction may also be seen.[3]

An unusual variant of secondary syphilis is lues maligna,[27,28] an ulcerative form characterized by severe thrombotic endarteritis obliterans involving vessels at the dermal-subcutaneous junction with resultant ischemic necrosis. A concomitant dense plasmacellular infiltrate with a variable admixture of histiocytes may be observed. Defective-cell-mediated immunity may play an integral role in the pathogenesis of lues maligna, particularly in cases where vascular alterations are minimal.[29,30] Several cases of lues maligna arising in the setting of HIV disease have been described with involvement of the oral cavity as the principal manifestation.

A case of secondary syphilis resembling bullous pemphigoid by both light microscopy and immunofluorescent studies has been described.[31]

The histopathology of the syphilis cornee/keratoderma punc-

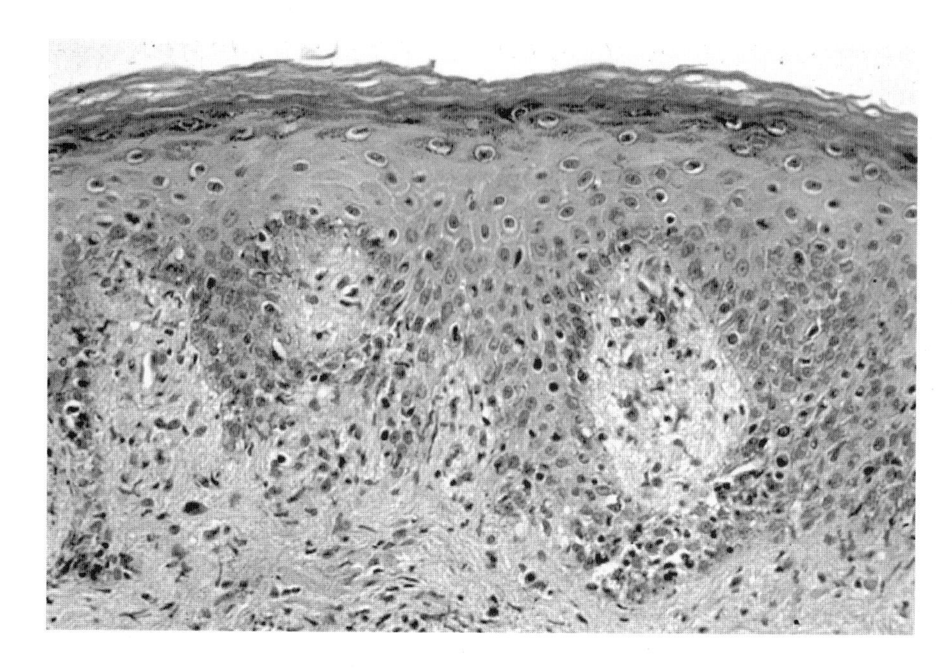

FIG. 22-5. Secondary syphilis There is psoriasiform epidermal hyperplasia with basilar vacuolopathy and focal lymphocyte tagging along the dermal-epidermal junction. The epidermis is surmounted by a hyperkeratotic scale. In contrast to the dense lichenoid morphology illustrated in Fig. 22-4, the infiltrate is less intense, and plasma cells are inconspicuous.

tatum associated with secondary syphilis is characterized by an epidermal invagination containing a horny plug composed of laminated layers of parakeratotic cells with loss of the granular cell layer and thinning of the subjacent prickle cell layer.[32] A moderately dense perivascular plasmacellular infiltrate with concomitant capillary wall thickening involves the cutaneous vasculature.

In the rare pustular lesions of secondary syphilis, a necrotizing pustular follicular reaction accompanied by noncaseating granulomata and a perivascular lymphoplasmacellular infiltrate characterizes the histopathology.[3]

In addition to small, sarcoidal granulomata in papular lesions of early secondary syphilis, late secondary syphilis may show extensive lymphoplasmacellular and histiocytic infiltrates resembling nodular tertiary syphilis.[33] Conversely, lesions of early tertiary syphilis may lack granulomata.[34]

Although often nonspecific, the hepatitis of secondary syphilis may produce a granulomatous or cholestatic morphol-

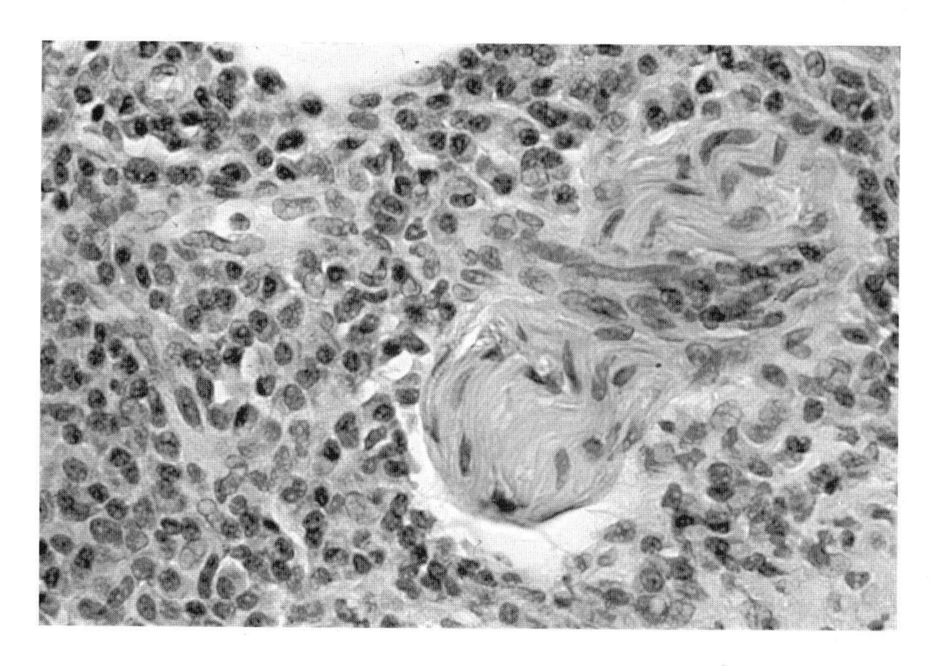

FIG. 22-6. Secondary syphilis A dense, plasma-cell-rich infiltrate surrounds the cutaneous nerves of the dermis.

ogy on liver biopsy; hepatic necrosis and spirochetes may also be observed.[35] The nephrosis or glomerulonephritis of secondary syphilis shows proliferative changes in the glomeruli.[36]

Histogenesis. It has been shown that the renal changes occurring in secondary syphilis relate to immune complexes containing treponemal antigen. Not only has direct immunofluorescence shown granular deposits of immunoglobulins and complement along the glomerular basement membrane,[36,37] but indirect immunofluorescence antibody studies employing rabbit treponemal antibody and sheep antirabbit globulin conjugate have demonstrated the presence of treponemal antigen in the glomerular deposits.[36]

Differential Diagnosis. The differential diagnosis of lesions of secondary syphilis includes other causes of lichenoid dermatitis including lichen planus, a lichenoid hypersensitivity reaction, pityriasis lichenoides and connective tissue disease, sarcoidosis, psoriasis, and psoriasiform drug eruptions.[10] Prominent spongiosis, suprabasilar dyskeratosis, a mid and deep perivascular component, and the presence of plasma cells are not histologic features of lichen planus or psoriasis. Although a middermal perivascular infiltrate, keratinocyte necrosis, and prominent lymphocytic exocytosis are present in pityriasis lichenoides, the infiltrate in this entity is purely mononuclear in nature; neither spongiform pustulation nor plasmacellular infiltration is observed. Although lichenoid hypersensitivity reactions and psoriasiform drug reactions may also demonstrate a perivascular infiltrate of plasma cells, tissue eosinophilia is typically observed as well.

Tertiary Syphilis

Tertiary syphilis is categorized into nodular tertiary syphilis confined to the skin; benign gummatous syphilis principally affecting skin, bone, and liver; cardiovascular syphilis; syphilitic hepatic cirrhosis; and neurosyphilis. In the first variant, the granulomas are small and may be absent in rare cases.[34] The granulomatous process is limited to the dermis, where scattered islands of epithelioid cells are usually intermingled with a few multinucleated giant cells amid an infiltrate of lymphoid and plasma cells. As a rule, necrosis is not a conspicuous finding. The vessels may show endothelial swelling.[30]

In benign gummatous syphilis, the main pathology, irrespective of which organ is involved, is one of granulomatous inflammation with large central zones of acellular necrosis. In cutaneous lesions, the blood vessels throughout the dermis and subcutaneous fat exhibit an endarteritis obliterans phenomenon along with angiocentric plasmacellular infiltrates of variable density. The skin lesions involve the subcutaneous fat as well as the dermis.[38]

In cardiovascular syphilis, elastic tissue fragmentation and reduplication with neovascularization and fibrosis of main arteries occurs. Neurosyphilis includes an asymptomatic form—meningovascular syphilis—and parenchymatous syphilis, which is divided into generalized paresis of the insane and tabes dorsalis.[39] In meningovascular syphilis, an inflammatory endarteritis involves the leptomeningeal vessels. In generalized paresis of the insane, gliosis with ventricular dilatation is observed; spirochetes are identified in the cortex in 50% of the cases. In tabes dorsalis, there is demyelinization of the posterior columns of the spinal cord, atrophy of the posterior spinal roots, and lymphoplasmacellular leptomeningitis.[4,39]

NONVENEREAL TREPONEMATOSES

Yaws (Frambesia Tropica)

Yaws is caused by *T pallidum*, subspecies *pertenue*, which is indistinguishable microscopically from *T pallidum* subspecies *pallidum*, but has been said to be distinctive by virtue of the substitution of a single nucleotide coding for a 19-kD polypeptide demonstrable by Southern blot analysis.[40] Spread by casual contact between 1° or 2° lesions and abraded skin, the disease is most prevalent in warm, moist, tropical climates; 95% of the studied population in one province of Ecuador proved seropositive in one series.[41] Children are particularly afflicted.[42] Sites of involvement include buttocks, legs, and feet.

Primary Yaws

The initial primary stage lesion, or "mother yaw," begins as an erythematous papule roughly 21 days postinoculation, which enlarges peripherally to form a 1- to 5-cm nodule surrounded by satellite pustules covered by an amber crust. A red, crusted appearance prompted German physicians to lend the appellation "frambesia" to the disease. Lesions may heal as pitted, hypopigmented scars. Fever, arthralgia, and lymphadenopathy may coexist.

Secondary Yaws

Similar constitutional symptoms weeks to months later may herald progression to the secondary stage, characterized by involvement of any or all skin, bones, joints, and cerebrospinal fluid. *Skin lesions* resemble the "mother yaw" but tend to be smaller and more numerous, hence the designation "daughter yaws." Periorificial lesions may mimic venereal syphilis. A circinate appearance ("tinea yaws") may be observed, as may a morbilliform eruption and/or condylomatous vegetations involving the axillae and groins. Macular, hyperkeratotic, and papillomatous lesions may be present on palmoplantar surfaces, and may cause the patient to walk with a painful, crablike gait ("crab yaws"). Papillomatous nail-fold lesions may give rise to "pianic onychia." Relapsing cutaneous disease occurs up to 5 years later, tending to involve periorificial and periaxillary sites. A lifelong noninfectious latent state may then eventuate. *Bone lesions* consist of painful, sometimes palpable periosteal thickening of arms and legs, occasionally accompanied by soft tissue swellings around the involved small bones of the hands and feet.

Tertiary Yaws

Roughly 10% of cases progress to *tertiary yaws*, the skin manifestations that comprise subcutaneous abscesses, ulcers that may coalesce to form serpiginous tracts, keloids, kerato-

Color Figures

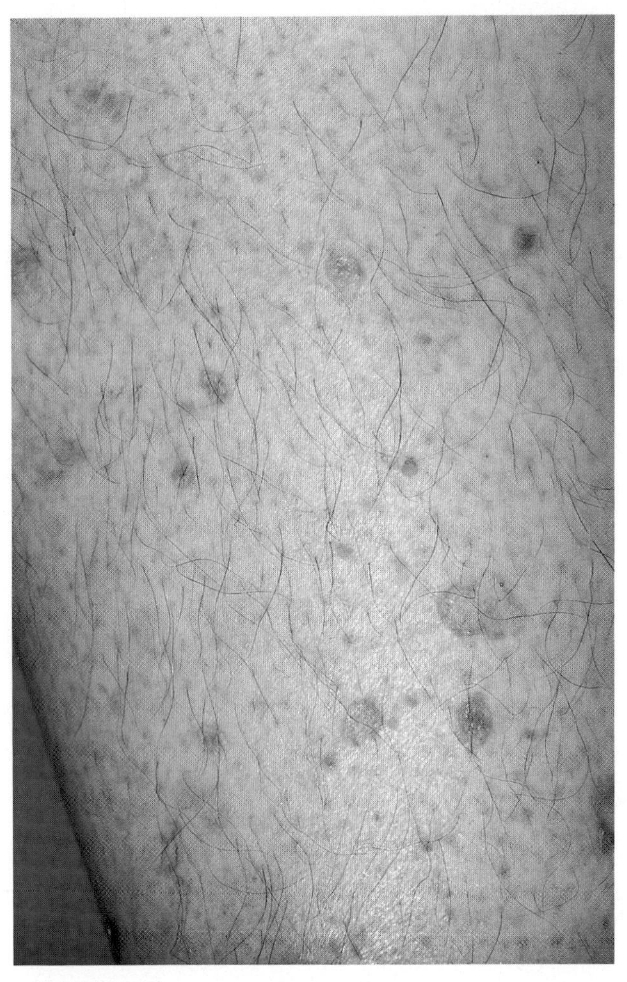

COLOR FIG. 6-1. Disseminated superficial actinic porokeratosis
Numerous pink-brown thin plaques are present on the leg. The individual lesions have a characteristic raised peripheral rim. (Photograph by William K. Witmer, University of Pennsylvania.)

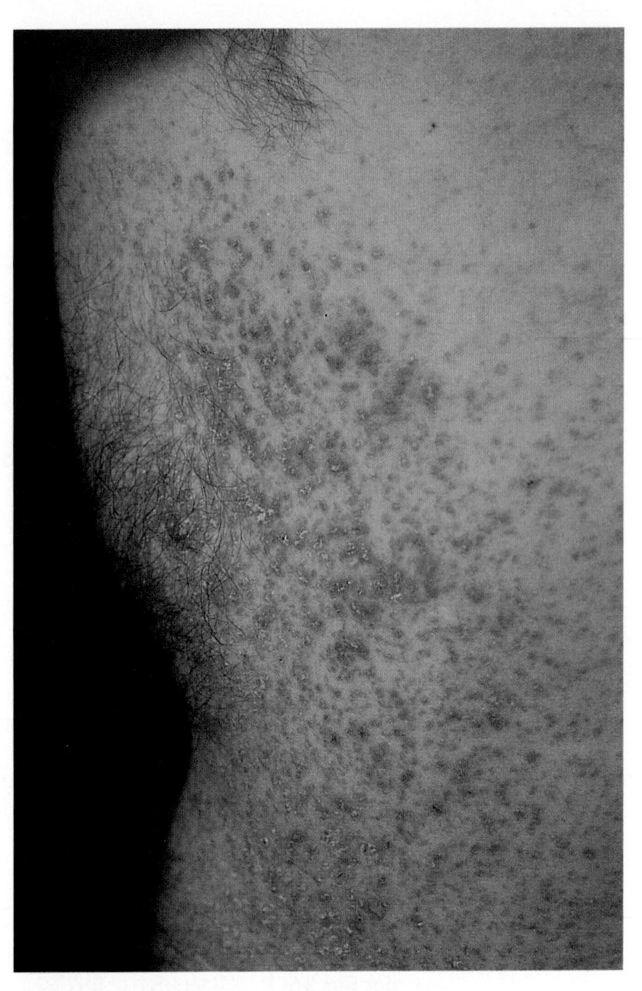

COLOR FIG. 6-2. Darier's disease
Multiple tiny hyperkeratotic papules that coalesce into plaques present on the trunk.

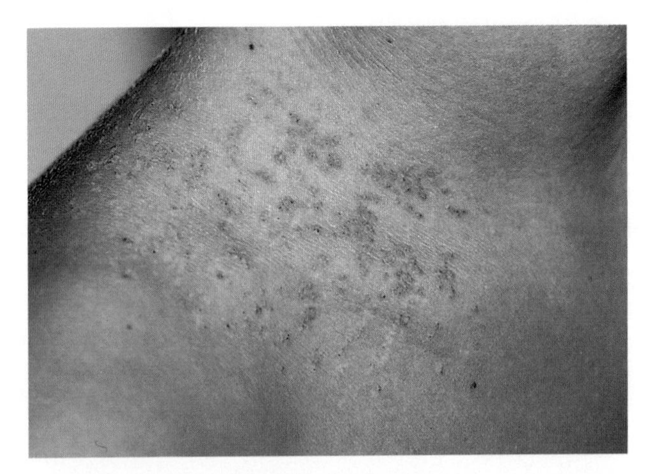

COLOR FIG. 6-3. Keratosis follicularis
Crusted papules in a follicular distribution at the base of the neck and upper chest.

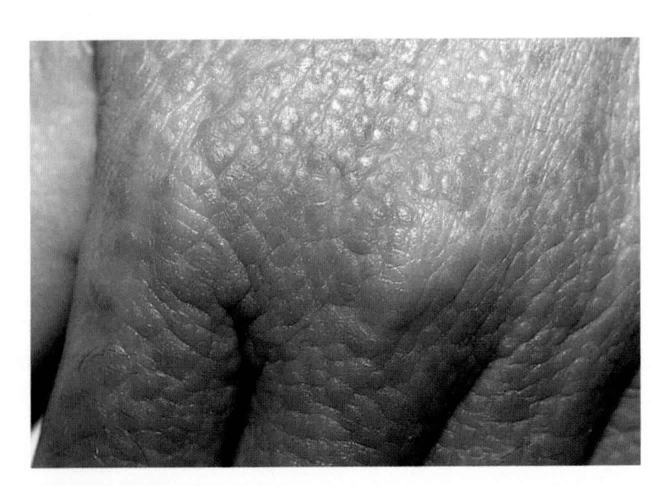

COLOR FIG. 6-4. Acrokeratosis verruciformis of Hopf
Flat papules on back of hands.

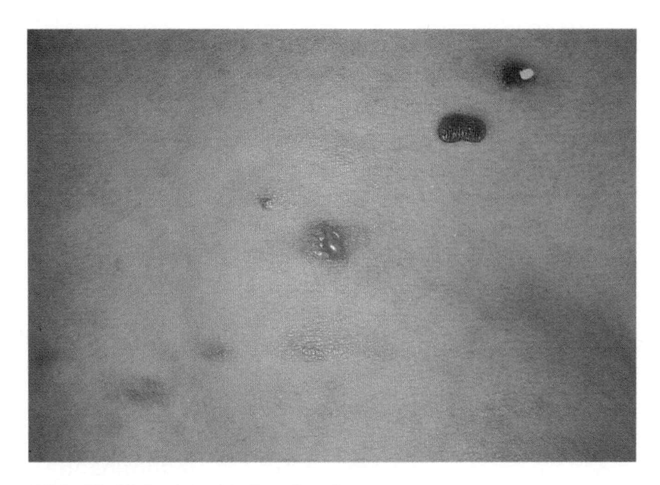

COLOR FIG. 6-5. Urticaria pigmentosa
Blister formation.

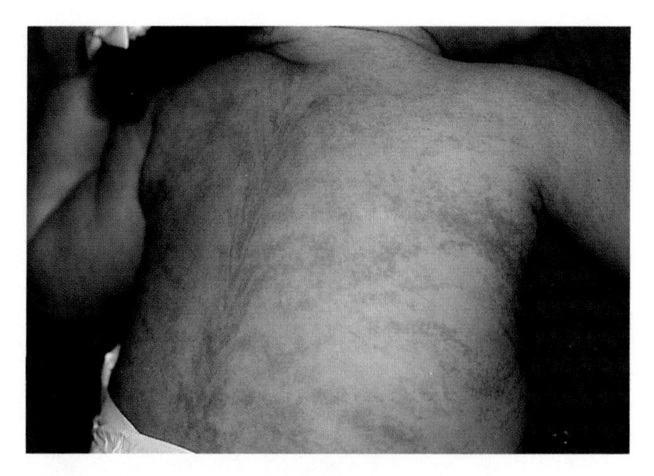

COLOR FIG. 6-6. Incontinentia pigmenti
Streaking and whorled pigmentation on the trunk.

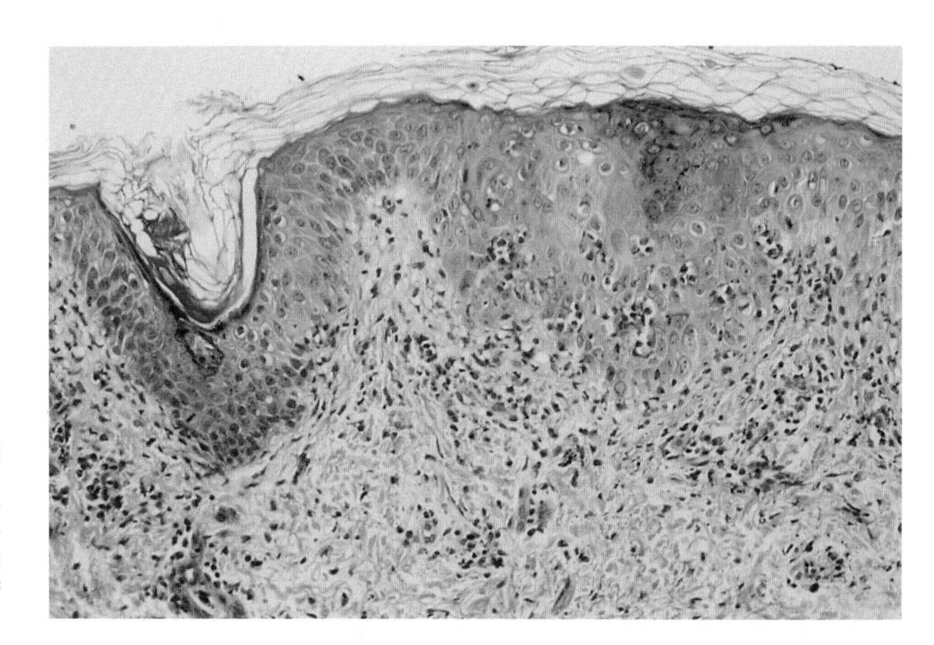

COLOR FIG. 6-7. Incontinentia pigmenti
The transition stage between vesicular and acanthotic. Many eosinophils are seen in the dermis and in the focally acanthotic and spongiotic epidermis (low magnification).

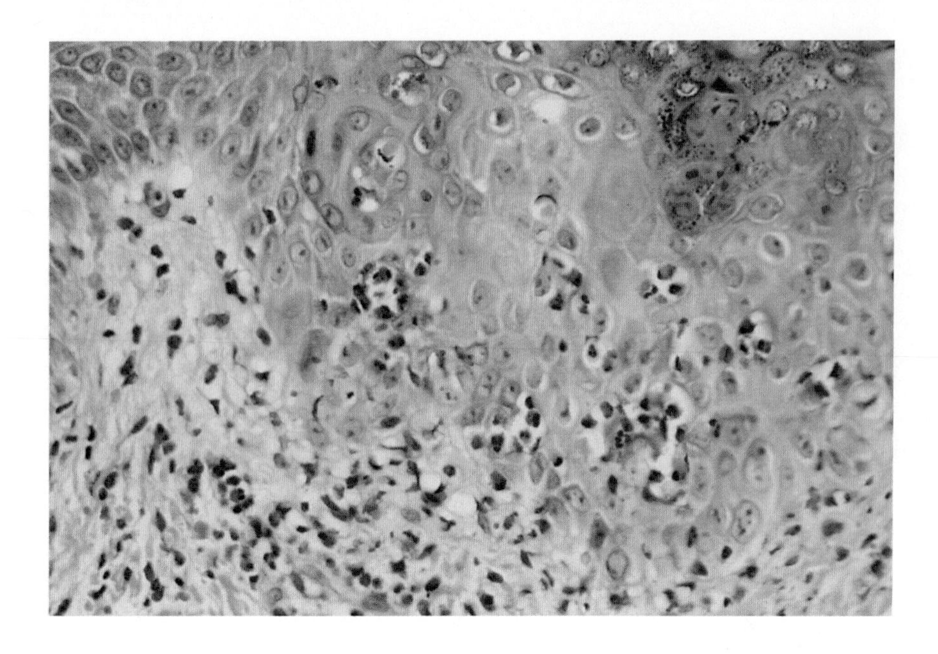

COLOR FIG. 6-8. Incontinentia pigmenti
High magnification of Color Fig. 6-7 showing eosinophilic spongiosis and acanthosis (original magnification × 400).

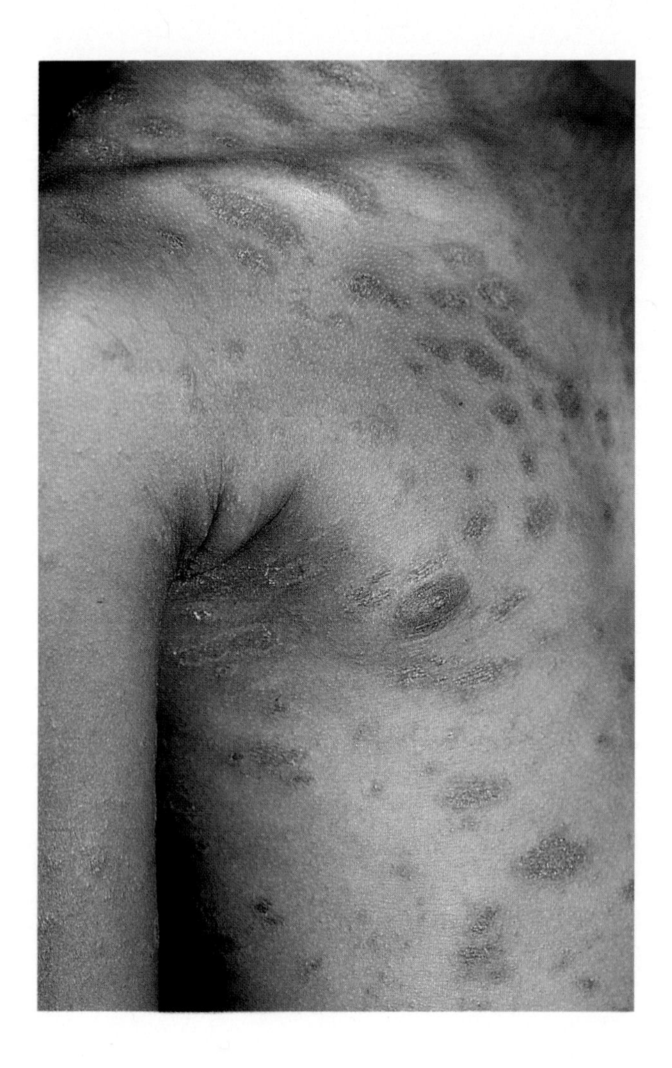

COLOR FIG. 7-1. Pityriasis rosea
Numerous oval-shaped macules on the trunk and upper extremities with a collarette of fine scale. (Photograph by William K. Witmer, University of Pennsylvania.)

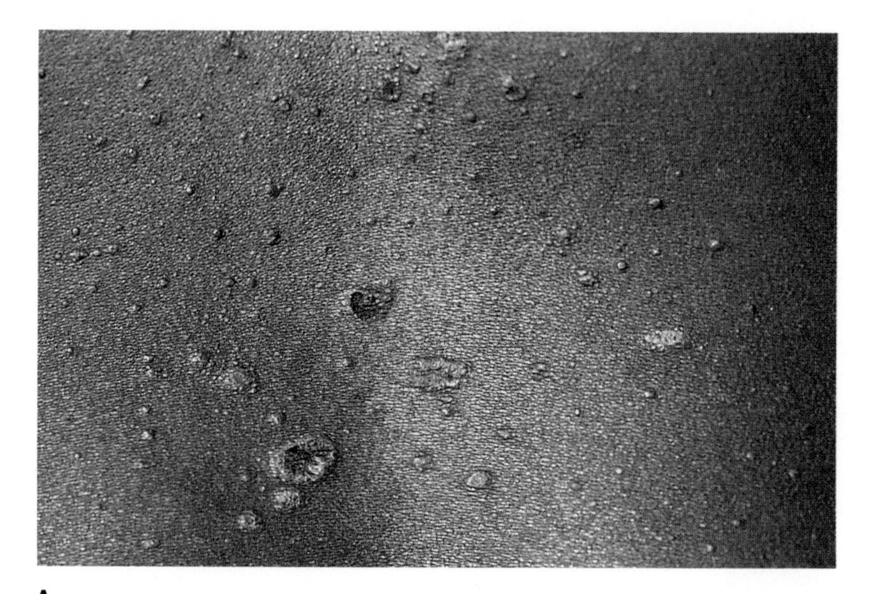

A

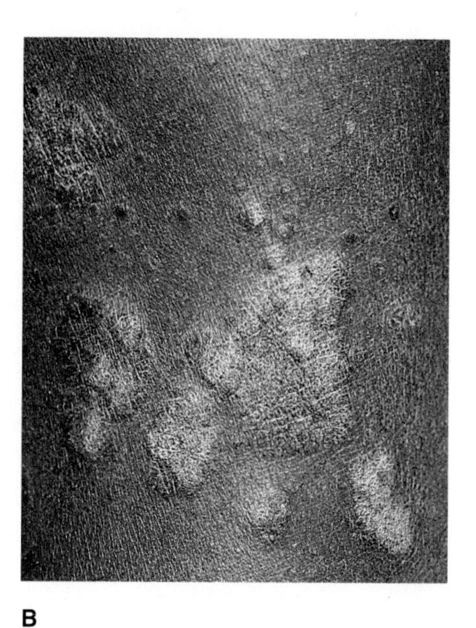

B

COLOR FIG. 7-2. Lichen planus
(**A**) Multiple flat-topped violaceous papules. (**B**) Hypertrophic variant of lichen planus shows verrucous hyperkeratotic plaques that may mimic deep fungal infections or cutaneous malignancies. (Photograph by William K. Witmer, University of Pennsylvania.)

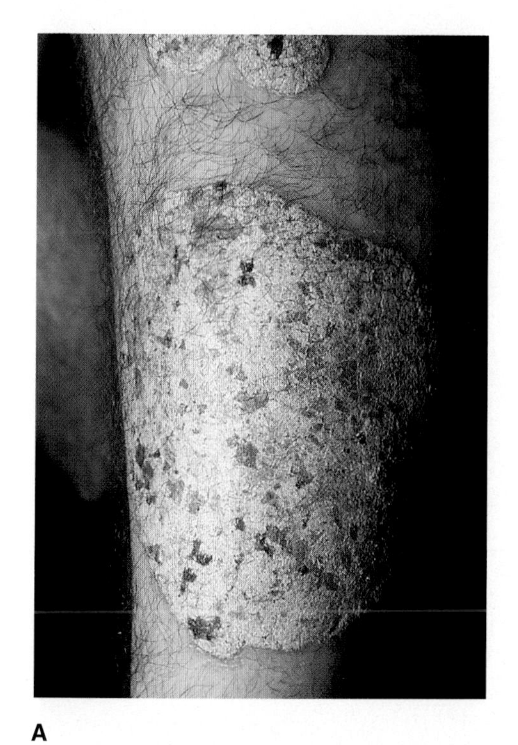

A

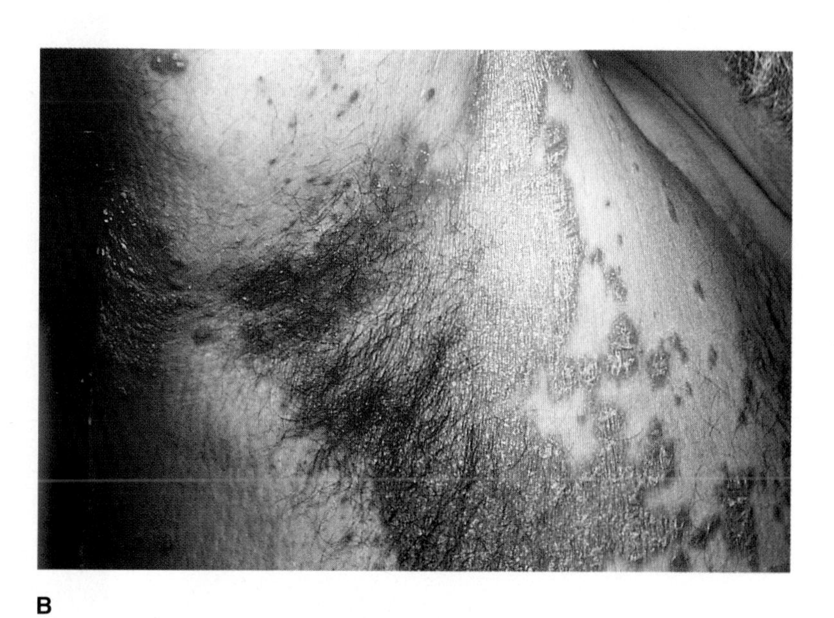

B

COLOR FIG. 7-3. Psoriasis
(**A**) Well-demarcated erythematous plaque with a thick, white silvery scale on extensor surfaces. (**B**) Inverse psoriasis is characterized by similar lesions in the axillary and groin regions. (Courtesy of Jeffrey Miller, MD.)

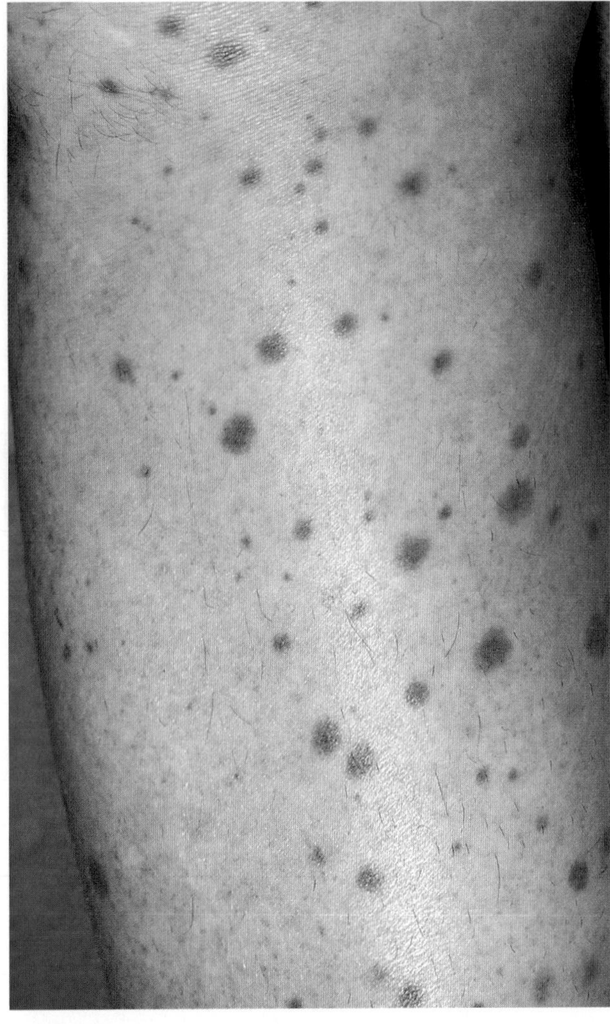

COLOR FIG. 8-1. Leukocytoclastic vasculitis
Multiple, small purpuric papules on the leg that do not blanch with pressure. (Photograph by William K. Witmer, University of Pennsylvania.)

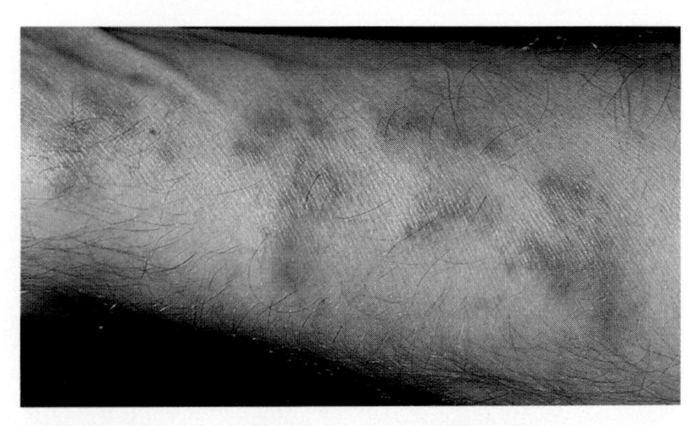

COLOR FIG. 9-1. Allergic contact dermatitis
Linear erythematous papules and plaques with small vesicles. Linear lesions of the extremities are characteristic of an allergic contact dermatitis to plants. (Photograph by William K. Witmer, University of Pennsylvania.)

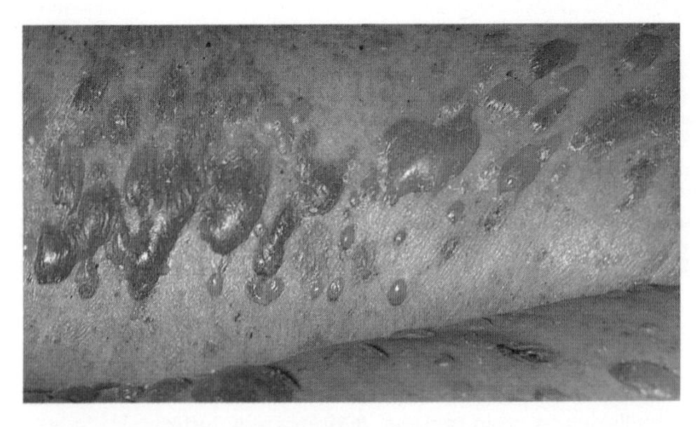

COLOR FIG. 9-2. Bullous pemphigoid
Tense blisters occurring within an erythematous or urticarial base. (Photograph by William K. Witmer, University of Pennsylvania.)

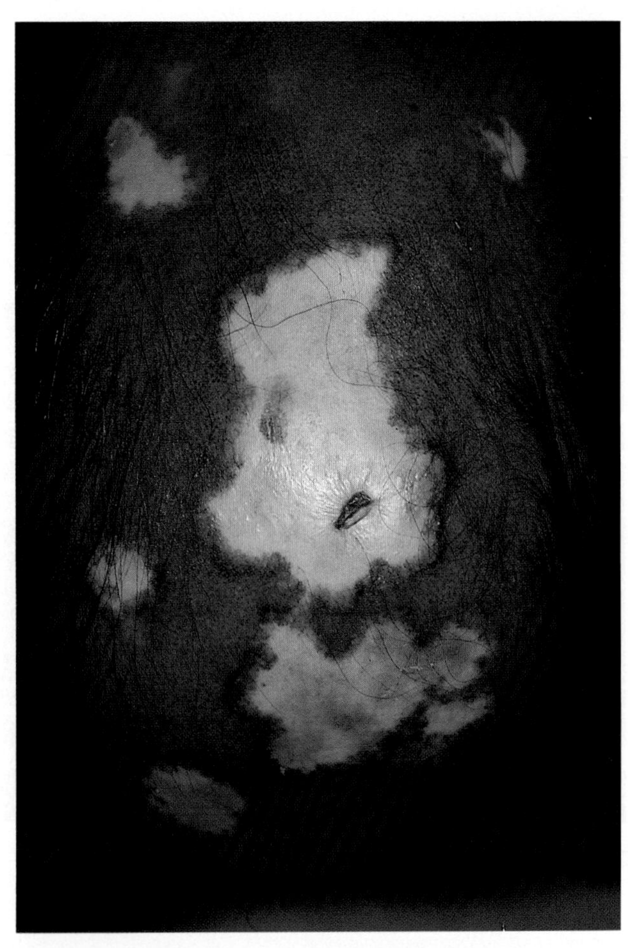

COLOR FIG. 10-1. Discoid lupus erythematosus
Erythematous and hypopigmented atrophic plaques on the scalp with peripheral hyperpigmentation.

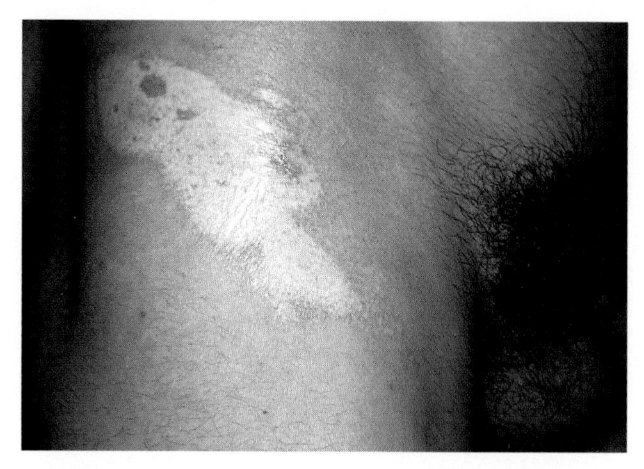

COLOR FIG. 10-2. Lichen sclerosus et atrophicus
Hypopigmented macule with atrophic, wrinkled surface.

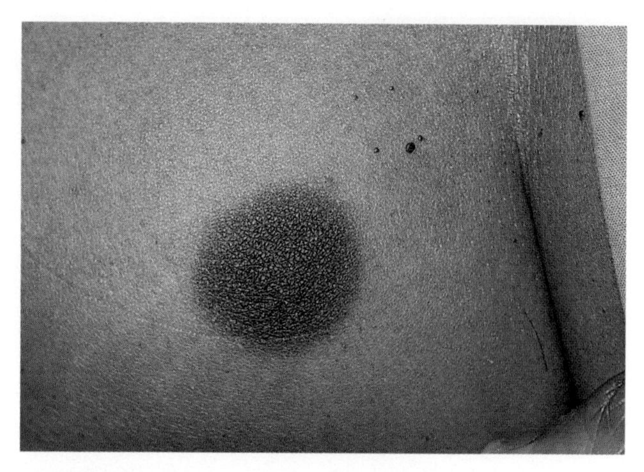

COLOR FIG. 11-1. Fixed drug eruption
A solitary gray-brown macule that recurs at the same site upon ingestion of the offending medication. (Photograph by William K. Witmer, University of Pennsylvania.)

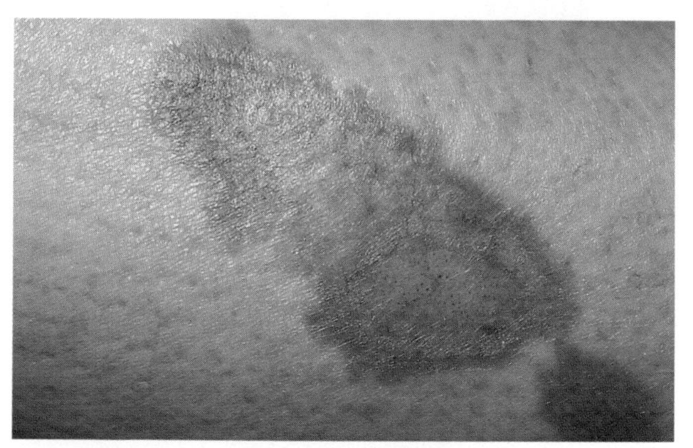

COLOR FIG. 14-1. Necrobiosis lipoidica
A solitary plaque of the pretibial region shows a pink-brown color, atrophy, and telangiectasia. (Photograph by William K. Witmer, University of Pennsylvania.)

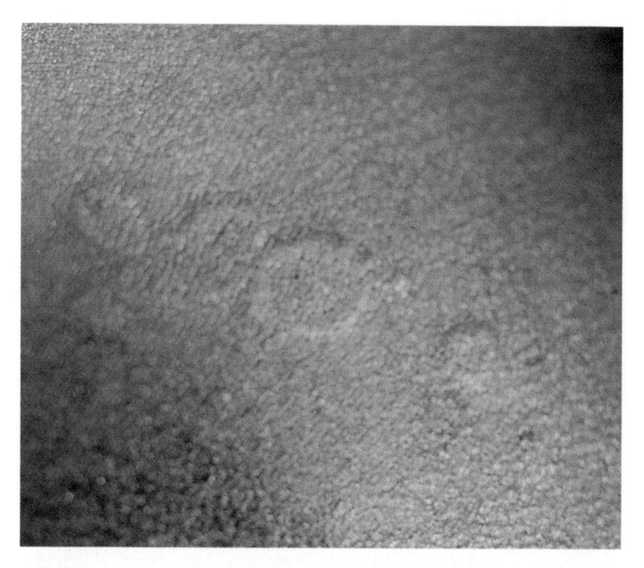

COLOR FIG. 14-2. Granuloma annulare
Annular plaque with a raised peripheral border. There is no scale or surface change. Granuloma annulare may be mistaken for tinea corporis.

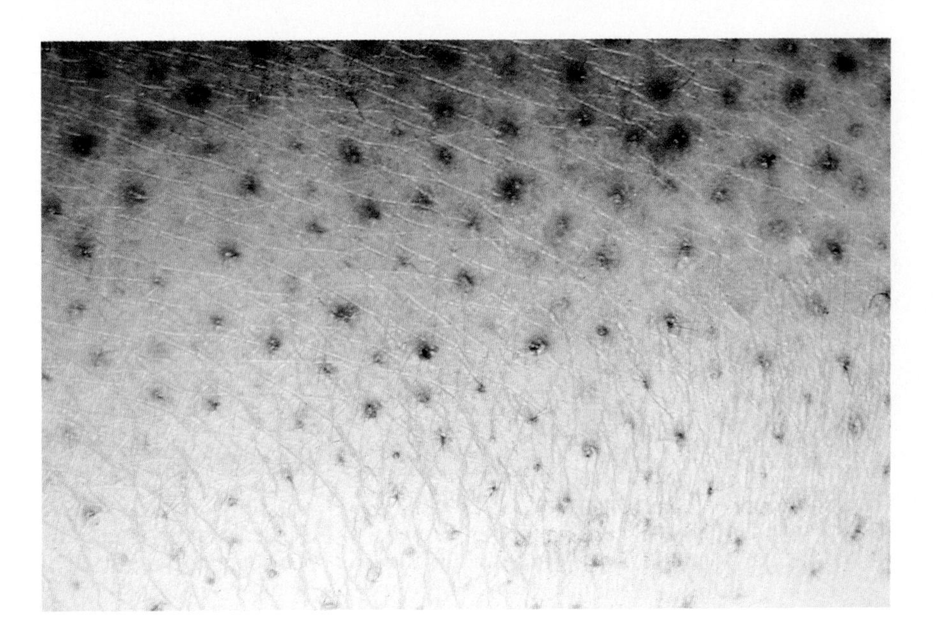

COLOR FIG. 16-1. Follicular purpuric macules characteristic of scurvy
(Courtesy of Dr. David Eslicker, Tennessee.)

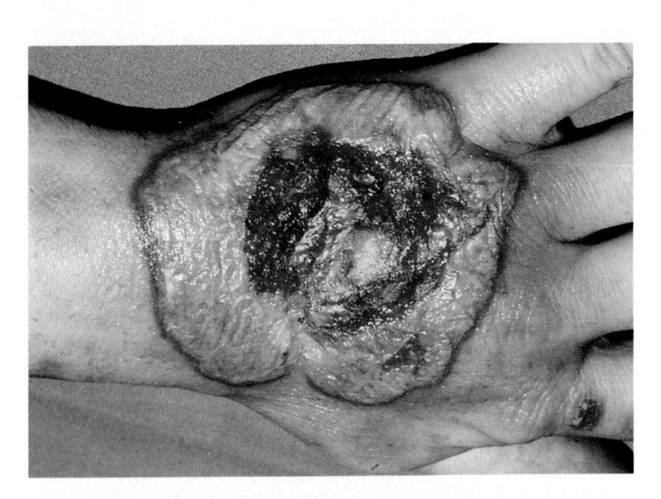

COLOR FIG. 16-2. Pyoderma gangrenosum
A tender fluctuant centrally necrotic plaque with a sharply circumscribed violaceous border.

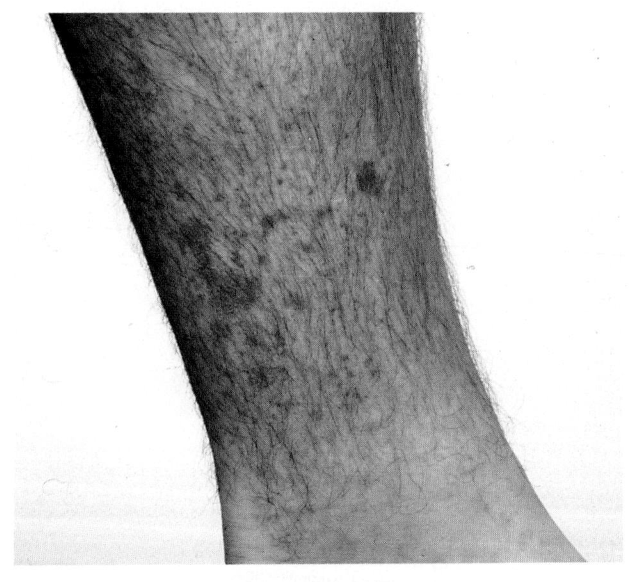

COLOR FIG. 16-3. Ulcerative colitis
This patient with ulcerative colitis developed an IgA–associated leukocytoclastic vasculitis.

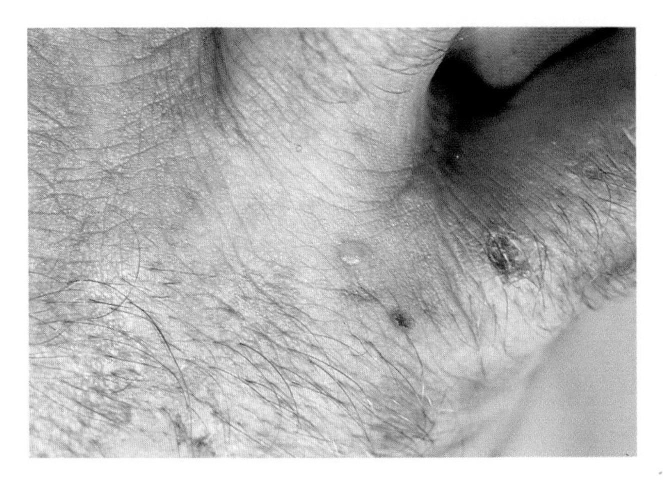

COLOR FIG. 17-1. Porphyria cutanea tarda
Tense blisters and erosions present on sun-exposed surfaces.

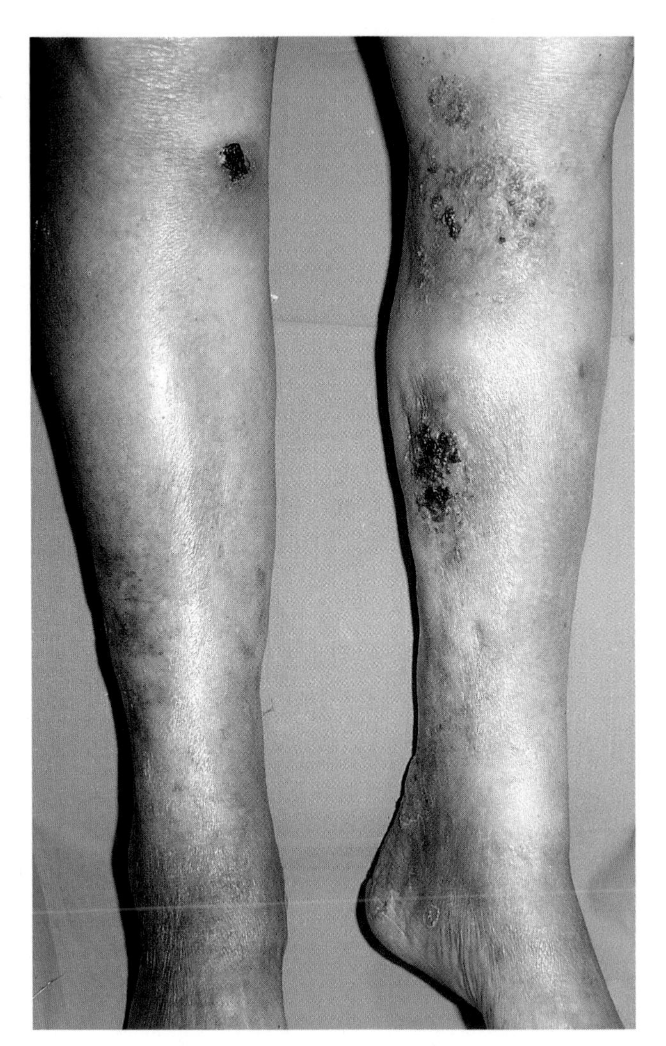

COLOR FIG. 20-2. Nodular vasculitis/erythema induratum
More advanced disease presents as hemorrhagic ulcers and depressed lesions with a predilection for the posterior calf region.

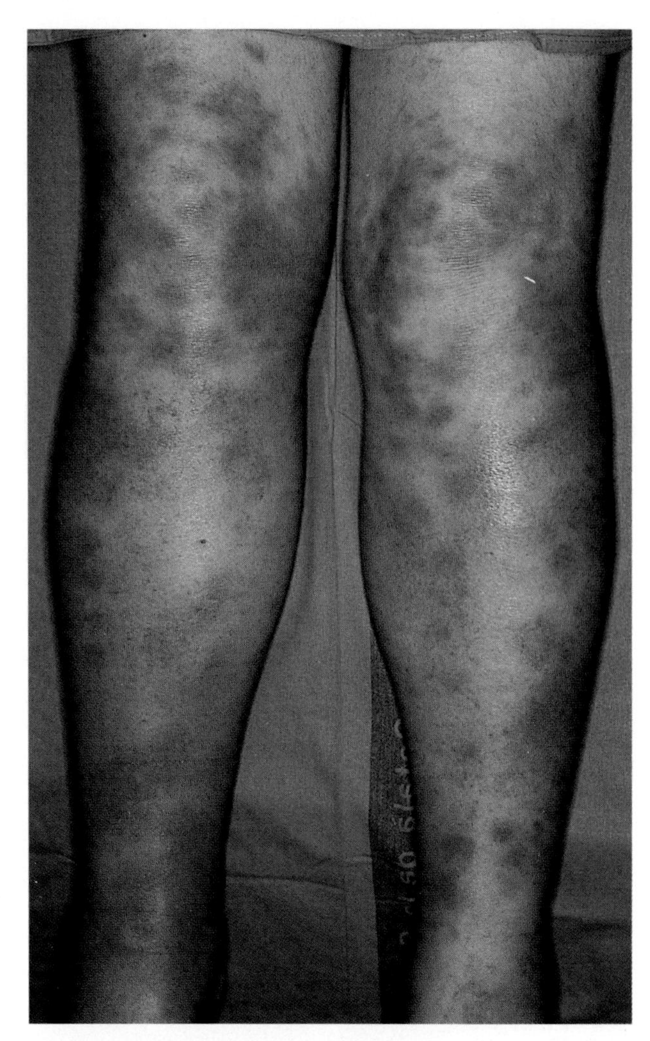

COLOR FIG. 20-1. Erythema nodosum
Erythematous nodules are abundant on the anterior shins bilaterally.

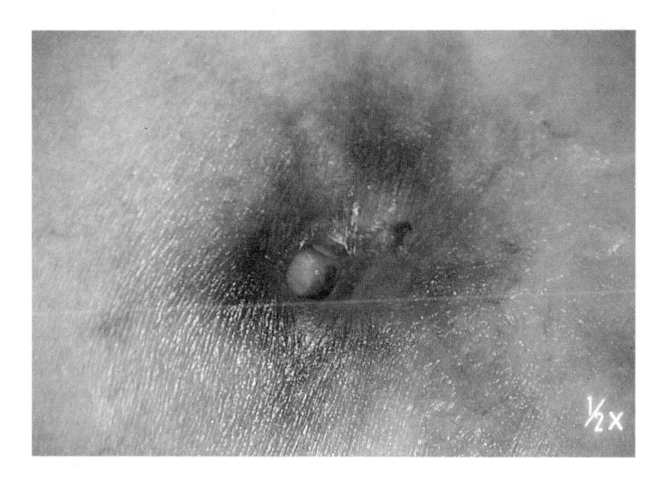

COLOR FIG. 20-3. Weber-Christian disease
An indurated nodule on the leg has developed a perforation and drains a turbid, sterile, oily fluid with necrotic tissue.

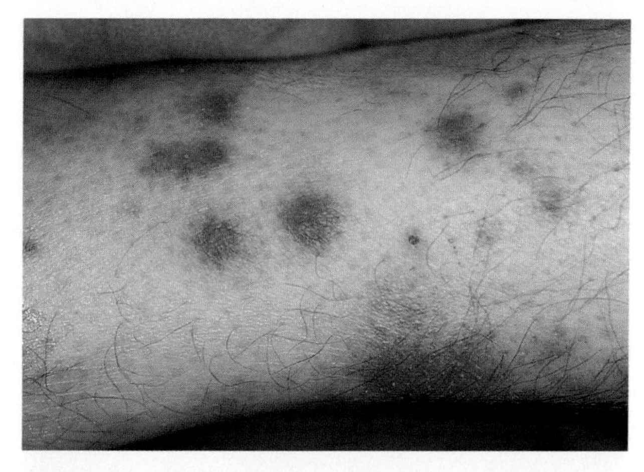

COLOR FIG. 20-4. Pancreatic enzyme panniculitis
Erythematous nodules appear most commonly on the lower legs.

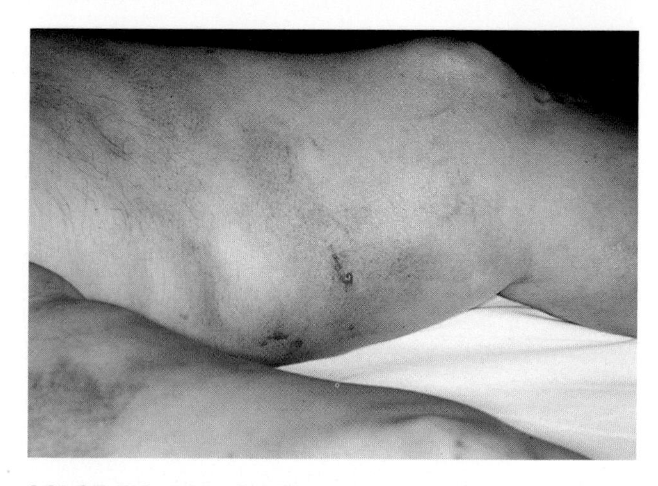

COLOR FIG. 20-5. Calcifying panniculitis
This patient with hyperparathyroidism developed erythematous, hemorrhagic, indurated plaques that were cold to touch.

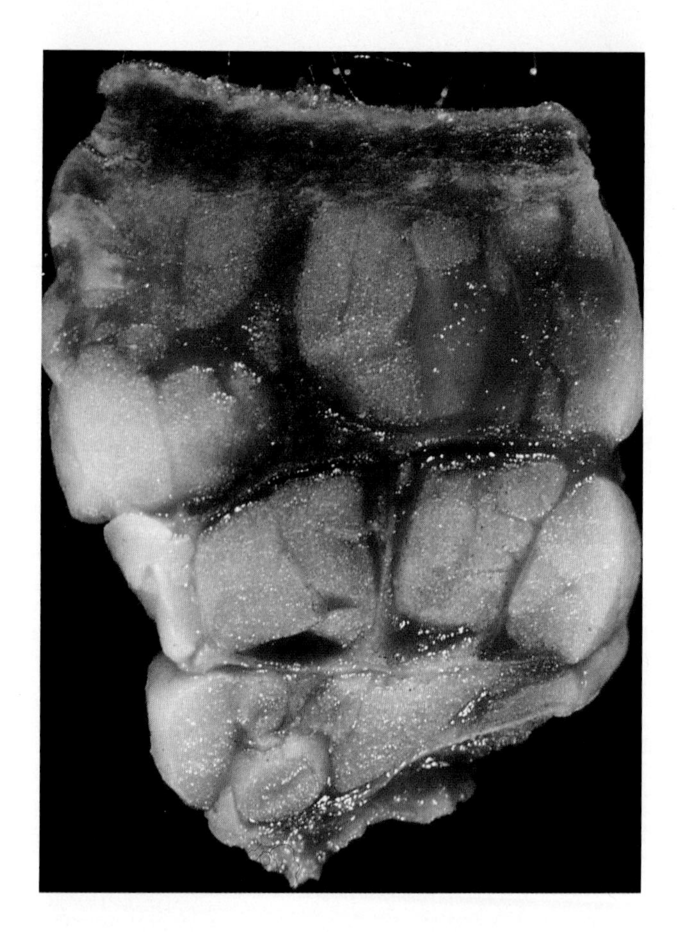

COLOR FIG. 20-6. Histiocytic cytophagic panniculitis
This cross-sectioned skin nodule shows both septal and lobular infiltration and hemorrhage. Note also the dermal hemorrhage.

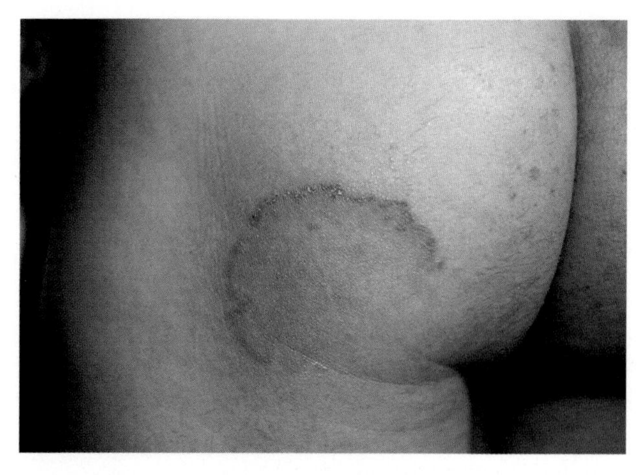

COLOR FIG. 23-1. Tinea corporis
Erythematous, annular patch with peripheral scale and central clearing.

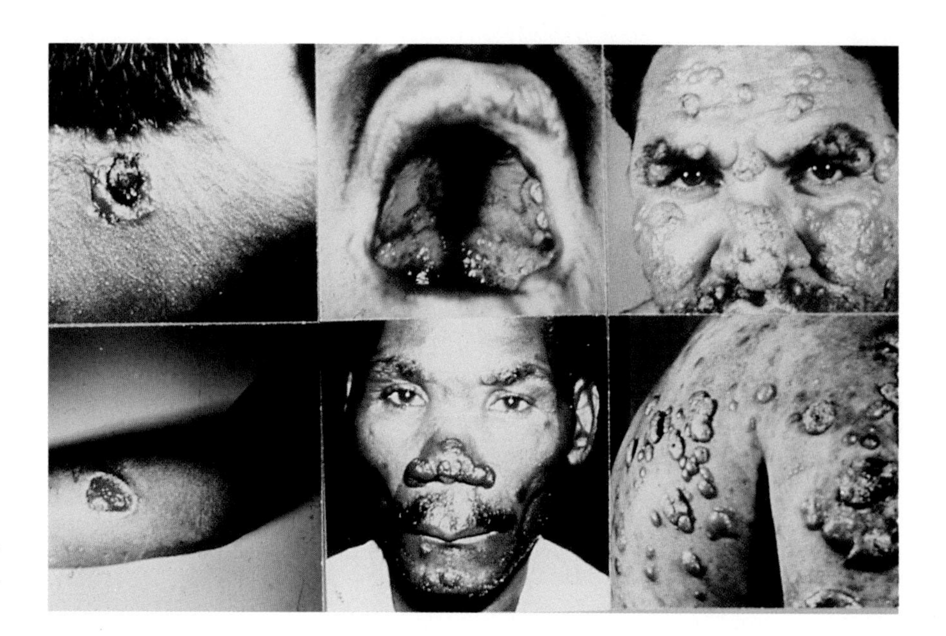

COLOR FIG. 24-1. Spectrum of American cutaneous leishmaniasis

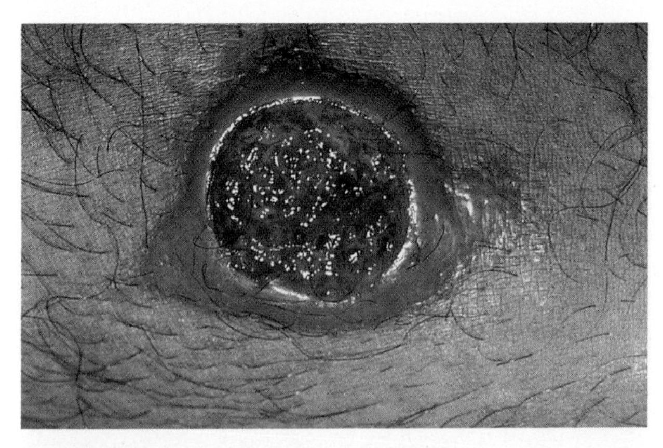

COLOR FIG. 24-2. American cutaneous leishmaniasis, ulcerated localized lesion

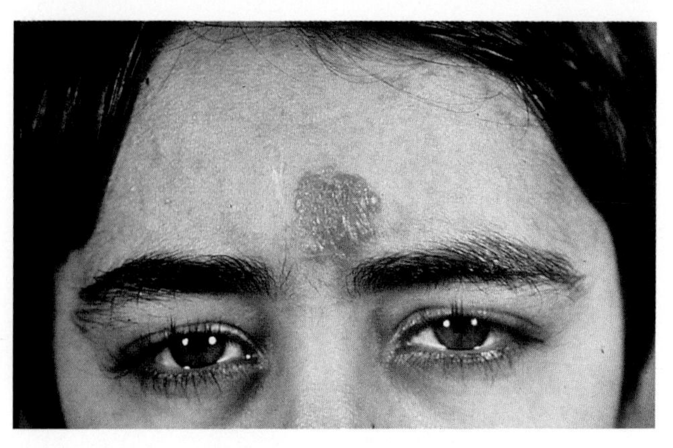

COLOR FIG. 24-3. American cutaneous leishmaniasis, nonulcerated lesion, infiltrated plaque

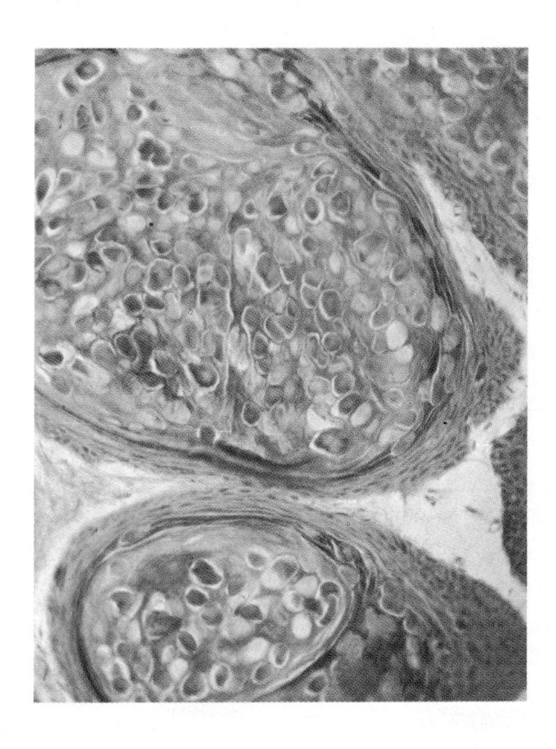

COLOR FIG. 26-1. Molluscum contagiosum
In the horny layer, numerous large basophilic molluscum bodies lie enmeshed in a network of eosinophilic horny fibers (original magnification ×350).

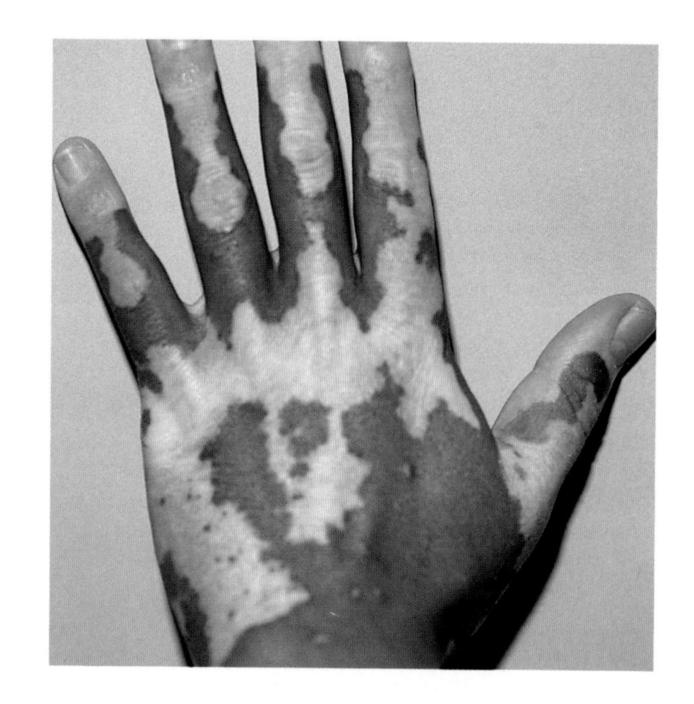

COLOR FIG. 28-1. Vitiligo
Well-demarcated areas of depigmentation adjacent to normal skin. (Photograph by William K. Witmer, University of Pennsylvania.)

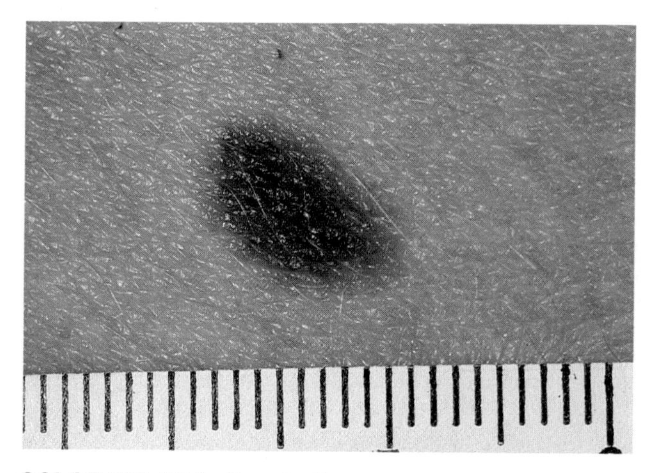

COLOR FIG. 29-1. Dysplastic nevus
Dysplastic nevi are larger than 5 mm and have a macular component or are entirely macular, as in this example. They have a "fuzzy," indefinite, and slightly irregular border with slight to moderate pigmentary variegation. These features when prominent, can overlap with those of an early in situ or microinvasive melanoma.

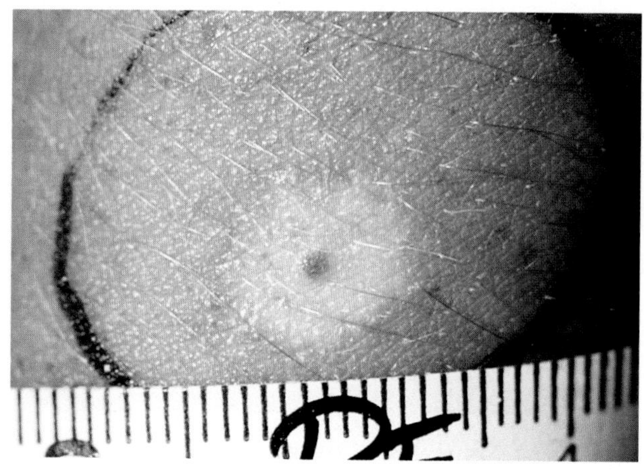

COLOR FIG. 29-2. Halo nevus
A common papular compound nevus is surrounded by a concentric area of depigmentation. In time, most such nevi will disappear, and the area will slowly repigment.

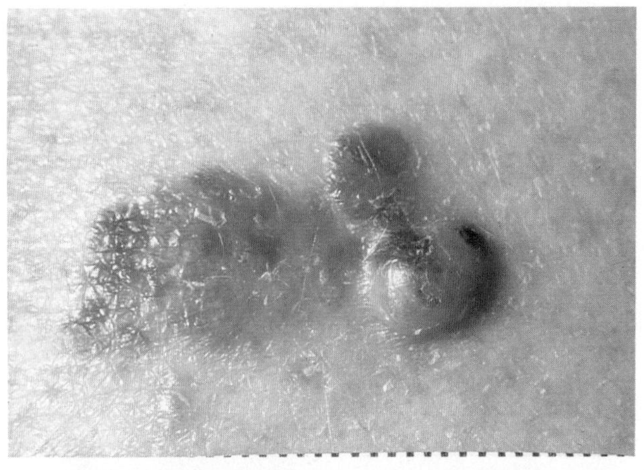

COLOR FIG. 29-3. Superficial spreading melanoma, with radial and vertical growth phases
The lesion as a whole demonstrates the ABCD clinical criteria for melanoma—Asymmetry, Border irregularity, Color variegation with shades of tan, brown, and pink, and a Diameter considerably greater than 6 mm. The tumorigenic compartment at the bottom right periphery of the lesion presents clinically as an expansile, more or less symmetrical mass. At upper right there is a papule that histologically was an associated nevus.

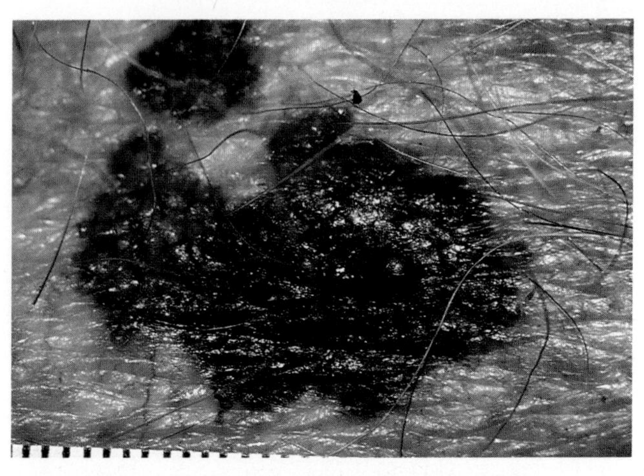

COLOR FIG. 29-4. Lentigo maligna melanoma
Radial *(upper left)* and vertical *(right)* growth phases are both present in this lesion. The radial growth phase shows a characteristic reticulated pattern of fine lines in a brown background. The vertical growth phase in this example is a black nodule. The lesion has arisen in chronically sun-damaged skin of an elderly subject.

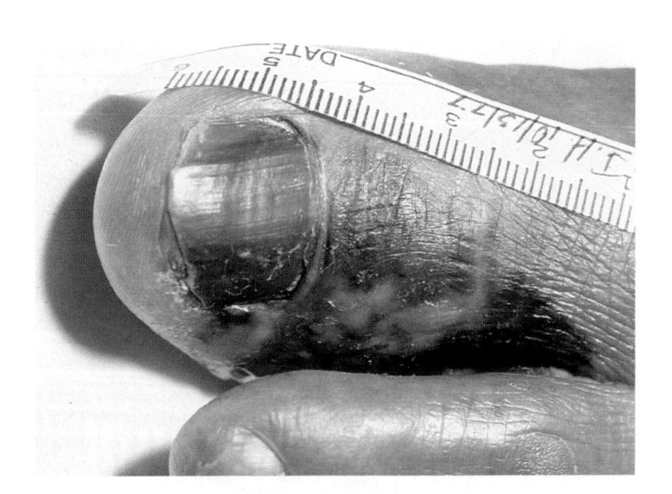

COLOR FIG. 29-5. Acral lentiginous subungual melanoma
Like the lesion in Color Fig. 29-3, this lesion presents the ABCD morphology. The lesion extends from under the nail to extensively involve the nail fold and surrounding skin. This pattern of pigment is not observed in subungual nevi or hematomas, and is known as Hutchinson's sign.

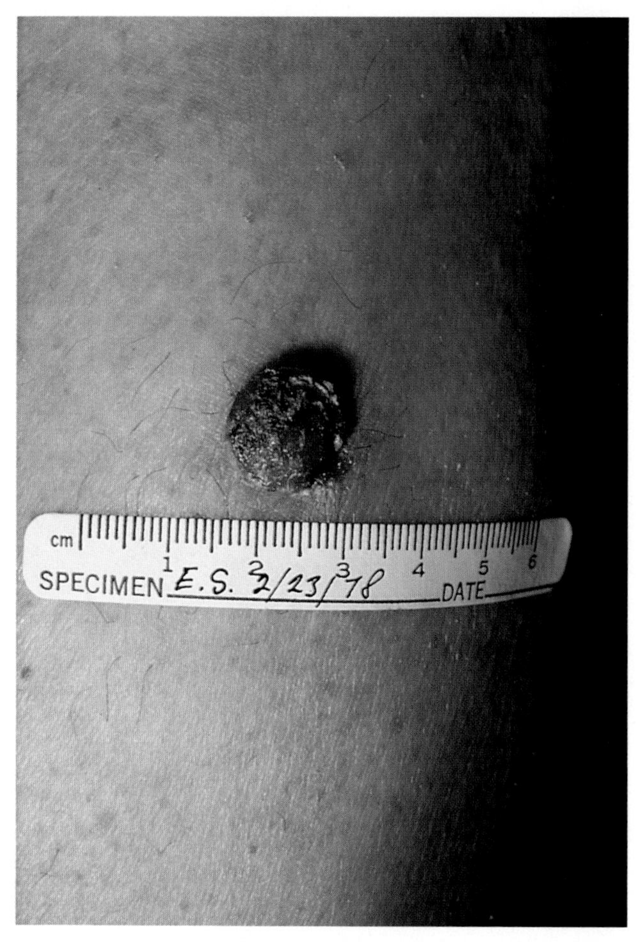

COLOR FIG. 29-6. Nodular melanoma
An early nodular melanoma may present as a seemingly innocuous papule. In a more advanced lesion, as shown here, there is evidence of ulceration and there may be a history of bleeding or oozing.

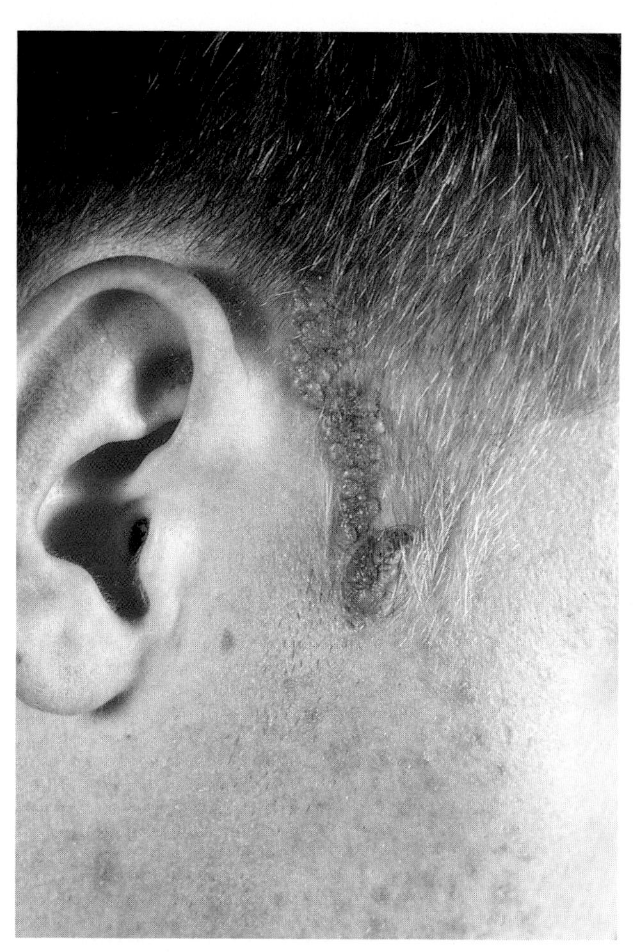

COLOR FIG. 31-1. Nevus sebaceus of Jadassohn
Well-defined, yellow-brown verrucous plaque on the scalp that is present at birth.

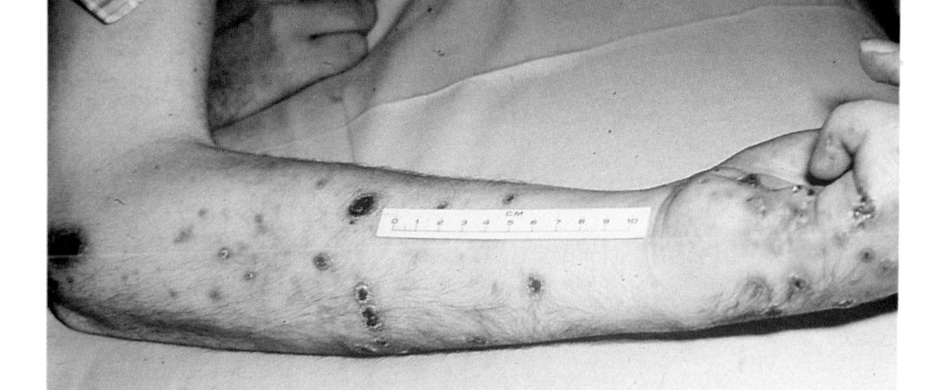

COLOR FIG. 33-1. Epithelioid sarcoma
Flexion contractures of the fingers with multiple ulcerating nodules of the hand and forearm.

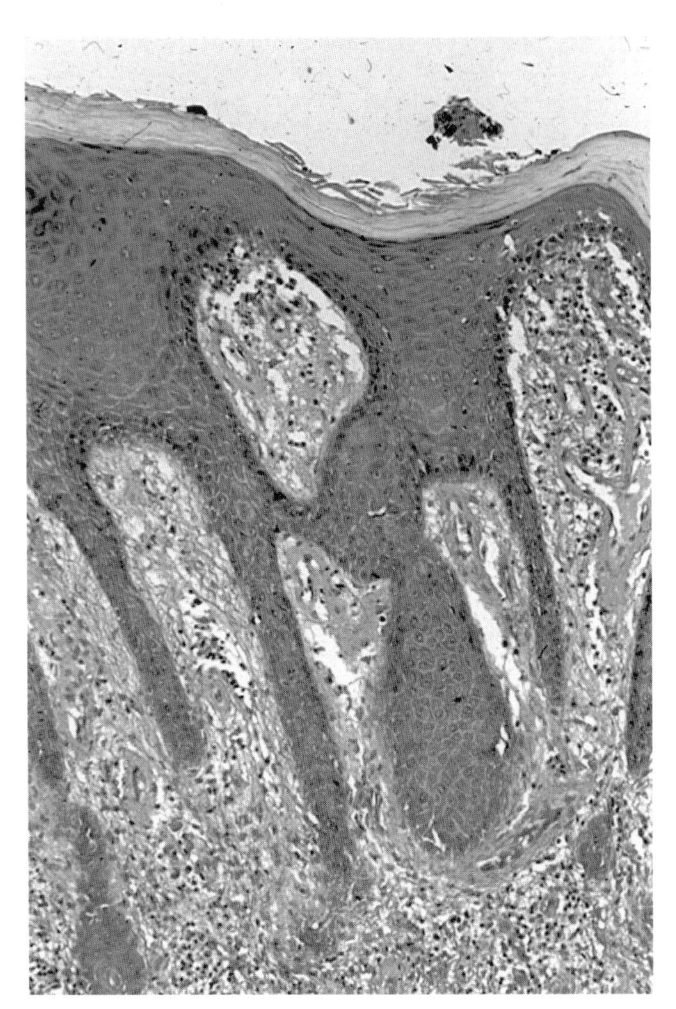

FIG. 22-7. Yaws, the primary lesion
The biopsy shows a psoriasiform hyperplasia of the epidermis, accompanied by slight spongiosis and an intense lymphohistiocytic and plasmacellular infiltrate in the subjacent corium.

derma, and palmoplantar hyperkeratosis. The bone and joint lesions of this stage include osteomyelitis, hypertrophic or gummatous periostitis, and chronic tibial osteitis, which may lead to "saber shin" deformities. Bilateral hypertrophy of the nasal processes of the maxilla produces the rare but characteristic "goundou," which obstructs the nasal passages and, if not treated with early antibiotic therapy, may require surgery. Another otorhinolaryngological complication is "gangosa," characterized by nasal septal or palatal perforation. Although neurological and ophthalmological involvement is not a universally accepted phenomenon, reports of macular atrophy and culture-positive aqueous humor suggest that yaws may exhibit neurophthalmological manifestations similar to those of venereal syphilis. A less virulent form of the disease, observed in lower-prevalence areas, is termed "attenuated yaws," the cutaneous manifestations of which comprise greasy gray lesions in the skin folds.

Histopathology. Primary lesions show acanthosis, papillomatosis, spongiosis, and neutrophilic exocytosis with intra-epidermal microabscess formation. A heavy, diffuse, dermal infiltrate of plasma cells, lymphocytes, histiocytes, and granulocytes is observed; unlike syphilis, blood vessels manifest little or no endothelial proliferation (Figs. 22-7 and 22-8).[43,44] The *secondary lesions* show the same histologic appearance, resembling condylomata lata in their epidermal changes, but differing by virtue of the dermal infiltrate being in a diffuse, as opposed to a perivascular, disposition. The ulcerative lesions of *tertiary yaws* greatly resemble those observed in late syphilis in histologic appearance.[44] The spirochetes can be demonstrated in primary and secondary lesions by dark-field examination. Silver stains demonstrate numerous organisms between keratinocytes. Unlike *T pallidum*, which is found in both epidermis and dermis, *T pertenue* is almost entirely epidermotropic.[44]

Differential Diagnosis. The distinction between yaws and syphilis is based on clinical features, although the location of the organism in a skin biopsy may be helpful, no histologic feature or laboratory test absolutely distinguishes the two diseases.[45]

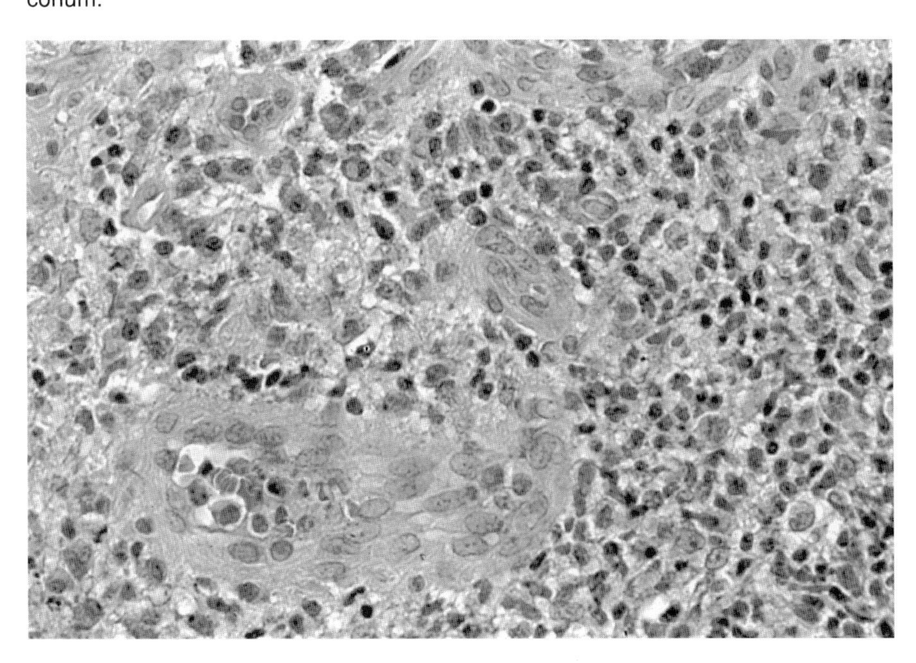

FIG. 22-8. Yaws, the primary lesion
The biopsy shows an intense angiocentric lymphohistiocytic and plasmacellular infiltrate without the characteristic endarteritis obliterans vascular alterations observed in syphilis.

Pinta

Unique among the treponematoses, pinta, caused by *T carateum*, demonstrates only skin manifestations.[46] The disorder is endemic to Central America and restricted to the Western Hemisphere. It affects no age group preferentially, and is the mildest of the treponematoses, with hypopigmentation being the only significant sequela. The incidence of pinta is declining precipitously for reasons unknown. Transmission appears to be from lesion to skin, classically between family members; the ritualistic whipping of diseased adults and unaffected youths is the putative mode of transmission in one aboriginal tribe in the Amazon basin.[46]

The *primary lesion* is characterized by an erythematous papule surrounded by a halo, and occurs 7 days to 2 months postinoculation. By direct extension or through fusion of satellite lesions, the primary site may grow to a diameter of 12 cm, forming an ill-defined erythematous plaque, most commonly on the legs or other exposed sites. In infants, the primary lesion classically occurs at the sites where the baby was most closely held to the affected mother. The *secondary lesions*, or "pintids," manifest months after inoculation as small, erythematous, scaly papules that coalesce to form psoriasiform plaques. Both primary and secondary lesions are highly infectious. In the tertiary stage, hypopigmented macules are present over bony prominences such as wrists, ankles, and elbows. Symmetrical areas of achromia, alternating with areas of normal or hyperpigmented skin, may result in a mottled appearance. Atrophy and/or hyperkeratoses may be present. An attenuated variant is not described.

Histopathology. Primary and *secondary* lesions show a similar morphology—namely, acanthosis with spongiosis and a sparse dermal infiltrate of lymphocytes, plasma cells, and neutrophils disposed about dilated blood vessels.[47] Endothelial swelling in the dermal vasculature is inconspicuous.[48] Lichenoid inflammation may be present, accompanied by hyperkeratosis, hypergranulosis, basal layer vacuolopathy, and pigmentary incontinence. Increased numbers of Langerhans' cells are present in the epidermis.[49] Lesions of the *tertiary stage* are hyperpigmented, characterized by large numbers of melanophages within the dermis, or depigmented, manifesting complete absence of epidermal melanin. Both lesions show epidermal atrophy and perivascular lymphocytic infiltrates. Organisms are present in all but late, longstanding lesions.

Histogenesis. Electron microscopy reveals absent melanocytes in depigmented lesions of tertiary or late pinta.[49]

Endemic Syphilis (Bejel)

Unlike yaws, endemic syphilis, caused by *T pallidum* subspecies *endemicum*, is largely confined to the arid climates of the Arabian peninsula and the southern border of the Sahara dessert,[46] whose seminomadic populations term the disease "bejel." Children 2 to 15 years of age constitute the principal reservoir. Infection occurs by skin-to-skin contact or by means of fomites such as communal pipes or drinking vessels.

Primary stage skin lesions are rare and are characterized by erythematous papules or ulcers of the oropharyngeal mucosa or the skin of the nipple of an uninfected mother nursing an infected infant.

More commonly, the initial manifestation is the *secondary stage* lesions, characteristically multiple, shallow, rather painless ulcers involving lips, buccal mucosa, tongue, fauces, or tonsils. Such lesions may be accompanied by hoarseness due to treponemal laryngitis and/or regional lymphadenopathy. Condylomata lata involving the axillae and anogenital regions are also observed. Rarely, the secondary stage manifests as erythematous, crusted papules, macules, or an annular papulosquamous eruption, which may be accompanied by generalized lymphadenopathy or periostitis.

The *tertiary stage* comprises gummatous lesions of nasopharynx, larynx, skin, and bone, which may progress to ulcers that heal as depigmented, sometimes geographic scars with peripheral hyperpigmentation. Bone and joint involvement may manifest as tibial periostitis, which mimics that of yaws, or as mutilating lesions involving the nasal septum and palate. Ophthalmological involvement comprises uveitis, chorioretinitis,

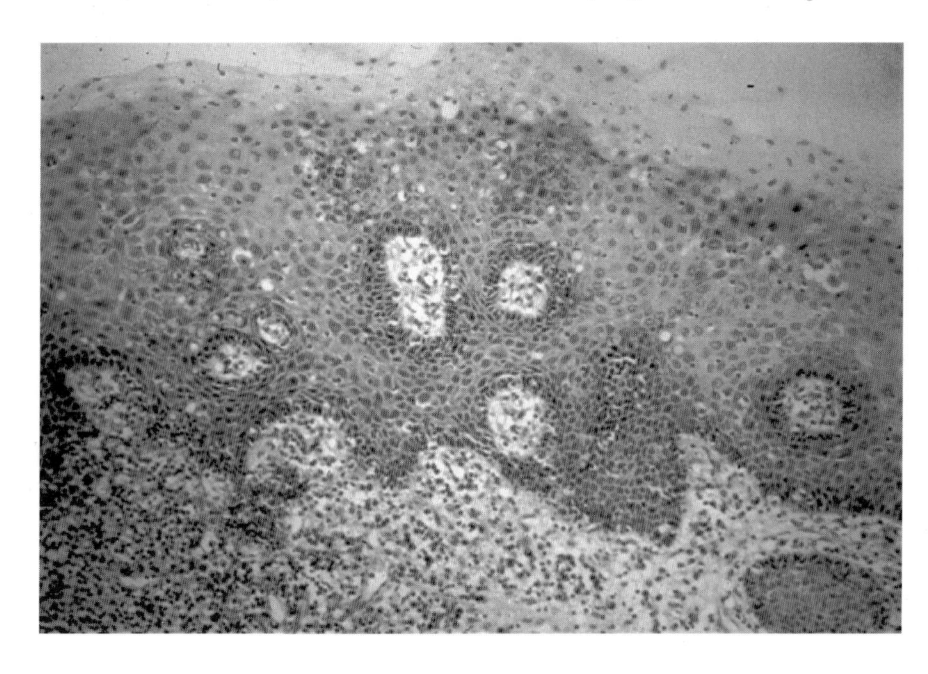

FIG. 22-9. Bejel
The biopsy is remarkable for an acanthotic epidermis with parakeratosis and a dense mononuclear cell infiltrate in the subjacent dermis.

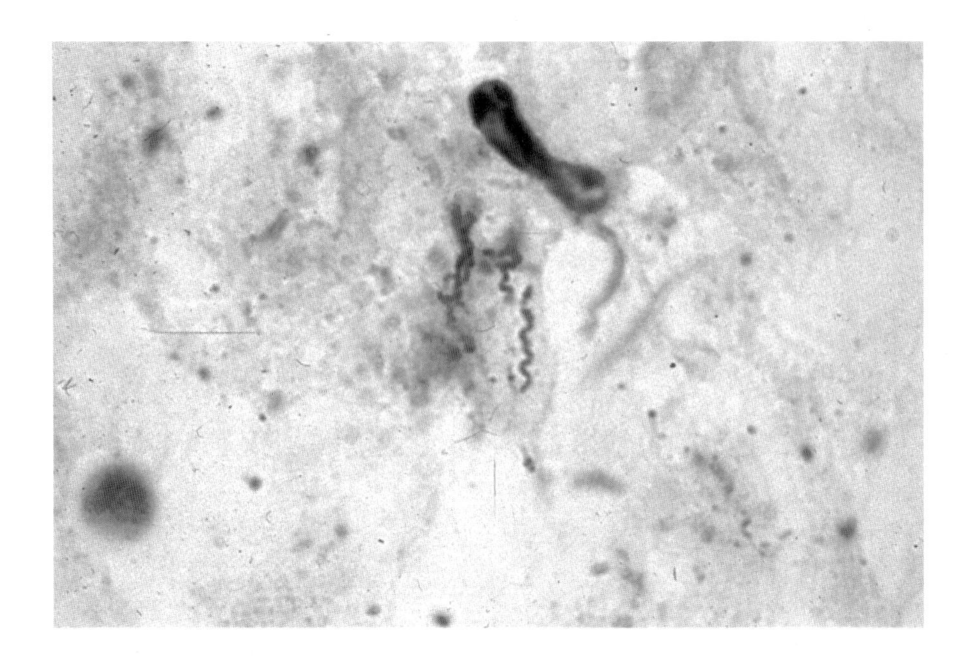

FIG. 22-10. Bejel
Characteristic organism is a silver-positive spirochete.

choroiditis, and optic atrophy; *T pallidum* has been cultured from intraocular fluid.

Histopathology. Although the pathology of early lesions of endemic syphilis is not well characterized, late lesions are said to show parakeratosis, acanthosis, spongiosis, pigmentary incontinence, and a dermal lymphohistiocytic and plasma cell infiltrate (Figs. 22-9 and 22-10).

Lyme Disease

Background

First described in patients from Lyme, Connecticut in 1975,[50] Lyme disease is a systemic spirochetosis caused by the spirochete *Borrelia burgdorferi* and transmitted by the soft ticks of the species *Ornithodorus*.[51] The disease in the index cases manifested as inflammatory arthritis and central nervous system and cardiac symptoms[52] preceded by cutaneous erythema.

Although the tick *Ixodes dammini* is the prototypic vector,[51,53] other species of ticks from the genus *Ixodes* can also be infected—namely, *I racinus*,[54] *I pacificus,* and *I scapularis*.[55,56] Lyme disease is the most common tick-borne disease in the United States and has been reported in 43 states, in Europe, elsewhere in North America, in Africa, and in Asia.[55] There are three phases. In stage I (early) Lyme disease, hematogenous dissemination from lesions of erythema chronicum migrans to other organs may occur, the effects of which are usually self-limited[57] and include orchitis, splenomegaly, lymphadenopathy, and mild pneumonitis. The two main systems involved in stage II are neural and cardiac.[57] The triad of meningitis, cranial neuritis, and radiculoneuritis is characteristic for neural involvement; Lyme cerebritis may also occur. Cardiac involvement manifests mainly as tachycardia and heart blocks, the basis of which is epi- and transmyocarditis. A biopsy of myocardium may show interstitial lymphoplasmacellular infiltrates, with a bandlike endocardial disposition said to be characteristic. A nonneutrophilic myocardial vasculitis has been described. Chronic disease at organ sites where spirochetes persist, most commonly the skin and nervous system in Europe and the musculoskeletal system in North America, constitutes stage III. Lyme arthritis and synovitis are characterized by a migratory oligoarthritis usually involving the knee joint, with the shoulder, wrist, temporomandibular, and ankle joints involved in some cases.

Erythema Chronicum Migrans

First described by Arvid Afzelius in 1909,[55] erythema chronicum migrans is the distinctive cutaneous manifestation of stage I Lyme disease in both Europe and America and represents the site of primary tick inoculation. Patients may not be aware of the often painless tick bite. The lesion starts as an area of scaly erythema or a distinct red papule within 3 to 30 days after the tick bite, before spreading centrifugally with central clearing after a few weeks, occasionally reaching a diameter of 25 centimeters.[58] The clinical presentation may be atypical by virtue of purpuric, vesicular, or linear lesions. Average lesional duration is 10 weeks in the European variant and 4 weeks in the American variant; in some cases, lesions persist for as long as 12 months. Females are affected more frequently in the European variant than in the American variant. The lesions may be solitary or multiple, the latter reflecting hematogenous dissemination of the spirochete, which may be accompanied by fever, fatigue, headaches, cough, and arthralgias.[51]

Histopathology. An intense superficial and deep angiocentric, neurotropic, and eccrinotropic infiltrate predominated by lymphocytes with a variable admixture of plasma cells and eosinophils is the principal histopathology (Fig. 22-11). Plasma cells have been identified most frequently in the peripheries of lesions of erythema chronicum migrans, whereas eosinophils are identified in the centers of the lesions.[59] Not infrequently, these florid dermal alterations are accompanied by eczematous epithelial alterations, and some cases exhibit edema of blood

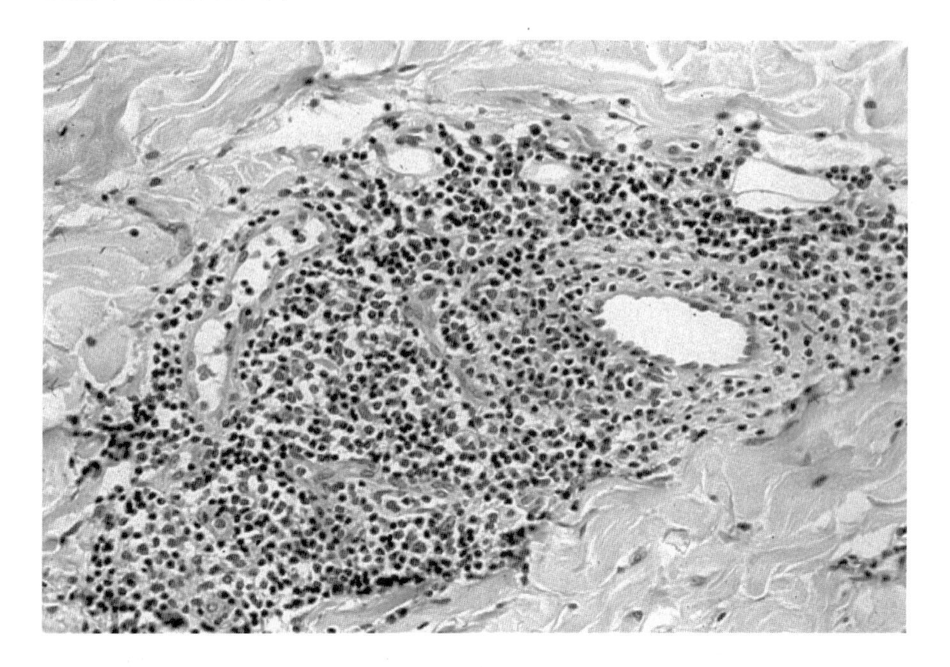

FIG. 22-11. Erythema chronicum migrans
The central nidus at the inoculation site demonstrates a necrotizing granulomatous vasculitis, whereas the periphery is predominated by an angiocentric mononuclear cell vascular reaction, shown here.

vessels with transmural migration of lymphocytes and plasma cells (personal observation of Mihm), granulomatous neuritis or vasculitis with luminal thrombosis (personal observations of Magro and Crowson), and interstitial infiltration of the reticular dermis with a concomitant incipient sclerosing reaction. A Warthin-Starry stain may be positive; one study demonstrated spirochetes by this technique in 41% of the cases, with approximately one to two spirochetes, measuring 10 to 25 μm by 0.2 to 0.3 μm, per section.[59] Spirochetes have been identified primarily from the advancing border of the lesion. Most patients have elevated IgM antibody titers.[57]

Differential Diagnosis. The differential diagnosis includes other causes of delayed hypersensitivity where potential antigenic stimuli include other forms of arthropod assaults, drugs, and contactants. A similar distribution of the dermal infiltrate is observed in connective tissue disease; however, tissue eosinophilia along with concomitant eczematous changes are not features of the latter. Differentiation from erythema annulare centrifugum may be impossible.

Dermal Atrophying and Sclerosing Lesions as Manifestations of Lyme Disease

Acrodermatitis Chronica Atrophicans

First described in 1883 in Germany and subsequently named by Herxheimer in 1902,[60] acrodermatitis chronica atrophicans usually begins as a diffuse or localized erythema on one extremity with the underlying dermis having a doughy consistency. After several months, the lesions become atrophic. The skin is frequently so thin that vessels and subcutaneous tissue can be easily visualized.[60] Appendageal structures disappear, resulting in hair loss and decreased sweat and sebum production. The lesions are located mainly on the upper and lower extremities, frequently around joints, and spare the palms, soles, face, and trunk.[61] Sclerosis may predominate in late stage lesions and take several distinct forms—namely, pseudosclerodermatous plaques over the dorsa of the feet; dense, fibrotic linear bands over ulnar and tibial areas; or localized fibromas overlying joint surfaces.[60] Antibodies against *B burgdorferi* are present in 100% of cases. Patients frequently have an elevated ESR and hypergammaglobulinemia. Either at the peripheries of lesions or distant from them, anetoderma, lymphocytoma, and morphea have also been described.[61]

Histopathology. Within a few months to a year, the epidermis appears atrophic with loss of the rete ridges (Fig. 22-12). There is granular layer diminution, and the epidermis is surmounted by a hyperkeratotic scale. In one study, a sparse interface dermatitis characterized by lymphocyte tagging along the dermal-epidermal junction, as well as basal layer cytolysis, was seen in 41% of cases (Fig. 22-12)[62] resulting in variable postinflammatory pigmentary alterations ranging from leukoderma to hyperpigmentation.[60] The papillary dermis appears edematous, with a grenz zone of collagen fibers oriented parallel to the epidermis[63] ranging from a few strands to a wide zone,[64] with subsequent eosinophilic homogenization.[63] A bandlike lymphocytic infiltrate is found in the mid- and upper dermis and in some cases may produce a lichenoid morphology, obscuring the dermal-epidermal junction. Occasionally it extends throughout the cutis and subcutis.[62,63] The infiltrate is predominantly in an angiocentric, eccrinotropic, and folliculotropic disposition and comprises mainly lymphocytes and histiocytes.[63] Eosinophils, neutrophils, and plasma cells form a minor cell populace.[63] The vessels amid the superficial infiltrate appear destroyed.[62] Within the infiltrate, there is piecemeal fragmentation of collagen and elastic tissue is lacking. Beneath the infiltrate, disorganization and destruction of the collagen, along with hyperplasia, fragmentation, and basophilia of the elastic fibers[62] are observed. An end-stage lesion exhibits a characteristic constellation of epidermal atrophy, large dilated dermal vessels, and an attenuated dermis composed of damaged and degenerated collagen and elastic fibers with lipoid phanerosis.[63] The collagen may appear homogenized and hypereosinophilic.[63] There is marked atrophy of adnexae with periadnexal fibrosis.

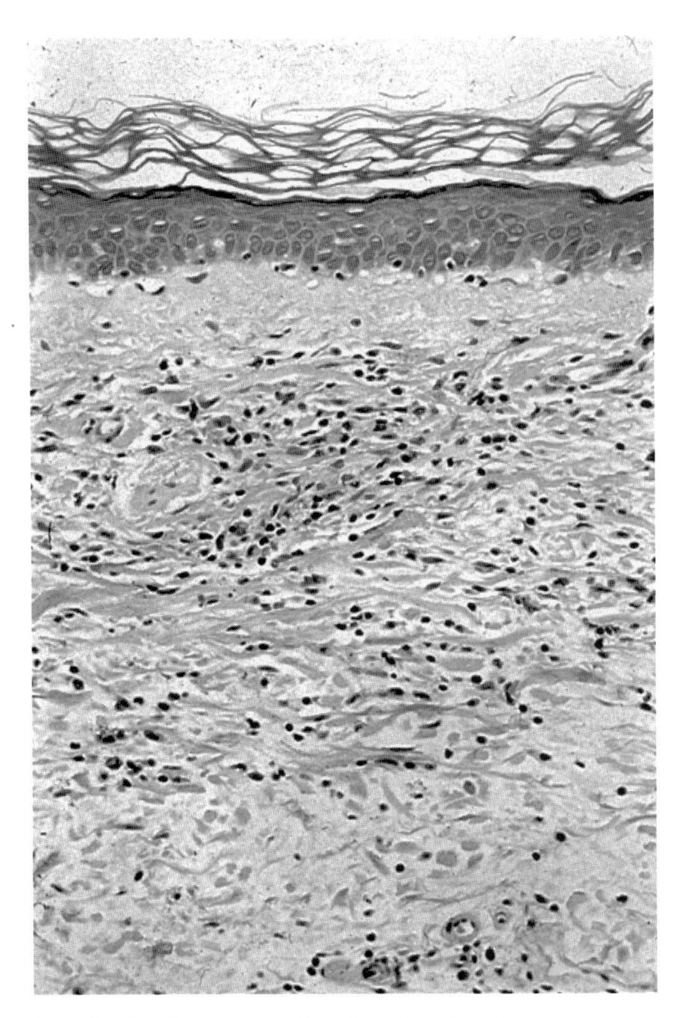

FIG. 22-12. Acrodermatitis chronica atrophicans
The epidermis is atrophic, with loss of the retiform pattern, granular cell layer diminution, and overlying basketweave orthohyperkeratosis. There is a sparse interface dermatitis with lymphocyte tagging along the dermal-epidermal junction. The papillary dermis is edematous and the reticular dermal collagen fibers appear thin, exhibiting an orientation parallel to the epidermis. A concomitant interstitial lymphohistiocytic infiltrate is found in intimate apposition to the attenuated collagen fibers.

Histogenesis. Acrodermatitis chronica atrophicans is mainly a stage III (late) cutaneous manifestation of the European variant of Lyme disease; the major vector is *I ricinus*[60] and hence the distribution of the lesion is worldwide, with middle Europe being the epicenter.[60] Most North American cases occur in European immigrants; *I racinus* is not an inhabitant of North America.[60] Immunophenotyping reveals that most of the lymphocytes are of T cell phenotype and that the elastic fibers express HLA-DR,[62] suggesting a role for cell-mediated immunity in lesional development.

Other Atrophying and Sclerosing Disorders Associated with Lyme Disease

Atrophoderma of Pasini and Pierini, facial hemiatrophy of Perry-Romberg, lichen sclerosus et atrophicus, eosinophilic fasciitis, and morphea (Fig. 22-13) are among the atrophying and sclerosing disorders of connective tissue that have been associated with *B burgdorferi* infection based on the positive serology for *B burgdorferi* in patients with these conditions, the isolation of spirochetal organisms in cultures of the respective skin lesions, and/or their identification in histologic sections.[55,56,64,65] In addition, acrodermatitis chronica atrophicans and morphea may coexist in the same patient. A possible etiologic basis of the sclerosis in all five entities—either as the inciting event (in morphea and eosinophilic fasciitis) or as an end-stage phenomenon (in atrophoderma, facial hemiatrophy, and lichen sclerosus)—may relate to increased production of interleukin I mediated by the *B burgdorferi* spirochete resulting in enhanced fibroblast production.[63] Only progressive facial hemiatrophy will be considered further, because all the conditions are covered in other sections (Chap. 10).

Facial hemiatrophy is an apposite term for an atrophying condition of the skin, subcutaneous fat, muscle, and bone involving either one division of the trigeminal nerve or half of the face.

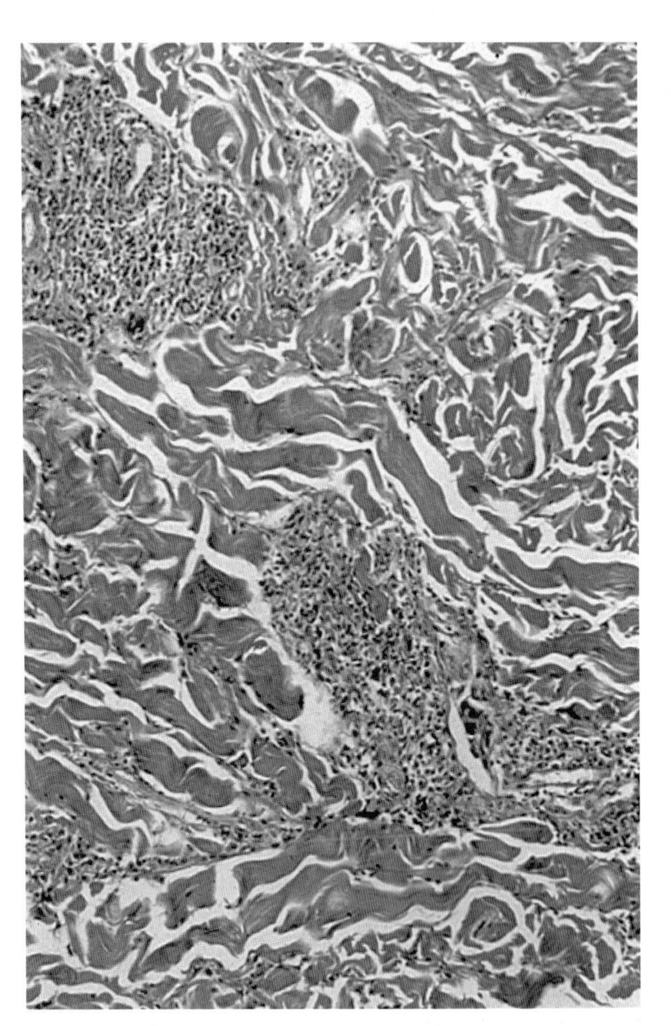

FIG. 22-13. *Borrelia burgdorferi*–associated morphea
The dermis exhibits a sclerodermoid tissue reaction characterized by widened hypereosinophilic collagen fibers with loss of the normal fibrillar architecture and an interstitial lymphohistiocytic infiltrate in close apposition to the altered collagen fibers. Special stains reveal spirochetal forms amid the inflammatory infiltrate.

Occasionally the entire ipsilateral side of the body may be affected or the atrophy may first manifest on the trunk or extremities.

Histopathology. A sclerodermoid tissue reaction mimicking morphea is observed, including the presence of adnexal atrophy and subcutaneous fibrosis. The muscles are atrophic, with loss of striations, edema, and vacuolation. Ocular and neurologic complications including iritis, keratitis, optic nerve atrophy, trigeminal neuralgia, and facial palsy may occur.[55]

Borrelial Lymphocytoma Cutis

Lymphocytoma cutis is a benign cutaneous lymphoid hyperplasia first described by Spiegler before the end of the nineteenth century and subsequently named lymphocytoma cutis in 1921 by Kaufmann-Wolff. Various triggering factors have been isolated, such as drugs, contactants, and infections, suggesting that an excessive immmune response to antigen may be its etiologic basis. The *B burgdorferi* spirochete transmitted by *I ricinus* has been implicated among the infectious agents. Evidence supportive of a spirochetal etiology of some cases of lymphocytoma cutis includes the identification of spirochete-like structures in mercury- and silver-stained sections of skin biopsies from patients with lymphocytoma cutis in whom increased serum titers of antibodies against *Borrelia* spirochetes are observed.[66] The term *borrelioma* has been coined to describe such lesions. Lymphocytoma cutis in association with *B burgdorferi* infection has the same clinical appearance as lesions arising in other settings—namely, as isolated or multiple violaceous, firm nodules and infiltrative plaques.[56] Sites of predilection for the solitary lesions are the earlobes, nipples, and areolae mammae. Lesions of lymphocytoma cutis may occur at sites of erythema chronicum migrans or in patients with stage II Lyme disease. Jessner's lymphocytic infiltrate of skin is considered by some authors to be a form of lymphocytoma cutis and has been reported in one patient whose biopsy showed spirochetes.[55]

Histopathology. Histologically, there is a dense diffuse and/or nodular pandermal infiltrate of well-differentiated lymphocytes with a variable admixture of immunoblasts, eosinophils, and plasma cells; the infiltrate may have a folliculotropic, eccrinotropic, and neurotropic disposition. Germinal centers may be observed (Fig. 22-14). A grenz zone of uninvolved dermis separates the dermal infiltrate from the epidermis.

Differential Diagnosis. Other causes of lymphocytoma cutis should be considered, such as drug therapy[67] or other infections (i.e., herpetic or mycobacterial). A well-differentiated lymphocytic lymphoma and chronic lymphocytic leukemia should be excluded, because both may mimic the diffuse type of lymphocytoma cutis. When eosinophils and plasma cells are present and when there are germinal centers, the distinction from malignant lymphoma is less challenging.

Histogenesis. Most ticks become infected with *B burgdorferi* by feeding on small animals, in particular the white-footed mouse. *B burgdorferi* is a long, narrow spirochete with flagella.[68] It has at least 30 different proteins, including two major outer-surface proteins—Osp A and Osp B, which elicit antibody responses late in the course of the disease.[68] It has been suggested that phagocytosis of the spirochete by macrophages leads to two different mechanisms of degradation: a phagolysosomal process, which may lead to MHC-class II–restricted antigen processing, and cytosolic degradation, which leads to MHC-class I–restricted antigen presentation. This disparity may in part explain the variable immunological aspects of Lyme disease.[69]

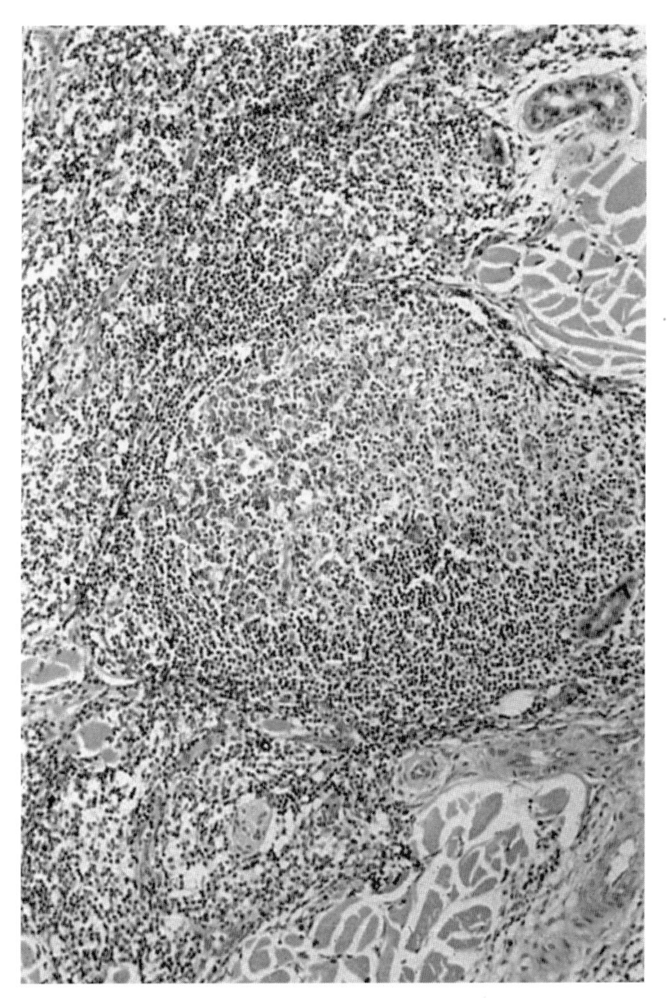

FIG. 22-14. Lymphocytoma cutis in association with *Borrelia burgdorferi* infection
The biopsy shows a dense, nodular, lymphohistiocytic infiltrate spanning the dermis; germinal centerlike foci are noted.

REFERENCES

1. Hook EW, Marra CM. Acquired syphilis in adults. N Engl J Med 1992; 326:1060.
2. Sparling PF. Natural history of syphilis. In: Homes KK, Mardh P-A, Sparling PF, et al. Sexually transmitted diseases. 2nd ed. New York: McGraw-Hill, 1990:213.
3. Noppakun N, Dinerart SM, Solomon AR. Pustular secondary syphilis. Int J Dermatol 1987;26:112.
4. Stockli HR. Neurosyphilis heute. Dermatologica 1982;165:232.
5. Moskovitz BL, Klimek JJ, Goldman RL, et al. Meningovascular syphilis after "appropriate" treatment of primary syphilis. Arch Intern Med 1982;142:139.
6. Janier M, Pertuiset EF, Poisson M, et al. Manifestations precoces de la syphilis neuro-meningee. Ann Derm Venereol (Stockh) 1985;112:133.
7. Tanabe JL, Huntley AC. Granulomatous tertiary syphilis. J Am Acad Dermatol 1986;15:341.

8. Johnson PC, Farnie MA. Testing for syphilis. Dermatol Clin 1994;12: 9.
9. Sanchez PJ. Congenital syphilis. Adv Pediatr Infect Dis 1992;7:161.
10. Jeerapaet P, Ackerman AS. Histologic patterns of secondary syphilis. Arch Dermatol 1973;107:373.
11. Hartsock RJ, Halling LW, King FM. Luetic lymphadenitis. Am J Clin Pathol 1970;53:304.
12. Yobs AR, Brown L, Hunter EF. Fluorescent antibody technique in early syphilis. Arch Pathol 1964;77:220.
13. Beckett JR, Bigbee JW. Immunoperoxidase localization of *Treponema pallidum*. Arch Pathol 1979;103:135.
14. Metz J, Metz G. Elektronenmikroskopischer nachweis von *Treponema pallidum* in hautefflorescenzen der unbehandelten lues I und II. Arch Dermatol Forsch 1972;243:241.
15. Sykes JA, Miller JN, Kalan AJ. *Treponema pallidum* within cells of a primary chancre from a human female. Br J Vener Dis 1974;50:40.
16. Wecke J, Bartunek J, Stuttgen G. *Treponema pallidum* in early syphilitic lesions in humans during high-dosage penicillin therapy: An electron microscopical study. Arch Dermatol Res 1976;257:1.
17. Poulsen A, Kobayasi T, Secher L et al. *Treponema pallidum* in macular and papular secondary syphilis skin eruptions. Acta Derm Venereol (Stockh) 1986;66:251.
18. Azar RH, Pham TD, Kurban AK. An electron microscopic study of a syphilitic chancre. Arch Pathol 1970;90:143.
19. Poulsen A, Kobayasi T, Secher L et al. The ultrastructure of *Treponema pallidum* isolated from human chancres. Acta Derm Venereol (Stockh) 1985;65:367.
20. Klingmuller G, Ishibashi Y, Radke K. Der elektronenmikroskopische Aufbau des *Treponema pallidum*. Arch Klin Exp Dermatol 1968;233: 197.
21. Crowson AN, Magro CM, Alfa M et al. A comparative histopathological, immunophenotypic, and ultrastructural study of penile chancroid lesions in HIV+ and HIV− African males. Lab Invest 1994;70:45A.
22. Abell E, Marks R, Wilson Jones E. Secondary syphilis. A clinicopathological review. Br J Dermatol 1975;93:53.
23. Paterou M, Stavrianeas N, Civatte J et al. Histologie de la syphilis secondaire. Ann Dermatol Venereol 1979;106:923.
24. Cochran RIE, Thomson J, Fleming KA et al. Histology simulating reticulosis in secondary syphilis. Br J Dermatol 1976;95:251.
25. Kahn LE, Gordon W. Sarcoid-like granulomas in secondary syphilis. Arch Pathol 1971;92:334.
26. Montgomery H. Dermatopathology. New York: Harper & Row, 1967: 417.
27. Fisher DA, Chang LW, Tuffanelli DL. Lues maligna. Arch Dermatol 1979;99:70.
28. Degos R, Touraine R, Collart P et al. Syphilis maligne precoce d'evolution mortelle (avec examen anatomique). Bull Soc Fr Dermatol Syphiligr 1970;77:10.
29. Adam W, Korting GW. Lues maligna. Arch Klin Exp Dermatol 1960; 210:14.
30. Petrozzi JW, Lockshin NA, Berger RI. Malignant syphilis. Arch Dermatol 1974;109:387.
31. Lawrence T, Saxe N. Bullous secondary syphilis. Clin Exp Dermatol 1992;17:44.
32. Kerdel-Vegas F, Kopf AW, Tolmach JA. Keratoderma punctatum syphiliticum: Report of a case. Br J Dermatol 1954;66:449.
33. Lantis LR, Petrozzi JW, Hurley HJ. Sarcoid granuloma in secondary syphilis. Arch Dermatol 1969;99:748.
34. Matsuda-John SS, McElgunn PST, Ellis CN. Nodular late syphilis. J Am Acad Dermatol 1983;9:269.
35. Longstreth P, Hoke AQ, McElroy C. Hepatitis and bone destruction as uncommon manifestations of early syphilis. Arch Dermatol 1976;112: 1451.
36. Tourville DR, Byrd LR, Kim DU et al. Treponemal antigen in immunopathogenesis of syphilitic glomerulonephritis. Am J Pathol 1976; 82:479.
37. Bansal RC, Cohn H, Fani K et al. Nephrotic syndrome and granulomatous hepatitis. Arch Dermatol 1978;114:1228.
38. Holtzmann H, Hassenpflug K. Tertiarsyphilitische lymphknotenbeteiligung vom granulierenden typ bei einem kranken mit plattenartigen gummen der haut. Arch Klin Exp Dermatol 1962;215:230.
39. Luxon LM. Neurosyphilis (review). Int J Dermatol 1980;19:310.
40. Noordhoek GT, Hermans PWM, Paul AN et al. *Treponema pallidum* subspecies *pallidum* (Nichols) and *Treponema pallidum* subspecies *pertenue* (CDC 2575) differ in at least one nucleotide: Comparison of two homologous antigens. Micro Pathog 1989;6:29.
41. Guderian RH, Guzman JR, Calvopina M, Cooper P. Studies on a focus of yaws in the Santiago Basin, province of Esmeraldas, Ecuador. Trop Geogr Med 1991;43:142.
42. Engelkens HJH, Judanarso J, Oranje AP et al. Endemic treponematoses: Part 1. Yaws. Int J Dermatol 1992;30:77.
43. Williams HU. Pathology of yaws. Arch Pathol 1935;20:596.
44. Hasselmann CM. Comparative studies on the histopathology of syphillis, yaws and pinta. Br J Vener Dis 1957;33:5.
45. Greene CA, Harman RRM. Yaws truly: A survey of patients indexed under "Yaws" and a review of the clinical and laboratory problems of diagnosis. Clin Exp Dermatol 1986;11:41.
46. Engelkens HJH, Niemel PLA, van der Sluis JL et al. Endemic treponematoses: Part II. Pinta and endemic syphilis. Int J Dermatol 1991;30: 231.
47. Pardo-Castello V, Ferrer I. Pinta. Arch Dermatol Syph 1942;45:843.
48. Hasselmann CM. Studien uber die histopathologie von pinta, frambosie und syphilis. Arch Klin Exp Dermatol 1955;201:1.
49. Rodriguez HA, Albores-Saavedra J, Lozano MM et al. Langerhans' cells in late pinta. Arch Pathol 1971;91:302.
50. Steere AC, Grodzicki RL, Kornblatt AN, et al. The spirochetal etiology of Lyme disease. N Engl J Med 1983;308:733.
51. Duray PH. Histopathology of clinical phases of human Lyme disease. Rheum Dis Clin North Am 1989;15:691.
52. Steere AC, Malawista SE, Snydman DR et al. Lyme arthritis: An epidemic of oligoarticular arthritis in children and adults in three Connecticut communities. Arthritis Rheum 1977;20:7.
53. Benach JL, Bosler EM, Hanrahan JP, et al. Spirochetes isolated from the blood of two patients with Lyme disease. N Engl J Med 1983;308: 740.
54. Barbour AB, Tessier SL, Todd WJ. Lyme disease spirochetes in Ixodid tick spirochetes share a common surface antigenic determinant defined by a monoclonal antibody. Infect Immun 1983;41:795.
55. Abele DC, Anders KH. The many faces and phases of borreliosis: I. Lyme disease. J Am Acad Dermatol 1990;23:167.
56. Asbrink E, Hovmark A. Cutaneous manifestations in *Ixodes*-borne *Borrelia* spirochetosis. Int J Dermatol 1987;26:215.
57. Sigel LH, Curran AS. Lyme disease: A multifocal worldwide disease. Ann Rev Public Health 1991;12:85.
58. Cote J. Lyme disease. Int J Dermatol 1991;30:500.
59. Berger BW. Erythema chronicum migrans of Lyme disease. Arch Dermatol 1984;120:1017.
60. Burgdorf WHS, Woret WI, Schultes O. Acrodermatitis chronica atrophicans. Int J Dermatol 1979;595.
61. Kaufman L, Gruber BL, Philips ME, Benach JL. Late cutaneous Lyme disease: Acrodermatitis chronica atrophicans. Am J Med 1989;86:828.
62. Aberer E, Klade H, Hobisch G. A clinical, histological, and immunohistochemical comparison of acrodermatitis chronica atrophicans and morphea. Am J Dermatopathol 1991;13:334.
63. Montgomery H. Montgomery H. Dermatopathology. New York: Harper & Row, 1967:766.
64. Aberer E, Klade H, Stanek G, Gebhart W. *Borrelia burgdorferi* and different types of morphea. Dermatologica 1991;182:145.
65. Aberer E, Stanek G, Ertl M, Neumann R. Evidence for spirochetal origin of circumscribed scleroderma (morphea). Acta Derm Venereol (Stockh) 1987;67:225.
66. Hovmark A, Asbrink E, Olsson I. The spirochetal etiology of lymphadenosis benign cutis solitaria. Acta Derm Venereol (Stockh) 1986; 66:479.
67. Magro CM, Crowson AN. Drug-induced immune dysregulation as a cause of atypical cutaneous lymphoid infiltrates: A hypothesis. Hum Pathol 1996;27:125.
68. Jantausch BA. Lyme disease, Rocky Mountain spotted fever, ehrlichiosis: Emerging and established challenges for the clinician. Ann Allergy 1994;73:4.
69. Rittig MG, Haupl T, Krause A et al. *Borrelia burgdorferi*-induced ultrastructural alterations in human phagocytes: A clue to pathogenicity? J Pathol 1994;173:269.

Lever's Histopathology of the Skin, eighth edition, edited by David Elder et al. Lippincott–Raven Publishers, Philadelphia © 1997.

CHAPTER 23

Fungal Diseases

B. Jack Longley

Some diseases, such as botryomycosis, actinomycosis, and erythrasma, have traditionally been included with the fungal diseases but are actually caused by bacteria. In the interest of clarity these will be discussed in the chapter on bacterial diseases. Protothecosis will continue to be included in this chapter because there is no separate chapter for infections by algae.

Since the terminology for fungal infections of the skin has been used in confusing ways, we will define our terms here. *Hyphae* are elongated filamentous forms of fungi that usually form an intertwining mass called a *mycelium. Yeasts* are single-celled, usually rounded fungi that reproduce by budding (blastospore formation). Yeast cells and their progeny sometimes adhere and form chains or *"pseudohyphae"* that may also form mycelia and that may be difficult to distinguish from true hyphae by light microscopy. *Dematiaceous fungi* are fungi that bear melaninlike pigment on their walls. *Tinea* is a clinical term that has been used since ancient times to describe superficial fungal infections of the skin; it is usually modified with an anatomic or other term to describe the location or color of the infection. The *dermatophytes* are fungi that were originally classified by Sabouraud[1] and redefined by Emmons,[2] and that include the three genera *Microsporum, Trichophyton,* and *Epidermophyton.* Thus *dermatophytosis* is inappropriate as a histologic diagnostic term unless a definite assignment of an organism to one of the three genera of dermatophytes can be made. *Dermatomycosis* refers to any fungal infection of the skin and may be caused by dermatophytes, yeast, or other fungi, including those that do not usually cause cutaneous disease.

The primary cutaneous fungal pathogens fall into two groups: those that tend to cause superficial infections and those that cause deep infections. Fungi that usually cause systemic disease, and only secondarily colonize the skin, form a third group of cutaneous pathogens. A number of factors, including the immune status of the host, may modify the cutaneous histologic reaction patterns, but the response to individual organisms within these groups tends to be similar. Thus infections with organisms causing superficial dermatomycoses, such as the dermatophytes, *Candida* species, *Malassezia (Pityrosporum) furfur,* and *Cladosporium (Exophialia* or *Phaeoannellomyces) werneckii,* are generally characterized by hyphae or pseudohyphae and sometimes yeast cells in the keratin layer of the epidermis and in follicles. The intensity of the tissue reaction is variable, with involvement of the epidermis and follicular epithelium ranging from an almost undetectable response, through very mild focal spongiosis, to a more exuberant or chronic spongiotic-psoriasiform pattern. Although they may provoke a mixed dermal inflammatory infiltrate, these organisms are not found in the dermis except in the case of follicular rupture. Histologic reactions in deep cutaneous fungal infections, including primary cutaneous aspergillosis, chromomycoses, phaeohyphomycosis, phaeomycetoma, rhinosporidiosis, and lobomycosis, typically consist of a mixed dermal infiltrate that is often associated with pseudoepitheliomatous hyperplasia and occasionally with dermal fibrosis. Incidental cutaneous infections by fungi that usually primarily involve other organs, such as blastomycosis or coccidioidomycosis, typically show a pattern similar to that seen with the deep primary cutaneous fungi: a mixed dermal infiltrate with multinucleated giant cells associated with pseudoepitheliomatous hyperplasia. A few organisms, such as *Histoplasma* and *Loboa loboi,* are more likely to be associated with epidermal thinning than with hyperplasia, and other systemic fungal infections, such as disseminated candidiasis with its microabscess formation, cryptococcosis with its gelatinous and granulomatous reaction patterns, or zygomycosis and aspergillosis with their tendency for vascular invasion and infarction, show special tissue reaction patterns.

DERMATOPHYTOSIS

The dermatophytes consist of three genera of imperfect fungi, *Epidermophyton, Trichophyton,* and *Microsporum,* that are capable of colonizing keratinized tissue such as the stratum corneum of the epidermis, the hair, and the nails. Thus, in immunocompetent hosts dermatophytes cause only superficial infections. Some fungi have characteristics similar to those of the dermatophytes and have been included in these genera but are more properly termed the "dermatophytelike fungi" because they have not been shown to cause human disease. The dermatophytes and dermatophytelike fungi are grouped according to their natural habitat as anthropophilic, zoophilic, and geophilic with primary reservoirs of infection in humans, ani-

B. J. Longley: Departments of Dermatology and Pathology, Yale University School of Medicine, New Haven, CT

mals, and the soil, respectively. Fungi in all three categories may cause human infections.[3] Although there are exceptions, anthropophilic fungi tend to produce the least vigorous host response and zoophilic fungi the greatest. Finally, certain species of dermatophytes tend to be associated with infection of certain tissues and with certain clinical forms of disease, although there may be considerable variation in different geographic and socioeconomic environments, and in different ethnic and age groups. Thus *Epidermophyton* species, as the name suggests, infect mainly the epidermis, although occasionally the nails are involved. *Trichophyton* and *Microsporum* species, however, may infect the hair and nails as well as the epidermis.

Clinically, fungal infections of seven anatomical regions are commonly recognized: tinea capitis (including tinea favosa or favus of the scalp), tinea barbae, tinea faciei, tinea corporis (including tinea imbricata), tinea cruris, tinea of the hands and feet, and tinea unguium.

Tinea capitis is dermatophytosis of the skin and hair of the scalp, and in the United States is most commonly caused by *T tonsurans*.[4] *M audouinii*, *M canis*, and much less commonly other *Microsporum* species may also cause tinea capitis. With the exception of favus, caused by *T schoenleinii*, cases caused by *Trichophyton* species other than *T tonsurans* are exceptional. Clinically, scalp infection with *Microsporum* is mostly confined to children and commonly shows a band of bright green fluorescence in the hair under a Wood light. *Trichophyton* species other than *T schoenleinii*, which shows subtle pale green fluorescence along the length of the hair, do not fluoresce in a Wood light. Occasional infections with *T tonsurans*, and more commonly *T schoenleinii*, may persist into adulthood. In most types of tinea capitis, the affected hairs tend to break off either at the level of the scalp or slightly above it. The anthropophilic fungi *M audouinii* and *T violaceum* usually produce only a slight inflammatory reaction, but the zoophilic fungus *M canis* often produces pronounced inflammation of the affected areas of the scalp, so-called kerion Celsi. The anthropophilic fungus *T tonsurans* may produce only slight scaling and broken-off hairs (black dot ringworm) in some patients, but stimulates a marked inflammatory reaction in others.[4] *T verrucosum* may also affect the scalp.

Favus, rare in the United States, is usually caused by *T schoenleinii*, although a similar clinical picture may occasionally be seen with other fungi. Favus affects mainly the scalp, where it produces inflammation with formation of perifollicular hyperkeratotic crusts, called scutula. Destruction of the hair occurs relatively late in the infection. Healing takes place with scarring.

Tinea faciei is a fungal infection of the glabrous skin of the face characterized by a persistent eruption of red macules, papules, and patches, the latter of which may show an arcuate border. It is caused usually by *T rubrum* and occasionally by *T mentagrophytes*[5] or *T tonsurans*.[6]

Tinea barbae, also rare in the United States, is a fungal infection limited to the coarse hair-bearing beard and mustache areas of men. Tinea barbae may be caused by *T mentagrophytes*, but usually is due to *T verrucosum (faviforme)*, an infection also often referred to as "cattle ringworm" because it is usually contracted from cattle. Both *T mentagrophytes* and *T verrucosum* are zoophilic and typically cause a kerionlike, soft, nodular inflammatory infiltration.[7]

Tinea corporis may be caused by any dermatophyte, but by far the most common cause in the United States is *T rubrum*, followed by *M canis* and *T mentagrophytes*. In *T rubrum* infection there are large patches showing central clearing and a polycyclic scaling border, which may be quite narrow and threadlike. Occasionally, *T rubrum* causes an asymptomatic nodular perifolliculitis in circumscribed areas, often called "Majocchi granuloma." It was first described as a scalp infection seen in children, but is seen most commonly on the legs in association with an infection of the soles, particularly in women who shave their legs.[8] In infections with *M canis*, tinea corporis manifests itself as several annular lesions with a raised papulovesicular border and central clearing. If the disease is caused by *T mentagrophytes*, one finds one or at the most a few annular lesions showing little or no central clearing. *T verrucosum* may occasionally cause tinea corporis, manifest as grouped follicular pustules referred to as "agminate folliculitis."[7]

Tinea cruris, usually caused by *T rubrum* and occasionally by *T mentagrophytes* or *Epidermophyton floccosum*, shows sharply demarcated areas, often with a raised border, on the upper and inner surfaces of the thighs. From there, the eruption can extend to the perineal and perianal regions, and to the scrotum in men.

Tinea of the feet and hands (tinea pedis et manus) is usually caused by *T rubrum* or *T mentagrophytes*. In cases of infection with *T rubrum*, the soles and sometimes also the palms show diffuse erythema and superficial scaling; in cases of infection with *T mentagrophytes*, the lesions consist of maceration between the toes and an erythematous, vesicular eruption on the soles and palms.

Tinea unguium refers to dermatophytic infection of the nails, usually caused by *T rubrum*. *Onychomycosis* is a broader term that encompasses any fungal infection involving the nails and that includes disease caused by yeasts or other nondermatophytic fungi, which may be responsible for 40% to 70% of nail infections.[9] Tinea unguium is characterized by yellowish gray or white discoloration of the nail and varying degrees of hyperkeratosis and thickening of the subungual region (pachyonychia) and disintegration or detachment of the nail plate (onycholysis). The most common clinical form is distal subungual onychomycosis; less common forms include lateral or proximal onychomycosis and white superficial onychomycosis.

Histopathology. In histologic sections, fungi may present as filamentous hyphae, arthrospores, yeast forms, or pseudohyphae. Hyphae are threadlike structures that may be septate or nonseptate; they grow by extending and branching and may form matlike structures called mycelia. Arthrospores are spores formed by fragmentation of septate hyphae at the septum, and may assume a number of different shapes but usually appear as rounded, boxlike, or short cylindrical forms. Yeast are single-celled forms that appear as round, elongated, or ovoid bodies; they grow by budding, and their progeny may adhere to each other and form elongated chains called pseudohyphae. It may be difficult to distinguish pseudohyphae from true hyphae by light microscopy.

For the demonstration of fungi in histologic sections, two stains can be used: the periodic acid–Schiff (PAS) reaction (Chap. 4), which stains fungi deeply red, and the Gomori methenamine silver nitrate (GMS) method, which stains fungi black. Fungi stain positively with the PAS reaction because of two substances rich in neutral polysaccharides in their cell walls: cellulose and chitin.[10] The fungal polysaccharides are diastase-resistant, unlike glycogen, so it is useful to clear the tissue sections of glycogen by diastase treatment, since glycogen granules in the dermis may resemble fungal spores.[11]

Tinea Capitis and Tinea Barbae

Infection of follicles usually starts with colonization of the stratum corneum of the perifollicular epidermis (Fig. 23-1). Hyphae extend down the follicle, growing on the surface of the hair shaft. Hyphae then invade the hair, penetrating the cuticle and then proliferating downward, first in the subcuticular portion of the cortex, just under the hair surface, and then more deeply in the hair cortex, extending to the upper limit of the zone of keratinization.[10] Rounded and boxlike arthrospores may be found mainly within the hair shaft in *endothrix* infections, or within the hair shaft and forming a sheath around it in *ectothrix* infections. *Endothrix* infections are caused by *T tonsurans* or *T violaceum*; except for *T schoenleinii* which causes favus, all other dermatophytes infecting hair shafts cause *ectothrix* infections. Although hyphae invade the shafts in both types of infections, they may not be evident in a hair plucked from an endothrix infection because the more superficial hyphae rapidly break up into arthrospores and destroy the keratin of the hair shaft. When plucked, the weakened shaft typically breaks at a relatively superficial point so that only the arthrospores are seen. The dermis, which almost never contains fungi, shows a perifollicular infiltrate of varying intensity, depending on the degree of reac-

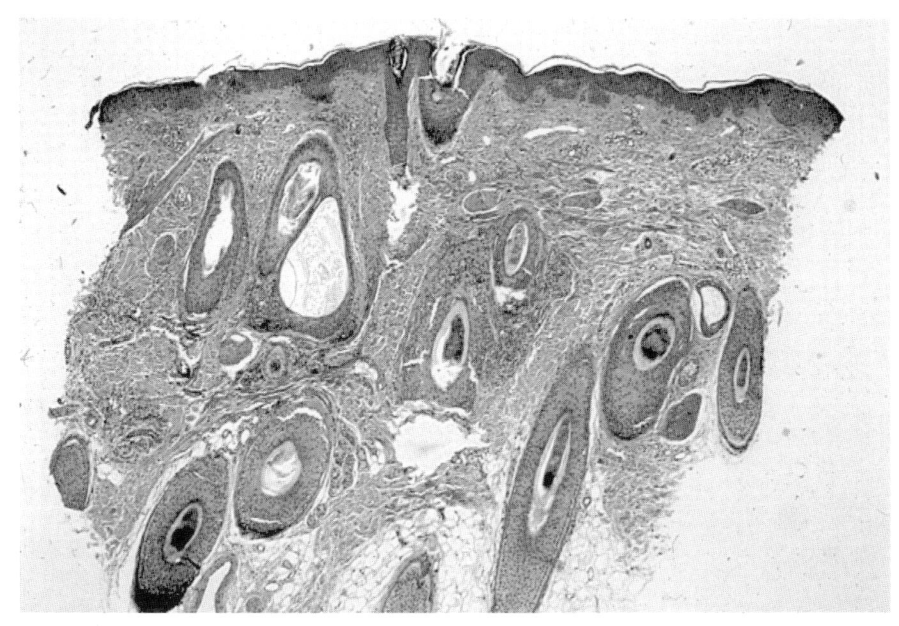

A

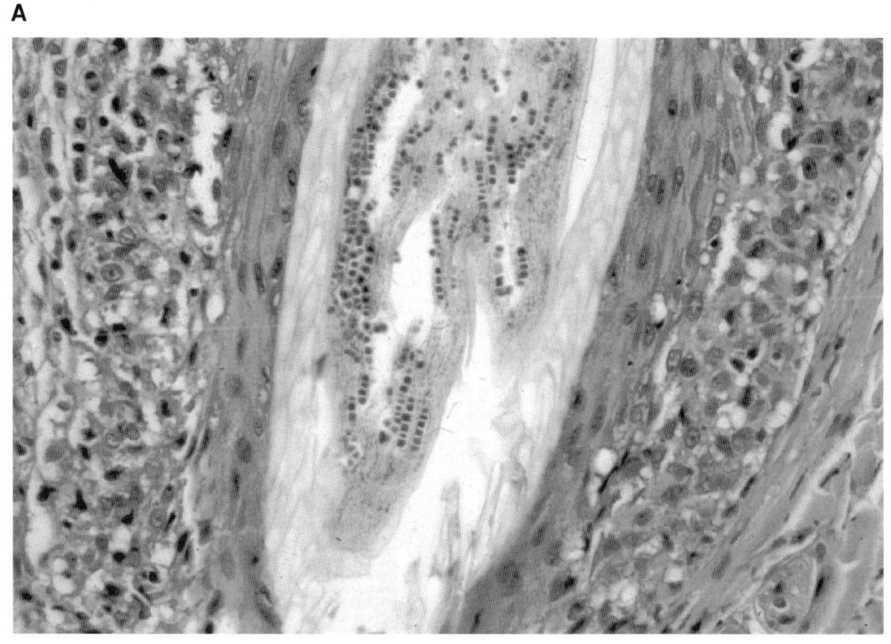

B

FIG. 23-1. Tinea capitis
(**A**) H&E stain shows arthrospores and hyphal elements in most follicles. A lymphohistiocytic, perifollicular infiltrate is present. (**B**) H&E stain shows arthrospores in endothrix infection.

tion of the patient. In addition to a chronic inflammatory infiltrate, multinucleated giant cells may be present in the vicinity of disrupted or degenerated hair follicles.[12] In some patients, those with the clinical form of infection known as "kerion Celsi," there is a pronounced inflammatory tissue reaction to the fungi with follicular pustule formation and interfollicular neutrophilic infiltration, as well as a marked chronic inflammatory infiltrate surrounding the hair follicles. Not infrequently, in cases with a severe inflammatory reaction, fungi can no longer be found, either by microscopic examination or by culture,[7,13] but may be demonstrated using fluorescein-labeled *T mentagrophytes* antiserum that cross-reacts with antigens of all dermatophyte species.[14]

Tinea of the Glabrous Skin

In tinea of the glabrous skin, which includes tinea faciei, tinea corporis, tinea cruris, and tinea of the feet and hands, fungi occur only in the horny layers of the epidermis and, with two exceptions, *T rubrum* and *T verrucosum* (see later), do not invade hairs and hair follicles. In histologic sections, even on staining with the PAS reaction or with methenamine silver nitrate, the number of fungi seen in the horny layer usually is small, so that they may be easily missed. In occasional instances, however, they are present in sufficient numbers that, even in sections stained with hematoxylin-eosin, they can be recognized as faintly basophilic, refractile structures (Fig. 23-2). Their identi-

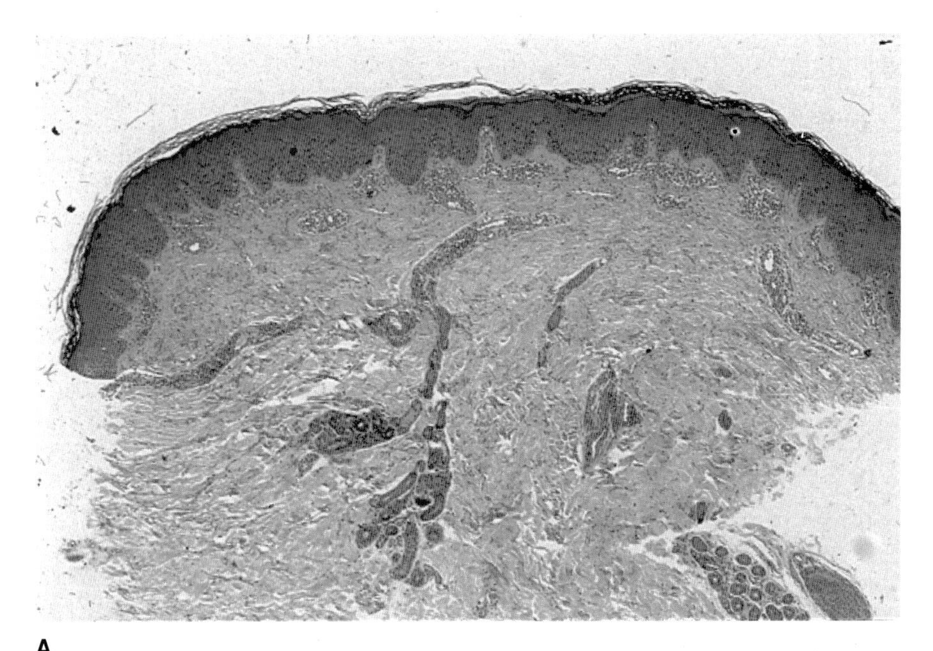

A

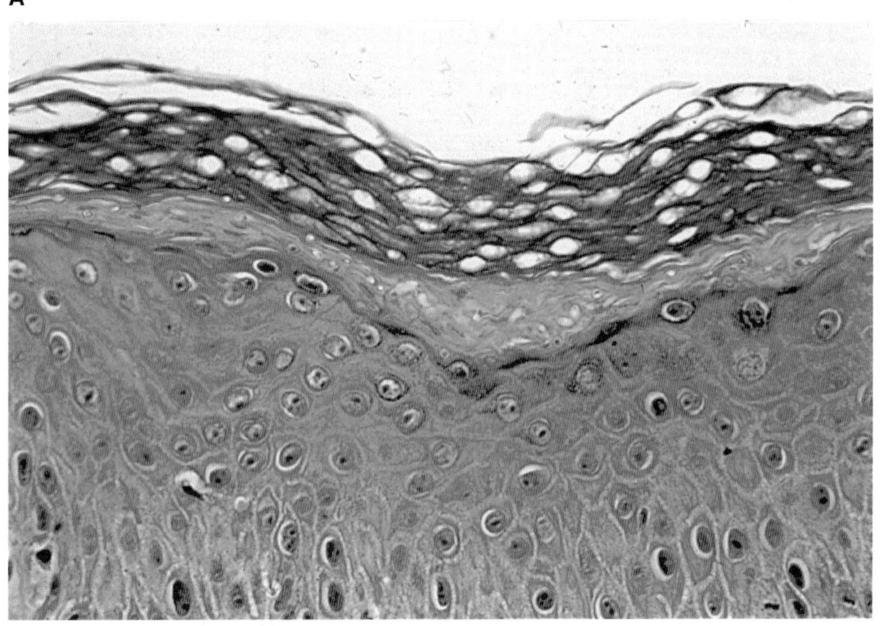

B

FIG. 23-2. Tinea corporis
(**A**) H&E stain shows a superficial perivascular, predominantly lymphoid infiltrate with mild psoriasiform epidermal hyperplasia and compact hyperkeratosis. (**B**) Cross sections of refractile hyphae are visible as clear spaces in parakeratotic stratum corneum (H&E stain).

fication in hematoxylin-eosin–stained sections may be aided by lowering the microscope condenser, which enhances the refractility of the fungal elements. In infections with *Microsporum* or *Trichophyton*, only hyphae are seen, and, in infections with *E floccosum*, chains of spores are present. If fungi are present in the horny layer, they usually are "sandwiched" between two zones of cornified cells, the upper being orthokeratotic and the lower consisting partially of parakeratotic cells. This "sandwich sign" should prompt the performance of a stain for fungi for verification. The presence of neutrophils in the stratum corneum is another valuable diagnostic clue.[15] In the absence of demonstrable fungi, the histologic picture of fungal infections of the glabrous skin is not diagnostic. Depending on the degree of reaction of the skin to the presence of fungi, one sees the histologic features of an acute, a subacute, or a chronic spongiotic dermatitis (Chap. 9).

Two fungal infections of the glabrous skin, those with *T rubrum* and with *T verrucosum,* occasionally are associated with an invasion of hairs and hair follicles and a subsequent perifolliculitis.

The nodular perifolliculitis ("Majocchi granuloma") caused by *T rubrum* shows, on staining with the PAS reaction or with methenamine silver nitrate, numerous hyphae and spores within hairs and hair follicles and in the inflammatory infiltrate of the dermis. Although the spores present within hairs or hair follicles measure about 2 μm in diameter, those located in the dermis, especially within multinucleated giant cells, may be larger, measuring up to 6 μm.[8] The fungal elements reach the dermis through a break in the follicular wall. The dermal infiltrate shows, besides central necrosis and occasionally also suppuration, lymphoid cells, macrophages, epithelioid cells, and scattered multinucleated giant cells.[16]

The agminate folliculitis caused by *T verrucosum (faviforme)* shows mycelia and spores within hairs and hair follicles in PAS-stained sections.[7] The dermis around the hair follicles, however, contains no fungi. Depending on the severity and on the stage of the inflammatory reaction, either an acute or a chronic inflammatory infiltrate is predominant around the hair follicles in the dermis. In well-established lesions, the inflammatory infiltrate contains many plasma cells, microabscesses, and small aggregates of foreign-body giant cells.[7]

Tinea Unguium

Although microscopic examination of potassium hydroxide mounts and cultures of nail scrapings often establish a diagnosis of onychomycosis, there are false-negative results if the fungus infection is in the nail bed or is situated in the lower portion of the nail plate. A nail biopsy taken by punch technique or scalpel under local anesthesia will often reveal the fungi.[17] *Trichophyton rubrum* is by far the most common fungus; occasionally *T mentagrophytes* is present. As described in following sections, *Candida* species may attack the soft tissue around the nail.[9]

Favus

Mainly hyphae and only a few spores of *T schoenleinii* are present in the stratum corneum of the epidermis around and within hairs. The scutula consist of keratinized as well as parakeratotic cells, exudate, and inflammatory cells intermingled with segmented hyphae and spores that are well preserved at the periphery but appear degenerated and granular in the center of the scutula.[18] In active areas, the dermis shows a pronounced inflammatory infiltrate containing multinucleated giant cells and many plasma cells in association with degenerating hair follicles. In old areas, there is fibrosis and an absence of pilosebaceous structures.[12]

DISEASES CAUSED BY *MALASSEZIA FURFUR*

Two dermatoses, pityriasis versicolor and *Malassezia (Pityrosporum)* folliculitis, are generally accepted as being caused by the genus *Malassezia.* The frequently used term "tinea versicolor" is not accurate since *Malassezia* are not dermatophytes. Pityriasis versicolor usually affects the upper trunk, where one finds areas of brown discoloration that may lighten in color to appear hypopigmented. On gentle scraping, the surface of the discolored areas shows fine, branny scaling. *Malassezia (Pityrosporum)* folliculitis is a chronic condition that may resemble acne vulgaris[19] and that consists of red follicular papules or pustules, predominantly on the upper back and anterior chest, measuring 2 to 4 mm.[20] Occasionally, pityriasis versicolor and *Pityrosporum* folliculitis occur together.[21]

In addition to these two diseases, it has been suggested that seborrheic dermatitis may be the result of colonization by *M furfur*. Seborrheic dermatitis has been reported to respond to antifungal therapy and has been associated with heavy colonization by *M furfur*.[22] These observations and their interpretation are controversial, however, and it has not been established that *M furfur* contributes to the pathogenesis of seborrheic dermatitis.[23]

Pityriasis (Tinea) Versicolor

In contrast to other fungal infections of the glabrous skin, the horny layer in lesions of pityriasis versicolor contains abundant amounts of fungal elements, which can often be visualized in sections stained with hematoxylin-eosin as faintly basophilic structures. *Malassezia (Pityrosporum)* is present as a combination of both hyphae and spores (Fig. 23-3), often referred to as "spaghetti and meatballs." The inflammatory response in pityriasis versicolor is usually minimal, although there may occasionally be slight hyperkeratosis,[24] slight spongiosis, or a minimal superficial perivascular lymphocytic infiltrate.

Histogenesis. The names *Pityrosporum orbiculare* and *P ovale*, are currently widely accepted as synonyms for *M furfur*.[25] The yeast phase of *M furfur* is widespread; in addition, a few short rods resembling hyphae may be seen in 8% of normal subjects.[26] In patients with pityriasis versicolor, *M furfur* becomes dimorphous by forming numerous true septate hyphae in addition to spores. The organism then becomes pathogenic.[27]

M furfur produces a substance that directly affects the normal mechanism of epidermal pigmentation.[28] Electron microscopic study has shown that melanocytes produce abnormally small melanosomes, which are not transferred to keratinocytes, in hypopigmented areas.[29] In areas of hyperpigmentation, in con-

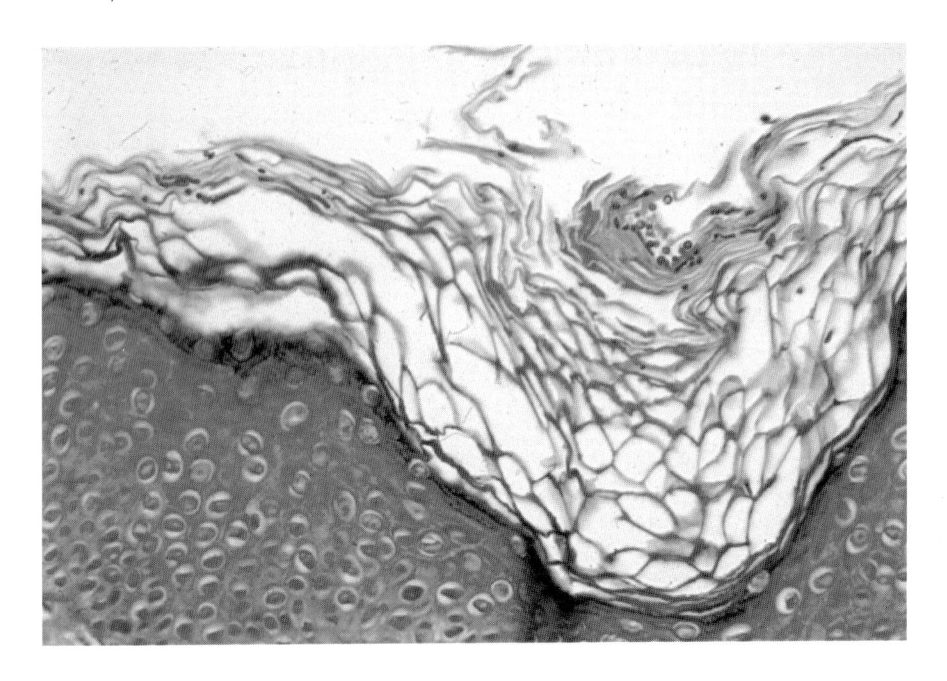

FIG. 23-3. Pityriasis (tinea) versicolor
A slightly hyperkeratotic stratum corneum contains numerous hyphae and spores (H&E stain).

trast, the melanosomes are large, unpackaged, and heavily melanized.[30]

Malassezia (*Pityrosporum*) Folliculitis

The involved pilosebaceous follicles show dilatation resulting from plugging of the infundibulum with keratinous material. Inflammatory cells are present both within and around the infundibulum.[19] In some instances, the follicular epithelium is disrupted with development of a peri-infundibular abscess (Fig. 23-4).[20,31] In every instance, PAS-stained sections show PAS-positive, diastase-resistant, spheric to oval, singly budding yeast organisms 2 to 4 μm in diameter. They are located predominantly within the infundibulum and at the dilated orifice of the follicular lumen but are occasionally observed also in the perifollicular dermis. No hyphae are seen.

Histogenesis. It has been assumed that *Malassezia* organisms cause hyperkeratosis in the follicular ostium, thereby preventing the normal flow of sebum and causing the follicular, acnelike lesions.[19]

Seborrheic Dermatitis

The histologic features of seborrheic dermatitis are described in Chap. 7.

CANDIDIASIS

Candida albicans is a dimorphous fungus growing in both yeast and filamentous forms on the skin. It exists in a commensal relationship with man. The spectrum of infection may be divided into three groups:[32] acute mucocutaneous candidiasis, chronic mucocutaneous candidiasis, and disseminated candidiasis.

Acute Mucocutaneous Candidiasis

Acute mucocutaneous candidiasis, the common, benign, self-limited form of candidiasis, is caused by environmental changes that act either locally, like heat and sweating, or systemically, like antibiotic or corticosteroid therapy. It results in a localized infection of intertriginous areas, either alone or in association with oral, vulvar, or paronychial lesions. Intertriginous lesions show erythematous, often eroded areas lined by a scaly epidermal fringe. Small, superficial pustules may be seen either along the fringe or peripheral to it as satellite lesions.

Acute candidiasis of the vagina is common in pregnancy and may cause, as a result of ascending intrauterine infection, *congenital cutaneous candidiasis* of the fetus characterized by widely scattered macules, papulovesicles, and pustules present at birth or within a few days after birth. It differs from *neonatal candidiasis*, which is acquired by the infant during passage through the birth canal, and is usually seen after the first week of life. Neonatal candidiasis usually manifests itself as oral candidiasis and less often as lesions confined to the diaper area.[33] In the absence of an immune defect, both congenital and neonatal candidiasis respond well to therapy.

Histopathology. If the primary lesion is a vesicle or pustule, it is usually located subcorneally, as in impetigo (Fig. 23-5).[34] In some instances, the pustules have a spongiform appearance, so that they are indistinguishable from the spongiform pustules of Kogoj seen in pustular psoriasis (Chap. 7).[35]

The fungal organisms are present, usually in small amounts only, in the stratum corneum. They consist of pseudohyphae, which predominate by far, and ovoid spores, some of the latter in the budding stage. The pseudohyphae, which are septate and show branching at a 90-degree angle, measure from 2 to 4 μm in diameter. The pseudohyphae tend to be constricted at their septa and tend to have septa at their branch points.[36] The ovoid spores vary from 3 to 6 μm in size (Table 23-1).

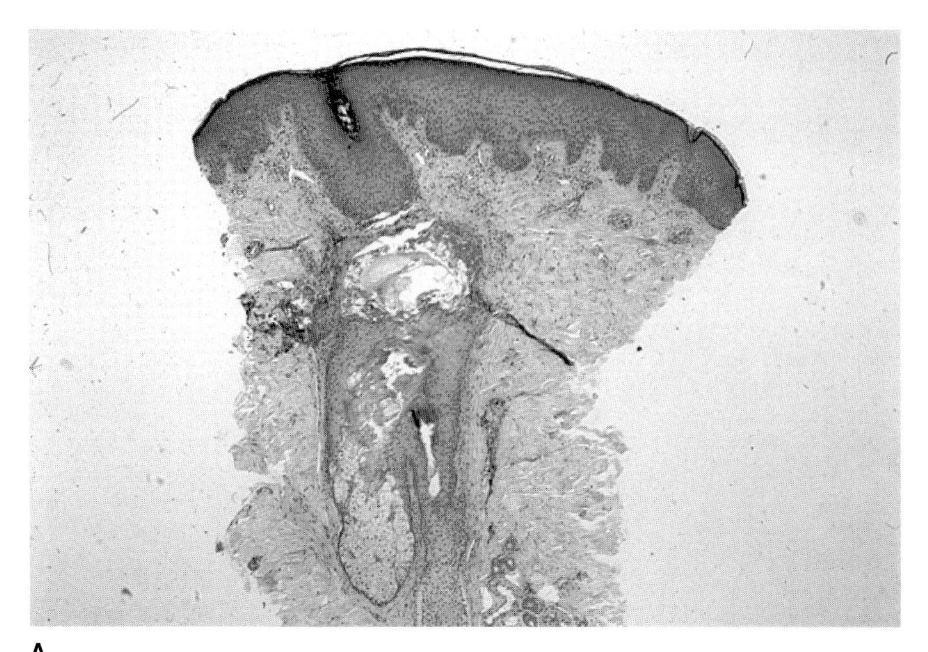

A

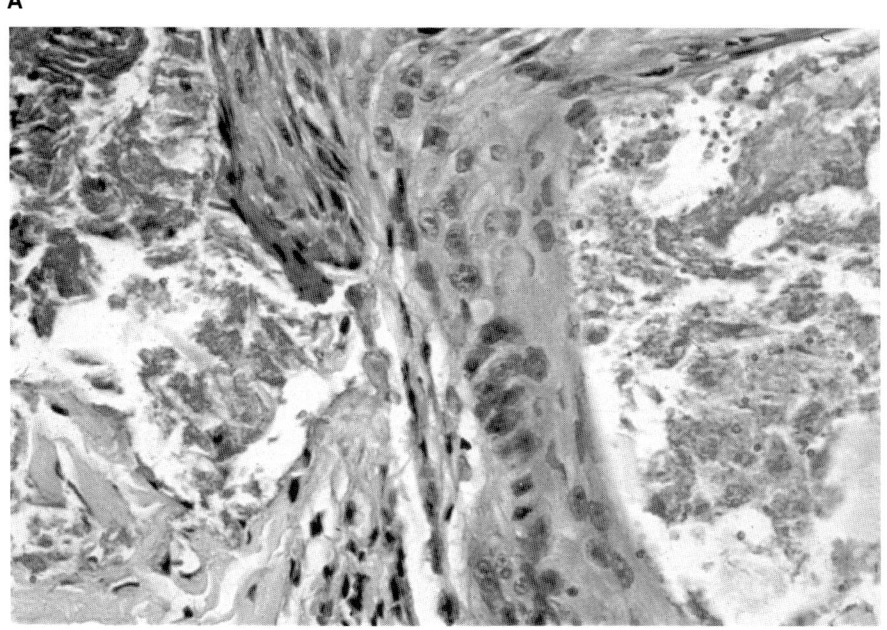

B

FIG. 23-4. *Malassezia (pityrosporum)* folliculitis
(**A**) A plugged and ruptured follicle contains numerous round yeast forms (H&E stain). (**B**) H&E stain shows round and budding yeast forms in follicle and surrounding dermis.

Pathogenesis. On electron microscopy, the majority of the mycelia and spores are found to be situated inside the cells of the stratum corneum, many of which are parakeratotic.[37]

Chronic Mucocutaneous Candidiasis

Chronic mucocutaneous candidiasis is a heterogeneous group of conditions in which patients have chronic and recurrent candidal infections of the skin, nails, and mucous membranes. In chronic mucocutaneous candidiasis beginning in childhood, a rare clinical variant called "candida granuloma" may develop. In this variant, numerous hyperkeratotic, crusted plaques are present, mainly on the face and scalp but also elsewhere.[38,39] Otherwise, the individual lesions seen in chronic mucocutaneous candidiasis are similar to those seen in acute forms of this disease, and systemic lesions do not occur.[40]

The type of chronic mucocutaneous candidiasis that is currently most commonly seen is probably the type associated with the acquired immunodeficiency syndrome (AIDS). This type consists of recurrent candidal infections of the mouth and perianal area. Oral candidiasis may occur as an early sign of immunosuppression before other symptoms have appeared.[41] If persistent, oral candidiasis may be an indication of esophageal candidiasis in AIDS.[42] In addition, *Candida* organisms are fre-

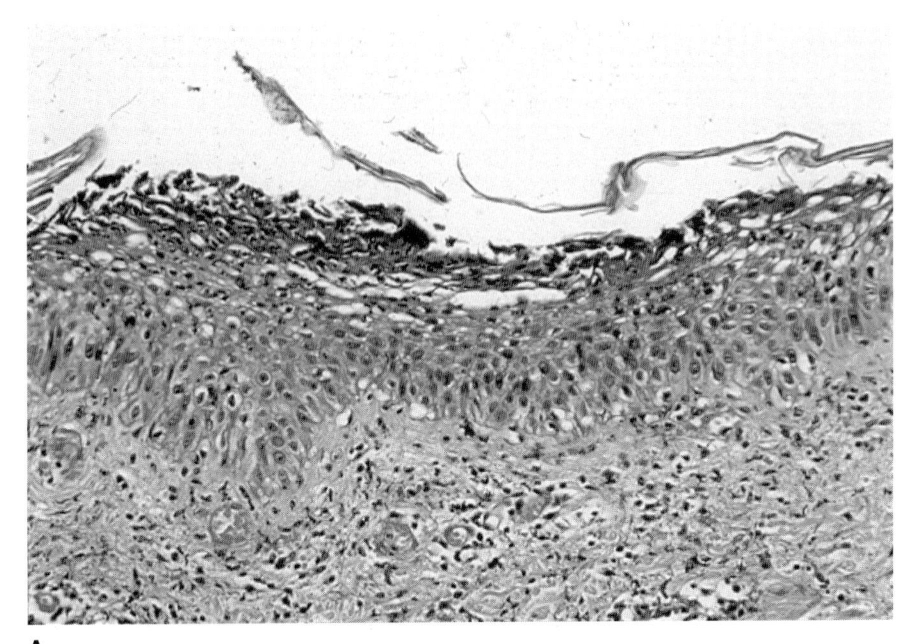

A

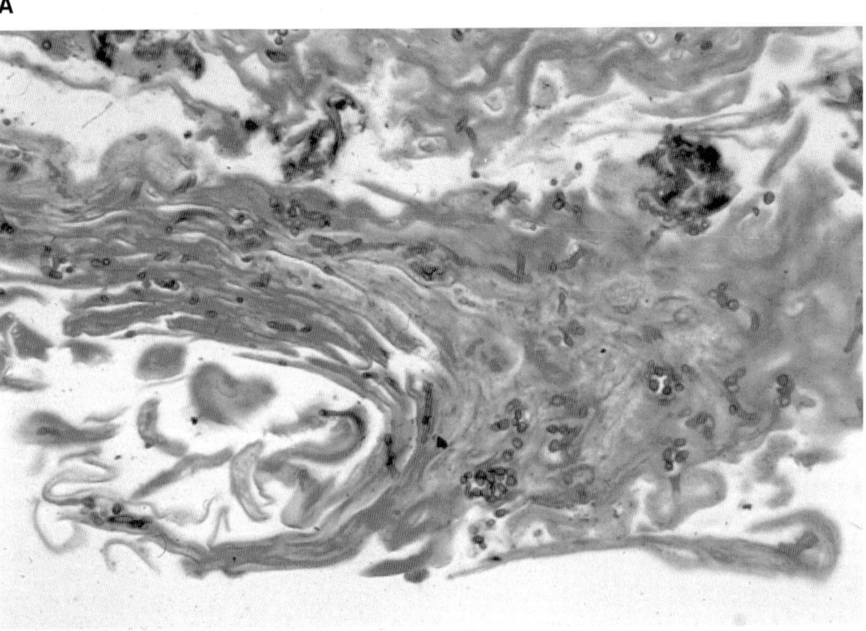

B

FIG. 23-5. Candidiasis
(**A**) H&E stain shows a subcorneal pustule with an underlying mixed dermal infiltrate. (**B**) GMS stain shows pseudohyphae and ovoid yeast in hyperkeratotic stratum corneum.

quently observed on the surface of lesions of oral hairy leukoplakia, which is a viral leukoplakia caused by Epstein-Barr virus, perhaps in combination with human papillomavirus (Chap. 26).[43]

Other types of chronic mucocutaneous candidiasis have been described in association with autoimmune diseases, inherited immune deficiencies or endocrinopathies, or thymomas.

Histopathology. The histologic findings are identical with those of acute mucocutaneous candidiasis, except in cases of candidal granuloma.

Candidal granuloma shows pronounced papillomatosis and hyperkeratosis and a dense infiltrate in the dermis composed of lymphoid cells, neutrophils, plasma cells, and multinucleated giant cells. The infiltrate may extend into the subcutis.[38] *Candida albicans* usually is present only in the stratum corneum.[35,38,39] In some instances, however, fungal elements are found also within hairs,[44] in the viable epidermis,[45] and in the dermis.[46,47]

Disseminated Candidiasis

Disseminated, or systemic, candidiasis is a not uncommon serious complication among patients with impaired host–defense mechanisms, particularly among those with hematologic malignancies. The diagnosis is often difficult to establish, since *Candida* organisms can be cultured from blood specimens in only 25% of the patients.[48] Unless treated, the disease is rapidly fatal. It has been emphasized that the triad of fever, papular rash, and diffuse muscle tenderness must be regarded as

TABLE 23-1. *Histological appearance of tissue and fungi in superficial dermatomycoses*

Disease	Histologic appearance	Fungal size and morphology
Dermatophytosis	Minimal to spongiotic-psoriasiform, pustular, or folliculitis pattern with mixed dermal infiltrate.	Refractile, 1–2 μm septate hyaline hyphae in stratum corneum, occasional chains of spores.
Pityriasis (tinea) versicolor	Slight hyperkeratosis.	2–8 μm round spores, 2–3 μm thick, short, sometimes curved hyphae.
Mallassezia (Pityrosporum) folliculitis	Plugged, sometimes ruptured follicle with follicular and perifollicular mixed infiltrate.	2–8 μm round spores within follicle, rarely in perifollicular tissue. Usually no hyphae.
Candidiasis	Spongiotic or subcorneal pustular dermatitis with mixed dermal infiltrate. Erosions may be present.	3–6 μm round to oval, sometimes budding spores, 2–4 μm thick pseudohyphae.

presumptive evidence of disseminated candidiasis.[49,50] Unfortunately, the characteristic skin lesions are seen in only 13% of the patients.[48]

Cutaneous lesions of disseminated candidiasis consist of single or, more commonly, multiple red or purpuric papulonodules 0.5 to 1.0 cm in diameter. They frequently have a pale center. These papulonodules are seen most commonly on the trunk and the proximal portions of the extremities.[50]

Histopathology. Histologic examination reveals one or several aggregates of hyphae and spores focally within the dermis, often at sites of vascular damage and generally visible only in sections stained with the PAS reaction or the GMS stain. Some of the spores, which are 3 to 6 μm in diameter, show budding.[48] The aggregates of hyphae and spores may lie in an area of leukocytoclastic vasculitis,[50] within a microabscess,[51] or in an area of only mild inflammation.[48] The aggregates of *Candida* often are small, and step sections through the biopsy specimen may be necessary to find them. The epidermis is usually unaffected.

Because the diffuse muscle tenderness is caused by infiltration of muscle tissue by yeast organisms, biopsy of a tender muscle area may also aid in establishing the diagnosis of disseminate candidiasis.[52]

Histogenesis. Only about half of the infections in disseminated candidiasis are caused by *Candida albicans*, with *Candida tropicalis* and *Candida krusei* causing the remainder.[48]

ASPERGILLOSIS

Aspergillus species are ubiquitous in the environment; humans are constantly exposed to and frequently colonized by these organisms, although they rarely cause disease. Severe, invasive disease typically involves the lungs and is usually seen only in immunocompromised hosts, particularly those with neutropenia, hematologic malignancy, or a history of chronic corticosteroid or antibiotic therapy.[53] *Aspergillus fumigatus* is the most common cause of both colonization and invasive aspergillosis, followed in frequency by *A flavus* and *A niger*.[54] Cutaneous aspergillosis may occur as a primary infection or may be secondary to disseminated aspergillosis (Table 23-2). The lesions of primary cutaneous aspergillosis are usually found at an intravenous infusion site: either at the actual access site[55,56] or where the unit has been secured with a colonized board or tape.[56–58] One observes either one or several macules, papules, plaques, or hemorrhagic bullae, which may rapidly progress into necrotic ulcers that are covered by a heavy black eschar. Death often results from secondary systemic dissemination of the aspergillosis.[59,60] However, rapid diagnosis and institution of intravenous treatment with amphotericin may prevent a fatal outcome.[56]

Primary cutaneous infection has been seen in patients with AIDS, but dissemination is not typical in these patients unless they have one or more of the previously mentioned risk factors.[61] Umbilicated papules resembling lesions of molluscum contagiosium, and representing "dermatophytelike" involvement of follicles, has been described in AIDS-related cases[58] and in a child with leukemia.[62] In addition, *Aspergillus* may colonize burn or surgical wounds and subsequently invade viable tissue; in these cases the prognosis is generally good.[63,64]

Secondary cutaneous aspergillosis, usually associated with invasive lung disease, shows multiple scattered lesions as a result of embolic, hematogenous spread, and has a poor prognosis.[53,65]

Histopathology. Unlike the case with most deep cutaneous fungal infections, pseudoepitheliomatous epidermal hyperplasia is not characteristic of cutaneous aspergillosis. In the more serious primary forms and in the secondary disseminated form, numerous *Aspergillus* hyphae are seen in the dermis (Fig. 23-6). Hyphae may be seen in hematoxylin-eosin–stained sections, but PAS or silver methenamine staining may be required. The hyphae, which measure 2 to 4 μm in diameter,[60] are often arranged in a radiate fashion, are septate, and show branching at an acute angle. Spores are absent. Hyphae may be seen invading blood vessels[59] and may be seen around areas of ischemic necrosis with very little inflammation in some instances. In other cases, there may be an acute inflammatory reaction with polymorphonuclear leukocytes in addition to lymphocytes and histiocytes.

In patients with primary cutaneous or subcutaneous aspergillosis who are otherwise in good health, the number of hyphae present is relatively small, and there may be a well-developed granulomatous reaction.[66,67]

ZYGOMYCOSIS (MUCORMYCOSIS, PHYCOMYCOSIS)

Infection of the skin with fungi of class *Zygomycetes* is rare and is usually caused by members of two genera, *Rhizopus* and *Mucor*. Infections with these organisms are clinically aggres-

TABLE 23-2. *Histologic appearance of tissue and fungi in deep and secondary dermatomycoses*

Disease	Histologic appearance	Fungal size and morphology
Aspergillosis	Primary infection: granulomatous infiltrate. Immunocompromised host (primary and secondary infection): angioinvasion, ischemic necrosis, and hemorrhage.	2–4 μm septate hyphae with dichotomous branching at 45-degree angle.
Zygomycosis (mucormycosis, phycomycosis)	Angioinvasion with thrombosis and infarction, necrosis, and variable, mild, neutrophilic infiltrate.	7–30 μm hyphae with branching at irregular angles and intervals. Variably thin, often collapsed or twisted walls.
Subcutaneous phaeohyphomycosis (phaeohyphomycotic cyst)	Deep, coalescing, suppurative granulomatous foci surrounded by fibrous capsule.	Loosely arranged, septate, occasionally branching pigmented hyphae varying from 2 to 25 μm in diameter.
Alternariosis	Pseudocarcinomatous epithelial hyperplasia with intraepidermal microabscesses and suppurative granulomatous dermal infiltrate.	5–7 μm septate hyphae with variable branching and brown pigmentation. 3–10 μm round to oval spores, often with double contours.
North American blastomycosis	Pseudocarcinomatous epithelial hyperplasia with intraepidermal microabscesses. Suppurative granulomatous dermal infiltrate with giant cells.	8–15 μm thick-walled spores with single broad-based buds.
Paracoccidioidomycosis	Like North American blastomycosis.	6–20 μm spores with narrow-necked, single or multiple buds. "Mariner's wheels" up to 60 μm in diameter.
Lobomycosis	Atrophic epidermis with dermal macrophage and giant cell infiltrate. Unstained organisms give sievelike appearance to dermis.	9–10 μm "lemon-shaped" spores with single budding, often in chains.
Chromoblastomycosis	Like North American blastomycosis.	6–12 μm thick-walled, dark brown spores, often in clusters. Some cells possess cross walls.
Coccidioidomycosis	Primary inoculation: mixed dermal infiltrate with granulocytes, lymphocytes, and occasional histiocytic giant cells. Systemic: like North American blastomycosis, but granulomas may be more tuberculoid in nature.	10–80 μm thick-walled spores with granular cytoplasm. The larger spores contain endospores.
Cryptococcosis	"Gelatinous reaction" with many spores; "granulomatous reaction" with fewer spores.	4–12 μm spore with wide capsule in "gelatinous reaction"; 2–4 μm spore in "granulomatous reaction."
Histoplasmosis		
var. *capsulatum*	Suppurative granulomatous infiltrate in ulcerative skin lesions, neutrophils and eosinophils in oral lesions. Histiocytes contain variable numbers of organisms.	2–4 μm round, narrow-necked budding spores with clear halo (pseudocapsule) in the cytoplasm of large histiocytes.
var. *duboisii* (African)	Granulomatous dermal infiltrate with focal suppuration.	8–15 μm ovoid spores in macrophages and free in tissue.
Sporotrichosis	Cutaneous lesions: epidermal hyperplasia with intraepidermal abscesses, suppurative granulomatous dermal infiltrate, occasional asteroid bodies. Subcutaneous nodules: central zone of neutrophils surrounded by zones of epithelioid macrophages and round cells.	4–6 μm round to oval spores.
Eumycetoma	Abscess in granulation tissue, fibrosis, and sinus tracts.	0.5–2.0 mm sulfur granules composed of 4–5 μm thick septate hyphae.
Rhinosporidiosis	Hyperplastic epithelium with papillomatosis, deep invagination with pseudocysts, and "Swiss cheese" corium.	7–12 μm spores, sporangia up to 300 μm.

sive and, since both types of fungi are of the order Mucorales, may also be referred to collectively as *mucormycoses*.[68] Chronic subcutaneous infections with members of the family Entomophthoraceae have also been classified as *Zygomycetes*.

Zygomycosis involving the skin occurs in three major forms. The rhinocerebral form is a fulminant, usually lethal infection that starts in a paranasal sinus and quickly spreads to contiguous structures, including the nose and paranasal skin, the orbit, and the brain.[68] Clinically, this form is seen in diabetics and immunosuppressed patients and is characterized by discharge and swelling with mucocutaneous ulceration and the formation of black eschars.

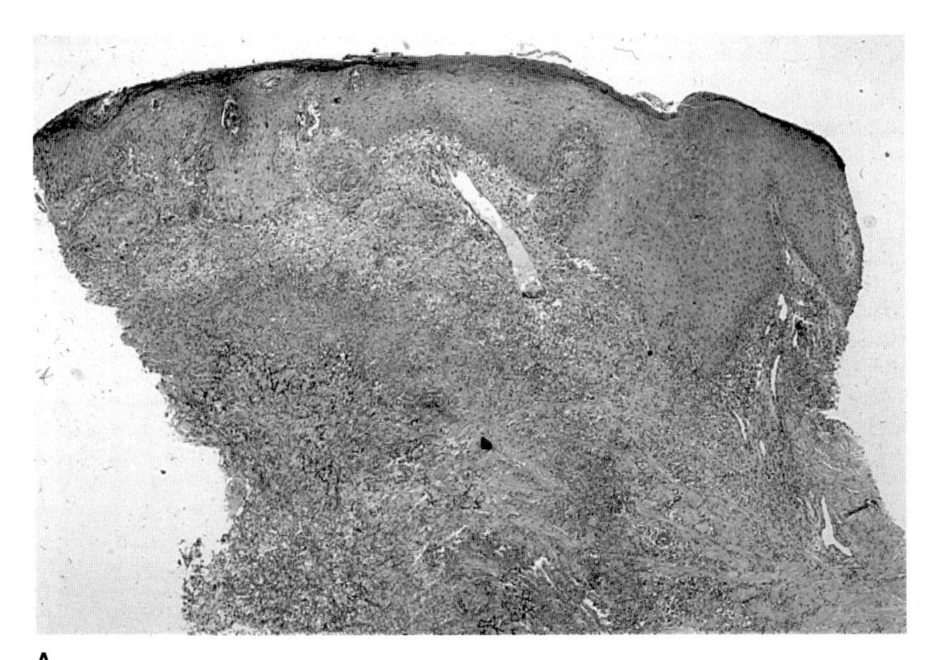

A

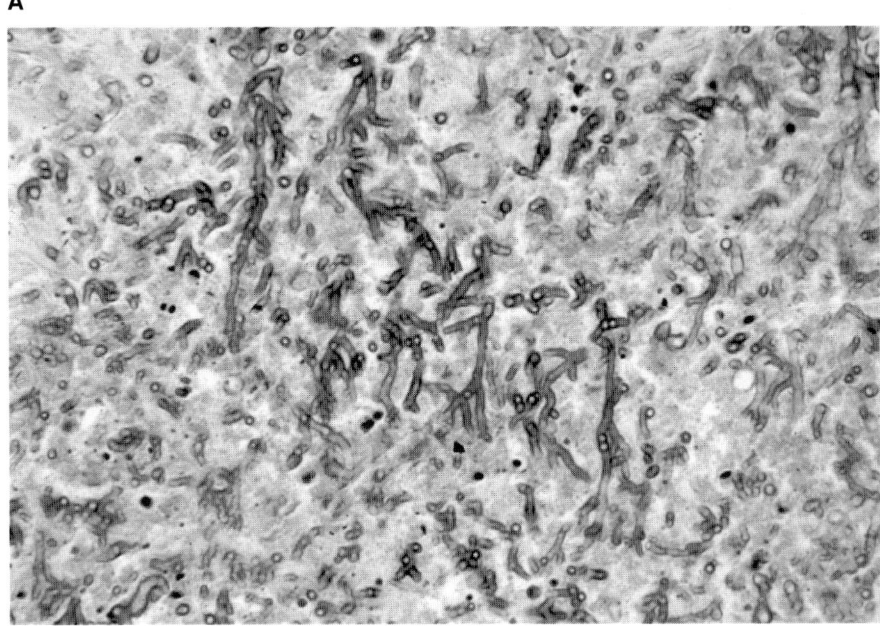

B

FIG. 23-6. Aspergillosis
(**A**) H&E stain shows a central area of dermal necrosis with branching hyphae. (**B**) H&E stain shows septate hyphae branching at an acute angle in a background of necrotic tissue.

Primary cutaneous zygomycosis may occur in patients suffering burns or major trauma, or following minor trauma in patients with diabetes or other metabolic or immunosuppressive systemic disorders.[68–70] Primary cutaneous infection has also been reported after the use of infected tape.[71,72] Zygomycosis has been seen in a few patients with human immunodeficiency virus (HIV) infection, almost all of whom used illicit intravenous drugs, but not in the general HIV-positive population.[73] Skin lesions of primary cutaneous zygomycosis may show early formation of pustules or blisters but are soon characterized by ulceration and eschar formation. The ulcers may heal or may lead to fatal systemic spreading of the infection.[74]

Cutaneous lesions may also be seen as a result of embolization and infarction in patients with systemic zygomycosis. The lesions may begin as erythematous macules that blister and ulcerate,[75] or may occur as an indurated nodule.[76]

Chronic subcutaneous zygomycosis occurs in tropical and subtropical areas in persons who are otherwise healthy, leading to slowly enlarging, painless, firm swelling, most commonly on the face.[68,77]

Histopathology. The histologic changes in zygomycosis are primarily dermal; the hallmark of zygomycosis is vascular invasion by very large, long, nonseptate hyphae with thrombosis and infarction (Fig. 23-7).[68,76] The hyphae may also be found in the surrounding tissue and show irregular branching.[74] The hyphae are thin-walled, so that they may be twisted or collapsed and often appear ring-shaped or oval in cross or tangential sections (see Fig. 23-7).[68,71] They are often easily located even in routinely stained sections because of their very large size, up to 30 μm in diameter, although they may be visualized even better in PAS- or silver methenamine–stained sections.[70] Spores are rarely seen.

SUBCUTANEOUS PHAEOHYPHOMYCOSIS

Phaeohyphomycosis has been defined as a subcutaneous or systemic infection by dematiaceous, mycelia-forming fungi, that is, those fungi having dark-walled hyphae.[78] This is a histopathologic definition of a disease process that can be caused by many different organisms and that can have multiple different clinical presentations. It includes several entities that have been called "chronic mycoses" in the past, but is distinct from chromoblastomycosis, which is characterized by pigmented spores without hyphal forms. Although eumycetoma caused by dematiaceous fungi could be included under this definition,[79] that has not generally been the case, probably since eumycetoma is such a distinctive clinical entity.[80]

Subcutaneous phaeohyphomycosis typically presents as a solitary abscess or nodule on the extremity of an adult male. A history of trauma or a splinter can sometimes be elicited. Systemic spread from a cutaneous infection has not been described. The other major clinical forms of phaeohyphomycosis are infection of the paranasal sinuses and of the central nervous system. Alternariosis (see next section) has also been considered a phaeohyphomycosis.

Histopathology. Lesions of subcutaneous phaeohyphomy-

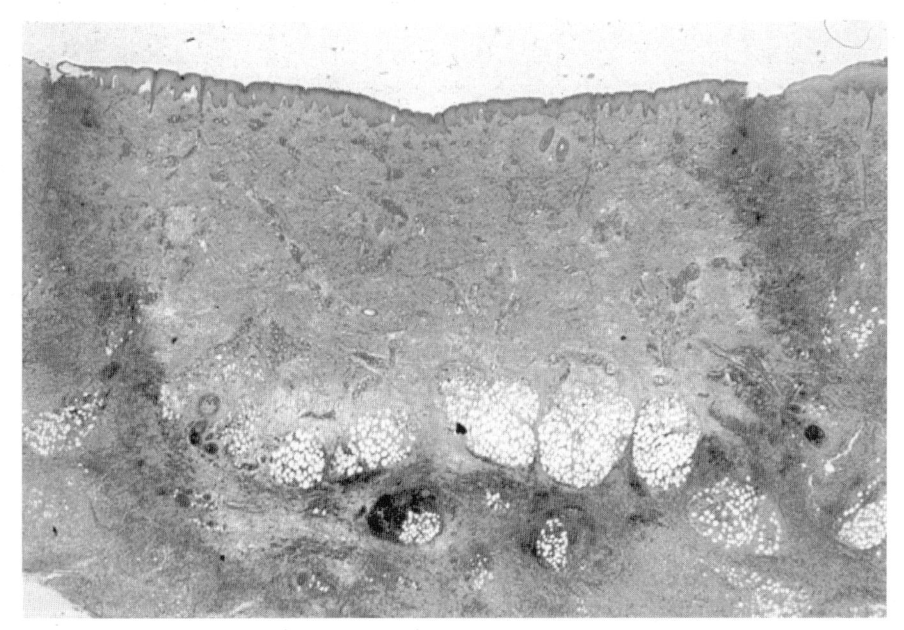

A

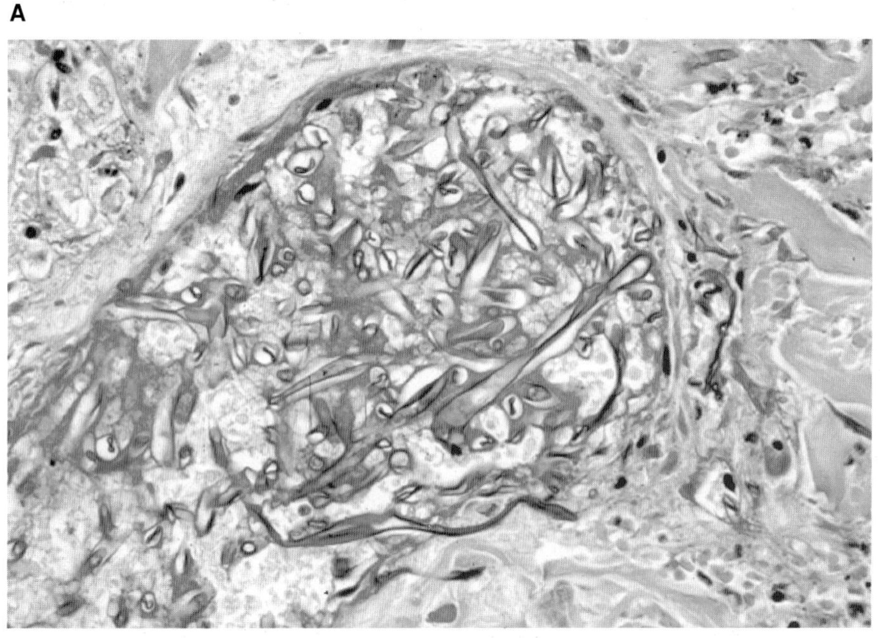

B

FIG. 23-7. Zygomycosis (mucormycosis)
(**A**) H&E stain shows infarction of dermis, epidermis, and subcutaneous fat with lymphohistiocytic and neutrophilic infiltrate, and angioinvasion by broad nonseptate hyphae. (**B**) H&E stain shows irregularly branching, twisted, and collapsed hyphae.

cosis start as small, often stellate foci of suppurative granulomatous inflammation. The area of inflammation gradually enlarges and usually forms a single large cavity with a surrounding fibrous capsule, the so-called phaeohyphomycotic cyst (Fig. 23-8A).[81] The central space is filled with pus formed of polymorphonuclear leukocytes and fibrin. There is a surrounding granulomatous reaction composed of histiocytes, including epithelioid cells and multinucleated giant cells, lymphocytes, and plasma cells. Diligent search may identify an associated splinter in the tissue or liquid pus. The organisms are found within the cavity and at its edge, often within histiocytes (see Fig. 23-8B). The hyphae often have irregularly placed branches and show constrictions around their septae that may cause them to resemble pseudohyphae or yeast forms, but true yeast forms are rare. Mycelia, if present, are more loosely arranged than the compact masses of hyphae seen in eumycetoma. Pigment is not always obvious, but the organisms of phaeohyphomycosis can be distinguished from *Aspergillus* species because the latter have hyphae with relatively uniform diameter and regular dichotomous branching.[80] Furthermore, disseminated aspergillosis is associated with vascular invasion, ischemic necrosis, and relatively less inflammation.

Pathogenesis. The subcutaneous cystic type of phaeohyphomycosis is usually caused by *Phialophora gougerotii* (formerly called *Sporotrichum gougerotii*).[82,83] In rare instances, it is due to *Exophiala (Fonsecaea, Wangiella)* dermatitidis.[84] Cerebral phaeohyphomycosis is caused by a fungus different from those causing cutaneous infection, and is not associated with skin lesions. This fungus, called *Cladosporium trichoides*, shows not only spores but also mycelia, in contrast to the organisms causing cutaneous phaeohyphomycosis.[85,86]

CUTANEOUS ALTERNARIOSIS

Because the hyphae of *Alternaria* species are pigmented, alternariosis may also be considered a phaeohyphomycosis. *Alternaria* species commonly colonize human skin[87] but are generally nonpathogenic for humans. Cutaneous alternariosis may occur following trauma,[88] by colonization of a preexisting lesion, which usually consists of dermatitis of the face that has been treated topically with corticosteroids,[89,90] or, rarely, by hematologic spread, most likely from pulmonary infection caused by inhalation of the organism. Patients with cutaneous alternariosis are often debilitated or immunocompromised or receiving immunosuppressive therapy.[80,91–93] Despite the increasing prevalence of HIV infection, however, only one case has been described in an AIDS patient.[94] Morphologically, the lesions of cutaneous alternariosis are so variable as to be nonspecific, and include crusted ulcers, verrucous or granulomatous and multilocular lesions,[90] and subcutaneous nodules.[88]

Histopathology. Although fungi are found mainly in the deeper layers of the dermis and in the subcutaneous region in the hematogenous and the traumatogenic forms, they are localized predominantly in the epidermis in cases in which *Alternaria* colonizes preexisting lesions.[90] The dermis shows a suppurative granulomatous reaction associated with variable pseudoepitheliomatous epidermal hyperplasia and ulceration. Organisms may be present both as broad, branching, brown septate hyphae, 5 to 7 μm thick (Fig. 23-9),[89] and as large, round to oval, often doubly contoured spores measuring 3 to 10 μm in diameter.[90] The spores may be seen both lying free in the tissue[87] and within macrophages and giant cells.[93] There may be intraepidermal microabscesses with hyphae in the stratum corneum and stratum spinosum.[87] The hyphae and spores stain deeply with PAS or silver methenamine.

NORTH AMERICAN BLASTOMYCOSIS

North American blastomycosis, caused by *Blastomyces dermatitidis*, occurs in three forms: primary cutaneous inoculation blastomycosis, pulmonary blastomycosis, and systemic blastomycosis.[95]

Primary cutaneous inoculation blastomycosis is very rare and occurs almost exclusively as a laboratory or autopsy room infection. It starts at the site of injury on a hand or wrist as an indurated, ulcerated, chancriform solitary lesion. Lymphangitis and lymphadenitis may develop in the affected arm. Small nodules may be present along the involved lymph vessel. Spontaneous healing takes place within a few weeks or months.[96,97]

Pulmonary blastomycosis, the usual route of acquisition of the infection, may be asymptomatic or may produce mild to moderately severe, acute pulmonary signs, such as fever, chest pain, cough, and hemoptysis. In rare instances, acute pulmonary blastomycosis is accompanied by erythema nodosum.[98] The pulmonary lesions either resolve or progress to chronic pulmonary blastomycosis with cavity formation.

In systemic blastomycosis, the lungs are the primary site of infection. Granulomatous and suppurative lesions may occur in many different organs, but, aside from the lungs, they are most commonly found in the skin, followed by the bones, the male genital system, the oral and nasal mucosa, and the central nervous system. Untreated systemic blastomycosis has a mortality rate in excess of 80%.[99] Although antimycotic therapy can reduce mortality to 10% in otherwise uncomplicated cases, systemic blastomycosis has a particularly aggressive course in immunosuppressed patients, including those with HIV infections.[100,101] In some cases, however, cutaneous lesions are the only clinical manifestation after pulmonary infection.[102] It may be pointed out that the same phenomenon of a benign systemic form with cutaneous lesions occurs, though rarely, after pulmonary infection in several other deep mycoses, for instance, in coccidioidomycosis, cryptococcosis, histoplasmosis, and sporotrichosis.[103]

Cutaneous lesions are very common in systemic blastomycosis, occurring in about 70% of the patients. They may be solitary or numerous. They occur in two types, either as verrucous lesions, the more common type, or as ulcerative lesions. Verrucous lesions show central healing with scarring and a slowly advancing, raised, verrucous border that is beset by a large number of pustules or small, crusted abscesses. Ulcerative lesions begin as pustules and rapidly develop into ulcers with a granulating base. In addition, subcutaneous abscesses may occur; they usually develop as an extension of bone lesions. Lesions of the oral or nasal mucosa may present either as ulcers or as heaped-up masses of friable tissue. In some instances, they are contiguous with cutaneous lesions.[99] An unusual early cutaneous manifestation of systemic blastomycosis is a pustular eruption that may be

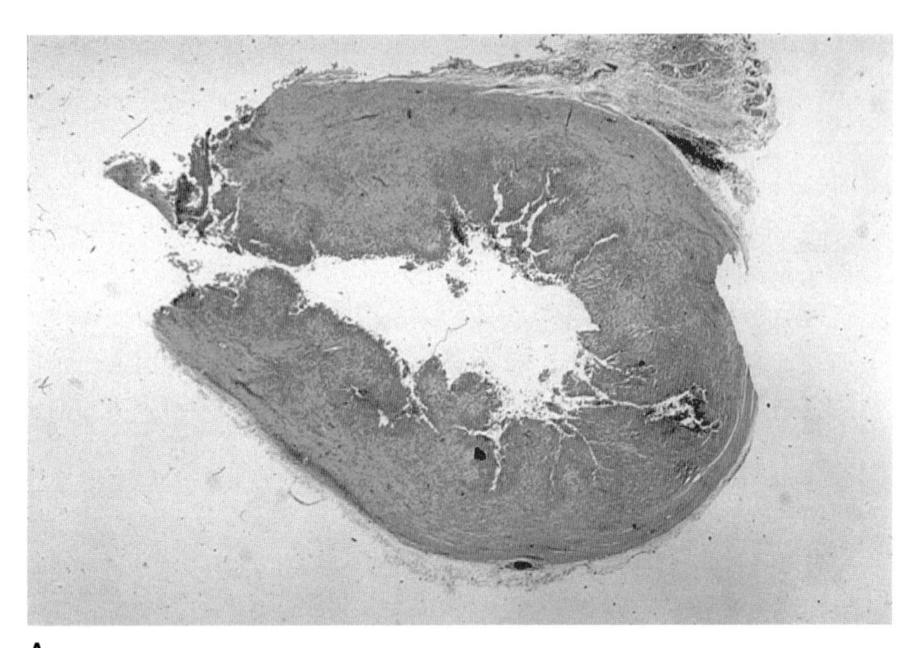

A

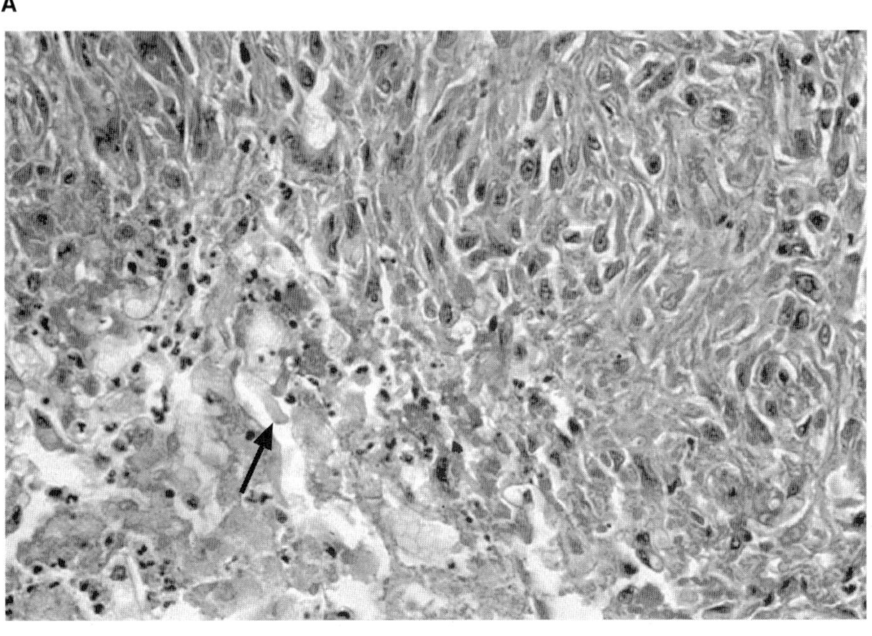

B

FIG. 23-8. Phaeohyphomycosis (**A**) H&E stain shows a pseudocyst with a large central cavity and a fibrous capsule. (**B**) H&E stain shows pigmented hyphal forms at edge of cavity.

widespread[104] or largely acral in distribution.[105] In the benign systemic form of blastomycosis with only cutaneous lesions, the lesions usually are on the face and are of the verrucous type.[106]

Histopathology. In primary cutaneous inoculation blastomycosis, the primary lesion shows at first a nonspecific inflammatory infiltrate without epithelioid or giant cells. Numerous organisms, many in a budding state, are present. After a few weeks occasional giant cells may be seen, and later on the primary lesion may show the verrucous histologic pattern usually seen in skin lesions of systemic blastomycosis (Fig. 23-10A). The small lymphangitic nodules show a partially necrotic inflammatory infiltrate with organisms.[97] The regional lymph nodes show a granulomatous reaction with numerous giant cells, in which the organisms are predominantly located.[96]

For an examination of the verrucous lesions of systemic blastomycosis, it is important that the specimen for biopsy be taken from the active border. There is considerable downward proliferation of the epidermis, often amounting to pseudocarcinomatous hyperplasia. Intraepidermal abscesses often are present. Occasionally, multinucleated giant cells are completely enclosed by the proliferating epidermis. The dermis is permeated by a polymorphous infiltrate. Neutrophils usually are present in large numbers and form small abscesses. Multinucleated giant cells are scattered throughout the dermis. Usually they lie alone and not within groups of epithelioid cells; occasionally, there are tuberculoid formations, although without evidence of caseation necrosis.[107] In the ulcerative lesions, the dermal changes are the same as in the verrucous lesions, but the epidermis is absent.[108]

The spores of *B dermatitidis* are found in histologic sections

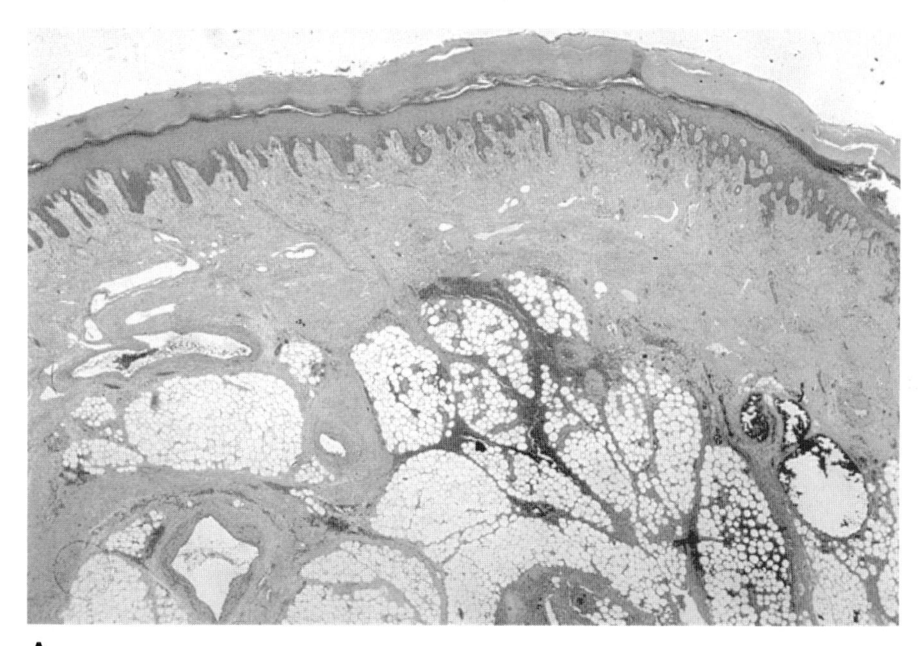

A

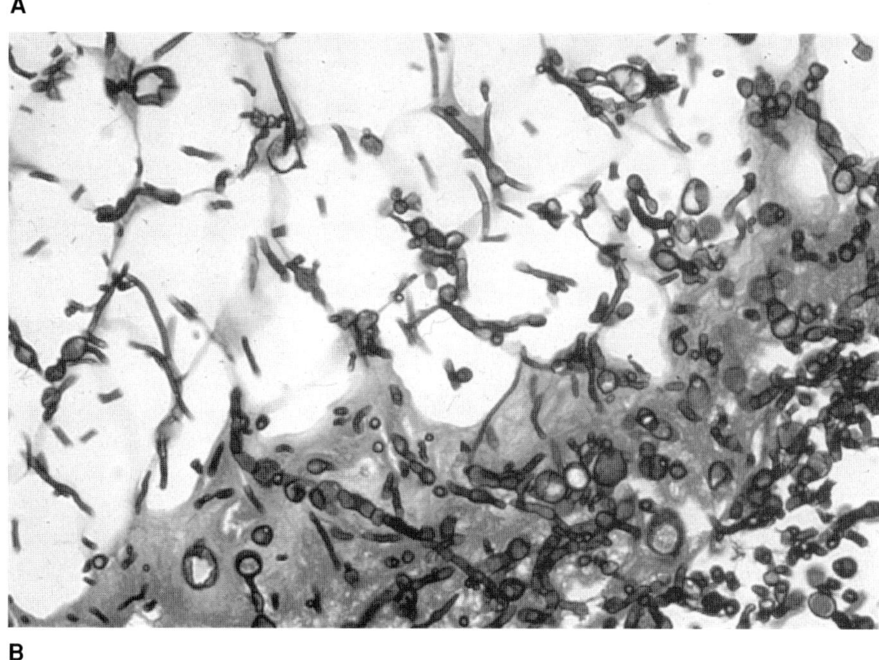

B

FIG. 23-9. Alternariosis
(**A**) H&E stain shows a mixed inflammatory infiltrate in the deep dermis and subcutaneous fat. (**B**) GMS stain shows broad branching hyphae.

often only after a diligent search, usually in clusters of neutrophils or within giant cells (see Fig. 23-10B). One or several spores may lie within a giant cell, where they are easily spotted, even in sections stained with routine stains. Unstained, the spores resemble small, round holes punched out of the cytoplasm of the giant cells. On high magnification, the spores are seen to have a thick wall, which gives them a double-contoured appearance. They measure 8 to 15 μm in diameter (average, 10 μm). Occasionally, spores showing a single broad-based bud are seen. As in most fungal infections, many more spores are visualized in sections stained with the PAS reaction or with methenamine silver than in routinely stained sections.

The histologic appearance of the visceral lesions in North American blastomycosis is analogous to that of the cutaneous lesions. The number of neutrophils is often great, and numerous abscesses may be present.[108]

Pathogenesis. Of great value is the demonstration of the spores of *B dermatitidis* in tissue sections either by direct immunofluorescence[109] or by immunoperoxidase.[110] The required antiserum is prepared in rabbits with pure cultures of fungi and is conjugated either with fluorescein isothiocyanate or with horseradish peroxide. The antiserum can be applied to fresh as well as to formalin-fixed, paraffin-embedded tissue sections. Prior staining with hematoxylin-eosin does not interfere with the procedure.

Corresponding antisera are valuable also for the demonstra-

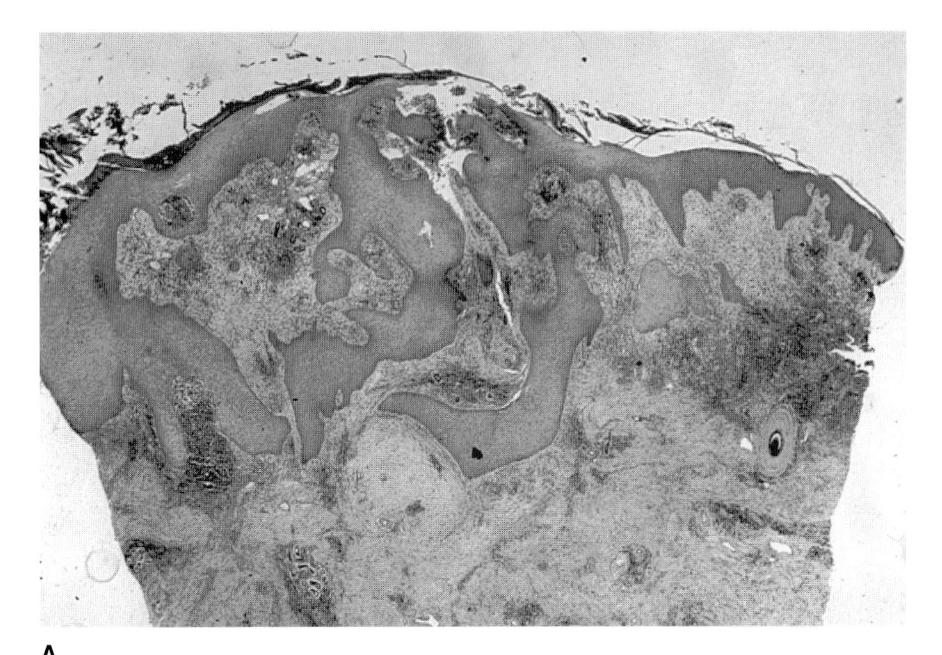

A

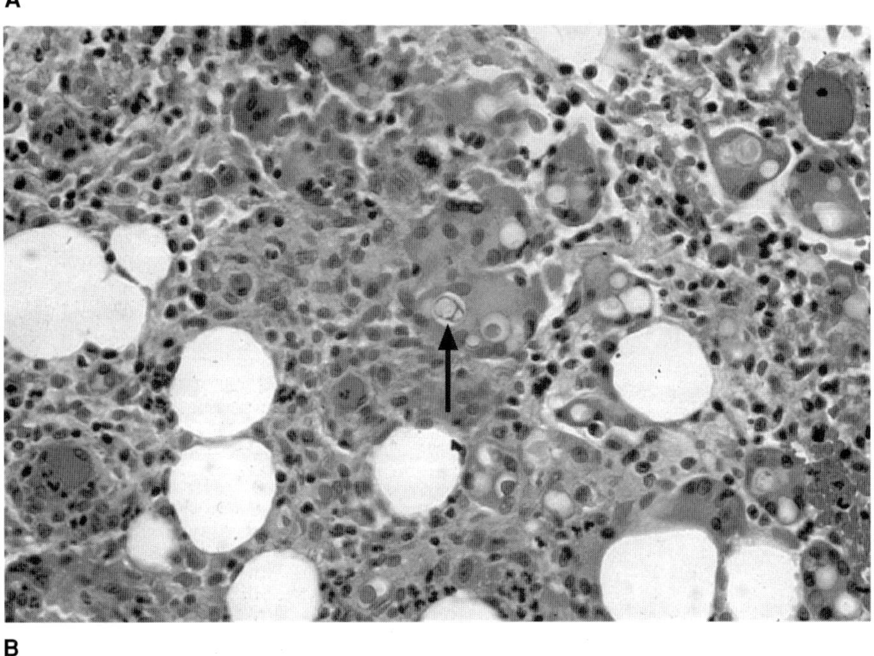

B

FIG. 23-10. North American blastomycosis
(**A**) H&E stain shows marked, pseudoepitheliomatous hyperplasia with intraepidermal microabscess formation. (**B**) H&E stain shows broad-based budding spore (*arrow*) in multinucleated giant cell.

tion of the spores of *Sporothrix schenckii*, *Cryptococcus neoformans*,[110] *Candida albicans*, *C tropicalis*, *C krusei*, *Aspergillus*, and *Histoplasma capsulatum*.[111]

Differential Diagnosis. The verrucous lesions of systemic blastomycosis must be differentiated from other deep fungal infections, tuberculosis verrucosa cutis, halogenodermas, and squamous cell carcinoma. Mucicarmine staining, which highlights the capsule of *C neoformans*, allows its differentiation from the spores of *B dermatitidis*, and the narrow-necked budding forms of *H capsulatum* can be distinguished from the broader-based buds of *B dermatitidis* without special stains. Tuberculosis verrucosa cutis shows no spores in the tissue, the number of neutrophils is smaller, and areas of caseation necrosis usually are present. Halogenodermas may be difficult to differentiate from a deep fungal infection without obvious organisms, but the presence of intraepidermal abscesses, a mixed dermal inflammatory infiltrate, and multinucleated giant cells is usually sufficient to rule out squamous cell carcinoma.

PARACOCCIDIOIDOMYCOSIS

Paracoccidioidomycosis, also called *South American blastomycosis* because it occurs almost exclusively in South and Central America, is a chronic granulomatous disease caused by *Paracoccidioides brasiliensis*.

P brasiliensis probably almost always gains entrance into the human body through inhalation and infects the lungs, where there is a subclinical infection that can be recognized only through a positive paracoccidioidin skin test.[112,113] The typical patient with clinical disease is an adult male with an indolent, slowly progressive course. The first clinical manifestation is usually lesions in the oropharynx and on the gingivae. The lesions in the mouth begin as papules and nodules that then ulcerate. Subsequently, extensive granulomatous, ulcerated lesions develop in the mouth, nose, larynx, and pharynx. Extensive cervical lymphadenopathy develops, with suppuration of some of the lymph nodes. The oral lesions may extend to the neighboring skin, with formation of similar granulomatous, ulcerated lesions around the mouth and nose.[112]

Through both lymphatic and hematogenous spread, the disease may subsequently involve many lymph nodes, both subcutaneous and visceral, and the lower gastrointestinal tract. In cases with wide dissemination, the lungs are clinically involved, presenting a picture greatly resembling chronic pulmonary tuberculosis.[114] Adrenal insufficiency due to destruction of the adrenal glands, uncommon in other systemic mycoses except histoplasmosis, is not infrequent.[115] Rarely, widely scattered cutaneous lesions resulting from hematogenous spread are observed during the stage of dissemination. The lesions may be papular, pustular, nodular, papillomatous, or ulcerated.[116]

The disease develops and disseminates more rapidly in children, the so-called subacute progressive juvenile form.[117] Although experience is limited, it appears that there is little effect on the course of paracoccidioidomycosis in early HIV infection,[118] but that HIV patients with severe immunosuppression are at risk for a more fulminant course.[119]

Histopathology. Examination of cutaneous or mucosal lesions reveals a granulomatous infiltrate showing epithelioid and giant cells in association with an acute inflammatory infiltrate and abscess formation.[120] Spores may lie within giant cells or free in the infiltrate, especially in the abscesses. They are best demonstrated with the PAS reaction or with methenamine silver. Pseudoepitheliomatous hyperplasia may be marked (Fig. 23-11A).

Many of the spores present in the tissue show only single, usually narrow-based buds or no buds at all.[114] In the rare spores with multiple budding, peripheral buds are distributed over the whole surface of the ball-shaped fungus cell (see Fig. 23-11B). Because of protrusion of the peripheral buds, such yeast cells in cross sections have the appearance of a marine pilot's wheel. Whereas nonbudding or singly budding spores measure from 6 to 20 μm in diameter, spores with multiple budding may measure up to 60 μm in size.

Occasionally, histologic examination does not reveal spores with multiple budding. The resemblance to North American blastomycosis may then be such that cultural studies are necessary for differentiation.[121]

LOBOMYCOSIS

Lobomycosis is an extremely indolent fungal infection characterized by asymptomatic, usually smooth, nodular lesions that resemble keloids on the ear, face, or extremity. The lesions may coalesce to form plaques, but generally are limited to one area. Although the lesions persist, the condition is limited to the skin, except for occasional involvement of a regional lymph node.[122] The infection, which is probably caused by a minor local injury, occurs sporadically in the South American tropics and in Panama.[123] The causative fungus is designated *Loboa loboi.*

Histopathology. The dermis shows an extensive infiltrate of macrophages and large giant cells separated from a usually atrophic epidermis by a Grenz zone. Scattered lymphocytes and plasma cells are present, but neutrophils are not typically present. Numerous fungus spores lie both within these cells and outside of them, and because the fungus does not stain with hematoxylin-eosin, there may be so many unstained areas that the section may have a sievelike appearance (Fig. 23-12).[123]

On staining with the PAS reaction or with methenamine silver, the fungus spores are on average 10 μm in diameter. They possess a thick capsule, about 1 μm in thickness, with a tip that gives the organisms a distinctive "lemonlike" appearance. The spores occasionally show single budding[124] and often form single chains joined together by small, tubular bridges.[125]

Pathogenesis. The macrophages contain abundant PAS-positive granular material that appears to consist of fragments of fungal capsules, indicating that the host macrophages are unable to digest the glycoproteins in the capsules.[124]

CHROMOBLASTOMYCOSIS

Chromoblastomycosis is a slowly progressive cutaneous mycosis caused by pigmented (dematiaceous) fungi that occur as round, nonbudding forms in tissue sections. Inasmuch as budding is absent, the designation chromo*blasto*mycosis is somewhat inappropriate. In the past, the related term *chromomycosis* has been used for these infections as well as for subcutaneous and cerebral infections by dematiaceous fungi in which hyphal forms almost always predominate. These two latter types of infections are clinically and histologically distinct and are best classified as phaeohyphomycoses.[126]

Chromoblastomycosis is usually caused by one of five closely related species: *Phialophora verrucosa, Fonsecaea pedrosoi, F compactum, Exophiala* (*Fonsecaea, Wangiella*) *dermatitidis,* and *Cladosporium carrionii.*[127] These fungi are saprophytes that can be found growing in soil, decaying vegetation, or rotten wood in subtropical and tropical countries. The primary lesion is thought to develop as a result of traumatic implantation of the fungus into the skin,[84,127,128] and the occasional occurrence of chromoblastomycosis in Finland and northern Russia is attributed to decaying wood in hot saunas.[129,130]

The cutaneous lesions are most commonly located on the lower extremities and consist of verrucous papules, nodules, and plaques that may itch. While some of the lesions heal with scarring, new ones may appear in the vicinity as a result of spreading of the fungus along superficial lymphatic vessels[131] or autoinoculation.[126] Lymphatic blockage with elephantiasis may occur.

Hematogenous dissemination may cause extensive cutaneous lesions,[130,132,133] but it is a rare event, even in immunocompromised persons, and the disease is not as aggressive as are some other fungal infections.[134]

Histopathology. The cutaneous type of chromoblastomycosis resembles North American blastomycosis in histologic appearance with a lichenoid-granulomatous inflammatory pattern. There are pseudoepitheliomatous epidermal hyperplasia and an extensive dermal infiltrate composed of many epithelioid histi-

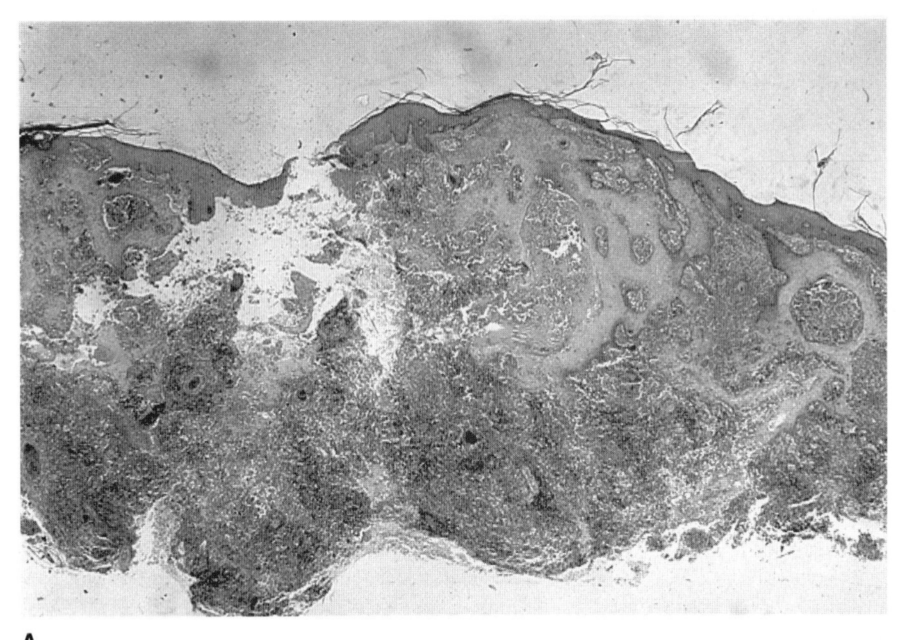

A

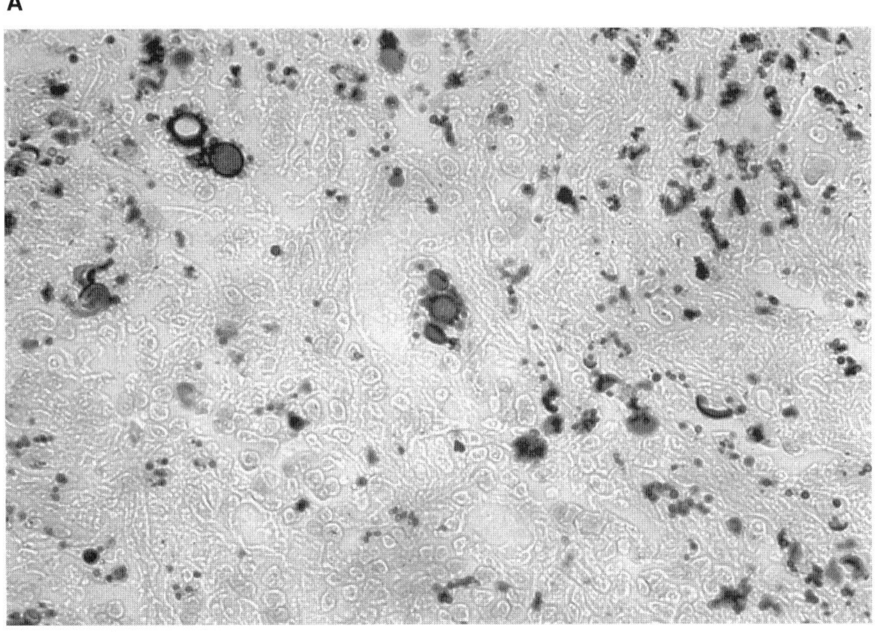

B

FIG. 23-11. Paracoccidioidomycosis
(**A**) H&E stain shows marked pseudoepitheliomatous epidermal hyperplasia with microabscess formation and a mixed dermal infiltrate. (**B**) GMS stain shows variably sized yeast, some with multiple buds.

ocytes,[135] as well as multinucleated giant cells, small abscesses and clusters of neutrophils, and variable numbers of lymphocytes, plasma cells, and eosinophils. Tuberculoid formations may be present, but caseation necrosis is absent.[136,137]

The causative organisms are found within giant cells as well as free in the tissue, especially in the abscesses. They appear as conspicuous, dark brown, thick-walled, ovoid or spheric spores varying in size from 6 to 12 μm[137] and lying either singly or in chains or clusters (Fig. 23-13). Because of their brown pigmentation, the spores can be easily seen without the use of special stains. Reproduction is by intracellular wall formation and septation, not by budding, and in some of the spores cross walls can be seen. In cases with marked hyperplasia of the epidermis, fungus spores can be seen, as in North American blastomycosis, within microabscesses or giant cells surrounded by epidermal proliferation; even transepidermal elimination of fungal spores may be observed, resulting in clinically visible black dots.[138,139]

Pathogenesis. Although percutaneous inoculation of the fungus is widely accepted as the mode of infection, the fact that the cutaneous manifestations show no chancriform syndrome but rather a granulomatous infiltrate resembling that of North American blastomycosis suggests that the cutaneous lesions of chromomycosis may arise by hematogenous dissemination from a silent primary pulmonary focus.[140] Though this view is supported by occasional reports of hematogenous dissemination (see earlier) and by the observation of multiple areas of calcification in the chest x-ray film of a patient with chromoblasto-

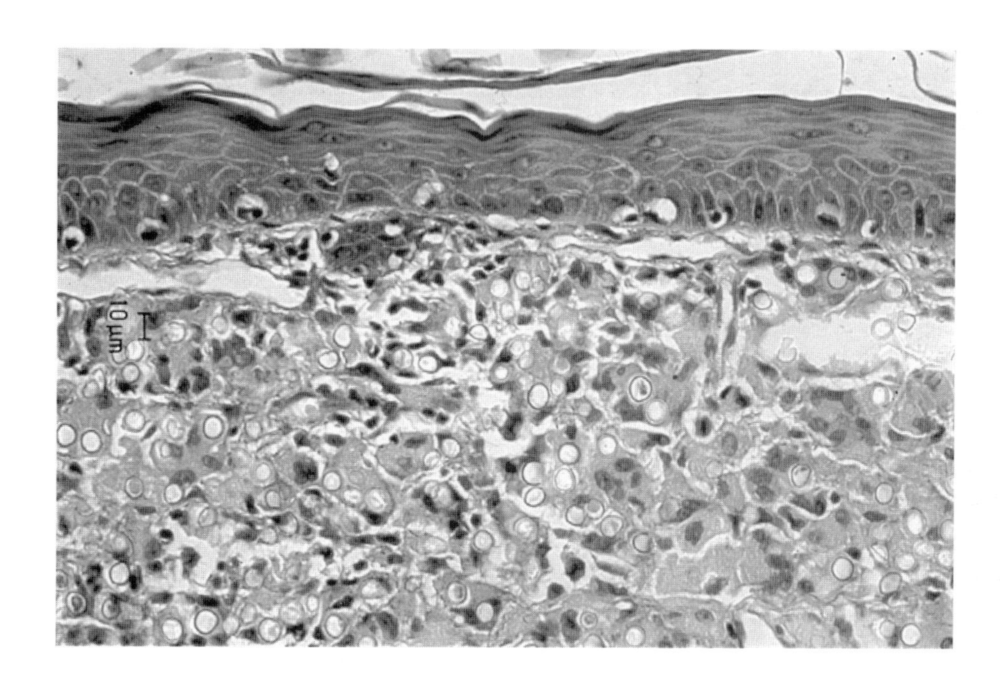

FIG. 23-12. Lobomycosis
A diffuse dermal infiltrate of multinucleated giant cells containing spores is present beneath a flattened epidermis (H&E stain).

mycosis,[133] convincing evidence is lacking. In support of the concept that cutaneous inoculation may cause cutaneous chromoblastomycosis, pigmented fungal elements were found on embedded wood splinters associated with a foreign-body reaction and in direct contact with the surrounding dermis in two patients,[141] and one patient developed classic cutaneous chromoblastomycosis caused by *F pedrosoi* after trauma with a tree branch containing the same organisms.[142]

COCCIDIOIDOMYCOSIS

Coccidioidomycosis is caused by *Coccidioides immitis*. Like blastomycosis, it occurs in three forms: primary cutaneous inoculation coccidioidomycosis, pulmonary coccidioidomycosis, and systemic coccidioidomycosis. The disease is endemic in certain regions of the Southwestern United States, especially in the San Joaquin and Sacramento valleys in southern California, in southern Arizona, and in the northwest of Mexico.[143] The fungus is resident in the soil of these areas, which have an arid or semiarid climate, and is inhaled with dust particles.

Primary cutaneous inoculation coccidioidomycosis is very rare. In a few instances, as in primary cutaneous inoculation blastomycosis, it has occurred as a laboratory or an autopsy room infection[144–146]; but, unlike primary cutaneous inoculation blastomycosis, it has also been found as a naturally occurring infection through injuries by thorns or splinters.[147–149] A tender, ulcerated nodule forms within 1 to 3 weeks at the site of inoculation and may enlarge into a granulomatous, ulcerated plaque. This is followed, as in the case of accidental inoculation with *B dermatitidis,* by regional lymphangitis and lymphadenitis. Healing usually takes place within a few months, but in one reported patient, meningitis developed, requiring prolonged intrathecal treatment with amphotericin B.[149]

Pulmonary coccidioidomycosis is the most common form of the infection; epidemiologic skin test studies suggest that between 30% and 90% of the population in the Southwestern United States have been infected.[150–152] Most immunocompetent infected individuals are asymptomatic, although about 40% will develop transient symptoms of an acute respiratory infection. The development of erythema nodosum is not uncommon, but most individuals recover without serious sequelae.[153] In 2% to 8% of the cases, however, the pulmonary lesions progress to chronic disease with cavity formation before finally healing.[147]

Systemic coccidioidomycosis follows the primary pulmonary infection in only about 1 of each 10,000 cases in otherwise immunocompetent, light-skinned persons. However, Mexicans are about 5 times, blacks 25 times, and Filipinos 175 times more likely to acquire systemic disease, which has a mortality rate of about 50% when untreated.[154] The risk of dissemination and a fatal outcome is greater in HIV-infected patients, particularly those with AIDS.[155,156] Disseminated coccidioidomycosis may occasionally represent the first manifestation of AIDS.[155]

Immunosuppressive therapy may cause activation of a latent pulmonary infection of coccidioidomycosis. Dissemination of the infection is frequently explosive and may be fatal.[154,157] Therefore, all patients with a history of travel or residence in endemic areas should receive a coccidioidin skin test and have a chest roentgenogram before immunosuppressive therapy is initiated.[143]

In systemic coccidioidomycosis, many organs, especially the meninges, the lungs, the bones, and the lymph nodes, may be involved. Coccidioidal fungemia often occurs in severe, acute forms of systemic coccidioidomycosis and is associated with a high mortality.[155]

Cutaneous lesions occur in 15% to 20% of the cases of systemic coccidioidomycosis.[158] They may consist of verrucous papules, nodules, or plaques, or of subcutaneous abscesses, which may break through the skin to form draining sinuses. One or a few cutaneous nodules or plaques may occasionally be the only clinical manifestation of systemic coccidioidomycosis, heralding a relatively good prognosis.[143,158] A rare manifestation is the sudden widespread appearance of small pustules on

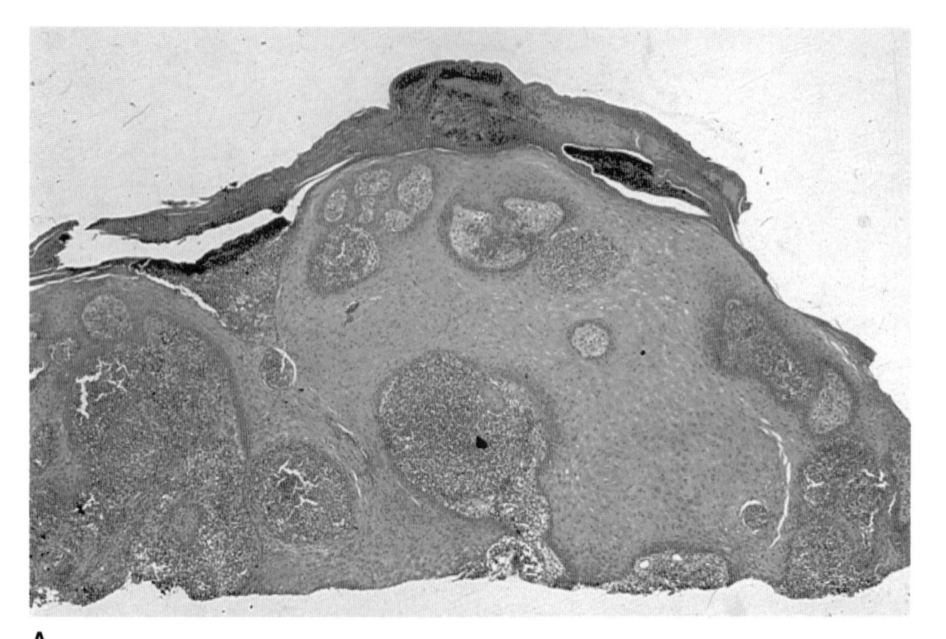

A

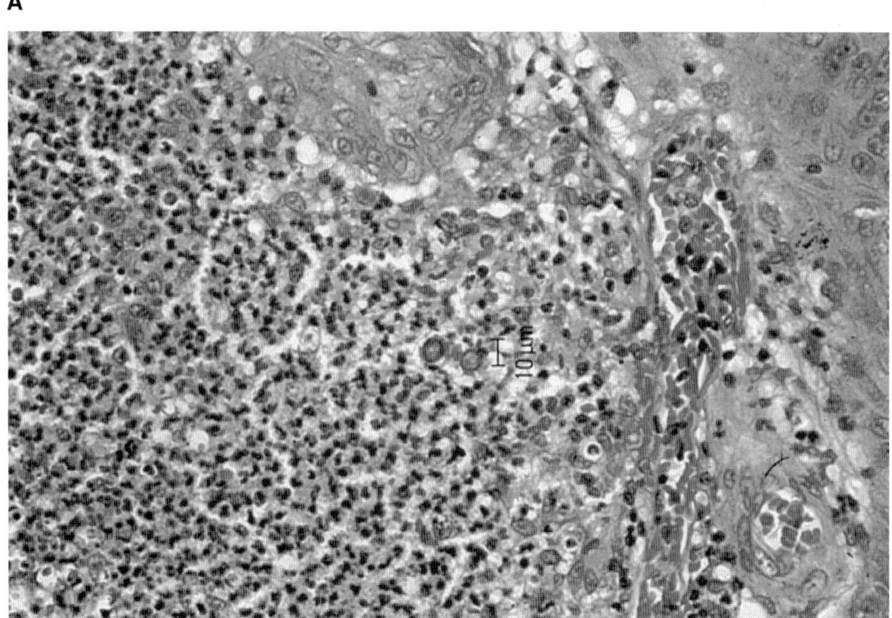

B

FIG. 23-13. Chromoblastomycosis
(**A**) H&E stain shows pseudoepitheliomatous epidermal hyperplasia with microabscess formation and a mixed inflammatory infiltrate. (**B**) Pigmented spores (adjacent to scale marker) resembling "copper pennies" are surrounded by a neutrophilic infiltrate (H&E stain).

an erythematous base,[159] just as has been described in North American blastomycosis.

Histopathology. In primary cutaneous inoculation coccidioidomycosis, one observes a dense inflammatory infiltrate of neutrophils, eosinophils, lymphoid cells, and plasma cells with an occasional giant cell. Small abscesses may be seen.[144] Spores, and in some cases also hyphae, are present.[158] The regional lymph nodes show a well-developed granulomatous reaction consisting of epithelioid and giant cells. Spores are found within and outside the giant cells.

The verrucous nodules and plaques of the skin in systemic coccidioidomycosis histologically resemble those of North American blastomycosis (Fig. 23-14A). However, they show less of a tendency toward abscess formation, and caseation necrosis may occur.[107] The causative organisms are found as spores free in the tissue and within multinucleated giant cells. As a rule, they are present in large numbers.

The subcutaneous abscesses show a central area of necrosis surrounded by a granulomatous infiltrate that is tuberculoid in type and composed of lymphoid cells, plasma cells, epithelioid cells, and some giant cells. Numerous spores are present extracellularly as well as intracellularly in the giant cells.[107] The pustules seen in a few cases show the presence of spores within them.[159]

The nodose skin lesions occurring in primary pulmonary coccidioidomycosis have the same histologic appearance as those in idiopathic erythema nodosum.[160]

The spores of *Coccidioides immitis* vary in size from 10 to 80 μm (Fig. 23-14B), the average size being about 40 μm. Thus the fungi of *Coccidioides* are much larger than those of *Blasto-*

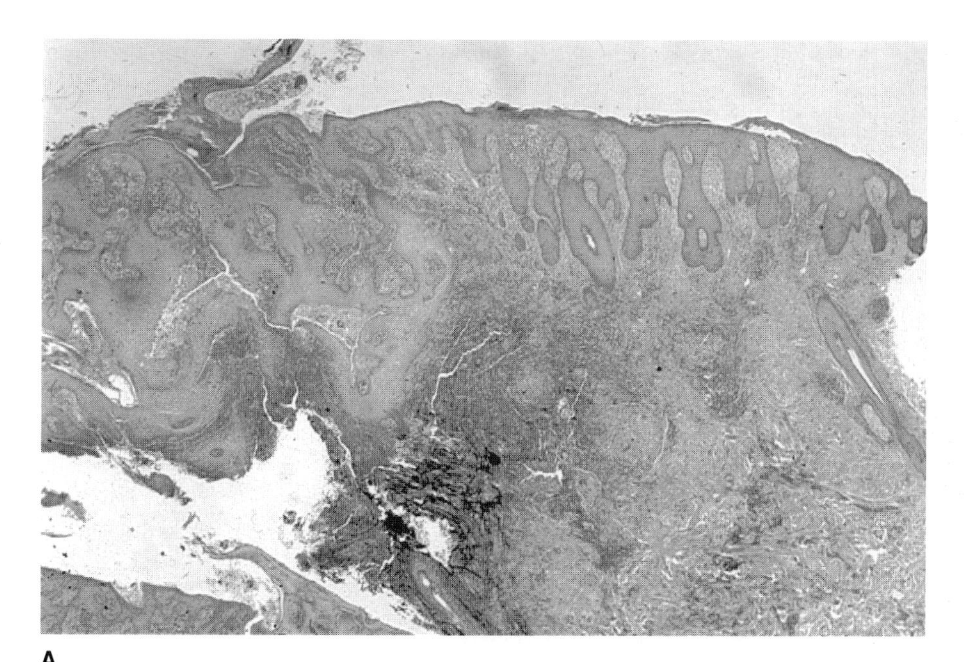

A

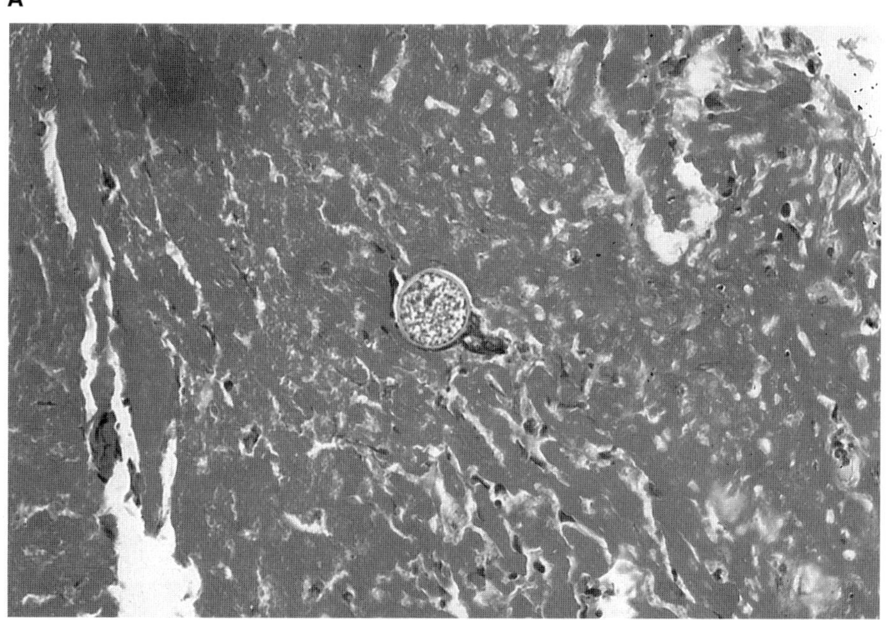

B

FIG. 23-14. Coccidioidomycosis (**A**) The low-power pattern is similar to that of North American blastomycosis with pseudoepitheliomatous epidermal hyperplasia and a mixed inflammatory infiltrate (H&E stain). (**B**) A large round thick-walled spore with granular cytoplasm is present in a background of necrotic tissue (H&E stain).

myces, Cryptococcus, or *Phialophora*. The spores are round and thick-walled and have a granular cytoplasm. Multiplication takes place by the formation of endospores, which may be seen lying inside the larger spores. The endospores are released into the tissue by rupture of the spore wall. Endospores may measure up to 10 μm in diameter.

Pathogenesis. The coccidioidin skin test, which consists of the intradermal injection of 0.1 mL of a 1:100 dilution of coccidioidin, is of value in distinguishing between primary pulmonary infection and systemic infection. The test converts from negative to positive within a few weeks of the primary pulmonary infection and remains positive in patients with adequate immunity. Patients with erythema multiforme or nodose lesions are exquisitely sensitive to coccidioidin, and even higher dilutions have been recommended for use in such cases.[161] In contrast, patients with disseminated disease tend to have a persistently negative skin test.[146]

CRYPTOCOCCOSIS

Cryptococcosis occurs throughout the world. *Cryptococcus neoformans*, the fungus that causes cryptococcosis, is found in the excreta of birds, mainly pigeons and chickens, and in soil contaminated by them. *C neoformans* is spread by aerosol, and transient colonization of the respiratory tract and skin of humans is not rare.[162] Primary cutaneous (inoculation) cryptococcosis is extremely rare.[163,164] The organism generally enters the body through the respiratory tract, where it can cause symptomatic or asymptomatic infection, either of which may be followed by hematogenous spread.[165] Although clinical disease occurs in some apparently normal individuals, it usually develops in immunocompromised hosts, especially those with AIDS,[166] but also in patients taking corticosteroids[167–169] and in patients with hematopoietic malignancies[170,171] or sarcoidosis.[171–173]

In patients with active disease, cryptococcosis often manifests itself as a widespread systemic disease with predominant involvement of the brain and meninges, and the presence of the fungus in the spinal fluid. In addition, there may be osseous lesions and involvement of the kidneys and prostate. Cutaneous lesions are found in 10% to 15% of the cases of systemic cryptococcosis.[174] In rare instances, lesions of the oral mucosa also occur.[170] Without adequate treatment, mortality with the systemic form is 70% to 80%; untreated cerebromeningeal cryptococcosis is almost invariably fatal. Cryptococcemia is an extremely grave prognostic sign.[175]

In some instances of systemic cryptococcosis, central nervous system involvement is not seen, and there are only one or a few lesions in the skin, the lymph nodes, bones, or the eyes.[165] In cases in which only cutaneous lesions are present, the disease may take a benign course, ending with healing of the lesions, even without treatment.[176,177] However, cutaneous lesions may be the presenting sign of systemic cryptococcosis and may be followed by wide dissemination of the disease with a fatal ending.[165,177]

The appearance of the cutaneous lesions is not diagnostic and is quite variable. The lesions may consist of papules, pustules, herpetiform vesicles, nodules, infiltrated plaques, subcutaneous swellings or abscesses, or ulcers.[174] Lesions resembling those of molluscum contagiosum, Kaposi's sarcoma, or acne have been described in patients with AIDS.[178–180] In infections limited to the skin, generally only one or possibly two lesions are present, but in cases with widespread systemic infection, there are often multiple cutaneous lesions.[168–170,174,181]

Cryptococcal cellulitis is a variant form that may occasionally be limited to the skin. This form has an abrupt onset and spreads rapidly. It is seen only in markedly immunosuppressed hosts, especially in renal transplant patients.[182] There may be multiple sites of involvement.[183]

Histopathology. Two types of histologic reaction to infection with *Cryptococcus neoformans* may occur in the skin as well as elsewhere: gelatinous and granulomatous. Both types may be seen in the same skin lesion.[169,184] Gelatinous lesions show numerous organisms in aggregates and only very little tissue reaction (Fig. 23-15A). In contrast, granulomatous lesions show a pronounced tissue reaction consisting of histiocytes, giant cells, lymphoid cells, and fibroblasts; areas of necrosis may also be seen. The organisms are present in a much smaller number than in gelatinous lesions. They are found mainly within giant cells and histiocytes but are encountered also free in the tissue.[185]

Cryptococcus neoformans, a round to ovoid spore, measures from 4 to 12 μm in diameter in the gelatinous reaction but often only 2 to 4 μm in the granulomatous reaction (Fig. 23-15B).[185] The spore stains with the PAS reaction and the methenamine silver stain and shows a dark brown or black color with the Fontana-Masson stain, which completely disappears with melanin bleach.[186] Like *Blastomyces dermatitidis,* it multiplies by budding. Usually it is surrounded by a wide capsule. The capsule does not stain with hematoxylin-eosin or with the PAS reaction, but because of the presence of acid mucopolysaccharides, it stains metachromatically purple with methylene blue,[187] blue with alcian blue,[188] and red with mucicarmine.[189] When the alcian blue stain and the PAS reaction are combined, the yeast cell stains red and the surrounding capsule blue. In areas in which *Cryptococcus neoformans* has a wide, gelatinous capsule, the inflammatory infiltrate is minimal, leading to the so-called gelatinous reaction. However, yeast cells that do not form a capsule elicit an intense inflammatory reaction.[186]

Cryptococcal cellulitis shows nonspecific acute and chronic inflammation in which cryptococcal organisms can be demonstrated with the PAS and mucicarmine stains.[182]

Pathogenesis. Cryptococcus neoformans is inhaled as a relatively small, nonencapsulated organism measuring approximately 3 μm in diameter. Under favorable nutrient conditions in the human host, the size of the organism increases up to 12 μm, and a wide gelatinous capsule forms. The lack of a tissue reaction to encapsulated *Cryptococcus neoformans* is best explained by the fact that the thick capsule prevents contact of the organism with the host tissue and thus inhibits phagocytosis of the organism.[185] Failure of the organism to form a capsule probably is the result of a defect in one of its metabolic pathways.[186]

On electron microscopy, the mucinous capsule of *Cryptococcus neoformans* is seen to consist of radially arranged fibrillary material, with the fibrils intertwining and having a beaded appearance.[190]

Ever since cases of cryptococcosis with only one or a few cutaneous lesions have been described, some authors have assumed that a purely cutaneous form of cryptococcosis produced by cutaneous inoculation exists.[191,192] However, the fact that purely cutaneous lesions show no chancriform syndrome with regional lymphadenopathy speaks against the theory of primary inoculation of the skin.[168] It has been recommended that all cases that seem to be purely cutaneous cryptococcosis should be considered potentially disseminated.[193] Cultural studies should include the spinal fluid, sputum, prostatic fluid, and urine to rule out disseminated disease.[167]

Differential Diagnosis. In the granulomatous type of reaction, *Cryptococcus neoformans* may have no capsule, may be small, with an average diameter of only 3 μm, and is found largely within macrophages and giant cells. Histologic differentiation from *Blastomyces dermatitidis, Histoplasma capsulatum,* and other fungi may then be difficult; but only *Crytococcus neoformans* stains black with the Fontana-Masson stain.[186]

HISTOPLASMOSIS

Histoplasmosis is caused by the fungus *Histoplasma capsulatum. H capsulatum* and histoplasmosis are found throughout the world, but the largest endemic focus is in the central eastern United States, especially the Ohio and lower Mississippi river valleys, where 85% to 90% of the population have positive skin tests for histoplasmin.[194] It has been estimated that 40 million persons have undergone pulmonary infection with *H capsulatum,* and that there are 200,000 new cases annually in the United States.[195,196]

Like blastomycosis and coccidioidomycosis, histoplasmosis may occur in three forms: primary cutaneous inoculation histoplasmosis, primary pulmonary histoplasmosis caused by inhalation, and disseminated histoplasmosis.

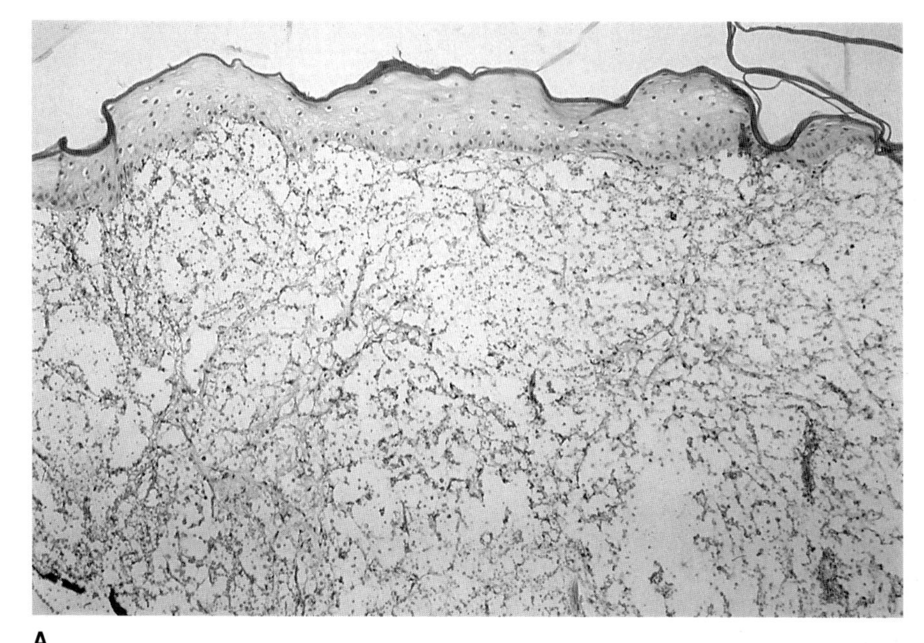

A

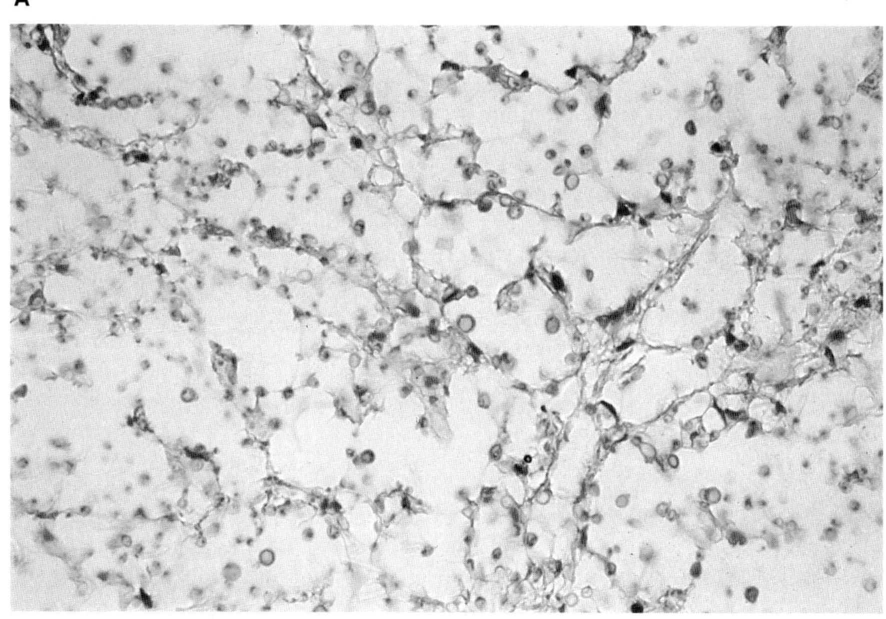

B

FIG. 23-15. Cryptococcosis (**A**) H&E stain shows spores surrounded by wide capsules with relatively little inflammatory reaction. (**B**) Spores, but not their capsules, can be visualized in routine stained sections (H&E stain).

Primary cutaneous inoculation histoplasmosis, a very rare event, is benign and self-limited in duration. It generally occurs as a laboratory infection and presents as a chancriform syndrome, with a nodule or ulcer at the site of inoculation and associated lymphangitis and lymphadenitis.[197,198]

Primary pulmonary histoplasmosis, the common form of infection, is usually asymptomatic, although acute pulmonary histoplasmosis with symptoms resembling those of influenza may develop in a minority of patients. Chronic pulmonary histoplasmosis usually occurs in patients with preexisting lung disease and may result in the formation of cavities.[194] It develops in about 1 of 2000 infections, resembles pulmonary tuberculosis in its symptoms, and may end fatally unless treated.

Before the advent of HIV, disseminated histoplasmosis developed in only 1 of 50,000 infections[199] and was usually found in infants, in patients with lymphoma,[200,201] or in those receiving immunosuppressive treatment.[202] Although not as frequent in the general AIDS population as coccidioidomycosis and cryptococcosis,[203] disseminated histoplasmosis can be the most frequent opportunistic infection in AIDS patients living in highly endemic areas.[204,205]

Disseminated histoplasmosis presents a variable clinical picture, depending on the degree of parasitization. Cases with severe degrees of parasitization (acute disseminated disease) occur principally in infants and immunosuppressed patients, and may be fatal. There is often high, persistent fever and extensive involvement of the reticuloendothelial system with hepatosplenomegaly; anemia, leukocytopenia, and thrombocytopenia may also be seen. Cases with moderate degrees of parasitization (subacute disseminated disease) occur in both adults and infants, who, if adequately treated, may survive. Fever, hepatosplenomegaly, and bone marrow depression are mild or moderate. Adrenal involvement leading to adrenal insufficiency, as well as gastrointestinal ulceration, meningitis, and endocarditis, are common. Cases with mild degrees of parasitization (chronic disseminated disease) are associated with destructive focal lesions in a number of organs, and occur almost exclusively in adults. There may or may not be fever, hepatosplenomegaly, bone marrow depression, adrenal insufficiency, meningitis, or endocarditis. In the chronic disseminated form, the response to treatment generally is good.[206] If no cutaneous or oral lesions are present, the most useful diagnostic method is a bone marrow biopsy and occasionally also biopsy of the liver or of a palpable lymph node.[202]

Cutaneous lesions occur in only 6% of patients with disseminated histoplasmosis, but may rarely be the presenting sign.[206–208] Cutaneous lesions occur in a wide variety of forms, none of which can be said to be characteristic. Most commonly they consist of primary ulcers,[207] often with annular, heaped-up borders.[209] They may also consist of papules, nodules, or large plaquelike lesions.[206,210] Papules may umbilicate, causing a resemblance to lesions of molluscum contagiosum.[211] Lesions may be purpuric or crusted, or may develop pustular caps and ulcerate.[209] There may be tender, red nodules due to panniculitis.[212] A rare cutaneous manifestation is a generalized pruritic erythroderma.[213,214] In addition, there may be a number of nonspecific cutaneous manifestations associated with histoplasmosis, including erythema nodosum and erythema multiforme.[215]

In contrast to the rarity of cutaneous lesions, lesions of the oral mucosa occur in about half of all cases of disseminated histoplasmosis and are not infrequently the presenting sign of the disease.[206] Lesions of the oral mucosa often start as painless papular swellings and usually ulcerate. The contiguous skin may also be involved. Biopsy of a mucosal or cutaneous lesion may be the most rapid method of arriving at a specific diagnosis of disseminated histoplasmosis, and may allow for the rapid institution of lifesaving therapy.[216]

Histopathology. Histologic examination of a lesion of primary cutaneous inoculation histoplasmosis stained with methenamine silver shows numerous yeast cells within the cytoplasm of histiocytes.[198]

In acute disseminated histoplasmosis, usually seen in infants or immunocompromised patients, lesions consist mostly of histiocytes heavily parasitized by organisms, with relatively little tissue reaction or infiltration by other inflammatory cells. Cutaneous lesions in the chronic form of the disease tend to be composed of better-differentiated macrophages with fewer organisms.[206] A suppurative granulomatous pattern may develop, especially in ulcerated lesions. There may be foci of necrosis, and giant cells may also be present.[209] Although well-developed tubercles are characteristic of pulmonary histoplasmosis, they are unusual in the skin. Oral lesions, especially when ulcerated, may show a more mixed infiltrate with neutrophils and eosinophils.[217]

The diagnostic feature in all types of cutaneous lesions is the presence of spores of *H capsulatum* within the cytoplasm of macrophages and occasionally also within giant cells.[210, 218] Similarly, in *Histoplasma* panniculitis, numerous spores of *H capsulatum* are seen within the cytoplasm of macrophages.[212]

The spores of *H capsulatum* usually can be recognized in sections stained with hematoxylin and eosin, Gram stain, or a Giemsa stain (Fig 23-16). They appear as round or oval bodies surrounded by a clear space that was originally interpreted as a capsule, giving rise to the name *H capsulatum*. The spores, not including the clear space surrounding them, measure from 2 to 4 μm in diameter. Silver impregnation stains and electron microscopic studies show, however, that *H capsulatum* does not possess a capsule and that the inner portion of the clear space represents the cell wall of the fungus, whereas the outer part of the clear space forms a halo separating the cell wall of the fungus from the cytoplasm of the macrophage.[218]

Pathogenesis. On *electron microscopy,* it can be seen that each spore of *H capsulatum,* including its halo, is located within a phagosome that is lined by a trilaminar membrane. The halo is partly filled with granular, cytoplasmic material.[218]

H capsulatum is a dimorphous fungus that grows in culture at temperatures below 35°C and on natural substrates in soil as a mycelial fungus elaborating macroaleuriospores (8–16 μm) and microaleuriospores (2–5 μm). When inhaled, the latter sprout and transform into small budding yeasts that are 2 to 5 μm in di-

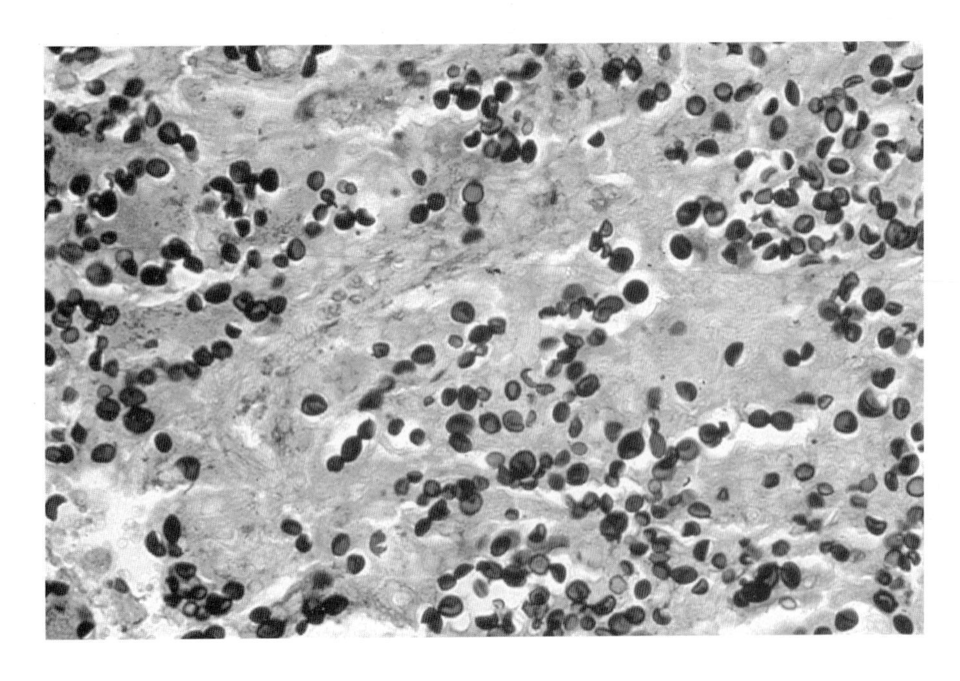

FIG. 23-16. Histoplasmosis Large spores of *H capsulatum* var. *duboisii* are seen extracellularly and in giant cells (GMS stain).

ameter. In cultures at a temperature of 37°C, the organism also grows in the yeastlike form.[219]

Differential Diagnosis. The histologic appearance of histoplasmosis, characterized by the presence of parasitized macrophages within a chronic inflammatory infiltrate, is much like that of rhinoscleroma, granuloma inguinale, and cutaneous leishmaniasis. For their differential diagnosis, see Table 24-1. It may be pointed out that, in addition, only in histoplasmosis is the causative organism stained by the usual fungal stains, such as the PAS reaction and methenamine silver. For a discussion of differential diagnosis from cryptococcosis, see page 537.

African Histoplasmosis

In addition to classical histoplasmosis caused by *H capsulatum*, there is a form of histoplasmosis that is caused by *H capsulatum* var. *duboisii*, and that has been called African histoplasmosis because it occurs almost exclusively in Central Africa. It usually occurs as a relatively indolent form involving the skin as well as the subcutaneous tissue, bones, and lymph nodes.[220,221] This organism relatively rarely causes a disseminated form of disease that involves many internal organs and that may be fatal, thus resembling more classical disseminated histoplasmosis.[222]

The cutaneous lesions may be one, a few, or many. They consist of papules, nodules, and plaques that often ulcerate.[223] There may be large, subcutaneous granulomas that develop into fluctuant, nontender abscesses.[220] Purulent bone lesions may result in draining sinus tracts extending through the skin.[221]

Histopathology. The cutaneous lesions show a dense, mixed cellular infiltrate containing numerous giant cells and scattered histiocytes, lymphocytes, and plasma cells. There are focal aggregates of neutrophils forming small abscesses.[223] Numerous yeast cells, 8 to 15 μm in diameter, are present mainly in the giant cells but also in histiocytes and extracellulary.[221]

Pathogenesis. In spite of the fact that African histoplasmosis differs in its clinical character and in the size of the organism from classic histoplasmosis, it is clear that *H capsulatum* and *H duboisii* are variants of the same species, since, after prolonged in vitro growth at 37°C, the small yeast cells of *H capsulatum* can assume the same size as those of *H duboisii*.[221] The primary portal of entry for African histoplasmosis is not known.

SPOROTRICHOSIS

Surveys with the sporotrichin skin test, showing a positive reaction in up to 10% of the population in certain areas, suggest that many infections with *Sporothrix schenckii* are minor or asymptomatic, and not recognized clinically.[224,225] Clinical sporotrichosis usually occurs as one of two primary cutaneous forms, either the fixed cutaneous or the lymphocutaneous form. Both result from direct inoculation at a site of minor trauma. Although the infection may rarely disseminate from either form by autoinnoculation to other skin sites or by hematogenous spread,[226–228] systemic sporotrichosis more commonly follows pulmonary infection. Development of systemic sporotrichosis, although rare, occurs particularly in persons with a depressed immune response, such as patients with lymphoma or persons receiving corticosteroids for a prolonged period of time.[229] *S schenckii* is not a common opportunist in HIV-infected individuals, but disseminated sporotrichosis has been seen in a few patients with AIDS.[230]

The lymphocutaneous form of sporotrichosis starts with a painless papule that grows into an ulcer, usually on a finger or hand. Subsequently, a chain of asymptomatic nodules appears along the lymph vessel draining the area. These lymphatic nodules may undergo suppuration with subsequent ulceration.

In the fixed cutaneous form, a solitary plaque or occasionally a group of lesions is seen, most commonly on an arm or the face. It may show superficial crusting[231] or a verrucous surface.[232–235] There is no tendency toward lymphatic spread.

Systemic sporotrichosis may be unifocal or multifocal, and usually develops subsequent to pulmonary infection. Unifocal systemic sporotrichosis may affect the lungs, a single joint or symmetric joints, the genitourinary tract, or, rarely, the brain.[236] Chronic pulmonary sporotrichosis greatly resembles pulmonary tuberculosis.[237] Multifocal systemic sporotrichosis nearly always shows widely scattered cutaneous lesions, which start as nodules or as subcutaneous abscesses and undergo ulceration.[238] In addition, one usually observes involvement of the lungs[228] or of several joints of the extremities.[238] The predilection of *S schenckii* for cooler parts of the body, such as the skin, lungs, and joints of the extremities has been attributed to the fact that the organism grows best at temperatures less than 37°C.

Histopathology. Primary cutaneous lesions of sporotrichosis that are only a few weeks old and are ulcerated usually show a nonspecific inflammatory infiltrate composed of neutrophils, lymphoid cells, plasma cells, and histiocytes.[11] If the lesion is older and possesses an elevated border or appears verrucous, small, intraepidermal abscesses are often found in the hyperplastic epidermis, and the dermis shows, scattered through a lymphoplasmacytic infiltrate, small abscesses, eosinophils, giant cells, and small granulomas often associated with asteroid bodies.[11,232,234] Later, through coalescence, a characteristic arrangement of the infiltrate in three zones may develop. These include a central "suppurative" zone composed of neutrophils; surrounding it, a "tuberculoid" zone with epithelioid cells and multinucleated histiocytes; and peripheral to it, a "round cell" zone of lymphoid cells and plasma cells.[232,238]

The lymphatic nodules of lymphocutaneous sporotrichosis, as well as the cutaneous nodules of multifocal systemic sporotrichosis, at first show scattered granulomas within an inflammatory infiltrate, predominantly in the deep dermis and subcutaneous fat.[232,239] These enlarge and run together to form irregularly shaped suppurative granulomata, and eventually a large abscess surrounded by zones of histiocytes and lymphocytes as described for primary lesions.[232]

In many instances, it is not possible to recognize the causative organisms of *S schenckii* in tissue sections, particularly in the two common forms, the lymphocutaneous and the fixed cutaneous forms. This seems to be true especially in cases of sporotrichosis reported from the United States[240] and from Europe.[239] In these areas, negative findings are common even with diastase digestion of glycogen granules prior to staining of sections with the PAS reaction. Nor has staining with methenamine silver increased the frequency of positive findings.[239] Even in cases with positive findings, numerous sections often have to be examined before one or a few organisms are visualized.[241] Immunohistochemical staining using primary antibodies directed against *S schenckii* may increase the percentage of cases in which the organism can be demonstrated to 83%, more than double that achieved with ordinary histochemical methods.[242] In addition, there are apparently significant geographic differences, since, in a series of cutaneous sporotrichosis reported from Japan, 98% of the cases showed spores in tissue sections on staining with the PAS reaction.[243] If present, the spores of *S schenckii* appear as round to oval bodies 4 to 6 μm in diameter that stain more strongly at the periphery than in the center (Fig. 23-17).[241] Single or occasionally multiple buds are present. In some instances, small, cigar-shaped bodies up to 8 μm long are also present.[227,238] In only very few cases can clumps of branching, nonseptate hyphae be demonstrated.[227,238]

Asteroid bodies may be seen in sporotrichosis as well as in a number of other infectious processes, and in sarcoidosis. Asteroid bodies are visible in sections stained with hematoxylin-eosin, and in sporotrichosis consist a central spore 5 to 10 μm in diameter surrounded by radiating elongations of a homogeneous eosinophilic material. The phenomenon of radiating eosinophilic material found around infectious agents, described in sporotrichosis by Splendore[244] and in schistosomiasis by Hoeppli,[245] has been thought to represent deposition of antigen-antibody complexes and debris from host inflammatory cells.[246] Measurements of the greatest diameter of asteroid bodies in sporotrichosis vary from 7 to 25 μm, with a mean of 20 μm.[232] Asteroid bodies have been observed in only a few cases of sporotrichosis occurring in the United States, and it may be difficult to demonstrate the central spore.[247,248] However, asteroid bodies are found frequently in cases of sporotrichosis from South Africa,[232] Japan,[243] and Australia,[249] with an incidence varying from 39% to 65%.

Pathogenesis. S schenckii occurs throughout the world and is commonly contracted through exposure to vegetal matter, often a splinter or thorn, although transmission by insects and animals has been reported.[250] In nearly all cases of sporotri-

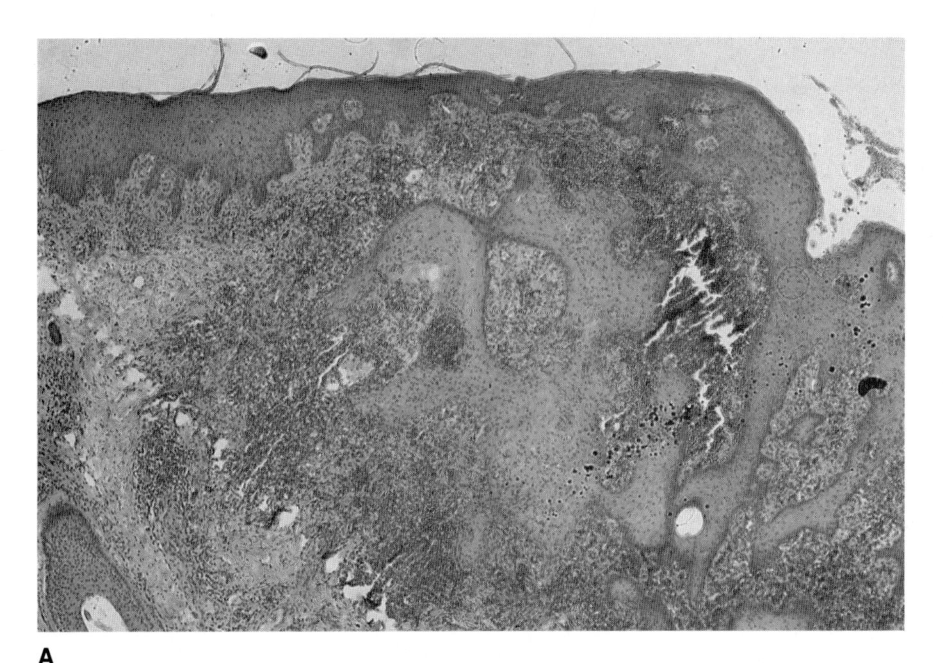

A

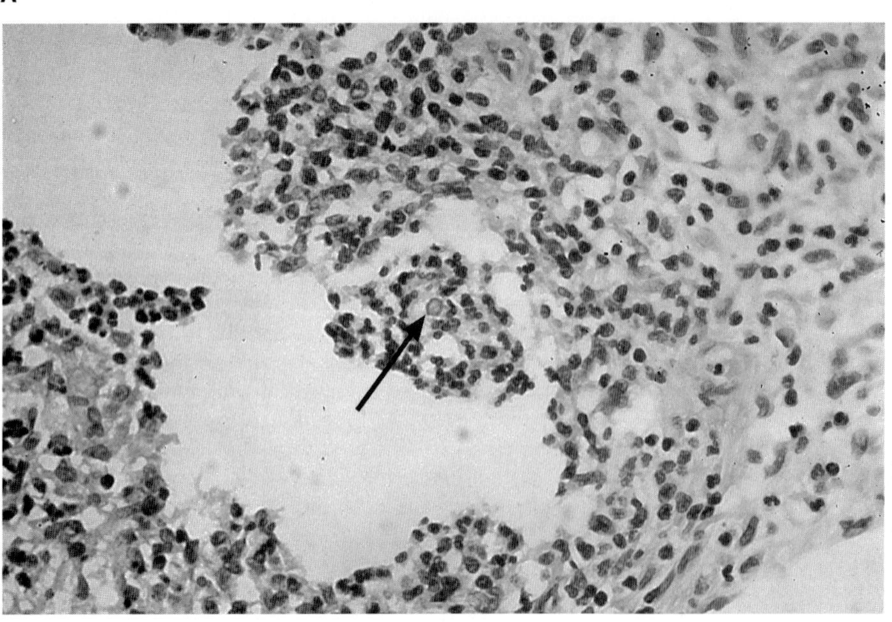

B

FIG. 23-17. Sporotrichosis
(**A**) H&E stain shows pseudoepitheliomatous epidermal hyperplasia with microabscess formation. (**B**) H&E stain. A round spore, staining more darkly at the periphery than centrally, is surrounded by a neutrophilic infiltrate.

chosis, even in those without demonstrable fungi in the tissue, *S schenkii* can be grown easily on Sabouraud medium. The fungus is dimorphic: At room temperature, it grows in a mycelial form with conidiophores bearing conidia as a "bouquet" at the tip; at 37°C, it grows in a yeast form.[240] At 39°C, there is no growth, a fact that has led to the use of local thermotherapy.[239,243]

Differential Diagnosis. If the fungus is not found in sections, a diagnosis of sporotrichosis can only be suspected; however, it can be excluded in dubious cases by a negative cutaneous sporotrichin test, which is almost always positive except in cases of disseminated disease.[239] The subcutaneous abscesses of tularemia and of infections with *Mycobacterium marinum* may have the same histologic appearance as the cutaneous and subcutaneous nodules and abscesses of sporotrichosis, and must be excluded.

EUMYCETOMA (FUNGAL MYCETOMA)

A number of fungi and filamentous bacteria may cause an indolent local infection, characterized by induration associated with draining sinuses. These diverse agents may have clinically identical presentations that have been collectively called mycetoma. The term *actinomycetoma* refers to such infections when they are caused by filamentous bacteria; they are discussed further in Chapter 17. *Eumycetoma*, however, is caused by a group of true fungi with thick septate hyphae, including *Petriellidium boydii* (*Allescheria boydii, Pseudoallescheria boydii*), *Madurella grisea,* and *M mycetomatis* (*mycetomi*).[251,252] Differentiation between actinomycetoma and eumycetoma is important because they respond to different treatments.

These infections occur most often in tropical and subtropical

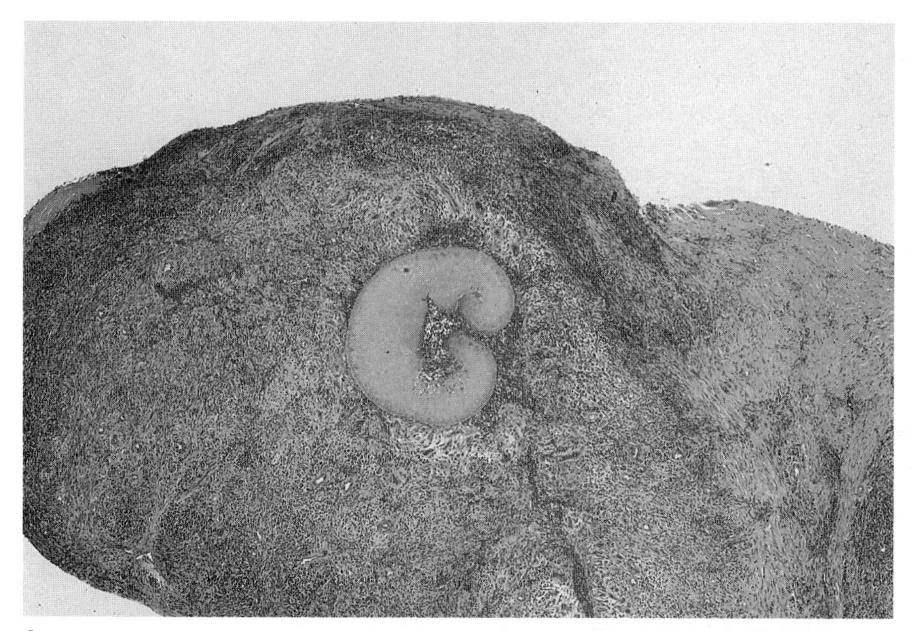

A

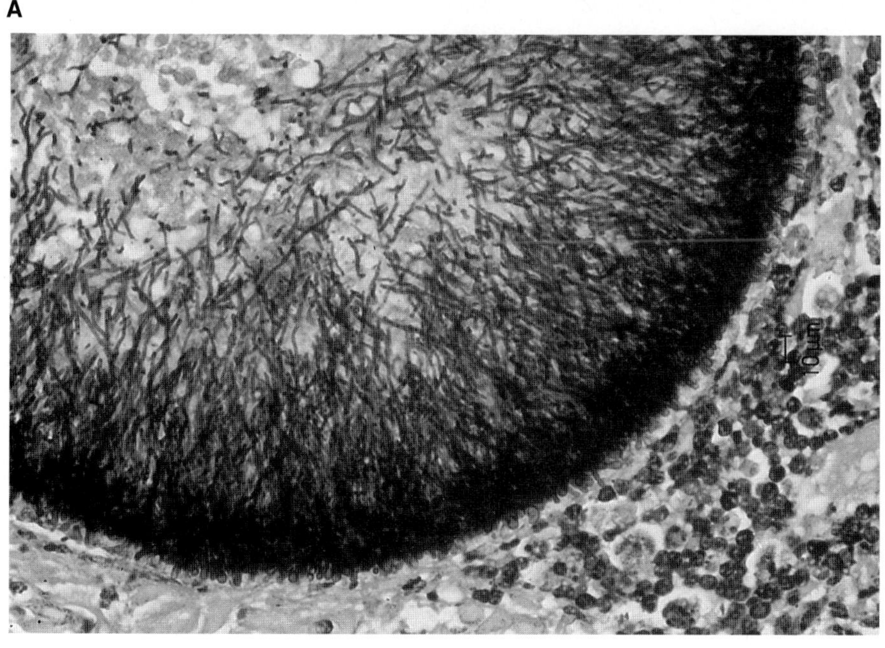

B

FIG. 23-18. Eumycetoma (**A**) H&E stain shows a "sulfur granule" in a purulent area of granulation tissue. (**B**) The sulfur granule is composed largely of septate hyphae of *P boydii* (GMS stain).

locations and are caused by subcutaneous inoculation at a site of trauma, often in the foot of unshod individuals; thus the term *Madura foot* has been used synonymously with mycetoma. There is no obvious association with immunosuppression. Although much more common in tropical regions, eumycetoma is seen occasionally in the United States, where the most common cause is *Petriellidium boydii*.[253] Eumycetoma is a persistent, relentlessly progressive local infection without a tendency to spread systemically. It starts as a subcutaneous nodule or nodules, usually on a foot but occasionally on a hand.[254] The nodules eventuate in abscesses and draining sinuses. Gradually, the muscles and tendons are damaged, and osteomyelitis develops. So-called sulfur granules or grains, which are tightly knit clusters of organisms, are discharged from the draining sinuses. These granules are black in cases of eumycetoma caused by the dematiaceous fungi *Madurella grisea* and *Madurella mycetomatis*,[255,256] whereas they are colorless in eumycetoma caused by *Petriellidium boydii*.[257]

Histopathology. Histologic examination of the indurated skin shows extensive granulation tissue containing abscesses that may lead into sinuses. The granulation tissue is nonspecific in appearance. In the early phase of the disease, the tissue surrounding the abscesses is composed of lymphoid cells, plasma cells, histiocytes, and fibroblasts, whereas in the late phase fibroblasts may predominate. The diagnosis can be established only by finding the "sulfur granules" (Fig. 23-18A). Because they occur almost exclusively in abscesses or sinuses, an area containing purulent material should be chosen as the site for biopsy.

Most granules measure between 0.5 and 2.0 mm in diameter,

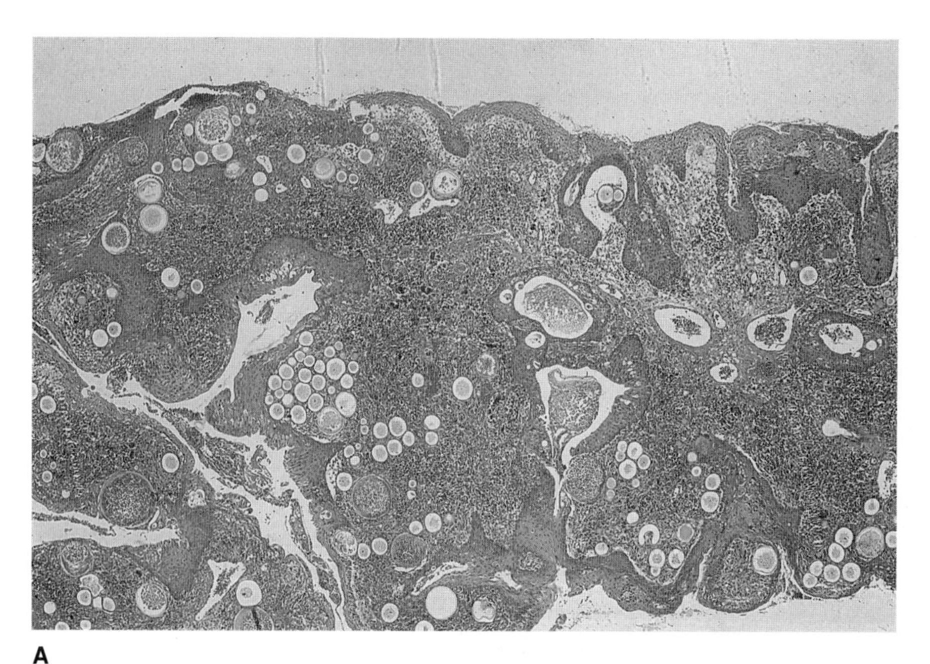

A

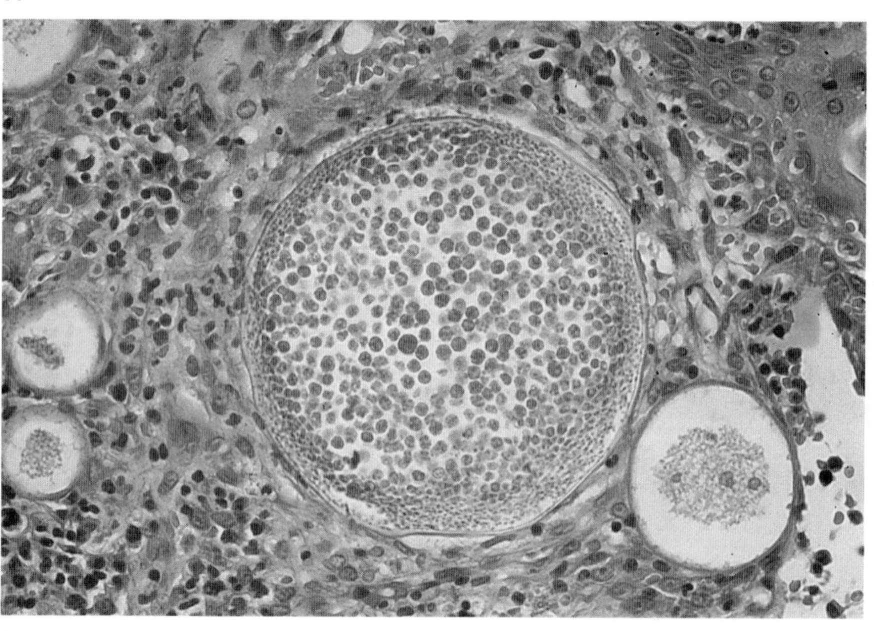

B

FIG. 23-19. Rhinosporidiosis (**A**) H&E stain shows marked papillomatosis and deep invaginations of the nasal mucosa. (**B**) A sporangium contains many individual spores (H&E stain).

and are thus large enough to be visible macroscopically.[255] The granules of both eumycetoma and actinomycetoma stain with the PAS reaction and with methenamine silver (see Fig. 23-18B); those of eumycetoma are composed of septate hyphae 4 to 5 μm thick, whereas the granules of actinomycetoma usually consist of fine, branching filaments or bacillary forms that are only about 1 μm thick.[256] A Gram stain is of considerable value in distinguishing between actinomycetoma and eumycetoma; filaments of actinomycetoma are gram-positive, whereas the hyphae in grains of eumycetoma are gram-negative.[258] The study of discharged granules crushed on a slide and stained with lactophenol blue also allows differentiation between the thin filaments of actinomycetoma and the thicker hyphae of eumycetoma.[258]

RHINOSPORIDIOSIS

Rhinosporidiosis is a chronic infection that is caused by *Rhinosporidium seeberi*. Rhinosporidiosis typically involves mucosal surfaces, most frequently the nasal mucosa, and may involve contiguous skin. This disease is seen primarily in India and Ceylon, but a number of cases have been seen in South America and a few in the United States.[259]

The mode of transmission is not known. Lesions start as a papule, often pruritic, that grows into an erythematous polypoid mass that may cause obstruction of the nose and nasopharynx. Small cysts and pseudocysts develop and may discharge a combination of mucus, pus, and organisms, creating

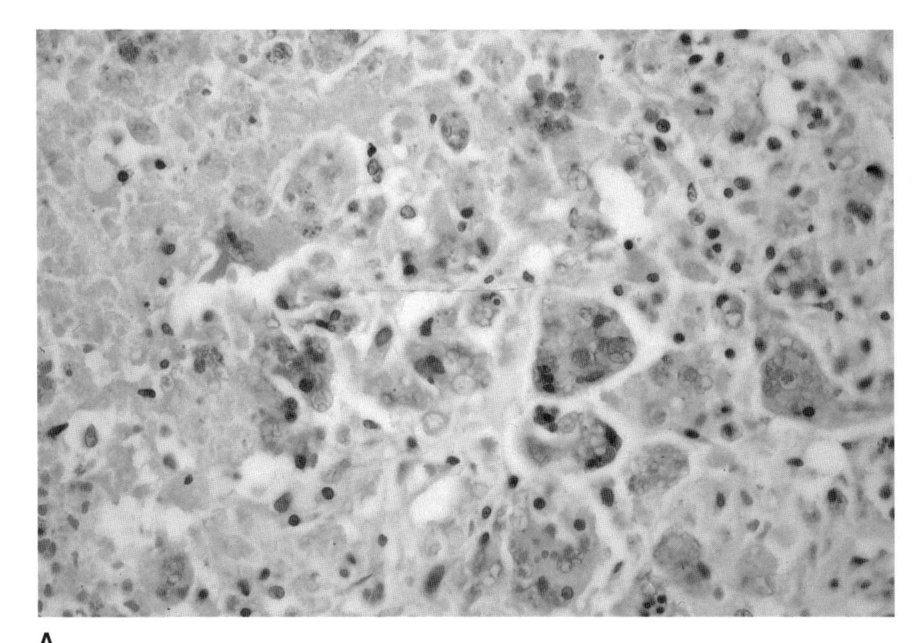
A

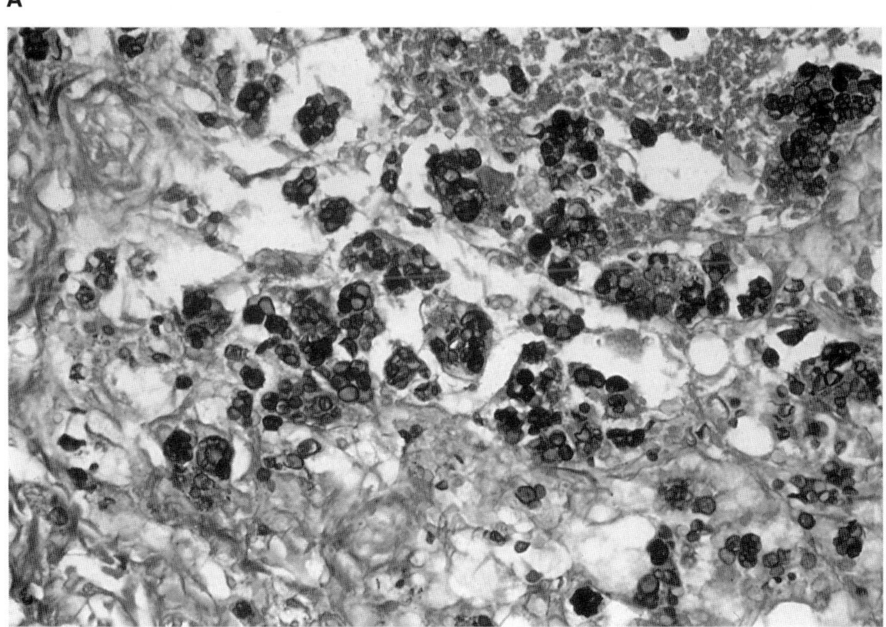
B

FIG. 23-20. Protothecosis
(**A**) H&E stain shows individual cells and clusters of organisms within giant cells. (**B**) The morula-like clusters in multinucleated giant cells are highlighted by silver impregnation (GMS stain).

tiny white dots and giving lesions a characteristic "strawberrylike" appearance.[260] Lesions of the ocular mucosa tend to be flatter, and skin lesions have a warty shape.[261] Involvement of the genital mucosa has also been reported.[262] Dissemination of the organism is extremely rare.[263]

Histopathology. The epithelium is hyperplastic with papillomatosis and deep invaginations, some of which form pseudocysts (Fig. 23-19A). Numerous globular cysts of varying shape, representing sporangia in different stages of development, give the corium a distinctive "Swiss cheese" appearance. There is a surrounding dense, mixed inflammatory infiltrate with lymphocytes and histiocytes, including occasional giant cells, plasma cells, neutrophils, and eosinophils.

R seeberi is a large, endosporulating organism with a distinctive morphology that can usually be recognized in hematoxylin- and eosin–stained sections (see Fig. 23-19B). Sporangia develop from individual spores about the size of an erythrocyte.[264] The spores develop into small uninucleate cysts that enlarge and develop a chitinous eosinophilic wall. With increasing size, nuclear divisions lead to the development of up to 16,000 spores in a sporangium. These distinctive structures may be 300 μm in diameter. Rupture of the cyst or release of the spores through a pore in the cyst wall results in individual spores into the surrounding tissue. The organisms stain with the PAS reaction at all stages, but GMS and mucicarmine stains are not effective for organisms less than 100 μm in diameter.[265]

Differential Diagnosis. The different clinical presentation of coccidioidomycoses and the smaller size of the spherical coccidioidal sporangia (less than 60 μm in diameter) allow for an easy distinction of that disease from rhinosporidiosis.

CUTANEOUS PROTOTHECOSIS

Prototheca is a genus of algae that causes cutaneous infections in humans. Discussion of *Prototheca* is included in this chapter because this organism may be isolated on Sabouraud's medium and has traditionally been discussed in mycology texts, and because this text has no separate chapter for diseases caused by algae. Although there is one report of cutaneous infection in a patient also infected with HIV,[94] cutaneous protothecosis usually occurs in otherwise healthy persons following trauma and wound contamination with water.[91] Lesions develop very slowly and may be single or multiple papules, plaques, or nodules with smooth, verrucous, or ulcerated surfaces.[91,266–271]

Histopathology. The histologic appearance, like the clinical appearance, is not characteristic, so that the diagnosis depends on the finding of the organisms. Usually there is a mixed inflammatory infiltrate with areas of necrosis and fairly numerous giant cells (Fig. 23-20). In sections stained with hematoxylin-eosin, the organisms stain faintly or not at all. On staining with PAS or silver methenamine, however, the organisms stain well and are seen both within giant cells and free in the tissue.[268]

Individual organisms are spheric and measure 6 to 10 μm in diameter.[271] However, as the result of septation, many contain endospores and then are considerably larger. Further subdivision of daughter cells within the parent cell leads to the formation of "sporangia" containing as many as 50 cells lying clustered together as morulalike structures.[266] Ultimately, such a sporangium breaks down into individual organisms.

Pathogenesis. Prototheca is a genus of saprophytic, achloric (nonpigmented) algae. These organisms reproduce asexually by way of internal septation, producing autospores identical to the parent cell. *Prototheca* forms creamy, yeastlike colonies on Sabouraud's medium between 25°C and 37°C. These colonies become visible within 48 hours.[268]

ACKNOWLEDGEMENTS

The author would like to acknowledge the help of Dr. Douglas Wear, Mr. Ronald Neafie, Dr. Wayne Meyers, and the rest of the Department of Infectious and Parasitic Disease Pathology at the Armed Forces Institute of Pathology, as well as of Kathy Boris for administrative assistance.

REFERENCES

1. Sabouraud R. Les teignes. Paris: Masson et Cie, 1910.
2. Emmons CW. Dermatophytes: Natural groupings based on the form of spores and accessory organs. Arch Dermatol Syphilol 1934;30:337.
3. Kwon-Chung KJ, Bennett JE. Dermatophytosis. In: Kwon-Chung KJ, Bennett JE. Medical mycology. Philadelphia: Lea & Febinger, 1992: 105.
4. Rasmussen JE, Ahmed AR. Trichophytin reactions in children with tinea capitis. Arch Dermatol 1978;114:371.
5. Pravda DJ, Pugliese MM. Tinea faciei. Arch Dermatol 1978;114:250.
6. Bronson DM, Desai DR, Barsky S, McMillen Foley S. An epidemic of infection with *Trichophyton tonsurans* revealed in a 20-year survey of fungal infections in Chicago. J Am Acad Dermatol 1983;8:322.
7. Birt AR, Wilt JC. Mycology, bacteriology, and histopathology of suppurative ring-worm. Arch Dermatol 1954;69:441.
8. Mikhail GR. *Trichophyton rubrum* granuloma. Int J Dermatol 1970;9:41.
9. André J, Achten G. Onychomycosis. Int J Dermatol 1987;26:481.
10. Kligman AM, Mescon H, DeLamater ED. The Hotchkiss-McManus stain for the histopathologic diagnosis of fungus diseases. Am J Clin Pathol 1951;21:86.
11. Fetter BF. Human cutaneous sporotrichosis due to *Sporotrichum schenckii*: Technique for demonstration of organisms in tissues. Arch Pathol 1961;71:416.
12. Graham JH, Johnson WC, Burgoon CF Jr, Helwig EB. Tinea capitis. Arch Dermatol 1964;89:528.
13. Zaslow I, Derbes VJ. The immunologic nature of kerion celsi formation. Dermatol Int 1971;8:1.
14. Imamura S, Tanaka M, Watanabe S. Use of immunofluorescence staining in kerion. Arch Dermatol 1975;111:906.
15. Gottlieb GJ, Ackerman AB. The "sandwich sign" of dermatophytosis. Am J Dermatopathol 1986;8:347.
16. Wilson JW, Plunkett OA, Gregersen A. Nodular granulomatous perifolliculitis of the legs caused by *Trichophyton rubrum.* Arch Dermatol 1954;69:258.
17. Scher RK, Ackerman AB. The value of nail biopsy for demonstrating fungi not demonstrable by microbiologic techniques. Am J Dermatopathol 1980;2:55.
18. Dvoretzky I, Fisher BK, Movshovitz M, Schewach-Millet M. Favus. Int J Dermatol 1980;19:89.
19. Berretty P, Neumann M, Hausman R, Dingemans K. Follikulitis, verursacht durch *Pityrosporum.* Hautarzt 1980;31:613.
20. Potter BS, Burgoon CFJ, Johnson WC. *Pityrosporum* folliculitis: Report of seven cases and review of the *Pityrosporum* organism relative to cutaneous disease. Arch Dermatol 1973;107:388.
21. Bäck O, Faergemann J, Hörnqvist R. *Pityrosporum* folliculitis: A common disease of the young and middle-aged. J Am Acad Dermatol 1985;12:56.
22. Heng MCY, Henderson CL, Barker DC, Haberfelde G. Correlation of *Pityrosporum ovale* density with clinical severity of seborrheic dermatitis as assessed by a simplified technique. J Am Acad Dermatol 1990;23:82.

23. Leyden JJ, McGinley KJ, Kligman AM. Role of microorganisms in dandruff. Arch Dermatol 1976;112:333.
24. Galadari I, el Komy M, Mousa A et al. Tinea versicolor: Histologic and ultrastructural investigation of pigmentary changes. Int J Dermatol 1992;31:253.
25. Porro MN, Passi S, Caprilli F, Mercantini R. Induction of hyphae in cultures of *Pityrosporum* by cholesterol and cholesterol esters. J Invest Dermatol 1977;69:531.
26. Roberts SOB. *Pityrosporum* orbiculare: Incidence and distribution of clinically normal skin. Br J Dermatol 1969;81:264.
27. McGinley KJ, Lantis LR, Marples RR. Microbiology of tinea versicolor. Arch Dermatol 1970;102:168.
28. Jung EG, Bohnert E. Mechanism of depigmentation in pityriasis versicolor alba. Arch Dermatol Res 1976;256:333.
29. Charles CR, Sire DJ, Johnson BL, Beidler JG. Hypopigmentation in tinea versicolor: A histochemical and electronmicroscopic study. Int J Dermatol 1973;12:48.
30. Allen HB, Charles CR, Johnson BL. Hyperpigmented tinea versicolor. Arch Dermatol 1976;112:1110.
31. Heid E, Grosshans E, Provencher D, Basset M. Folliculites *Pityrosporiques*. Ann Dermatol Venereol 1978;105:133.
32. Maize JC, Lynch PJ. Chronic mucocutaneous candidiasis of the adult: A report of a patient with an associated thymoma. Arch Dermatol 1972;105:96.
33. Chapel TA, Gagliardi C, Nichols W. Congenital cutaneous candidiasis. J Am Acad Dermatol 1982;6:926.
34. Maibach HI, Kligman AM. The biology of experimental human cutaneous moniliasis (*Candida albicans*). Arch Dermatol 1962;85:233.
35. Degos R, Garnier G, Civatte J. Pustulose par *Candida albicans* avec lésions psoriasiformes rappelant le psoriasis pustuleux. Bull Soc Fr Dermatol Syphiligr 1962;69:231.
36. Kwon-Chung KJ, Bennett JE. Candidiasis. In: Kwong-Chung KJ, Bennett JE. Medical mycology. Philadelphia: Lea & Febinger, 1992: 280.
37. Scherwitz C. Ultrastructure of human cutaneous candiosis. J Invest Dermatol 1982;78:200.
38. Hauser FV, Rothman S. Monilial granuloma: Report of a case and review of the literature. Arch Dermatol Syphil 1950;61:297.
39. Kugelman TP, Cripps DJ, Harrell ER Jr. *Candida* granuloma with epidermophytosis: Report of a case and review of the literature. Arch Dermatol 1963;88:150.
40. Kirkpatrick CH. Chronic mucocutaneous candidiasis. J Am Acad Dermatol 1994;31:S14.
41. Conant MA. Hairy leukoplakia: A new disease of the oral mucosa. Arch Dermatol 1987;123:585.
42. Tavitian A, Raufman J-P, Rosenthal LE. Oral candidiasis as a marker for esophageal candidiasis in the acquired immunodeficiency syndrome. Ann Intern Med 1986;104:54.
43. Lupton GP, James WD, Redfield RR et al. Oral hairy leukoplakia: A distinctive marker of human T-cell lymphotropic virus type III (HTLV-III) infection. Arch Dermatol 1987;123:624.
44. Hellier FF, La Touche CJ, Rowell NR. Monilial granuloma treated with amphotericin B in an achondroplastic with bronchiectasis. Br J Dermatol 1963;75:375.
45. Engel MF. Monilial granuloma with hypergammaglobulineamia: Treatment with amphotericin B and dermabrasion. Arch Dermatol 1961;84:192.
46. Papazian CE, Koch R. Monilial granuloma with hypothyroidism: Report of a case treated with amphotericin B. N Engl J Med 1960;262: 16.
47. Ezold M, Schönborn C. Über ein granuloma candidamyceticum des erwachsenen, behandelt mit amphotericin B. Z Hautkr 1964;37:379.
48. Bodey GP, Luna M. Skin lesions associated with disseminated candidiasis. JAMA 1974;229:1466.
49. Jarowski CI, Fialk MA, Murray HW et al. Fever, rash, and muscle tenderness: A distinctive clinical presentation of disseminated candidiasis. Arch Int Med 1978;138:544.
50. Grossman ME, Silvers DN, Walther RR. Cutaneous manifestations of disseminated candidiasis. J Am Acad Dermatol 1980;2:111.
51. Jacobs MI, Magid MS, Jarowski CI. Disseminated candidiasis: Newer approaches to early recognition and treatment. Arch Dermatol 1980; 116:1277.
52. Kressel B, Szewczyk C, Tuazon CU. Early clinical recognition of disseminated candidiasis by muscle and skin biopsy. Arch Int Med 1978; 138:429.
53. Young RC, Bennett JE, Vogel CL et al. Aspergillosis: The spectrum of the disease in 98 patients. Medicine (Baltimore) 1970;49:147.
54. Kwon-Chung KJ, Bennett JE. Aspergillosis. In: Kwong-Chung KJ, Bennett JE. Medical mycology. Philadelphia: Lea & Febinger, 1992: 201.
55. Allo MD, Miller J, Townsend T, Tan C. Primary cutaneous aspergillosis associated with Hickman intravenous catheters. N Engl J Med 1987;317:1105.
56. Grossman ME, Fithian EC, Behrens C et al. Primary cutaneous aspergillosis in six leukemic children. J Am Acad Dermatol 1985;12: 313.
57. Estes SE, Hendricks AA, Merz WG, Prystowsky SD. Primary cutaneous aspergillosis. J Am Acad Dermatol 1980;3:397.
58. Hunt SJ, Nagi C, Gross KG et al. Primary cutaneous aspergillosis near central venous catheters in patients with the acquired immunodeficiency syndrome. Arch Dermatol 1992;128:1229.
59. Prystowsky SD, Vogelstein B, Ettinger DS et al. Invasive aspergillosis. N Engl J Med 1976;295:655.
60. Carlile JR, Millet RE, Cho CT, Vats TS. Primary cutaneous aspergillosis in a leukemic child. Arch Dermatol 1978;114:78.
61. Pursell KJ, Telzak EE, Armstrong D. *Aspergillus* species colonization and invasive disease in patients with AIDS. Clin Infect Dis 1992;14: 141.
62. Googe PB, DeCoste SD, Herold WH, Mihm MC Jr. Primary cutaneous aspergillosis mimicking dermatophytosis. Arch Pathol Lab Med 1989;113:1284.
63. Panke TW, McManus AT, Spebar MJ. Infection of a burn wound by *Aspergillus niger*: Gross appearance simulating ecthyma gangrenosa. Am J Clin Pathol 1979;72:230.
64. Lai C-S, Lin S-D, Chou C-K, Lin H-J. Aspergillosis complicating the grafted skin and free muscle flap in a diabetic. Plast Reconstr Surg 1993;92:532.
65. Findlay GH, Roux HF, Simson IW. Skin manifestations in disseminated aspergillosis. Br J Dermatol 1971;85:94.
66. Caro I, Dogliotti M. Aspergillosis of the skin: Report of a case. Dermatologica 1973;146:244.
67. Cahill KM, El Mofty AM, Kawaguchi TP. Primary cutaneous aspergillosis. Arch Dermatol 1967;96:545.
68. Kwon-Chung KJ, Bennett JE. Mucormycosis. In: Kwon-Chung KJ, Bennett JE. Medical mycology. Philadelphia: Lea & Febinger, 1992: 524.
69. Adam RD, Hunter G, DiTomasso J, Comerci G Jr. Mucormycosis: Emerging prominence of cutaneous infections. Clin Inf Dis 1994;19: 67.
70. Rabin ER, Lundberg GD, Mitchell ET. Mucormycosis in severely burned patients: Report of two cases with extensive destruction of the face and naval cavity. N Engl J Med 1961;264:1286.
71. Hammond DE, Winkelmann RK. Cutaneous phycomycosis: Report of three cases with identification of *Rhizopus*. Arch Dermatol 1979;115: 990.
72. Gartenberg G, Bottone EJ, Keusch GT, Weitzman I. Hospital-acquired mucormycosis (*Rhizopus rhizopodiformis*) of skin and subcutaneous tissue. N Engl J Med 1978;299:1115.
73. Sanchez MR, Ponge-Wilson I, Moy JA, Rosenthal S. Zygomycosis and HIV infection. J Am Acad Dermatol 1994;30:904.
74. Veliath AJ, Rao R, Prabhu MR, Aurora AL. Cutaneous phycomycosis (mucormycosis) with fatal pulmonary dissemination. Arch Dermatol 1976;112:509.
75. Kramer BS, Hernandez AD, Reddick RL et al. Cutaneous infarction: Manifestation of disseminated mucormycosis. Arch Dermatol 1977; 113:1075.
76. Meyer RD, Kaplan MH, Ong M, Armstrong D. Cutaneous lesions in disseminated mucormycosis. JAMA 1973;225:737.
77. Herstoff JK, Bogaars H, McDonald CJ. Rhinophycomycosis entomophthorae. Arch Dermatol 1978;114:1674.
78. Ajello L. The gamut of human infections caused by dematiaceous fungi. Japan J Med Mycol 1981;22:1.
79. McGinnis MR. Chromoblastomycosis and phaeohyphomycosis: New concepts, diagnosis, and mycology. J Am Acad Dermatol 1983;8:1.
80. Kwon-Chung KJ, Bennett JE. Phaeohyphomycosis. In: Kwon-Chung KJ, Bennett JE. Medical mycology. Philadelphia: Lea & Febinger, 1992:620.

81. Ziefer A, Connor DH. Phaeomycotic cyst: A clinicopathologic study of twenty-five patients. Am J Trop Med Hyg 1980;29:901.
82. Young JM, Ulrich E. Sporotrichosis produced by *Sporotrichum gougeroti*. Arch Dermatol 1953;67:44.
83. Kempson RL, Sternberg WH. Chronic subcutaneous abscesses caused by pigmented fungi, a lesion distinguishable from cutaneous chromoblastomycosis. Am J Clin Pathol 1963;39:598.
84. Greer KE, Gross GP, Cooper PH, Harding SA. Cystic chromomycosis due to *Wangiella dermatitidis*. Arch Dermatol 1979;115:1433.
85. Symmers WSC. A case of cerebral chromoblastomycosis (cladosporiosis) occurring in Britain as a complication of polyarteritis treated with cortisone. Brain 1960;83:37.
86. Watson KC. Cerebral chromoblastomycosis. J Pathol Bacteriol 1962; 84:233.
87. Pedersen NB, Mardh PA, Hallberg T et al. Cutaneous alternariosis. Br J Dermatol 1976;94:201.
88. Mitchell AJ, Solomon AR, Beneke ES, Anderson TF. Subcutaneous alternariosis. J Am Acad Dermatol 1983;8:673.
89. Higashi N, Asada Y. Cutaneous alternariosis with mixed infection of *Candida albicans:* Report of a patient responding to Natamycin. Arch Dermatol 1973;108:558.
90. Male O, Pehamberger H. Sekundäre kutanmykosen durch alternariaarten. Hautarzt 1986;37:94.
91. Nelson AM, Neafie RC, Connor DH. Cutaneous protothecosis and chlorellosis, extraordinary "aquatic-borne" algal infections. Clin Dermatol 1987;5:76.
92. Chevrant-Breton J, Boisseau-Lebreuil M, Fréour E et al. Les alternarioses cutanées humaines: A propos de 3 cas. Revue de la littérature. Ann Dermatol Venereol 1981;108:653.
93. Bourlond A, Alexandre G. Dermal alternariosis in a kidney transplant recipient. Dermatologica 1984;168:152.
94. Woolrich A, Koestenblatt E, Don P, Szaniawski W. Cutaneous protothecosis and AIDS. J Am Acad Dermatol 1994;31:920.
95. Harrell ER, Curtis AC. North American blastomycosis. Am J Med 1959;27:750.
96. Wilson JW, Cawley EP, Weidman FD, Gilmer WS. Primary cutaneous North American blastomycosis. Arch Dermatol 1955;71:39.
97. Larson DM, Eckman MR, Alber RL, Goldschmidt VG. Primary cutaneous (inoculation) blastomycosis: An occupational hazard to pathologists. Am J Clin Pathol 1983;79:253.
98. Miller DD, Davies SF, Sarosi GA. Erythema nodosum and blastomycosis. Arch Int Med 1982;142:1839.
99. Witorsch P, Utz JP. North American blastomycosis: A study of 40 patients. Medicine (Baltimore) 1968;47:169.
100. Witzig RS, Hoadley DJ, Greer DL, Abriola KP, Hernandez RL. Blastomycosis and human immunodeficiency virus: Three new cases and review. South Med J 1994;87:715.
101. Pappas PG, Threlkeld MG, Bedsole GD et al. Blastomycosis in immunocompromised patients. Medicine (Baltimore) 1993;72:311.
102. Mercurio MG, Elewski BE. Cutaneous blastomycosis. Cutis 1992;50: 422.
103. Procknow JJ, Loosli CG. Treatment of the deep mycoses. Arch Intern Med 1958;101:765.
104. Hashimoto K, Kaplan RJ, Daman LA et al. Pustular blastomycosis. Int J Dermatol 1977;16:277.
105. Henchy FP III, Daniel CR III, Omura EF, Kheir SM. North American blastomycosis: An unusual clinical manifestation. Arch Dermatol 1982;118:287.
106. Klapman MH, Superfon NP, Solomon LM. North American blastomycosis. Arch Dermatol 1970;101:653.
107. Moore M. Mycotic granulomata and cutaneous tuberculosis: A comparison of the histopathologic response. J Invest Dermatol 1945; 6:149.
108. Littman ML, Wicker EH, Warren AS. Systemic North American blastomycosis: Report of a case with cultural studies of the etiologic agent and observations on the effect of streptomycin and penicillin in vitro. Am J Pathol 1948;24:339.
109. Kaplan W, Kraft DE. Demonstration of pathogenic fungi in formalin-fixed tissues by immunofluorescence. Am J Clin Pathol 1969;52:420.
110. Russell B, Beckett JH, Jacobs PH. Immunoperoxidase localization of *Sporothrix schenckii* and *Cryptococcus neoformans*. Arch Dermatol 1979;115:433.
111. Moskowitz LB, Ganjei P, Ziegels-Weissman J et al. Immunohistologic identification of fungi in systemic and cutaneous mycoses. Arch Pathol Lab Med 1986;110:433.
112. Londero AT, Ramos CD. Paracoccidioidomycosis: A clinical and mycologic study of forty-one cases observed in Santa Maria, RS, Brazil. Am J Med 1972;52:771.
113. Restrepo A, Robledo M, Ospina S et al. Distribution of paracoccidioidin sensitivity in Columbia. Am J Trop Med Hyg 1968;17:25.
114. Salfelder K, Doehnert G, Doehnert H-R. Paracoccidioidomycosis: Anatomic study with complete autopsies. Virchows Arch 1969;348: 51.
115. Murray HW, Littman ML, Roberts RB. Disseminated paracoccidioidomycosis (South American blastomycosis) in the United States. Am J Med 1974;56:209.
116. Furtado TA. Mechanism of infection in South American blastomyocosis. Dermatol Tropica 1963;2:27.
117. Kwon-Chung KJ, Bennett JE. Paracoccidioidomycosis. In: Kwon-Chung KJ, Bennett JE. Medical mycology. Philadelphia: Lea & Febinger, 1992:594.
118. Bakos L, Kronfeld M, Hampe S et al. Disseminated paracoccidioidomycosis with skin lesions in a patient with acquired immunodeficiency syndrome. J Am Acad Dermatol 1989;20:854.
119. Goldani LZ, Martinez R, Landell GAM et al. Paracoccidioidomycosis in a patient with acquired immunodeficiency syndrome. Mycopathologia 1989;105:71.
120. Götz H. Klinische und experimentelle studien über das granuloma paracoccidioides. Arch Dermatol Syphiligr 1954;198:507.
121. Perry HO, Weed LA, Kierland RR. South American blastomycosis: Report of case and review of laboratory features. Arch Dermatol Syphiligr 1954;70:477.
122. Azulay RD, Carneiro JA, Cunha MDG, Reis LT. Keloidal blastomycosis (Lobo's disease) with lymphatic involvement: A case report. Int J Dermatol 1976;15:40.
123. Tapia A, Torres-Calcindo A, Arosemena R. Keloidal blastomycosis (Lobo's disease) in Panama. Int J Dermatol 1978;17:572.
124. Bhawan J, Bain RW, Purtilo DT et al. Lobomycosis: An electronmicroscopic, histochemical and immunologic study. J Cutan Pathol 1976;3:5.
125. Jaramillo D, Cortés A et al. Lobomycosis: Report of the eighth Colombian case and review of the literature. J Cutan Pathol 1976; 3:180.
126. Kwon-Chung KJ, Bennett JE. Chromoblastomycosis. In: Kwon-Chung KJ, Bennett JE. Medical mycology. Philadelphia: Lea & Febinger, 1992:337.
127. Vollum DI. Chromomycosis: A review. Br J Dermatol 1977;96:454.
128. Carrión AL. Chromoblastomycosis and related infections: New concepts, differential diagnosis, and nomenclatorial implications. Int J Dermatol 1975;14:27.
129. Putkonen T. Die chromomykose in Finnland: Der mögliche anteil der finnischen sauna an ihrer verbreitung. Hautarzt 1966;17:507.
130. Ariewitsch AM. Über die metastasierung der chromomykose infection. Dermatol Wochenschr 1967;153:685.
131. Derbes VJ, Friedman I. Chromoblastomycosis. Dermatol Tropica 1964;3:201.
132. Azulay RD, Serruya J. Hematogenous dissemination in chromoblastomycosis. Arch Dermatol 1967;95:57.
133. Caplan RM. Epidermoid carcinoma arising in extensive chromoblastomycosis. Arch Dermatol 1968;97:38.
134. Wackym PA, Gray GF Jr, Richie RE, Gregg CR. Cutaneous chromomycosis in renal transplant recipients: Successful management in two cases. Arch Intern Med 1985;145:1036.
135. Nödl F. Zue histologie der chromomykose. Z Hautkr 1963;35:305.
136. Moore M, Cooper ZK, Weiss RS. Chromomycosis (chromoblastomycosis). JAMA 1943;122:1237.
137. French AJ, Russell SR. Chromoblastomycosis: Report of first case recognized in Michigan, apparently conducted in South Carolina. Arch Dermatol Syphil 1953;67:129.
138. Batres E, Wolf JE Jr, Rudolph AH, Knox JM. Transepithelial elimination of cutaneous chromomycosis. Arch Dermatol 1978;114:1231.
139. Goette DK, Robertson D. Transepithelial elimination in chromomycosis. Arch Dermatol 1984;120:400.
140. Wilson JW. Therapy of systemic fungus infections in 1961. Arch Intern Med 1961;108:292.
141. Tschen JA, Knox JM, McGavran MH, Duncan WC. Chromomycosis:

The association of fungal elements and wood splinters. Arch Dermatol 1984;120:107.
142. Rubin HA, Bruce S, Rosen T, McBride ME. Evidence for percutaneous inoculation as the mode of transmission for chromoblastomycosis: J Am Acad Dermatol 1991;25:951.
143. Schwartz RA, Lamberts RJ. Isolated nodular cutaneous coccidioidomycosis: The initial manifestation of disseminated disease. J Am Acad Dermatol 1981;4:38.
144. Trimble JR, Doucette J. Primary cutaneous coccidioidomycosis: Report of a case of a laboratory infection. Arch Dermatol 1956;74:405.
145. Overholt EL, Hornick RB. Primary cutaneous coccidioidomycosis. Arch Intern Med 1964;114:149.
146. Carroll GF, Haley LD, Brown JM. Primary cutaneous coccidioidomycosis. Arch Dermatol 1977;113:933.
147. Harrell ER, Honeycutt WM. Coccidioidomycosis: A traveling fungus disease. Arch Dermatol 1963;87:188.
148. Levan NE, Huntington RW Jr. Primary cutaneous coccidioidomycosis in agricultural workers. Arch Dermatol 1965;92:215.
149. Winn WA. Primary cutaneous coccidioidomycosis: Reevaluation of its potentiality based on study of three new cases. Arch Dermatol 1965;92:221.
150. Drutz DJ, Catanzaro A. Coccidioidomycosis. Part I. Am Rev Respir Dis 1978;117:559.
151. Drutz DJ, Catanzaro A. Coccidioidomycosis. Part II. Am Rev Respir Dis 1978;117:727.
152. Dodge RR, Lebowitz MD, Barbee R, Burrows B. Estimates of *C. immitis* infection by skin test reactivity in an endemic community. Am J Public Health 1985;75:863.
153. Medoff G, Kobayashi GS. Strategies in the treatment of systemic fungal infections. N Engl J Med 1980;302:145.
154. Deresinski SC, Stevens DA. Coccidioidomycosis in compromised hosts: Experience at Stanford University Hospital. Medicine (Baltimore) 1974;54:377.
155. Ampel NM, Dols CL, Galgiani JN. Coccidioidomycosis during human immunodeficiency virus infection: Results of a prospective study in a coccidioidal endemic area. Am J Med 1993;94:235.
156. Wheat J. Histoplasmosis and coccidioidomycosis in individuals with AIDS: A clinical review. Infect Dis Clin North Am 1994;8:467.
157. Lynch PJ, Rather EP, Rutala PJ. Pemphigus and coccidioidomycosis. Cutis 1978;22:581.
158. Levan NE, Kwong MQ. Coccidioidomycosis: Persistent pulmonary lesion, solitary "disseminated" lesion of face, occupational aspects. Arch Dermatol 1963;87:511.
159. Bayer AS, Yoshikawa TT, Galpin JE, Guze LB. Unusual syndromes of coccidioidomycosis: Diagnostic and therapeutic considerations. Medicine (Baltimore) 1976;55:131.
160. Winer LH. Histopathology of the nodose lesion of acute coccidioidomycosis. Arch Dermatol Syphil 1950;61:1010.
161. Kwon-Chung KJ, Bennett JE. Coccidioidomycosis. In: Kwon-Chung KJ, Bennett JE. Medical mycology. Philadelphia: Lea & Febinger, 1992:356.
162. Randhawa HS, Paliwal DK. Occurrence and significance of *Cryptococcus neoformans* in the oropharynx and on the skin of a healthy human population. J Clin Microbiol 1977;6:325.
163. Glaser JB, Garden A. Inoculation of cryptococcosis without transmission of the acquired immunodeficiency syndrome. N Engl J Med 1985;313:266.
164. Ng WF, Loo KT. Cutaneous cryptococcosis—primary versus secondary disease: Report of two cases with review of literature. Am J Dermatopathol 1993;15:372.
165. Kwon-Chung KJ, Bennett JE. Cryptococcosis. In: Kwon-Chung KJ, Bennett JE. Medical mycology. Philadelphia: Lea & Febinger, 1992: 397.
166. Dismukes WE. Cryptococcal meningitis in patients with AIDS. J Infect Dis 1988;157:624.
167. Sarosi GA, Silberfarb PM, Tosh FE. Cutaneous cryptococcosis: A sentinel of disseminated disease. Arch Dermatol 1971;104:1.
168. Schupbach CW, Wheeler CE Jr, Briggaman RA et al. Cutaneous manifestations of disseminated cryptococcosis. Arch Dermatol 1976;112: 1734.
169. Chu AC, Hay RJ, MacDonald DM. Cutaneous cryptococcosis. Br J Dermatol 1980;103:95.
170. Cawley EP, Grekin RH, Curtis AC. Torulosis: A review of the cutaneous and adjoining mucous membrane manifestations. J Invest Dermatol 1950;14:327.
171. Frieden TR, Bia FJ, Heald PW et al. Cutaneous cryptococcosis in a patient with cutaneous T cell lymphoma receiving therapy with photopheresis and methotrexate. Clin Infect Dis 1993;17:776.
172. Diamond RD, Bennett JE. Prognostic factors in cryptococcal meningitis: A study of 111 cases. Ann Intern Med 1974;80:176.
173. Kaplan MH, Rosen PP, Armstrong D. Cryptococcosis in a cancer hospital: Clinical and pathological correlates in forty-six patients. Cancer 1977;39:2265.
174. Pema K, Diaz J, Guerra LG et al. Disseminated cutaneous cryptococcosis: Comparison of clinical manifestations in the pre-AIDS and AIDS eras. Arch Intern Med 1994;154:1032.
175. Perfect JR, Durack DT, Gallis HA. Cryptococcemia. Medicine (Baltimore) 1983;62:98.
176. Sussman EJ, McMahon F, Wright D, Friedman HM. Cutaneous cryptococcosis without evidence of systemic involvement. J Am Acad Dermatol 1984;11:371.
177. Gordon PM, Ormerod AD, Harvey G et al. Cutaneous cryptococcal infection without immunodeficiency. Clin Exp Dermatol 1993;19: 181.
178. Penneys NS, Hicks B. Unusual cutaneous lesions associated with acquired immunodeficiency syndrome. J Am Acad Dermatol 1985;13: 845.
179. Manrique P, Mayo J, Alvarez JA et al. Polymorphous cutaneous cryptococcosis: Nodular, herpes-like, and molluscum-like lesions in a patient with the acquired immunodeficiency syndrome. J Am Acad Dermatol 1992;26:122.
180. Blauvelt A, Kerdel FA. Cutaneous cryptococcosis mimicking Kaposi's sarcoma as the initial manifestation of disseminated disease. Int J Dermatol 1992;31:279.
181. Crounse RG, Lerner AB. Cryptococcosis: Case with unusual skin lesions and favorable response to amphotericin B therapy. Arch Dermatol 1958;77:210.
182. Carlson KC, Mehlmauer M, Evans S, Chandrasoma P. Cryptococcal cellulitis in renal transplant recipients. J Am Acad Dermatol 1987;17: 469.
183. Hall JC, Brewer JH, Crouch TT, Watson KR. Cryptococcal cellulitis with multiple sites of involvement. J Am Acad Dermatol 1987;17: 329.
184. Moore M. Cryptococcosis with cutaneous manifestations: Four cases with a review of published reports. J Invest Dermatol 1957;28:159.
185. Gutierrez F, Fu YS, Lurie HI. Cryptococcosis histologically resembling histoplasmosis: A light and electron microscopical study. Arch Pathol 1975;99:347.
186. Ro JY, Lee SS, Ayala AG. Advantage of Fontana-Masson stain in capsule-deficient cryptococcal infection. Arch Pathol Lab Med 1987; 111:53.
187. Linell F, Magnusson B, Nordén Å. Cryptococcosis: Review and report of a case. Acta Derm Venereol (Stockh) 1953;33:103.
188. Ruiter M, Ensink GJ. Acute primary cutaneous cryptococcosis. Dermatologica 1964;128:185.
189. Littman ML, Walter JE. Cryptococcosis: Current status. Am J Med 1968;45:922.
190. Collins DN, Oppenheim IA, Edwards MR. Cryptococcosis associated with systemic lupus erythematosus: Light and electron microscopic observations on a morphologic variant. Arch Pathol 1971;91:78.
191. Brier RL, Mopper C, Stone J. Cutaneous cryptococcosis: Presentation of a case and a review of previously reported cases. Arch Dermatol 1957;75:262.
192. Miura T, Akiba H, Saito N, Seiji M. Primary cutaneous cryptococcosis. Dermatologica 1971;142:374.
193. Noble RC, Fajardo LF. Primary cutaneous cryptococcosis: Review and morphologic study. Am J Clin Pathol 1972;57:13.
194. Goodwin RA Jr, Des Prez RM. Histoplasmosis. Am Rev Respir Dis 1978;117:929.
195. Kwon-Chung KJ, Bennett JE. Histoplasmosis. In: Kwon-Chung KJ, Bennett JE. Medical mycology. Philadelphia: Lea & Febinger, 1992: 464.
196. U.S. National Communicable Disease Center. Morbidity and mortality weekly report annual supplement: Summary. 1968, MMWR, 17, 1969.
197. Tosh FE, Balhuizen J, Yates JL, Brasher CA. Primary cutaneous histoplasmosis. Arch Intern Med 1964;114:118.

198. Tesh RB, Schneidau JD Jr. Primary cutaneous histoplasmosis. N Engl J Med 1966;275:597.
199. Goodwin RA Jr, Owens FT, Snell JD et al. Chronic pulmonary histoplasmosis. Medicine (Baltimore) 1976;413.
200. Cawley EP, Curtis AC. Histoplasmosis and lymphoblastoma: Are these diseases related? J Invest Dermatol 1948;11:443.
201. Ende N, Pizzolato P, Ziskind J. Hodgkin's disease associated with histoplasmosis. Cancer 1952;5:763.
202. Kauffman CA, Israel KS, Smith JW et al. Histoplasmosis in immunosuppressed patients. Am J Med 1978;64:923.
203. Bonner JR, Alexander WJ, Dismukes WE et al. Disseminated histoplasmosis in patients with the acquired immune deficiency syndrome. Arch Intern Med 1984;144:2178.
204. Wheat LJ. Histoplasmosis in Indianapolis. Clin Infect Dis 1992; 14:S91.
205. Neubauer MA, Bodensteiner DC. Disseminated histoplasmosis in patients with AIDS. South Med J 1992;85:1166.
206. Goodwin RA Jr, Shapiro JL, Thurman GH et al. Disseminated histoplasmosis: Clinical and pathologic correlations. Medicine (Baltimore) 1980;59:1.
207. Studdard J, Sneed WF, Taylor MR Jr, Campbell GD. Cutaneous histoplasmosis. Am Rev Respir Dis 1976;113:689.
208. Curtis AC, Grekin JN. Histoplasmosis: A review of the cutaneous and adjacent mucous membrane manifestations with a report of three cases. JAMA 1947;134:1217.
209. Miller HE, Keddie FM, Johnstone HG, Bostick WL. Histoplasmosis: Cutaneous and mucomembranous lesions, mycologic and pathologic observations. Arch Dermatol Syphil 1947;56:715.
210. Chanda JJ, Callen JP. Isolated nodular cutaneous histoplasmosis: The initial manifestation of recurrent disseminated disease. Arch Dermatol 1978;114:1197.
211. Barton EN, Ince RWE, Patrick AL, et al. Cutaneous histoplasmosis in the acquired immune deficiency syndrome: A report of three cases from Trinidad. Trop Geogr Med 1988;40:153.
212. Abildgaard WH Jr, Hargrove RH, Kalivas J. *Histoplasma* panniculitis. Arch Dermatol 1985;121:914.
213. Samovitz M, Dillon TK. Disseminated histoplasmosis presenting as exfoliative erythroderma. Arch Dermatol 1970;101:216.
214. Cramer HJ. Erythrodermatische hauthistoplasmose. Dermatologica 1973;146:249.
215. Sellers TF Jr, Price WN Jr, Newberry WM Jr. An epidemic of erythema multiforme and erythema nodosum caused by histoplasmosis. Ann Intern Med 1965;62:1244.
216. Zarabi CM, Thomas R, Adesokan A. Diagnosis of systemic histoplasmosis in patients with AIDS. South Med J 1992;85:1171.
217. Nejedly RF, Baker LA. Treatment of localized histoplasmosis with 2-hydroxstilbamidine. Arch Intern Med 1955;95:37.
218. Dumont A, Piché C. Electron microscopic study of human histoplasmosis. Arch Pathol 1969;87:168.
219. Rippon JW. Medical mycology. Philadelphia: Saunders, 1974.
220. Lucas AO. Cutaneous manifestations of African histoplasmosis. Br J Dermatol 1970;82:435.
221. Nethercott JR, Schachter RK, Givan KF, Ryder DE. Histoplasmosis due to *Histoplasma capsulatum* var *duboisii* in a Canadian immigrant. Arch Dermatol 1978;114:595.
222. Williams AO, Lawson EA, Lucas AO. African histoplasmosis due to *Histoplasma duboisii*. Arch Pathol 1971;92:306.
223. Flegel H, Kaben U, Westphal H-J. Afrikanische histoplasmose. Hautarzt 1980;31:50.
224. Schneidau JD Jr, Lamar LM, Hairston MA Jr. Cutaneous hypersensitivity to sporotrichin in Louisiana. JAMA 1964;188:371.
225. Ingrish FM, Schneidau JD Jr. Cutaneous hypersensitivity to sporotrichin in Maricopa county, Arizona. J Invest Dermatol 1967;49: 146.
226. Urabe H, Honbo S. Sporotrichosis. Int J Dermatol 1986;25:255.
227. Shelley WB, Sica PA Jr. Disseminate sporotrichosis of skin and bone cured with 5-fluorocytosine: Photosensitivity as a complication. J Am Acad Dermatol 1983;8:229.
228. Smith PW, Loomis GW, Luckasen JL, Osterholm RK. Disseminated cutaneous sporotrichosis: Three illustrated cases. Arch Dermatol 1981;117:143.
229. Lynch PJ, Voorhees JJ, Harrell ER. Systemic sporotrichosis. Ann Intern Med 1970;73:23.
230. Shaw JC, Levinson W, Montanaro A. Sporotrichosis in the acquired immunodeficiency syndrome. J Am Acad Dermatol 1989;21:1145.
231. Dellatorre DL, Lattanand A, Buckley HR, Urbach F. Fixed cutaneous sporotrichosis of the face: Successful treatment of a case and review of the literature. J Am Acad Dermatol 1982;6:97.
232. Lurie HI. Histopathology of sporotrichosis: Notes on the nature of the asteroid body. Arch Pathol 1963;75:421.
233. Carr RD, Storkan MA, Wilson JW, Swatek FE. Extensive verrucous sporotrichosis of long duration: Report of a case resembling cutaneous blastomycosis. Arch Dermatol 1964;89:124.
234. Itani Z. Die sporotrichose. Hautarzt 1971;22:110.
235. Dolezal JF. Blastomycoid sporotrichosis: Response to low-dose amphotericin B. J Am Acad Dermatol 1981;4:523.
236. Wilson DE, Mann JJ, Bennett JE, Utz JP. Clinical features of extracutaneous sporotrichosis. Medicine (Baltimore) 1967;46:265.
237. Baum GL, Donnerberg RL, Stewart D et al. Pulmonary sporotrichosis. N Engl J Med 1969;280:410.
238. Stroud JD. Sporotrichosis presenting as pyoderma gangrenosum. Arch Dermatol 1968;97:667.
239. Male O. Diagnostische und therapeutische probleme bei der kutanen sporotrichose. Z Hautkr 1974;49:505.
240. Segal RJ, Jacobs PH. Sporotrichosis. Int J Dermatol 1979;18:639.
241. Fetter BF, Tindall JP. Cutaneous sporotrichosis: Clinical study of nine cases utilizing an improved technique for demonstration of organisms. Arch Pathol 1964;78:613.
242. Marques MEA, Coelho KIR, Sotto MN, Bacchi CE. Comparison between histochemical and immunohistochemical methods for diagnosis of sporotrichosis. J Clin Pathol 1992;45:1089.
243. Kariya H, Iwatsu T. Statistical survey of 100 cases of sporotrichosis. J Dermatol 1979;6:211.
244. Splendore A. Sobre a cultura d'uma nova especiale de cogumello pathogenico (sporotrichose de Splendore). Revista de Sociedade Scientifa de São Paulo 1908;3:62.
245. Hoeppli R. Histological observations in experimental schistosomiasis Japonica. Chin Med J 1932;46:1179.
246. Hiruma M, Kawada A, Ishibashi A. Ultrastructure of asteroid bodies in sporotrichosis. Mycoses 1991;34:103.
247. Moore M, Ackerman LV. Sporotrichosis with radiate formation in tissue. Arch Dermatol 1946;53:253.
248. Pinkus H, Grekin JN. Sporotrichosis with asteroid tissue forms: Report of a case. Arch Dermatol Syphil 1950;61:813.
249. Auld JC, Beardsmore GL. Sporotrichosis in Queensland: A review of 37 cases at the Royal Brisbane Hospital. Australas J Dermatol 1979; 20:14.
250. Reed KD, Moore FM, Geiger GE, Stemper ME. Zoonotic transmission of sporotrichosis: Case report and review. Clin Infect Dis 1993; 16:384.
251. Palestine RF, Rogers RS III. Diagnosis and treatment of mycetoma. J Am Acad Dermatol 1982;6:107.
252. Hay RJ, MacKenzie DWR. Mycetoma (Madura foot) in the United Kingdom: A survey of forty-four cases. Clin Exp Dermatol 1983; 8:553.
253. Green WO Jr, Adams TE. Mycetoma in the United States: A review and report of seven additional cases. Am J Clin Pathol 1964;42:75.
254. Go IH, Neering H. Actinomycosis. Br J Dermatol 1986;115:592.
255. Butz WC, Ajello L. Black grain mycetoma: A case due to *Madurella grisea*. Arch Dermatol 1971;104:197.
256. Taralakshmi VV, Pankajalakshmi VV, Arumugam S et al. Mycetoma caused by *Madurella mycetomii* in Madras. Australas J Dermatol 1978;19:125.
257. Barnetson RSC, Milne LJR. Mycetoma. Br J Dermatol 1978;99:227.
258. Zaias N, Taplin D, Rebell G. Mycetoma. Arch Dermatol 1969;99:215.
259. Karunaratne WAE. Rhinosporidiosis in man. London: The Athlone Press of the University of London, 1964.
260. Prins LC, Tange RA, Dingemans KP. Rhinosporidiosis in the Netherlands: A case report including ultramicroscopic features. ORL J Otorhinolaryngol Relat Spec 1983;45:237.
261. Prevost E, Kreutner A Jr, Vollotton WW, Walker EM Jr. Conjunctival lesion caused by *Rhinosporidium seeberi*. South Med J 1980;73:1077.
262. Kwon-Chung KJ, Bennett JE. Rhinosporidiosis. In: Kwon-Chung KJ, Bennett JE. Medical mycology. Philadelphia: Lea & Febinger, 1992; 695.
263. Rajam RV, Viswanathan GS, Rao AR, Rangiah PN. Rhinosporidiosis: A study with report of a fatal case of systemic dissemination. Ind J Surg 1955;17:269.
264. Binford CH, Connor DH. Pathology of tropical and extraordinary dis-

eases. Vol 2, Washington, D.C.: Armed Forces Institute of Pathology, 1976;597.
265. Easley JR, Meuten DJ, Levy MG et al. Nasal rhinosporidiosis in the dog. Vet Pathol 1986;23:50.
266. Nabai H, Mehregan AH. Cutaneous protothecosis: Report of a case from Iran. J Cutan Pathol 1974;1:180.
267. Mayhall CG, Miller CW, Eisen AZ et al. Cutaneous protothecosis: Successful treatment with amphotericin B. Arch Dermatol 1976;112: 1749.
268. Wolfe ID, Sacks HG, Samorodin CS, Robinson HM. Cutaneous protothecosis in a patient receiving immunosuppressive therapy. Arch Dermatol 1976;112:829.
269. Venezio FR, Lavoo E, Williams JE et al. Progressive cutaneous protothecosis. Am J Clin Pathol 1982;77:485.
270. Tindall JP, Fetter BF. Infections caused by achloric algae: Protothecosis. Arch Dermatol 1971;104:490.
271. Mars PW, Rabson AR, Rippey JJ, Ajello L. Cutaneous protothecosis. Br J Dermatol 1971;85:76.

Lever's Histopathology of the Skin, eighth edition,
edited by David Elder et al. Lippincott–
Raven Publishers, Philadelphia © 1997.

CHAPTER 24

Protozoan Diseases of the Skin

Jacinto Convit

LEISHMANIASIS

Leishmaniasis is transmitted by a protozoan parasite that causes three different major forms of the disease in humans:

1. *Cutaneous leishmaniasis* (CL), with two varieties: (a) American cutaneous leishmaniasis (ACL) produced by either the *Leishmania brasiliensis* complex or the *L mexicana* complex, which occur in vast areas of the American continent; and (b) Oriental cutaneous leishmaniasis (OCL), produced by *L tropica* or by two strains that have been considered as its subspecies, *L major* and *L aethiopia*, which occur in certain areas of the European continent, Middle East, Asia, and Africa.[1] In either variety, the initial cutaneous lesions generally occur as single or multiple erythematous papules on exposed areas of the body, weeks to months after the bite of an infected sandfly. The papules may enlarge to form indurated nodules, which frequently ulcerate to form a central crater.[2]

2. *Mucocutaneous leishmaniasis* (MCL; espundia), seemingly unique to the spectrum of American disease, may involve the upper respiratory system and oropharynx sometimes years after a primary lesion has healed. The involvement may cause considerable deformity and may progress to involve the palate, tongue, mouth, and pharynx to produce an extensive midline facial defect.[2]

3. *Visceral leishmaniasis*, also with two varieties: (a) Kala-Azar, produced by *L donovani*, which occurs in the African and Asian continents and certain areas of Brazil and is characterized by epidemic outbreaks that involve large population groups; and (b) a variety known as Mediterranean Kala-Azar, which is characterized by the occurrence of isolated cases in certain areas of Europe and Latin American countries.[3] In Europe the parasite causing this type of disease has been identified as *L infantum* and in Latin America the causative parasite has been identified as *L chagasi*.

The American and the Oriental varieties of cutaneous leishmaniasis can both be placed along a clinical and immunopathological spectrum in which the clinical features depend on the response of the host to the parasite. At one pole of the spectrum is the localized form (LCL), characterized by the occurrence of one or a few lesions with very few parasites and a well-developed immunological response. These cases generally respond very well to treatment. At the other pole is the diffuse form (DCL), characterized by multiple lesions, large numbers of parasites, absence of immunological response, and a poor response to treatment. Between these poles are the *mucocutaneous leishmaniasis* mentioned above, the *chronic* or *verrucous* form, which refers to primary lesions lasting more than two years and presenting as raised plaques,[4] and the *relapse* (recidivans) form, which may present as circinate papules at the edge of the scars of previously healed lesions.[5] These intermediate forms of the disease generally are very resistant to treatment even though they have a moderate number of parasites and exhibit delayed hypersensitivity-type immune phenomena directed towards leishmania parasites (Color Fig. 24-1). More than 90% of cutaneous leishmaniasis cases can be placed in the localized end of the spectrum (Color Figs. 24-2 and 24-3). The intermediate mucocutaneous, verrucous, or relapse forms taken together account for about 8% of ACL, and are very rare in OCL. Diffuse cases are extremely rare.

At the pole of the spectrum represented by localized cutaneous leishmaniasis, both in ACL and OCL, secondary infection is an important component of the disease. These infections are due to ulceration of lesions and secondary contamination by environmental materials, especially in inhabitants of rural areas. They are produced by a varied microbial flora. These infections greatly influence the evolution of lesions since they can disorganize and even destroy the granuloma induced by the leishmania parasite and, if not adequately treated, can induce chronicity of lesions. Published reports tend to consider that the occurrence of lesions of variable seriousness both in ACL and in OCL can be attributed to different parasite strains, but in our view the diversity of lesions relates more importantly to the immunological response of the host and to the intensity of secondary infections.

Histopathology. The morphology of cutaneous lesions is similar in the two cutaneous varieties (ACL and OCL).

J. Convit: Instituto Nacional de Dermatologia, Caracas, Venezuela

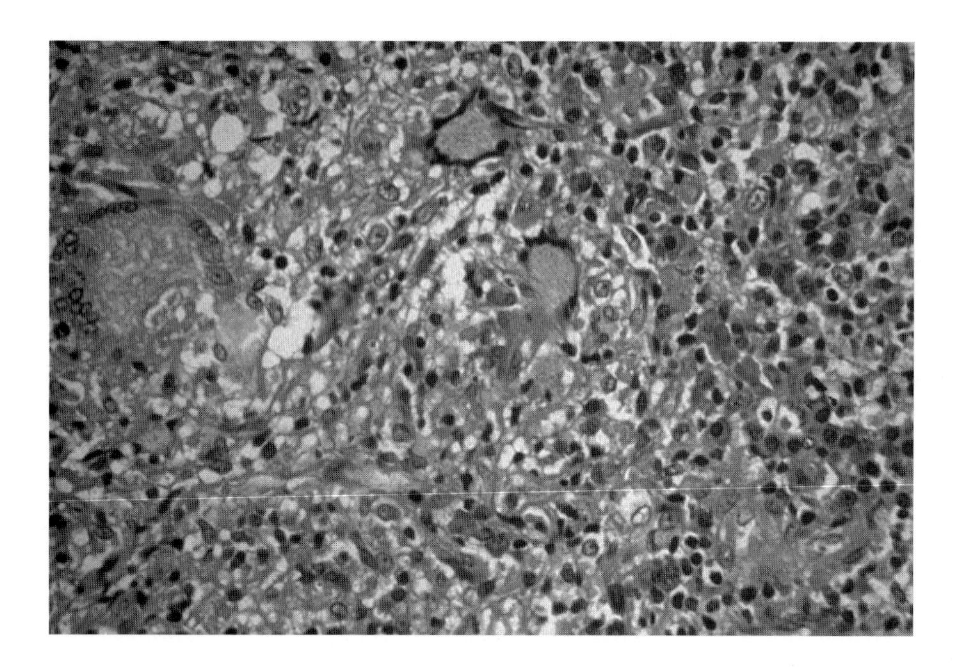

FIG. 24-1. Histologic structure of granuloma produced by *Leishmania*

Localized Cutaneous Leishmaniasis

Early lesions are characterized by a macrophagic infiltrate with a slight tendency to epithelioid differentiation (related to time of evolution), with associated infiltration by lymphoid cells. In this stage there are variably abundant parasites inside macrophages, facilitating diagnosis both through direct lesional touch smears and in biopsy sections. At this time the Montenegro reaction to leishmania antigen is frequently negative or weakly positive, and lesions usually have not yet become ulcerated (Fig. 24-1).

In the intermediate or late stages most lesions are ulcerated. In the few lesions that are not ulcerated the morphology is characterized by a tuberculoid-type granuloma with prominent lymphoid infiltration. An interesting finding in this stage is the relationship between CD4 and CD8 T cells, where CD4 cells predominate but the CD8 cells are located at the periphery of tuberculoid nodules, while CD4 cells are scattered within the granuloma as well as separate from it.[6] When the lesions are ulcerated, they show nonspecific inflammatory changes related both to time of evolution and to secondary infections. In these cases, biopsies should be taken from the periphery of ulcerated lesions to include the non-ulcerated edge of the lesion (Fig. 24-2).

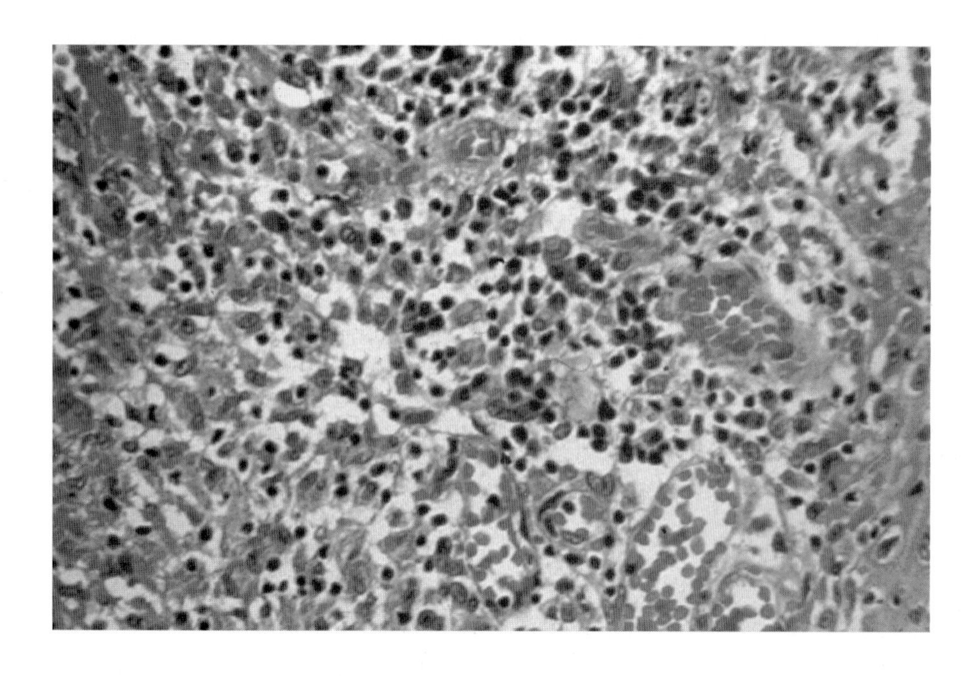

FIG. 24-2. Histologic structure of granuloma produced by secondary infection over a lesion produced by *Leishmania*

The histopathology of acute lesions is usually characterized by epithelial loss, but in chronic lesions there can be a variable degree of epithelial hypertrophy. In the dermis there is granulomatous inflammation influenced by the time of evolution and by secondary infection. As a result of these two factors there is great variation in morphology. The appearances may range from predominance of a leishmanial granuloma with macrophages showing epithelioid differentiation, abundant Langerhans-type and foreign-body type giant cells and lymphocytes, to complete absence of epithelioid cell granulomas, but with a subacute or chronic mixed-cell reaction provoked by secondary infection. The latter may present with macrophagic infiltrates, formation of small abscesses, necrotic areas, plasma-cell infiltrates, and proliferation of small vessels as evolution time becomes more prolonged. In this stage, parasites in lesions become increasingly difficult to find. Usually only a few isolated parasites can be found in direct lesion smears, many of them atypical. Culture of these parasites is extremely difficult both due to their scarcity and to secondary infection. Sometimes previous intensive treatment of secondary infection can favor detection of parasites in this type of lesion.

In ulcerated lesions the CD4 and CD8 T cells lose the distribution seen in non-ulcerated lesions, and both types are seen scattered diffusely in the infiltrates. In this stage the Montenegro reaction is strongly positive, with a greater than 30 mm diameter in some cases. In this type of disease, due to the scarcity of parasites, molecular biology techniques (PCR) have been very helpful for obtaining a parasitological diagnosis in more than 90% of cases.[6]

Mucocutaneous, Chronic Verrucous, and Relapse Leishmaniasis

In these lesions that occupy the intermediate area of the leishmaniasis spectrum, the microscopic morphology is quite variable. In *chronic cutaneous leishmaniasis*, which refers to lesions having a duration of greater than two years, there is variable epithelial hypertrophy, which in some cases can be pseudoepitheliomatous. There may be well-formed granulomas resembling lupus vulgaris but lacking caseation necrosis. Leishmania organisms may be difficult to find in these lesions.[7] In *leishmaniasis recidivans* the histologic changes combine features of both the acute and the chronic forms. The dermis shows an infiltrate of macrophages, lymphoid cells, and some plasma cells as well as tuberculoid granulomas. The number of leishmania organisms is variable. They are difficult to find in some cases.[7]

The other forms that occupy the interpolar area of the spectrum, *verrucous* and *relapse leishmaniasis* (leishmaniasis recidivans), have a variable structure, with a predominant leishmanial granuloma in some cases, while in others the mixed response to secondary infection predominates. In verrucous forms of both varieties (ACL and OCL) the structure is reminiscent of verrucous tuberculosis and parasites are extremely few.

In early *mucocutaneous leishmaniasis* there may be macrophagic infiltration with abundant giant-cell reactivity and a lymphoid infiltrate. Parasites are frequently seen in early lesions, becoming more difficult to find as the lesion progresses. In ulcerated mucosal lesions the inflammatory infiltrate may be nonspecific and diagnosis may be difficult. This type of lesion can occur jointly with cutaneous lesions or can develop many years after cutaneous lesions have healed.[2] In the late stages of mucous lesions secondary infection appears and the reaction to that infection suppresses the "in situ" response to leishmania parasites, becoming a chronic mixed-cell inflammatory lesion with, in some cases, very few giant cells. As a consequence of this process, parasites become extremely rare and biopsies, smears, and even cultures appear parasitologically negative. It is in these cases that molecular biology techniques such as PCR become very important, since they allow parasitologic confirmation in a high percentage of cases. It is also in these late stages that mucous ACL lesions may invade the palate, pharynx, and larynx. Parasites isolated from these lesions always belong to the *L brasiliensis* complex, whereas in localized cutaneous forms, they can belong either to the *L brasiliensis* or to the *L mexicana* complexes. In mucosal ACL lesions the Montenegro reaction is positive and it can be greater than 30 mm in diameter in 50% of cases. In this stage confusion with paracoccidiomycosis, epithelial or lymphomatous neoplasms, and rhinoscleroma is possible, but the histopathological examination clarifies the diagnosis.

Diffuse Cutaneous Leishmaniasis

The diffuse pole of both varieties of cutaneous leishmaniasis is characterized by plaque-like or nodular lesions that can be localized in a single area of the body in the early stages and then extend until they cover most of the skin and start to slowly compromise nasal, buccal, and laryngeal mucous tissue in very advanced cases. Clinically, lesions can be confused with lepromatous leprosy or with cutaneous lymphomas. The Montenegro reaction is negative. We also have observed the visceralization of cutaneous leishmaniasis lesions, both in ACL and in OCL, as a consequence of HIV-induced immunodefficiency.

The microscopic morphology of DCL is a macrophagic infiltrate with sparse lymphocytes and with enormous numbers of parasites inside macrophages (Figs. 24-3 and 24-4).

Differential Diagnosis of the Various Forms of Leishmaniasis

Leishmania parasites can be easily identified in skin smears and in histopathological sections when parasites are abundant. When parasites are few, diagnosis can be done through direct lesion smears after careful search by an experienced observer. In other cases with very few parasites, identification is very difficult or almost impossible. Leishmaniasis is one of four cutaneous diseases that are characterized by an infiltrate containing large parasitized macrophages. The others are *rhinoscleroma* and *granuloma inguinale*, caused by bacteria, and *histoplasmosis*, caused by a fungus. In spite of great similarities, these four diseases have points of differentiation that in most instances make a histologic diagnosis possible. Leishmania parasites are differentiated from *Histoplasma capsulatum* by their oval form and by the presence of a nucleus and a kinetoplast; this last body is not present in *histoplasma*. The leishmania parasite is more easily differentiated from the organisms that produce rhinoscleroma and granuloma inguinale (Table 24-1).

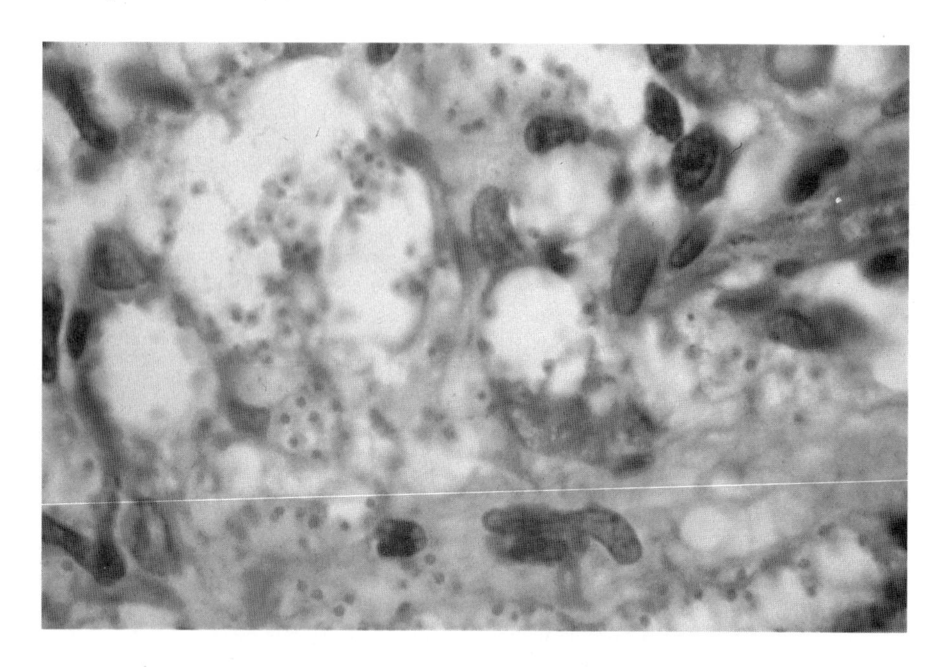

FIG. 24-3. Diffuse cutaneous leishmaniasis case with nodules and plaque on face

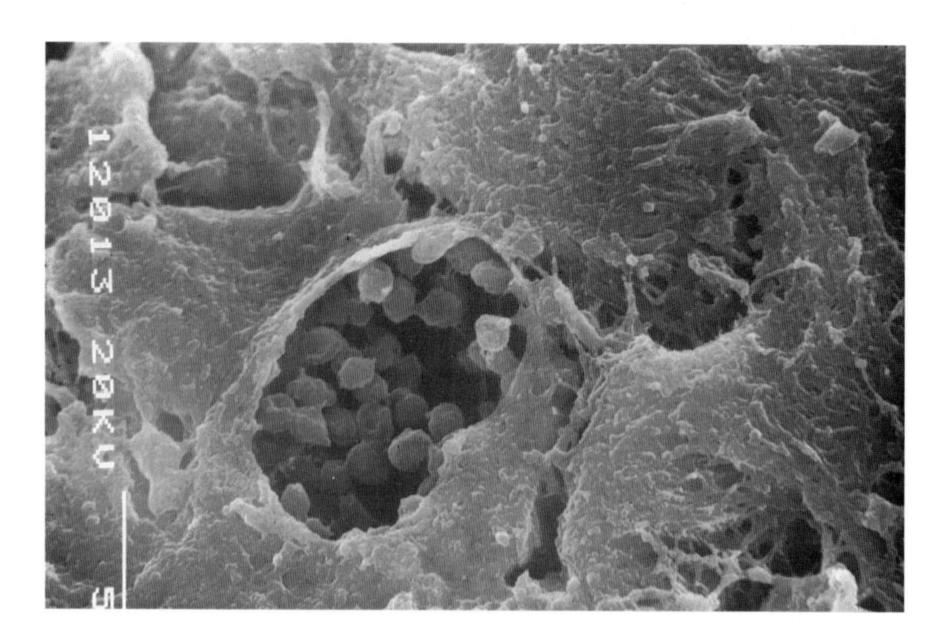

FIG. 24-4. Diffuse cutaneous leishmaniasis
Cytoplasmic vacuole filled with *Leishmania* amastigotes (microphotograph with scanning electron microscope). (Courtesy of Professors Nishiura and Bretaña.)

TABLE 24-1. *Points of differentiation among four cutaneous disease characterized by parasitized histiocytes*

Disease	Distinctive histologic features	Size of organism (μm)	Appearance of organism in tissue
Rhinoscleroma	Mikulicz cells larger than other parasitized histiocytes. Plasma cells and Russell bodies prominent	*Klebsiela pneumoniae rhinoscleromatis* 2–3 μm	Round or oval
Granuloma inguinale	Small abscesses scattered through infiltrate	Calymmato-bacterium granulomatis (Donovan bodies) 1–2 μm	Encapsulated round or oval bodies
Histoplasmosis	Foci of necrosis common	Histoplasma capsulatum 2–4 μm	Round or oval bodies surrounded by a clear halo
Leishmaniasis	Variable: granulomas, mixed infiltrates, abscesses, sheets of histiocytes	*Leishmania* species 2–4 μm	Nonencapsulated round/oval bodies containing a nucleus and a paranucleus (kinetoplast)

Dermal Post-Kala-Azar Leishmaniasis

There are two Kala-Azar varieties. One that compromises large population groups is seen in Asia and Africa and is produced by *L donovani*. The other variety, Mediterranean Kala-Azar, produced by *L chagasi* or *L infantum*, is found as isolated cases in Europe and Latin America. These disorders are characterized by chronic, irregular fever, anemia, weight loss, and hepatosplenomegaly. Cutaneous lesions (dermal Kala-Azar) may occur either during the visceral disease or later in cases where visceral disease seems to be extinguished. These latter manifestations are very frequent in India (20%) and in some areas of East Africa (5%), but are very rare in Latin America.

Histopathology. The cutaneous manifestations are characterized by macules, plaques, and nodular lesions, which can mimic lepromatous leprosy. Macular lesions show a structure formed by an upper-dermal infiltrate formed by histiocytes, lymphoid cells, and plasma cells. Leishmania parasites are frequently rare and often have to be searched for in direct lesion smears. In plaque lesions cellular infiltration is more dense and is formed by histiocytes, lymphoid cells, and plasma cells; these last cells are more abundant. There are many more parasites than in macular lesions. In nodular lesions there is a granuloma that extends down to the subcutis, formed by macrophages and some giant cells, with infiltration by lymphoid and plasma cells. Parasites are very abundant inside macrophages in most cases, but in others, the parasite population is low.

REFERENCES

1. Walton BC. Leishmaniasis: A world-wide problem. Int J Dermatol 1989;28:305.
2. Keeling JH. Tropical parasitic infections. In: James WD, ed. Military dermatology. Washington, D.C.: Armed Forces Institute of Pathology, 1994;255.
3. Marsden PD. Current concepts in parasitology: Leishmaniasis. N Engl J Med 1979;300:350.
4. Hart M, Livingood CS, Goltz RW et al. Late cutaneous leishmaniasis. Arch Dermatol 1969;99:455.
5. Strick RA, Borok M, Gasiorowski HC. Recurrent cutaneous leishmaniasis. J Am Acad Dermatol 1983;9:437.
6. Convit J, Ulrich M, Fernandez CT et al. The clinical and immunological spectrum of American cutaneous leishmaniasis. Trans R Soc Trop Med Hyg 1993;87:444.
7. Farah FS, Malak JA. Cutaneous leishmaniasis. Arch Dermatol 1971;103:467.

Lever's Histopathology of the Skin, eighth edition,
edited by David Elder et al. Lippincott–
Raven Publishers, Philadelphia © 1997.

CHAPTER 25

Parasitic Infestations of the Skin

David Elder, Rosalie Elenitsas, Bernett Johnson Jr., and Christine Jaworsky

SCABIES

Burrows are the characteristic lesions of scabies, which is caused by the eight-legged itch mite *Sarcoptes scabiei*. The burrows, which are produced by female mites, occur mainly on the palms, the palmar and lateral aspects of the fingers, the web spaces between the fingers, the flexor surfaces of the wrists, the nipples of women, and the genitals of men. They appear as fine, tortuous, blackish threads a few millimeters long. Often, a vesicle is visible near the blind end of the burrow. The mite is situated in this vesicle and often is visible as a tiny gray speck. In addition, there is a papular pruritic eruption, usually without recognizable burrows. It is most pronounced on the abdomen, the lower portions of the buttocks, and the anterior axillary folds. In some patients, itching nodules persist for several months after successful treatment. They are found most commonly on the scrotum and are thought to represent lesions that at one time harbored mites but no longer contain them.

In a rare variant, the so-called Norwegian scabies, innumerable mites are present. Patients with this variant show widespread erythema, hyperkeratosis, and crusting, but no obvious burrows. An "exaggerated" form of scabies with generalized papulosquamous lesions may occur in patients with the acquired immunodeficiency syndrome.[1]

Histopathology. A definitive diagnosis of scabies can be made only by demonstration of the mite or its products. A very superficial epidermal shave biopsy of an early papule or, preferably, of an entire burrow may be carried out with a scalpel blade.[2] Local anesthesia is not required. The biopsy specimen is placed on a glass slide, and a drop of immersion oil and then a cover slip are placed on top of it.

Histologic examination of a specimen containing a burrow reveals that the burrow in almost its entire length is located within the horny layer. Only the extreme, blind end of the burrow, where the female mite is situated, extends into the stratum malpighii.[3] The mite has a rounded body and measures about 400 μm in length (Fig. 25-1).[4]

Spongiosis is present in the stratum malpighii near the mite to such an extent that formation of a vesicle is often the result. Even if no mite is found in the sections, the presence of eggs containing larvae, of egg shells, or of fecal deposits within the horny layer is indicative of scabies.[5] The dermal infiltrate in sections containing mites shows varying numbers of eosinophils. Papular lesions not containing mites show a nonspecific picture in which eosinophils generally are absent.[6]

In *persistent nodular scabies*, there is a dense, chronic inflammatory infiltrate in which eosinophils may be present. The blood vessels may have thickened walls, and there may even be vasculitis with fibrinoid deposits and inflammatory cells within the vessel walls.[5] Atypical mononuclear cells may be found, and in some instances, the nodules show, as in persistent arthropod bites or stings (see later), a histologic picture resembling lymphoma.[7] Mites are hardly ever found in the nodules.

In Norwegian scabies, the thickened horny layer is riddled with innumerable mites, so that nearly every section shows several parasites (Fig. 25-2).[5]

Pathogenesis. Scanning electron microscopy reveals the keratinocytes around the burrow to be compacted, indicating that the mite physically forces its way in between the keratinocytes, rather than chewing a passage. The burrow is essentially a tunnel within the stratum corneum, formed as the mite burrows down to the live stratum granulosum for nourishment.[8]

Both cell-mediated and humoral hypersensitivities are activated in scabies. The acute eczematoid reaction in the epidermis is indicative of cell-mediated hypersensitivity. A role for humoral hypersensitivity is suggested by the presence of immunoglobulin M (IgM) and the third component of complement (C3) in vessel walls and occasionally also along the dermal-epidermal junction.[9] Norwegian scabies is observed generally in persons who have a congenital or iatrogenic impairment of the immune responses but also in the mentally deficient and the physically debilitated.[10]

D. Elder: Department of Pathology and Laboratory Medicine, University of Pennsylvania, Philadelphia, PA

R. Elenitsas: Department of Dermatology, University of Pennsylvania, Philadelphia, PA

B. Johnson Jr.: Department of Dermatology, University of Pennsylvania, Philadelphia, PA

C. Jaworsky: Departments of Dermatology and Pathology, Case Western Reserve University, Cleveland, OH; Department of Dermatology, University of Pennsylvania, Philadelphia, PA

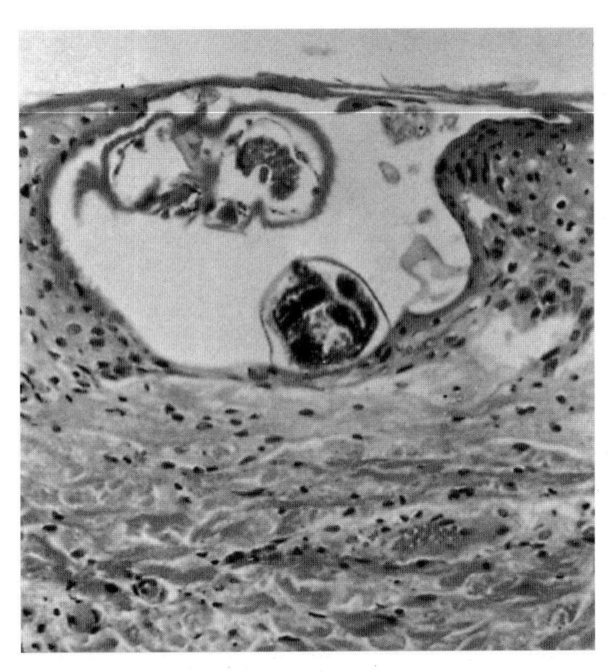

FIG. 25-1. Scabies
A female mite is located within a subcorneal burrow.

LARVA MIGRANS ERUPTION

Larva migrans eruption is caused by filariform larvae of the dog and cat hookworms *Ancylostoma braziliensis* and *A. caninum*. It is commonly known as creeping eruption. Migration is manifested by an irregularly linear, thin, raised burrow, 2 to 3 mm wide. The larva moves a few millimeters per day. The eruption is self-limited because humans are abnormal hosts. The feet and buttocks are the areas most commonly involved.

Histopathology. The larva is found in a specimen taken from just beyond the leading edge of the track. It is located in a burrow in the epidermis (Fig. 25-3). The lesion, aside from the larva which is often not observed in the biopsies, shows spongiosis and intraepidermal vesicles in which necrotic keratinocytes can be seen. The epidermis and the upper dermis contain a chronic inflammatory infiltrate with many eosinophils.[11]

SUBCUTANEOUS DIROFILARIASIS

Subcutaneous infection of humans by *Dirofilaria* is rare. This infection, transmitted by mosquitoes, may occur throughout the southern, eastern, and midwestern states of the United States. One or, occasionally, several well-defined, firm, slightly red, tender nodules 1 to 2 cm in diameter are present.

Histopathology. At the center of the subcutaneous nodule, there is a tightly convoluted worm seen in multiple transverse and diagonal sections. Transverse sections measure 125 to 250 μm in diameter. The worm, often partially degenerated, possesses a thick, laminated cuticle. It is embedded in eosinophilic, fibrinoid material and surrounded by an inflammatory reaction that includes mononuclear cells, many eosinophils, and often foreign-body giant cells[12–14] (Fig. 25-4).

Pathogenesis. The usual hosts of *Dirofilaria* are animals. In dogs, the worm *Dirofilaria immitis* causes the so-called heartworm disease. This organism may cause pulmonary dirofilariasis in a human as an accidental host. Subcutaneous dirofilariasis is usually caused in the United States by *D tenuis* and in Europe, Africa, and Asia by *D repens*, parasites of the American opossum and of dogs and cats, respectively.[15] From these animals,

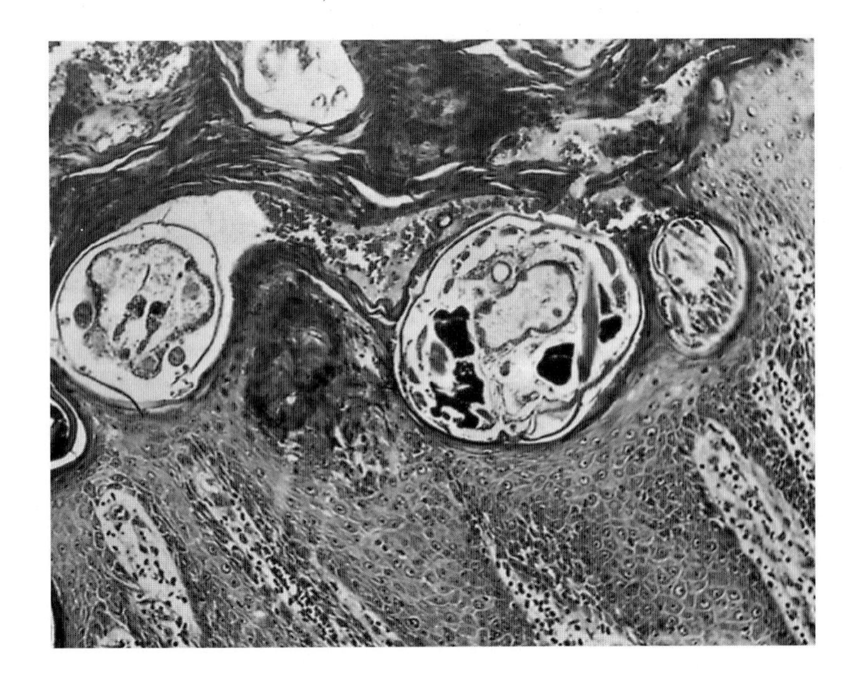

FIG. 25-2. Scabies (Norwegian scabies)
Multiple subcorneal burrows containing female mites are present. There are also hyperkeratosis, acanthosis, and a marked dermal cellular infiltrate. (Courtesy of Robert N. Buchanan Jr., MD.)

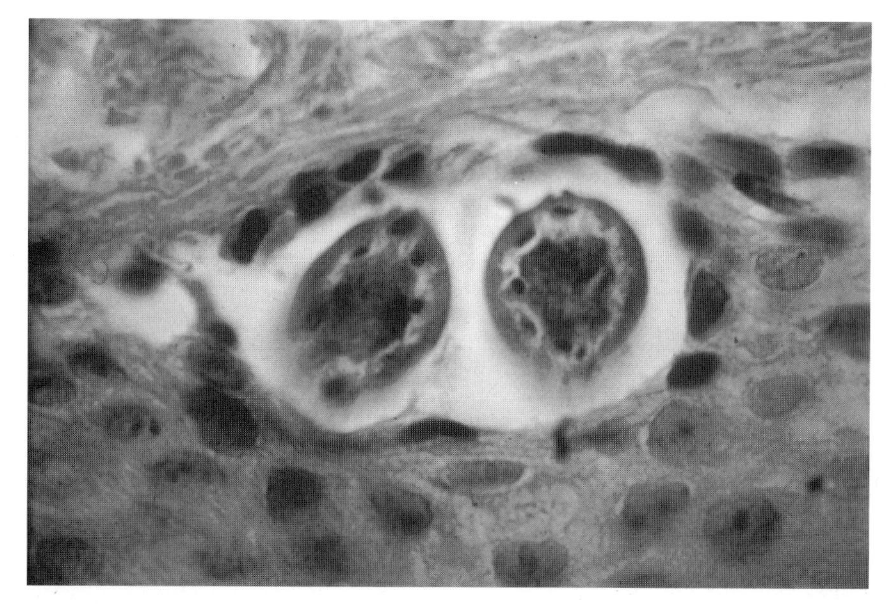

FIG. 25-3. Larva migrans
Cross section of larvae of *Ancylostoma* in the superficial epidermis (PAS stain). (From Johnson BJ Jr., Honig P, Jaworsky C, eds., Pediatric dermatopathology, Newton, MA: Butterworth-Heineman, 1994. Reprinted with permission.)

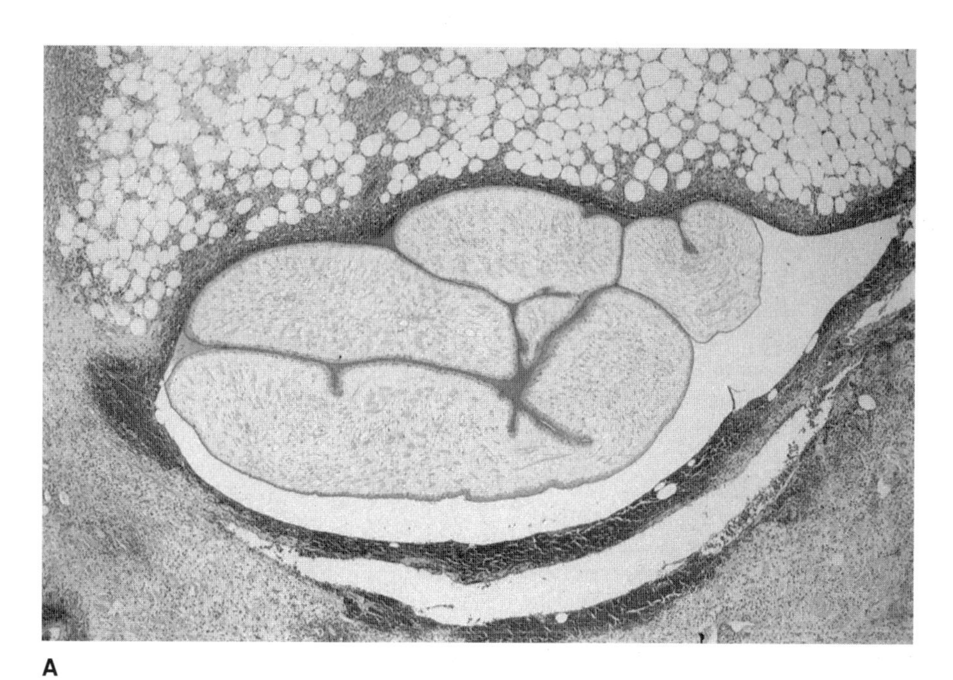

A

FIG. 25-4. Dirofilariasis
(**A**) The worm can be seen coiled in the center of an inflammatory nodule in the subcutis. *(continued on next page)*

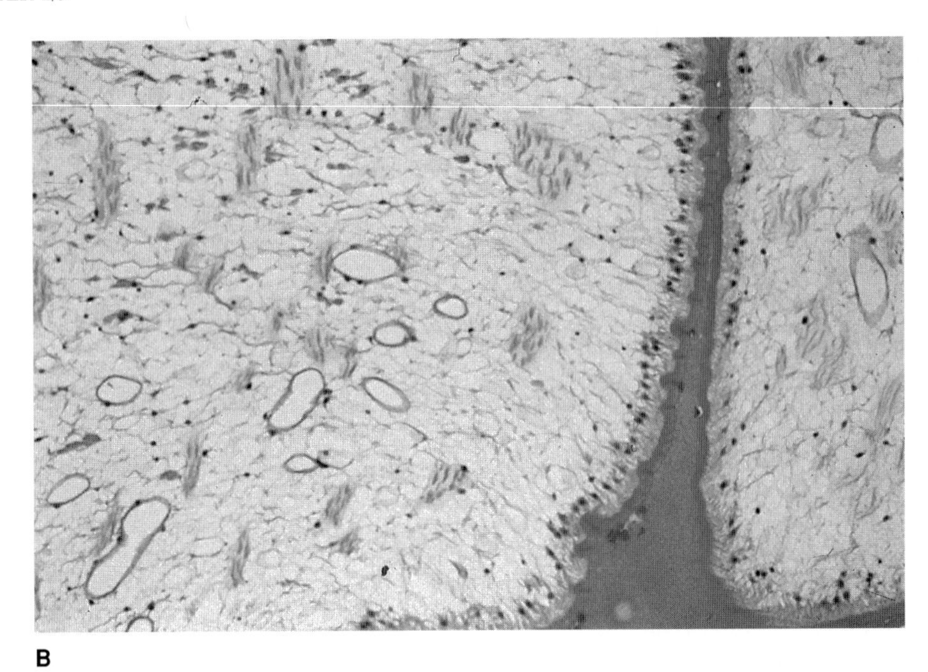

B

FIG. 25-4. *Continued*
(**B**) The worm has a cuticle with internal and external longitudinal ridges, and internal organs.

mosquitoes may transmit microfilariae to humans, who act as terminal hosts.[12]

ONCHOCERCIASIS

Onchocerciasis is common in certain regions of Central America, Venezuela, and tropical Africa. It is transmitted by black flies of the genus *Simulium*, which breed in fast-flowing rivers; through their proboscises, the infective larvae of *Onchocerca volvulus*, a filarial nematode, enter the human skin. They mature to the adult stage in the subcutaneous tissue. The adult filariae or worms live in the deep dermis and subcutis and become clinically apparent as asymptomatic subcutaneous nodules called onchocercomas, of which there are usually only a few, ranging in size from 0.5 to 2.0 cm. The adult worms do not cause any harm; however, their progeny, consisting of millions of microfilariae, live in the dermis and the aqueous humor of the eyes, where they provoke inflammatory changes after several years. Clinically, onchocercal dermatitis is characterized by itching, edema, lichenification, and pigment shifting. Later on, the skin becomes atrophic. In the eyes, iritis may result in blindness. On slit lamp examination, the microfilariae in the anterior chamber of the eyes may be seen to be moving actively.[16] *Onchocerca volvulus*, like *Wucheria bancrofti*, may also be a cause of lymphatic filariasis, in which massive numbers of microfilariae may occlude lymphatics and result in elephantiasis.[17]

Histopathology. The onchocercomas show at their peripheries a chronic inflammatory infiltrate and fibrosis. Their centers consist of dense fibrous tissue containing transverse and diagonal sections of adult worms measuring from 100 to 500 μm in transverse diameter (Fig. 25-5B). Some of them are alive at the time of biopsy. Dead worms are surrounded by an inflammatory reaction containing foreign-body giant cells. Microfilariae, hatched by female worms, are occasionally observed within lymphatic vessels of the onchocercomas, through which they are disseminated in the skin. They are from 5 to 9 μm in diameter and from 150 to 360 μm in length[18] (Fig. 25-5A and B).

In onchocercal dermatitis, many undulating microfilariae are present within the dermis, mainly close to the epidermis (Fig. 25-5C). Their number decreases greatly with time, and thus they may be difficult to find in old lesions.[19] In early infections, reactive changes in the dermis are minimal, but, in the course of years, chronic inflammatory cells and eosinophils accumulate

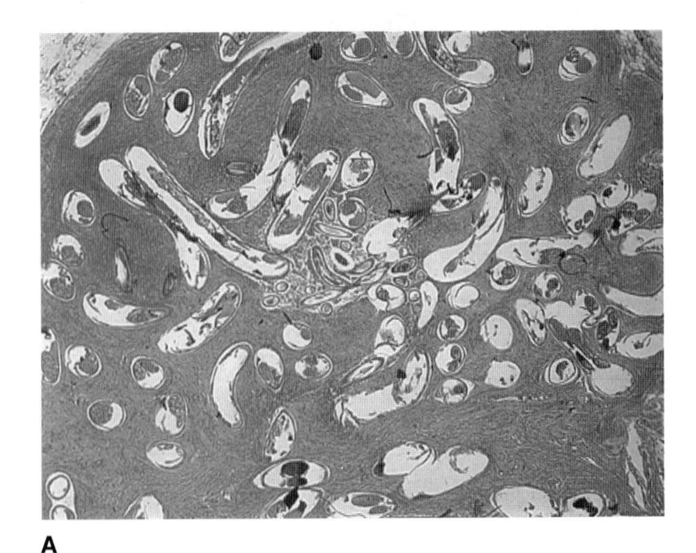

A

FIG. 25-5. Onchocercal nodule (onchocercoma)
(**A**) Cross sections of adult female worms embedded in a fibrous reaction.

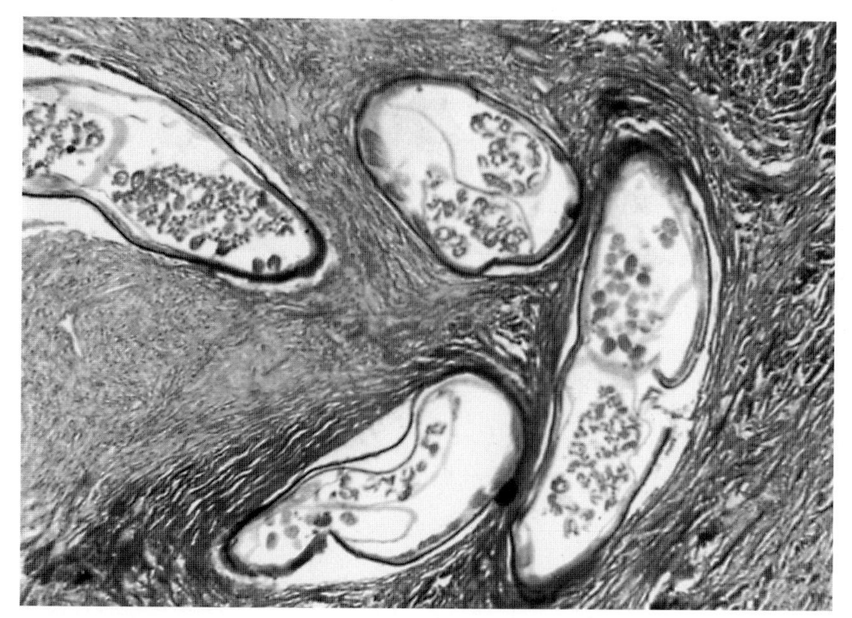

B

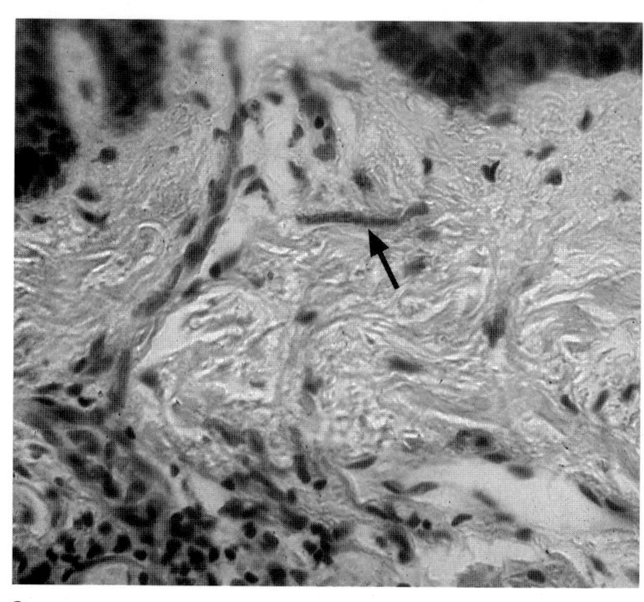

C

FIG. 25-5. *Continued*
(B) Adult worms in a fibrous stroma. (**C**) Onchocercal dermatitis. Microfilariae are present in the superficial dermis. They have the appearance of narrow, elongated fibroblast-like cells with multiple tiny nuclei *(arrow)*.

around the vessels, and, ultimately, fibrosis of the dermis and flattening of the epidermis result.[16]

Pathogenesis. The slow development of the cutaneous changes and also of the ocular changes suggests that microfilariae, as they gradually disintegrate, act as a source of foreign protein and that the dermatitis and iritis are the result of a delayed hypersensitivity.[16]

STRONGYLOIDIASIS

Strongyloides stercoralis is a small intestinal nematode that has the ability to multiply within the human host. It affects the skin very rarely except in immunocompromised patients who may develop a fatal disseminated infection showing extensive purpura associated with massive invasion of the skin by larvae. In addition, there may be linear streaks caused by the rapidly migrating larvae.

Histopathology. Cross and oblique sections of *S. stercoralis* are observed at all levels of the dermis. The larvae measure from 9 to 15 μm in diameter. In addition, there are numerous extravasated erythrocytes.[20]

SCHISTOSOMIASIS

Schistosomiasis is acquired through exposure to a schistosome pathogenic to humans that has been discharged by a freshwater snail and is in the cercarial stage. The cercariae burrow through the skin and migrate to venous plexuses, where they mature. The initial penetration causes a pruritic papular eruption referred to as a swimmer's itch. Several weeks after penetration, the schistosomes have matured into worms 15 to 25 mm in length. The female then releases thousands of eggs. Their release may be accompanied by urticaria and a serum-sickness-like syndrome manifested by fever and/or urticaria sometimes with purpura called bilharzides or schistosomides.[21–23]

Three species of *Schistosoma* are pathogenic to humans. *Schistosoma mansoni* is common in the Caribbean islands and in northeastern South America; *S japonicum* is found in Eastern Asia; and *S haematobium* is common in the Middle East and in Africa. The usual habitats of *S mansoni* are the portal circulation and mesenteric venules of the large intestines, with discharge of the eggs in the stool. The usual habitat of *S japonicum* is the small gut, also resulting in discharge of the eggs with the stool. The usual habitats of *S haematobium* are the pelvic and vesical venules, with passage of the eggs with the urine. *S mansoni* and *S japonicum,* through granulomas in the liver, may cause portal hypertension and esophageal varices, and *S haematobium,* through granulomas in the bladder, may lead to hematuria and hydronephrosis.[24] In Africa, mixed infections with both *S mansoni* and *S haematobium* are not uncommon.[22]

Specific cutaneous involvement (known as *bilharziasis cutanea tarda*) may occur as papular, verrucous, ulcerative, or granulomatous lesions in the genital or perianal skin secondary to the deposition of eggs in dermal vessels connecting with deeper vessels.[23,25,26] Cutaneous lesions in the genital and perianal regions are caused usually by *S haematobium*. This is due in part to the much greater production of eggs by *S haematobium* than by *S mansoni*. *S haematobium* is also found in the more superficial hemorrhoidal and vesical plexuses, and *S mansoni* is found in the deeper mesenteric plexuses.[23] In rare instances, there is "ectopic" involvement of the skin elsewhere when ova have become dislodged from their natural habitat in the venous circulation. One observes in such cases either slightly erythematous grouped papules on the thorax[22] or, rarely, a solitary plaque on the face.[27]

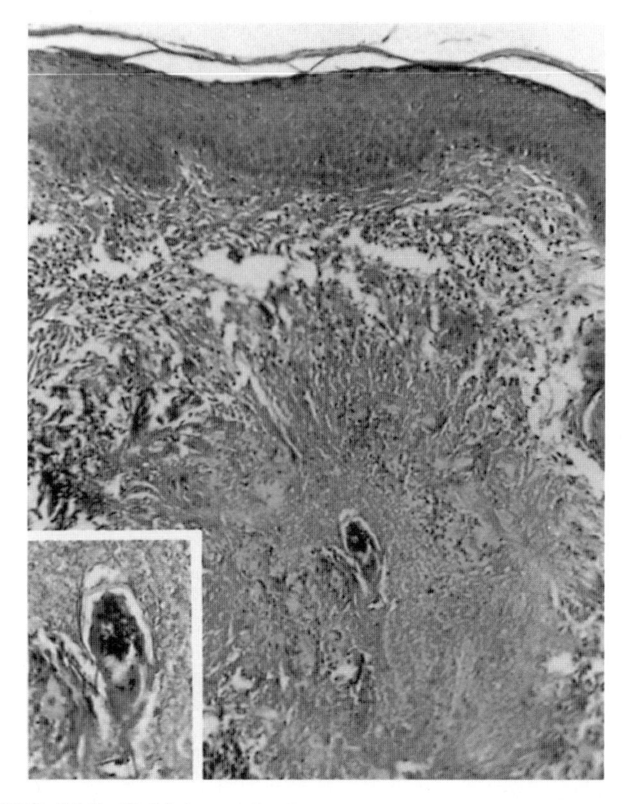

FIG. 25-6. Schistosomiasis
An ovum of *S mansoni*, showing a spine on its lateral aspect, is located in an area of necrosis. Inset shows the ovum at a higher magnification.

Dermatitis schistosomica (swimmer's itch) is caused usually by the cercaria of nonhuman species of Schistosoma (usually avian species primarily affecting ducks or other water birds). These cercaria can penetrate the skin but go no further. The dermatitis produced by human species of Schistosoma is milder than that caused by nonhuman species.[21]

Histopathology. The main pathologic feature in schistosomiasis is the schistosomal egg granuloma. In genital and perianal lesions, numerous ova are found within a granulomatous infiltrate or within microabscesses.[25] The ova measure up to 1 mm in greatest dimension and possess a chitinous outer shell staining positively with the periodic acid-Schiff (PAS) stain. The presence and position of a spine on the shell of the ova permit their classification within the tissue. *S haematobium* ova have a spine in the apical position, whereas the spine of *S mansoni* ova is on the lateral aspect (Fig. 25-6), and *S japonicum* ova have no spine. Ova may be seen crossing the epithelium toward the surface. In rare instances, one may also see adult worms within distended blood vessels in the dermis.[25,26]

In ectopic papules or plaques, many palisading, necrotizing granulomas extend throughout the dermis and may cause perforation of the epidermis. Within the necrotic area, one or several ova may be observed (see Fig. 25-6). The infiltrate at the periphery of the necrotic area shows epithelioid cells, histiocytes, lymphocytes, and numerous plasma cells[22] ; in some instances, it shows eosinophils and giant cells.[27]

Pathogenesis. The eggs and embryos are said to release soluble substances that act as antigens sensitizing T lymphocytes. These, in turn, release lymphokines leading to migration of macrophages and eosinophils, and to granuloma formation.[21]

SUBCUTANEOUS CYSTICERCOSIS

The pork tapeworm *Taenia solium* develops in the human intestinal tract following the ingestion of inadequately cooked pork containing *T solium* larvae. The tapeworm discharges its eggs in the feces. When these eggs are ingested by humans, usually through contamination of hands and food by the subject's own feces, they hatch, and larvae are borne by blood or lymph to various tissues, where they develop into cysticerci. These organisms are encountered most often in the subcutaneous tissue, eye, brain, skeletal muscle, and heart.[28]

Clinically, one or several, or, rarely, numerous firm, asymptomatic nodules are present in the subcutaneous tissue. They usually measure 1 to 2 cm in diameter.[29] They persist for many years. In some patients with subcutaneous cysticercosis, there is a preceding or simultaneous intestinal infection with *T solium* (taeniasis).[30]

The subcutaneously located cysts of cysticercosis do not carry any risk to the patient's health; but the cysts possess great value in the diagnosis of cysticercosis of the brain, which causes seizures.[31]

Histopathology. A thick, fibrous capsule surrounds a cystic cavity containing clear fluid and a white, irregularly shaped membranous structure representing a cysticercus larva and referred to as *Cysticercus cellulosae*.[32] It shows, on careful step sectioning, the scolex of the larva with suckers and hooks visible.[31]

MYIASIS

The order Diptera (having two wings) includes flies, gnats, and mosquitoes. When fly larvae inhabit the human body, the condition is called myiasis (from the Greek word for fly, *myia*). The distribution of myiasis is worldwide, with greater abundance of cases and of causative species in the tropics. The responsible agents may be obligatory, as in the case of the human botfly, *Dermatobia hominis*, or opportunistic. The opportunistic organisms do not depend on a human host. Examples of these include *Musca domestica*, the common housefly, and the screw worm *Cochliomyia hominovorax*, which is distributed in the southern United States and tropical Americas.

Myiasis may be classified by location in the body. Cutaneous myiasis includes wound myiasis and furuncular myiasis in which larvae develop and penetrate into the skin and subcutis to form an inflammatory mass. In nasopharyngeal myiasis, which may be caused by *C hominovorax*, the nose, sinuses, nasopharynx, and orbit may be infested by deeply burrowing larvae, which are about an inch long and may be present in large numbers in a single lesion. Infestation of the nose or ears may lead to penetration of the brain with a high fatality rate.[33]

Histopathology. The larvae are usually grossly visible and are usually alive at the time of biopsy. *Furuncular myiasis* presents as a subdermal inflammatory mass containing larvae. In the American tropics, a furuncular lesion known as a "warble" is caused by the human botfly, *D hominis*, whose eggs are transmitted by a mosquito or other vector. There is an intense mixed inflammatory infiltrate of neutrophils, lymphocytes, plasma cells, and giant cells surrounding the cavity, which is occupied by the larva. When the larva is mature, it moves actively, enlarging the superficial opening, and escapes, leaving an empty inflammatory sinus cavity, which is prone to secondary infection.

In *wound myiasis*, which may be caused by many different fly species including *M domestica*, the maggots are deposited on necrotic flesh. Generally, they remain superficial and can be recognized grossly.[33]

ARTHROPOD BITES AND STINGS

Mosquito bites evoke an early toxic response that is urticarial and a later allergic response that is characterized by papules.[34]

Stings of bees, wasps, or hornets may produce one of three types of reaction: an acute necrotic response, a subacute inflammatory response, or a chronic lymphoid response.[35] The latter is referred to as a persistent arthropod sting. The bites of ticks may similarly result in persistent papular or nodular lesions that cause a diagnostic problem clinically and histologically.

Bites by the black recluse spider are common in the south central United States. The bites are often painless. After early nonspecific changes, nonhealing necrotic ulcers may form.

Hypersensitivity to insect bites, especially from fleas, mosquitoes, or bedbugs, may result in papular urticaria.

Histopathology. Mosquito bites show mainly neutrophils during the early toxic response and a mononuclear infiltrate of lymphoid cells and plasma cells during the later allergic response. Eosinophils are few or absent.[34]

The acute necrotic response and the subacute inflammatory response to the stings of bees, wasps, or hornets have a nonspecific histologic appearance. The chronic lymphoid response to these stings and also to the bites of ticks may have a pseudolymphomatous appearance because of the presence of large transformed lymphoid cells.

In the chronic lymphoid response, the dermis presents a dense inflammatory infiltrate that may even extend into the subcutaneous fat. It consists of lymphoid cells and histiocytes with an admixture of eosinophils and plasma cells. Some of the cells may show hyperchromatic nuclei indicative of transformed cells. Multinucleated cells may also occur. Frequently, there are large lymphoid follicles with germinal centers, a reassuring feature.[36] In the case of tick bites, parts of the tick are occasionally found in the dermis (Fig. 25-7). Bites of black recluse spiders initially show neutrophilic perivasculitis with hemorrhage. Later on, in cases of necrotic ulcers one finds arterial wall necrosis and an infiltrate containing many eosinophils.[37]

Differential Diagnosis. In the chronic lymphoid response, the dense infiltrate and the presence of hyperchromatic nuclei

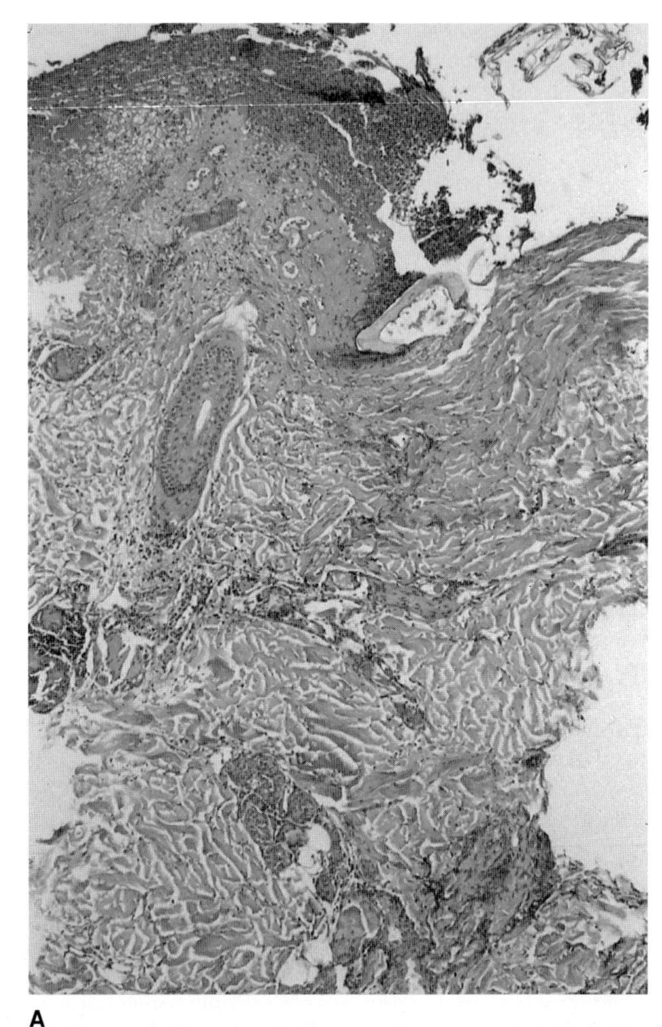

A

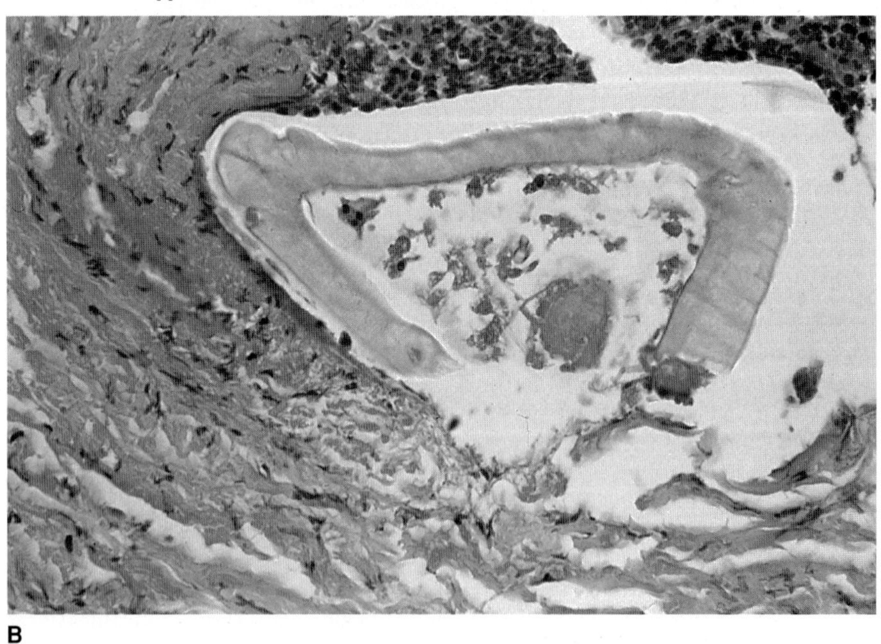

B

FIG. 25-7. (**A**) Mouthparts of a tick are visible at the site of a recent tick bite. In other examples, the mouthparts may be deeper in the dermis and associated with a more cellular persistent tick bite reaction. (**B**) High-magnification view of tick mouthparts in the superficial dermis. The reaction is minimal, indicating that the bite is recent.

may suggest mycosis fungoides, or the multinucleated cells, if present, may suggest Hodgkin's disease because of their resemblance to Reed-Sternberg cells. However, the presence of lymphoid follicles like those seen in lymphocytoma points toward a benign, reactive process such as arthropod bites or stings.

PAPULAR URTICARIA

Papular urticaria, also known as lichen urticatus, is the result of hypersensitivity to bites from certain insects, especially mosquitoes, fleas, and bedbugs. One observes edematous papules and papulovesicles, which, because of severe itching, usually are excoriated. The eruption is more commonly found in children than adults, and, if caused by mosquitoes, is limited to the summer months. The lesions of papular urticaria are clinically and often also histologically indistinguishable from those of prurigo simplex (Chap. 7).

Histopathology. The stratum malpighii shows intercellular and intracellular edema and occasionally a spongiotic vesicle. A chronic inflammatory infiltrate is present around the vessels of the dermis, often extending into the lower dermis and containing a significant admixture of eosinophils (Fig. 25-8).[38]

Differential Diagnosis. Eosinophils, if present in significant numbers, favor a diagnosis of papular urticaria rather than prurigo simplex.

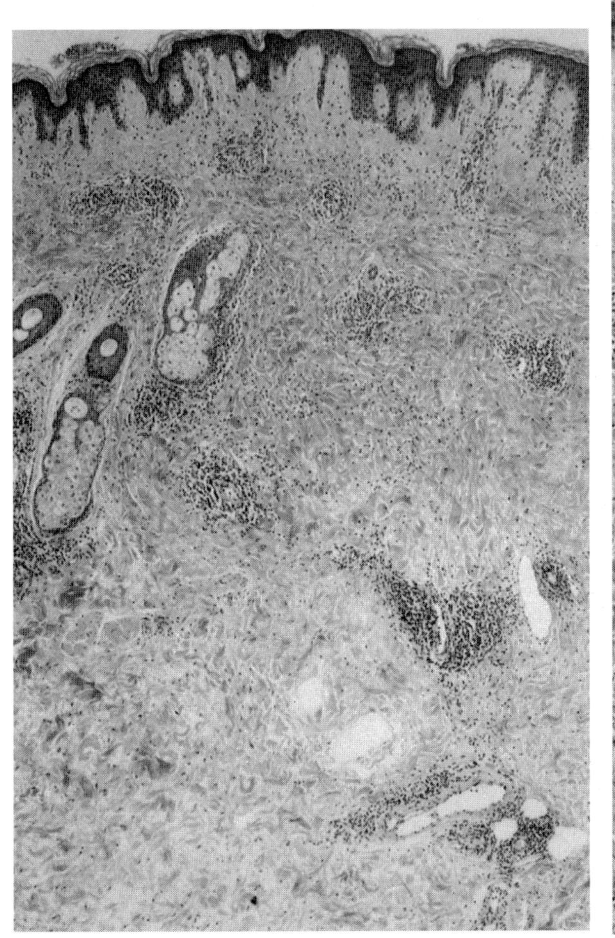

A

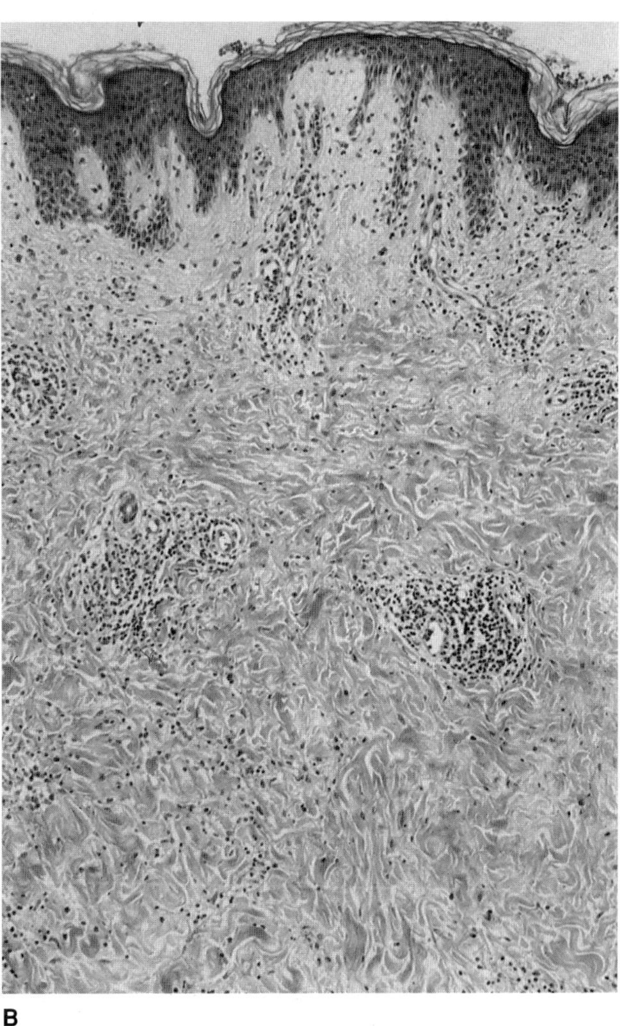

B

FIG. 25-8. Papular urticaria (insect bite reaction)
(**A**) Superficial and deep inflammation. The reaction is broader superficially than at its base. (**B**) There may be slight spongiosis or, as in this example, little or no epidermal reaction. (**C**) Perivascular lymphocytes and eosinophils. *(continued on next page)*

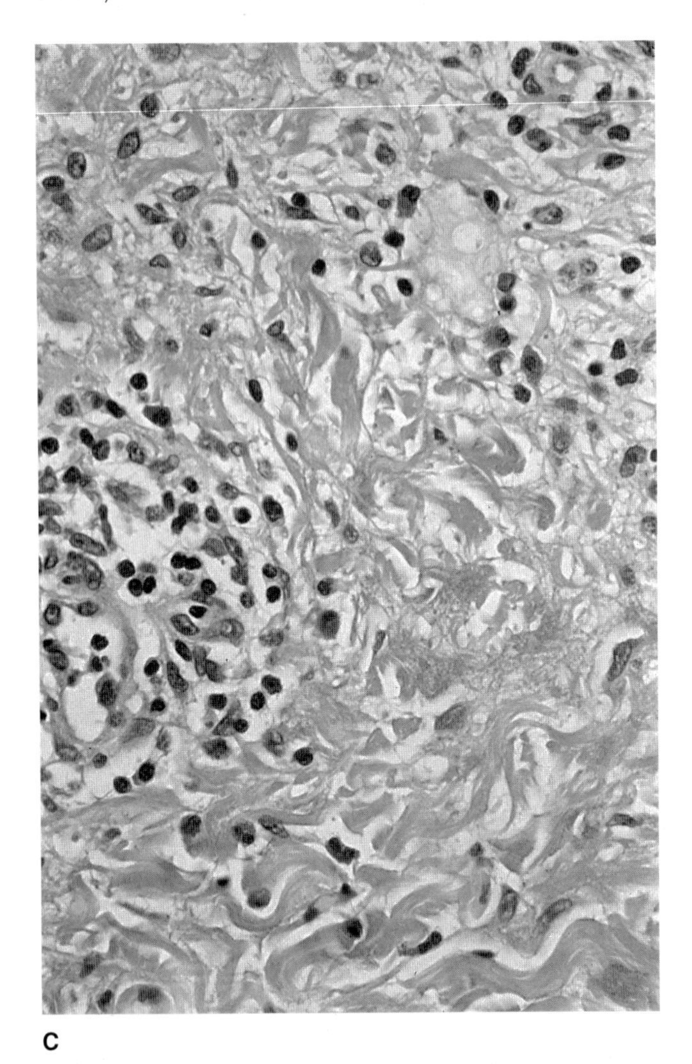

C

FIG. 25-8. ***Continued***

REFERENCES

1. Sadick N, Kaplan MA, Pahwa SG et al. Unusual features of scabies complicating human T-lymphotropic virus type III infection. J Am Acad Dermatol 1986;15:482.
2. Martin WC, Wheeler CE Jr. Diagnosis of human scabies by epidermal shave biopsy. J Am Acad Dermatol 1979;1:335.
3. Hejazi N, Mehregan AH. Scabies: Histological study of inflammatory lesions. Arch Dermatol 1975;111:37.
4. Orkin M, Maibach HI. This scabies pandemic. N Engl J Med 1978;298: 496.
5. Fernandez N, Torres A, Ackerman AB. Pathological findings in human scabies. Arch Dermatol 1977;113:320.
6. Falk ES, Eide TJ. Histologic and clinical findings in human scabies. Int J Dermatol 1981;20:600.
7. Thomson J, Cochrane T, Cochran R et al. Histology simulating reticulosis in persistent nodular scabies. Br J Dermatol 1974;90:421.
8. Shelley WB, Shelley ED. Scanning electron microscopy of the scabies burrow and its contents, with special reference to the *Sarcoptes scabiei* egg. J Am Acad Dermatol 1983;9:673.
9. Hoefling KK, Schroeter AL. Dermatoimmunopathology of scabies. J Am Acad Dermatol 1980;3:237.
10. Dick GF, Burgdorf WHC, Gentry WC Jr. Norwegian scabies in Bloom's syndrome. Arch Dermatol 1979;115:212.
11. Sulica VJ, Berberian B, Kao GF. Histopathologic findings in cutaneous larva migrans (abstr). J Cutan Pathol 1988;15:346.
12. Billups J, Schenken JR, Beaver PC. Subcutaneous dirofilariasis in Nebraska. Arch Pathol 1980;104:11.
13. Payan HM. Human infection with *Dirofilaria*. Arch Dermatol 1978; 114:593.
14. Fisher BK, Homayouni M, Orihel TC. Subcutaneous infections with *Dirofilaria*. Arch Dermatol 1964;89:837.
15. Neaffie RC, Connor DH, Meyers WM. Dirofilariasis. In: Binford CH, Connor DH, eds. Pathology of tropical and extraordinary diseases. Washington, D.C.: Armed Forces Institute of Pathology, 1976:391.
16. Connor DH, Williams PH, Helwig EB et al. Dermal changes in onchocerciasis. Arch Pathol 1969;87:193.
17. Routh HB, Bhowmik KR. Filariasis. Dermatol Clin 1994;12:719.
18. Connor DH, Neaffie RC. Onchocerciasis. In: Binford CH, Connor DH, eds. Pathology of tropical and extraordinary diseases. Washington, DC: Armed Forces Institute of Pathology, 1976:360.
19. Rozenman D, Kremer M, Zuckerman F. Onchocerciasis in Israel. Arch Dermatol 1984;120:505.
20. Von Kuster LC, Genta RM. Cutaneous manifestations of strongyloidiasis. Arch Dermatol 1988;124:1826.
21. Amer M. Cutaneous schistosomiasis. Dermatol Clin 1994;12:713.
22. Wood MG, Srolovitz H, Schetman D. Schistosomiasis. Arch Dermatol 1976;112:690.
23. Walther RR. Chronic papular dermatitis of the scrotum due to *Schistosoma mansoni*. Arch Dermatol 1979;115:869.
24. Mahmoud AA. Schistosomiasis. N Engl J Med 1977;297:1329.
25. Torres VM. Dermatologic manifestations of schistosomiasis mansoni. Arch Dermatol 1976;112:1539.
26. McKee PH, Wright E, Hutt MSR. Vulval schistosomiasis. Clin Exp Dermatol 1983;8:189.
27. Jacyk WK, Lawande RW, Tulpule SS. Unusual presentation of extragenital cutaneous schistosomiasis mansoni. Br J Dermatol 1980;103: 205.
28. Raimer S, Wolf JE Jr. Subcutaneous cysticercosis. Arch Dermatol 1978;114:107.
29. Tschen EH, Tschen EA, Smith EB. Cutaneous cysticercosis treated with metrifonate. Arch Dermatol 1981;117:507.
30. Schlossberg D, Mader JT. *Cysticercus cellulosae* cutis. Arch Dermatol 1978;114:459.
31. Falanga V, Kapoor W. Cerebral cysticercosis: Diagnostic value of subcutaneous nodules. J Am Acad Dermatol 1985;12:304.
32. King DT, Gilbert DJ, Gurevitch AW et al. Subcutaneous cysticercosis. Arch Dermatol 1979;115:236.
33. Noutsis C, Millikan LE. Myiasis. Dermatol Clin 1994;12:729.
34. Bandman HJ, Bosse K. Histologie des Mückenstiches (*Aedes aegypti*). Arch Klin Exp Dermatol 1967;231:59.
35. Horen WP. Insect and scorpion sting. JAMA 1972;221:894.
36. Allen AC. Persistent "insect bites" (dermal eosinophilic granulomas) simulating lymphoblastomas, histiocytoses, and squamous cell carcinomas. Am J Pathol 1948;24:367.
37. Pucevich MV, Chesney TMCC. Histopathologic analysis of human bites by the brown recluse spider (abstr). Arch Dermatol 1983;119:851.
38. Shaffer B, Jacobsen C, Beerman H. Histopathologic correlation of lesions of papular urticaria and positive skin test reactions to insect antigens. Arch Dermatol 1954;70:437.

Lever's Histopathology of the Skin, eighth edition,
edited by David Elder et al. Lippincott–
Raven Publishers, Philadelphia © 1997.

CHAPTER 26

Diseases Caused by Viruses

Neal Penneys

Viruses are obligatory intracellular parasites that lack organelles, such as ribosomes and mitochondria, have no metabolism of their own, and consequently must use the organelles, the energy, and many of the enzymes of the host cell to replicate. In doing so, viruses may disturb the metabolism of the host cell and act as pathogens.

Viruses are composed of a central core of nucleoprotein called the *nucleoid,* which contains either deoxyribonucleic acid (DNA) or ribonucleic acid (RNA). The nucleoid is surrounded by the capsid, the subunits of which, called *capsomers,* contain the major antigenic components of the virus. The nucleoid and the capsid form the essential part of the virus or virion. Viruses that replicate in the nucleus of the host cell, on leaving the nucleus, may acquire an outer coat derived from the nuclear membrane, whereas virions that replicate in the cytoplasm may derive an outer coat from the plasma membrane.

Before viruses can enter a cell, they must attach themselves to specific receptors of the plasma membrane; thus, they are species-specific. Viruses enter the cytoplasm of a cell by a process akin to phagocytosis, acquiring an outer coat of plasma membrane. Once inside the cell, the viruses induce the synthesis of an "uncoating" protein. As the outer coat and the capsid are being digested by the uncoating protein, the exposed nucleoids lose their characteristic structure. The viruses now are in "eclipse" and do not become apparent until replication has taken place and new virions or viruses, each composed of a nucleoid and a capsid, have been formed. During the process of replication, the proteins of the cell follow the genetic code of the specific virus nucleic acid, and the proteins that are formed are characteristic of the virus rather than of the cell. The first proteins formed after the uncoating are specific enzymes needed for replication of the virus nucleic acids. The proteins constituting the capsid are also synthesized. Myriads of virus may be released from an infected cell.

The diameters of viruses infecting the skin vary from 20 nm for the echoviruses to 300 nm for the poxviruses. Under favorable conditions, poxviruses may be recognizable under a light microscope—for example, variola viruses as Paschen bodies. As a rule, however, viruses can be resolved by light microscopy only when aggregated into inclusion bodies.

Inclusion bodies are roughly spherical. Their average size is about 7 μm, the size of an erythrocyte. Electron microscopy has shown that inclusion bodies represent sites at which virus replication is occurring or has occurred. They are observed in three groups of viruses: in the herpesvirus and papillomavirus groups, where they are found within the nuclei of cells, and in the poxvirus group, where they occur within the cytoplasm. In the nucleus, they are surrounded by a clear halo as a result of margination of the nuclear chromatin. In some viral infections, such as molluscum contagiosum, inclusion bodies contain masses of virions and are basophilic and Feulgen-positive; in contrast, herpesviruses have left the inclusion bodies, except for a few residual nucleoids, and the inclusion bodies are then eosinophilic and Feulgen-negative.

Five groups of viruses can affect the skin or the adjoining mucous surfaces: (1) the herpesvirus group, including herpes simplex types 1 and 2 and the varicella-zoster virus, which are DNA-containing organisms that multiply within the nucleus of the host cell; (2) the poxvirus group, including smallpox, milkers' nodules, orf, and molluscum contagiosum, which are DNA-containing agents that multiply within the cytoplasm; (3) the papovavirus group, including the various types of verrucae, which contain DNA and replicate in the nucleus; (4) the picornavirus group, including coxsackievirus group A, causing hand-foot-and-mouth disease, which contain RNA rather than DNA in their nucleoids; and (5) retroviruses, including human immunodeficiency virus (HIV), the cause of acquired immunodeficiency syndrome (AIDS). Primary HIV infection may be associated with both an exanthem and an enanthem, which are histologically nondescript. The array of skin lesions associated with HIV is generally a consequence of eventual immunosuppression.

HERPES SIMPLEX

Two immunologically distinct viruses can cause herpes simplex: herpes simplex virus type 1 (orofacial type) and herpes simplex virus type 2 (genital type), often referred to as HSV-1

N. Penneys: Department of Dermatology, St. Louis School of Medicine, St. Louis, MO

and HSV-2, respectively. Primary infection with HSV-1 is subclinical in childhood. In about 10% of the cases, acute gingivostomatitis occurs, usually in childhood and only rarely in early adult life. Primary infection may also occur in rare instances as a respiratory infection, as Kaposi's varicelliform eruption, as keratoconjunctivitis, or as a fatal visceral disease of the newborn. HSV-2 generally is acquired venereally. Occasionally, an infant contracts HSV-2 in utero or by direct contact in the birth canal.

Primary infections with herpes simplex are always acquired from another person. The incubation period for HSV-2 ranges from 3 to 14 days, with an average of 5 days. Recurrent infections of the oral cavity, the skin, or the genitals can result either from reactivation of a latent infection or from a new infection.

Recurrent HSV-1 infections occur most commonly on or near the vermilion border of the lips. Recurrences may be spontaneously triggered by sunlight or by febrile illness. Besides the lips, any part of the skin or oral mucosa can be affected by HSV-1. Even though most infections of the genitalia and adjoining skin are caused by HSV-2, some infections in this area are caused by HSV-1. However, genital HSV-1 infections are less likely to recur than HSV-2 infections: the rate of recurrence in one series was 14% for HSV-1 infections compared with 60% for HSV-2 infections.[1]

Both primary and recurrent herpes simplex, in their earliest stages, show one or several groups of vesicles on an inflamed base. If located on a mucous surface, the vesicles erode quickly, whereas, if located on the skin, they may become pustular before crusting.

The following are special forms of cutaneous herpes simplex: *Kaposi's varicelliform eruption* (eczema herpeticum); *herpetic folliculitis of the bearded region,* characterized by grouped vesiculofollicular lesions that heal within a few weeks; and *herpetic whitlow,* which is manifested by painful, deep-seated vesicles limited to the paronychial or volar aspects of the distal phalanx of a finger. Herpetic whitlow occurs largely in medical and dental personnel following minor injuries and may be caused by either HSV-1 or HSV-2. Noncutaneous forms of herpes simplex infection include herpetic oropharyngitis, pneumonia, encephalitis, esophagitis, and proctitis.

Herpes Simplex in Compromised Hosts

Three forms of herpes simplex are characteristically found in children or adults with impairment of the cellular immune system. Impairment may be caused by (1) congenital diseases such as the Wiskott-Aldrich syndrome or dysplasia of the thymus, (2) lymphoma or leukemia, (3) severe burns, (4) prolonged immunosuppressive therapy, or (5) the acquired immunodeficiency syndrome (AIDS). The most common of the three forms is chronic ulcerative herpes simplex. Generalized acute mucocutaneous herpes simplex or systemic herpes simplex.

Chronic ulcerative herpes simplex exhibits persistent ulcers and erosions, usually starting on the face or in the perineal region. Without treatment, gradual widespread extension is the rule. The infection may progress into systemic herpes simplex.

Generalized acute mucocutaneous herpes simplex follows a localized vesicular eruption. Dissemination associated with fever takes place, suggestive of smallpox or varicella. In some instances, death results without the presence of visceral lesions.

Systemic herpes simplex usually follows oral or genital lesions of herpes simplex. Areas of necrosis—particularly in the liver, adrenals, and pancreas—lead rapidly to death. In some patients, a few cutaneous lesions of herpes simplex also exist.

Congenital Herpes Simplex

Because almost 1% of patients in prenatal clinics have HSV-2 infections by culture of the vagina and one-third of these have lesions, there exists the potential of congenital herpes simplex infection. It is important, however, to distinguish primary HSV-2 infection of the mother from recurrent infection. In recurrent infection, the presence of neutralizing antibody to HSV-2 results in a low rate of attack of the fetus.[2] In maternal HSV-2 *primary infection,* the mode of infection of the infant is important. *Transplacental infection* of the fetus occurs during the first 8 weeks of gestation and produces severe congenital malformation. If infection occurs at a later time, malformations are less severe and consist of growth and psychomotor retardation, microcephaly, and a widespread, recurrent vesicular eruption that can mimic a mechanobullous disorder.

Localized herpetic lesions several days after delivery are the initial manifestation if infection is acquired in the birth canal. In vertex deliveries, the scalp is a common site for the development of initial herpetic vesicles. It is rare for transplacental or neonatal infection to remain limited to the skin. It can be followed by systemic herpetic infection, such as encephalitis, hepatoadrenal necrosis, or pneumonia, resulting in death.

Herpes Simplex Associated with Erythema Multiforme

Herpes simplex virus is the most common identified etiologic agent in recurrent erythema multiforme.[3] Molecular diagnostic methods, primarily the polymerase chain reaction, have been used to detect herpetic DNA in the skin lesions of recurrent erythema multiforme in both adults and children.[4,5] The association is further supported by suppression of recurrent lesions in this group by therapy directed at herpes simplex virus.

Histopathology of Herpes Simplex

Herpes simplex of the skin produces profound degeneration of keratinocytes, resulting in acantholysis. Degeneration of epidermal cells occurs in two forms: ballooning degeneration and reticular degeneration, both of which are changes typical of viral vesicles. As in all vesiculobullous diseases, an early lesion should be selected for biopsy; otherwise, secondary changes, especially invasion of inflammatory cells, may obscure the diagnostic features. The earliest changes include nuclear swelling of keratinocytes. With hematoxylin and eosin stains, these nuclei appear slate gray and homogeneous. Ballooning degeneration then follows.

Ballooning degeneration is swelling of epidermal cells. Balloon cells have a homogeneous, eosinophilic cytoplasm (Figs. 26-1 and 26-2). They may be multinucleate. Balloon cells lose their intercellular bridges and become separated from one another, and unilocular vesicles result. Ballooning degeneration occurs mainly at the bases of viral vesicles, so that the vesicle that formed intraepidermally ultimately may be subepidermal.

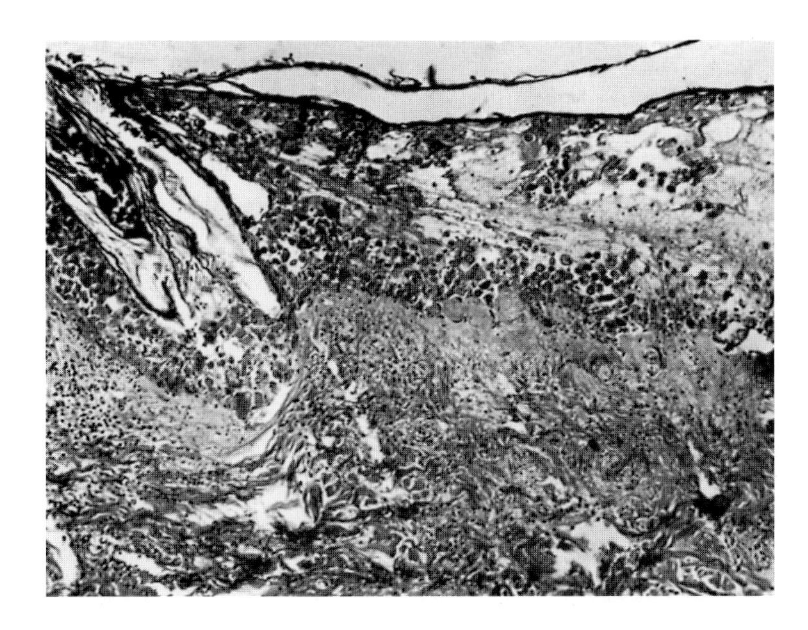

FIG. 26-1. Herpes simplex
There is marked ballooning degeneration of the cells at the floor of the vesicle. The cells of a hair follicle shown at the left also exhibit ballooning degeneration. Reticular degeneration, observed at the top of the vesicle, is only slight (low magnification).

Ballooning degeneration can affect epithelial cells of hair follicles and sebaceous glands. Inclusion bodies are frequently observed in the centers of enlarged, round nuclei of balloon cells. The inclusion bodies are eosinophilic and surrounded by a clear space or halo (see Fig. 26-2). They measure from 3 to 8 μm in diameter.

Reticular degeneration is a process in which epidermal cells are distended by intracellular edema, so that cell walls rupture. Through coalescence, a multilocular vesicle results, the septa of which are formed by resistant cellular walls (Fig. 26-3). Reticular degeneration occurs in the upper portions and at the peripheries of viral vesicles. In older vesicles, the cellular walls disappear. In this way, the originally multilocular portions of the vesicle may become unilocular. Reticular degeneration is not specific for viral vesicles, because it also occurs in the vesicles of dermatitis.

The upper dermis beneath viral vesicles contains an inflammatory infiltrate of variable density. In some cases of herpes simplex, vascular damage is present, showing necrosis of vessel walls, microthrombi, and hemorrhage. In addition, eosinophilic inclusions may be found in endothelial cells and fibroblasts.

Chronic ulcerative herpes simplex may be difficult to recognize as being of viral genesis if epidermis is absent. However, viral cytopathic changes may be observed in keratinocytes at the margin of the ulcer. Viral cultures or typing of HSV-1 and HSV-2 by direct immunofluorescence or immunoperoxidase technique can be used to prove the diagnosis. However, the most rapid and accurate method may be the use of molecular diagnostic methods such as the polymerase chain reaction.[6]

Tzanck Smear. Cytologic examination of a stained smear taken from the floor of an early, freshly opened vesicle is often useful. Many acantholytic balloon cells with one or several

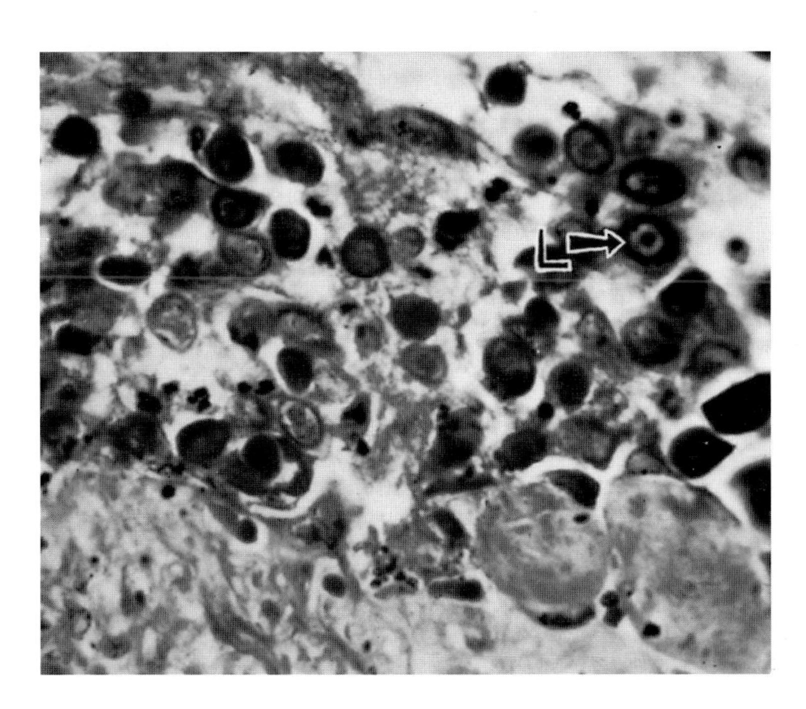

FIG. 26-2. Herpes simplex
Same as Fig. 26-1, but at high magnification. Balloon cells at the floor of a vesicle are shown. On the right, an eosinophilic inclusion body surrounded by a halo lies in the nucleus of a balloon cell. Other cells exhibit the more characteristic pattern of homogeneous pale chromatin without inclusion bodies.

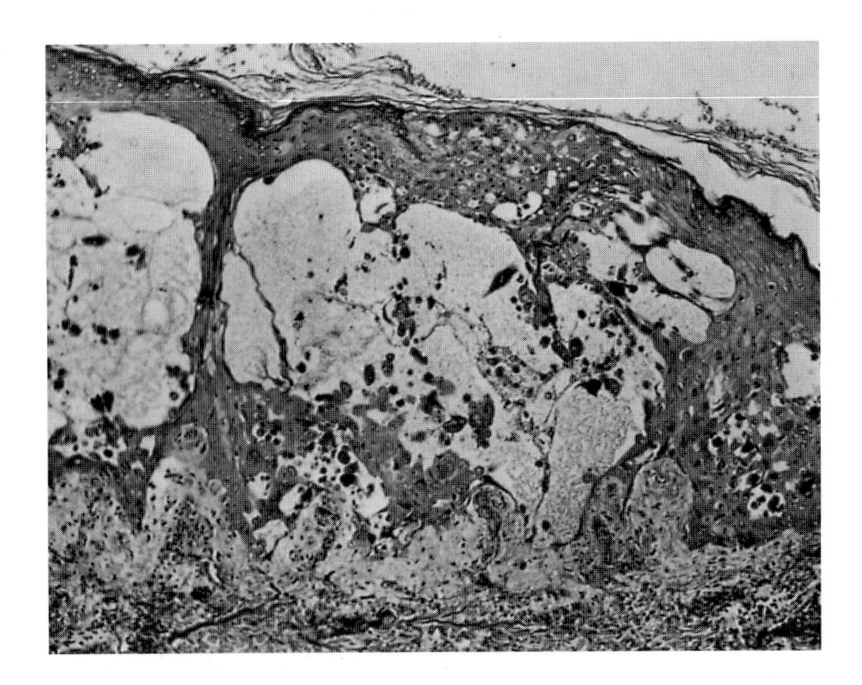

FIG. 26-3. Herpes simplex
Reticular degeneration is present, especially at the top of the vesicle, resulting in a multilocular vesicle. In addition, ballooning degeneration can be seen at the floor of the vesicle.

nuclei may be seen. The presence of many balloon cells results from the fact that the smear is taken from the floor of the blister, where ballooning degeneration is most pronounced. In one study, the accuracy of interpretation of Tzanck preparations by practicing dermatologists declined as the length of time in practice increased.[7]

Viral Identification. The herpes simplex virus can be directly identified by culture, by direct immunofluorescence testing, or by molecular diagnostic tests. For culture, material from the floor of a blister or other infected material is inoculated onto HeLa cells, human amnion cells, or fibroblasts. The virus has a cytopathogenic effect on the culture cells. Direct immunofluorescence examination for the presence of the viral antigen in cells infected with herpes simplex virus is then performed. Herpes simplex DNA can be extracted and amplified by the polymerase chain reaction from stained and unstained Tzanck smears, crusts, fresh tissue, and paraffin sections of suspected lesions. With appropriate probes, each herpes-type virus can be specifically identified from the amplified product.

For distinction between the two types of HSV, immunoperoxidase staining may be performed on sections of the lesions using two monoclonal antibodies, one directed against HSV-1 and the other against HSV-2, or DNA can be amplified and unique portions of the genome used for specific identification of the virus. In situ hybridization can be used for visual demonstration of genomic material in tissue.[8,9] For determination of the antibody titer in the patient's serum, the complement fixation reaction is usually used.

On electron microscopy, the herpes simplex virus is spheric. Its DNA-containing core measures approximately 40 nm in diameter. The virion has a diameter of about 100 nm and together with its outer coat measures around 135 nm.[10] Ultrastructurally, the virion of herpes simplex is indistinguishable from that of varicella.

HSV-1 and HSV-2 differ not only in their antigenicity, because each type is preferentially neutralized by its own specific antibody, but also in their effects on tissue cultures and in their growth characteristics.

Recurrent Infection. Primary infection with either HSV-1 or HSV-2 is often subclinical and is followed by emergence of specific circulating antibodies and latency of the infection. In some persons infected with either HSV-1 or HSV-2, the virus can become activated intermittently and give rise to recurrent lesions. The first few recurrences usually are accompanied by increases in the antibody titer; thereafter, the appearance of lesions is unrelated to the antibody titer.

Although recurrences, particularly of HSV-2, can be based on reinfection, they are often based on reactivation of a latent infection of the regional sensory ganglia, where the virus exists in a latent, nonreplicative state. One proposal is that trigger factors activate virus in the ganglia. Virus then migrates along nerves to epithelium.

Differential Diagnosis. Viral vesicles produced by the herpes simplex virus and by the varicella-zoster virus are identical. Furthermore, an incompletely developed case of herpes zoster can mimic herpes simplex infection, both clinically and histologically. In the context of immunosuppression, chronic cutaneous forms of both viruses exist and their specific identification may not be possible by clinical morphology or light microscopy. Molecular diagnostic methods are the quickest and most reliable way to separate and identify the specific viruses in these situations.

VARICELLA AND HERPES ZOSTER

Varicella (chickenpox) and herpes zoster are produced by the same virus, the varicella-zoster virus. Varicella results from contact of a nonimmune person with this virus, whereas herpes zoster occurs in persons who have had previous varicella, either clinically or subclinically. Although varicella occasionally develops in children exposed to herpes zoster, exogenous infection very rarely causes herpes zoster. As a rule, herpes zoster is caused by reactivation of a latent infection in either a spinal or a cranial sensory ganglion. On reactivation, the virus spreads from the ganglion along the corresponding sensory nerve or nerves to the skin.

Varicella

In varicella, a generalized eruption develops after an incubation period of about 2 weeks. About 95% of patients are children. Serious complications are very rare in normal children. The lesions of varicella begin as small papules, which develop into vesicles. In mild cases, most vesicles become crusted without changing into pustules. In severe cases, the vesicles may have slightly hemorrhagic bases ("dew drops on rose petals"). New lesions continue to develop for several days, and so lesions in different stages of development can be observed.

Three systemic complications can occur in varicella without the existence of immunosuppression: primary varicella pneumonia, Reye's syndrome, and varicella of the fetus and newborn. Primary varicella pneumonia occurs in approximately 14% of adults with varicella and carries a significant mortality. Reye's syndrome is an acute, severe, and usually fatal encephalopathy associated with fatty degeneration of the viscera, particularly of the liver. It follows mainly varicella but also other viral infections. Although usually observed in children, it also may occur in adults.[11] Varicella in the first 20 weeks of pregnancy has a 2% risk of producing embryopathy or other congenital malformations.[12] Maternal varicella late in pregnancy may be transmitted to the fetus transplacentally or may contaminate the baby during passage through the birth canal, resulting in neonatal varicella.

Varicella in Compromised Hosts

In patients with impairment of the cellular immune system, such as in lymphoma and as a result of treatment with immunosuppressants, continued viral replication may lead to a prolonged course and to dissemination to various organs. Varicella pneumonia is not uncommon, even in children, and death may result from dissemination. The varicella-zoster virus may produce particularly severe problems for patients with AIDS. There may be continuous dissemination of vesicular lesions, formation of chronic vegetative lesions, or development of chickenpox pneumonia or of herpes zoster.

Herpes Zoster

Although herpes zoster occurs largely in adults, particularly in those of advanced age, about 5% of patients with herpes zoster are children less than 15 years of age. The course in children without immune defects usually is mild. The eruption in herpes zoster consists of grouped vesicles on inflammatory bases and arranged along the course of a sensory nerve. The bases of the lesions frequently are hemorrhagic, and some may become necrotic and ulcerate. Not infrequently, there are a few scattered nondermatomal lesions, and rarely there is a generalized eruption, including mucosal lesions, indistinguishable from that of varicella.

Herpes Zoster in Compromised Hosts

Both the incidence and the severity of herpes zoster are greater in patients with impaired cellular immunity. The incidence of herpes zoster is particularly high in patients with advanced Hodgkin's disease who are receiving chemotherapy or radiation, and in persons infected with HIV. In the context of HIV infection, herpes zoster may fail to resolve, disseminate, or produce atypical vegetative and ulcerative lesions.[13]

Although patients with disseminated herpes zoster but without associated serious illness have good prognoses, patients with impaired cellular immunity may develop widespread, fatal systemic manifestations, such as pneumonia, gastroenteritis, or encephalitis.

Histopathology. Lesions of varicella and herpes zoster are histologically indistinguishable from those of herpes simplex. Frequently, however, the degree of vessel damage, microthrombi, and hemorrhage are more pronounced in varicella and, particularly, in herpes zoster than in herpes simplex. In severe cases of varicella and in disseminated herpes zoster, eosinophilic inclusion bodies have also been observed in the dermis within the nuclei of capillary endothelial cells and of fibroblasts bordering the affected vessels. In contrast, in localized herpes zoster, in which the virus reaches the epidermis by way of the cutaneous nerves rather than the capillaries, inclusion bodies have been demonstrated within neurilemmal cells of the small nerves in the dermis underlying the vesicles. Immunohistochemical methods using specific monoclonal antibodies may have some utility in separating varicella-zoster virus from herpes simplex virus.[14] Using an antibody specific for an envelope glycoprotein, Nikkels and colleagues demonstrated reactivity in sebaceous cells, endothelial cells, mononuclear phagocytes, and factor XIIIa-positive dendrocytes.[14]

Visceral Lesions. The visceral lesions caused by hematogenous dissemination in varicella and herpes zoster are indistinguishable from one another and from those produced by herpes simplex. However, the neural lesions in herpes zoster are quite specific for that disease (see text following).

In fatal cases of *pneumonia due to varicella* or *herpes zoster,* the autopsy reveals intranuclear eosinophilic inclusion bodies in bronchiolar epithelial cells and alveolar cells.

Fatal *systemic varicella* or *herpes zoster* usually occurs in children or adults with inherited, acquired, or induced defects in cellular immunity. There are areas of focal necrosis containing intranuclear eosinophilic inclusion bodies in various organs, especially the liver, the kidneys, the adrenals, and the lungs. However, in varicella, even in the case of widespread lesions with inclusion bodies in many internal organs, invasion of the central nervous system is rare except in neonates.

In fatal cases of *neonatal varicella,* widespread lesions are the rule. These lesions may even involve the brain. In contrast, in Reye's syndrome occurring in conjunction with varicella and presenting as acute and severe encephalopathy and fatty degeneration of the viscera, particularly of the liver, no inclusion bodies are found, and no virus can be isolated from either the brain or the viscera.

The *neural lesions in herpes zoster* begin either in a dorsal root ganglion or in a cranial nerve ganglion with a severe inflammatory infiltrate that can be associated with necrosis of ganglion cells, with intranuclear inclusions in ganglion cells and nerve fibers, and with hemorrhage. Inflammatory and degenerative changes extend from the involved ganglia along the sensory nerves to the skin. In addition, inflammatory and degenerative changes extend proximally from the ganglion to the posterior nerve root and into the spinal cord, producing a unilateral, segmental myelitis in the posterior columns.

Asymptomatic upward extension of the virus along the spinal cord from the dorsal root ganglion to the brain apparently is not uncommon, considering that about one-fourth of the patients with herpes zoster have pleocytosis of the spinal fluid and that varicella-zoster virus occasionally can be isolated from spinal fluid. However, fatal cases of encephalomyelitis or encephalitis are rare in herpes zoster and occur only in compromised hosts.

Tzanck Smear. Cytologic examination of the contents of vesicles is carried out for varicella and herpes zoster in the same way as for herpes simplex. It is a very useful diagnostic test, confirming the diagnosis in 80% to 100% of the cases, whereas cultures can confirm it in only 60% to 64%.[15]

Viral Identification. The herpes simplex virus and the varicella-zoster virus are indistinguishable by electron microscopy. However, in contrast with herpes simplex, the varicella-zoster virus does not grow in ordinary tissue cultures, although it does grow in tissue cultures containing human fetal diploid kidney cells or human foreskin fibroblasts. Specific antibodies are available for serologic or immunohistochemical viral identification.

Histogenesis. Electron microscopic examination of the cutaneous lesions of varicella and herpes zoster reveals virus particles in the capillary endothelium in varicella and sporadically in the axons of dermal nerves in herpes zoster. If present in sufficient numbers, the virions within epidermal nuclei may lie partially in crystalloid aggregates. On leaving the nucleus for the cytoplasm, most virions are enveloped by an outer coat derived from the nuclear membrane, increasing the size of the virus particle from about 100 nm to about 150 nm. Subsequently, the virions are extruded into the intercellular space, where they are phagocytized by macrophages. As a result of this phagocytosis, the phagolysosomes of the macrophages may contain numerous virions.

HUMAN COWPOX INFECTION

The main carriers of human cowpox are cats and rodents, rather than cattle. Infection in these animals is usually manifested as a single, small, crusted ulcer. In unvaccinated patients it occasionally causes crusted ulcers located in exposed areas, such as on the hands or face, occasionally with lymphangitis and regional lymphadenopathy.

Histopathology. Early lesions of human cowpox infection show prominent reticular degeneration. Eosinophilic, intracytoplasmic inclusion bodies are present, a valuable feature in distinguishing poxvirus from herpesvirus infections.

Histogenesis. Like the virus of variola, the virus causing human cowpox infection is an orthopox virus (Orthopox bovis). Under electron microscopic examination, it is rectangular and morphologically indistinguishable from the virus of variola.

KAPOSI'S VARICELLIFORM ERUPTION

Eczema herpeticum and eczema vaccinatum (Kaposi's varicelliform eruption) occur in patients with preexisting dermatoses, usually atopic dermatitis. Occasionally, seborrheic dermatitis or other dermatosis, such as Darier's disease, benign familial pemphigus, pemphigus foliaceus, mycosis fungoides, Sézary's syndrome, or ichthyosis vulgaris, provide the "soil" in which Kaposi's varicelliform eruption develops.

Eczema herpeticum is usually caused by HSV-1 and on rare occasions by HSV-2. Eczema herpeticum can occur as either a primary or a recurrent type of infection. A primary infection with HSV-1 occurs in persons without circulating HSV-1 antibodies. The great majority of patients with the primary type of eczema herpeticum are infants and children. The recurrent type of eczema herpeticum occurs in patients with circulating HSV-1 antibodies. The first attack of eczema herpeticum, whether of the primary or the recurrent type, may be the result of exogenous infection, whereas subsequent attacks may result from either reinfection or reactivation (see section on Herpes Simplex). The primary type of eczema herpeticum can be a serious disease with viremia and potential internal organ involvement resulting in death. In contrast, the recurrent type of eczema herpeticum generally shows no viremia and internal organ involvement except in immunologically compromised patients. Occasionally, secondary bacterial infection with subsequent septicemia may cause death.

Clinically, all forms of eczema herpeticum and eczema vaccinatum look alike, but eczema vaccinatum is rarely if ever seen in modern practice because vaccinia virus is no longer used for smallpox prevention. Both show a more or less extensive eruption composed of vesicles and pustules that may be umbilicated. These vesicles and pustules occur chiefly in the areas of the preexisting dermatosis but also on normal skin. The face is usually severely affected and may be edematous. There may be fever and prostration. The mortality of eczema herpeticum is approximately 10%, with most fatalities occurring in infants and children with a primary type of herpetic infection and in adults with inadequate cellular immunity.

Histopathology. Both eczema herpeticum and eczema vaccinatum show vesicles and pustules of the viral type. Even though the pustules exhibit only necrotic epidermis in their centers, one may still see reticular and ballooning degeneration at their peripheries. In eczema herpeticum, but not in eczema vaccinatum, multinucleated epithelial giant cells often are present.

Differential Diagnosis. Because eczema herpeticum and eczema vaccinatum look alike clinically, and because the histologic similarity is great in the absence of inclusion bodies and of multinucleated epithelial cells, differentiation of the two diseases may have to depend on nonhistologic means, such as a history of possible exposure to the vaccinia virus. The most efficient and rapid means of identifying the viral agent is to use DNA amplification methods and appropriate probes.

CYTOMEGALOVIRUS INCLUSION DISEASE

Immunosuppression provides a setting in which cytomegalovirus (CMV) can produce a widespread, potentially fatal, systemic infection. The skin is rarely affected. Skin lesions consist of a more or less widespread, exanthematous eruption of macules and papules that may become purpuric. Perianal le-

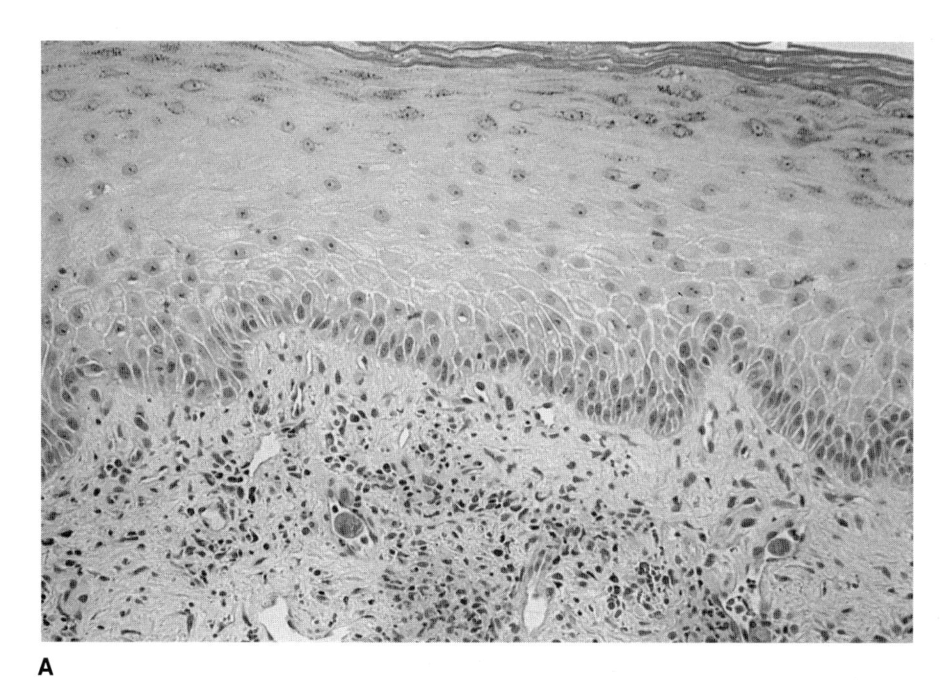

A

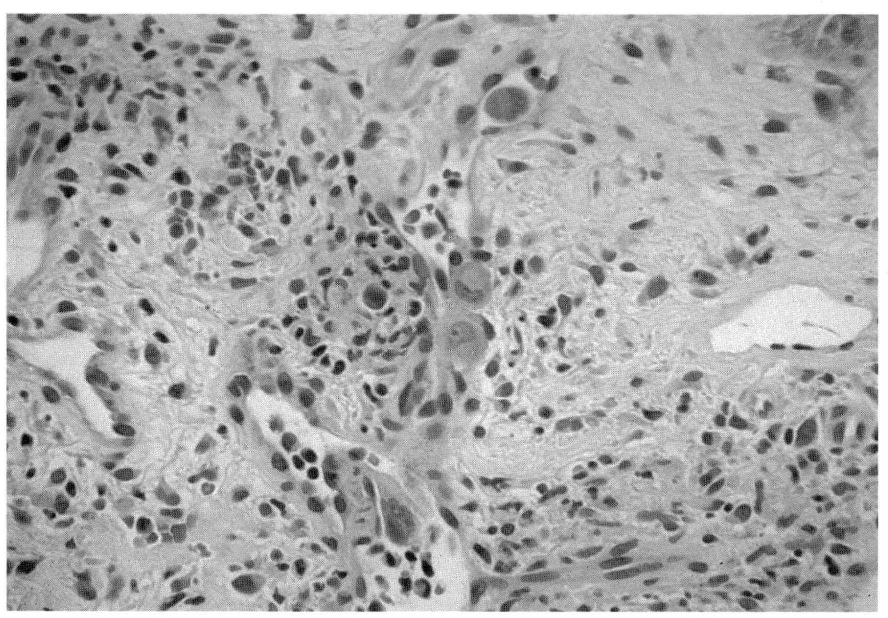

B

FIG. 26-4. Cytomegalic inclusion disease
(**A**) Scanning magnification shows superficial perivascular and diffuse inflammation with prominent vessels. Enlarged endothelial cells may be apparent at this magnification. (**B**) In the dilated dermal vessels, among normal endothelial cells, there are large, irregularly shaped endothelial cells. *(continued on next page)*

sions may be ulcerated. In the context of HIV infection, CMV-associated viral cytopathic changes can be observed as epiphenomena in skin biopsies in that they do not appear to be the primary pathogen in the specimen and the cause of the skin eruption. CMV infection commonly coexists with HIV (a large percentage of homosexual men have evidence of CMV infection in the context of HIV), but less than half of all AIDS patients are diagnosed with end-organ disease caused by CMV before death.

Histopathology. Dilated dermal vessels exhibit, among normal endothelial cells, large, irregularly shaped endothelial cells with large, hyperchromatic, basophilic, intranuclear inclusions (Fig. 26-4). Some of the inclusions are surrounded by clear halos. A polymorphous inflammatory infiltrate with focal leukocytoclastic changes may also be present. In the context of HIV infection, other pathologic processes may also be present in the same tissue section. Immunohistochemical studies using monoclonal or polyclonal antibodies to CMV antigens can be used in paraffin-embedded sections to reveal viral proteins and confirm the presence of the virus. CMV DNA can also be amplified from skin biopsy specimens with polymerase chain reaction techniques and specific primers and probes for CMV, or can be identified by in situ hybridization.

Histogenesis. Electron microscopy shows intranuclear viral

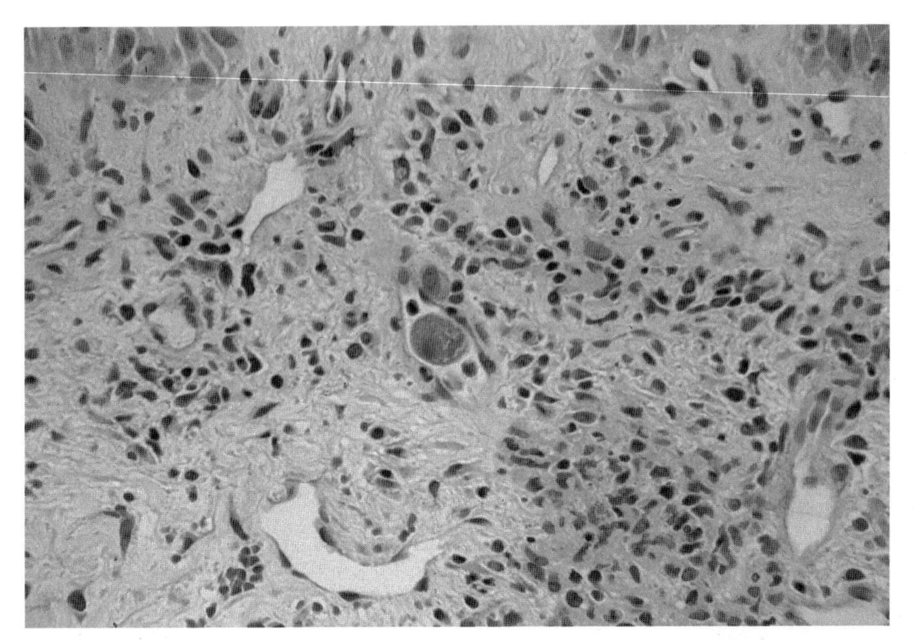

C

FIG. 26-4. *Continued*
(**C**) The enlarged endothelial cells contain large, hyperchromatic, basophilic, intranuclear inclusions. Some of the inclusions are surrounded by clear halos. There may be basophilic cytoplasmic inclusions also.

particles approximately 110 nm in diameter. The virus greatly resembles that of herpes simplex.

PARAPOX VIRUS INFECTIONS (MILKERS' NODULES, ORF)

Milkers' nodules, orf, and bovine papular stomatitis pox are clinically identical in humans and are induced by indistinguishable parapox viruses.

Milkers' nodules are acquired from udders infected with pseudocowpox or paravaccinia (parapox). This disease is called bovine papular stomatitis pox when the source of the infection is calves with oral sores contracted through sucking infected udders.

Orf (ecthyma contagiosum) is acquired from infected sheep or goats with crusted lesions on the lips and in the mouth.

After an incubation period of 3 to 7 days, parapox virus infections produce one to three (rarely more) painful lesions measuring 1 to 2 cm in diameter on the fingers, or occasionally elsewhere as a result of autoinoculation. During a period of approximately 6 weeks, they pass through six clinical stages, each lasting about 1 week[16]: (1) the maculopapular stage; (2) the target stage, during which the lesions have red centers, white rings, and red halos; (3) the acute weeping stage; (4) the nodular stage, which shows hard, nontender nodules; (5) the papillomatous stage, in which the nodules have irregular surfaces; and (6) the regressive stage, during which the lesions involute without scarring.

Histopathology. During the maculopapular and target stages, there is vacuolization of cells in the upper third of the stratum malpighii, leading to multilocular vesicles. Eosinophilic inclusion bodies are in the cytoplasm of vacuolated epidermal cells, a distinguishing feature from herpes virus infections. Intranuclear eosinophilic inclusion bodies are also present in some cases. During the target stage, vacuolated epidermal cells with inclusion bodies are only in the surrounding white ring.[16] The epidermis shows elongation of the rete ridges,

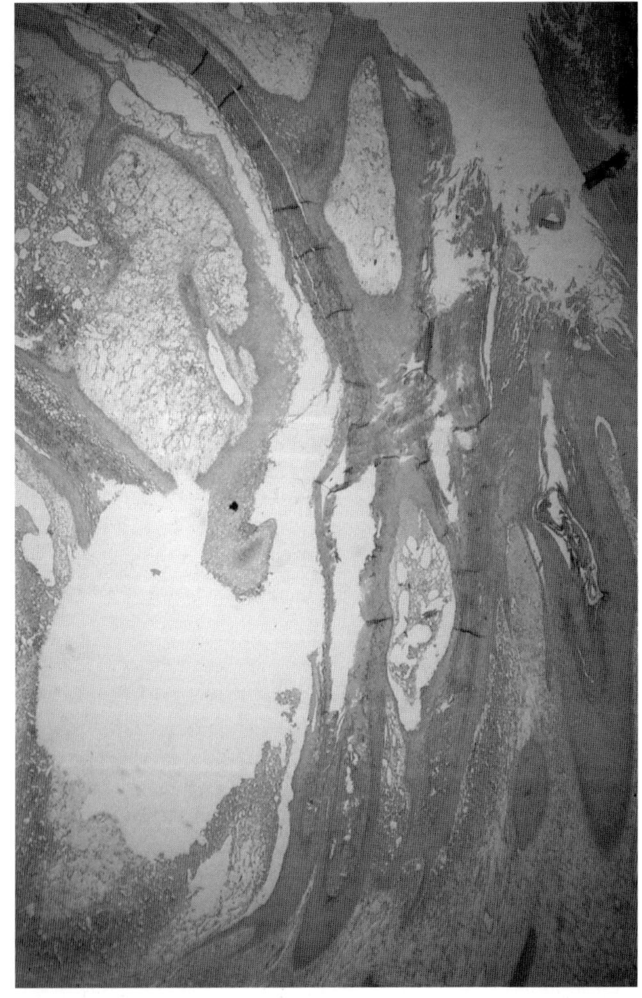

A

FIG. 26-5. Orf
(**A**) At scanning magnification, in the papillomatous stage, the epidermis shows acanthosis with fingerlike downward projections.

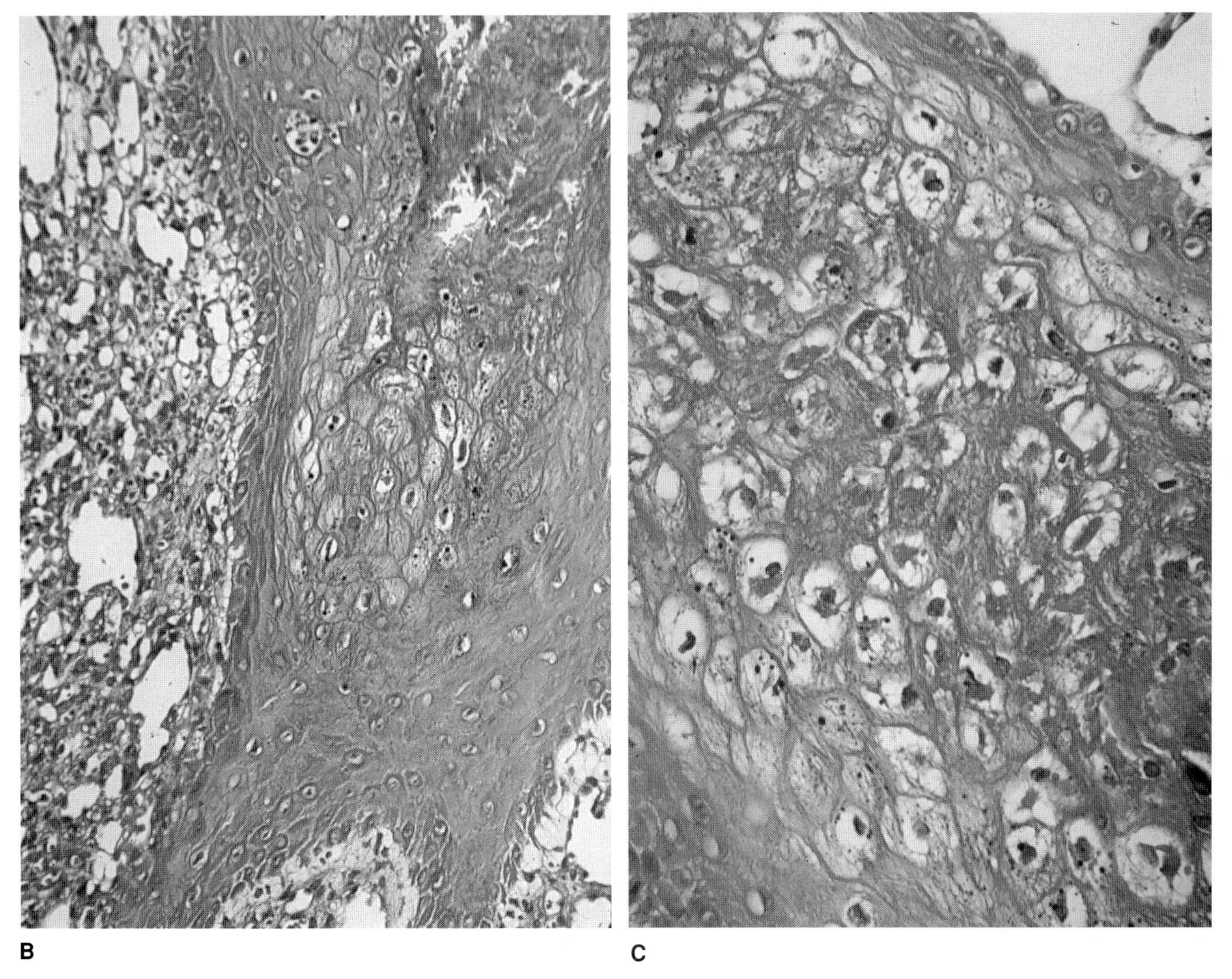

FIG. 26-5. ***Continued***
(**B**) There is vacuolization of cells in the upper third of the stratum malpighii, and the dermis shows vasodilatation and chronic inflammation. (**C**) Eosinophilic inclusion bodies in the cytoplasm of vacuolated epidermal cells distinguish orf from herpesvirus infections. Intranuclear eosinophilic inclusion bodies are also present in some cases.

and the dermis contains many newly formed, dilated capillaries and a mononuclear infiltrate.

In the acute weeping stage, the epidermis is necrotic throughout. A massive infiltrate of mononuclear cells extends throughout the dermis.

In the later stages, the epidermis shows acanthosis with fingerlike downward projections, and the dermis shows vasodilatation and chronic inflammation, followed by resolution (Fig. 26-5).

Viral Identification. In lesions less than 2 weeks old, the virus can be grown in tissue cultures of various cell types, including bovine or rhesus monkey kidney cells and human amnion cells or fibroblasts. In older lesions, one has to rely on serologic changes or on viral antigen demonstration in lesional material.

Electron microscopy reveals that the parapox virus is cylindrical in shape and has convex ends. It consists of a dense DNA core surrounded by a less dense, wide capsid and by two narrow, electron-dense outer layers. On the average, the virion measures 140 by 310 nm.

MOLLUSCUM CONTAGIOSUM

Molluscum contagiosum occurs most frequently in the pediatric age group and consists of a variable number of small, discrete, waxy, skin-colored, delled, dome-shaped papules, usually 2 to 4 mm in size. In adults, molluscum contagiosum is primarily a sexually transmitted disease. A papule of molluscum contagiosum may appear inflamed. In immunocompetent patients, the lesions involute spontaneously. During involution, there may be mild inflammation and tenderness. In the setting of immunosuppression, such as in HIV infection, molluscum contagiosum can attain considerable size and be widely disseminated.

In immunocompromised patients, particularly those with AIDS, hundreds of lesions of molluscum contagiosum may be observed, showing little tendency toward involution. Furthermore, clinically normal skin in the vicinity of molluscum lesions in HIV-infected persons may be infected by molluscum virus.[17] In the context of AIDS, a variety of systemic fungal diseases, including cryptococcosis, histoplasmosis, and penicillium marnefei, can disseminate and produce skin lesions that resemble molluscum contagiosum.

Histopathology. In molluscum contagiosum, the epidermis is acanthotic. Many epidermal cells contain large, intracytoplasmic inclusion bodies—the so-called molluscum bodies (Fig. 26-6). These bodies first appear as single, minute, ovoid eosinophilic structures in the lower cells of the stratum malpighii at a level one or two layers above the basal cell layer. The molluscum bodies increase in size as infected cells move toward the surface. The molluscum bodies in the upper layers of the epidermis displace and compress the nucleus so that it appears as a thin crescent at the periphery of the cell. At the level of the granular layer, the staining reaction of the molluscum bodies changes from eosinophilic to basophilic. In the horny layer, basophilic molluscum bodies measuring up to 35 μm in diameter lie enmeshed in a network of eosinophilic horny fibers (Color Fig. 26-1). In the center of the lesion, the stratum corneum ultimately disintegrates, releasing the molluscum bodies. Thus, a central crater forms.

The surrounding dermis usually shows little or no inflammatory reaction, except in instances in which the lesion of molluscum contagiosum ruptures and discharges molluscum bodies and horny material into the dermis.

During the period of spontaneous involution, a mononuclear infiltrate may be observed in close apposition to the lesion infiltrating between the infected epidermal cells.

Electron microscopic examination reveals that the molluscum inclusion bodies contain, embedded in a protein matrix, large numbers of molluscum contagiosum viruses (EM 14). The virus of molluscum contagiosum belongs to the poxvirus group. Like the viruses of variola, vaccinia, and cowpox, it is "brick-shaped" and measures approximately 300 by 240 nm. The virus of molluscum contagiosum has not been grown in tissue culture. Molluscum contagiosum virus can be detected directly in tissue specimens using in situ hybridization.[18]

The spontaneous disappearance of molluscum contagiosum may well represent a cell-mediated immune rejection of the lesion by the host.

VERRUCA

The traditional clinical classification of human papillomavirus (HPV) infection is based on appearance and location. Clinical patterns include: (1) verruca vulgaris or common wart, including filiform wart; (2) palmoplantar wart; (3) mosaic-type palmoplantar wart; (4) verruca plana; and (5) condyloma acuminatum or anogenital wart. Uncommon presentations include epidermodysplasia verruciformis and the intraoral lesions of Heck's disease.

Although there is a significant variation in clinical morphology, all represent infection by HPV, a member of the papova group. In turn, modern molecular methods have identified large numbers of human papillomavirus types, with as many as 67 being recognized by 1994. Classification of HPV type is based on the extent of DNA homology and not on serologic analysis. A new genotype is described if its DNA is less than 50% homologous to the DNA of other known types. HPV types have evolved with specific cellular tropisms and the ability to produce type-specific morphologic changes. Although more than one type can share the same cellular tropism, certain HPV types are commonly found in certain types of lesions. There exists a fairly good association of the viral type with the lesions listed below:

Verruca vulgaris: HPV types 2, 4, 7
Verruca plana: HPV type 3
Palmoplantar warts: HPV types 1, 2, 4
Condyloma acuminatum (low cancer risk): HPV types 6, 11

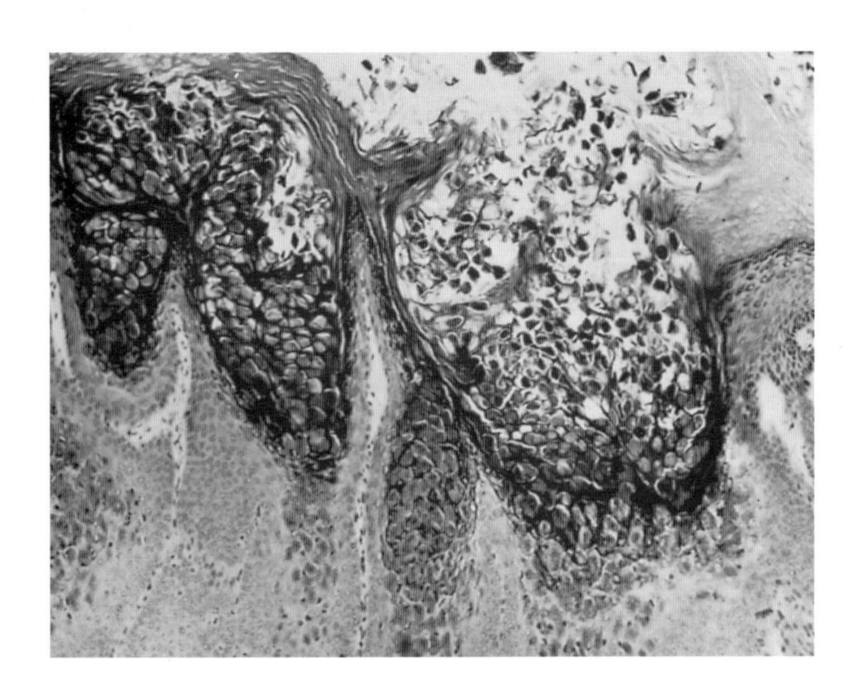

FIG. 26-6. Molluscum contagiosum Numerous intracytoplasmic inclusion bodies, so-called molluscum bodies, can be seen forming in the lower epidermis. They increase in size as they move toward the surface.

Condyloma acuminatum (high cancer risk): HPV types 16, 18, 31, 33, 51
Focal epithelial hyperplasia (Heck's disease): HPV types 13, 32
Bowenoid papulosis: HPV types 16, 18, 31, 33, 51
Butcher's warts: HPV type 7
Epidermodysplasia verruciformis: HPV types 3, 5, 8–10, 12, 14, 15, 17, 19–29, 38, 47
Laryngeal carcinoma: HPV type 30
Giant condyloma of Buschke and Loewenstein: HPV type 6
Cervical and vaginal atypias: HPV types 16, 18, 31, 33, 51

The association of particular HPV types with specific groups of warts, however, is not absolute; HPV-1 has been found in verrucae vulgares and condylomata acuminata, HPV-2 in condylomata acuminata, and HPV-3 in verrucae vulgares. HPV-7, in addition to occurring in verrucae vulgares on the hands of butchers, has been encountered in the verrucae vulgares of nonbutchers.

The value of HPV typing in the clinical setting is not clear. Definitive HPV typing can be obtained through DNA hybridization or amplification of HPV genomic material by the polymerase chain reaction. However, positive results cannot be considered definitive in predicting outcome. High-risk HPV types can be missed through sampling errors. In the end, close follow-up is important in the management of HPV infection, particularly when the patient has clinical exposure to potentially high-risk HPV types.[19]

Verruca Vulgaris

Verrucae vulgares are circumscribed, firm, elevated papules with papillomatous ("verrucous") hyperkeratotic surfaces. They occur singly or in groups. Generally, they are associated with little or no tenderness. Verrucae vulgares occur most commonly on the dorsal aspects of the fingers and hands. They are also found on the soles of the feet and less often on the palms as mosaic warts. Rarely, verrucae vulgares occur on the oral mucosa. Filiform warts, variants of verruca vulgaris, show threadlike, keratinous projections arising from horny bases. They are most commonly found on the face and scalp.

Histopathology. Verrucae vulgares show acanthosis, papillomatosis, and hyperkeratosis. The rete ridges are elongated and, at the periphery of the verruca, are often bent inward so that they appear to point radially toward the center (arborization). The characteristic features that distinguish verruca vulgaris from other papillomas are foci of vacuolated cells, referred to as koilocytotic cells, vertical tiers of parakeratotic cells, and foci of clumped keratohyaline granules. These three changes are quite pronounced in young verrucae vulgares. The foci of koilocytes are located in the upper stratum malpighii and in the granular layer (Fig. 26-7). The koilocytes possess small, round, deeply basophilic nuclei surrounded by a clear halo and pale-staining cytoplasm. These cells contain few or no keratohyaline granules, even when they are located in the granular layer. The ver-

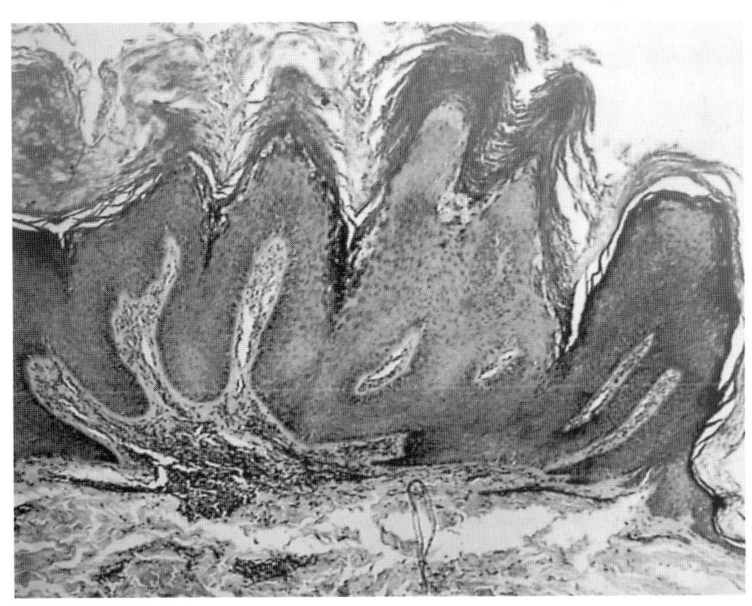
A

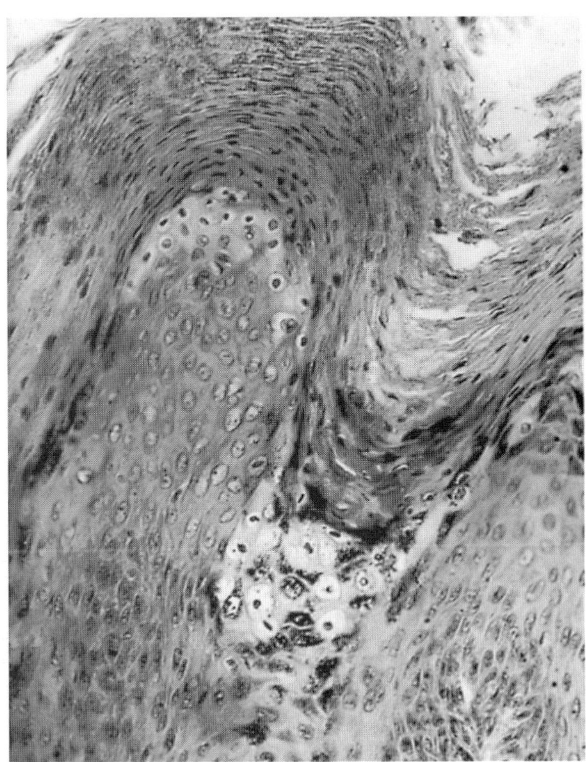
B

FIG. 26-7. Verruca vulgaris
(**A**) Low magnification. One observes hyperkeratosis, acanthosis, and papillomatosis. The rete ridges are elongated and bent inward at both margins and thus appear to point radially to the center. (**B**) Same as Fig. 26-7A, but at high magnification. Groups of large, vacuolated cells lie in the upper stratum malpighii and in the granular layer. A tier of parakeratotic cells lies over the crest of a papillomatous elevation.

tical tiers of parakeratotic cells are often located at the crests of papillomatous elevations of the rete malpighii overlying a focus of vacuolated cells. Compared with ordinary parakeratotic nuclei, the nuclei of the parakeratotic cells in verrucae vulgares are larger and more deeply basophilic, and many of them appear rounded rather than elongated. Although no granular cells are seen overlying the papillomatous crests, they are increased in number and size in the intervening valleys and contain heavy, irregular clumps of keratohyaline granules (see Fig. 26-7).

In filiform warts, the papillae are more elongated than in verrucae vulgares. They contain dilated capillaries, and small areas of hemorrhage may be seen in the thickened horny layer at the tip of the filiform wart.

Histogenesis. The wart virus, or HPV, is a DNA virus belonging to the papova group. No difference has been noted in electron microscopic appearance among the virus particles in the various types of HPV. However, the quantity varies with the different types. Frequently, virus particles are absent in verrucae vulgares on electron microscopic examination.

Negative results of electron microscopic examination do not exclude the presence of HPV. Viral antigens, such as papillomavirus common antigen, can be detected using immunohistochemistry, and HPV DNA can be amplified from lesions using the polymerase chain reaction and appropriate primers. Viral genomic material can also be identified by in situ hybridization. Viral DNA replication occurs in proliferating basal cells, but structural capsid protein forms in the midepidermis, so that mature HPV viral structures, if present, are observed only in the upper epidermis.

The virus particles are spherical bodies with a diameter of about 50 nm. Each particle consists of an electron-dense nucleoid with a stippled appearance surrounded by a less dense capsid. The wart virus replicates in the nucleus, where the viral particles are located as dense aggregates in a crystalloid arrangement. Eosinophilic intranuclear bodies are very rare in verrucae vulgares. The wart virus does not grow in tissue cultures and is not pathogenic for any animal.

Although warts are very common, especially in children and adolescents, defective cell-mediated immunity predisposes to the development of some types of warts. The frequency of warts in persons with renal transplants receiving immunosuppressive therapy is greater than that of the general population. In the context of HIV infection, a variety of papillomavirus infections have been reported. Eradication of cutaneous infection becomes increasingly difficult as the degree of immunosuppression becomes more profound.

Differential Diagnosis. For a discussion of differentiation of verruca vulgaris from other papillomas, see Chap. 30.

Deep Palmoplantar Warts

Deep palmoplantar warts can be tender and occasionally swollen and red. Although they may be multiple, they do not coalesce as do mosaic warts, which are verrucae vulgares. Deep palmoplantar warts occur not only on the palms and soles but also on the lateral aspects and tips of the fingers and toes. Unlike superficial, mosaic-type palmoplantar warts, deep palmoplantar warts usually are covered with a thick callus. When the callus is removed with a scalpel, the wart becomes apparent. Verrucous carcinoma of the foot has been reported in association with HPV-2.[20]

Histopathology. Whereas superficial, mosaic-type palmoplantar warts have a histologic appearance analogous to that of verruca vulgaris and represent HPV-2 or HPV-4, deep palmoplantar warts represent type HPV-1. These lesions, also known as myrmecia ("anthill") or inclusion warts, are characterized by abundant keratohyalin, which differs from normal keratohyalin by being eosinophilic. Starting in the lower epidermis, the cytoplasm of many cells contains numerous eosinophilic granules, which enlarge in the upper stratum malpighii and coalesce to form large, irregularly shaped, homogeneous "inclusion bodies." They either encase the vacuolated nucleus or are separated from it by perinuclear vacuolization. It has been pointed out that these homogeneous eosinophilic bodies resemble molluscum bodies, except that they do not displace the nucleus laterally. An actual granular layer does not exist. The homogeneous, eosinophilic intracytoplasmic material seems to merge with the

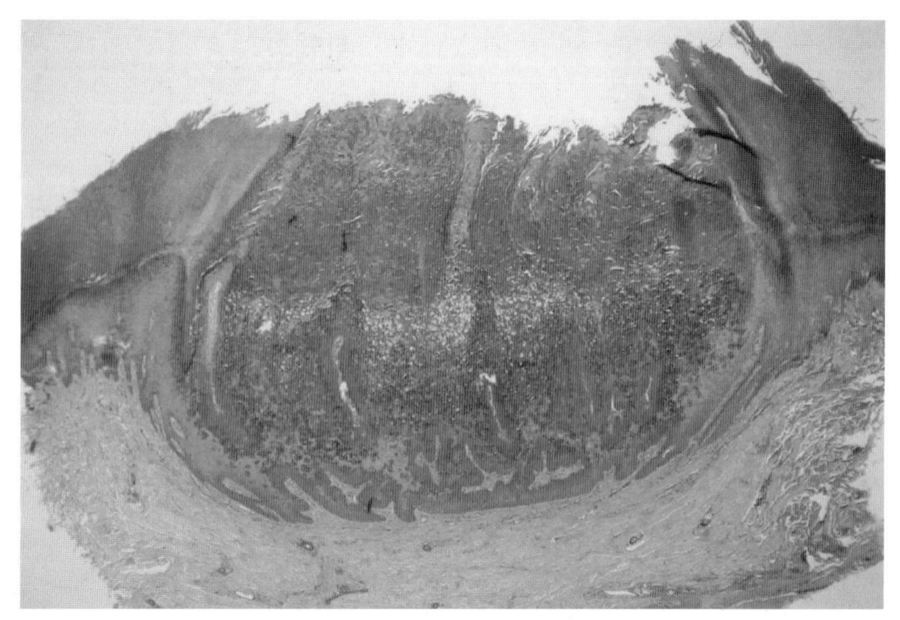
A

Fig. 26-8. Deep palmoplantar wart (myrmecia)
(**A**) Virally induced proliferation of keratinocytes results in greatly elongated dermal papillae (papillomatous or "verrucous" proliferation). Superficially, the elongated retia are displaced laterally while their tips point to the center in the deep portion of the lesion. The lesion is covered by thickened keratin, resulting in a tendency to grow inward rather than outward from the surface.

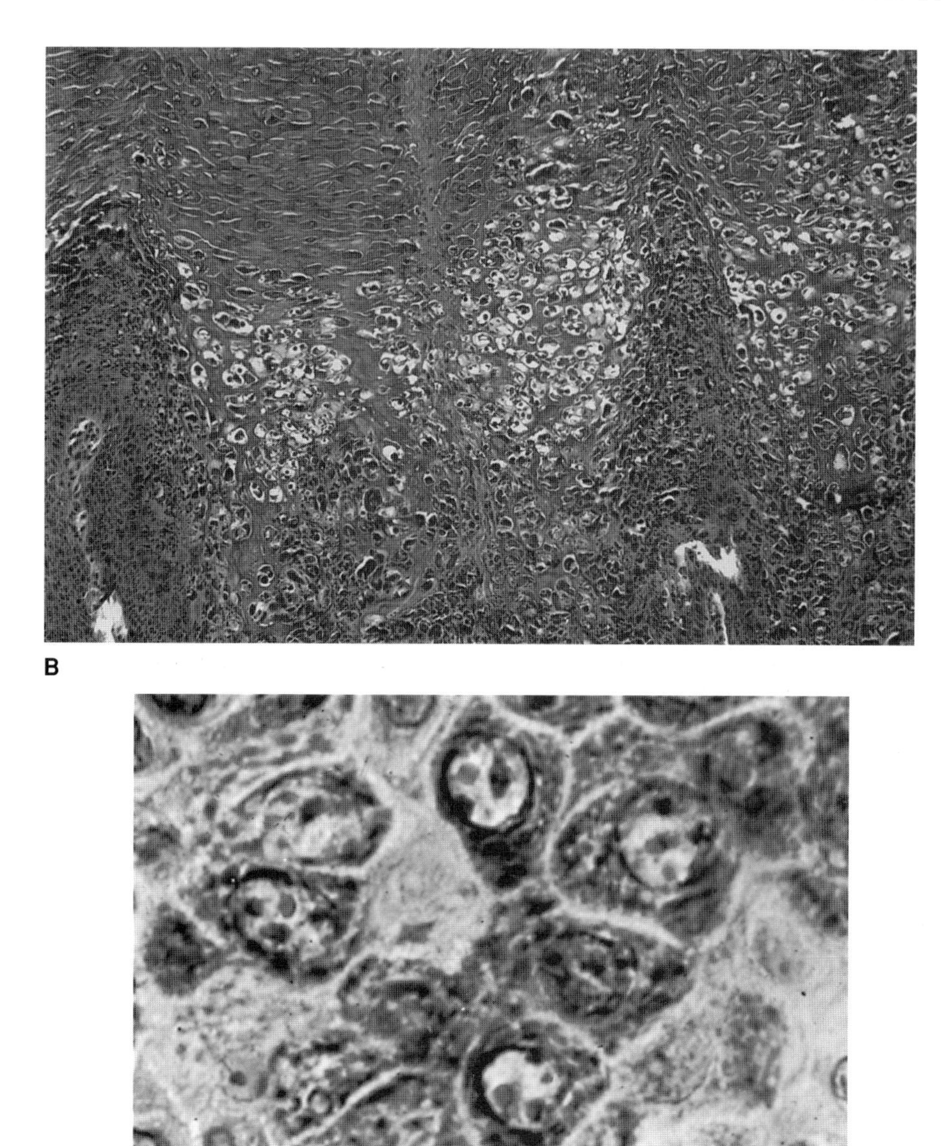

Fig. 26-8. ***Continued***
(**B**) The proliferating keratinocytes are vacuolated and contain prominent eosinophilic keratohyaline granules. (**C**) The epidermal cells have large, vacuolated nuclei. Five of the nuclei contain round eosinophilic bodies, formerly thought to represent inclusion bodies but actually representing keratohyalin. The darker, basophilic particles in the nuclei are nucleoli.

keratin formed by less altered cells. The nuclei in the stratum corneum persist, appearing as deeply basophilic round bodies surrounded by a wide, clear zone (Fig. 26-8). In addition to the large intracytoplasmic eosinophilic inclusion bodies, some of the cells in the upper stratum malpighii with vacuolated nuclei contain a small intranuclear eosinophilic "inclusion body." It is round and of about the same size as the nucleolus, which, however, is basophilic (see Fig. 26-8). Both the intranuclear eosinophilic inclusion body and the basophilic nucleolus disappear as the vacuolated nucleus changes into a smaller, deeply basophilic structure.

Histogenesis. Under electron microscopic examination, viral particles are first observed in the upper portion of the stratum malpighii within and around the nucleolus. Their number increases, and in cells just beneath the stratum corneum, nucleoli are no longer detected. In many instances, the material of the nucleus appears to be entirely replaced by virus particles except for a thin rim of chromatin closely applied to the nuclear membrane. The particles tend to be arranged in regular or crystalline formations. In the stratum corneum, no normal cell structures are recognizable, but there remain large, compact aggregates of virus particles surrounded by keratinous matter.

Verruca Plana

Verrucae planae are slightly elevated, flat, smooth papules. They may be hyperpigmented. The face and the dorsa of the hands are affected most commonly. In rare instances, there is extensive involvement, with lesions also on the extremities and

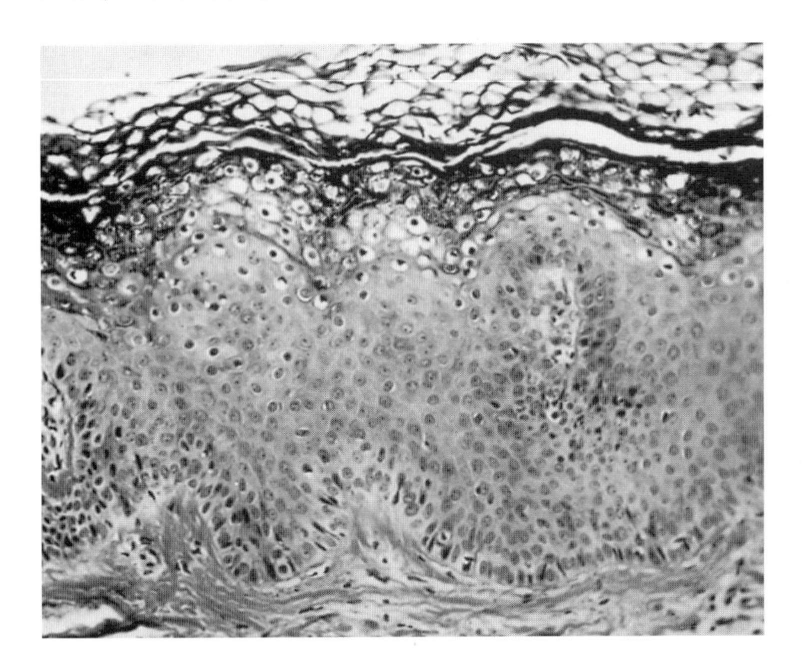

FIG. 26-9. Verruca plana
One observes hyperkeratosis and acanthosis but no papillomatosis or parakeratosis. Numerous vacuolated cells lie in the upper stratum malpighii, including the granular layer. The horny layer has a pronounced basket-weave appearance resulting from the vacuolization of the horny cells.

trunk. If starting in childhood and occurring in several members of the family, such disseminate cases of verruca plana have been mistakenly held to be instances of epidermodysplasia verruciformis, from which they differ by the absence of red, "tinea versicolor-like" patches and lack of malignant transformation of some of the exposed lesions.

Histopathology. Verrucae planae show hyperkeratosis and acanthosis but, unlike verrucae vulgares, have no papillomatosis, only slight elongation of the rete ridges, and no areas of parakeratosis.

In the upper stratum malpighii, including the granular layer, there is diffuse vacuolization of the cells (Fig. 26-9). Some of the vacuolated cells are enlarged to about twice their normal size. The nuclei of the vacuolated cells lie at the centers of the cells, and some of them appear deeply basophilic. The granular layer is uniformly thickened, and the stratum corneum has a pronounced basket-weave appearance resulting from vacuolization of the horny cells. The dermis appears normal.

Histogenesis. Verrucae planae are induced by HPV-3. Electron microscopic examination reveals marked cytoplasmic edema. The tonofilaments are dislodged to the periphery of the cell. The keratohyaline granules appear normal. Viral particles are numerous in the nuclei of vacuolated cells.

Epidermodysplasia Verruciformis

In epidermodysplasia verruciformis (EV), there is a widespread eruption resembling verrucae planae with a tendency toward confluence into patches. Also, there are irregu-

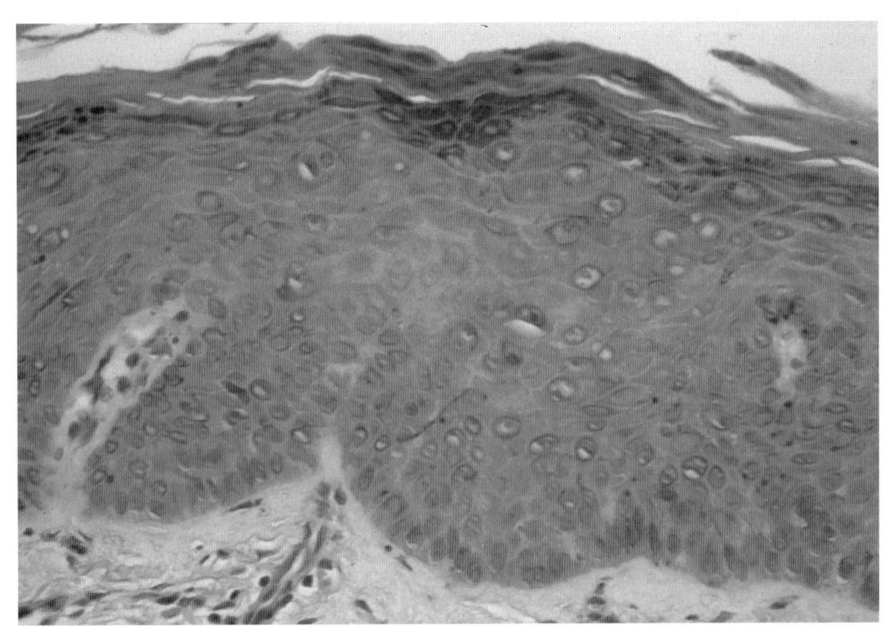

A

FIG. 26-10. Epidermodysplasia verruciformis
(**A**) The epidermis is hyperkeratotic and slightly acanthotic. Vacuolated cells are present in the upper stratum malpighii and granular layer.

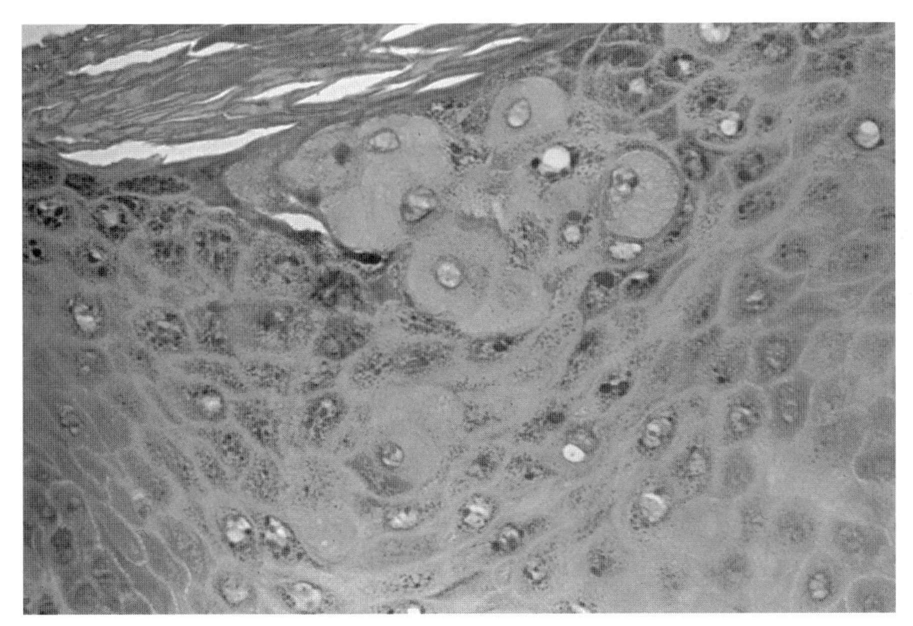

B

FIG. 26-10. *Continued*
(**B**) Affected keratinocytes have abundant, slightly basophilic cytoplasm. Keratohyalin granules may be prominent, although not in this example. Although some nuclei may appear pyknotic, others appear large, round, and empty.

larly outlined, slightly scaling macules of various shades of brown, red, and white that are tinea versicolor-like. Skin lesions resembling seborrheic keratosis have been noted.[21] The eruption usually begins in childhood and may be familial. Development of Bowen's disease (squamous cell carcinoma in situ) within lesions in exposed areas is a common occurrence, and invasive lesions of squamous cell carcinoma are occasionally found. EV-like lesions can develop in renal transplant patients[22] and in HIV-infected persons.[23]

Histopathology. The epidermal changes, although similar to those observed in verruca plana, often differ by being more pronounced and more extensive (Fig. 26-10). Affected keratinocytes are swollen and irregularly shaped. They show abundant, slightly basophilic cytoplasm and contain numerous round, basophilic keratohyalin granules. A few dyskeratotic cells may be seen in the lower part of the epidermis. Although some nuclei appear pyknotic, others appear large, round, and empty owing to marginal distribution of the chromatin.

Histogenesis. In epidermodysplasia verruciformis skin lesions, many HPV types have been found, and in some individual patients, several types have been identified. Electron microscopic examination shows viral particles, often in a semicrystalline pattern within nuclei located in the stratum granulosum. In contrast, the swollen cells in the stratum malpighii show virions in their nuclei in small aggregates only in some cases but none at all in others.

Viral particles are absent in lesions of Bowen's disease or squamous cell carcinoma arising within lesions of EV but rarely are observed in the upper layers of the epidermis overlying malignant lesions. However, HPV-5-specific DNA or HPV-8-specific DNA has been demonstrated on several occasions in squamous cell carcinomas arising in lesions of EV.

The underlying defect in EV is not known but may involve oncogene or immunologic misfunction.

Condyloma Acuminatum

Condylomata acuminata, or anogenital warts, can occur on the penis, on the female genitals, and in the anal region. Condylomata acuminata of the skin consist of fairly soft, verrucous papules that occasionally coalesce into cauliflower-like masses. Condyloma are flatter on mucosal surfaces.

Malignant progression is associated with infection by certain HPV types. In particular, HPV types 16, 18, 31, 33, and 51 have been associated with both in situ and invasive processes of the male and female genital regions as well as the vagina and cervix in women. This alteration may cover a spectrum from Bowen's disease to squamous cell carcinoma, potentially with extension to metastasis. (Concerning the development of bowenoid papulosis in patients with condylomata acuminata, see next page.)

Giant condyloma of Buschke and Loewenstein (Buschke-Loewenstein tumor) is regarded as representing verrucous carcinoma (Chap. 30). Recently, HPV-6 DNA has been found in this lesion.[24] Therefore, it is likely that giant condylomata begin as viral condylomata acuminata before developing into verrucous carcinoma. Clinically, the resemblance to a large aggregate of condylomata acuminata is very great, especially in the early stage. The most frequent location is the glans penis and foreskin (where urethral fistulae may result), but they may occur also on the vulva and in the anal region.

Histopathology. In condyloma acuminatum, the stratum corneum is only slightly thickened. Lesions located on mucosal surfaces show parakeratosis. The stratum malpighii shows papillomatosis and considerable acanthosis, with thickening and elongation of the rete ridges. Mitotic figures may be present. Usually, invasive squamous cell carcinoma can be ruled out because the epithelial cells show an orderly arrangement and the border between the epithelial proliferations and the dermis is sharp (Fig. 26-11). The most characteristic feature, important for the diagnosis, is the presence of areas in which the epithelial cells show distinct perinuclear vacuolization. These vacuolated

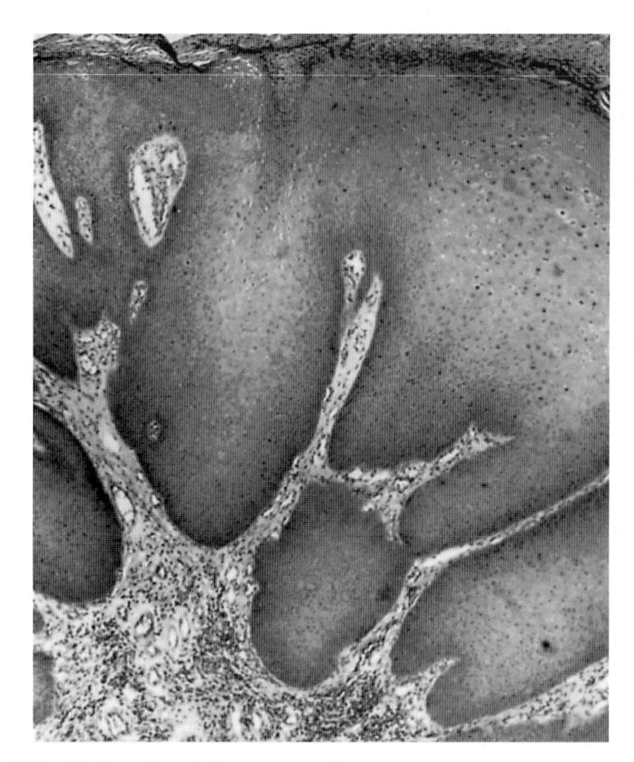

FIG. 26-11. Condyloma acuminatum
There is pronounced acanthosis. Many cells of the stratum malpighii appear vacuolated and have round, hyperchromatic nuclei.

epithelial cells are relatively large and possess hyperchromatic, round nuclei resembling the nuclei seen in the upper portion of the epidermis in verrucae vulgares. It must be kept in mind, however, that vacuolization is a normal occurrence in the upper portions of all mucosal surfaces, so that vacuolization in condylomata acuminata can be regarded as being possibly of viral genesis only if it extends into the deeper portions of the stratum malpighii. Koilocytotic ("raisin") nuclei, double nuclei, and apoptotic keratinocytes may be present but are often less prominent than in uterine cervical lesions.

Giant Condylomata Acuminata of Buschke and Loewenstein

Generally, vacuolization of keratinocytes is mild or absent, in contrast to condyloma acuminatum. There is tremendous proliferation of the epidermis with displacement of the underlying tissue, but the ratio of nucleus to cytoplasm is low. The invasive strands of tumor usually possess a well-developed basal cell layer. (For further discussion of verrucous carcinoma, see Chap. 30.)

Histogenesis. Papillomaviruses induce a variety of proliferative lesions in humans. Of the many types of human papillomaviruses that have been identified, a subset that includes types 16, 18, 31, 33, and 51 is associated with anogenital cancers.[25,26] These cancers develop from precursor lesions such as condylomata acuminata on the external genitalia, vaginal intraepithelial neoplasia in the vagina (VIN), and cervical intraepithelial neoplasia on the cervix (CIN). Viral production occurs in low-grade lesions that are only slightly altered in their pattern of differentiation from normal cells, but the concentration of mature virions in condylomata acuminata is low. The production of viral particles, genome amplification, capsid protein synthesis, and virion assembly is dependent on differentiation and is restricted to suprabasal cells. In more atypical lesions, viral DNA is usually found integrated into host chromosomes and no viral production is noted. Recent advances suggest that the E6 and E7 HPV oncoproteins function by inactivation of cell cycle regulators, thus providing the initial step in progression to malignancy. Condylomata acuminata can also be associated with HPV types 6 and 11; these types have less oncogenic potential.

BOWENOID PAPULOSIS OF THE GENITALIA

Bowenoid papuloses are small, red papules of the genitalia. Some lesions are distinctly verrucous in appearance. The lesions are located in men on the glans and shaft of the penis and in women in the perineal and vulvar areas. Generally, the lesions are diagnosed clinically as genital warts, and the histologic finding of "Bowen's disease" appears incongruous.

The lesions have a definite tendency toward spontaneous resolution; some lesions regress, but others may appear and in turn also regress. Still, in some patients, lesions have persisted for prolonged periods. In rare cases, invasive squamous cell carcinoma has been described as arising in a bowenoid papule.

Some authors regard the disorder as benign and, in particular, as different from Bowen's disease,[27] but others have found that bowenoid papulosis presents a high risk for cervical neoplasia both for female patients and for sexual partners of male patients[28] (see section on Histogenesis).

Histopathology. Bowenoid papulosis shows the typical features of Bowen's disease. These features consist of crowding and an irregular, "windblown" arrangement of the nuclei, many of which are large, hyperchromatic, and pleomorphic (Fig. 26-12). Dyskeratotic and multinucleated keratinocytes are also present, as are atypical mitoses. (For a detailed description of Bowen's disease, see Chap. 30.) Some researchers believe that bowenoid papulosis differs from Bowen's disease by virtue of a lesser degree of cytologic atypia. In a few instances, bowenoid papulosis and condylomata acuminata have been found coexisting in the same patient.

Histogenesis. Bowenoid papulosis represents infection by HPV types associated with high risk of malignancy evolution, such as HPV types 16, 18, 31, 33, and 51. As noted above, these types elaborate oncoproteins that interfere with normal cellular homeostasis. A significant fact is that HPV types associated with oncogenesis are commonly found in other genital areas and can be associated with malignancies in these areas, such as carcinoma of the vagina, cervix, penis, and anus. Precursor lesions can be found in these sites. The development of carcinoma in situ lesions of the cervix has been noted.

Differential Diagnosis. Bowenoid papulosis of the genitalia in most instances is differentiated from Bowen's disease on the basis of clinical data, such as onset at an earlier average age, multiplicity of lesions, smaller size of lesions, verrucoid appearance of some lesions, and tendency toward spontaneous regression. Thus, Bowen's disease or squamous cell carcinoma in situ cannot be ruled out by biopsy alone in most cases.

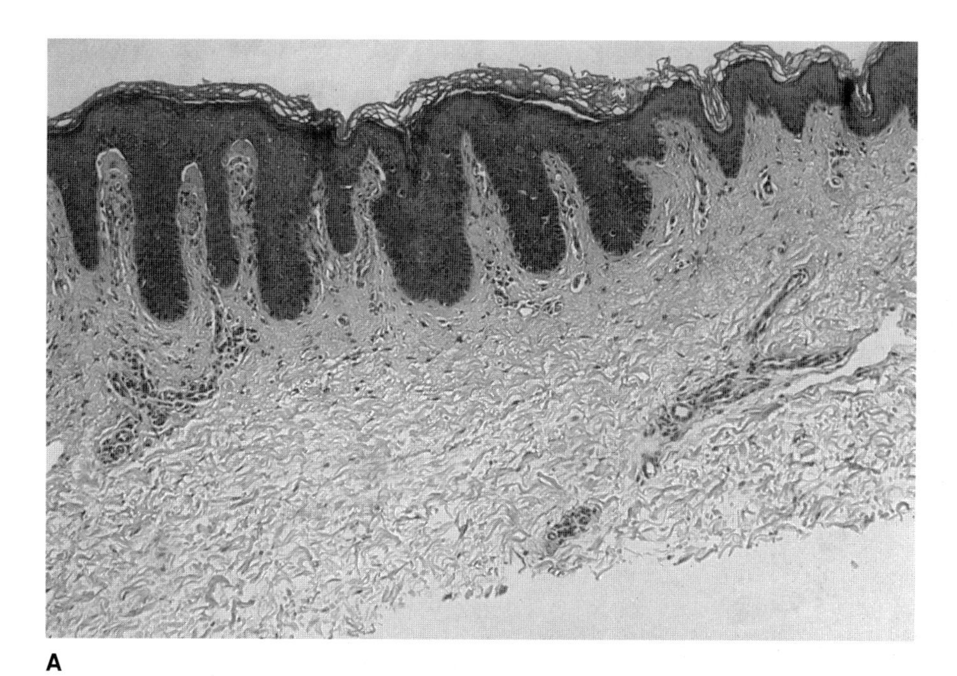

A

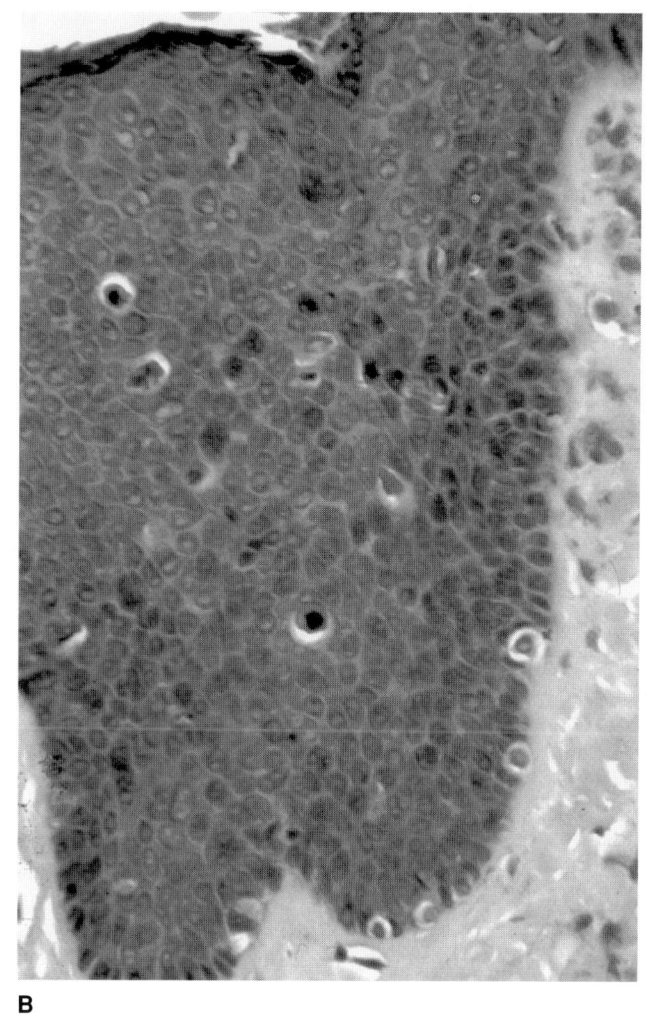

B

FIG. 26-12. Bowenoid papulosis
(**A**) The epithelium is irregularly thickened with disorderly maturation, which may impart a "windblown" look at scanning or intermediate magnification. (**B**) The keratinocytic nuclei are crowded and there is partial arrest of maturation. Mitoses are present above the basal layers, and the nuclei tend to be hyperchromatic and irregular, sometimes with nucleoli.

Changes induced by recent application of podophyllum resin need to be considered. The changes induced by podophyllum resin consist of necrotic keratinocytes and bizarre mitotic figures and are most pronounced during the first 72 hours after application.

ORAL FOCAL EPITHELIAL HYPERPLASIA

A rare condition described in Native Americans, oral focal epithelial hyperplasia (Heck's disease), has since been found to occur in many countries and races, but most commonly among the Eskimos of Greenland.[29] It occurs mainly in children, often in small endemic foci. Although the disease is chronic, spontaneous remissions occur. Oral focal hyperplasia has been described in the context of HIV infection.[30]

The lesions are limited to the oral mucosa—most commonly, the mucosa of the lower lip. There are numerous soft, white papules 2 to 4 mm in diameter. Most are discrete, but some are confluent. The lesions are asymptomatic.

Histopathology. The oral epithelium shows acanthosis with thickening and elongation of the rete ridges. Throughout the epithelium, there are areas where the cells show marked vacuolization and stain only faintly. Vacuolization is most pronounced in the upper portion of the epithelium, but it may extend into the broadened rete ridges.

Histogenesis. Electron microscopic examination reveals viral particles with the size of the human papillomavirus arranged in a crystalline pattern. HPV types 13 and 32 are typical for oral focal epithelial hyperplasia.

Differential Diagnosis. The histologic appearance of the affected oral epithelium in focal epithelial hyperplasia is identical to that of oral epithelial nevus, or white sponge nevus (Chap. 30).

HAND-FOOT-AND-MOUTH DISEASE

Hand-foot-and-mouth disease occurs in small epidemics, affecting mainly children and having a mild course that usually lasts less than a week. Small vesicles may be confined to the mouth, where they evolve into small ulcers. Only scattered vesicles surrounded by an erythematous halo are observed on the palms of the hands, the soles of the feet, and the ventral surfaces and sides of the fingers and toes.

Hand-foot-and-mouth disease is caused by a coxsackievirus, which is an enterovirus and a member of the picornavirus group. In most instances, coxsackievirus type A16 has been isolated; only rarely has another type, such as A5 or A9, been found.

Histopathology. Early vesicles are intraepidermal, whereas old vesicles may be subepidermal in location. There is pronounced reticular degeneration of the epidermis, resulting in multilocular vesiculation. In the deep layers of the epidermis, some ballooning degeneration may be found. Neither inclusion bodies nor multinucleated giant cells are present.

Histogenesis. Electron microscopic examination reveals that some keratinocytes contain within their cytoplasm aggregates of virus particles exhibiting a crystalloid pattern. The coxsackievirus can be cultured from the stool and occasionally also from the vesicles. The virus grows well on human epithelial cell cultures and on monkey kidney tissue cultures.

ACQUIRED IMMUNODEFICIENCY SYNDROME (AIDS)

Since 1981, AIDS, as a gradually spreading epidemic, initially affected certain risk groups such as male homosexuals, recipients of blood transfusions, and intravenous drug abusers, but has since extended to involve heterosexuals and newborns of infected mothers. AIDS is caused by infection with a retrovirus called human immunodeficiency virus (HIV). The virus is spread almost exclusively through blood and semen.

HIV infects T helper cells or their precursors, leading to their destruction. The result is an irreversible state of cellular immune deficiency, causing death by predisposing the patient to a variety of opportunistic infections, especially to *Pneumocystis carinii* pneumonia and the uncontrolled development of tumors, most notably Kaposi's sarcoma (Chap. 34) and lymphoma. Lymphomas often are high-grade B-cell lymphomas, presenting frequently in extranodal sites such as the central nervous system. Recently, DNA sequences of a new herpesvirus have been detected in AIDS-associated Kaposi's sarcoma, classic Kaposi's sarcoma, and AIDS-related body-cavity-based lymphoma.[31,32] It seems likely that the presence of this organism is associated with the development of these neoplasms.

Among the opportunistic infections affecting the skin and mucous membranes of patients with AIDS are many that commonly occur in immunologically intact persons but are atypical in the context of HIV infection.[13] Examples are bacterial infections, such as impetigo and folliculitis (Chap. 21); viral infections, such as herpes simplex and HPV; and fungal infections, such as candidiasis and dermatophytosis (Chap. 23). Oral candidiasis is often an early clinical manifestation of AIDS and in progressing may cause painful esophagitis. Severe herpes zoster with subsequent scarring in a young individual may reflect HIV-seropositivity. Some infections occur in clinically obscure forms because they do not have recognizable morphologic features. In addition, systemic infectious disease can produce skin lesions, even though the classic organs of involvement for that agent may not include the skin. Among these are cytomegalovirus, *Cryptococcus, Mycobacterium, Histoplasma*, and others.

A rather characteristic clinical manifestation, highly suggestive of AIDS, is *oral hairy leukoplakia.* There are white, corrugated, "hairy" lesions commonly on the lateral aspects of the tongue. Epstein-Barr virus appears to be necessary for production of this lesion, although HPV and candida are also frequently present. Another unique infectious disease first recognized in the context of HIV infection is *bacillary angiomatosis.* Bacillary angiomatosis is a systemic infectious disease caused by *R henselae* or *R quintana.*[33] Cutaneous lesions resemble Kaposi's sarcoma or hemangioma but resolve with appropriate antibiotic therapy.

Nonspecific inflammatory skin disorders are common in patients with AIDS and include *seborrheic dermatitis*, a pruritic follicular eruption, and a poorly characterized *interface dermatitis.*

Seborrheic dermatitis occurs commonly in HIV infection. It can be quite severe, with the severity correlating with the patient's clinical status and CD4 count.[34] The histopathology of this eruption is similar to that of idiopathic seborrheic dermatitis, although some feel that distinctive histologic patterns are present.[35]

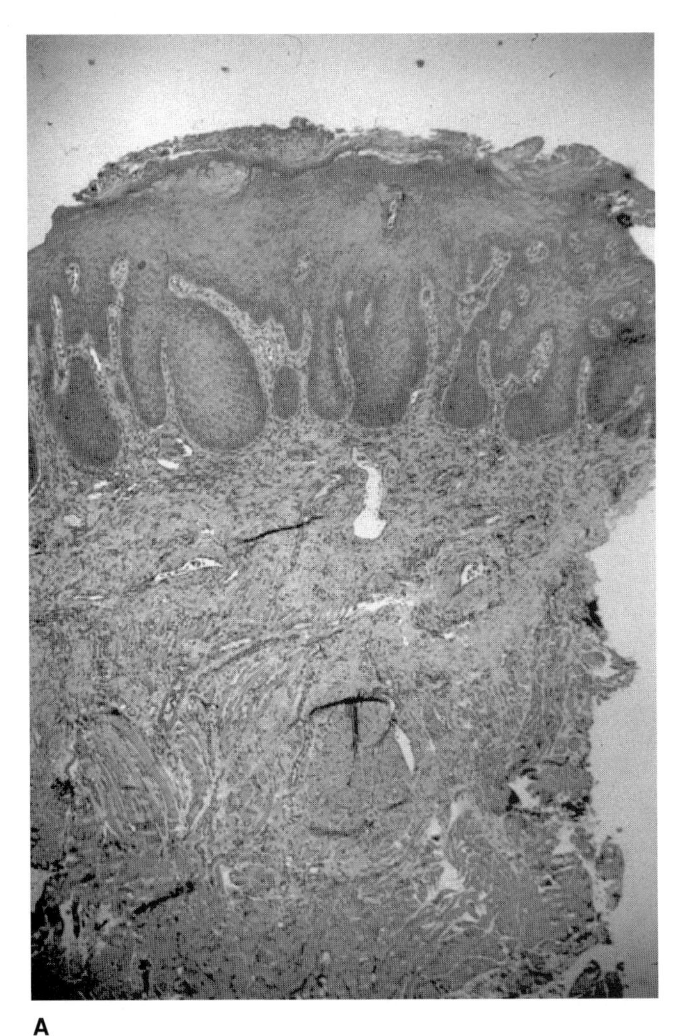

A

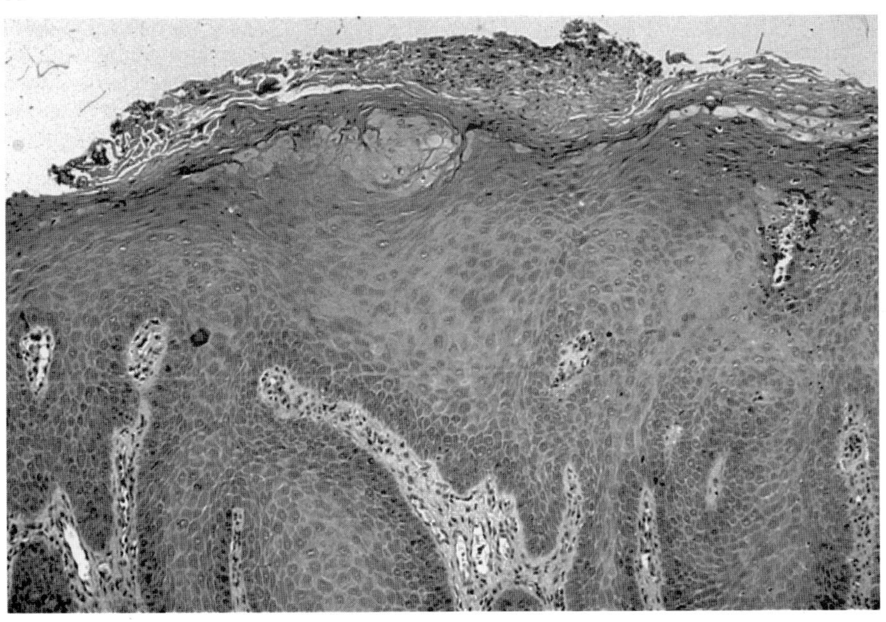

B

FIG. 26-13. Oral hairy leukoplakia (**A**) Scanning magnification shows the characteristic complex rete pattern of lingual epithelium. There is hyperkeratosis and parakeratosis, and there may be neutrophils in the stratum corneum. Pallor of superficial keratinocytes is focally apparent. (**B**) Hyperkeratosis and parakeratosis, epithelial pallor, and scant inflammation in the superficial lamina propria. *(continued on next page)*

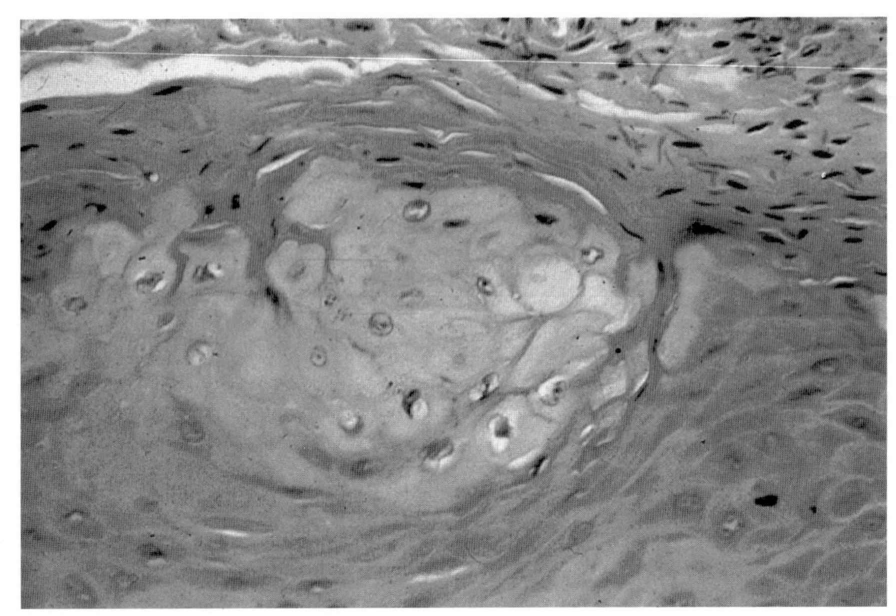

C

FIG. 26-13. *Continued*
(**C**) Detail of swollen, pale superficial keratinocytes, with open pale nuclei, but without specific viral cytopathic changes.

A nonspecific follicular eruption, named *eosinophilic pustular folliculitis*, is present in a significant number of patients with HIV infection.[36] There is some confusion over the descriptive terminology used to identify the eruption clinically. The eruption is chronic and pruritic. Histologically, there may be folliculitis with transmigration of eosinophils into the follicular epithelium, mimicking the changes observed in Ofuji's disease. However, in many cases, the histologic picture is less specific, showing only a polymorphous inflammatory response and mild folliculitis (*papular eruption of AIDS*).[37]

The interface dermatitis, observed in a series of 25 patients with AIDS, presents as a more or less widespread eruption of pink or red macules, papules, or plaques. It resembles and may represent a form of drug eruption or erythema multiforme.[38]

Histopathology. There is no unique histology of HIV infection in the skin. Primary exanthems of HIV show nonspecific lymphocytoid infiltrates with mild epidermal changes, primarily spongiosis.[39] Biopsies of AIDS-related eruptions are often nonspecific. The histologies of the myriad of subsequent consequences of HIV infection will be examined in other sections of this text.

The lesions of oral hairy leukoplakia show irregular keratin projections, parakeratosis, and acanthosis.[40] A characteristic finding within the epithelium is vacuolar change of superficial keratinocytes (Fig. 26-13). Candida organisms may be demonstrable.[41]

Seborrheic dermatitis in patients with AIDS may show nonspecific changes, including spotty keratinocytic necrosis, leukoexocytosis, and plasma cells in a superficial perivascular infiltrate.[35]

The papular eruption may exhibit nonspecific perivascular eosinophils with mild folliculitis,[37] although epithelioid cell granulomas have also been reported.[42,43]

The interface dermatitis shows, as the name implies, vacuolar alteration of the basal cell layer, scattered necrotic keratinocytes, and a superficial perivascular lymphohistiocytic infiltrate. The vacuolar alteration and number of necrotic keratinocytes tend to be more pronounced than in drug eruptions.[38]

REFERENCES

1. Reeves WC, Corey L, Adams HG et al. Risk of recurrence after first episode of genital herpes. N Engl J Med 1981;305:315.
2. Prober CG, Sullender WM, Yasukawa LL et al. Low risk of herpes simplex virus infections in neonates exposed to the virus at the time of vaginal delivery to mothers with recurrent genital herpes simplex infections. N Engl J Med 1987;316:240.
3. Schofield JK, Tatnall FM, Leigh IM. Recurrent erythema multiforme: Clinical features and treatment in a large series of patients. Brit J Dermatol 1993;128:542.
4. Darragh TM, Egbert BM, Berger TG, Yen TS. Identification of herpes simplex virus DNA in lesions of erythema multiforme by the polymerase chain reaction. J Am Acad Dermatol 1991;24:23.
5. Weston WL, Brice SL, Jester JD et al. Herpes simplex virus in childhood erythema multiforme. Pediatrics 1992;89:32.
6. Nahass GT, Goldstein BA, Zhu WY et al. Comparison of Tzanck smear, viral culture, and DNA diagnostic methods in detection of herpes simplex and varicella-zoster infection. JAMA 1992;268:2541.
7. Grossman MC, Silvers DN. The Tzanck smear: Can dermatologists accurately interpret it? J Am Acad Dermatol 1992;27:403.
8. Montone KT, Brigati DJ. In situ molecular pathology: Instrumentation, oligonucleotides, and viral nucleic acid detection. J Histotech 1994;17:195.
9. Xwang JY, Montone KT. A rapid simple in situ hybridization method for herpes simplex virus employing a synthetic biotin-labeled oligonucleotide probe: A comparison with immunohistochemical methods for HSV detection. J Clin Lab Anal 1994;8:105.
10. Morecki R, Becker NH. Human herpesvirus infection: Its fine structure identification in paraffin-embedded tissue. Arch Pathol 1968;86:292.
11. Meythaler JM, Varma RR. Reye's syndrome in adults. Arch Intern Med 1987;147:61.
12. Pastuszak AL, Levy M, Schick B et al. Outcome after maternal varicella infection in the first 20 weeks. New Engl J Med 1994;330:901.
13. Penneys NS. Skin manifestations of AIDS. London: Martin Dunitz, 1995;102.

14. Nikkels AF, Debrus S, Sadzot-Delvaux C et al. Comparative immunohistochemical study of herpes simplex and varicella-zoster infections. Virchows Arch A Pathol Anat Histopathol 1993;42:121.
15. Solomon AR, Rasmussen JE, Weiss JS. A comparison of the Tzanck smear and viral isolation in varicella and herpes zoster. Arch Dermatol 1986;122:282.
16. Leavell UW Jr, Phillips JA. Milker's nodules. Arch Dermatol 1975; 111:1307.
17. Smith KJ, Skelton HG, Yeager J et al. Molluscum contagiosum: Ultrastructural evidence for its presence in skin adjacent to clinical lesions in patients infected with human immunodeficiency virus type 1. Arch Dermatol 1992;128:223.
18. Forghani B, Oshiro LS, Chan CS et al. Direct detection of Molluscum contagiosum virus in clinical specimens by in situ hybridization using biotinylated probe. Mol Cell Probes 1992;6:67.
19. Rock B, Shah KV, Farmer ER. A morphologic, pathologic, and virologic study of anogenital warts in men. Arch Dermatol 1992;127:495.
20. Noel JC, Peny MO, Detremmerie O et al. Demonstration of human papillomavirus type 2 in a verrucous carcinoma of the foot. Dermatology 1993;187:58.
21. Tomasini C, Aloi F, Pippione M. Seborrheic keratosis-like lesions in epidermodysplasia verruciformis. J Cutan Pathol 1993;20:237.
22. Tieben LM, Berkhout RJ, Smits HL et al. Detection of epidermodysplasia verruciformis-like human papillomavirus types in malignant and premalignant skin lesions of renal transplant recipients. Brit J Dermatol 1994;131:226.
23. Berger T, Sawchuk WS, Leonardi C et al. Epidermodysplasia verruciformis-associated papillomavirus infection complicating human immunodeficiency virus disease. Brit J Dermatol 1991;124:79.
24. Noel JC, Vandenbossche M, Peny MO et al. Verrucous carcinoma of the penis: Importance of human papillomavirus typing for diagnosis and therapeutic decision. Eur Urol 1992;22:83.
25. Della Torre G, Donghi R, Longoni A et al. HPV DNA in intraepithelial neoplasia and carcinoma of the vulva and penis. Diagn Molec Pathol 1992;1:25.
26. Ikenberg H, Spitz C, Schmitt B et al. Human papillomavirus DNA in locally recurrent cervical cancer. Gynecol Oncol 1994;52:332.
27. Patterson JW, Kao GF, Graham JH et al. Bowenoid papulosis: A clinicopathologic study with ultrastructural observations. Cancer 1986;57: 823.
28. Obalek S, Jablonska S, Beaudenon S et al. Bowenoid papulosis of the male and female genitalia: Risk of cervical neoplasia. J Am Acad Dermatol 1986;14:433.
29. Archard HO, Heck JW, Stanley HR. Focal epithelial hyperplasia. Oral Surg 1965;20:201.
30. Vilmer C, Cavelier-Bally B, Pinquier L et al. Focal epithelial hyperplasia and multifocal human papillomavirus infection in an HIV-seropositive man. J Am Acad Dermatol 1994;30:497.
31. Moore PS, Chang Y. Detection of herpesvirus-like DNA sequences in Kaposi's sarcoma in patients with and those without HIV infection. New Engl J Med 1995;332:1181.
32. Cesarman E, Chang Y, Moore PS et al. Kaposi's sarcoma-associated herpesvirus-like DNA sequences in AIDS-related body-cavity-based lymphoma. New Engl J Med 1995;332:1186.
33. Koehler JE, Quinn FD, Berger TG et al. Isolation of rochalimaea species from cutaneous and osseous lesions of bacillary angiomatosis. New Engl J Med 1992;327:1625.
34. Llifson AR, Hessol NA, Buchbinder SP, Holmberg SD. The association of clinical conditions and serologic tests with CD4+ lymphocyte counts in HIV-infected subjects without AIDS. AIDS 1991;5:1209.
35. Soeprono FF, Schinella RA, Cockerell CJ et al. Seborrheic-like dermatitis of acquired immunodeficiency syndrome. J Am Acad Dermatol 1986;14:242.
36. Buchness MR, Lim HW, Hatcher VA et al. Eosinophilic pustular folliculitis in the acquired immunodeficiency syndrome. New Engl J Med 1988;318:1183.
37. Hevia O, Jimenez-Acosta F, Ceballos PI et al. Pruritic papular eruption of the acquired immunodeficiency syndrome: A clinicopathologic study. J Am Acad Dermatol 1991;24:231.
38. Rico MJ, Kory WP, Gould EW et al. Interface dermatitis in patients with the acquired immunodeficiency syndrome. J Am Acad Dermatol 1987;16:1209.
39. Hulsebosch HJ, Claessen FAP, Van Ginkel CJW et al. Human immunodeficiency virus exanthem. J Am Acad Dermatol 1990;23:483.
40. Lupton GP, James WD, Redfield RR et al. Oral hairy leukoplakia. Arch Dermatol 1987;123:624.
41. Winzer M, Gilliar U, Ackerman AB. Hairy lesions of the oral cavity. Am J Dermatopathol 1988;10:155.
42. Goodman DS, Teplitz ED, Wishner A et al. Prevalence of cutaneous disease in patients with acquired immunodeficiency syndrome (AIDS) or AIDS-related complex. J Am Acad Dermatol 1987;17:210.
43. James WD, Redfield RR, Lupton GP et al. A papular eruption associated with human T-cell lymphotropic virus type III disease. J Am Acad Dermatol 1985;13:563.

Lever's Histopathology of the Skin, eighth edition,
edited by David Elder et al. Lippincott–
Raven Publishers, Philadelphia © 1997.

CHAPTER 27

The Histiocytoses

Walter H. C. Burgdorf

The histiocytic disorders cover a wide range of primary and secondary, solitary and multiple, benign and malignant disorders unified only by being for the most part uncommon and poorly understood. The "X" in histiocytosis X as originally proposed by Liechtenstein was designed to reflect the unknown; even though we have drifted away from the designation, it to some degree still reflects our knowledge.

The histiocytoses can be classified many ways; three convenient methods use the cell of origin, the histologic pattern, and the clinical disease entities. Although these three schemas are beginning to correlate (i.e., a given cell type produces a single pattern that leads to the diagnosis of a single disease), for the most part one is confronted by a morass of overlapping and contradicting terms. As Headington pointed out in an oft-cited "obituary," the concept of the histiocyte has hindered our approach to many diseases.[1] Or, as the Foucars suggested, no one would be foolhardy enough to write about a group of disorders known as the "lymphocytoses," but we still struggle with histiocytoses.[2]

Starting at the cellular level, the Foucars have suggested the term *M-PIRE system* (Mononuclear Phagocyte and ImmunoRegulatory Effector cells) as a neutral and relatively all-encompassing designation for histiocytes.[2] Two other elegant reviews still use the designation of histiocyte.[3,4] All agree that there are two basic subdivisions of this family of cells:

1. The bone marrow–derived monocytes, which migrate to tissue, where they differentiate into macrophages, fixed histiocytes, or professional phagocytes. Apparently the immature macrophages (i.e., monocytes that have just entered the skin) are still quite responsive to cytokines, but they soon become fixed, not so much in a physical sense as in that their biologic role is limited. Free or migrating histiocytes are quite rare, found primarily in the spleen and tonsils. These professional phagocytes are known by many names, based on their site, such as Kupffer cells in the liver or tingible body macrophages in lymph nodes. They are capable of phagocytosis, are rich in lysosomal enzymes, and are very active metabolically. There are a number of monoclonal antibodies available to identify macrophages, including KP1 (CD68), MAC 387, KiM1P, and Leu-M1 (CD15). Older markers of phagocytic activity such as lysozyme and α_1-antitrypsin are identified by polyclonal antibodies and not as helpful.[5]

2. The dendritic cells are also for the most part bone marrow–derived and reside in the skin or lymph nodes. They are primarily involved in antigen presentation to lymphocytes and rarely show marked phagocytosis. In the skin, the prominent dendritic cell is the Langerhans cell (LC), characterized by Birbeck granules, S-100, and CD1a positivity. The indeterminate cell is closely related, perhaps an LC variant that lacks Birbeck granules.

Other antigen-processing dendritic cells in the lymph nodes include the interdigitating dendritic cells (old name: interdigitating reticulum cell), which present antigens to T cells in the cortex, and the follicular dendritic cells (old name: dendritic reticulum cell), which interact with B cells in the germinal centers. Both of these cells lack Birbeck granules and do not express CD1a; although both are S-100–positive, the reaction is usually minimal with the follicular dendritic cells. Instead they express a cell-specific antigen usually recognized by the monoclonal antibody R4/23.

There are also dendritic cells in the skin that are not involved in antigen processing. One is the dermal dendrocyte, recognized by XIIIa positivity and a failure to stain for S-100. The monoclonal antibody CD34 (QBEnd 10) also identifies dermal dendrocytes and endothelial cells. Another closely related cell is the dendritic perivascular cell, identified by the MS-1 antigen.[6] This antigen was initially used as a marker for discontinuous endothelial cells; it may serve to attach perivascular dendritic cells to the microvasculature. Most of the idiopathic strictly cutaneous histiocytoses stain positively for MS-1, whereas systemic disorders such as sarcoidosis and necrobiotic disorders such as granuloma annulare lack positivity.

These two basic categories of histiocytes have given rise to the most widely used but unfortunately somewhat crude classification. Winkelmann[7] initially suggested the categories "X" and "non-X," in which "X" referred to histiocytosis X and "non-X" to all the rest. Gianotti and Caputo[8] expanded the classification but still retained Winkelmann's split. The Writing Group of the Histiocyte Society[9] suggested the following terms: class I, or Langerhans cell histiocytosis (LCH); class II, or histiocytoses of mononuclear phagocytes other than Langerhans cells—in

W. H. C. Burgdorf: Clinical Lecturer, Department of Dermatology, Ludwig Maximilian University, Munich, Germany

TABLE 27-1. *Classification of histiocytoses*

S-100+, CD1a+, and Birbeck granules	
Langerhans' cell histiocytosis	(LCH)
Congenital self-healing reticulohistiocytosis	(CSHRH)
S-100+, CD1a+, no Birbeck granules	
Indeterminate cell histiocytosis	(ICH)
S-100+, CD1a−, no Birbeck granules	
Sinus histiocytosis with massive lymphadenopathy	(SHML)
MS1+, macrophage markers +, S-100−, CD1a−, no Birbeck granules	
Xanthoma disseminatum	(XD)
Diffuse normolipemic plane xanthoma	(DNLX)
Necrobiotic xanthogranuloma	(NXG)
Papular xanthoma	(PX)
Verruciform xanthoma	(VX)
Juvenile xanthogranuloma	(JXG)
Giant cell reticulohistiocytoma	(GCRH)
Multicentric reticulohistiocytosis	(MR)
Progressive nodular histiocytoma	(PNH)
Hereditary progressive mucinous histiocytosis	(HPMH)
Eruptive histiocytomas	(EH)
Benign cephalic histiocytosis	(BCH)

short, non–Langerhans cell histiocytosis (non-LCH); and class III, or malignant histiocytic disorders. We will employ a modification of this scheme, shown in Table 27-1, which uses primarily the presence or absence of S-100, CD1a, and Birbeck granules to subdivide the disorders. In addition, Table 27-2 offers an overview of the disorders using a variety of other markers. Reference 10 is an annotated synopsis of the literature.

The histiocyte may have a variety of morphologic characteristics, including vacuolated, xanthomatized, spindle-shaped, scalloped, and oncocytic cells.[11] These cells, along with their associated giant cells, produce a bewildering array of histologic patterns as shown in Table 27-3, some of which will be covered in the chapter and others of which are dispersed throughout the text. Included are the following:

1. Xanthomas. Phagocytic cells take up lipids or other clear material, producing foamy cellular accumulations. Xanthomas may be associated with systemic disorders or with trauma, or may be idiopathic.
2. Fibromas. Fibrous or spindle cell proliferations, such as seen in a dermatofibroma, may develop in many of the histiocytic disorders. Although trauma is the usual cause, some are also idiopathic.
3. Cellular infiltrates, which can be further subdivided based on the presence of zonality (i.e., a granuloma), giant cells, necrobiosis, and the presence of infectious agents or foreign-bodies. The giant cells themselves may be subdivided into foreign-body, Touton, ground glass, and nonspecific types.
4. Almost normal skin. A variety of metabolic diseases can be identified through skin biopsy in which abnormal storage products are identified at the electron microscopic level.

Finally, one can consider the baffling array of diseases that may be associated with the above-mentioned cells and patterns. They include the following:

1. Metabolic disorders, including hyperlipoproteinemias, other disorders of fat metabolism, and a diverse array of storage disorders. Typically papular or nodular xanthomas are produced. In previous editions of this text, diseases such as Tangier disease, Niemann-Pick disease, Gaucher disease, and Farber disease (lipogranulomatosis) were covered in detail. They typically present either with normal skin, pigmentary changes, or nodules in which the abnormal metabolic accumulations can be identified, usually by electron microscopy. The diagnosis of these disorders is not a practical question for the dermatopathologist, and they will not be further considered.
2. Infectious diseases. Tuberculosis, Hansen disease, other mycobacterial infections, and leishmaniasis may produce granulomas. Histoid Hansen disease in particular may mimic fibrohistiocytic processes.[12] In addition, the infection-associated hemophagocytic syndrome leads to cutaneous infiltrates displaying erythrophagocytosis. Malakoplakia is a chronic granu-

TABLE 27-2. *Antigenic markers in histiocytic disorders*

Disease	S-100	CD1a	Birbeck	MS-1	KP1	MAC 387	CD34	Factor XIIIa
LCH	+	+	+	−	−	−	−	−
CSHRH	+	+	+	−	−	−	−	−
ICH	+	+	−	−	−	−	−	−
SHML	+	−	−	−	−	−	−	+/−
XD	−	−	−	+	+	−	−	+
NXG	−	−	−	?	?	?	−	−
PX	−	−	−	+/−	+/−	+/−	−	−
VX	−	−	−	?	+	+	−	−
JXG	−	−	−	+	+	−	−	+/−
MR	−	−	−	+	+	−	−	−
GCRH	−	−	−	+	+	−	−	+/−
EH	−	−	−	+	+	−	+/−	−
BCH	−	−	−	?	?	?	?	?
DerDendr	−	−	−	−	−	−	?	+
DF/His	−	−	−	−	+/−	−	+	+
GA	−	−	−	−	+	+	−	−

+ = positive; − = negative; +/− = variable or conflicting data; ? = little or no data.

TABLE 27-3. *Patterns of histiocytic infiltrates*

Foamy
True xanthomas
Cholestanolemia, phytosterolemia
Verruciform xanthoma
Xanthoma disseminatum
Diffuse normolipemic plane xanthoma
Papular xanthoma
Eruptive normolipemic xanthoma
Progressive nodular histiocytoma (superficial lesions)
Langerhans' cell histiocytosis (very rarely)
Fibrous
Dermatofibroma/histiocytoma
Juvenile xanthogranuloma (spindle cell variant)
Progressive nodular histiocytoma (deep lesions)
Dermal dendrocytoma
Xanthoma disseminatum (disseminated xanthosiderohistiocytosis)
Hereditary progressive mucinous histiocytosis
Cellular
Dermatofibroma/histiocytoma
Langerhans' cell histiocytosis
Congenital self-healing reticulohistiocytosis
Indeterminate cell histiocytosis
Juvenile xanthogranuloma
Benign cephalic histiocytosis
Granuloma annulare
Eruptive histiocytomas
Progressive nodular histiocytoma (all lesions)
Sinus histiocytosis with massive lymphadenopathy
Giant Cell Predominance
Juvenile xanthogranuloma (most lesions)
Mutlicentric reticulohistiocytosis
Giant cell reticulohistiocytoma
Necrobiotic xanthogranuloma
Unusual Features
Necrobiosis
Granuloma annulare
Necrobiotic xanthogranuloma
Mucin
Hereditary progressive mucinous histiocytosis

lomatous histiocytic response, presumably to an infectious agent, that occurs occasionally in the skin. The key histologic finding is the presence of intracellular Michaelis-Gutmann bodies.

3. Tumors. Some lymphomas present with cutaneous granulomatous infiltrates; included in this group are Hodgkin disease and Lennert lymphoma. Most if not all of the diseases diagnosed in the past as histiocytic malignancies are lymphomas.[13] Malignant fibrous histiocytoma and its more superficial cutaneous variant, atypical fibroxanthoma, are established diagnoses, but the cell or cells of origin remain unclear.

4. Trauma. Most dermatofibromas and verruciform xanthomas are probably the result of trauma, be it an insect bite, folliculitis, or another insult. More diffuse types of plane and papular xanthoma have also been reported secondary to cutaneous damage from light or following marked inflammation.

5. Foreign bodies. External objects, such as glass fragments, silica, and many others, may produce cutaneous granulomas, often of the sarcoidal type. Patients with sarcoidosis not only have idiopathic granulomatous infiltrates, but are more likely to react to foreign bodies. A ruptured follicular cyst is also accompanied by a histiocytic response.

6. Idiopathic. Unfortunately, most diseases fit here, and there is little logic to what has been considered a histiocytic disorder and what has been cubbyholed elsewhere. For example, granuloma annulare consists of a cutaneous histiocytic infiltrate but is considered a necrobiotic disorder, along with many histologically similar lesions.[14] Granuloma faciale has surprisingly little granuloma formation but has retained its name. Both rheumatoid arthritis and sarcoidosis are characterized by histiocytic reaction patterns not only in the skin but also in other organs; nonetheless, they are not considered histiocytoses.

A number of systemic idiopathic histiocytic disorders will not be further considered because they rarely come to the attention of the dermatopathologist. Included in this list is a group where lymphocytic and histiocytic proliferations are intimately related, such as infection-associated hemophagocytic syndrome, familial hemophagocytic lymphohistiocytosis, malignant lymphoma, with reactive benign erythrophagocytosis, erythrophagocytic T-gamma lymphoma, and histiocytic necrotizing lymphadenitis (Kikuchi syndrome).[4,15,16] Other entities that could be placed here include the various syndromes with sea blue histiocytes and the X-linked lymphoproliferative syndrome (Purtilo syndrome).[6] Finally, two extremely rare syndromes, familial histiocytic dermatoarthritis[17] and dermatochondrocorneal dystrophy (Francois syndrome),[18] present with dermatofibroma- or histiocytoma-like cutaneous changes.

Even the question of benign versus malignant is clouded when considering the histiocytic disorders. In considering Langerhans cell histiocytosis, the clonality of the lesions and the occasional fatal outcome probably warrant a malignant diagnosis, although one must recognize the tendency to self-healing and the efficacy of relatively innocuous therapeutic regimens. When evaluating macrophage disorders, the distinctions are somewhat more clear. Most cutaneous processes are reactive, as are storage disorders, hemophagocytic syndromes, and sinus histiocytosis with massive lymphadenopathy. True malignant histiocytoses are rare but include malignant hemophagocytic histiocytosis, malignant histiocytosis with 5q35 gene rearrangement, the occasional but extremely rare true histiocytic lymphoma, and the well-established monocytic and myelomonocytic leukemias, which may have skin involvement.[13]

XANTHOMAS

Xanthomas are a cutaneous clue to the possible presence of hyperlipidemia, defined as an elevated fasting cholesterol level of over 240 mg/dL or a triglyceride level of over 200 mg/dL. Hyperlipidemia may be unexpectedly identified during routine evaluations or searched for because of a family history of lipid abnormalities, cardiovascular disease, or the presence of one of its many secondary causes. Once hyperlipidemia is identified, one must first exclude these secondary causes, which include diabetes mellitus, hypothyroidism, nephrotic syndrome, biliary disease, alcohol abuse, and a variety of medications, including estrogens, corticosteroids, and retinoids. In the 1960s Frederickson classified the primary hyperlipidemias on the basis of their electrophoretic lipoprotein phenotype. He considered not just cholesterol and triglycerides, but the basic packages in which they were transported throughout the body—chylomicrons, very-low-density lipoproteins (VLDL), low-density lipoproteins (LDL), and high-density lipoproteins (HDL)—to produce initially five and then six diagnostic categories. This classification has undergone major modifications because of advances in two areas:

1. The protein component of lipoproteins, known as apoproteins, has been extensively characterized and subdivided. The different apoproteins serve to bind lipids, regulate enzymes, and identify cell receptors. For example, a patient may have normal amounts of cholesterol but decreased levels of HDL, which is essential for the removal of intracellular cholesterol.
2. The specific genetic defect has been identified for a number of disorders, the best known of which is familial hypercholesterolemia, in which there is a defective LDL receptor.

Most patients with lipoprotein abnormalities do not have xanthomas, but the presence of xanthomas should alert the clinician to the need for an internal evaluation. The type of xanthoma is primarily a clinical diagnosis and correlates poorly with the exact lipid abnormality. With these limitations in mind, Table 27-4 gives a brief overview of the relationship between xanthomas and hyperlipidemias, as do references 19–21. One must also consider normocholesterolemic (or normolipemic) xanthomas.[22] Parker has divided this group into the following categories[23]:

Type IA: a lipoprotein containing another source of excess sterol (such as cholestanol in cerebrotendinous xanthomatosis or sitosterol in phytosterolemia).
Type IB: a lipoprotein containing abnormal apoprotein, which selectively binds cholesterol or triglyceride that is present nonetheless in normal amounts.
Type II: associated with lymphoproliferative disease (diffuse plane xanthomas).
Type III: no lipoprotein abnormality or associated lymphoproliferative disease; many are idiopathic and others posttraumatic. Typical examples include xanthoma disseminatum and papular xanthoma, although other non–Langerhans cell histiocytoses may also have a xanthomatized appearance.

Type II and Type III disorders are reviewed in greater detail later.

The xanthomas may be subdivided into eruptive xanthomas, tuberous xanthomas, tendon xanthomas, xanthelasmata, and plane xanthomas. Eruptive xanthomas are almost always associated with chylomicronemia and are most commonly seen in secondary forms of hyperlipoproteinemia. Eruptive xanthomas consist of small, soft, yellow papules with a predilection for the buttocks and the posterior aspects of the thighs. They come and go with fluctuations in the chylomicron level in the plasma. The lipid in these lesions is primarily triglycerides.

Tuberous and tuberoeruptive xanthomas are found predominantly in cases with an increase in chylomicron and VLDL remnants. They are large nodes or plaques located most commonly on the elbows, knees, fingers, and buttocks. Most of the lipid in these xanthomas is in the form of cholesterol.

Tendon xanthomas occur in patients with excessive plasma LDL levels as well as in phytosterolemia and cholestanolemia (cerebrotendinous xanthomatosis). The Achilles tendons and the extensor tendons of the fingers are most frequently affected.

Xanthelasmata consist of slightly raised, yellow, soft plaques on the eyelids. Although xanthelasmata are the commonest of the cutaneous xanthomas, they are also the least specific because they occur frequently in persons with normal lipoprotein levels. It is estimated that about 50% of persons with xanthelasma have normal serum lipid levels.

Plane xanthomas typically develop in skin folds and especially in the palmar creases. Diffuse plane xanthomas are typically seen as multiple grouped papules and poorly defined yellowish plaques in normolipemic patients, often with paraproteinemia, lymphoma, or leukemia. On the other hand, intertriginous plane xanthomas suggest homozygous familial hypercholesterolemia, whereas palmar crease xanthomas are virtually specific for remnant removal disease. The palmar xanthomas associated with cholestasis (primary biliary cirrhosis

TABLE 27-4. *Types of xanthomas*

Type	Typical location	Histology	Associated diseases
Eruptive	Buttocks, limbs	Subtle; few foam cells; extracellular lipid may be present	Genetic: lipoprotein lipase deficiency, familial hypertriglyceridemia, familial combined hyperlipidemia, remnant removal disease Secondary: diabetes, alcohol, estrogen, retinoids
Tuberous	Pressure points (knees, elbows, buttocks)	Large deposits with clefts and fibrosis	Genetic: remnant removal disease Secondary: hypothyroidism
Tendinous	Achilles tendon, extensor tendons of hands, feet	Large deposits with clefts and fibrosis	Genetic: heterozygous familial hypercholesterolemia, familial defective apo B, cholestanolemia, phytosterolemia
Plane	Intertriginous areas, palmar creases	Numerous foam cells	Genetic: homozygous familial hypercholesterolemia (intertriginous), remnant removal disease (palmar crease) Secondary: cholestasis, myeloma (normolipemic)
Xanthelasma	Eyelids	Foam cells; usually adjacent skeletal muscle	Not specific

Source: Cruz PD Jr., East C, Bergstresser PR. Dermal, subcutaneous and tendon xanthomas: Diagnostic markers for specific lipoprotein disorders. J Am Acad Dermatol 1988;19:95–111.

and biliary atresia) are plaquelike and tend to extend past the creases. Eruptive plane xanthomas have also been described in normolipemic patients.

Histopathology. The histologic appearance of xanthomas of the skin and the tendons is characterized by foam cells, macrophages that have engulfed lipid droplets. There may be varying degrees of fibrosis, giant cells, and clefts, depending on the type and site of xanthoma sampled, but most are surprisingly similar (Fig. 27–1A and B). All xanthomas are characterized by a degree of fixation artifact. Formalin fixation and paraffin embedding remove lipids so that only their shadows are left behind. Histiocytes take up the lipid released into the tissue, developing a foamy or vacuolated cytoplasm, depending on the size of the deposit. However, the lipid droplets can be seen if frozen or formalin-fixed sections are stained with fat stains such as scarlet red or Sudan red. Most of the xanthoma cells are mononuclear, but giant cells, especially of the Touton type with a wreath of nuclei, may be found. Larger extracellular deposits of cholesterol and other sterols leave behind clefts (Fig. 27-2). In the past, much emphasis was placed on the refractile nature of xanthomatous deposits. Frozen or formalin-fixed frozen sections can be examined under polarized light. Cholesterol esters are doubly refractile, whereas other lipids are not. Thus tendon and tuberous xanthomas tend to be doubly refractile, whereas

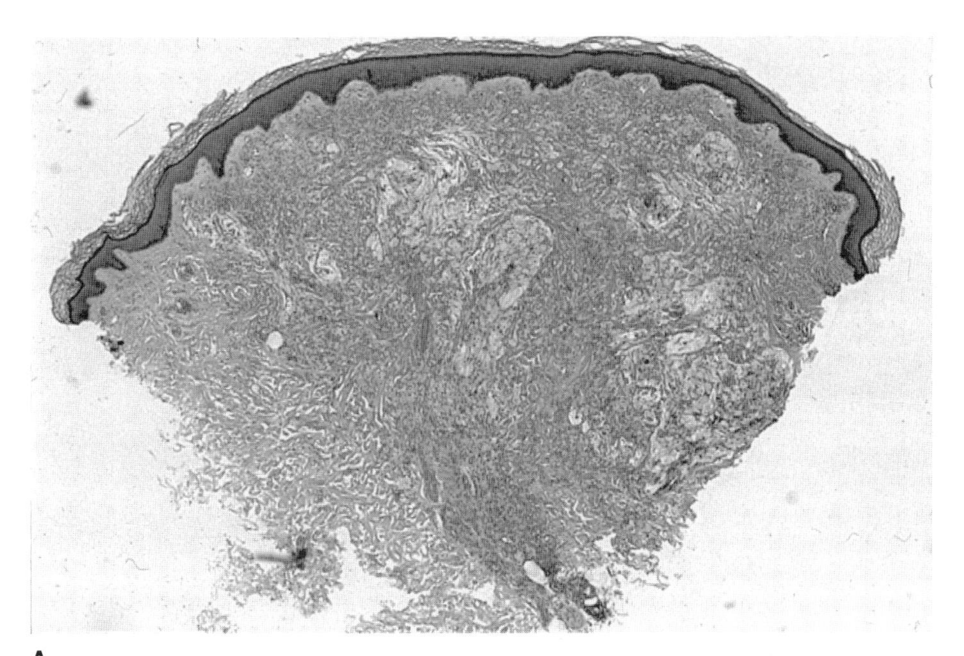

A

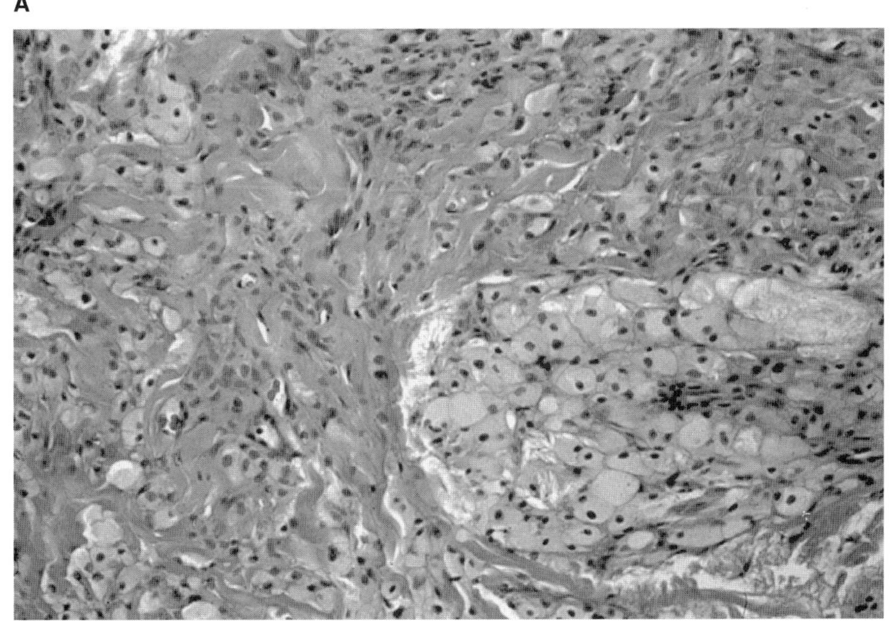

B

FIG. 27-1. Plane xanthoma
(**A**) Numerous foam cells are admixed with fibrotic areas. In the upper and middermis the infiltrate is cellular with few foam cells. (**B**) Same lesion as *A* at higher magnification, showing histiocytes, foam cells, both individually between strands of collagen and in a larger packet, and fibrosis.

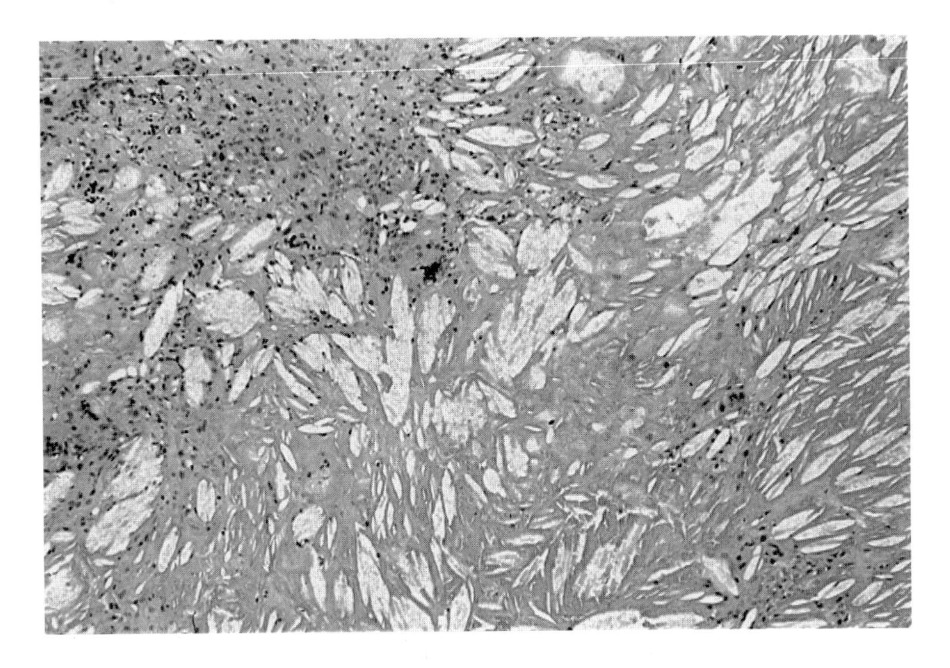

FIG. 27-2. Tuberous xanthoma Cholesterol clefts are most prominent, but there is also a collection of histiocytes in the upper left corner. Foam cells are not seen.

other xanthomas are not. Triglycerides are more rapidly metabolized than cholesterol. This may explain the more transient nature of eruptive xanthomas as compared to tuberous xanthomas. Similarly, the more chronic lesions are far more likely to show fibrosis.[20] Some differences exist in the histologic appearance of the various types of xanthoma.

Eruptive xanthomas, when of recent origin, often show a considerable admixture of nonfoamy cells, among them lymphoid cells, histiocytes, and neutrophils, whereas the number of well-developed foam cells may still be small. Because the rapid transport of lipid, especially triglycerides, into the tissue overwhelms the capacity of the histiocytes, free or extracellular lipid may be seen. These pools of lipid surrounded by histiocytes mimic granuloma annulare histologically.[24] Fully developed eruptive xanthomas are rich in foamy cells. Some may show uratelike crystals, causing confusion with gout.[25]

Tuberous xanthomas consist of large and small aggregates of xanthoma or foam cells. In early lesions, there usually is a slight admixture of nonfoamy cells, among them lymphoid cells, histiocytes, and neutrophils. In well-developed lesions, the infiltrate is composed almost entirely of foam cells. Ultimately, collagen bundles replace many of the foam cells. Cholesterol clefts may be found. Tendon xanthomas are identical to tuberous xanthomas in histologic appearance but may be even larger and are often submitted without their overlying skin.

Xanthelasmata located on the eyelids differ from tuberous xanthomas by the fairly superficial location of the foam cells and the nearly complete absence of fibrosis. Superficial striated muscles, vellus hairs, small vessels, and a thinned epidermis all suggest location on the eyelid and serve as clues to the histologic diagnosis of xanthelasma (Fig. 27-3).

Plane xanthomas should be suspected when the overlying

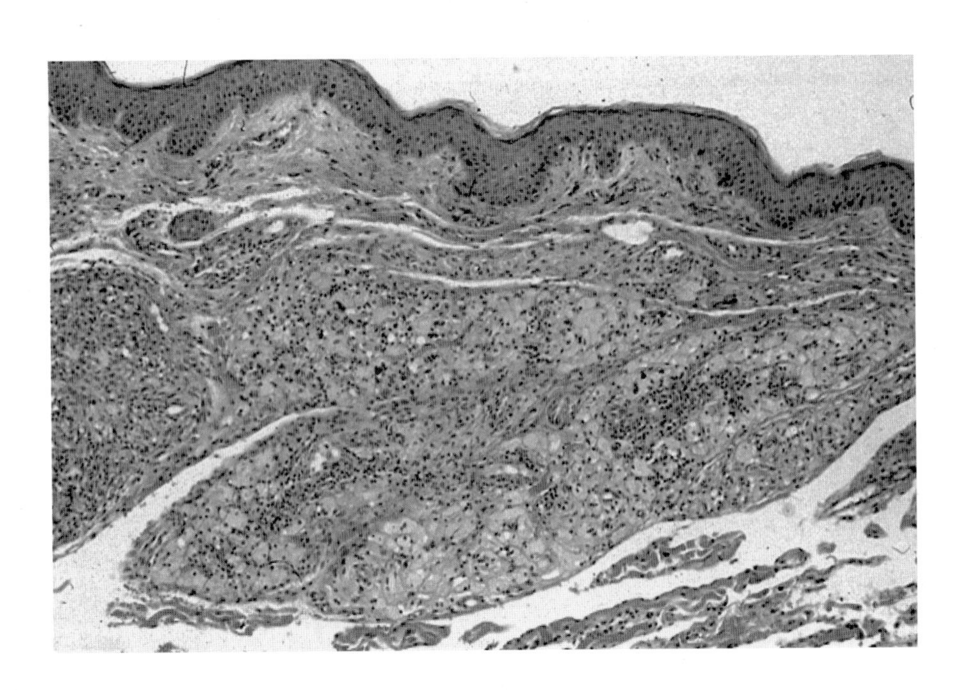

FIG. 27-3. Xanthelasma The thin epidermis and muscle fibers at base are a clue to the eyelid location. Lobules of foamy cells in this location allow the specific diagnosis of xanthelasma.

epidermis is thickened with hyperkeratosis and a stratum lucidum, indicating a palmar location. Plane xanthomas from other sites have no unique features.

Pathogenesis. Whereas the pathogenesis of many forms of hyperlipidemia is well understood, the formation of xanthomas remains unclear. Although only a small percentage of hyperlipidemic patients have xanthomas, there are few clues to who develops the lesions and why. Elevated levels of LDL and VLDL tend to predispose to xanthomas. These lipoproteins carry cholesterol. In high plasma concentrations, they permeate the walls of dermal capillaries and are phagocytosed by histiocytes producing foam cells. Parker has compared this process to the similar one of atheroma formation.[23] In addition, HDL is essential in the scavenging of tissue cholesterol, so low levels of this lipoprotein also contribute to xanthoma formation.

LANGERHANS CELL HISTIOCYTOSIS (HISTIOCYTOSIS X)

Langerhans cell histiocytosis (LCH) or histiocytosis X is characterized by a proliferation of dendritic or Langerhans histiocytes.[4,26] If LCH occurs during the first year of life, it is usually characterized by significant, potentially fatal visceral involvement and classified as acute disseminated LCH (Letterer-Siwe disease). If LCH develops during early childhood, the disease is manifested predominantly by osseous lesions with less extensive visceral involvement and known as chronic multifocal LCH or Hand-Schüller-Christian disease. In older children and adults, LCH is usually of the chronic focal type, often presenting one or few bone lesions known as eosinophilic granuloma. Cutaneous lesions are very commonly encountered in Letterer-Siwe disease and occur occasionally in the two other forms.

The clinical course and the prognosis of LCH are difficult to predict. The most important parameters are the age of the patient, the number of organs involved, and the degree of organ dysfunction. Abnormalities of the bone marrow, liver, or lungs suggest a poor prognosis. Skin and bone involvement are usually good signs; in some studies, the absence of bone involvement has been a poor sign.[26] Paradoxically, the presence of skin disease at birth is a good sign (see congenital self-healing reticulohistiocytosis), but involvement before the age of 2, a bad one. Histology is in general a poor way to stage LCH.[27] Patients with disseminated LCH seem to be at risk for a variety of systemic tumors, including lymphomas, leukemias, and lung tumors.[28] In general, about 10% of patients with multifocal disease die, 30% undergo complete remission, and the remaining 60% embark upon a chronic, shifting course.[26]

Acute disseminated LCH usually occurs in infants. Rarely, it is seen in older children or adults. The prognosis generally is serious, particularly if the disease is extensive. The most common manifestations are fever, anemia, thrombocytopenia, enlargement of the liver and spleen, lymphadenopathy, and pulmonary infiltrates. Osteolytic lesions are uncommon except in the mastoid region of the temporal bone, resulting in a clinical picture of otitis media. In about 80% of the cases, cutaneous lesions are present. They often are the first sign of the disease and are therefore of considerable diagnostic importance.

The cutaneous lesions usually consist of petechiae and papules. In some cases, one observes numerous closely set, brownish papules covered with scales or crusts. This type of eruption may be extensive, involving particularly the scalp, face, and trunk. The resemblance of this eruption to seborrheic dermatitis or Darier disease often is striking. In rare instances, a widespread cutaneous eruption is the only clinical manifestation in infants and even in the elderly.[29] The prognosis in such cases is good. Other adults may have similar cutaneous findings but multisystem disease and do poorly.[30]

In chronic multifocal LCH, diabetes insipidus, exophthalmos, and multiple defects of the bones, especially of the cranium, represent the classic triad of Hand-Schüller-Christian disease. However, any one or even all three of the cardinal symptoms may be absent, and involvement may occur in entirely different organs. For example, enlargement of the liver, spleen, or lymph nodes may be found. Pulmonary involvement is common but often resolves or stabilizes. Osteolytic lesions of the long bones may result in a spontaneous fracture.

Cutaneous lesions occur in about one third of the cases. Three types of skin lesions may occur. Most common are infiltrated nodules and plaques undergoing ulceration, especially in the axillae, the anogenital region, and the mouth.[31] Next in frequency is an extensive eruption of coalescing, scaling, or crusted papules. Finally, in rare instances only, one observes scattered, soft, yellow, papular xanthomas. The xanthomatous form of LCH is most uncommon in the skin but is seen more often in other organs.[32] A complicating issue is that patients with LCH tend to develop more juvenile xanthogranulomas than expected.[26]

Chronic focal or multifocal LCH or eosinophilic granuloma represents the third and least severe disease in this group. The lesions are either solitary or few. Most common are lesions of the bones, but the skin or the oral mucosa is occasionally involved, either with or without osseous lesions. Involvement of the jaw leading to a loose or floating tooth is a fairly typical occurrence. Eosinophilic ulcer of the oral mucosa has a similar name but is not otherwise related; it usually involves the tongue, is often triggered by trauma, resolves spontaneously, and does not contain LC. Although the disease is chronic, there is a tendency toward spontaneous healing, and simple surgery is generally curative. In rare instances, however, cases originally diagnosed as chronic focal disease may progress into multifocal or even disseminated disease.

The biggest problem in classifying LCH involves cases limited to the skin. Congenital self-healing reticulohistiocytosis (CSHRH) is a form of LCH generally present at birth or in the first few weeks of life that typically resolves spontaneously. However, acute disseminated LCH may also be present at birth but is rarely nodular.[33] If there is a diffuse cutaneous eruption, one must anticipate multiorgan involvement; one or several nodules suggest CSHRH. Another unusual clinical picture is that of infantile LCH,[34] in which patients under the age of 14 have a limited number of papules or nodules without systemic involvement. They, too, do well. Finally, cutaneous LCH is very pleomorphic; lesions may be vesicular,[35] ulcerated,[36] or urticarial.[37] Not surprisingly, small papular lesions may resemble granuloma annulare, both clinically and histological. Nail bed involvement is not uncommon.[38]

A final question is that of malignant LCH (malignant histiocytosis X; not to be confused with malignant histiocytosis). There are rare cases of a solitary tumor[39,40] or a lymphomalike picture[13] featuring cytologically atypical dendritic histiocytes, in which cases the diagnosis seems entirely appropriate. However, when the skin is diffusely involved, the problem becomes cloudy. Acute disseminated LCH can reasonably be argued to be a malignancy because it is progressive, destructive, potentially fatal, and shows clonality. Some cases have been identified with marked cytological atypia, including mitoses, and a poor clinical outcome.[41,42] Unfortunately, most often the diagnosis has been made retrospectively. It is unclear if malignant LCH is simply a "bad case" of LCH or if it represents a different biologic process.

Other dendritic cells may also produce tumors; those associated with indeterminate cells are considered later. Follicular dendritic cell sarcoma has been described as a spindle cell proliferation found in enlarged cervical or axillary lymph nodes, rarely showing a fatal course. Tumors of interdigitating dendritic cells have also been described, but with a less uniform clinical pattern.[4]

Histopathology. The histologic picture unites the many varied forms of LCH. The key to diagnosis is identifying the typical LCH or histiocytosis X cell in the appropriate surroundings. The cell has a distinct folded or lobulated, often kidney-shaped nucleus. Nucleoli are not prominent, and the slightly eosinophilic cytoplasm is unremarkable. Since this cell's appearance on light microscopy is not unique, other methods must be employed to identify it. For years the gold standard has been electron microscopy to find the typical Birbeck or Langerhans cell granules. Today additional techniques are available. Using paraffin-fixed tissue, either the S-100 antigen or the peanut agglutinin (PNA) can be sought. The LCH cell has a typical halo and/or dot pattern with the latter. Although CD1a was previously only applicable to frozen sections, it can now be applied to formalin-fixed, paraffin-embedded specimens. The degree of certainty with which the infiltrative histiocyte is identified determines the type of diagnosis. According to the Histiocyte Society, a typical clinical and light microscopic picture leads to a presumptive diagnosis; confirmation by typical S-100 or PNA staining produces a diagnosis; a definite diagnosis requires either a positive CD1a stain or electron microscopic demonstration of Birbeck granules.[9]

Although three kinds of histologic reactions have been described in LCH histiocytosis—proliferative, granulomatous, and xanthomatous—only the first two are commonly seen. A relationship exists between the type of histologic reaction and the clinical type of disease. In general, the proliferative reaction with its almost purely histiocytic infiltrate is typical of acute disseminated LCH and the granulomatous reaction of chronic focal or multifocal LCH, as the name *eosinophilic granuloma* suggests. The xanthomatous reaction is seen in Hand-Schüller-Christian disease but also in other organs, especially the meninges and bones. Xanthomatous lesions in the skin are decidedly rare. The histologic reaction present in the skin depends on the type of skin lesion. Because more than one type of skin lesion is occasionally present, different types of histologic reactions may be found in the same patient.

The proliferative reaction is encountered in the skin in petechiae, in both hemorrhagic and nonhemorrhagic papules, and in scaling and crusting eruptions. It is characterized by the presence of an extensive infiltrate of histiocytes. The infiltrate usually lies close to or involves the epidermis, resulting in ulceration and crusting (Fig. 27-4A and B). Inflammatory cells are also present, most often lymphocytes but also eosinophils (see Fig. 27-4C). Extravasated erythrocytes may also be present. In this stage, cytology is quite distinctive,[43] and a touch preparation from an ulcerated or weeping lesion, stained with a hematologic stain, can often provide a rapid diagnosis.

The granulomatous reaction is found most commonly in infiltrated plaques and nodules in the genital area, in the axillary region, or on the scalp, as well as in the soft tissue and bone lesions. Histologically, it shows extensive aggregates of histiocytes often extending deep into the dermis. Eosinophils are present in various quantities (see Fig. 27-4D). Generally, they lie in clusters instead of being diffusely scattered, and may develop into microabscesses. Irregularly shaped, multinucleated giant cells are occasionally seen. In addition, some neutrophils, lymphoid cells, and plasma cells may be present. Frequently, extravasation of erythrocytes is found. True foam cells are usually absent; occasionally, however, some of the histiocytes possess a vacuolated cytoplasm.

Histologically, the uncommon xanthomatous reaction reveals in the dermis numerous foam cells, as well as varying numbers of histiocytes and some eosinophils. Multinucleated giant cells are frequently present. They are mainly of the foreign-body type but occasionally have the appearance of Touton giant cells.

In malignant LCH (malignant histiocytosis X), by definition there is frank cytological atypia with larger pleomorphic histiocytes, with atypia and mitoses.[41,42] It must be reemphasized that cellular morphology is a poor way to predict the course of LCH, except in the case of nodular frankly anaplastic tumors or lymphomas, both of which are rare.

Visceral Lesions. The visceral lesions seen in histiocytosis X show the same three types of reactions just described for the skin. The organs most commonly affected are the spleen, liver, lungs, lymph nodes, and bones. In Hand-Schüller-Christian disease, the diabetes insipidus is caused by granulomatous infiltration of the posterior pituitary gland, the tuber cinereum, or the hypothalamus; the exophthalmos, by retroorbital accumulations of granulomatous tissue; and the multiple defects in the skull, by the osteolytic effect of granulomatous infiltrates.

Pathogenesis. A unique feature of LCH is its relationship to the normal Langerhans cell. Although the key cell of LCH, the old histiocyte X, is very similar to a normal Langerhans cell, there are subtle differences.[44] Birbeck granules are convincing proof of the relationship, but they are present in varying amounts in LCH. Particularly when dealing with a sparsely infiltrated dermatitic picture, the search can be frustrating. In larger infiltrates, one can usually readily find the characteristic organelles.

In addition to the S-100, PNA, and CD1a stains, which are part of the diagnostic approach to LCH, many other special stains have been employed. Of particular interest is the PCNA,[45] which may have prognostic value. Other indicators of proliferation may also be positive, suggesting that LCH cells have an aberrant phenotype and are not under ordinary growth control.

A series of studies have shown that LCH is most often a clonal proliferation. Different groups have studied female patients with the disease and used a variety of x-linked polymorphisms to demonstrate clonality.[46,47] Despite the clonality studies, most clinicians view LCH as primarily a reactive process because of its tendency toward spontaneous remissions and its relatively good response to mild, relatively nontoxic therapeutic regimens.

Differential Diagnosis. The differential diagnosis for LCH varies with the histologic pattern. The most difficult situation is an early proliferative dermatitic lesion with little epidermotropism and few characteristic cells. Without adequate clinical background, it is easy to make the mistaken diagnosis of superficial perivascular dermatitis. One should keep LCH in mind in all biopsies of dermatitis from infants and freely employ the S-100 stain. When a nodule or tumor is present, the presence of eosinophils and the sheets of characteristic cells usually allow a confident diagnosis. The cutaneous xanthomas are identical to juvenile xanthogranuloma or xanthoma disseminatum, but neither of these disorders should be rich in S-100–positive cells, and the clinical setting should be different.

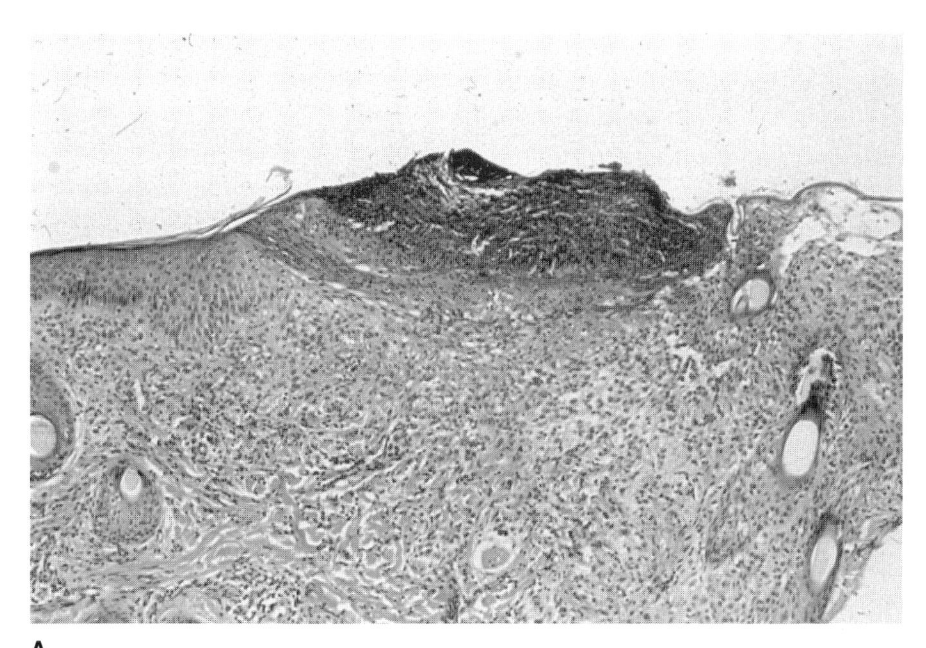

A

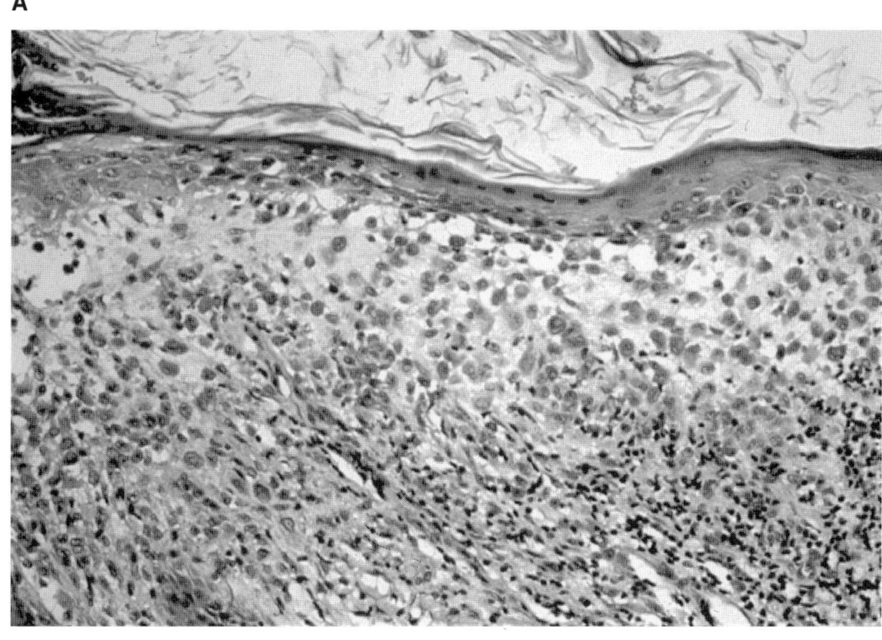

B

FIG. 27-4. Langerhans cell histiocytosis
(**A**) Crusted papular lesion in a young infant. A dense cellular infiltrate is seen beneath the crust. (**B**) Another lesion from the same patient as *A*. Here the large kidney-shaped histiocytes are dispersed along the epidermal-dermal junction. (*continued on next page*)

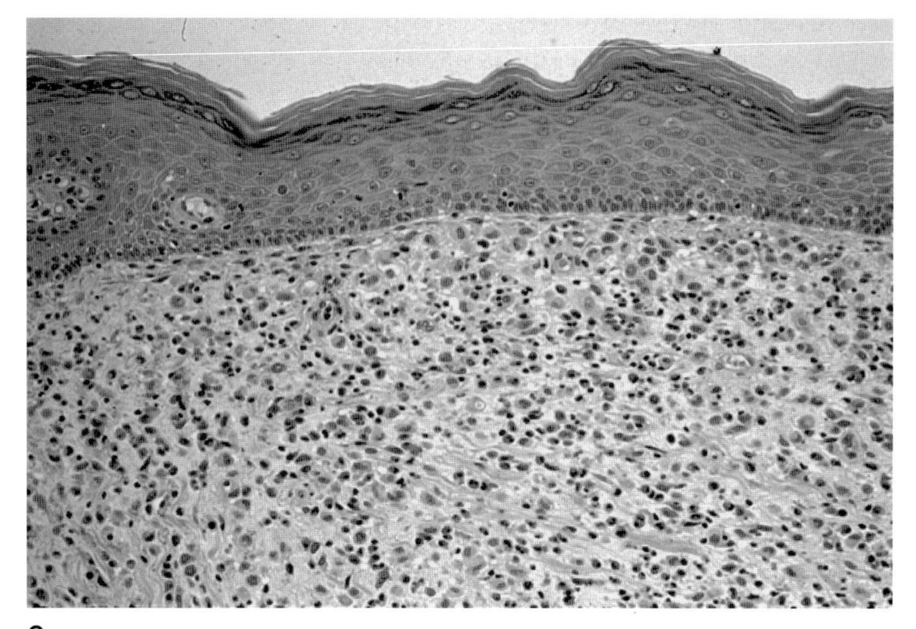

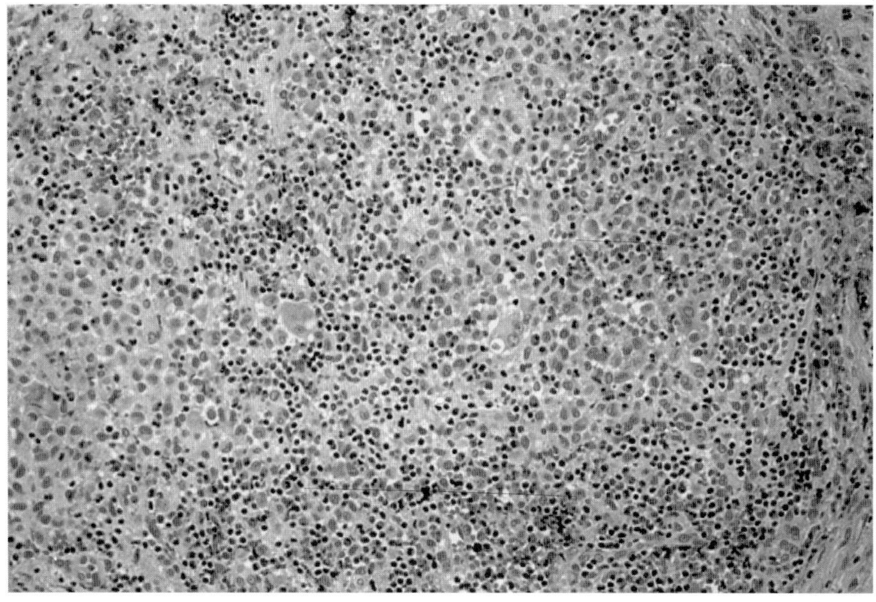

D

FIG. 27-4. *Continued*
(**C**) An infiltrate of histiocytes admixed with numerous eosinophils. There is no epidermal destruction. (**D**) A deep nodular cutaneous infiltrate rich in eosinophils with clusters of typical large histiocytes.

CONGENITAL SELF-HEALING RETICULOHISTIOCYTOSIS

Congenital self-healing reticulohistiocytosis (CSHRH) was first described in 1973 by Hashimoto and Pritzker.[48] It usually is present at birth but may not appear until several days or weeks after delivery. Affected infants have scattered papules and nodules. Large nodules tend to break down in the center and form crater-shaped ulcers. Usually, the number of lesions varies from several to a dozen; on rare occasions, numerous lesions are widely scattered over the entire skin. In about 25% of cases, a solitary nodule is present at birth.[49] The lesions begin to involute within 2 to 3 months and have completely regressed within 12 months. But the patients should be carefully followed; relapses may occur, including bone involvement, and the occasional case may behave as LCH, requiring a "new" diagnosis.[50]

In some classification schemes, Hashimoto-Pritzker disease has been limited to patients with multiple papules and nodules. Other variants are then the solitary nodule and the lesions that are not present at birth but appear soon thereafter (Illig-Fanconi syndrome).[51]

Histopathology. The lesions show densely aggregated histiocytes with abundant eosinophilic cytoplasm (Fig. 27-5). Some of the histiocytes are large and form giant cells, with diameters up to 50 μm. In some cells, the cytoplasm has a "ground glass" appearance. There is also an admixture of lymphocytes, neu-

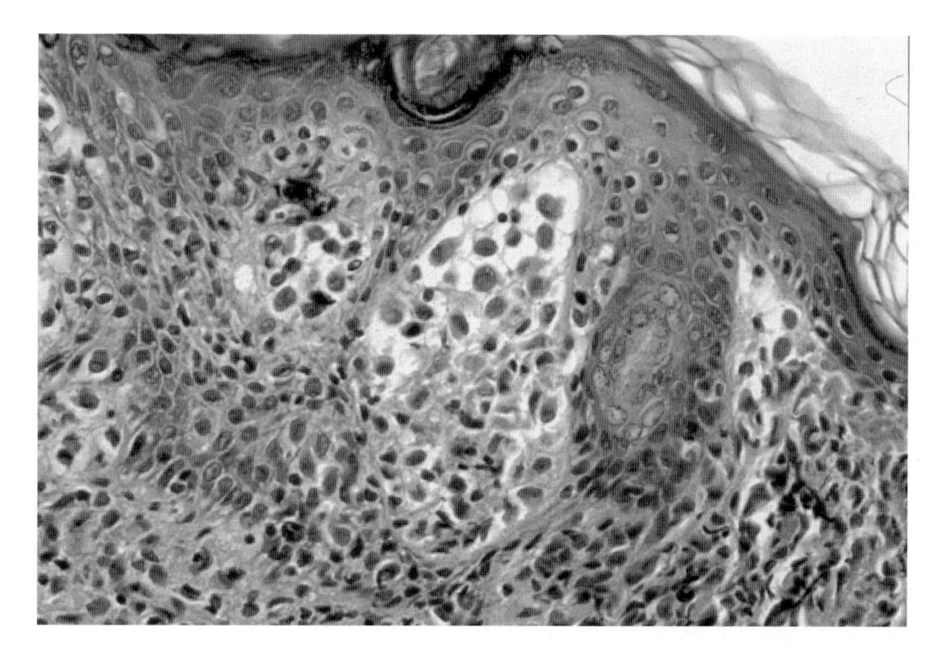

FIG. 27-5. Congenital self-healing reticulohistiocytosis
The central dermal papilla is filled by "reticulohistiocytes," large cells with eosinophilic cytoplasm. Although this same picture is also seen in Langerhans' cell histiocytosis, the lack of epidermal damage supports the diagnosis of congenital self-healing histiocytosis. The lesion was congenital and regressed promptly.

trophils, and eosinophils. Moderate numbers of foam cells may be found. The histiocytes may rarely invade and damage the epidermis.[52] In many cells, portions of the cytoplasm are periodic acid–Schiff (PAS)–positive and diastase-resistant.[48,53] The histologic picture may somewhat resemble giant cell reticulohistiocytosis, but giant cells are less common and mitoses more common.[54,55]

The term *reticulohistiocyte* has caused some confusion. Hashimoto and Pritzker originally used it as a histiocyte with abundant ground glass cytoplasm, occasionally in the form of a giant cell.[48] They chose the term in part at least because of the large size of the cells, which reminded them of the cells of reticulum cell sarcoma (an old name for large-cell or anaplastic lymphoma). However, reticulohistiocytes are benign. Others have confused the issue by suggesting that reticulohistiocytes are connected either with the fibrosis or increased "reticulin" seen in many histiocytic proliferations or with blood reticulocytes, which have a stippled or reticular basophilic cytoplasm. The latter two explanations both sound attractive but are incorrect. The reticulohistiocyte is simply one morphologic pattern for a histiocyte; it can develop from both Langerhans cell histiocytes and macrophages. The latter cells have also been designated oncocytic macrophages.[56]

There are many similarities between CSHRH and LCH. Immunohistochemical stains give the same pattern of positivity for S-100, CD1a, and PNA. Although there are qualitative ultrastructural differences reported, such as fewer Birbeck granules and the presence of laminated dense bodies, the bottom line is that CSHRH cannot be distinguished with certainty from LCH by histologic criteria alone.[54,55,57]

Pathogenesis. The laminated dense bodies probably represent degenerating histiocytes and thus are an ultrastructural clue to the self-healing process. Otherwise CSHRH can be viewed as a variant of LCH with the immune system ruling sovereign over the aberrant histiocytes, leading to a spontaneous cure in almost all cases. Cases of CSHRH that progress or do not regress should logically be viewed as chronic focal or multifocal LCH limited to skin, which also has an excellent prognosis.

Differential Diagnosis. If there are sheets of histiocytes with abundant cytoplasm, one can suggest the diagnosis of CSHRH, especially in the appropriate clinical setting. For nodular lesions the only histologic differential diagnostic is LCH. The papules may be somewhat less distinctive. A biopsy is needed in newborns with ulcerated nodules to exclude a congenital leukemia or extramedullary hematopoesis with sepsis (blueberry muffin syndrome). Some cases may behave similarly but on histologic examination have no Langerhans cell markers[58]; their etiology is unclear.

INDETERMINATE CELL HISTIOCYTOSIS

In the past decade a few cases have been described in which electron microscopy reveals no Birbeck granules but in which many cells are positive for S-100 and CD1a and thus can be regarded as indeterminate cells. The diagnosis of indeterminate cell histiocytosis (ICH) was first proposed by Wood and colleagues[59] in 1985 when they reassessed a previously reported case.[60]

Clinically, such cases show no characteristic features; patients may have numerous papules or nodules that may coalesce.[61,62] One patient has been described with a single congenital regressing nodule, identical in appearance to CSHRH.[63] No systemic lesions have been found. Solitary tumors have also been identified with overlap features.[64] The disorder is too rare to allow generalizations about the clinical course.

Histopathology. Either a monomorphous infiltrate of histiocytes or histiocytes intermingled with some giant cells and foam cells are found.

Pathogenesis. Indeterminate cells are most likely a variant of normal Langerhans' cells. Most authors have extrapolated from the features of the indeterminate cell to define ICH. Zelger and colleagues have approached the problem slightly differently,[65] defining ICH as an overlap between LCH and non-LCH, in which the cells are S-100 + but also have macrophage markers. Since there are overlaps between normal LC and macrophages, this too is a reasonable definition.

SINUS HISTIOCYTOSIS WITH MASSIVE LYMPHADENOPATHY

Sinus histiocytosis with massive lymphadenopathy (SHML) was first described by Rosai and Dorfman in 1969.[66] Massive cervical lymphadenopathy, usually bilateral and painless, is the most common manifestation. SHML is generally a benign disorder in spite of its propensity to form large masses and to disseminate to both nodal and extranodal sites. In most patients the disease resolves spontaneously, others have persistent problems, and very few die.[67,68] Skin is the most common extranodal

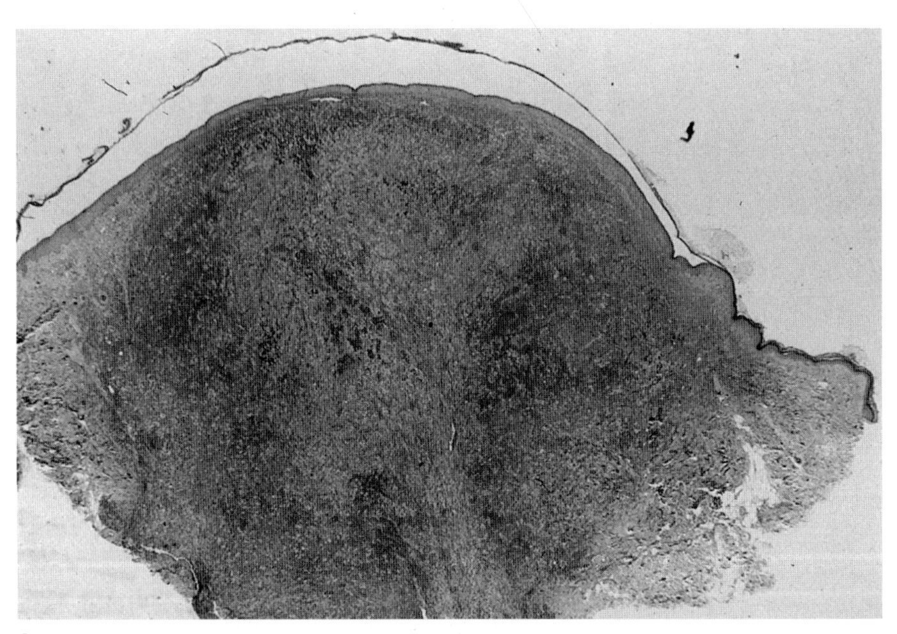

A

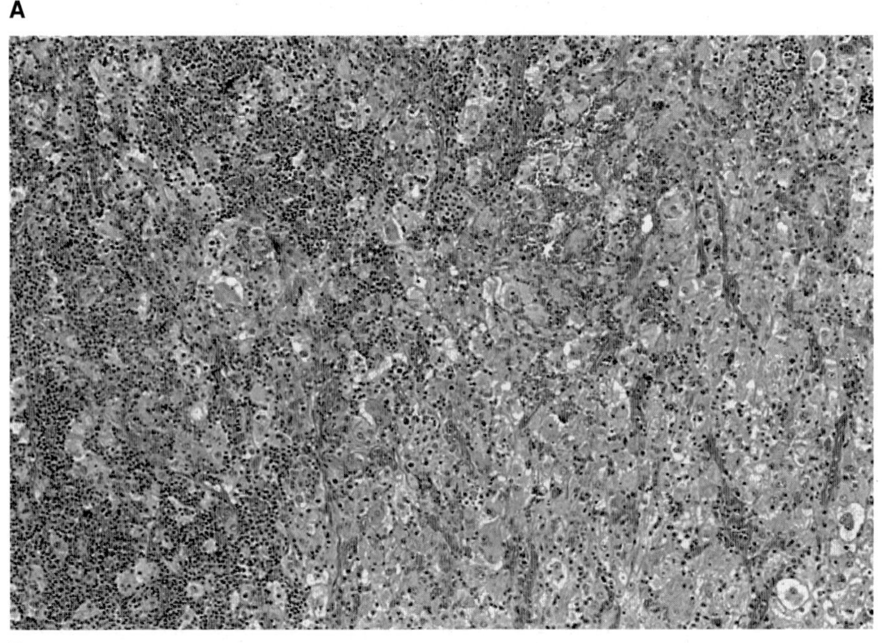

B

FIG. 27-6. Sinus histiocytosis with massive lymphadenopathy (**A**) Nodular infiltrate rich in pale-staining cells centrally. (**B**) Typical pattern of strands of pale sinus histiocytes admixed with darker-staining lymphocytes.

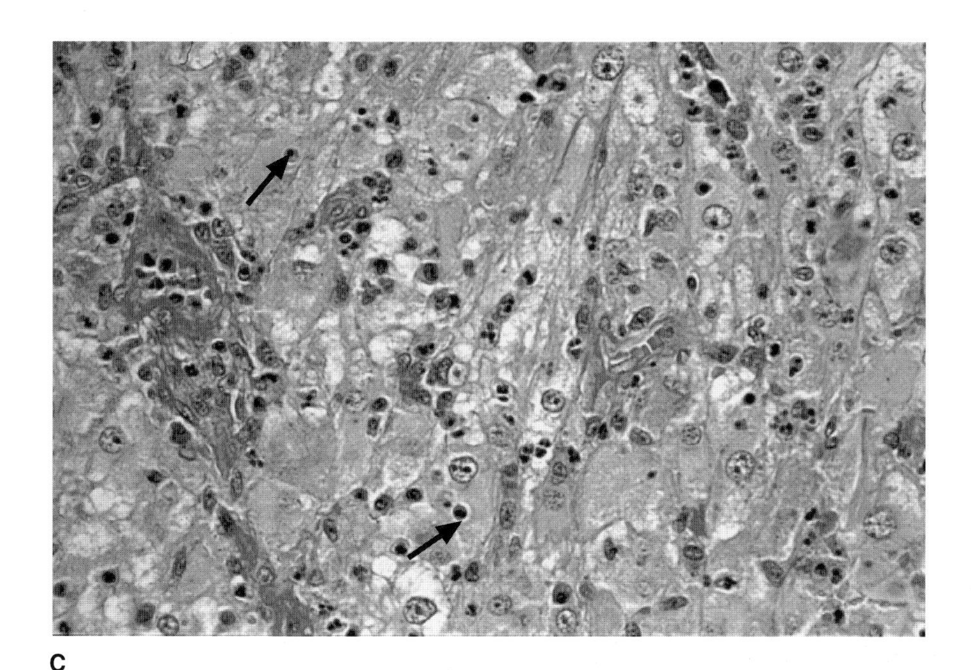

C

FIG. 27-6. ***Continued***
(C) Numerous large histiocytes, several of which have ingested lymphocytes, demonstrating emperipolesis.

site, with over 10% of patients having cutaneous involvement. The lesions are typically papules or nodules. A similar percentage have soft tissue involvement, usually of the subcutaneous tissue.[68–70] Occasionally the soft tissue lesion may present as a breast mass[71] or panniculitis.[72]

Histopathology. The skin lesions contain a polymorphous infiltrate in which histiocytes with abundant cytoplasm are the most prominent element (Fig. 27-6A). Occasionally they may be multi-nucleated or have a foamy cytoplasm (see Fig. 27-6B). However, the hallmark histologic feature is emperipolesis of lymphocytes (see Fig. 27-6C).[68] Emperipolesis differs slightly from phagocytosis in that the lymphocytes are taken up but not attacked by enzymes, leading to particle ingestion. Thus they appear intact. On occasion, red cells can also be taken up.[69,73]

In the lymph nodes, the sinuses are greatly dilated and crowded with inflammatory cells, particularly histiocytes. Here they tend to have an abundant foamy cytoplasm and also display emperipolesis.

Pathogenesis. The histiocytes are S-100-positive but CD1a-negative, and do not contain Birbeck granules. About 50% are CD30-positive.[74] Factor XIIIa–positive cells have also been identified,[75] but in most cases they are in the minority and seem to be innocent bystanders and not part of the active proliferation.[68]

XANTHOMA DISSEMINATUM

In the rare condition of xanthoma disseminatum (XD), numerous widely disseminated but often closely set and even coalescing, round to oval, orange or yellow-brown papules and nodules are found mainly on the flexor surfaces, such as the neck, axillae, antecubital fossae, groin, and perianal region.[76] Often there are lesions around the eyes. The mucous membranes are affected in 40% to 60% of cases. In addition to oral lesions, there may be pharyngeal and laryngeal involvement.[77] Three patterns have been identified[78]; the most typical is the persistent form; rarely lesions may regress spontaneously and even more infrequently in the progressive form there may systemic involvement. About 60% of cases begin between the ages of 5 and 25.

Diabetes insipidus is encountered in about 40% of cases but usually is mild and transitory, in contrast to that seen with LCH. It results from the infiltration of the hypothalamic-pituitary axis by xanthomatous cells. Characteristically, internal lesions other than diabetes insipidus are absent. In a few instances multiple osteolytic lesions have been found, especially in the long bones, as well as lung and CNS infiltrates.[79] In one case there was an association with Waldenström's macroglobulinemia.[80]

A possible variant of XD, disseminated xanthosiderohistiocytosis, has been described in patients with hematologic malignancies.[81] This disorder may also be related to disseminated dermal dendrocytomas,[82] since the clinical photographs from the two most recent cases[81,82] are almost interchangeable, with multiple papules and nodules on the chest and highly distinctive keloidal lesions on the extremities. The lesions are not truly xanthomatous but instead fibrohistiocytic, staining positively with factor XIIIa, and may represent a variation on the theme of multiple dermatofibromas in immunosuppressed patients. These unique patients also resemble the spindle cell variant of juvenile xanthogranuloma and its disseminated form, progressive nodular histiocytomas.

Histopathology. In early lesions, scalloped histiocytes dominate the histologic picture.[11] This histiocytic precursor has been used by the Mayo group to characterize XD; papular xanthoma and diffuse plane xanthoma rarely show histiocytes. Even when a bandlike pattern is present, epidermal involvement does not occur.[78] More developed lesions may still be primarily histiocytic, but xanthomatization occurs in most cases. These mature forms show a histologic picture that is regarded as typical for XD, namely, a mixture of histiocytes, xanthoma cells, inflammatory cells, and numerous Touton and foreign-body giant cells. Occasionally, however, only few Touton giant cells are present. Some lesions consist almost exclusively of foam cells.[76]

Pathogenesis. In the past, some authors have assumed a relationship between XD and LCH. Although in both conditions xanthomatous lesions and diabetes insipidus may occur, XD occurs in older patients, often has mucosal involvement, and only rarely involves bone. In addition, the pituitary involvement is different. Finally xanthomatous lesions are expected in XD and rare in LCH.

Immunohistochemistry also supports this clinical view, since the histiocytes in XD fail to stain with S-100 and CD1a, and Birbeck granules are not present. Some cells are positive for KP1, especially the foamy and giant cells, whereas others show factor XIIIa positivity, suggesting a relationship to dermal dendrocytes.[83]

DIFFUSE NORMOLIPEMIC PLANE XANTHOMA

In diffuse normolipemic plane xanthoma (DNPX), another rare disorder, one observes papules, patches, or, most commonly, even larger diffuse areas of orange-yellow discoloration of the skin. Whereas the smaller lesions are distinct, the diffuse areas have a poorly defined border. The face, particularly the periorbital areas, and the upper trunk are sites of predilection. The disorder may mimic xanthelasma initially but progresses to involve wide areas of skin. The lesions usually persist indefinitely. By definition, the patient has no lipid abnormalities.[84,85]

Most cases of diffuse normolipemic plane xanthoma are associated with hematologic disorders, most commonly paraproteinemias, including multiple myeloma, benign monoclonal gammopathy (often IgA), Castleman's disease,[86] and cryoglobulinemia. In other instances, diffuse normolipemic plane xanthoma has developed in areas of chronic inflammation, such as atopic dermatitis or persistent light eruption. In Parker's classification, the diagnosis of DNPX is restricted to lesions associated with hematologic malignancies, and the other clinically similar lesions are classified as idiopathic.[23] This diagnosis should be rendered cautiously because the skin disorder may precede the hematologic problem by many years.

There is clinical overlap with papular xanthoma, since generalized papular xanthomas have also been reported with many of the conditions associated with diffuse normolipemic plane xanthomas. There are also cases that begin as papular xanthomas, but the lesions evolve and coalesce into diffuse plane xanthomas.[87] In addition, DNPX has many features in common with necrobiotic xanthogranuloma,[88] including the presence of large patches and plaques, periorbital involvement, association with paraproteinemias, and a similar histology. In one case the disease evolved from DNPX into necrobiotic xanthogranuloma.[89]

Histopathology. Histologic examination reveals large sheets and clusters of foam cells, as well as foam cells singly and in small groups, diffusely scattered throughout the dermis. In some areas, the foam cells lie in thin streaks between collagen bundles, and occasionally a perivascular arrangement is noted. There may be an admixture of histiocytes and lymphoid cells; rarely, Touton giant cells are seen. Scattered foam cells have been observed even in clinically normal skin.

Pathogenesis. The mechanism of xanthoma formation is unclear. Possible explanations include the secretion of cytokines or immunoglobulins by the underlying lymphocytic proliferation, which in turn could stimulate macrophages or alter lipoprotein activity. This theory fails to explain why the skin involvement so often occurs first. The immunohistochemical phenotyping of the histiocytic cells has yielded variable results.

Differential Diagnosis. A single lesion cannot be distinguished from other small xanthomas. If marked necrobiosis or giant cell formation is present, necrobiotic xanthogranuloma should be considered.

A

FIG. 27-7. Necrobiotic xanthogranuloma
(**A**) Low-power view showing a diffuse infiltrate with amorphous necrobiotic areas, cellular regions rich in giant cells, and a nodular lymphoid infiltrate (lower right). (**B**) Higher magnification of panel *A*, showing a cellular infiltrate with numerous giants, mostly of the Touton type, and marked pale necrobiotic regions. (**C**) Another view showing a prominent lymphoid follicle and focal necrobiosis.

NECROBIOTIC XANTHOGRANULOMA WITH PARAPROTEINEMIA

A rare disorder, necrobiotic xanthogranuloma with paraproteinemia (NXG) can usually be recognized histologically but may show clinical similarities to DNPX. Large, often yellow, indurated plaques are found with atrophy, telangiectasia, and occasionally also ulceration.[90] The most common location is periorbital[91]; in one review, 21 of 22 patients had skin findings in this area.[92] The thorax is also commonly involved.

Histopathology. Granulomatous masses are present either as focal aggregates or as large, intersecting bands occupying the dermis and subcutaneous tissue (Fig. 27-7A). The intervening tissue separating the granulomas shows extensive necrobiosis (see Fig. 27-7B). The granulomas contain histiocytes, foam cells, and often also an admixture of inflammatory cells, often arranged as lymphoid follicles (see Fig. 27-7C). A distinctive feature is the presence of numerous large giant cells, both of the Touton type with a peripheral rim of foamy cytoplasm and of the foreign-body type. Aggregates of cholesterol clefts are also common.[93,94]

Pathogenesis. In most patients, serum protein electrophoresis shows an IgG monoclonal gammopathy that usually consists of kappa light chains.[92] In several patients, bone marrow examination has revealed multiple myeloma.[90,95]

Differential Diagnosis. Other necrobiotic disorders, especially necrobiosis lipoidica diabeticorum and subcutaneous granuloma annulare or rheumatoid nodule, may be considered. In necrobiotic xanthogranuloma, the necrobiosis is far more extensive and often occurs in broad bands, associated

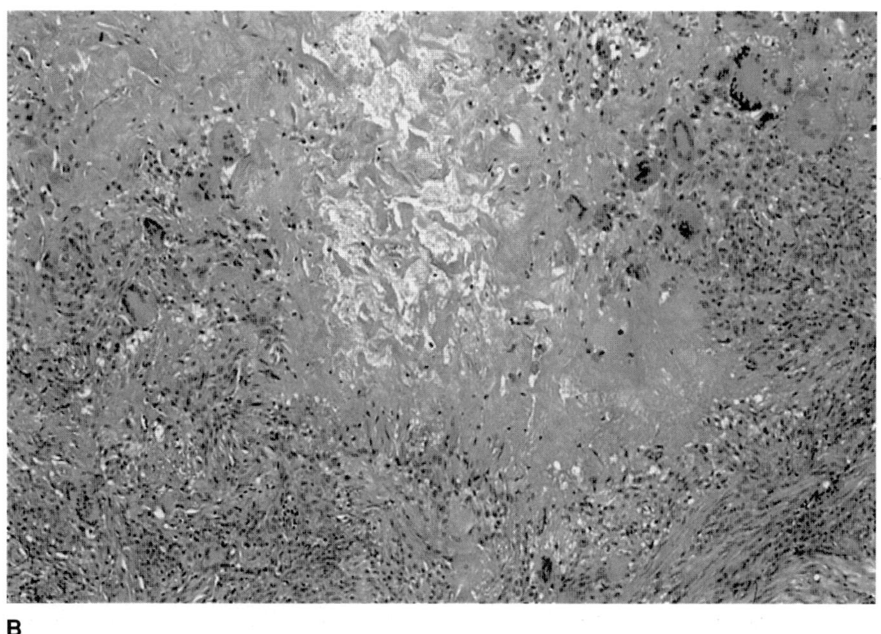

B

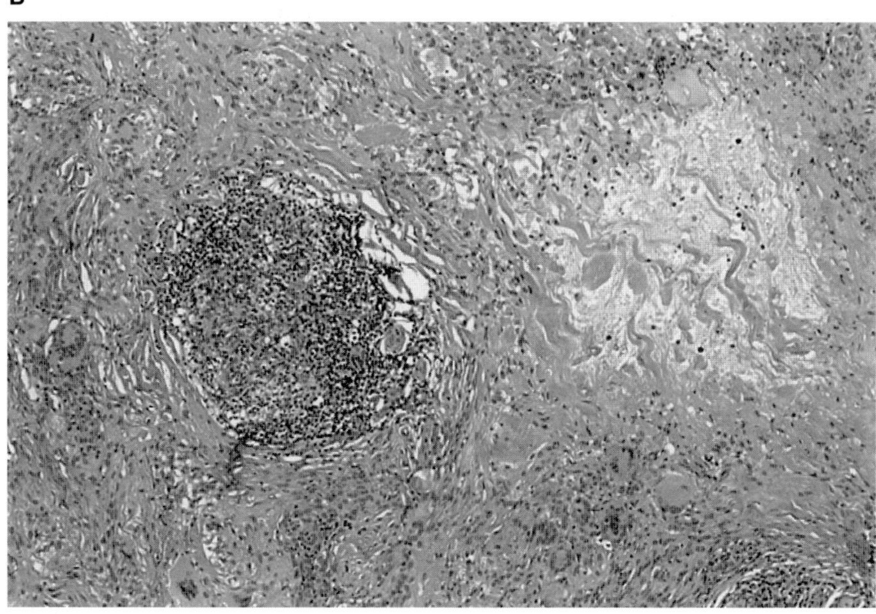

C

FIG. 27-7. ***Continued***

with extensive infiltrates of Touton giant cells, foamy histiocytes, and lymphocytes. Vascular involvement is rare, but panniculitis is common. Thus the cellularity and extent of necrobiosis usually serve as reliable clues, as does the periorbital location.

PAPULAR XANTHOMAS

Papular xanthomas (PX) are not clinically distinct. Patients present with multiple papules, sometimes with a yellow hue.[96] Although the lesions may be generalized, they have neither the distribution pattern of xanthoma disseminatum nor the confluence of diffuse normolipemic plane xanthoma. Plaques are not seen. Individual lesions may also be somewhat larger than in the related disorders. The patients show no abnormalities of lipid metabolism. Most patients have been adults, but occasional cases have been seen in children.[97,98] The oral mucosa may be involved.

Cases of eruptive normolipemic xanthomas[99] have also been described. Here the lesions appear suddenly, as in eruptive xanthoma associated with chylomicronemia, but with a more random distribution not favoring the extremities. A similar case has been described in an infant.[87] Diffuse papular xanthomas have also been described in association with mycosis fungoides[100] and erythrodermic atopic dermatitis.[101]

Histopathology. Small accumulations of foam cells are seen in the dermis. Even when early lesions are biopsied, a cellular or histiocytic phase is not seen.[102] An unusual solitary plexiform xanthoma has been described in a normolipemic patient[103]; the tumor had multiple dermal nodules consisting of foamy cells with some fibrosis and few giant cells. The relationship of this rare tumor to the non-LCH is unclear, but perhaps it fits best in this group.

Pathogenesis. PX is a heterogeneous group, not a single disease. Some cases have contained factor XIIIa–positive cells.[98] The presence or absence of a histiocytic precursor phase is a criterion that is hard to employ in daily practice. There must be histiocytic cells present initially that rapidly become xanthomatized.

Differential Diagnosis. Plane, papular, and eruptive normolipemic xanthomas are a clinical diagnosis of exclusion. Histologically, the lesions have no unique features; one sees accumulations of foam cells in the dermis with varying degrees of inflammation. Giant cells are uncommon. The differences between postinflammatory diffuse plane and papular xanthomas are minimal; surely plane and papular lesions occur in the same patient.

VERRUCIFORM XANTHOMA

Verruciform xanthoma (VX) occurs most commonly in the oral cavity, where it was first described by Shafer.[104] Lesions are typically solitary, asymptomatic hyperkeratotic papillomatous nodules. Most cases involve the gingival or alveolar mucosa, although other oral sites may be affected.[105] Although the process is usually benign, it has been associated with carcinoma in situ.[106]

In addition, VX may occur in the skin in several settings (reviewed in references 107–108). Idiopathic cutaneous VX is usually anogenital or perioral; trauma is probably the triggering agent. Similar changes have been seen in sun-damaged skin, again associated with carcinoma in situ.[109] VX has been reported secondary to a variety of inflammatory lesions, including discoid lupus erythematosus,[107] lichen planus, bullous diseases, epidermal nevus, especially inflammatory linear verrucous epidermal nevus (ILVEN), and following psoriasiform inflammation in AIDS.[108]

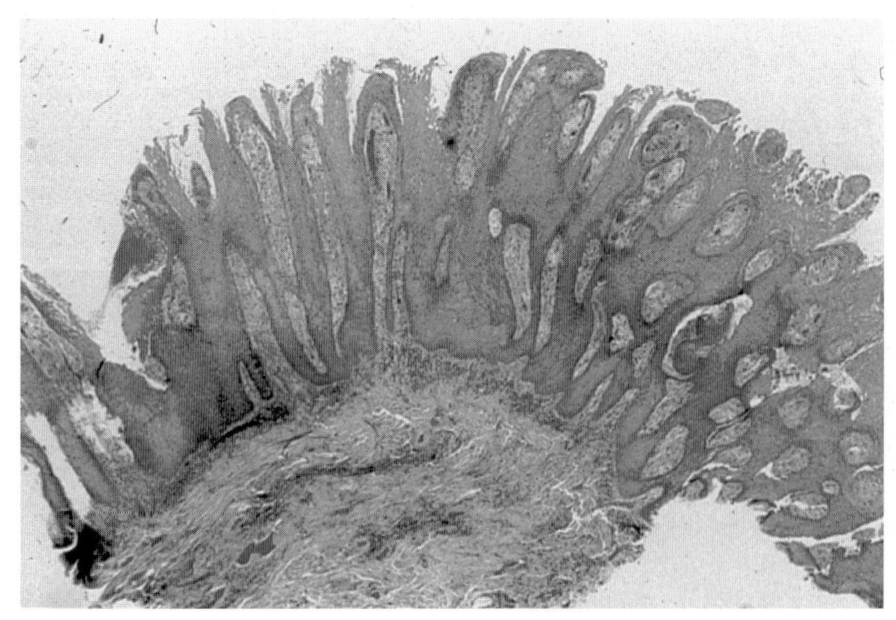

FIG. 27-8. Verruciform xanthoma (**A**) Papilloma with marked elongation and thinning of the dermal papillae. There is prominent hyperkeratosis with a modest lymphohistiocytic infiltrate at base. (**B**) Higher magnification showing foamy cells in the papillae with inflammatory cells in the adjacent crust.

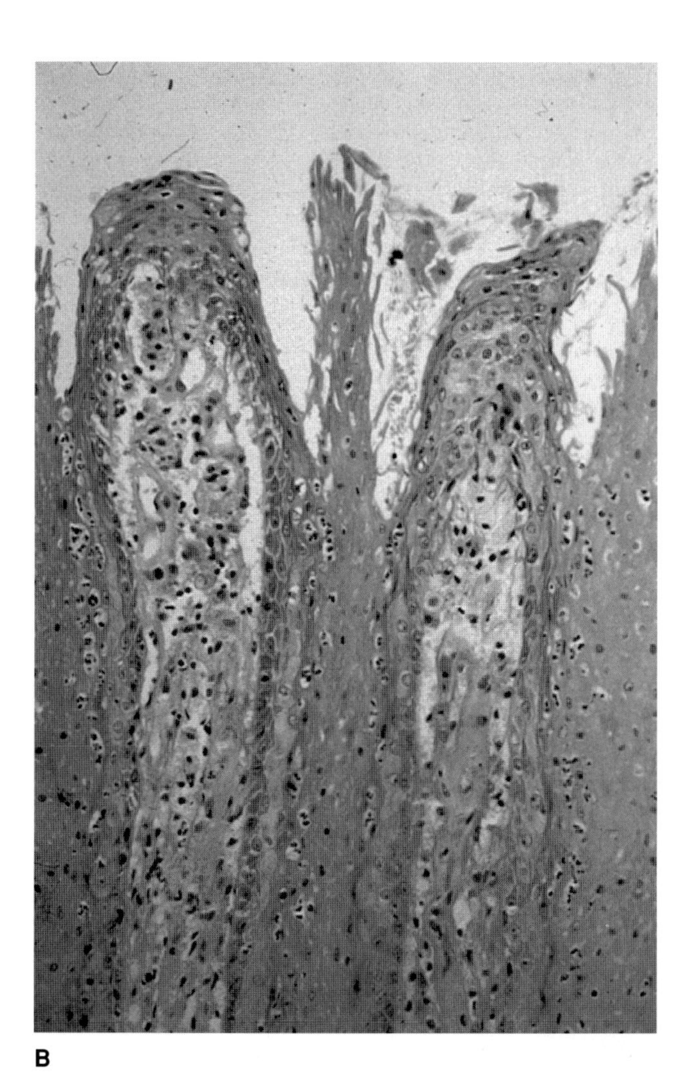

B

FIG. 27-8. *Continued*

Histopathology. The low-power picture is that of a verruca, often leading to a mistaken diagnosis. There is marked elongation of the rete ridges extending to a uniform level in the dermis (Fig. 27-8A). An infiltrate of foam cells is confined to the elongated dermal papillae located between the rete ridges (see Fig. 27-8B). Sometimes the xanthomatous cells may appear granular. The vessels in the papillae are also more prominent. The overlying epithelium is parakeratotic, and candidal hyphae or bacteria may be found.

Pathogenesis. Degenerating keratinocytes[110] or perhaps even melanocytes[111] are felt to be the source of the lipid material. Trauma and inflammation are the two best-established triggers. The foamy cells are positive for macrophage markers.

JUVENILE XANTHOGRANULOMA

Juvenile xanthogranuloma (JXG) is a benign disorder in which one, several, or occasionally numerous red to yellow nodules are present.[112–114] Because the lesions are also seen in adults *JXG* is admittedly an imperfect term. However, since xanthogranuloma alone has a variety of connotations in the pathology of different organ systems, we prefer to retain the designation *JXG*.

The papules and nodules are usually 0.5 to 1.0 cm in diameter. Most lesions appear during the first year of life; 20% are present at birth. In children the lesions may grow rapidly but almost always regress within a year. Lesions in adults are not uncommon[115] but are usually solitary and persistent.

JXG may be clinically subdivided into several forms. The micronodular form is most common; patients are infants with many small nodules. Occasionally a macronodular form is seen with only a few lesions, but these are often several centimeters in diameter. There are frequently clinical overlaps between the micro- and macronodular forms. Plaques may also be seen, as well as prominent nasal involvement (the Cyrano form).[116] A lichenoid variant has also been reported.[117] When adults have multiple lesions, the diagnosis is less clear, since multicentric reticulohistiocytosis as well as progressive nodular histiocytomas must be considered.[118] The spindle cell JXG presents as a deep dermal or subcutaneous nodule; it is usually solitary but is also seen in progressive nodular histiocytomas.[119] Finally, there are subcutaneous or deep JXGs.[120–122]

A number of systemic complications are associated with JXG. Ocular involvement including glaucoma and bleeding into the anterior chamber is the most common; it occurs in about 10% of young patients, most often with micronodular disease. Oral lesions may occur.[123] An association between JXG, cafe-au-lait macules, neurofibromatosis I, and juvenile chronic myelogenous leukemia has been identified.[124] JXG have also been identified in many other organ systems, usually in association with macronodular lesions. Included in the list of potential sites are the CNS,[125,126] kidney,[127] lungs, liver, testes, and pericardium. As one attempts to assess the types of systemic involvement with JXG, the picture becomes cloudy. *Xanthogranulomatous inflammation* simply refers to the presence of both foam cells and giant cells; it is not specific for one disease. Thus, in the absence of skin involvement, the diagnosis of JXG lacks specificity.

Bone involvement with JXG is most confusing of all. Erdheim-Chester disease consists of sclerotic bone lesions associated with soft tissue xanthogranulomatous inflammation. It is almost always seen in adults.[128] Thus when soft tissue "JXG" is diagnosed, the skeletal system should be surveyed and the diagnosis of Erdheim-Chester disease considered. The combination of a histiocytic skin lesion and radiological evidence of bone lesions does not always mean LCH.

Histopathology. The typical JXG contains histiocytes with a variety of cellular features. Zelger and colleagues have described five types: vacuolated, xanthomatized, scalloped, oncocytic, and spindle-shaped.[11] Early lesions may show large accumulations of histiocytes without any lipid infiltration intermingled with only a few lymphoid cells and eosinophils. When no foam cells or giant cells are seen, the possibility of JXG is often overlooked.[129] Usually some degree of lipidization is present, even in very early lesions, manifested by pale-staining histiocytes. In mature lesions, a granulomatous infiltrate is usually present containing foam cells, foreign-body giant cells, and Touton giant cells as well as histiocytes, lymphocytes, and eosinophils (Figs. 27-9A and B). The presence of giant cells, most of them Touton giant cells, showing a perfect "wreath" of nuclei surrounded by foamy cytoplasm is quite typical for JXG (see Fig. 27-9C). Occasionally, Touton giant cells are absent even in mature lesions.[113] Older, regressing lesions show proliferation of fibroblasts and fibrosis replacing part of the infiltrate. Two types of spindle cells have been identified[130]: dendritic and fusiform. The dendritic cells tend to be at the periphery of lesions and are usually S-100–positive. The fusiform cells are the macrophages.

Lesions from children and adults are quite similar histologically. The oncocytic or reticulohistiocytic type of histiocyte with an eosinophilic cytoplasm is uncommon in childhood lesions but may be seen in adult lesions.[56] The spindle cell variant is also more common in adults. Here one sees predominantly a spindle cell proliferation, similar to blue nevus or dermatofibroma, with few foamy or giant cells. The overlying epidermal changes and entrapment of collagen seen with dermatofibromas are absent.[119]

The deep or soft tissue lesions tend to be well circumscribed, but may infiltrate muscle. Giant cells are relatively less common and spindle cells are present. In one study, cells were CD1a-positive.[121]

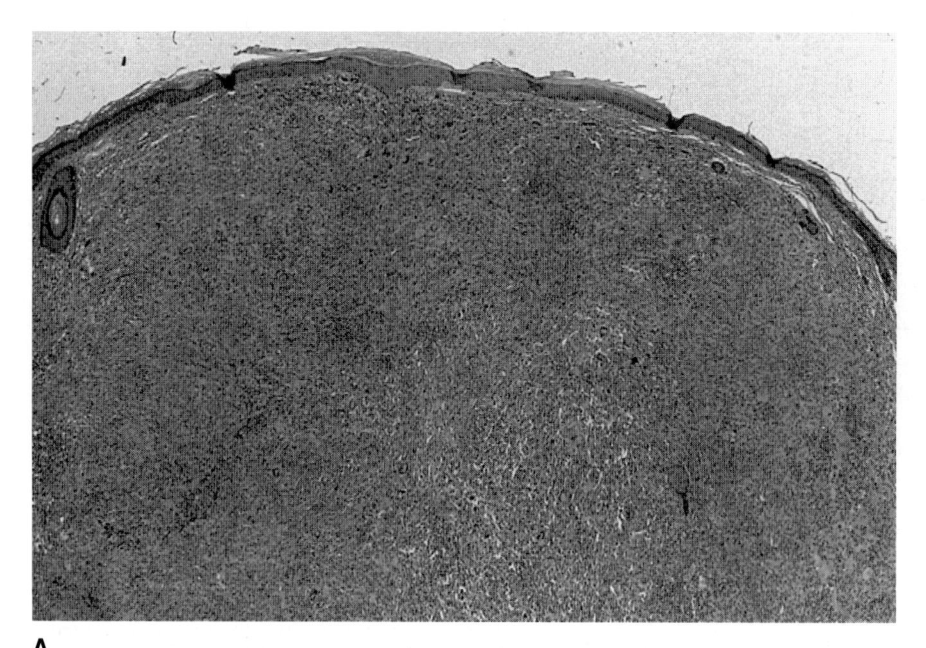

A

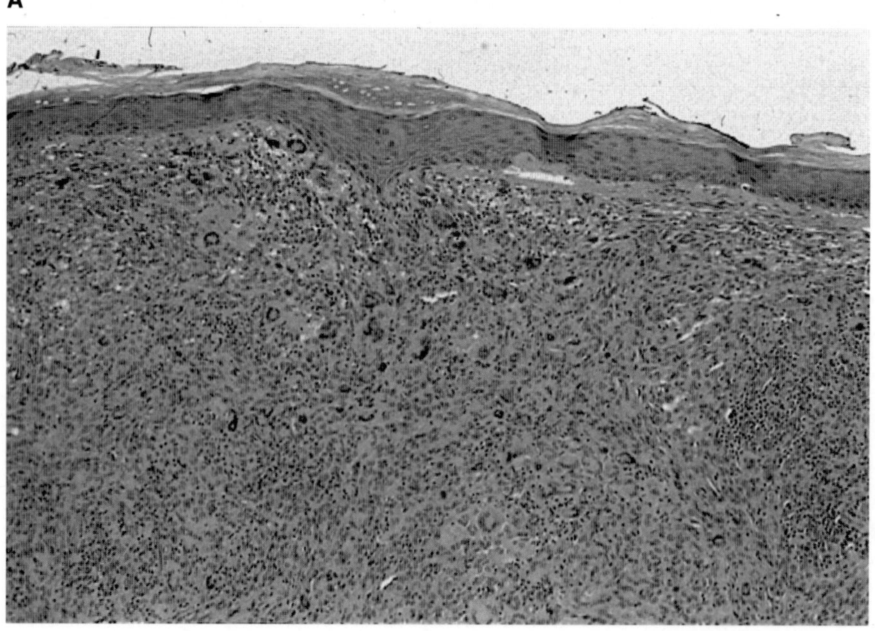

B

FIG. 27-9. Juvenile xanthogranuloma
(**A**) A dome-shaped papule with a rich cellular infiltrate filling the dermis but sparing the epidermis with a thin Grenz zone. (**B**) Higher magnification of *A*, showing a thin Grenz zone, a cellular infiltrate, and numerous Touton giant cells.

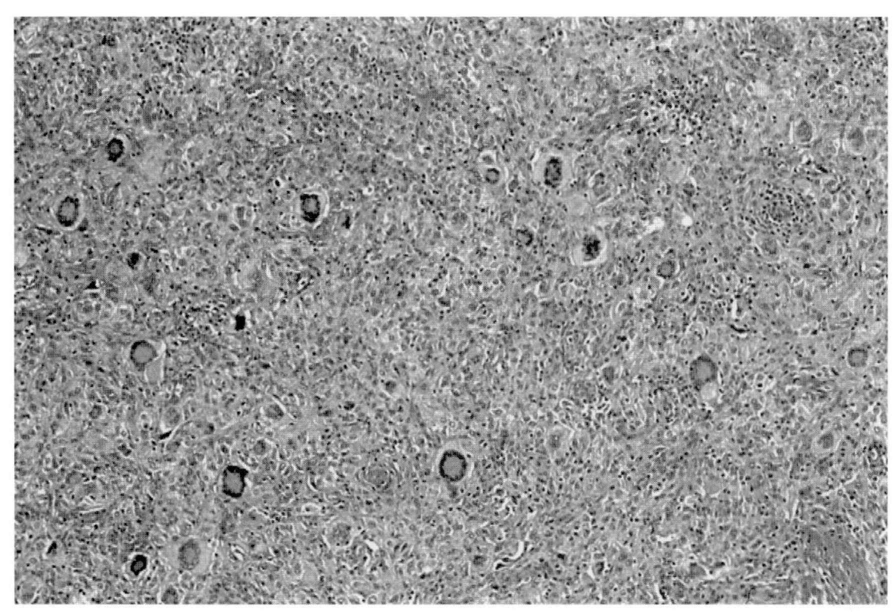

C

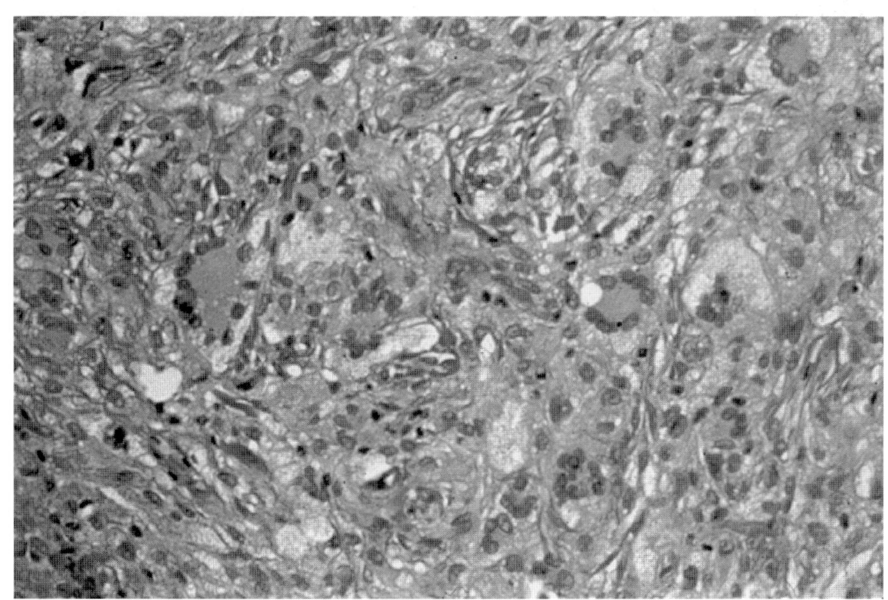

D

FIG. 27-9. *Continued*
(**C**) Another view showing multiple Touton giant cells. (**D**) Touton giants have central eosinophilic cytoplasm surrounded by a ring of nuclei, outside of which the cytoplasm is foamy.

Pathogenesis. The cause of JXG is unknown. The histiocytes carry macrophage markers. Both S-100 and CD1a positivity have been rarely reported[121,131]; these findings remain unexplained. Passenger dendritic cells are present in many dermal inflammatory processes.

The morphological subtypes seen in JXG may help explain the broad spectrum of non-LCH.[11] The typical solitary JXG contains a varying mixture of all types. Other lesions consist of a more monomorphous population and may present as solitary tumors or diffuse disorders. For example, oncocytic histiocytes are found in reticulohistiocytoma and multicentric reticulohistiocytosis, whereas xanthomatized histiocytes dominate in papular xanthoma and xanthoma disseminatum; in the latter disorder, scalloped histiocytes are also common.

There is marked overlap among these histologic patterns. In a study of 60 cases of childhood histiocytic tumors, including classic JXG, transitional or spindle cell JXG, histiocytomas, and dermatofibromas, not only did the JXG forms overlap, but the clinically distinct histiocytomas and dermatofibromas also had similar antigen profiles. The latter lesions tended to have been present for a much longer period of time, suggesting that histologic patterns may reflect the age of the lesion.[132]

Differential Diagnosis. The typical histologic picture of JXG is unmistakable. However, the many variants lead to a baffling array of diagnostic possibilities:

1. Cellular or vacuolated pattern. An infiltrate of unremarkable small cells, similar to LCH but S-100–negative and not epidermotropic. Identical to benign cephalic histiocytosis.

2. Foamy pattern. Identical to the rare xanthomatous form of LCH but S-100 and CD1a–negative. Also indistinguishable histologically from papular xanthoma.
3. Spindle cell pattern. Similar to blue nevus (but S-100–negative) and to dermatofibroma (but lacking epidermal changes and factor XIIIa positivity). Identical to progressive nodular histiocytoma.
4. Oncocytic pattern. Shows overlaps with reticulohistiocytosis. When Touton giant cells and eosinophils dominate, JXG is generally diagnosed; when ground glass cytoplasm dominate, reticulohistiocytosis is preferred.

RETICULOHISTIOCYTOSIS

Two types of reticulohistiocytosis are recognized: giant cell reticulohistiocytoma (GCRH) and multicentric reticulohistiocytosis (MRH). Both types occur almost exclusively in adults. The histologic picture is very similar in the two types. In GCRH one observes a single nodule in over 90% of cases, but occasionally multiple lesions are seen.[133] The lesions are seen most commonly on the head and neck. The nodules are smooth and 0.5 to 2.0 cm in diameter.[134] They may involute spontaneously. Even patients with multiple lesions show no sign of systemic involvement.

In multicentric reticulohistiocytosis, a name first coined by Goltz and Laymon in 1954,[135] the patients tend to be females, usually in the fifth or sixth decade of life, with widespread cutaneous involvement and a destructive arthritis.[136,137] Nodules ranging in size from a few millimeters to several centimeters are most common on the extremities; they resemble GCRH. Multiple papules on the face may coalesce, producing a leonine facies.[138] The small papules also create the "coral bead sign," many tiny reticulohistiocytomas along the nail fold. In about half of the patients, nodules are present also on the oral or nasal mucosa.[136] Finally, about 25% also have xanthelasmata.[137]

The polyarthritis may be mild or severe, but it has been absent in only a few cases. If severe, it may be mutilating, especially on the hands, through destruction of articular cartilage and subarticular bone. In addition, there is an association with hyperlipidemia (30%–50%), a variety of internal malignancies (15%–30%), and autoimmune diseases (5%–15%).[136,138] The disease tends to wax and wane over many years, with mutilating arthritis and disfigurement real possibilities.

Histopathology. The characteristic histologic feature in both GCRH and MRH is the presence of numerous multinucleate giant cells and oncocytic histiocytes showing abundant eosinophilic, finely granular cytoplasm, often with a "ground glass" appearance (Fig. 27-10A and B). In older lesions giant cells and fibrosis are more common. There may be subtle differences between the two lesions.[139] In GCRH the giant cells may be larger than 200μm, tend to have more than 20 often irregular nuclei, and are found in a background of eosinophilic mononuclear cells with scalloped outlines (see Fig. 27-10C). Transition cells with 2 to 3 nuclei suggest that the giant cells do arise from the oncocytic histiocytes. In contrast, in MRH the giant cells are smaller (50–100μm), have perhaps 10 regular nuclei, and are almost always strikingly PAS-positive (Fig. 27-11). In addition, factor XIIIa-positive dendritic cells are more likely to be found at the periphery of GCRH. Although these possible differences are intriguing, the two conditions often cannot be separated microscopically.

The polyarthritis present in nearly all instances of MRH is caused by the same type of infiltrate as found in the cutaneous lesions. In early or mild cases, the granulomatous infiltrate is confined to the synovial membrane. In patients with mutilating arthritis, the granulomatous infiltrate is found also in the subarticular cartilage and bone, leading to fragmentation and degeneration. Although similar infiltrates have been described in other organs, their clinical significance is unclear.[137]

Pathogenesis. Both disorders are non-LCH, so the cells are S-100 and CD1a–negative and have no Birbeck granules. Instead, ultrastructural examination shows abundant mitochondria and lysosomes, which correlate with the ground glass ap-

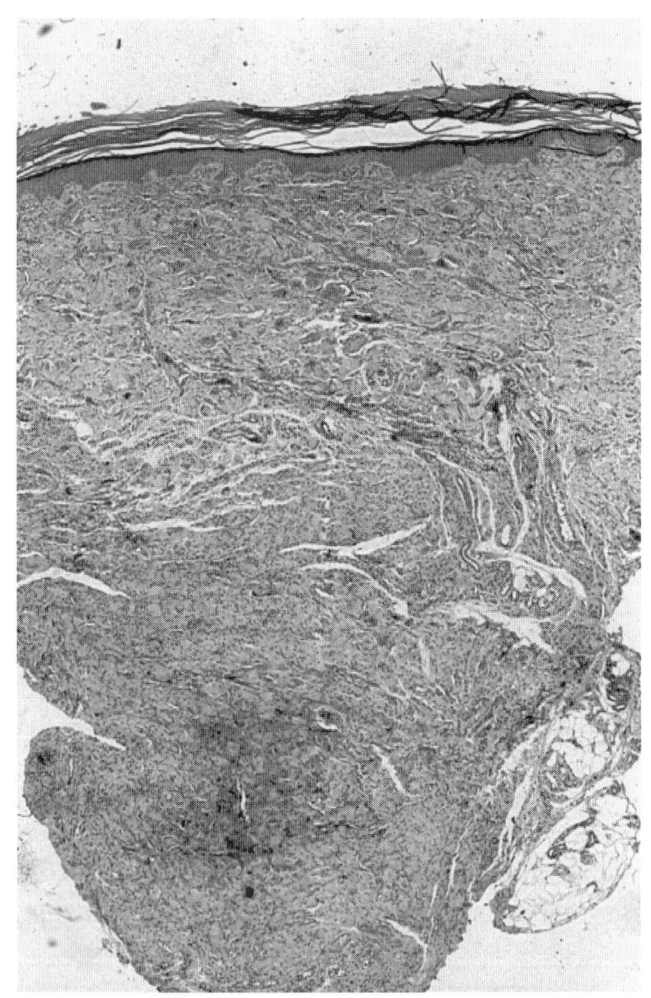

A

FIG. 27-10. Giant cell reticulohistiocytoma
(**A**) A diffuse dermal giant cell infiltrate with sparse inflammation. (**B**) A thinned epidermis and relatively clear giant cells replacing the upper dermis. (**C**) The giant cells are large and irregular and contain large numbers of haphazardly arranged nuclei.

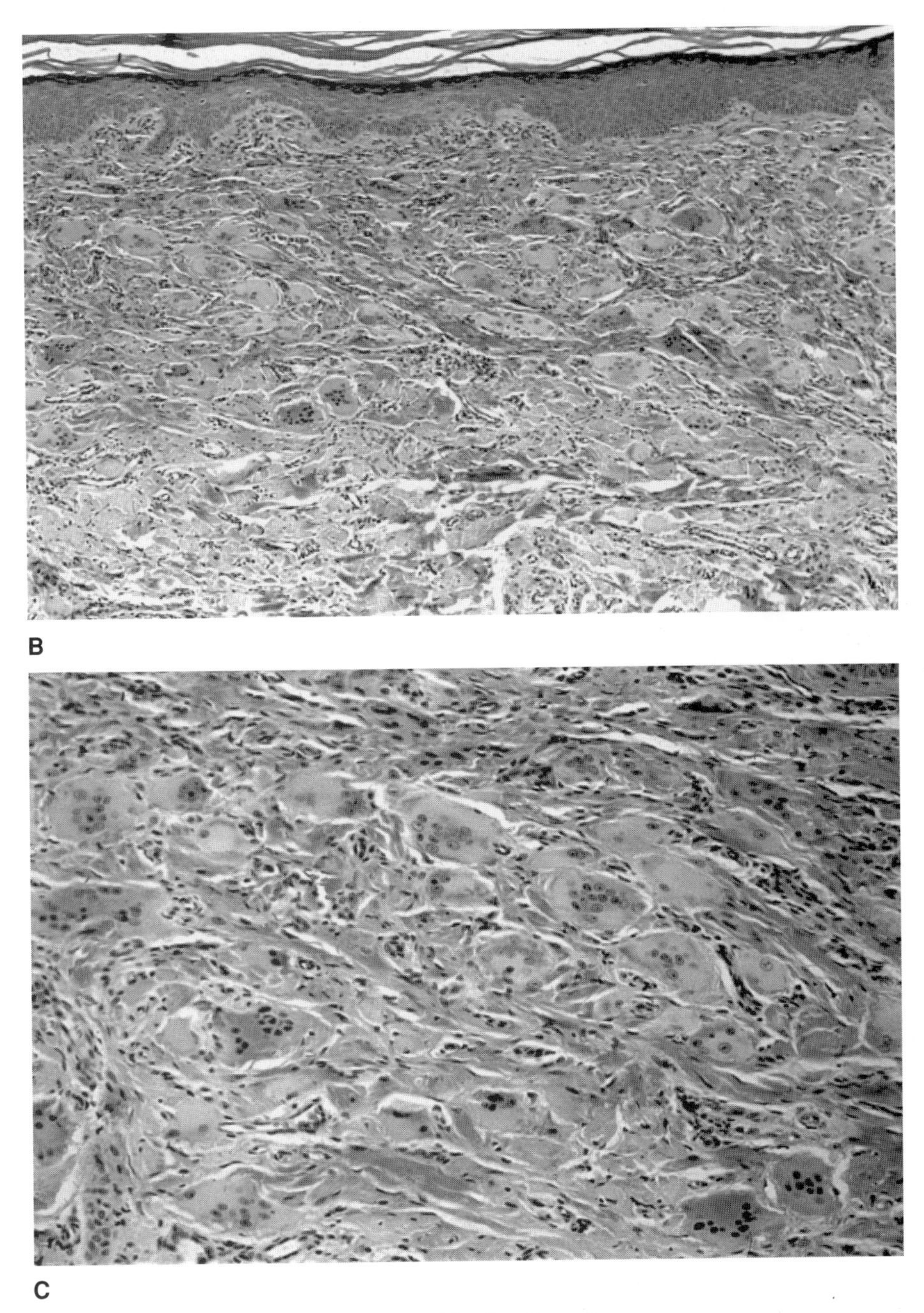

FIG. 27-10. ***Continued***

pearance. In addition, ingestion of collagen may been seen, resembling the Luse bodies seen in Hodgkin's disease.[140] The cells are also positive for most macrophage markers, including KP1, but negative for factor XIIIa.[141] Occasional cases have been described with both S-100 and factor XIII positivity; exactly how to explain and classify these cases remains a problem.[142,143]

The solitary lesions are felt to be reactive, perhaps with trauma as a trigger in some cases. In MRH, the concept of superantigen stimulation has been brought forward; a cytokine may selectively stimulate the oncocytic histiocytes, resulting in their proliferation and the subsequent tissue destruction. There may also be an underlying abnormality of lipid metabolism as manifested by the frequent xanthelasmata and lipoprotein abnormalities.

Differential Diagnosis. There are histologic overlaps between GCRH and JXG. In JXG there are more foamy cells and fewer oncocytic or ground glass cells. In addition, JXG usually contains some Touton giant cells, which show a regular arrangement of nuclei in a wreathlike fashion and, peripheral to them, foamy cytoplasm. This contrasts with the irregular arrangement of nuclei in the giant cells of GCRH.

The clinical differential diagnosis of MRH is lengthy, but a skin biopsy is quite helpful in pointing one in the right direction. Gout, rheumatoid arthritis, sarcoidosis, and even lepromatous leprosy may be considered.

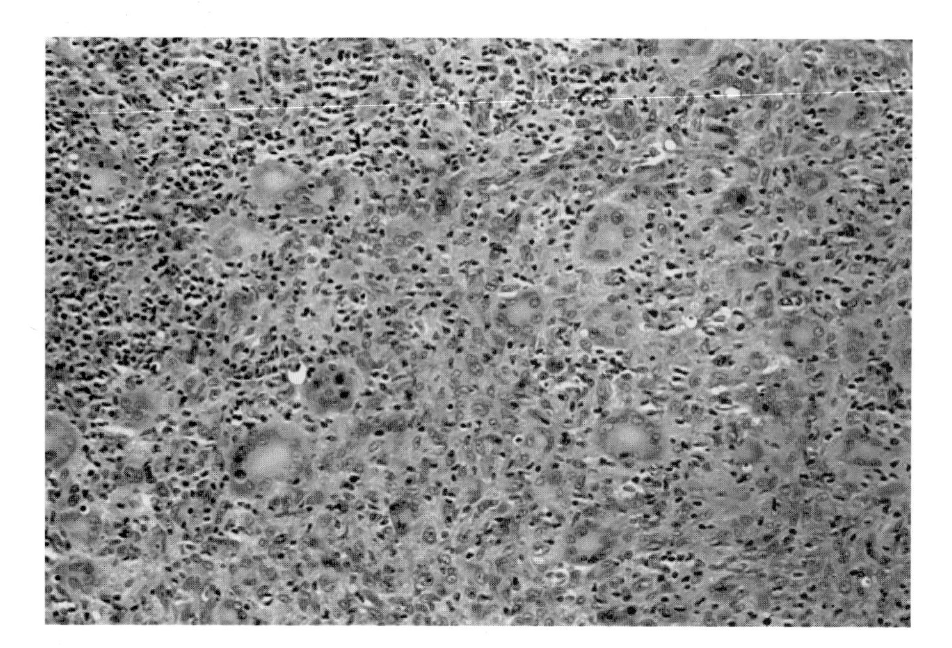

FIG. 27-11. Multicentric reticulohistiocytoma
Compare to Fig. 27-10C. Here the giant cells are smaller and more uniform and have fewer uniformly arranged nuclei. These two illustrations were chosen to exaggerate the possible differences between giant cell reticulohistiocytoma and multicentric reticulohistiocytoma.

PROGRESSIVE NODULAR HISTIOCYTOMA

Only a small number of cases of progressive nodular histiocytoma, a clinically distinct histiocytic proliferation, have been described.[22,144] Patients typically have hundreds of lesions of two distinct types: superficial xanthomatous papules 2 to 10 mm in diameter and deep fibrous nodules 1 to 3 cm in diameter. The key to diagnosis is these two distinct lesions. Conjunctival, oral, or laryngeal lesions may occur. Lesions rarely if ever regress. Familial or congenital cases have not been reported.

Histopathology. The histologic picture, in contrast to the clinical picture, is not diagnostic. Two patterns can be recognized that correlate with the clinical lesions. The smaller papules are xanthomatous, rich in foam cells and occasional Touton giant cells. The larger nodules contain a spindle cell proliferation that is identical to spindle cell JXG.[119]

Differential Diagnosis. Progressive nodular histiocytomas are probably a variant of multiple JXG. When the distinctive clinical picture is present, the diagnosis should be considered. Some authors have used the term *progressive nodular histiocytosis* as a synonym,[119] whereas others employ the same term for the leonine phase of multicentric reticulohistiocytosis,[138] causing further confusion.

HEREDITARY PROGRESSIVE MUCINOUS HISTIOCYTOSIS

This extremely uncommon eruption shows autosomal dominant inheritance and begins in early adolescence. All reported cases have been females, and the disease is confined to the skin. There are nodules that are generalized in distribution. They do not exceed 1 cm in diameter and increase in number, without spontaneous regression.[145,146]

Histopathology. The nodules show spindle-shaped and stellate histiocytes, with only an occasional giant cell. The stroma shows collagen bundles separated by abundant mucin that stains with toluidine blue and shows marked metachromasia, indicating the presence of acid mucopolysaccharides.

Pathogenesis. The nature of both the mucinous material and the histiocytic cell is unclear. Early lesions do not show a cellular or histiocytic phase.

Differential Diagnosis. Clinically the lesions appear similar to progressive nodular histiocytomas. Histologically, they must be separated from other forms of cutaneous mucinosis, none of which typically have a spindle cell component.

ERUPTIVE HISTIOCYTOMAS

Eruptive histiocytomas (EH) are characterized by the presence of innumerable flesh-colored to red macules and papules that develop in crops and that may involute spontaneously.[147–150] The disease takes a variable course; it may persist, remit, or relapse. As the infiltrates regress, the lesions may evolve into hyperpigmented macules.[151] Although most patients are adults, the condition may arise already in infancy.[152,153] In rare instances, oral lesions have been observed. There may be an associated underlying disorder, such as a malignancy; the histiocytic eruption may improve when the malignancy is treated.[154]

Histopathology. Histologic examination reveals an infiltrate composed of various types of histiocytes; most often small vacuolated cells are seen in a perivascular arrangement, but other morphological variants may be represented or even dominate.[65] Multinucleated giant cells are usually absent but have been described.[155] In some lesions, an inflammatory infiltrate is also present.

Pathogenesis. The etiology is unknown. As a matter of definition, one is dealing with a proliferation of histiocytes that are not actively phagocytic. Most cases are non-LCH, although eruptive cases of CSHRH and ICH have been described.[65] These cells appear so rapidly that it is not surprising that they are often undifferentiated. Older lesions may show fibrosis or giant cells. The histiocytes may in some cases appear in response to cytokines released by tumors, but in general their appearance remains unexplained. In one instance, lesions stained with antibodies to CD34, a marker usually found on fibroblasts but also present on bone marrow stem cells.[156]

Differential Diagnosis. Even though the histologic picture of this condition is indistinguishable from the earlier stages of JXG, XD, PNH, and even MRH, the sudden onset and the failure of the lesions to become foamy is characteristic. The paucity of histiocytes with ground glass cytoplasm and of giant cells distinguishes this disorder from MRH.

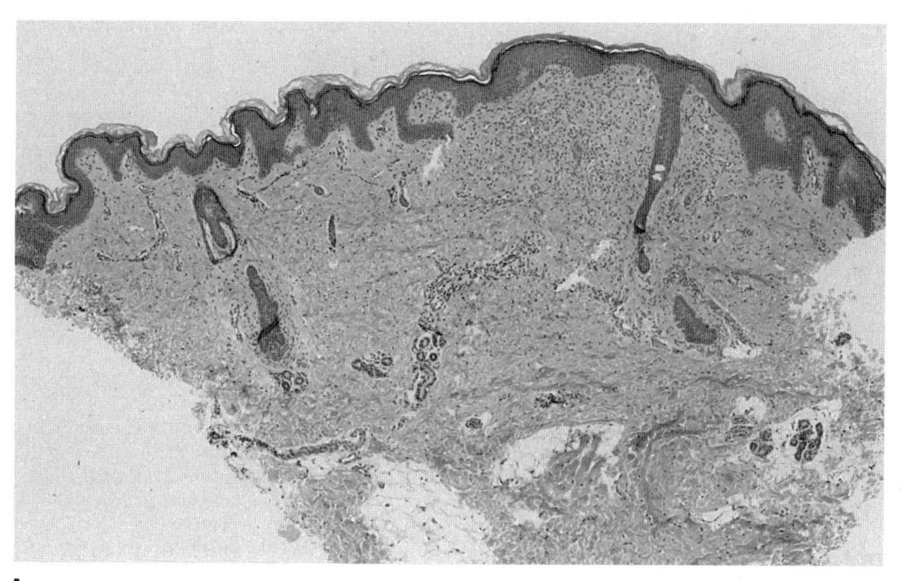

A

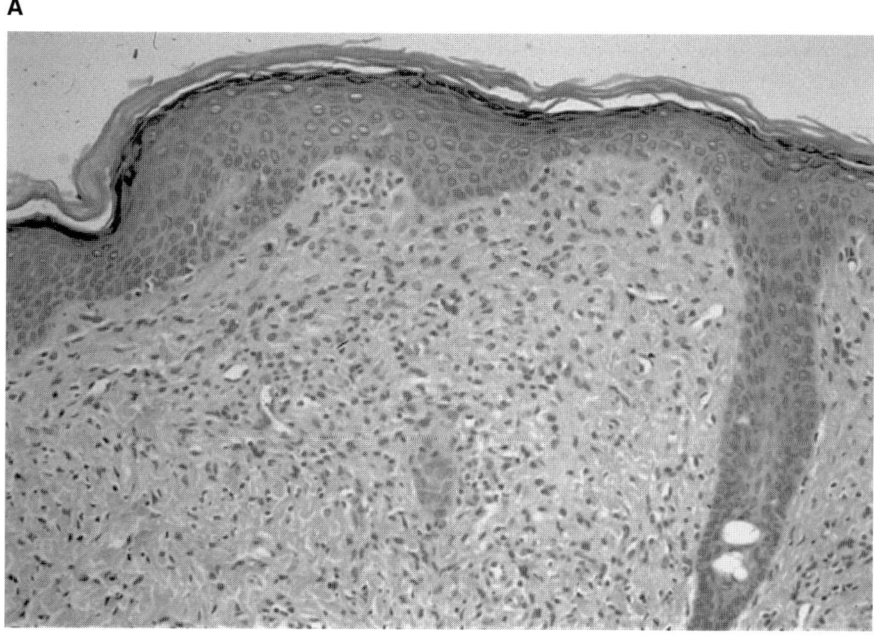

B

FIG. 27-12. Benign cephalic histiocytosis
(**A**) A sparse lichenoid infiltrate without foamy cells. (**B**) The epidermis is normal. The histiocytes are smaller than in Langerhans' cell histiocytosis and more round. No eosinophils are present. This histologic picture is not specific; it is the prototype of a pure histiocytic infiltrate as seen in eruptive histiocytoma, early juvenile xanthogranuloma, and benign cephalic histiocytosis.

BENIGN CEPHALIC HISTIOCYTOSIS

Benign cephalic histiocytosis, first described in 1971 by Gianotti, Caputo, and Ermacora,[157] is a self-healing histiocytosis limited to the skin. The eruption usually starts during the first 3 years of life and is almost always on the face, although it may become generalized. The lesions consist of red to yellow papules, which after a few years become flat and pigmented and finally resolve.[158–161]

Histopathology. The infiltrate tends to be sparse and consists of histiocytes with regularly shaped nuclei and sparse cytoplasm. Three patterns have been observed: papillary dermal, lichenoid, and diffuse.[162] The papillary dermal pattern is most common; there is a cohesive infiltrate of histiocytes in the upper dermis. The cells tend to be large and have an eosinophilic cytoplasm. Foam cells and epidermotropism are rare; eosinophils are often seen. The diffuse pattern is a minor variant in which the histiocytes are sparser and spread throughout the dermis. The lichenoid pattern is easily confused with LCH, but the nuclear changes seen in the latter are not present; crusting and ulceration are also uncommon (Fig. 27-12A and B).

Pathogenesis. The cause of BCH is unknown. Rare cases may be S-100–positive but CD1a–negative.

Differential Diagnosis. Benign cephalic histiocytosis overlaps with eruptive histiocytomas, progressive nodular histiocytomas, papular xanthomas, and multiple JXG.[162,163] If the lesions are clinically typical, the diagnosis can be made with some confidence.

REFERENCES

1. Headington JT. The histiocyte: In memoriam. Arch Dermatol 1986; 122:532.
2. Foucar K, Foucar E. The mononuclear phagocyte and immunoregulatory effector (M-PIRE) system: Evolving concepts. Semin Diagn Pathol 1990;7:4.
3. Wood GS, Haber RS. Novel histiocytoses considered in the context of histiocyte subset differentiation. Arch Dermatol 1993;129:210.
4. Weiss LM. Histiocytic and dendritic cell proliferations. in Neoplastic Hematopathology. Knowles DM, ed. Baltimore: Williams and Wilkins, 1992:1459.
5. Fartasch M, Goerdt S, Hornstein OP. Chancen und Grenzen paraffingängiger Zellmarker in der diagnostik primärer kutaner Histiozytosen. Hautarzt 1995;46:144.
6. Goerdt S, Kolde G, Bonsmann G et al. Immunohistochemical comparison of cutaneous histiocytoses and related skin disorders: Diagnostic and histogenetic relevance of MS-1 high molecular weight protein expression. J Pathol 1993;170:421.
7. Winkelmann RK. Cutaneous syndromes of non-X histiocytosis: A review of the macrophage-histiocyte diseases of the skin. Arch Dermatol 1981;117:667.
8. Gianotti F, Caputo R. Histiocytic syndromes: A review. J Am Acad Dermatol 1985;13:383.
9. Writing Group of the Histiocyte Society. Histiocytosis syndromes in children. Lancet 1987;1:208.
10. Snow JL, Su WPD. Histiocytic diseases. J Am Acad Dermatol 1995; 33:111.
11. Zelger BWH, Sidoroff A, Orchard G, Cerio R. Non-Langerhans' cell histiocytoses: A new unifying concept. Am J Dermatopathol 1996; 18:(in press).
12. Triscott JA, Nappi O, Ferrara G, Wick MR. "Pseudoneoplastic" leprosy: Leprosy revisited. Am J Dermatopathol 1995;17:297.
13. Cline MJ. Histiocytes and histiocytosis: Blood 1994;84:2840.
14. Guitart J, Zemtsov A, Bergfeld WF, Tomecki KJ. Diffuse dermal histiocytosis: A variant of generalized granuloma annulare. Am J Dermatopathol 1991;13:174.
15. Ben-Ezra JM, Koo CH. Langerhans' cell histiocytosis and malignancies of the M-PIRE system. Am J Clin Pathol 1993;99:464.
16. Burgdorf WHC. Malignant histiocytic infiltrates. In Lymphoproliferative Disorders of the Skin, Murphy GF, Mihm MC Jr, eds. Boston: Butterworth, 1986:217.
17. Valente M, Parenti A, Cipriani R, Peserico A. Familial histiocytic dermatoarthritis: Histological and ultrastructural findings in two cases. Am J Dermatopathol 1987;9:491.
18. Caputo R, Sambvani N, Monti M et al. Dermochondrocorneal dystrophy (François syndrome). Arch Dermatol 1988;124:424.
19. Parker F. Xanthomas and hyperlipidemias. J Am Acad Dermatol 1985;13:1.
20. Cruz PD Jr, East C, Bergstresser PR. Dermal, subcutaneous and tendon xanthomas: Diagnostic markers for specific lipoprotein disorders. J Am Acad Dermatol 1988;19:95.
21. Cruz PD Jr. Xanthomas. In: Demis DJ (ed). Clinical Dermatology. Vol. 2. Philadelphia: Lippincott–Raven, 1994;1.
22. Burgdorf WHC, Kusch SL, Nix TE Jr, Pitha J. Progressive nodular histiocytoma. Arch Dermatol 1981;117:644.
23. Parker F. Normocholesterolemic xanthomatosis. Arch Dermatol 1986;122:1253.
24. Cooper PH. Eruptive xanthoma: A microscopic simulant of granuloma annulare. J Cutan Pathol 1986;13:207.
25. Walsh NMG, Murray S, D'Intino Y. Eruptive xanthomata with uratelike crystals. J Cutan Pathol 1994;21:350.
26. Malone M. The histiocytoses of childhood. Histopathology 1991;19: 105.
27. Risdall RJ, Dehner LP, Duray P et al. Histiocytosis X (Langerhans' cell histiocytosis): Prognostic role of histopathology. Arch Pathol Lab Med 1983;107:59.
28. Maarten Egeler R, Neglia JP, Puccetti DM et al. Association of Langerhans' cell histiocytosis with malignant neoplasms. Cancer 1993;71:865.
29. Lichtenwald DJ, Jakubovic HR, Rosenthal D. Primary cutaneous Langerhans' cell histiocytosis in an adult. Arch Dermatol 1991;127: 1545.
30. Novice FM, Collison DW, Kleinsmith DM et al. Letterer-Siwe disease in adults. Cancer 1989;63:166.
31. Curtis AC, Cawley EP. Eosinophilic granuloma of bone with cutaneous manifestations. Arch Dermatol 1947;55:810.
32. Altman J, Winkelmann RK. Xanthomatous cutaneous lesions of histiocytosis X. Arch Dermatol 1963;87:164.
33. Esterly NB, Maurer HS, Gonzalez-Crussi F. Histiocytosis X: A seven-year experience at a children's hospital. J Am Acad Dermatol 1985; 13:481.
34. Bonifazi E. Place des histiocytoses auto-involutives au sein des histiocytoses Langerhansiennes'. Ann Dermatol Venereol 1992;119:397.
35. Higgins CR, Tatnall FM, Leigh IM. Vesicular Langerhans' cell histiocytosis: An uncommon variant. Clin Exp Dermatol 1994;19:350.
36. Modi D, Schultz EJ. Skin ulceration as sole manifestation of Langerhans' cell histiocytosis. Clin Exp Dermatol 1991;16:212.
37. Foucar E, Piette WW, Tse DT et al. Urticating histiocytosis: A mast cell-rich variant of histiocytosis X. J Am Acad Dermatol 1986;14:867.
38. Holzberg M, Spraker MK. Nail pathology in histiocytosis X. J Am Acad Dermatol 1985;13:522.
39. Delabie J, DeWolf-Peeters C, DeVos R et al. True histiocytic neoplasm of Langerhans' cell type. J Pathol 1991;163:217.
40. Tani M, Ishii N, Kumagai M et al. Malignant Langerhans' cell tumor. Br J Dermatol 1992;126:398.
41. Wood C, Wood GS, Deneau DG et al. Malignant histiocytosis X: Report of a rapidly fatal case in an elderly man. Cancer 1984;54:347.
42. Ben-Ezra J, Bailey A, Azumi N et al. Malignant histiocytosis X: A distinct clinicopathologic entity. Cancer 1991;68:1050.
43. Van Heerde P, Maarten Egeler R. The cytology of Langerhans' cell histiocytosis (histiocytosis X). Cytopathology 1991;2:149.
44. Hage C, Willman CL, Favara BE, Isaacson PG. Langerhans' cell histiocytosis (histiocytosis X): Immunophenotype and growth fraction. Hum Pathol 1993;24:840.
45. Helm KF, Lookingbill DP, Marks JG Jr. A clinical and pathological study of histiocytosis X in adults. J Am Acad Dermatol 1993;29:166.
46. Willman CL, Busque L, Griffith BB et al. Langerhans' cell histiocytosis (histiocytosis X): A clonal proliferative disease. N Engl J Med 1994;331:154.
47. Yu RC, Chu C, Buluwela L, Chu AC. Clonal proliferation of Langerhans' cells in Langerhans' cell histiocytosis. Lancet 1994;343:767.
48. Hashimoto K, Pritzker MS. Electron microscopic study of reticulohistiocytoma: An unusual case of congenital self-healing reticulohistiocytosis. Arch Dermatol 1973;107:263.

49. Bernstein EF, Resnik KS, Loose JH et al. Solitary congenital self-healing reticulohistiocytosis. Br J Dermatol 1993;129:449.
50. Longaker MA, Frieden IJ, LeBoit PE, Sherertz EF. Congenital "self-healing" Langerhans' cell histiocytosis: The need for long-term followup. J Am Acad Dermatol 1994;31:910.
51. Bonifazi E, Caputo R, Ceci A, Meneghini C. Congenital self-healing reticulohistiocytosis: Clinical, histologic, and ultrastructural study. Arch Dermatol 1982;118:267.
52. Hashimoto K, Griffin D, Kohsbaki M. Self-healing reticulohistiocytosis. Cancer 1982;49:331.
53. Ikeda M, Yamamoto Y, Kitagawa N et al. Solitary nodular Langerhans' cell histiocytosis. Br J Dermatol 1993;128:220.
54. Hashimoto K, Kagetsu N, Taniguchi Y et al. Immunohistochemistry and electron microscopy in Langerhans' cell histiocytosis confined to the skin. J Am Acad Dermatol 1991;25:1044.
55. Divaris DXG, Ling FCK, Prentice RSA. Congenital self-healing histiocytosis: Report of two cases with histochemical and ultrastructural studies. Am J Dermatopathol 1991;13:481.
56. Zelger B, Cerio R, Orchard G, Wilson-Jones E. Juvenile and adult xanthogranuloma: A histological and immunohistochemical comparison. Am J Surg Pathol 1994;18:126.
57. Schaumberg-Lever G, Rechowicz E, Fehrenbacher B et al. Congenital self-healing reticulohistiocytosis: A benign Langerhans' cell disease. J Cutan Pathol 1994;21:59.
58. Shimizu H, Komatsu T, Harada T et al. An immunohistochemical and ultrastructural study of an unusual case of multiple non-X histiocytoma. Arch Dermatol 1988;124:1254.
59. Wood GS, Hu C-H, Beckstead JH, Turner RR, Winkelmann RK. The indeterminate cell proliferative disorder: Report of a case manifesting as an unusual cutaneous histiocytosis. J Dermatol Surg Oncol 1985; 11:1111.
60. Winkelmann RK, Hu C-H, Kossard S. Response of nodular non-X histiocytosis to vinblastine. Arch Dermatol 1982;118:913.
61. Kolde G, Bröcker EB. Multiple skin tumors of indeterminate cells in an adult. J Am Acad Dermatol 1986;15:591.
62. Saijo S, Hara M, Kuramoto Y, Tagami H. Generalized eruptive histiocytoma: A report of a case showing the presence of indeterminate cells. J Cutan Pathol 1991;18:134.
63. Levisohn D, Seidel D, Phelps A, Burgdorf W. Solitary congenital indeterminate cell histiocytoma. Arch Dermatol 1993;129:81.
64. Berti E, Gianotti R, Alessi E. Unusual cutaneous histiocytosis expressing an intermediate immunophenotype between Langerhans' cells and dermal macrophages. Arch Dermatol 1988;124:1250.
65. Sidoroff A, Zelger B, Steiner H, Smith N. Indeterminate cell histiocytosis: A clinicopathological entity with features of both X- and non-X histiocytosis. Br J Dermatol 1996;134:525.
66. Rosai J, Dorfman RF. Sinus histiocytosis with massive lymphadenopathy: A newly recognized benign clinicopathological entity. Arch Pathol 1969;87:63.
67. Rosai J, Dorfman RF. Sinus histiocytosis with massive lymphadenopathy: A pseudolymphomatous benign disorder: Analysis of 34 cases. Cancer 1972;30:1174.
68. Foucar E, Rosai J, Dorfman R. Sinus histiocytosis with massive lymphadenopathy: Review of the entity. Semin Diagn Pathol 1990;7:19.
69. Thawerani H, Sanchez RL, Rosai J, Dorfman RF. The cutaneous manifestations of sinus histiocytosis with massive lymphadenopathy. Arch Dermatol 1978;114:191.
70. Pérez A, Rodríguez M, Febrer I, Aliaga A. Sinus histiocytosis confined to the skin: Case report and review of the literature. Am J Dermatopathol 1995;17:384.
71. Mac-Moune Lai F, Lam WY, Chin CW, Ng WL. Cutaneous Rosai-Dorfman disease presenting as a suspicious breast mass. J Cutan Pathol 1994;21:377.
72. Suster S, Cartagena N, Cabello-Inchausti B, Robinson MJ. Histiocytic lymphophagocytic panniculitis: An unusual extranodal presentation of sinus histiocytosis with massive lymphadenopathy (Rosai-Dorfman disease). Arch Dermatol 1988;124:1246.
73. Chu P, LeBoit P. Histologic features of cutaneous sinus histiocytosis (Rosai-Dorfman disease): Study of cases both with and without systemic involvement. J Cutan Pathol 1992;19:201.
74. Eisen RN, Buckley PJ, Rosai J. Immunophenotypic characterization of sinus histiocytosis with massive lymphadenopathy (Rosai-Dorfman disease). Semin Diagn Pathol 1990;7:74.
75. Perrin C, Michiels JF, Lacour JP et al. Sinus histiocytosis (Rosai-Dorfman disease) clinically limited to the skin: An immunohistochemical and ultrastructural study. J Cutan Pathol 1993;20:368.
76. Altman J, Winkelmann RK. Xanthoma disseminatum. Arch Dermatol 1962;86:582.
77. Varotti C, Bettoli V, Berti E et al. Xanthoma disseminatum: A case with extensive mucous membrane involvement. J Am Acad Dermatol 1991;25:433.
78. Caputo R, Veraldi S, Grimalt R et al. The various clinical patterns of xanthoma disseminatum: Considerations on seven cases and review of the literature. Dermatology 1995;190:19.
79. Blobstein SH, Caldwell D, Carter DM. Bone lesions in xanthoma disseminatum. Arch Dermatol 1985;121:1313.
80. Goodenberger ME, Piette WW, Macfarlane DE, Argenyi ZB. Xanthoma disseminatum and Waldenström's macroglobulinemia. J Am Acad Dermatol 1990;23:1015.
81. Battaglini J, Olsen TG. Disseminated xanthosiderohistiocytosis, a variant of xanthoma disseminatum, in a patient with a plasma cell dyscrasia. J Am Acad Dermatol 1984;11:750.
82. Nickoloff BJ, Wood GS, Chu M et al. Disseminated dermal dendrocytomas: A new cutaneous fibrohistiocytic disorder? Am J Surg Pathol 1990;14:867.
83. Zelger B, Cerio R, Orchard G et al. Histologic and immunohistochemical study comparing xanthoma disseminatum and histiocytosis X. Arch Dermatol 1992;128:1207.
84. Altman J, Winkelmann RK. Diffuse normolipemic plane xanthoma. Arch Dermatol 1962:85:633.
85. Lynch PJ, Winkelmann RK. Generalized plane xanthoma and systemic disease. Arch Dermatol 1966;93:639.
86. Sherman D, Ramsay B, Theodorou NA et al. Reversible plane xanthoma, vasculitis and peliosis hepatitis in giant lymph node hyperplasia (Castleman's disease): A case report and review of the cutaneous manifestations of giant lymph node hyperplasia. J Am Acad Dermatol 1992;26:105.
87. Horiuchi Y, Ito A. Normolipemic papuloeruptive xanthomatosis in an infant. J Dermatol 1991;18:235.
88. Williford PM, White WL, Jorizzo JL, Greer K. The spectrum of normolipemic plane xanthoma. Am J Dermatopathol 1993;15:572.
89. Umbert I, Winkelmann RK, Cavender P. Plane normolipemic xanthoma developing necrobiotic xanthogranuloma with leukopenia, monoclonal gammopathy, and low complement (abstr). J Cutan Pathol 1992;19:556.
90. Kossard S, Winkelmann RK. Necrobiotic xanthogranuloma with paraproteinemia. J Am Acad Dermatol 1980;3:257.
91. McGregor JM, Miller J, Smith NP, Hay RJ. Necrobiotic xanthogranuloma without periorbital lesions. J Am Acad Dermatol 1993;29:466.
92. Finan MC, Winkelmann RK. Necrobiotic xanthogranuloma with paraproteinemia: A review of 22 cases. Medicine (Baltimore) 1986;65: 376.
93. Finan MC, Winkelmann RK. Histopathology of necrobiotic xanthogranuloma with paraproteinemia. J Cutan Pathol 1987;14:92.
94. Mehregan DA, Winkelmann RK. Necrobiotic xanthogranuloma. Arch Dermatol 1992;128:94.
95. Venencie PY, Puissant A, Verola O et al. Necrobiotic xanthogranuloma with myeloma. Cancer 1987;59:588.
96. Sanchez RL, Raimer SS, Peltier F, Swedo J. Papular xanthoma: A clinical, histologic, and ultrastructural study. Arch Dermatol 1985; 121:626.
97. Caputo R, Gianni E, Imondi D et al. Papular xanthoma in children. J Am Acad Dermatol 1990;22:1052.
98. Fonseca E, Contreras F, Cuevas J. Papular xanthoma in children: Report and immunohistochemical study. Pediatr Dermatol 1993;10:139.
99. Caputo R, Monti M, Berti E et al. Normolipemic eruptive cutaneous xanthomatosis. Arch Dermatol 1986;122:1294.
100. Darwin BS, Herzberg AJ, Murray JC, Olsen EA. Generalized papular xanthomatosis in mycosis fungoides. J Am Acad Dermatol 1992;26: 828.
101. Goerdt S, Kretzschmar L, Bonsmann G et al. Normolipemic papular xanthomatosis in erythrodermic atopic dermatitis. J Am Acad Dermatol 1995;32:326.
102. Bundino S, Zina AM, Aloi F. Papular xanthoma: Clinical, histological, and ultrastructural study. Dermatologica 1988;177:382.
103. Beham A, Fletcher CDM. Plexiform xanthoma: An unusual variant. Histopathology 1991;19:565.
104. Shafer WB. Verruciform xanthoma. Oral Surg 1971;31:784.
105. Mostafa KA, Takata T, Ogawa I et al. Verruciform xanthoma of the oral mucosa: A clinicopathological study with immunohistochemical findings relating to pathogenesis. Virchows Arch A Pathol Anat 1993; 423:243.

106. Drummond JF, White DK, Damm DD, Cramer JR. Verruciform xanthoma with carcinoma in situ. J Oral Maxillofac Surg 1989;47:396.
107. Meyers DC, Woosley JT, Reddick RL. Verruciform xanthoma in association with discoid lupus erythematosus. J Cutan Pathol 1992;19:156.
108. Smith KJ, Skelton HG, Angritt P. Changes of verruciform xanthoma in an HIV-1+ patient with diffuse psoriasiform skin disease. Am J Dermatopathol 1995;17:185.
109. Jensen JL, Liao S-Y, Jeffes EWB III. Verruciform xanthoma of the ear with coexisting epidermal dysplasia. Am J Dermatopathol 1992;14:426.
110. Zegarelli DJ, Zegarelli-Schmidt ED, Zegarelli EV. Verruciform xanthoma: Further light and electron microscopic studies with addition of a third case. Oral Surg 1975;40:246.
111. Balus S, Breathnach AS, O'Grady AJ. Ultrastructural observations on "foam cells" and the source of their lipid in verruciform xanthoma. J Am Acad Dermatol 1991;24:760.
112. Helwig EB, Hackney VC. Juvenile xanthogranuloma (nevoxanthoendothelioma). Am J Pathol 1954;30:625.
113. Sonoda T, Hashimoto H, Enjoji M. Juvenile xanthogranuloma: Clinicopathologic analysis and immunohistochemical study of 57 patients. Cancer 1985;56:2280.
114. Sangüeza OP, Salmon JK, White CR Jr, Beckstead JH. Juvenile xanthogranuloma: A clinical, histopathologic, and immunohistochemical study. J Cutan Pathol 1995;22:327.
115. Rodriguez J, Ackerman AB. Xanthogranuloma in adults. Arch Dermatol 1976;112:43.
116. Caputo R, Grimalt R, Gelmetti R, Cottoni F. Unusual aspects of juvenile xanthogranuloma. J Am Acad Dermatol 1993;29:868.
117. Kolde G, Bonsmann G. Generalized lichenoid juvenile xanthogranuloma. Br J Dermatol 1992;126:66.
118. Whitmore SE. Multiple xanthogranulomas in an adult: Case report and literature review. Br J Dermatol 1992;127:177.
119. Zelger BWH, Staudacher C, Orchard G et al. Solitary and generalized variants of spindle cell xanthogranuloma (progressive nodular histiocytosis). Histopathology 1995;27:11.
120. Janney CG, Hurt MA, Santa Cruz DJ. Deep juvenile xanthogranuloma: Subcutaneous and intramuscular forms. Am J Surg Pathol 1991;15:150.
121. De Graaf JH, Timens W, Tamminga RYJ, Molenaar WM. Deep juvenile xanthogranuloma: A lesion related to dermal indeterminate cells. Hum Pathol 1992;23:905.
122. Sánchez Yus E, Requena L, Villegas C, Valle P. Subcutaneous juvenile xanthogranuloma. J Cutan Pathol 1995;22:460.
123. Satow SJ, Zee S, Dawson KH et al. Juvenile xanthogranuloma of the tongue. J Am Acad Dermatol 1995;33:376.
124. Zvulunov A, Barak Y, Metzker A. Juvenile xanthogranuloma, neurofibromatosis, and juvenile chronic myelogenous leukemia: World statistical analysis. Arch Dermatol 1995;131:904.
125. Paulus W, Kirchner T, Ott MM et al. Histiocytic tumor of Meckel's cave: An intracranial equivalent of juvenile xanthogranuloma of the skin. Am J Surg Pathol 1992;16:76.
126. Botella-Estrada R, Sanmartin O, Grau M, Alegre V, Mas C, Aliaga A. Juvenile xanthogranuloma with central nervous system involvement. Pediatr Dermatol 1993;10:64.
127. Kodet R, Elleder M, DeWolf-Peeters C, Mottl H. Congenital histiocytosis: A heterogenous group of diseases, one presenting as so-called congenital self-healing histiocytosis. Pathol Res Pract 1991;187:458.
128. Miller RL, Sheeler LR, Bauer TW, Bukowski RM. Erdheim-Chester disease: Case report and review of the literature. Am J Med 1986;80:1230.
129. Claudy AL, Misery L, Serre D, Boucheron S. Mulitple juvenile xanthogranulomas without foam cells and giant cells. Pediatr Dermatol 1993;10:61.
130. Tahan S, Pastel-Levy C, Bhan AK, Mihm MC Jr. Juvenile xanthogranuloma: Clinical and pathologic characterization. Arch Pathol Lab Med 1989;113:1057.
131. Andersen WK, Knowles DM, Silvers DN. CD1 (OKT6)-positive juvenile xanthogranuloma: OKT6 is not specific for Langerhans' cell histiocytosis (histiocytosis X). J Am Acad Dermatol 1992;26:850.
132. Marrogi AJ, Dehner LP, Coffin CM, Wick MR. Benign cutaneous histiocytic tumors in childhood and adolescence, excluding Langerhans' cell proliferations: A clinicopathologic and immunohistiochemical analysis. Am J Dermatopathol 1992;14:8.
133. Toporcer MB, Kantor GR, Benedetto AV. Multiple cutaneous reticulohistiocytomas (reticulohistiocytic granulomas). J Am Acad Dermatol 1991;25:948.
134. Purvis WE III, Helwig EB. Reticulohistiocytic granuloma ("reticulohistiocytoma") of the skin. Am J Clin Pathol 1954;24:1005.
135. Goltz RW, Laymon CW. Multicentric reticulohistiocytosis of the skin and synovia. Arch Dermatol 1954;69:717.
136. Barrow MV, Holubar K. Multiple reticulohistiocytosis: A review of 33 patients. Medicine (Baltimore) 1969;48:287.
137. Campbell DA, Edwards NL. Multicentric reticulohistiocytosis: Systemic macrophage disorder. Bailliere's Clin Rheumatol 1991;5:301.
138. Torres L, Sanchez JL, Rivera A, Gonzâlez A. Progressive nodular histiocytosis. J Am Acad Dermatol 1993;29:278.
139. Zelger B, Cerio R, Soyer HP et al. Reticulohistiocytoma and multicentric reticulohistiocytosis: Histopathologic and immunophenotypic distinct entities. Am J Dermatopathol 1994;16:577.
140. Fortier-Beaulieu M, Thomine E, Boullie M-C et al. New electron microscopic findings in a case of multicentric reticulohistiocytosis: Long spacing collagen inclusions. Am J Dermatopathol 1993;15:587.
141. Salisbury JR, Hall PA, Williams HC et al. Multicentric reticulohistiocytosis: Detailed immunophenotyping confirms macrophage origin. Am J Surg Pathol 1990;14:687.
142. Perrin C, Lacour JP, Michiels JF et al. Multicentric reticulohistiocytosis. Immunohistological and ultrastructural study: A pathology of dendritic cell lineage. Am J Dermatopathol 1992;14:418.
143. Hunt SJ, Shin SS. Solitary reticulohistiocytoma in pregnancy: Immunohistochemical and ultrastructural study of a case with unusual immunophenotype. J Cutan Pathol 1995;22:177.
144. Taunton OD, Yeshurun D, Jarratt M. Progressive nodular histiocytoma. Arch Dermatol 1978;114:1505.
145. Bork K, Hoede N. Hereditary progressive mucinous histiocytosis in women. Arch Dermatol 1988;124:1225.
146. Bork K. Hereditary progressive mucinous histiocytosis: Immunohistochemical and ultrastructural studies in an additional family. Arch Dermatol 1994;130:1300.
147. Winkelmann RK, Muller SA. Generalized eruptive histiocytoma. Arch Dermatol 1963;88:586.
148. Caputo R, Alessi E, Allegra F. Generalized eruptive histiocytoma. Arch Dermatol 1981;117:216.
149. Ashworth J, Archard L, Woodrow D, Cream JJ. Multiple eruptive histiocytoma cutis in an atopic. Clin Exp Dermatol 1990;15:454.
150. Stables GI, MacKie RM. Generalized eruptive histiocytoma. Br J Dermatol 1992;126:196.
151. Umbert IJ, Winkelmann RK. Eruptive histiocytoma. J Am Acad Dermatol 1989;20:958.
152. Winkelmann RK, Kossard S, Fraga S. Eruptive histiocytoma of childhood. Arch Dermatol 1980;116:565.
153. Caputo R, Ermacora E, Gelmetti C et al. Generalized eruptive histiocytoma in children. J Am Acad Dermatol 1987;17:449.
154. Arnold M-L, Anton-Lamprecht I. Multiple eruptive cephalic histiocytomas in a case of T-cell lymphoma: A xanthomatous stage of benign cephalic histiocytosis in an adult patient? Am J Dermatopathol 1993;15:581.
155. Shimizu N, Ito M, Sato Y. Generalized eruptive histiocytoma: An ultrastructural study. J Cutan Pathol 1987;14:100.
156. Goerdt S, Bonsmann G, Sunderkötter C et al. A unique non-Langerhans' cell histiocytosis with some features of generalized eruptive histiocytoma. J Am Acad Dermatol 1994;31:322.
157. Gianotti F, Caputo R, Ermacora E. Singulière histiocytose infantile à cellules avec particules vermiformes intracytoplasmiques. Bull Soc Fr Dermatol Syphiligra 1971;78:232.
158. Gianotti F, Caputo R, Ermacora E, Gianni E. Benign cephalic histiocytosis. Arch Dermatol 1986;122:1038.
159. Larralde de Luna M, Glikin I, Golberg J et al. Benign cephalic histiocytosis: Report of four cases. Pediatr Dermatol 1989;6:198.
160. Goday JJ, Raton JA, Landa N et al. Benign cephalic histiocytosis: Study of a case. Clin Exp Dermatol 1993;18:280.
161. Peña-Penabad C, Unamuno P, Garcia-Silva J et al. Benign cephalic histiocytosis: Case report and literature review. Pediatr Dermatol 1994;11:164.
162. Gianotti R, Alessi E, Caputo R. Benign cephalic histiocytosis: A distinct entity or part of a wide spectrum of histiocytic proliferative disorders of children? Am J Dermatopathol 1993;15:315.
163. Zelger BG, Zelger B, Steiner H, Mikuz G. Solitary giant xanthogranuloma and benign cephalic histiocytosis: Variants of juvenile xanthogranuloma. Br J Dermatol 1995;133:598.

Lever's Histopathology of the Skin, eighth edition,
edited by David Elder et al. Lippincott–
Raven Publishers, Philadelphia © 1997.

CHAPTER 28

Pigmentary Disorders of the Skin

Richard L. Spielvogel and Gary R. Kantor

CONGENITAL DIFFUSE MELANOSIS

This condition, also termed *melanosis diffusa congenita*[1] or *generalized cutaneous melanosis*,[2,3] is thought to be recessively inherited, appears at or shortly after birth, and demonstrates progressive diffuse hyperpigmentation. The pigmentation is most intense on the abdomen and back and may be reticulate in the axillae and groin. Thin nails[3] and yellow-white hair[1] have been noted.

Histopathology. Increased melanization is seen in both the basalar and midepidermal keratinocytes, along with melanophages in the superficial dermis.

Histogenesis. On electron microscopic examination, Braun-Falco et al[2] noted increased numbers of single melanosomes in the keratinocytes and Klint et al[3] described dispersion of melanosomes throughout the keratinocyte cytoplasm.

RETICULATE PIGMENTARY ANOMALIES

Numerous cutaneous disorders have been documented that are characterized by hyperpigmentation that is clinically seen in a reticulate, retiform, or fishnet-like pattern. These disorders are unified by increased melanin in the epidermis and exclude post-inflammatory pigmentary alterations and conditions displaying reticulation secondary to vascular phenomena such as livedo reticularis.

Macular amyloidosis in the interscapular region may demonstrate a reticulate pattern.[4] Progressive cribriform and zosteriform hyperpigmentation begins in the second decade of life with reticulate pigmentation of the lower half of the trunk or thighs in a dermatomal distribution.[5] *Acropigmentation symmetrica of Dohi* (dyschromatosis symmetrica hereditaria) is a progressive autosomal dominant disorder that appears as hyperpigmented and hypopigmented macules on the dorsa of the hands and feet, progressing to cover the acral areas.[6] *Reticulate acropigmentation of Kitamura* presents as slightly depressed hyperpigmented macules on the dorsal hands and feet that evolve to a reticulate pattern as the individual ages. There is progression to involve the extremities, lateral neck, and occasionally the trunk and face. There has been an association with palmar and plantar pits.[7] Reticulate acropigmentation of Kitamura and *Dowling-Degos disease* (reticulate pigmented anomaly of the flexures) may appear together,[8] supporting the concept that they are different expressions of one disorder. In Dowling-Degos disease, a dominantly inherited dermatosis, heavily pigmented macules arranged in a reticulate pattern with a tendency to coalesce appear on flexural skin, axillae, lateral neck, inframammary and inguinal folds, antecubital and popliteal fossae, and intergluteal cleft, but may also be seen on the genitalia, inner thighs, chest, face, and abdomen.[9] Extensive areas of the skin may be affected. Pitted perioral scars, hyperpigmented comedones, hidradenitis suppurativa, multiple cysts and abscesses, keratoacanthomas and squamous cell carcinomas have been associated.

The *Naegeli-Franceschetti-Jadassohn syndrome* (Naegeli's reticular pigmented dermatosis) is an inherited disorder with reticulate pigmentation involving the neck and flexural skin along with perioral and periocular skin.[10] There are numerous associated findings including hypohidrosis, keratoderma, hypoplasia of fingerpad dermatoglyphics, and teeth and nail abnormalities. *Dermatopathia pigmentosa reticularis*[11] is similar to Naegeli's reticular pigmented dermatosis and the X-linked recessive syndrome of dyskeratosis congenita may also demonstrate reticulate hyperpigmentation.

Histopathology. The histologic findings in these conditions are quite similar. There is hyperpigmentation of the basalar keratinocytes with either a normal or slightly increased number of melanocytes. Reticulate acropigmentation of Kitamura and to a greater degree, Dowling-Degos disease, demonstrate digitated elongations of the hyperpigmented rete ridges with a tendency to spare the suprapapillary epithelium. In Dowling-Degos disease these thin, branching, heavily pigmented downward proliferations also involve the infundibula of follicles and in some instances horn cysts may be seen.[9] Although there is no preceding inflammatory dermatosis in dermatopathia pigmentosa reticularis, clumps of melanin-laden melanophages are seen in the papillary dermis in a patchy distribution without overlying epi-

R. L. Spielvogel: Department of Dermatology, Allegheny University of Health Sciences, Philadelphia, PA

G. R. Kantor: Department of Dermatology, Allegheny University of the Health Sciences, Philadelphia, PA

dermal hyperpigmentation.[12] Finally, reticulate macular amyloidosis demonstrates a patchy distribution of melanin within the amyloid globules, which are seen in the dermal papillae.

Histogenesis. These conditions are thought to be inherited, although the genes responsible for their expression have not been identified.

MELASMA

Melasma is an acquired, localized, usually symmetrical hyperpigmentation of the face occurring in women. The forehead, cheeks, upper lip, and chin are affected. It often is associated with pregnancy or the ingestion of oral contraceptives and is aggravated by sunlight.

Histopathology. An epidermal and a dermal type can be recognized, although frequently there is a combination of the two types. Light and histochemical (DOPA) studies reveal an increase in the number and activity of melanocytes that are engaged in increased formation, melanization, and transfer of pigment granules to keratinocytes and melanophages.[13]

ADDISON'S DISEASE

Addison's disease represents a hypofunction of the adrenal cortex and is characterized by progressive weakness, hypotension, and hyperpigmentation of the skin and oral mucous membranes. In some cases hyperpigmentation is the initial clinical manifestation.[14] The hyperpigmentation is generalized but is most pronounced on sun-exposed skin, at sites of pressure, and on the genitalia. Patchy oral mucosal pigmentation is often present.

Histopathology. The histologic findings simulate the normal findings in patients with naturally dark skin and are therefore not diagnostic. Increased amounts of melanin are seen in the basalar keratinocytes and often in the keratinocytes in the upper spinous layer. The number of melanocytes is not increased. Variable numbers of melanophages may be seen in the papillary dermis.[15]

Histogenesis. Most commonly, Addison's disease is the result of an idiopathic atrophy of the adrenal glands on an autoimmune basis, with subsequent inadequate production of cortisol and aldosterone.

Addison's disease is often associated with other autoimmune diseases. Other causes of adrenal hypofunction include damage of adrenal glands by tuberculosis, metastatic carcinoma, and deep fungal infections.

The hyperpigmentation in Addison's disease is caused by an increased release of melanocyte-stimulating hormone (MSH) from the pituitary gland. Adrenocorticotropic hormone (ACTH) and MSH synthesis and secretion in the pituitary gland are linked. The increased production of ACTH and MSH in Addison's disease is a compensatory, feedback-controlled response to low adrenal gland activity.

POSTINFLAMMATORY PIGMENTARY ALTERATION

Pigment alteration in the skin from a preceding inflammatory disorder can produce clinical hypopigmentation, hyperpigmentation, or both. It occurs commonly in processes that affect the dermal-epidermal interface such as fixed drug eruptions, lichen planus, benign lichenoid keratosis, and erythema multiforme. In some individuals the alteration can be dramatic, producing dark pigmentation resembling primary melanocytic lesions or marked hypopigmentation resembling vitiligo. Wood's light accentuates epidermal melanin and is useful as a clinical tool in defining the nature and extent of pigmentary alteration.

Histopathology. Epidermal melanin is increased in clinical hyperpigmentation and decreased in clinical hypopigmentation. In both clinical forms of pigmentary alteration, melanophages are present in the superficial dermis, along with a variably dense infiltrate of lymphohistiocytes around superficial blood vessels and in dermal papillae (Fig. 28-1).[16] Necrotic keratinocytes and coarse collagen bundles in the papillary dermis are occasionally seen.[16,17]

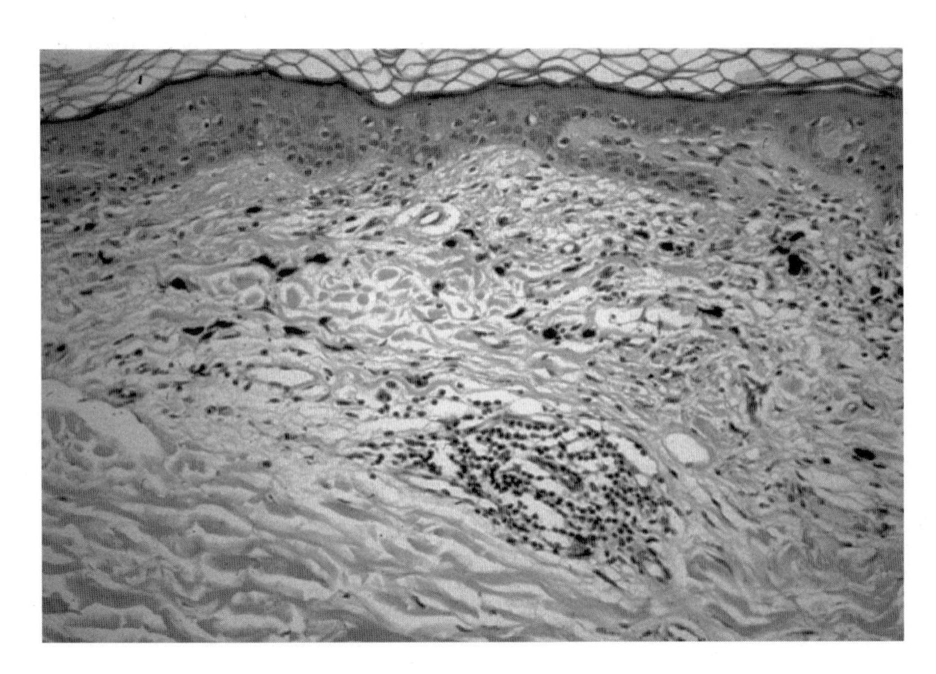

FIG. 28-1. Postinflammatory hyperpigmentation
There are numerous melanophages in the papillary dermis along with a mild perivascular lymphocytic infiltrate. The epidermis is normal.

BERLOQUE DERMATITIS AND PHYTOPHOTODERMATITIS

Localized hyperpigmented patches produced by furocoumarin-containing oil of bergamot found in perfumes have a distinctive clinical presentation. The patches assume drop-like shapes resembling pendants (French: *berloque*) and are usually located on the sides of the neck or retroauricular areas. Plants containing furocoumarins produce a postinflammatory hyperpigmentation and include lime, wild and cow parsnip, wild carrot, bergamot orange, and fig.[18] The dermatitis produced by celery results from a furocoumarin produced by a fungus infecting the celery.

Histopathology. Features identical to postinflammatory hyperpigmentation are found, including increased epidermal melanin and melanophages in the superficial dermis. Variable chronic inflammation is present.

CHEMICAL DEPIGMENTATION

Chemicals are capable of producing depigmentation resembling vitiligo. Hydroquinones and phenols are the most common causes and are found in bleaching agents, adhesives, cosmetics, photographic processing materials, and antioxidants used in the manufacture of rubber.[19,20] Depigmentation may also occur in body sites remote from chemical contact, presumably from systemic absorption or inhalation.

Histopathology. Features indistinguishable from vitiligo are found.[19] Decreased or absent melanocytes are present with a variable superficial perivascular lymphocytic infiltrate.

IDIOPATHIC GUTTATE HYPOMELANOSIS

This common disorder of unknown cause produces a few or numerous sharply circumscribed white macules predominantly on the sun-exposed extensor surfaces of the extremities. They measure 2 to 6 mm in diameter and, once formed, do not enlarge.[21]

Histopathology. In sections stained with the Fontana-Masson method, the melanin content in lesional skin is markedly reduced and there is either a significant reduction or an absence of dopa-positive melanocytes. The lesional borders are sharply demarcated. Within the hypomelanotic epidermis, the melanin granules are irregularly distributed.[22]

Histogenesis. On electron microscopic examination, the scattered residual melanocytes in lesional skin are round and less dendritic with fewer melanosomes that are incompletely melanized.[23]

PUVA-INDUCED PIGMENT ALTERATIONS

PUVA therapy consists of the oral ingestion or topical application of a furocoumarin-containing psoralen compound followed by patient exposure to high-intensity UVA radiation in a controlled-light-box setting. It is widely used for treating psoriasis and cutaneous T-cell lymphoma and less commonly used for a variety of other dermatoses including repigmentation therapy of vitiligo.

A spectrum of clinical and histologic changes are seen during and after PUVA therapy. Acutely, the phototoxic erythema peaks at 48 to 72 hours. Hyperpigmentation (tanning) is delayed for several days and is more pronounced and longer lasting than that induced by UVB exposure.[24] Prolonged therapy leads to photoaging with cutaneous atrophy, fine wrinkling, mottled hyperpigmentation and hypopigmentation, telangiectasias, and loss of elasticity.[25] Stellate lentigines or PUVA freckles often develop after prolonged therapy.[26] There is also a dose-dependent increase in the risk of squamous cell carcinoma,[27] especially in the genital areas.[28]

Histopathology. The histologic changes of PUVA-induced acute phytotoxicity are similar to sunburn with numerous pink apoptotic cells ("sunburn cells") scattered throughout the epidermis. Early in the therapeutic course, the melanocytes in the basalar epidermis and keratinocytes in the mid spinous layer are heavily melanized. Prolonged therapy leads to gradual flattening of the rete ridges, telangiectasias, increased papillary dermal acid mucopolysaccharide deposition, thinning and basophilic degeneration of elastic fibers, and hyperplasia and fragmentation of elastic fibers.[29] Hyperpigmented skin without other clinical changes frequently demonstrates small foci of keratinocytic nuclear atypia and loss of the normal maturation pattern.[30] Actinic keratoses, Bowen's disease, and squamous cell carcinomas may develop. PUVA freckles or lentigines show increased numbers of melanocytes and elongation of the rete ridges with focal atypical melanocytes.[31]

Histogenesis. On election microscopy melanosomes are diffusely distributed throughout the epidermis.[32] There is basement membrane thickening with focal dissolution. Elastic fibers in the dermis appear homogenized and fragmented.[33] In the deep dermis there is reduplication of the basal layer of capillaries and increased pinocytosis of endothelial cells.[34]

ALBINISM

Albinism is a heritable disorder causing a generalized lack of pigmentation of the skin, hair, and eyes. Involvement of the eyes only is called ocular albinism and is X-linked recessive. Oculocutaneous albinism (OCA) affects both eyes and skin and is autosomal recessive.

There are at least 10 types of OCA based on the degree of tyrosinase activity, hair color, and associated systemic disorders. Tyrosinase is a copper-containing enzyme responsible for the biosynthesis of melanin. Mutations to the tyrosinase gene result in inactivity of the enzyme (tyrosinase-negative OCA) and cause the most severe subtype.[35] Tyrosinase activity can be detected in plucked anagen hair bulbs by radioisotope assay[36] or by incubation in tyrosine solution and examination for pigment formation. In tyrosinase-positive OCA, synthesis of melanin pigment is reduced but present and patients acquire some melanin pigment in hair, skin, and eyes beginning in childhood. Hair color varies from yellow (yellow-mutant OCA) to red (rufous OCA) to platinum (pt OCA) to brown (brown OCA) to black (black-locks-albinism-deafness syndrome [BADS]). Associated systemic disorders include platelet defect and ceroid storage (Hermansky-Pudlak syndrome), defects in immunity (Chédiak-Higashi syndrome), and microphthalmia and mental retardation (Cross syndrome).

Prenatal diagnosis of OCA can be made by analysis of fetal

skin biopsy or the tyrosinase gene in fetal cells obtained by amniocentesis.[37]

Histopathology. Histologic examination shows the presence of basal melanocytes in skin and hair bulb; however, Fontana-Masson's stain fails to show any melanin. In patients with the tyrosinase-positive type of albinism, the epidermal melanocytes form pigment if sections of skin are incubated with dopa.

Histogenesis. Electron microscopic examination in albinism shows normally structured melanocytes in the epidermis.[38] In tyrosinase-positive albinism some melanosomes contain melanin, thus representing stage III and IV melanosomes. In contrast, in tyrosinase-negative albinism, the melanosomes contain no melanin and are present as stage I and II premelanosomes. Melanosome transfer to keratinocytes is not altered.

The tyrosinase gene has been localized in the long arm of chromosome 11.[39] Mutations in the protein-coding region of the gene are responsible for the defect. Tyrosinase-positive OCA has been mapped to chromosome 15 and mutations of this gene produce a wide range of clinical manifestations.[40] Molecular genetics has uncovered the gene mutations in some forms of albinism and will likely provide more accurate prognostic information and genetic counselling to families at risk.

PIEBALDISM (PATTERNED LEUKODERMA)

Piebaldism is an autosomally dominant disorder characterized by irregularly shaped depigmented patches that are present from birth and are associated in about 85% of the cases with a white forelock arising from a depigmented area in the center of the forehead. The depigmented areas have a predilection for the ventral skin, that is, the center of the face, the ventral chest, and the abdomen. Small islands of hyperpigmentation, 1 to 5 cm in diameter, are present, usually within the depigmented areas. The condition used to be called partial albinism, but this term is no longer used because of the difference in pathogenesis between oculocutaneous albinism and piebaldism.

A variant of piebaldism is *Klein-Waardenburg syndrome*, also dominantly inherited, in which one observes lateral displacement of the inner canthi of the eyes, heterochromia of the irides, and congenital deafness. About half of the patients have a white forelock, and about 12% have patches of depigmentation from birth.

Histopathology. The depigmented skin and hair usually have no melanocytes.[41] Also, hair from the white forelock does not show darkening of the hair bulb on incubation in tyrosinase solution. In some cases forelock epidermis may show a few melanocytes that are dopa positive.[42]

Histogenesis. Electron microscopic examination of the depigmented skin usually reveals a complete absence of melanocytes.[42] In contrast, Langerhans' cells are normal in appearance and distribution. In some instances only, an occasional melanocyte is seen with unmelanized ellipsoidal or spherical melanosomes. Electron microscopy of plucked forelock hair reveals absence of melanin in the cortex, cuticle, and inner root sheath.[42] The small hyperpigmented islands show many abnormal spherical, granular melanosomes.

A mutation of the gene that encodes melanocytic migration into the hair follicle and epidermis in affected areas of the body during embryonic development has been implicated.[39]

VITILIGO

Vitiligo is an acquired, disfiguring, patchy, total loss of skin pigment. Stable patches often have an irregular border but are sharply demarcated from the surrounding skin. There may be surrounding hyperpigmented skin. In expanding lesions, there may rarely be a slight rim of erythema at the border and a thin zone of transitory partial depigmentation. Hairs in patches of vitiligo usually become white. The scalp and eyelashes are rarely affected. In generalized vitiligo, the face, upper trunk, dorsal hands, periorificial areas, and the genitals are most commonly affected. Localized disease includes a linear, segmented pattern. There is a strong familial association.

In *Vogt-Koyanagi-Harada syndrome*, an aseptic meningitis is often the initial symptom, followed by uveitis and dysacousia. Patches of vitiligo involving the skin and frequently also the eyelashes and scalp develop. There is often an association with alopecia areata.

Histopathology. The central process in vitiligo is the destruction of melanocytes at the dermo–epidermal junction. With silver stains or the dopa reaction, well-established lesions of vitiligo are totally devoid of melanocytes. The periphery of expanding lesions that are hypopigmented rather than completely depigmented still show a few dopa-positive melanocytes and some melanin granules in the basal layer.[43] In the outer border of patches of vitiligo, melanocytes are often prominent and demonstrate long dendritic processes filled with melanin granules. Rarely, a superficial perivascular and somewhat lichenoid mononuclear cell infiltrate is observed at the border of the depigmented areas. Focal areas of vacuolar change at the dermal-epidermal junction in association with a mild mononuclear cell infiltrate have been seen in the normal-appearing skin adjacent to vitiliginous areas.[44,45]

Histogenesis. Electron microscopic studies[45,46] and immunohistochemistry studies using a panel of 17 monoclonal antibodies directed against melanocytes[47] confirm the complete absence of melanocytes in areas of stable vitiligo (Fig. 28-2). In the hypopigmented zone of expanding lesions, most melanocytes show signs of degeneration. Some studies have demonstrated peripheral damage to keratinocytes and melanocytes, suggesting that a cytoxic agent, possibly an auto antibody, is directed against these cells.[48] A combination of hair follicle split-dopa stains and hair follicle split-scanning electron microscopy demonstrated inactive, dopa-negative melanocytes in the outer root sheaths of normal hair follicles. These inactive melanocytes are also seen in the outer root sheaths of hair follicle from vitiliginous patches. Treatment of vitiligo stimulated these inactive melanocytes in the middle and lower parts of the outer root sheaths to divide, proliferate, and migrate upward to the dermal-epidermal junction of overlying skin. Melanocytes then radiate to form the pigmented islands clinically visible in repigmented lesions.[49,50]

Autoimmune mechanisms with an underlying genetic predisposition are the most likely cause of vitiligo, although neurohumoral, autocytotoxicity, and exogenous chemical exposure are alternative theories or contributing mechanisms. Antibodies to melanocytes have been found by immunoprecipitation in the sera of patients with vitiligo but not in normal sera.[51] Also, sera from patients with vitiligo causes damage to melanocytes in cell cultures, suggesting that the antibodies present in these sera are involved in the pathogenesis of vitiligo.[52] Vitiligo patients also

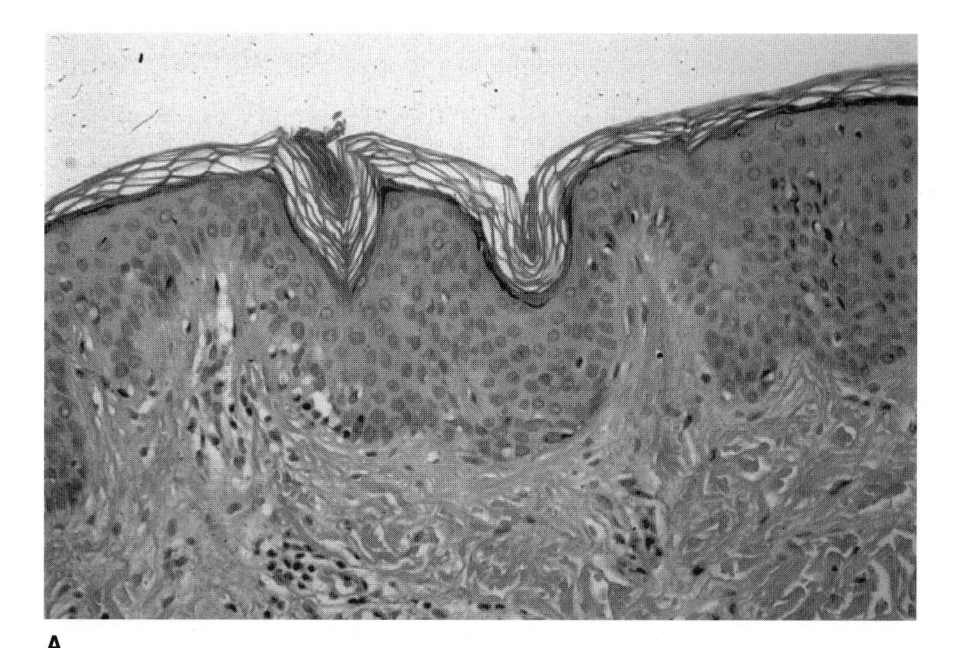

A

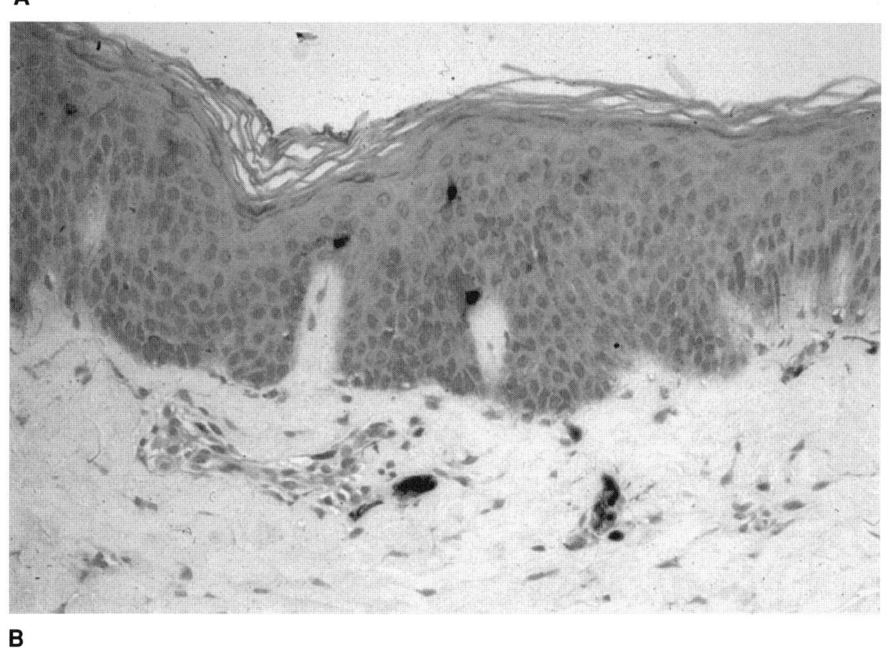

B

FIG. 28-2. Vitiligo
(**A**) There is a total loss of melanocytes in the depigmented skin near the border of this patch. (**B**) S-100 protein immunoperoxidase staining confirms the loss of melanocytes although Langerhans' and dermal dendritic cells stain positively.

have an increased incidence of antibodies against adrenal and thyroid cells, thyroglobulin, gastric parietal cells, and pancreatic islet cells. Although the epidermal density of Langerhans' cells is normal in vitiligo,[53] contact sensitivity reactions to dinitrochlorobenzene are weaker in vitiligo than in the adjacent uninvolved skin, suggesting a possible functional impairment of Langerhans' cells in the lesions of vitiligo.[54] T cells expressing a cutaneous lymphocyte-associated antigen typical of skin-homing T cells are present at the edge of vitiligo patches. These findings are consistent with a hypothesis that lesional T cells rather than circulating antimelanocytic antibody may be responsible for the patchy destruction of cutaneous melanocytes in vitiligo.[55] Other studies have shown more striking aberrations of T-cell subtypes in active areas of vitiligo than in static patches of vitiligo.[56]

Additional evidence for an autoimmune phenomenon includes the occasional coexistence of vitiligo and idiopathic uveitis[57] and the frequent presence of vitiligo in the Vogt-Koyanagi-Harada syndrome.

Finally, patients with metastatic melanoma may develop vitiligo, which portends a slightly longer survival and suggests an immunologic mechanism.[58]

CHÉDIAK-HIGASHI SYNDROME

The Chédiak-Higashi syndrome is a rare autosomally recessive disorder characterized by cutaneous, ocular, neurologic, and hematologic abnormalities. There is a greatly increased susceptibility to bacterial infections and a unique "accelerated phase" that often leads to death.[59] The accelerated phase is manifested by fever, jaundice, hepatosplenomegaly, lymphadenopathy, pancytopenia, and widespread lymphohistiocytic organ infiltrates. Giant lysosomal granules in the cytoplasm of circulating white blood cells are typical for the syndrome.

The Chédiak-Higashi syndrome is a subtype of oculocutaneous albinism (see earlier), and patients demonstrate fair skin with susceptibility to severe sunburn, silvery colored hair, and pale irides with photophobia and nystagmus. Severe and recurrent infections of the respiratory tract and skin are common.

Histopathology. Light microscopic features of skin sections show normal findings.[60] Fontana-Masson's stain shows sparse melanin granules, some of which are grouped and others of which are larger than normal.[60] Similar large, irregularly shaped melanin granules are scattered in the upper dermis within melanophages. Hair shafts also demonstrate abnormal aggregates of melanin.[61]

The giant lysosomal granules can be demonstrated in peripheral blood, in skin (melanocytes or Langerhans' cells), and other organs. A blood smear stained with Giemsa or Wright's stain shows the granules are azurophilic. They are found in all white blood cell lines but are most easily seen in neutrophils.

Histogenesis. Electron microscopic examination reveals within melanocytes giant melanosomes of irregular shape surrounded by a limiting membrane. They further increase in size by fusing with other giant particles. Within the giant melanosomes, one observes a granular matrix and filaments showing periodicity and varying degrees of pigmentation. The largest melanosomes show signs of degeneration leading to vacuolization and the formation of residual bodies. In addition, normal melanosomes are present in the melanocytes and are transferred to keratinocytes; however, they are packaged into abnormally large lysosomes. Similar abnormally large, membrane-bound lysosomes are found in the hair. The giant melanosomes in melanocytes and the giant lysosomes in keratinocytes form because of a defect in membrane or microtubule function. Hypopigmentation occurs because melanosomes within keratinocytes are found within a relatively few large lysosomes rather than being dispersed in the cell cytoplasm.

The giant granules in the cytoplasm of white blood cells develop by the fusion of primary lysosomes with one another and with cytoplasmic material. Even though microorganisms are phagocytized into phagocytic vacuoles in a normal fashion, their intracellular killing is delayed because of the unavailability of primary lysosomes to discharge their bacterial enzymes into the phagocytic vacuoles. Also, cathepsin G, a potent antimicrobial protease in neutrophils, is absent in Chédiak-Higashi syndrome.

Prenatal diagnosis of Chédiak-Higashi syndrome may be made by fetal blood sampling or study of amniotic fluid or chorionic villus cells.[62]

REFERENCES

1. Braun-Falco O, Burg G, Selzle D et al. Melanosis diffusa congenita. Hautarzt 1980;31:324.
2. Platin P, Sassolas B, Garanov J, Guillet G. What is your diagnosis? Generalized cutaneous melanosis. Ann Dermatol Venereol 1990;117: 739.
3. Klint A, Oomen C, Geerts ML, Brevillard F. Congenital diffuse melanosis. Ann Dermatol Venereol 1987;114:11.
4. Brownstein MH, Hashimoto K. Macular amyloidosis. Arch Dermatol 1972;106:50.
5. Rower JM, Carr RD, Lowney ED. Progressive cribriform and zosteriform hyperpigmentation. Arch Dermatol 1978;114:98.
6. Kim NI, Park SY, Youn JI, Lim SD. Dyschromatosis symmetrica hereditaria affecting two families. Korean J Dermatol 1980;18:585.
7. Kanwar AJ, Kaur S, Rajagopalan M. Reticulate acropigmentation of Kitamura. Int J Dermatol 1990;29:219.
8. Tappero JW, Kershenovich J, Berger TG. Combined acral and flexural reticulate pigmentary anomaly. Arch Dermatol 1992;128:1411.
9. Wilson Jones E, Grice K. Reticulate pigmented anomaly of the flexures: Dowling-Degos disease, a new genodermatosis. Arch Dermatol 1978;114:1150.
10. Whiting DA. Naegeli's reticular pigmented dermatosis. Br J Dermatol 1971;85:71.
11. Maso MJ, Schwartz RA, Lambert C. Dermatopathia pigmentosa reticularis. Arch Dermatol 1990;126:935.
12. Rycroft RG, Calnan CD, Allenby CF. Dermatopathia pigmentosa reticularis. Clin Exp Dermatol 1977;2:39.
13. Sanchez NP, Pathuk MA, Sato S et al. Melasma: A clinical, light microscopic, ultrastructural and immunofluorescence study. J Am Acad Dermatol 1981;4:698.
14. Clerkin EP, Sayegh S. Melanosis as the initial symptom of Addison's disease. Lahey Clin Found Bull 1966;15:173.
15. Montgomery H, O'Leary PA. Pigmentation of the skin in Addison's disease, acanthosis nigricans, and hemochromatosis. Arch Dermatol 1930;21:970.
16. Ackerman AB. Histologic diagnosis of inflammatory skin diseases. Philadelphia: Lea & Febiger, 1978;178.
17. Murphy GF. Dermatopathology: A practical guide to common disorders. Philadelphia: Saunders, 1995;322.
18. Storer JG, Rasmussen JE. Plant dermatitis. J Am Acad Dermatol 1983; 9:1.
19. Fisher AA. Differential diagnosis of idiopathic vitiligo: Part III. Occupational leukoderma. Cutis 1994;53:278.
20. Fisher AA. Differential diagnosis of idiopathic vitiligo from contact leukoderma: Part II. Leukoderma due to cosmetics and bleaching creams. Cutis 1994;53:232.
21. Cummings KI, Cottel WI. Idiopathic guttate hypomelanosis. Arch Dermatol 1966;93:184.
22. Ortonne JP, Perrot H. Idiopathic guttate hypomelanosis: Ultrastructural study. Arch Dermatol 1980;116:664.
23. Ploysangam T, Dee-Ananlap S, Suvanprakorn P. Treatment of idiopathic guttate hypomelanosis with liquid nitrogen: Light and electron microscopic studies. J Am Acad Dermatol 1990;23:681.
24. Abel EA. Acute and chronic side effects of PUVA therapy: Clinical and histologic changes. In Abel EA, ed. Photochemotherapy in psoriasis. New York:Igaku-Shoin, 1992.
25. Pfau RG, Hood AF, Morrison WC. Photoaging: The role of UVB, solar-simulated UVB, visible, and psoralen UVA radiation. Br J Dermatol 1986;114:318.
26. Miller RA. Psoralens and UVA-indicated stellate hyperpigmented freckling. Arch Dermatol 1982;118:619.
27. Stern RS, Laird N, Melski J et al. Cutaneous squamous cell carcinoma in patients treated with PUVA. N Engl J Med 1984;310:1156.
28. Stern RS and members of the Photo Chemotherapy Follow-up Study. Genital tumors among men with psoriasis exposed to psoralens and ultraviolet A radiation (PUVA) and ultraviolet B radiation. N Engl J Med 1990;322:1093.
29. Bergfeld WF. Histologic changes in skin after photo chemotherapy. Cutis 1977;20:504.
30. Abel EA, Cox AJ, Farber EM. Epidermal dystrophy and actinic keratoses in psoriasis patients following oral psoralen photo chemotherapy (PUVA). J Am Acad Dermatol 1982;7:333.
31. Rhodes AR, Harrist TJ, Momtaz TK. The PUVA-induced pigmented macule: A lentiginous proliferation of large, sometimes cytologically atypical melanocytes. J Am Acad Dermatol 1983;9:47.
32. Hashimoto K. Psoralen-UVA treated psoriatic lesions: Ultrastructural changes. Arch Dermatol 1978;114:711.

33. Zelickson AS, Mottaz JH, Zelickson BD et al. Elastic tissue changes in skin following PUVA therapy. J Am Acad Dermatol 1980;3:186.
34. Torras H, Bombi JA. PUVA therapy: Long term degenerative effects. II. Study of ultrastructural changes in the skin induced by PUVA therapy. Med Cutan Ibero Lat Am 1987;15:179.
35. Spritz RA, Strunk KM, Biebel LB, King RA. Detection of mutations in the tyrosinase gene in a patient with type IA oculocutaneous albinism. N Engl J Med 1990;322;1724.
36. King RA, Olds DP. Hair bulb tyrosinase activity in oculocutaneous albinism: Suggestions for pathway control and block location. Am J Med Genet 1985;20:49.
37. Shimizu H, Nizeki H, Suzumori K et al. Prenatal diagnosis of oculocutaneous albinism by analysis of the fetal tyrosinase gene. J Invest Dermatol 1994;103:104.
38. Hishida H. Electron microscopic studies of melanosomes in oculo-cutaneous albinism. Jpn J Dermatol [A] 1973;83:119.
39. Tomita Y. The molecular genetics of albinism and piebaldism. Arch Dermatol 1994;130:355.
40. Lee S, Nicholls RD, Bundey S et al. Mutations of the P gene in oculocutaneous albinism, ocular albinism, and Prader-Willi syndrome plus albinism. N Engl J Med 1994;330:529.
41. Winship I, Young K, Martell R. Piebaldism: An autonomous autosomal dominant entity. Clin Genet 1991;39:330.
42. Chang T, McGrae JD, Hashimoto K. Ultrastructural study of two patients with both piebaldism and neurofibromatosis I. Pediatr Dermatol 1993;10:224.
43. Brown J, Winkelmann RK, Wolfe K. Langerhans' cells in vitiligo. J Invest Dermatol 1967;49:386.
44. Moellmann G, Klein-Angerer S, Scollay DA et al. Extra cellular granular material and degeneration of keratinocytes in the normally pigmented epidermis of patients with vitiligo. J Invest Dermatol 1982;79: 321.
45. Galadari E, Mehregan AH, Hashimoto K. Ultrastructural study of vitiligo. Int J Dermatol 1993;32:269.
46. Birbeck MS, Breathnach AS, Everall JD. An electron microscope study of basal melanocytes and high-level clear cells (Langerhans' cells) in vitiligo. J Invest Dermatol 1961;37:51.
47. LePoole IC, van den Wijngaard RM, Westerhof W et al. Presence or absence of melanocytes in vitiligo lesions: An immunohistochemical investigation. J Invest Dermatol 1993;100:816.
48. Bhawan J, Bhutani LK. Keratinocyte damage in vitiligo. J Cutan Pathol 1983;10:207.
49. Cui J, Shen LY, Wang GC. Role of hair follicles in the repigmentation of vitiligo. J Invest Dermatol 1991;97:410.
50. Arrunategui A, Arroyo C, Garcia L et al. Melanocyte reservoir in vitiligo. Int J Dermatol 1994;33:484.
51. Naughton GK, Eisinger M, Bystryn J. Detection of antibodies to melanocytes in vitiligo by specific immunoprecipitation. J Invest Dermatol 1983;81:540.
52. Norris DA, Kissinger RM, Naughton GM et al. Evidence for immunologic mechanisms in human vitiligo: Patients' sera induce damage to human melanocytes in vitro. J Invest Dermatol 1988;90:783.
53. Claudy AL, Rouchouse B. Langerhans' cells and vitiligo: Quantitative study of T6 and HLA-DR antigen-expressing cells. Acta Derm Venereol (Stockh) 1984;64:334.
54. Uehara M, Myauchi H, Tanaka S. Diminished contact sensitivity response in vitiliginous skin. Arch Dermatol 1984;120:195.
55. Badri AM, Todd PM, Garioch JJ et al. An immunohistological study of cutaneous lymphocytes in vitiligo. J Pathol 1993;170:149.
56. Mozzanica N, Frigerio V, Finzi AF et al. T-cell subpopulations in vitiligo: A chronobiologic study. J Am Acad Dermatol 1990;22:223.
57. Nordlund JJ, Taylor NT, Albert DM et al. The prevalence of vitiligo and poliosis in patients with uveitis. J Am Acad Dermatol 1981;4:528.
58. Nordlund JJ, Kirkwood JM, Forget BM et al. Vitiligo in patients with metastatic melanoma: A good prognostic sign. J Am Acad Dermatol 1983;9:689.
59. Barak Y, Nir E. Chédiak-Higashi syndrome. Am J Pediatr Hematol Oncol 1987;9:42.
60. Carillo-Farga J, Gutierrez-Palomera G, Ruiz-Maldonado R et al. Giant cytoplasmic granules in Langerhans' cells of Chédiak-Higashi syndrome. Am J Dermatopathol 1990;12:81.
61. Anderson LL, Paller AS, Malpass D et al. Chédiak-Higashi syndrome in a black child. Pediatr Dermatol 1992;9:31.
62. Diukman R, Tanigawara A, Cowan MJ, Golbus MS. Prenatal diagnosis of Chédiak-Higashi syndrome. Prenat Diagn 1992;12:877.

Lever's Histopathology of the Skin, eighth edition,
edited by David Elder et al. Lippincott–
Raven Publishers, Philadelphia © 1997.

CHAPTER 29

Benign Pigmented Lesions and Malignant Melanoma

David Elder and Rosalie Elenitsas

Melanocytic proliferations are composed of one or more of three types of cells: melanocytes, nevus cells, and melanoma cells, each of which may be located in the epidermis or in the dermis. Melanocytes are solitary dendritic cells that generally are separated from one another by other cells (keratinocytes or fibroblasts). Nevus cells and melanoma cells differ from melanocytes in that they have undergone proliferation to lie in contiguity with their neighbors. Melanoma cells, in turn, acquire nuclear abnormalities constituting "uniform cytologic atypia." The lesions may be benign or malignant. Malignant tumors of melanocytes are called malignant melanomas. Although "melanoma" was at one time taken to include benign pigmented lesions, this term is now considered to be synonymous with "malignant melanoma," and the two terms will be used interchangeably in this chapter. Major morphological differences among melanocytes, nevus cells, and melanoma cells are summarized in Table 29-1.

BENIGN PIGMENTED LESIONS

Benign pigmented lesions composed of epidermal melanocytes include freckles, solar lentigines ("actinic" or, formerly, senile lentigo), the melanotic macules of Albright's syndrome, and Becker's melanosis. The café-au-lait patches of neurofibromatosis have been described elsewhere. Benign pigmented lesions derived from dermal melanocytes include the Mongolian spot, the nevi of Ota and of Ito, and the blue nevus. Benign tumors of nevus cells are called melanocytic nevi. They can be divided into junctional nevi, inlcuding lentigo simplex; compound nevi; and intradermal nevi. There are special variants of melanocytic nevi, the more important of which include the Spitz nevus, the pigmented spindle cell nevus, the congenital melanocytic nevus, and the dysplastic nevus.

D. Elder: Department of Pathology and Laboratory Medicine, University of Pennsylvania, Philadelphia, PA
R. Elenitsas: Department of Dermatology, University of Pennsylvania, Philadelphia, PA

Dermal Melanocytoses and Hamartomas

Mongolian Spot

The typical Mongolian spot occurs in the sacrococcygeal region as a uniformly blue discoloration resembling a bruise. It consists of a noninfiltrated, round or ovoid, rather ill-defined patch of varying size. It is found very frequently in Mongoloid and Negroid infants, but it also occurs occasionally in Caucasoid infants. It is present at birth and usually disappears spontaneously within 3 to 4 years.[1]

Occasionally, Mongolian spots occur outside the lumbosacral region as aberrant Mongolian spots, such as on the middle or upper part of the back; they may then be multiple and bilateral and persist. Extensive and persistent Mongolian spots are commonly observed in patients with bilateral nevus of Ota.[2]

Histopathology. In the Mongolian spot, the dermis shows in its lower half or two-thirds greatly elongated, slender, often slightly wavy dendritic cells containing melanin granules. These cells, which are present in a low concentration, lie widely scattered between the collagen bundles and, like the collagen bundles, generally lie parallel to the skin surface. Even though they are melanocytes, these cells show little or no increase in their pigment content on incubation with dopa compared with unincubated sections, probably as a result of complete utilization or down-regulation of the melanogenic enzymes in the process of forming melanin. No melanophages are observed.

Nevi of Ota and Ito and Dermal Melanocyte Hamartoma

Nevi of Ota and Ito and dermal melanocyte hamartoma are types of dermal melanocytosis that differ from the Mongolian spot by usually having a speckled rather than a uniform blue appearance and by showing a greater concentration of dermal melanocytes, with location in the upper rather than the lower portion of the dermis.[3]

The *nevus of Ota* represents a usually unilateral discoloration of the face composed of blue and brown, partially confluent macular lesions. The periorbital region, temple, forehead, malar

TABLE 29-1. *Morphological differences among melanocytes, nevus cells, and melanoma cells*

Melanocytes	Nevus cells	Melanoma cells
Cytoplasm is dendritic.	Cytoplasm is rounded or spindle-shaped.	Cytoplasm is rounded or spindle-shaped.
Cells are solitary.	Cells are arranged in clusters.	Cells are arranged in clusters and large sheets.
Nuclei are small and regular.	Nuclei of most cells are small and regular.	Most nuclei are large, irregular, and hyperchromatic.
Mitoses are rare.	Mitoses are rare.	Mitoses are usually present.

area, and nose are usually involved. Because of this usual distribution, Ota has called the lesion nevus fuscocaeruleus ophthalmomaxillaris. There is frequently also a patchy blue discoloration of the sclera of the ipsilateral eye and occasionally also of the conjunctiva, cornea, and retina.[4] In some instances, the oral and nasal mucosae are similarly affected.[5] In about 10% of the cases, the lesions of the nevus of Ota are bilateral rather than unilateral. They may be present at birth and may also appear during the first year of life or during adolescence, but they rarely occur in childhood. They have a tendency toward gradual extension. Malignant change in the cutaneous lesions of a nevus of Ota is extremely rare.

In the nevus of Ota, the involved areas of the skin show a brown to slate-blue even or mottled discoloration, usually without any infiltration. Occasionally, some areas are slightly raised. In some patients, discrete nodules varying in size from a few millimeters to a few centimeters and having the appearance of blue nevi are found within the areas of discoloration. Persistent Mongolian spots are quite common in association with the nevus of Ota. Extensive Mongolian spots are always found in bilateral cases of nevus of Ota.[6]

The *nevus of Ito* differs from the nevus of Ota by its location in the supraclavicular, scapular, and deltoid regions. It may occur alone or in association with an ipsilateral or bilateral nevus of Ota.[5] Like the nevus of Ota, it has a mottled, macular appearance.

In the *dermal melanocyte hamartoma,* a single, very extensive area of gray-blue pigmentation may be present from the time of birth.[3] The involvement may be nearly generalized.[7] In other instances, there are several coalescing blue macules that have gradually extended within a circumscribed area from the time of childhood.[8]

Histopathology. The noninfiltrated areas of the nevus of Ota, as well as the nevus of Ito and the dermal melanocyte hamartoma, show, like the Mongolian spot, elongated, dendritic melanocytes scattered among the collagen bundles. However, in these three forms of dermal melanocytosis, the melanocytes generally are more numerous and more superficially located than in the Mongolian spot. Although most of the fusiform melanocytes lie in the upper third of the reticular dermis, melanocytes may also occur in the papillary layer, and may extend as far down as the subcutaneous tissue. Melanophages are observed in only a few lesions.[3,5]

Slightly raised and infiltrated areas show a larger number of elongated, dendritic melanocytes than do noninfiltrated areas, thus approaching the histologic picture of a blue nevus, and nodular areas are indistinguishable histologically from a blue nevus.[9]

Malignant changes in lesions of nevus of Ota have been reported in a handful of cases. The histologic appearance of the tumors is typically that of a malignant or cellular blue nevus.[10,11] In a few instances, a primary melanoma of the choroid, iris, orbit, or brain has developed in patients with a nevus of Ota involving an eye.[12]

Histogenesis of Dermal Melanocytoses

The blue color of the dermal melanocytoses depends on the phenomenon in which light passing through the skin is scattered as it strikes dark particles, such as melanin. Owing to the Tyndall effect, the colors of light that have longer wavelengths such as red, orange, and yellow, tend to be less scattered and therefore continue to travel in a forward direction, but the colors of shorter wavelength, such as blue, indigo, and violet, are scattered to the side and backward to the skin surface. This phenomenon is also responsible for the distinctive color of blue nevi.

The Mongolian spot is a result of the delayed disappearance of dermal melanocytes. Under electron microscopy, the dermal melanocytes can be seen to contain numerous fully melanized melanosomes. Only a few melanocytes show premelanosomes as evidence of ongoing melanoneogenesis.[1]

Because the concentration of melanocytes in the nevi of Ota and Ito and in the dermal melanocyte hamartoma is greater than in the Mongolian spot, it has been suggested that these lesions are nevoid or hamartomatous, analogous to the blue nevus.[3] Although the lesional cells are considered to be melanocytes, the dopa reaction may be negative, probably as a result of all melanogenic enzyme having been consumed in heavily pigmented melanocytes.[3]

Blue Nevi

Blue nevi generally occur on the skin, although, in rare instances, they have been observed in mucous membranes.[13] On the skin, three types of blue nevi are recognized: the common blue nevus, the cellular blue nevus, and the combined nevus.

Histologically, the common feature of blue nevi is the presence of pigmented spindle and dendritic melanocytes in a focal area of the reticular dermis, associated, unlike the dermal melanocytoses, with alterations in the dermal collagen architecture.

Common Blue Nevus

The *common blue nevus* occurs as a small, well-circumscribed, dome-shaped nodule of slate-blue or blue-black color.

The lesion rarely exceeds 1 cm in diameter. Common blue nevi are frequently found on or near the dorsa of the hands and feet. Usually, there is only one lesion, but there may be several. A rare manifestation is the plaque type of blue nevus, which shows within a circumscribed area numerous macules and papules. This type of lesion may be present at birth[14] or may appear later in life.[15] Malignant degeneration does not occur in the common blue nevus.

Histopathology. In the common blue nevus, the melanocytes have the same appearance as those in the Mongolian spot and in the nevus of Ota, but their density is much greater. Greatly elongated, slender, often slightly wavy melanocytes with long, occasionally branching dendritic processes lie grouped in irregular bundles in the dermis (Fig. 29-1). The bundles of cells may extend into the subcutaneous tissue or lie close to the epidermis. However, the epidermis is normal, except in the combined nevus (see later). The greatly elongated melanocytes lie predominantly with their long axes parallel to the epidermis. Most of

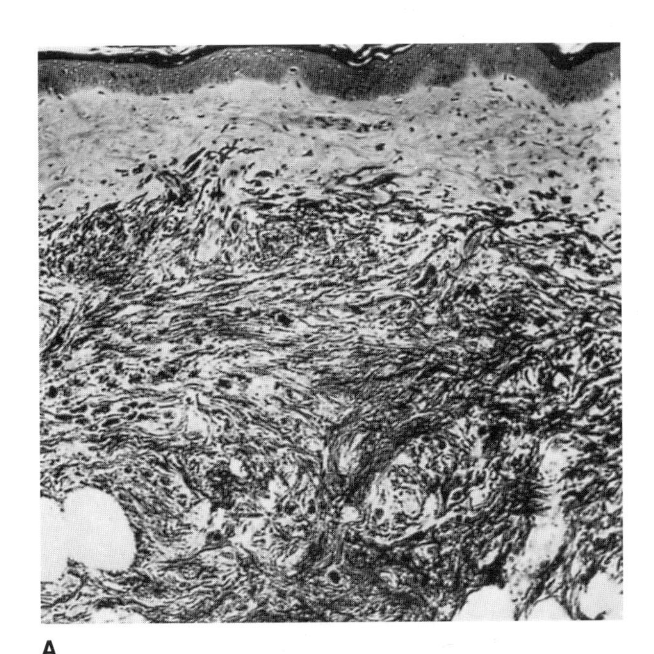

A

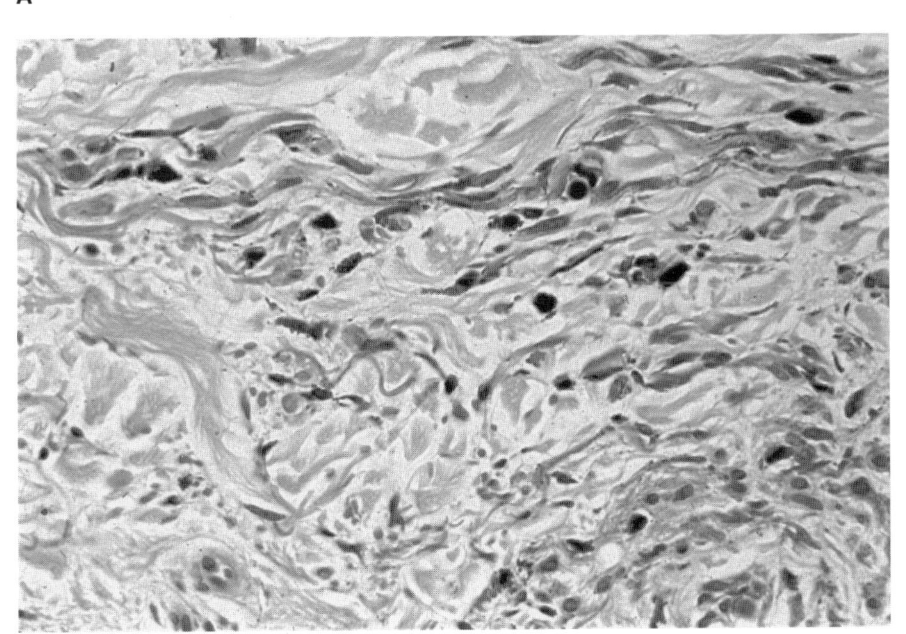

B

FIG. 29-1. Blue nevus, common type
(**A**) Low magnification. Numerous greatly elongated, slender, often slightly wavy melanocytes show dendritic processes and are filled with melanin. They lie grouped in irregular bundles in the lower dermis and in the subcutaneous fat. (**B**) Spindle-shaped or dendritic melanocytes are distributed among reticular dermis collagen bundles, which are often slightly thickened. Unlike the cells of most common or congenital nevi that involve the reticular dermis, the cells of blue nevi are heavily pigmented.

them are filled with numerous fine granules of melanin, often so completely that their nuclei cannot be seen. The melanin granules may also fill the long, often wavy, occasionally branching dendritic processes. Wavy fiber bundles similar to nerves may be present, indicative of Schwannian differentiation. Occasionally, lesional cells are seen in the perineurium of authentic nerves, a finding that is not indicative of malignancy.

Melanophages are frequently observed near the bundles of melanocytes. The melanophages differ from the melanocytes by being shorter and thicker, by showing no dendritic processes, and by containing larger granules. In contrast to the melanocytes, the melanophages are dopa-negative. The number of fibroblasts and the amount of collagen are often also increased, resulting in disruption of the normal architecture of the connective tissue.

Cellular Blue Nevus

The *cellular blue nevus* consists of a blue nodule that is usually larger than the common blue nevus. It generally measures 1 to 3 cm in diameter, but it may be larger. It shows either a smooth or an irregular surface. About half of all cellular blue nevi have been located over the buttocks or in the sacrococcygeal region.[13] Although rare, malignant degeneration of cellular blue nevi can occur (see section on Malignant Blue Nevus).

Histopathology. Areas of deeply pigmented dendritic melanocytes, as observed also in the common type of blue nevus, are admixed with cellular islands composed of closely aggregated, rather large spindle-shaped cells with ovoid nuclei and abundant pale cytoplasm often containing little or no melanin[1] (Fig. 29-2). Melanophages with abundant melanin may be present between the islands. The spindle-shaped lesional cells are occasionally pigmented, at least in some areas. The diagnosis of cellular blue nevus is generally easy in "biphasic" lesions with both dendritic and spindle-shaped cells, but it can be difficult in occasional lesions without dendritic cells and without melanin, which, however, often becomes apparent when a silver stain is used.

Larger islands composed of spindle-shaped cells may consist of many intersecting bundles of cells extending in various directions and resembling the storiform pattern observed in a neurofibroma.[16] In some of the intersecting bundles, the cells appear rounded, perhaps as a result of cross sectioning. Not infrequently, the cellular islands penetrate into the subcutaneous fat, often forming a bulbous expansion there that is highly characteristic of cellular blue nevi. If, in addition, the nuclei show pleomorphism, and if bizarre, atypical-appearing cells, including multinucleated giant cells, are present together with a surrounding inflammatory infiltrate, differentiation from a malignant blue nevus or a melanoma can be difficult. These "atypical" blue nevi have become recognized as a rare but distinct variant of cellular blue nevi.[17,18] Although most of these lesions have a benign course, a few have been locally aggressive or have metastasized at least to regional lymph nodes,[19] and a guarded prognosis is appropriate in the presence of more than a few mitoses (see section on Melanocytic Tumors of Uncertain Malignant Potential). The absence or scarcity of mitotic figures and the absence of areas of necrosis are evidence against a diagnosis of malignant blue nevus, and the presence of areas of

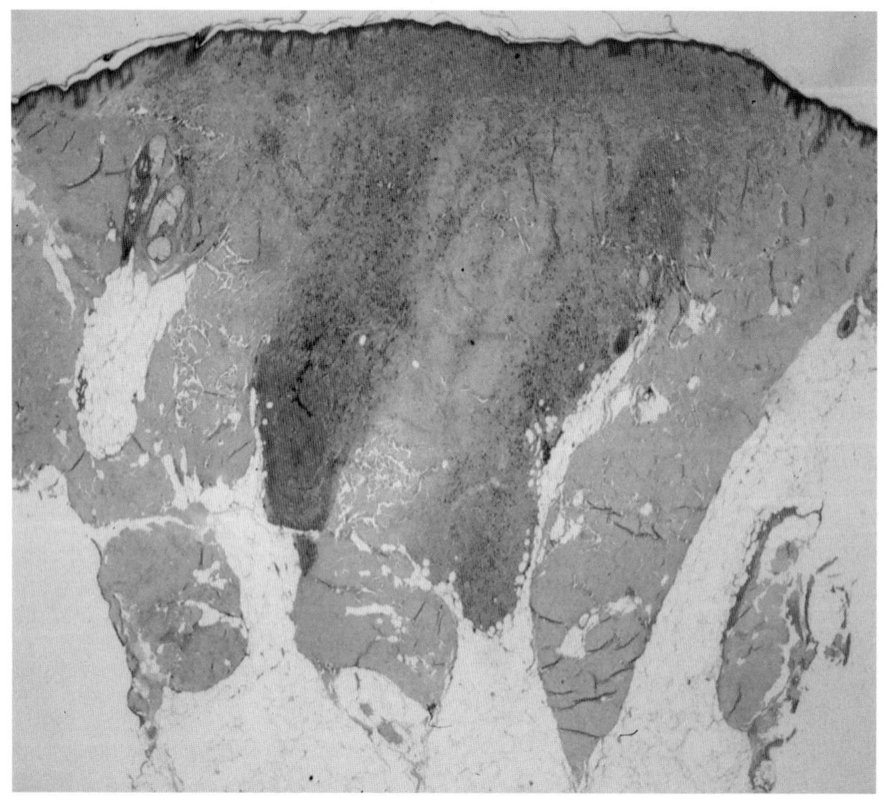

A

FIG. 29-2. Cellular blue nevus (**A**) Usually broader at the surface than at the base, the cellular blue nevus spans the reticular dermis, usually involving the superficial panniculus. Often there is a region of increased cellularity that may form a bulbous expansion at the base.

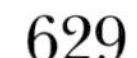

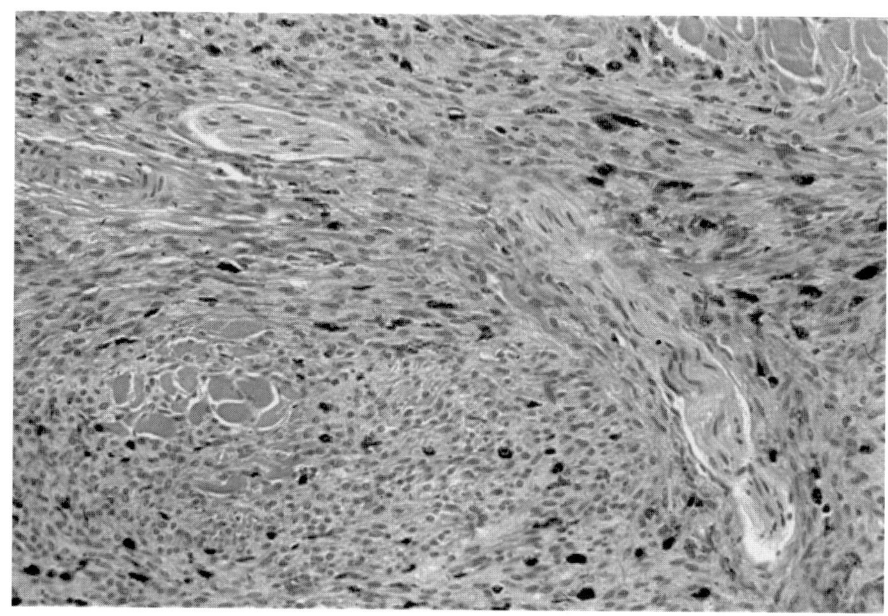

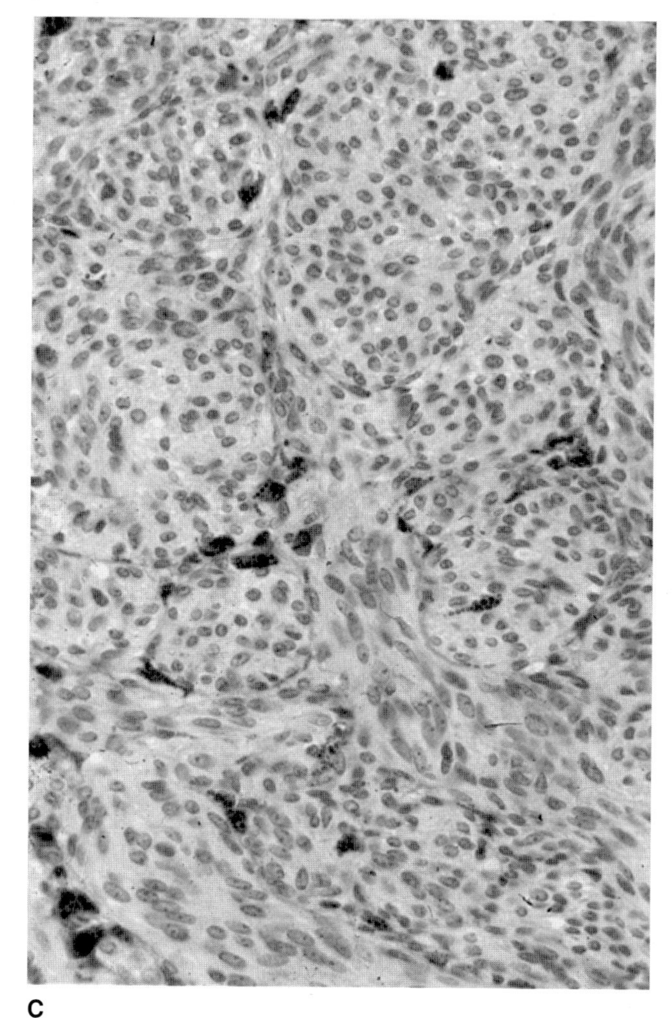

C

FIG. 29-2. *Continued*
(**B**)Spindle cells usually predominate in cellular blue nevi. They lie in contiguity with one another, unlike the cells of common blue nevi, most of which are separated from one another by collagen bundles. (**C**) The "mixed-biphasic" pattern is the most frequent in cellular blue nevi, with ovoid islands of polygonal cells with somewhat clear cytoplasm alternating with bundles of spindle cells, the latter often pigmented. Mitoses are very rare in most examples.

dendritic cells elsewhere in the tumor, as well as the lack of a characteristic intraepidermal component, speak against a diagnosis of melanoma.

In several instances in which cellular blue nevi were excised with regional lymph nodes under the mistaken diagnosis of melanoma, moderately pleomorphic cells of cellular nevus have been found in the regional lymph nodes, either in the marginal sinuses[13] or in the capsule.[20] It is sometimes assumed that these cells do not represent true metastases but were passively transported to the lymph nodes and lodged there as inert deposits. However, some examples of this phenomenon in our experience have shown high-grade uniform atypia, necrosis, and fairly numerous mitoses, apparently indicative of an active neoplasm.

Combined Nevus

The term *combined nevus* is applied to the association of a blue nevus with an overlying melanocytic nevus,[21] or to other combinations of benign nevi.[22] Clinically, combined nevi often present with a focal area of deep pigmentation.

Histopathology. In a combined nevus, one component is often a blue nevus that may be either a common or a cellular blue nevus. The other component may be an overlying nevus of the junctional, compound, intradermal or, rarely, Spitz nevus type.[23] Such lesions may simulate melanoma clinically, because of the appearance of a very darkly pigmented spot within a background nevus. Histologically, the pigmented spindle cells of the blue nevus component may give rise to suspicion, but mitoses and high-grade atypia are absent, and the pigmented cells often blend with the background nevus rather than displacing or destroying it. Further, it is extremely unusual for a melanoma to arise in the dermal component of a nevus in the absence of a characteristic intraepidermal component.

Histogenesis of Blue Nevi

There is general agreement that the cells of the common blue nevus are melanocytes, which may show evidence of Schwannian differentiation. This occasional resemblance to neural tumors had led in the past to suggestions of neural origin for blue nevi.[24] However, the lesional cells of blue nevi and their variants react positively with antibodies to the S-100 and HMB-45 antigens, the latter in this context being quite specific for melanocytic differentiation.[25] Also, melanosomes are resolved by electron microscopy (EM 1), and the electron microscopic dopa reaction indicates that the spindle-shaped cells of the cellular blue nevus have melanogenic potential.[26]

Freckles and Hyperpigmentations

By definition, a freckle (ephelid) is a small, flat, tan or brown lesion that histologically shows increased pigment in keratinocytes, but no increase in the number of melanocytes. Hyperpigmentations may be described as larger macular pigmented lesions that show hyperpigmentation of keratinocytes without melanocytic proliferation. Lentigines are macular hyperpigmentations that differ from freckles and hyperpigmentations in that the number of epidermal melanocytes is greater.

Ephelids (Freckles)

Freckles, or ephelids, are small, brown macules scattered over skin exposed to the sun. Exposure to the sun deepens the pigmentation of freckles, in contrast to lentigo simplex, whose already deep pigment does not change. Freckles, simple lentigines, and solar lentigines are difficult to distinguish from one another clinically, and are considered together in most clinical and epidemiological studies. Taken together, these lesions constitute a significant risk factor for the developmemt of melanoma.[27]

Histopathology. Freckles show hyperpigmentation of the basal cell layer, but in contrast to lentigo simplex, there is no elongation of the rete ridges and, by definition, no obvious increase in the concentration of melanocytes. In fact, in epidermal spreads of freckled skin, the number of dopa-positive melanocytes within the freckles may appear decreased on comparison with the adjacent epidermis. However, the melanocytes that are present may be larger, and they may show more numerous and longer dendritic processes than the melanocytes of the surrounding epidermis.

Histogenesis. Under electron microscopy, the melanocytes within freckles are found to be essentially similar to those of dark-skinned persons. Melanocytes of the surrounding epidermis, by contrast, show constitutionally few and minimally melanized melanosomes, many of which are rounded rather than elongated,[28] characteristic of the skin of individuals who have the fair-skinned phenotype, often associated with red hair and/or blue eyes, that is prone to freckles.[27]

Melanotic Macules of Albright's Syndrome

Albright's syndrome is characterized by usually unilateral polyostotic fibrous dysplasia, precocious puberty in females, and melanotic patches. The patches usually are large in size and few in number, are located on only one side of the midline, often on the same side as the bone lesions, and have a jagged, irregular border, like the "coast of Maine," in contrast to the smooth "coast of California" type of border of the café-au-lait patches of neurofibromatosis.

Histopathology. Except for hyperpigmentation of the basal layer, there is no abnormality, and both the number and the size of the melanocytes are normal.[29]

Differential Diagnosis. The melanotic macules of Albright's syndrome only rarely show the "giant" melanin granules that are commonly seen in some of the melanocytes and keratinocytes within the café-au-lait patches of neurofibromatosis.[29]

Mucosal Melanotic Macules

These benign lesions present as a pigmented patch on a mucous membrane. Common locations include the vermilion border of the lower lip, the oral cavity, the vulva, and, less often, the penis. These lesions may simulate melanoma clinically but histologically there is no contiguous melanocytic proliferation and no significant atypia. Because there may be a slight increase in the number of melanocytes, although there is no nest formation, the term "genital lentiginosis" has recently been proposed for these lesions.[30] The lesions may be synonymously referred to as "mucosal lentigo" or "mucosal melanotic macule." In the common location on the vulva ("vulvar lentigo"), this process may appear quite alarming clinically, presenting as a broad, irregular, and asymmetric patch of brown to blue-black hyperpigmentation, easily meeting the "ABCD" criteria for melanoma discussed later.[31] The lesion may be multicentric with alternating areas of normal and pigmented mucosa resembling areas of partial regression of a melanoma. The lesions are entirely macular, which would be unusual in an invasive melanoma. The so-called *"labial lentigo" ("labial melanotic macule")*, a hyperpigmented macule of the lip, is closely related to the lesions of genital skin. It is rarely biopsied because the clinical appearances are characteristic and do not suggest malignancy. These lesions are uniformly pigmented light brown, usually completely macular, and usually less than about 6 mm in diameter.

Histopathology. At first glance, a biopsy specimen may appear normal. The findings include mild acanthosis without elongation of rete ridges, and hyperpigmentation of basal keratinocytes, recognized in comparison with surrounding epithelium, with scattered melanophages in the dermis. Although melanocytes may be normal in number, in most instances the number is slightly increased.[32] In contrast to true melanocytic neoplasms (nevi or melanomas), the cell bodies of the lesional melanocytes are separated by those of keratinocytes—that is, there is no contiguous proliferation of melanocytes. Occasionally, especially in the penile and vulvar lesions, there are prominent dendrites of melanocytes ramifying among the hyperpigmented keratinocytes. There may be associated mild keratinocytic hyperplasia, and scattered melanophages in the papillary dermis may account for the blue-black color that may simulate melanoma clinically.

Differential Diagnosis. The histologic distinction from radial growth melanoma is easy because of the absence of neoplastic (contiguous) melanocytic proliferation.

Pathobiology. The process appears to be one of reactive hyperplasia with some features of postinflammatory hyperpigmentation, rather than a neoplasm. The phenomenon appears to be completely benign.

Becker's Melanosis

Becker's melanosis, also called Becker's pigmented hairy nevus, occurs most commonly as a large, unilateral patch showing hyperpigmentation and hypertrichosis on the shoulder, back, or chest of a man.[33] Usually, the patch is sharply but irregularly demarcated, but occasionally the lesion presents as coalescing macules instead of a patch. The lesion commonly appears during the second decade of life. In some instances, Becker's melanosis affects areas other than the shoulder and chest. Also, it may be multiple and bilateral, and may be found in women.

In a recent report, nine cases of melanoma in association with Becker's nevus were described.[34] Five of these were on the same body site as the nevus. It remains to be seen whether these reports represent a greater incidence than chance would suggest.

The hairiness always appears after the pigmentation, and quite frequently no hypertrichosis is observed. It is therefore possible that cases described as progressive cribriform and zosteriform hyperpigmentation represent a variant of Becker's melanosis without hypertrichosis.[35]

Of interest is the association of a pilar smooth muscle hamartoma with Becker's melanosis. In such cases, the area of Becker's melanosis may exhibit slight perifollicular papular elevations or slight induration.[36]

Histopathology. The epidermis shows slight acanthosis and regular elongation of the rete ridges. There is hyperpigmentation of the basal layer, and melanophages are seen in the upper dermis.[33] The number of melanocytes is increased. This increase is particularly evident when melanocytes are stained for dopa-oxidase activity in both involved and uninvolved skin nearby.[37] The hair structures appear normal, or increased in number.

In cases with associated smooth muscle hamartomas, irregularly arranged, thick bundles of smooth muscle are present in the dermis.[36] An increase in smooth muscle fibers exists in nearly all cases, although it may be slight.

The melanomas that have been described in association with Becker's nevus have been of the superficial spreading type, originating in the epidermis.[34]

Lentigines

Lentigines are macular hyperpigmentations in which the number of epidermal melanocytes is increased and there are no nests of melanocytes such as those present, by definition, in nevi. The term "lentigo" is derived from the Latin "lenz," meaning lens or lentil.[38] Thus, the term in its original usage is clinical, referring to a small ovoid or lens-shaped pigmented spot. The term has come to be applied to larger pigmented lesions, especially those that recapitulate to a greater or lesser extent the histologic features of a lentigo simplex: basal proliferation of melanocytes arranged as single cells rather than in nests, typically but not always associated with elongation of the rete ridges. This pattern of melanocytic proliferation is termed "lentiginous." Lentiginous melanocytic proliferation is observed in the macules of solar lentigo and lentigo simplex, and in the macular or plaque components of lentiginous junctional and compound nevi, of lentiginous dysplastic nevi, and of melanomas of the lentigo maligna, acral, and mucosal-lentiginous types.

Solar Lentigines (Actinic Lentigo)

Solar lentigines commonly occur as multiple lesions in areas exposed to the sun, such as the face and extensor surfaces of the forearms, but most commonly on the dorsa of the hands. The lesions rarely occur before the fifth decade and therefore were often referred to as senile lentigo.[39] However, sun exposure, rather than age, is the eliciting factor. Thus, the lesions do not occur on sun-protected skin, even in the elderly. Solar lentigines commonly occur in elderly Caucasoids. They are not infiltrated, possess a uniform dark brown color, and have an irregular outline. They vary in diameter from minute to more than 1 cm and may coalesce. Solar lentigines are risk markers for the development of melanoma,[27] and are commonly numerous in the skin around melanomas, as observed in melanoma reexcision specimens. Lesions termed "sunburn freckles" by some clinicians may overlap clinically and histologically with actinic lentigines. They are blotchy macular areas of tan hyperpigmentation, usually on the order of 1 cm in diameter, that often appear on the shoulders or other sun-exposed areas of young persons after severe sunburn. Other perhaps related lesions are intensely dark, perfectly macular reticulated lesions that have been called "reticulated lentigo" or "ink spot lentigo."[40]

Solar lentigines and seborrheic keratoses may resemble each other in clinical appearance, and both are commonly referred to as "liver spots" or "age spots." Seborrheic keratoses in general show more hyperkeratosis clinically. In contrast, lentigo maligna differs from solar lentigo in clinical appearance by its irregular distribution of pigment, often in a finely reticulated pattern, and by its greater asymmetry, border irregularity and larger size.

Prolonged treatment with psoralen and ultraviolet light A (PUVA) can induce formation of pigmented macules ("PUVA lentigines") in the irradiated areas, which are similar to solar lentigines except that their color is darker and their pigment is more irregularly distributed.[41]

Histopathology. The rete ridges are significantly elongated. They either appear club-shaped or are tortuous and show small, budlike extensions. The elongated rete ridges are composed, especially in their lower portions, of deeply pigmented basaloid cells intermingled with melanocytes. The melanocytes appear significantly increased in number in some cases,[42] but only slightly or not at all increased in others.[39] They possess an increased capacity for melanin production, as shown by the fact that, on staining with dopa, they show more numerous as well as longer and thicker dendritic processes than the melanocytes of control skin.[43] The upper dermis often contains a few melanophages and sometimes a mild, perivascular lymphoid infiltrate.

Solar lentigines differ from ephelids by definition, in having an increased number of epidermal melanocytes. However, in some lesions, the proliferation may be demonstrable only by formal counting.[41] In contrast to lentigo simplex, lentiginous nevi, and lentiginous melanomas, the melanocytic proliferation is "noncontiguous" (see Lentigo Simplex section).

In some lesions, the rete ridges are elongated to such an extent that strands of basaloid cells form anastomosing branches, resulting in a reticulated pattern closely resembling that observed in the reticulated pigmented type of seborrheic keratosis from which they differ by the absence of horn cysts.[39]

PUVA-induced pigmented macules represent solar lentigines on the basis of irregular elongation of their rete ridges. They show an increased number of large melanocytes that may appear slightly atypical.[41]

Histogenesis. Under electron microscopy, the basal layer of keratinocytes exhibits increased melanosomes and melanosome complexes, and the melanosome complexes inside the keratinocytes appear larger than those found in uninvolved skin.[42] Even in the upper layers of the epidermis, including the horny layer, numerous melanosomes are present largely in a dispersed state rather than as complexes.

Differential Diagnosis. In lentigo simplex, the lesional melanocytes are more obviously increased in number and lie in contiguity with one another. Lentigo maligna is typically much broader and shows flattening or even absence of the rete ridges together with contiguous proliferation and uniform atypia of its melanocytes, and, like lentigo simplex, it may possess a dermal lymphocytic infiltrate. In actinic lentigo, the lesional melanocytes do not lie in contiguity with one another, even though they may be increased in number. There is little or no evidence of cytologic atypia, or of pagetoid proliferation (melanocytes above the basal layer; see Fig. 29-19B).

Lentigo Simplex and Related Lesions

Lentigines are macular hyperpigmentations in which the number of epidermal melanocytes is increased. In solar lentigines, as described earlier, the cell bodies are separated from one another by those of keratinocytes, and the proliferation may be termed "noncontiguous." The proliferation may be described as "contiguous" if the cell bodies touch one another, as in lentigo simplex (and also in lentiginous nevi and lentiginous melanomas).

Lentigo simplex arises most frequently in childhood, but it may appear at any age.[44] In lentigo simplex, there are usually only a few scattered lesions without predilection to areas of sun exposure. They are small, symmetrical, and well-circumscribed macules that are evenly pigmented but vary individually from brown to black. They are not infiltrated and usually measure only a few millimeters in diameter. Clinically, lentigo simplex is indistinguishable from a junctional nevus. Special forms of lentigo simplex are lentiginosis profusa, the multiple lentigines syndrome or leopard syndrome, and speckled lentiginous nevus, also referred to as nevus spilus.

Lentiginosis profusa shows innumerable small, pigmented macules either from birth or starting in childhood or early adulthood without any other abnormalities.[45] The mucous membranes are spared. There is no family history. *Agminated* or *segmental lentigines* have been defined as a circumscribed group of small pigmented macules arranged in a small or large group, often in a segmental pattern, with each macule consisting of a lentiginous intraepidermal proliferation of melanocytes.[46] The *speckled lentiginous nevus,* or *nevus spilus,* consists of a light brown patch or band present from the time of birth that in childhood becomes dotted with small, dark brown macules.[47,48]

The *multiple lentigines syndrome,* a dominant trait, is characterized by the presence of thousands of flat, dark brown macules on the skin but not on the mucous surfaces. The lentigines begin to appear in infancy and gradually increase in number. Although most macules vary from pinpoint size to 5 mm in diameter, some dark spots are much larger, up to 5 cm in diameter. Features of this rare syndrome, known also by the mnemonic *leopard syndrome,* besides the lentigines (L), may include electrocardiographic conduction defects (E), ocular hypertelorism (O), pulmonary stenosis (P), and abnormalities of the genitalia (A), consisting of gonadal or ovarian hypoplasia, retardation of growth (R), and neural deafness (D). Not all of these manifestations are present in every case.[49] Another syndrome associated with lentigines is known under the acronyms *NAME* or *LAMB* or *myxoma* syndrome (lentiginous nevi, atrial and/or mucocutaneous myxomas, myxoid neurofibromas, ephelides, blue nevi).[46]

The *Peutz-Jeghers syndrome* shows dark brown macules clinically resembling lentigines in the perioral region. Similar macules are observed on the vermilion border of the mouth and the oral mucosa, and often on the dorsa of the fingers. Although a few cases of this dominantly inherited disorder have shown only the pigmentary anomaly, there are usually multiple polyps in the gastrointestinal tract, mainly in the small intestine.[50] The polyps may cause episodes of intussusception and intestinal bleeding, but they rarely become malignant.

Histopathology. Lentigines, in general, show a slight or moderate elongation of the rete ridges, an increase in the concentration of melanocytes in the basal layer, an increase in the amount of melanin in both the melanocytes and the basal keratinocytes, and the presence of melanophages in the upper dermis. In some instances, melanin is also present in the upper layers of the epidermis, including the stratum corneum. A mild inflammatory infiltrate may be intermingled with the melanophages.[44] In lesions otherwise clinically characteristic of lentigo simplex, small nests of nevus cells are commonly observed at the epidermal-dermal junction, especially at the lowest pole of rete ridges. The lesions then combine features of a lentigo simplex and a junctional nevus (lentiginous junctional nevus, or "jentigo").[44] Because of the existence of these transitional forms, the lentigo simplex is regarded as a form of evolving melanocytic nevus, and is discussed as such in a later section.

In *lentiginosis profusa* and the *multiple lentiginines syndrome,* as a rule, the lesions are "pure" lentigines without the formation of nevus cell nests. In large spots, however, there may be junctional nevus cell nests, and there may even be nevus cell nests in the upper dermis.[51]

In *speckled lentiginous nevus,* or nevus spilus, the light brown patch or band shows the histologic features of lentigo simplex. The speckled areas show junctional nests of nevus cells at the lowest poles of some of the rete ridges and diffuse junctional activity and dermal aggregates of nevus cells.[47]

In the lesions of *Peutz-Jeghers syndrome,* the basal cell layer shows marked hyperpigmentation. Although the number of melanocytes may appear to be slightly increased, no increase has been found in dopa-stained sections.[52] The intestinal polyps appear to be hamartomas, because glands are intermingled with smooth muscle bundles.[52]

Histogenesis of Lentigines

The presence of occasional giant melanin granules has been reported in various forms of lentigines and lentiginous nevi, as well as in other conditions associated with hyperpigmentation, including the café-au-lait spots of neurofibromatosis,[53] less commonly in café-au-lait spots without neurofibromatosis, and on occasion even in normal skin of healthy persons.[54] Thus, they have no diagnostic specificity.

Giant melanin granules vary in size from 1 to 6 μm. Because of their size and heavy melanization, the larger granules are readily recognized by light microscopy. Although observed largely within melanocytes, they also occur in keratinocytes and melanophages to which they have been transferred.[49] Under electron microscopy, the giant melanin granules have been regarded as macromelanosomes, or alternatively as autolysosomes referred to as "melanin macroglobules."[55]

Melanocytic Nevi

Common Melanocytic Nevus

Although the term "nevus" may refer to a variety of hamartomatous and/or neoplastic lesions in the skin, the unqualified term in common usage and in this chapter refers to a *melanocytic nevus,* generally considered to be a benign neoplastic proliferation of melanocytes. Nevi vary considerably in their clinical appearance. In addition to the pathological variants, which will be discussed separately, five clinical types can be recognized: (1) flat lesions, (2) slightly elevated lesions often with raised centers, and flat peripheries, (3) papillomatous lesions, (4) dome-shaped lesions, and (5) pedunculated lesions. The first three types are always pigmented; the latter two may or may not be pigmented. Dome-shaped lesions often exhibit several coarse hairs. Although exceptions occur, one can predict to a certain degree from the clinical appearance of a nevus whether on histologic examination it will prove to be a junctional nevus, a compound nevus, or an intradermal nevus. Most small, flat lesions represent either a lentigo simplex or a junctional nevus; flat lesions or lesions with flat peripheries greater than 5 mm in diameter with irregular indefinite borders and pigment variegation are clinically dysplastic nevi, although, if these changes are severe, melanoma may need to be ruled out; most slightly elevated lesions and some papillomatous lesions represent compound nevi; and most papillomatous lesions and nearly all dome-shaped, and pedunculated lesions represent intradermal nevi.[56]

Melanocytic nevi are only rarely present at birth (see section on Congenital Melanocytic Nevus). Most nevi appear in adolescence and early adulthood. In this age period, they may occur episodically and, rarely, as widespread eruptive nevi.[57] Occasionally, new nevi arise in midlife and rarely in later life. Except for occasional cosmetic significance, nevi are important only in relation to melanoma, for which they are risk markers, simulants, and potential precursors.[58,59]

Histopathology. Melanocytic nevi are defined and recognized by the presence of nevus cells, which, even though they are melanocytes, differ from ordinary melanocytes by being arranged at least partially in clusters or "nests." Other defining characteristics of nevus cells include a tendency toward rounded rather than dendritic cell shape, and a propensity to retain pigment in their cytoplasm rather than to transfer it to neighboring keratinocytes. Nevus cells show considerable variation in their appearance, so that they are often recognizable as nevus cells more by their arrangement in clusters or nests than by their cellular characteristics. As the result of a shrinkage artifact, nevus cell nests often appear partially separated from their surrounding stroma.

Although a histologic subdivision of nevi into junctional, compound, and intradermal nevi is generally accepted, it should be realized that these are transitional stages in the "life cycle" of nevi, which start out as junctional nevi and, after having become intradermal nevi, undergo involution.

Lentigo simplex. The lentigo simplex described earlier may be regarded as an early or evolving form of melanocytic nevus. The lack of nests at the histological level distinguishes the lentigo from a nevus. However, transitional forms between a simple lentigo and a lentiginous junctional nevus are commonly observed, and the two histological "entities" are indistinguishable clinically, giving rise to the term "nevoid lentigo"[44,59] (Fig. 29-3).

Junctional nevus. In a junctional nevus, nevus cells may lie in well-circumscribed nests either entirely within the lower epidermis or bulging downward into the dermis but still in contact with the epidermis, perhaps in a stage of "dropping off" to form a compound nevus. The nevus cells in these nests generally have a regular, cuboidal appearance, although they are occa-

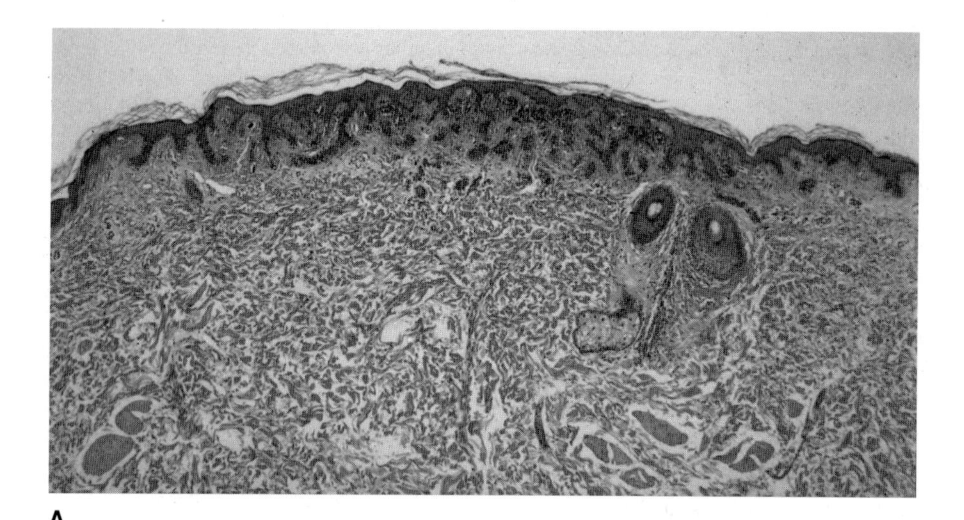

A

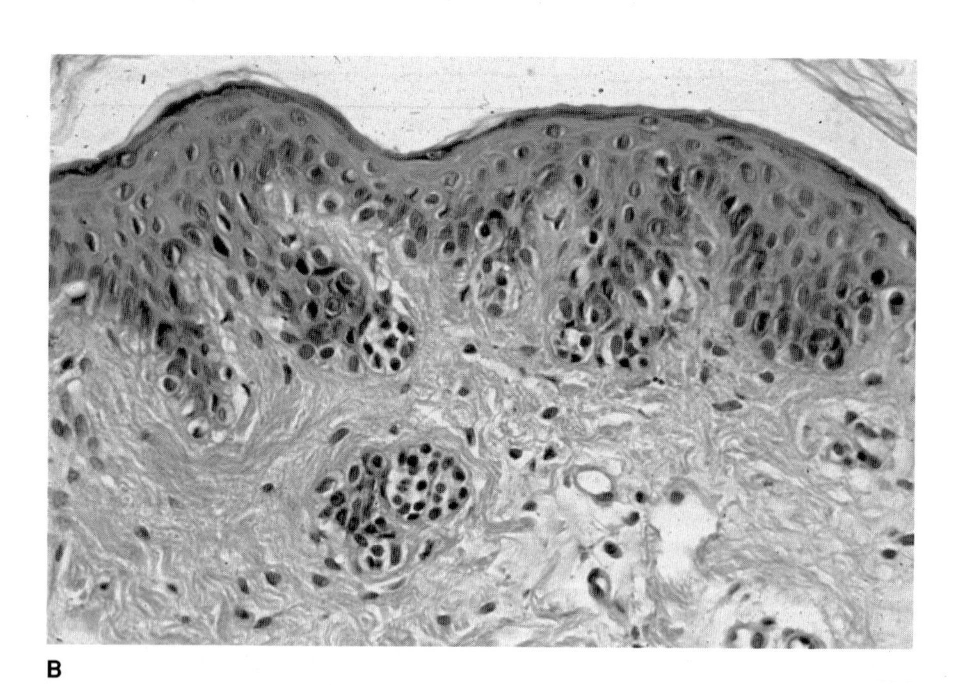

B

FIG. 29-3. Lentiginous compound nevus
(**A**) Most examples are less than 4 mm in diameter, usually about 2 to 3 mm. In the epidermis, single cells are arranged near the dermal-epidermal junction about elongated rete ridges (a "lentiginous" pattern). A dermal component, if present, lies at the center of the lesion, and the epidermal component extends beyond its "shoulder." (**B**) In a nevus, by definition, at least a few nests (cluster of five or more melanocytes) are present in the epidermis. A lentigo simplex may appear identical at scanning magnification to a lentiginous junctional nevus, but nests are absent. Many lentiginous nevi, as shown here, have a few nevus cells in the dermis, and thus are compound nevi. There is minimal or no atypia. These architectural features are repeated but exaggerated in dysplastic nevi, which in addition exhibit mild to moderate random cytologic atypia and are broader.

sionally spindle-shaped. In addition, varying numbers of diffusely arranged nevus cells are seen in the lowermost epidermis, especially in the basal cell layer. Varying amounts of melanin granules are present in the nevus cells. Some of the nevus cells, on staining with silver, show dendritic processes containing melanin granules, making them indistinguishable from melanocytes.

Although nevus cells only occasionally penetrate into the upper layers of the epidermis, there may be aggregates of melanin granules in the stratum corneum in deeply pigmented junctional nevi. Often, the rete ridges are elongated as in lentigo simplex and single cells as well as nests of nevus cells are observed at the bases of the rete ridges. Not infrequently, as in lentigo simplex, the upper dermis contains an infiltrate of melanophages and mononuclear cells. These lesions that combine features of lentigo simplex and junctional nevus are exceedingly common, and may be termed "lentiginous junctional nevi." Lesions with these features larger than 5 mm clinically or 4 to 5 mm in histologic section are often dysplastic nevi.

In children, some junctional nevi may show considerable cellularity with some pleomorphism and with some pagetoid cells above the basal layer. They may also often show fine dusty melanin particles and a dense inflammatory infiltrate.[60] Some of these lesions may represent Spitz nevi or dysplastic nevi. The small size of the lesion, the sharp lateral demarcation, the lack of severe or uniform atypia and of mitoses, and the fact that melanomas are very rare in children help in the distinction from melanoma. However, if the criteria mentioned above are met, the diagnosis of melanoma should be considered, even in a child.

Compound nevus. A compound nevus possesses features of both a junctional and an intradermal nevus. Nevus cell nests may be present in the epidermis, as well as in the dermis and "dropping off" from the epidermis into the dermis. Nevus cells in the upper, middle, and lower dermis may present characteristic morphological variations called *types A, B,* and *C,* respectively.[61] Usually, the *Type A* nevus cells in the upper dermis are cuboidal and show abundant cytoplasm containing varying amounts of melanin granules. Type A cells with especially abundant cytoplasm may be termed "epithelioid cells." Melanophages are occasionally seen in the surrounding stroma. The cells in the middermis usually are *type B* cells; they are distinctly smaller than type A cells, display less cytoplasm and less melanin, and generally lie in well-defined aggregates. They may to some extent resemble lymphoid cells. *Type C* nevus cells in the lower dermis tend to resemble fibroblasts or Schwann cells, because they are usually elongated and have spindle-shaped nuclei. They often lie in strands and only rarely contain melanin (Figs. 29-4, 29-5, and 29-6).

The decrease in size and good nesting observed in nevi are often referred to as maturation and are regarded as evidence of benignity, because the cell size in a melanoma usually does not decrease with depth. If dermal nevus cells are confined to the papillary dermis, they often retain a discrete, or "pushing" border with the stroma. However, nevus cells that enter the reticular dermis tend to disperse among collagen fiber bundles as single cells or attenuated single files of cells. This pattern of infiltration of the dermis differs from that in melanomas, where groups of cells tend to dissect and displace the collagen bundles in a more "expansive" pattern.[62] Lesions where nevus cells extend into the lower reticular dermis and the subcutaneous fat, or are located within nerves, hair follicles, sweat ducts, and sebaceous glands, may be termed "congenital pattern nevi"[63] (see Fig. 29-4).

Intradermal nevus. Intradermal nevi show essentially no junctional activity. The upper dermis contains nests and cords of nevus cells. Multinucleated nevus cells in which small nuclei lie either in a rosettelike arrangement or close together in the center of the cell may be present. These giant nevus cells differ sig-

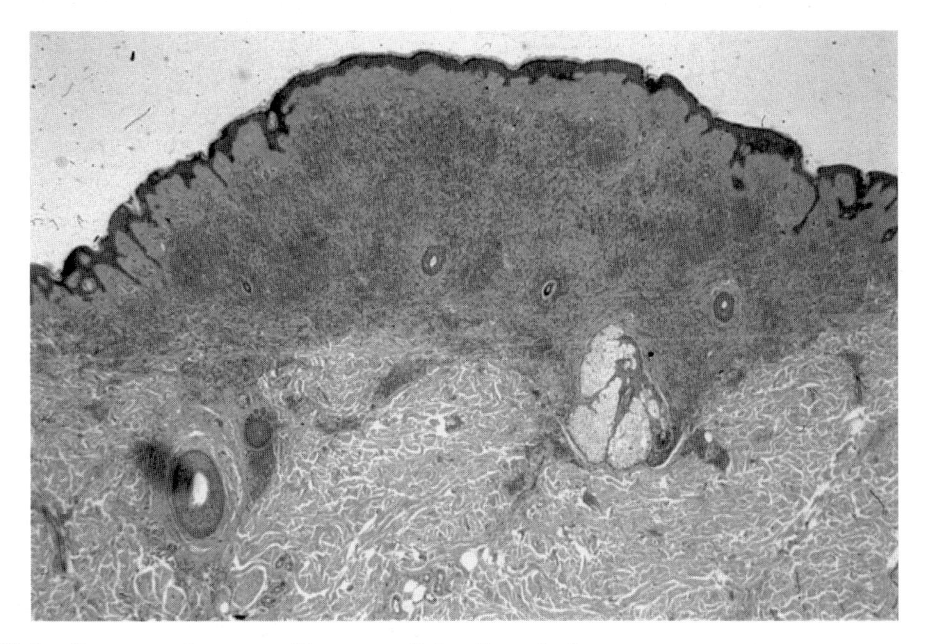

FIG. 29-4. Compound nevus with congenital pattern features
The extension of nevus cells into the upper reticular dermis and around skin appendages is a pattern that is quite characteristic of giant or nongiant congenital nevi. However, acquired nevi may also exhibit this "deep" pattern, and, conversely, congenital nevi are not always "deep."

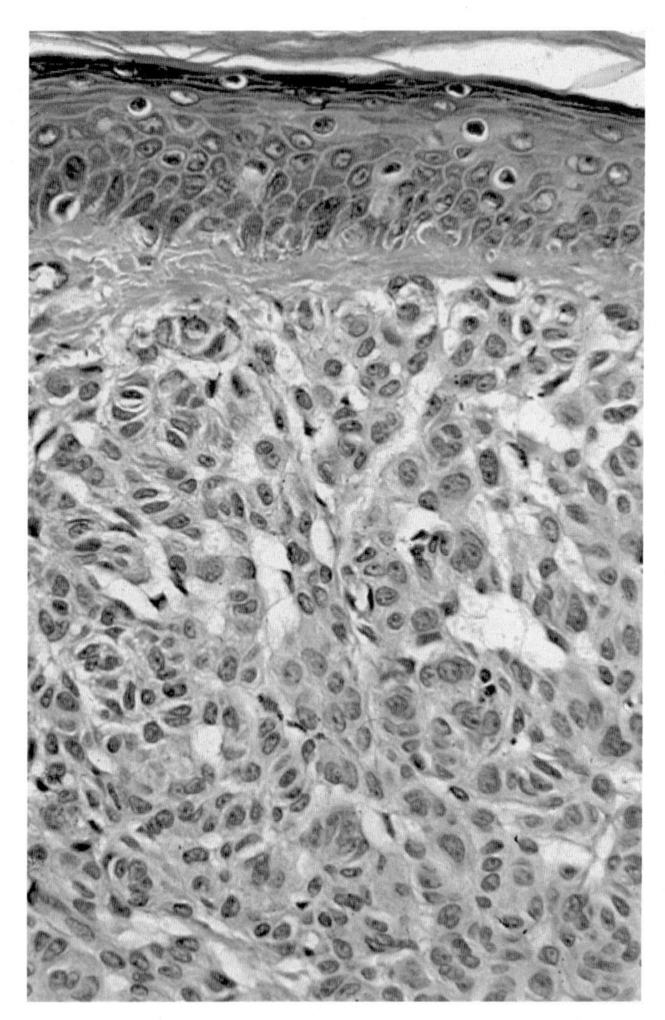

FIG. 29-5. Dermal nevus with type A nevus cells
Nevus cells are present in the dermis, but there are none in the epidermis. The "type A" cells contain visible cytoplasm, which is in contact with that of neighboring nevus cells. The nuclei are small, without atypia or prominent nucleoli. There are no mitoses.

nificantly in appearance from the irregularly and even bizarrely shaped giant cells frequently observed in Spitz nevi and occasionally in melanomas. As a result of shrinkage during tissue processing, clefts may form between some nests of nevus cells and the surrounding stroma, leaving a space that simulates a lymphatic space. This may simulate lymphatic invasion (see Fig. 29-6).[64]

Whereas the nevus cell nests located in the upper dermis often contain a moderate amount of melanin, the type C nevus cells in the midportion and the lower dermis rarely contain melanin. These type C cells appear spindle-shaped, are arranged in bundles, and are embedded in collagenous fibers having a loose, pale, wavy appearance similar to that of the fibers in a neurofibroma ("neurotized nevus") (Fig. 29-7). Such formations have been referred to as neuroid tubes. In other areas, the nevus cells lie within concentrically arranged, loosely layered filamentous tissue, forming so-called nevic corpuscles that resemble Meissner's tactile bodies (Fig. 29-8).

Occasional intradermal nevi are devoid of nevus cell nests in the upper dermis and contain only spindle-shaped nevus cells embedded in abundant, loosely arranged collagenous tissue. These nevi may be referred to as neural nevi. The differentiation from a solitary neurofibroma may be difficult in routinely stained sections, but distinction may be possible with an immunohistochemical technique employing myelin basic protein, which is positive only in neurofibroma[65] (see section on Histogenesis).

Some intradermal and, less commonly, compound nevi show hyperkeratosis and papillomatosis, which may be associated with a lacelike, downward growth of epidermal strands and with horn cysts. Such nevi resemble seborrheic keratoses in their epidermal architecture. In other instances, large hair follicles are observed. Rupture of a large hair follicle may manifest itself clinically as an increase in the size of the nevus associated with an inflammatory reaction, leading to suspicion of a melanoma. Histologic examination in such instances shows a partially destroyed epidermal follicular lining with a pronounced inflammatory infiltrate containing foreign-body giant cells as a reaction to the presence of keratin in the dermis.[66] Occasionally,

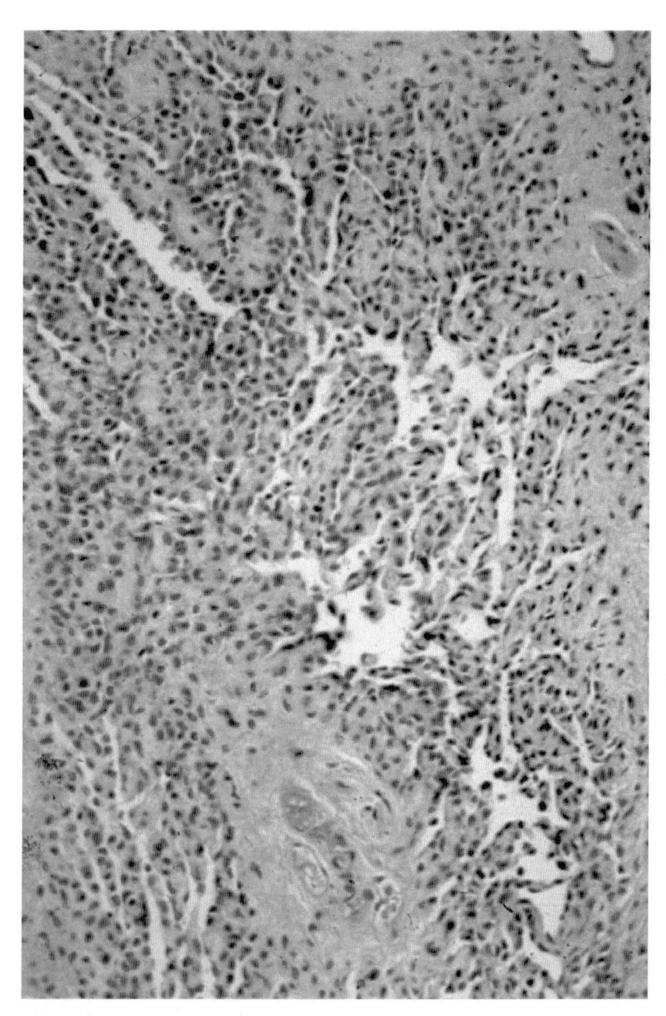

FIG. 29-6. Type B nevus cells with pseudolymphatic spaces in a dermal nevus
The type B nevus cells have small nuclei and scant cytoplasm, reminiscent of lymphocytes. The spaces are a common artifact in dermal or compound nevi. They may simulate lymphatic invasion of a melanoma but are completely benign.

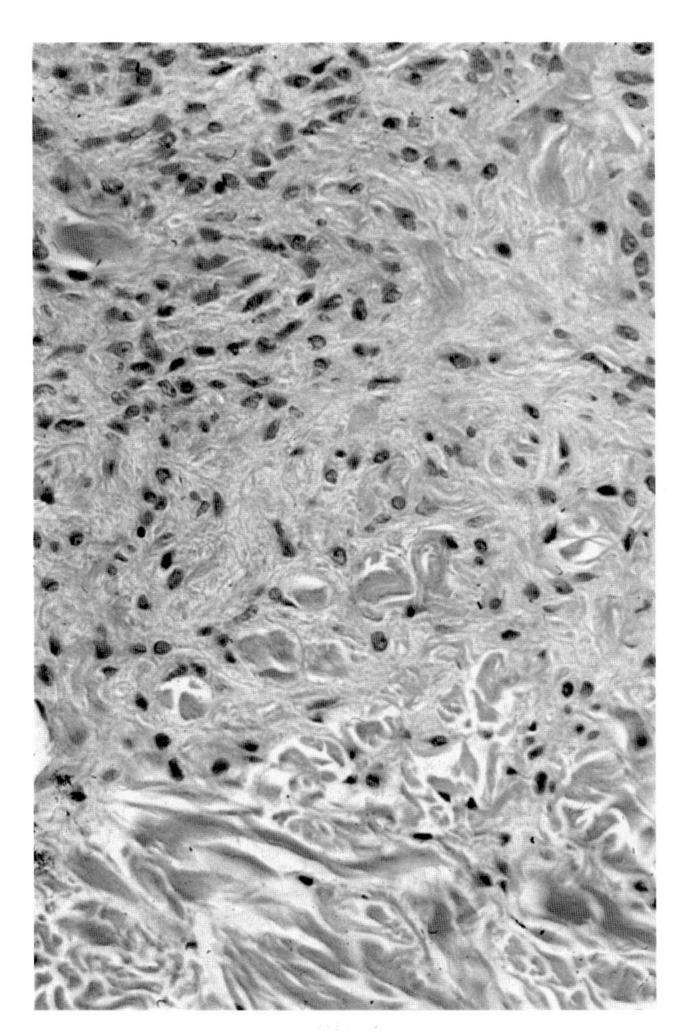

FIG. 29-7. Type C dermal nevus cells
The cells at the base of a nevus tend to be spindle-shaped and to have collagen between the individual cells. If they extend into the reticular dermis, they tend to "disperse" as individual cells among the superficial collagen fibers, a pattern that is also characteristic of Spitz nevi.

intradermal nevi contain scattered, large fat cells within the aggregates of nevus cells. This is likely to be a regressive phenomenon in which fat cells replace involuting nevus cells.[67]

Pathogenesis of Acquired Melanocytic Nevi

For many years, Masson's theory of the dual origin of nevus cells was widely accepted.[68] He believed that the nevus cells in the upper dermis developed from epidermal melanocytes, whereas the nevus cells in the lower dermis developed from Schwann cells, as suggested by the frequent presence of nerve-like structures in the latter. The fact that both melanocytes and Schwann cells are derived from the neural crest seemed to support Masson's view, as did the presence of a nonspecific cholinesterase reaction in both deep nevus cells and Schwann cells, and the absence of melanin in the deep nevus cells.[69] However, in favor of a melanocytic origin of these deep dermal nevus cells was the presence of melanosomes with dopa-oxidase activity even in nevus cells deep in the dermis that had a neuroid appearance under light microscopy.[70] An electron microscopic examination of neuroid structures in nevi revealed that these "nevic corpuscles" contained no Schwann cells or axons, but were instead composed exclusively of nevus cells containing premelanosome-like dense bodies in the perikaryon.[71] Furthermore, myelin basic protein has been found to be regularly present by immunoperoxidase in Schwann cells and absent in all types of melanocytic nevi.[65]

Another important point in favor of a single origin of the nevus cell is to be found in the life cycle of nevi. Although there are exceptions, most nevi appear in childhood, adolescence, and early adulthood, and, with advancing age, there is a progressive decrease in the number of nevi.[67] The evolution and regression of nevi correlate with their histologic appearance. Junctional proliferation of nevus cells is present in almost every nevus in children, but decreases with age. Intradermal nevi, by contrast, are most unusual in the first decade of life, and their proportion increases progressively with age. The incidences of fibrosis, fatty infiltration, and neuroid changes increase with age. Thus, the formation of cylindrical neuroid structures represents the

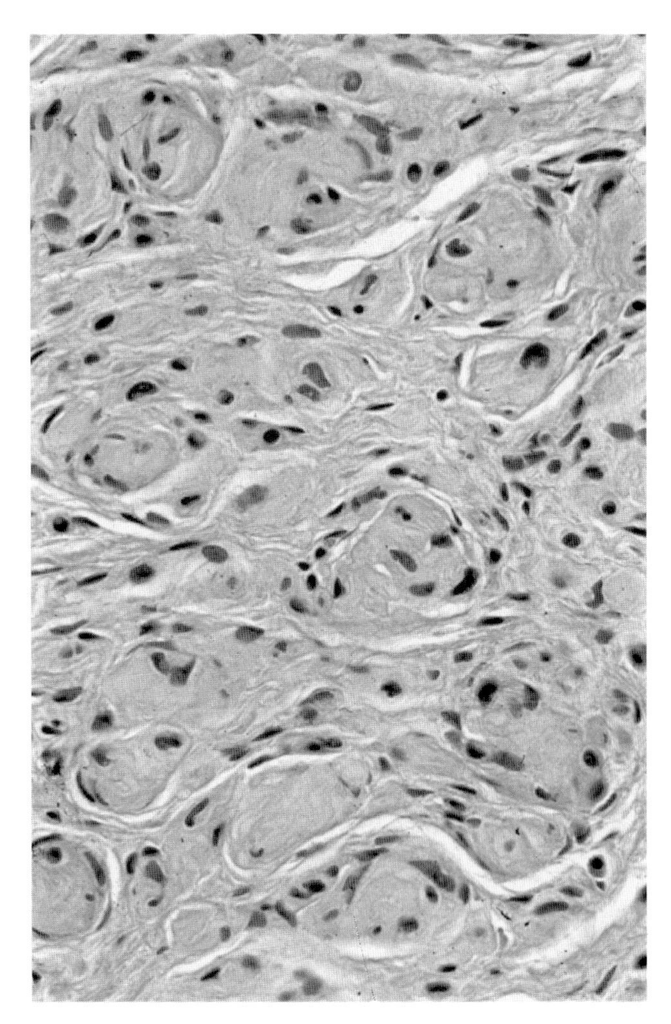

FIG. 29-8. Neurotized dermal nevus cells
The structures at the base of a "neurotized" dermal nevus may be reminiscent of nerve fibers or neural organs such as Wagner-Meissner corpuscles.

end stage of differentiation and not a source of origin of intradermal nevi.[67,72,73]

Concerning the relationship between epidermal melanocytes and nevus cells, some authors believe that these two types of cells differ in embryological genesis, the nevus cell originating from a neural crest precursor cell referred to as a nevoblast.[74] Most authors, however, regard the two types of cells as identical.[73,75] It would seem that the morphologic features by which nevus cells differ from melanocytes, such as their absence of dendrites under light microscopy, their arrangement in cell nests, their larger size, and their tendency to retain pigment, are secondary adjustments of the cells. Electron microscopy has shown that the fine structure of nevus cells is comparable to that of epidermal melanocytes.[75] Cultured nevus cells, whether derived from congenital or acquired lesions, have been found to be highly dendritic, just as epidermal melanocytes are.[76] In conclusion, it seems established that nevus cells differ from Schwann cells and are variant forms of melanocytes.

Balloon Cell Nevus

Balloon cell nevi are histologic curiosities that possess no clinical features by which they can be differentiated from other nevi. They are quite rare.[77,78]

Histopathology. Balloon cells may be seen within the epidermis singly or in groups, or may be absent from the epidermis. In the dermis, they are arranged in lobules of varying size, often with an admixture of ordinary nevus cells, and often with transitional forms between the ordinary and balloon nevus cells. The balloon cells may be multinucleated, and are considerably larger than ordinary nevus cells. Their nuclei are small, round, and usually centrally placed. Their cytoplasm appears either empty or finely granular, often with a few small melanin granules. There may be melanophages that are solidly packed with pigment.[77] Stains for lipids, glycogen, and acidic or neutral mucopolysaccharides are negative in balloon cells. Electron microscopic examination reveals in balloon cells numerous large vacuoles formed by enlargement and coalescence of melanosomes.[78,79] Balloon cell nevi are differentiated from balloon cell melanomas by the usual criteria. The large fat cells present in some intradermal nevi as a result of fatty infiltration differ from balloon cells by having flattened nuclei at their peripheries. In differentiation from clear cell hidradenoma and other clear cell tumors, the presence of *S*-100 protein and absence of keratin in balloon cell nevi might be helpful.

Nevus of Acral Skin

Melanocytic nevi are present on the skin of the palms or soles in as many as 4% to 9% of the population.[80] Clinically, they are usually small, symmetrical, well-circumscribed brown macules, with a tendency toward dark ridging along dermoglyphics that can be clinically striking and may impart a seemingly irregular border. They are usually stable, and are more often junctional than are nevi of the trunk.

Histopathology. Acral nevi tend to be more cellular than most common nevi, and the nevus cells may be arranged in predominantly lentiginous rather than nested patterns in the epidermis. Recently, pagetoid proliferation of lesional nevus cells in the epidermis above the basal layer was described in benign acral nevi.[81] These features may perhaps account for recommendations in the older literature to remove acral nevi because of suspicion of melanoma. However, there is no evidence that these lesions are common precursors or risk markers for acral melanomas.

Acral nevi may simulate and must be differentiated from melanomas, and this may be difficult especially in small biopsies. An acral lentiginous lesion that extends to specimen borders should be evaluated carefully, and clinicopathologic correlation should be obtained to ensure that the specimen does not represent the periphery of a larger lesion. In compound acral nevi, the nevus cells in the dermis, unlike melanoma cells, mature to the lesional base. There may be patchy lymphocytes and occasional melanophages in the dermis. Some of these features may suggest dysplastic nevus. However, the rete ridge pattern of keratinocytes in most acral nevi does not show the uniform elongation with occasional anastomosing retia that characterizes dysplastic nevi, the stromal changes of dysplastic nevi are not observed in most acral nevi, and atypia of melanocytes, as a rule, is minimal or absent.

Melanonychia Striata

Melanonychia striata refers to a pigmented band extending parallel to the long axis of the nail. Such bands are common in blacks and Asians and therefore regarded as normal.[82] However, the sudden appearance of melanonychia striata in whites is cause for concern, requiring a punch biopsy of the nail matrix. An exception is the melanonychia striata seen in the Laugier-Hunziker syndrome, which may affect one, several, or all fingernails in association with pigmented macules of the lips or the buccal mucosa. This type of melanonychia is always benign.[83]

The biopsy is performed by making longitudinal bilateral releasing incisions along the medial and lateral sides of the posterior nail fold. Next, the entire posterior nail fold is reflected proximally in order to expose and make visible the very end of the pigmented streak, which is usually within the matrix of the nail. The biopsy specimen is then taken with a 3- or 4-mm punch through the nail plate and matrix down to the phalangeal bone.[84]

Histopathology. Histologic examination in most instances shows merely hyperpigmentation without an obvious increase in the number of melanocytes.[82] Such lesions have been termed "melanotic macules."[85] In a recent study of 18 cases, 10 were melanotic macules, one was melanoma in situ, another showed keratinocytic atypia, and three were subungual hemorrhages.[86] In some cases, a junctional nevus or a compound nevus of acral type, as described earlier, or an acral lentiginous melanoma, either in situ or invasive, may be found.

Nevus of Genital Skin

Some clinically unremarkable nevi located on or near genital skin may present with histologic features that simulate some aspects of melanomas. The lesions have no clinical significance except the possibility of diagnostic error. They are most often observed on the vulva of young (premenopausal) women.[87]

Similar lesions also occur, although uncommonly, on the male genitalia.[88] The lesions are often removed incidentally. They are typically symmetrical papular lesions, usually less than 1 cm in diameter, and uniformly pigmented with discrete, well-circumscribed borders. The atypical features appear to represent a histologic curiosity observed in a minority of vulvar nevi. In a comparative histologic study of vulvar and common nevi, most of the vulvar lesions were unremarkable.[89] Vulvar nevi themselves are quite uncommon; among patients in a gynecology practice, the prevalence was only 2.3%.[90] The clinical differential diagnosis also includes early "genital lentigines," as described earlier.

Histopathology. At scanning magnification, the nevus typically appears as a small, well-circumscribed papular lesion composed of nevus cells arranged in clusters in the papillary dermis and arranged mainly in nests in the epidermis, where the cells do not extend beyond the shoulder of the dermal component (Fig. 29-9). The nevus cells may be large, with prominent nucleoli and abundant cytoplasm with finely divided melanin pigment. The epidermal nests may vary considerably in size and

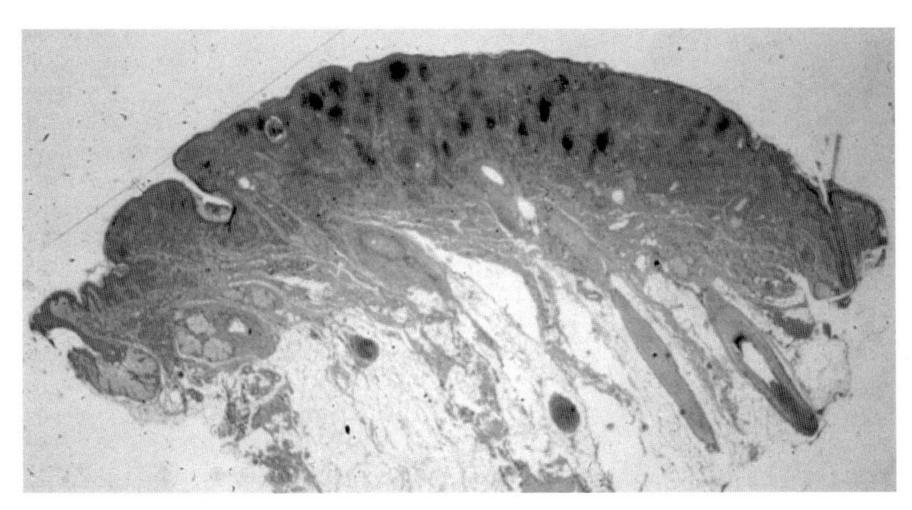

A

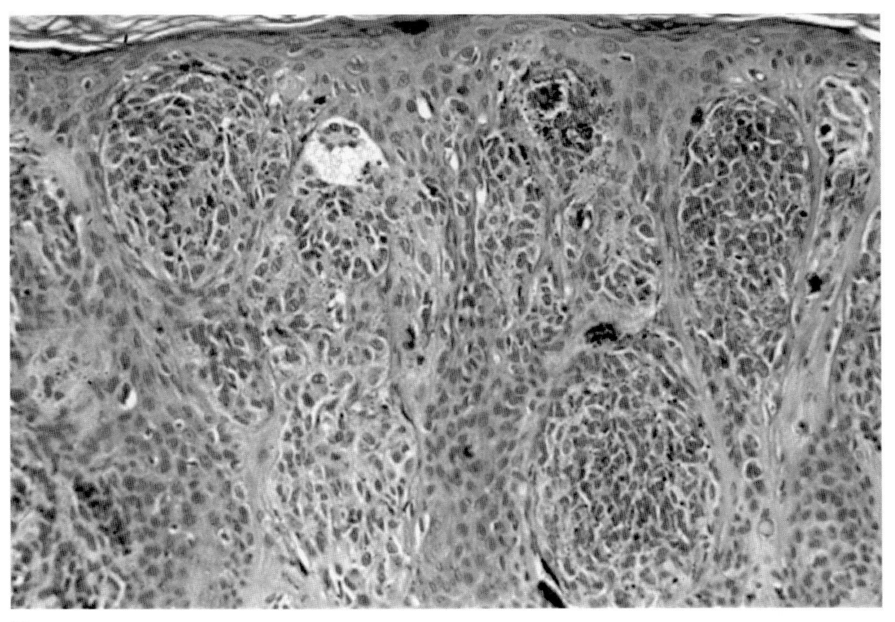

B

FIG. 29-9. Nevus of genital skin (**A**) Nevi on genital skin may exhibit atypical features at high magnification but are usually relatively small and symmetrical and thus benign in their appearance at scanning magnification, and also clinically. (**B**) Atypical features in genital nevi may include nests that tend to be large and confluent, and to vary a good deal in size and shape, and cells that tend to be large, with macronucleoli. Mitoses are rare or absent, and there is no adjacent in situ or microinvasive radial growth phase component.

shape, tending to become confluent. The nests also tend to vary in terms of position, originating from the sides as well as the tips of retia, and often oriented parallel to the surface. Single cells and nests of nevus cells may occasionally be present within the epithelia of skin adnexa. The epidermis may be irregularly thickened, resulting in an asymmetrical silhouette. Some of the features observed in atypical vulvar nevi may arouse a suspicion of melanoma. Unlike most mucosal melanomas, however, the lesions are comparatively small and well-circumscribed, without extensive radial growth phase proliferation of atypical melanocytes beyond the major dermal component. Moreover, there is little or no pagetoid spread of single or nested melanocytes into the epidermis, there is no necrosis and usually no ulcer, and, most importantly, there is no mitotic activity in the dermis.[89] The diagnosis of melanoma in vulvar skin should be made with caution in a premenopausal woman.

Spitz Nevus

The Spitz nevus, now generally named after Sophie Spitz, who first described it in 1948,[91] is known also as *benign juvenile melanoma* and as *spindle and epithelioid cell nevus*. The lesion was originally thought to occur largely in children, but it is now well recognized in young to early middle-aged adults.[92,93] Only rarely is it present at birth.[94]

The lesion usually is solitary and is encountered most commonly on the lower extremities and face.[95] In most instances, it consists of a dome-shaped, hairless pink nodule. Most Spitz nevi are small: in 95% of the patients, the size of the tumor is less than 1 cm, and in 75% it is 6 mm or less.[96] The color is usually pink because of a scarcity of melanin, and the nevus is then often diagnosed clinically as granuloma pyogenicum, angioma, or dermal nevus. However, it may be tan, brown, or even black. Ulceration is observed only rarely. After an initial period of growth, most Spitz nevi are stable.

In rare instances, multiple tumors are encountered either agminated (grouped) in one area or widely disseminated.[97]

Histopathology. Because of the large size of the lesional cells, often with considerable nuclear and cytoplasmic pleomorphism and the frequent presence of an inflammatory infiltrate, the histologic picture often resembles that of a nodular melanoma. There is no doubt that, before the recognition of the Spitz nevus as an entity, many cases were misdiagnosed as melanomas. Even today, differentiation between Spitz nevus and melanoma can often be very difficult and occasionally even impossible. Features that aid in the distinction may be summarized as architectural pattern and cytologic features (Fig. 29-10).

In terms of their *architectural pattern,* Spitz nevi resemble common nevi. They are usually compound, but they can be intradermal or entirely junctional. They are small, symmetrical, and well circumscribed. It is quite unusual for the intraepidermal component to extend beyond the dermal component, and such a finding should prompt serious consideration of melanoma.[98] The epidermal component is arranged in nests that tend to be oriented vertically and, although large, do not vary a great deal in size and shape or tend to become confluent. In Spitz nevi with junctional activity, there are often artifactual clefts above the nests of nevus cells at the epidermal-dermal junction. Rarely seen in melanoma, this represents a useful diagnostic feature.[96]

Although there may be diffuse junctional activity, permeation of the epidermis by tumor cells is relatively slight. If present, it usually consists of single nevus cells or small groups of cells and is generally limited to the lower part of the epidermis.[93] In a few Spitz nevi, however, this pagetoid proliferation may be quite marked, especially in young children (Fig. 29-11).[99] Involvement of the suprabasal epidermis is not a common feature of Spitz nevi in adults; in such cases, the diagnosis of melanoma should be considered.[100] Occasionally, nests of lesional cells are observed in transit through the epidermis, a phenomenon described as transepidermal elimination of nevus cells.[101]

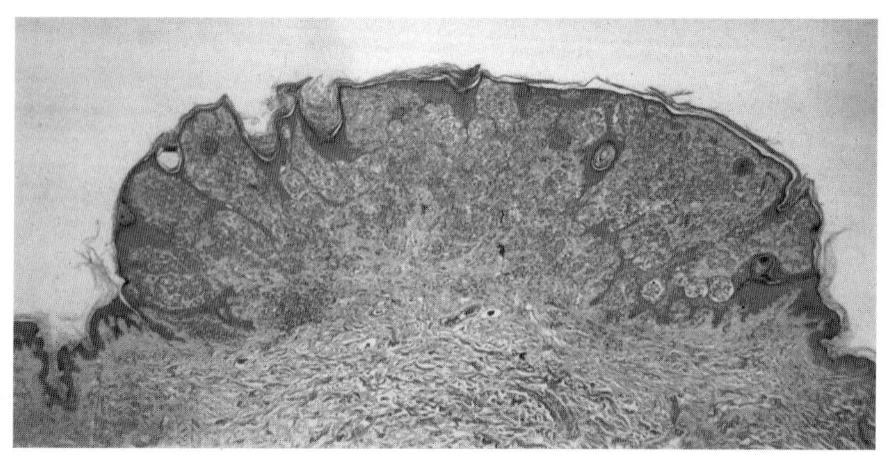

A

FIG. 29-10. Spitz nevus
(**A**) Most Spitz nevi are small, circumscribed, symmetrical papules at scanning magnification and clinically.

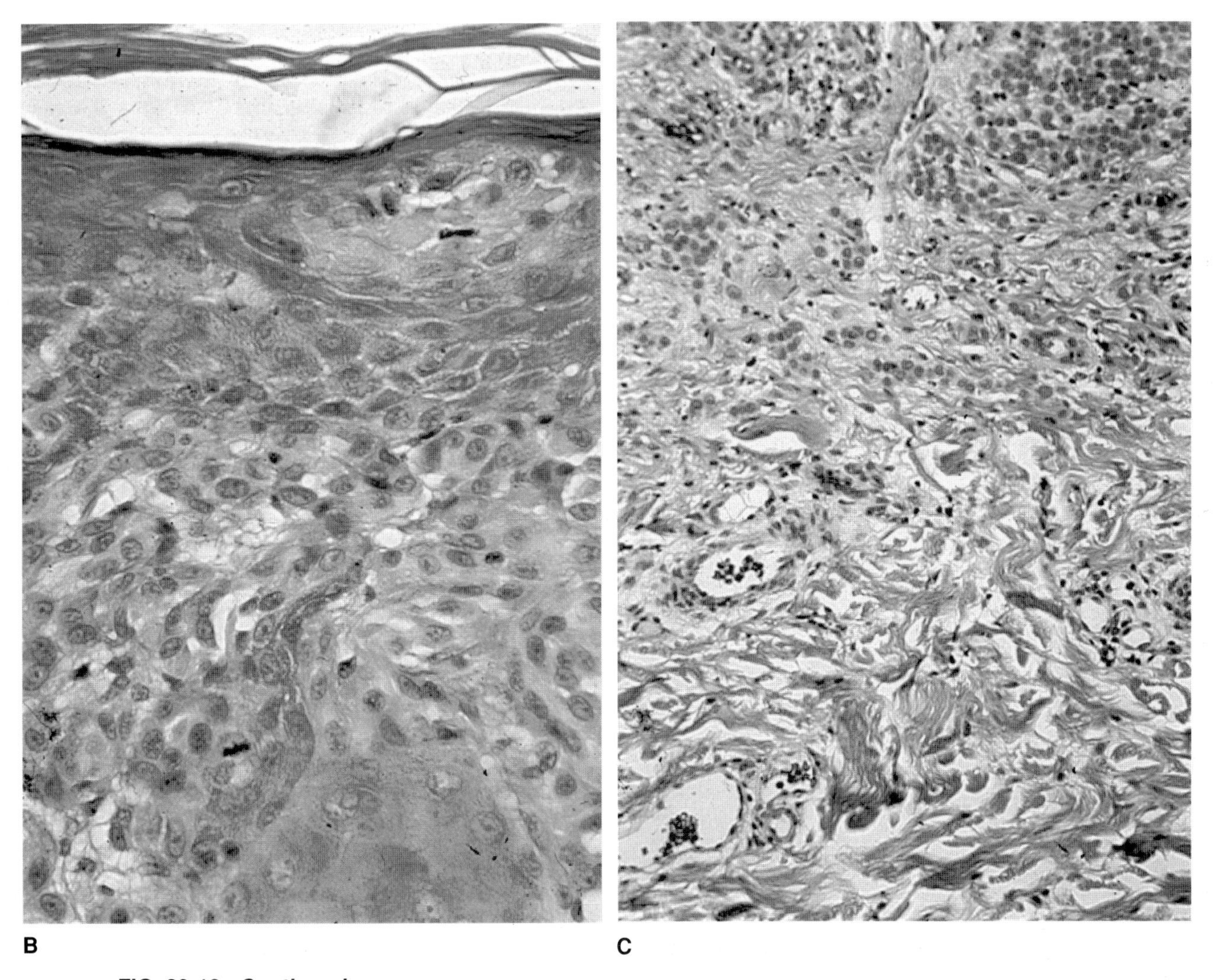

FIG. 29-10. ***Continued***
(**B**) Spitz nevi are defined by the presence of large cells, with abundant amphophilic cytoplasm, which may be spindle-shaped or polygonal. The nuclei in a given Spitz nevus are homogeneous, usually large but with smooth nuclear membranes, and with prominent nucleoli. (**C**) At the base of a Spitz nevus, the lesional cells become smaller and "dispersed" among the reticular dermis collagen fibers.

The epidermis is often hyperplastic with elongated rete ridges. Occasionally, this hyperplasia is sufficiently florid to be termed pseudoepitheliomatous, representing a possible source of confusion with squamous cell carcinoma, especially in a superficial biopsy.[102] However, the epidermis may be thinned and even ulcerated, especially in very young children. Found in fewer than half of the patients, diffuse edema and telangiectasia in the papillary dermis, if present, are of slight diagnostic importance. The edema may cause a loose arrangement of the nevus cell nests.[96]

Important *cytologic features* of Spitz nevi include especially the presence of large spindle cells and epithelioid cells. Spindle cells or epithelioid cells may predominate, or the two types of cells may be intermingled.[93] Apart from the shape of their cell bodies, the spindle cells and epithelioid cells in any given Spitz nevus resemble one another in nuclear and cytoplasmic consistency, suggesting that they may represent dimorphic expression of a single cell type. The cells are large, with abundant amphophilic cytoplasm and prominent eosinophilic or amphophilic nucleoli. The size of the lesional cells, more than any other feature, sets the Spitz nevus apart from the common nevus,[103] and also from most melanomas. Bizarre giant cells may be present in both melanomas and Spitz nevi, the difference being that, in the latter, they usually have regular nuclei of similar size, whereas in melanomas the nuclei are usually more pleomorphic.[98] Mitoses are found in about half of the cases. Usually, there are only a few, but occasionally they are quite numerous. However, atypical mitoses are uncommon, and, if they are found, the lesion should be interpreted with great caution.[96] The complete absence of mitoses in 50% of Spitz nevi is very helpful in ruling out melanoma in these cases.

Of special importance is *maturation* of the cells with increasing depth, so that they become smaller and look more like the cells of a common nevus.[96] Also important is the *uniformity* of the lesional cells from one side of the lesion to the other: at any given level of the lesion from the epidermis to its base, the

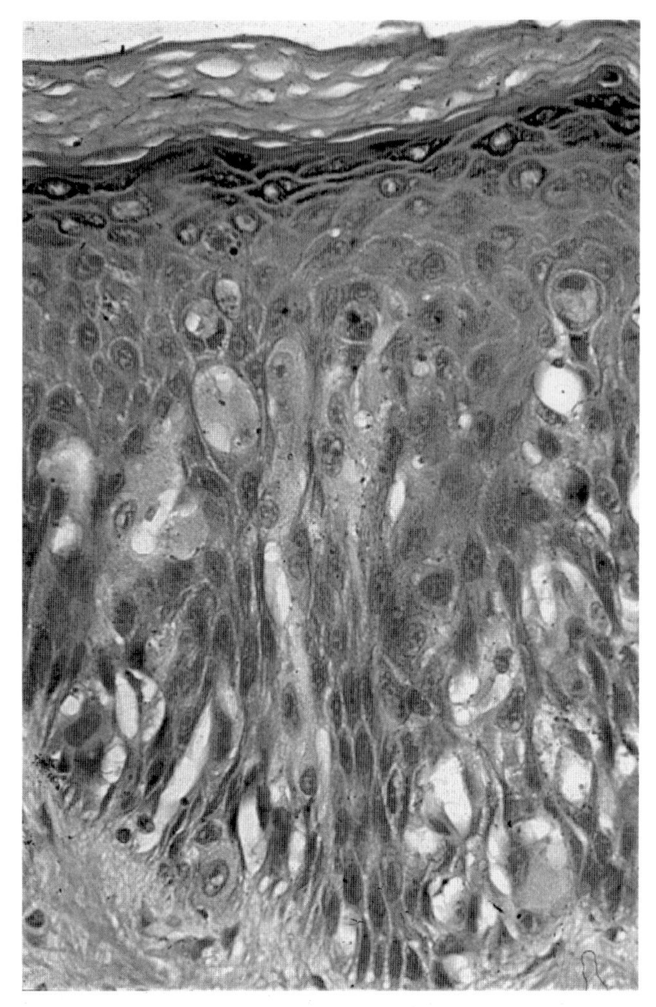

FIG. 29-11. Spitz nevus
Pagetoid extension of the cells of a Spitz nevus into the epidermis, as shown here, is not diagnostic of a melanoma if other attributes of melanoma are not observed. This pagetoid proliferation is not uncommon, at least focally, in lesions of young children.

lesional cells look the same. Although large superficially, the cells at the bases of most Spitz nevi are small, and they tend to disperse as single cells or files of single cells among reticular dermis collagen bundles. Other benign nevi also tend to infiltrate in this way if they involve the reticular dermis.[62] Involvement of the reticular dermis is highly characteristic of Spitz nevi, and as they descend into this part of the dermis, some of the cells become separated from the apparent border of the lesion to form "outlier cells"[96] that can be revealed by a stain for S-100 antigen. Melanomas, in contrast, tend to form solid tongues or fascicles of tumor cells that separate and displace the collagen bundles in the reticular dermis without forming outlier cells.

A useful although not pathognomonic cytologic criterion for Spitz nevi is the presence within the epidermis of red globules resembling colloid bodies in 60% to 80% of the cases. They may form fairly large bodies through coalescence. These "Kamino bodies," which likely represent apoptotic lesional cells, are most commonly observed in the basal layer above the tips of dermal papillae (see Fig. 29-13). Similar-appearing eosinophilic globules have been noted in the epidermis in only 2% of melanomas and 0.9% of ordinary nevi, in which they are, however, less conspicuous because they do not coalesce.[104,105]

Melanin is in many instances completely or nearly absent in Spitz nevi. In a few cases, melanin is moderate or dense.[93] Some of these "pigmented Spitz nevi" are better classified as pigmented spindle cell nevi, related lesions that are discussed in the next section. An inflammatory infiltrate is found in many Spitz nevi and may be quite heavy. Its distribution can be bandlike, mainly at the base, as in some melanomas. Often, however, the infiltrate is patchy around blood vessels and is present throughout the lesion.[92,93,96]

On comparing Spitz nevi occurring in adults with those observed in children, it appears that pure epithelioid cell Spitz nevi are rare in adults. Also, lesions in adults often are more pigmented than those in children.[106] Furthermore, desmoplastic Spitz nevi occur predominantly in adults.[93]

Desmoplastic Spitz nevi. In some examples of Spitz nevi, diffuse fibrosis is present. These desmoplastic Spitz nevi generally show no junctional activity, nesting, or pigmentation. The nevus cells are predominantly spindle-shaped and compressed by a desmoplastic stroma. However, they differ from dermatofibromas by the presence of epithelioid and often also multinucleated cells. Desmoplastic melanomas almost always show associated lentiginous melanomas, in contrast to the rarity of junctional activity in desmoplastic Spitz nevi.[107]

Hyalinizing Spitz nevi. Hyalinizing Spitz nevi present with spindle or epithelioid nevus cells embedded in a paucicellular hyalinized collagenous stroma. Some of these lesions have been mistaken histologically for metastatic carcinomas.[108]

Histogenesis. Under electron microscopic examination, Spitz nevi show, in their upper portions, melanocytes with numerous melanosomes; in their lower portions, the number of melanosomes in the melanocytes decreases. Melanization is incomplete in most melanosomes, and there is evidence of lysosomal degradation of melanosome complexes.[109] The paucity of melanin in most Spitz nevi is thus explained. Biological marker studies have shed little or no light on the mechanisms whereby Spitz nevi appear to have the capacities for invasive and tumorigenic proliferation in the dermis, but to lack the capacity for metastasis.

Differential Diagnosis. Differentiation of a Spitz nevus from a nodular melanoma can be difficult and even impossible in some cases, because all of the changes seen in the Spitz nevus may also be observed in melanoma. There are cases on record that were diagnosed as instances of Spitz nevus but later proved to be melanomas.[110] Other cases, regarded by some as "malignant Spitz nevi," have metastasized to regional lymph nodes but not beyond.[111] These lesions, often large, ulcerated, deeply infiltrative, and mitotically active, might alternatively be regarded as "melanocytic tumors of uncertain potential." The diagnosis of a Spitz nevus depends on an assessment of multiple morphological features, which are summarized earlier and in Table 29-2.

Morphometric and immunohistochemical studies have shown differences between Spitz nevi and melanomas, but none of these adjuncts to histological diagnosis is in standard use. By immunohistochemistry, Spitz nevi react not only with differen-

TABLE 29-2. *Morphological features of Spitz nevus versus melanoma*

Spitz nevus	Melanoma
Pattern features	
Usually less than 6 mm in diameter	Usually greater than 6 mm in diameter
Usually symmetrical	Often but not always asymmetrical
Epidermal hyperplasia, hyperkeratosis, and hypergranulosis may be prominent.	Epidermal reaction is often minimal.
Usually little or no pagetoid spread of lesional cells into epidermis	Usually obvious pagetoid spread into epidermis
Epidermal component does not extend beyond the lateral border.	Lateral extension (radial growth phase) is common except in nodular melanoma.
Ovoid nests of lesional cells oriented perpendicular to epidermis.	Nests variable in size, shape, and orientation
Discontinuous junctional proliferation	May be continuous proliferation
Little or no pigment	Often heavily pigmented, or irregularly scattered pigmented cells within lesion
Small, uniform nests in dermis at base	Larger variable nests at base
Single attenuated cells dispersed between reticular dermis collagen bundles at base	Nests and fascicles rather than single cells in the reticular dermis
Cytologic features	
Nuclear chromatin is open, with prominent nucleoli.	Nuclei may be hyperchromatic.
Single and confluent eosinophilic globoid bodies in epidermis and superficial dermis	If present, globoid "Kamino" bodies are inconspicuous and usually single.
Mitoses absent or low mitotic rate	Mitoses rarely absent, rate often high
Atypical mitoses rare or absent	Atypical mitoses common
Mitoses rare in lower third of lesion	Mitoses common in lower third
Cells uniform from side to side	Greater tendency toward cellular variability
Cells mature with descent to base	Little or no maturation

tiation markers for melanocytes such as S-100 antigen, but also with HMB-45, a melanosomal antigen often expressed in proliferating melanocytic lesions. Like nevi and unlike melanomas, Spitz nevi show a tendency toward diminution of nuclear size and/or DNA content,[112,113] and of reactivity with certain antigens,[114] from the superficial to the deep portions of the nevus. This stratification may be regarded as an expression of maturation that is diagnostically and no doubt also biologically important in the distinction between Spitz nevi and melanomas. Nuclear size or volume measured morphometrically has provided fairly good discrimination in some hands,[115] especially when measured at the base of the tumor or when combined with a "maturation parameter"—namely, the ratio of nuclear area in the deep and superficial portions.[113] Cell proliferation marker studies using PCNA have in general shown Spitz nevi to be intermediate between common nevi and melanomas, but the specificity has been insufficient for diagnostic use.[116–118] Perhaps of greatest potential practical utility, the absence of aneuploidy as judged by cytofluorometry[119] or DNA in situ hybridization (FISH)[110,120] has been quite specifically associated with Spitz nevi as opposed to melanomas in several studies. Few of these methods, however, have been applied to series of difficult cases, in which they are most needed but where their utility is likely to be most limited. In one such study, De Wit et al., using FISH, were able to identify only three of five lesions that had been originally diagnosed as Spitz nevi but later reclassified as melanoma because of the occurrence of metastasis.[110]

Because of the difficulty of making an absolutely certain differentiation between Spitz nevus and melanoma, it is advisable as a precautionary measure that all lesions diagnosed as Spitz nevi be excised in persons at or beyond puberty, particularly because such lesions are usually small. Although the issue is debatable,[121] exceptions to this general rule might include those lesions where there are cosmetic or other contraindications to excision, and where the diagnosis of Spitz nevus is certain despite the partial nature of the biopsy.[122] Also, one should never exclude a diagnosis of melanoma based on age alone, because melanomas may arise in children, although this is rare.

Pigmented Spindle Cell Nevus

The pigmented spindle cell nevus, first described by Richard Reed in 1973,[123] may be regarded as a variant of the Spitz nevus[93,124] or as a distinctive clinicopathologic entity.[125] In our experience and that of others, most cases differ significantly from classical Spitz nevi, but some present with overlapping features, indicative of a close relationship between the two entities.[126,127] Although this distinction has no clinical significance in that each is a benign lesion, it is important to rule out melanoma, and this is facilitated by an understanding of the differences between these two common melanoma simulants.

The lesions are usually 3 to 6 mm in diameter, deeply pigmented, and either flat or slightly raised. Most patients are young adults, and the most common location is on the lower extremities. Pigmented spindle cell nevi are uncommon after the age of 35. A classical presentation is that of a newly evolved black plaque on the thigh of a young woman. Because of the heavy pigment and the history of sudden appearance, a clinical diagnosis of melanoma is often suspected clinically. In contrast, Spitz nevi are usually submitted with a benign clinical diagnosis, such as an angioma or a dermal nevus. Like the Spitz nevi, the lesions are generally stable after a relatively sudden appearance and a short-lived period of growth.

Histopathology. The pigmented spindle cell nevus is characterized by its relatively small size and its symmetry, and by a proliferation of uniform, narrow, elongated, spindle-shaped, often heavily pigmented melanocytes at the dermal-epidermal junction. The nests of spindle cells are vertically oriented, and tend to blend with adjacent keratinocytes rather than forming clefts as in Spitz nevi (Fig. 29-12). Kamino bodies may be present as in Spitz nevi (Fig. 29-13). The tumor cells often form bundles that are separated by elongated rete ridges. In the papillary dermis, the nevus cells lie in a compact cluster pattern, pushing the connective tissue aside. Involvement of the reticular dermis, common in Spitz nevi, is unusual in pigmented spindle cell nevi. Some lesions show upward epidermal extension of junctional nests of melanocytes. Single-cell upward invasion of the epidermis in a pagetoid pattern may be present but is usually not prominent.[125,128] The features that may lead to a diagnosis qualified as "atypical pigmented spindle cell nevus" include architectural abnormalities such as poor circumscription and pagetoid proliferation, prominent cytological atypia, and a prominent epithelioid cell component.[127] The significance of these "atypical" variants appears to lie in their greater chance of being misdiagnosed as melanomas, because all reports of pigmented spindle cell nevi emphasize their benign behavior after excision.[126,127]

Differential Diagnosis. The major differential is with melanoma of the superficial spreading type. In contrast to these melanomas, pigmented spindle cell nevi are smaller, symmetrical, and show sharply demarcated lateral margins. The tumor cells appear strikingly uniform "from side to side." If lesional cells descend into the papillary dermis, they mature along nevus lines in pigmented spindle cell nevi, in contrast to melanomas. Mitoses may be present in the epidermis in either lesion, but are uncommon in the dermis in pigmented spindle cell nevi. Abnormal mitoses are very uncommon indeed. Pagetoid proliferation is usually not prominent, and the spindle cell type differs from the epithelioid cells that predominate in most superficial spreading melanomas. Lentigo maligna melanomas may have spindle cells in their vertical growth phase components, but the epidermal component is usually composed of smaller, nevoid, but atypical cells. Some rare examples of lesions with larger expansile nodules may be difficult to distinguish from melanomas, and a descriptive diagnosis may be appropriate (see section on Melanocytic Tumor of Uncertain Malignant Potential). Some cases may present overlapping features with dysplastic nevi, but may usually be distinguished on the basis of their irregularly thickened epidermis, their vertically oriented nests, and their uniformity of cell type. In some cases, this distinction may be more difficult. Such lesions can be signed out descriptively, with a recommendation for additional clinical assessment of the patient to rule out other melanoma risk factors. If such factors are absent, the significance of an isolated lesion is likely to be minimal.

Congenital Melanocytic Nevus

A congenital melanocytic nevus may be defined as a lesion present at birth and containing nevus cells. Congenital nevi are

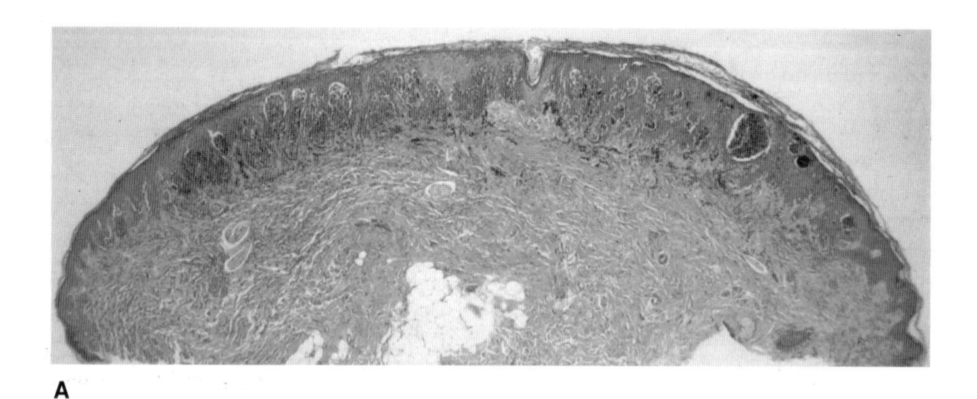

A

FIG. 29-12. Pigmented spindle cell nevus
(**A**) The typical configuration of this lesion is that of a plaque whose breadth is considerably greater than its height. The lesional cells are typically junctional or confined to the epidermis and the papillary dermis. (**B**) As in the classic Spitz nevus, the lesional cells are arranged in nests that tend to be vertically oriented. Unlike those of the Spitz nevus, the cells are narrow, elongated spindle cells without epithelioid cells, and they contain abundant, usually coarse melanin pigment. (**C**) As in Spitz nevi, some (usually a slight) degree of pagetoid proliferation is not unexpected. Mitoses may be numerous in the epidermis, but the lesional cells in the dermis tend to be mature, with few mitoses.

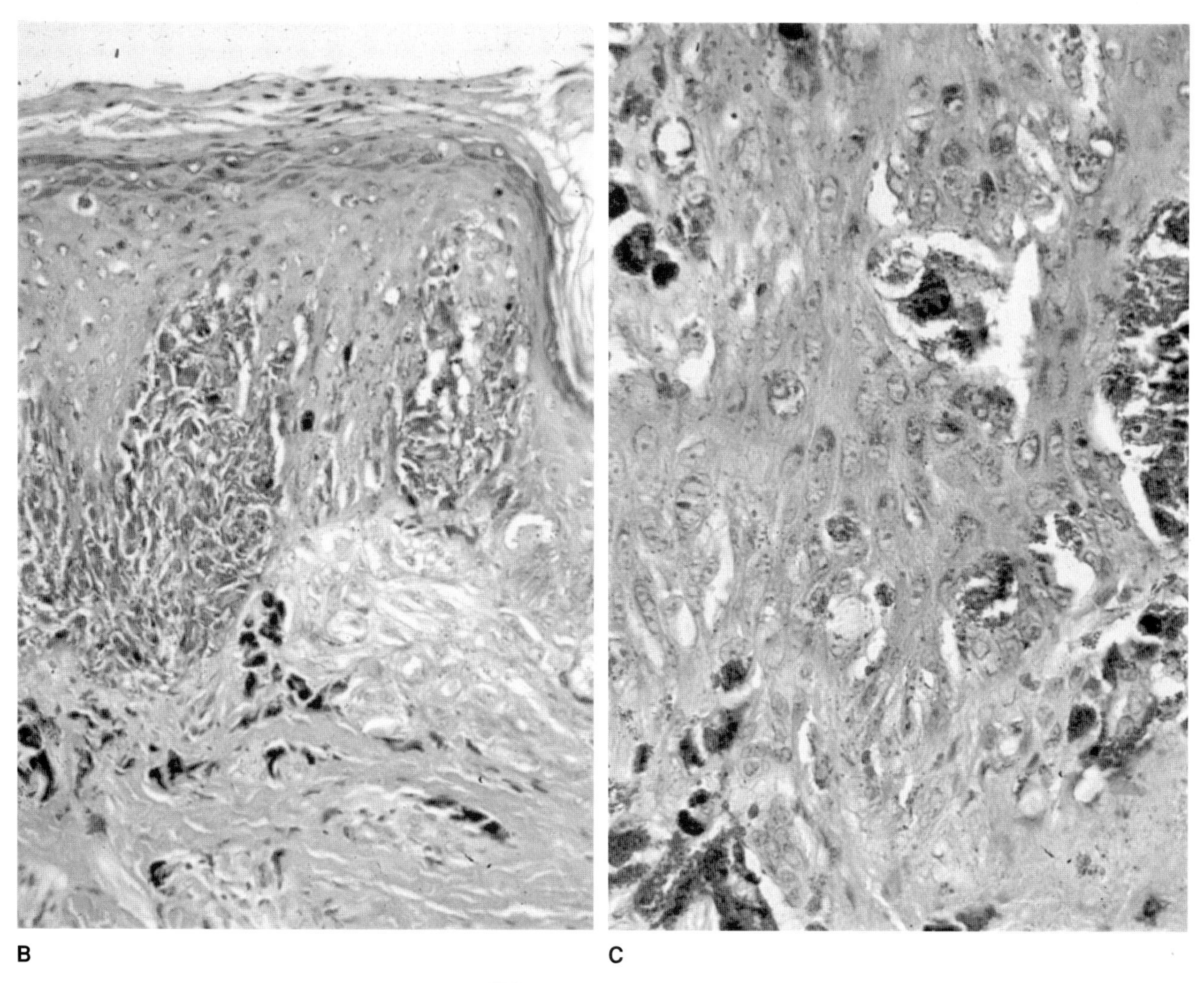

FIG. 29-12. ***Continued***

found in about 1% to 2% of newborn infants.[129,130] In many instances, congenital nevi are larger than acquired nevi, measuring more than 1.5 cm in diameter.[131] However, only a few are of considerable size. Those measuring more than 20 cm in greatest diameter are referred to as giant congenital melanocytic nevi.[132] *Nongiant congenital melanocytic nevi* are usually slightly raised and often pigmented, and they may show a moderate growth of hair. Special forms are the *cerebriform congenital nevus,* which is found on the scalp as a skin-colored, convoluted mass[133]; the *spotted grouped pigmented nevus,* showing closely set brown to black papules[134]; and the *congenital acral melanocytic nevus,* which consists of a blue-black patch on the sole or the distal portion of a finger clinically resembling an acral lentiginous melanoma.[135] *Giant congenital melanocytic nevi* often have the distribution of a garment ("garment nevi"). They usually are deeply pigmented and are covered with a moderate growth of hair. Often, there are many scattered "satellite" lesions of a similar appearance.[136] These satellite nevi are benign, in contrast to the satellite mestatases that may be associated with melanomas. Leptomeningeal melanocytosis is occasionally found in cases in which the giant congenital nevus involves the neck and scalp. There may be not only epilepsy and mental retardation but also a primary leptomeningeal melanoma.[137]

Incidence of Cutaneous Melanoma

The lifetime incidence of melanoma arising either in a giant nevus or, as seen occasionally, in one of the many smaller satellite nevi is estimated to lie between 6.3% and 12%.[132,138] Thus, the majority of patients with congenital nevi will never develop melanoma. The melanoma may be present at birth, or it may arise in infancy or at any time later in life. The mortality of such melanomas is high.[137] In a recent cohort study in which 33 patients with giant congenital nevi were followed, two fatal melanomas developed, representing a relative risk approximately 1000 times greater than that in the general population.[139] In another study of 92 cases, the relative risk for melanoma was increased 239-fold,[140] and in a third study of 80 cases, three melanomas occurred after an average follow-up of about 5

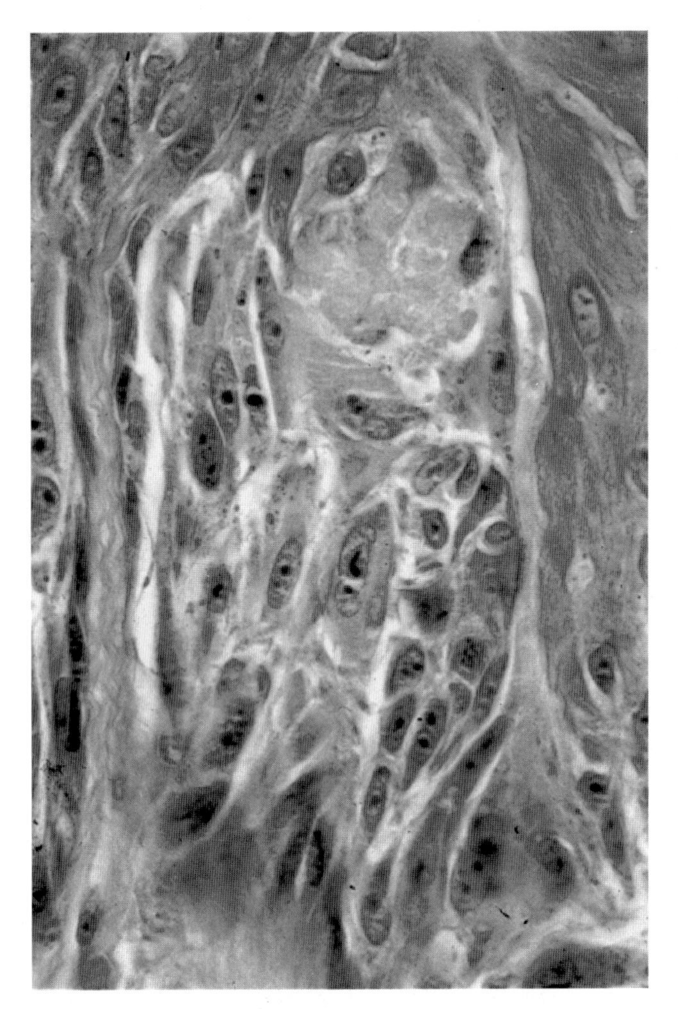

FIG. 29-13. Kamino bodies in a spindle cell nevus This nevus has prominent eosinophilic globoid Kamino bodies in its epidermal compartment. These may also be seen in Spitz nevi.

years.[141] A review of the literature shows that approximately 70% of the melanomas that have occurred in patients with giant congenital nevi have occurred before puberty; some of these melanomas have occurred in extracutaneous sites, especially the central nervous system.[137,140] It is therefore generally agreed that it would be desirable for giant melanocytic nevi to be excised, if feasible. However, complete excision is often not possible, and melanomas may develop in extracutaneous sites. Thus, clinical surveillance is an acceptable alternative.[142]

The incidence of melanoma in nongiant congenital nevi—that is, in those less than 20 cm in greatest diameter—is unknown, but it is probably greater than that in a comparable area of normal skin. It is likely that the risk is related to the lesion's size.[142] The excision of all nongiant congenital nevi where feasible is advised by many,[143,144] although not by all, authors.[132] Most of the melanomas observed in these nongiant lesions have occurred after puberty.[145]

Histopathology. The histologic appearance of giant congenital nevi generally differs from that of acquired nevi. Nongiant congenital nevi may have the same histologic appearance as acquired nevi, or may show specific diagnostic features of congenital nevi.[63,146,147]

Nongiant congenital melanocytic nevi. At one time, these nevi were thought to be superficial at birth and to show deep involvement later.[131] However, a serial study showed no change in pattern in follow-up biopsies.[147] This and other studies have shown various patterns in the distribution of the nevus cells independent of the age of the patient. Thus, nongiant congenital nevi may be junctional, compound, or intradermal nevi, and their location in the dermis may be either superficial, which may include junctional involvement, or superficial and deep.[148,149] They may differ from acquired nevi by one or more of the following features: (1) presence of melanocytes around and within hair follicles, in sweat ducts and glands, in sebaceous glands, in vessel walls, and in the perineurium of nerves; (2) extension of melanocytes between collagen bundles singly or in double rows; and (3) extension into the deepest reticular dermis and into the subcutis (see Fig. 29-4).[131] However, many nongiant congenital nevi show none of these features. For example, some documented congenital nevi have been entirely junctional,[147] whereas the likelihood of deep dermal involvement appears to increase with the size of the lesion and is actually uncommon in lesions smaller than 1.5 cm.[146] Conversely, the presence of most of the features mentioned above has been documented in nevi that were indubitably acquired after birth ("tardive" congenital nevi).[150] Thus, nevi with the constellation of features described above may be characterized as "nevi with congenital pattern features," but not all of these lesions are truly congenital in origin. It remains to be seen whether such nevi have any significance as risk markers or potential precursors of melanoma (see Fig. 29-4).

Among the special forms of nongiant congenital nevi, the *cerebriform congenital nevus* usually presents as an intradermal nevus with neuroid changes simulating those observed in neurofibroma.[133] The *spotted grouped pigmented nevi* also are intradermal nevi. They are either eccrine-centered or follicle-centered. If they are eccrine-centered, each eccrine sweat duct is tightly enveloped by nevus cells, whereas hair follicles are involved only slightly.[151] If they are follicle-centered, nevus cell nests are found mainly around the hair follicles.[134] In the *acral nevus,* a compound nevus is observed with considerable pigmentation in the upper dermis, and aggregates of nonpigmented nevus cells are present around blood vessels and eccrine glands in the lower dermis.[135]

Giant congenital melanocytic nevi. These nevi often are more complex than nongiant congenital nevi. Three patterns may be found within them: a compound or intradermal nevus, a "neural nevus," and a blue nevus pattern.[137] In most instances, the compound or intradermal nevus component predominates, whereas in others the "neural nevus" component predominates. In the latter case, formations such as neuroid tubes and nevic corpuscles are present. These areas may show considerable similarity to a neurofibroma. A component resembling a blue nevus or a cellular blue nevus is found in some of the giant pigmented nevi, usually as a minor component.[137] In rare instances, however, the entire congenital scalp lesion consists of a giant blue nevus, one of which was reported to have extended to the dura[152] and another to have infiltrated the brain[19] (Fig. 29-14).

Melanoma in congenital nevi. If a melanoma arises in a congenital nevus, it usually originates at the epidermal-dermal junction and has the appearance of an ordinary form of melanoma, usually of the superficial spreading type (see section

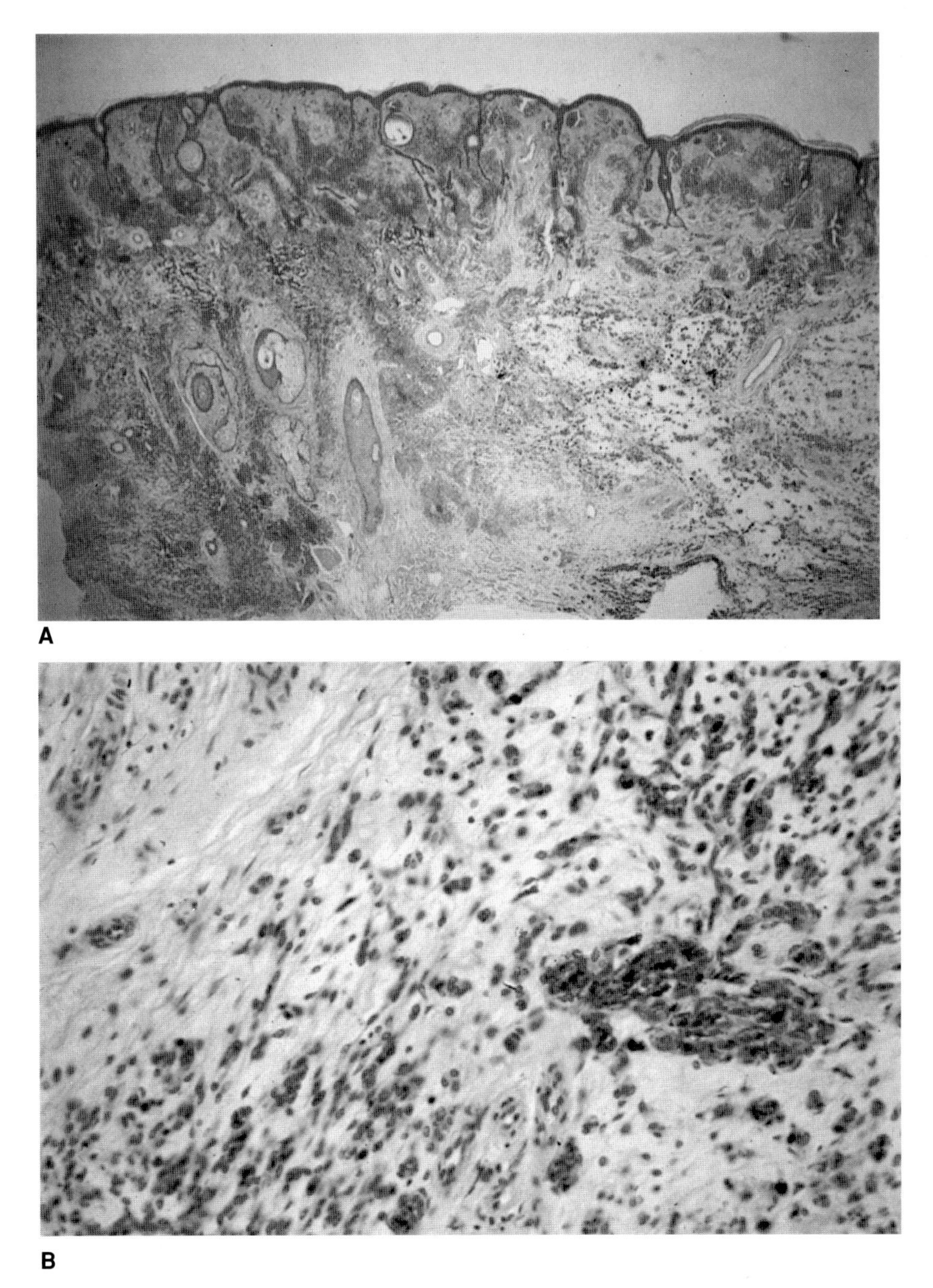

FIG. 29-14. Giant congenital nevus
(**A**) This nevus is very broad (many centimeters, extending well beyond the borders of the image, and "deep"—that is the lesional cells extend from the epidermis through the reticular dermis and into the fat. (**B**) Sheets of nevus cells are distributed among reticular dermis collagen bundles. The dermal component of giant congenital nevi is often variably cellular, and in addition to nevic differentiation there may be evidence of Schwannian or even heterotopic elements.

on Superficial Spreading Melanoma). Occasionally, however, the melanoma in a giant congenital nevus, in contrast with nearly all other cutaneous melanomas, arises deep in the dermis.[137,153] In such cases, it usually consists largely of undifferentiated "blastic" cells resembling lymphoblasts and containing little or no melanin.[137] Other patterns of malignancy that have been described in congenital nevi have included neoplasms with the appearance of neurosarcomas,[154] lesions that have been termed malignant blue nevi,[155,156] neoplasms with heterologous mesenchymal elements including rhabdomyoblasts and lipoblasts, undifferentiated spindle cell cancers, and well-differentiated neoplasms termed minimal deviation melanomas.[157] It has been emphasized that peculiar differentiation is to be expected in neoplasms of congenital nevi, and that alarmingly cellular neoplasms may not behave aggressively.[157] Thus, pathology does not always readily predict outcome. This is especially true, in our experience, in the first few months of life.

Proliferative nodules in congenital nevi. Although melanomas may occur in the dermal components of congenital nevi, cellular proliferative nodules that occur in these nevi often do not behave in a clinically aggressive fashion. Indications of a likely benign course in such nodules include (1) low mitotic rate, (2) absence of necrosis, (3) absence of high-grade uniform nuclear atypia, and (4) evidence of maturation in the form of "blending" or transitional forms between the cells in the nodule and the adjacent nevus cells. If some of these features are present in slight degree, the descriptive diagnosis of "melanocytic tumor of uncertain potential" may be appropriate.

Leptomeningeal melanocytosis. There is a diffuse infiltration of the leptomeninges with pigmented melanocytes. Also, the blood vessels entering the brain and spinal cord may be surrounded by melanocytes, and there may be areas of infiltration of the brain or spinal cord with melanocytes. Leptomeningeal melanoma can infiltrate the leptomeninx and form multiple nodules in the brain.[158]

Deep Penetrating Nevus

The deep penetrating nevus is a distinctive entity that has some features of combined, blue, and Spitz nevi.[159,160] In the first report of 70 cases from a referral center, many cases had previously been misdiagnosed as melanomas. Similar lesions had been previously described using different terminology.[161,162] Most of the lesions occurred in the second and third decades (range 3 to 63 years).[159] The head, neck, and shoulder were the most frequent sites, with no occurrences on the hands or feet. The lesions ranged from 2 to 9 mm in diameter, and were darkly pigmented papules and nodules, often diagnosed clinically as blue nevi or cellular blue nevi. In a mean follow-up of 7 years, none recurred or metastasized. However, a prospective follow-up series has not been reported. In cross section, the lesions extended at least halfway into the dermis, with a smooth, dome-shaped elevation of the epidermis.

Histopathology. At scanning magnification, the lesions are circumscribed and pyramidal in shape, with a broad base abutting the epidermis and an apex extending into or toward the fat (Fig. 29-15). Nests of nevus cells at the dermal-epidermal junction are usually present. The dermal component is composed of loosely arranged nests or fascicles of large pigmented spindle and epithelioid cells interspersed with melanophages. In many cases there is an admixture of smaller, more conventional nevus cells. The lesional cell nests tend to surround skin appendages and to infiltrate the collagen at the periphery of the lesion. The cells do not "mature" much with descent into the dermis. Some lesions have a patchy mild lymphocytic infiltrate.

At higher magnification, nuclear pleomorphism may be striking in some lesions, with variation in size and shape, hyperchromasia, and nuclear pseudoinclusions. Nucleoli are usually inconspicuous, but a few large eosinophilic nucleoli may be observed. Importantly, mitoses are absent or very rare, with no more than one or two in multiple sections of any given lesion. The cytoplasm is abundant, and contains finely divided brown melanin pigment. The lesional cells react positively for S-100 protein and HMB-45 antigen.[25]

Differential Diagnosis. Deep penetrating nevi can be distinguished from *nodular melanoma* by architectural and cytologic features. Most bulky tumorigenic melanomas exhibit a more striking pattern of epidermal involvement with spread of atypical cells into the epidermis and, often, with ulceration. Melanomas are often asymmetrical and likely to be broader than they are deep, whereas deep penetrating nevi tend to be vertically oriented like Spitz nevi. Tumorigenic melanomas usually exhibit a more destructive pattern of infiltration, with displacement and compression of the stroma, and often with necrosis. Most also exhibit marked nuclear atypia with frequent, and often abnormal, mitoses. A few nodular spindle cell melanomas have lower-grade nuclei, and in these cases the presence of more than a few mitoses may be decisive. A recent study found rates of expression of a cell cycle proliferation marker to be somewhat higher than in banal nevi, but considerably lower than in melanomas.[163]

Benign lesions that may show some tendency toward overlapping features with deep penetrating nevi include *common and cellular blue nevi,* as well as *spindle and epithelioid cell nevi.* Although deep penetrating nevi can usually be distinguished from these benign lesions, the distinction from melanoma is of greatest importance. Neural involvement is not an indicator of malignancy in these lesions.

Dysplastic Nevus

Dysplastic nevi were first described under the designations of *B-K mole syndrome* and *atypical mole syndrome* as multiple lesions occurring in patients with one or several melanomas and in some of their relatives.[164,165] It soon became apparent that multiple moles, in addition to their familial occurrence, could occur as a sporadic phenomenon in patients with melanomas. This was referred to as the *dysplastic nevus syndrome.*[166] Subsequently, cases of multiple dysplastic nevi without melanoma were reported.[167] This was followed by the recognition that dysplastic nevi frequently occur as solitary lesions, and are quite common, being found in 5% to 20% of various populations, depending on the criteria used.[59]

Dysplastic nevi form, clinically and histologically, a continuum extending from a common nevus to a superficial spreading melanoma.[168] They may be located anywhere on the body but are found most commonly on the trunk. A suitable rigorous definition of a clinically dysplastic nevus includes (1) the presence of a macular component either as the entire lesion or surrounding a papular center; (2) large size, exceeding 5 mm; (3) irregular or ill-defined "fuzzy" border; and (4) irregular pigmentation within the lesion[169] (Color Fig. 29-1).

Histopathology. When dysplastic nevi were first described in association with melanoma, it was considered that dysplastic nevi by definition always contained cytologically atypical melanocytes.[59,164] Later, it was argued by a National Institutes of Health panel that an abnormal pattern of melanocytic growth was a sufficient criterion without requiring atypia.[168] It was even stated that "most compound nevi that are confined to the epidermis and the papillary dermis are dysplastic nevi."[170] Subsequently, the term "Clark's nevus" was coined to encompass all nevi with a purely junctional component (either alone or adjacent to a dermal component), irrespective of lesion size or the presence or absence of cytologic atypia.[171] This definition would include the very common small lentiginous junctional and compound nevi. Thus, the term "Clark's nevus" is not synonymous with the term "dysplastic nevus." Because of controversy regarding its use and definition, use of the term "dysplastic nevus" was discouraged by another NIH panel, which

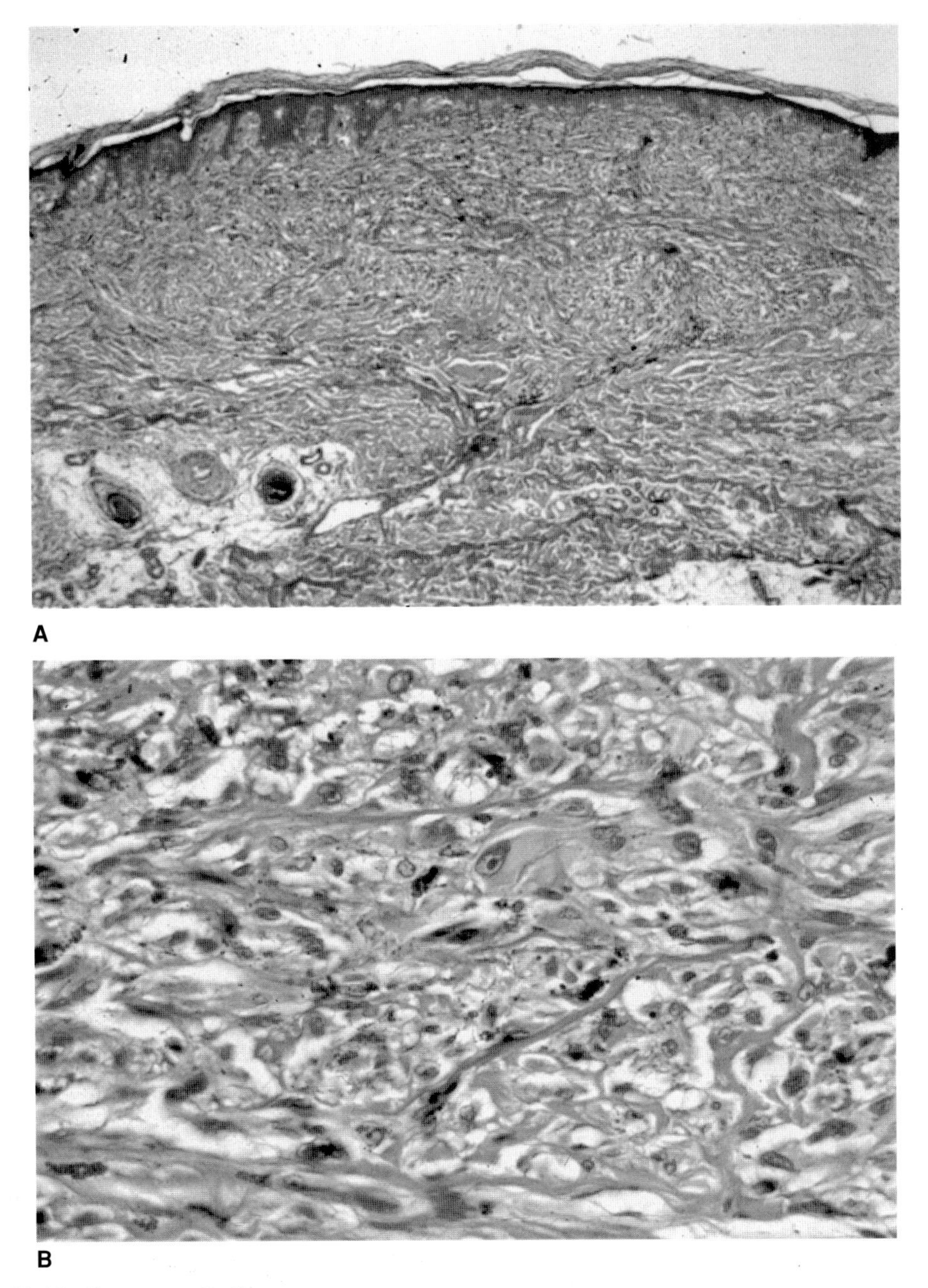

FIG. 29-15. Deep penetrating nevus
(**A**) At scanning magnification, the lesion is pyramidal, with its base applied to the epidermis and its apex in the reticular dermis. (**B**) The lesional cells in the dermis are arranged in clusters. They may be heavily pigmented, and their nuclei may be large, hyperchromatic, and pleomorphic. Mitoses are absent.

proposed the synonymous term "nevus with architectural disorder and melanocytic atypia."[172] This clumsy term has not been widely used. Specificity in distinguishing dysplastic from nondysplastic nevi is likely to be increased by the inclusion of size and cytologic atypia as criteria, as was done in the original reports. Small lesions or lesions with architectural features of dysplastic nevi but without atypia may be reported as "compound nevi" or as "lentiginous compound nevi," or the NIH descriptive terminology may be used.[58,168] Criteria for assessing melanocytic dysplasia may be summarized in two categories: *architectural features* and *cytologic features*[59] (Fig. 29-16).

In the *architectural pattern* of melanocytic dysplasia, lentiginous proliferation of nevus cells in the epidermis is the dominant feature. There is elongation of the rete ridges and an increase in the number of melanocytes, which are arranged as single cells and in nests whose long axes tend to lie parallel to the epidermal surface and that tend to form "bridges" between adjacent retia. The melanocytes in the junctional nests are frequently spindle-shaped, but they may be large and epithelioid and show abundant cytoplasm with fine, dusty melanin particles. If the lesion is compound, nests of melanocytes in the papillary dermis show a uniform appearance and evidence of maturation with

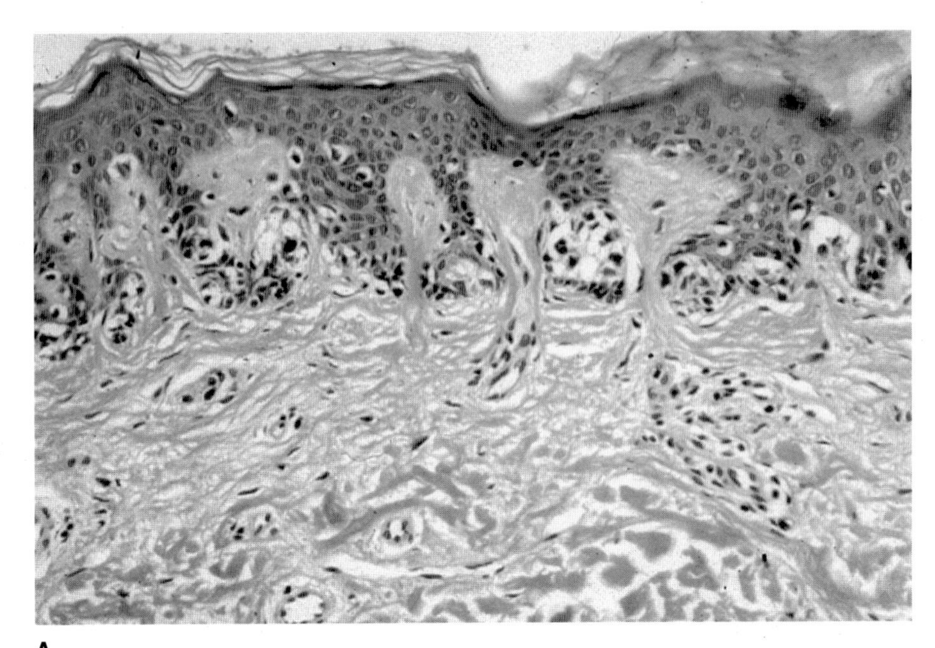

A

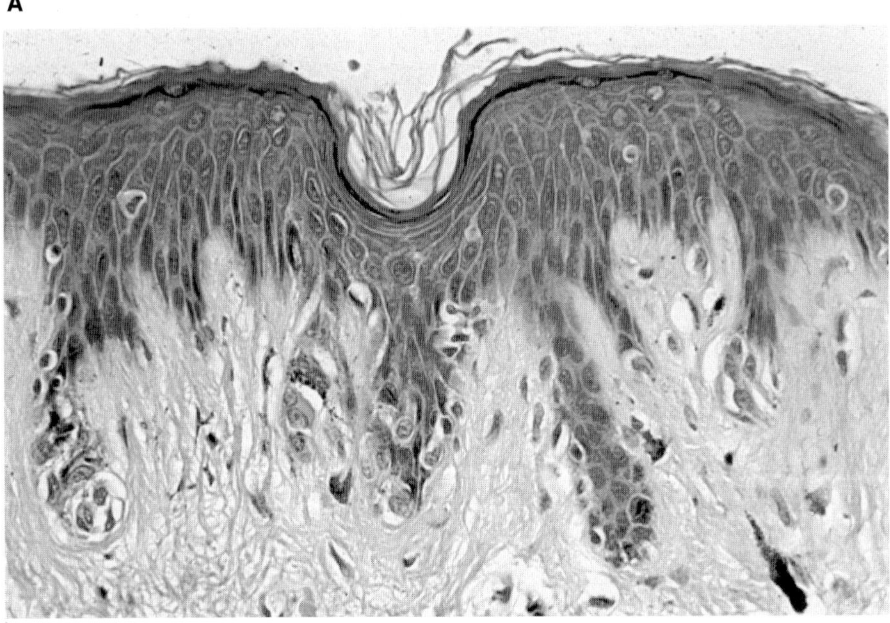

B

FIG. 29-16. Compound dysplastic nevus
(**A**) At scanning magnification, the lesions are broad and symmetrical. If a dermal component is present, the epidermal component shown here (which is always present) extends beyond its "shoulder." (**B** and **C**) In the junctional compartment of the nevus (the "shoulder"), the epidermal rete ridges are elongated but delicate, and there are nests of lesional cells that tend to be oriented parallel to the surface and to bridge between adjacent elongated retia. The lesional cell nuclei tend to be moderately enlarged in comparison with most banal type A nevus cells, and a minority of them have irregular nuclei that are irregular, hyperchromatic, or have prominent nucleoli ("random" mild to moderate cytologic atypia).

descent into the dermis, as in an ordinary compound nevus. In these compound dysplastic nevi, the intraepidermal component extends by definition beyond the lateral border of the dermal component, forming a "shoulder" to the lesion histologically, and a "target-like" or "fried-egg" pattern clinically. An inflammatory infiltrate, usually only of a mild or moderate degree and intermingled with melanophages, is present in the dermis beneath areas of junctional activity. Extension of melanocytes into the epidermis is absent or slight and is limited to the lowermost layers. Most dysplastic nevi are clinically stable,[173] so that they are not "active" in the sense of continuing growth.

Cytologically, in addition to the lentiginous melanocytic hyperplasia, melanocytic nuclear atypia is required for the diagnosis, characterized by irregularly shaped, large, hyperchro-

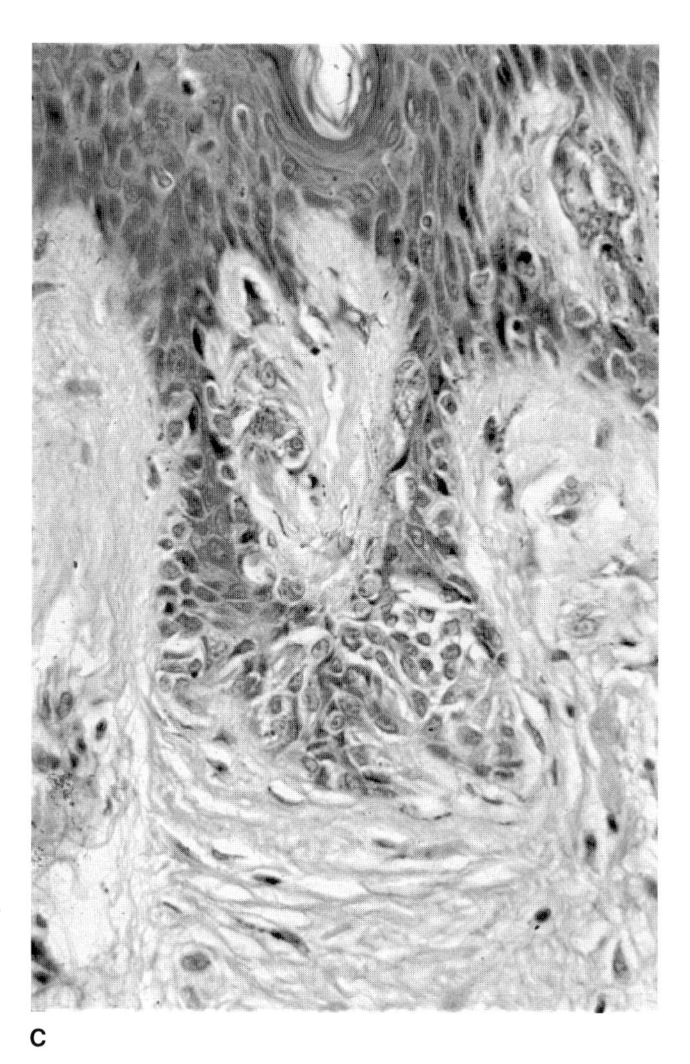

FIG. 29-16. ***Continued***

matic nuclei in some melanocytes.[58] Most atypical melanocytes lie singly or in small groups, and the atypia involves only a minority of the lesional cells ("random" cytologic atypia) (see Fig. 29-16). Focal extension of atypical-appearing melanocytes into the lower spinous layer may occur, but if this is prominent, transformation into melanoma in situ may have occurred.[167] A borderline lesion may be a dysplastic nevus or an early superficial spreading melanoma that is still in situ or microinvasive. Because such early melanomas are curable after simple excision,[174] this distinction does not carry the implication of increased mortality, so long as the lesion is entirely removed. For lesions with severe dysplasia where the differential diagnosis includes the possibility of early melanoma, conservative reexcision is recommended for lesions that have been minimally or incompletely excised.

The diagnosis of melanocytic dysplasia was found to be reproducible by two international multidisciplinary groups that used agreed-upon criteria.[175,176] In another study, including participants whose published criteria differed in their requirements for atypia and for a size criterion, it was concluded that the participating pathologists used different diagnostic criteria, but that their usage was consistent.[177] It has been suggested that histologic criteria may be more specific when applied to larger lesions, and that cytologic atypia may play a key role in the identification and significance of these lesions. Slight melanocytic atypia may be subtle and poorly reproducible, and may be of modest significance. On the other hand, the diagnosis of severe atypia is likely to be both more reproducible and of substantially greater biological significance.[178]

Pathobiology. After the early descriptions of dysplastic nevi as markers of high risk for melanoma in hereditary melanoma kindreds, it was widely assumed that identification of individuals in the community at high risk for melanoma required biopsies of nevi to "rule out dysplasia." Subsequent studies have shown that risk is best assessed by clinical evaluation of the patient's history and cutaneous phenotype. The total number of nevi and the number of large nevi,[179] light skin color, and high freckle density[27] are all risk factors for development of melanoma. Family history of melanoma is another significant risk factor,[180] as is a personal history of prior melanoma.[181] The strongest single risk factor is the presence and number of dysplastic nevi. In members of hereditary melanoma kindreds, the lifetime risk for melanoma approaches 100% in members who have clinically dysplastic nevi, corresponding to approximately a 100-fold relative risk compared with the general population.[181–183] In people without a family history of melanoma, the relative risk as determined in multiple cohort and case-control studies from different geographic regions is on the order of 3- to 10-fold, depending on the number of dysplastic (clinically atypical) nevi on their skin.[179,184–190] These data are based on clinical evaluation of nevi. Formal case-control studies of the risk associated with *histologically* dysplastic nevi do not exist, because of the difficulty of obtaining biopsies in adequate numbers of cases and controls. Even when a biopsy can be obtained, usually only one or two nevi are sampled, whereas clinical examination considers the entire phenotype. In one study, histologically verified clinically dysplastic nevi were associated with a relative risk of 4.6 for melanoma.[191] In a multiobserver study where biopsies had been taken from 24 melanoma cases and 21 random controls, four of six observers (who used different criteria) found an increased prevalence of histologic dysplasia ranging up to a 3.5-fold increase in cases compared with controls.[177]

Although melanomas in patients with dysplastic nevi may arise within preexisting dysplastic nevi, the majority arise de novo. Histologic changes indistinguishable from those in dysplastic nevi are observed at the peripheries of melanomas in approximately 20% to 30% of the cases,[58,192,193] supporting the view that at least some cutaneous melanomas take origin in dysplastic nevi. Even so, most dysplastic nevi are clinically stable[173] and will never evolve into melanomas. This paradox is explained by the fact that dysplastic nevi are vastly more common than melanomas in the general population, and provides a rationale against indiscriminate excision of dysplastic nevi for prophylaxis of melanoma.

In keeping with their role as potential precursors and as simulants of melanoma, dysplastic nevi tend to occupy an intermediate position between nevi and melanomas in laboratory studies. In cell cycle proliferation marker studies, the reactivity of dysplastic nevi is intermediate, although closer to that of common nevi than to that of melanoma.[194,195] Electron microscopic studies of dysplastic nevi have show abnormal spherical and partially melanized melanosomes similar to those observed in superficial spreading melanomas.[196,197] Although most in situ hybridization or immunohistochemical studies have shown reactivity similar to that of common nevi, dysplastic nevi have reacted in an intermediate manner with some markers,[198] whereas the reactivity with others has been more akin to that of melanomas,[197,199] or to nevi.[200] Interesting recent studies have shown that the amount of red pheomelanin is greater in dysplastic nevi than in common nevi or normal skin.[201] Because pheomelanin may be a generator of toxic-free radicals after UV irradiation, this attribute may increase the risk of genetic mutations in these lesions, which may contribute to continued tumor progression.

Management. The major importance of biopsy in an individual with dysplastic nevi is to rule out the possibility of melanoma in a problematic lesion. Key features in making this distinction are reviewed in Table 29-3. Lesions in which some features of dysplasia are observed but not judged to be diagnostic may be reported as "lentiginous (junctional or compound) nevi," or "nevus with architectural disorder," with an interpretive note. Such a note may indicate that additional evaluation of the patient could be appropriate for assessment of melanoma risk, and that periodic surveillance could be appropriate, especially if there are other clinically atypical nevi, or a family or personal history of melanoma.

In conclusion, in patients with dysplastic nevi, periodic surveillance of the patient, and evaluation of first-degree relatives, may be indicated. This is especially true if the clinically dysplastic lesions are numerous, and for patients who have personal or family histories of melanoma. There is evidence that surveillance and/or education of persons at increased risk for melanoma can result in the diagnosis of melanomas in their early, curable stages.[202] The major role of biopsy and of histologic examination of nevi in such persons is to rule out melanoma in a clinically suspicious or changing lesion. Lesions whose biopsies show severe dysplasia or changes suggestive of evolving melanoma in situ (see Table 29-3) should be considered for conservative reexcision if their margins are close or involved.

Halo Nevus

A halo nevus, also known as Sutton's nevus or nevus depigmentosa centrifugum, represents a pigmented nevus surrounded by a depigmented zone, or halo (Color Fig. 29-2). The nevus may be of almost any of the types described in the preceding sections, and a similar halo reaction may be seen in relation to a primary or metastatic melanoma.[203] In the common type of halo nevus, which is characterized histologically by an inflammatory infiltrate and is therefore referred to as *inflammatory halo nevus,* the central nevus only rarely shows erythema or crusting; however, it undergoes involution in most instances, a process that extends over a period of several months. The area of depigmentation shows no clinical signs of inflammation and, even though it may persist for many months or even years, ultimately disappears in most cases. However, there are well-document examples in which a halo nevus fails to involute, even though an inflammatory infiltrate is present, and repigmentation of the halo takes place.[204] Most persons with halo nevi are children or young adults, and the back is the most common site. Not infrequently, halo nevi are multiple, occurring either simultaneously or successively.

Besides the more common inflammatory halo nevus with histologically apparent inflammation, there also are cases of *noninflammatory halo nevi* in which histologic examination shows no inflammatory infiltrate.[205] In such instances, the nevus does not involute. In addition, there is the so-called *halo nevus phenomenon,* also referred to as *halo nevus without halo.* In these instances, the nevus shows histologic signs of inflammation analogous to a halo nevus but without presenting a halo clinically.[205,206] Such nevi may involute.

Halo dermatitis around a melanocytic nevus refers to a tem-

TABLE 29-3. *Key features of dysplastic nevus versus radial growth phase melanoma*

Dysplastic nevus	Radial growth phase melanoma
Pattern features	
May be less than 6 mm in diameter, not often more than 10 mm	Usually greater than 6 mm in diameter, often much greater than 10 mm
Somewhat symmetrical	Often highly asymmetrical
Often symmetrically arranged about "shoulders" of a mature dermal nevus	If dermal nevus is present, it is likely to be asymmetrically placed.
Uniformly elongated, narrow, delicate rete ridges	Irregularly thickened epidermis, often with effaced rete ridges
No alteration of stratum corneum	May be hyperkeratotic
Nests predominate over single cells in the epidermis.	Single cells predominate except in late lesions.
Little or no pagetoid spread of lesional cells into epidermis	Usually obvious pagetoid spread into epidermis, extending to stratum corneum
Patchy lymphocytic infiltrate in papillary dermis	Brisk bandlike infiltrate
No regression	Regression common
Last lesional cells at lateral border are often in a nest.	Last cells are often single, and may be above the basal zone.
Cytologic features	
Scattered atypical epithelioid cells with dusty melanin pigment, nucleoli, and anisokaryosis ("random atypia")	Epithelioid cells with dusty pigment, nucleoli, and anisokaryosis predominate ("uniform atypia")
Most cells are not atypical.	Most cells are atypical.
No mitoses in epidermis or dermis	Intraepidermal mitoses in about one-third of cases; no mitoses in dermis
Cells in dermis, if any, are smaller than those in epidermis.	Cells in dermis are similar to those in epidermis.

porary banal inflammatory reaction surrounding a nevus (Meyerson's *eczematous nevus*).[207] There is a papular compound nevus that becomes surrounded by an eczematous halo. Histologically, the epidermis adjacent to the nevus is spongiotic. An analogous phenomenon of "nevocentric" erythema multiforme has also been described.[208]

Histopathology. An inflammatory halo nevus in its early stage shows nests of nevus cells embedded in a dense inflammatory infiltrate, in the upper dermis and at the epidermal-dermal junction (Fig. 29-17). Later, more scattered nevus cells than nests are observed. Even when melanin is still present in the nevus cells, these cells often show evidence of damage to their nuclei and cytoplasm, and some frankly apoptotic nevus cells are commonly observed. Some cells, especially superficially, may have enlarged ovoid nucleoli, changes that may be regarded as a form of "reactive atypia." High-grade nuclear atypia is not observed. Importantly, the lesional cells tend to show evidence of "maturation," becoming smaller with descent from superficial to deep within the lesion. Lesional cell mitoses are rare, but if present should prompt consideration of the possibility of melanoma. Most of the cells in the dense inflammatory infiltrate are lymphocytes. However, some of them are macrophages

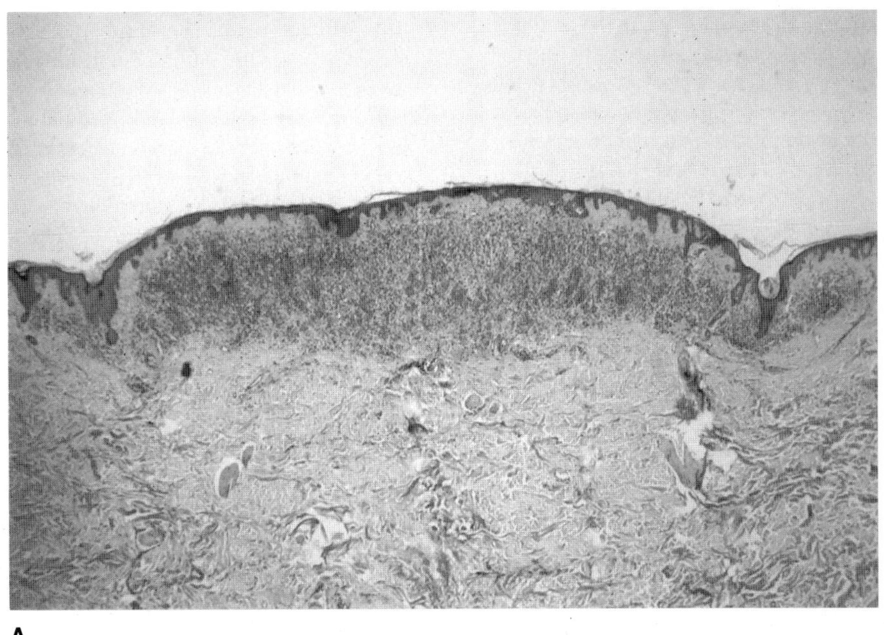

A

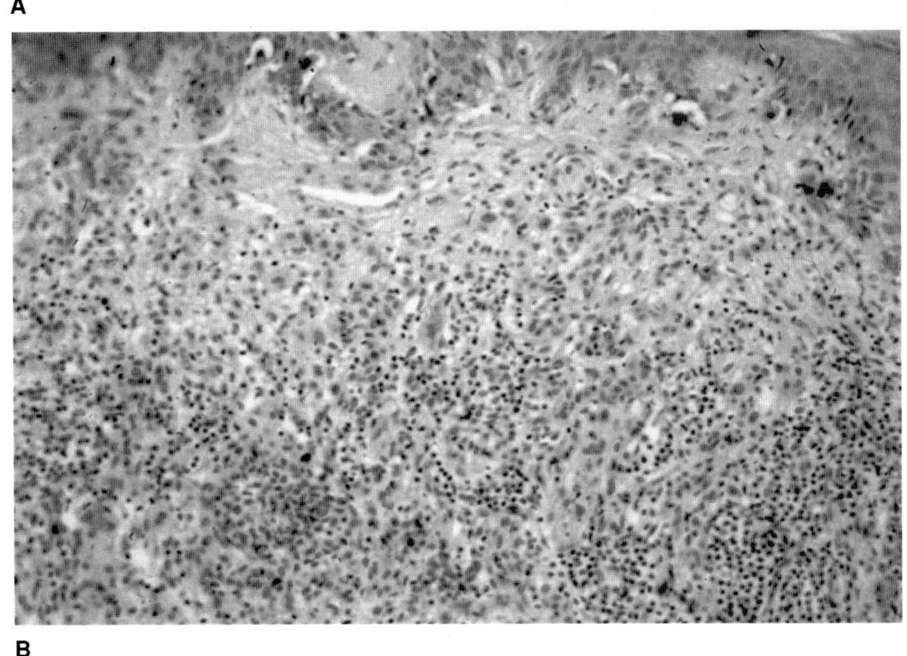

B

FIG. 29-17. Halo nevus
(**A**) These nevi are usually small and symmetrical. A dense infiltrative lymphocytic response blurs the silhouettes of the lesional nevus cells in the dermis at scanning magnification. (**B**) Small lymphocytes are diffusely placed among the dermal nevus cells, which may appear swollen and slightly atypical ("reactive" atypia). Severe or uniform atypia or mitotic activity should suggest the possibility of melanoma.

containing various amounts of melanin. As the infiltrate invades the nevus cell nests, it often is difficult to distinguish between the lymphoid cells of the infiltrate and the type B nevus cells in the middermis, because they, too, have the appearance of lymphoid cells. The infiltrate tends to extend upward into the lower portion of the epidermis. In most instances, the infiltrate is characterized by dense cellular packing without vasodilatation or intercellular edema and by sharp demarcation along its lower border.

At a later stage, only a few and finally no distinct nevus cells can be identified. Gradually, after all nevus cells have disappeared, the inflammatory infiltrate subsides.

In both the inflammatory and noninflammatory halo nevi, the epidermis of the halo at first shows a reduction in the amount of melanin on staining with silver and fewer dopa-positive melanocytes than are observed in the normal epidermis. Ultimately, there is complete absence of melanin and also a negative dopa reaction. Especially in early lesions, lymphocytes may be seen rosetting around damaged melanocytes in the halo.

Histogenesis. Immunohistochemical staining for S-100 protein helps in the identification of nevus cells within the inflammatory infiltrate, because their number may be small and it may be difficult to differentiate them from the lymphocytes of the infiltrate.[209] However, Langerhans' cells and some histiocytes also react with S-100 protein. Electron microscopic study reveals that, under the influence of the lymphocytic infiltrate, all nevus cells and melanocytes within reach of the infiltrate at first are damaged and ultimately disappear. In the nevus, many nevus cells appear vacuolated and contain only few melanosomes, but large aggregates of melanosomes are observed within macrophages.[210]

In the depigmenting halo, the melanocytes show various kinds of degeneration, such as vacuolization and coagulation of the cytoplasm and autophagocytosis of melanosomes. The melanocytes are observed partially in the upper layers of the epidermis and are apparently shed from the epidermis.[211] Both in halo nevi and in vitiligo, the depigmentation takes place through disappearance of the melanocytes. However, the association of vitiligo and halo nevus is not sufficiently common for halo nevus to be regarded as a form of vitiligo.

Differential Diagnosis. It can be difficult to differentiate the early lesions of an inflammatory halo nevus from a melanoma; both types of lesions may have a dense cellular infiltrate in the dermis, and, in halo nevi, the nevus cell nests, as a result of having been invaded by the cellular infiltrate, may appear atypical. The danger of misinterpretation is greatest in halo nevi without halos, the so-called halo nevus phenomenon. However, the inflammatory infiltrate in halo nevi is more pronounced than in melanoma and extends diffusely through the lesion, rather than being concentrated at the periphery as in most examples of tumorigenic melanoma. The diagnosis of melanoma rather than halo nevus is likely for a complex lesion that has an adjacent in situ or microinvasive component. Whether or not such an adjacent component is present, attributes of the nodule itself that should prompt consideration of melanoma include larger size, asymmetry, lack of lesional cell maturation, uniform high-grade nuclear atypia, and mitotic activity.

If no identifiable nevus cells are present, the diagnosis of halo nevus is suggested by the presence of melanophages in the dense cellular infiltrate and by the absence of melanin in the epidermis on staining with silver.

Recurrent Nevus (Pseudomelanoma)

Recurrence of a nevus may show clinical hyperpigmentation that on biopsy may exhibit histological changes suggestive of melanoma.[212–214] Recurrence may follow incomplete removal of a nevus, particularly by a shave biopsy or electrodesiccation, or the nevus may apparently have been completely excised. The pigmentation in recurrent nevi is confined to the region of the scar, and typically presents within a few weeks of the surgical procedure. After this rapid appearance, the pigment is stable. In contrast, recurrent melanoma does not respect the border of the scar, and extends over time into the adjacent skin. Paradoxically, recurrent melanoma occurs more slowly, over months or years, but progresses inexorably.

Histopathology. Although most recurrent nevi are not atypical, in a few instances they contain slightly atypical melanocyte, both singly and in nests, arranged mainly along the epidermal-dermal junction, but occasionally also extending into the upper dermis and also extending up into the epidermis in a pagetoid pattern[128] (Fig. 29-18). Deep remnants of the nevus may be seen in the reticular dermis beneath the scar.[213] A lymphocytic infiltrate with melanophages may be observed in the upper dermis. Distinction from melanoma may be difficult without a pertinent history. However, the presence of fibrosis in the upper dermis and often of remnants of a melanocytic nevus beneath the zone of fibrosis, as well as the sharp lateral demarcation, usually make a correct diagnosis possible. As is true clinically, the recurrent nevus is confined to the epidermis above the scar, whereas recurrent melanoma may extend into the adjacent epidermis. However, persistent nevus, after a partial biopsy, may also involve skin adjacent to a scar. In this instance, ordinary criteria for the distinction between melanomas and nevi apply, as discussed later. In any problematic case in which the diagnosis is in doubt, the original biopsy should be obtained for review.

Histogenesis. The nevus cells in some recurrent lesions may originate from residual nevus cells located either at the periphery of the lesion or along the outer root sheaths of hairs. Recurrences that follow complete excision may result from activation of melanocytes. The confinement of these reactive changes to the regenerating epidermis above the biopsy scar suggests that the process may be related to growth factors involved in wound healing. Some of these, such as fibroblast growth factors, are known to be trophic for melanocytes in vitro.[215]

MALIGNANT MELANOMA

Malignant melanoma may be located in situ or may be invasive. Invasive melanoma may be tumorigenic ("vertical growth phase") or nontumorigenic ("radial growth phase"). Melanoma in situ and nontumorigenic invasive melanoma can be divided into (1) lentigo maligna, (2) superficial spreading, (3) acral lentiginous, and (4) mucosal lentiginous types. Tumorigenic melanoma may arise in relation to a preexisting nontumorigenic component of any of the types listed earlier, in which case it is named accordingly. Alternatively, tumorigenic melanoma may arise de novo, in which case it is termed "nodular melanoma." Important variants of tumorigenic melanoma include desmoplastic melanoma and neurotropic melanoma. Other unusual forms of tumorigenic melanoma will be discussed later.

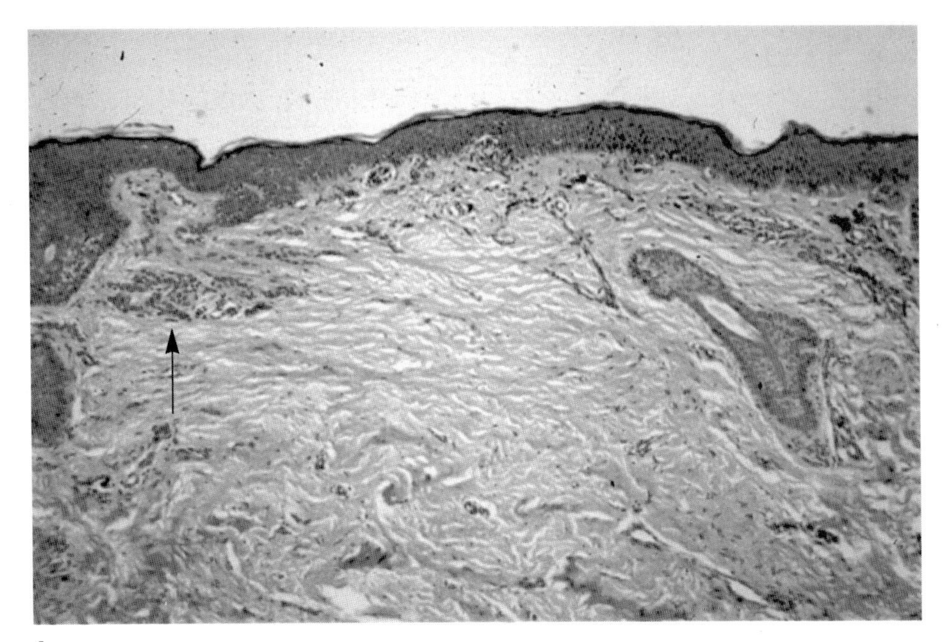

A

B

FIG. 29-18. Recurrent and persistent melanocytic nevus
(**A**) Recurrent pigmentation may occur after complete excision of a nevus, or may occur in the scar of a partial removal, as in this example, where the pathology of the recurrent nevus is visible only above the scar, and residual dermal nevus cells of the persistent original nevus are present *(arrow)* adjacent to the scar *(center and right)*. (**B**) The cells of the recurrent nevus in the epidermis are variably enlarged, and they may be arranged with single cells predominating in foci and extending up into the epidermis in a pagetoid pattern, usually confined to the lower portions of the epidermis.

All major types of melanoma originate almost invariably from melanocytes at the epidermal-dermal junction. Although the lesions are commonly associated with a preexisting nevus, more than half of them arise de novo, or completely supplant the precursor. The majority of melanomas are thought to be caused by sunlight exposure, either intermittent (sunburn episodes) in the more common superficial spreading melanomas, or chronic in the lentigo maligna melanomas.

Classification of Melanoma

There are two major categories of melanoma, which represent sequential stages or "phases" of stepwise tumor progression.[216] In the nontumorigenic *radial* or *horizontal growth phase,* the neoplastic melanocytes (melanoma cells) are confined to the epidermis (melanoma in situ) or to the epidermis and papillary dermis without formation of a tumor mass

TABLE 29-4. *Classification of melanoma*

Radial Growth Phase (RGP)
Nontumorigenic Melanoma
In Situ or Microinvasive
  Superficial spreading melanoma (SSM)
  Lentigo maligna melanoma (LMM)
  Acral lentiginous melanoma (ALM)
  Unclassified radial growth phase (URGP)
Vertical Growth Phase (VGP)
Tumorigenic Melanoma
No RGP Compartment
  Nodular melanoma (NM, 10% of all melanomas[219])
RGP Compartment Present (may be SSM, LMM, ALM, URGP)
  Usual vertical growth phase
  Desmoplastic
  Neurotropic
    Other variants (e.g., nevoid/minimal deviation, "balloon cell," "amelanotic," "spindle cell")

(microinvasive melanoma). This phase may be followed after varying lengths of time by the focal appearance of the tumorigenic *vertical growth phase*—a phase of dermal invasion with tumor formation. Thus, a fully evolved melanoma may have two major lesional compartments: the nontumorigenic, in situ or microinvasive radial growth phase; and a contiguous tumorigenic vertical growth phase compartment. In addition, dermal and/or epidermal compartments of an associated nevus may be recognized in some melanomas. Variants of each of the major compartments have been described and are listed in Table 29-4.[217–219]

About 5% to 10% of melanomas fall into "unclassified" or "other" categories.[220] The fact that categorization of an individual case is occasionally difficut does not mean that classification of melanoma, after accounting for tumor thickness and site, is unnecessary, as has been stated.[221] Even though in the tumorigenic stage, the prognosis is similar for all four types of melanoma, depending largely on the depth of invasion, the duration of the in situ phase preceding lentigo maligna melanoma is, on the average, longer than that of superficial spreading melanoma.[222] Furthermore, there are differences in the apparent etiology of the various forms of melanoma. Finally, the separate descriptions of the morphological variants have nosological and pedagogical value, facilitating accurate diagnosis by enabling the recognition of the variant patterns.

Morphology of Tumorigenic and Nontumorigenic Melanoma

In their nontumorigenic stage, melanomas tend to expand more or less inexorably along the radii of an imperfect circle as viewed clinically. The clinically derived term "radial growth" has no intuitive histologic meaning, and the histologic term "horizontal growth phase" has been suggested as an alternative. The major clinical diagnostic criteria have been summarized as "ABCD criteria," which include lesional Asymmetry (one half of a lesion does not match the other half in shape or in color distribution), lesional Border irregularity (the lesion tends to have an indented coastline like the map of a small island), lesional Color variegation (the surface is multicolored and may include shades of tan, brown, blue-black, gray-white, and other variations), and lesional Diameter (generally greater than 6 mm, although some melanomas are smaller[223] (Color Figs. 29-3, 29-4, and 29-5).

Histologically, most of the lesional cells in the nontumorigenic melanomas are located in the epidermis. Microinvasion is defined as the presence of a few lesional cells in the papillary dermis, without "tumorigenic proliferation," which is defined later. Microinvasive lesions are not specifically distinguishable from in situ melanomas on clinical grounds. Whether microinvasive or in situ, nontumorigenic melanomas appear to lack competence for metastasis. In a database of 624 clinical stage I invasive melanoma cases followed for 10 years or more, the 8-year survival rate among 161 patients with microinvasive or in situ (pure RGP) melanomas was 100 ± 1%. In the same database, the patients with lesions in only the radial growth phase were 4.3 years younger than those who also exhibited lesions in the vertical growth phase, which is consistent with the hypothesis that the radial growth phase is antecedent and relatively indolent.[174]

Clinically, the tumorigenic vertical growth phase is qualitatively different from the plaquelike radial growth phase. The tumor appears as an expanding papule within a previously indolent plaque lesion, and grows in three dimensions in a balloonlike fashion to form a nodule. Typicallly, the ABCD criteria do not apply to the tumor nodule itself, which is commonly symmetrical with smooth borders. The color is often quite uniform, and may be pink rather than blue-black, and the diameter is often less than 6 mm, even in a quite high-risk lesion (Color Fig. 29-6). For these reasons, diagnosis of melanoma may be subtle in a nodular melanoma that lacks an adjacent nontumorigenic compartment.

The major histologic feature that distinguishes a tumorigenic melanoma is the capacity for proliferation of melanoma cells in the extracellular matrix of the dermis to form an expansile mass.[224] In contrast, nontumorigenic melanoma cells may proliferate inexorably in the epidermal compartment, and may invade the dermis, but do not proliferate there. The lack of metastatic capacity in nontumorigenic melanomas may be explained by considering that cell proliferation in the matrix of a distant site is essential to the development of a metastasis. Thus, it is likely that a tumor that cannot proliferate in the matrix at its local site of origin will not do so in a metastatic site either. Operational definitions of tumorigenic and nontumorigenic melanoma are as follows.[224,225]

Tumorigenic Melanoma (Vertical Growth Phase)

A. A *mass* of melanoma cells is present in the dermis, defined as at least one cluster (nest) in the dermis that is larger than the largest intraepidermal cluster (indicative of a tumor with the capacity for expansile growth in the dermis), *or*
B. The presence of any mitoses in the dermal component of the melanoma is also indicative of a tumor with the capacity for expansile growth in the dermis and defines a typical vertical growth phase even in the absence of criterion A.

Nontumorigenic Melanoma (Radial Growth Phase)

A. No mass of melanoma cells is present in the dermis (no cluster larger than the largest intraepidermal cluster), *and*
B. There are no mitoses in the dermal component of the melanoma.

Radial growth phase may be "pure," or may be recognized as a "compartment" of a complex primary melanoma in which the earlier listed histologic criteria apply only to that portion of the melanoma adjacent to the VGP (see Fig. 29-3). "Pure" RGP melanoma may be defined as "the absence of VGP in a primary melanoma."

In a recent study conducted by the Pathology Panel of the Cancer Research Campaign in the United Kingdom, the level of agreement for recognition of vertical growth phase was "good" as judged by formal kappa analysis, and was improved after discussion of standardized criteria among members of the reviewing panel.[226]

The Nontumorigenic Compartment of Primary Malignant Melanoma (Radial Growth Phase)

In this section, the morphology of the nontumorigenic compartments of the different forms of melanoma will be described. Next, the morphology of the tumorigenic vertical growth phase, which tends to be similar among the different forms, will be discussed. Typically, about 90% of all melanomas have a nontumorigenic compartment, and about half of these also have a tumorigenic focus. About 10% of melanomas, termed "nodular melanomas," have a tumorigenic but no in situ or invasive compartment.

Superficial Spreading Melanoma

Superficial spreading melanoma (SSM), also referred to as pagetoid melanoma,[218] is the most frequent form of melanoma (about 70% of all cases), and may therefore be regarded as "common" or "usual" melanoma. These lesions have been described in the past as "atypical melanocytic hyperplasia"[227] or as "precancerous melanosis," a term that dates back to one of the earliest descriptions of melanoma.[228] The lesions may occur on exposed skin but are rather more commonly found on intermittently exposed skin and are rare on unexposed skin. The most frequently involved sites are the upper back, especially in men, and the lower legs, especially in women. The lesions are slightly or definitely elevated, with palpable borders and irregular, partly arciform outlines (see Fig. 29-3). There is often variation in color that includes not only tan, brown, and black, but also pink, blue, and gray. White areas may be observed at sites of spontaneous regression. Microinvasion may be clinically inapparent, but the onset of tumorigenic vertical growth is indicated by the development of a papule followed by nodularity and sometimes also ulceration, the latter usually being a late feature. In rare instances the lesion has a verrucous surface, in which case differentiation from a seborrheic keratosis may be difficult.[229] In its early stage of development, superficial spreading melanoma may be indistinguishable clinically from a dysplastic nevus. Histologic examination is thus the "gold standard" and is necessary for accurate diagnosis.

Histopathology. Architectural pattern features of importance in the diagnosis include the large diameter of the lesions, poor circumscription (the last cells at the edge of the lesion tend to be small, single, and scattered), and asymmetry (one half of the lesion does not mirror the other half).[230] The epidermis is irregularly thickened and thinned. Rather uniformly rounded, large melanocytes are scattered in a pagetoid pattern throughout the epidermis. The large cells lie predominantly in nests in the lower epidermis and singly in the upper epidermis. The nests tend to vary a good deal in size and shape, and to become confluent.[88] Dermal melanophages and a dermal infiltrate are regularly present. The lymphocytic infiltrate is typically dense and bandlike, especially in invasive lesions. This contrasts with the patchy perivascular infiltrate of dysplastic nevi (Fig. 29-19).

Cytologically, the lesional cells are rather uniform and have atypical, hyperchromatic nuclei and abundant cytoplasm containing varying amounts of melanin that often consists of small, "dusty" particles. The tumor cells are almost entirely devoid of dendrites. This "uniform cytological atypia" is of considerable diagnostic importance and contrasts with the random atypia of dysplastic nevi.

Histogenesis. Electron microscopic examination reveals melanosomes in great numbers in the large pagetoid tumor cells. Their shape is largely spheroid, rather than ellipsoid as in normal melanocytes and in the tumor cells of lentigo maligna. They often also show other abnormalities, such as an absence of cross-linkages of the filaments within the melanosomes.[231] Melanization within the melanosomes is variable but often incomplete.

Differential Diagnosis. A junctional nevus differs from superficial spreading melanoma in the radial growth phase by a lack of atypicality in the tumor cells, particularly in their nuclei, by a lack of pagetoid upward extension of tumor cells, by the absence of a significant inflammatory infiltrate in the upper dermis, and by a sharper lateral demarcation. Salient features in the important distinction from junctional melanocytic dysplasia have been reviewed (see Table 29-3) and include, at scanning magnification, larger size, asymmetry, an irregularly thickened and thinned epidermis, and a bandlike lymphocytic infiltrate. At higher magnification, indicators of melanoma include the presence of high-level pagetoid proliferation (large neoplastic cells scattered among benign keratinocytes), high-grade and/or uniform cytologic atypia, and lesional cell mitoses (which are present in about one-third of the cases). The differential diagnostic distinction from lentiginous melanoma is of lesser consequence, because the management is the same. In lentigo maligna, the epidermis is atrophic, and pagetoid proliferation is less prominent. Problematic cases can be reported as "malignant melanoma" (e.g., in situ or microinvasive) without designation as to type.

When the tumorigenic vertical growth phase is present, it does not differ appreciably from that in any other form of melanoma, except for the adjacent radial growth phase. Classification of such "complex" primary melanomas is based on the morphology of the radial growth phase (Fig. 29-20).

Among the nonmelanocytic neoplasms that must be differentiated from a superficial spreading melanoma in situ are Paget's disease and pagetoid examples of Bowen's disease. Paget's dis-

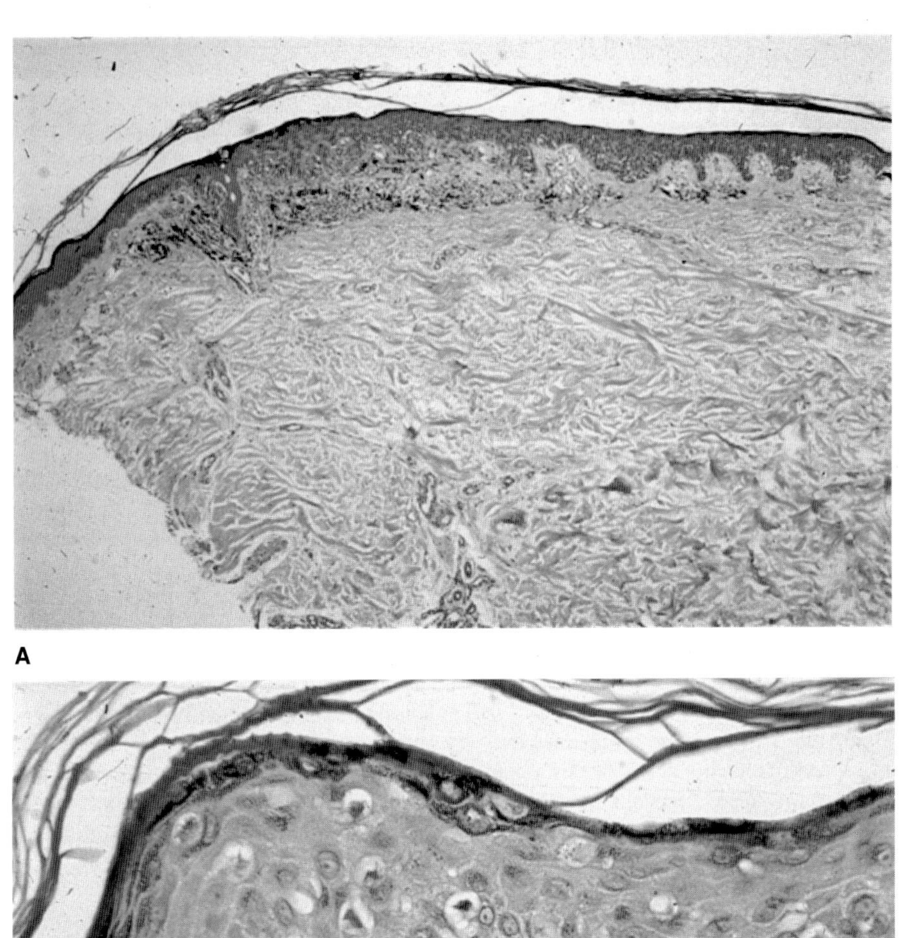

A

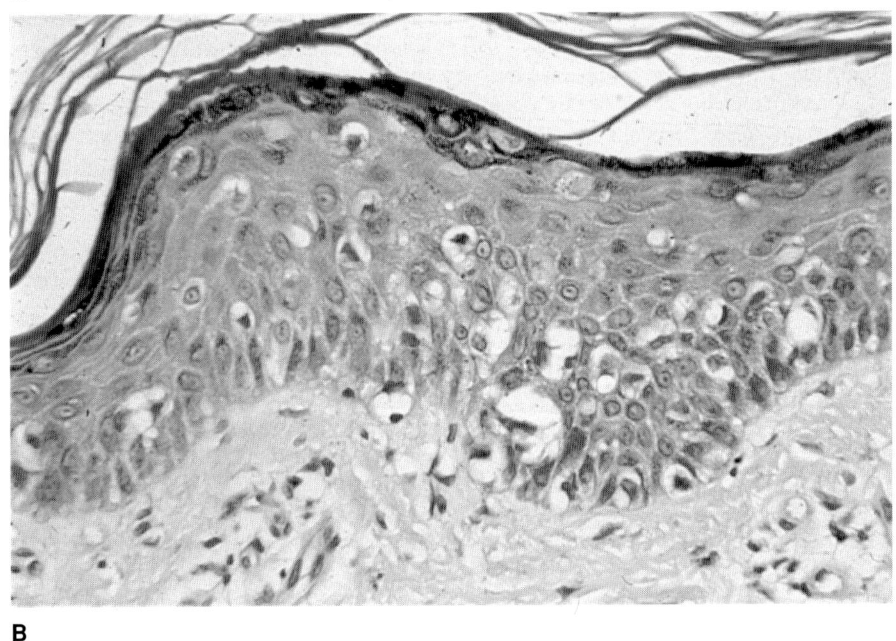

B

FIG. 29-19. Superficial spreading melanoma, microinvasive
(**A**) Scanning magnification reveals a broad plaque that is asymmetrical in the distribution of the lesional cells and responding lymphocytes and keratinocytes. (**B**) The lesional cells are uniformly atypical, and they tend to be arranged at least focally with single cells predominating and extending up into the epidermis in a pagetoid pattern. In this view, the basement membrane is intact (in situ).

ease usually shows remnants of compressed basal cells beneath the tumor cells, whereas in superficial spreading melanoma the lesional cells extend to the basement membrane. In Paget's disease, the tumor cells may stain positively for carcinoembryonic antigen and keratin, and are negative for HMB-45. S-100 reactivity, although unusual, may be observed in Paget's disease. Pagetoid Bowen's disease shows, as a rule, a well-preserved basal cell layer, except in areas in which dermal invasion has taken place, and, immunohistochemically, it stains positively for antikeratin antibodies (e.g., AE1/AE3[232]). As a rule, it does not stain with S-100 or HMB-45. It should be noted that the cells of Paget's disease and of Bowen's disease may contain melanin pigment, because of transfer from reactive melanocytes in the adjacent skin (see also Chap. 30).

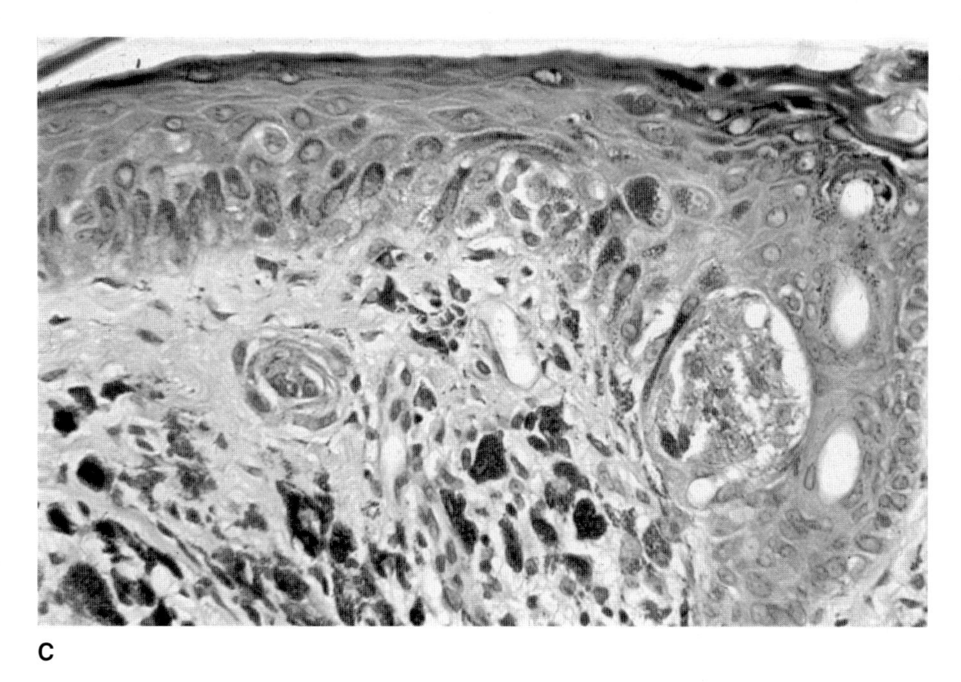

C

FIG. 29-19. *Continued*
(**C**) In another portion of the lesion, there is a cluster of cells in the dermis that is smaller than the largest intraepidermal cluster, and there are no dermal mitoses. These attributes define a focus of "microinvasive" nontumorigenic melanoma (radial growth phase).

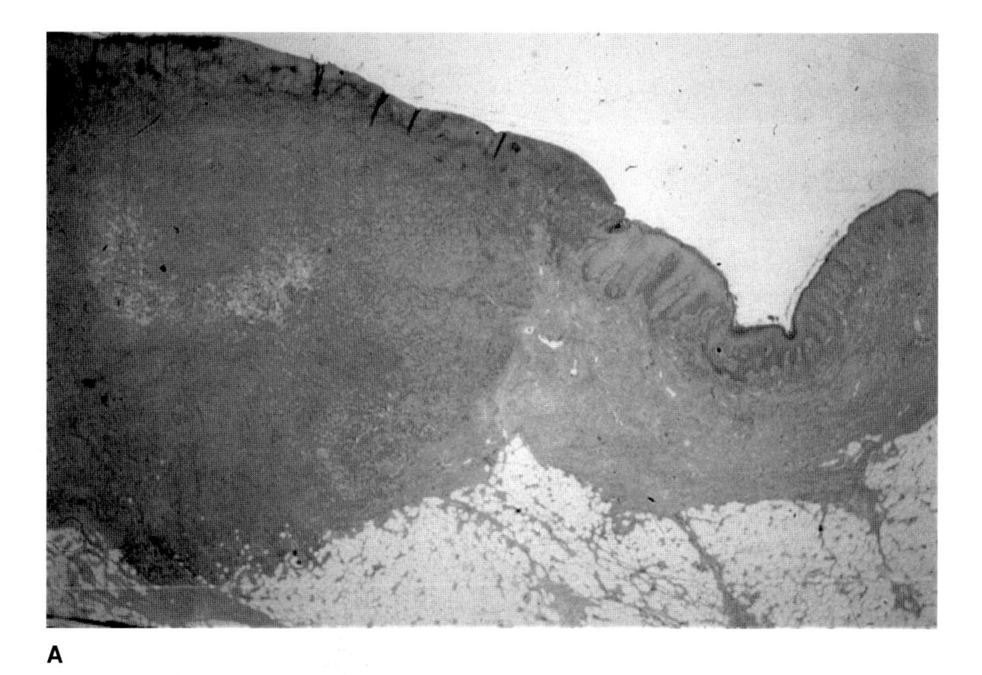

A

FIG. 29-20. Malignant melanoma, tumorigenic (radial and vertical growth phases)
(**A**) At scanning magnification, a bulky ulcerated tumor nodule *(left)* is eccentrically placed in contiguity with a broad plaque, the nontumorigenic radial growth phase compartment. (*continued on next page*)

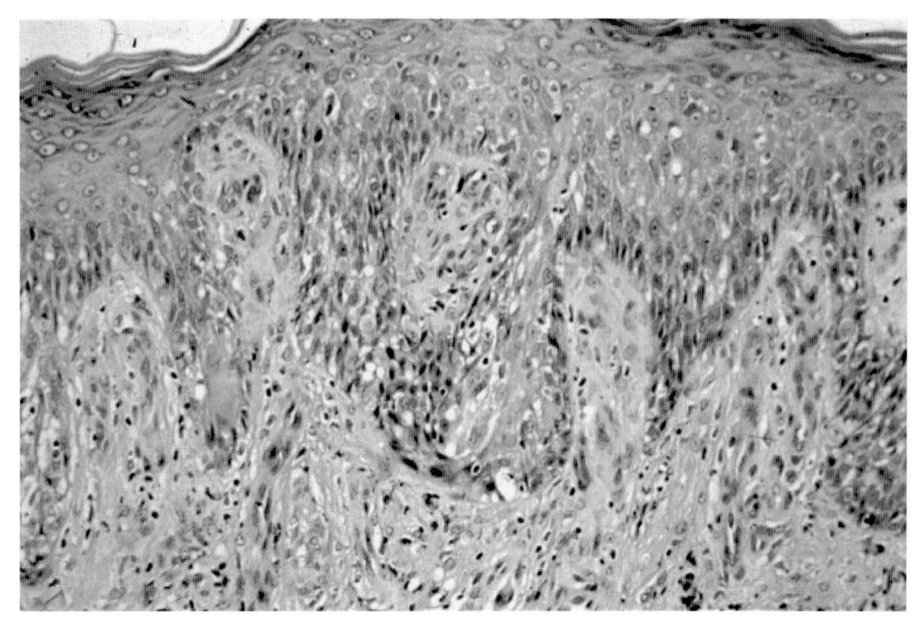

B

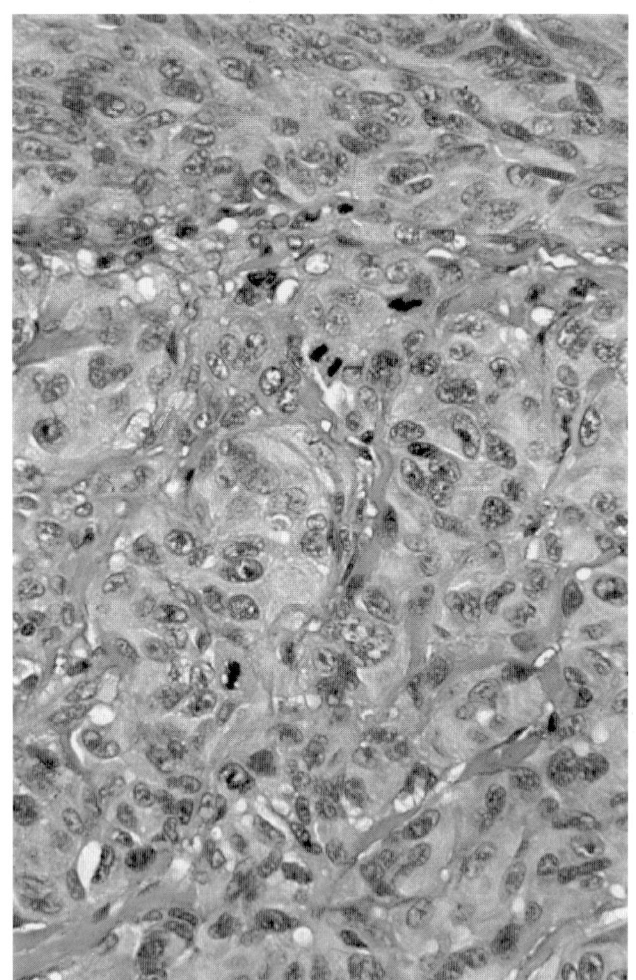

C

FIG. 29-20. *Continued*
(**B**) The nontumorigenic compartment adjacent to the nodule is composed of uniformly atypical large epithelioid melanocytes in a hyperplastic epidermis. Pagetoid proliferation, although present, is less prominent than in many examples. This lesion has some features of both superficial spreading and lentigo maligna melanoma, and may appropriately be regarded as an example of tumorigenic melanoma, unclassified as to type. (**C**) The tumorigenic nodule is composed of uniformly atypical mitotically active malignant melanocytes (melanoma cells).

Lentigo Maligna Melanoma

Lentigo maligna melanoma (LMM), previously referred to as melanosis circumscripta preblastomatosa of Debreuilh and also as melanotic freckle of Hutchinson, accounts for about 10% of all melanomas and typically occurs on the chronically exposed cutaneous surfaces of the elderly, most commonly on the face, and occasionally on the back, forearms, or lower legs.[233] The term "lentigo maligna" may be regarded as synonymous with "lentigo maligna melanoma in situ" for most purposes. However, "lentigo maligna" is preferred by many because these lesions, like other melanomas in situ, do not metastasize after complete excision, although they may persist and recur if not adequately excised. The lesion evolves slowly over many years, starting as an unevenly pigmented macule that gradually extends peripherally and may attain a diameter of several centimeters. It has an irregular border and, as long as it remains in situ or microinvasive, shows no induration. Although extending in some areas, it may show spontaneous regression in others, resulting in irregular depigmented areas. The color varies from light brown to brown, with minute dark brown or black flecks. Fine reticulated lines are usually also present and are helpful in distinguishing the lesions from actinic lentigines (see Color Fig. 29-4). In contrast to SSM, the border is usually impalpable and indistinct. For this reason, the accurate clinical delineation of the border of an LMM can be problematic, and this not uncommonly results in unexpected positive or close margins in resection specimens. Occasionally, a lesion of lentigo maligna lacks melanin pigmentation.[234] The clinical appearance then resembles that of a solar keratosis or Bowen's disease, or of an inflammatory patch, such as lupus.

It has been suggested that the risk of progression from lentigo maligna to invasive lentigo maligna melanoma may be about 5%,[235] although some cases may progress rapidly.[236,237] After adjustment for tumor thickness and other factors, lentigo maligna melanoma has the same prognosis as other forms of melanoma.[238]

Histopathology—Architectural features. In its earliest stage, lentigo maligna may show at its periphery only hyperpigmentation with slight melanocytic proliferation, mainly in the basal cell layer. Toward the center of the lesion, there is a more pronounced increase in the concentration of basal melanocytes and some irregularity in their arrangement. Until there is contiguous proliferation of lesional melanocytes, these changes are not specific and may overlap with those of actinic lentigines. The epidermis is frequently flattened, in contrast to SSM, where it is irregularly thickened and thinned, or to actinic lentigines, where there is elongation of the rete. This feature, although of diagnostic importance, is less prominent than in SSM (Fig. 29-21).

Some nesting of melanocytes in the basal layer may be observed, but this is not usually pronounced until invasion of the dermis has begun to develop.[239] The atypical melanocytes within the nests usually retain their spindle shape, and they often "hang down" like teardrops from the interface.[219] Except in areas of nesting, the melanocytes tend to retain their dendritic processes. If the melanocytes are heavily melanized, some

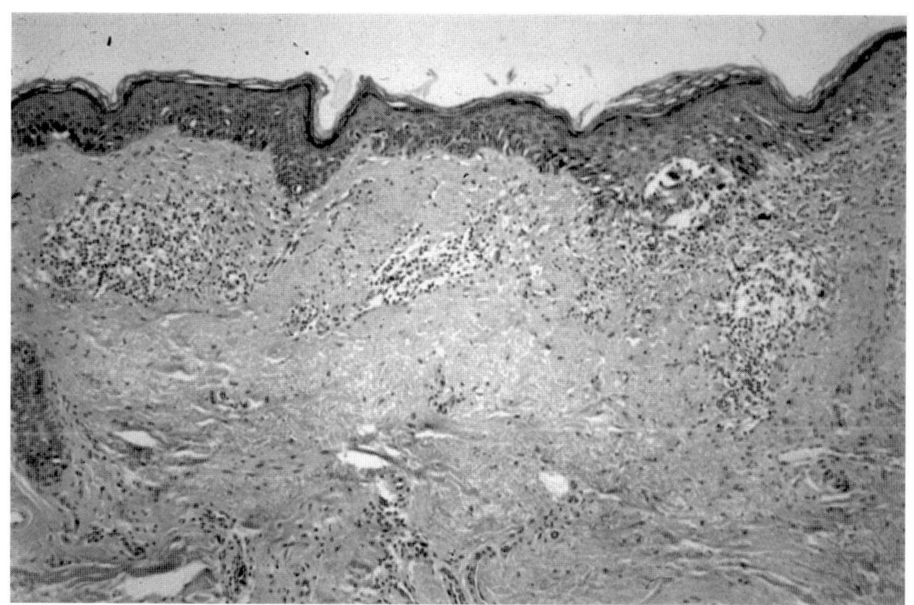

A

FIG. 29-21. Lentigo maligna melanoma, in situ
(**A**) At low magnification, the lesions are broad and asymmetrical in the distribution of lesional and host responding cells. The epidermis is atrophic, and there is usually severe actinic elastosis in the dermis. (*continued on next page*)

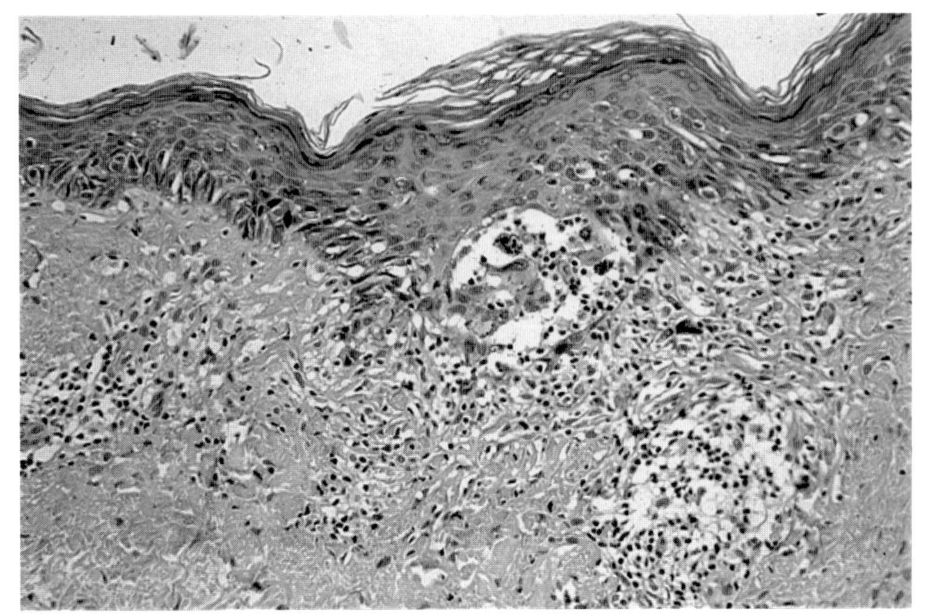
B

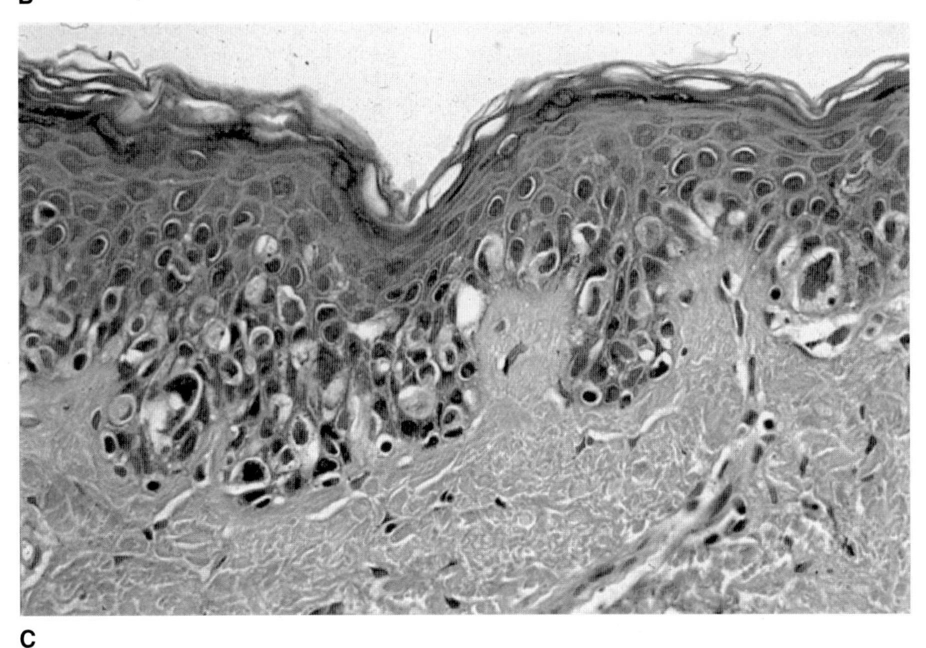
C

FIG. 29-21. ***Continued***
(**B**) In a focal area, the basement membrane is disrupted by the lymphocytic infiltrate in the dermis. However, there is no clear evidence of lesional cells extending into the dermis. (**C**) As in superficial spreading melanoma, the lesional cells exhibit moderate to severe uniform cytological atypia. There is usually some evidence of pagetoid proliferation in lentigo maligna melanoma, especially near areas of invasion. However, especially at the periphery of the lesion, this is much less prominent, and the lesional cells are smaller than in superficial spreading melanoma.

dendrites may be visible even in sections stained with hematoxylin-eosin; otherwise, staining with silver demonstrates the dendrites.

The upper dermis, which almost always shows severe elastotic solar degeneration, contains numerous melanophages and a rather pronounced, often bandlike, inflammatory infiltrate. Invasion may be demonstrable in these areas of dermal inflammation. Because invasion in a lentigo maligna melanoma is a focal process, it is advisable to cut step sections throughout the block of tissue in order not to miss such areas. The presence or absence of tumorigenic vertical growth phase is recognized using criteria already presented.

Cytologic features. In fully evolved lesions of lentigo maligna, the lesional melanocytes in the epidermis show a marked increase in concentration, so that they come to lie in contiguity with one another, and their number in some areas exceeds that of the basal keratinocytes. Many of them are elongated and spindle-shaped. Their nuclei appear atypical, being enlarged, hyperchromatic, and pleomorphic. Frequently, atypical melanocytes extend along the basal cell layer of hair follicles, often for a considerable distance and frequently extending to the base of a shave biopsy specimen. Usually, the proliferating melanocytes contain moderate amounts of melanin, and melanin is present also in keratinocytes. There is usually some upward pagetoid extension of atypical melanocytes.

The properties of contiguous proliferation, and uniform cytologic atypia, in a broad, poorly circumscribed lesion are of major importance in the diagnosis of in situ or microinvasive lentigo maligna melanoma. These features are shared also with superficial spreading melanoma, whereas focal pagetoid proliferation, although often present, is less prominent. Mitotic figures are not commonly present in the epidermal compartment; if present in the dermis they are indicative of tumorigenic vertical growth.

Pathogenesis. As an explanation for the somewhat distinctive behavior of lentigo maligna, the theory has been offered that it is derived from spindle-shaped junctional melanocytes and thus represents a melanocytic melanoma, in contrast to the superficial spreading melanoma, which is derived from rounded junctional nevus cells and thus can be regarded as a nevocytic melanoma.[240] Electron microscopy provides some support for this theory. The melanocytes of lentigo maligna are large, synthetically active cells with many dendrites. The melanosomes are essentially normal, except that they appear somewhat more elongated than those in normal melanocytes.[241] This is in contrast to superficial spreading melanomas, in which the melanosomes show considerable abnormalities.

Acral Lentiginous Melanoma

Acral lentiginous melanoma (ALM) occurs on the hairless skin of the palms and soles and in the ungual and periungual regions, the soles being the most common site.[219,242,243] Acral melanoma is uncommon in all ethnic groups, but it is the predominant form of melanoma in persons with darker skin. In groups such as Asians, Hispanics, Polynesians, and blacks, for whom the overall incidence of melanoma is low, most melanomas are of the acral type. However, the absolute incidence of acral melanoma in these groups is similar to that in Caucasians who have a much higher overall incidence of melanoma.[244] These considerations suggest that different etiologic factors, probably not involving sunlight, are operative in acral than in other sites. Although the survival rate of patients with acral melanomas in most series is poor,[245] this is probably a result of their typically advanced microstage and/or stage at diagnosis.

Clinically, in situ or microinvasive acral lentiginous melanoma shows uneven pigmentation with an irregular, often indefinite border (see Color Fig. 29-5). The soles of the feet are most commonly involved.[245] If the tumor is situated in the nail matrix, the nail and nail bed may show a longitudinal pigmented band, and the pigment may extend onto the nail fold (Hutchinson's sign). Tumorigenic vertical growth may be heralded by the onset of a nodule, with development of ulceration (Fig. 29-22). However, some acral melanomas may be deeply invasive while remaining quite flat, because the thick stratum corneum acts as a barrier to exophytic growth.

Histopathology. The lesions are termed "lentiginous" because the majority of the lesional cells are single and located near the dermal-epidermal junction, especially at the periphery of the lesion. Usually, however, some tumor cells can be found in the upper layers of the epidermis, especially near areas of invasion in the centers of the lesions. The histologic picture differs from that of lentigo maligna, because of irregular acanthosis, the lack of elastosis in the dermis, and the frequently dendritic character of the lesional cells.[219,246] Early in situ or microinvasive lesions may show, especially at the periphery, a deceptively benign histologic picture consisting of an increase in basal melanocytes and hyperpigmentation with only focal

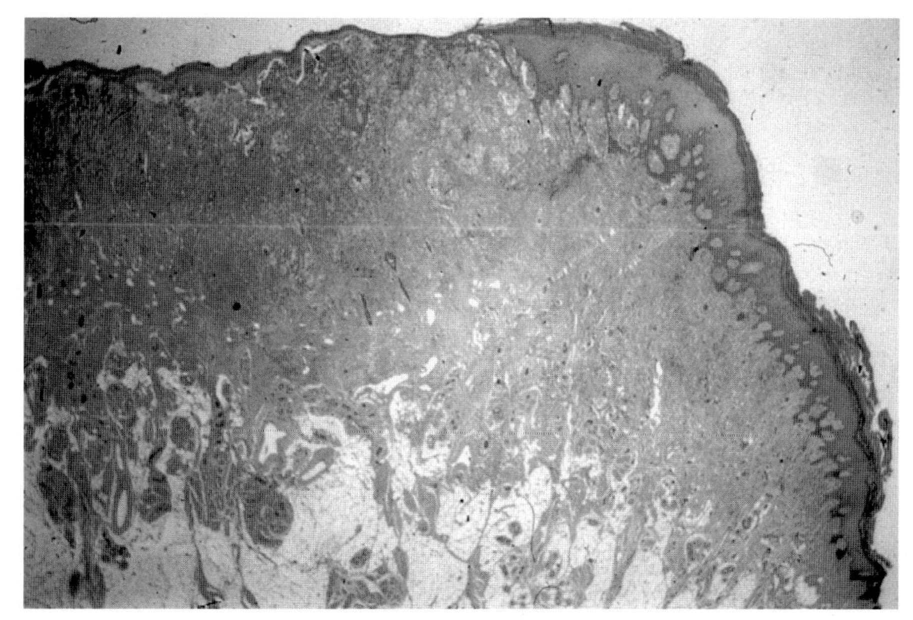

A

FIG. 29-22. Acral lentiginous melanoma, tumorigenic (radial and vertical growth phases)
(**A**) The lesion is broad and cellular. In this example from a finger, a bulky tumor nodule at the left of the image is in contiguity with an in situ radial growth phase at the right. (*continued on next page*)

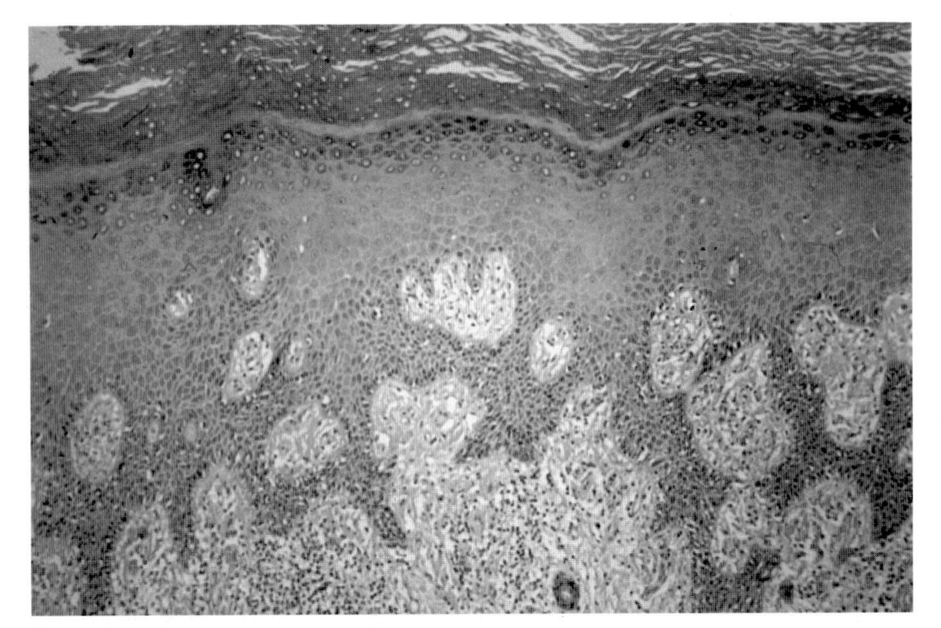

B

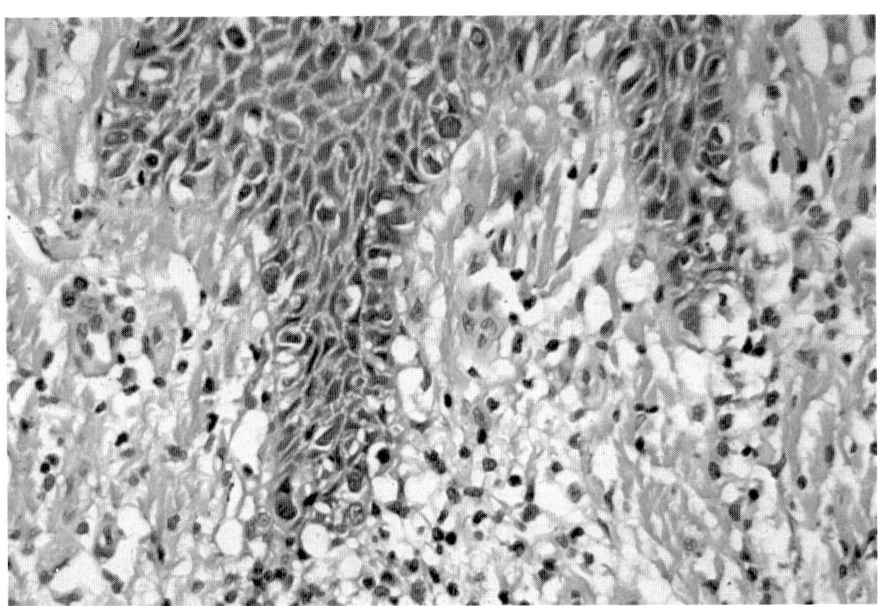

C

FIG. 29-22. ***Continued***
(**B**) As in lentigo maligna and other lentiginous melanocytic proliferations, the lesional cells in acral lentiginous melanoma tend to be arranged as single cells near the dermal-epidermal junction ("lentiginous" pattern), especially at the periphery of the lesion. There may a brisk lichenoid inflammatory infiltrate, which, in some lesions or in a partial biopsy, may simulate a reactive process. (**C**) As in any melanoma, there is moderate to severe uniform cytologic atypia. Pagetoid proliferation may be present near the center of the lesion, but this is less prominent than in superficial spreading melanoma. The neoplastic cells may be difficult to identify because of "masking" by the inflammatory infiltrate, as in this example.

atypia of the melanocytes. However, in the centers of the lesions, uniform, severe cytologic atypia is usually readily evident. There may be a lichenoid lymphocytic infiltrate that may largely obscure the dermal-epidermal junction, and in some cases this may be so dense as to simulate an inflammatory process. In most of the lesions, both spindle-shaped and rounded, pagetoid tumor cells are observed, and, in many cases, pigmented dendritic cells are prominent. Pigmentation is often pronounced, resulting in the presence of melanophages in the upper dermis and of large aggregates of melanin in the broad stratum corneum. As in lentigo maligna, when tumorigenic vertical growth phase is present, it is often of the spindle cell type and not uncommonly desmoplastic and/or neurotropic. In other instances, the invasive and tumorigenic cells in the dermis may be deceptively differentiated along nevus lines.

Mucosal Lentiginous Melanoma

Next to the skin and eyes, mucosal lentiginous melanoma is most apt to arise in the juxtacutaneous mucous membranes, such as the oral mucosa,[247] nose and nasal sinuses,[248] vagina,[249] and anorectal mucosa.[250] Mucosal melanomas are analogous to acral melanomas in histologic appearance and aggressiveness, which has led to the use of the histologic term "mucosal-lentiginous" melanoma.[219]

The Tumorigenic Compartment of Primary Malignant Melanoma (Vertical Growth Phase)

The morphologies of the variant forms of nontumorigenic melanoma have been discussed earlier. A tumorigenic vertical growth phase may develop in association with any of these to form a "complex" primary melanoma. In such cases, the histology shows a tumorigenic compartment adjacent to or within the confines of a nontumorigenic compartment. Nodular melanoma differs from these complex melanomas in that it is a tumorigenic melanoma with no clinically or histologically evident adjacent nontumorigenic compartment.[219] The morphologies of the "usual" or "common" forms of vertical growth phase will be described below in the section "Common Tumorigenic Melanoma, Including Nodular Melanoma."

Occasional melanomas exhibit variant patterns that may lead to diagnostic confusion because they may be characteristically observed in nonmelanocytic tumors. Several variants of melanoma—desmoplastic, neurotropic, polypoidal, verrucous, balloon cell, signet cell, myxoid, and minimal deviation melanoma—deserve brief description. Other variants that will not be described here include small cell, adenoid/papillary, pleomorphic (fibrohistiocytic),[251] and the rare bone-forming or "osteogenic" melanoma.[252]

Common Tumorigenic Melanoma, Including Nodular Melanoma

Nodular melanoma, by definition, contains only tumorigenic vertical growth (sometimes associated with a precursor) and thus has a poorer prognosis on the average than superficial spreading melanoma. However, when other risk factors such as thickness are controlled, the prognosis of nodular melanoma is not worse than that of other forms of melanoma.[253] Nodular melanomas occur in slightly older patients than the common superficial spreading melanoma and are relatively more frequent in men.[219] A nodular melanoma starts as an elevated, variably pigmented papule that increases in size quite rapidly to become a nodule and often undergoes ulceration (see Color Fig. 29-6). The ABCD criteria reviewed earlier do not apply to nodular melanomas, which often present clinically as quite small, symmetrical, and well-circumscribed papules or nodules. These may be conspicuously pigmented, oligomelanotic, or even amelanotic. The tumorigenic nodule that may develop in nodular melanoma does not differ clinically or histologically from the nodule that may occur in relation to a preexisting nontumorigenic melanoma. Indeed, nodular melanomas may represent examples of "telescoped" tumor progression in which the antecedent radial phase has been so short-lived as to be inapparent.[254]

Histopathology—Architectural features. In a typical tumorigenic melanoma, there is contiguous growth of uniformly atypical melanocytes in the dermis, forming an often asymmetrical tumor mass that is larger (usually much larger) than the largest nest in the overlying epidermis. Asymmetry is often apparent at the cytologic level as variation in cell size, shape, and pigmentation, and in the distribution of the host response, such that one half of the lesion is not a mirror image of the other half. However, the silhouette of the entire lesion may be quite symmetrical, especially in a nodular melanoma that lacks an adjacent component (Fig. 29-23). Conversely, if a nontumorigenic radial growth phase compartment is present, asymmetry is likely to be more apparent, both at the clinical and histologic levels. Usually, the tumor mass fills and expands the papillary dermis (level III) or invades between coarse collagen fibers of the reticular dermis (level IV). Most level III melanomas and most melanomas greater than 0.75 mm in thickness are tumorigenic. The epidermis is frequently ulcerated, or there is an adherent scale-crust. It is often stetched and attenuated or, alternatively, may be irregularly hyperplastic and even pseudoepitheliomatous.

Perhaps the best-known single criterion for melanoma is the upward "pagetoid" extension of tumor cells into the epidermis overlying the melanoma. However, this "pagetoid melanocytosis" is not specific for melanoma.[128] Whereas in nodular melanoma, permeation of the epidermis with tumor cells is limited to that portion overlying the dermal tumor, lateral extension of melanoma cells in the epidermis and papillary dermis beyond the confines of the dermal tumor is observed in the adjacent nontumorigenic compartment of complex primary melanomas (SSM, LMM, ALM). This phenomenon greatly aids in histologic recognition of these tumors, and, conversely, the recognition of nodular melanomas, which lack this adjacent component, may be difficult. For this reason, nodular melanoma may be difficult or impossible to distinguish from a metastatic melanoma in the skin, and when such a tumor is amelanotic, the distinction from other cutaneous malignancies may be impossible without immunohistochemistry.

The amount of *inflammatory infiltrate* in melanomas varies. As a rule, early invasive malignant and many in situ melanomas show a bandlike inflammatory infiltrate, often itermingled with melanophages, at the base of the tumor. In tumors that extend deep into the dermis, the inflammatory infiltrate is quite variable, but it is often only slight to moderate rather than pronounced. Lymphocytes extending among tumor cells are often associated with morphologic evidence of damage to individual tumor cells (apoptosis). These *tumor-infiltrating lymphocytes* (TIL) have been shown to have independent favorable prognostic significance.[253] The lymphocytic infiltrate around melanomas is a T-cell response.[255] Tumor-infiltrating lymphocytes extracted from melanomas (mostly metastatic cases) may be cytotoxic and may be directed against immunogenic melanoma-associated antigens.[256]

Cytologic features. The tumor cells in the dermis show great variation in size and shape. Nevertheless, two major types of cells—epithelioid and spindle-shaped—can be recognized. Many tumors show both types of cells, but usually one type predominates. Generally, the "lentiginous" forms of melanoma (e.g., LMM and ALM) tend to show a predominance of spindle-shaped cells, whereas superficial spreading and nodular melanomas are composed largely of epithelioid cells.[253] The epithelioid cells tend to lie in alveolar formations, and the spindle-shaped cells in irregulary branching formations. The alveolar formations of the epithelioid cells are surrounded by thin fibers of collagen containing a few fibroblasts. Tumors in which spindle cells predominate may resemble sarcomas or other spindle cell tumors but in most cases differ from them by the presence of junctional melanocytic activity.

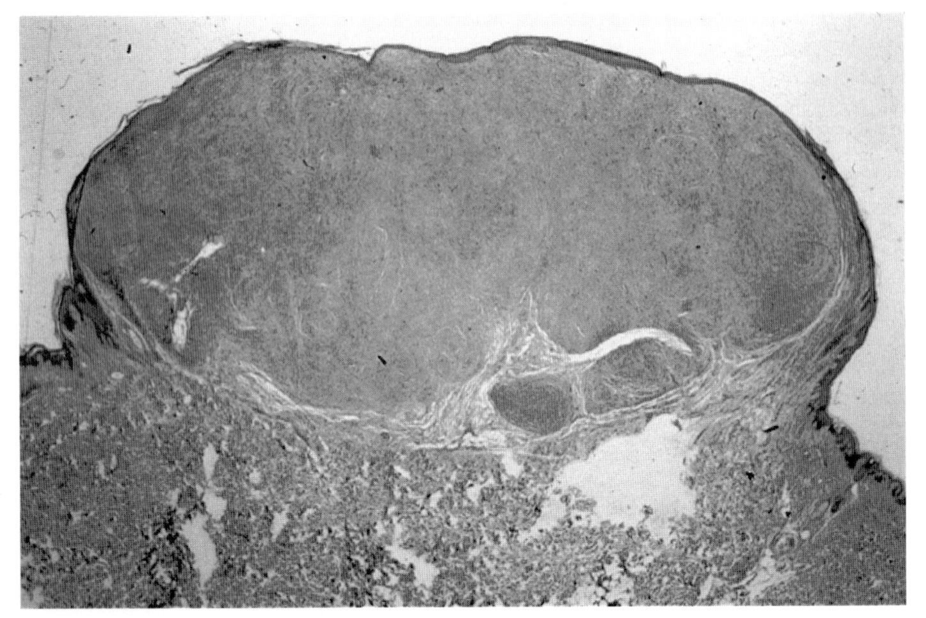

A

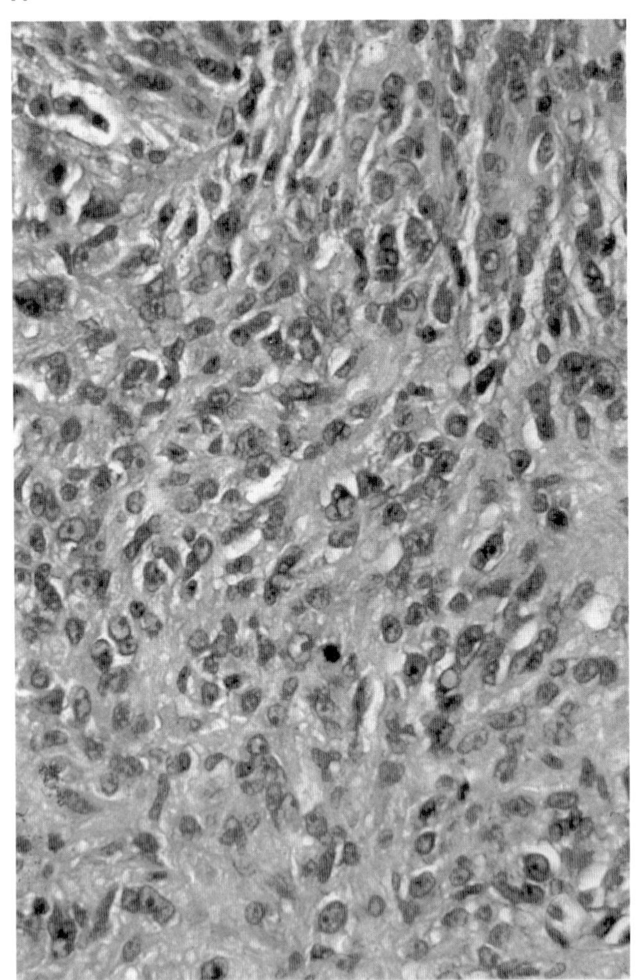

B

FIG. 29-23. Tumorigenic melanoma, nodular type (verticle growth phase without radial growth phase)
(**A**) The nodules of tumorigenic melanomas tend to be symmetrical at scanning magnification, although there may be uneven distribution of pigment and of the lymphocytic response within many of the lesions. When there is no adjacent nontumorigenic radial growth phase component, as here, the lesion is termed "nodular melanoma." If a radial growth phase component is present, the melanoma is classified according to the type of that compartment (e.g., "superficial spreading melanoma with vertical growth phase"). (**B**) The lesional cells of nodular melanoma exhibit severe uniform cytologic atypia, usually with readily evident mitoses. In any given high magnification field such as this, the appearances are indistinguishable from those of a vertical growth phase associated with a superficial spreading melanoma or lentigo maligna melanoma, or from those of a metastasis.

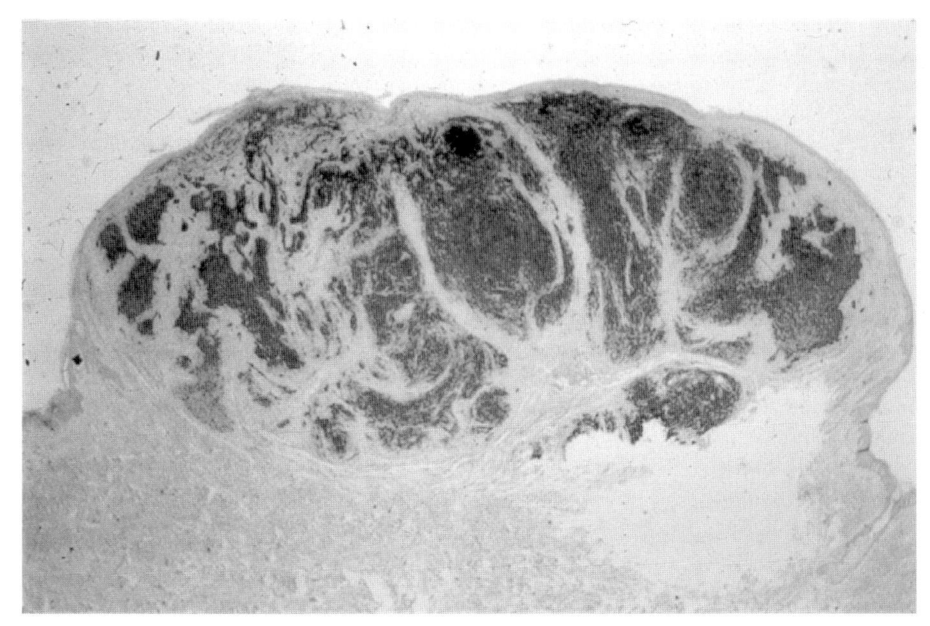

FIG. 29-23. *Continued*
(**C**) The brown reaction product in the lesional cells, as shown by S-100 immunohistochemical staining, is striking, even at scanning magnification.

The uniformly atypical nuclei of the cells that constitute the tumor nodule are larger than those of melanocytes or nevus cells, with irregular nuclear membranes, hyperchromatic chromatin, and often prominent nucleoli that tend to be irregular in size, shape, and number. The atypia is considered to be "uniform" if more than 50% of the cells have these characteristics, but more often than not, all or most of the cells are atypical. In additional to this uniform moderate or severe cytologic atypia, there is also a diagnostically important failure of the melanocytes in the deeper layers of the dermis to decrease in size (absence of "maturation"; see Figs. 29-20C and 29-23B). This must not be confused, however, with the presence of an intradermal nevus beneath a melanoma, a fairly common feature.

Mitotic figures are usually present in the lesional cells of the dermal and epidermal compartments of tumorigenic melanomas (they are present in the epidermal lesional cells in about one-third of nontumorigenic melanomas[257]; see Figs. 29-20C and 29-23B). The nuclei of epidermal keratinocytes may be enlarged, with prominent nucleoli, although they are not irregular or hyperchromatic. Mitoses may also be observed in adjacent hyperplastic keratinocytes. In contrast, mitotic figures are rarely present in benign nevi other than Spitz nevi, and even in the latter lesions the rate is usually low or zero.[96]

Differential Diagnosis. Great difficulty may be encountered in differentiating a melanoma from a junctional or compound nevus. The actual incidence of a wrong diagnosis is not inconsiderable, judging from the frequency with which pathologists disagree in their opinions. When there is doubt, the differential diagnosis should be clearly indicated, so that appropriate therapeutic intervention can be planned. Melanocytic lesions that have been partially removed by shave biopsy should be entirely excised if there is any doubt at all about the diagnosis.

The most important attributes that differentiate the tumorigenic vertical growth phase of melanoma from nevi include *asymmetry, lack of maturation* of lesional cells with descent into the dermis, and *uniform cytologic atypia.*

Considerations in the important distinction between thin melanomas and dysplastic nevi are listed in Table 29-3. The most important differential diagnostic consideration for nodular melanoma is the Spitz nevus. The criteria for this distinction are presented in Table 29-2.

In some instances, it may be difficult to recognize a highly undifferentiated melanoma as such. The specific identification of a tumor as melanoma depends on the identification of melanin or on appropriate immunohistochemical reactivity in an appropriate setting. The *amount* of melanin present varies greatly in melanomas. In some tumors, considerable melanin is found not only within the tumor cells but also within melanophages located in the stroma. In others, hematoxylin-eosin staining may show no evidence of melanin. However, a Fontana-Masson silver stain usually reveals at least a few cells containing melanin.[258] If appropriate tissue is available, the dopa reaction is always positive in at least part of the tumor, and electron microscopy shows some melanosomes and premelanosomes in nearly all cases.[258] However, in practice today, these methods have been largely supplanted by immunohistochemical techniques.

Immunohistochemistry. Most of the problems in diagnosis of amelanotic melanomas can be resolved by immunohistochemistry, using a panel of antibodies including S-100, HMB-45, keratin (low and intermediate molecular weight), and LCA.[259,260] Immunohistochemical testing for S-100 protein is nearly always positive in melanomas.[261] A keratin stain should be done in addition to staining for S-100 protein, to rule out rare S-100-positive carcinomas.[262] A few studies have reported positive keratin reactivity in melanomas, but this is very unusual when standard methods are used in paraffin section.[263] Reactivity of melanomas, mostly metastatic, has been described with polyclonal but not monoclonal CEA, and occasional melanomas react with the epithelial marker EMA.[264] Melanomas, unlike carcinomas, express vimentin, an intermediate filament that is usually associated with mesenchymal tissues.[265] Lymphomas are usually positive for LCA, whereas they are negative for S-100 and HMB-45. The anaplastic large cell type of non-Hodgkin's lymphoma, which may present primarily in the skin, is quite likely to be confused with melanoma, and these tumors are frequently positive for the CD30 (Ki-1) antigen, and usually for LCA.[266]

The HMB-45 antigen is also very useful in making the distinction between melanomas and nonmelanoma tumors. Like S-100, HMB-45 is positive in many benign melanocytic tumors and thus is not specific for melanoma. Its overall sensitivity of about 70% is less than that of S-100 (close to 100%[267]), especially in spindle cell melanomas, where HMB-45 is usually negative.[268] The specificity of the HMB-45 antigen depends on the context in which it is used. Benign melanocytic lesions that may react with HMB-45 include the junctional components of most nevi and the dermal components of dysplastic nevi, blue nevi, cellular blue nevi, deep penetrating nevi, and Spitz nevi. Thus, HMB-45 cannot be used to distinguish benign from malignant melanocytic neoplasms. If the diagnostic differential is between melanoma and carcinoma, on the other hand, the diagnostic specificity of a positive test is very high (see also Table 4-3).

Desmoplastic and Neurotropic Melanomas

Desmoplastic melanoma presents attributes of melanocytic, fibroblastic, and Schwannian differentiation, often mixed within a single lesion.[269] Desmoplasia is most often observed in a spindle cell vertical growth phase of lentigo maligna melanoma[270] or acral lentiginous melanoma.[271] However, desmoplastic changes are occasionally seen in tumors with rounded or undifferentiated melanoma cells.[272] The collagen in desmoplastic melanoma is arranged as delicate fibrils that extend between the tumor cells and separate them from one another. The relationship between tumor cells and stroma is thus similar to that observed in sarcomas, in contrast to most melanomas, where an epithelial pattern of collagen fibers surrounding groups or clusters of tumor cells may be demonstrated—for example, with a reticulin stain. Interestingly, neurotized nevi may also show the pattern of individual cells surrounded by collagen that characterizes desmoplastic melanoma, and the arrangement of the cells of desmoplastic melanoma in "wavy" fiber bundles may also recall the "Schwannian" patterns of neurofibromas, neurotized nevi, and malignant schwannomas.

Histopathology. In desmoplastic melanoma, the melanoma cells are usually elongated and amelanotic and are embedded in a markedly fibrotic stroma, so that it is often difficult to decide which are fibroblasts and which are melanoma cells. Because of the frequent absence of melanin, differentiation from a fibrohistiocytic or neural lesion may be difficult. Staining with S-100 protein antibody usually marks many of the spindle-shaped cells, indicating that they are not fibroblastic,[273] but nevi, neurofibromas, and neurogenic sarcomas are also typically S-100-positive. The HMB-45 antigen is usually not demonstrable in these spindle-cell melanomas.[25] The distinction from a neurogenic sarcoma may be very difficult or impossible in cases where there is no pigment and there is no characteristic superficial radial growth phase component.[274] Some of these lesions might alternatively be regarded as superficial malignant epithelioid schwannomas. The prognostic implications are similar, whichever diagnostic term is used (Fig. 29-24).

Although the reported survival rate for desmoplastic melanoma is poor, this is because many of the cases reported in the earlier literature had already recurred at the time the diagnoses were made. A recent report of a series of desmoplastic melanomas that had been prospectively diagnosed and definitively treated at their initial presentation showed that the survival rate was no different than that for the usual forms of melanoma when thickness, mitotic rate, host response, and other risk factors were controlled. Indeed, the probability of survival is relatively good for prospectively diagnosed and definitively treated desmoplastic melanoma, because, despite the considerable thickness of many of these lesions, the prognostically important mitotic rate and lymphocytic responses are often favorable.[275]

Neurotropic melanoma is often a variant of desmoplastic melanoma.[276–278] There are fascicles of desmoplastic melanoma that have invaded cutaneous nerves, usually in a spindle-cell vertical component with fibrosis. However, some neurotropic melanomas lack these latter features of desmoplastic melanoma. Many of these are spindle cell tumorigenic melanomas of acral lentiginous or lentigo maligna type, but some are composed of epithelioid cells. Neurotropism in a primary melanoma is associated with increased risk for local recurrence, even after standard "definitive" therapy, and also with increased mortality.[275]

Differential Diagnosis. It is very important to differentiate desmoplastic melanoma from benign conditions, including neurotized nevi and neurofibromas, as well as fibrohistiocytic lesions such as cellular dermatofibromas. Other considerations include low-grade malignancies, such as fibromatoses and dermatofibrosarcoma protruberans, and fully malignant lesions such as malignant schwannoma. The latter group of lesions may overlap biologically as well as morphologically, and their management is the same—namely, complete excision and follow-up. Misdiagnosis of desmoplastic melanoma as one or another of the benign lesions listed earlier is not uncommon, because attributes of malignancy, such as anaplasia and frequent mitoses, are often not prominent features of these lesions. The large size and asymmetrical silhouette of many of these lesions differ from those of most benign lesions. One subtle clue to the diagnosis at low magnification is the frequent presence of a lymphocytic infiltrate, distributed as nodular aggregates of infiltrating lymphocytes throughout the tumor, which are not present in neurofibromas, nevi, or most fibrohistiocytic lesions. Lymphocytes may also be clustered about nerves involved by tumor cells in neurotropic melanomas. Other helpful diagnostic attributes, which may not be readily evident unless sought because of a high index of suspicion, include the presence of an atypical intraepidermal melanocytic component that may be subtle and not always diagnostic of frank melanoma, and usually the presence of at least a few mitoses in the dermal component of the lesion.

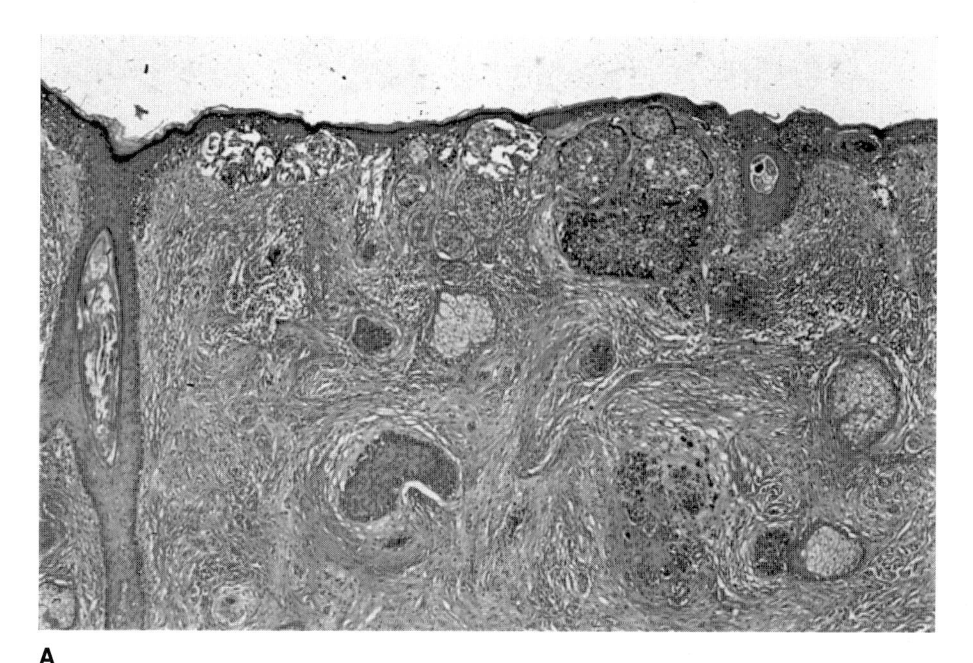

A

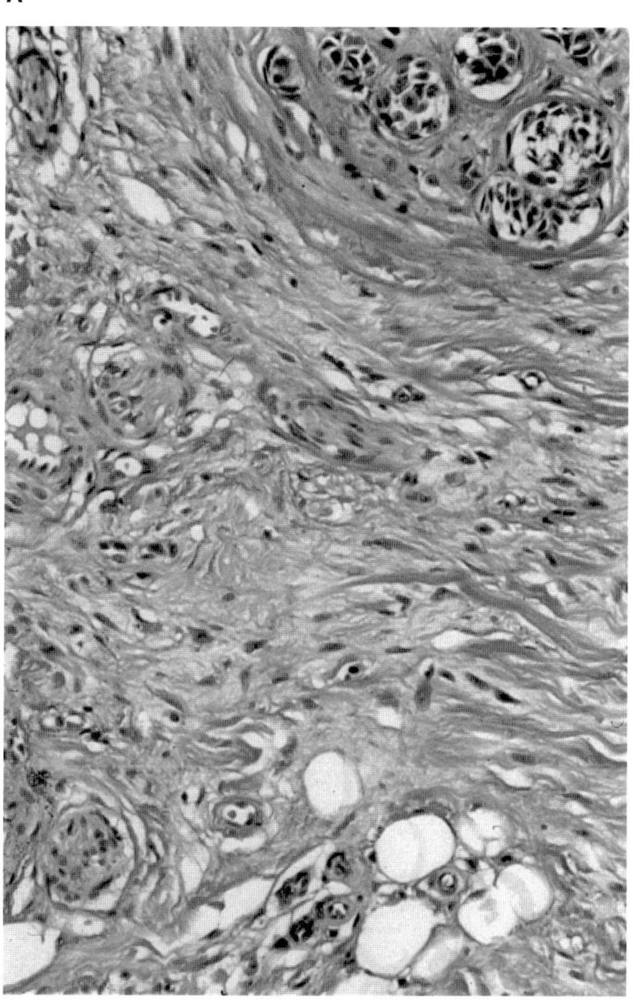

B

FIG. 29-24. Desmoplastic and neurotropic melanomas (**A**) At scanning magnification, there is a lentigo maligna melanoma in the epidermis and superficial dermis, with large nests of invasive epithelioid and pigmented melanocytes. Although not present in every desmoplastic melanoma, these atypical epithelioid cells greatly facilitate the recognition of the lesion as a melanoma. (**B**) Atypical spindle cells arranged in loose fascicles extend into the deeper dermis and subcutis, beneath the epithelioid cell component. This subtle proliferation is easily overlooked, resulting in potential "undercalling" of the diagnosis and microstage. (*continued on next page*)

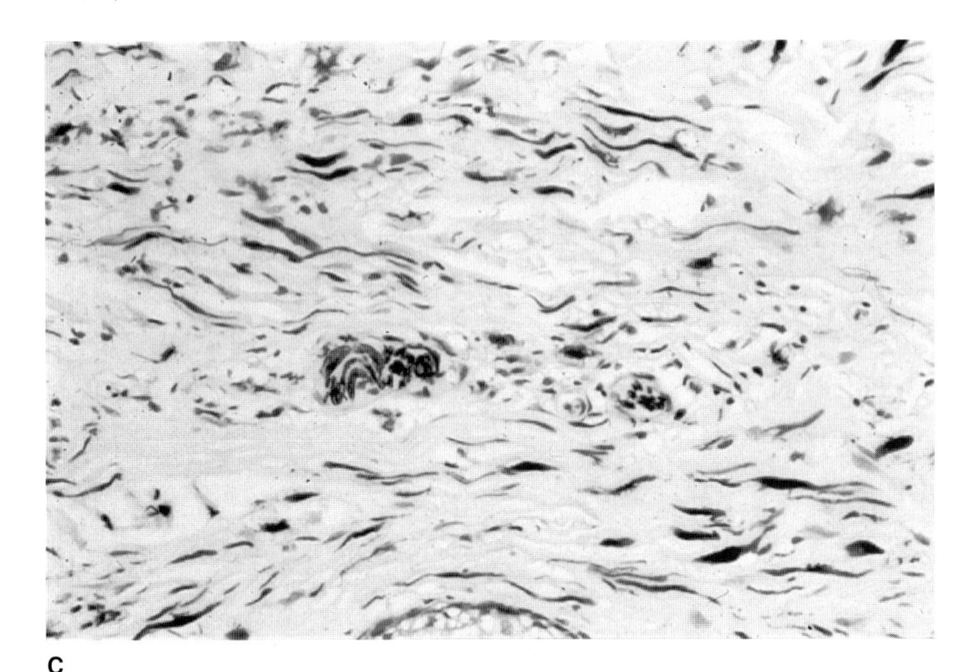

C

FIG. 29-24. *Continued*
(**C**) The spindle cells are S-100-positive. S-100 stain is of great value in delineating the boundaries of desmoplastic melanomas, but should be interpreted cautiously because it is not specific for melanoma cells.

Polypoidal Melanoma

Also termed "pedunculated" melanoma, polypoidal melanoma is confined, at least at first, to a nodule connected to the underlying skin by a pedicle or stalk.[279] The surface of the nodule often shows erosion or ulceration.[280] Because these tumors are bulky, the prognosis is often poor, but not worse than predicted by other risk factors.[253] By convention, polypoidal melanomas are considered to represent level III invasion unless tumor cells extend into the reticular dermis (level IV).

On histologic examination, the protruding nodule is filled with melanoma cells, whereas the underlying stalk or pedicle is initially free of tumor cells. Later, the tumor may infiltrate the pedicle and the dermis adjacent to the pedicle.

Verrucous Melanomas

A verrucous melanoma presents as a markedly hyperkeratotic, tumorigenic nodule that may simulate a verruca or a verrucous carcinoma clinically.[281–283] Histologically as well, the lesions are associated with marked keratosis and verrucous hyperplasia of kertinocytes that may assume pseudoepitheliomatous proportions and raise a question of squamous cell carcinoma unless the underlying neoplastic melanocytes are appreciated.[284] Some other lesions are misdiagnosed histologically as benign nevi or seborrheic keratoses.[282] "Verrucous" changes of adjacent keratinocytes are sometimes observed adjacent to acral and especially subungual melanomas, which are often mistaken clinically for warts on initial presentation if pigment is not prominent. In such instances, an inadequate biopsy that does not include the underlying neoplasm could appear to be consistent with a wart.

Balloon Cell Melanoma

Usually, in addition to more characteristic melanoma cells of the epithelioid type, some melanomas contain aggregates of "balloon cells." These balloon cells, characterized by their abundant, clear cytoplasm, may show relatively little nuclear atypia and thus may resemble those observed in a balloon cell nevus. The overall architecture of the lesion, in conjunction with cytologic atypia, identifies the tumor as a melanoma. Transitions from the ordinary melanoma cells to the balloon cells are usually evident. The metastases of a balloon cell melanoma may or may not be composed largely of balloon cells, and balloon cell metastases have been reported in a melanoma that did not contain them in the primary tumor.[285] Therefore, this possibility should be considered in the differential diagnosis of metastatic clear cell tumors. The cells exhibit immunopathologic reactivity characteristic of melanoma.

Signet Cell Melanoma

Melanomas that contain prominent signet-ring cells may be confusing and must be distinguished from adenocarcinomas, tumors of vascular endothelium or adipose tissue, lymphomas, and epithelioid smooth muscle tumors. The signet cell morphology may be recognized in the primary tumors,[286] or only in metastatic sites.[287] Similar cells may be seen in benign nevi, and may also occur as a result of freezing artifact.[286] Immunohistochemistry may be used to confirm the diagnosis of a melanocytic lesion and rule out competing possibilities. In evaluating these results, it should be recognized that both CEA and keratin expression have been reported in melanomas.[288,289]

Myxoid Melanoma

A histologic pattern of prominent myxoid stroma has been described in some primary and metastatic melanomas.[290,291] The differential diagnosis may be very broad, including lipoblastic, myoblastic, fibroblastic, neurogenic, or chondroblastic tumors with myxoid stroma.[290] If the diagnosis is suspected, immunohistochemistry can be done to support the diagnosis. Fontana stain may reveal melanin pigment, and electron microscopy has shown melanosomes in a few cases.

Minimal Deviation Melanoma

Recognized by only some authors, this lesion is referred to as "borderline type" when it is limited to the papillary dermis and as "minimal deviation type" when it extends into the reticular dermis.[292] These tumors are considered to exhibit less cytologic atypia than the common forms of melanoma. The lesions in their vertical phase consist of uniformly expansile nodules, and the cells in the nodules tend to be arranged in uniform patterns. If the tumor cells are epithelioid in type, they may resemble cells of the ordinary acquired nevus. In the spindle cell variants, the tumor cells may resemble the cells of a Spitz nevus or, if pigmented or arranged in compact fascicles, a pigmented spindle cell nevus. Because of the resemblance to nevus cells, the term "nevoid melanoma" has also been used.[293] Even though recurrences, metastases, and death may occur, minimal deviation melanomas are said to be biologically not as aggressive as common melanomas. However, in our opinion, prognosis by multivariable prognostic models is advisable.

Epidemiology, Prognosis, and Management of Melanomas

Risk Factors for the Development of Melanomas

The major phenotypic risk factors for the development of melanomas have been discussed in previous sections. These include freckles, the total number of banal nevi, and, especially, the presence and number of dysplastic nevi. In addition, type I skin that burns easily and tans poorly is a risk factor, as are other indicators of acute sun exposure, such as living in a sunny climate, a history of weekend and vacation sun exposure, and a history of sunburn episodes. Among these risk factors, melanocytic nevi and indicators of "acute, intermittent" sun exposure are more strongly related to superficial spreading and nodular melanomas, whereas skin type, ethnic background, and measures of total accumulated exposure to the sun ("chronic, continuous sun exposure") are more strongly related to lentigo maligna melanoma.[294] Age is also a strong risk factor, operating in a continuously progressive fashion in lentigo maligna melanoma in contrast to a more complex pattern for superficial and nodular melanomas.[244] The etiologic factors that may be related to acral and mucosal melanomas are unknown.

Preexisting Melanocytic Nevus

It is well known that melanomas can develop in congenital nevi and in dysplastic nevi. Histologically, remnants of banal nevi are found in about 10% to 35% of all melanomas, and evidence of associated melanocytic dysplasia is observed in up to about 40%.[59] Remnants of a dysplastic nevus adjacent to a radial growth phase (usually of the superficial spreading type) can be distinguished from the latter using the criteria presented in Table 29-3. Remnants of a dermal component of a nevus deep in a melanoma can be distinguished from the melanoma cells by the following criteria: (1) the dermal nevus cells are smaller; (2) they are arranged in nests that tend to be small and uniform in size and shape; (3) there is evidence of maturation from superficial to deep within the nevus but not within the melanoma cell population; and (4) there are no mitoses in the dermal nevus cells. Occasional examples of differentiated dermal melanoma cells may meet some of these criteria and thus present difficulties of interpretation. In addition to the earlier listed criteria, (5) there is evidence in these melanoma cells of continuous differentiation from a more obviously malignant superficial component.

An exception to the general rule that melanomas arise at the epidermal-dermal border is observed occasionally in congenital nevi, in which a melanoma may arise deep in the dermis.[137] In very rare instances, a melanoma may develop within or beneath an intradermal nevus, resulting in a large nodular growth.[295]

Multiple Primary Melanomas

People who have had cutaneous melanomas are at risk of developing additional melanomas, with an incidence of approximately 5% in the first 10 years after diagnosis.[296] The occurrence of multiple and familial melanomas has already been pointed out in relation to dysplastic nevi. A prior melanoma is a strong risk factor for subsequent melanoma, especially in young patients and in familial melanoma kindreds.[181,183] It is important to differentiate an additional melanoma from a metastatic melanoma—especially from an epidermotropic metastasis,[297] because the prognosis of an independent primary is likely to be much better than that of a metastasis.

Malignant Melanoma in Infancy and Childhood

Malignant melanoma is a disease primarily of adults. The incidence of prepubertal melanoma is very low. In a few instances, it has occurred as multiple metastases resulting from transplacental transmission.[298] Occasionally, a melanoma arises in infancy or childhood in a giant congenital nevus. Three patterns of primary melanoma can occur in children.[299] In most instances, the melanoma shows a histologic picture similar to that in adults and the prognosis depends on thickness and other "microstaging" attributes. In other cases, the tumors are composed of small "blastic" malignant cells, and the course is usually aggressive, although sometimes unpredictably so, especially in tumors that arise in congenital nevi. In a few instances, the histologic picture is reminiscent of that observed in Spitz nevi. In some of these cases, metastases occur that are limited to the regional lymph nodes, and the child survives after adequate treatment.[111,299] However, at least one example of a "Spitzean" melanoma with a fatal outcome has been reported.[299]

Biopsy of Melanoma

The question of whether an incisional biopsy is permissible in a lesion that is strongly suspected of being a melanoma has been widely discussed. Several authors, especially authors from Europe, have opposed the performance of an incisional biopsy, because they believe it may cause metastatic spread.[300,301] In other studies, no deleterious effects of preceding punch biopsies were noted.[302,303] It is difficult in studies of this sort to control for other risk factors, which might be expected to be more prevalent in the larger tumors for which incisional biopsies might be contemplated.

Because a correct diagnosis is more likely when the entire tumor can be studied, excisional biopsy is advisable whenever feasible, and only for large lesions is incisional biopsy indicated.[304] If a tumorigenic vertical growth phase is present, it should be entirely contained within the biopsy, if possible. Shave biopsy or curetting is not optimal, because it may result in inadequate material for diagnosis; it may also make impossible a determination of the depth of penetration of the tumor, which is very important for prognosis and for planning of the extent of surgical procedures.

Staging of Melanoma

The purpose of staging is to define subsets of cases with similar prognoses for management and investigational purposes. The five-stage (stages 0 to IV) clinicopathologic staging system of the American Joint Committee on Cancer (AJCC) primarily considers aspects of the tumor (T), the presence and size of nodal metastases (N), and the presence and sites of distant metastases (M) to determine a stage based on all three attributes (TNM).[305] The 5-year survival rate for newly diagnosed localized primary melanoma cases (stages 0 to II) is about 80%, compared with a 35% survival rate when lymph nodes are involved (stage III). Using the prognostic models discussed later, subsets of cases with more or less favorable prognoses can be identified. When distant metastases are present, the 5-year survival rate is on the order of 10%.[306]

Levels of Invasion

Although tumor thickness is now considered to be the single most important prognostic attribute, the levels of invasion suggested by Clark[216] have prognostic value in certain subsets of cases.[307] They also have descriptive value. The different levels appear to reflect the sequential acquisiton of new properties by evolving tumors. They are defined as follows, with survival rates for prospectively diagnosed and definitively treated clinical stage I cases in parentheses.[308]

In level I tumors (100% 10-year disease-free survival), the melanoma cells are confined to the epidermis and its appendages. These in situ melanomas (AJCC stage 0) presumably lack the capacity to invade through a basement membrane. In level II tumors (96% survival), there is extension into the papillary dermis, with at most only a few melanoma cells extending to the interface between papillary and reticular dermis. These melanomas are "microinvasive," but they lack the capacity to form tumors in all but a few cases. The level II tumors that metastasize all have small tumorigenic papules (VGP), as previously defined. In level III tumors (86%), there is extension of the tumor cells throughout the papillary dermis, filling it and impinging on the reticular dermis but without invading it. These melanomas are competent to form tumors in the papillary dermis, a loose mesenchyme that is specialized to support epithelium. Level IV tumors (66%) not only are invasive and tumorigenic, but also have the capacity to invade the dense, sparsely vascular mesenchyme of the reticular dermis. Level V tumors (53%) invade the subcutaneous fat.

Thickness of the Tumor

Tumor thickness is the single most important factor in predicting survival for stage I patients. Breslow, in 1970, first measured tumor thickness objectively with a micrometer.[309] The depth of invasion is measured from the top of the granular layer to the deepest extension of the tumor; in ulcerated lesions, measurement is from the ulcer base overlying the deepest point of invasion. In the initial report, metastasis did not occur in lesions less than 0.76 mm in greatest thickness. Since then, there have been reports of metastases from "thin" melanomas although this continues to be rare. Metastasis from "thin" melanomas, or from level II melanomas, appears to be explained by the presence of tumorigenic melanoma (vertical growth phase). In one series, metastases occurred in 2% of melanomas less than 0.76 mm thick. All cases that metastasized were tumorigenic. The rate of metastasis for tumorigenic melanomas less than 0.76 mm thick was 15%, whereas in nontumorigenic (radial growth phase) melanoma of any thickness (most are thinner than 1 mm), the metastatic rate was zero.[174]

In determining the depth of penetration, whether by level or by measurement, the following rules apply: (1) Melanocytes in junctional nests are not considered invasive, even though they may "push" into the papillary dermis. (2) If deep nests of melanoma cells arise from the epithelium of cutaneous appendages, they are not used in measurement from the surface. (3) A column of melanocytes extending from the lower border of the lesion into the deep dermis at nearly a right angle is not measured, because it is likely that the column arises from an appendage; this supposition can usually be verified by serial sectioning or keratin staining[310] (Fig. 29-25).

Partial and Complete Regression of Melanoma

Partial regression is common in melanomas. Usually, it is observed in the nontumorigenic compartment ("radial growth phase regression"). Regression is defined as a focal area in which there is delicate fibroplasia of the papillary dermis, usually with a sprinkling of melanophages and lymphocytes, with melanoma present in the epidermis and/or papillary dermis to one or both sides, but not within the area of regression (Fig. 29-26). Paradoxically, partial regression of the radial growth phase has been associated in some series with poorer prognosis. In

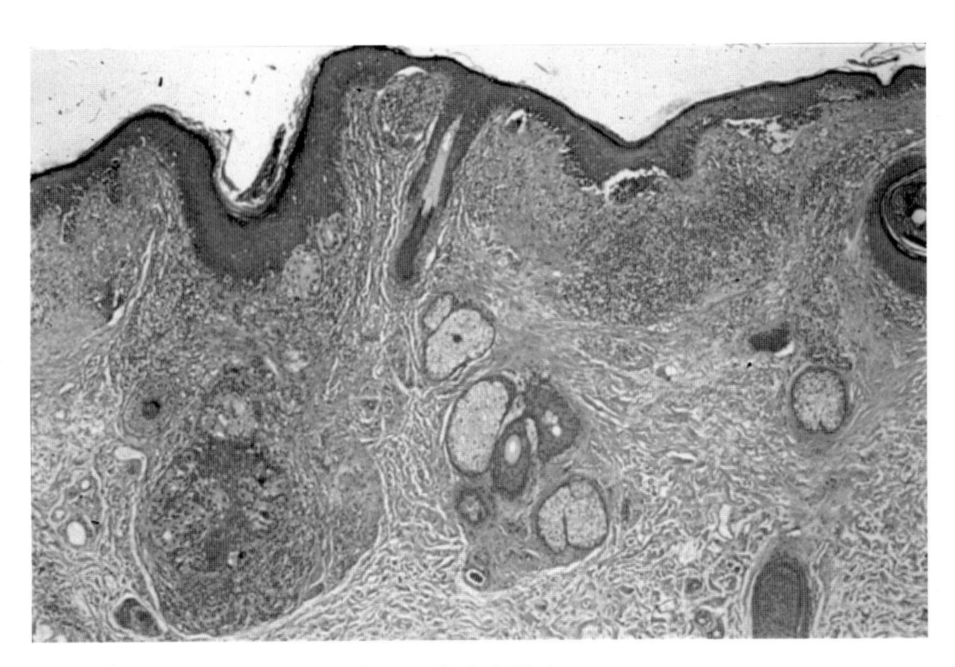

FIG. 29-25. Extension of melanoma down a hair follicle
Lentigo maligna melanoma, characterized by single and nested uniformly atypical melanocytes near the dermal-epidermal junction. At left center, a hair follicle is largely replaced by melanoma cells, which are confined to the epidermis and adventitial dermis of the follicle. This melanoma is nontumorigenic. Invasive cells at the base of the follicle should not be used for thickness measurement.

contrast, tumor-infiltrating lymphocytes within the vertical growth phase are associated with improved survival rates[253] (Fig. 29-27). Regression of the vertical growth phase has not been well described. Occasionally, one sees an area of fibrosis and melanophages apparently partial replacing a portion of a tumor nodule, and, very infrequently, this process may proceed to completion, resulting in a collection of melanophages in the dermis that could represent the residual evidence of a preexisting tumor nodule. This phenomenon has been aptly referred to as "tumoral melanosis."[311]

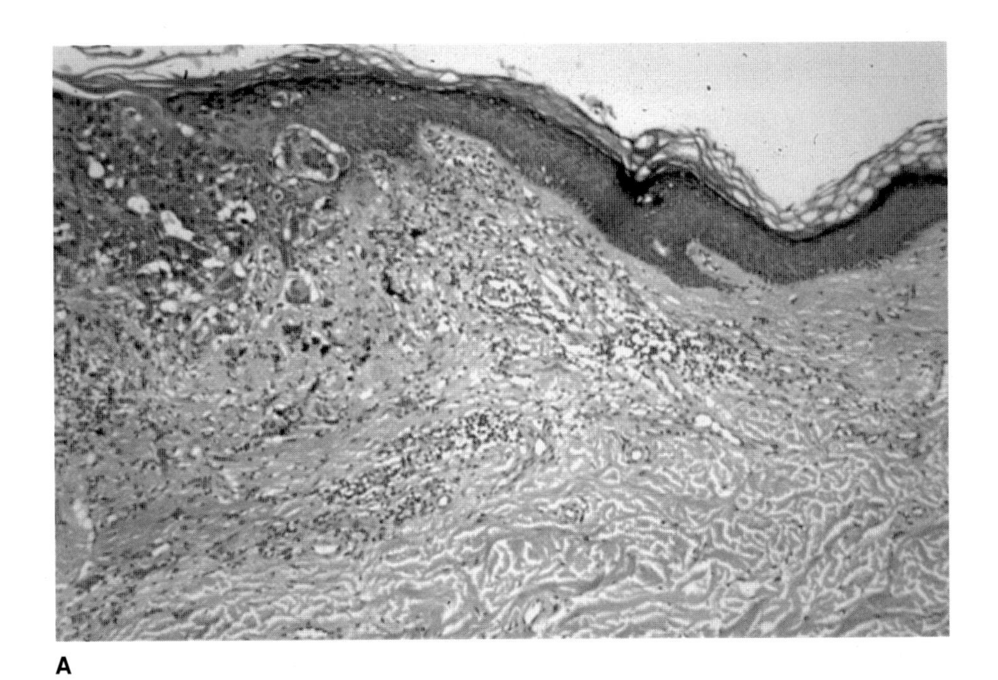

A

FIG. 29-26. Partial regression of the radial growth phase
(**A**) At left, there are melanoma cells in the epidermis and papillary dermis. To the right, there is fibrosis with lymphocytes and melanophages in the papillary dermis. (*continued on next page*)

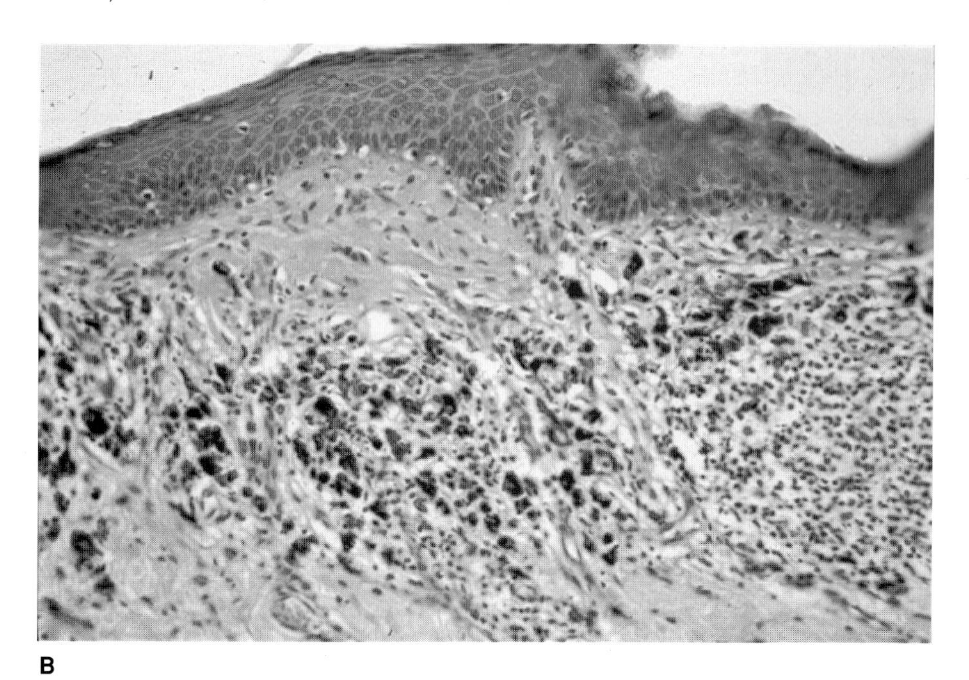

B

FIG. 29-26. *Continued*
(**B**) In another area of partial radial growth phase regression, the papillary dermis is widened by fibroblasts with lymphocytes and melanophages.

In occasional cases of metastatic melanoma with no obvious primary tumor, clinical examination may reveal a hypopigmented or irregularly hyperpigmented atrophic patch in the skin of the nodal drainage region.[312] Some other cases of apparently regressed primary melanoma may present as clinically pigmented, variegated lesions, clinically suspicious for melanoma. Some of these cases have presented with concomitant metastases, but others, in our experience, have not been associated with metastasis. Although the diagnosis of melanoma cannot be made with certainty in these latter cases, we have seen at least one case in which a metastatic melanoma developed after a period of follow-up. Histologic examination shows, in the case of depigmented lesions, telangiectasia and some pigmented macrophages in the papillary dermis, and, in the case of still-pigmented lesions, an irregular band of melanophages and inflammatory cells in the upper part of the dermis. In some cases, serial sections may reveal a few melanoma cells in the dermis or in the subcutaneous tissue.

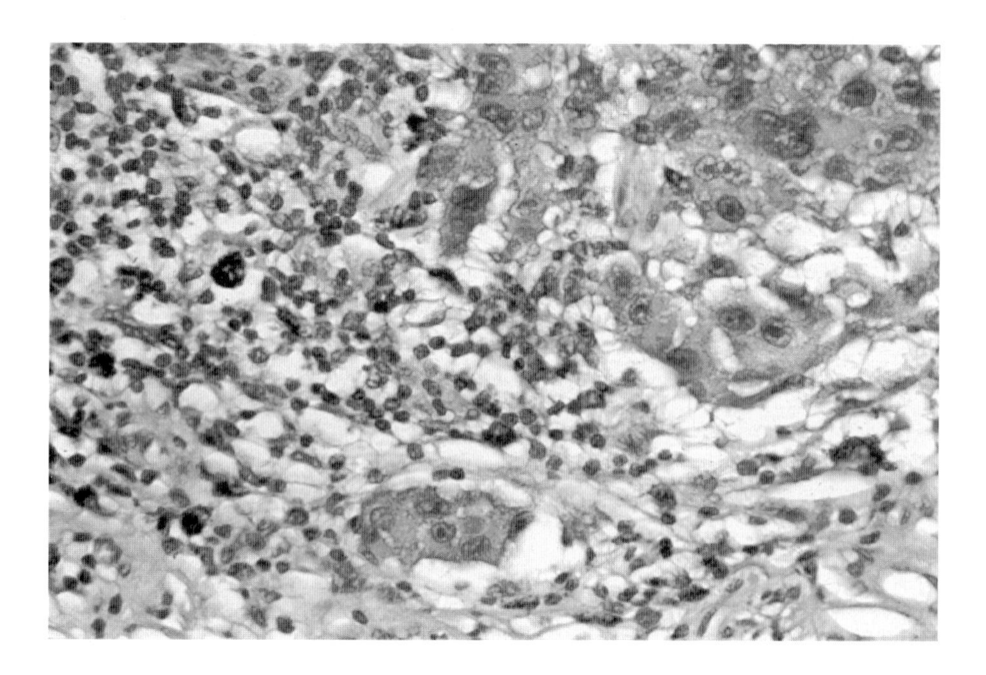

FIG. 29-27. Tumor-infiltrating lymphocytes (TIL) at the base of the vertical growth phase of a primary melanoma
Lymphocytes that are "among" the tumor cells, often associated with evidence of apoptosis of the cells, are a favorable prognostic attribute.

Tumor-Infiltrating Lymphocytes

The presence of tumor-infiltrating lymphocytes (TIL) that are actually among and in contact with the tumor cells of the vertical growth phase has been shown to have powerful independent prognostic significance[253,313,314] (see Fig. 29-27). The prognosis is best for tumors with a "brisk" TIL response, defined as lymphocytes forming a continuous band beneath the tumor or diffusely throughout its substance. Tumors with "absent" TIL have the worst prognosis, and a "nonbrisk" response is associated with an intermediate prognosis. The presence of a noninfiltrative lymphocytic infiltrate around the tumor, usually at its base, is unassociated with prognosis. Lymphocytosis decreases with the depth of penetration and is usually scant in deeply invasive tumors.

Mitotic Rate

Mitotic rate has been associated with prognosis in several studies.[253,315,316] The mitotic rate, determined in the tumorigenic compartments of primary melanomas, has been shown to have powerful independent significance.[253] The prognosis is best when the mitotic rate is zero and worst when the rate is greater than six mitoses per square millimeter.

Ulceration

Ulceration, the loss of continuity of the epithelium over the surface of the tumor, has prognostic significance in some series. In one series, ulceration in stage I reduces the 5-year survival rate from 80% to 55%.[317] In other series, ulceration is not an independent prognostic attribute in multivariable analyses, even though it is significant as a single variable.[253] A potentially useful prognostic algorithm has recently been published in which ulceration is the primary stratifying variable.[318]

Other Clinicopathologic Prognostic Factors

Various factors in additon to tumor thickness have been cited as influencing the prognosis of clinical stage I melanoma, but many of them are directly related to thickness. In different clinicopathologic databases, multivariate analyses have led to prognostic models that differ somewhat in the predictive variables that are shown to have independent significance. Several features, however, have appeared in two or more of the studies. Among the favorable clinical factors is *location* of the tumor on the hair-bearing portions of the limbs, in contrast to location on the trunk, neck and head, or palms and soles.[253,317] There is general agreement that women have better prognoses than men, owing partly, but not entirely, to the higher incidence in women of lesions on the extremities, for which the prognosis is more favorable than that for lesions on the trunk.[319] The age of the patient has an adverse prognostic effect in some series.[253]

Among the histologic factors, the type of tumor—nodular or superficial spreading—does not independently affect the prognosis.[253] Nodular melanomas, on average, are thicker than superficial spreading melanomas and thus have worse prognoses overall. However, at similar thicknesses, the two types of tumors have similar mortality rates.[320] The presence of vascular or lymphatic invasion and the scarcity or absence of melanin in the tumor cells, indicative of poor differentiation, affect the prognosis adversely in some series, but they do so at least in part because they correlate with tumor thickness and other variables[253] (Fig. 29-28).

Biological Markers

Biological markers derived from the study of primary tumors or of host attributes may be expected to add to the precision of present prognostic models. Most such studies to date have been pilot studies of small series of cases, lacking the statistical power needed to draw confident conclusions. A more definitive recent matched-pair analysis of the proliferation marker Mib-1 found its expression to be significantly related to mortality risk.[321] In another matched-pair analyses, tumor vascularity was found not to correlate with survival rate.[322]

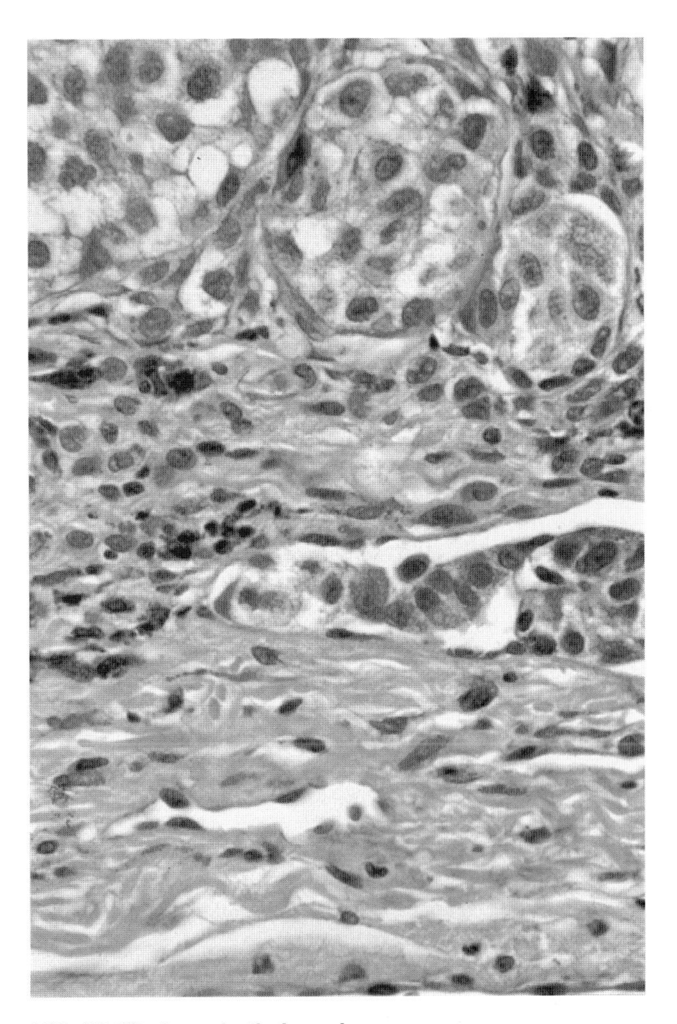

FIG. 29-28. Lymphatic invasion
Although not often recognized, except in very thick tumors, lymphatic invasion is probably an adverse prognostic attribute.

Multivariable Prognostic Models

The "gold standard" for considering any putative prognostic marker to be clinically important is its inclusion as an independent variable in a multivariable analysis. So far, no such studies have been published for other than the traditional histopathological and clinical variables reviewed earlier. Based on these multivariable analyses, prognostic models have been published, either requiring the use of a calculator to determine regression functions or, more simply, using published tables to provide quantitative probability estimates.[224,253,323] Although these models are useful in planning of therapy, and especially in the development and execution of clinical trials, determination of thickness remains in predominant use for planning of therapy for stage I melanoma.

Local Excision

Formerly, the margin of resection of the primary tumor was regarded by most authors as optimal at about 5 cm beyond the perimeter of the lesion. However, a narrower margin has become acceptable. Margin width recommendations were recently reviewed by an NIH Consensus Conference.[172] A margin of 0.5 to 1.0 cm is recommended for excision of a melanoma in situ, with a margin of 1 cm for melanomas less than 1.0 mm thick, and a 2- to 3-cm skin margin for lesions thicker than 1.0 mm.[324] A recent worldwide cooperative study has shown that in patients with primary melanomas no thicker than 2 mm, excisions with margins of 1 cm gave results as good as those of excisions with margins of 3 cm.[325] Naturally, histologic examination of the excised tumor and its margins is mandatory, because margins may be involved in spite of a clinically normal appearance. The dermis should be evaluated carefully for the presence of satellites, which may have prognostic significance. Satellites are rare in relation to thin tumors, but in one study they were detected in 22% of the reexcision specimens from melanomas greater than 2.25 mm in thickness.[326]

Elective Lymph Node Dissection

A clinically positive lymph node in a patient with primary cutaneous melanoma should be biopsied, and if the node is histologically positive, a full regional node dissection should be done as a "therapeutic" procedure with curative intent and to gain local control. For clinically negative lymph nodes, the role of "elective regional lymph node dissection" (ERLND) is controversial. Theoretically, regional nodes could be regarded as necessary filters that must be bypassed by all melanomas that metastasize systematically. However, it is clear that many melanomas metastasize by the hematogenous route to distant organs without ever involving regional nodes. Thus, lymph node involvement in many cases may be simply a marker of a melanoma that has already metastasized.

The incidence of regional lymph node involvement increases with the thickness of the tumor. Involvement of the regional lymph nodes is extremely rare in melanomas less than 0.76 mm thick. It is therefore generally agreed that elective regional lymph node dissection is not indicated for these melanomas (most of which are nontumorigenic). For tumors 0.76 mm thick or thicker, the data are conflicting,[313,324,327,328] and therapeutic trials are in progress to resolve the issues.

AJCC stage III melanoma patients with palpable lymph nodes are at high risk of having distant metastases. The number of involved lymph nodes and the depth of the tumor are important prognostic factors. Patients who have metastases in less than 20% of their resected regional lymph nodes and a tumor thickness of less than 3.5 mm have a 5-year disease-free survival rate of 80%, compared with 18% for patients who have a tumor thickness greater than 3.5 mm or metastases in 20% or more of their resected lymph nodes.[329] The size of involved nodes is not related to survival[330] (a defect in the AJCC staging system is its use of node size rather than the number and proportion of involved nodes). In an interesting recent study, the presence of brisk tumor-infiltrating lymphocytes (TIL) in a lymph node metastasis was associated with a survival rate of 83%, compared to 29% in patients whose metastases lacked TIL.[331]

Malignant Blue Nevus

Malignant blue nevus is a rare tumor. It may arise in a blue nevus,[332,333] a giant congenital nevus,[157] or a nevus of Ota,[9] or it may be malignant from the start.[334] A malignant blue nevus may involve the dermis and may be ulcerated, or may present as a deep-seated expansile mass.[334] In some lesions classified as malignant blue nevus, metastases occur that are limited to the regional lymph nodes, and the patient survives after removal of the tumor and the involved lymph nodes.[333] In other cases, however, death occurs as a result of widespread metastases.[26,332,334,335] Unfortunately, reliable distinction between these two groups of cases is not possible.

Histopathology. Recognition of a lesion as a malignant blue nevus rather than a common melanoma is based on the absence of junctional activity and the presence of at least some bipolar tumor cells with branching dendritic processes containing melanin granules.[26,333,334] This may require silver staining, because melanin is often scanty in malignant blue nevi arising from areas of cellular blue nevus. However, considerable amounts of melanin are present in some malignant blue nevi.[334]

In addition to showing the standard features of malignancy, such as invasiveness of the tumor, atypicality and pleomorphism of the nuclei, and presence of atypical mitoses, malignant blue nevi often show areas of necrosis as evidence of their malignant nature.[333,334] The combination of uniform cytologic atypia, high-grade atypia, spontaneous tumor necrosis, and more than a few mitoses may be considered diagnostic of malignant blue nevus in a lesion with a characteristic associated blue nevus pattern. Some lesions that have not met all these criteria—for example, lesions that have lacked necrosis—have metastasized. Tumors with the overall appearance of cellular blue nevus that show only some of these features, in minor degree, may be signed out descriptively as "melanocytic tumor of uncertain malignant potential" (MELTUMP) (see later).

Histogenesis. Although some authors have regarded the tumor cells as being related to Schwann cells,[333] electron microscopic studies have shown the presence of melanosomes in the cells and a lack of cytoplasmic enclosures of unmyelinated axons, which would be present if the tumor cells were Schwann cells. Although the melanosomes in many cells are devoid of melanin,[334] incubation with dopa has shown that they are strongly dopa-positive.[26] Thus, it is evident that the tumor cells are melanocytes.

Differential Diagnosis. Malignant blue nevus differs from primary melanoma by the absence of junctional activity and by the presence of associated common and/or cellular blue nevus. However, distinction of a malignant blue nevus from a metastatic melanoma can be difficult, because metastatic melanoma is occasionally found without a demonstrable primary melanoma. The primary melanoma may have involuted or may be located at an obscure internal site. The presence of dendritic cells indicative of an associated blue nevus or cellular blue nevus component is then the most reliable criterion favoring a diagnosis of malignant blue nevus instead of a metastatic melanoma. In doubtful cases, the differential diagnosis of metastatic melanoma should be expressed, and a workup for another primary should be considered clinically.

Melanocytic Tumors of Uncertain Malignant Potential (MELTUMPs)

This is a descriptive term for a heterogeneous group of melanocytic tumors that exhibit some features indicative of possible malignancy, such as nuclear atypia, macronucleoli, mitotic activity, necrosis, or ulceration, but in number or degree insufficient to justify a malignant diagnosis.

Histopathology. Tumors appropriately placed in this descriptive category may be quite bulky neoplasms on the order of several millimeters in diameter and thickness, composed of pigmented, often spindle-shaped cells. The overall cellularity may be relatively low compared with that of fully malignant melanoma. There may be occasional mitoses, but not more than one or a few per section plane. Abnormal mitoses, if present, are usually indicative of frank malignancy. Focal areas of individual-cell necrosis may be present, but if there are areas of confluent geographic necrosis, or if an ulcer is present, a frankly malignant diagnosis is appropriate. There may be a few enlarged melanocytes in the epidermis, but if there is an intraepidermal component that can be identified as a radial growth phase of melanoma of any of the common types, a diagnosis of melanoma should be made.

Differential Diagnosis. This descriptive diagnosis is one of exclusion, and the differential diagnosis includes specific neoplasms described elsewhere in this chapter, including atypical and malignant Spitz nevi, minimal deviation melanomas, deep penetrating nevi, cellular neurothekeoma (discussed Chap. 36, Tumors of Neural Tissue in the Skin), atypical cellular blue nevi, and melanomas.

Some lesions that may be placed in this descriptive category that have not been discussed elsewhere are composed of dendritic cells stuffed with abundant and coarsely divided pigment that obscures the nuclei.[224] Sometimes these cells are difficult to distinguish from melanophages. Some of these lesions may have prominent epidermal involvement, with pagetoid spread of the heavily pigmented lesional cells into the epidermis, and a dermal component that is broader in the papillary than in the reticular dermis. These lesions, despite their unusual cytology, have pattern features that are relatively characteristic of melanoma. Some related lesions, where criteria for malignancy are not deemed to have been fully met, may be placed in the descriptive category of "uncertain malignant potential." Yet other very rare lesions present as nodular clusters of authentic melanophages ("tumoral melanosis"[311]). These lesions may be examples of complete regression of a pigmented vertical growth phase nodule, a very rare phenomenon that is quite differential from the partial regression frequently observed in the radial growth phase compartments of common melanomas.

Metastatic Melanoma

Metastatic spread, uncommon in thin melanomas, is quite common in tumors thicker than 2 mm. Lymph node metastases usually present earlier than hematogenous metastases. Although metastases usually occur within 5 years after onset of the disease, their appearance may be delayed, especially in "thin" melanomas.[336] Late metastases, beyond 10 years, are rare.[337]

The prognosis for patients with distant metastatic disease is very poor. In a recent study, the overall median survival period was 7.5 months; patients with non-regional cutaneous, nodal, or gastrointestinal metastases had a median survival period of 12.5 months and an estimated 5-year survival rate of 14%.[338]

In about 4% to 10% of the patients who present initially with metastases of melanoma, no primary tumor can be found.[339] Although the primary tumor may in some instances be in an internal organ, it can be assumed that it was in most instances located in the skin and regressed spontaneously. In some instances, there is a history of a spontaneously resolving pigmented lesion, and one may see at that site either a hypopigmented area[340] or an irregular, flat, pigmented lesion.[341]

Histopathology. The histologic appearance of *melanoma metastases in the skin* usually differs from that of a primary melanoma by the absence of an inflammatory infiltrate and of junctional activity (Fig. 29-29). However, primary melanomas may occasionally fail to involve the epidermis, and may also not show an inflammatory infiltrate, particularly when they are deeply invasive. Furthermore, in occasional instances, even metastases exhibit a prominent lymphocytic infiltrate,[331] and can contact the overlying epidermis in a way that is suggestive of junctional activity, with nests of atypical melanocytes in the epidermis.

Epidermotropic metastatic melanoma refers to a metastatic deposit that is initially localized in the papillary dermis and involves the overlying epidermis. Most of these lesions occur in an extremity regional to a distal primary melanoma. Epidermotropic metastasis is characterized by (1) thinning of the epidermis by aggregates of atypical melanocytes within the dermis, (2) inward turning of the rete ridges at the periphery of the lesion, and (3) usually no lateral extension of atypical melanocytes within the epidermis beyond the concentration of the metastasis in the dermis.[342] However, this distinction can be very difficult at times, and cases have recently been reported in which there was lateral extension beyond the dermal component.[343] In some other cases, the metastatic cells are small and nevoid, with few if any mitoses, and in these instances of *differentiated epidermotropic metastatic melanoma* the lesions can be mistaken for compound nevi.

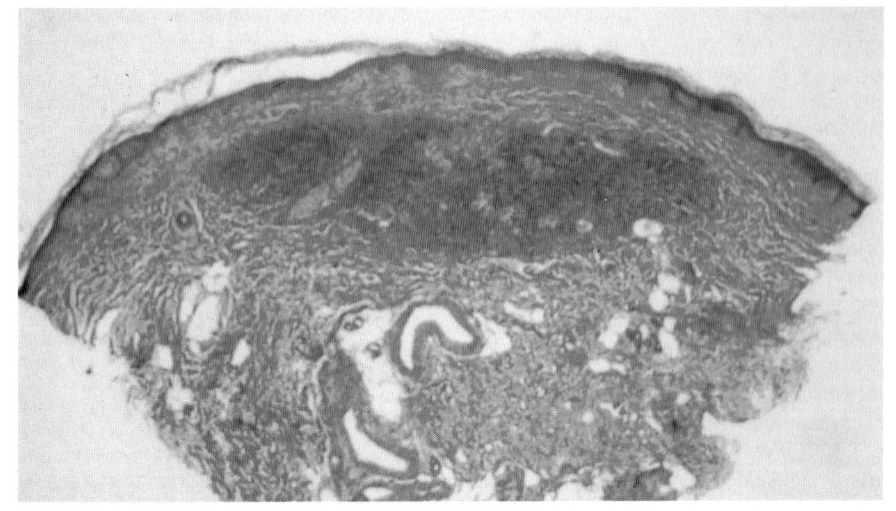

A

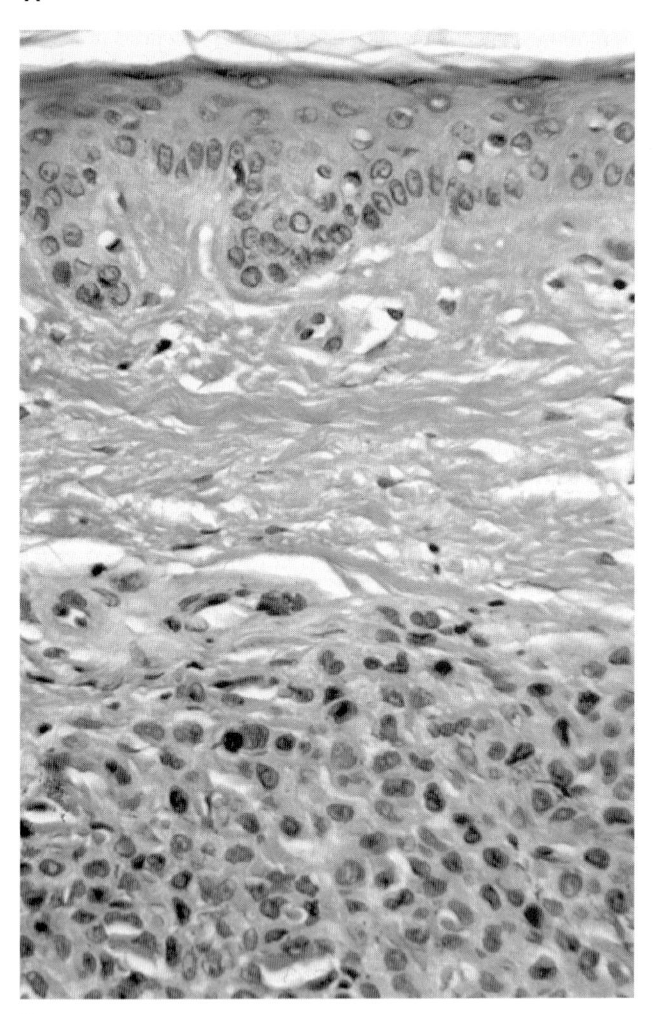

B

FIG. 29-29. Dermal metastatic melanoma
(**A**) Metastatic melanoma often presents as a fairly symmetrical cellular nodule in the reticular dermis or subcutis. The lesions are often quite small, as here, at the time they are excised and presented for an initial diagnosis of metastatic spread. (**B**) Cytologically, the cells are uniformly atypical, as in tumorigenic primary melanomas. Sometimes, especially in superficial or epidermotropic cutaneous metastases, atypia is deceptively minimal. The identification of mitotic activity, and of lymphatic invasion, may be very helpful in making the diagnosis.

Generalized Melanosis in Metastatic Melanoma

This is a rare phenomenon that may be associated with widespread melanoma metastases. It is characterized by diffuse slate-blue discoloration of the entire skin, the conjunctivae, and the oral and pharyngeal mucous membranes, often with melanuria. Melanin granules have been observed also in blood smears within neutrophils and monocytes. Autopsy reveals a similar discoloration in the intima of the large arteries and of many visceral organs.[344]

Histologically, numerous melanin granules are located within macrophages throughout the dermis, especially around capillaries. They stain with the Fontana-Masson stain and are dopa-positive. In addition, some dermal vessels are focally plugged with dark, amorphous dopa-positive material. In most instances, only melanophages have been found. It is assumed that the melanin is produced by distant melanoma cells and then carried by the blood to the skin, to be deposited within dermal melanophages.[344] In a few cases, two types of pigmented cells have been identified in the dermis, particularly in semithin sections: melanophages and individually scattered melanoma cells appearing larger and less pigmented than the melanophages. On autopsy, melanin phagocytosis is observed in many organs, especially in the Kupffer cells of the liver and the cells lining the sinusoids of the lymph nodes, spleen, and adrenal glands.[345]

REFERENCES

1. Kikuchi I, Inoue S. Natural history of the Mongolian spot. J Dermatol 1980;7:449.
2. Hidano A, Kajima H, Ikeda S et al. Natural history of nevus of Ota. Arch Dermatol 1967;95:187.
3. Burkhart CG, Gohara A. Dermal melanocyte hamartoma. Arch Dermatol 1981;117:102.
4. Kopf AW, Weidman AI. Nevus of Ota. Arch Dermatol 1962;85:195.
5. Mishima Y, Mevorah B. Nevus Ota and Nevus Ito in American Negroes. J Invest Dermatol 1961;36:133.
6. Hidano A, Kajima H, Ikeda S et al. Natural history of nevus of Ota. Arch Dermatol 1967;95:187.
7. Bashiti HM, Blair JD, Triska RA et al. Generalized dermal melanocytosis. Arch Dermatol 1981;117:791.
8. Mevorah B, Frenk E, Delacrétaz J. Dermal melanocytosis. Dermatologica 1977;154:107.
9. Dorsey CS, Montgomery H. Blue nevus and its distinction from Mongolian spot and the nevus of Ota. J Invest Dermatol 1954;22:225.
10. Kopf AW, Bart RS. Malignant blue (Ota's) nevus. J Dermatol Surg Oncol 1982;8:442.
11. Nödl F, Krüger R. Maligner blauer Nävus bei Nävus Ota. Hautarzt 1984;35:421.
12. Enriquez R, Egbert B, Bullock J. Primary malignant melanoma of the central nervous system. Arch Pathol 1973;95:392.
13. Rodriguez HA, Ackerman LV. Cellular blue nevus. Cancer 1968; 21: 393.
14. Pittman JL, Fisher BK. Plaque-type of blue nevus. Arch Dermatol 1976;112:1127.
15. Hendricks WM. Eruptive blue nevi. J Am Acad Dermatol 1981;4:50.
16. Santa Cruz DJ, Yates AJ. Pigmented storiform neurofibroma. J Cutan Pathol 1977;4:9.
17. Avidor I, Kessler E. "Atypical" blue nevus: A benign variety of cellular blue nevus. Dermatologica 1977;154:39.
18. Temple-Camp CRE, Saxe N, King H. Benign and malignant cellular blue nevus. Am J Dermatopathol 1988;10:289.
19. Silverberg GD, Kadin ME, Dorfman RF et al. Invasion of the brain by a cellular blue nevus of the scalp. Cancer 1971;27:349.
20. Lambert WC, Brodkin RH. Nodal and subcutaneous cellular blue nevi: A pseudometastasizing pseudomelanoma. Arch Dermatol 1984; 120:367.
21. Leopold JG, Richards DB. The interrelationship of blue and common nevi. J Pathol 1968;95:37.
22. Pulitzer DR, Martin PC, Cohen AP, Reed RJ. Histologic classification of the combined nevus: Analysis of the variable expression of melanocytic nevi. Am J Surg Pathol 1991;15:1111.
23. Pulitzer DR, Martin PC, Cohen AP, Reed RJ. Histologic classification of the combined nevus: Analysis of the variable expression of melanocytic nevi. Am J Surg Pathol 1991;15:1111.
24. Masson P. My conception of cellular nevi. Cancer 1951;4:19.
25. Skelton H III, Smith KJ, Barrett TL et al. HMB-45 staining in benign and malignant melanocytic lesions: A reflection of cellular activation. Am J Dermatopathol 1991;13:543.
26. Mishima Y. Cellular blue nevus: Melanogenic activity and malignant transformation. Arch Dermatol 1970;101:104.
27. Bliss JM, Ford D, Swerdlow AJ et al. Risk of cutaneous melanoma associated with pigmentation characteristics and freckling: Systematic overview of 10 case-control studies. Int J Cancer 1995;62:367.
28. Breathnach AS, Wyllie LM. Electron microscopy of melanocytes and melanosomes in freckled human epidermis. J Invest Dermatol 1964; 42:389.
29. Benedict PH, Szabo G, Fitzpatrick TB. Melanotic macules in Albright's syndrome and in neurofibromatosis. JAMA 1968;205:618.
30. Barnhill RL, Albert LS, Shama SK et al. Genital lentiginosis: A clinical and histopathologic study. J Am Acad Dermatol 1990;22:453.
31. Maize JC. Mucosal melanosis. Dermatol Clin 1988;6:283.
32. Sexton FM, Maize JC. Melanotic macules and melanoacanthomas of the lip: A comparative study with census of the basal melanocyte population. Am J Dermatopathol 1987;9:438.
33. Becker SW. Concurrent melanosis and hypertrichosis in the distribution of nevus unius lateris. Arch Dermatol Syph 1949;60:155.
34. Fehr B, Panizzon RG, Schnyder UW. Becker's nevus and malignant melanoma. Dermatologica 1991;182:77.
35. Rower JM, Carr RD, Lowney ED. Progressive cribriform and zosteriform hyperpigmentation. Arch Dermatol 1978;114:98.
36. Urbanek RW, Johnson WC. Smooth muscle hamartoma associated with Becker's nevus. Arch Dermatol 1978;114:98.
37. Tate PR, Hodge SJ, Owen LG. A quantitative study of melanocytes in Becker's nevus. J Cutan Pathol 1980;7:404.
38. Taylor EJ, ed. Dorland's Illustrated Medical Dictionary, 27th ed. Philadelphia: Saunders, 1988;910.
39. Mehregan AH. Lentigo senilis and its evolution. J Invest Dermatol 1975;65:429.
40. Bolognia JL. Reticulated black solar lentigo: "Ink spot lentigo." Arch Dermatol 1992;128:934.
41. Rhodes AR, Harrist TJ, Momtaz TK. The PUVA-induced pigmented macule: A lentiginous proliferation of large, sometimes cytologically atypical melanocytes. J Am Acad Dermatol 1983;9:47.
42. Montagna W, Hu F, Carlisle K. A reinvestigation of solar lentigines. Arch Dermatol 1980;116:1151.
43. Hodgson C. Lentigo senilis. Arch Dermatol 1963;87:197.
44. Gartmann H. Zur dignitätder naevoiden lentigo. Z Hautkr 1978;53:91.
45. Kaufmann J, Eichmann A, Neves C et al. Lentiginosis profusa. Dermatologica 1976;153:116.
46. Rhodes AR. Neoplasms: Benign neoplasias, hyperplasias, and dysplasias of melanocytes. In: Fitzpatrick TB, Eisen AZ, Wolff K, eds. Dermatology in general medicine. 4th ed. New York: McGraw-Hill, 1993;996.
47. Stewart DM, Altman J, Mehregan AH. Speckled lentiginous nevus. Arch Dermatol 1978;114:895.
48. Van der Horst JC, Dirksen HJ. Zosteriform lentiginous nevus. Br J Dermatol 1981;104:104.
49. Weiss LW, Zelickson AS. Giant melanosomes in multiple lentigines syndrome. Arch Dermatol 1977;113:491.
50. Jeghers H, McKusick BA, Katz KH. Generalized intestinal polyposis and melanin spots of the oral mucosa, lips and digits. N Engl J Med 1949;241:993, 1031, 1036.
51. Selmanowitz VJ. Lentiginosis profusa syndrome (multiple lentigines syndrome). Acta Derm Venereol (Stockh) 1971;51:387.
52. Yamada K, Matsukawa A, Hori Y et al. Ultrastructural studies on pigmented macules of Peutz-Jeghers syndrome. J Dermatol 1981;8:367.
53. Jimbow K, Szabo G, Fitzpatrick TB. Ultrastructure of giant pigment granules (macromelanosomes) in the cutaneous pigmented macules of neurofibromatosis. J Invest Dermatol 1973;61:300.
54. Konrad K, Wolff K, Hönigsmann H. The giant melanosome: A model of deranged melanosome-morphogenesis. J Ultrastruct Mol Struct Res 1974b;48:102.

55. Nakagawa H, Hori Y, Sato S et al. The nature and origin of the melanin macroglobule. J Invest Dermatol 1984;83:134.
56. Shaffer B. Pigmented nevi. Arch Dermatol 1955;72:120.
57. Eady RAJ, Gilkes JJH, Wilson Jones E. Eruptive naevi: Report of two cases. Br J Dermatol 1977;97:267.
58. Clark WH Jr, Elder DE, Guerry D IV et al. A study of tumor progression: The precursor lesions of superficial spreading and nodular melanoma. Hum Pathol 1984;15:1147.
59. Elder DE, Clark WH Jr, Elenitsas R et al. The early and intermediate precursor lesions of tumor progression in the melanocytic system: Common acquired nevi and atypical (dysplastic) nevi. Semin Diagn Pathol 1993;10:18.
60. Eng AM. Solitary small active junctional nevi in juvenile patients. Arch Dermatol 1983;119:33.
61. Miescher G, Von Albertini A. Histologie de 100 cas de naevi pigmentaires d'après les méthodes de masson. Bull Soc Fr Dermatol Syphiligr 1935;42:1265.
62. Smolle J, Smolle-Juettner FM, Stettner H, Kerl H. Relationship of tumor cell motility and morphologic patterns. Am J Dermatopathol 1992;14:231.
63. Rhodes AR, Silverman RA, Harrist TJ et al. A histologic comparison of congenital and acquired nevomelanocytic nevi. Arch Dermatol 1985;121:1266.
64. Sagebiel RW. Histologic artifacts of benign pigmented nevi. Arch Dermatol 1972;106:691.
65. Penneys NS, Mogollon R, Kowalczyk A. A survey of cutaneous neural lesions for the presence of myelin basic protein. Arch Dermatol 1984;120:210.
66. Freeman RG, Knox JM. Epidermal cysts associated with pigmented nevi. Arch Dermatol 1962;85:590.
67. Stegmaier OC. Natural regression of the melanocytic nevus. J Invest Dermatol 1959;32:413.
68. Masson P. My conception of cellular nevi. Cancer 1951;4:9.
69. Winkelmann RK. Cholinesterase nevus: Cholinesterases in pigmented tumors of the skin. Arch Dermatol 1960;82:17.
70. Thorne EG, Mottaz JH, Zelickson AS. Tyrosinase activity in dermal nevus cells. Arch Dermatol 1971;104:619.
71. Niizuma K. Electron microscopic study of nevic corpuscle. Acta Derm Venereol (Stockh) 1975;55:283.
72. Lund HZ, Stobbe GD. The natural history of the pigmented nevus: Factors of age and anatomic location. Am J Pathol 1949;25:1117.
73. Maize JC, Foster G. Age-related changes in melanocytic nevi. Clin Exp Dermatol 1979;15:49.
74. Mishima Y. Macromolecular changes in pigmentary disorders. Arch Dermatol 1965;91:519.
75. Gottlieb B, Brown AL Jr., Winkelmann RK. Fine structure of the nevus cell. Arch Dermatol 1965;92:81.
76. Gilchrest BA, Treloar V, Grassi AM et al. Characteristics of cultivated adult human nevocellular nevus cells. J Invest Dermatol 1986;87:102.
77. Goette DK, Doty RD. Balloon cell nevus. Arch Dermatol 1978;114: 109.
78. Schrader WA, Helwig EB. Balloon cell nevi. Cancer 1967;20:1502.
79. Okun MR, Donnellan B, Edelstein L. An ultrastructural study of balloon cell nevus. Cancer 1974;34:615.
80. MacKie RM, English J, Aitchison TC et al. The number and distribution of benign pigmented moles (melanocytic nevi) in a healthy British population. Brit J Dermatol 1985;113:167.
81. Boyd AS, Rapini RP. Acral melanocytic neoplasms: A histological analysis of 158 lesions. J Am Acad Dermatol 1994;31:740.
82. Kouskoukis CE, Scher RK, Hatcher VA. Melanonychia striata longitudinalis. J Dermatol Surg Oncol 1982;8:284.
83. Baran R, Barrière H. Longitudinal melanonychia with spreading pigmentation in Laugier-Hunziker syndrome. Br J Dermatol 1986;115: 707.
84. Kopf AW, Albom M, Ackermann AB. Biopsy technique for longitudinal streaks of pigmentation in nails. Am J Dermatopathol 1984;6: 309.
85. Scher RK, Silvers DN. Longitudinal melanonychia striata. J Am Acad Dermatol 1991;24:1035.
86. Molina D, Sanchez JL. Pigmented longitudinal bands of the nail: A clincopathologic study. Am J Dermatopathol 1995;17:539.
87. Friedman RJ, Ackerman AB. Difficulties in the histologic diagnosis of melanocytic nevi on the vulvae of premenopausal women. In: Pathology of malignant melanoma. Ackerman AB, ed. New York: Masson, 1981;119.
88. Maize JC, Ackerman AB. Pigmented lesions of the skin: Clinicopathologic correlations. Philadelphia: Lea & Febiger, 1987.
89. Christensen WN, Friedman KF, Woodruff JD, Hood AF. Histologic characteristics of vulval nevocellular nevi. J Cutan Pathol 1987;14:87.
90. Rock B, Hood AF, Rock JA. Prospective study of vulvar nevi. J Am Acad Dermatol 1990;22:104.
91. Spitz S. Melanomas of childhood. Am J Pathol 1948;24:591.
92. Allen AC. Juvenile melanomas of children and adults and melanocarcinomas of children. Arch Dermatol 1960;82:325.
93. Paniago-Pereira C, Maize JC, Ackerman AB. Nevus of large spindle and/or epithelioid cells: Spitz's nevus. Arch Dermatol 1978;114:1811.
94. Stanka F, Lechner W. Benignes juveniles melanom (spindelzellnävus) in atypischer ausprägung. Hautarzt 1985;36:113.
95. Gartmann H, Ganser M. Der Spitz-naevus, spindelzellen- und/oder epitheloidzellennaevus: Eine klinische analyse von 652 tumoren. Z Hautkr 1985;60:22.
96. Weedon D, Little JH. Spindle and epithelioid cell nevi in children and adults: A review of 211 cases of the Spitz nevus. Cancer 1977;40:217.
97. Smith SA, Day CL, Van Der Ploeg DE. Eruptive widespread Spitz nevi. J Am Acad Dermatol 1986;15:1155.
98. McGovern VJ. Spitz Nevus. In: McGovern VJ ed. Melanoma: Histological diagnosis and prognosis. New York: Raven Press, 1983;37.
99. Busam KJ, Barnhill RL. Pagetoid Spitz nevus: Intraepidermal Spitz tumor with prominent pagetoid spread. Am J Surg Pathol 1995;19: 1061.
100. Mérot Y, Frenk E. Spitz nevus (large spindle cell and/or epithelioid cell nevus): Age-related involvement of the suprabasal epidermis. Virchows Arch [A] 1989;415:97.
101. Mérot Y. Transepidermal elimination of nevus cells in spindle and epithelioid cell (Spitz) nevi [letter]. Arch Dermatol 1988;124:1441.
102. Scott G, Chen KTK, Rosai J. Pseudoepitheliomatous hyperplasia in Spitz nevi. Arch Pathol 1989;113:61.
103. McWhorter HE, Woolner LB. Pigmented nevi, juvenile melanomas and malignant melanomas in children. JAMA 1954;156:695.
104. Kamino H, Misheloff E, Ackerman AB et al. Eosinophilic globules in Spitz's nevi: New findings and a diagnostic sign. Am J Dermatopathol 1979;1:319.
105. Arbuckle S, Weedon D. Eosinophilic globules in the Spitz nevus. J Am Acad Dermatol 1982;7:324.
106. Echevarria R, Ackerman LV. Spindle and epithelioid cell nevi in the adult. Cancer 1967;20:175.
107. Barr RJ, Morales RV, Graham JH. Desmoplastic nevus: A distinct variant of mixed spindle cell and epithelioid cell nevus. Cancer 1980; 46:557.
108. Suster S. Hyalinizing spindle and epithelioid cell nevus: A study of five cases of a distinctive histologic variant of Spitz's nevus. Am J Dermatopathol 1994;16:593.
109. Schreiner E, Wolff K. Die ultrastruktur des benignen juvenilen melanoms. Arch Klin Exp Dermatol 1970;237:749.
110. De Wit PEJ, Kerstens HMJ, Poddighe PJ et al. DNA in situ hybridization as a diagnostic tool in the discrimination of melanoma and Spitz naevus. J Pathol 1994;173:227.
111. Smith KJ, Barett TL, Skelton HG et al. Spindle cell and epithelioid cell nevi with atypia and metastasis: Malignant Spitz tumor. Am J Surg Pathol 1989;13:931.
112. LeBoit PE, Van Fletcher H. A comparative study of Spitz nevus and nodular malignant melanoma using image analysis cytometry. J Invest Dermatol 1987;88:753.
113. Leitinger G, Cerroni L, Soyer HP et al. Morphometric diagnosis of melanocytic skin tumors. Am J Dermatopathol 1990;12:441.
114. Lazzaro B, Rebers A, Herlyn M et al. Immunophenotyping of compound and Spitz nevi and vertical growth phase melanomas using a panel of monoclonal antibodies reactive in paraffin sections. J Invest Dermatol 1993;100:313S.
115. Steiner A, Binder M, Mossbacher U et al. Estimation of the volume-weighted mean nuclear volume discriminates Spitz's nevi from nodular malignant melanomas. Lab Invest 1994;70:381.
116. Hofmann Wellenhof R, Rieger E, Smolle J, Kerl H. Proliferative activity in Spitz's nevi compared with other melanocytic skin lesions. Melanoma Research 1993;3:313.
117. Niemann TH, Argenyi ZB. Immunohistochemical study of Spitz nevi

and malignant melanoma with use of antibody to proliferating cell nuclear antigen. Am J Dermatopathol 1993;15:441.
118. Tu P, Mitauchi S, Miki Y. Proliferative activities in Spitz nevus compared with melanocytic nevus and malignant melanoma using expression of PCNA/cyclin and mitotic rate. Am J Dermatopathol 1993;15: 311.
119. Chi H-I, Ishibashi Y, Shima A et al. Use of DAPI cytofluorometric analysis of cellular DNA content to differentiate Spitz nevus from malignant melanoma. J Invest Dermatol 1990;95:154.
120. Matsuta M, Kon S, Thompson C et al. Interphase cytogenetics of melanocytic neoplasms: Numerical aberrations of chromosomes can be detected in interphase nuclei using centromeric DNA probes. J Cutan Pathol 1994;21:1.
121. Casso EM, Grin-Jorgensen CM, Grant-Kels JM. Spitz nevi. J Am Acad Dermatol 1992;27:901.
122. Shapiro PE. Spitz nevi. J Am Acad Dermatol 1993;29:667.
123. Reed RJ, Ichinose H, Clark WH et al. Common and uncommon melanocytic nevi and borderline melanomas. Semin Oncol 1973;2:119.
124. Maize JC, Ackerman AB. Spitz's nevus. In: Maize JC, Ackerman AB, eds. Pigmented lesions of the skin. Philadelphia: Lea & Febiger, 1987; 228.
125. Guillen FJ, Murphy GF. Nevomelanocytic lesions with spindle cell differentiation. J Dermatol Surg Oncol 1985;11:225.
126. Sagebiel RW, Chinn EK, Egbert BM. Pigmented spindle cell nevus: Clinical and histologic review of 90 cases. Am J Surg Pathol 1984;8: 645.
127. Barnhill RL, Barnhill MA, Berwick M, Mihm MC Jr. The histologic spectrum of pigmented spindle cell nevus: A review of 120 cases with emphasis on atypical variants. Hum Pathol 1991;22:52.
128. Haupt HM, Stern JB. Pagetoid melanocytosis: Histologic features in benign and malignant lesions. Am J Surg Pathol 1995;19:792.
129. Walton RG, Jacobs AH, Cox AJ. Pigmented lesions in newborn infants. Br J Dermatol 1976;95:389.
130. Rivers JK, Frederiksen PC, Dibdin C. A prevalence survey of dermatoses in the Australian neonate. J Am Acad Dermatol 1990;23:77.
131. Mark GJ, Mihm MC, Liteplo MG et al. Congenital melanocytic nevi of the small and garment type. Hum Pathol 1973;4:395.
132. Kopf AW, Bart RS, Hennessey P. Congenital nevocytic nevi and malignant melanomas. J Am Acad Dermatol 1979;1:123.
133. Orkin M, Frichot BC III, Zelickson AS. Cerebriform intradermal nevus. Arch Dermatol 1974;110:575.
134. Morishima T, Endo M, Imagawa I et al. Clinical and histopathological studies on spotted grouped pigmented nevi with special reference to eccrine-centered nevus. Acta Derm Venereol (Stockh) 1976;56: 345.
135. Botet MV, Caro FR, Sánchez JL. Congenital acral melanocytic nevi clinically resembling acral lentiginous melanoma. J Am Acad Dermatol 1981;5:406.
136. Slaughter JC, Hardman JM, Kempe LG et al. Neurocutaneous melanosis and leptomeningeal melanomatosis in children. Arch Pathol 1969;88:298.
137. Reed WB, Becker WS Jr, Becker WS Sr et al. Giant pigmented nevi, melanoma, and leptomeningeal melanocytosis. Arch Dermatol 1965; 91:100.
138. Rhodes AR, Wood WC, Sober AJ et al. Nonepidermal origin of malignant melanoma associated with a giant congenital nevocellular nevus. Plast Reconstr Surg 1981;67:766.
139. Swerdlow AJ, English JSC, Qiao Z. The risk of melanoma in patients with congenital nevi: A cohort study. J Am Acad Dermatol 1995;32: 595.
140. Marghoob AA, Schoenbach SP, Kopf AW et al. Large congenital nevi and the risk for the development of malignant melanoma. Arch Dermatol 1996;132:170.
141. Ruiz-Maldomnado R, Tamayo L, Duran C. Giant pigmented nevi: Clinical, histopathologic and therapeutic considerations. J Pediatr 1992;120:906.
142. Rhodes AR. Congenital nevomelanocytic nevi: Histologic patterns in the first year of life and evolution during childhood. Arch Dermatol 1986;122:1257.
143. Solomon LM. The management of congenital melanocytic nevi. Arch Dermatol 1980;116:1017.
144. Rhodes AR, Sober AJ, Day CL et al. The malignant potential of small congenital nevocellular nevi. J Am Acad Dermatol 1982;6:230.
145. Illig L, Weidner F, Hundeiker M et al. Congenital nevi smaller than 10 cm as precursors of melanoma. Arch Dermatol 1985;121:1274.
146. Everett MA. Histopathology of congenital pigmented nevi. Am J Dermatopathol 1989;11:11.
147. Zitelli JA, Grant MG, Abell E et al. Histologic patterns of congenital nevocytic nevi and implications for treatment. J Am Acad Dermatol 1984;11:402.
148. Kuehnl-Petzoldt C, Kunze J, Mueller R. Histology of congenital nevi during the first year of life. Am J Dermatopathol 1984;6:81.
149. Stenn KS, Arons M, Hurwitz S. Patterns of congenital nevocellular nevi. J Am Acad Dermatol 1983;9:388.
150. Clemmensen OJ, Kroon S. The histology of "congenital features" in early acquired melanocytic nevi. J Am Acad Dermatol 1988;19:742.
151. Mishima Y. Eccrine-centered nevus. Arch Dermatol 1973;107:59.
152. Menter MA, Griessel PJC, De Klerk DJ. Giant blue naevus of the scalp with underlying scalp defect. Br J Dermatol 1971;85:73.
153. Penman HG, Stringer HCW. Malignant transformation in giant congenital pigmented nevus. Arch Dermatol 1971;103:428.
154. Weidner N, Flanders DJ, Jochimsen PR et al. Neurosarcomatous malignant melanoma arising in a neuroid giant congenital melanocytic nevus. Arch Dermatol 1985;121:1302.
155. Pack GT, Davis J. Nevus giganticus pigmentosus with malignant transformation. Surgery 1961;49:347.
156. Grouls V, Helpap B, Crnic A. Kombination eines malignen blauen naevus mit einem congenitalen tierfellnaevus. Z Hautkr 1981;56:943.
157. Hendrickson MR, Ross JC. Neoplasms arising in congenital giant nevi: Morphologic study of seven cases and a review of the literature. Am J Surg Pathol 1981;5:109.
158. Williams HI. Primary malignant meningeal melanoma associated with benign hairy nevi. J Pathol 1969;99:171.
159. Seab JA Jr, Graham JH, Helwig EB. Deep penetrating nevus. Am J Surg Pathol 1989;13:39.
160. Mehregan DA, Mehregan AH. Deep penetrating nevus. Arch Dermatol 1993;129:328.
161. Barnhill RL, Mihm MC Jr, Magro CM. Plexiform spindle cell naevus: A distinctive variant of plexiform melanocytic naevus. Histopathology 1991;18:243.
162. Pulitzer DR, Martin PC, Cohen AP, Reed RJ. Histologic classification of the combined nevus: Analysis of the variable expression of melanocytic nevi. Am J Surg Pathol 1991;15:1111.
163. Mehregan DR, Mehregan DA, Mehregan AH. Proliferating cell nuclear antigen staining in deep-penetrating nevi. J Am Acad Dermatol 1995;33:685.
164. Clark WH Jr, Reimer RR, Greene M et al. Origin of familial malignant melanomas from heritable melanocytic lesions. Arch Dermatol 1978; 114:732.
165. Lynch HT, Frichot BC III, Lynch JF. Familial atypical multiple mole-melanoma syndrome. J Med Genet 1978;15:352.
166. Elder DE, Goldman LI, Goldman SC et al. Dysplastic nevus syndrome. Cancer 1980;46:1787.
167. Rahbari H, Mehregan AH. Sporadic atypical mole syndrome. Arch Dermatol 1981;117:329.
168. National Institutes of Health Consensus Development Conference. Precursors to malignant melanoma. J Am Acad Dermatol 1984;10: 683.
169. Kelly JW, Crutcher WA, Sagebiel RW. Clinical diagnosis of dysplastic melanocytic nevi. J Am Acad Dermatol 1986;14:1044.
170. Ackerman AB, Mihara I. Dysplasia, dysplastic melanocytes, dysplastic nevi, the dysplastic nevus syndrome, and the relation between dysplastic nevi and malignant melanomas. Hum Pathol 1985;16:87.
171. Ackerman AB, Briggs PL, Bravo F. Dysplastic nevus, compound type vs. Clark's nevus, compound type. In: Ackerman AB, Briggs PL, Bravo F, eds. Differential diagnosis in dermatopathology. Vol. III. Philadelphia: Lea & Febiger, 1993;158.
172. National Institutes of Health: Consensus Development Conference. Diagnosis and treatment of early melanoma. JAMA 1992;268:1314.
173. Halpern AC, Guerry D IV, Elder DE et al. Natural history of dysplastic nevi. J Am Acad Dermatol 1993;29:51.
174. Guerry D IV, Synnestvedt M, Elder DE, Schultz D. Lessons from tumor progression: The invasive radial growth phase of melanoma is common, incapable of metastasis, and indolent. J Invest Dermatol 1993;100:342S.
175. De Wit PEJ, Van't Hof-Grootenboer B, Ruiter DJ et al. Validity of the histopathological criteria used for diagnosing dysplastic naevi. Eur J Cancer [A] 1993;29A:831.

176. Clemente C, Cochran AJ, Elder DE et al. Histopathologic diagnosis of dysplastic nevi: Concordance among pathologists convened by the World Health Organization Melanoma Programme. Hum Pathol 1991;22:313.
177. Piepkorn MW, Barnhill RL, Cannon-Albright LA et al. A multiobserver, population-based analysis of histologic dysplasia in melanocytic nevi. J Am Acad Dermatol 1994;30:707.
178. Weinstock MA. Dysplastic nevi revisited. J Am Acad Dermatol 1994; 30:807.
179. Holly EA, Kelly JW, Shpall SN, Chiu S-H: Number of melanocytic nevi as a risk factor for malignant melanoma. J Am Acad Dermatol 1987;17:459.
180. Ford D, Bliss JM, Swerdlow AJ et al. Risk of cutaneous melanoma associated with a family history of the disease. Int J Cancer 1995;62: 377.
181. Carey WP Jr, Thompson CJ, Synnestvedt M et al. Dysplastic nevi as a melanoma risk factor in patients with familial melanoma. Cancer 1994;74:3118.
182. Greene M, Clark WH Jr, Tucker MA et al. High risk of malignant melanoma in melanoma-prone families with dysplastic nevi. Ann Intern Med 1985;102:458.
183. Halpern AC, Guerry D, Elder DE et al. A cohort study of melanoma in patients with dysplastic nevi. J Invest Dermatol 1993;100:346S.
184. Swerdlow AJ, English J, MacKie RM et al. Benign melanocytic naevi as a risk factor for malignant melanoma. Brit Med J 1986;292:1555.
185. Nordlund JJ, Kirkwood J, Forget BM et al. Demographic study of clinically atypical (dysplastic) nevi in patients with melanoma and comparison subjects. Cancer Res 1985;45:1855.
186. Roush GC, Nordlund JJ, Forget B et al. Independence of dysplastic nevi from total nevi in determining risk for nonfamilial melanoma. Prev Med 1988;17:273.
187. Halpern AC, Guerry D IV, Elder DE et al. Dysplastic nevi as risk markers of sporadic (non-familial) melanoma: A case-control study. Arch Dermatol 1991;127:995.
188. Garbe C, Büttner P, Weiss J et al. Risk factors for developing cutaneous melanoma and criteria for identifying persons at risk: Multicenter case-control study of the Central Malignant Melanoma Registry of the German Dermatological Society. J Invest Dermatol 1994;102:695.
189. Schneider JS, Moore DH II, Sagebiel RW. Risk factors for melanoma incidence in prospective follow-up: The importance of atypical (dysplastic) nevi. Arch Dermatol 1994;130:1002.
190. Marghoob AA, Kopf AW, Rigel DS et al. Risk of cutaneous malignant melanoma in patients with "classic" atypical-mole syndrome: A case-control study. Arch Dermatol 1994;130:993.
191. Augustsson A, Stierner U, Rosdahl I, Suurküla M. Common and dysplastic naevi as risk factors for cutaneous malignant melanoma in a Swedish population. Acta Derm Venereol (Stockh) 1991;71:518.
192. Rhodes AR, Harrist TJ, Day CL et al. Dysplastic melanocytic nevi in histologic association with 234 primary cutaneous melanomas. J Am Acad Dermatol 1983;9:563.
193. Black WC. Residual dysplastic and other nevi in superficial spreading melanoma. Cancer 1988;62:163.
194. Takahashi H, Strutton GM, Parsons PG. Determination of proliferating fractions in malignant melanomas by anti-PCNA/cyclin monoclonal antibody. Histopathology 1991;18:221.
195. Urso C, Bondi R, Balzi M. Cell kinetics of melanocytes in common and dysplastic nevi and in primary and metastatic cutaneous melanoma. Pathol Res Pract 1992;323:329.
196. Rhodes AR, Seki Y, Fitzpatrick TB, Stern RS. Melanosomal alterations in dysplastic melanocytic nevi: A quantitative, ultrastructrual investigation. Cancer 1988;61:358.
197. Jimbow K, Horikoshi T, Takahashi H et al. Fine structural and immunohistochemical properties of dysplastic melanocytic nevi: Comparison with malignant melanoma. J Invest Dermatol 1989;92:304S.
198. Elder DE, Rodeck U, Thurin J et al. Antigenic profile of tumor progression stages in human melanocytic nevi and melanomas. Cancer Res 1989;49:5091.
199. Smoller BR, McNutt NS, Hsu A. HMB-45 staining of dysplastic nevi: Support for a spectrum of progression toward melanoma. Am J Surg Pathol 1989;13:680.
200. Fogt F, Vortmeyer AO, Tahan SR. Nucleolar organizer regions (AgNOR) and Ki-67 reactivity in cutaneous melanocytic lesions. Am J Dermatopathol 1995;17:12.
201. Yamada K, Salopek T, Jimbow K, Ito S. An extremely high content of pheomelanin in dysplastic nevi. J Invest Dermatol 1989;92:544a.
202. Masri GD, Clark WH Jr, Guerry D IV et al. Screening and surveillance of patients at high risk for malignant melanoma results in detection of earlier disease. J Am Acad Dermatol 1990;22:1042.
203. Kopf AW, Morrill SD, Silberberg I. Broad spectrum of leukoderma acquisitum centrifugum. Arch Dermatol 1965;92:14.
204. Berman A. Halo nevus with exceptional clinical features. Arch Dermatol 1978;114:1081.
205. Brownstein MH. Halo nevi without dermal infiltrate. J Invest Dermatol 1978;114:1718.
206. Happle R, Echternacht K, Schotola I. Halonaevus ohne halo. Hautarzt 1975;26:44.
207. Nicholls DSH, Mason GH. Halo dermatitis around a melanocytic nevus: Meyerson's naevus. Br J Dermatol 1988;118:125.
208. Pariser RJ. "Nevocentric" erythema multiforme. J Am Acad Dermatol 1994;31:491.
209. Penneys NS, Mayoral F, Barnhill R et al. Delineation of nevus cell nests in inflammatory infiltrates by immunohistochemical staining for the presence of S-100 protein. J Cutan Pathol 1985;12:28.
210. Swanson JL Wayte DM, Helwig EB. Ultrastructure of halo nevi. J Invest Dermatol 1968;50:434.
211. Cashimoto K. A case of halo nevus with effete melanocytes. Acta Derm Venereol (Stockh) 1975;55:87.
212. Kornberg R, Ackerman AB. Pseudomelanoma: Recurrent melanocytic nevus following partial surgical removal. Arch Dermatol 1975;111:1588.
213. Park HK, Leonard DM, Arrington JH III et al. Recurrent melanocytic nevi: Clinical and histologic review of 175 cases. J Am Acad Dermatol 1987;17:285.
214. Goldenhersh MA, Scheflan M, Zeligovsky A. Recurrent melanocytic nevi after Solcoderm therapy: A new cause of pseudomelanoma. J Am Acad Dermatol 1992;27:1012.
215. Herlyn M. Molecular and cellular biology of melanoma. Austin/Georgetown: R. G. Landes Company, 1993.
216. Clark WH Jr, From L, Bernardino EA, Mihm MC Jr. The histogenesis and biologic behavior of primary human malignant melanomas of the skin. Cancer Res 1969;29:705.
217. Clark WH Jr. A classification of malignant melanoma in man correlated with histogenesis and biologic behavior. In: Montagna W, Hu F, eds. Advances in biology of skin. Vol 8. The pigmentary system. New York: Pergamon Press, 1966;621.
218. McGovern VJ. The classification of melanoma and its histologic reporting. Pathology 1970;2:85.
219. Clark WH Jr, Elder DE, Van Horn M. The biologic forms of malignant melanoma. Hum Pathol 1986;5:443.
220. McGovern VJ, Mihm MC Jr, Bailly C et al. The classification of malignant melanoma and its histologic reporting. Cancer 1973;32:1446.
221. Ackerman AB, David KM. A unifying concept of malignant melanoma. Hum Pathol 1986;17:438.
222. Flotte TJ, Mihm MC Jr. Melanoma: The art versus the science of dermatopathology. Hum Pathol 1986;17:441.
223. Rigel DS, Friedman RJ. The rationale of the ABCDs of early melanoma. J Am Acad Dermatol 1993;29:1060.
224. Elder DE, Murphy GF. Malignant tumors: Melanomas and related lesions. In: Elder DE, Murphy GF, eds. Melanocytic tumors of the skin. Washington, DC, Armed Forces Institute of Pathology, 1991;103.
225. Elder DE, Guerry D IV, Epstein MN et al. Invasive malignant melanomas lacking competence for metastasis. Am J Dermatopathol 1984;6:55.
226. Cook MG, Clarke TJ, Humphreys S et al. The evaluation of diagnostic and prognostic criteria and the terminology of thin cutaneous malignant melanoma. Histopathology, in press, 1996.
227. Sagebiel RW. Histopathology of borderline and early malignant melanomas. Am J Surg Pathol 1979;3:543.
228. Dubreuilh MW. De la melanose circonscrite precancereuse. Ann Dermatol Syphiligr 1912;3:129.
229. Steiner A, Konrad K, Pehamberger H et al. Verrucous malignant melanoma. Arch Dermatol 1988;124:1534.
230. Price NM, Rywlin AM, Ackerman AB. Histologic criteria for the diagnosis of superficial spreading malignant melanoma. Cancer 1976; 38:2434.
231. Clark WH Jr, Ainsworth AM, Bernardino EA et al. The developmental biology of malignant melanomas. Semin Oncol 1975;2:83.
232. Guldhammer B, Norgaard T. The differential diagnosis of ontraepidermal malignant lesions using immunohistochemistry. Am J Dermatopathol 1986;8:295.

233. Clark WH Jr, Mihm MC Jr. Lentigo maligna and lentigo-maligna melanoma. Am J Pathol 1969;55:39.
234. Paver K, Stewart M, Kossard S et al. Amelanotic lentigo maligna. Australas J Dermatol 1981;22:106.
235. Weinstock MA, Sober AJ. The risk of progression of lentigo maligna to lentigo maligna melanoma. Br J Dermatol 1987;116:303.
236. Michalik EE, Fitzpatrick TB, Sober AJ. Rapid progress of lentigo maligna to deeply invasive lentigo maligna melanoma. Arch Dermatol 1983;119:831.
237. McGovern VJ, Mihm MC Jr, Bailly C et al. The classification of malignant melanoma and its histologic reporting. Cancer 1973;32:1446.
238. Koh HK, Michalik E, Sober AJ et al. Lentigo maligna melanoma has no better prognosis than other types of melanoma. J Clin Oncol 1984; 2:994.
239. Cramer SF, Kiehn CL. Sequential histologic study of evolving lentigo maligna melanoma. Arch Pathol 1982;106:121.
240. Mishima Y, Matsunaka M. Pagetoid premalignant melanosis and melanoma: Differentiation from Hutchinson's melanotic freckle. J Invest Dermatol 1975;65:434.
241. Anton-Lamprecht I, Tilgen W. Zur ultrastruktur der melanotischen präcancerose. Arch Dermatol Forsch 1972;244:264.
242. Arrington JH III, Reed RJ, Ichinose H, Krementz ET. Plantar lentiginous melanoma: A distinctive variant of human cutaneous malignant melanoma. Am J Surg Pathol 1977;1:131.
243. McGovern VJ, Cochran AJ, Van der Esch EP et al. The classification of malignant melanoma, its histological reporting and registration: A revison of the 1972 Sydney classification. Pathology 1986;18:12.
244. Elder DE. Skin cancer: Melanoma and other specific nonmelanoma skin cancers. Cancer 1995;75:245.
245. Coleman WP III, Loria PR, Reed RJ et al. Acral lentiginous melanoma. Arch Dermatol 1980;116:773.
246. Paladugu RR, Winberg CD, Yonemoto RH. Acral lentiginous melanoma: A clinicopathologic study of 36 patients. Cancer 1983;52: 161.
247. Rapini RP, Golitz LE, Greer RO et al. Primary malignant melanoma of the oral cavity: A review of 177 cases. Cancer 1985;55:1543.
248. Mesara BW, Burton WD. Primary malignant melanoma of the upper respiratory tract. Cancer 1968;21:217.
249. Norris HJ, Taylor HB. Melanomas of the vagina. Am J Clin Pathol 1966;46:420.
250. Wanebo HJ, Woodruff JM, Farr GH et al. Anorectal melanoma. Cancer 1981;47:1891.
251. Nakhleh RE, Wick MR, Rocamora A et al. Morphologic diversity in malignant melanomas. Am J Clin Pathol 1990;93:731.
252. Lucas DR, Tazelaar HD, Unni KK et al. Osteogenic melanoma: A rare variant of malignant melanoma. Am J Surg Pathol 1993;17:400.
253. Clark WH Jr, Elder DE, Guerry D IV et al. Model predicting survival in stage I melanoma based on tumor progression. J Natl Cancer Inst 1989;81:1893.
254. Heenan PJ, Holman CD. Nodular malignant melanoma: A distinct entity or a common end stage? Am J Dermatopathol 1982;4:477.
255. Kornstein MJ, Brooks JS, Elder DE. Immunoperoxidase localization of lymphocyte subsets in the host response to melanoma and nevi. Cancer Res 1983;43:2749.
256. Spagnoli GC, Schaefer C, Willimann TE et al. Peptide-specific CTL in tumor-infiltrating lymphocytes from metastatic melanomas expressing MART-I/Melan-A, gp100 and tyrosinase genes: A study in an unselected group of HLA-A2.1-positive patients. Int J Cancer. 1995;64:309.
257. Stolz W, Schmoeckel C, Welkovich B, Braun-Falco O. Semiquantitative analysis of histologic criteria in thin malignant melanomas. J Am Acad Dermatol 1989;20:1115.
258. Azar HA, Espinoza CG, Richman AV et al. "Undifferentiated" large cell malignancies: An ultrastructural and immunocytochemical study. Hum Pathol 1982;13:323.
259. DeLellis RA, Dayal Y. The role of immunohistochemistry in the diagnosis of poorly differentiated malignant neoplasms. Semin Oncol 1987;14:173.
260. Thomson W, MacKie RM. Comparison of five antimelanoma antibodies for identification of melanocytic cells on tissue sections in routine dermatopathology. J Am Acad Dermatol 1989;21:1280.
261. Nakajima T, Watanabe S, Sato Y et al. Immunohistochemical demonstration of S-100 protein in malignant melanoma and pigmented nevus, and its diagnostic application. Cancer 1982;50:912.
262. Drier JK, Swanson PE, Cherwitz DL, Wick MR. S-100 protein immunoreactivity in poorly differentiated carcinomas: Immunohistochemical comparison with malignant melanoma. Arch Pathol Lab Med 1987;111:447.
263. Zarbo RJ, Gown AM, Nagle RB et al. Anomalous cytokeratin expression in malignant melanoma: One- and two-dimensional Western blot analysis and immunohistochemical survey of 100 melanomas. Mod Pathol 1990;3:494.
264. Ben-Izhak O, Stark P, Levy R et al. Epithelial markers in malignant melanoma: A study of primary lesions and their metastases. Am J Dermatopathol 1994;16:241.
265. Drier JK, Swanson PE, Cherwitz DL et al. S-100 protein immunoreactivity in poorly differentiated carcinoma. Arch Pathol 1987;111: 447.
266. Kurtin PJ, DiCaudo DJ, Habermann TM et al. Primary cutaneous large cell lymphomas: Morphologic, immunophenotypic, and clinical features of 20 cases. Am J Surg Pathol 1994;18:1183.
267. Argenyi ZB, Cain C, Bromley C et al. S-100 protein-negative malignant melanoma: Fact or fiction? A light microscopic and immunohistochemical study. Am J Dermatopathol 1994;16:233.
268. Wick MR, Swanson PE, Rocamora A. Recognition of malignant melanoma by monoclonal antibody HMB-45. J Cutan Pathol 1988;15: 201.
269. Conley J, Lattes R, Orr W. Desmoplastic malignant melanoma. Cancer 1971;28:914.
270. Labrecque PG, Hu CH, Winkelmann RK. On the nature of desmoplastic melanoma. Cancer 1976;38:1205.
271. Arrington JR III, Reed RJ, Ichinose H et al. Plantar lentiginous melanoma. Am J Surg Pathol 1977;1:131.
272. Frolow GR, Shapiro L, Brownstein MH. Desmoplastic malignant melanoma. Arch Dermatol 1975;111:753.
273. Reiman HM, Goellner JR, Woods JE et al. Desmoplastic melanoma of the head and neck. Cancer 1987;60:2269.
274. Jain S, Allen PW. Desmoplastic malignant melanoma and its variants: A study of 45 cases. Am J Surg Pathol 1989;13:358.
275. Baer S, Raymond AK, Schultz D et al. Desmoplasia and neurotropism as prognostic variables in survival outcome for malignant melanoma. Cancer 1995;76:2242.
276. Reed RJ, Leonard DD. Neurotropic melanoma: A variant of desmoplastic melanoma. Am J Surg Pathol 1979;3:301.
277. Carlson JA, Dickersin GR, Sober AJ, Barnhill RL. Desmoplastic neurotropic melanoma: A clinicopathologic analysis of 28 cases. Cancer 1995;75:478.
278. Smithers BM, McLeod GR, Little JH. Desmoplastic, neural transforming and neurotropic melanoma: A review of 45 cases. Aust N Z J Surg 1990;60:967.
279. Kiene P, Petres-Dunsche C, Fölster-Holst R. Pigmented pedunculated malignant melanoma: A rare variant of nodular melanoma. Br J Dermatol 1995;133:300.
280. Rosenberg L, Golstein J, Ben-Yakar Y et al. The pedunculated malignant melanoma. J Dermatol Surg Oncol 1981;7:123.
281. Clark WH Jr. A classification of malignant melanoma in man correlated with histogenesis and biologic behavior. In: Montagna W, Hu F, eds. Advances in the biology of the skin. Vol. VIII. New York: Pergamon Press, 1967;621.
282. Blessing K, Evans AT, Al-Nafussi A. Verrucous naevoid and keratotic malignant melanoma: A clinico-pathological study of 20 cases. Histopathology 1993;23:453.
283. Steiner A, Konrad K, Pehamberger H, Wolff K. Verrucous malignant melanoma. Arch Dermatol 1988;124:1534.
284. Kamino H, Tam ST, Alvarez L. Malignant melanoma with pseudocarcinomatous hyperplasia—an entity that can simulate squamous cell carcinoma: A light-microscopic and immunohistochemical study of four cases. Am J Dermatopathol 1990;12:446.
285. Mowat A, Reid R, MacKie R. Balloon cell metastatic melanoma: An important differential in the diagnosis of clear cell tumours. Histopathology 1994;24:469.
286. Livolsi VA, Brooks JJ, Soslow R et al. Signet cell melanocytic lesions. Mod Pathol 1992;5:515.
287. Sheibani K, Battifora H. Signet-ring cell melanoma: A rare morphologic variant of malignant melanoma. Am J Surg Pathol 1988;12:28.
288. Selby WL, Nance KV, Park HK. CEA immunoreactivity in metastatic malignant melanoma. Mod Pathol 1992;5:415.
289. Sanders DSA, Evans AT, Allen CA et al. Classification of CEA-re-

lated positivity in primary and metastatic malignant melanoma. J Pathol 1994;172:343.
290. Bhuta S, Mirra JM, Cochran AJ. Myxoid malignant melanoma: A previously undescribed histologic pattern noted in metastatic lesions and a report of four cases. Am J Surg Pathol 1986;10:203.
291. Prieto VG, Kanik A, Salob S, McNutt NS. Primary cutaneous myxoid melanoma: Immunohistologic clues to a difficult diagnosis. J Am Acad Dermatol 1994;30:335.
292. Murphy G, Lopansri S, Mihm MC Jr. Clincopathologic type of malignant melanoma. Relevance to biologic behavior and diagnostic surgical approach. J Dermatol Surg Oncol 1985;11:674.
293. Schmoeckel C, Castro CE, Braun-Falco O. Nevoid malignant melanoma. Arch Dermatol Res 1985;277:362.
294. Heenan PJ, Armstrong BK, English DR, Holman CDJ. Pathological and epidemiological variants of cutaneous malignant melanoma. In: Elder DE, ed. Pigment cell. Vol. 8. Basel: Karger, 1987;107.
295. Tajima Y, Nakahima T, Sugano I et al. Malignant melanoma within an intradermal nevus. Am J Dermatopathol 1994;16:301.
296. Slingluff CL Jr, Vollmer RT, Seigler HF. Multiple primary melanoma: Incidence and risk factors in 283 patients. Surgery 1993;113: 330.
297. Abernethy JL, Soyer HP, Kerl H et al. Epidermotropic metastatic malignant melanoma simulating melanoma in situ: A report of 10 examples from two patients. Am J Surg Pathol 1994;18:1140.
298. Skov-Jensen T, Hastrup J, Lambrethsen E. Malignant melanoma in children. Cancer 1966;19:620.
299. Barnhill RLW, Flotte TJ, Fleischli M, Perez-Atayde A. Cutaneous melanoma and atypical Spitz tumors in childhood. Cancer 1995;76: 1833.
300. Ironside P, Pitt TTE, Rank BK. Malignant melanoma: Some aspects of pathology and prognosis. Aust N Z Surg 1977;47:70.
301. Rampen FHJ, Van der Esch EP. Biopsy and survival of malignant melanoma. J Am Acad Dermatol 1985;12:385.
302. Epstein E, Bragg K, Linden G. Biopsy and prognosis of malignant melanoma. JAMA 1969;208:1369.
303. Lederman JS, Sober AJ. Does biopsy type influence survival in clinical stage I cutaneous melanoma? J Am Acad Dermatol 1985;13:983.
304. Harris MN, Gumport SL. Biopsy technique for malignant melanoma. J Dermatol Surg Oncol 1975;1:24.
305. Beahrs OH, Henson DE, Hutter RVP, Kennedy BJ. Handbook for staging of cancer. Philadelphia: Lippincott, 1993;155.
306. Balch CM, Cascinelli N, Drzewiecki KT et al. A comparison of prognostic factors worldwide. In: Balch CM, Houghton AN, Milton GW et al., eds. Cutaneous melanoma. 2nd ed. Philadelphia: Lippincott, 1985; 188.
307. Kelly JW, Sagebiel RW, Clyman S, Blois MS. Thin level IV malignant melanoma: A subset in which level is the major prognostic indicator. Ann Surg 1985;202:98.
308. Buttner P, Garbe C, Bertz J et al. Primary cutaneous melanoma: Optimized cutoff points of tumor thickness and importance of Clark's level for prognostic classification. Cancer 1995;75:2499.
309. Breslow A. Thickness, cross-sectional areas and depth of invasion in the prognosis of cutaneous melanoma. Ann Surg 1970;172:902.
310. Breslow A. Prognostic factors in the treatment of cutaneous melanoma. J Cutan Pathol 1979;6:208.
311. Barr RJ. The many faces of completely regressed primary melanoma. In: LeBoit, PE. Malignant melanoma and melanocytic lesions. Philadelphia: Hanley & Belfus, 1994;359.
312. Jonk A, Kroon BBR, Rümke P et al. Lymph node metastasis from melanoma with an unknown primary site. Br J Surg 1990;77:665.
313. Elder DE, Guerry D IV, Van Horn M et al. The role of lymph node dissection for clinical stage I malignant melanoma of intermediate thickness (1.51–3.99 mm). Cancer 1985;56:413.
314. Clemente CG, Mihm MC Jr, Bufalino R et al. Prognostic value of tumor-infiltrating lymphocytes in the vertical growth phase of stage I cutaneous melanoma. Cancer 1996 (in press).
315. Cochran AJ. Histology and prognosis in malignant melanoma. J Pathol 1969;97:459.
316. Schmoeckel C, Braun-Falco O. The prognostic index in malignant melanoma. Arch Dermatol 1978;114:871.
317. Balch CM, Wilkerson JA, Murad TM et al. The prognostic significance of ulceration of cutaneous melanoma. Cancer 1980;45:3012.
318. MacKie RM, Aitchison T, Sirel JM et al. Prognostic models for subgroups of melanoma patients from the Scottish Melanoma Group database 1979–86, and their subsequent validation. Br J Cancer 1996; 71:173.
319. Shaw HM, McGovern VJ, Milton GW et al. Malignant melanoma: Influence of site of lesion and age of patient in the female superiority in survival. Cancer 1980;46:2731.
320. Larsen TE, Grude TH. A retrospective histological study of 669 cases of primary cutaneous malignant melanoma in clinical stage I. Acta Pathol Microbiol Scand [A] 1979;87:131.
321. Ramsay JA, From L, Iscoe NA, Kahn HJ. MIB-1 proliferative activity is a significant prognostic factor in primary thick cutaneous melanomas. J Invest Dermatol 1995;105:22.
322. Busam KJ, Berwick M, Blessing K et al. Tumor vascularity is not a prognostic factor for malignant melanoma of the skin. Am J Pathol 1995;147:1049.
323. Schuchter LM, Schultz DJ, Synnestvedt M et al. A simple prognostic model predicting ten year survival in patients with stage I melanoma JAMA, 1996 (in press).
324. Balch CM, Murad TM, Soong SJ et al. Tumor thickness as a guide to surgical management of clinical stage I melanoma patients. Cancer 1979;43:883.
325. Veronesi U, Cascinelli N, Adamus J et al. Thin stage I primary cutaneous malignant melanoma. N Engl J Med 1988;318:1159.
326. Elder DE, Guerry D IV, Heiberger RM et al. Optimal resection margin for cutaneous malignant melanoma. Plast Reconst Surg 1983;71: 66.
327. Sim FH, Taylor WF, Ivins JC et al. A prospective randomized study of the efficacy of routine elective lymphadenectomy in management of malignant melanoma: Preliminary results. Cancer 1978;41:948.
328. Veronesi U, Adamus J, Bandiera DC et al. Inefficacy of immediate node dissection in stage I melanoma of the limbs. N Engl J Med 1977; 297:627.
329. Day CL Jr, Sober AJ, Lew RA et al. Malignant melanoma patients with positive nodes and relatively good prognosis. Cancer 1981;47: 955.
330. Buzaid AC, Tinoco LA, Jendiroba D et al. Prognostic value of size of lymph node metastases in patients with cutaneous melanoma. J Clin Oncol 1995;13:2361.
331. Mihm MC Jr, Clemente CG, Cascinelli N. Tumor infiltrating lymphocytes in lymph node melanoma metastases: A histopathologic prognostic indicator and an expression of local immune response. Lab Invest 1996;74:43.
332. Kwittken J, Negri L. Malignant blue nevus. Arch Dermatol 1966;94: 64.
333. Merkow LP, Burt RC, Hayeslip DW et al. A cellular and malignant blue nevus. Cancer 1969;24:888.
334. Hernandez FJ. Malignant blue nevus. Arch Dermatol 1973;107:741.
335. Goldenhersh MA, Savin RC, Barnhill RL et al. Malignant blue nevus. J Am Acad Dermatol 1988;19:712.
336. Rogers GS, Kopf AW, Rigel DS et al. Hazard-rate analysis in stage I malignant melanoma. Arch Dermatol 1986;122:999.
337. Raderman O, Giles S, Rothem AJ et al. Late metastases (beyond ten years) of cutaneous malignant melanoma. J Am Acad Dermatol 1986; 15:374.
338. Barth A, Wanek LA, Morton DL. Prognostic factors in 1,521 melanoma patients with distant metastases. J Am Coll Surgeons 1995; 181:A193.
339. Baab GH, McBride CM. Malignant melanoma: The patient with an unknown site of primary origin. Arch Surg 1975;110:896.
340. Smith JL, Stehlin JS Jr. Spontaneous regression of primary malignant melanomas with regional metastases. Cancer 1965;18:1399.
341. Pellegrini AE. Regressed primary malignant melanoma with regional metastases. J Dermatol 1980;116:585.
342. Kornberg R, Harris M, Ackerman AB. Epidermotropically metastatic malignant melanoma. Arch Dermatol 1978;114:67.
343. Abernethy JL, Soyer HP, Kerl H et al. Epidermotropic metastatic malignant melanoma simulating melanoma in situ: A report of 10 examples from two patients. Am J Dermatopathol 1994;18:1140.
344. Konrad K, Wolff K. Pathogenesis of diffuse melanosis secondary to malignant melanoma. Br J Dermatol 1974;91:635.
345. Adrian RM, Murphy GF, Sato S et al. Diffuse melanosis secondary to metastatic malignant melanoma. J Am Acad Dermatol 1981;5:308.

Lever's Histopathology of the Skin, eighth edition,
edited by David Elder et al. Lippincott–
Raven Publishers, Philadelphia © 1997.

CHAPTER 30

Tumors and Cysts of the Epidermis

Nigel Kirkham

CLASSIFICATION OF TUMORS OF THE EPIDERMIS

Epidermal tumors can be divided into tumors of the surface epidermis and tumors of the epidermal appendages. In each of the two classes, benign and malignant tumors occur.

Benign tumors in general are characterized by (1) a symmetrical architecture and a circumscribed profile; (2) a tendency to differentiate along organized tissue lines; (3) uniformity in the appearance of the tumor cell nuclei; (4) architectural order in the arrangement of the tumor cell nuclei; (5) restraint in the rate of growth; and (6) absence of metastases.

Malignant tumors, in contrast, are characterized by (1) a less symmetrical architecture and a poorly circumscribed profile; (2) a variable but often poorly differentiated phenotype; (3) atypicality in the appearance of the tumor cell nuclei, which show pleomorphism, that is, great variability in size and shape, and anaplasia, that is, hyperplasia and hyperchromasia; (4) architectural disorder in the arrangement of the tumor cell nuclei with loss of polarity; (5) rapid growth with the presence of mitoses, including atypical mitoses; and (6) potentiality to give rise to metastases.

Of the criteria of malignancy just cited, only the potentiality to give rise to metastases is decisive evidence for the malignancy of a tumor. For metastases to form, the tumor cells must possess a degree of autonomy that nonmalignant cells do not have. This autonomy enables malignant tumor cells to induce foreign tissue to furnish the necessary stroma in which they can multiply.

In addition to malignant tumors, one finds in the surface epidermis so-called premalignant tumors, better regarded as tumors located largely in situ. Although cytologically malignant, they are biologically still benign.

The tumors of the surface epidermis have been classified by the World Health Organization as follows:[1]

N. Kirkham: Department of Pathology, Royal Sussex County Hospital, Brighton, United Kingdom

Epithelial Tumors

Benign

- Epidermal
  - Epidermal nevus
  - Seborrhoeic keratosis
    - Irritated
    - Adenoid
    - Plane
    - With an intraepidermal epithelioma pattern
    - Melanoacanthoma
    - Inverted follicular keratosis
    - Benign squamous keratosis
  - Clear cell acanthoma
    - (also nevus comedonicus, epidermolytic acanthoma, acantholytic acanthoma, oral white sponge nevus)
  - Fibroepithelial polyp
  - Warty dyskeratoma
  - Actinic keratosis
    - (also precancerous leukoplakia, oral florid papillomatosis, Bowen's disease, erythroplasia of Queyrat)
  - Keratoacanthoma
    - Giant keratoacanthoma
    - Keratoacanthoma centrifugum marginatum
    - Subungual keratoacanthoma
    - Multiple keratoacanthomas
    - Multiple eruptive keratoacanthomas
  - Benign lichenoid keratosis

Malignant

- Squamous cell carcinoma
  - Spindle cell
  - Acantholytic
  - Verrucous
  - Horn forming
  - Lymphoepithelial
- Basal cell carcinoma
  - Multifocal superficial (superficial multicentric)
  - Nodular (solid, adenoid cystic)
  - Infiltrating

Nonsclerosing
Sclerosing (desmoplastic morpheic)
Fibroepithelial
Basal cell carcinoma with adnexal differentiation
Follicular
Eccrine
Basosquamous carcinoma
Keratotic basal cell carcinoma
Pigmented basal cell carcinoma
Basal cell carcinoma in basal cell nevus syndrome
Micronodular basal cell carcinoma

This chapter also includes details on cysts that are classified as follows:

Follicular cysts
Infundibular cyst
Trichilemmal cyst
Steatocystoma multiplex
Dermoid cyst
Eruptive vellus hair cyst
Milia
Bronchogenic and thyroglossal duct cysts
Cutaneous ciliated cyst
Median raphe cyst of the penis

LINEAR EPIDERMAL NEVUS

Linear epidermal nevi, or verrucous nevi, may be either localized or systematized.

In the *localized type,* which is present usually but not invariably at birth, only one linear lesion is present. It consists of closely set, papillomatous, hyperkeratotic papules. It may be located anywhere—on the head, trunk, or extremities. Being located on only one side of the patient, it is often referred to as *nevus unius lateris.* In its configuration, the localized type of linear epidermal nevus resembles the inflammatory linear verrucous epidermal nevus (ILVEN), but the latter differs clinically by the presence of erythema and pruritus and histologically by the presence of inflammation and parakeratosis (see Chap. 7).

In the *systematized type,* papillomatous hyperkeratotic papules in a linear configuration are present not just as one linear lesion, as in the localized type, but as many linear lesions. These linear lesions often show a parallel arrangement, particularly on the trunk. They may be limited to one side of the patient or may have a bilateral, symmetric distribution. The term *ichthyosis hystrix* is occasionally used, perhaps unnecessarily, for instances of extensive bilateral lesions.[2]

Localized and, more commonly, systematized linear epidermal nevi may be associated with skeletal deformities and central nervous system deficiencies, such as mental retardation, epilepsy, and neural deafness.[3]

The presence of a basal cell epithelioma within a linear epidermal nevus has been observed occasionally, particularly on the head in cases in which the linear epidermal nevus has been associated with either a nevus sebaceus or a syringocystadenoma papilliferum (see Chap. 31).[4] In areas other than the head, it is very rare.[5] Similarly, development of a squamous cell carcinoma has been described only rarely,[6,7] but in one instance the squamous cell carcinoma had metastasized to a regional lymph node.[8]

Histopathology. Nearly all cases of the localized type of linear epidermal nevus and some cases of the systematized type show the histologic picture of a benign papilloma.[2,9] One observes considerable hyperkeratosis, papillomatosis, and acanthosis with elongation of the rete ridges resembling seborrheic keratosis (Fig. 30-1).

Occasionally in cases of the localized type, but quite frequently in cases of the systematized type, particularly those with a widespread distribution, one observes the rather striking histologic picture referred to either as *epidermolytic hyperkeratosis*[10] or as *granular degeneration of the epidermis.*[11] It is the same process that was first recognized in all cases of bullous congenital ichthyosiform erythroderma, a disorder that is often referred to as *epidermolytic hyperkeratosis* (Chap. 6). It has since been found to occur in several other conditions as well (see Isolated and Disseminated Epidermolytic Acanthoma).

The salient histologic features of epidermolytic hyperkeratosis are (1) perinuclear vacuolization of the cells in the stratum spinosum and in the stratum granulosum; (2) peripheral to the vacuolization, irregular cellular boundaries; (3) an increased number of irregularly shaped, large keratohyaline granules; and (4) compact hyperkeratosis in the stratum corneum.[11,12]

In some instances, histologic examination of unilateral linear lesions reveals features of acantholytic dyskeratosis as seen in Darier's disease (see Chap. 6). In some patients, these linear lesions have been present since birth or infancy,[13] but in most instances they have arisen in adult life.[14] Because acantholytic

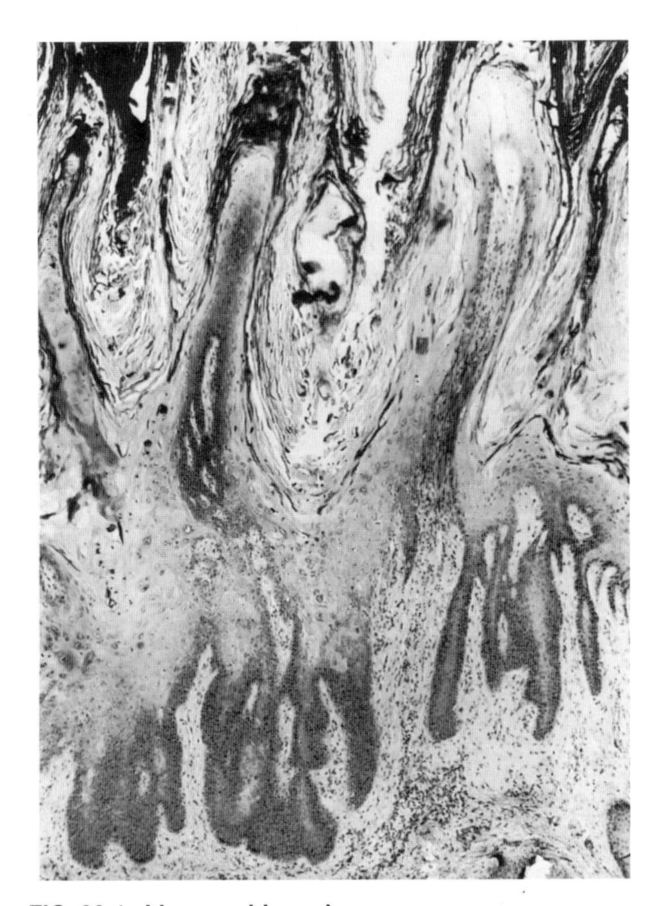

FIG. 30-1. Linear epidermal nevus
There are considerable hyperkeratosis, papillomatosis, and acanthosis with elongation of the rete ridges.

dyskeratosis is not specific for Darier's disease, the proposal has been made to designate such cases not as Darier's disease but as acantholytic dyskeratotic epidermal nevus.[14]

Differential Diagnosis. The histologic picture of a benign papilloma, as found in most cases of linear epidermal nevus, can also be seen in seborrheic keratosis, verruca vulgaris, and acanthosis nigricans. Even though these four conditions have in common hyperkeratosis and papillomatosis, they can be differentiated easily in typical cases; however, one is occasionally unable to make a diagnosis any more specific than benign papilloma. Thus, in the following three situations, clinical data are required for differentiation from linear epidermal nevus: (1) the hyperkeratotic type of seborrheic keratosis, which is characterized by the absence of basaloid cells and horn cysts and instead shows upward extension of epidermis-lined papillae; (2) old verrucae vulgares, which no longer show vacuolization of epidermal cells or columns of parakeratosis (see Chap. 26); and (3) acanthosis nigricans showing more pronounced acanthosis and greater elongation of the rete ridges than usual (see Chap. 17).

HYPERKERATOSIS OF NIPPLE AND AREOLA

Hyperkeratosis and papillomatosis of nipples and areola appear at puberty or during pregnancy and persist unchanged.

Histopathology. There are papillomatous elongations of the epidermis with hyperkeratosis and areas of keratotic plugging.[15] This condition represents a nevoid form of hyperkeratosis.[16]

NEVUS COMEDONICUS

A nevus comedonicus consists of closely set, slightly elevated papules that have in their center a dark, firm hyperkeratotic plug resembling a comedo. Nevus comedonicus, like linear epidermal nevus, usually has a linear configuration and occurs as a single lesion. In some instances, however, there are multiple bilateral linear lesions[17] or lesions that are randomly distributed rather than linear.[18] Lesions may be present on the palms or soles in addition to other areas.[19,20] Such cases may represent a combination of nevus comedonicus with a porokeratotic eccrine duct nevus (see text following).

Histopathology. Each comedo is represented by a wide, deep invagination of the epidermis filled with keratin. These invaginations resemble dilated hair follicles; in fact, as evidence that they actually represent rudimentary hair follicles, one occasionally finds in the lower portion of an invagination one or even several hair shafts.[17] One or two small sebaceous gland lobules may also be seen opening into the lower pole of invaginations.[18]

In several instances, the keratinocytes composing the follicular epithelial wall have shown the typical changes of epidermolytic hyperkeratosis (see text following),[21] indicative of a relationship of nevus comedonicus to systematized nevus verrucosus (see Chap. 31).

POROKERATOTIC ECCRINE DUCT NEVUS

Porokeratotic eccrine duct nevus may be limited to a palm[22] or to a sole[23] but may be present on both hands and feet and elsewhere.[24] It also may involve not only eccrine ducts but also involve hair follicles on the hairy parts of the body.[25]

Histopathology. In the porokeratotic eccrine duct nevus, each invagination consists of a dilated eccrine duct containing a parakeratotic plug. The absence of the granular layer at the base of the plug together with the presence of keratinocytes showing vacuolization of their cytoplasm results in a histologic picture resembling that of porokeratosis (see Chap. 6).[22–24]

ISOLATED AND DISSEMINATED EPIDERMOLYTIC ACANTHOMA

Isolated epidermolytic acanthoma, histologically characterized by the presence of "epidermolytic hyperkeratosis," does not have a characteristic clinical appearance or location. Usually it occurs as a solitary papillomatous lesion less than 1 cm in diameter.[26–28] Occasionally, several lesions are seen in a localized area.[29,30]

Disseminated epidermolytic acanthoma occurs as numerous discrete, flat, brownish papules 2 to 6 mm in diameter, resembling seborrheic keratoses. The upper trunk, especially the back, is the site of predilection.[31,32]

Histopathology. In addition to hyperkeratosis and papillomatosis, one observes pronounced epidermolytic hyperkeratosis, also referred to as *granular degeneration*, throughout the stratum malpighii, sparing only the basal layer, just as seen in linear epidermal nevi with epidermolytic changes. One observes both intracellular and intercellular edema of the epidermal cells and keratohyaline granules that are coarser than normal and extend to a greater depth in the stratum malpighii.[26]

Differential Diagnosis. Myrmecia warts, caused by human papilloma virus type 1 (HPV-1), also show perinuclear vacuolization and an abundance of keratohyaline granules, representing a type of "granular degeneration" similar to that seen in epidermolytic hyperkeratosis. However, in myrmecia warts, the keratohyaline granules are eosinophilic and coalesce in the upper layers of the epidermis to form large, homogeneous, eosinophilic "inclusion bodies." In verrucae vulgares, usually caused by HPV-2, foci of vacuolated cells and clumped basophilic keratohyaline granules may be present, but these changes are limited to the upper layers of the epidermis. In addition, both myrmecia warts and verrucae vulgares show focal parakeratosis, rather than orthokeratosis as seen in epidermolytic hyperkeratosis (see Chap. 26).

INCIDENTAL EPIDERMOLYTIC HYPERKERATOSIS

Epidermolytic hyperkeratosis is seen not only in isolated and disseminated epidermolytic hyperkeratosis (see text preceding) but also as a *regular* finding in epidermolytic hyperkeratosis, or bullous congenital ichthyosiform erythroderma (Chap. 6), and in epidermolytic keratosis palmaris et plantaris and as an *occasional* finding in linear epidermal nevus and nevus comedonicus. In addition, epidermolytic hyperkeratosis may represent an *incidental* histologic finding in many different types of lesions, largely but not exclusively tumors. It has also been observed in normal oral mucosa adjacent to lesions of squamous cell carcinoma and basal cell epithelioma.[33]

Histopathology. Epidermolytic hyperkeratosis may be seen throughout an entire lesion of solar keratosis[34] and in the entire lining of trichilemmal cyst.[35] More commonly, however, the histologic features of epidermolytic hyperkeratosis are seen as a small focus, often limited to a single epidermal rete ridge, in such diverse lesions as sebaceous hyperplasia,[36] intradermal nevus, hypertrophic scar,[37] superficial basal cell epithelioma,[38] seborrheic keratosis, the margin of a squamous cell carcinoma, lichenoid amyloidosis, and granuloma annulare.[10] In some instances, the process is limited to one or two intraepidermal sweat duct units.[37]

ISOLATED AND DISSEMINATED ACANTHOLYTIC ACANTHOMA

This condition usually occurs as a solitary papule or small nodule,[39] although there may be multiple lesions.[40,41] No characteristic clinical appearance or location exists, although multiple lesions have been seen largely in the genital region.[23,42]

Histopathology. Acantholysis is the most prominent feature. The pattern may resemble that of pemphigus vulgaris, pemphigus vegetans, pemphigus foliaceus, or benign familial pemphigus.[39] Acantholysis may be combined with dyskeratosis, in which case the histologic picture resembles that of Darier's disease as the result of the presence of corps ronds and grains.[10,40,41]

INCIDENTAL FOCAL ACANTHOLYTIC DYSKERATOSIS

Analogous to epidermolytic hyperkeratosis, acantholytic dyskeratosis is seen as a *regular* histologic feature in Darier's disease (see Chap. 6), transient acantholytic dermatosis, and warty dyskeratoma. It also is an *occasional* finding in acantholytic dyskeratotic epidermal nevus, a variant of linear epidermal nevus. In addition, again like epidermolytic hyperkeratosis, focal acantholytic dyskeratosis is observed occasionally as an *incidental* histologic finding in a variety of lesions.

Histopathology. Focal suprabasal clefts with overlying acantholytic and dyskeratotic cells, some of which have the appearance of corps ronds, have been seen as a single focus in the epidermis overlying such diverse lesions as dermatofibroma, basal cell epithelioma, melanocytic nevus, and chondrodermatitis nodularis helicis,[35] as well as in pityriasis rosea[43] and acral lentiginous malignant melanoma.[44]

ORAL WHITE SPONGE NEVUS

First described in 1935,[45] oral white sponge nevus is a benign autosomal dominant disorder that affects noncornifying stratified squamous epithelia. It may be present at birth or have its onset in infancy, childhood, or adolescence.[46] Extensive areas of the oral mucosa and sometimes the entire oral mucosa have a thickened, folded, creamy white appearance. In some instances, the rectal mucosa,[45] vagina,[47] nasal mucosa,[48] or esophagus[49] is also involved. This distribution of lesions suggests that mutations in the epithelial keratins K4 and/or K13 may be responsible: a three base-pair deletion in the helix initiation peptide of K4 has been reported in affected members of two families.[50]

The oral lesions seen in pachyonychia congenita are both clinically and histologically indistinguishable from a white sponge nevus (Chap. 6).[48]

Histopathology. The oral epithelium shows hyperplasia with much more pronounced hydropic swelling of the epithelial cells than is normal for the oral mucosa. The swelling, though extensive, is focal.[51] It extends into the rete ridges but spares the basal layer.[52] The nuclei appear smaller than normal.[46] The surface shows parakeratosis, as does the normal oral mucosa, and only rarely are there small accumulations of keratohyaline granules.[47]

Pathogenesis. On electron microscopic examination, large cytoplasmic areas of the epithelial cells appear optically empty or contain only faint granular material. Tonofilaments are limited to the perinuclear and peripheral areas. The intercellular areas show irregular dilatation, and large, irregularly shaped vacuoles are present within the cytoplasm.[53] A possibly fundamental disturbance is the presence of numerous intracellular Odland bodies or membrane-coating granules (Chap. 3), which are not extruded into the intercellular spaces.[54]

Differential Diagnosis. The histologic picture of oral white sponge nevus is identical to that seen in pachyonychia congenita (see text preceding) and to that of oral focal epithelial hyperplasia[53] and of leukoedema of the oral mucosa (see text following).

LEUKOEDEMA OF THE ORAL MUCOSA

Leukoedema of the oral mucosa is a common condition that, when pronounced, shows a clinical and histologic resemblance to oral white sponge nevus. However, leukoedema differs from white sponge nevus by being patchy rather than diffuse, by having exacerbations and remissions and adult onset, and by not being inherited.[55]

Histopathology. In leukoedema of the oral mucosa, as in oral white sponge nevus, the suprabasal epithelial cells show marked intracellular edema. The nuclei appear smaller than normal.

LINGUA GEOGRAPHICA

In geographic tongue, also referred to as superficial migratory glossitis, the dorsum of the tongue shows irregularly shaped red patches surrounded by a whitish, raised border a few millimeters wide. The patches change configuration from day to day.[56]

Histopathology. Whereas the dorsum of the tongue normally shows a granular and a horny layer, these layers are absent in the red patches of lingua geographica. Along the whitish border, the epithelium shows irregular thickening and infiltration of neutrophils. In its upper portion, the epithelium shows collections of neutrophils within the interstices of a spongelike network formed by degenerated and thinned epithelial cells.[57,58] The histologic picture thus shows Kogoj's spongiform pustules, which are indistinguishable from those seen in pustular psoriasis.

Pathogenesis. The presence of spongiform pustules generally is regarded as diagnostic of pustular psoriasis and as almost specific for it (see Chap. 8), even though it rarely occurs in other pustules, such as those caused by *Candida albicans.*[59] It has

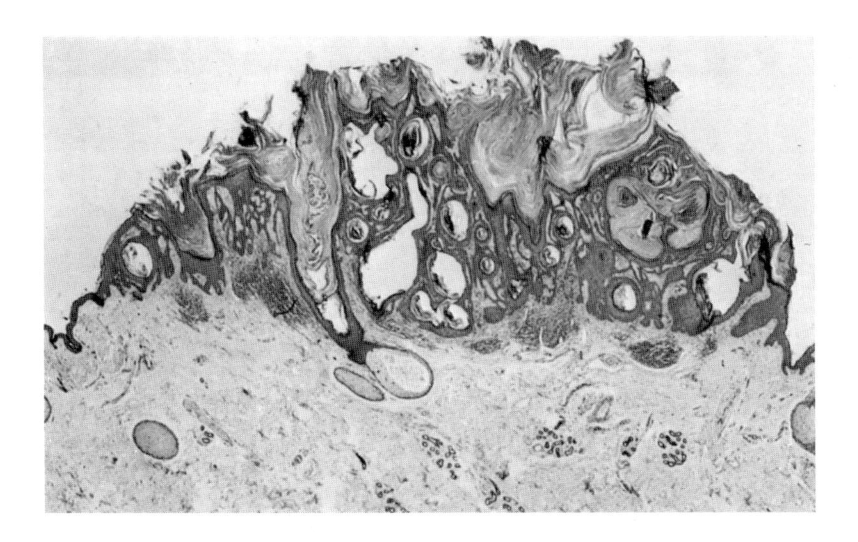

FIG. 30-2. Seborrheic keratosis, low magnification
The lower border of the tumor in general follows a straight line from the normal epidermis at one end of the tumor to the normal epidermis at the other end.

therefore been suggested that geographic tongue represents a localized form of pustular psoriasis.[60] However, even though pustular psoriasis and lingua geographica may both show annular lesions on the tongue, pustular psoriasis of the mouth generally shows clinical evidence of pustules and is usually seen also in other areas of the mouth. It is therefore best to regard lingua geographica as a separate entity.

SEBORRHEIC KERATOSIS

Seborrheic keratoses are very common lesions: sometimes single but often multiple. They occur mainly on the trunk and face but also on the extremities, with the exception of the palms and soles. Seborrheic keratoses usually do not appear before middle age. They are sharply demarcated, brownish in color, and slightly raised, so that they often look as if they are stuck on the surface of the skin. Most of them have a verrucous surface, which has a soft, friable consistency. Some, however, have a smooth surface but characteristically show keratotic plugs. Although most lesions measure only a few millimeters in diameter, a lesion may occasionally reach a size of several centimeters. Crusting and an inflammatory base are found if the lesion has been subjected to trauma. Occasionally, small seborrheic keratoses are pedunculated, especially on the neck and upper chest, and then clinically resemble soft fibromas (see Chap. 33).

Histopathology. Seborrheic keratoses show a considerable variety of histologic appearances. Six types are generally recognized: irritated, adenoid or reticulated, plane, clonal, melanoacanthoma, inverted follicular keratosis, and benign squamous keratosis (Figs. 30-2 to 30-6). Often more than one type is found in the same lesion. In addition, two clinical variants of seborrheic keratosis will be described. They are dermatosis papulosa nigra and stucco keratosis.

All types of seborrheic keratosis have in common hyperkeratosis, acanthosis, and papillomatosis. The acanthosis in most instances is due entirely to upward extension of the tumor. Thus the lower border of the tumor is even and generally lies on a straight line that may be drawn from the normal epidermis at one end of the tumor to the normal epidermis at the other end (see Fig. 30-2). Two types of cells are usually seen in the acanthotic epidermis: squamous cells and basaloid cells. The former have the appearance of squamous cells normally found in the epidermis; the basaloid cells are small and uniform in appearance and have a relatively large nucleus. In areas of slight intercellular edema, intercellular bridges can be easily recognized.[61] Thus they resemble the basal cells found normally in the basal layer of the epidermis.

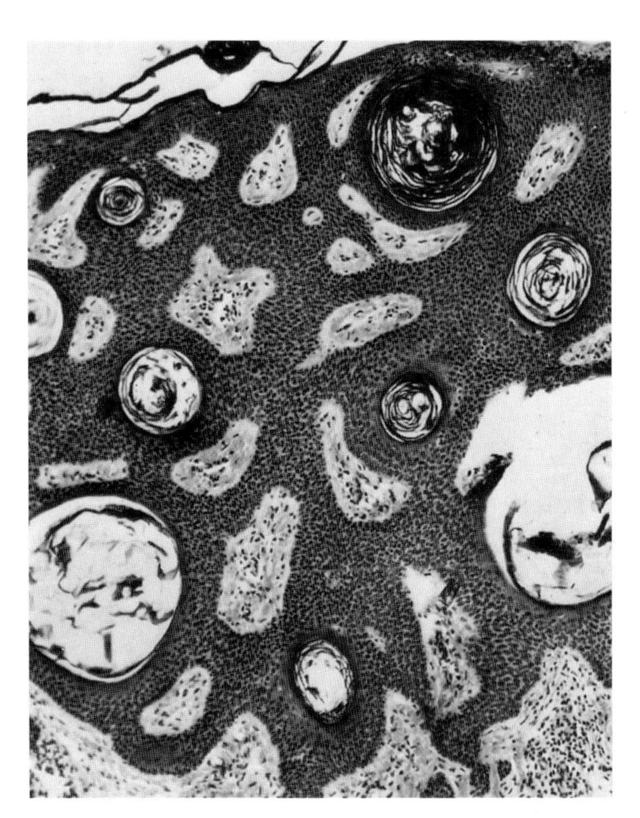

FIG. 30-3. Seborrheic keratosis, high magnification
Thick, interwoven tracts of epidermal cells compose the tumor. Most of the epidermal cells have the appearance of epidermal basal cells and are referred to as basaloid cells. Interspersed are cystic inclusions of horny material representing either horn cysts, when they form within the tumor, or pseudohorn cysts, when they consist of horny invaginations.

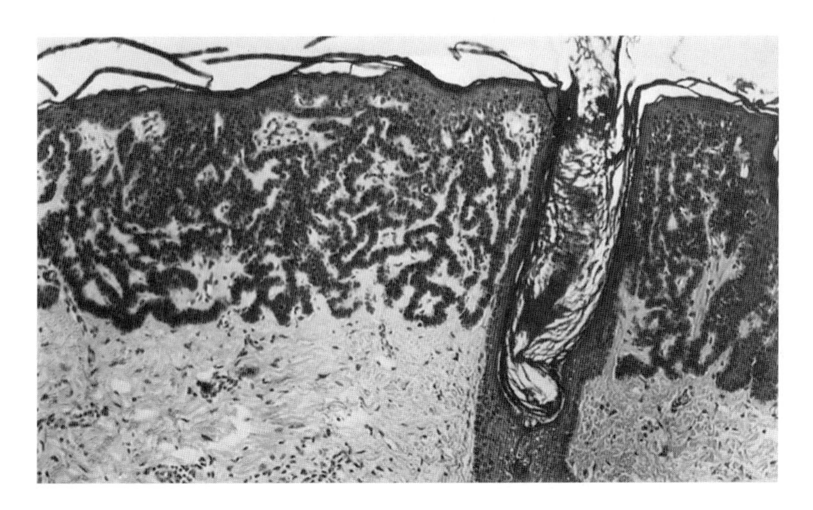

FIG. 30-4. Seborrheic keratosis
Thin interwoven tracts composed of a double row of epidermal basal cells compose the tumor. No cystic inclusions of horny material are present.

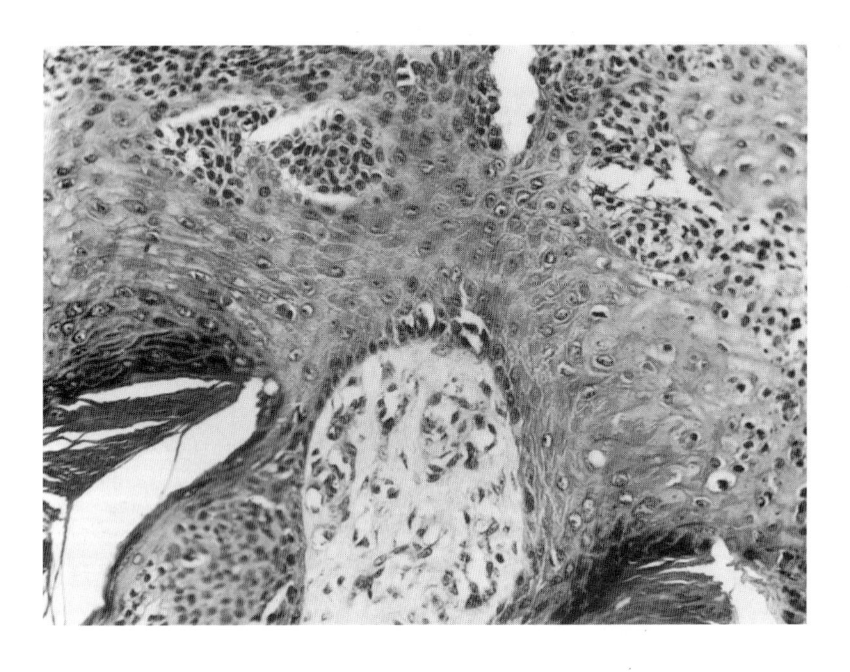

FIG. 30-5. Seborrheic keratosis
Well-defined nests of small basaloid cells are present. The nests resemble foci of basal cell epithelioma, but intercellular bridges can be recognized in some areas.

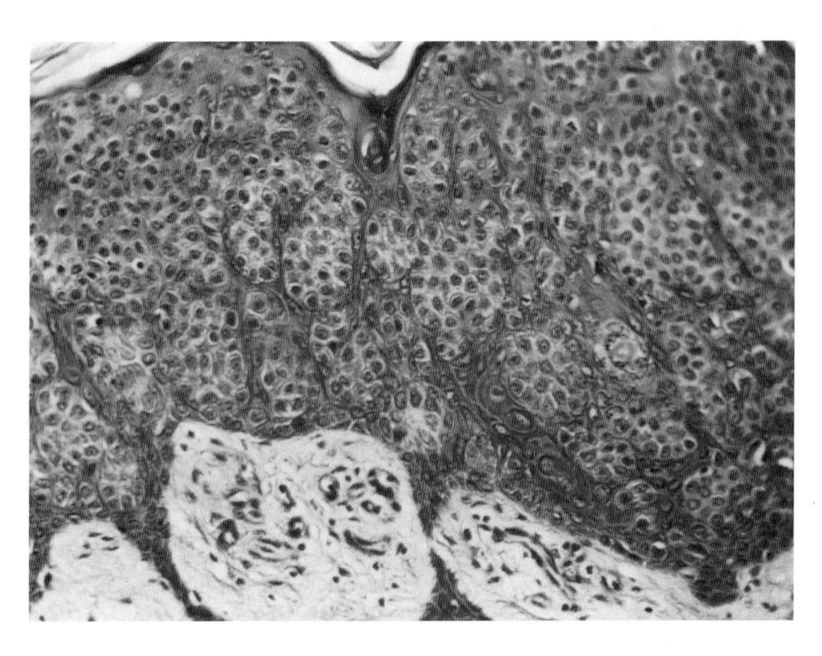

FIG. 30-6. Seborrheic keratosis
Well-defined nests of large cells with distinct intercellular bridges are present.

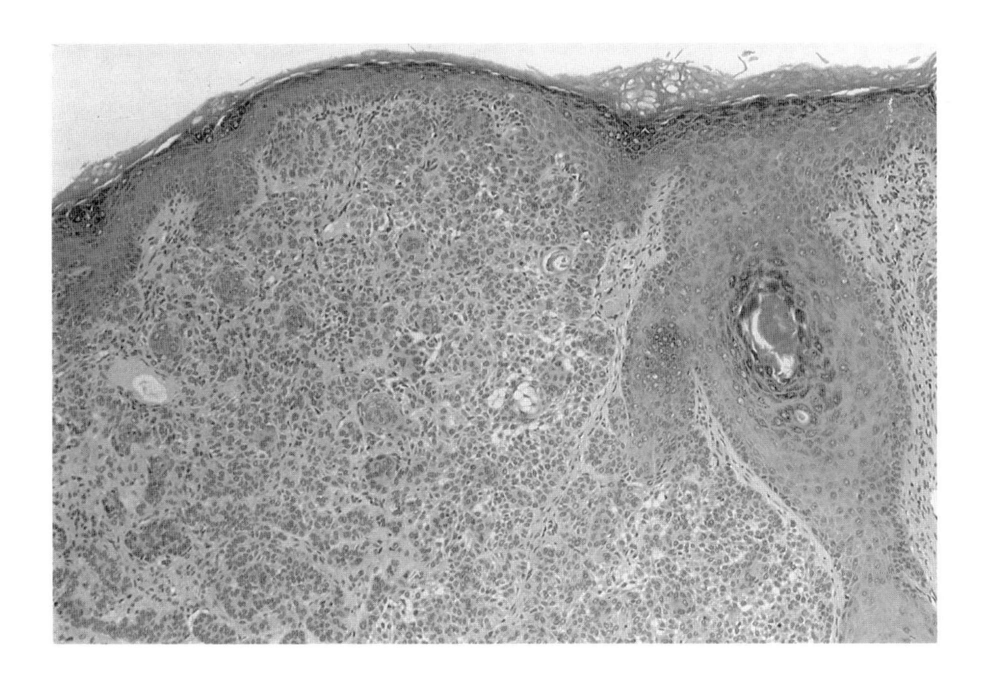

FIG. 30-7. Inverted follicular keratosis
An endophytic proliferation of mature squamous epithelium with "squamous eddies."

Irritated Type and Inverted Follicular Keratosis

In the irritated, or activated, type of seborrheic keratosis, squamous cells outnumber basaloid cells. The characteristic feature is the presence of numerous whorls or eddies composed of eosinophilic flattened squamous cells arranged in an onion-peel fashion, resembling poorly differentiated horn pearls (Figs. 30-7 and 30-8). These "squamous eddies" are easily differentiated from the horn pearls of squamous cell carcinoma by their large number, small size, and circumscribed configuration. Irritated seborrheic keratoses, in addition, may show areas of downward proliferation breaking through the horizontal demarcation generally present in nonirritated seborrheic keratoses.[62,63] Frequently, some of these proliferations are seen to originate from the walls of keratin-filled invaginations. Inflammation beneath irritated seborrheic keratoses usually is mild or absent, indicating that irritated seborrheic keratoses are different from inflamed seborrheic keratoses.

In a few instances, acantholysis has been observed within tumor nests composed of squamous cells.[64] These acantholytic changes differ from those occurring in incidental focal acantholytic dyskeratosis by not showing suprabasal location or dyskeratotic cells resembling corps ronds.[65]

Pathogenesis. The formation of numerous squamous eddies is the result of the "activation" of resting basaloid cells into squamous cells. This unique and highly diagnostic feature of irritated or activated seborrheic keratoses, as well as their downward proliferation, is the result of irritation. This has been proved experimentally by the excision of seborrheic keratoses either after a previous biopsy[66] or after irritation with croton oil.[67]

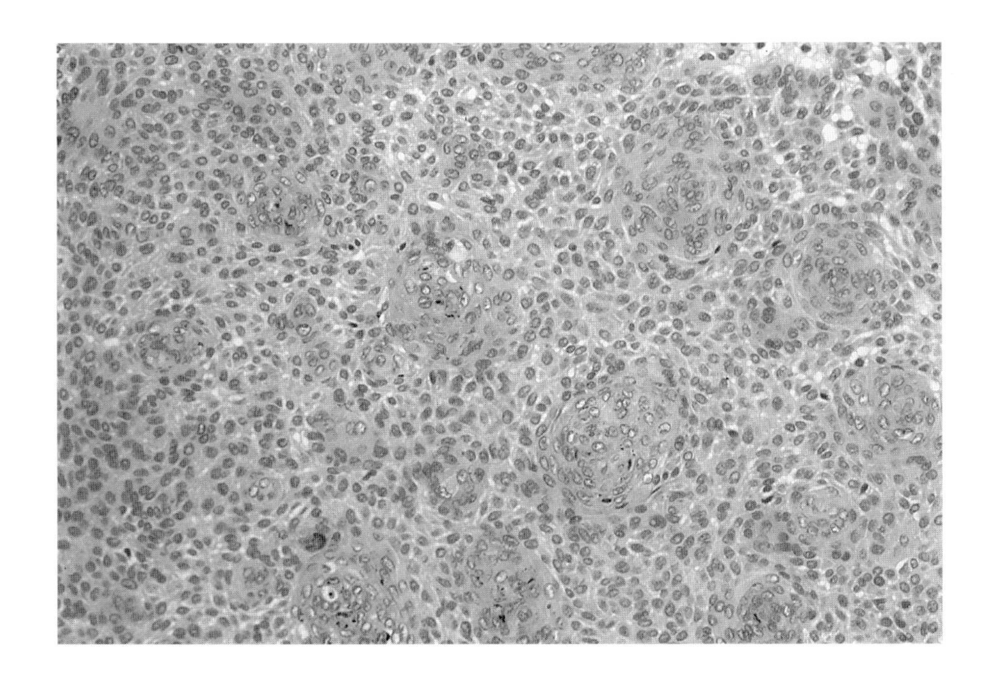

FIG. 30-8. Inverted follicular keratosis
Numerous whorls of eosinophilic flattened squamous cells, so-called squamous eddies, are present. They differ from the horn pearls of squamous cell carcinoma by their large number, small size, and circumscribed configuration. The lesional cells lack significant cytologic atypia.

The identical histologic picture as seen in irritated seborrheic keratosis has been described under the designations of *inverted follicular keratosis*[68,69] and *follicular poroma*.[70,71] As these terms indicate, the authors regard the keratin-filled invaginations as follicular infundibula and the proliferations arising from them as composed of cells of the follicular infundibulum. The follicular infundibulum consists of cells with the same type of keratinization as the surface epidermis, and there is evidence that seborrheic keratoses incorporate cells of the infundibular portion of the hair follicle and are partially derived from these cells. Seborrheic keratoses, like inverted follicular keratoses, occur exclusively on hair-bearing skin. Some seborrheic keratoses even contain aggregates of vellus hairs within the keratinous invaginations, an occurrence analogous to trichostasis spinulosa (see Chap. 18).[72] Although some authors merely concede that irritated seborrheic keratoses and inverted follicular keratoses may be histologically indistinguishable,[63,73,74] others regard the two disorders as identical.[62,72,75] Because of their histologic similarity and particularly because of the highly specific appearance of the squamous eddies that occur in these two conditions, they are best regarded as identical.

Adenoid or Reticulated Type

In the adenoid or reticulated type of seborrheic keratosis, numerous thin tracts of epidermal cells extend from the epidermis and show branching and interweaving in the dermis. Many tracts are composed of only a double row of basaloid cells (see Fig. 30-4). Horn cysts and pseudo–horn cysts are absent in purely reticulated lesions; however, the reticulated type often also shows areas of the acanthotic type, and horn cysts and pseudo–horn cysts are commonly seen in these areas. The basaloid cells of the reticulated type of seborrheic keratosis usually show marked hyperpigmentation.

There is both clinical and histologic evidence of a close relationship between lentigo senilis (lentigo solaris) and the reticulated type of seborrheic keratosis. A lesion of lentigo solaris may even become a reticulated seborrheic keratosis through exaggeration of the process of downward budding of pigmented basaloid cells (see Chap. 29).[76]

Acanthotic Type

In the acanthotic type, the most common type of seborrheic keratosis, hyperkeratosis and papillomatosis often are slight, but the epidermis is greatly thickened. Although only narrow papillae are included in the thickened epidermis in some cases, one can see in other lesions a retiform pattern composed of thick, interwoven tracts of epithelial cells surrounding islands of connective tissue (see Fig. 30-3). Horny invaginations that on cross sections appear as pseudo–horn cysts are numerous. In addition, there also are true horn cysts, which, like the pseudo–horn cysts, show sudden and complete keratinization with only a very thin granular layer.

The true horn cysts begin as foci of orthokeratosis within the substance of the lesion.[77] In time, they enlarge and are carried by the current of epidermal cells toward the surface of the lesion, where they unite with the invaginations of surface keratin. In the greatly thickened epidermis, basaloid cells usually outnumber squamous cells.

The amount of melanin in seborrheic keratoses of the acanthotic type is often greater than normal. Excess amounts of melanin are seen in about one third of the specimens stained with hematoxylin-eosin[78]; staining with silver reveals excess amounts in about two thirds of the cases.[79] In dopa-stained sections, melanocytes are limited to the dermal-epidermal junctional layer present at the base of the tumor and at the interfaces between the tumor tracts and the islands of dermal stroma.[67] The melanin, largely present in keratinocytes, is in most instances also limited to keratinocytes located at the dermal-epidermal junction. Only deeply pigmented lesions show melanin widely distributed throughout the tumor within basaloid cells.[80]

A mononuclear inflammatory infiltrate is seen quite frequently in the dermis underlying a seborrheic keratosis. The inflammation may impinge on the tumor in a lichenoid or eczematous pattern. In the lichenoid pattern, a bandlike infiltrate is seen hugging the basal cell layer of the tumor. In the eczematous pattern, there is exocytosis leading to spongiosis. Squamous eddies, typical of irritated seborrheic keratoses, are only rarely seen in inflamed seborrheic keratoses.[81]

Formation of an in situ carcinoma within an acanthotic seborrheic keratosis, so-called bowenoid transformation, is seen occasionally.[82,83] It seems to occur predominantly in lesions located in sun-exposed areas of the skin, so that sun damage may be a factor.[84] In one reported case, a metastasis in a regional lymph node was found.[85] On rare occasions, a basal cell epithelioma may form within an acanthotic seborrheic keratosis and may extend from there into the underlying dermis.[86,87]

Pathogenesis. Electron microscopic examination has confirmed the light microscopic impression that the small basaloid cells seen in the acanthotic type of seborrheic keratosis are related to cells of the epidermal basal cell layer rather than to the basaloma cells of basal cell epithelioma. They possess a fair number of desmosomes and a moderate number of tonofilaments that differ from those present in cells of the epidermal basal cell layer only by showing less orientation.[88]

Hyperkeratotic Type

In the hyperkeratotic type, also referred to as the digitate or serrated type, hyperkeratosis and papillomatosis are pronounced, whereas acanthosis is not very conspicuous. The numerous digitate upward extensions of epidermis-lined papillae often resemble church spires. The histologic picture then resembles that seen in acrokeratosis verruciformis of Hopf (see Chap. 6). The epidermis consists largely of squamous cells, although small aggregates of basaloid cells may be seen here and there. As a rule, no excess amounts of melanin are found.

Clonal Type

In the clonal, or nesting, type of seborrheic keratosis, well-defined nests of cells are located within the epidermis. In some instances, the nests resemble foci of basal cell epithelioma, since the nuclei appear small and dark-staining and intercellular bridges are seen in only a few areas (see Fig. 30-5).[89] The histologic picture in such cases has been erroneously interpreted by some authors as representing an intraepidermal epithelioma of Borst-Jadassohn (see Chap. 31).[90] In other instances of clonal seborrheic keratosis, the nests are composed of fairly large cells showing distinct intercellular bridges, with the nests separated from one another by strands of cells exhibiting small, dark nuclei (see Fig. 30-6).

Melanoacanthoma

This rather rare variant of pigmented seborrheic keratosis[80] differs from the usual type of pigmented seborrheic keratosis by showing a marked increase in the concentration of melanocytes. Rather than being confined to the basal layer of the tumor lobules, many melanocytes are scattered throughout the tumor lobules.[80,91] In some instances, well-defined islands of basaloid cells intermingled with many melanocytes are distributed through the tumor.[92] The melanocytes are large and richly dendritic and contain variable amounts of melanin. The block in transfer of melanin from melanocytes to keratinocytes often is only partial,[91] although in some instances nearly all the melanin is retained in the melanocytes.[93]

Pathogenesis. Melanoacanthoma is a benign mixed tumor of melanocytes and keratinocytes.[80]

DERMATOSIS PAPULOSA NIGRA

Dermatosis papulosa nigra is found in about 35% of all adult blacks, often has its onset during adolescence,[94] and has been described in a 3-year-old child.[95] The lesions are located predominantly on the face, especially in the malar regions, but may also occur on the neck and upper trunk. They usually consist of small, smooth, pigmented papules, except on the neck and trunk, where some of them may be pedunculated.

Histopathology. The lesions have the histologic appearance of seborrheic keratoses but are smaller. Most lesions are of the acanthotic type and show thick interwoven tracts of epithelial cells. The cells are largely squamous in appearance, with only a few basaloid cells.[94] Horn cysts are quite common. An occasional lesion shows a reticulated pattern, in which the tracts are composed of a double row of basaloid cells. Melanin pigmentation is pronounced in all lesions.

STUCCO KERATOSIS

Stucco keratoses are small, gray-white seborrheic keratoses 1 to 3 mm in diameter, located in symmetric arrangement on the distal portions of the extremities, especially the ankles. They can easily be scraped off without any resultant bleeding.

Histopathology. Stucco keratoses have the appearance of the hyperkeratotic type of seborrheic keratosis, showing the church-spire pattern of upward-extending papillae.[96,97] Horn cysts and basaloid cells are usually absent.[98]

LESER-TRÉLAT SIGN

The Leser-Trélat sign is characterized by the sudden appearance of numerous seborrheic keratoses in association with a malignant tumor. Although many reports have appeared in recent years concerning this sign and although its existence is accepted, it is not always easy to decide which cases should be included. In some instances, numerous seborrheic keratoses develop on inflamed skin, but this does not represent the Leser-Trélat sign.[81] A review of 40 cases that were accepted as representing the Leser-Trélat sign[99] showed that 30% had "malignant" acanthosis nigricans (Chap. 17) either accompanying[100] or following the sign.[101] Thus the Leser-Trélat sign has been interpreted as "an incomplete form of acanthosis nigricans"[102] or as "potentially representing an early stage of acanthosis nigricans."[101]

Although the malignant tumor in 67% of the reported cases consisted of an abdominal adenocarcinoma,[99,103] the remaining 33% included many different types of malignancies, including leukemia[104] or mycosis fungoides.[105] More controversially a case-control study failed to demonstrate a specific association between eruptive seborrhoeic keratoses and internal cancer risk.[106]

Histopathology. The seborrheic keratoses in the Leser-Trélat sign are the same as other seborrheic keratoses. The hyperkeratotic form is indistinguishable from malignant acanthosis nigricans.[99,107]

LARGE CELL ACANTHOMA

Large cell acanthoma occurs as a slightly hyperkeratotic, sharply demarcated patch, usually on sun-exposed skin of the head or extremities. As a rule, it measures less than 1 cm in size. Generally, it is a solitary lesion: occasionally multiple lesions are observed.[108–110]

Histopathology. Within a well-demarcated area of the epidermis, the scattered large keratinocytes are about twice the normal size and have proportionally large nuclei. There may be a disordered arrangement of the keratinocytes.

Pathogenesis. The lesion is aneuploid, with various stages of development, and is probably related to stucco keratosis.[108,110]

CLEAR CELL ACANTHOMA

Clear cell acanthoma, a tumor that is clinically and histologically quite distinct, was first described in 1962.[111] It is not rare. Typically the lesions are solitary and occur on the legs. They are slowly growing, sharply delineated, red nodules or plaques 1 to 2 cm in diameter and usually covered with a thin crust and exuding some moisture. A collarette is often seen at the periphery. It has been said that the lesion appears stuck on, like a seborrheic keratosis, and is vascular, like a granuloma pyogenicum.[112,113]

Histopathology. Within a sharply demarcated area of the epidermis, all epidermal cells, with the exception of cells of the basal cell layer, appear strikingly clear and slightly enlarged (Fig. 30-9). The nuclei of the clear epidermal cells appear normal. When staining is carried out with the periodic acid–Schiff (PAS) reaction, the presence of large amounts of glycogen is revealed within the cells.[111,114]

Slight spongiosis is present between the clear cells. The rete ridges are elongated and may show intertwining.[115] The surface shows parakeratosis with few or no granular cells. The acrosy-

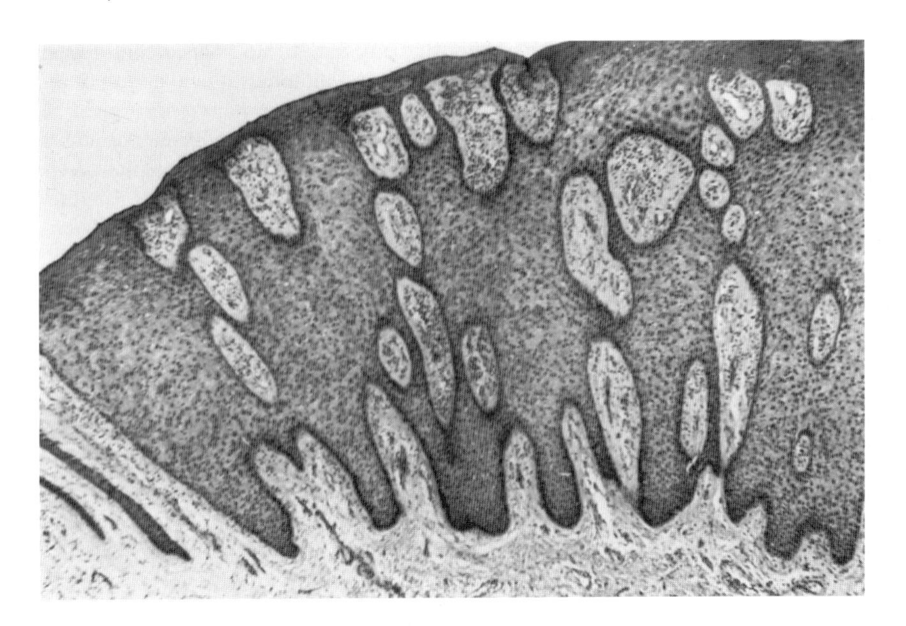

FIG. 30-9. Clear cell acanthoma, low magnification
The cells within the thickened epidermis appear strikingly clear because of the presence of large amounts of glycogen.

ringia and acrotrichia within the tumor retain their normal stainability.[116] There is an absence of melanin within the tumor cells, but dendritic melanocytes containing melanin are occasionally seen interspersed between the clear cells.[114,117]

A conspicuous feature in most lesions is the presence throughout the epidermis of numerous neutrophils, many of which show fragmentation of their nuclei (Fig. 30-10). The neutrophils often form microabscesses in the parakeratotic horny layer.[118,119] Dilated capillaries are seen in the elongated papillae and often also in the dermis underlying the tumor.[114] In addition, a mild to moderately severe cellular infiltrate composed largely of lymphoid cells is present in the dermis. Some clear cell acanthomas appear papillomatous, so that they have the configuration of a seborrheic keratosis.[120]

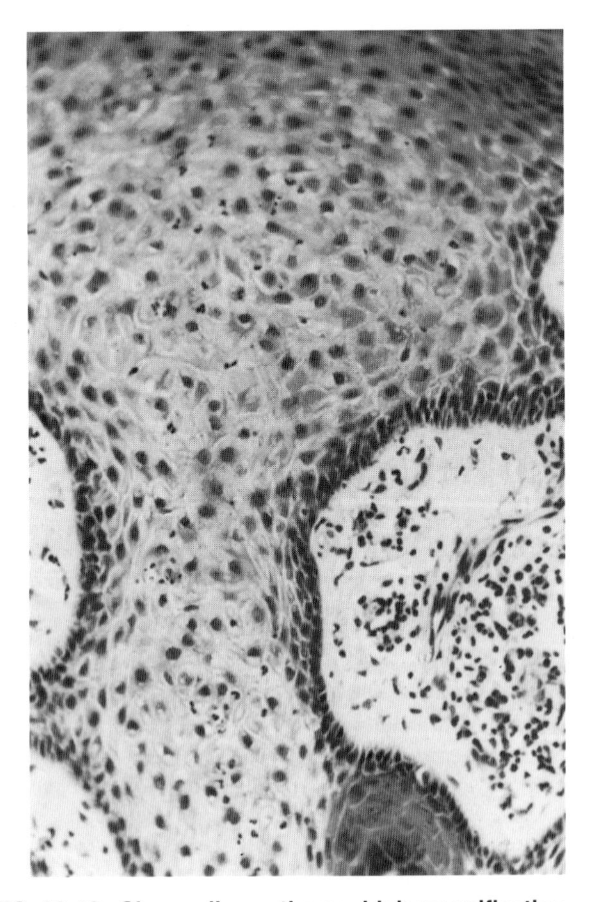

FIG. 30-10. Clear cell acanthoma, high magnification
Neutrophils and nuclear dust are scattered through the tumor. At the lower border, part of an acrosyringium is visible with cells that have retained their normal stainability.

Beneath the tumor, some cases have shown hyperplasia of sweat ducts[118] or syringoma-like proliferations.[121]

Pathogenesis. On histochemical examination, phosphorylase is absent in clear cell acanthoma except for the basal cell layer. This enzyme normally is present in the epidermis and is necessary for the degradation of glycogen.[122]

Electron microscopy reveals glycogen granules in the tumor cells, except in the cells of the basal cell layer. In the lower portion of the tumor, the glycogen granules are seen largely around the nuclei. In the upper portion, however, the amount of glycogen is increased, and the granules are seen to infiltrate between the tonofilaments.[122]

Although the melanocytes, including their dendrites, contain melanosomes, hardly any melanosomes are present within the tumor cells, indicating a blockage in the transfer of melanosomes from the melanocytes to the tumor cells.[123]

EPIDERMAL OR INFUNDIBULAR CYST

Epidermal cysts are slowly growing, elevated, round, firm, intradermal or subcutaneous tumors that cease growing after having reached 1 to 5 cm in diameter. They occur most commonly on the face, scalp, neck, and trunk. Although most epidermal cysts arise spontaneously in hair-bearing areas, occasionally they occur on the palms or soles[124,125] or form as the result of trauma.[126] Usually a patient has only one or a few epidermal cysts, rarely many. In Gardner's syndrome, however, numerous epidermal cysts occur, especially on the scalp and face (Chap. 33).

Histopathology. Epidermal cysts have a wall composed of

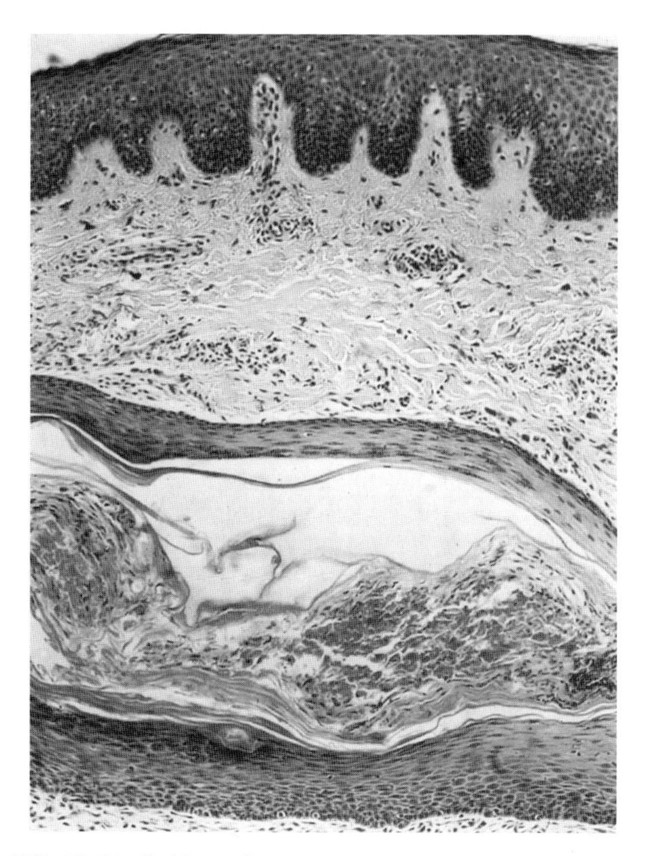

FIG. 30-11. Epidermal cyst
The wall of the cyst is composed of true epidermis, that is, squamous, granular, and horn cells. The cyst is filled with horny material arranged in laminated layers.

true epidermis, as seen on the skin surface and in the infundibulum of hair follicles, the infundibulum being the uppermost part of the hair follicle that extends down to the entry of the sebaceous duct. In young epidermal cysts, several layers of squamous and granular cells can usually be recognized (Fig. 30-11). In older epidermal cysts, the wall often is markedly atrophic, either in some areas or in the entire cyst, and may consist of only one or two rows of greatly flattened cells. The cyst is filled with horny material arranged in laminated layers. In sections stained with hematoxylin-eosin, melanocytes and melanin pigmentation of keratinocytes can be seen only rarely in epidermal cysts of whites but frequently in epidermal cysts of blacks. Silver stains reveal that most of the melanin is located in the basal layer of the cyst lining, but some melanin is seen also in the contents of the cyst.[127]

When an epidermal cyst ruptures and the contents of the cyst are released into the dermis, a considerable foreign-body reaction with numerous multinucleated giant cells results, forming a *keratin granuloma*. The foreign-body reaction usually causes disintegration of the cyst wall. However, it may lead to a pseudocarcinomatous proliferation in remnants of the cyst wall, simulating a squamous cell carcinoma.[128]

Development of a basal cell epithelioma,[129] a lesion of Bowen's disease,[130] or a squamous cell carcinoma[131] in epidermal cysts is a rare event. In cases of squamous cell carcinoma, the tumor is apt to be of low malignancy and does not metastasize. It is likely that some cases that were regarded in the past as malignant degeneration of epidermal cysts now are interpreted either as pseudocarcinomatous hyperplasia in a ruptured epidermal cyst[128] or as proliferating trichilemmal tumor (Chap. 31).[132]

Pathogenesis. It is widely assumed that most spontaneously arising epidermal cysts are related to the follicular infundibulum. The occurrence of hybrid cysts with partially epidermal and partially trichilemmal lining favors this assumption.[133] Epidermal cysts in nonfollicular regions, such as the palms or soles, probably form as a result of the traumatic implantation of epidermis into the dermis or subcutis.[124,125]

As seen by electron microscopy, the keratinization in epidermal cysts is identical to that in the surface epidermis and in the pilosebaceous infundibulum, since the keratin located within the keratinized cells consists of relatively electron-lucent tonofilaments embedded in an electron-dense interfilamentous substance derived from keratohyaline granules. The keratinized cells of the cyst content have a markedly flattened, elongated appearance and are surrounded by a thick marginal band rather than by a plasma membrane. Desmosomes are no longer present.[134]

MILIA

Milia are multiple, superficially located, white, globoid, firm lesions, generally only 1 to 2 mm in diameter. A distinction is made between primary milia, which arise spontaneously on the face in predisposed individuals, and secondary milia, which occur either in diseases associated with subepidermal bullae, such as bullous pemphigoid, dystrophic epidermolysis bullosa,[135] and porphyria cutanea tarda, or after dermabrasion[136] and other trauma.

Histopathology. Primary milia of the face are derived from the lowest portion of the infundibulum of vellus hairs at about the level of the sebaceous duct. The milia often are still connected with the vellus hair follicle by an epithelial pedicle. Primary milia are small cysts differing from epidermal cysts only in size. They are lined by a stratified epithelium a few cell layers thick and contain concentric lamellae of keratin.[136]

Secondary milia have the same histologic appearance as primary milia.[136] They may develop from any epithelial structure and on serial sections may still show a connection to the parent structure, whether a hair follicle, sweat duct, sebaceous duct, or epidermis.[137] Secondary milia that follow blistering arise in most instances from the eccrine sweat duct and very rarely from a hair follicle. In a certain percentage, however, no connection is found with any skin appendage, suggesting that the milia have developed from aberrant epidermis.[138] In milia derived from eccrine sweat ducts, the sweat ducts are frequently seen to enter the cyst wall at the bottom of the milium.[136,138]

Pathogenesis. Primary milia of the face represent a keratinizing type of benign tumor.[136] In contrast, secondary milia represent retention cysts caused by proliferative tendencies of the epithelium after injury.[139]

TRICHILEMMAL OR PILAR CYST

Trichilemmal or pilar cysts are clinically indistinguishable from epidermal cysts. They differ from epidermal cysts, however, in frequency and distribution. They are less common than epidermal cysts, constituting only about 25% of the combined material; about 90% of trichilemmal cysts occur on the scalp. Trichilemmal cysts often show an autosomal dominant inheritance pattern and are solitary in only 30% of the cases, with 10% of patients having more than 10 cysts.[140] Furthermore, in contrast to epidermal cysts, trichilemmal cysts are easily enucleated and appear as firm, smooth, white-walled cysts.[141]

Histopathology. The wall of trichilemmal cysts is composed of epithelial cells possessing no clearly visible intercellular bridges. The peripheral layer of cells shows a distinct palisade arrangement not seen in epidermal cysts. The epithelial cells close to the cystic cavity appear swollen and are filled with pale cytoplasm (Fig. 30-12). These swollen cells do not produce a granular layer but generally undergo abrupt keratinization, although nuclear remnants are occasionally retained in a few cells. The content of the cysts consists of homogeneous eosinophilic material.[134]

Whereas focal calcification of the cyst content does not occur in epidermal cysts, foci of calcification are seen in approximately one quarter of trichilemmal cysts (Fig. 30-13).[140] A considerable foreign-body reaction results when the wall of a trichilemmal cyst ruptures, and the cyst may then undergo partial or complete disintegration (Fig. 30-14).

Trichilemmal cysts frequently disclose small, acanthotic foci in their walls that are indistinguishable from solid areas, as seen in a proliferating trichilemmal cyst.[142] The association of a trichilemmal cyst with tumor lobules of a proliferating trichilemmal cyst is also seen occasionally (Chap. 31).[140]

Pathogenesis. Trichilemmal cysts, also referred to as pilar cysts, originally were called sebaceous cysts. The name was changed when it became apparent that the keratinization in them is analogous to the keratinization that takes place in the outer root sheath of the hair, or trichilemma.[143] The outer root sheath of the hair does not keratinize wherever it covers the inner root sheath. It keratinizes normally in two areas, the follicular isthmus of anagen hairs and the sac surrounding catagen and telogen hairs, because in these two regions the inner root sheath has disappeared. The follicular isthmus of anagen hairs is the short, middle portion of the hair follicle, extending upward from the attachment of the arrector pili muscle to the entrance of the sebaceous duct. At the lower end of the follicular isthmus, the inner root sheath sloughs off, exposing the outer root sheath, which, in its exposed portion, undergoes a specific type of homogeneous keratinization without the interposition of a granular layer. This type of trichilemmal keratinization also takes place in the sac surrounding catagen and telogen hairs, because hairs in these stages have lost their inner root sheath. The differentiation toward hair keratin in trichilemmal cysts has been confirmed by immunohistochemical staining because they stain with antikeratin antibodies derived from human hair, in contrast to epidermal cysts, which stain with antikeratin antibodies obtained from human callus.[144]

Electron microscopic examination of the epithelial lining of trichilemmal cysts shows that, on their way from the peripheral layer toward the center, the epithelial cells have an increasing number of filaments in their cytoplasm. The transition from nucleate to anucleate cells is abrupt and is associated with the loss of all cytoplasmic organelles. The junction between the keratinizing and keratinized cells shows interdigitations.[145] The keratinized cells are filled with tonofilaments and, unlike those in epidermal cysts, retain their desmosomal connections.[134]

Differential Diagnosis. Even though both the trichilemmal cyst and the proliferating trichilemmal cyst show trichilemmal types of keratinization and can occur together, one is essentially a cyst and the other essentially a solid, tumorlike proliferation.

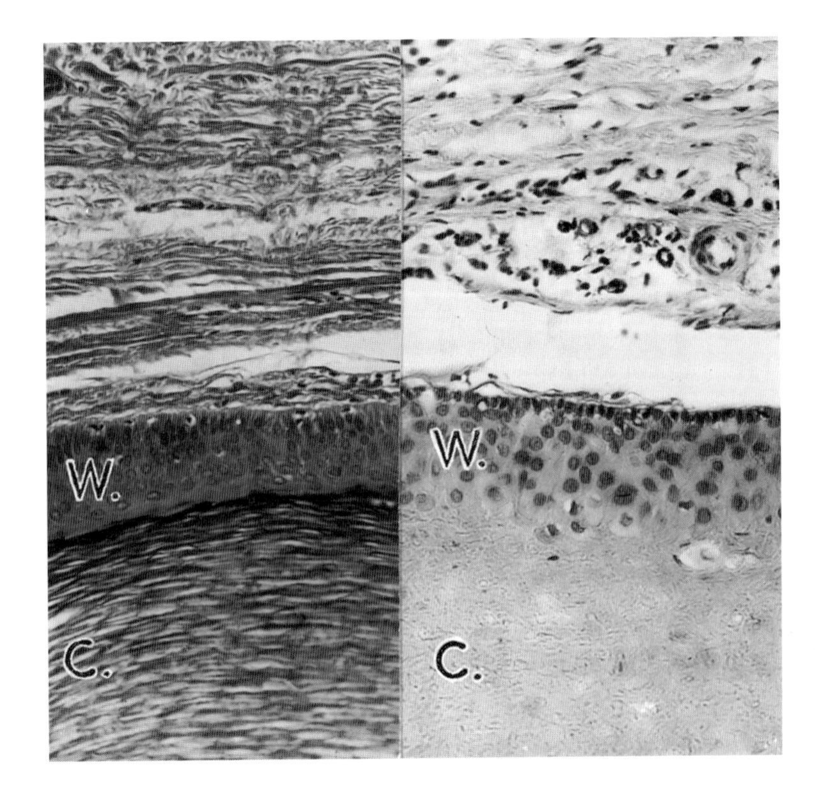

FIG. 30-12. Epidermal and trichilemmal cysts (*Left*) The wall (*W.*) of the epidermal cyst is composed of epidermis; the cystic cavity (*C.*) contains horny material arranged in laminated layers. (*Right*) The wall (*W.*) of the trichilemmal cyst shows distinct palisading of the peripheral cell layer and swelling of the cells close to the cystic cavity (*C.*). The content of the cysts consists of homogeneous horny material.

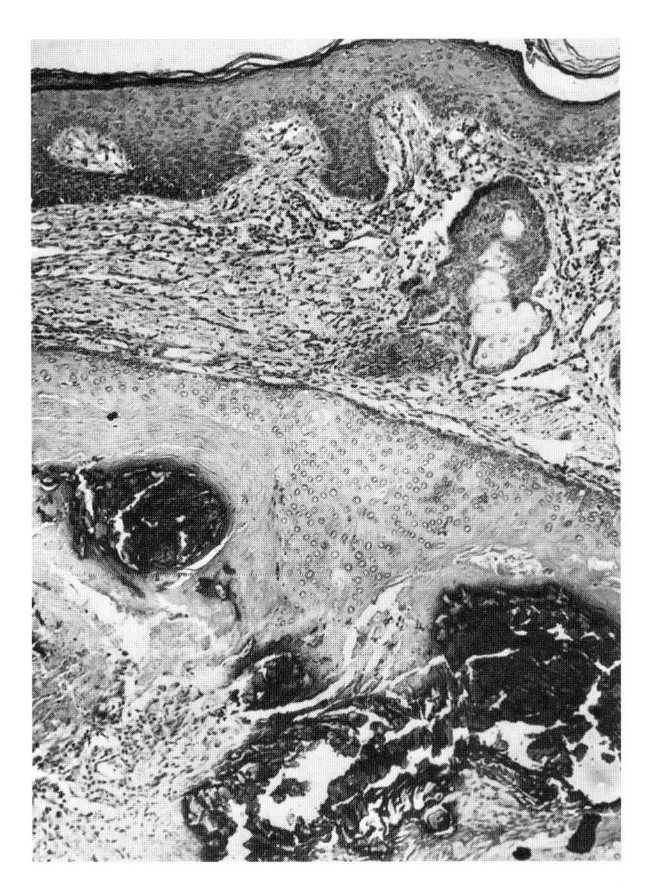

FIG. 30-13. Trichilemmal cyst
The palisading of the basal layer makes it evident that this is a trichilemmal cyst. The cyst has ruptured, and fibrous tissue has proliferated into the lumen.

The latter is therefore discussed under Tumors With Differentiation Toward Hair Structures (see Chap. 31).

STEATOCYSTOMA MULTIPLEX

Steatocystoma multiplex is inherited in an autosomal dominant pattern. One observes numerous small, rounded, moderately firm, cystic nodules that are adherent to the overlying skin and usually measure 1 to 3 cm in diameter. When punctured, the cysts discharge an oily or creamy fluid and, in some instances, also small hairs.[146] They are found most commonly in the axillae, in the sternal region, and on the arms. Steatocystoma also occurs occasionally as a solitary, noninherited tumor in adults, where it is referred to as *steatocystoma simplex.*[147]

Histopathology. The cysts have walls that are intricately folded with several layers of epithelial cells, although in atrophic areas only two or three layers of flat cells may be present. Elsewhere is a basal layer in palisade arrangement, above which are two or three layers of swollen cells without recognizable intercellular bridges. Central to these cells there is a thick, homogeneous, eosinophilic horny layer that forms without an intervening granular layer. It protrudes irregularly into the lumen in a fashion simulating the decapitation secretion of apocrine glands (Fig. 30-15).[148]

A characteristic feature seen in most lesions of steatocystoma is the presence of flattened sebaceous gland lobules either within or close to the cyst wall.[149] In some cysts, invaginations resembling hair follicles extend from the cyst wall into the surrounding stroma, and in rare instances true hair shafts are seen within them, indicating that the invaginations represent the outer root sheath of hairs. In a few cysts, the lumen contains clusters of hair, mainly of lanugo size but partially of interme-

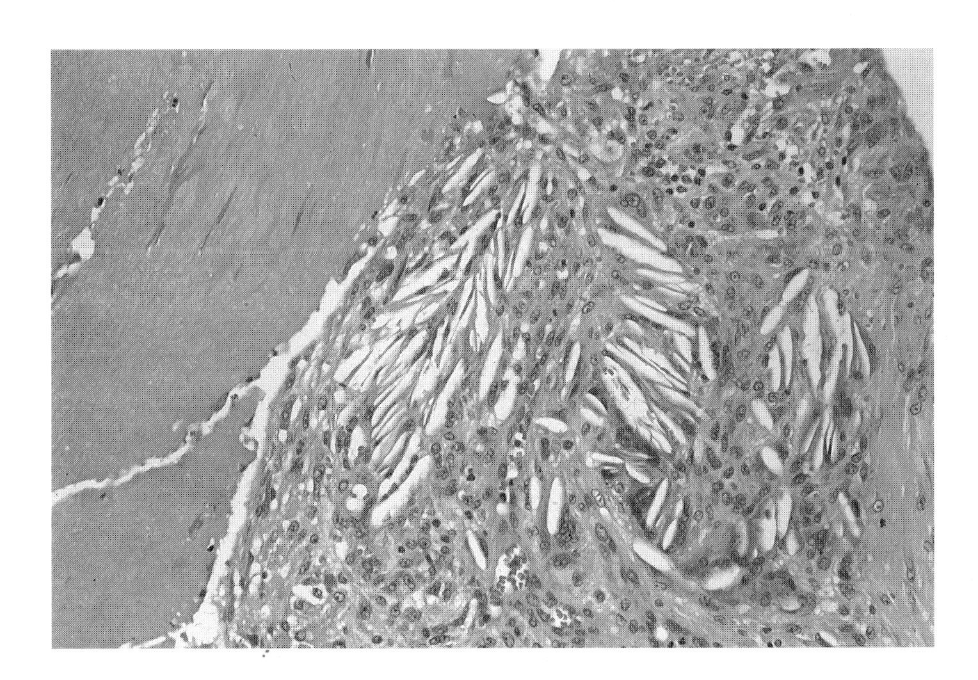

FIG. 30-14. Keratin granuloma
At the edge of a partially ruptured pilar cyst, cholesterol clefts form a prominent part of a keratin granuloma.

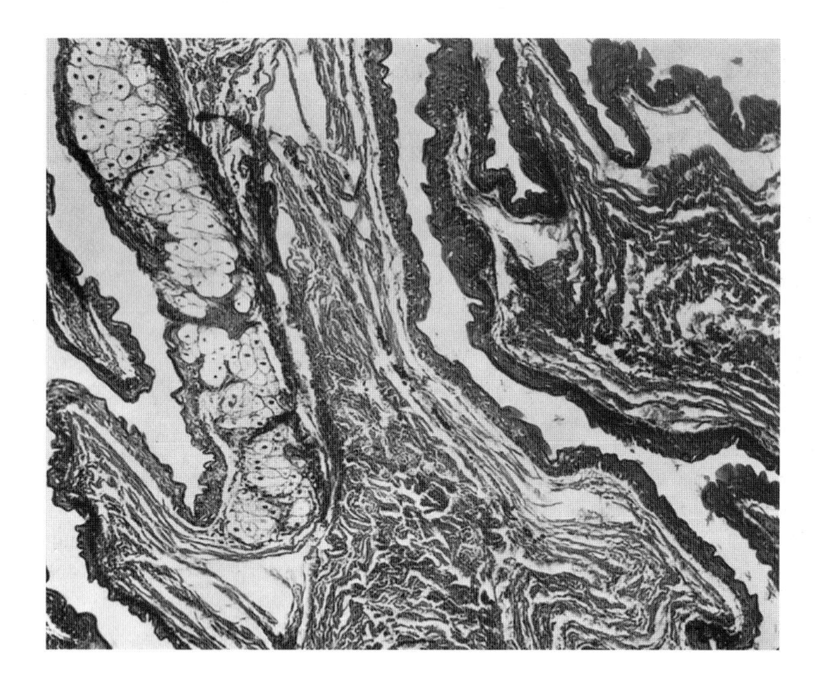

FIG. 30-15. Steatocystoma multiplex
The cyst wall shows intricate folding. The lining of the cyst consists of a homogeneous horny layer that protrudes irregularly into the lumen. On the left, flattened sebaceous gland lobules lie within, or close to, the cyst wall.

diate character.[150] When stained with the PAS reaction, the cells of the cyst wall are found to be rich in glycogen.

Pathogenesis. Electron microscopic examination has shown that the cyst wall consists of keratinizing cells. Nearest to the lumen, the cyst wall consists of several layers of flattened, very elongated horny cells interconnected by desmosomes.

It appears likely that differentiation in the cyst wall of steatocystoma multiplex is to a large extent in the direction of the sebaceous duct.[151,152] The sebaceous duct and the outer root sheath are composed of similar cells, but undulation and thinning of the horny layer and the existence of sebaceous cells in the cyst wall are characteristic features of the sebaceous gland side of the sebaceous duct.[152] Sebaceous duct cells, like outer root sheath cells, contain abundant glycogen and amylophosphorylase, keratinize without the interposition of keratohyaline granules, and on electron microscopic examination, after keratinization retain their desmosomes.[148]

PIGMENTED FOLLICULAR CYST

This is an uncommon pigmented lesion resembling a nevus.

Histopathology. The cyst wall consists of infundibular epidermis. The cyst contains, in addition to laminated keratin, numerous large pigmented hair shafts. One or two growing hair follicles are seen in the wall of the cyst.[153]

DERMOID CYST

Dermoid cysts are subcutaneous cysts that usually are present at birth. They occur most commonly on the head, mainly around the eyes, and occasionally on the neck. When located on the head, they often are adherent to the periosteum. Usually they measure between 1 and 4 cm in diameter.

Histopathology. Dermoid cysts, in contrast to epidermal cysts, are lined by an epidermis that possesses various epidermal appendages that are usually fully matured (Fig. 30-16). Hair follicles containing hairs that project into the lumen of the cyst are often present. In addition, the dermis of dermoid cysts usually contains sebaceous glands, often eccrine glands, and in about 20% of the cases, apocrine glands that have matured (Fig. 30-17).[154]

Pathogenesis. Dermoid cysts are a result of the sequestration of skin along lines of embryonic closure.

BRONCHOGENIC AND THYROGLOSSAL DUCT CYSTS

Bronchogenic cysts are rare. They are small, solitary lesions seen most commonly in the skin or subcutaneous tissue just above the sternal notch. Rarely, they are located on the anterior aspect of the neck or on the chin. As a rule, they are discovered shortly after birth. They may show a draining sinus.

Thyroglossal duct cysts are clinically indistinguishable from bronchogenic cysts, except that they are usually located on the anterior aspect of the neck.

Histopathology. Bronchogenic cysts are lined by a mucosa consisting of pseudostratified columnar epithelium (Fig. 30-18). Some of the epithelial cells show cilia extending into the lumen (Fig. 30-19). Goblet cells may be interspersed. The wall frequently contains smooth muscle and mucous glands but only rarely contains cartilage.[153]

Thyroglossal duct cysts differ from bronchogenic cysts in that they do not contain smooth muscle and they frequently contain thyroid follicles.[155]

Pathogenesis. On electron microscopy the cilia show two central microtubules surrounded by nine paired microtubules.[156]

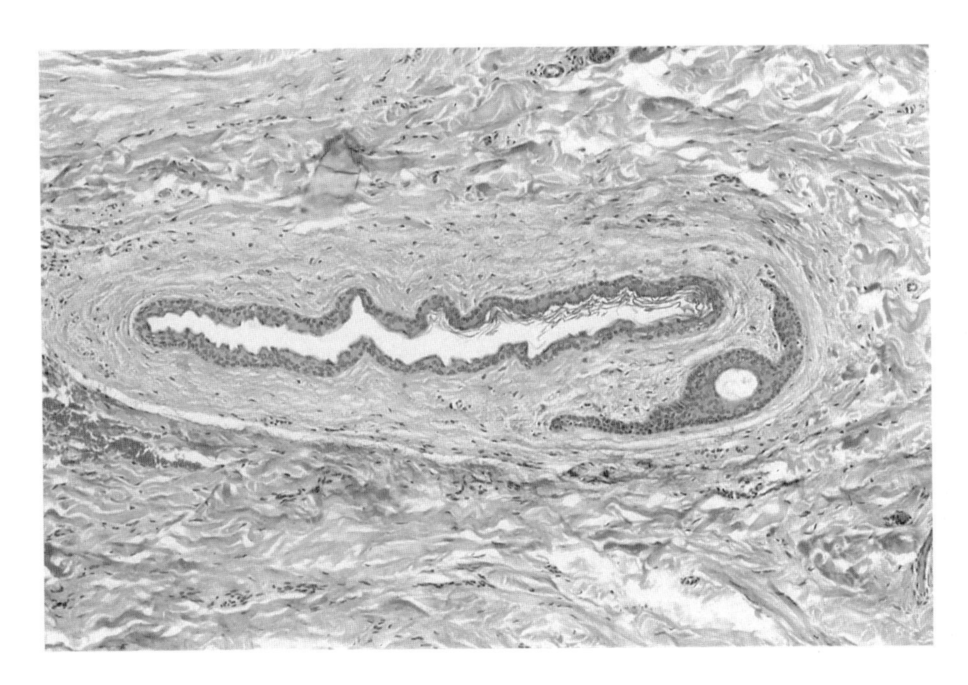

FIG. 30-16. External angular dermoid cyst
The cyst is small and well defined, with adnexal structures in its wall.

CUTANEOUS CILIATED CYST

Cutaneous ciliated cysts are found very rarely in females as a single lesion, largely on the lower extremities, and even more rarely in males and on the back.[157–159] They usually measure several centimeters in diameter. They are either unilocular or multilocular and are filled with clear or amber fluid.

Histopathology. Cutaneous ciliated cysts show numerous papillary projections lined by a simple cuboidal or columnar ciliated epithelium. Mucin-secreting cells are absent.[159]

Pathogenesis. The epithelial lining of the cysts resembles that seen in the fallopian tube. On electron microscopy, the cilia show two central filaments encircled by nine pairs of filaments.[160]

MEDIAN RAPHE CYST OF THE PENIS

Median raphe cysts of the penis arise usually in young adults. They are located on the ventral aspect of the penis, most com-

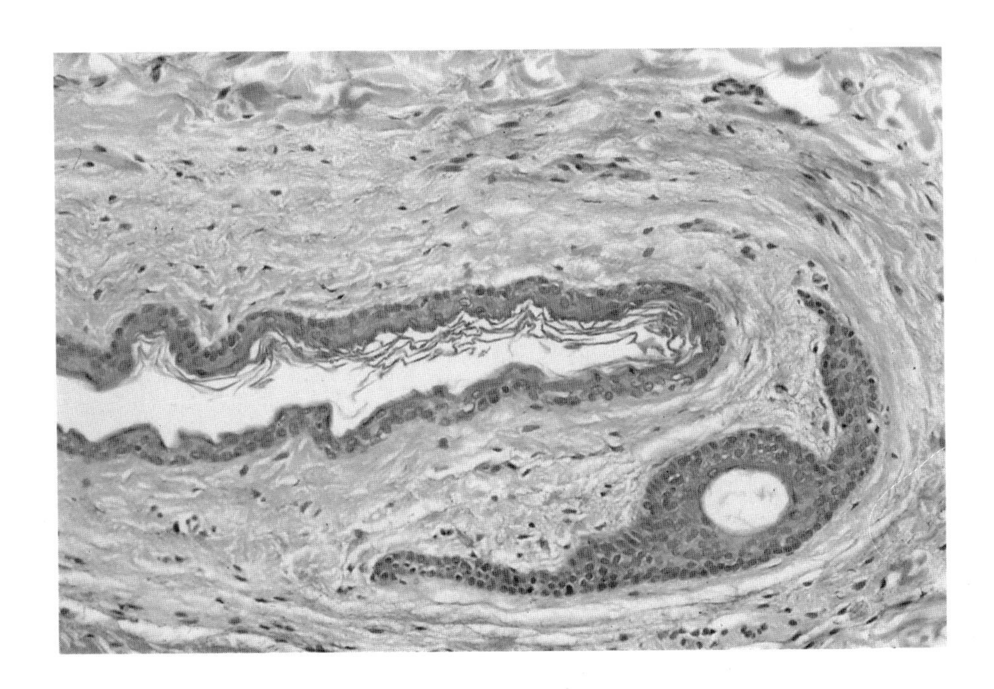

FIG. 30-17. External angular dermoid cyst
Higher power shows adnexal differentiation in the cyst wall.

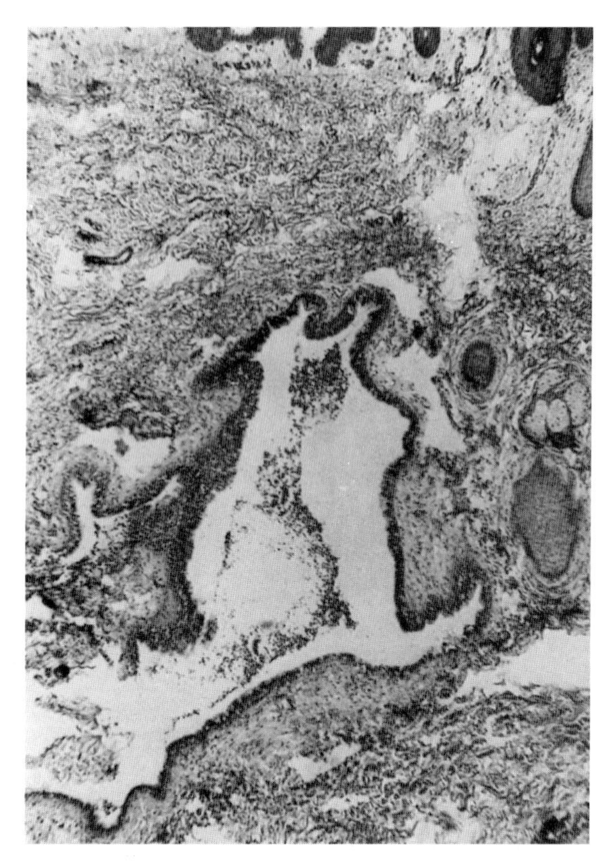

FIG. 30-18. Bronchogenic cyst, low magnification
The cyst located in the dermis is lined by a pseudostratified columnar epithelium.

monly on the glans. They are solitary and measure only a few millimeters in diameter.[161] However, they may extend over several centimeters in a linear fashion.[162] It seems that, in some instances, median raphe cysts have been erroneously reported as apocrine cystadenoma of the penis.[163,164]

Histopathology. The cysts are lined by pseudostratified columnar epithelium varying from one to four cells in thickness, mimicking the transitional epithelium of the urethra. Some of the epithelial cells have clear cytoplasm, mucin-containing cells are uncommon, and a case lined by ciliated epithelium has been described.[165]

Pathogenesis. It is likely that median raphe cysts do not represent a defective closure of the median raphe, but rather the anomalous budding and separation of urethral columnar epithelium from the urethra.[166]

ERUPTIVE VELLUS HAIR CYSTS

In eruptive vellus hair cysts, a condition first described in 1977,[167] asymptomatic follicular papules 1 to 2 mm in diameter occur, most commonly on the chest but in some instances elsewhere. Some of the papules have a crusted or umbilicated surface. The condition is usually seen in children and young adults but can develop at any age. Spontaneous clearing may take place in a few years. Autosomal dominant inheritance has been described.[168,169]

Histopathology. A cystic structure is usually seen in the middermis lined by squamous epithelium. It contains laminated keratinous material and varying numbers of transversely and obliquely cut vellus hairs.[167] In some cysts, vellus hairs are seen emerging from follicle-like invaginations of the cyst wall.[170] In other cysts, a telogen hair follicle is seen extending from the lower surface toward the subcutis.[167] Crusted or umbilicated lesions show either a cyst communicating with the surface and extruding its contents[169,171] or partial destruction of a cyst by a granulomatous infiltrate and elimination of vellus hairs to the surface of the skin.[172]

Pathogenesis. Eruptive vellus hair cysts represent a developmental abnormality of vellus hair follicles that predisposes them to occlusion at their infundibular level. This results in retention of hairs, cystic dilatation of the proximal part of the follicle, and secondary atrophy of the hair bulbs.[167,171] There is a close relationship with steatocystoma multiplex.[173] Both processes could be described as multiple pilosebaceous cysts.[174]

WARTY DYSKERATOMA

Warty dyskeratoma, first described in 1957,[175] usually occurs as a solitary lesion, most commonly on the scalp, face, or neck, although a case with multiple lesions has been described.[176] It has also been reported in non–sun-exposed skin including the oral mucosa, usually on the hard palate or an alveolar ridge.[177,178] Although its clinical appearance is not always distinctive, it often occurs as a slightly elevated papule or nodule with a keratotic umbilicated center.[179] The lesion, after having reached a certain size, persists indefinitely.

Histopathology. The center of the lesion is occupied by a large, cup-shaped invagination connected with the surface by a channel filled with keratinous material (Fig. 30-20). The large invagination contains numerous acantholytic, dyskeratotic cells in its upper portion. The lower portion of the invagination is occupied by numerous villi, that is, markedly elongated dermal papillae that are often lined with only a single layer of basal

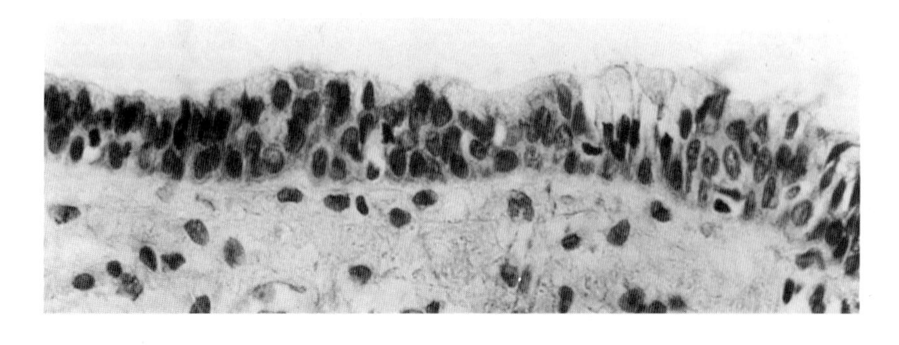

FIG. 30-19. Bronchogenic cyst, high magnification
Cilia are recognizable on several of the lining cells.

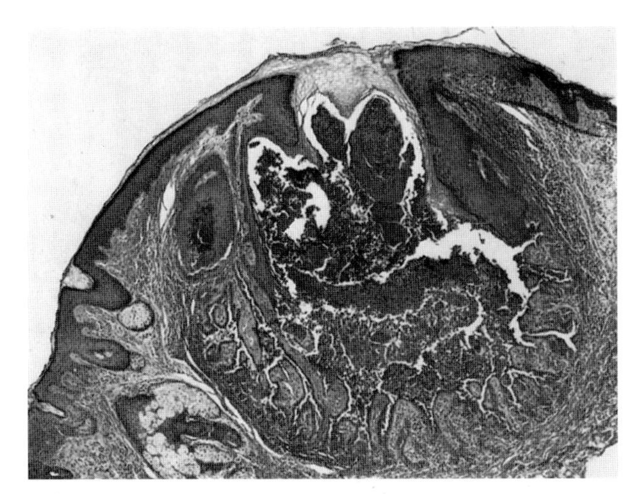

FIG. 30-20. Warty dyskeratoma, low magnification
A large invagination is connected with the surface by a channel containing keratinous material. (Courtesy of Armed Forces Institute of Pathology, No. 57-6202.)

cells and project upward from the base of the cup-shaped invagination (Fig. 30-21).[175,180–182] Typical corps ronds can usually be seen in the thickened granular layer lining the channel at the entrance to the invagination (Fig. 30-22).[179,183]

Pathogenesis. The central cup-shaped invagination has been interpreted by several observers as a greatly dilated hair follicle, because in early lesions a hair follicle or sebaceous gland is often connected with the invagination.[180] Occasionally, two or three adjoining follicles seem to be involved.[179] The fact, however, that warty dyskeratoma can arise on the oral mucosa indicates that, as in Darier's disease, the dyskeratotic, acantholytic process is not always derived from a pilosebaceous structure.

Although attempts were made at first to correlate warty dyskeratoma with Darier's disease, it is now generally agreed that warty dyskeratoma represents an entity, "a benign cutaneous tumor that resembles Darier's disease microscopically."[175]

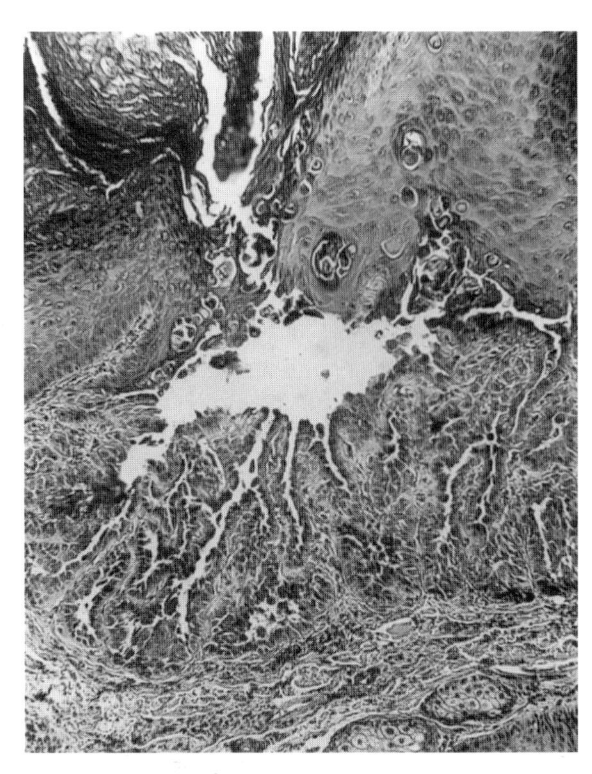

FIG. 30-22. Warty dyskeratoma
Typical corps ronds are located in the thickened granular layer lining the channel that leads into the invagination.

ACTINIC KERATOSIS

Solar keratoses are also known as actinic keratoses. The adjective *solar* is more specific, because it refers to the sun as the cause, whereas the adjective *actinic* refers to a variety of rays.[184] Even among the sun rays, action spectrum evaluations indicate that the ultraviolet B (UVB) rays (290–320 nm)

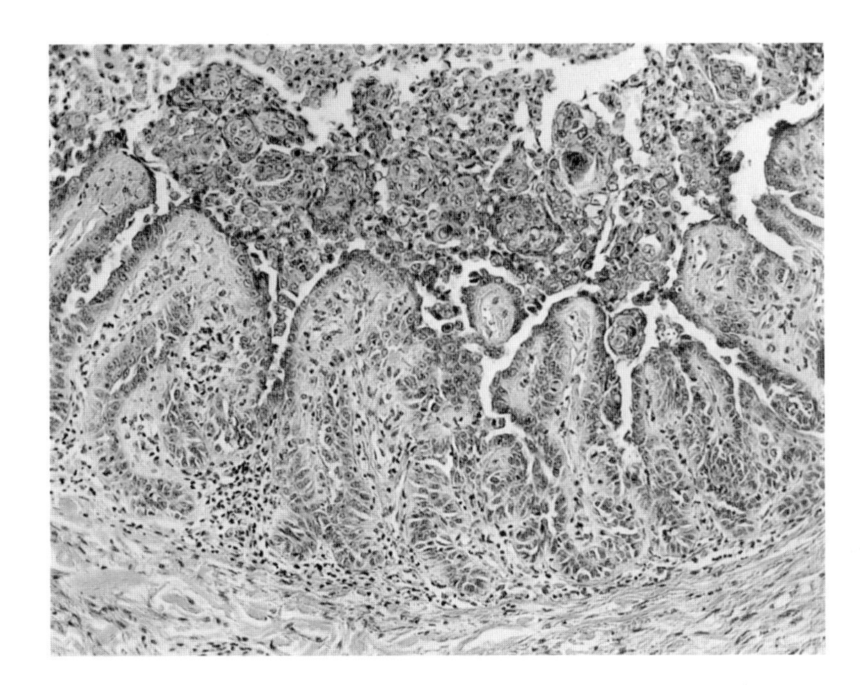

FIG. 30-21. Warty dyskeratoma
The villi at the base of the invagination are covered with a single layer of epidermal cells. Acantholytic, dyskeratotic cells lie above the villi. (Courtesy of Armed Forces Institute of Pathology, No. 57-6203.)

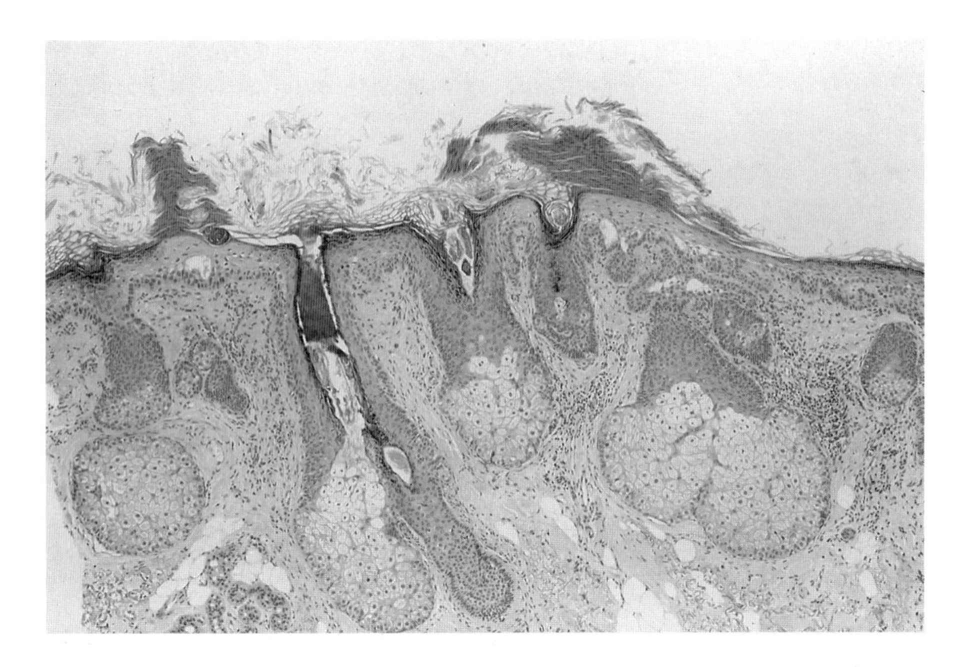

FIG. 30-23. Actinic keratosis
Tall columns of parakeratotic keratin alternate with bands of orthokeratotic keratin in this mildly atypical keratosis.

are the most damaging ("carcinogenic") rays, although UVA rays (320–400 nm) can augment the damaging effects of UVB rays.[185]

Actinic keratoses are usually seen as multiple lesions in sun-exposed areas of the skin in persons in or past middle life who have fair complexions. Excessive exposure to sunlight over many years and inadequate protection against it are the essential predisposing factors. Actinic keratoses are seen most commonly on the face and the dorsa of the hands and in the bald portions of the scalp in men.[186]

Usually, the lesions measure less than 1 cm in diameter. They are erythematous, are often covered by adherent scales, and except in their hypertrophic form, show little or no infiltration. Some actinic keratoses are pigmented and show peripheral spreading, making clinical differentiation from lentigo maligna difficult.[187] Occasionally, lesions show marked hyperkeratosis and then have the clinical aspect of cutaneous horns. A lesion analogous to actinic keratosis occurs on the vermilion border of the lower lip as *solar cheilitis* and may show areas of erosion and hyperkeratosis.[188–190]

Actinic keratosis and solar cheilitis can develop into squamous cell carcinoma. However, the incidence of this transformation is difficult to determine, because the borderline between actinic keratosis and squamous cell carcinoma is not clear-cut (see Histopathology). It has been estimated that in 20% of patients with actinic keratoses squamous cell carcinoma develops in one or more of the lesions.[191] Usually, squamous cell carcinomas arising either in actinic keratoses or de novo in sun-damaged skin do not metastasize. The incidence of metastasis in different series varies from 0.5%[192] to 3%.[193] In carcinoma of the

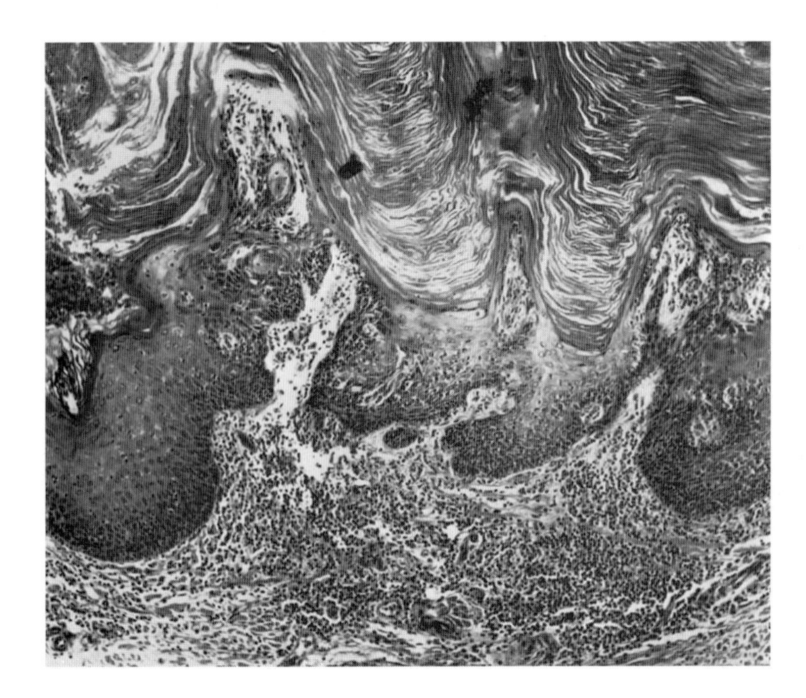

FIG. 30-24. Actinic keratosis, hypertrophic type
One observes hyperkeratosis and papillomatosis. The stratum malpighii demonstrates irregular hyperplasia in which the epidermal cells show a rather disorderly arrangement and some of the nuclei appear pleomorphic and atypical. The upper dermis shows a rather pronounced chronic inflammatory infiltrate.

vermilion border of the lip, however, metastases have been found in 11% of the cases.[193]

Histopathology. Actinic keratoses are keratinocytic dysplasias or squamous cell carcinomas in situ. This definition is preferable to their designation as precancerosis, because most of them never progress to cancers. Biologically, the lesions are still benign; invasion into the dermis, if present at all, is limited to the most superficial portion, the papillary dermis (see Differential Diagnosis).

Five types of actinic keratosis can be recognized histologically: hypertrophic, atrophic, bowenoid, acantholytic, and pigmented. Transitions and combinations among these five types occur. In addition, many cutaneous horns prove on histologic examination to be actinic keratoses.

In the *hypertrophic type* of actinic keratosis, hyperkeratosis is pronounced and is usually intermingled with areas of parakeratosis.[194] This variety of keratosis, sometimes referred to as *florid keratosis*, may easily be overdiagnosed as invasive squamous cell carcinoma by the unwary. Mild or moderate papillomatosis may be present. The epidermis is thickened in most areas and shows irregular downward proliferation that is limited to the uppermost dermis and does not represent frank invasion (Fig. 30-23). A varying proportion of the keratinocytes in the stratum malpighii show a loss of polarity and thus a disorderly arrangement. Some of these cells show pleomorphism and atypicality ("anaplasia") of their nuclei, which appear large, irregular, and hyperchromatic. Often the nuclei in the basal layer are closely crowded together (Fig. 30-24). Some of the cells in the midportion of the epidermis show premature keratinization, resulting in dyskeratotic cells or apoptotic bodies characterized by homogeneous, eosinophilic cytoplasm with or without a nucleus. In contrast to the epidermal keratinocytes, the cells of the hair follicles and eccrine ducts that penetrate the epidermis within actinic keratoses retain their normal appearance and keratinize normally.[195,196] Occasionally, cells of the normal adnexal epithelium extend over the atypical cells of the epidermis in an umbrella-like fashion. In some cases, abnormal keratinocytes extend downward on the outside of the follicular infundibulum to the level of the sebaceous duct and, less commonly, along the eccrine duct.[196]

A variant of the hypertrophic type of actinic keratosis is the lichenoid actinic keratosis, which demonstrates nuclear atypia, irregular acanthosis and hyperkeratosis, the presence of basal cell liquefaction, degeneration of the basal cell layer, and a bandlike "lichenoid" infiltrate in close apposition to the epidermis.[197] Fairly numerous eosinophilic, homogeneous apoptotic bodies are seen in the upper dermis as so-called Civatte bodies. Aside from the presence of nuclear atypicality, there is considerable resemblance to lichen planus and benign lichenoid keratosis (see Chap. 7).

In rare instances of actinic keratosis of the hypertrophic type, in addition to finding anaplastic nuclei in the lower epidermis, one finds areas of epidermolytic hyperkeratosis in the upper epidermis (Fig. 30-25). These changes are like those seen in bullous congenital ichthyosiform erythroderma, in linear epidermal nevus, and as incidental epidermolytic hyperkeratosis in a variety of lesions. In areas of epidermolytic hyperkeratosis, one observes in the upper epidermis clear spaces around the nuclei and a thickened granular layer with large, irregularly shaped keratohyaline granules.[34] Epidermolytic hyperkeratosis may occur also in lesions of solar cheilitis.[198]

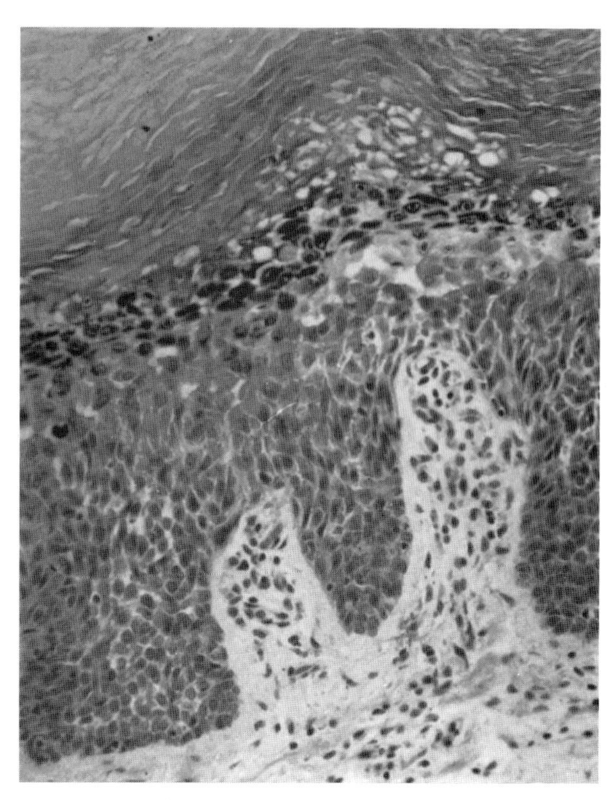

FIG. 30-25. Actinic keratosis, hypertrophic type, with epidermolytic hyperkeratosis
In addition to disorderly arrangement and anaplasia of the nuclei in the lower epidermis, epidermolytic hyperkeratosis, also referred to as *granular degeneration*, is present in the upper epidermis. One observes clear spaces around the nuclei and a thickened granular layer with large, irregularly shaped keratohyaline granules.

In the *atrophic type* of actinic keratosis, hyperkeratosis usually is slight. The epidermis is thinned and devoid of rete ridges. Atypicality of the cells is found predominantly in the basal cell layer, which consists of cells with large hyperchromatic nuclei that lie close together (Fig. 30-26). The atypical basal layer may proliferate into the dermis as buds and ductlike structures. It may also surround as cell mantles the upper portion of pilosebaceous follicles and sweat ducts, the epithelium of which otherwise appears normal.[196]

The *bowenoid type* of actinic keratosis is histologically indistinguishable from Bowen's disease. As in Bowen's disease, there is within the epidermis considerable disorder in the arrangement of the nuclei, as well as clumping of nuclei and dyskeratosis (Fig. 30-27).

In the *acantholytic type* of actinic keratosis, immediately above the atypical cells composing the basal cell layer there are clefts or lacunae similar to those seen in Darier's disease (Chap. 6).[199] These clefts form as a result of anaplastic changes in the lowermost epidermis, resulting in dyskeratosis and loss of the intercellular bridges (Fig. 30-28). A few acantholytic cells may be present within the clefts (Fig. 3-29). Because the acantholysis is preceded by cellular changes, it is referred to as *secondary acantholysis*, in contrast to the primary acantholysis seen in the "acantholytic" diseases, such as pemphigus vulgaris and Darier's disease. Above the acantholytic clefts, the epider-

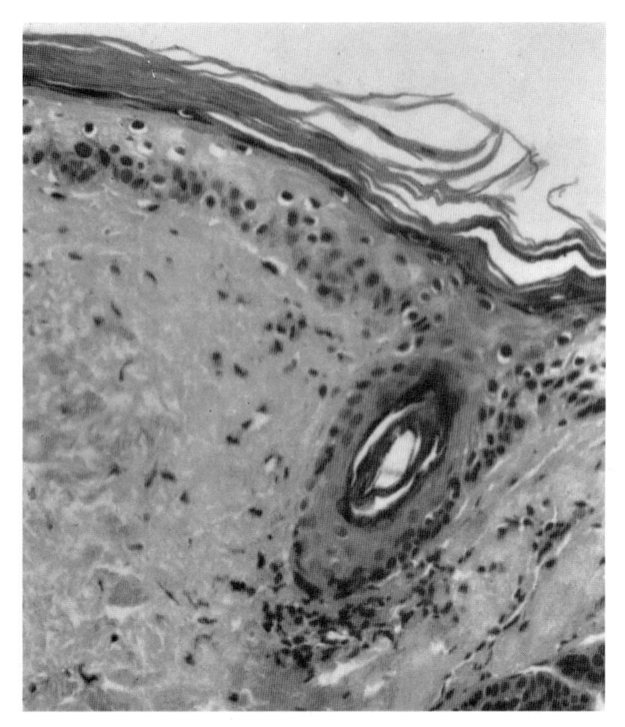

FIG. 30-26. Actinic keratosis, atrophic type
Hyperkeratosis is mild. The epidermis is atrophic. The nuclei of the basal cells are anaplastic and appear crowded together. Anaplastic basal cells also line a hair follicle as a cell mantle.

mis shows varying degrees of atypicality but generally less atypicality than is seen in the basal cell layer. The anaplastic cells of the basal cell layer frequently show extensions into the upper dermis as buds or short, ductlike structures. Suprabasal acantholysis may be seen also around hair follicles and sweat ducts in the upper dermis. When atypia is full-thickness or high-grade, the term *acantholytic squamous cell carcinoma in situ* may be applied.

In the *pigmented type* of actinic keratosis, excessive amounts of melanin are present, especially in the basal cell layer. In some cases, the atypical keratinocytes are well melanized.[200] In others, almost all the melanin is retained within the cell bodies and dendrites of the melanocytes, indicating some block in melanin transfer. Numerous melanophages are seen in most cases in the superficial dermis.[187]

In all five types of actinic keratosis, the upper dermis usually shows a fairly dense, chronic inflammatory infiltrate composed predominantly of lymphoid cells but often also containing plasma cells. Solar cheilitis, more frequently than actinic keratosis of the skin, shows an inflammatory infiltrate in which plasma cells predominate.[188] Although the upper dermis usually shows solar or basophilic degeneration, this may be absent in areas with a pronounced inflammatory reaction, probably because the inflammation has resulted in a regeneration of collagen.

In instances in which the histologic diagnosis is actinic keratosis but the clinical diagnosis is squamous cell carcinoma, it is advisable to section more deeply into the block of tissue, because progression into squamous cell carcinoma may have taken place in another area. Because no sharp line of demarcation exists between the two conditions, it is not always possible to decide whether a lesion can still be regarded as a actinic keratosis or should be classified as an early squamous cell carcinoma. Thus some authors regard squamous cell carcinoma as a lesion in which irregular aggregates of atypical keratinocytes are found in the papillary dermis, not in continuity with the overlying epidermis[201]; others call a lesion that does not extend downward to the level of the reticular dermis an actinic keratosis without qualification.[202] This decision is rarely a vital one, because early squamous cell carcinoma arising in an actinic keratosis rarely causes metastases, although it may become deeply invasive and destructive through further growth. Because carcinomas arising in solar cheilitis have a significantly higher tendency to metastasize than carcinomas arising in actinic keratosis, and because invasion of the dermis in solar cheilitis may be focal, lesions of solar cheilitis require thorough examination by means of step sections.[189]

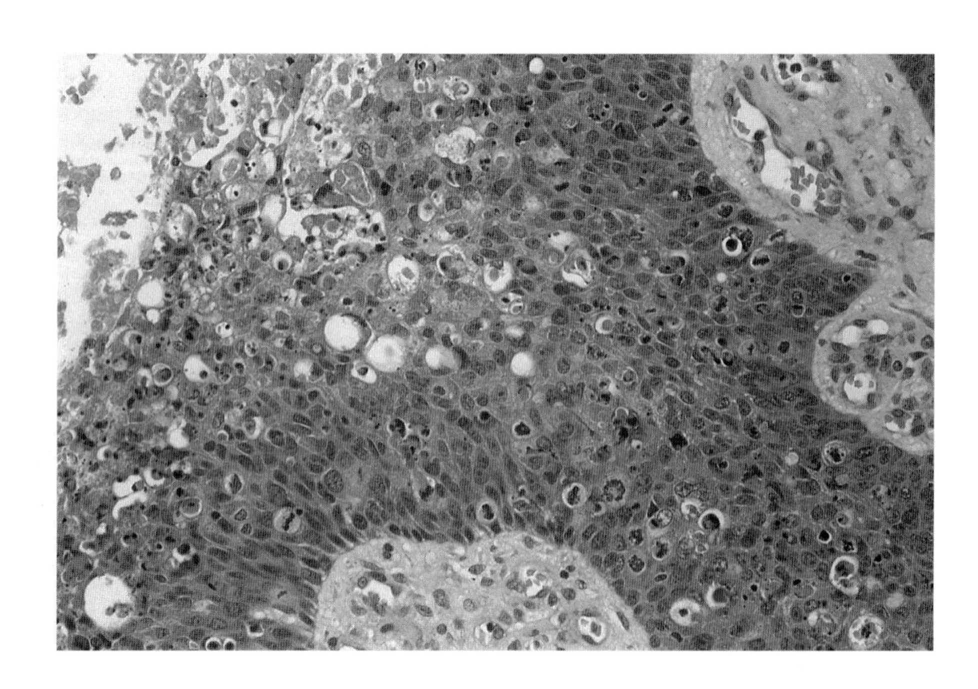

FIG. 30-27. Actinic keratosis, Bowenoid type
Marked cellular and nuclear pleomorphism are present together with frequent and atypical mitoses in a Bowenoid actinic keratosis (squamous cell carcinoma in situ).

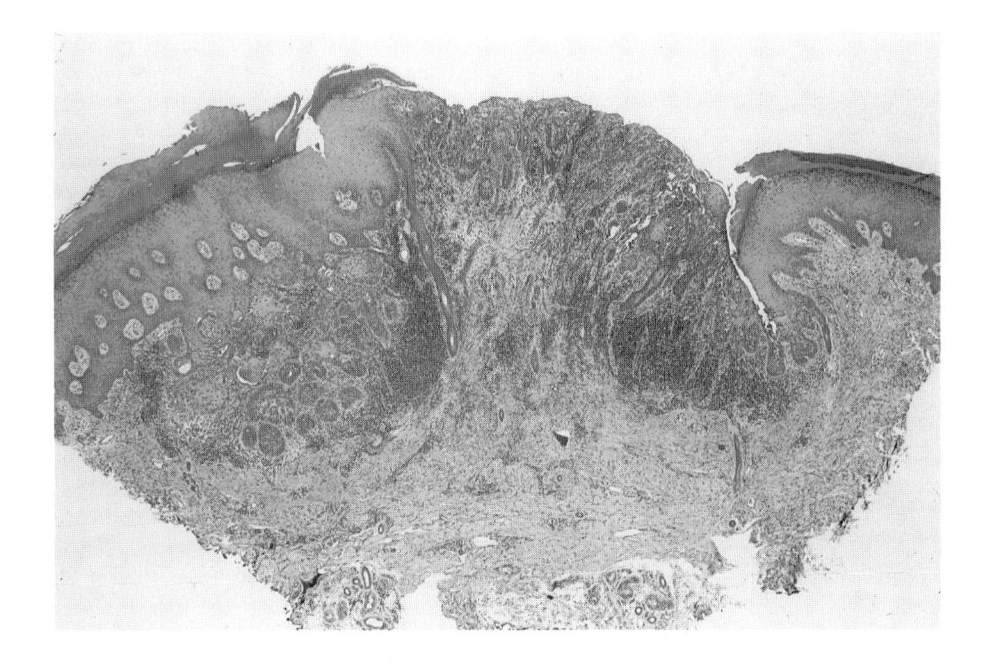

FIG. 30-28. Actinic keratosis, acantholytic type
There are hyperkeratosis and parakeratosis, and the epidermis is irregularly thickened. In the dermis, there is elastosis and a dense lichenoid inflammatory infiltrate. The keratosis is partly ulcerated and shows focal acantholytic change.

Pathogenesis. On electron microscopic examination, only a difference in degree was found to exist between actinic keratosis and squamous cell carcinoma.[203] In applying blood group antigens as indicators of malignancy to sections of actinic keratosis, areas of positive staining alternate with areas showing no staining, the lack of staining being indicative of anaplasia. Areas of irregular downward proliferation or early invasion are consistently negative.[204]

Differential Diagnosis. In actinic keratoses showing relatively slight atypicality, or anaplasia, of the tumor cells, diagnosis may be difficult. Thus a hypertrophic actinic keratosis with a lichenoid inflammatory infiltrate may show a close histologic resemblance to the lesion known as *benign lichenoid keratosis.* In fact, this lesion was at one time thought to be a variant of actinic keratosis.[205] Benign lichenoid keratosis differs from actinic keratosis by showing dissolution rather than atypicality of the basal cell layer, analogous to lichen planus (Chap. 7).[206,207]

An atrophic actinic keratosis may closely resemble lupus erythematosus, because both types of lesions show flattening of the epidermis. Although lupus erythematosus shows vacuolization and actinic keratosis shows atypicality of the cells in the basal layer, these two changes are not always easily distinguished from one another. Therefore, other findings, such as follicular plugging and a patchy, periappendageal infiltrate in lupus erythematosus, are necessary for differentiation (Chap. 10).

A pigmented actinic keratosis may resemble lentigo maligna, particularly if the melanin is seen largely within the melanocytes.[187] Usually, however, lentigo maligna shows more flattening of the epidermis than pigmented actinic keratosis and, more important, a great increase in the number of melanocytes, together with atypicality in the melanocytes but not in the basal keratinocytes (Chap. 29).

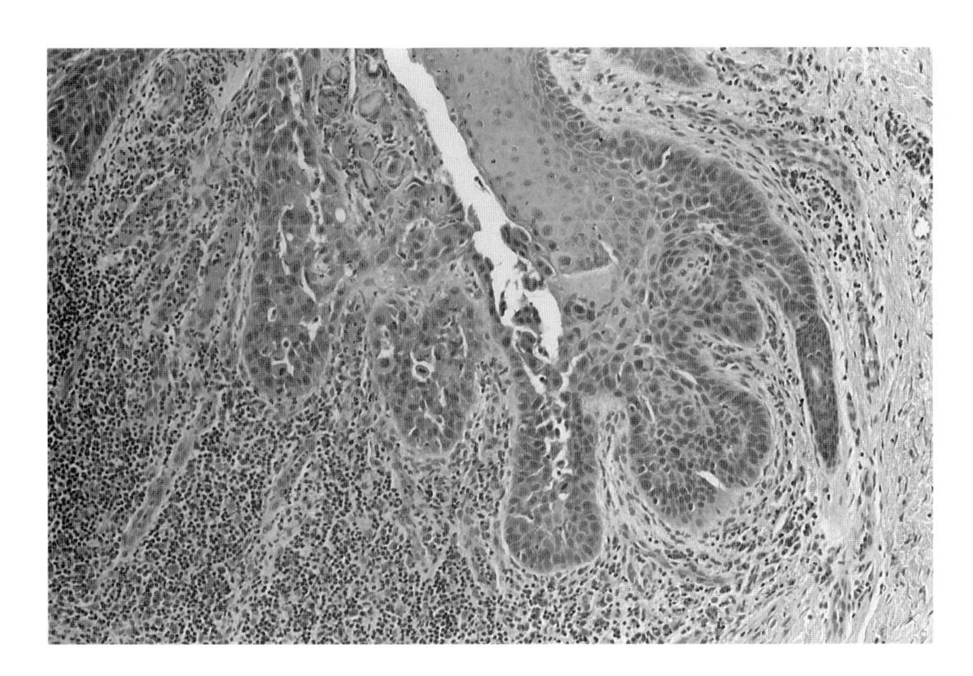

FIG. 30-29. Actinic keratosis, acantholytic type
Keratinocytes in the basal layer are crowded, with an increased nuclear-cytoplasmic ratio, and they tend to become separated from one another and to adopt a rounded configuration. This process of "secondary acantholysis" may in some instances result in the formation of pseudoglandular spaces that may mimic a glandular pattern of differentiation.

CUTANEOUS HORN

Cutaneous horn, or *cornu cutaneum,* is the clinical term for a circumscribed, conical, markedly hyperkeratotic lesion in which the height of the keratotic mass amounts to at least half of its largest diameter.[208] The term refers to a reaction pattern and not to a specific lesion.[209]

Histopathology. On histologic examination, different types of lesions can be seen at the base of the conical hyperkeratosis of a cornu cutaneum. Most commonly, an actinic keratosis is encountered.[210] In some instances, a filiform verruca, a seborrheic keratosis, or a squamous cell carcinoma is found.[208] On rare occasions, a trichilemmoma[209] or a basal cell epithelioma is seen.[211] For a description of trichilemmal horn, see Chap. 31.

ORAL LEUKOPLAKIA

The term *leukoplakia* was used in the past by dermatologists and gynecologists[212] to designate white patches of the oral mucosa or the vulva that showed early, in situ, anaplastic changes; the term *leukokeratosis* was used for patches with a histologically benign appearance. However, leukoplakia has been redefined on the basis of the concept proposed by oral pathologists,[213] and this concept has been accepted by the World Health Association.[214]

According to this concept, the term *leukoplakia* carries no histologic connotation and is used only as a clinical description. It is defined as a white patch or plaque that will not rub off and that cannot be characterized clinically or histologically as any specific disease (e.g., lichen planus, lupus erythematosus, candidiasis, white sponge nevus).[215] The reason for using the term *leukoplakia* as a purely clinical designation is that a distinction between benign leukoplakia and leukoplakia with dysplastic changes cannot be made on clinical grounds. It is therefore essential that all white plaques that either are idiopathic in origin or persist for 3 to 4 weeks after any existing irritation has been eliminated be examined histologically.[216] In many cases of oral leukoplakia, either chemical irritation through tobacco or mechanical irritation through dental stumps or ill-fitting dentures plays a role. Although the leukoplakia clears in some instances after the irritation has been removed, it persists in others. However, the transformation of a benign leukoplakia into a malignant leukoplakia is regarded as rare.[217] Still, any leukoplakia that is growing or altering its appearance requires a repeat biopsy.[28]

Clinically, lesions of leukoplakia on the oral mucosa consist of one or several white patches that may not be raised and that appear ill defined. However, if they are slightly elevated, they appear sharply demarcated, with an irregular outline.

Erythroplakia of the oral mucosa consists of red, sharply delineated patches that vary greatly in size. Some of these lesions are sprinkled or intermingled with patches of leukoplakia and are then referred to as *speckled erythroplakia.*[218]

On examination by histology, scraping, or culture, both leukoplakia and erythroplakia frequently show *Candida albicans* as a secondary invader, a finding that may give rise to an incorrect diagnosis of candidiasis.[219] However, infection with *C albicans* may cause oral lesions that are clinically indistinguishable from leukoplakia.[220]

The analysis of oral leukoplakias and oral invasive carcinomas for human papillomavirus-related DNA has shown a significant percentage of these lesions to be reactive with papillomavirus antibodies, allowing the conclusion that they are induced by papillomaviruses, especially by HPV-11 and HPV-16[221,222] (Chap. 26).

For a discussion of leukoplakia of the vulva, see p. 711, and of oral hairy leukoplakia, see Chap. 26.

Histopathology. The white color of leukoplakia is the result of hydration of a thickened horny layer. On histologic examination, about 80% of the lesions of oral leukoplakia are found to be benign.[215,219] Such lesions show hyperkeratotic or parakeratotic thickening of the horny layer, acanthosis, and a chronic inflammatory infiltrate. Of the remaining 20% of the cases, 17% show varying degrees of dysplasia or in situ carcinoma, and 3% show infiltrating squamous cell carcinoma.[215] Ultimate development of carcinoma has been observed in 7% to 13% of all cases of leukoplakia.[214] Localization of the leukoplakia seems to play an important role in the presence of malignancy. Leukoplakias on the buccal mucosa were found to be benign in 96% of the cases; whereas on the floor of the mouth, only 32% of the leukoplakias were benign, 31% showed a carcinoma in situ, and 37% an invasive carcinoma.[223]

In situ carcinoma, also referred to as precancerous leukoplakia, usually has the same histologic appearance as the hypertrophic type of actinic keratosis. Thus the most important features observed within a moderately acanthotic epithelium are, first, pleomorphism and atypicality of the nuclei, which appear large, irregular, and hyperchromatic, and, second, loss of polarity, resulting in a disorderly arrangement of the cells (Fig. 30-30). In some instances, one finds as additional features premature keratinization resulting in dyskeratotic cells in the midportion of the epithelium, crowding of nuclei in the basal cell layer, and irregular downward proliferations of the epithelium.

Erythroplakia of the oral mucosa, in contrast to leukoplakia, invariably shows nuclear atypicality. One observes in situ carcinoma in half of the cases and invasive carcinoma in the other half.[218] The red appearance is explained by the absence of the normal surface covering of orthokeratin or parakeratin.

Differential Diagnosis. A decision as to whether in situ carcinoma exists in a leukoplakia can be difficult, since some pleomorphism of nuclei and some loss of polarity of the cells can be seen occasionally also in various inflammatory conditions, including benign leukoplakia.[216] In cases of doubt, step sections throughout the biopsy specimen are required, as well as, possibly, examination of additional biopsy specimens. The decision as to whether a leukoplakia is benign or is a carcinoma in situ is of great importance. In comparison with squamous cell carcinoma of the skin developing in an actinic keratosis, squamous cell carcinoma of the oral mucosa developing in a leukoplakia with in situ carcinoma has a much greater tendency to metastasize.

Also, differentiation of leukoplakia from oral lichen planus may cause difficulties both clinically and histologically. In lichen planus no atypia is seen and there often is partial absence of basal cells. In addition, the prevalence of Langerhans' cells in lesions of lichen planus may aid in the differentiation.[224]

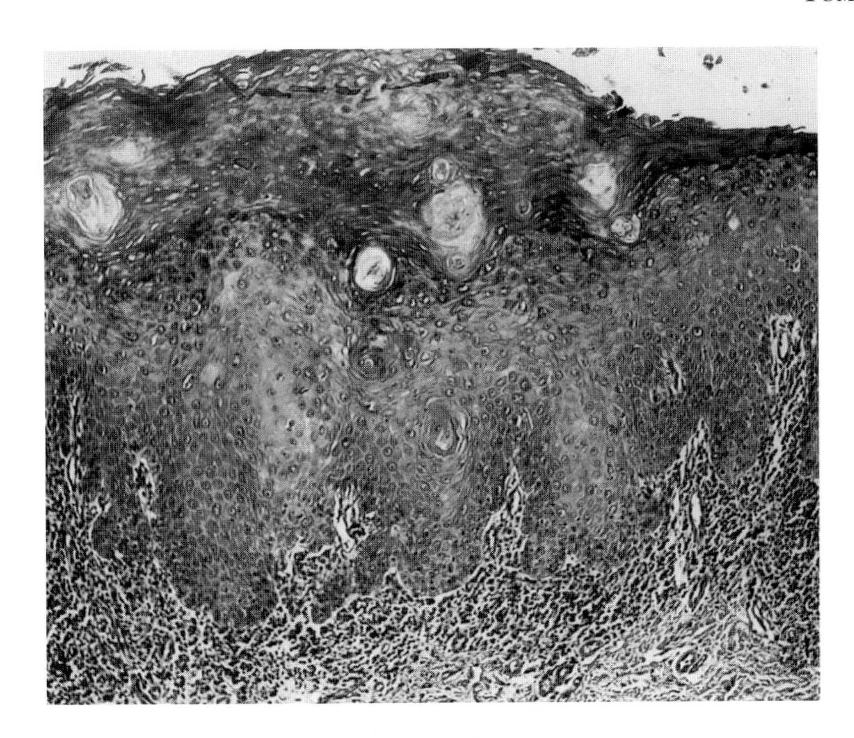

FIG. 30-30. Leukoplakia of the oral mucosa with in situ anaplasia
The lesion shows hyperkeratosis and acanthosis. In addition to disorderly arrangement of the cells, there is nuclear atypicality.

VERRUCOUS HYPERPLASIA, VERRUCOUS CARCINOMA OF THE ORAL MUCOSA

Verrucous hyperplasia of the oral mucosa consists of extensive verrucous, white patches that may arise as such or develop from lesions of leukoplakia. Verrucous hyperplasia and verrucous carcinoma are indistinguishable clinically. They may coexist, or verrucous carcinoma may develop from verrucous hyperplasia. In some instances, verrucous hyperplasia develops into frank squamous cell carcinoma rather than into verrucous carcinoma.[225]

Verrucous carcinoma of the oral mucosa is also known as *oral florid papillomatosis*. Clinically, one observes white, cauliflower-like lesions that may involve large areas of the oral mucosa and that gradually extend and coalesce. Extensive local tissue destruction may occur. However, metastases are rare and, if they occur, remain limited to the regional lymph nodes.[226–228]

Histopathology. Verrucous hyperplasia shows a hyperplastic epithelium with upward extension of verrucous projections located predominantly superficial to the adjacent epithelium.[225]

Verrucous carcinoma (oral florid papillomatosis) differs in its early stage from verrucous hyperplasia by showing, in addition to the surface verrucous projections, extension of the lesion into the underlying connective tissue.[225] The downward extensions of the epithelium are round and club-shaped and appear well demarcated from the surrounding stroma. Nuclear pleomorphism or hyperchromasia and formation of horn pearls are absent.

Some lesions of verrucous carcinoma persist in this stage for many years, although ultimately they show in the areas of deepest extension a moderate loss of polarity, increased cytoplasmic basophilia, nuclear hyperchromasia, and frequent mitotic figures. These features, however, do not suffice for a diagnosis of squamous cell carcinoma.[229] Other lesions show sufficient nuclear atypicality and loss of polarity in the downward proliferations to indicate the presence of a well-differentiated squamous cell carcinoma.[230] In about 10% of the cases of verrucous carcinoma, transformation into a classic squamous cell carcinoma takes place.[227,228] (For a more detailed discussion of verrucous carcinoma, see p. 716.)

NECROTIZING SIALOMETAPLASIA

One or occasionally two ulcers showing a rolled border and measuring 1 to 2 cm in diameter are found usually on the hard palate, but occasionally on the soft palate. If located on the hard palate, bone may be exposed at the base of the ulcer. Spontaneous healing takes place within 6 to 12 weeks. The importance of necrotizing sialometaplasia, a rare condition first reported in 1973,[231] lies in its clinical and histologic resemblance to carcinoma.[186]

Histopathology. Histologic examination shows coagulative necrosis of salivary gland lobules and squamous metaplasia within adjacent viable lobules. The connective tissue framework of the necrotic glands remains intact, thereby preserving the lobular architecture of the salivary gland. Faintly basophilic material representing sialomucin is seen within the necrotic glands. This is both PAS-positive and alcian-blue–positive. Adjacent to the necrotic glands, one may see normal-appearing salivary gland acini. Other salivary gland structures show either partial squamous metaplasia, with a peripheral rim of squamous cells, or complete replacement by squamous epithelium. The squamous metaplasia also involves the salivary ducts.[232,233]

Pathogenesis. The abrupt clinical onset and rapid spontaneous healing suggest that an acute vascular insult results in infarction and coagulation necrosis of the salivary acini.[232]

Differential Diagnosis. To pathologists not familiar with this condition, the apparent irregular proliferation and deep extension of squamous epithelium may suggest a diagnosis of carcinoma. However, the confinement of cytologically benign squamous epithelium to the preexisting lobular pattern of salivary glands should permit the correct diagnosis.[234]

EOSINOPHILIC ULCER OF THE TONGUE

One or two asymptomatic ulcers measuring 0.8 to 2.0 cm in diameter arise suddenly on the tongue. Spontaneous healing takes place within a few weeks.

Histopathology. A dense cellular infiltrate is present at the base of the ulcer, extending through the submucosa into the striated muscle bundles of the tongue. Most of the cells are eosinophils, but there are also lymphocytes and histiocytes.[235,236] In one case, focal leukocytoclastic vasculitis was present.[237]

Differential Diagnosis. This lesion differs from eosinophilic granuloma of histiocytosis X (see Chap. 27) clinically by its tendency to arise and heal rapidly, and histologically by the smaller number and smaller size of the histiocytes.[235]

BOWEN'S DISEASE

Bowen's disease usually consists of a solitary lesion. It may occur on exposed or on unexposed skin. It may be caused on exposed skin by exposure to the sun and on unexposed skin by the ingestion of arsenic (see Pathogenesis, following and Arsenical Keratosis and Carcinoma). Lesions of Bowen's disease can form in lesions of epidermodysplasia verruciformis caused by HPV-5 (see Chap. 26). Not infrequently the fingers, including the nail fold or nail bed, are involved.[238]

Bowen's disease manifests itself as a slowly enlarging erythematous patch of sharp but irregular outline, showing little or no infiltration. Within the patch are generally areas of scaling and crusting. Although Bowen's disease may resemble a superficial basal cell epithelioma, it differs from it by the absence of a fine pearly border and lack of a tendency to heal with central atrophy. Lesions of Bowen's disease can occur on the glans penis, where they are referred to also as erythroplasia of Queyrat.

Bowenoid papulosis of the genitalia, because of its probable relationship to genital warts, is discussed in Chap. 26.

Histopathology. Bowen's disease is an intraepidermal squamous cell carcinoma referred to also as squamous cell carcinoma in situ. Thus it represents biologically but not morphologically a *precancerous dermatosis,* under which designation it was described originally in 1912.[239]

The epidermis shows acanthosis with elongation and thickening of the rete ridges, often to such a degree that the papillae located between the rete ridges are reduced to thin strands (Fig. 30-31). Throughout the epidermis, the cells lie in complete disorder, resulting in a "windblown" appearance (Fig. 30-32). Many cells appear highly atypical, showing large, hyperchromatic nuclei. Multinucleated epidermal cells containing clusters of nuclei are often present (Fig. 30-33). The horny layer usually is thickened and consists largely of parakeratotic cells with atypical, hyperchromatic nuclei.[240]

A common and rather characteristic feature is the presence of cells showing atypical individual cell keratinization (Fig. 30-34). Such dyskeratotic cells are large and round and have a homogeneous, strongly eosinophilic cytoplasm and a hyperchromatic nucleus. The infiltrate of atypical cells in Bowen's disease frequently extends into follicular infundibula and causes replacement of the follicular epithelium by atypical cells down to the entrance of the sebaceous duct.[184]

Even though the marked atypicality of the epidermal cells includes the cells of the basal layer, the border between the epidermis and dermis everywhere appears sharp, and the basement membrane remains intact. The upper dermis usually shows a moderate amount of a chronic inflammatory infiltrate.

An occasional finding in Bowen's disease is vacuolization of the cells, especially in the upper portion of the epidermis.[241] Also, in exceptional cases, multiple nests of atypical cells are scattered through a normal epidermis, sometimes with sparing of the basal cell layer. This results in a histologic picture that

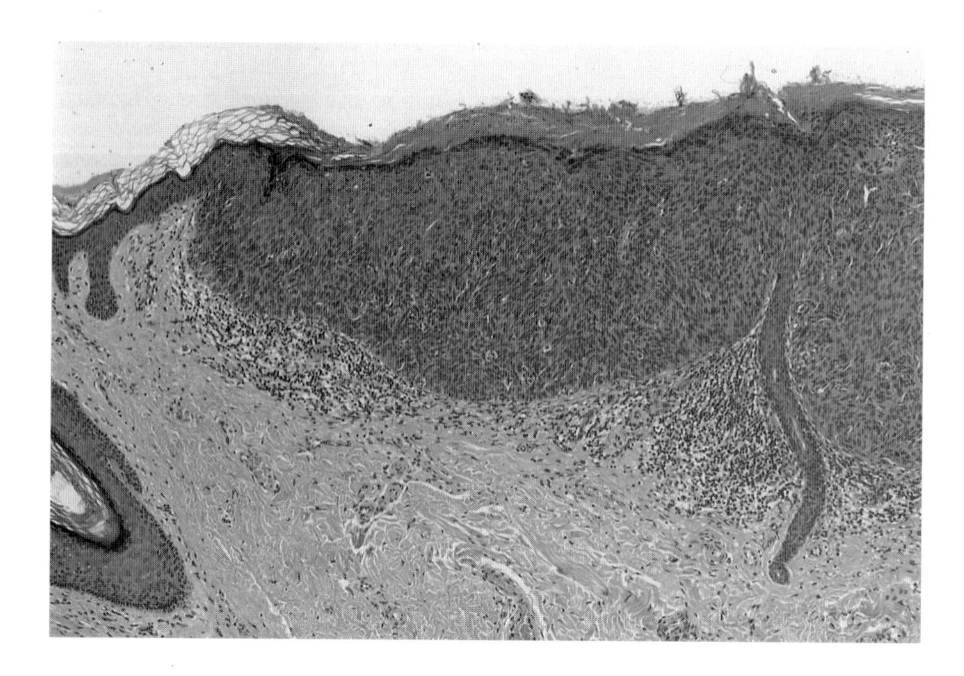

FIG. 30-31. Bowen's disease The epidermis is irregularly thickened with obliteration of the rete ridges. The normal maturation pattern is effaced.

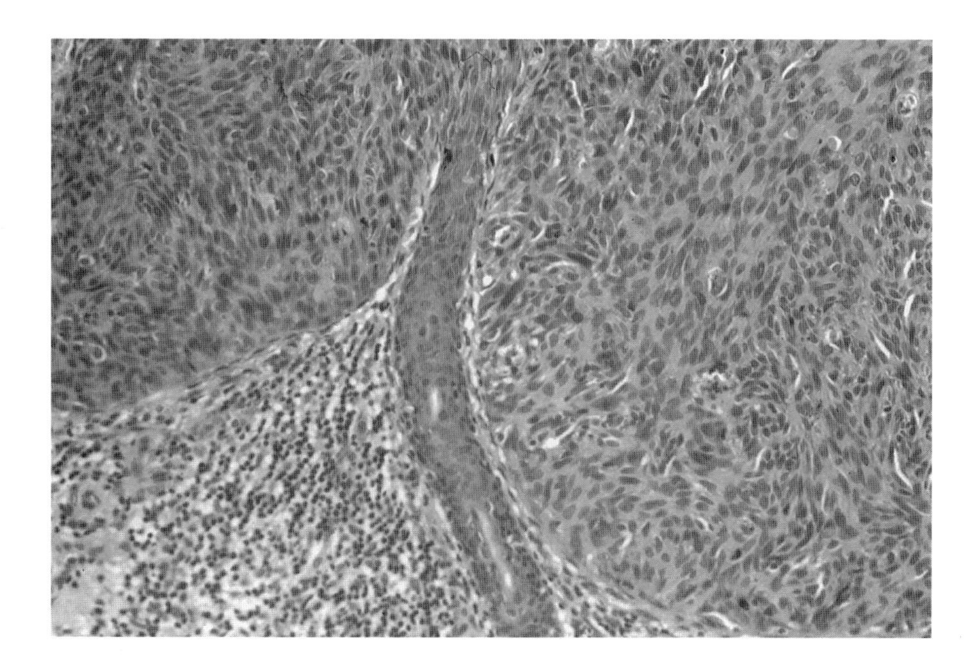

FIG. 30-32. Bowen's disease Throughout the epidermis, the cells lie in disarray, resulting in a "wind-blown" appearance. The Bowenoid proliferation extends downward into the dermis but does not invade an eccrine sweat duct.

used to be interpreted as intraepidermal epithelioma of Borst-Jadassohn (Chap. 31).[184,242]

In a small percentage of cases of Bowen's disease, an invasive squamous cell carcinoma develops. The usual figure quoted is 3% to 5%.[243] The highest incidence given is 11%.[244] On the opposite end is a statement that, in the vast majority of cases, Bowen's disease remains a carcinoma in situ during the lives of those affected.[245] If invasion happens, it usually takes place after many years' duration of the disease. The invasive tumor retains the cytologic characteristics of the intraepidermal tumor, and invasion may occur at first in only a limited area. To avoid missing such an area, it is advisable to examine representative sections throughout the entire tissue block. As soon as invasion has taken place, the prognosis changes. So long as Bowen's disease remains in its intraepidermal stage, metastases do not occur. However, once invasion of the dermis has occurred, there exists the possibility of regional and even visceral metastases.[244]

Pathogenesis. No agreement exists about the frequency with which visceral carcinoma develops in patients with Bowen's disease. The first authors to point out an association between Bowen's disease and visceral cancer found that, of 35 patients with Bowen's disease who were known to have died, 20 (57%) had an associated internal cancer.[244] In a subsequent series, however, a significant increase in the incidence of associated internal cancer was observed only in patients in whom the lesions of Bowen's disease were located in areas not exposed to the sun (33%); in patients in whom the lesions were in exposed areas, the incidence of visceral cancer was low (5%).[246] Subsequent studies, with one exception,[247] have not demonstrated in patients with Bowen's disease a significantly increased risk of internal malignancy.[184,248–250]

Electron microscopic examination of lesions of Bowen's disease has demonstrated the presence of many dyskeratotic cells. The perinuclear aggregation and condensation of tonofilaments in these dyskeratotic cells are similar to but more pronounced

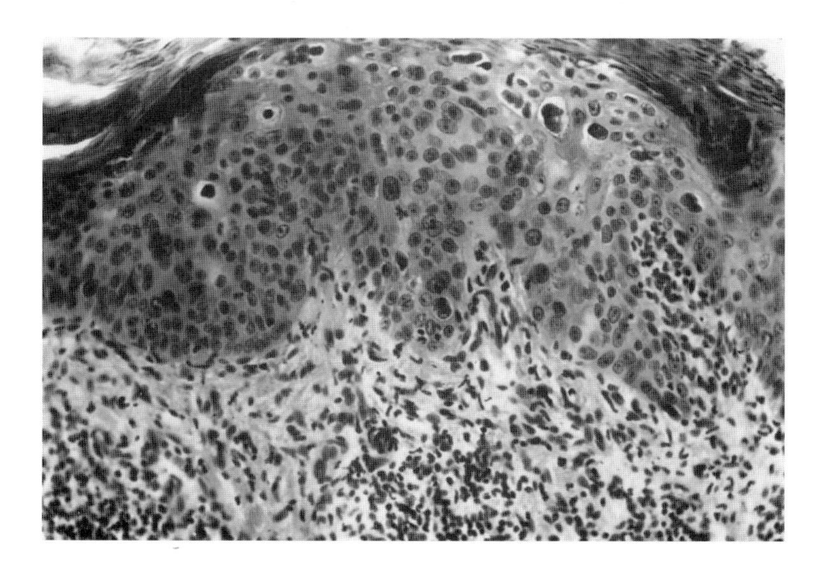

FIG. 30-33. Bowen's disease The epidermis is thickened. The border between the epidermis and dermis appears sharp. The cells of the stratum malpighii lie in complete disorder, and many of them appear atypical, showing large, hyperchromatic nuclei. Several multinucleated epidermal cells are present. The stratum corneum shows parakeratosis.

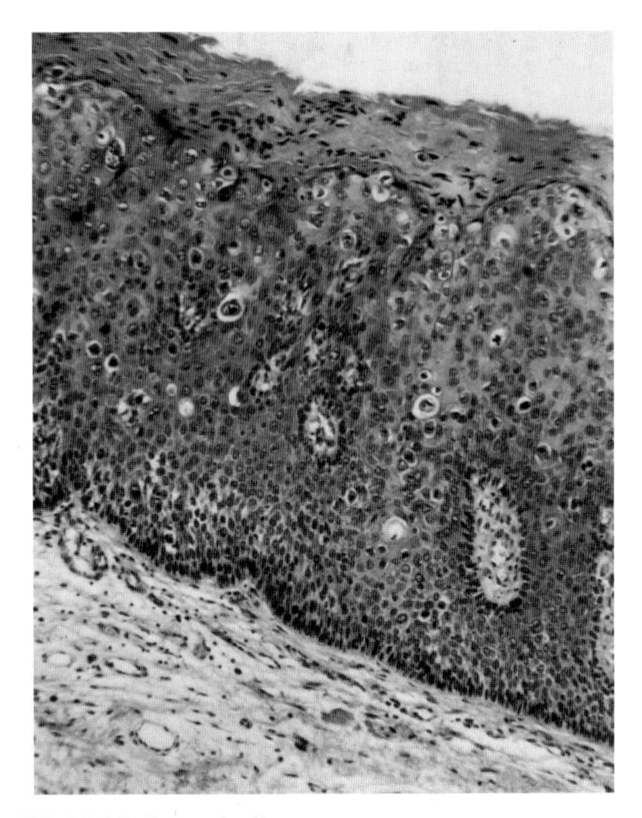

FIG. 30-34. Bowen's disease
In addition to the changes described for Fig. 30-33, there are scattered cells within the stratum malpighii showing atypical individual cell keratinization or dyskeratosis.

than in the dyskeratotic cells of Darier's disease.[251] Some of the markedly dyskeratotic cells in Bowen's disease disintegrate, and portions of such cells are phagocytized by other epidermal cells, which may contain, in addition to the phagocytized dyskeratotic material, phagocytized desmosomes in their cytoplasm.[251,252] In other instances, the intracellularly located desmosomes are not phagocytized but are drawn into the dyskeratotic cells of Bowen's disease together with aggregating tonofilaments.[253] The phenomenon of intracytoplasmic desmosomes, however, is not specific for Bowen's disease, although it is found most commonly in this condition. Thus intracytoplasmic desmosomes have been observed within dyskeratotic keratinocytes in Darier's disease,[254] squamous cell carcinoma,[255] and keratoacanthoma[256]; within nondyskeratotic keratinocytes in extramammary Paget's disease[257] and malignant melanoma[258]; and even within normal keratinocytes in both the epidermis[259] and the oral mucosa.[260] It can be assumed that the occasional occurrence of invaginations of the plasma membrane is a normal event in keratinocytes and that the invaginated plasma membrane can contain desmosomal structures. These structures are more resistant to enzymatic destruction than the plasma membrane and thus may be found free in the cytoplasm.[260]

Two types of epidermal giant cells can be recognized in Bowen's disease. In one type, an entire dyskeratotic cell has been "cannibalized" by another keratinocyte and is located within the cytoplasm of the phagocytizing cell.[261] In the second type, multiple nuclei lie in the center of the giant cell surrounded by dyskeratotic tonofilaments. It seems that, by becoming entangled with the spindles of the mitotic apparatus, the dyskeratotic tonofilaments interfere with the normal division of the cell so that nuclear division can take place but cellular division cannot.[251,252]

Differential Diagnosis. No histologic difference exists between bowenoid actinic keratosis and Bowen's disease. They differ merely in size, the bowenoid actinic keratosis usually being smaller than Bowen's disease.

Paget's disease may share with Bowen's disease the presence of vacuolated cells, but, in contrast with Bowen's disease, it shows no dyskeratosis. In addition, the material contained in Paget cells is often PAS-positive and diastase-resistant, whereas the PAS-positive material that is sometimes present in the vacuolated cells of Bowen's disease is glycogen and therefore diastase-labile.[262]

ERYTHROPLASIA OF QUEYRAT (BOWEN'S DISEASE OF THE GLANS PENIS, CARCINOMA IN SITU)

Erythroplasia of Queyrat is the term often used for carcinoma in situ located on the glans penis. Clinically and histologically, it is identical to Bowen's disease, and this designation would seem preferable for simplicity's sake. The only reason for keeping the term *erythroplasia of Queyrat* alive is that it was introduced in 1911,[263] 1 year before the description of Bowen's disease.[239]

Erythroplasia or Bowen's disease of the glans penis is seen almost exclusively in uncircumcised men. It manifests itself as an asymptomatic, sharply demarcated, bright red, shiny, very slightly infiltrated plaque on the glans penis, or less often, in the coronal sulcus or on the inner surface of the prepuce.[264]

Histopathology. Erythroplasia of Queyrat of the glans penis has the same histologic appearance as Bowen's disease. Progression into an invasive squamous cell carcinoma has been observed in up to 30% of the patients,[265] with metastases in about 20% of the patients with invasive erythroplasia.[266] It thus has a greater tendency toward invasion and metastasis than Bowen's disease of the skin.[265]

Differential Diagnosis. A clinical diagnosis of erythroplasia of Queyrat requires histologic examination of an adequate biopsy for confirmation, since differentiation from balanitis circumscripta plasmacellularis is not possible on a clinical basis.

BALANITIS CIRCUMSCRIPTA PLASMACELLULARIS

A disorder first described by Zoon in 1952,[267] balanitis circumscripta plasmacellularis has the same clinical appearance as erythroplasia of Queyrat or Bowen's disease of the glans penis. In some instances, erosions with a tendency to bleed are present.[268] Like erythroplasia, this disorder is seen almost exclusively in uncircumcised males.[269] On rare occasions, an analogous lesion referred to as *vulvitis circumscripta plasmacellularis* is observed on the vulva.[270,271]

Histopathology. The epidermis appears thinned and often shows absence of its upper layers.[272] It may be partially detached as a result of subepidermal cleavage or even absent.[268,273] If present, the epidermis often has a rather distinctive appearance; in addition to being thinned and flattened, it is composed of diamond- or lozenge-shaped, flattened keratinocytes that are separated from each other by uniform intercellular edema.[269] Erythrocytes may be seen permeating the epidermis. In some cases, the keratinocytes appear degenerated or necrotic.[272]

The upper dermis shows a bandlike infiltrate in which numerous plasma cells are often seen.[267,272] In some cases, however, their number is only moderate[269] or even small.[273] In addition, the capillaries are dilated, and there may be extravasations of erythrocytes and deposits of hemosiderin.[274]

Pathogenesis. It has been pointed out that plasma cells frequently predominate in the inflammatory response at mucocutaneous junctions in a variety of benign and malignant processes. Thus the term *circumorificial plasmacytosis* was introduced for benign plasma cell infiltrates on the glans penis, vulva, and lips.[275–277] However, the combination of histologic and clinical features seen in balanitis circumscripta plasmacellularis, and probably also in vulvitis circumscripta plasmacellularis, is unique and deserves recognition as an entity.[269,270,272]

LEUKOPLAKIA OF THE VULVA

As in the case of oral leukoplakia, leukoplakia of the vulva is purely a clinical designation requiring histologic examination for clarification of the diagnosis, especially to decide whether or not atypicality of the epithelial cells exists. The clinical aspect of leukoplakia of the vulva is more variable than that of oral leukoplakia because it does not always consist just of white patches as in the mouth but may have a papular or verrucous appearance. The reason is that on the vulva, human papilloma virus (HPV) infections can occur as flat papular condylomas,[278] often in association with similar lesions on the cervix. Also, bowenoid papulosis, in the presence of multiple, coalescing papules, may result in a verrucous aspect of the leukoplakia (Chap. 26).[279] A clear-cut histologic decision often is not possible unless adequate clinical data are available.

Histopathology. Flat condylomas show intracellular vacuolization that may result in a somewhat atypical appearance of the epithelium referred to as *koilocytotic atypia*. This may be difficult to differentiate from true atypia.[278] In the case of bowenoid papulosis, clinical data are needed for a differentiation from true Bowen's disease (Chap. 26).

ARSENICAL KERATOSIS AND CARCINOMA

Inorganic arsenic was a frequently used oral medication for a number of dermatoses until evidence accumulated in the 1930s that, besides its long-known tendency to form arsenical keratoses on the palms and soles, inorganic arsenic quite frequently causes carcinoma of the skin.[280] In the 1950s, it became apparent that inorganic arsenic could cause visceral carcinoma. The most common form in which inorganic arsenic has been administered was Fowler's solution containing 1% potassium arsenite.

Careless handling of industrial wastes can introduce arsenic into well water used for domestic consumption, resulting in "epidemic" occurrences of arsenical keratoses and cutaneous carcinomas.[281,282]

Arsenical keratoses of the palms and soles, consisting of verrucous papules without surrounding inflammation, are a common manifestation of prolonged arsenic ingestion. Thus, in a follow-up study of 262 patients who had been taking Fowler's solution for 6 to 26 years before this study, arsenical keratoses of the palms and soles were observed in 40%, and arsenic-induced carcinomas of the skin in 8%.[283] In the study from Taiwan, 80% of the 428 patients with arsenical carcinomas of the skin had arsenical keratoses of the palms and soles.[284] The minimal latent period between the beginning of arsenic intake and the onset of arsenical keratoses of the palms and soles has been found to be 2.5 years, and the average latent period 6 years.[283]

Cutaneous carcinomas following arsenic ingestion are usually multiple, and about three quarters of them are located on the trunk.[284] They consist of erythematous, scaling, occasionally crusted patches that slowly increase in size. Carcinomas can also arise in arsenical keratoses of the palms and soles.[283,284] The average latency between the beginning of arsenic intake and the onset of carcinoma has been 18 years, with a range from 3 to 40 years.[285]

Visceral carcinoma can be caused by arsenic intake, but the actual incidence is difficult to determine because of the long latent period, which may vary from 13 to 50 years, with an average of 24 years.[286] The most common locations appear to be bronchi and the genitourinary system.[283,286] There are on record two incidences of prolonged arsenic intake in which lung cancer occurred in a high percentage of the patients: one report concerned vineyard workers exposed to an arsenic insecticide[287] and the other dealt with villagers exposed to arsenic-containing drinking water.[288] In the latter series, the onset of pulmonary cancer started 30 years after the arsenic exposure.

Because Bowen's disease is the most common cutaneous carcinoma produced by arsenic, the possibility of a relationship between Bowen's disease and visceral carcinoma is of interest. This association, first pointed out in 1959,[244] appears to be greatest in those cases of Bowen's disease in which the lesions are located in unexposed areas and thus are not caused by sun exposure. In one report, an association with internal carcinoma was found in about one third of the cases.[246] It has been suggested that arsenic is the common denominator in such cases, causing both Bowen's disease and internal carcinoma. However, subsequent studies have shown no significant relationship between Bowen's disease in covered areas and internal malignancy[248]; or, if such a relationship has been found to exist, no arsenic ingestion has been found in most of the patients.[247]

Histopathology. In arsenical keratoses of the palms and soles, one may find, in some instances, only hyperkeratosis and acanthosis without evidence of nuclear atypicality.[284] However, when one cuts deeper into the tissue block, atypicality may become apparent. Whereas some arsenical keratoses show only mild nuclear atypicality, the findings in others are those of a squamous cell carcinoma in situ and are analogous to Bowen's disease or an actinic keratosis. One observes disorder in the arrangement of the squamous cells and nuclear atypicalities, such as hyperchromasia, clumping, or dyskeratosis.[289] Atrophy of the epidermis and basophilic degeneration of the upper dermis, as seen in some actinic keratoses, are absent in arsenical keratoses. Evidence of development into an invasive squamous cell carcinoma may be seen in some arsenical keratoses.[283,284,289]

The type of cutaneous carcinoma that follows arsenic ingestion can be either squamous cell carcinoma or basal cell carcinoma, usually as multiple lesions. Squamous cell carcinomas usually occur as in situ lesions analogous to Bowen's disease, and basal cell carcinomas occur most commonly as superficial basal cell carcinomas, although invasive squamous cell carcinomas and basal cell carcinomas occur occasionally. Invasive tumors may arise de novo or may develop within preexisting lesions of Bowen's disease or superficial basal cell carcinoma.

A matter of controversy has been whether arsenical carcinomas occur more commonly as lesions of Bowen's disease or as superficial basal cell carcinomas. For many years, it was accepted that lesions of Bowen's disease were the usual reaction.[241] However, two more publications have stated that superficial basal cell carcinomas are far more prevalent than lesions of Bowen's disease[283,290]; yet, in two other publications, Bowen's disease was found to be much more common.[284,289] The most likely explanation for this discrepancy appears to be that, in many instances, lesions of Bowen's disease have been misinterpreted as superficial basal cell carcinoma.[289] The distinction can indeed be difficult; one author who found mainly superficial basal cell carcinomas conceded that 25% of them showed "squamous metaplasia,"[290] and another author has proposed the concept of "combined forms" consisting of a "mixture of superficial basal cell carcinoma and intraepidermal carcinoma."[284] It appears likely that lesions designated as superficial basal cell carcinoma with squamous metaplasia or as combined forms represent lesions of Bowen's disease. (For histologic descriptions of Bowen's disease and superficial basal cell carcinoma, see pp. 708 and 719, respectively.)

Pathogenesis. In vitro experiments concerning the effects of inorganic arsenic on human epidermal cells have shown that arsenic depresses premitotic DNA replication. Furthermore, incubation with inorganic arsenic and subsequent exposure of the cell cultures to ultraviolet light causes interruption of the enzymatic "dark repair mechanism" in the epidermal cells. Among other enzymes, arsenic seems to block predominantly DNA polymerase by attaching itself to sulfhydryl groups. The damaging effect of arsenic on DNA may explain its carcinogenic effect.[291]

SQUAMOUS CELL CARCINOMA

Squamous cell carcinoma may occur anywhere on the skin and on mucous membranes with squamous epithelium. It rarely arises from normal-appearing skin. Most commonly, it arises in sun-damaged skin, either as such or from an actinic keratosis. Next to sun-damaged skin, squamous cell carcinomas arise most commonly in scars from burns and in stasis ulcers, termed *Marjolin's ulcers.*[292] In regard to metastases, carcinomas arising in sun-damaged skin have a very low propensity to metastasize, the incidence amounting to only about 0.5%.[192] This is in contrast to a metastatic rate of 2% to 3% for all patients with squamous cell carcinoma of the skin, with death resulting in about three quarters of the patients with metastases.[193,293] Carcinomas of the lower lip, even though in most cases also induced by exposure to the sun, have a much higher incidence of metastasis, about 16%, with death occurring in about half of these patients as the result of metastases.[294] Also, the rate of metastases is higher in adenoid and mucin-producing squamous cell carcinomas of the skin than in the common type.

Cutaneous squamous cell carcinomas that arise secondary to inflammatory and degenerative processes have a much higher rate of metastasis than those developing in sun-damaged skin. Thus the rate of metastasis was found to be 31% in squamous cell carcinomas arising in osteomyelitic sinuses,[295] 20% in radiation-induced skin cancer,[296] and 18% in carcinomas developing in burn scars.[297] Furthermore, carcinomas arising from modified skin, such as the glans penis and the vulva, and from the oral mucosa have a rather high rate of metastasis unless recognized and adequately treated at an early stage.

The incidence of squamous cell carcinomas, like that of other malignant neoplasms, is significantly increased in immunosuppressed patients.[298] The incidence of cutaneous squamous cell carcinoma has been found to be 18 times greater in patients with a renal transplant and immunosuppression than in the average population.[299] Squamous cell carcinomas may also show greater aggressiveness in such patients.[300]

Clinically, squamous cell carcinoma of the skin most commonly consists of a shallow ulcer surrounded by a wide, elevated, indurated border. Often the ulcer is covered by a crust that conceals a red, granular base. Occasionally, raised, fungoid, verrucous lesions without ulceration occur.

Three variants of squamous cell carcinoma, *adenoid squamous cell carcinoma, mucin-producing squamous cell carcinoma,* and *verrucous carcinoma,* will be discussed later.

Histopathology. Squamous cell carcinoma of the skin is a true, invasive carcinoma of the surface epidermis. On histologic examination, one finds the tumor to consist of irregular masses

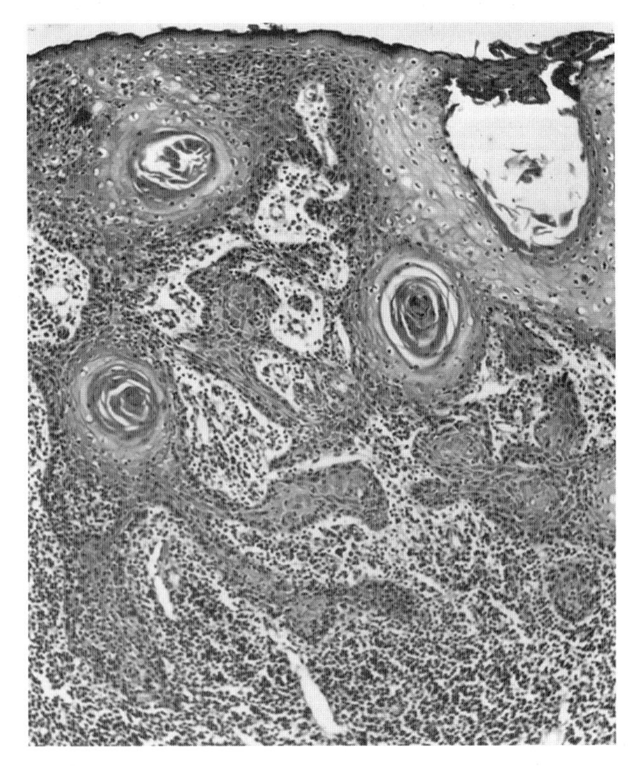

FIG. 30-35. Squamous cell carcinoma
There is invasion of the dermis by epidermal masses, the cells of which are predominantly mature squamous cells showing relatively slight atypicality. Several horn pearls are present. The dermis shows a marked inflammatory reaction.

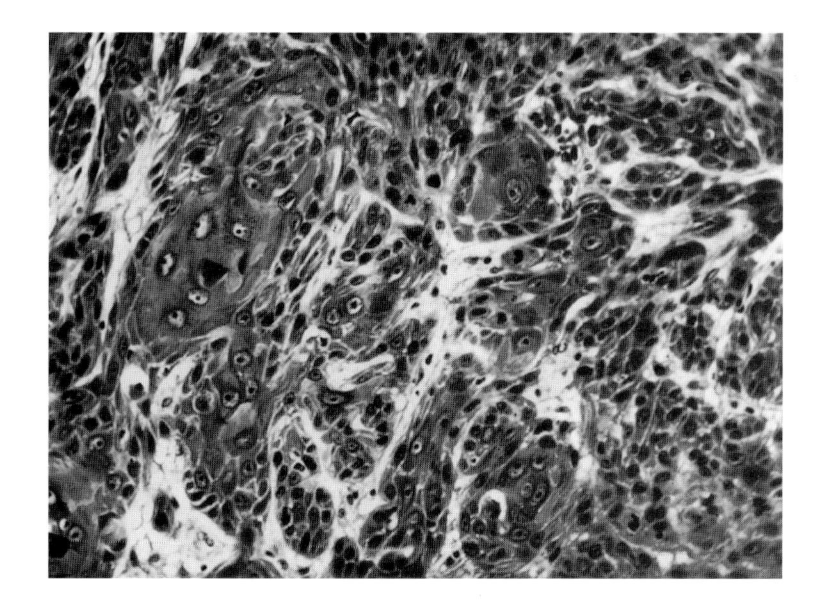

FIG. 30-36. Squamous cell carcinoma, moderately differentiated
The cell masses show much less keratinization than in a well-differentiated tumor. There are only a few horn pearls, and those present show incompletely keratinized centers. Atypical cells are conspicuous.

of epidermal cells that proliferate downward into the dermis (Fig. 30-35). The invading tumor masses are composed in varying proportions of normal squamous cells and of atypical (anaplastic) squamous cells. The number of atypical squamous cells is higher in the more poorly differentiated tumors (Fig. 30-36). Atypicality of squamous cells expresses itself in such changes as great variation in the size and shape of the cells, hyperplasia and hyperchromasia of the nuclei, absence of intercellular bridges, keratinization of individual cells, and the presence of atypical mitotic figures (Fig. 30-37).

Differentiation in squamous cell carcinoma is in the direction of keratinization. Keratinization often takes place in the form of horn pearls, which are very characteristic structures composed of concentric layers of squamous cells showing gradually increasing keratinization toward the center. The center shows usually incomplete and only rarely complete keratinization. Keratohyaline granules within the horn pearls are sparse or absent.

Marjolin's ulcer is a term applied to tumors that arise at the periphery of a chronic ulcer or a scar.[292] The scar may be due to a remote burn or to radiation, or there may be a chronic inflammatory process such as a draining osteomyelitis sinus. The tumors often are well differentiated and may arise in a background of pseudoepitheliomatous hyperplasia, making diagnosis difficult (Fig. 30-38). The tumors may be deeply invasive (Fig. 3-39).

Spindle cell squamous cell carcinoma in particular may show a great resemblance to atypical fibroxanthoma.[301] In some instances, spindle cell squamous cell carcinomas contain areas in which the cells either show intercellular bridges and beginning keratinization or show evidence of origin from the epidermis. In other cases, however, such areas cannot be detected. The spindle cells are intermingled with collagen and may be arranged in whorls.[302] Not infrequently, pleomorphic giant cells are seen (Fig. 30-40).[301] In such instances, distinction from atypical fibroxanthoma may be difficult: differential diagnosis by immunohistochemical examination is required (see Pathogenesis).

Raised, verrucous lesions of squamous cell carcinoma may show a considerable histologic resemblance to keratoacanthoma by having a central keratin-filled crater with peripheral buttresses. In most instances, however, one finds less cellular maturation and evidence of nuclear atypicality (Fig. 30-41).

Pathogenesis. Electron microscopy of squamous cell carcinoma, in comparison with normal epidermal squamous cells, shows a reduction in the number of desmosomes on the cell surface. In their place, microvilli extend into the widened intercellular spaces. Desmosomes can be seen within the cytoplasm of some of the tumor cells, either by themselves or attached to bundles of tonofilaments.[255] Their intracytoplasmic loca-

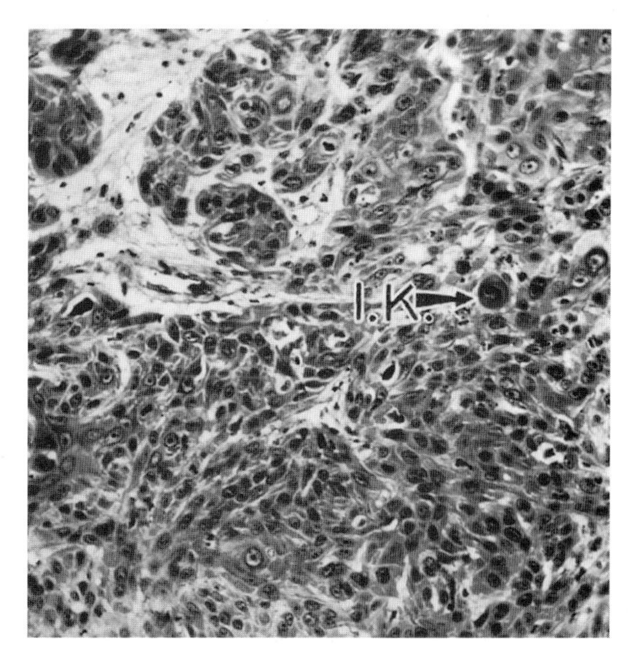

FIG. 30-37. Squamous cell carcinoma, poorly differentiated
No horn pearls are present. Keratinization occurs only in small cell groups. Many cells are atypical and devoid of prickles. To the right, a cell shows individual cell keratinization (*I.K.*).

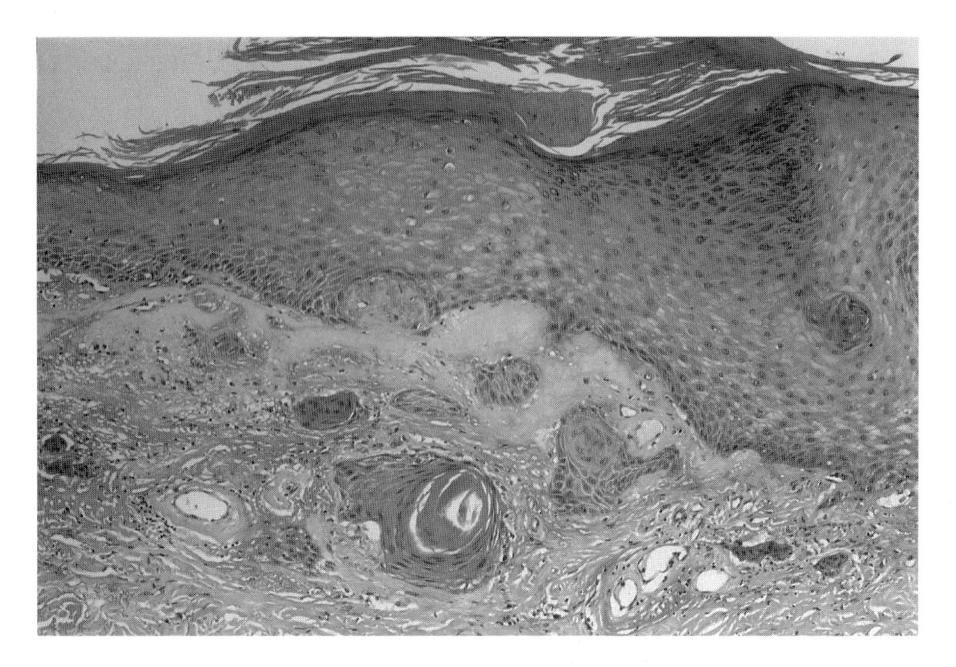

FIG. 30-38. Postradiotherapy squamous cell carcinoma
This lesion, arising in an area treated many years previously with radiotherapy, shows a combination of invasive keratinizing squamous cell carcinoma and stromal damage secondary to radiotherapy.

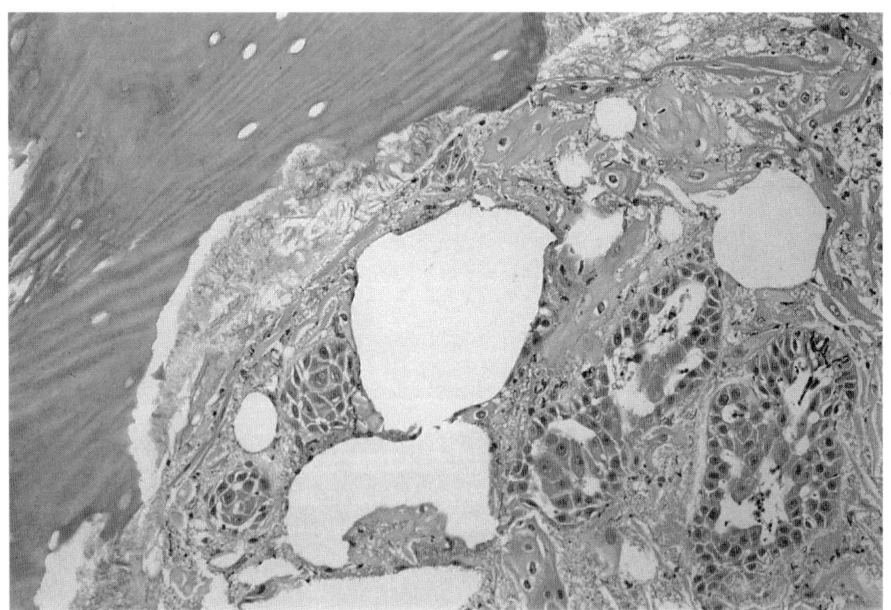

FIG. 30-39. Squamous cell carcinoma invading bone
This tumor arose in a Marjolin's ulcer. A curetting specimen from bone at the base of the ulcer shows squamous cell carcinoma invading the marrow space in association with necrotic bone.

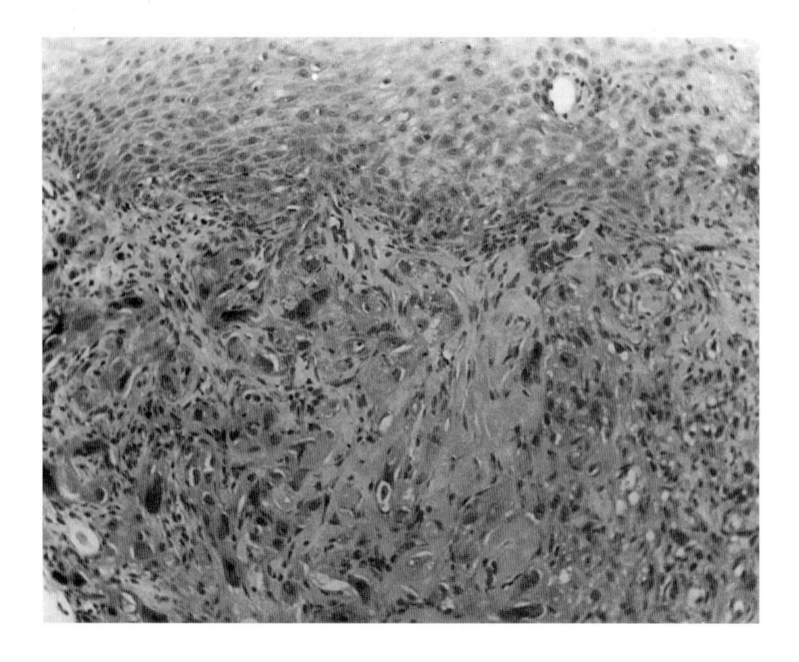

FIG. 30-40. Spindle cell squamous cell carcinoma with pleomorphic giant cells
The tumor resembles an atypical fibroxanthoma but in a few areas shows evidence of origin from the epidermis.

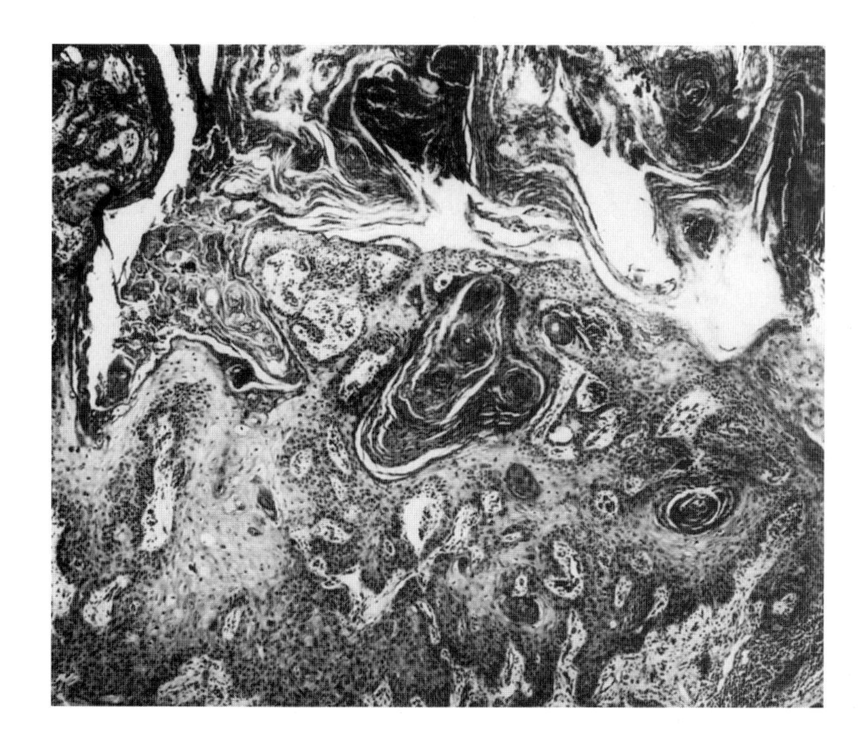

FIG. 30-41. Squamous cell carcinoma The tumor resembles a keratoacanthoma but shows less maturation and nuclear atypicality.

tion may be the result of either phagocytosis or invagination of the plasma membrane. However, it is not a specific finding for squamous cell carcinoma; intracytoplasmic desmosomes can be found also in keratoacanthoma and Bowen's disease, as well as in several unrelated epidermal proliferations and even in normal keratinocytes.

At the dermal-epidermal junction, the basement membrane shows sporadic discontinuities through which long cytoplasmic protrusions penetrate, indicating invasion of the dermis by epidermal keratinocytes.[303]

In early squamous cell carcinoma, lymphocytes are often seen in close contact with tumor cells, some of which show degenerative changes such as disruption of the plasma membrane, as well as fragmentation and subsequent release of organelles into the intercellular spaces. This can be interpreted as the cellular expression of an immune reaction against tumor cells.[304]

The epithelial nature of the sarcoma-like cells in *spindle cell squamous cell carcinoma* is supported by electron microscopic findings, which have shown that these cells contain tonofilaments and occasional desmosome-like structures.[302,305] Electron microscopy has also shown that structures diagnosed by light microscopy as atypical fibroxanthomas represent a heterogeneous group of neoplasms and that some are in actuality spindle cell squamous cell carcinomas.[301,306]

Immunohistochemical methods are of considerable value in the differentiation of squamous cell carcinoma from mesodermal tumors, such as atypical fibroxanthoma and malignant fibrous histiocytoma, and from malignant melanoma. For the identification of keratinocytes, primary antibodies directed against high-molecular-weight cytokeratins may be used. In contrast, atypical fibroxanthoma and malignant fibrous histiocytomas react with vimentin (see Chap. 35) and malignant melanoma with S-100 protein (see Chap. 29). At times, even differentiation of a squamous cell carcinoma from a lymphoma may be difficult, in which case a positive reaction with monoclonal antileukocyte antibody would favor lymphoma[307] (see Chap. 32). The immunohistochemistry may also be valuable in identifying tumor cells of a squamous cell carcinoma in the midst of an inflammatory infiltrate and can thus aid in deciding whether or not the margins of an excised specimen are free of tumor cells.[308] The immunohistochemical differential diagnosis of spindle cell neoplasms in the skin is discussed also in Chapters 4, 29, and 35.

Differential Diagnosis. The diagnosis of squamous cell carcinoma, although easily made in typical cases, may sometimes be difficult.

The differences between squamous cell carcinoma and actinic keratosis lie in the degree rather than the type of changes. In both conditions, one finds atypicality of cells, with dyskeratosis of individual cells and downward proliferation of the epidermis. However, only in squamous cell carcinoma is there invasion of the reticular dermis. No sharp line of demarcation exists between the two conditions, and not infrequently, on step sectioning for a lesion, the histologic appearance of actinic keratosis reveals one or several areas in which the changes have progressed to squamous cell carcinoma.

For discussions of differentiation of squamous cell carcinoma from pseudocarcinomatous hyperplasia, see p. 717; from keratoacanthoma, p. 731; and from basal cell carcinoma, p. 719.

ACANTHOLYTIC (ADENOID) SQUAMOUS CELL CARCINOMA

As a result of dyskeratosis and subsequent acantholysis, squamous cell carcinomas occasionally show what may appear to be tubular and alveolar formations on histologic examination. Such lesions have been termed *adenoid* or *pseudoglandular* squamous cell carcinomas, but they are better termed *acantholytic*. Clinically, they are found almost exclusively in sun-damaged skin of elderly patients, especially on the face and ears.[309,310] They have also been seen on the vermilion border of the lower lip.[311] Two instances of occurrence on the oral mucosa have been reported, but both were recurrences after radiation therapy.[312]

On sun-exposed skin, acantholytic squamous cell carcinomas may arise as such or may develop from an actinic keratosis.[310,313] In most instances, they do not differ in clinical appearance from the usual type of squamous cell carcinoma and thus commonly show a central ulceration surrounded by a raised, indurated border. Occasionally, they greatly resemble a keratoacanthoma in clinical appearance.[314] The incidence of metastases varies. In one series it was only 2%,[310] but in another series 14% of the patients had fatal metastases.[315] Tumor size of greater than 1.5 cm correlates with the risk of an adverse outcome.

Histopathology. The adenoid changes may be seen in only a portion of a squamous cell carcinoma or throughout the lesion. Not infrequently, an actinic keratosis of the acantholytic type is seen overlying the lesion. There are tubular and alveolar lumina lined with one or several layers of epithelium (Fig. 30-42). In areas in which the lumina are lined with a single layer of epithelium, the epithelial cells resemble glandular cells, but in areas with several layers of epithelium, squamous and partially keratinized cells usually form the inner layers. The lumina are filled with desquamated acantholytic cells, many of which are partially or fully keratinized.[310,314,316] In some cases, the eccrine ducts at the periphery of these tumors show signs of dilatation and proliferation (Fig. 30-43).[309,316] These ductal changes probably are induced by the surrounding inflammatory infiltrate.

Pathogenesis. These tumors represent squamous cell carcinomas of lobular growth in which there is considerable dyskeratosis with individual cell keratinization resulting in acantholysis in the center of the lobular formations. This process is analogous to the suprabasal clefts seen in some actinic keratoses.[314] Acantholytic squamous cell carcinomas differ from sweat gland carcinomas (see Chap. 31), in which the single row of cuboidal cells lining the lumina consists of true glandular cells.[317,318] These latter tumors may in some instances be highly malignant.

MUCIN-PRODUCING SQUAMOUS CELL CARCINOMA

This rare variant of squamous cell carcinoma is associated with a more aggressive clinical course than are most cutaneous squamous cell carcinomas.[319] The 11 cases have been reported under different designations, such as mucoepidermoid carcinoma[320] and adenosquamous carcinoma of the skin.[319] The latter designation may lead to confusion with adenoid squamous cell carcinoma.

Histopathology. Varying numbers of mucin-producing cells are found within tumors that have the appearance of a squamous cell carcinoma. These cells generally appear large and pale and stain positively with the PAS method and with mucicarmine.[319,321] Treatment of sections with sialidase eliminates the mucicarmine staining material, whereas treatment with hyaluronidase fails to do so. Thus the material is epithelial mucin (sialomucin).[319] Occasionally, true glandular lumina are present.[319,322] Some of the lumina resemble distorted eccrine ducts and stain positively for carcinoembryonic antigen.[322]

VERRUCOUS CARCINOMA

Verrucous carcinoma is a low-grade squamous cell carcinoma first described in 1948[323] as occurring in the oral cavity. The diagnosis of verrucous carcinoma requires evaluation of the clinical and microscopic appearance and biologic behavior of the neoplasm. It is a slowly growing, at first exophytic, verrucous, and fungating tumor that may ultimately penetrate deep into the tissue. However, it causes regional metastases only very late, if at all. Because of its high degree of histologic differentiation, it is often not recognized as a carcinoma for a long time.

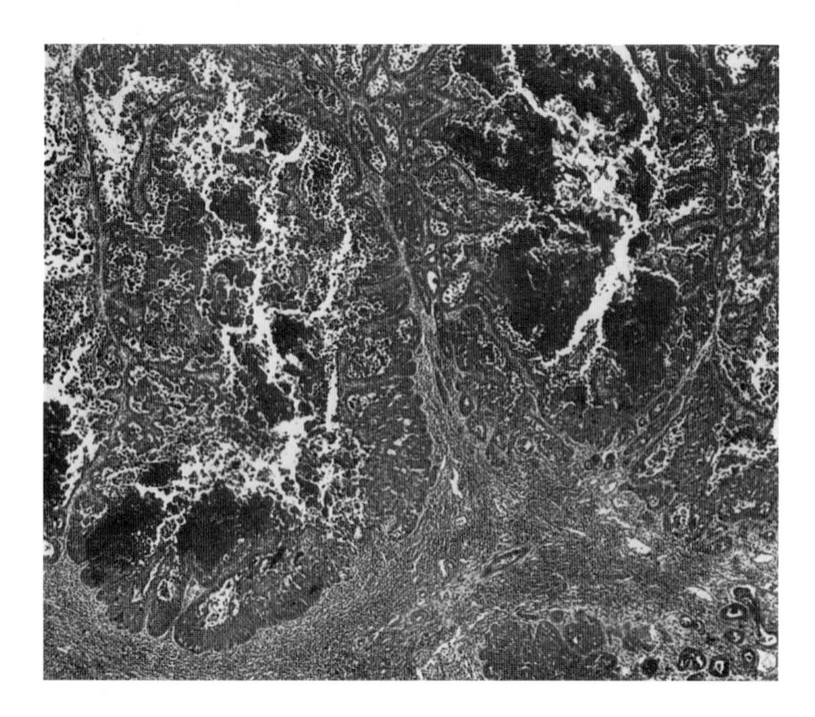

FIG. 30-42. Acantholytic squamous cell carcinoma, low magnification
The tumor shows large alveolar spaces into which papillary projections protrude. The alveolar spaces contain many desquamated acantholytic cells, many of which appear dyskeratotic.

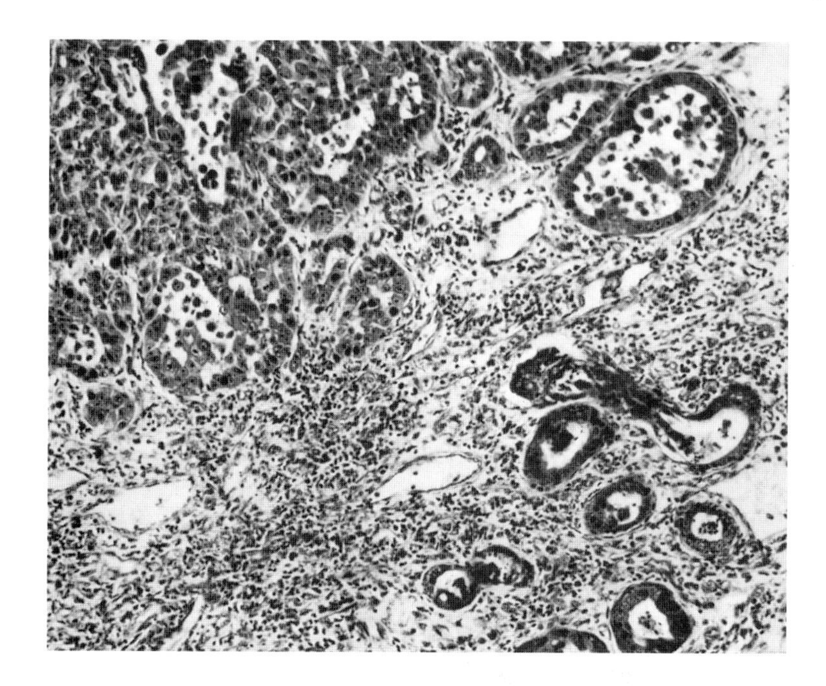

FIG. 30-43. Acantholytic squamous cell carcinoma
High magnification of the base of the tumor shown in Fig. 30-42. The tabular lumina of the tumor contain acantholytic, dyskeratotic cells. The sweat glands in the lower right corner show some epithelial proliferation, probably induced by the inflammatory infiltrate.

Three major forms of verrucous carcinoma are recognized, all of them occurring in areas of maceration.

Verrucous carcinoma of the oral cavity, also called oral florid papillomatosis, shows white, cauliflower-like lesions that may involve large areas of the oral mucosa.

Verrucous carcinoma of the genitoanal region, also called giant condylomata acuminata of Buschke and Loewenstein, most commonly occurs on the glans penis and foreskin of uncircumcised males, where it consists of papillomatous proliferations. Ultimately, it may penetrate into the urethra. It may also occur on the vulva in females and in the anal region (Chap. 26).

Plantar verrucous carcinoma, also called epithelioma cuniculatum,[324] at first shows a striking resemblance to an intractable plantar wart. As the exophytic mass grows, it shows a great tendency toward deep, penetrating growth, resulting in numerous deep crypts filled with horny material and pus. The crypts resemble the burrows of rabbits, hence the name *cuniculatum.* The tumor ultimately penetrates the plantar fascia[325] and may even destroy metatarsal bones and invade the skin of the dorsum of the foot.[326]

The occurrence of verrucous carcinoma has been described occasionally in many other areas, such as the face[327] and back,[328] as well as in preexisting lesions, such as chronic ulcers and draining sinuses of hidradenitis suppurativa.[329]

Histopathology. For the diagnosis of verrucous carcinoma, a large, deep biopsy is essential. The superficial portions generally resemble a verruca by showing hyperkeratosis, parakeratosis, and acanthosis. The keratinocytes appear well differentiated, stain lightly with eosin, and possess a small nucleus. The tumor invades with broad strands that often contain keratin-filled cysts in their center. There are large, bulbous, downward proliferations that compress the collagen bundles and push them aside. Thus the tumor has been said to invade by "bulldozing rather than stabbing."[330] Even in the deep portions of the tumor, nuclear atypia, individual cell keratinization, and horn pearls are absent.[331]

However, in some instances, particularly in the oral cavity[227,230] but occasionally also in the genitoanal region[332] and on the plantar surface,[333,334] verrucous carcinoma may ultimately show sufficient nuclear atypicality and loss of polarity to indicate the development of a true squamous cell carcinoma. In rare instances, the development of regional lymph node metastases has been observed in verrucous carcinoma of the mouth,[228] the genitals,[332] and the soles of the feet.[334] Radiation therapy has led in some instances of oral verrucous carcinoma to anaplastic transformation and extensive metastases.[335]

Pathogenesis. Although a viral cause of verrucous carcinoma has been suspected for a long time, demonstration of viral particles by electron microscopy has been possible in only a few instances of verrucous carcinoma. Viruslike particles were demonstrated in 1 case of plantar verrucous carcinoma presumed to be associated with a plantar wart,[336] in the superficial epithelium of 5 of 13 cases of plantar verrucous carcinoma,[337] and in 1 case of verrucous carcinoma of the vagina. The recently introduced, more sensitive, and more specific method of demonstrating various types of human papilloma viruses by means of DNA hybridization has succeeded in proving the presence of HPV-6, and less frequently of HPV-11, in Buschke-Loewenstein tumors of the external genitals in both sexes.[338] Similarly, HPV-6 was found in a vulvar tumor of Buschke-Loewenstein through molecular hybridization.[339]

PSEUDOCARCINOMATOUS HYPERPLASIA

Pseudocarcinomatous hyperplasia or *pseudoepitheliomatous hyperplasia,* as it is often called, represents a considerable downward proliferation of the epidermis into the dermis. Clinically and histologically, this downward proliferation may suggest a squamous cell carcinoma. It occurs occasionally (1) in chronic proliferative inflammatory processes, such as bromoderma, blastomycosis, blastomycosis-like pyoderma (pyoderma vegetans),[340] or hidradenitis suppurativa,[341] and (2) at the edges of chronic ulcers, as seen in the following conditions: after burns or in stasis dermatitis,[342] pyoderma gangrenosum, basal cell epithelioma,[343] lupus vulgaris, osteomyelitis, scrofulo-

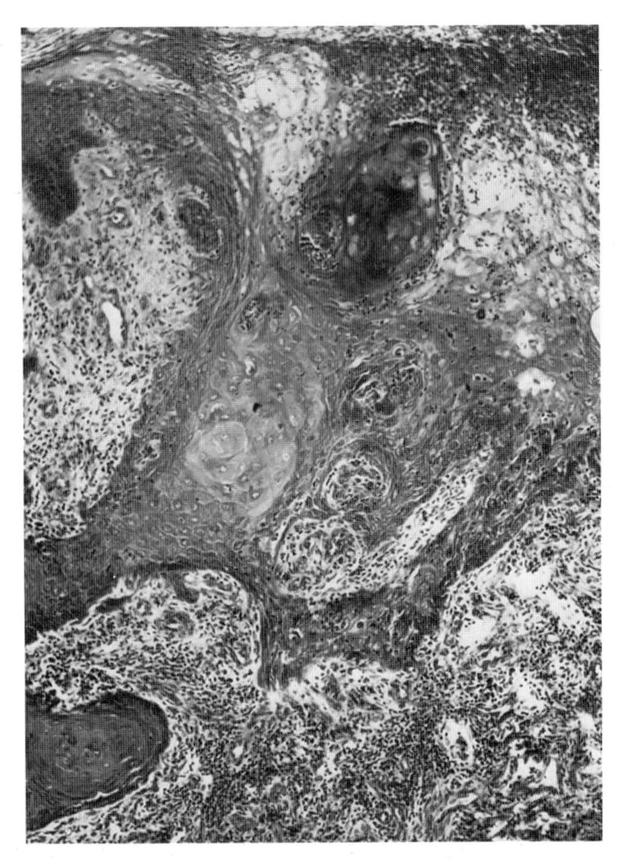

FIG. 30-44. Pseudocarcinomatous hyperplasia in bromoderma
There is downward proliferation of the epidermis analogous to squamous cell carcinoma, grade 1. In the field shown, it is impossible to rule out carcinoma. Note, however, the permeation of the epidermis in many areas by inflammatory cells.

derma, gumma, and granuloma inguinale. In addition, granular cell tumor is known to evoke quite frequently a pseudocarcinomatous hyperplasia.

Histopathology. Histologically, pseudocarcinomatous hyperplasia shows an epithelial hyperplasia that often closely resembles moderately or well-differentiated squamous cell carcinoma. Although squamous cell carcinoma may develop at the edges of chronic ulcers, it is likely that some cases that are regarded as such actually represent pseudocarcinomatous hyperplasia. Nevertheless, a lesion starting out as pseudocarcinomatous hyperplasia at the edge of an ulcer may eventually develop into a squamous cell carcinoma and even metastasize.[344,345]

The histologic picture of pseudocarcinomatous hyperplasia shows irregular invasion of the dermis by uneven, jagged, often sharply pointed epidermal cell masses and strands with horn-pearl formation and often numerous mitotic figures (Fig. 30-44). These irregular proliferations of the epidermis may extend below the level of the sweat glands, where they appear in sections as isolated islands of epidermal tissue.[341] However, the squamous cells usually are well differentiated, and atypicalities, such as individual cell keratinization and nuclear hyperplasia and hyperchromasia, are minimal or absent (Fig. 30-45). Furthermore, one often sees invasion of the epithelial proliferations by leukocytes and disintegration of some of the epidermal cells in pseudocarcinomatous hyperplasia, findings that usually are absent in squamous cell carcinoma.[342] Nevertheless, even when all of these criteria are taken into account, it may still be difficult to differentiate squamous cell carcinoma from pseudocarcinomatous hyperplasia by the study of just one histologic section.[341] Multiple biopsies and detailed clinical data may be necessary for differentiation.

In every section in which a diagnosis of squamous cell carcinoma is contemplated, it is worthwhile to study the inflammatory infiltrate for the possible presence of granulomas, as seen in tuberculosis and the deep mycoses, or of intraepidermal abscesses, as seen in bromoderma. If such evidence is found, one

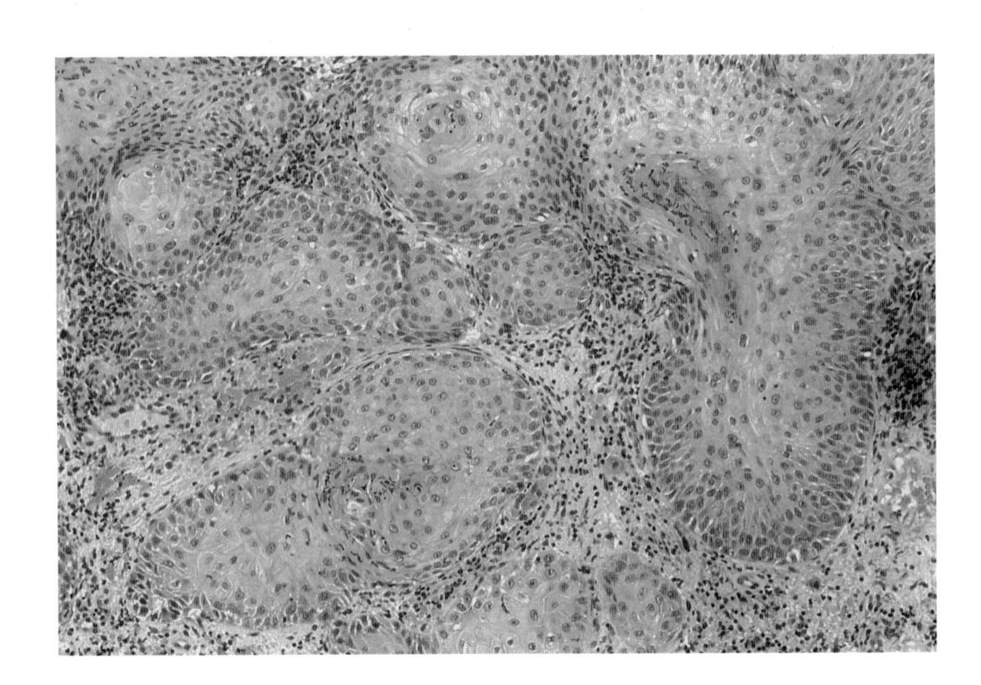

FIG. 30-45. Pseudocarcinomatous hyperplasia
This curetting specimen shows a proliferative squamous lesion without substantial atypia and mimicking an invasive lesion.

may be dealing with pseudocarcinomatous hyperplasia instead of squamous cell carcinoma.

Differential Diagnosis. Differentiation of pseudocarcinomatous hyperplasia from verrucous carcinoma rarely causes difficulties, because in verrucous carcinoma there is verrucous upward proliferation and downward proliferation. Also, verrucous carcinoma shows more pronounced keratinization in the downward extensions, which appear bulbous rather than sharply pointed.

BASAL CELL CARCINOMA

Basal cell carcinomas are seen almost exclusively on hair-bearing skin, especially on the face. Except in the nevoid basal cell carcinoma syndrome (see Chap. 31), they rarely occur on the palms[346,347] or on the soles.[348,349] Their occurrence on the mucous membrane is doubted; instances of basal cell carcinoma of the oral mucosa reported in the literature[350] probably are ameloblastomas.[351]

Basal cell carcinomas usually occur as single lesions, although the occurrence of several lesions, either simultaneously or subsequently, is not infrequent. About 40% of patients who have had a basal cell carcinoma will have one or more basal cell carcinomas within 10 years.[352] Basal cell carcinomas generally occur in adults, although they may be seen in children.[353–355] However, there are three rare forms of basal cell carcinoma with early onset. In the linear, unilateral basal cell nevus, all lesions are present at birth. In the nevoid basal cell syndrome and the Bazex syndrome, some patients manifest lesions before puberty.

Predisposing Factors. Although basal cell carcinomas may arise without apparent reason, there are several predisposing factors. The most common of them is a light skin color in association with prolonged exposure to strong sunlight.[356] The predisposing effect of sun exposure is particularly evident in patients with xeroderma pigmentosum, in whom both basal cell carcinoma and squamous cell carcinoma are common (see Chap. 6). That prolonged sun exposure alone does not suffice to produce basal cell carcinomas is suggested by their great rarity on the dorsa of hands and fingers.[357] Additional factors that predispose a person to develop both basal cell carcinoma and squamous cell carcinoma are large or numerous doses of roentgen rays[358,359] and, less commonly, burn scars[360,361] and other scars.[362] In contrast, most carcinomas of the skin caused by the prolonged intake of inorganic arsenic are squamous cell carcinomas, which often, like Bowen's disease, are located in situ.[241,289] Occasionally, however, basal cell carcinomas, particularly superficial basal cell carcinomas, can result[283,284] (see Arsenical Keratosis and Carcinoma).

Occurrence of Metastases. As a rule, basal cell carcinomas do not metastasize. However, there are exceptions. The incidence of metastasis ranges from 0.01% in pathologic specimens[363] through 0.028% in dermatologic patients[364] to 0.1% in patients from surgical centers.[365] A review published in 1984 described 175 cases with histologically proven metastases.[366]

The typical case history of a metastatic basal cell carcinoma is that of a large, ulcerated, locally invasive and destructive primary lesion that has recurred despite repeated surgical procedures or radiotherapy.[367] However, massive size, ulceration, or history of multiple recurrences are not absolute prerequisites for metastasis.[368] Most observers have found no specific histologic type of basal cell carcinoma that is more capable of metastasizing than others.[369–371] Also, no evidence exists that the hosts' immunologic defenses are severely compromised.[366] However, some authors assert that the metatypical or basosquamous type of basal cell carcinoma is the most likely to metastasize.[372]

In contrast to metastatic squamous cell carcinoma of the skin, which shows lymphogenic metastases to lymph nodes in 80% to 90% of cases, in metastatic basal cell carcinoma, hematogenic and lymphogenic spread show about an even distribution.[366] Although about 50% of the patients with metastatic basal cell carcinoma have metastases to lymph nodes as their first site of spread, lungs and bones also are frequently the first site of involvement. Metastases to the liver, other viscera, and to the skin or subcutaneous tissues have occurred. However, these areas were usually involved only when at least one of the three major sites of metastasis was also affected.[373] The average survival time after metastasis to the lungs, bones, or internal organs is about 10 months.[374]

Clinical Appearance. Five clinical types of basal cell carcinoma occur: (1) noduloulcerative basal cell carcinoma, including rodent ulcer, by far the most common type; (2) pigmented basal cell carcinoma; (3) morphea-like or fibrosing basal cell carcinoma; (4) superficial basal cell carcinoma; and (5) fibroepithelioma. In addition, there are three clinical syndromes in which basal cell carcinomas play an important part. They are (1) the nevoid basal cell carcinoma syndrome; (2) the linear unilateral basal cell nevus; and (3) the Bazex syndrome, showing follicular atrophoderma with multiple basal cell carcinomas.

Noduloulcerative basal cell carcinoma begins as a small, waxy nodule that often shows a few small telangiectatic vessels on its surface. The nodule usually increases slowly in size and often undergoes central ulceration. A typical lesion then consists of a slowly enlarging ulcer surrounded by a pearly, rolled border. This represents the so-called rodent ulcer.

Most rodent ulcers possess a limited potential for growth; however, occasionally they can be infiltrative and aggressive and then can reach considerable size and invade deeply. On the face, they may destroy the eyes and nose,[375] or they may penetrate the skull and invade the dura mater.[376] Death may then ensue. (Such destructive basal cell carcinomas are seen occasionally also in the nevoid basal cell carcinoma syndrome; see text following.)

Pigmented basal cell carcinoma differs from the noduloulcerative type only by the brown pigmentation of the lesion.

Morphea-like or fibrosing basal cell carcinoma manifests itself as a solitary, flat or slightly depressed, indurated, yellowish plaque. The surface is smooth and shiny. The border is often ill defined. The overlying skin remains intact for a long time before ulceration finally occurs.

Superficial basal cell carcinoma consists of one or several erythematous, scaling, only slightly infiltrated patches that slowly increase in size by peripheral extension. The patches are often surrounded, at least in part, by a fine, threadlike, pearly border. The patches usually show small areas of superficial ulceration and crusting. In addition, their center may show smooth, atrophic scarring. In contrast to the first three types of basal cell carcinoma that are commonly situated on the face, superficial basal cell carcinoma occurs predominantly on the trunk.

Fibroepithelioma consists of usually only one but occasionally of several raised, moderately firm, slightly pedunculated nodules, covered by smooth, slightly reddened skin. Clinically, they resemble fibromas. The most common location is the back.

The *nevoid basal cell carcinoma syndrome* is an autosomal dominant disorder with low penetration. Small nodules appear between puberty and 35 years of age, and there may be hundreds or thousands of them.[377] During the "nevoid" stage, the nodules slowly increase in number and size. They are haphazardly distributed over the face and body. During adulthood, many of the basal cell carcinomas undergo ulceration, and later in life, the disease sometimes enters a "neoplastic" stage, in which some of the basal cell carcinomas, especially of the face, become invasive, destructive, and mutilating. Occasionally, even death occurs as the result of invasion of an orbit and of the brain.[378–380] There also may be metastases to the lung.[378]

Half of the adult patients with the nevoid basal cell carcinoma syndrome show numerous palmar and plantar pits 1 to 3 mm in diameter. These pits usually develop during the second decade of life and represent *formes frustes* of basal cell carcinoma (see Histopathology).[381] Also, epidermal cysts are quite common.[382]

Most patients show multiple skeletal and central nervous system anomalies,[379] among which are odontogenic keratocysts of the jaws, anomalies of the ribs, scoliosis, mental retardation, and calcification of the falx cerebri. In several reported cases, there were also cerebellar medulloblastomas[383] or fibrosarcomas of a mandible or maxilla.[384] In the jaw cysts, an ameloblastoma may arise.[385]

The *linear unilateral basal cell nevus* is very rare. There is an extensive unilateral linear or zosteriform eruption, usually present since birth, consisting of closely set nodules of basal cell carcinoma.[386] They may be interspersed with comedones[387,388] and striaelike areas of atrophy.[389] The lesions do not increase in size with aging of the patient.

The *Bazex syndrome,* first described in 1966,[390] is dominantly inherited and shows as its main features (1) follicular atrophoderma characterized by widened follicular openings like "ice-pick marks" mainly on the extremities and (2) multiple, small basal cell carcinomas on the face, usually arising first in adolescence or early adulthood[391] but occasionally in late childhood.[392] In addition, there may be localized anhidrosis or generalized hypohidrosis, and congenital hypotrichosis on the scalp and elsewhere.[392]

Histopathology. In the common solid type of basal cell carcinoma, nodular masses of basaloid cells are formed that extend into the dermis in relation to a delicate, specialized tumor stroma (Fig. 30-46). Cystic spaces may form as a result of tumor necrosis or cellular dyshesion (Fig. 30-47). The characteristic cells of basal cell carcinoma, referred to by some as basaloma cells, have a large, oval, or elongated nucleus and relatively little cytoplasm. Often, the cytoplasm of individual cells is poorly defined, so that it may appear as if their nuclei are embedded in a symplasmatic mass. The nuclei resemble those of basal cells of the epidermis, but basaloma cells differ from basal cells by having a larger ratio of nucleus to cytoplasm[393] and by not showing intercellular bridges. The nuclei in basal cell carcinomas as a rule have a rather uniform, nonanaplastic appearance. They usually show no pronounced variation in size or intensity of staining and no abnormal mitoses, even in the rare instances

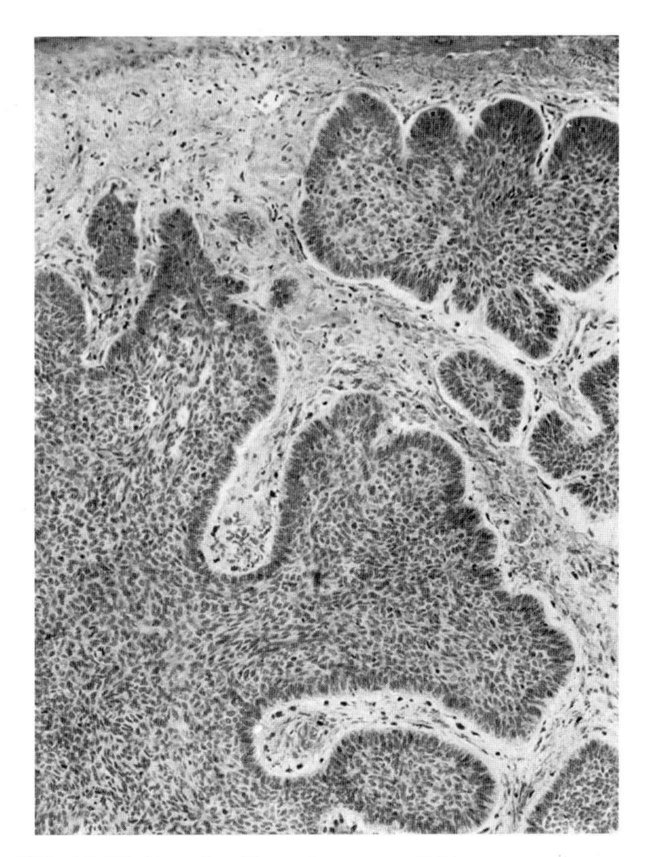

FIG. 30-46. Basal cell carcinoma, solid type
There are masses of various shapes and sizes composed of basal cell carcinoma cells or basalioma cells. The peripheral cell layer of the tumor masses shows a palisade arrangement of the nuclei.

of basal cell carcinoma with metastases. In the exceptional cases of basal cell carcinoma in which one finds, interspersed among the usual cells of basal cell carcinoma, cells with large hyperchromatic nuclei, multiple nuclei, and bizarre "starburst" mitoses, the clinical course is not different from that of the usual basal cell carcinoma[394,395] (Fig. 30-48). Although most basal cell carcinomas appear well demarcated, some show an infiltrative growth. They are now widely recognized as a distinct histologic subtype (Figs. 30-49 and 30-50).

The connective tissue stroma proliferates with the tumor and is arranged in parallel bundles around the tumor masses, so that a mutual relationship seems to exist between the parenchyma of the tumor and its stroma.[396,397] The stroma adjacent to the tumor masses often shows numerous young fibroblasts; in addition, it may appear mucinous.[398,399] Frequently there are areas of retraction of the stroma from tumor islands, resulting in peritumoral lacunae (Fig. 30-51). These lacunae once were regarded as a fixation artifact, but peritumoral lacunae can be observed also on cryostat sections. Immunostaining with antibodies to laminin, type IV collagen, and bullous pemphigoid has revealed the presence of laminin and type IV collagen on the stroma side of the lacunae, but bullous pemphigoid antigen is absent at the site of lacunae.[400] Even though bullous pemphigoid antigen is diminished in other areas of basal cell carcinoma,[401] it is likely that loss of this antigen contributes to the formation of peritumoral lacunae.[400] Because these lacunae are quite typical for

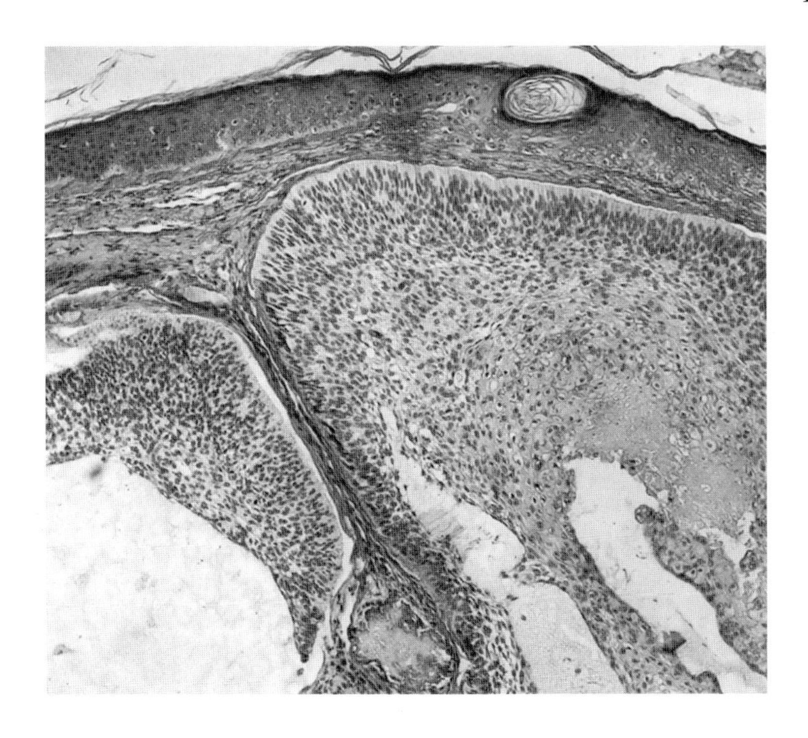

FIG. 30-47. Basal cell carcinoma, solid type with cystic degeneration
In an originally solid basal cell carcinoma cystic spaces have formed within the large cell masses as the result of tumor cell disintegration.

some basal cell carcinomas, their presence aids in the differentiation of basal cell carcinoma from other tumors, such as squamous cell carcinoma. Also, stromal or intratumor deposits of amyloid are found quite frequently (see Pathogenesis).[402] A mild inflammatory infiltrate is often seen in the stroma of nonulcerated basal cell carcinomas but may be entirely lacking. If ulceration occurs, there usually is a rather pronounced inflammatory reaction.

From a histologic point of view, basal cell carcinomas can be divided into two groups: undifferentiated and differentiated. Those of the latter group show a slight degree of differentiation toward the cutaneous appendages of hair, sebaceous glands, apocrine glands, or eccrine glands. A sharp dividing line between the two groups cannot be drawn, because many undifferentiated basal cell carcinomas show differentiation in some areas, and most differentiated basal cell carcinomas show areas lacking differentiation. By correlating the clinical classification with the histologic classification, it can be stated that the noduloulcerative type of basal cell carcinoma, as well as the lesions of the nevoid basal cell carcinoma syndrome, the linear unilateral basal cell nevus, and the Bazex syndrome, may show differentiation or no differentiation, but the other four types of basal cell carcinoma—pigmented basal cell carcinoma, fibrosing basal cell carcinoma, superficial basal cell carcinoma, and fibroepithelioma—usually show little or no differentiation.

Basal cell carcinomas showing no differentiation are called *solid* basal cell carcinomas. They can be subdivided into *circumscribed* and *infiltrative*. Those with differentiation toward hair structures are called *keratotic;* toward sebaceous glands, *basal cell carcinomas with sebaceous differentiation;* and to-

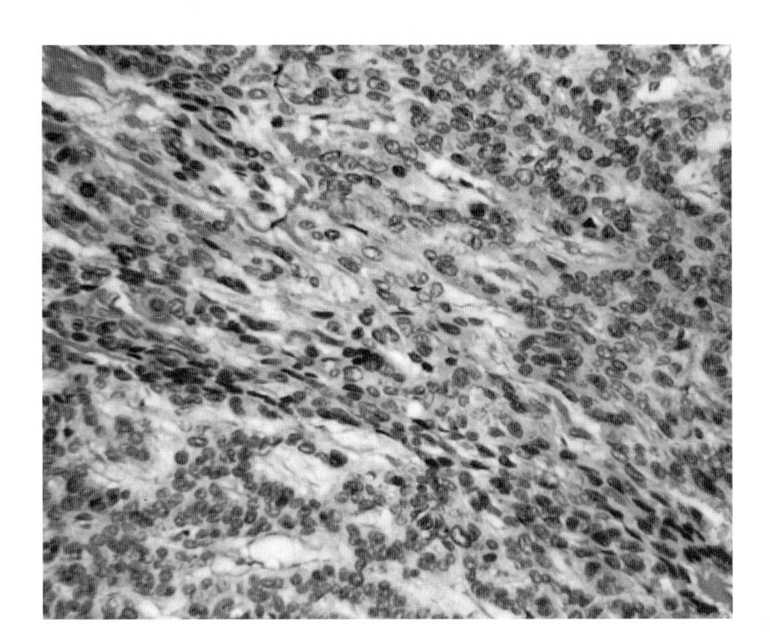

FIG. 30-48. Basal cell carcinoma with differentiation into two types of cells
One type of cell is large and has an oval pale nucleus; the other type of cell is small and has an elongated dark nucleus.

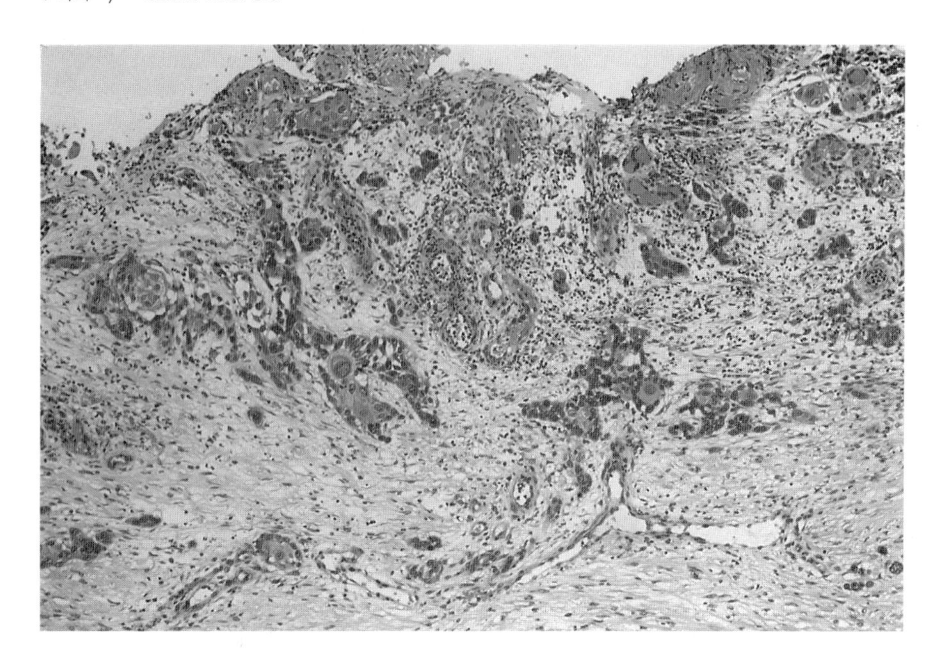

FIG. 30-49. Basal cell carcinoma, infiltrative
Basaloid cells infiltrate the dermis in an excision specimen taken from the base of a previously curetted recurrent lesion.

ward tubular glands, *adenoid* basal cell carcinomas. In many differentiated basal cell carcinomas, differentiation is directed toward more than one of these cutaneous appendages. For example, areas of keratinization may be found in a tumor that also shows adenoid structures. No difference exists in the rate of growth between undifferentiated and differentiated basal cell carcinomas.

Solid basal cell carcinoma of the *circumscribed* type shows tumor masses of various sizes and shapes embedded in the dermis (see Fig. 30-46). In more than 90% of basal cell carcinomas, a connection between tumor cell formations and the surface epidermis can be shown to exist.[403] Occasionally, a tumor mass is found in contact with an outer root sheath. The peripheral cell layer of the tumor masses often shows a palisade arrangement, whereas the nuclei of the cells inside lie in a haphazard fashion. Solid basal cell carcinomas containing large aggregates of tumor cells occasionally show disintegration of their cells in the center of the tumor masses, resulting in cyst formation (see Fig. 30-51).[404] Some solid basal cell carcinomas, though they show little or no structural differentiation toward any of the epidermal appendages, nevertheless show two types of cells: a large cell with an oval, pale nucleus, and a small cell with an elongated, dark nucleus (see Fig. 30-48).[404]

Solid basal cell carcinomas of the *infiltrative* type, also referred to as *aggressive* basal cell carcinomas, show the basaloid cells predominantly arranged as elongated strands, only a few layers thick and with little or no palisading of the peripheral cells. Such strands can invade deeply. The demarcation of the tumor from the stroma is often poor.[405] There are cell aggregates that display an irregular, spiky configuration.[406] The cells and their nuclei show great variations in size and shape[407] (see Figs. 30-49 and 30-50). There is little or no increase in the density of stroma

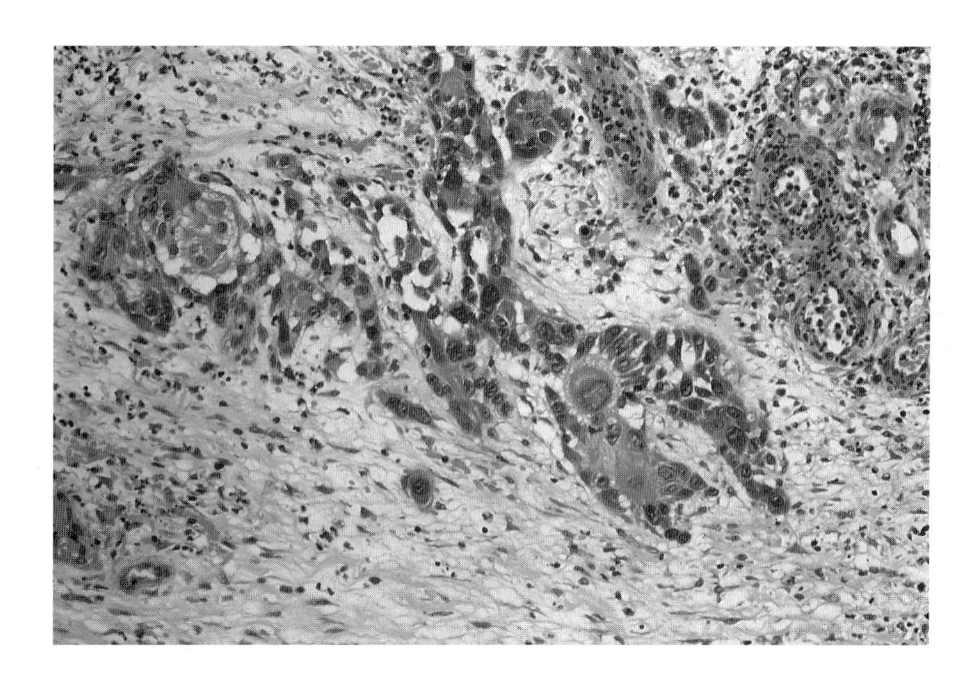

FIG. 30-50. Basal cell carcinoma, infiltrative
There is more atypia than in most basal cell carcinomas, and there is focal squamous differentiation within the infiltrating cords of basaloid cells, consistent with the so-called metatypical variant of basal cell carcinoma.

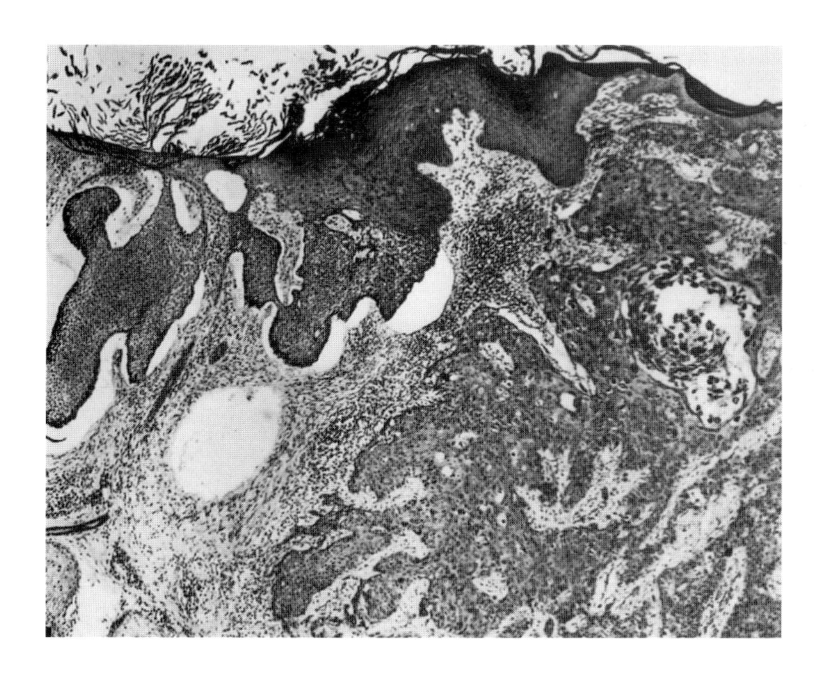

FIG. 30-51. Mixed carcinoma
A basal cell carcinoma (*left*) and a squamous cell carcinoma (*right*) lie side by side.

collagen and no significant increase in the number of fibroblasts. There may be foci of squamous differentiation (see Fig. 30-50). The number of inflammatory cells depends to some degree on the extent of ulceration. There often is perineural infiltration[405] and, on the face, there may be invasion of bone.[376]

Keratotic basal cell carcinoma shows parakeratotic cells and horn cysts in addition to undifferentiated cells (Fig. 30-52). The parakeratotic cells possess elongated nuclei and a slightly eosinophilic cytoplasm, in contrast to the deeply basophilic cytoplasm of undifferentiated cells. The parakeratotic cells may lie in strands, in concentric whorls, or around the horn cysts (Fig. 30-53). It is likely that they are cells with initial keratinization somewhat similar to the nucleated cells in the keratogenic zone of normal hair shafts. The horn cysts, which are composed of fully keratinized cells, represent attempts at hair shaft formation.[408] Just as in the keratinization of the hair shaft, the horn cysts form without the interposition of granular cells. Some keratotic basal cell carcinomas possess horn cysts of considerable size (Fig. 30-54).

Keratotic basal cell carcinoma shares with trichoepithelioma the presence of horn cysts, and it is sometimes difficult to decide whether a lesion represents a keratotic basal cell carcinoma or a trichoepithelioma (see Chap. 31). Clinical data may be necessary for a decision to be reached. The horn cysts must not be confused with the horn pearls that occur in squamous cell carcinoma (see Differential Diagnosis).

Basal cell carcinoma with sebaceous differentiation shows essentially a basal cell carcinoma in which there are interspersed aggregates of sebaceous cells and cells transitional from basaloma cells to sebaceous cells. The transitional cells have

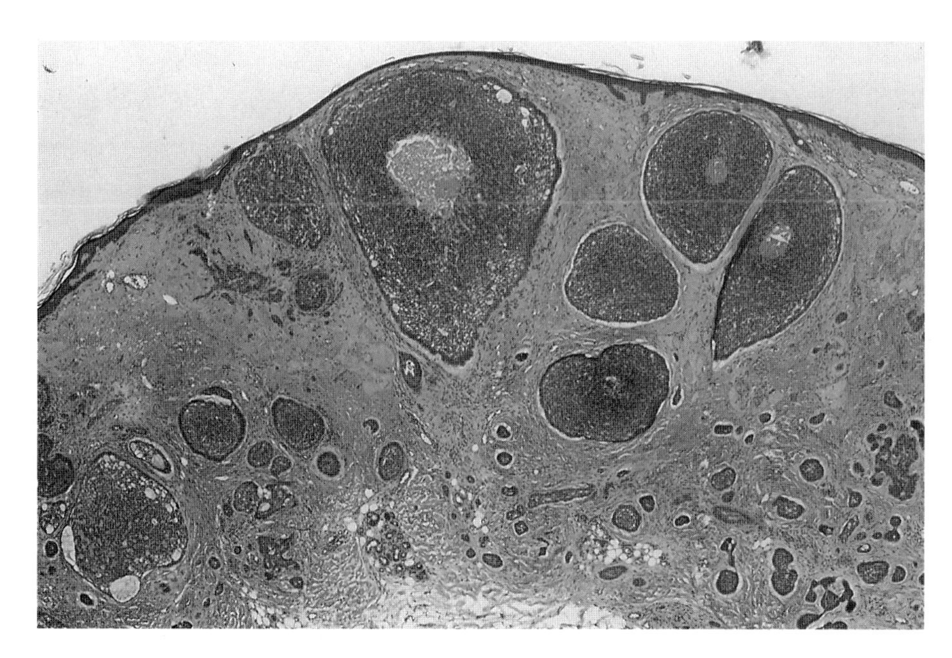

FIG. 30-52. Keratotic basal cell carcinoma
The lesion shows solid nodules of tumor similar to a common basal cell carcinoma but with central foci of pronounced squamous differentiation with keratinization.

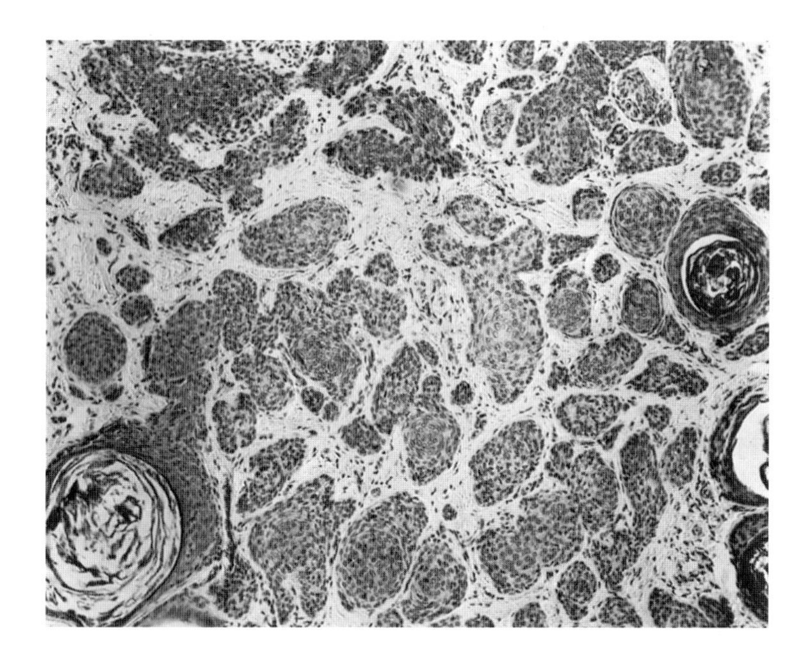

FIG. 30-53. Keratotic basal cell carcinoma
In addition to undifferentiated tumor cells, there are parakeratotic cells and horn cysts. The parakeratotic cells possess an elongated nucleus and a slightly eosinophilic cytoplasm; they lie in strands, in concentric whorls, or around the horn cyst.

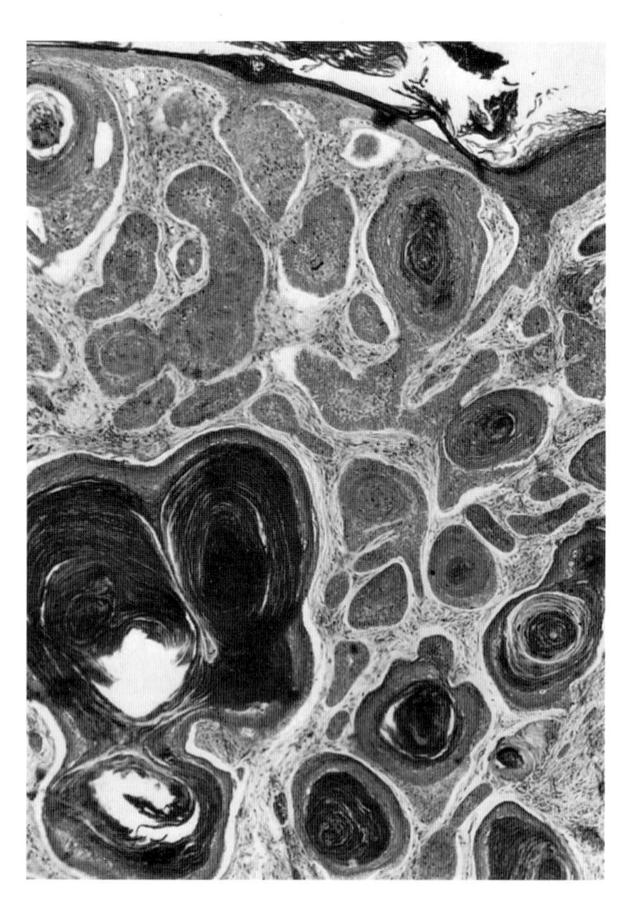

FIG. 30-54. Keratotic basal cell carcinoma
This tumor contains unusually large horn cysts.

granules that stain positive with Sudan III and other lipid stains[388] (see Chap. 4). A clear-cut separation from sebaceoma (sebaceous epithelioma) is at times impossible because transitions exist. Most examples of lesions thought to represent basal cell carcinomas with sebaceous differentiation are probably actually sebaceomas.[409]

Adenoid basal cell carcinoma shows formations suggesting tubular, glandlike structures. The cells are arranged in intertwining strands and radially around islands of connective tissue, resulting in a tumor with a lacelike pattern (Fig. 30-55). In rare instances, lumina may be surrounded by cells that have the appearance of secretory cells (Fig. 30-56). The lumina may be filled with a colloidal substance or with an amorphous granular material, but definite evidence of secretory activity of the cells lining the lumina cannot be obtained, even with histochemical methods. Similarly, because of the low degree of differentiation of the cells, histochemical reactions that would indicate either apocrine or eccrine differentiation are negative.[410] The tumor originally described as basal cell tumor with eccrine differentiation[411] is now regarded as an eccrine carcinoma and referred to as *syringoid eccrine carcinoma* (see Chap. 31).

Four uncommon histologic variants of basal cell carcinoma have been described: an adamantinoid type, a granular type, a clear cell type, and a type with matricial differentiation. *Adamantinoid basal cell carcinoma* shows a great histologic resemblance to dental ameloblastoma or adamantinoma.[412] One observes solid masses of basaloma cells with palisading at the periphery. Inside this layer, the cells show elongated nuclei and stellate cytoplasm stretched as thin, connecting bridges across empty spaces, as seen in adamantinoma. In *granular basal cell carcinoma,* some of the tumor cells have the usual appearance of basaloma cells, whereas others show a gradual transition to

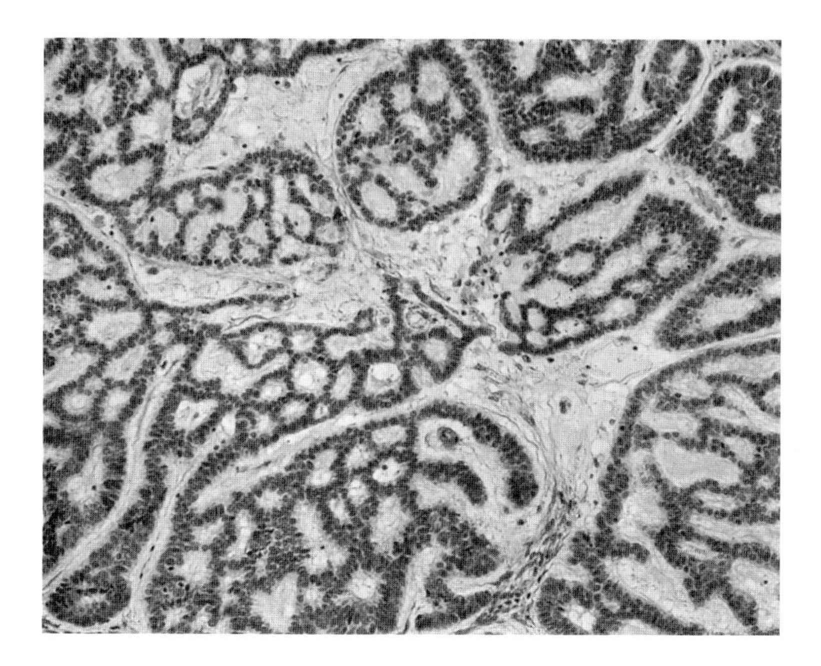

FIG. 30-55. Adenoid basal cell carcinoma
The strands of epithelial cells present a lacelike pattern. The stroma has a mucoid appearance.

granular cells. The granular cells show in their cytoplasm numerous eosinophilic granules with a tendency to coalesce.[413,414] The eosinophilic lysosome-like granules greatly resemble those seen in granular cell tumor (see Chap. 36). In the *clear cell basal cell carcinoma,* the clear cell pattern may occupy all or part of the tumor islands. The clear cells contain vacuoles of different sizes filled with glycogen.[415] The vacuoles often cause peripheral displacement of the nucleus, giving the cells a signet-ring appearance.[416] In *basal cell carcinoma with matricial differentiation,* islands of shadow cells, as seen in pilomatricoma, are located within a basal cell carcinoma.[417]

Noduloulcerative basal cell carcinoma, clinically the most common type of basal cell carcinoma, may on histologic examination appear solid, keratotic, or adenoid. The histologic descriptions given in text preceding for solid, keratotic, and adenoid basal cell carcinoma apply in general to the noduloulcerative type of basal cell carcinoma.

Although about 75% of basal cell carcinomas are found on staining with dopa to contain melanocytes, and melanin is present in about 25% of them,[418] large amounts of melanin are encountered only rarely (Fig. 30-57). The melanin is produced by benign melanocytes that colonize the tumor. These tumors are called *pigmented basal cell carcinomas.*

Basal cell carcinomas with large amounts of melanin are shown on staining with silver to contain melanocytes interspersed between the tumor cells. These melanocytes have nu-

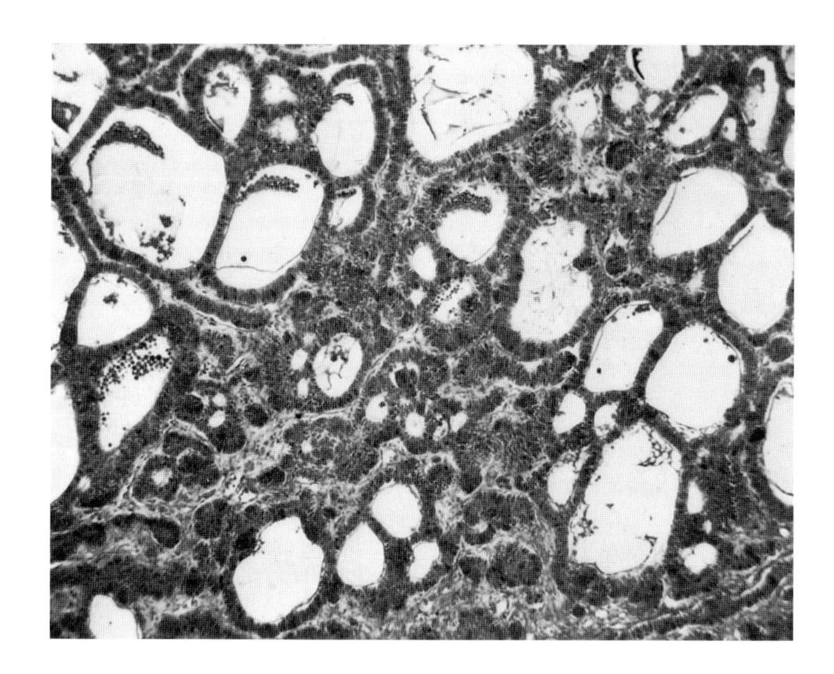

FIG. 30-56. Adenoid basal cell carcinoma
The tumor contains lumina surrounded by cells that look like glandular cells.

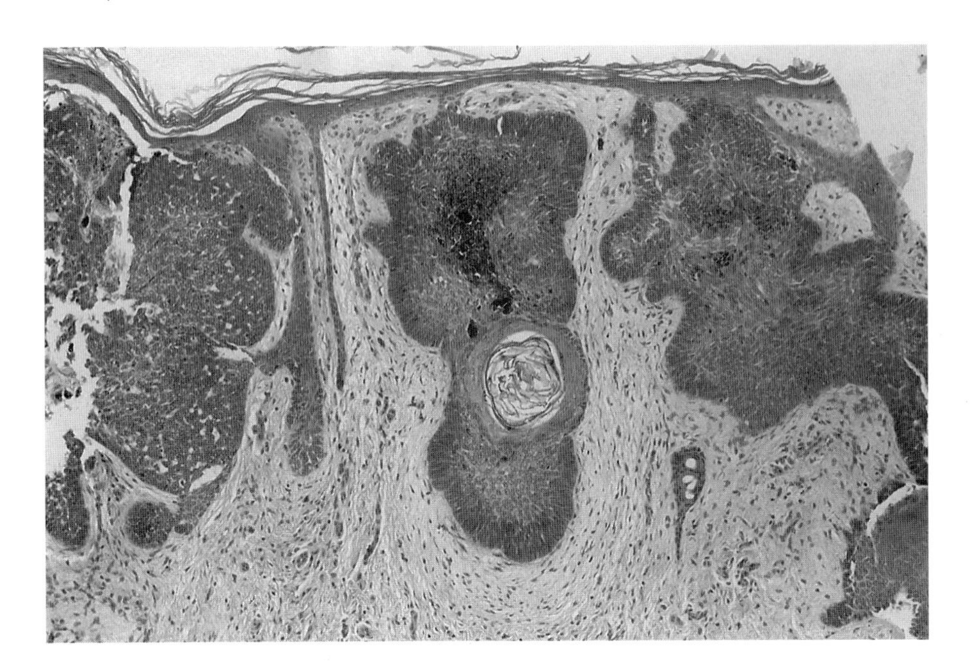

FIG. 30-57. Pigmented basal cell carcinoma
Melanin pigment is present within solid islands of basal cell carcinoma. In this example pigment is not present in substantial amounts in macrophages between the islands of tumor cells.

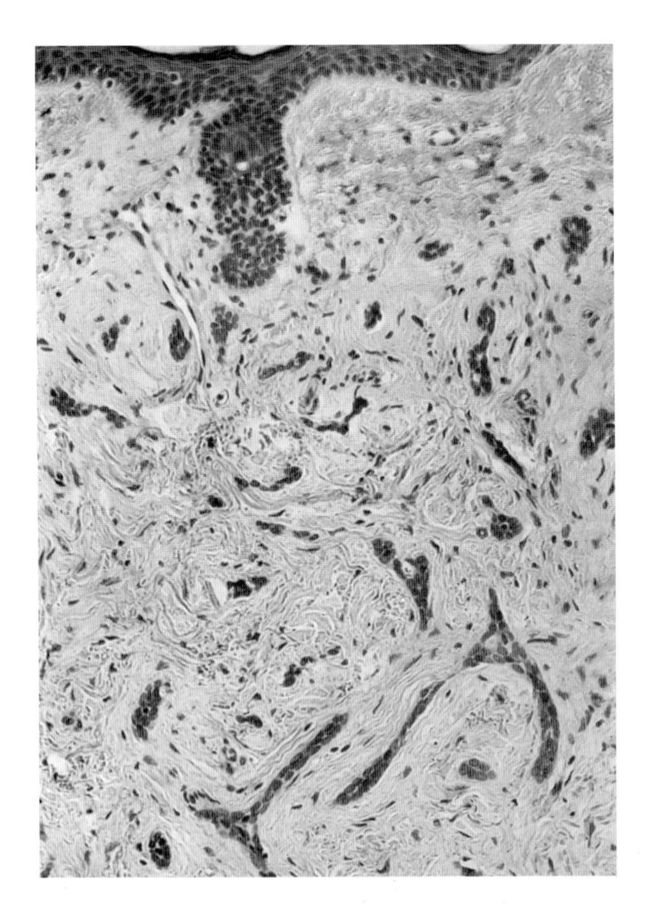

FIG. 30-58. Morphea-like or fibrosing basal cell carcinoma
Innumerable small groups of closely packed tumor cells, many of them arranged in elongated strands, are embedded in a dense fibrous stroma.

merous melanin granules in their cytoplasm and dendrites.[418] This contrasts with normal epidermal melanocytes of whites, in which there are only a few rather small melanin granules because most of the melanin is located within the keratinocytes.[419] The tumor cells in some pigmented basal cell carcinomas may contain very little melanin, but there are many melanophages in the connective tissue stroma surrounding the tumor masses. (For details, see Electron Microscopy.)

Connective tissue participation is much greater in the *morphea-like or fibrosing* variant than in the other types of basal cell carcinoma. Embedded in a dense fibrous stroma are innumerable groups of tumor cells arranged in elongated strands (Fig. 30-58).[420] Most of the strands are narrow, often only one cell thick, so that they resemble the narrow strands of tumor cells seen in the skin in metastatic scirrhous carcinoma of the breast. However, on searching, one usually finds at least a few larger aggregates of tumor cells and some strands of tumor cells showing branching. The strands of tumor cells often extend deep into the dermis.

Superficial basal cell carcinoma shows buds and irregular proliferations of tumor tissue attached to the undersurface of the epidermis (Fig. 30-59). The peripheral cell layer of the tumor formations often shows palisading. In most cases, there is little penetration into the dermis. The overlying epidermis usually shows atrophy. Fibroblasts, often in a fairly large number, are arranged around the tumor cell proliferations. In addition, a mild or moderate amount of a nonspecific chronic inflammatory infiltrate is present in the upper dermis.

Some superficial basal cell carcinomas, after having persisted as such for various lengths of time, become invasive basal cell carcinomas. Because this change may be limited at first to a few areas, representative sections throughout the entire block should be examined. For a discussion of the evidence that superficial basal cell carcinoma is unicentric, see Pathogenesis.

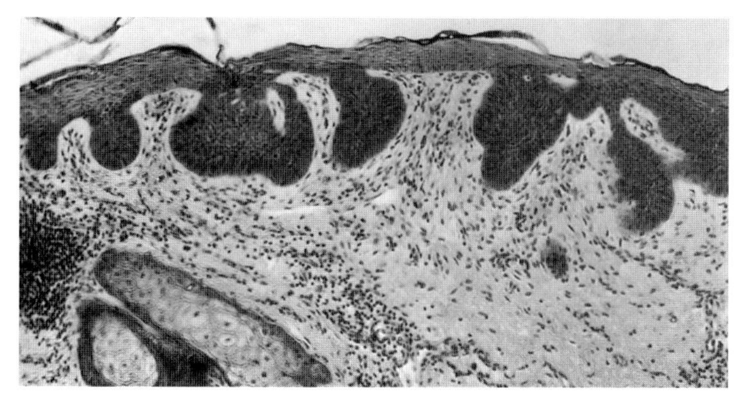

FIG. 30-59. Superficial basal cell carcinoma
The tumor shows buds and irregular proliferations of tumor tissue attached to the undersurface of the epidermis. Note the similarlity between the tumor buds in this illustration and the primary epithelial germ buds in the embryonal skin shown in Fig. 3-2 in Chap. 3.

In *fibroepithelioma,* first described in 1953,[396] long, thin, branching, anastomosing strands of basal cell carcinoma are embedded in a fibrous stroma (Figs. 30-60 and 30-61).[396,421] Many of the strands show connections with the surface epidermis. Here and there, small groups of dark-staining cells showing a palisade arrangement of the peripheral cell layer may be seen along the epithelial strands, like buds on a branch. Usually, the tumor is quite superficial and is well demarcated at its lower border. Fibroepithelioma combines features of the intracanalicular fibroadenoma of the breast, the reticulated type of seborrheic keratosis, and superficial basal cell carcinoma.[396] Fibroepithelioma can change into an invasive and ulcerating basal cell carcinoma.[422]

The multiple basal cell carcinomas seen in the *nevoid basal cell carcinoma syndrome* present no features that distinguish them from ordinary basal cell carcinoma, even while they are still in the early nevoid stage and have not yet become invasive and destructive, as they may be later in the neoplastic stage.[423] All the diverse features of basal cell carcinoma, such as solid, adenoid, cystic, keratotic, superficial, and fibrosing formations, can be seen in the lesions of the nevoid basal cell carcinoma syndrome.[424] Usually, a histologic distinction between the nevoid basal cell carcinoma syndrome and typical trichoepithelioma is easy, because keratotic cysts are more prominent in the latter. However, some lesions of trichoepithelioma show relatively few horn cysts. A histologic distinction in such cases may be impossible,[425] and clinical data will be necessary (see Chap. 31).

The palmar and plantar pits are a result of the premature desquamation of most of the horny layer.[426] On histologic examination, the epidermal rete ridges beneath the pits are found to be crowded with cells resembling those of basal cell carcinoma. Overlying these rete ridges, there is a markedly thinned granular layer topped by a very thin layer of loose keratin.[381] In some patients, the pits actually show at their base the presence of small basal cell carcinomas.[427] In rare instances, one or several clinically visible basal cell carcinomas arise on the palms or soles in patients with palmar and plantar pits.[426,428,429]

The jaw cysts represent odontogenic keratocysts. They are lined by a festooned epithelium consisting of two to five layers of squamous cells that form keratin without the presence of a granular cell layer.[430] Each jaw cyst may consist of either one large cyst or multiple microcysts.[424] Some of the cutaneous cysts, instead of being epidermal cysts, have the appearance of the jaw cysts and are similar to those cysts seen in steatocystoma multiplex but without showing sebaceous lobules.[430]

The basal cell carcinomas in *linear unilateral basal cell nevus* have a variable histologic appearance. The tumor formations may be solid, adenoid, keratotic, or cystic.[387,431] In addition, there may be areas resembling trichoepithelioma[386] or

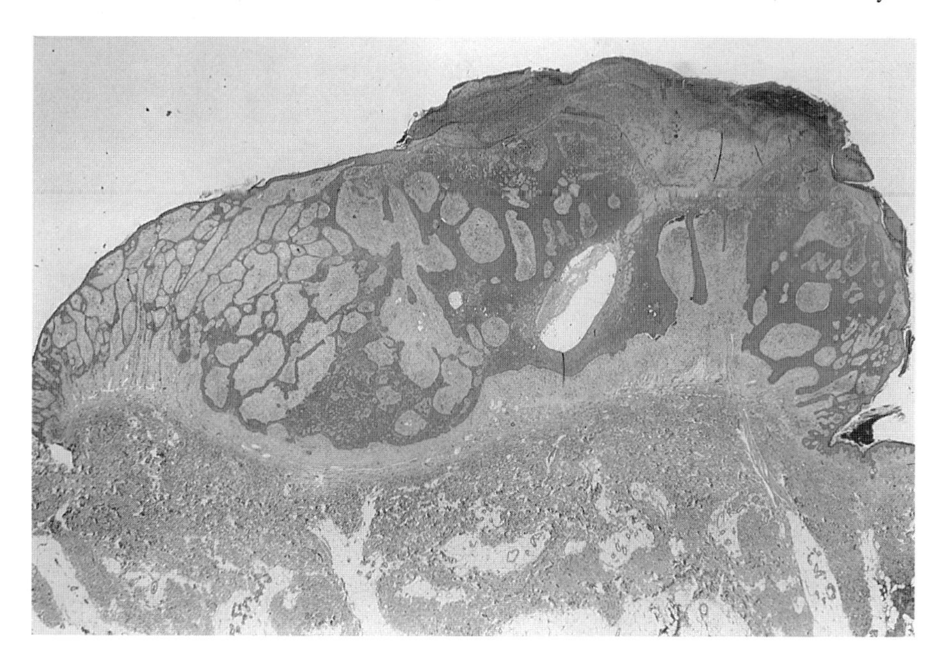

FIG. 30-60. Fibroepithelioma of Pinkus (fibroepithelial basal cell carcinoma)
The tumor has an elevated nodular appearance with, in this instance, a focus of superficial ulceration and hemorrhage.

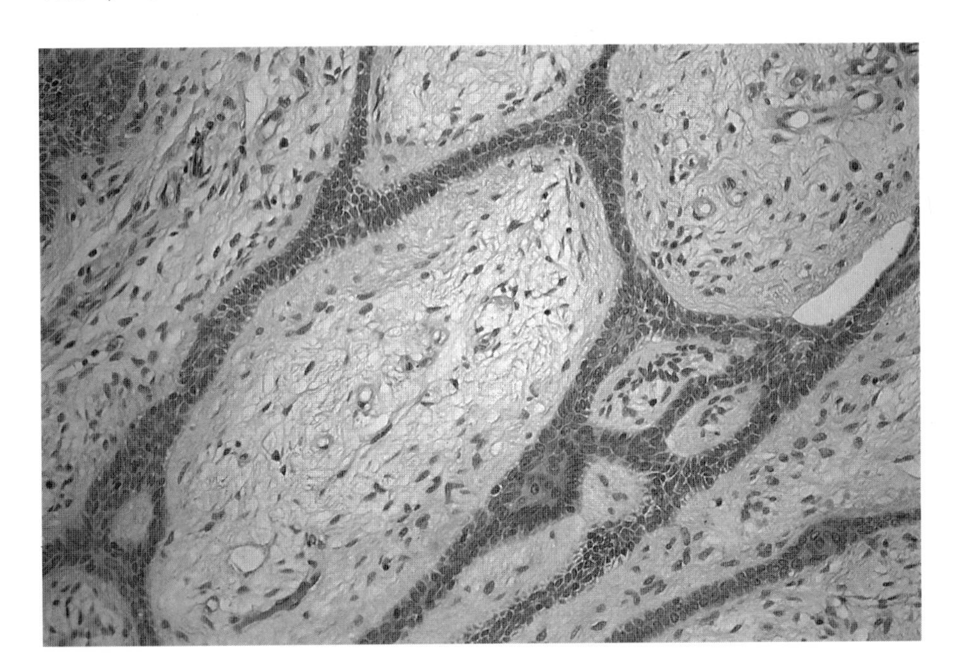

FIG. 30-61. Fibroepithelioma of Pinkus (fibroepithelial basal cell carcinoma)
Long, thin, branching, anastomosing strands of basal cell carcinoma are embedded in a fibrous stroma.

eccrine spiradenoma.[432] The walls of the comedones show numerous buds of basal cell carcinoma extending into the surrounding dermis.[387,389]

The basal cell carcinomas encountered in the *Bazex syndrome* have a variable histologic appearance. Some of them are indistinguishable from trichoepithelioma.[391,392] The areas of follicular atrophoderma show a dilated follicular ostium leading into a distorted and underdeveloped pilosebaceous unit.[392]

The tumor described in 1926 by Jadassohn and regarded by him as an intraepidermal epithelioma analogous to one previously reported by Borst has been referred to subsequently as *Borst-Jadassohn epithelioma.* For a long time this tumor and similar tumors subsequently described were thought to be intraepidermal basal cell carcinomas, because the cells composing the intraepidermal islands usually are small and have a deeply basophilic cytoplasm.[433] However, on careful examination, it became evident that the cells composing the intraepidermal islands in the presumed intraepidermal basal cell carcinomas possess intercellular bridges and are seborrheic keratoses of the clonal type.[66,434] The existence of an intraepidermal basal cell carcinoma is also unlikely because the close relationship that exists between tumor and stroma in basal cell carcinoma excludes the formation of intraepidermal nests, which would lack any contact with the stroma.[435]

However, there are several types of tumors, some benign and some malignant, that on occasion show well-defined islands of cells within the epidermis that differ in their appearance from the surrounding epidermal cells.[90] This is referred to as the *Jadassohn phenomenon.* Among the tumors that occasionally have an intraepidermal location are the following:

Clonal seborrheic keratosis. Some of these tumors show intraepidermal aggregates of basaloid cells suggestive of a basal cell carcinoma in situ (see Fig. 30-5),[66] whereas others show intraepidermal islands of an irritated seborrheic keratosis simulating a squamous cell carcinoma in situ.

Bowen's disease. Occasionally, one observes clonal aggregates of Bowen's disease within the epidermis.[436] At a later stage, there may be dermal invasion.[437]

Intraepidermal poroma, also referred to as *hidroacanthoma simplex (*Chap. 31).[438,439]

Intraepidermal malignant eccrine poroma.[440] In cases of intraepidermal metastases of malignant eccrine poroma, the tumor masses extend through the superficial lymphatics from the dermis into the epidermis (see Chap. 31).[441]

The concept of intraepidermal tumors has been extended also to include Paget's disease of the breast, extramammary Paget's disease (Chap. 31), intraepidermal junction nevus (see Chap. 29), and malignant melanoma in situ (see Chap. 29).[90]

Some authors still regard the intraepidermal epithelioma of Jadassohn as a distinct entity that may invade the dermis and occasionally cause metastases.[442] It has been postulated that this tumor arises from acrosyringium keratinocytes or pluripotential adnexal cells and represents an adnexal carcinoma.[442]

The existence of *basal cell carcinomas with features of squamous cell carcinoma* was first postulated in 1922.[443] Two types of basal squamous cell epitheliomas, referred to as *metatypical epitheliomas,* were recognized: a mixed and an intermediary type. The mixed type was described as showing focal keratinization consisting of pearls with a colloidal or parakeratotic center, and the intermediary type as showing within a network of narrow strands two kinds of cells, an outer row of dark-staining basal cells and an inner layer of cells appearing larger, lighter, and better defined than the basal cells and regarded as intermediate in character between basal and squamous cells (see Figs. 30-49 and 30-50).

Several authors have accepted the existence of basal squamous cell epitheliomas or metatypical epitheliomas.[372,444–446] They are considered by some to represent a transition from basal cell carcinoma to squamous cell carcinoma. It has been stated that a continuum extends from basal cell carcinoma at one extreme to squamous cell carcinoma at the other.[446] The incidence of basal squamous cell carcinomas among basal cell carcinomas has been judged to be 3%,[446] 8%,[445] and even 12%.[444] It has also been stated that basal squamous cell epitheliomas show a greater tendency to metastasize than basal cell carcinomas.[372,444,446]

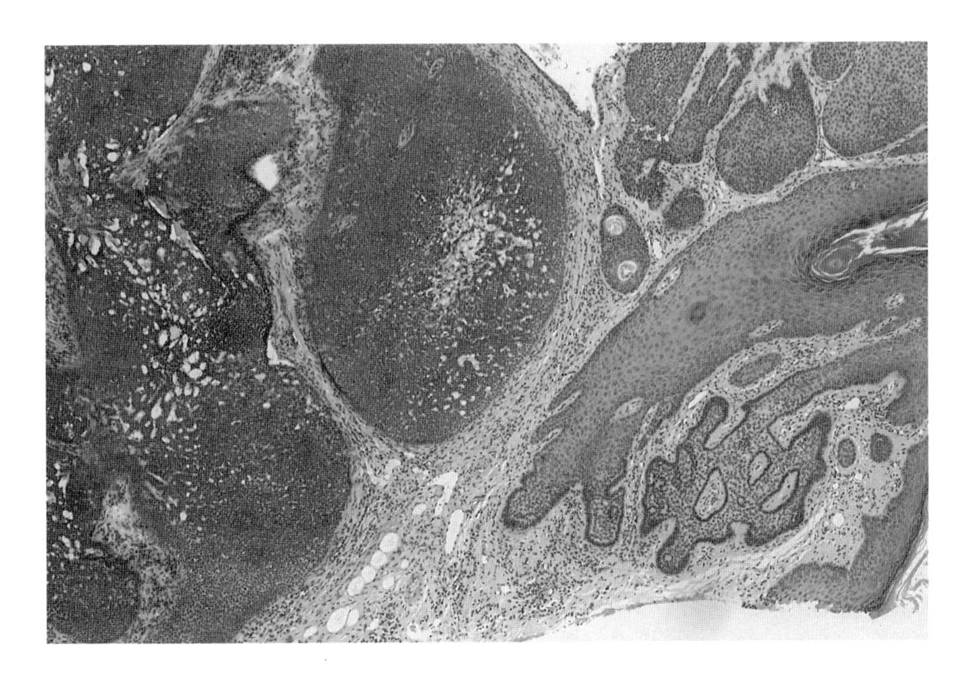

FIG. 30-62. Basal cell carcinoma showing follicular differentiation Nodular islands of basaloid cells are associated with a focal proliferation of basaloid cells in association with a hair follicle.

However, the existence of basal squamous cell epitheliomas is questioned by many.[397,447–451] It would seem that the entirely different genesis of squamous cell carcinoma, a true anaplastic carcinoma of the epidermis, and basal cell carcinoma, a tumor composed of immature rather than anaplastic cells, makes the occurrence of transitional forms quite unlikely (see Pathogenesis). It can be assumed that the so-called mixed type of basal squamous cell epithelioma represents a keratotic basal cell carcinoma (see Fig. 30-53) and that the intermediate type represents a basal cell carcinoma with differentiation into two types of cells (see Fig. 30-48). Other putative examples of basosquamous differentiation are better interpreted as *basal cell carcinoma with follicular differentiation* (Figs. 30-62 and 30-63).

Mixed carcinoma shows a squamous cell carcinoma contiguous to a basal cell carcinoma as a so-called collision tumor (see Fig. 30-51). It is likely that, in most instances, the squamous cell carcinoma develops secondary to the basal cell carcinoma. Like other chronic ulcerative lesions, such as burns and stasis ulcers, basal cell carcinoma may stimulate the development of a squamous cell carcinoma. Before making a diagnosis of mixed carcinoma, however, one must rule out the possibility of pseudocarcinomatous hyperplasia occurring in a basal cell carcinoma.

Pathogenesis. Krompecher, the original describer of basal cell carcinoma, stated in 1903 that he regarded this tumor as a carcinoma of the basal cells of the epidermis and that those tumors that show a tendency toward gland formation are imitating the potential of the basal cells to form cutaneous glands.[452] Krompecher's view is still supported by some.[453–455] According to Geschickter and Koehler, only those basal cells with a potential to develop into glandular cells give rise to basal cell carcinoma. They suggested the designation *appendage cell carcinoma*. Mallory held the opinion that basal cell carcinomas are

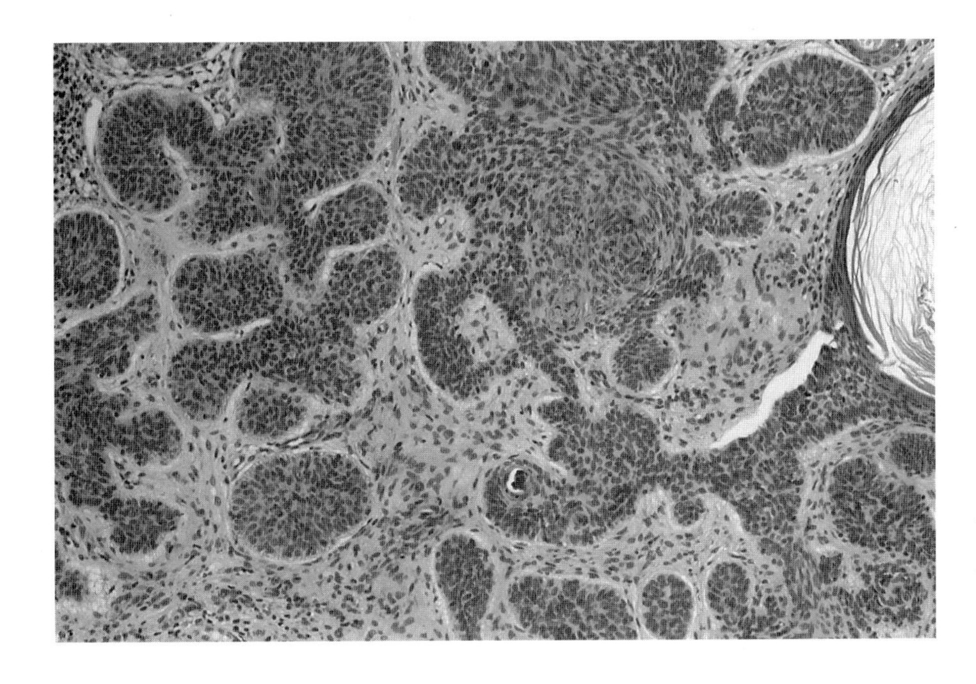

FIG. 30-63. Basal cell carcinoma with follicular differentiation Epithelium and stroma form structures reminiscent of follicular germs, and there is formation of a horn cyst resembling a follicular structure.

carcinomas of hair matrix cells. In 1947, Foot expressed the view that basal cell carcinomas are carcinomas that have developed from distorted primordia of dermal adnexa rather than from ordinary epidermal basal cells.[408] He stated that the tumors imitate the embryonal development of one or all three types of adnexal primordia, that is, hair, sebaceous gland, and sweat gland.

The first author to express doubts that basal cell carcinomas are carcinomas was Adamson; in 1914, he stated that, in his opinion, basal cell carcinomas are nevoid tumors originating "from latent embryonic foci aroused from their dormant state at a later period in life."[456] He believed that the latent embryonic foci usually are embryonic pilosebaceous follicles but occasionally are embryonic sweat ducts. Several other authors have since reached similar conclusions, among them Wallace and Halpert, who stated in 1950 that they regarded basal cell carcinomas as benign tumors arising from cells destined to form hair follicles.[457] They proposed the term *trichoma* for them.

In 1948, Lever expressed his belief that basal cell carcinomas are not carcinomas and are not derived from basal cells, but rather are nevoid tumors, or hamartomas, derived from primary epithelial germ cells. In other words, basal cell carcinomas originate from incompletely differentiated, immature cells and not from anaplastic cells. Although gamma-glutamyl transpeptidase activity is observed in the atypical cells in squamous cell carcinoma, Bowen's disease, and actinic keratoses, no gamma-glutamyl transpeptidase activity is expressed in the cells of basal cell carcinoma.[458] In this view, basal cell carcinoma represents the least differentiated of the appendage tumors.

It was originally assumed, analogous to Adamson's view, that the primary epithelial germ cells giving rise to basal cell carcinoma are in all instances embryonic cells that lay dormant until the onset of neoplasia. Even though this view applies to the linear unilateral basal cell nevus, which is usually present from birth, it is likely that, as suggested by Pinkus, basal cell carcinomas occurring later in life arise not from dormant embryonic primary epithelial germ cells but from pluripotential cells that form continuously during life and, like embryonic primary epithelial germ cells, have the potential of forming hair, sebaceous glands, and apocrine glands.[396] The fact that basal cell carcinomas may arise in sun-exposed areas and in areas of radiodermatitis supports this view. Their tendency to local invasion and tissue destruction, their capacity for local persistence and recurrence if not ablated, and their occasional capacity for metastasis support the concept that these lesions are carcinomas, albeit in most instances with little or no capacity for metastasis.

Pilar differentiation. Differentiation in basal cell carcinoma is predominantly toward pilar keratin. The presence of citrulline in keratinized structures indicates that the origin of the keratin is the hair matrix, because epidermal keratin contains no citrulline.[449] Studies with monoclonal cytokeratin antibodies support the assumption of pilar differentiation in basal cell carcinoma. Thus a cytokeratin antibody binding to the follicular epithelium but not to the interfollicular epidermis stains all cells of basal cell carcinoma.[459] Also, a monoclonal antibody against basal cell carcinoma keratin stains, in addition to the cells of basal cell carcinoma, all follicular cells below the isthmus portion of normal anagen hair follicles.[460]

Stromal factor. The importance of stroma in the development of basal cell carcinomas is borne out by the fact that autotransplants of basal cell carcinomas survive only when they include connective tissue stroma.[461] Also, the rarity of basal cell carcinomas on the palms and soles and the fact that the palmar and plantar pits of the nevoid basal cell carcinoma syndrome very rarely show a full-fledged basal cell carcinoma suggest that the palms and soles do not possess the stromal factor necessary for the formation of basal cell carcinomas.[462]

Lack of autonomy. Basal cell carcinomas, when transplanted to the anterior chamber of the rabbit's eye together with their connective tissue stroma, fail to grow, in contrast to squamous cell carcinoma.[463] Furthermore, basal cell carcinomas, in contrast to many human tumors, do not grow when transplanted subcutaneously to athymic nude mice.[464] These observations suggest a lack of autonomy of the cells of at least some basal cell carcinomas. Because autonomy of the tumor cell is a prerequisite for the formation of metastases and represents a characteristic feature of malignant tumors,[465] the absence of autonomy in basal cell carcinoma is consistent with its inability to metastasize in most instances.

Site of origin. The usual site of origin of basal cell carcinoma appears to be the surface epidermis. Occasionally, however, the tumor may originate from the outer root sheath of a hair follicle.[466,467]

Of particular interest is the manner of growth of *superficial basal cell carcinoma.* Routine sectioning carried out perpendicular to the skin surface shows seemingly independent nests of basal cell carcinoma suggestive at times of the growth of primary epithelial germs in the embryonic skin (see Fig. 2-1). Thus it was at one time widely assumed that the peripheral extension seen in superficial basal cell carcinoma was based on a "multicentric" growth characterized by the formation of new buds of tumor tissue at the periphery. However, on the basis of findings in serial sections and in wax reconstructions of superficial basal cell carcinomas, Madsen has favored the theory of a "unicentric" origin.[468–469] Madsen was able to show that the tumor strands are continuous but are attached to the undersurface of the epidermis only at intervals, like garlands. Madsen found not only in his wax reconstructions but also in sections cut parallel to the surface of the skin that individual tumor islands are interconnected. Oberste-Lehn,[470] using a technique of separating the epidermis from the dermis by maceration, could not find such interconnections, but the possibility could not be excluded, as Madsen pointed out, that the interconnections had ruptured as a result of the maceration. It was subsequently shown when trypsin was used for the separation of the epidermis from the dermis that interconnections exist between tumor cell nests in superficial basal cell carcinoma. Similarly, three-dimensional reconstruction by means of serial horizontal microscopic sections and a special computer confirmed a unicentric origin.[471]

Electron Microscopy. The predominant cell in undifferentiated basal cell carcinoma is characterized by a large nucleus, poorly developed desmosomes, and rather sparse tonofilaments. Thus the tumor cells differ from normal epidermal basal cells. They resemble the cells of the undifferentiated hair matrix[472] or the immature basal cells of the embryonic epidermis, particularly those of the primary epithelial germ.[473,474] In addition to the prevalent large, light cells, a few cells that are smaller, darker, and more irregularly shaped can be found.[404,473] The darkness of the latter cells is due to the abundance of ribonucleoprotein particles in their cytoplasm. A well-developed basement membrane separates the tumor from the dermis.[472] Processes from the tumor cells do not usually penetrate the basement membrane in basal cell carcinoma, in contrast to squamous cell carcinoma, in which processes extend through a fragmented basement membrane into the stroma.[475]

Keratinization is commonly observed by electron microscopy in basal cell carcinoma, especially in the keratotic type. In addition to well-developed desmosomes and many thick bundles of tonofilaments, dense clumps of homogeneous, dyskeratotic material are present in many keratinizing cells. A small number of keratohyaline granules are often seen. They probably represent trichohyaline granules, which occur in the process of keratinization of the inner root sheath and its cuticle.[473]

Some basal cell carcinomas show areas of adenoid differentiation in which cells are grouped around glandlike lumina. Such cells may show pronounced infolding of the plasma membrane at their lateral borders as seen normally in eccrine ductal cells.[404]

In pigmented basal cell carcinomas, most of the melanin is found within melanocytes of the tumor and in melanophages located in the connective tissue stroma. Although numerous melanosomes are present in the dendrites of the melanocytes, the tumor cells generally do not phagocytize the melanin-containing dendrites, resulting in a blockage of the transfer of melanin from melanocytes to the tumor cells.[476,477] This is analogous to the blocked transfer from melanocytes to tumor cells in some pigmented seborrheic keratoses referred to as *melanoacanthoma*. Nevertheless, in occasional instances of pigmented basal cell carcinoma, some transfer of melanosomes to the tumor cells takes place. The tumor cells then contain melanosomes, which are located largely as melanosome complexes within lysosomes.[473]

Presence of Amyloid. Cell proliferation in basal cell carcinoma is considerable. The experimentally determined cell-doubling time of 9 days, however, does not conform with the clinical observation that basal cell carcinoma, as a rule, is a very slowly growing tumor.[478] This suggests that there must be cell death. In addition to phagocytosis by neighboring tumor cells and macrophages, apoptosis of tumor cells also often takes place, with transformation of the cells into colloid bodies and subsequently into amyloid.[402,479] This conversion of epithelial cells into amyloid is analogous to that occurring in lichenoid and macular amyloidosis. Colloid bodies, demonstrable by direct immunofluorescence for immunoglobulin M (IgM), have been found in 89% of basal cell carcinomas.[402] Amyloid has been observed in the stroma and inside the tumor islands both by histochemistry and by electron microscopy in as many as 65% of basal cell carcinomas.[402,480] This amyloid shows positive staining with antikeratin antiserum, indicating that it is derived from tonofilaments.[481] The fact that the amyloid is permanganate-resistant indicates that it is not secondary amyloid.[482]

Differential Diagnosis. Differentiation of basal cell carcinoma from squamous cell carcinoma can sometimes be difficult, so difficult that some authors believe that intermediate forms (basal squamous cell epitheliomas) occur. However, as a rule, differentiation is fairly easy. One of the best points of differentiation is that most cells of basal cell carcinoma stain deeply basophilic, whereas most cells of squamous cell carcinoma, at least in low-grade lesions, have an eosinophilic tint due to partial keratinization. The cells in high-grade squamous cell carcinoma may appear basophilic because of the absence of keratinization. However, they differ from basal cell carcinoma by showing much greater atypicality of their nuclei and their mitotic figures. It is important to remember that keratinization is not a prerogative of squamous cell carcinoma; it occurs also in basal cell carcinoma with differentiation toward hair structures (see Keratotic Basal Cell Carcinoma). Keratinization in basal cell carcinomas may be partial and then result in parakeratotic bands and whorls, or it may be complete and result in horn cysts. The keratinization seen in the horn cysts differs from that seen in the horn pearls of squamous cell carcinomas by being abrupt and complete rather than gradual and incomplete. The fairly common presence in basal cell carcinoma of areas of retraction of the tumor cell masses from the surrounding connective tissue also aids in the differentiation of this tumor from squamous cell carcinoma, in which such areas of retraction are rarely found.

The differential diagnosis of basal cell carcinoma from trichoepithelioma is discussed in Chap. 31. Of particular importance is the differentiation of fibrosing basal cell carcinoma from the only recently described desmoplastic trichoepithelioma. Both tumors have in common thin strands of small basaloid cells embedded in a dense, fibrous stroma, but desmoplastic trichoepithelioma also shows a considerable number of horn cysts. Many tumors originally diagnosed as basal cell carcinomas in children and teenagers could be reclassified as desmoplastic trichoepithelioma.[483]

EPIDERMAL TUMORS IN IMMUNOSUPPRESSED HOSTS

The widespread use of immunosuppressive therapy as part of organ transplantation and in the treatment of some immunologically mediated diseases has led to a new phenomenon of rapidly developing warts and epidermal tumors. There is a spectrum of squamous atypia ranging from typical viral warts through dysplastic or atypical warts to squamous cell carcinomas. The squamous cell carcinomas have been shown to have similar proliferative potential to similar lesions in hosts with normal immune function,[484] although they lack the host immune response that would normally be present.[485] They also share the same early expression of keratin 17 seen in a number of epidermal hyperproliferative states.[486] Mutations of p53 may play a part in the development of the tumors.[487] Rapidly progressing multiple squamous cell carcinomas have also been reported in association with chronic myeloid leukemia.[488] Basal cell carcinomas tend to show an infiltrative rather than a nodular growth pattern more frequently in the immunosuppressed.[489] Kaposi's sarcoma can also present as a fulminant process following liver or kidney transplantation[490,491] and may recur with the introduction of cyclosporin A therapy.[492] It has also been suggested that HIV-positive hosts have an increased risk of developing malignant melanoma.[493]

KERATOACANTHOMA

Two types of keratoacanthoma exist: solitary and multiple.

Solitary Keratoacanthoma

Since 1950, solitary keratoacanthoma, a common lesion, has been recognized as an entity and differentiated from squamous cell carcinoma, which it often resembles clinically and histologically.[494,495] Solitary keratoacanthoma occurs in elderly persons usually as a single lesion; however, occasionally, there are several lesions, or new lesions develop. The lesion consists of a firm, dome-shaped nodule 1.0 to 2.5 cm in diameter with a horn-filled crater in its center. The sites of predilection are exposed areas, where about 95% of solitary keratoacanthomas occur, but they may occur on any hairy cutaneous site.[496] They have not been reported on the palms, soles, or mucous surfaces, although, in rare instances, they occur subungually (see text following). Keratoacanthomas located on the vermilion border of the lip probably arise from hair follicles in the adjacent skin.[497] Keratoacanthomas usually reach their full size within 6 to 8 weeks and involute spontaneously, generally in less than 6 months. Healing takes place with a slightly depressed scar. In some instances, a keratoacanthoma increases in size for more than 2 months and takes up to 1 year to involute.[496]

An increased incidence of keratoacanthoma is observed in immunosuppressed patients.[498] Also, keratoacanthomas commonly occur in the Muir-Torre syndrome of sebaceous neoplasms and keratoacanthomas associated with visceral carcinomas (Chap. 31). Keratoacanthomas may be the only type of cutaneous tumor present in this syndrome.[499,500]

There are three rare clinical variants of solitary keratoacanthoma. In two forms, giant keratoacanthoma and keratoacanthoma centrifugum marginatum, the keratoacanthoma attains a large size. In *giant keratoacanthoma,* the growth rapidly reaches a size of 5 cm or more and may cause destruction of underlying tissues. Nevertheless, spontaneous involution takes place after several months, often accompanied by detachment of a large keratotic plaque. The most common sites are the nose[501,502] and the eyelids.[498,503,504] In *keratoacanthoma centrifugum marginatum,* the lesion may reach a size of 20 cm in diameter. There is no tendency toward spontaneous involution; instead, there is peripheral extension with a raised, rolled border and atrophy in the center of the lesion. The most common locations are the dorsa of the hands[505,506] and the legs.[507,508] The third rare variant is *subungual keratoacanthoma,* which shows a destructive crateriform lesion with keratotic excrescences under the distal portion of a fingernail. It fails to regress spontaneously, is tender, and by roentgenogram shows damage to the terminal phalanx by pressure erosion.[509–511]

Claims have been made that keratoacanthoma can undergo transformation into a squamous cell carcinoma either spontaneously[505,512] or as a result of immunosuppression.[498,513] It appears more likely, however, that the squamous cell carcinoma existed from the beginning in such instances (see Differential Diagnosis).[496,514]

Histopathology. The architecture of the lesion in a keratoacanthoma is as important to the diagnosis as the cellular characteristics. Therefore, if the lesion cannot be excised in its entirety, it is advisable that a fusiform specimen be excised for biopsy from the center of the lesion and that this specimen include the edge at least of one side and preferably of both sides of the lesion.[515] A shave biopsy is inadvisable, since the histologic changes at the base of the lesion are often of great importance in the differentiation from squamous cell carcinoma.

In the early proliferative stage, one observes a horn-filled invagination of the epidermis from which strands of epidermis protrude into the dermis. These strands are poorly demarcated from the surrounding stroma in many areas and may contain cells showing nuclear atypia[516] as well as many mitotic figures.[517] Even atypical mitoses may be seen occasionally.[518] Dyskeratotic cells, that is, cells showing individual cell keratinization, may also be seen in areas that otherwise do not show advanced keratinization. However, even at this early stage, some of the tumor areas show a fairly pronounced degree of keratinization, giving them an eosinophilic, glassy appearance. In the dermis, a rather pronounced inflammatory infiltrate is present.[517] Perineural invasion is occasionally seen in the proliferative phase of keratoacanthoma and should not be misinterpreted as evidence of malignancy.[519,520]

A fully developed lesion shows in its center a large, irregularly shaped crater filled with keratin (Fig. 30-64). The epidermis extends like a lip or a buttress over the sides of the crater. At the base of the crater, irregular epidermal proliferations extend both upward into the crater and downward from the base of the crater. These proliferations may still appear somewhat atypical, but less so than in the initial stage; the keratinization is extensive and fairly advanced, with only a thin shell of one or two layers of basophilic, nonkeratinized cells at the periphery of the proliferations, whereas the cells within this shell appear eosinophilic and glassy as a result of keratinization (Fig. 30-65). There are many horn pearls, most of which show complete keratinization in their center. The base of a fully developed keratoacanthoma appears regular and well demarcated and usually does not extend below the level of the sweat glands. A rather dense inflammatory infiltrate is present at the base of the lesion.[496,521]

In the involuting stage, proliferation has ceased, and most cells at the base of the crater have undergone keratinization. There may be shrunken, eosinophilic cells analogous to colloid or Civatte bodies among the tumor cells located nearest to the stroma as well as in the stroma, suggesting that cell degeneration followed by apoptosis contributes to the involution of the keratoacanthoma.[507] Gradually, the crater flattens and finally disappears during healing.

Pathogenesis. It is generally agreed that the lesion starts with hyperplasia of the infundibulum of one or several adjoining hair follicles and with squamous metaplasia of the attached sebaceous glands.[522] The application of cutaneous carcinogens to the skin of animals frequently produces, among other tumors, lesions with the histologic appearance of keratoacanthomas, and these tumors also have their origin in the infundibulum of one or several hair follicles.[523]

The cause of keratoacanthoma is not known. The theory of a viral genesis has not been confirmed. The electron microscopic findings are largely nonspecific. However, keratoacanthomas, like squamous cell carcinomas and lesions of Bowen's disease, often show the presence of fairly numerous intracytoplasmic desmosomes.[524,525]

Differential Diagnosis. Differentiation of typical, mature lesions of keratoacanthoma from squamous cell carcinoma generally is not difficult. In favor of a diagnosis of keratoacanthoma are the architecture of a crater surrounded by buttresses and the high degree of keratinization, which is manifested by the eosinophilic, glassy appearance of many of the cells. Clinical data are also of great value: rapid development of an exophytic lesion showing a central, horn-filled crater speaks for keratoacanthoma rather than for squamous cell carcinoma.

The greatest difficulties in the differentiation of a keratoacanthoma from a squamous cell carcinoma are encountered in very early lesions, because a horn-filled invagination may be

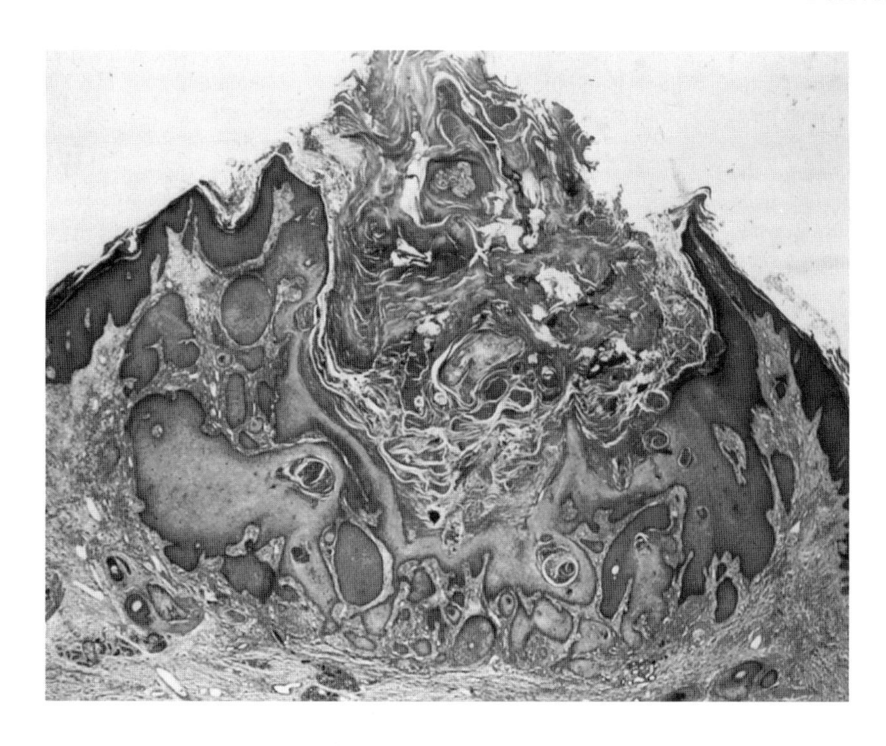

FIG. 30-64. Keratoacanthoma, low magnification
There is a large, central keratin-filled crater. On the right, the epidermis extends like a buttress over the side of the crater. Irregular epidermal proliferations extend downward from the base of the crater into the dermis.

seen in squamous cell carcinoma (see Fig. 30-41) and cells with an atypical appearance may occur in a keratoacanthoma. Occasionally, an early keratoacanthoma shows a greater degree of nuclear atypia than do some squamous cell carcinomas.[526] Also, individual cell keratinization can occur in keratoacanthoma. On rare occasions, even adenoid formations caused by dyskeratosis and acantholysis can occur in keratoacanthoma.[527] Thus it was found on reclassification in one study that in only 81% of the cases of keratoacanthoma could a diagnosis of squamous cell carcinoma be fully excluded and that in only 86% of the cases of squamous cell carcinoma could keratoacanthoma be ruled out with certainty. These findings explain why, on rare occasions, lesions classified as keratoacanthoma cause metastases.[514] Great caution is indicated in the diagnosis of giant keratoacanthomas. Several cases diagnosed as such turned out to be squamous cell carcinomas either by metastasizing[528] or by deep invasion into muscle.[529]

Because it is widely agreed that squamous cell carcinomas can masquerade as keratoacanthomas clinically and histologically,[496,530] it is best to err on the safe side in a case of doubt and to proceed on the assumption that the lesion is a squamous cell carcinoma.

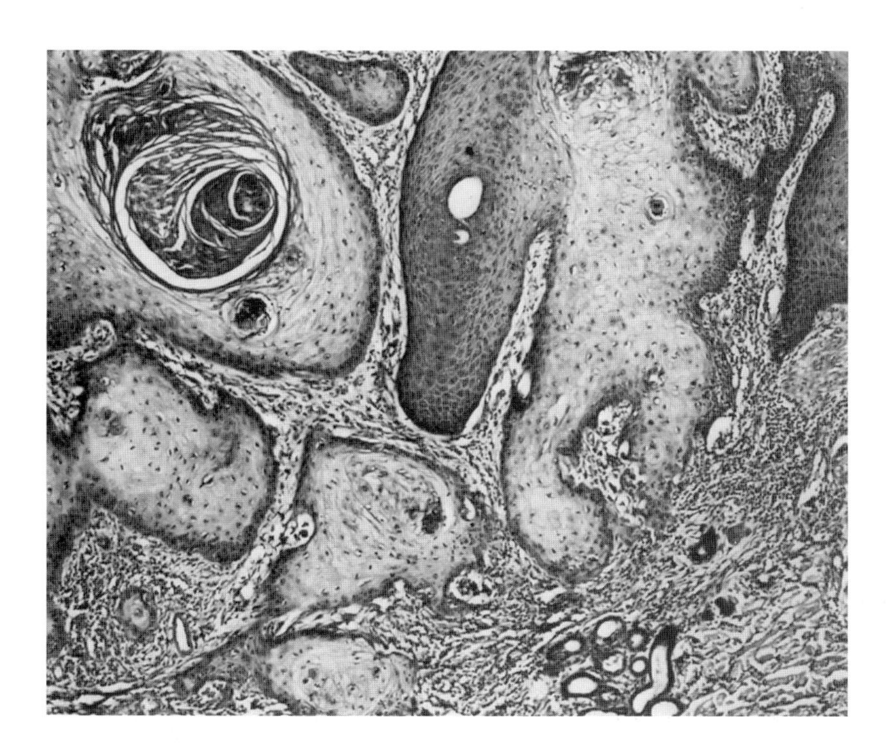

FIG. 30-65. Keratoacanthoma
Higher magnification of the epidermal proliferations at the base of the crater shows their resemblance to squamous cell carcinoma. However, there is more keratinization than is usually seen in squamous cell carcinoma, giving the tumor islands a glassy appearance.

Attempts at differentiating between keratoacanthoma and squamous cell carcinoma by histochemical or immunohistochemical methods have shown distinct differences in typical cases but not necessarily in borderline cases.

There are two variants of *multiple keratoacanthoma*: the multiple self-healing epitheliomas of the skin, or Ferguson Smith type, and the eruptive keratoacanthomas, or Grzybowski type. Both variants are rare in comparison with solitary keratoacanthoma.

In *multiple self-healing epitheliomas* of the skin, lesions begin to appear in childhood or adolescence on any part of the skin, including the palms and soles, but especially on the face and the extremities. Subungual lesions have also been described.[510] Generally, there are no more than a dozen lesions at any one time.[531] The lesions may reach the same size as solitary keratoacanthomas and after a few months heal with a depressed scar.[532,533] In some cases, however, the lesions do not heal.[534] In some patients, the condition is inherited.[534,535]

In *eruptive keratoacanthoma,* lesions do not appear until adult life. Many hundreds of follicular papules are present, measuring from 2 to 3 mm in diameter.[536,537] The oral mucosa and larynx may be involved.[538,539]

Histopathology. The histologic appearance of the lesions of multiple self-healing epitheliomas of the skin is similar to that of solitary keratoacanthoma.[531,533] More frequently than in solitary keratoacanthoma, the cutaneous proliferations in multiple self-healing epitheliomas of the skin are seen to be continuous with the follicular epithelium.[540] The cutaneous lesions in eruptive keratoacanthoma show less crater formation than those in solitary keratoacanthoma. The mucosal lesions lack a crater and can easily be misinterpreted as squamous cell carcinoma.[538,539]

Pathogenesis. It appears likely that multiple keratoacanthoma basically represents the same condition as solitary keratoacanthoma and that predisposition or genetic factors are responsible for the greater number of lesions.[541] In multiple as in solitary keratoacanthoma, lesions arising in hair-bearing parts of the skin have their onset in the upper portion of a hair follicle, whereas the site of origin of lesions arising on the palms, the soles, and the mucous membranes is not apparent.[538]

PAGET'S DISEASE

Paget's disease of the breast occurs almost exclusively in women. Only a few instances of its occurrence in the male breast have been described.[542] Of interest is its occurrence in the male breast after treatment of a carcinoma of the prostate with estrogen.[543] The cutaneous lesion in Paget's disease of the breast begins either on the nipple or the areola of the breast and extends slowly to the surrounding skin. It is always unilateral and consists of a sharply defined, slightly infiltrated area of erythema showing scaling, oozing, and crusting. There may or may not be ulceration or retraction of the nipple.

The cutaneous lesion is nearly always associated with carcinoma of the breast, and in more than half of the patients, a mass can be felt on palpation of the breast. Metastases in the axillary lymph nodes were found by one group of investigators in about 67% of their patients with a palpable mass of the breast and in 33% of those without a palpable mass.[544] This contrasts with the experience of others, who encountered no axillary metastases in the absence of a palpable mass of the breast.[545]

A clinical picture indistinguishable from that of early Paget's disease of the nipple may be seen in erosive adenomatosis of the nipple, a benign neoplasm of the major nipple ducts (see Chap. 31).[546]

Histopathology. In early lesions of Paget's disease of the breast, the epidermis usually shows only a few scattered Paget cells (Fig. 30-66). They are large, rounded cells that are devoid of intercellular bridges and contain a large nucleus and ample cytoplasm. The cytoplasm of these cells stains much lighter than that of the adjacent squamous cells. As the number of Paget cells increases, they compress the squamous cells to such an extent that the latter may merely form a network, the meshes of which are filled with Paget cells lying singly and in groups. In

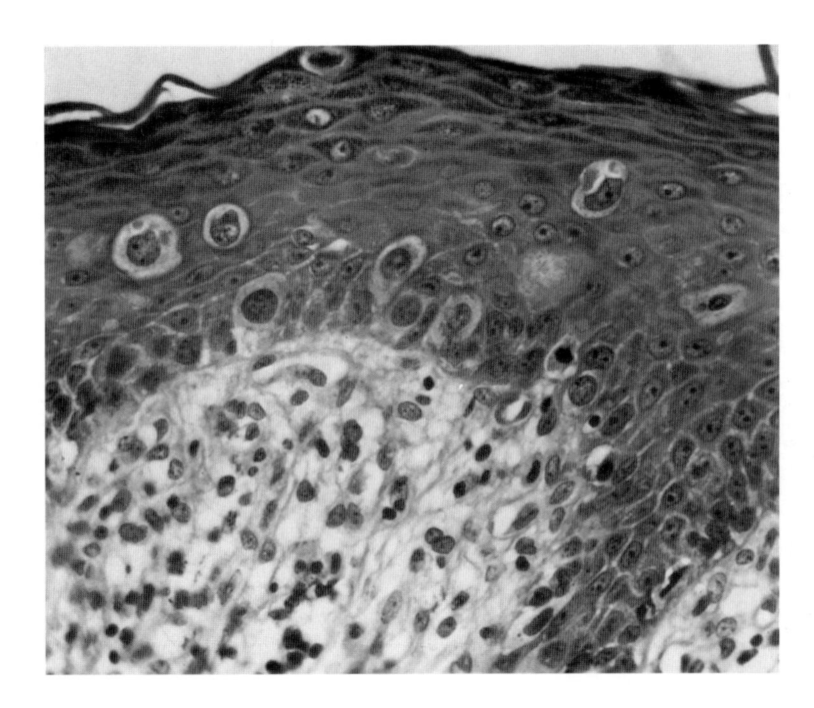

FIG. 30-66. Paget's disease
Only a few Paget cells are scattered through the epidermis. They are large rounded cells devoid of intercellular bridges, with ample pale-staining cytoplasm.

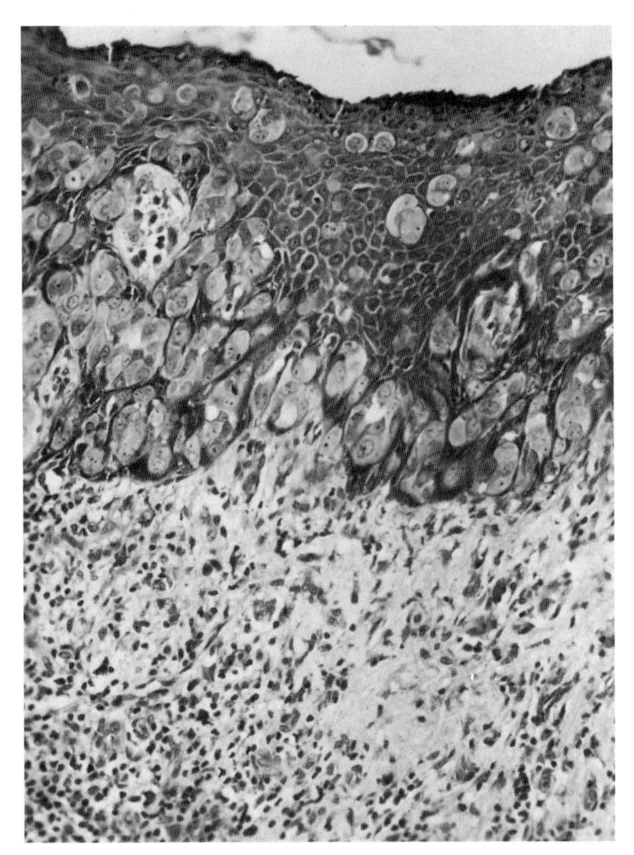

FIG. 30-67. Paget's disease, low magnification
The epidermis is permeated with numerous Paget cells lying singly and in groups. There is no invasion of the dermis by Paget cells. Flattened basal cells lie between the tumor cells and the dermis in many places, a finding that aids in the differentiation of Paget's disease from malignant melanoma in situ.

particular, one often observes flattened basal cells lying between Paget cells and the underlying dermis (Fig. 30-67).

Histochemical staining of the Paget cells within the epidermis in Paget's disease of the breast has given inconsistent results. In contrast with extramammary Paget's disease in which the presence of sialomucin can be demonstrated in abundance in nearly all cases, the Paget cells in Paget's disease of the breast stain with the PAS reaction in only some of the cases (Fig. 30-68),[547] and if positive, the number of positively staining cells is rather small.[548] The PAS-positive cells may be diastase-resistant, but often they are not.[549] Similarly, the alcian blue stain at pH 2.5 is only weakly positive in scattered Paget cells in some of the cases and negative in others.[549] Occasionally, Paget cells contain some melanin[550]; however, they are dopa-negative.[551]

The dermis in Paget's disease shows a moderately severe chronic inflammatory reaction. Although Paget cells do not invade the dermis from the epidermis, they may be seen extending from the epidermis into the epithelium of hair follicles.[552]

Histologic examination of the mammary ducts and glands nearly always shows malignant changes in some of them. At first, the carcinoma is confined within the walls of the ducts and glands (Fig. 30-69), but the tumor cells ultimately invade the connective tissue. From then on, lymphatic spread and metastases occur, just as in other types of mammary carcinoma. In mammary Paget's disease, the malignant changes have their onset in the lactiferous ducts and from there extend into the epidermis,[547] but there are rare instances in which the malignant cells are confined to the epidermis of the nipple or involve only the most distal portion of one lactiferous duct.[553]

Pathogenesis. As long as *electron microscopic examination* constituted the major factor in analyzing the derivation or the direction of differentiation of the cells in Paget's disease of the nipple, no clear decision could be reached whether the constituting cells were keratinocytes or glandular cells. The presence of desmosomes between neighboring Paget cells and between

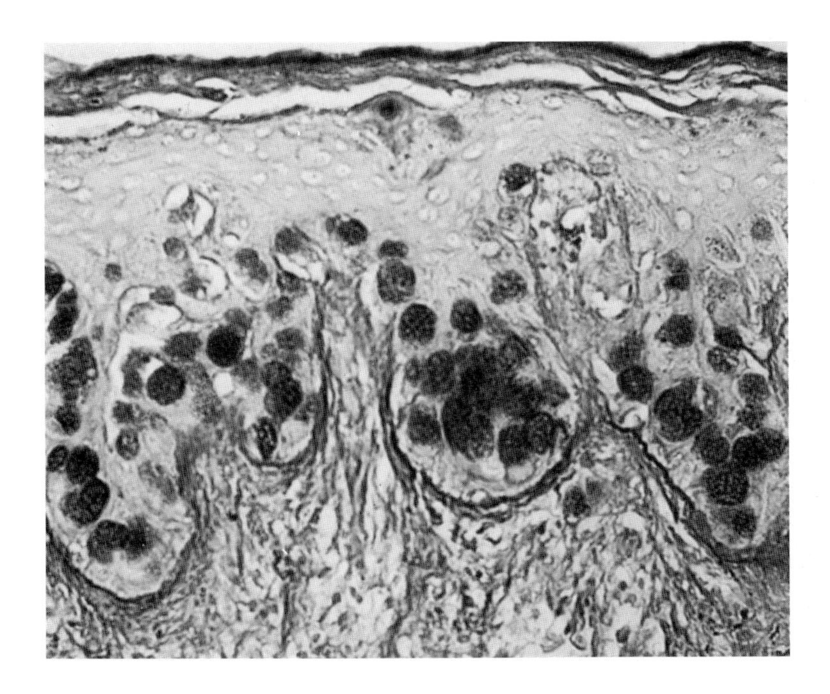

FIG. 30-68. Paget's disease, PAS stain
The cytoplasm of the Paget cells gives a positive PAS reaction that is diastase-resistant.

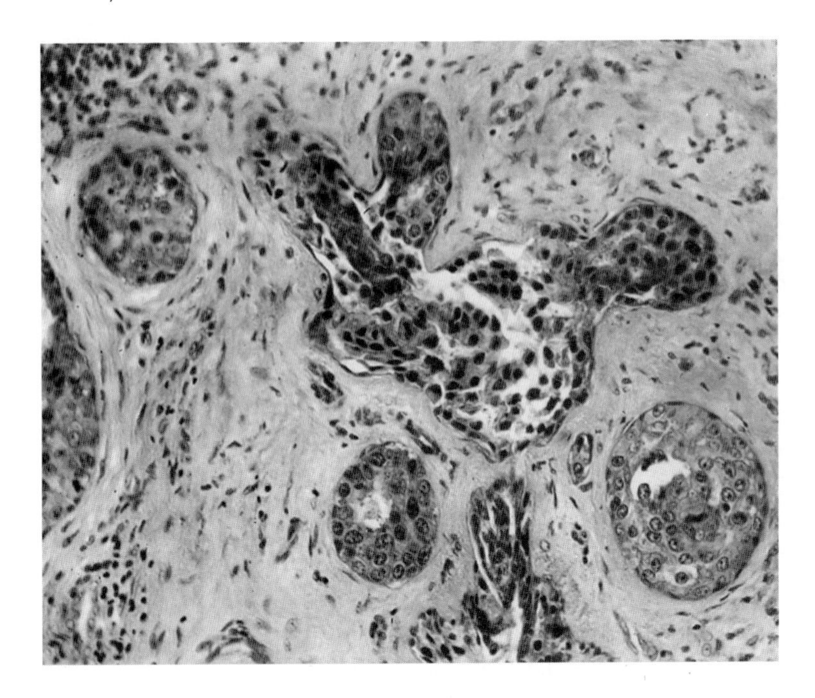

FIG. 30-69. Paget's disease
Intraductal carcinoma is present in the mammary ducts.

Paget cells and keratinocytes seemed to support a derivation from keratinocytes.[554] On the other hand, scattered desmosomes are normally found connecting the cells of the lactiferous ducts,[555] and wherever cytoplasmic processes of Paget cells lie in contact with the basal lamina, no hemidesmosomes are present, as they would be in the case of keratinocytes.[549] Also, Paget cells can be found bordering small lumina in areas in which groups of Paget cells lie together.[549,555,556]

Immunohistochemical studies in recent years have proved beyond any doubt the glandular derivation of the Paget cells of both mammary and extramammary Paget's disease. Thus carcinoembryonic antigen is regularly found in Paget cells. Whereas intervening keratinocytes and melanocytes do not stain, carcinoembryogenic antigen is present in the cells of normal eccrine and apocrine glands.[557] Furthermore, Paget cells express cytokeratins typical of glandular epithelia but do not react with antibodies to epidermal keratin.[558]

Enzyme histochemistry in Paget's disease of the breast has shown the presence of an apocrine enzymatic pattern in the intraepidermal Paget cells consisting of a strong reactivity for acid phosphatase and esterase and only a weakly positive reaction for aminopeptidase and succinic dehydrogenase.[559] This finding suggests that the intraepidermal Paget cells in Paget's disease of the breast are derived from mammary gland cells, because the mammary gland represents a modified apocrine gland.

Differential Diagnosis. Paget's disease of the breast must be differentiated from Bowen's disease and the superficial spreading or "pagetoid" type of malignant melanoma in situ. Although vacuolated cells may occur in both Paget's disease and Bowen's disease, one observes clear-cut transitions between the vacuolated cells and epidermal cells only in Bowen's disease. Furthermore, one may observe in Bowen's disease, but not in Paget's disease, clumping of nuclei within multinucleated epidermal cells and individual cell keratinization. In addition, the cells in Bowen's disease do not contain carcinoembryonic antigen but react with prekeratin contained in rabbit antihuman prekeratin antiserum.[560]

In the superficial spreading or pagetoid type of malignant melanoma in situ, as in the epidermis of Paget's disease of the breast, there are large, vacuolated cells scattered through the epidermis.[548] The difficulty in distinguishing between the two types of cells may be increased by the fact that Paget cells occasionally also contain melanin.[550] The most important points to remember in differentiating the two types of cells are as follows: (1) Paget cells are separated in many areas from the dermis by flattened basal cells, whereas melanoma cells border directly on the dermis; (2) Paget cells do not invade the dermis, whereas melanoma cells often do; (3) the tumor cells of malignant melanoma contain abundant cytoplasmic S-100 protein, but in tissues from Paget's disease, S-100 protein is usually absent in the tumor cells, although it may be seen in myoepithelial cells, Langerhans' cells, and Schwann cells of cutaneous nerves[561]; (4) Paget cells are dopa-negative, unlike melanoma cells; and (5) Melanoma cells unlike Paget cells may be positive for the HMB-45 antigen.

EXTRAMAMMARY PAGET'S DISEASE

Extramammary Paget's disease most commonly affects the vulva, less commonly the male genital area[562] or the perianal area,[551] and, in exceptional cases only, the axillae, the region of the ceruminal glands,[563] or that of Moll's glands.[564] In cases with involvement of the axillae, the genital area may also be affected.[565] Thus extramammary Paget's disease involves areas in which apocrine glands are normally encountered. Only very few cases of an association between mammary and vulvar Paget's disease have been described.[566] In rare instances, extramammary Paget's disease is a secondary event caused by extension of an adenocarcinoma either of the rectum to the perianal region,[551] of the cervix to the vulvar region,[567] or of the urinary bladder to the urethra and glans penis[568] or to the groin.[569] On the other hand, long-standing genital Paget's disease can extend inward to the cervix and urinary tract.[570]

In extramammary Paget's disease, the clinical picture shows a slowly enlarging reddish patch with oozing and crusting. The patch resembles an eczematous lesion but has a sharp, irregular border. In extramammary Paget's disease, in contrast to the mammary type, itching is common.

Histopathology. Extramammary Paget's disease shares with Paget's disease the presence of varying numbers of Paget cells within the epidermis. In some instances, the Paget cells are found to be limited to the epidermis. Frequently, Paget cells can also be identified within the epithelium of some hair follicles or eccrine sweat ducts.[571] Such in situ malignancy associated with extramammary Paget's disease has the same favorable prognosis as does extramammary Paget's disease limited to the epidermis. However, the prognosis is much more serious in cases in which the Paget cells have invaded the dermis from the epidermis[571,572] or from an underlying sweat gland carcinoma.[573] In this respect, extramammary Paget's disease differs from mammary Paget's disease, in which invasion of the dermis from the overlying epidermis does not occur.[552] Glandular clusters with a central lumen, absent in mammary Paget's disease, may be seen in the lower epidermis in extramammary Paget's disease.[571,574]

On histochemical staining, the Paget cells seen in the epidermis and in the adnexa show a positive reaction for sialomucinin in almost all cases of extramammary Paget's disease. Thus, the cytoplasm of the Paget cells is PAS-positive, diastase-resistant, stains with alcian blue at pH 2.5 but not at pH 0.4, and is hyaluronidase-resistant (Chap. 4). It usually stains positive also with colloidal iron and mucicarmine.[547] Nevertheless, these stains can be negative in cases of extramammary and of mammary Paget's disease.[548]

In cases of "secondary" extramammary Paget's disease, the process extends either from a mucus-secreting adenocarcinoma of the rectum to the perianal skin,[551,575,576] from a mucus-secreting endocervical carcinoma to the vulva,[567] or from a transitional cell carcinoma of the urinary bladder with urethral extension.[568,569] In such cases, the Paget cells in the perianal or vulvar skin are derived from the preexisting carcinoma and contain mucus that always is PAS-positive and diastase-resistant and always shows a positive staining reaction with alcian blue at pH 2.5 that is hyaluronidase-resistant. The mucus represents sialomucin, a nonsulfated acid mucopolysaccharide.[551] The prognosis in secondary extramammary Paget's disease is poor.

The prognosis of "primary" extramammary Paget's disease generally is better than that of mammary Paget's disease. In two large combined series of 123 patients with vulvar Paget's disease, only 26 patients (21%) showed an underlying invasive carcinoma in the dermis at the time of operation.[571,572] In the other 79%, the Paget cells were present only within the epidermis and the epithelium of the cutaneous appendages, so that the process was still in situ. Thus one author observed only two examples of invasive sweat gland carcinoma among more than 100 cases of extramammary Paget's disease,[573] and another author reported none among 12 cases.[558] However, the rate of local recurrence is high even after seemingly adequate excision. The reasons for this are that (1) the extent of histologically demonstrable disease is often far greater than that of the clinically visible lesion and (2) extramammary Paget's disease, in contrast to mammary Paget's disease, can arise multifocally even in clinically normal-appearing areas of the skin.[577]

Pathogenesis. At one time, the view was widely accepted that in primary extramammary Paget's disease the Paget cells in the epidermis are there as a result of an in situ upward extension of an in situ adenocarcinoma of sweat glands along eccrine or apocrine ducts.[574,578] This view is analogous to the generally accepted views that secondary extramammary Paget's disease represents an extension of a rectal, cervical, or urinary bladder adenocarcinoma and that the development of mammary Paget's disease is an extension of an epidermotropic lactiferous duct carcinoma. The fact that an underlying in situ adenocarcinoma often could not be demonstrated was explained by the anatomic differences between the breast, which has only 20 large, conspicuous lactiferous ducts, and the genital skin, which has thousands of small apocrine and eccrine glands, making location of the particular small gland involved by carcinoma technically difficult.[574] Staining with antikeratin monoclonal antibodies has indicated that upward extension of an in situ adenocarcinoma derived from malignant secretory cells present within sweat ducts can occur.[579]

Even though in some cases extramammary Paget's disease is the result of extension of an underlying apocrine or eccrine sweat gland carcinoma to the overlying epidermis, in most instances it has its origin within the epidermis.[572] Careful subserial total sectioning of excised lesions of vulvar Paget's disease has shown that the lesions within the epidermis and its appendages have a multifocal origin.[577] Another pertinent argument in favor of the independence of the epidermal foci from any appendageal foci is the observation that in cases with extensive epidermal lesions, involvement of eccrine ducts and glands is often sparse and involvement of apocrine ducts and glands almost invariably absent, even though some Paget cells form apocrine glandular structures in the epidermis.[571] Even if there is continuity between the epidermal and the ductal foci, there is no certain way of determining whether the extension is in an upward or downward direction. However, the clinching argument in favor of the autonomy of the epidermal foci in primary extramammary Paget's disease is the fact that, in contrast to mammary Paget's disease, dermal invasion generally originates from the epidermis not ductal or glandular structures.[571,572]

In cases in which the extramammary Paget's disease arises within the epidermis and extends from there at a later date into the adnexa and still later from the epidermis into the dermis, the question is: Which cell gives rise to the Paget cell? Two possibilities have been suggested, although proof for either is lacking. The first is that the Paget cell arises within the poral portion of an apocrine duct.[580] The second is that, because the disease tends to occur in areas rich in apocrine glands and because there is in some cases unequivocal evidence of apocrine differentiation in the epidermis, intraepidermal Paget cells may be formed by pluripotential germinative cells within the epidermis that go awry trying to form apocrine structures.[562,571]

Immunohistochemical studies indicate an apocrine genesis of extramammary Paget's disease. It is true that carcinoembryonic antigen merely indicates that the extramammary Paget cells are glandular rather than epidermal cells and does not decide whether they are apocrine or eccrine.[557,558] However, two immunoreactants for apocrine glands, gross cystic disease fluid protein[581] and apocrine epithelial antigen,[558] have been shown to react with the Paget cells of extramammary Paget's disease, providing evidence for an apocrine derivation.

Differential Diagnosis. Extramammary Paget's disease, like

Paget's disease of the breast, must be differentiated from Bowen's disease and especially from superficial spreading or pagetoid malignant melanoma in situ (see Paget's Disease, Differential Diagnosis).

REFERENCES

1. Heenan PJ, Elder DE, Sobin LH. Histological typing of skin tumours. Berlin: Springer-Verlag, 1996;39.
2. Basler RSW, Jacobs SI, Taylor WB. Ichthyosis hystrix. Arch Dermatol 1978;114:1059.
3. Solomon LM, Fretzin DF, Dewald RL. The epidermal nevus syndrome. Arch Dermatol 1968;97:273.
4. Winer LH, Levin GH. Pigmented basal-cell carcinoma in verrucous nevi. Arch Dermatol 1961;83:960.
5. Horn MS, Sausker WF, Pierson DL. Basal cell epithelioma arising in a linear epidermal nevus. Arch Dermatol 1981;117:247.
6. Dogliotti M, Frenkel A. Malignant change in a verrucous nevus. Int J Dermatol 1978;17:225.
7. Cramer SF, Mandel MA, Hauler R et al. Squamous cell carcinoma arising in linear epidermal nevus. Arch Dermatol 1981;117:222.
8. Levin A, Amazon K, Rywlin AM. A squamous cell carcinoma that developed in an epidermal nevus. Am J Dermatopathol 1984;6:51.
9. Su WPD. Histopathologic varieties of epidermal nevus. Am J Dermatopathol 1982;4:161.
10. Ackerman AB. Histopathologic concept of epidermolytic hyperkeratosis. Arch Dermatol 1970;102:253.
11. Braun-Falco O, Petzoldt D, Christophers E et al. Die granulöse degeneration bei naevus verrucosus bilateralis. Arch Klin Exp Dermatol 1969;235:115.
12. Zeligman I, Pomeranz J. Variations of congenital ichthyosiform erythroderma. Arch Dermatol 1965;91:120.
13. Demetree JW, Lang PG, St Clair JT. Unilateral linear zosteriform epidermal nevus with acantholytic dyskeratosis. Arch Dermatol 1979;115:875.
14. Starink TM, Woerdeman MJ. Unilateral systematized keratosis follicularis: A variant of Darier's disease or an epidermal nevus (acantholytic dyskeratotic epidermal naevus)? Br J Dermatol 1981;105:207.
15. Mehregan AH, Rahbari H. Hyperkeratosis of nipple and areola. Arch Dermatol 1977;113:1691.
16. Ortonne JP, El Baze P, Juhlin L. Nevoid hyperkeratosis of the nipple and areola mammae. Acta Derm Venereol (Stockh) 1986;66:175.
17. Fritsch P, Wittels W. Ein fall von bilateralem naevus comedonicus. Hautarzt 1971;22:409.
18. Paige TN, Mendelson CG. Bilateral nevus comedonicus. Arch Dermatol 1967;96:172.
19. Wood MG, Thew MA. Nevus comedonicus. Arch Dermatol 1968;98:111.
20. Harper KE, Spielvogel RL. Nevus comedonicus of the palm and wrist. J Am Acad Dermatol 1985;12:185.
21. Barsky S, Doyle JA, Winkelmann RK. Nevus comedonicus with epidermolytic hyperkeratosis. Arch Dermatol 1981;117:86.
22. Marsden RA, Fleming K, Dawber RPR. Comedo naevus of the palm: A sweat duct naevus? Br J Dermatol 1979;101:717.
23. Abell E, Read SI. Porokeratotic eccrine ostial and dermal duct nevus. Br J Dermatol 1980;103:435.
24. Aloi FG, Pippione M. Porokeratotic eccrine ostial and dermal duct nevus. Arch Dermatol 1986;122:892.
25. Coskey RJ, Mehregan AH, Hashimoto K. Porokeratotic eccrine duct and hair follicle nevus. J Am Acad Dermatol 1982;6:940.
26. Shapiro L, Baraf CS. Isolated epidermolytic acanthoma. Arch Dermatol 1970;101:220.
27. Gebhart W, Kidd RL. Das solitäre epidermolytische akanthom. Z Hautkr 1972;47:1.
28. Niizuma K. Isolated epidermolytic acanthoma. Dermatologica 1979;159:30.
29. De Coninck A, Willemsen M, De Dobbeleer G et al. Vulvar localization of epidermolytic acanthoma. Dermatologica 1986;172:276.
30. Zina AM, Bundino S, Pippione MG. Acrosyringial epidermolytic papulosis neviformis. Dermatologica 1985;171:122.
31. Hirone T, Fukushiro R. Disseminated epidermolytic acanthoma. Acta Derm Venereol (Stockh) 1973;53:393.
32. Miyamoto Y, Ueda K, Sato M et al. Disseminated epidermolytic acanthoma. J Cutan Pathol 1979;6:272.
33. Goette DK, Lapins NA. Epidermolytic hyperkeratosis as an incidental finding in normal oral mucosa. J Am Acad Dermatol 1984;10:246.
34. Ackerman AB, Reed RJ. Epidermolytic variant of solar keratosis. Arch Dermatol 1973;107:104.
35. Ackerman AB. Focal acantholytic dyskeratosis. Arch Dermatol 1972;106:702.
36. Nagashima M, Matsuoka S. So-called granular degeneration as incidental histopathological finding. Jpn J Dermatol (Series B) 1971;81:494.
37. Mehregan A. Epidermolytic hyperkeratosis. J Cutan Pathol 1978;5:76.
38. González SB. Epidermolytic hyperkeratosis associated with superficial basal cell carcinoma. Arch Dermatol 1983;119:186.
39. Brownstein MH. Acantholytic acanthoma. J Am Acad Dermatol 1988;19:783.
40. Chorzelski TP, Kudejko J, Jablonska S. Is papular acantholytic dyskeratosis of the vulva a new entity? Am J Dermatopathol 1984;6:557.
41. Coppola G, Muscardin LM, Piazza P. Papular acantholytic dyskeratosis. Am J Dermatopathol 1986;8:364.
42. Megahed M, Scharffetter-Kochanek K. Acantholytic acanthoma. Am J Dermatopathol 1993;15:283.
43. Stern JK, Wolf JE Jr, Rosan T. Focal acantholytic dyskeratosis in pityriasis rosea. Arch Dermatol 1979;115:497.
44. Botet MV, Sánchez JL. Vesiculation of focal acantholytic dyskeratosis in acral lentiginous malignant melanoma. J Dermatol Surg Oncol 1979;5:798.
45. Cannon AB. White sponge nevus of the mucosa: Naevus spongiosus albus mucosae. Arch Dermatol Syph 1935;31:365.
46. Jorgenson RJ, Levin S. White sponge nevus. Arch Dermatol 1981;117:73.
47. Zegarelli EV, Everett FG, Kutscher AH et al. Familial white folded dysplasia of the mucous membranes. Arch Dermatol 1959;80:59.
48. Witkop CJ Jr, Gorlin RJ. Four hereditary mucosal syndromes. Arch Dermatol 1961;84:762.
49. Haye KR, Whitehead FIH. Hereditary leukokeratosis of the mucous membranes. Br J Dermatol 1968;80:529.
50. Rugg EL, McLean WH, Allison WE et al. A mutation in the mucosal keratin K4 is associated with oral white sponge nevus. Nature Genet 1995;11:450.
51. Cooke BED, Morgan J. Oral epithelial nevi. Br J Dermatol 1959;71:134.
52. Stüttgen G, Berres HH, Will W. Leukoplakische epitheliale naevi der mundschleimhuat. Arch Klin Exp Dermatol 1965;221:433.
53. Kuhlwein A, Nasemann T, Jänner M. Nachweis von papillomviren bei fokaler epithelialer hyperplasie heck und die differentialdiagnose zum weissen schleimhautnävus. Hautarzt 1981;32:617.
54. Metz J, Metz G. Der naevus spongiosus albus mucosae. Z Hautkr 1979;54:604.
55. Duncan SC, Su WPD. Leukoedema of the oral mucosa. Arch Dermatol 1980;116:906.
56. Sigal MJ, Mock D. Symptomatic benign migratory glossitis: Report of two cases and literature review. Pediatr Dent 1992;14:392.
57. Dawson TAJ. Microscopic appearance of geographic tongue. Br J Dermatol 1969;81:827.
58. Marks R, Radden BG. Geographic tongue. Australas J Dermatol 1981;22:75.
59. Degos R, Garnier G, Civatte J. Pustulose par *Candida albicans* avec lésions psoriasiformes rappelant le psoriasis pustuleux. Bull Soc Fr Dermatol Syphiligr 1962;69:231.
60. O'Keefe E, Braverman IM, Cohen I. Annulus migrans: Identical lesions in pustular psoriasis, Reiter's syndrome, and geographic tongue. Arch Dermatol 1973;107:240.
61. Andrade R, Steigleder GK. Contribution à l'étude histologique et histochimique de la verrue seborrhéique (papillome basocellulaire). Ann Dermatol Syphiligr 1959;86:495.
62. Sim-Davis D, Marks R, Wilson Jones E. The inverted follicular keratosis. Acta Derm Venereol (Stockh) 1976;56:337.
63. Indianer L. Controversies in dermatopathology. J Dermatol Surg Oncol 1979;5:321.
64. Uchiyama N, Shindo Y. An acantholytic variant of seborrheic keratosis. J Dermatol 1986;13:222.

65. Tagami H, Yamada M. Seborrheic keratosis: An acantholytic variant. J Cutan Pathol 1978;5:145.
66. Morales A, Hu F. Seborrheic verruca and intraepidermal basal cell epithelioma of Jadassohn. Arch Dermatol 1965;91:342.
67. Mevorah B, Mishima Y. Cellular response of seborrheic keratosis following croton oil irritation and surgical trauma. Dermatologica 1965; 131:452.
68. Helwig EB. Inverted follicular keratosis. In: Proceedings of the 20th Seminar of the American Society of Clinical Pathologists, Washington, DC, 1954. Seminar on the skin: Neoplasms and dermatoses. Washington, DC: American Society of Clinical Pathologists, 1955; 38.
69. Mehregan AH. Inverted follicular keratosis. Arch Dermatol 1964;89: 229.
70. Duperrat B, Mascaro JM. Une tumeur développée aux dépens de l'acrotrichium ou partie intraépidermique du follicule pilaire: Porome folliculaire. Dermatologica 1963;126:291.
71. Grosshans E, Hanau D. L'adénome infundibulaire: Un porome folliculaire à différenciation sebacée et apocrine. Ann Dermatol Venereol 1981;108:59.
72. Kossard S, Berman A, Winkelmann RK. Seborrheic keratoses and trichostasis spinulosa. J Cutan Pathol 1979;6:492.
73. Headington JT. Tumors of the hair follicle: A review. Am J Pathol 1976;85:480.
74. Brownstein MH, Shapiro L. The pilosebaceous tumors. Int J Dermatol 1977;16:340.
75. Lever WF. Inverted follicular keratosis is an irritated seborrheic keratosis. Am J Dermatopathol 1983;5:474.
76. Mehregan AH. Lentigo senilis and its evolutions. J Invest Dermatol 1975;65:429.
77. Sanderson KF. The structure of seborrheic keratoses. Br J Dermatol 1968;80:588.
78. Becker SW. Seborrheic keratosis and verruca with special reference to the melanotic variety. Arch Dermatol Syphiligr 1951;63:358.
79. Lennox B. Pigment patterns in epithelial tumors of the skin. J Pathol Bacteriol 1949;61:587.
80. Mishima Y, Pinkus H. Benign mixed tumor of melanocytes and malpighian cells. Arch Dermatol 1960;81:539.
81. Berman A, Winkelmann RK. Inflammatory seborrheic keratoses with mononuclear cell infiltration. J Cutan Pathol 1978;5:353.
82. Rahbari H. Bowenoid transformation of seborrheic verrucae (keratoses). Br J Dermatol 1979;101:459.
83. Baer RL, Garcia RL, Partsalidou V et al. Papillated squamous cell carcinoma in situ arising in a seborrheic keratosis. J Am Acad Dermatol 1981;5:561.
84. Booth JC. Atypical seborrheic keratosis. Australas J Dermatol 1977; 18:10.
85. Christeler A, Delacrétaz J. Verrues séborrhéiques et transformation maligne. Dermatologica 1966;133:33.
86. Mikhail GR, Mehregan AH. Basal cell carcinoma in seborrheic keratosis. J Am Acad Dermatol 1982;6:500.
87. Goette DK. Basal cell carcinoma arising in seborrheic keratosis. J Dermatol Surg Oncol 1985;11:1014.
88. Braun-Falco O, Kint A, Vogell W. Zur histogenese der verruca seborrhoica: II. Mitteilung. Elektronenmikroskopische befunde. Arch Klin Exp Dermatol 1963;217:627.
89. Okun MF, Edelstein LM. Clonal seborrheic keratosis. In: Okun MF, Edelstein LM. Gross and microscopic pathology of the skin. Vol 2. Boston: Dermatopathology Foundation Press, 1976;576.
90. Mehregan AH, Pinkus H. Intraepidermal carcinoma: A critical study. Cancer 1964;17:609.
91. Schlappner OLA, Rowden G, Phillips TM et al. Melanoacanthoma: Ultrastructural and immunological studies. J Cutan Pathol 1978; 5:127.
92. Prince C, Mehregan AH, Hashimoto K et al. Large melanoacanthomas: A report of five cases. J Cutan Pathol 1984;11:309.
93. Delacrétaz J. Mélano-acanthome. Dermatologica 1975;151:236.
94. Hairston MA Jr, Reed RJ, Derbes VJ. Dermatosis papulosa nigra. Arch Dermatol 1964;89:655.
95. Babapour R, Leach J, Levy H. Dermatosis papulosa nigra in a young child. Pediatr Dermatol 1993;10:356.
96. Willoughby C, Soter NA. Stucco keratosis. Arch Dermatol 1972;105: 859.
97. Braun-Falco O, Weissmann I. Stukkokeratosen. Hautarzt 1978;29: 573.
98. Kocsard E, Carter JJ. The papillomatous keratoses: The nature and differential diagnosis of stucco keratosis. Australas J Dermatol 1971; 12:80.
99. Stieler W, Plewig G. Acanthosis nigricans maligna und Leser-Trélat-Zeichen bei doppelmalignom von mamma und magen. Z Hautkr 1987; 62:344.
100. Schwartz RA, Burgess GH. Florid cutaneous papillomatosis. Arch Dermatol 1978;114:1803.
101. Ronchese F. Keratoses, cancer and the sign of Leser-Trélat. Cancer 1965;18:1003.
102. Sneddon IB, Roberts JBM. An incomplete form of acanthosis nigricans. Gut 1962;3:269.
103. Liddell K, White JE, Caldwell JW. Seborrheic keratoses and carcinoma of the large bowel. Br J Dermatol 1975;92:449.
104. Kechijian P, Sadick NS, Mariglio J et al. Cytarabine-induced inflammation in the seborrheic keratoses of Leser-Trélat. Ann Intern Med 1979;91:868.
105. Lambert D, Fort M, Legoux A et al. Le signe de Leser-Trélat. Ann Dermatol Venereol 1980;107:1035.
106. Lindelof B, Sigurgeirsson B, Melander S. Seborrheic keratoses and cancer. J Am Acad Dermatol 1992;26:947.
107. Venencie PY, Perry HO. Sign of Leser-Trélat. J Am Acad Dermatol 1984;10:83.
108. Argenyi ZB, Huston BM, Argenyi EE et al. Large-cell acanthoma of the skin: A study by image analysis cytometry and immunohistochemistry. Am J Dermatopathol 1994;16:140.
109. Rabinowitz AD, Inghirami G. Large-cell acanthoma: A distinctive keratosis. Am J Dermatopathol 1992;14:136.
110. Sanchez Yus E, Del Rio E, Requena L. Large-cell acanthoma is a distinctive condition. Am J Dermatopathol 1992;14:140.
111. Degos R, Civatte J. Clear-cell acanthoma: Experience of 8 years. Br J Dermatol 1970;83:248.
112. Fine RM, Chernosky ME. Clinical recognition of clear-cell acanthoma (Degos). Arch Dermatol 1969;100:559.
113. Innocenzi D, Barduagni F, Cerio R, Wolter M. Disseminated eruptive clear cell acanthoma: A case report with review of the literature. Clin Exp Dermatol 1994;19:249.
114. Wells GC, Wilson Jones E. Degos' acanthoma: Acanthome à cellules claires. Br J Dermatol 1967;79:249.
115. Kerl H: Das klarzellenakanthom. Hautarzt 1977;28:456.
116. Zak FG, Girerd RJ. Das blasszellige akanthom (Degos). Hautarzt 1968;19:559.
117. Pierard GE. Mélanoacanthome à cellules claires. Ann Dermatol Venereol 1986;113:253.
118. Wilson Jones E, Wells GC. Degos' acanthoma: Acanthome à cellules claires. Arch Dermatol 1966;94:286.
119. Trau H, Fisher BK, Schewach-Millet M. Multiple clear cell acanthomas. Arch Dermatol 1980;116:433.
120. Fukushiro S, Takei Y, Ackerman AB. Pale-cell acanthosis. Am J Dermatopathol 1985;7:515.
121. Cramer HJ. Klarzellenakanthom (Degos) mit syringomatösen und naevus-sebaceus-artigen anteilen. Dermatologica 1971;143:265.
122. Desmons F, Breuillard F, Thomas P et al. Multiple clear-cell acanthoma (Degos). Int J Dermatol 1977;16:203.
123. Hu F, Sisson JK. The ultrastructure of pale cell acanthoma. J Invest Dermatol 1969;52:185.
124. Leonforte JF. Palmoplantare epidermiszyste. Hautarzt 1978;29:657.
125. Fisher BK, MacPherson M. Epidermoid cyst of the sole. J Am Acad Dermatol 1986;15:1127.
126. Onuigbo WIB. Vulval epidermoid cysts in the Igbos of Nigeria. Arch Dermatol 1976;112:1405.
127. Fieselman DW, Reed RJ, Ichinose H. Pigmented epidermal cyst. J Cutan Pathol 1974;1:256.
128. Raab W, Steigleder GK. Fehldiagnosen bei horncysten. Arch Klin Exp Dermatol 1961;212:606.
129. Delacrétaz J. Keratotic basal-cell carcinoma arising from an epidermoid cyst. J Dermatol Surg Oncol 1977;3:310.
130. Shelley WB, Wood MG. Occult Bowen's disease in keratinous cysts. Br J Dermatol 1981;105:105.
131. McDonald LW. Carcinomatous change in cysts of skin. Arch Dermatol 1963;87:208.
132. Wilson Jones E. Proliferating epidermoid cysts. Arch Dermatol 1966; 94:11.
133. Brownstein MH. Hybrid cyst: A combined epidermoid and trichilemmal cyst. J Am Acad Dermatol 1983;9:872.

134. McGavran MH, Binnington B. Keratinous cysts of the skin. Arch Dermatol 1966;94:499.
135. McGrath JA, Schofield OM, Eady RA. Epidermolysis bullosa pruriginosa: Dystrophic epidermolysis bullosa with distinctive clinicopathological features. Br J Dermatol 1994;130:617.
136. Epstein W, Kligman AM. The pathogenesis of milia and benign tumors of the skin. J Invest Dermatol 1956;26:1.
137. Leppard B, Sneddon IB. Milia occurring in lichen sclerosus et atrophicus. Br J Dermatol 1975;92:711.
138. Tsuji T, Sugai T, Suzuki S. The mode of growth of eccrine duct milia. J Invest Dermatol 1975;65:388.
139. Pinkus H. In discussion of Epstein W, Kligman AM. J Invest Dermatol 1956;26:10.
140. Leppard BJ, Sanderson KV. The natural history of trichilemmal cysts. Br J Dermatol 1976;94:379.
141. Leppard BJ, Sanderson KV, Wells RS. Hereditary trichilemmal cysts. Clin Exp Dermatol 1977;2:23.
142. Brownstein MH, Arluk DJ. Proliferating trichilemmal cyst: A simulant of squamous cell carcinoma. Cancer 1981;48:1207.
143. Pinkus H. "Sebaceous cysts" are trichilemmal cysts. Arch Dermatol 1969;99:544.
144. Cotton DWK, Kirkham N, Young BJJ. Immunoperoxidase anti-keratin staining of epidermal and pilar cysts. Br J Dermatol 1984;111:63.
145. Kimura S. Trichilemmal cysts. Dermatologica 1978;157:164.
146. Contreras MA, Costello MJ. Steatocystoma multiplex with embryonal hair formation. Arch Dermatol 1957;76:720.
147. Brownstein MH. Steatocystoma simplex: A solitary steatocystoma. Arch Dermatol 1982;118:409.
148. Hashimoto K, Fisher BK, Lever WF. Steatocystoma multiplex. Hautarzt 1964;15:299.
149. Oyal H, Nikolowski W. Sebocystomatosen. Arch Klin Exp Dermatol 1957;204:361.
150. Kligman AM, Kirschbaum JD. Steatocystoma multiplex: A dermoid tumor. J Invest Dermatol 1964;42:383.
151. Plewig G, Wolff HH, Braun-Falco O. Steatocystoma multiplex: Anatomic reevaluation, electron microscopy, and autoradiography. Arch Dermatol Res 1982;272:363.
152. Kimura S. An ultrastructural study of steatocystoma multiplex and the normal pilosebaceous apparatus. J Dermatol 1981;8:459.
153. Sandoval R, Urbina F. Pigmented follicular cyst. Br J Dermatol 1994; 131:130.
154. Brownstein MH, Helwig EB. Subcutaneous dermoid cysts. Arch Dermatol 1973;107:237.
155. Ambiavagar PC, Rosen Y. Cutaneous ciliated cyst on the chin: Probable bronchogenic cyst. Arch Dermatol 1979;115:895.
156. Van der Putte SCJ, Toonstra J. Cutaneous "bronchogenic" cyst. J Cutan Pathol 1985;12:404.
157. Ashton MA. Cutaneous ciliated cyst of the lower limb in a male. Histopathology 1995;26:467.
158. Sickel JZ. Cutaneous ciliated cyst of the scalp: A case report with immunohistochemical evidence for estrogen and progesterone receptors. Am J Dermatopathol 1994;16:76.
159. Tresser NJ, Dahms B, Berner JJ. Cutaneous bronchogenic cyst of the back: A case report and review of the literature. Pediatr Pathol 1994; 14:207.
160. Clark JV. Ciliated epithelium in a cyst of the lower limb. J Pathol 1969;98:289.
161. Cole LA, Helwig EB. Mucoid cysts of the penile skin. J Urol 1976; 115:397.
162. Dupré A, Lassère J, Christol B et al. Canaux et kystes dysembryoplasiques du raphé génito-périnéal. Ann Dermatol Venereol 1982; 109:81.
163. Ahmed A, Jones AW. Apocrine cystadenoma. Br J Dermatol 1969;81: 899.
164. Powell RF, Palmer CH, Smith EB. Apocrine cystadenoma of the penile shaft. Arch Dermatol 1977;113:1250.
165. Romani J, Barnadas MA, Miralles J et al. Median raphe cyst of the penis with ciliated cells. J Cutan Pathol 1995;22:378.
166. Paslin D. Urethroid cyst. Arch Dermatol 1983;119:89.
167. Esterly NB, Fretzin DF, Pinkus H. Eruptive vellus hair cysts. Arch Dermatol 1977;113:500.
168. Stiefler RE, Bergfeld WF. Eruptive vellus hair cysts: An inherited disorder. J Am Acad Dermatol 1980;3:425.
169. Piepkorn MW, Clark L, Lombardi DL. A kindred with congenital vellus hair cysts. J Am Acad Dermatol 1981;5:661.
170. Lee S, Kim JG. Eruptive vellus hair cyst. Arch Dermatol 1979;115: 744.
171. Burns DA, Calnan CD. Eruptive vellus hair cysts. Clin Exp Dermatol 1981;6:209.
172. Bovenmyer DA. Eruptive vellus hair cysts. Arch Dermatol 1979;115: 338.
173. Redondo P, Vazquez-Doval J, Idoate M et al. Multiple pilosebaceous cysts. Clin Exp Dermatol 1995;20:328.
174. Ohtake N, Kubota Y, Takayama O et al. Relationship between steatocystoma multiplex and eruptive vellus hair cysts. J Am Acad Dermatol 1992;26:876.
175. Szymanski FJ. Warty dyskeratoma. Arch Dermatol 1957;75:567.
176. Azuma Y, Matsukawa A. Warty dyskeratoma with multiple lesions. J Dermatol 1993;20:374.
177. Gorlin RJ, Peterson WC Jr. Warty dyskeratoma: A note concerning its occurrence in the oral mucosa. Arch Dermatol 1967;95:292.
178. Harrist TJ, Murphy GF, Mihm MC Jr. Oral warty dyskeratoma. Arch Dermatol 1980;116:929.
179. Tanay A, Mehregan AH. Warty dyskeratoma (review). Dermatologica 1969;138:155.
180. Graham JH, Helwig EB. Isolated dyskeratosis follicularis. Arch Dermatol 1958;77:377.
181. Delacrétaz J. Dyskératomes verruqueux et kératoses séniles dyskératosiques. Dermatologica 1963;127:23.
182. Metz J, Schröpl F. Zur nosologie des dyskeratoma segregans: "Warty dyskeratoma". Arch Klin Exp Dermatol 1970;238:21.
183. Furtado TA, Szymanski FJ. Étude histologique du dyskératose verruqueux. Ann Dermatol Syphiligr 1961;88:633.
184. Brownstein MH, Rabinowitz AD. The precursors of cutaneous squamous cell carcinoma. Int J Dermatol 1979;18:1.
185. Epstein JH. Photocarcinogenesis, skin cancer, and aging. J Am Acad Dermatol 1983;9:487.
186. Sober AJ, Burstein JM. Precursors to skin cancer. Cancer 1995;75: 645.
187. James MP, Wells GC, Whimster IW. Spreading pigmented actinic keratosis. Br J Dermatol 1978;98:373.
188. Koten JW, Verhagen ARHB, Frank GL. Histopathology of actinic cheilitis. Dermatologica 1967;135:465.
189. Cataldo E, Doku HC. Solar cheilitis. J Dermatol Surg Oncol 1981; 7:989.
190. Piscascia DD, Robinson JK. Actinic cheilitis: A review of the etiology, differential diagnosis, and treatment. J Am Acad Dermatol 1987; 17:255.
191. Montgomery H, Dörffel J. Verruca senilis und keratoma senile. Arch Dermatol Syph 1932;166:286.
192. Lund HZ. How often does squamous cell carcinoma of the skin metastasize? Arch Dermatol 1965;92:635.
193. MØller R, Reymann F, Hou-Jensen K. Metastases in dermatological patients with squamous cell carcinoma. Arch Dermatol 1979;115:703.
194. Billano RA, Little WP. Hypertrophic solar keratosis. J Am Acad Dermatol 1983;7:484.
195. Halter K. Uber ein wenig beachtetes histologisches kennzeichen des keratoma senile. Hautarzt 1952;3:215.
196. Pinkus H. Keratosis senilis. Am J Clin Pathol 1958;29:193.
197. Tan CY, Marks R. Lichenoid solar keratosis: Prevalence and immunologic findings. J Invest Dermatol 1982;79:365.
198. Vakilzadeh F, Happle R. Epidermolytic leukoplakia. J Cutan Pathol 1982;9:267.
199. Carapeto FJ, García-Pérez A. Acantholytic keratosis. Dermatologica 1974;148:233.
200. Braun-Falco O, Schmoeckel C, Geyer C. Pigmentierte aktinische keratosen. Hautarzt 1986;37:676.
201. Kerl H. What is the boundary that separates a thick solar keratosis and a thin squamous cell carcinoma? Am J Dermatopathol 1984;6:305.
202. Ackerman AB. What is the boundary that separates a thick solar keratosis and a thin squamous cell carcinoma? Am J Dermatopathol 1984;6:306.
203. Mahrle G, Thiele B. Epidermal dysplasia in solar keratosis (abstr). J Cutan Pathol 1983;10:295.
204. Schaumburg-Lever G, Alroy J, Gavris V et al. Cell-surface carbohydrates in proliferative epidermal lesions. Am J Dermatopathol 1984; 6:583.
205. Hirsch P, Marmelzat WL. Lichenoid actinic keratosis. Dermatol Int 1967;6:101.

206. Shapiro L, Ackerman AB. Solitary lichen planus-like keratosis. Dermatologica 1966;132:386.
207. Scott MA, Johnson WC. Lichenoid benign keratosis. J Cutan Pathol 1976;3:217.
208. Bart RS, Andrade R, Kopf AW. Cutaneous horn. Acta Derm Venereol (Stockh) 1968;48:507.
209. Brownstein MH, Shapiro EE. Trichilemmal horn: Cutaneous horn overlying trichilemmoma. Clin Exp Dermatol 1979;4:59.
210. Cramer HJ, Kahlert G. Das cornu cutaneum: Selbständiges krankheitsbild oder klinisches symptom? Dermatol Wochenschr 1964;150: 521.
211. Sandbank M. Basal cell carcinoma at the base of cutaneous horn: Cornu cutaneum. Arch Dermatol 1971;104:97.
212. McAdams AJ Jr, Kistner RW. The relationship of chronic vulvar disease, leukoplakia, and carcinoma in situ to carcinoma of the vulva. Cancer 1958;11:740.
213. Shklar G. Oral leukoplakia: Studies in enzyme histochemistry. J Invest Dermatol 1967;48:153.
214. Pindborg JJ. Pathology of oral leukoplakia. Am J Dermatopathol 1980;2:277.
215. Waldron CA, Shafer WG. Leukoplakia revisited: A clinicopathologic study of 3256 leukoplakias. Cancer 1975;36:1386.
216. Hornstein OP. Klinik, ätiologie und therapie der oralen leukoplakien. Hautarzt 1979;30:40.
217. Shklar G. Modern studies and concepts of leukoplakia in the mouth. J Dermatol Surg Oncol 1981;7:996.
218. Shafer WG, Waldron CA. Erythroplakia of the oral cavity. Cancer 1975;36:1021.
219. Grässel-Pietrusky R, Hornstein OP. Histologische untersuchungen zur häufigkeit des *Candidabefalls* präkanzeröser oraler leukoplakien. Hautarzt 1980;31:21.
220. Cawson RA, Lehner T. Chronic hyperplastic candidiasis: Candidal leukoplakia. Br J Dermatol 1968;80:9.
221. Löning T, Ikenberg H, Becker J et al. Analysis of oral papillomas, leukoplakias, and invasive carcinomas for human papillomavirus type related DNA. J Invest Dermatol 1985;84:417.
222. Gassenmaier A, Hornstein OP. Presence of papillomavirus DNA in benign and precancerous oral leukoplakias and squamous cell carcinomas. Dermatologica 1988;176:224.
223. Schell H, Schönberger A. Zur lokalisationshäufigkeit von benignen und präkanzerösen leukoplakien und von karzinomen in der mundhöhle. Z Hautkr 1987;62:798.
224. Rich AM, Reade PC. A quantitative assessment of Langerhans' cells in oral mucosal lichen planus and leukoplakia. Br J Dermatol 1989; 120:223.
225. Shear M, Pindborg JJ. Verrucous hyperplasia of the oral mucosa. Cancer 1980;46:1855.
226. Kraus FT, Perez-Mesa C. Verrucous carcinoma. Cancer 1966;19:26.
227. Samitz MH, Ackerman AB, Lantis LR. Squamous cell carcinoma arising at the site of oral florid papillomatosis. Arch Dermatol 1967;96: 286.
228. Grinspan D, Abulafia J. Oral florid papillomatosis: Verrucous carcinoma. Int J Dermatol 1979;18:608.
229. Wechsler HL, Fisher ER. Oral florid papillomatosis. Arch Dermatol 1962;86:480.
230. Kanee B. Oral florid papillomatosis complicated by verrucous squamous carcinoma. Arch Dermatol 1969;99:196.
231. Abrams AM, Melrose RJ, Howell FV. Necrotizing sialometaplasia: A disease simulating malignancy. Cancer 1973;32:130.
232. Raugi GJ, Kessler S. Necrotizing sialometaplasia: A condition simulating malignancy. Arch Dermatol 1979;115:329.
233. Piette F, Sauque E, Pellerin P et al. Sialométaplasie nécrosante. Ann Dermatol Venereol 1980;107:821.
234. Fechner RE. Necrotizing sialometaplasia: A source of confusion with carcinoma of the palate. Am J Clin Pathol 1977;67:315.
235. Shapiro L, Juhlin EA. Eosinophilic ulcer of the tongue. Dermatologica 1970;140:242.
236. Burgess GH, Mehregan AH, Drinnan AJ. Eosinophilic ulcer of the tongue. Arch Dermatol 1977;113:644.
237. Borroni G, Pericoli R, Gabba P et al. Eosinophilic ulcers of the tongue. J Cutan Pathol 1984;11:322.
238. Baran RL, Gormley DE. Polydactylous Bowen's disease of the nail. J Am Acad Dermatol 1987;17:201.
239. Bowen JT. Precancerous dermatosis. J Cutan Dis 1912;30:241.
240. Montgomery H. Precancerous dermatosis and epithelioma in situ. Arch Dermatol Syph 1939;39:387.
241. Montgomery H, Waisman M. Epithelioma attributable to arsenic. J Invest Dermatol 1941;4:365.
242. Strayer DS, Santa Cruz DJ. Carcinoma in situ of the skin: A review of histopathology. J Cutan Pathol 1980;7:244.
243. Kao GF. Editorial: Carcinoma arising in Bowen's disease. Arch Dermatol 1986;122:1124.
244. Graham JH, Helwig EB. Bowen's disease and its relationship to systemic cancer. Arch Dermatol 1959;80:133.
245. Ackerman AB. Reply to Mascaro JM: Bowenoid papulosis. J Am Acad Dermatol 1981;4:608.
246. Peterka ES, Lynch FW, Goltz RW. An association between Bowen's disease and internal cancer. Arch Dermatol 1961;84:623.
247. Callen JP, Headington J. Bowen's and non-Bowen's squamous intraepidermal neoplasia of the skin. Arch Dermatol 1980;116:422.
248. Andersen SL, Nielsen H, Raymann F. Relationship between Bowen's disease and internal malignant tumors. Arch Dermatol 1973;108:367.
249. Reymann F, Ravnborg L, Schon G et al. Bowen's disease and internal malignant disease. Arch Dermatol 1988;124:677.
250. Chuang TY, Reizner GT. Bowen's disease and internal malignancy. J Am Acad Dermatol 1988;19:47.
251. Seiji M, Mizuno F. Electron microscopic study of Bowen's disease. Arch Dermatol 1969;99:3.
252. Olson RL, Nordquist R, Everett MA. Dyskeratosis in Bowen's disease. Br J Dermatol 1969;81:676.
253. Sato A, Seiji M. Electron microscopic observations of malignant dyskeratosis in leukoplakia and Bowen's disease. Acta Derm Venereol Suppl (Stockh) 1973;53:101.
254. Arai H, Hori Y. An ultrastructural observation of intracytoplasmic desmosomes in Darier's disease. J Dermatol 1977;4:223.
255. Klingmüller G, Klehr HU, Ishibashi Y. Desmosomen im cytoplasma entdifferenzierter keratinocyten des plattenepithelcarcinoms. Arch Klin Exp Dermatol 1970;238:356.
256. Fisher ER, McCoy MM II, Wechsler HL. Analysis of histopathologic and electron microscopic determinants of keratoacanthoma and squamous cell carcinoma. Cancer 1972;29:1387.
257. Ishibashi Y, Niimura M, Klingmüller G. Elektronenmikroskopischer beitrag zur morphologie von Paget-Zellen. Arch Dermatol Forsch 1972;245:402.
258. Klug H, Haustein UF. Vorkommen von intrazytoplasmatischen desmosomen in keratinozyten. Dermatologica 1974;148:143.
259. Komura J, Watanabe S. Desmosome-like structures in the cytoplasm of normal human keratinocyte. Arch Dermatol Res 1975;253:145.
260. Schenk P. Desmosomale strukturen im cytoplasma normaler und pathologischer keratinocyten. Arch Dermatol Res 1975;253:23.
261. Olson RL, Nordquist R, Everett MA. An electron microscopic study of Bowen's disease. Cancer Res 1968;28:2078.
262. Raiten K, Paniago-Pereira C, Ackerman AB. Pagetoid Bowen's disease vs. extramammary Paget's disease. J Dermatol Surg Oncol 1976; 2:24.
263. Queyrat L. Erythroplasie du gland. Bull Soc Fr Dermatol Syphiligr 1911;22:378.
264. Goette DK. Erythroplasia of Queyrat. Arch Dermatol 1974;110:271.
265. Mikhail GR. Cancers, precancers, and pseudocancers on the male genitalia. J Dermatol Surg Oncol 1980;6:1027.
266. Graham JH, Helwig EB. Erythroplasia of Queyrat. In: Graham JH, Johnson WC, Helwig EB, eds. Dermal pathology. Hagerstown, MD: Harper & Row, 1972;597.
267. Zoon JJ. Balanoposthite chronique circonscrite bénigne à plasmocytes. Dermatologica 1952;105:1.
268. Eberhartinger C, Bergmann M. Balanoposthitis chronica circumscripta plasmacellularis Zoon und Phimose. Z Hautkr 1971;46:251.
269. Souteyrand P, Wong E, MacDonald DM. Zoon's balanitis: Balanitis circumscripta plasmacellularis. Br J Dermatol 1981;105:195.
270. Mensing H, Jänner M. Vulvitis plasmacellularis Zoon. Z Hautkr 1981; 56:728.
271. Davis J, Shapiro L, Baral J. Vulvitis circumscripta plasmacellularis. J Am Acad Dermatol 1983;8:413.
272. Brodin M. Balanitis circumscripta plasmacellularis. J Am Acad Dermatol 1980;2:33.
273. Jonquières EDL, De Lutzky FK. Balanites et vulvites pseudoérythroplasiques chroniques. Ann Dermatol Venereol 1980;107:173.
274. Nödl F. Zur klinik und histologie der balanoposthitis chronica cir-

cumscripta benigna plasmacellularis. Arch Dermatol Syph 1954;198: 557.
275. Schuermann H. Plasmocytosis circumorificialis. Dtsch Zahnarztl Z 1960;15:601.
276. Moldenhauer E. Die cheilitis plasmacellularis: Ein beitrag zur plasmocytosis circumorificialis. Dermatol Wochenschr 1966;152:636.
277. Baughman RD, Berger P, Pringle WM. Plasma cell cheilitis. Arch Dermatol 1974;110:725.
278. Crum CP, Liskow A, Petras P et al. Vulvar intraepithelial neoplasia: Severe atypia and carcinoma in situ. Cancer 1984;54:1429.
279. Ulbright TM, Stehman FB, Roth LM et al. Bowenoid dysplasia of the vulva. Cancer 1982;50:2910.
280. Montgomery H. Arsenic as an etiologic agent in certain types of epithelioma. Arch Dermatol Syph 1935;32:218.
281. Mazumder DN, Das Gupta J, Chakraborty AK et al. Environmental pollution and chronic arsenicosis in south Calcutta. Bull World Health Organ 1992;70:481.
282. Das D, Chatterjee A, Mandal BK et al. Arsenic in ground water in six districts of West Bengal, India: The biggest arsenic calamity in the world. Part 2. Arsenic concentration in drinking water, hair, nails, urine, skin-scale and liver tissue (biopsy) of the affected people. Analyst 1995;120:917.
283. Fierz U. Katamnestische untersuchungen über die nebenwirkungen der therapie mit anorganischem arsen bei hautkrankheiten. Dermatologica 1965;131:41.
284. Yeh S. Skin cancer in chronic arsenicism. Hum Pathol 1973;4:469.
285. Neubauer O. Arsenical cancer. Br J Cancer 1947;1:192.
286. Sommers SC, McManus RG. Multiple arsenical cancers of skin and internal organs. Cancer 1953;6:347.
287. Roth F. Über die chronische arsenvergiftung der moselwinzer unter besonderer berücksichtigung des arsenkrebses. Z Krebsforsch 1956; 61:287.
288. Miki Y, Kawatsu T, Matsuda K et al. Cutaneous and pulmonary cancers associated with Bowen's disease. J Am Acad Dermatol 1982;6:26.
289. Hundeiker M, Petres J. Morphogenese und formenreichtum der arseninduzierten Präkanzerosen. Arch Klin Exp Dermatol 1968;231:355.
290. Ehlers G. Klinische und histologische untersuchungen zur frage arzneimittelbedingter arsen-tumoren. Z Hautkr 1968;43:763.
291. Jung EG, Trachsel B. Molekularbiologische untersuchungen zur arsencarcinogenese. Arch Klin Exp Dermatol 1970;237:819.
292. Barr LH, Menard JW. Marjolin's ulcer. Cancer 1983;52:173.
293. Epstein E, Epstein NN, Bragg K et al. Metastases from squamous cell carcinomas of the skin. Arch Dermatol 1968;97:245.
294. Frierson HF Jr, Cooper PH. Prognostic factors in squamous cell carcinoma of the lower lip. Hum Pathol 1986;17:346.
295. Sedlin ED, Fleming JL. Epidermal carcinoma arising in chronic osteomyelitic foci. J Bone Joint Surg 1963;45:827.
296. Martin H, Strong E, Spiro RH. Radiation-induced skin cancer of the head and neck. Cancer 1970;25:61.
297. Arons MS, Lynch JB, Lewis SR et al. Scar tissue carcinoma: I. A clinical study with special reference to burn scar carcinoma. Ann Surg 1965;161:170.
298. Hoxtell EO, Mandel JS, Murray SS et al. Incidence of skin carcinoma after renal transplantation. Arch Dermatol 1977;113:436.
299. Gupta AK, Cardella CJ, Haberman HF. Cutaneous malignant neoplasms in patients with renal transplants. Arch Dermatol 1986;122: 1288.
300. Turner JE, Callen JP. Aggressive behavior of squamous cell carcinoma in a patient with preceding lymphocytic lymphoma. J Am Acad Dermatol 1981;4:446.
301. Evans HL, Smith JL. Spindle cell squamous carcinoma and sarcoma-like tumors of the skin. Cancer 1980;45:2687.
302. Manglani KS, Manaligod JR, Ray B. Spindle cell carcinoma of the glans penis. Cancer 1980;46:2266.
303. Kobayasi T. Dermo-epidermal junction in invasive squamous cell carcinoma. Acta Derm Venereol (Stockh) 1969;49:445.
304. Boncinelli U, Fornieri C, Muscatello U. Relationship between leukocytes and tumor cells in precancerous and cancerous lesions of the lip: A possible expression of immune reaction. J Invest Dermatol 1978;71: 407.
305. Battifora H. Spindle cell carcinoma: Ultrastructural evidence of squamous origin and collagen production by the tumor cells. Cancer 1976; 37:2275.
306. Barr RJ, Wuerker RB, Graham JH. Ultrastructure of atypical fibroxanthoma. Cancer 1977;40:736.
307. Gatter KC, Alcock C, Heryet A. The differential diagnosis of routinely processed anaplastic tumors using monoclonal antibodies. Am J Clin Pathol 1984;82:33.
308. Robinson JK, Gottschalk R. Immunofluorescent and immunoperoxidase staining of antibodies to fibrous keratin. Arch Dermatol 1984; 120:199.
309. Lever WF. Adenoacanthoma of sweat glands. Arch Dermatol Syph 1947;56:157.
310. Johnson WC, Helwig EB. Adenoid squamous cell carcinoma: Adenoacanthoma. Cancer 1966;19:1639.
311. Borelli D. Aspetti pseudoglandolari nell'epithelioma discheratosico: "Adenoacanthoma of sweat glands" di Lever. Dermatologica 1948; 97:193.
312. Takagi M, Sakota Y, Takayama S et al. Adenoid squamous cell carcinoma of the oral mucosa: Report of two autopsy cases. Cancer 1977; 40:2250.
313. Chorzelski T. Ein fall von übergang einer keratosis senilis mit dyskeratose vom typ des morbus Darier in ein dyskeratotisches spinaliom. Hautarzt 1963;14:37.
314. Muller SA, Wilhelmj CM Jr, Harrison EG Jr et al. Adenoid squamous cell carcinoma: Adenoacanthoma of Lever. Arch Dermatol 1964;89: 589.
315. Wick MR, Pettinato G, Nappi O. Adenoid (acantholytic) squamous carcinoma of the skin (abstr). J Cutan Pathol 1988;15:351.
316. Delacrétaz J, Madjedi AS, Loretan R. Epithelioma spinocellulare segregans: Über die sogenannten "adenoacanthome der schweissdrüsen" (Lever). Hautarzt 1957;8:512.
317. Lasser A, Cornog JL, Morris J MCL. Adenoid squamous cell carcinoma of the vulva. Cancer 1974;33:224.
318. Underwood JW, Adcock LL, Okagari T. Adenosquamous carcinoma of skin appendages (adenoid squamous cell carcinoma, pseudoglandular squamous cell carcinoma, adenoacanthoma of sweat glands of Lever) of the vulva. Cancer 1978;42:1851.
319. Weidner N, Foucar E. Adenosquamous carcinoma of the skin: An aggressive mucin- and gland-forming carcinoma. Arch Dermatol 1985; 121:775.
320. Gallager HS, Miller GV, Grampa G. Primary mucoepidermoid carcinoma of the skin. Cancer 1959;12:286.
321. Fulling KH, Strayer DS, Santa Cruz DJ. Adnexal metaplasia in carcinoma in situ of the skin. J Cutan Pathol 1981;8:79.
322. Friedman KJ. Low-grade primary cutaneous adenosquamous (mucoepidermoid) carcinoma. Am J Dermatopathol 1989;11:43.
323. Ackerman LV. Verrucous carcinoma of the oral cavity. Surgery 1948; 23:670.
324. Aird I, Johnson HD, Lennox B et al. Epithelioma cuniculatum: A variety of squamous carcinoma peculiar to the foot. Br J Surg 1954;42:245.
325. Brown SM, Freeman RG. Epithelioma cuniculatum. Arch Dermatol 1976;112:1295.
326. Reingold IM, Smith BP, Graham JH. Epithelioma cuniculatum pedis: A variant of squamous cell carcinoma. Am J Clin Pathol 1978;69:561.
327. Nguyen KQ, McMarlin SL. Verrucous carcinoma of the face. Arch Dermatol 1984;120:383.
328. Sanchez-Yus E, Velasco E, Robledo A. Verrucous carcinoma of the back. J Am Acad Dermatol 1986;14:947.
329. Klima M, Kurtis B, Jordan PH Jr. Verrucous carcinoma of the skin. J Cutan Pathol 1980;7:88.
330. Mohs FE, Sahl WJ. Chemosurgery for verrucous carcinoma. J Dermatol Surg Oncol 1979;5:302.
331. Brodin MB, Mehregan AH. Verrucous carcinoma. Arch Dermatol 1980;116:987.
332. Dawson DF, Duckworth JK, Bernhardt H et al. Giant condyloma and verrucous carcinoma of the genital area. Arch Pathol 1965;79:225.
333. Seehafer JR, Muller SA, Dicken CH et al. Bilateral verrucous carcinoma of the feet. Arch Dermatol 1979;115:1222.
334. McKee PH, Wilkinson JD, Corbett MF et al. Carcinoma cuniculatum: A case metastasizing to skin and lymph nodes. Clin Exp Dermatol 1981;6:613.
335. Perez CA, Kraus FT, Evans JC et al. Anaplastic transformation in verrucous carcinoma of the oral cavity after radiation therapy. Radiology 1966;86:108.
336. Wilkinson JD, McKee PH, Black MM et al. A case of carcinoma cuniculatum with coexistent viral plantar wart. Clin Exp Dermatol 1981; 6:619.
337. McKee PH, Wilkinson JD, Black MM et al. Carcinoma (epithelioma) cuniculatum. Histopathology 1981;5:425.

338. Gross G, Gissmann L. Urogenitale und anale papillomvirusinfektionen. Hautarzt 1986;37:587.
339. Mathieu A, Avril MF, Duvillard P et al. Tumeurs de Buschke-Löwenstein: Trois localisations vulvaires. Association à l'HPV6 dans un cas. Ann Dermatol Venereol 1985;112:745.
340. Su WPD, Duncan SC, Perry HO. Blastomycosis-like pyoderma. Arch Dermatol 1979;115:170.
341. Sommerville J. Pseudo-epitheliomatous hyperplasia. Acta Derm Venereol (Stockh) 1953;33:236.
342. Winer LH. Pseudoepitheliomatous hyperplasia. Arch Dermatol Syph 1940;42:856.
343. Freeman RG. On the pathogenesis of pseudoepitheliomatous hyperplasia. J Cutan Pathol 1974;1:231.
344. Ju DMC. Pseudoepitheliomatous hyperplasia of the skin. Dermatol Int 1967;6:82.
345. Wagner RF Jr, Grande DJ. Pseudoepitheliomatous hyperplasia vs. squamous cell carcinoma. J Dermatol Surg Oncol 1986;12:632.
346. Johnson DE. Basal-cell epithelioma of the palm. Arch Dermatol 1960; 82:253.
347. Hyman AB, Barsky AJ. Basal cell epithelioma of the palm. Arch Dermatol 1965;92:571.
348. Hyman AB, Michaelides P. Basal-cell epithelioma of the sole. Arch Dermatol 1963;87:481.
349. Lewis HM, Stensaas CO, Okun MR. Basal cell epithelioma of the sole. Arch Dermatol 1965;91:623.
350. Williamson JJ, Cohney BC, Henderson BM. Basal cell carcinoma of the mandibular gingiva. Arch Dermatol 1967;95:76.
351. Urmacher C, Pearlman S. An uncommon neoplasm of the oral mucosa. Am J Dermatopathol 1983;5:601.
352. Schubert H, Wolfram G, Güldner G. Basaliomrezidive nach behandlung. Dermatol Monatsschr 1979;165:89.
353. Murray JE, Cannon B. Basal-cell cancer in children and young adults. N Engl J Med 1960;262:440.
354. Maron H. Basaliom bei kindern. Dermatol Wochenschr 1963;147: 545.
355. Milstone EB, Helwig EB. Basal cell carcinoma in children. Arch Dermatol 1973;108:523.
356. Gellin GA, Kopf AW, Garfinkel L. Basal cell epithelioma. Arch Dermatol 1965;91:38.
357. Schubert H. Häufigkeit und lokalisation von basaliomen im Kopf-Hals-Bereich. Dermatol Monatsschr 1984;170:453.
358. Anderson NP, Anderson HE. Development of basal cell epithelioma as a consequence of radiodermatitis. Arch Dermatol Syph 1951;63: 586.
359. Schwartz RA, Burgess GH, Milgrom H. Breast carcinoma and basal cell epitheliomas after x-ray therapy for hirsutism. Cancer 1979;44: 1601.
360. Gaughan LJ, Bergeron JR, Mullins JF. Giant basal cell epithelioma developing in acute burn site. Arch Dermatol 1969;99:594.
361. Margolis MH. Superficial multicentric basal cell epithelioma arising in thermal burn scar. Arch Dermatol 1970;102:474.
362. Wechsler HL, Krugh FJ, Domonkos AN et al. Polydysplastic epidermolysis bullosa and development of epidermal neoplasms. Arch Dermatol 1970;102:374.
363. Weedon D, Wall D. Metastatic basal cell carcinoma. Med J Aust 1975; 2:177.
364. Paver K, Poyzen K, Burry N et al. The incidence of basal cell carcinoma and their metastases in Australia and New Zealand. Australas J Dermatol 1973;14:53.
365. Cotran RS. Metastasizing basal cell carcinomas. Cancer 1961;14: 1036.
366. Von Domarus H, Stevens PJ. Metastatic basal cell carcinoma: Report of five cases and review of 170 cases in the literature. J Am Acad Dermatol 1984;10:1043.
367. Amonette RA, Salasche SJ, Chesney T McC et al. Metastatic basal cell carcinoma. J Dermatol Surg 1981;7:397.
368. Dzubow LM. Metastatic basal cell carcinoma originating in the supraparotid region. J Dermatol Surg Oncol 1986;12:1306.
369. Assor D. Basal cell carcinoma with metastasis to bone. Cancer 1967; 20:2125.
370. Wermuth BM, Fajardo LF. Metastatic basal cell carcinoma. Arch Pathol 1970;90:458.
371. Soffer D, Kaplan H, Weshler Z. Meningeal carcinomatosis due to basal cell carcinoma. Hum Pathol 1985;16:530.
372. Farmer ER, Helwig EB. Metastatic basal cell carcinoma: A clinicopathologic study of 17 cases. Cancer 1980;46:748.
373. Mikhail GR, Nims LP, Kelly AP Jr et al. Metastatic basal cell carcinoma. (review) Arch Dermatol 1977;113:1261.
374. Safai B, Good RA. Basal cell carcinoma with metastasis. Arch Pathol 1977;101:327.
375. Dvoretzky I, Fisher BK, Haker O. Mutilating basal cell epithelioma. Arch Dermatol 1978;114:239.
376. Gormley DE, Hirsch P. Aggressive basal cell carcinoma of the scalp. Arch Dermatol 1978;114:782.
377. Gorlin RJ. Nevoid basal-cell carcinoma syndrome. Medicine (Baltimore) 1987;66:98.
378. Taylor WB, Anderson DE, Howell JB et al. The nevoid basal cell carcinoma syndrome. Arch Dermatol 1968;98:612.
379. Southwick GJ, Schwartz RA. The basal cell nevus syndrome: Disasters occurring among a series of 36 patients. Cancer 1979;44:2294.
380. Berendes U. Die klinische bedeutung der onkotischen phase des basalzellnaevus-syndroms. Hautarzt 1971;22:261.
381. Howell JB, Mehregan AH. Pursuit of the pits in the nevoid basal cell carcinoma syndrome. Arch Dermatol 1970;102:586.
382. Leppard BJ. Skin cysts in the basal cell naevus syndrome. Clin Exp Dermatol 1983;8:603.
383. Hermans EH, Grosfeld JCM, Spaas JAJ. The fifth phakomatosis. Dermatologica 1965;130:446.
384. Reed JC. Nevoid basal cell carcinoma syndrome with associated fibrosarcoma of the maxilla. Arch Dermatol 1968;97:304.
385. Happle R. Naevobasaliom und ameloblastom. Hautarzt 1973;24:290.
386. Anderson TE, Best PV. Linear basal cell nevus. Br J Dermatol 1962; 74:20.
387. Carney RG. Linear unilateral basal cell nevus with comedones. Arch Dermatol Syph 1952;65:471.
388. Horio M, Egami K, Maejima K et al. Electron microscopic study of sebaceous epithelioma. J Dermatol 1978;5:139.
389. Bleiberg J, Brodkin RH. Linear unilateral basal cell nevus with comedones. Arch Dermatol 1969;100:187.
390. Bazex A, Dupré A, Christol B. Atrophodermie folliculaire, proliférations basocellulaires et hypotrichose. Ann Dermatol Syphiligr (Paris) 1966;93:241.
391. Viksnins P, Berlin A. Follicular atrophoderma and basal cell carcinomas. Arch Dermatol 1977;113:948.
392. Plosila M, Kiistala R, Niemi KM. The Bazex syndrome: Follicular atrophoderma with multiple basal cell carcinoma, hypotrichosis and hypohidrosis. Clin Exp Dermatol 1981;6:31.
393. Rupec M, Kint A, Himmelmann GW et al. Zur ultrastruktur des soliden basalioms. Dermatologica 1975;151:288.
394. Okun MR, Blumental G. Basal cell epithelioma with giant cells and nuclear atypicality. Arch Dermatol 1964;89:598.
395. Rupec M, Vakilzadeh F, Korb G. Über das vorkommen von mehrkernigen riesenzellen in basaliomen. Arch Klin Exp Dermatol 1969; 235:198.
396. Pinkus H. Premalignant fibroepithelial tumors of the skin. Arch Dermatol Syph 1953;67:598.
397. Pinkus H. Epithelial and fibroepithelial tumors. Arch Dermatol 1965; 91:24.
398. Fanger H, Barker BE. Histochemical studies of some keratotic and proliferating skin lesions. Arch Pathol 1957;64:143.
399. Moore RD, Stevenson J, Schoenberg MD. The response of connective tissue associated with tumors of the skin. Am J Clin Pathol 1960;34: 125.
400. Mérot Y, Faucher F, Didierjean L et al. Loss of bullous pemphigoid antigen in peritumoral lacunae of basal cell epitheliomas. Acta Derm Venereol (Stockh) 1984;64:209.
401. Stanley JR, Beckwith JB, Fuller RP et al. A specific antigenic defect of the basement membrane is found in basal cell carcinoma but not in other epidermal tumors. Cancer 1982;50:1486.
402. Weedon D, Shand E. Amyloid in basal cell carcinomas. Br J Dermatol 1979;101:141.
403. Hundeiker M, Berger H. Zur morphogenese der basaliome. Arch Klin Exp Dermatol 1968;231:161.
404. Reidbord HE, Wechsler HL, Fisher ER. Ultrastructural study of basal cell carcinoma and its variants with comments on histogenesis. Arch Dermatol 1971;104:132.
405. Mehregan AH. Aggressive basal cell epithelioma on sunlight-protected skin. Am J Dermatopathol 1983;5:221.

406. Jacobs GH, Rippey JJ, Altini M. Prediction of aggressive behavior in basal cell carcinoma. Cancer 1982;49:533.
407. Lang PJ Jr, Maize JC. Histologic evaluation of recurrent basal cell carcinoma and treatment implications. J Am Acad Dermatol 1986;14:186.
408. Foot NC. Adnexal carcinoma of the skin. Am J Pathol 1947;23:1.
409. Troy JL, Ackerman AB. Sebaceoma: A distinctive benign neoplasm of adnexal epithelium differentiating toward sebaceous cells. Am J Dermatopathol 1984;6:7.
410. Wood MG, Pranich K, Beerman H. Investigation of possible apocrine gland component in basal-cell epithelioma. J Invest Dermatol 1958;30:273.
411. Freeman RG, Winkelmann RK. Basal cell tumor with eccrine differentiation. Arch Dermatol 1969;100:234.
412. Lerchin E, Rahbari H. Adamantinoid basal cell epithelioma. Arch Dermatol 1975;111:586.
413. Barr RJ, Graham JH. Granular cell basal cell carcinoma. Arch Dermatol 1979;115:1064.
414. Mrak RE, Baker GF. Granular basal cell carcinoma. J Cutan Pathol 1987;14:37.
415. Barnadas MA, Freeman RG. Clear cell basal cell epithelioma. J Cutan Pathol 1988;15:1.
416. Cohen RE, Zaim MT. Signet-ring clear-cell basal cell carcinoma. J Cutan Pathol 1988;15:183.
417. Aloi FG, Molinero A, Pippione M. Basal cell epithelioma with matricial differentiation. Am J Dermatopathol 1988;10:509.
418. Deppe R, Pullmann H, Steigleder GK. Dopa-positive cells and melanin in basal cell epithelioma. Arch Dermatol Res 1976;256:79.
419. Zelickson AS, Goltz RW, Hartmann JF. A histologic and electron microscopic study of a pigmenting basal cell epithelioma. J Invest Dermatol 1961;36:299.
420. Caro MR, Howell JB. Morphea-like epithelioma. Arch Dermatol Syph 1952;63:471.
421. Hornstein O. Über die Pinkussche varietät der basaliome. Hautarzt 1957;8:406.
422. Degos R, Hewitt J. Tumeurs fibro-épithéliales prémalignes de Pinkus et épithélioma baso-cellulaire. Ann Dermatol Syphiligr (Paris) 1955;82:124.
423. Howell JB, Caro MR. The basal-cell nevus. Arch Dermatol 1959;79:67.
424. Mason JK, Helwig EB, Graham JH. Pathology of the nevoid basal cell carcinoma syndrome. Arch Pathol 1965;79:401.
425. Jablonska S. Basaliome naevoider abkunft. Hautarzt 1961;12:147.
426. Howell JB, Freeman RG. Structure and significance of the pits with their tumors in the nevoid basal cell carcinoma syndrome. J Am Acad Dermatol 1980;2:224.
427. Holubar K, Matras H, Smalik AV. Multiple palmar basal cell epitheliomas in basal cell nevus syndrome. Arch Dermatol 1970;101:679.
428. Ward WH. Nevoid basal cell carcinoma associated with a dyskeratosis of the palms and soles. Australas J Dermatol 1960;5:204.
429. Taylor WB, Wilkins JW Jr. Nevoid basal cell carcinoma of the palm. Arch Dermatol 1970;102:654.
430. Barr RJ, Headley JL, Jensen JL et al. Cutaneous keratocysts of nevoid basal cell carcinoma syndrome. J Am Acad Dermatol 1986;14:572.
431. Horio T, Komura J. Linear unilateral basal cell nevus with comedo-like lesions. Arch Dermatol 1978;114:95.
432. Blanchard L, Hodge SJ, Owen LG. Linear eccrine nevus with comedones. Arch Dermatol 1981;117:357.
433. Sims CF, Parker RL. Intraepidermal basal cell epithelioma. Arch Dermatol Syph 1949;59:45.
434. Steffen C, Ackerman AB. Intraepidermal epithelioma of Borst-Jadassohn. Am J Dermatopathol 1985;7:5.
435. Holubar K, Wolff K. Intraepidermal eccrine poroma. Cancer 1969;23:626.
436. Okun MR, Edelstein LM. Gross and microscopic pathology of the skin. Vol. 2. Boston: Dermatopathology Foundation Press, 1976;618.
437. Berger P, Baughman R. Intra-epidermal epithelioma: Report of a case with invasion after many years. Br J Dermatol 1974;90:343.
438. Smith JLS, Coburn JG. Hidroacanthoma simplex. Br J Dermatol 1956;68:400.
439. Mehregan AH, Levson DN. Hidroacanthoma simplex. Arch Dermatol 1969;100:303.
440. Bardach H. Hidroacanthoma simplex with in situ porocarcinoma. J Cutan Pathol 1978;5:236.
441. Pinkus H, Mehregan AH. Epidermotropic eccrine carcinoma. Arch Dermatol 1963;88:597.
442. Graham JH, Johnson WC, Helwig EB, eds. Dermal pathology. Hagerstown, MD: Harper & Row, 1972.
443. Darier J, Ferrand M. L'épithéliome pavimenteux mixte et intermédiaire. Ann Dermatol Syphiligr (Paris) 1955;82:124.
444. Montgomery H. Basal squamous cell epithelioma. Arch Dermatol Syph 1928;18:50.
445. Gertler W. Zur epithelverbundenheit der basaliome. Dermatol Wochenschr 1965;151:673.
446. Borel DM. Cutaneous basosquamous carcinoma: Review of the literature and report of 35 cases. Arch Pathol 1973;95:293.
447. Welton DG, Elliott JA, Kimmelstiel P. Epithelioma. Arch Dermatol Syph 1949;60:277.
448. Lennox B, Wells AL. Differentiation in the rodent ulcer group of tumours. Br J Cancer 1951;5:195.
449. Holmes EJ, Bennington JL, Haber SL. Citrulline-containing basal cell carcinomas. Cancer 1968;22:663.
450. Smith OD, Swerdlow MA. Histogenesis of basal-cell epithelioma. Arch Dermatol 1956;74:286.
451. Freeman RG. Histopathologic considerations in the management of skin cancer. J Dermatol Surg 1976;2:215.
452. Krompecher E. Der basalzellenkrebs. Jena: Gustav Fischer, 1903.
453. Montgomery H. Dermatopathology. New York: Harper & Row, 1967;923.
454. Teloh HA, Wheelock MC. Histogenesis of basal cell carcinoma. Arch Pathol 1949;48:447.
455. Ten Seldam REJ, Helwig EB. Histological typing of skin tumours, Geneva: World Health Organization, 1974;48.
456. Adamson HG. On the nature of rodent ulcer: Its relationship to epithelioma adenoides cysticum of Brooke and to other trichoepitheliomata of benign nevoid character; its distinction from malignant carcinoma. Lancet 1914;1:810.
457. Wallace SA, Halpert B. Trichoma: Tumor of hair anlage. Arch Pathol 1950;50:199.
458. Chiba M, Jimbow K. Expression of gamma-glutamyl transpeptidase in normal and neoplastic epithelial cells of human skin. Br J Dermatol 1986;114:459.
459. Kariniemi AL, Holthöfer H, Vartto T et al. Cellular differentiation of basal cell carcinoma studies with fluorescent lectins and cytokeratin antibodies. J Cutan Pathol 1984;11:541.
460. Shimizu N, Ito M, Tazawa T et al. Anti-keratin monoclonal antibody against basal cell epithelioma keratin: BKN-1. J Dermatol 1987;14:359.
461. Van Scott EJ, Reinertson RP. The modulating influence of stromal environment on epithelial cells studied in human autotransplants. J Invest Dermatol 1961;36:109.
462. Covo JA. The pits in the nevoid basal cell carcinoma syndrome. Arch Dermatol 1971;103:568.
463. Gerstein W. Transplantation of basal cell epithelioma to the rabbit. Arch Dermatol 1963;88:834.
464. Grimwood RE, Johnson CA, Ferris CF et al. Transplantation of human basal cell carcinoma to athymic mice. Cancer 1985;56:519.
465. Greene HSN. The heterologous transplantation of embryonic mammalian tissue. Cancer Res 1943;3:809.
466. Zackheim HS. Origin of the human basal cell epithelioma. J Invest Dermatol 1963;40:283.
467. Brown AC, Crounse RB, Winkelmann RK. Generalized hair-follicle hamartoma. Arch Dermatol 1969;99:478.
468. Madsen A. De l'épithélioma baso-cellulaire superficiel. Acta Derm Venereol (Stockh) 22 Suppl 1941;7:1.
469. Madsen A. Studies on basal-cell epithelioma of the skin. Acta Pathol Microbiol 1965;65(Suppl)177:7.
470. Oberste-Lehn H. Zur histogense des Basalioms. Z Hautkr 1954;16:334.
471. Lang PG Jr, McKelvey AC, Nicholson JH. Three dimensional reconstruction of the superficial multicentric basal cell carcinoma. Am J Dermatopathol 1987;9:198.
472. Zelickson AS. An electron microscope study of the basal cell epithelioma. J Invest Dermatol 1962;39:183.
473. Lever WF, Hashimoto K. Electron microscopic and histochemical findings in basal cell epithelioma, squamous cell carcinoma and some appendage tumors. XIII Congressus Internat Dermatol. Vol 1. Berlin: Springer-Verlag, 1968;3.

474. Kumakiri M, Hashimoto K. Ultrastructural resemblance of basal cell epithelioma to primary epithelial germ. J Cutan Pathol 1978;5:53.
475. Cutler B, Posalaky Z, Katz I. Cell processes in basal cell carcinoma. J Cutan Pathol 1980;7:310.
476. Zelickson AS. The pigmented basal cell epithelioma. Arch Dermatol 1967;96:524.
477. Bleehen SS. Pigmented basal cell epithelioma. Br J Dermatol 1975; 93:361.
478. Weinstein GO, Frost P. Cell proliferation in human basal cell carcinoma. Cancer Res 1970;30:724.
479. Hashimoto K, Kobayashi H. Histogenesis of amyloid in the skin. Am J Dermatopathol 1980;2:165.
480. Hashimoto K, Brownstein MH. Localized amyloidosis in basal cell epithelioma. Acta Derm Venereol (Stockh) 1973;53:331.
481. Masu S, Hosokawa M, Seiji M. Amyloid in localized cutaneous amyloidosis: Immunofluorescence studies with anti-keratin antiserum especially concerning the difference between systemic and localized cutaneous amyloidosis. Acta Derm Venereol (Stockh) 1981;61:381.
482. Looi LM. Localized amyloidosis in basal cell carcinoma. Cancer 1983;52:1833.
483. Rahbari H, Mehregan AH. Basal cell epithelioma (carcinoma) in children and teenagers. Cancer 1982;49:350.
484. Hoyo E, Kanitakis J, Euvrard S, Thivolet J. Proliferation characteristics of cutaneous squamous cell carcinomas developing in organ graft recipients: Comparison with squamous cell carcinomas of nonimmunocompromised hosts by counting argyrophilic proteins associated with nucleolar organizer regions. Arch Dermatol 1993;129:324.
485. Viac J, Chardonnet Y, Euvrard S et al. Langerhans' cells, inflammation markers and human papillomavirus infections in benign and malignant epithelial tumors from transplant recipients. J Dermatol 1992; 19:67.
486. Proby CM, Churchill L, Purkis PE et al. Keratin 17 expression as a marker for epithelial transformation in viral warts. Am J Pathol 1993; 143:1667.
487. McGregor JM, Farthing A, Crook T et al. Posttransplant skin cancer: A possible role for p53 gene mutation but not for oncogenic human papillomaviruses. J Am Acad Dermatol 1994;30:701.
488. Angeli-Besson C, Koeppel MC, Jacquet P et al. Multiple squamous-cell carcinomas of the scalp and chronic myeloid leukemia. Dermatology 1995;191:321.
489. Oram Y, Orengo I, Griego RD et al. Histologic patterns of basal cell carcinoma based upon patient immunostatus. Dermatologic Surgery 1995;21:611.
490. Hertzler G, Gordon SM, Piratzky J et al. Case report: Fulminant Kaposi's sarcoma after orthotopic liver transplantation. Am J Med Sci 1995;309:278.
491. Abouna GM, Kumar MS, Samhan M. Kaposi's sarcoma in renal transplant recipients: a case report. Transplant Sci 1994;4:20.
492. Al-Sulaiman MH, Mousa DH, Dhar JM, Al-Khader AA. Does regressed posttransplantation Kaposi's sarcoma recur following reintroduction of immunosuppression? Am J Nephrol 1992;12:384.
493. McGregor JM, Newell M, Ross J et al. Cutaneous malignant melanoma and human immunodeficiency virus (HIV) infection: A report of three cases. Br J Dermatol 1992;126:516.
494. Musso L, Gordon H. Spontaneous resolution of molluscum sebaceum. Proc R Soc Med 1950;43:838.
495. Rook A, Whimster IW. Le kératoacanthome. Arch Belg Dermatol Syphiligr 1950;6:137.
496. Ghadially FN. Keratoacanthoma. In: Fitzpatrick TB, Eisen AZ, Wolff K et al., eds. Dermatology in general medicine, 2nd ed. New York: McGraw-Hill, 1979;383.
497. Silberberg I, Kopf A, Baer RL. Recurrent keratoacanthoma of the lip. Arch Dermatol 1962;86:44.
498. Sullivan JJ, Colditz GA. Keratoacanthoma in a subtropical climate. Australas J Dermatol 1979;20:34.
499. Muir EG, Bell AJY, Barlow KA. Multiple primary carcinomata of the colon, duodenum, and larynx associated with keratoacanthomata of the face. Br J Surg 1967;54:191.
500. Poleksic S. Keratoacanthoma and multiple carcinomas. Br J Dermatol 1974;91:461.
501. Rapaport J. Giant keratoacanthoma of the nose. Arch Dermatol 1975; 111:73.
502. Bart RS, Popkin GL, Kopf AW et al. Giant keratoacanthoma. J Dermatol Surg 1975;1:49.
503. Kallos A. Giant keratoacanthoma. Arch Dermatol 1958;78:207.
504. Obermayer ME. Das keratoakanthom: Seine zur gewebsdestruktion führende wachstumskapazität. Hautarzt 1964;15:628.
505. Belisario JC. Brief review of keratoacanthoma and description of keratoacanthoma centrifugum marginatum. Australas J Dermatol 1965; 8:65.
506. Miedzinski F, Kozakiewicz J. Das keratoakanthoma centrifugum: Eine besondere varietät des keratoakanthoms. Hautarzt 1962;13:348.
507. Weedon D, Barnett L. Keratoacanthoma centrifugum marginatum. Arch Dermatol 1975;111:1024.
508. Heid E, Grosshans E, Lazrak B et al. Keratoacanthoma centrifugum marginatum. Ann Dermatol Venereol 1979;106:367.
509. Macaulay WL. Subungual keratoacanthoma. Arch Dermatol 1976; 112:1004.
510. Stoll DM, Ackerman AB. Subungual keratoacanthoma. Am J Dermatopathol 1980;2:265.
511. Keeney GL, Banks PM, Linscheid RL. Subungual keratoacanthoma. Arch Dermatol 1988;124:1074.
512. Rook A, Whimster I. Keratoacanthoma: A 30-year retrospect. Br J Dermatol 1979;100:41.
513. Poleksic S, Yeung KY. Rapid development of keratoacanthoma and accelerated transformation into squamous cell carcinoma of the skin. Cancer 1978;41:12.
514. Kern WH, McGray MK. The histopathologic differentiation of keratoacanthoma and squamous cell carcinoma of the skin. J Cutan Pathol 1980;7:318.
515. Popkin GL, Brodie SJ, Hyman AB et al. A technique of biopsy recommended for keratoacanthoma. Arch Dermatol 1966;94:191.
516. Wade TR, Ackerman AB. The many faces of keratoacanthoma. J Dermatol Surg Oncol 1978;4:498.
517. De Moragas JM, Montgomery H, McDonald JR. Keratoacanthoma versus squamous-cell carcinoma. Arch Dermatol 1957;77:390.
518. Giltman LI. Tripolar mitosis in a keratoacanthoma. Acta Derm Venereol (Stockh) 1981;61:362.
519. Janecka IP, Wolff M, Crikelair GF et al. Aggressive histological features of keratoacanthoma. J Cutan Pathol 1978;4:342.
520. Lapins NA, Helwig EB. Perineural invasion by keratoacanthoma. Arch Dermatol 1980;116:791.
521. Levy EJ, Cahn MM, Shaffer B et al. Keratoacanthoma. JAMA 1954; 155:562.
522. Calnan CD, Haber H. Molluscum sebaceum. J Pathol Bacteriol 1955; 69:61.
523. Ghadially FN. The role of the hair follicle in the origin and evolution of some cutaneous neoplasms of man and experimental animals. Cancer 1961;14:801.
524. Takaki Y, Masutani M, Kawada A. Electron microscopic study of keratoacanthoma. Acta Derm Venereol (Stockh) 1971;51:21.
525. Von Bülow M, Klingmüller G. Elektronenmikroskopische untersuchungen des keratoakanthoms. Arch Dermatol Forsch 1971;241: 292.
526. Chalet MD, Connors RC, Ackerman AB. Squamous cell carcinoma vs. keratoacanthoma: Criteria for histologic differentiation. J Dermatol Surg 1975;1:16.
527. Stevanovic DV. Keratoacanthoma dyskeratoticum and segregans. Arch Dermatol 1965;92:666.
528. Piscioli F, Boi S, Zumiani G et al. A gigantic, metastasizing keratoacanthoma. Am J Dermatopathol 1984;6:123.
529. Goldenhersh MA, Olsen TG. Invasive squamous cell carcinoma initially diagnosed as giant keratoacanthoma. J Am Acad Dermatol 1984;10:372.
530. Nikolowski W. Zur problematik des keratoakanthoms. Dermatol Monatsschr 1970;156:148.
531. Sullivan JJ, Donoghue MF, Kynaston B et al. Multiple keratoacanthomas. Australas J Dermatol 1980;21:16.
532. Ferguson Smith J. A case of multiple primary squamous-celled carcinomata of the skin in a young man with spontaneous healing. Br J Dermatol 1934;46:267.
533. Tarnowski WM. Multiple keratoacanthomata. Arch Dermatol 1966; 94:74.
534. Hilker O, Winterscheidt M. Familiäre multiple keratoakanthome. Z Hautkr 1987;62:280.
535. Sommerville J, Milne JA. Familial primary self-healing squamous epithelioma of the skin (Ferguson Smith type). Br J Dermatol 1950;62: 485.

536. Grzybowski M. A case of peculiar generalized epithelial tumours of the skin. Br J Dermatol 1950;62:310.
537. Sterry W, Steigleder GK, Pullmann H et al. Eruptive keratoakanthome. Hautarzt 1981;32:119.
538. Rossman RE, Freeman RG, Knox JM. Multiple keratoacanthomas. Arch Dermatol 1964;89:374.
539. Winkelmann RK, Brown J. Generalized eruptive keratoacanthoma. Arch Dermatol 1968;97:615.
540. Wright AL, Gawkrodger DJ, Branford WA et al. Self-healing epitheliomata of Ferguson-Smith. Dermatologica 1988;176:22.
541. Rook A, Moffat JL. Multiple self-healing epithelioma of Ferguson Smith type. Arch Dermatol 1956;74:525.
542. Lancer HA, Moschella SL. Paget's disease of the male breast. J Am Acad Dermatol 1982;7:393.
543. Hadlich J, Göring HD, Linse R. Morbus Paget beim mann nach Östrogenbehandlung. Dermatol Monatsschr 1981;167:305.
544. Ashikari R, Park K, Huvos AG et al. Paget's disease of the breast. Cancer 1970;26:680.
545. Paone JF, Baker RR. Pathogenesis and treatment of Paget's disease of the breast. Cancer 1981;48:825.
546. Lewis HM, Ovitz ML, Golitz LE. Erosive adenomatosis of the nipple. Arch Dermatol 1976;112:1427.
547. Sitakalin C, Ackerman AB. Mammary and extramammary Paget's disease. Am J Dermatopathol 1985;7:335.
548. Hopsu-Havu VK, Sonck CE. The problem of extramammary Paget's disease: Report of four cases with "pagetoid" cells. Z Hautkr 1971;46: 41.
549. Ordoñez NG, Awalt H, MacKay B. Mammary and extramammary Paget's disease. Cancer 1987;59:1173.
550. Culberson JD, Horn RC Jr. Paget's disease of the nipple. Arch Surg 1956;72:224.
551. Helwig EB, Graham JH. Anogenital (extramammary) Paget's disease: A clinicopathologic study. Cancer 1963;16:387.
552. Orr JW, Parish DJ. The nature of the nipple changes in Paget's disease. J Pathol Bacteriol 1962;84:201.
553. Lagios MD, Westdahl PR, Rose MR et al. Alternative management in cases without or with minimal extent of underlying breast carcinoma. Cancer 1984;54:545.
554. Sagebiel RW. Ultrastructural observations on epidermal cells in Paget's disease of the breast. Am J Pathol 1969;57:49.
555. Ebner H. Zur ultrastruktur des morbus Paget mamillae. Z Hautkr 1969;44:297.
556. Caputo R, Califano A. Ultrastructural features of extramammary Paget's disease. Arch Klin Exp Dermatol 1970;236:121.
557. Nadji M, Morales AR, Girtanner RE et al. Paget's disease of the skin: A unifying concept of histogenesis. Cancer 1982;50:2203.
558. Kariniemi AL, Forsman L, Wahlström T et al. Expression of differentiation antigen in mammary and extramammary Paget's disease. Br J Dermatol 1984;110:203.
559. Belcher RW. Extramammary Paget's disease: Enzyme histochemical and electron microscopic study. Arch Pathol 1972;94:59.
560. Penneys NS, Nadji M, Morales A. Carcinoembryonic antigen in benign sweat gland tumors. Arch Dermatol 1982;118:225.
561. Glasgow BJ, Wen DR, Al-Jitawi S et al. Antibody to S-100 protein aids the separation of pagetoid melanoma from mammary and extramammary Paget's disease. J Cutan Pathol 1987;14:223.
562. Murrell TW Jr, McMullan FH. Extramammary Paget's disease. Arch Dermatol 1962;85:600.
563. Fligiel Z, Kaneko M. Extramammary Paget's disease of the external ear canal in association with ceruminous gland carcinoma. Cancer 1975;36:1072.
564. Whorton CM, Patterson JB. Carcinoma of Moll's glands with extramammary Paget's disease of the eyelid. Cancer 1955;8:1009.
565. Duperrat B, Mascaro JM. Maladie de Paget abdomino-scrotale (3e présentation): Apparition d'un épithéliome apocrine de l'aisselle et de lésions de maladie de Paget sur la peau axillaire sus-jacente. Bull Soc Fr Dermatol Syphiligr 1964;71:176.
566. Fetissoff F, Arbeille-Brassart B, Lansac J et al. Association d'une maladie de Paget mammaire et vulvaire. Ann Dermatol Venereol 1981; 109:43.
567. McKee PH, Hertogs KT. Endocervical adenocarcinoma and vulval Paget's disease: A significant association. Br J Dermatol 1980;103: 443.
568. Metcalf JS, Lee RE, Maize JC. Epidermotropic urothelial carcinoma involving the glans penis. Arch Dermatol 1985;121:532.
569. Ojeda VJ, Heenan PJ, Watson SH. Paget's disease of the groin associated with adenocarcinoma of the urinary bladder. J Cutan Pathol 1987;14:227.
570. Powell FC, Bjornsson J, Doyle JA et al. Genital Paget's disease and urinary tract malignancy. J Am Acad Dermatol 1985;13:84.
571. Jones RE Jr, Austin C, Ackerman AB. Extramammary Paget's disease. Am J Dermatopathol 1979;1:101.
572. Hart WR, Millman JB. Progression of intraepithelial Paget's disease of the vulva to invasive carcinoma. Cancer 1977;40:2333.
573. Wick MR, Goellner JR, Wolfe JT III et al. Vulvar sweat gland carcinomas. Arch Pathol 1985;109:43.
574. Lee SC, Roth LM, Ehrlich C et al. Extramammary Paget's disease of the vulva. Cancer 1977;39:2540.
575. Yoell JH, Price WG. Paget's disease of the perianal skin with associated adenocarcinoma. Arch Dermatol 1960;82:986.
576. Wood WS, Culling CFA. Perianal Paget disease. Arch Pathol 1975; 99:442.
577. Gunn RA, Gallager HS. Vulvar Paget's disease. Cancer 1980;46:590.
578. Koss LG, Brockunier A Jr. Ultrastructural aspects of Paget's disease of the vulva. Arch Pathol 1969;87:592.
579. Tazawa T, Ito M, Fujiwara H et al. Immunologic characteristics of keratin in extramammary Paget's disease. Arch Dermatol 1988;124: 1063.
580. Pinkus H, Mehregan AH. A guide to dermatopathology. 3rd ed. New York: Appleton-Century-Crofts, 1981;471.
581. Mérot Y, Mazoujian G, Pinkus G et al. Extramammary Paget's disease of perianal and perineal regions: Evidence of apocrine derivation. Arch Dermatol 1985;121:750.

Lever's Histopathology of the Skin, eighth edition,
edited by David Elder et al. Lippincott–
Raven Publishers, Philadelphia © 1997.

CHAPTER 31

Tumors of the Epidermal Appendages

David Elder, Rosalie Elenitsas, and Bruce D. Ragsdale

CLASSIFICATION OF THE APPENDAGE TUMORS

The benign tumors differentiating in the direction of epidermal appendages can be divided into four groups: those differentiating toward hair follicles, toward sebaceous glands, toward apocrine glands, and toward eccrine glands.

Diagnosis of adnexal neoplasms presents difficulties related to the large variety of different tumors and their variant forms, the frequency of differentiation along two or more adnexal lines in the same tumor,[1–3] and the complicated nomenclature.[4] The term *histogenesis* implies that the appearance of a tumor is indicative of the cell type of the tissue from which it arose ("cell of origin"). This concept has historical importance, but today the phenotypes that a proliferating neoplastic population is differentiating toward constitute the basis for assigning terms according to how closely the patterns resemble some recognizable normal cell or structure. In general, tumors do not derive directly from mature (differentiated) cells; rather, they are believed to originate from multipotential undifferentiated stem cells and to differentiate along particular pathways, which may be multiple. This concept predicts that tumors, including adnexal tumors, will imprecisely resemble their mature counterparts and also that multiple differentiation pathways may be expressed simultaneously in the same tumor. Benign adnexal tumors in which there is an admixture of follicular, eccrine, sebaceous, and/or apocrine adnexal differentiation, such as sebaceous units in combination with either eccrine and/or apocrine elements,[5] are a source of diagnostic confusion that likely results from multidirectional differentiation involving pluripotential cells of the epidermis or of adnexal structures.[4] Differentiation is probably influenced not only by genetic potential, but also by field effects such as regional vascularity and microenvironmental attributes of the epidermis, dermis, or subcutis.

Besides the benign tumors, there are carcinomas of epidermal appendages. Three types of glandular carcinoma are recognized: carcinoma of sebaceous glands, of eccrine sweat glands, and of apocrine glands. A few instances of malignant tumors of hair follicle structures have been reported, such as pilomatrix carcinoma, malignant proliferating trichilemmal cyst, trichilemmal carcinoma, and trichoblastic carcinoma.

Histopathology often can be interpreted in terms of normal differentiation of skin appendages. Clear or pale cell change due to cytoplasmic glycogen may recapitulate the embryonic acrosyringium in a nodular hidradenoma or the normally glycogenated follicular outer root sheath in a trichilemmoma. Cytoplasmic fat vacuoles that indent the nucleus are typical of sebaceous differentiation. Many adnexal tumors contain a distinctive, fibrotic, eosinophilic hyaline collagenous stroma that envelops the epithelial elements. This typical stroma assists in differentiating many basaloid adnexal neoplasms from basal cell carcinoma. Eccrine tumors commonly sport a nearly acellular hyalinized eosinophilic stroma with dilated thin-walled vessels (e.g., nodular hidradenoma). Tubule formation and focal keratinization occurring in eccrine tumors tend to differentiate them from renal cell or other metastatic clear cell carcinomas. Immunohistochemistry is of little value in distinguishing among the phenotypic patterns of adnexal neoplasms.[6]

Histology often changes with time and in response to local effects. For example, a trichilemmal cyst, possibly stimulated by inflammatory mediators, may as it ages transform into a proliferating trichilemmal cyst and ultimately into the solid pilar tumor of the scalp. It is likely that tumor progression, the "process whereby tumors go from bad to worse" also operates in adnexal tumors, as it does in other neoplastic systems. From a clinical point of view, however, adnexal neoplasms should not be regarded as precursors of malignancy.

Classification of the Benign Appendage Tumors

The four groups of benign appendage tumors with differentiation toward hair, sebaceous glands, apocrine glands, and eccrine glands can be divided, according to the decreasing degree of differentiation observed in them, into three major subgroups: a group of benign nonneoplastic conditions including hyperplasias, hamartomas, and cysts; a second group of benign neoplasms; and a third group of malignant neoplasms (Table 31-1). This classification is a simplification of the previous classification, which included lesions with intermediate degrees of dif-

D. Elder: Department of Pathology and Laboratory Medicine, University of Pennsylvania, Philadelphia, PA

R. Elenitsas: Department of Dermatology, University of Pennsylvania, Philadelphia, PA

B. D. Ragsdale: Department of Dermatology, University of Alabama, Birmingham, AL; Central Coast Pathology Consultants, San Luis Obispo, CA

ferentiation in a category of "epitheliomas,"[7,8] and is similar to the approach of the recent World Health Organization International Histological Classification of Tumours monograph.[9]

Of the three subgroups into which the benign appendage tumors can be divided, the hyperplasias, hamartomas, and cysts are composed of mature or nearly mature structures. The benign neoplasms in general show less differentiation than the hyperplasias; nonetheless, well-developed, differentiated or partially differentiated structures are present. The malignant neoplasms are a further step down with regard to degree of differentiation, and it may be difficult to recognize the type of structure that the tumor is attempting to form. The term *epithelioma* has been used in a number of different ways, variously including neoplasms considered currently to be either benign or malignant, and this term will not be used except for historical reasons. Basal cell carcinomas, which may have adnexal differentiation, are considered to be the least differentiated of the benign appendage tumors. In this volume, however, these neoplasms are discussed in the chapter on surface tumors of the skin (see Chap. 30).

Although most of the benign appendage tumors fit well into one of the entities listed in Table 31-1, tumors in an intermediate stage of differentiation are occasionally encountered.[10] Also, because of differentiation in more than one direction, combinations of several tumor types occur, so that one may find within the same tumor, for instance, differentiation toward sebaceous and apocrine structures.[11]

Histogenesis of the Benign Appendage Tumors

Three possibilities exist for the development of benign appendage tumors: they may develop from primary epithelial germs, from pluripotential cells, or from cells of preexisting structures. In 1948, the thesis was advanced that cutaneous tumors differentiating toward hair, sebaceous glands, or apocrine glands developed from primary epithelial germ cells and were primary epithelial germ tumors; further, that the hyperplasias, adenomas, and benign epitheliomas arose from primary epithelial germ cells that had attained a certain degree of differentiation before the onset of neoplasia.[8]

In the case of benign appendage tumors that are present at birth, such as the nevus sebaceus, (see Chap. 30) and syringocystadenoma papilliferum, it may be assumed that such tumors are actually derived from embryonic *primary epithelial germ cells*. In other instances, it is likely that the benign appendage tumors arise from *pluripotential cells* that have formed during life and possess the potential of differentiating into tumors with hair, sebaceous gland, or apocrine structures.[12] In genetically determined appendage tumors, such as multiple cylindromas, multiple trichoepitheliomas, and the nevoid basal cell carcinoma syndrome, it may be assumed that the genes regulating the development of pluripotential cells into cutaneous appendages are abnormal and sooner or later modify the growth of pluripotential cells into appendage tumors rather than into mature appendages. In some instances, primary epithelial germ cells and pluripotential cells differentiate in more than one direction, as is seen most commonly on the scalp, where a syringocystadenoma may differentiate into all three appendage structures. In many instances, particularly in solitary tumors arising after birth, adnexal tumors of the skin arise from the cells (likely the germ cells) of their corresponding structures.[13] This is likely to be true also of the adnexal tumors, that, in addition to occurring as multiple lesions with an autosomal dominant inheritance pattern, also occur as solitary, not inherited, lesions, such as trichoepithelioma and cylindroma.[14]

Terminology

The terms *nevus, hamartoma,* and *carcinoma* used in the classification of the benign appendage tumors require definition.

The term *nevus* is used in the literature in two different ways, referring (1) to a tumor composed of nevus cells derived from melanocytes (nevocellular nevus, melanocytic nevus, pigmented nevus) or (2) to a lesion that is usually present at birth and is composed of mature or nearly mature structures, such as nevus sebaceus, eccrine nevus, nevus verrucosus, and nevus flammeus. To avoid confusion, it is advisable to use the term *nevus* with a qualifying adjective, and to assume that *nevus* with-

TABLE 31-1. *Classification of the benign appendage tumors*

Lesions	Follicular differentiation	Sebaceous differentiation	Apocrine differentiation	Eccrine differentiation
Hyperplasias, hamartomas, cysts	Hair follicle nevus Dilated pore	Nevus sebaceus Sebaceous hyperplasia	Apocrine nevus	Eccrine nevus
Benign neoplasms	Trichofolliculoma Pilar sheath acanthoma Fibrofolliculoma Trichodiscoma Trichoepithelioma Trichoadenoma Pilomatricoma Proliferating trichilemmal cyst Trichilemmoma Tumor of the follicular infundibulum	Sebaceous adenoma Sebaceoma	Apocrine hidrocystoma Hidradenoma papilliferum Apocrine syringocystadenoma Tubular apocrine adenoma Erosive adenomatosis of the nipple Apocrine cylindroma	Eccrine hidrocystoma Syringoma Eccrine cylindroma Eccrine poroma Mucinous syringometaplasia Eccrine spiradenoma Nodular hidradenoma Chondroid syringoma

out a qualifying adjective designates a tumor composed of melanocytic nevus cells.

The term *hamartoma* is appropriate for those nevi that have no melanocytic nevus cells and, like congenital hyperplasias, are composed of mature or nearly mature structures. *Hamartoma,* derived from the Greek word *hamartanein* (to fail, to err), was chosen as the designation for "tumor-like malformations showing a faulty mixture of the normal components of the organ in which they occur."[15]

The term *epithelioma* has been used by many authors as a synonym for *carcinoma*. However, since the literal meaning of the word is "tumor of the epithelium," the term may be employed as a designation of benign as well as of malignant tumors of the epithelium, provided that a qualifying adjective is added.[16] Because the term has been used for both benign and malignant neoplasms, it seems best to avoid its use except in a clearly defined historical context. The term *carcinoma* is used for malignant epithelial tumors, including those that are characterized by a tendency to inexorable growth with local invasion and tissue destruction as well as those that may in addition have capacity for distant metastasis. Not all of the terminology used in this chapter conforms exactly to the above schema; we have selected terms that are widely understood and used, not necessarily those that are above all semantic scrutiny.[17]

TUMORS WITH DIFFERENTIATION TOWARD HAIR STRUCTURES

Hair Follicle Nevus

This rare, small tumor consists of a small nodule on the face and is usually present at birth.

Histopathology. There are numerous, small, well-differentiated hair follicles, occasionally accompanied by a few small sebaceous glands.[18]

Differential Diagnosis. The small vellus hair follicles present in the central part of the face greatly resemble the hair follicles in a hair follicle nevus.

Trichofolliculoma

Trichofolliculoma occurs in adults as a solitary lesion, usually on the face but occasionally on the scalp or neck. It consists of a small, skin-colored, dome-shaped nodule. Frequently, there is a central pore. If such a central pore is present, a wool-like tuft of immature, usually white hairs may be seen emerging from it, a highly diagnostic clinical feature.[19]

Histopathology. On histologic examination, the dermis contains a large cystic space that is lined by squamous epithelium and contains horny material and frequently also fragments of birefringent hair shafts.[20] In cases with a central pore, the large cystic space is continuous with the surface epidermis, an indication that it represents an enlarged, distorted hair follicle. In some cases, one or two additional cystic spaces are present in the dermis. Radiating from the wall of these "primary" hair follicles, one sees many small but usually fairly well differentiated "secondary" hair follicles. Well-developed secondary hair follicles often show a hair papilla. Furthermore, they usually show an outer and an inner root sheath, the latter of which may contain eosinophilic trichohyaline granules and, located in the center, a fine hair (Fig. 31-1). These fine hairs are visualized best where the secondary hair follicles appear in cross sections. Small groups of sebaceous gland cells may be embedded in the walls of the secondary hair follicles.[21] In some of the more rudi-

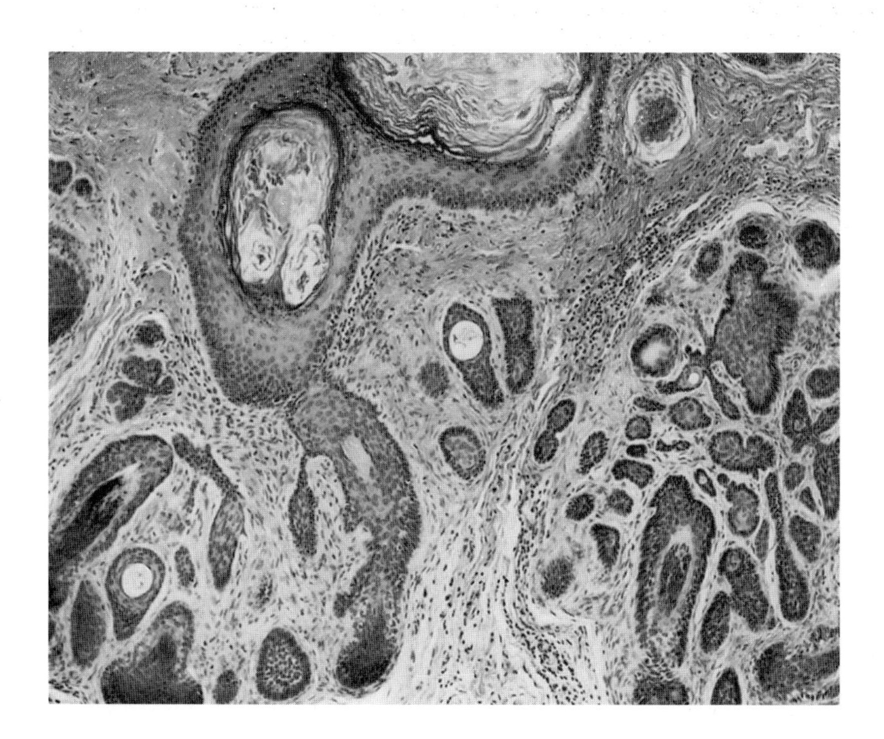

FIG. 31-1. Trichofolliculoma
At the top, one sees part of a keratin-filled cyst lined by squamous epithelium and representing a "primary" hair follicle. Grouped around the cyst are numerous small "secondary" hair follicles, some of which show, in addition to a hair and an outer root sheath, an inner root sheath with trichohyalin granules.

mentary secondary follicles, one observes a central horn cyst in place of a hair, as seen also in trichoepithelioma.[22] The stroma is rich in fibroblasts and is oriented in parallel bundles of fibers that encapsulate the epithelial proliferations in a manner resembling that of the normal fibrous root sheath.[7] Glycogen can be demonstrated in the outer root sheath of the secondary hair follicles, just as it is seen in the outer root sheath of mature hair structures.[20]

In all trichofolliculomas, epithelial strands interconnect the secondary hair follicles. Since these epithelial strands differentiate in the direction of the outer root sheath, the peripheral cell row is palisaded, and because of their glycogen content, the cells within the strands appear large and vacuolated.[7]

Sebaceous Trichofolliculoma

A variant of trichofolliculoma, sebaceous trichofolliculoma occurs in areas rich in sebaceous follicles, such as the nose. It is a centrally depressed lesion with a fistula-like opening from which terminal hairs and vellus hairs protrude.[23]

Histopathology. There is a rather large, irregularly shaped, centrally located cavity lined by squamous epithelium. Many radially arranged pilosebaceous follicles connect to the cavity. These contain sebaceous ducts and numerous well-differentiated, large sebaceous lobules, as well as hair follicles containing partially terminal and partially vellus hairs.[23]

Dilated Pore and Pilar Sheath Acanthoma

Dilated pore and pilar sheath acanthoma share with trichofolliculoma and sebaceous trichofolliculoma clinically the presence of a central pore and histologically the presence of a large cystic space that is continuous with the surface epidermis, lined by squamous epithelium, and filled with keratinous material.

The *dilated pore,* described in 1954 by Winer,[24] occurs on the face, usually as a solitary lesion and predominantly in adult males. It has the appearance of a giant comedo and does not possess any palpable induration.

The *pilar sheath acanthoma,* described in 1978,[25] is usually found on the skin of the upper lip of adults. It is seen elsewhere on the face only rarely. It occurs as a solitary skin-colored nodule with a central porelike opening.

Histopathology. The *dilated pore* shows a markedly dilated pilar infundibulum lined by an epidermis that is atrophic near the ostium but hypertrophic deeper in the cystic cavity, where it shows many rete ridges and irregular thin proliferations into the surrounding stroma. The keratin-filled cystic cavity may extend into the subcutaneous fat. In the lower portion, small sebaceous gland lobules and vellus hair follicles may be attached to the lining epidermis.[24]

The *pilar sheath acanthoma* differs from the dilated pore by showing a larger, irregularly branching cystic cavity. In place of thin proliferations, as seen in the dilated pore, numerous lobulated masses of tumor cells radiate from the wall of the cystic cavity into the dermis and the subcutaneous tissue.[25] The tumor cells in some areas show peripheral palisading and contain varying amounts of glycogen. They resemble outer root sheath epithelium.[26]

Multiple Fibrofolliculomas; Multiple Trichodiscomas

Multiple fibrofolliculomas have been described not only in association with trichodiscomas and acrochordons[27,28] but also in association with a large connective tissue nevus.[29]

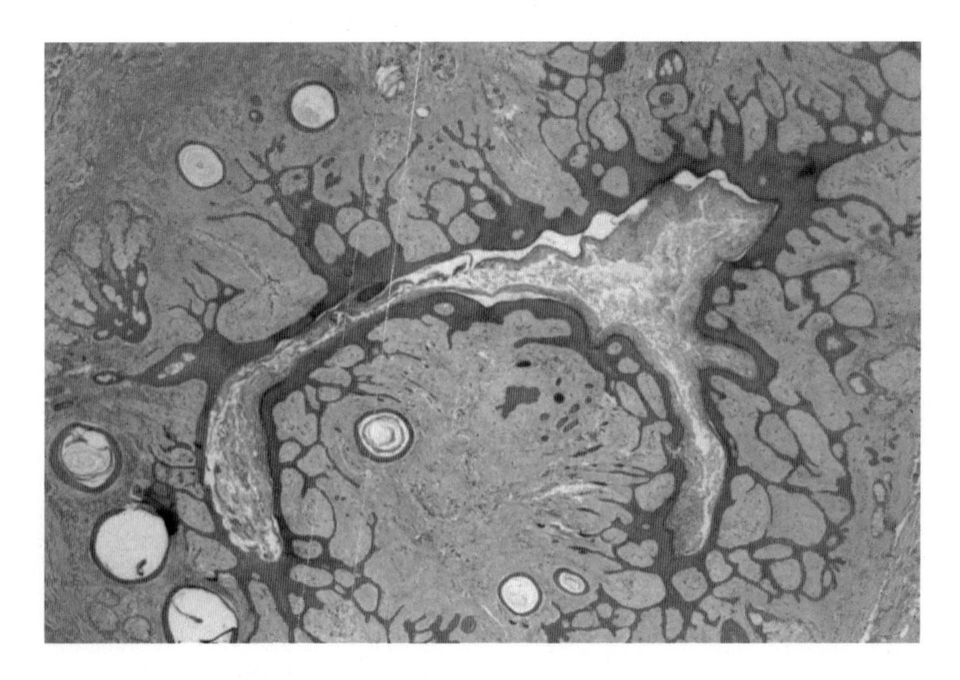

FIG. 31-2. Fibrofolliculoma
In the center of the lesion, a distorted hair follicle is surrounded by an amphophilic, mucoid, and fibrous stroma (see also Fig. 31-3).

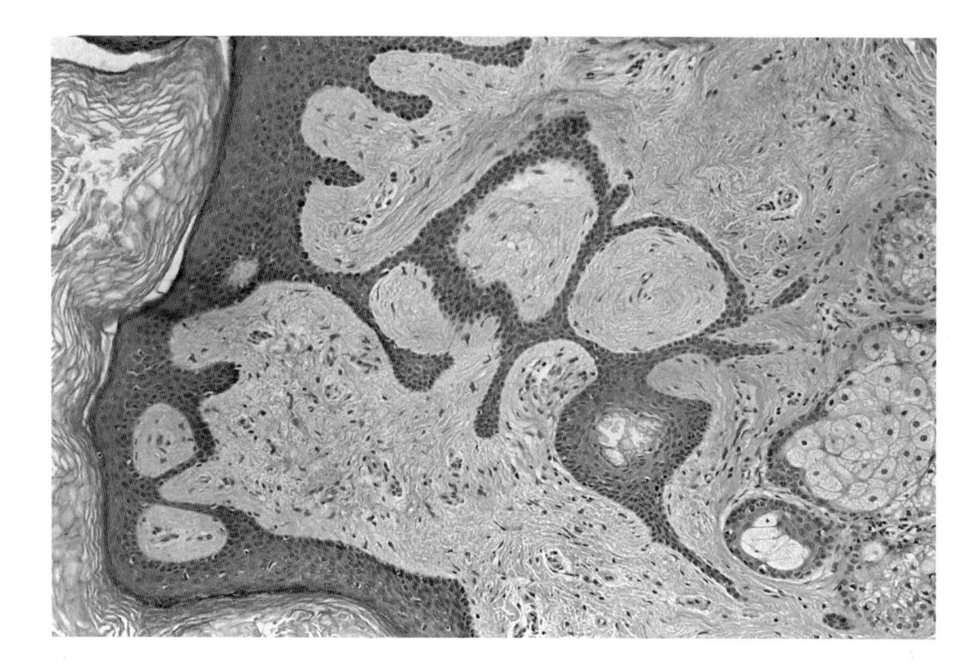

FIG. 31-3. Fibrofolliculoma Numerous thin, anastomosing bands of follicular epithelium extend into the stroma.

Fibrofolliculomas consist of multiple 2- to 4-mm large, yellow-white, smooth, dome-shaped lesions. In patients who also have trichodiscomas and acrochordons, the lesions are present in considerable number mainly on the face and neck. In such cases, the trichodiscomas are clinically indistinguishable from the fibrofolliculomas.[27] In a reported patient with a large connective tissue nevus, fibrofolliculomas were present in large numbers within as well as around the connective tissue nevus.[29]

Multiple trichodiscomas are clinically indistinguishable from fibrofolliculomas. Besides occurring in association with multiple fibrofolliculomas, multiple trichodiscomas also occur without them, as small papules either widely disseminated[30] or localized to one area.[31]

Histopathology. Fibrofolliculomas show in their center a hair follicle that often appears distorted. It is surrounded by a thick mantle of basophilic, mucoid stroma. Numerous thin, anastomosing bands of follicular epithelium extend into this stroma (Figs. 31-2 and 31-3).[27,29]

Trichodiscomas show in a subepidermal location within a circumscribed area fine fibrillary connective tissue thick-walled blood vessels with a small lumen. A hair follicle is usually found at the margin of the lesion.[29] Trichodiscomas are regarded as hamartomas of the mesodermal component of hair disks.[30]

The pedunculated acrochordons seen in association with multiple fibrofolliculomas may contain only dermal connective tissue. However, in some instances, they contain thin, anastomosing strands of epithelium; they are then fibrofolliculomas displaying the configuration of an acrochordon.[28]

Solitary fibrofolliculoma occurs as a rare, solitary papule on the face of elderly persons.

The histologic picture is the same as that seen in the multiple variant: multiple anastomosing strands of basaloid cells proliferate from the basal layer of a hair follicle into the surrounding fibromucinous stroma.[32]

Trichoepithelioma

The name *trichoepithelioma* is preferable to other designations, such as *epithelioma adenoides cysticum* and *multiple benign cystic epithelioma,* because it indicates that the differentiation in this tumor is directed toward hair structures. Trichoepithelioma occurs either in multiple lesions or as a solitary lesion.

Multiple trichoepithelioma is transmitted as an autosomal dominant trait.[33] In most instances, the first lesions appear in childhood and gradually increase in number.[34] One observes numerous rounded, skin-colored, firm papules and nodules usually between 2 and 8 mm in diameter and located mainly in the nasolabial folds but also on the nose, forehead, and upper lip. Occasionally, lesions are seen also on the scalp, neck, and upper trunk. Ulceration of the lesions occurs rarely. Transformation of one or several lesions into basal cell carcinomas is a very rare event.[35] Most of the cases reported as such in the past are now regarded as instances of nevoid basal cell carcinoma syndrome.[36] The simultaneous presence of lesions of trichoepithelioma and cylindroma, the latter of which is also dominantly inherited, has been observed repeatedly (see Cylindroma).

Solitary trichoepithelioma occurs more commonly than multiple trichoepitheliomas.[34] It is not inherited and consists of a firm, elevated, flesh-colored nodule usually less than 2 cm in diameter. Its onset usually is in childhood or early adult life.[37] Most commonly, the lesion is seen on the face, but it may occur elsewhere. The presence within the same tumor of a solitary trichoepithelioma and an apocrine adenoma has been described.[38]

Giant solitary trichoepithelioma, measuring several centimeters in diameter, is a distinct variant of trichoepithelioma.[39] It arises in later life and occurs most commonly on a thigh[40] and in the perianal region.[39]

Histopathology. As a rule, the lesions of multiple trichoepithelioma are superficial, and they appear well circumscribed,

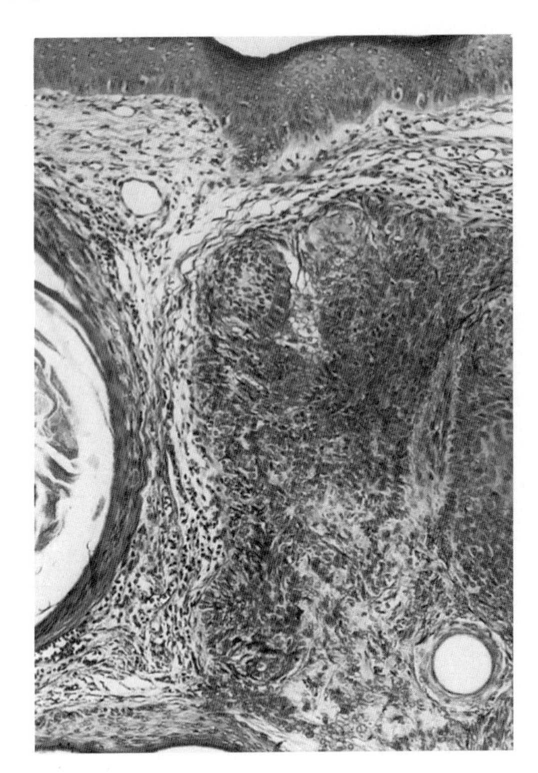

FIG. 31-4. Trichoepithelioma
The two major components are horn cysts of varying sizes and formations resembling basal cell epithelioma.

small, and symmetrical on histologic examination. Horn cysts are the most characteristic histologic feature, although they may be absent in some lesions. They consist of a fully keratinized center surrounded by basophilic cells that have the same appearance as the cells in the basal cell carcinoma ("basalioma cells"), except that they tend to lack high-grade atypia and mitoses, as are prominent in some but not all carcinomas (Fig. 31-4). The keratinization is abrupt and complete, in the manner of so-called "trichilemmal" keratinization, not gradual and incomplete as in the horn pearls of squamous cell carcinoma. Quite frequently, one observes one or a few layers of cells with eosinophilic cytoplasm and large, oval, pale, vesicular nuclei situated between the basophilic cells and the horn cysts.[34]

As the second major component of multiple trichoepitheliomas, tumor islands composed of basophilic cells of the same appearance as epidermal or skin appendage basal cells are arranged usually in a lacelike or adenoid network but occasionally also as solid aggregates. These tumor islands show peripheral palisading of their cells and are surrounded by a stroma with a moderate number of fibroblasts. The fibroblasts encircle and are tightly associated with the basaloid islands, lacking the retraction artifact typical of basal cell carcinoma (Fig. 31-5). Both the adenoid and the solid aggregates show invaginations, which contain numerous fibroblasts and thus resemble follicular papillae (Fig. 31-6).

Additional findings, observed in some but not all multiple trichoepitheliomas, are the presence of a foreign-body giant cell reaction in the vicinity of ruptured horn cysts and of calcium deposits either within the foci of the foreign-body reaction or within intact horn cysts.[34]

Occasionally, some lesions in patients with multiple trichoepithelioma show relatively little differentiation toward hair structures. Then they contain only a few horn cysts but many areas with the appearance of basal cell carcinoma.[34] Such lesions are indistinguishable from those of a keratotic basal cell carcinoma, which may also show horn cysts (Fig. 31-7). Thus, on a histologic basis, no sharp line of demarcation can be drawn between multiple trichoepithelioma and basal cell carcinoma. Diagnosis may be assisted in a given case by clinical data, such as the number and distribution of the lesions and the presence of hereditary transmission.

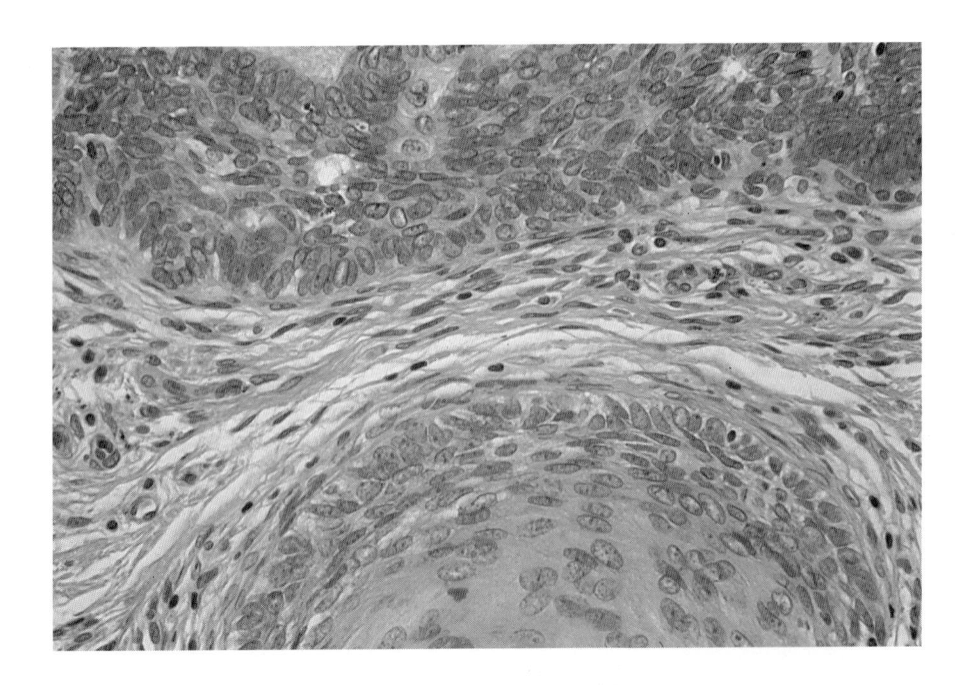

FIG. 31-5. Trichoepithelioma
Fibroblasts encircle and are tightly associated with the basaloid epithelial islands, lacking the retraction artifact typical of basal cell carcinoma.

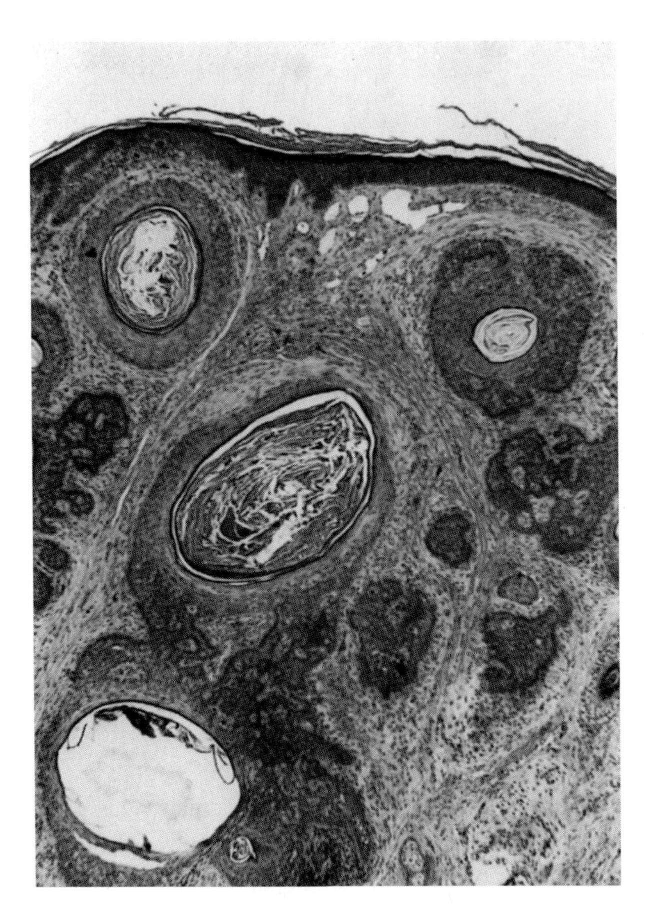

FIG. 31-6. Trichoepithelioma
In this case the walls of the horn cysts are formed by a few layers of cells with eosinophilic cytoplasm and large vesicular nuclei. Some of the basophilic cells are arranged in an adenoid network.

Solitary trichoepithelioma is used as histologic designation only for lesions showing a high degree of differentiation toward hair structures. Solitary lesions with relatively little differentiation toward hair structures are best classified as keratotic basal cell carcinoma. If a lesion is to qualify for the diagnosis of solitary trichoepithelioma, it should contain numerous horn cysts and abortive hair papillae and show only few areas with the appearance of basal cell carcinoma.[37] Mitotic figures should be very rare or absent, and the lesion should not be unduly large, asymmetrical, or infiltrative. Large and deep-seated lesions that otherwise have attributes of trichoepitheliomas have been termed *trichoblastomas* (Figs. 31-8, 31-9, and 31-10).[41,42] It has been argued that trichoblastoma (also known as trichoblastic fibroma) should be distinguished from trichoepithelioma because of its size, location (usually trunk versus face and neck in trichoepithelioma), and lack of keratinizing cysts.[43] Similar lesions that are infiltrative and that exhibit cytologic atypia and mitotic activity may be termed *trichoblastic carcinoma,* but these lesions overlap extensively with basal cell carcinoma. Such problematical lesions may be signed out descriptively as *malignant adnexal neoplasm* with a description of the apparent differentiation of the lesion. Criteria enumerated by Ackerman et al. that may have value in distinguishing trichoblastomas and trichilemmomas from basal cell carcinomas include the following: the presence in the former of symmetry, of circumscription with smooth margins and "shelling out" of the normal tissue, of follicular and "racemiform" patterns of lesional cells, the lack of a clefting artifact between stroma and epithelium that is characteristic of basal cell carcinoma, the lack of stromal edema and lymphocytes, the formation of a delicate stroma reminiscent of that formed around immature hair follicles, and the lack of ulceration.[42]

Histogenesis. It is assumed that the basophilic cells surrounding horn cysts are analogous to hair matrix cells and that the horn cysts represent attempts at hair shaft formation. The

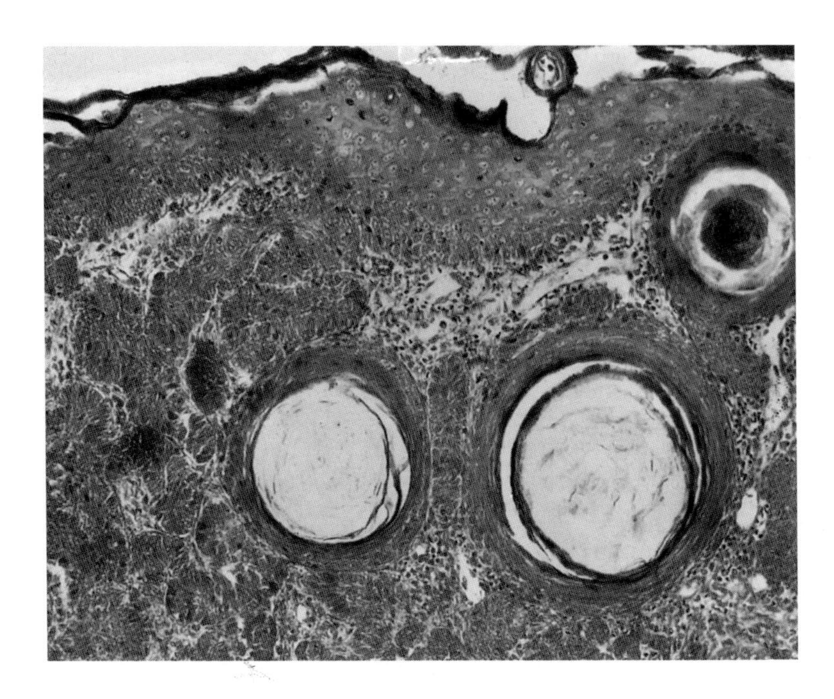

FIG. 31-7. Basal cell carcinoma with horn cysts
Histologically, this tumor is in an intermediate stage of differentiation between basal cell carcinoma and trichoepithelioma. Clinically, the lesion was a basal cell carcinoma.

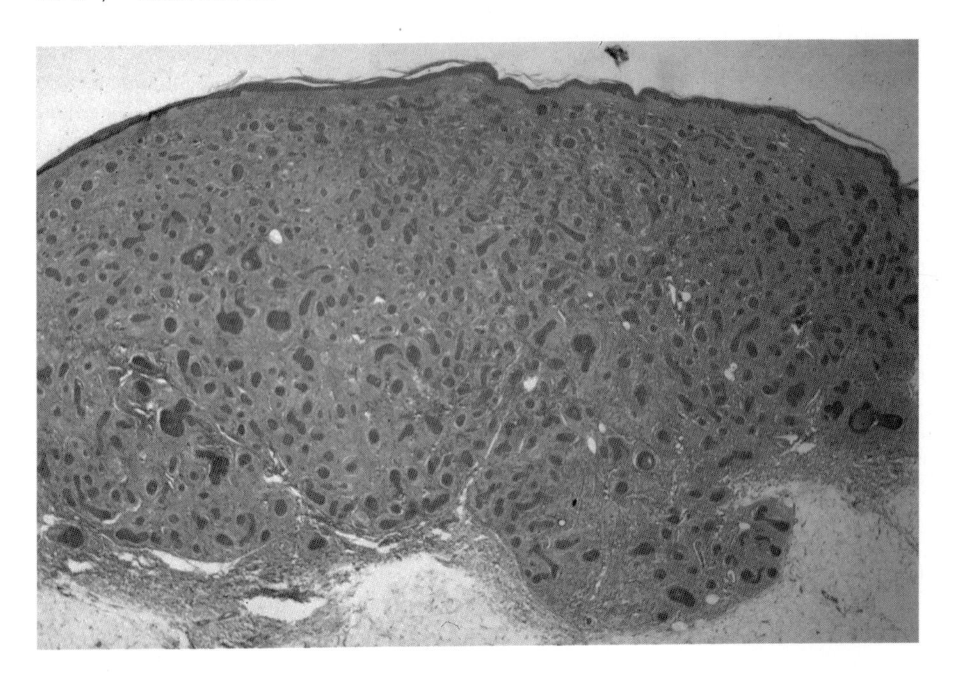

FIG. 31-8. Trichoblastoma
This is a bulky tumor that spans the dermis and involves the fat. The profile is generally symmetrical and the borders are quite well circumscribed.

eosinophilic cells seen occasionally around horn cysts probably represent cells with initial keratinization and are similar to the nucleated cells seen in normal hair shafts at the keratogenous zone.

Electron microscopic study has confirmed that the horn cysts of trichoepithelioma represent immature hair structures, with abrupt development of the horn cells from hair matrix cells.[44]

Histochemical staining with the Gomori stain for alkaline phosphatase has shown positive staining in many invaginations at the periphery of tumor islands and strands, indicative of a differentiation toward hair papillae (see Chap. 3).[45]

The close relationship between trichoepithelioma and basal cell carcinoma has been explained on the basis of the assumption that they have a common genesis from pluripotential cells, which, like primary epithelial germ cells, may develop toward hair structures.[8] Thus the two types of tumors differ, merely in the degree of maturity of their cells. Because cells of various degrees of maturity may occur in the same lesion, trichoepithe-

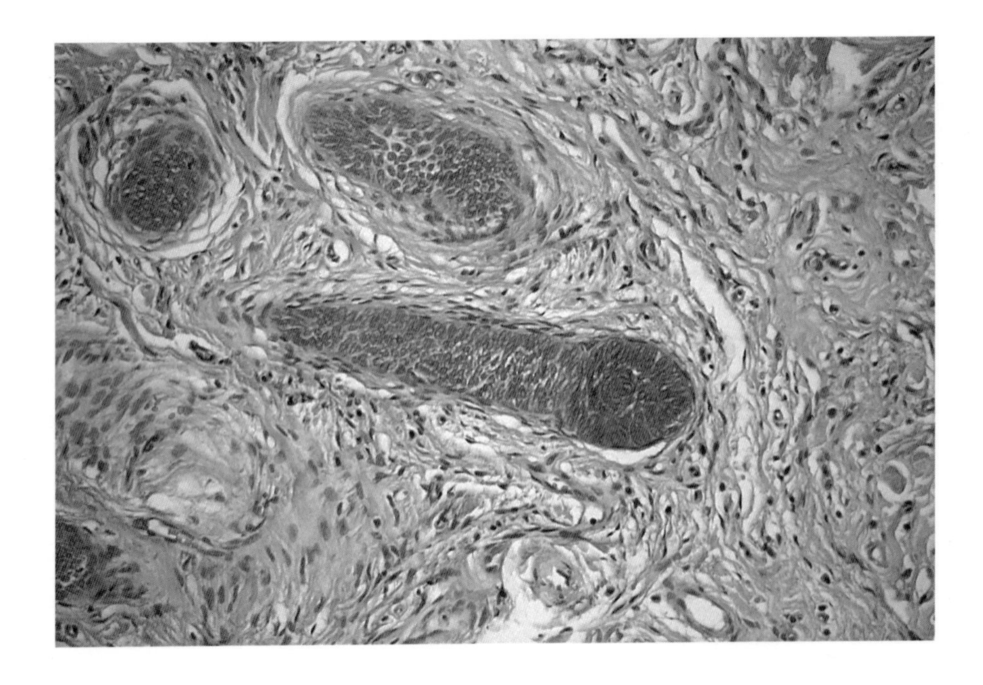

FIG. 31-9. Trichoblastoma
Higher power showing epithelial structures reminiscent of follicular germs (see also Fig. 31-10).

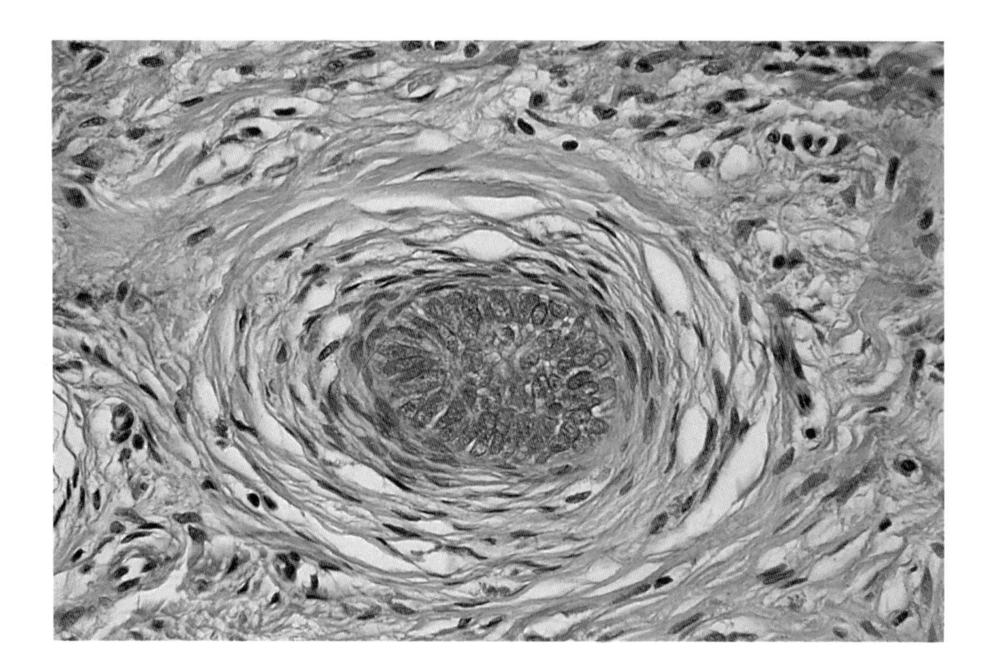

FIG. 31-10. Trichoblastoma
The follicular epithelium is surrounded by mesenchyme, reminiscent of that which may surround a developing hair follicle.

lioma may have areas consistent with the histologic picture of basal cell carcinoma and vice versa.

The occasional association of multiple trichoepithelioma with cylindroma, an appendage tumor with differentiation probably toward apocrine structures, and of a solitary trichoepithelioma with an apocrine adenoma also speaks in favor of the development of trichoepithelioma from immature cells with the potential to differentiate toward primary epithelial germ structures.

Differential Diagnosis. The difficulty of differentiating multiple trichoepithelioma from keratotic basal cell carcinoma on histologic grounds has been pointed out, and the need for clinical data has been stressed.

The differentiation of multiple trichoepithelioma from the nevoid basal cell carcinoma syndrome on histologic grounds can be just as difficult. This, too, often requires clinical data. Although both diseases are dominantly inherited and have multiple lesions, the lesions in trichoepithelioma are present mainly in the nasolabial fold, remain small, and hardly ever ulcerate, whereas the lesions in the nevoid basal cell carcinoma syndrome are haphazardly distributed and, especially in the late, "neoplastic" phase, can grow to considerable size, ulcerate deeply, and show severely destructive growth. In addition, patients with the nevoid basal cell carcinoma syndrome almost invariably show mutliple skeletal and central nervous system anomalies and frequently show multiple palmar and plantar pits (see Nevoid Basal Cell Carcinoma Syndrome, Chap. 30).

Desmoplastic Trichoepithelioma

Desmoplastic trichoepithelioma, a nonfamilial and usually solitary lesion, was formerly considered a solitary trichoepithelioma.[34,37] However, it has sufficient clinical and histologic characteristics to be regarded as a distinct variant of trichoepithelioma. The term *desmoplastic trichoepithelioma*[46] appears preferable to the designation *sclerosing epithelial hamartoma*[47] because it stresses the relationship of the lesion to solitary trichoepithelioma.

Clinically, the tumor almost always is located on the face, measures from 3 to 8 mm in diameter, and is markedly indurated. In many instances, there is a raised, annular border and a depressed nonulcerated center, causing the lesion to resemble granuloma annulare.[46] Most commonly, the lesion appears in early adulthood, but it quite frequently appears in the second decade of life.[47] It is much more common in females than in males.[46]

Histopathology. The three characteristic histologic features are narrow strands of tumor cells, horn cysts, and a desmoplastic stroma (Fig. 31-11).[46] The tumor strands usually are from one to three cells thick and are composed of small basaloid cells with prominent oval nuclei and scant cytoplasm. Usually there are numerous horn cysts, which in some cases are large.[48] Considerable amounts of densely collagenous and hypocellular stroma are present. Large aggregates of tumor cells are not seen. Foreign-body granulomas at the site of ruptured horn cysts and areas of calcification within some of the horn cysts are seen in many tumors.

Differential Diagnosis. The resemblance to microcystic adnexal (eccrine) carcinoma may be considerable, especially if a superficial specimen is taken for biopsy. Like desmoplastic trichoepithelioma, it shows horn cysts, strands of basaloid cells, and a dense desmoplastic stroma. It differs, however, by showing ductal structures and a deeply infiltrating growth.[49] The diagnosis of microcystic adnexal carcinoma should be considered in any tumor resembling a trichoepithelioma or a syringoma in which the lesional cells extend to the base of the specimen.

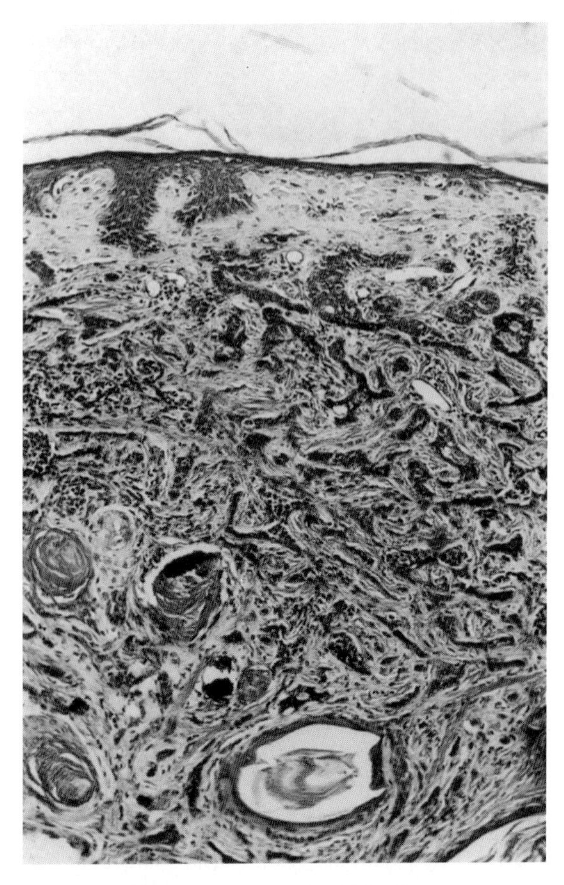

FIG. 31-11. Desmoplastic trichoepithelioma
The three characteristic features are narrow strands of basaloid tumor cells, horn cysts, and desmoplastic stroma.

The resemblance of desmoplastic trichoepithelioma to fibrosing basal cell carcinoma is great; however, in fibrosing basal cell carcinoma, horn cysts are absent. Of value in ruling out basal cell carcinoma, especially the morphea-like form,[50] are the absence of mitoses, individual cell necrosis, and mucinous stroma and the lack of foci of separation artifact of lesional epithelium and stroma. Epithelial membrane antigen (EMA) is positive in 75% of cases, whereas basal cell carcinomas in contrast are typically negative.

Occasional lesions of solitary or desmoplastic trichoepithelioma cannot reliably be distinguished from keratotic or fibrosing basal cell carcinomas, respectively. A descriptive report and a recommendation for complete excision are appropriate in such cases.

Trichoadenoma

A rare, solitary tumor first described in 1958,[51] trichoadenoma usually occurs on the face and varies from 3 to 15 mm in diameter. It may arise anytime during adult life.

Histopathology. Numerous horn cysts are present. They are surrounded by eosinophilic cells, which greatly resemble the eosinophilic cells that are often seen in trichoepithelioma located between the basophilic cells and the central horn cysts (Fig. 31-12). In some instances, a single layer of flattened granular cells is interpolated between the horn cysts and the surrounding eosinophilic cells.[52–54] Some islands consist only of eosinophilic epithelial cells without central keratinization. Sparse intercellular bridges have been observed between the eosinophilic cells. Foci of foreign-body granuloma are present at the sites of ruptured horn cysts.[51]

Histogenesis. The general architecture of trichoadenoma greatly resembles that of trichoepithelioma and thus suggests

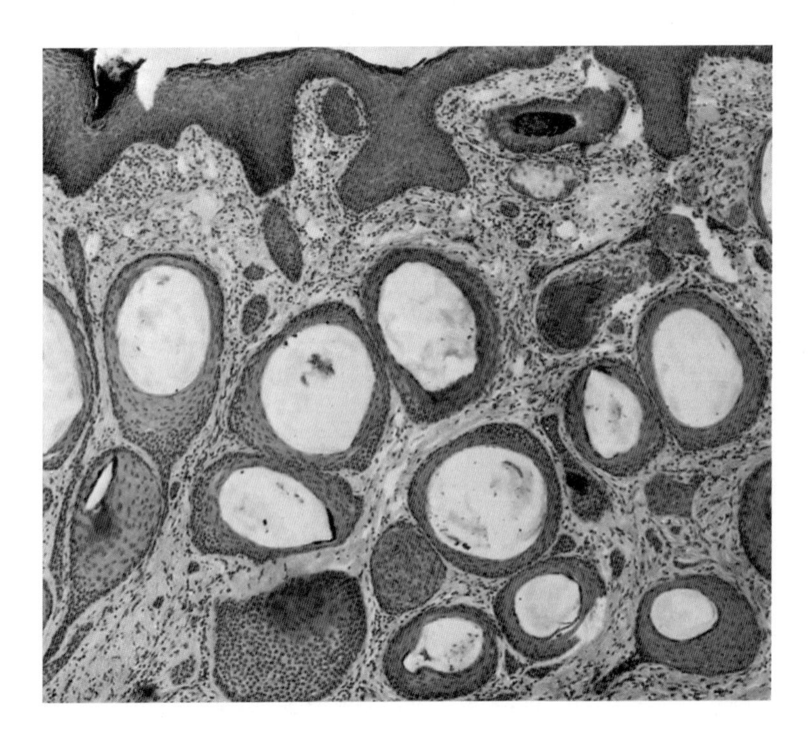

FIG. 31-12. Trichoadenoma
Numerous horn cysts are present surrounded by eosinophilic cells. Some islands consist entirely of eosinophilic epithelial cells.

the development of immature hair structures. However, because the cyst wall consists of epidermoid cells and the keratinization may take place with formation of keratohyalin, it has been suggested that the tumor differentiates largely toward the infundibular portion of the pilosebaceous canal.[52]

Immature Trichoepithelioma

An immature form of trichoepithelioma at the opposite end of the spectrum from trichoadenoma, immature trichoepithelioma is a neoplasm with differentiation toward the primitive hair germ.[55] Often it is not located on the face.

Histopathology. The tumor is well circumscribed and consists of numerous small tumor lobules composed of basaloid cells with invaginations resembling dermal hair papillae. Horn cysts and adenoid formations are absent.

Generalized and Localized Hair Follicle Hamartoma

Only a few cases have been described of generalized hair follicle hamartoma, a distinctive condition characterized by progressive alopecia starting in adulthood and by diffuse papules and plaques of the face, and by associated myasthenia gravis.[56–59]

A localized form has been described in which a hairless patch in the scalp appeared in adult life without myasthenia gravis.[60]

Histopathology. In both the generalized and localized forms, the hair loss is the result of damage inflicted on each hair follicle by gradually growing "hair follicle hamartomas."

Areas of alopecia without papules or plaques reveal more or less advanced replacement of the hair follicles by a lacelike network of basaloid cells with follicular differentiation resembling trichoepithelioma.[56,58]

The papules and plaques of the face show a complete lack of hair structures and extensive proliferations of basaloid cells embedded in a cellular stroma with formation of horn cysts in some areas. The histologic appearance is indistinguishable from that of trichoepithelioma.[57]

Differential Diagnosis. Linear unilateral basal cell nevus (see Chap. 30) shows similar basaloid proliferations, some of which may resemble trichoepithelioma; but the clinical picture is different because the lesion is congenital, unilateral, and nonprogressive. Similar changes affecting individual follicles may be seen as an incidental finding that must be dinstiguished from basal cell carcinoma, especially in reexcision specimens.

Pilomatricoma

Pilomatricoma, or calcifying epithelioma of Malherbe, is a tumor with differentiation toward hair cells, particularly hair cortex cells. Most commonly, it manifests itself as a firm, deep-seated nodule that is covered by normal skin. Occasionally, however, the tumor is more superficially located, causing a blue-red discoloration of the overlying skin, and, rarely, it protrudes as a sharply demarcated, dark red nodule. Rapid enlargement of a pilomatricoma may occur as the result of formation of a hematoma.[61] Perforation may take place with extrusion of parts of the contents.[62] Pilomatricoma occurs usually as a solitary lesion. The face and the upper extremities are the most common sites. Generally, the tumor varies in diameter from 0.5 to 3.0 cm, but it may be as large as 5 cm. The tumors may arise in persons of any age, but about 40% of them arise in children younger than 10, and about 60% in persons in the first two decades of life.[63] Although, as a rule, pilomatricoma is not hereditary, there are a few instances of familial occurrence, and in some of these cases the tumor is associated with myotonic dystrophy.[64] Unusual clinical variants include large, extruding, or perforating examples, multiple eruptive cases, familial cases, and malignant examples termed *pilomatrix carcinoma* (see text following).[65–68]

Histopathology. The tumor is sharply demarcated and often surrounded by a connective tissue capsule. It is usually located in the lower dermis and extends into the subcutaneous fat. Embedded in a rather cellular stroma, irregularly shaped islands of epithelial cells are present. As a rule, two types of cells, *basophilic cells* and *shadow cells,* compose the islands (Fig. 31-13).[69] In some tumors, however, basophilic cells are absent. The basophilic cells possess round or elongated, deeply basophilic nuclei and scanty cytoplasm, so that the nuclei lie close together. The cellular borders of the basophilic cells often are indistinct, so that it appears as if the nuclei were embedded in a symplasmic mass. The basophilic cells are arranged either on one side or along the periphery of the tumor islands. In some areas, the transition of basophilic cells into shadow cells is abrupt, whereas in others the transition is gradual. In areas of gradual transition there are cells showing a gradual loss of nuclei and ultimately appearing as faintly eosinophilic, keratinized shadow cells. The shadow cells have distinct border and possess a central unstained area as a shadow of the lost nucleus. In tumors of recent origin, numerous areas of basophilic cells usually are present. As the lesion ages, the number of basophilic cells decreases because of development into shadow cells, and in tumors of long standing few or no basophilic cells remain.

In many tumors, small, round, eosinophilic centers of keratinization are seen within areas of basophilic cells or within aggregates of shadow cells. The keratinization within these centers is abrupt and complete.[70] In some tumors, melanin is present, as can be expected in tumors with differentiation toward hair bulbs. It is found most commonly in shadow cells or within melanophages of the stroma, but in some instances is seen also in dendritic melanocytes located in islands of basophilic cells.[71] The stroma of the tumor usually shows a considerable foreign-body reaction containing many giant cells adjacent to the shadow cells.

With the von Kossa stain, calcium deposits are found in approximately 75% of the tumors.[72] Usually, the calcium is already apparent as deeply basophilic deposits in sections stained with hematoxylin-eosin. Most of the tumors containing clacium are composed largely of shadow cells. The calcium is seen either as fine basophilic granules within the cytoplasm of the shadow cells or as large sheets of amorphous, basophilic material replacing the shadow cells (Fig. 31-14). Occasionally, foci of calcification are seen in the stroma of the tumors. Areas of ossification are seen in 15% to 20% of the cases.[73] Ossification takes place in the stroma next to areas of shadow cells, probably through metaplasia of fibroblasts into osteoblasts (Fig. 31-15). Calcium-rich shadow cells may act as inducing factors.[74]

Histogenesis. Pilomatricoma was originally described in 1880 as calcified epithelioma of sebaceous glands[75]; however,

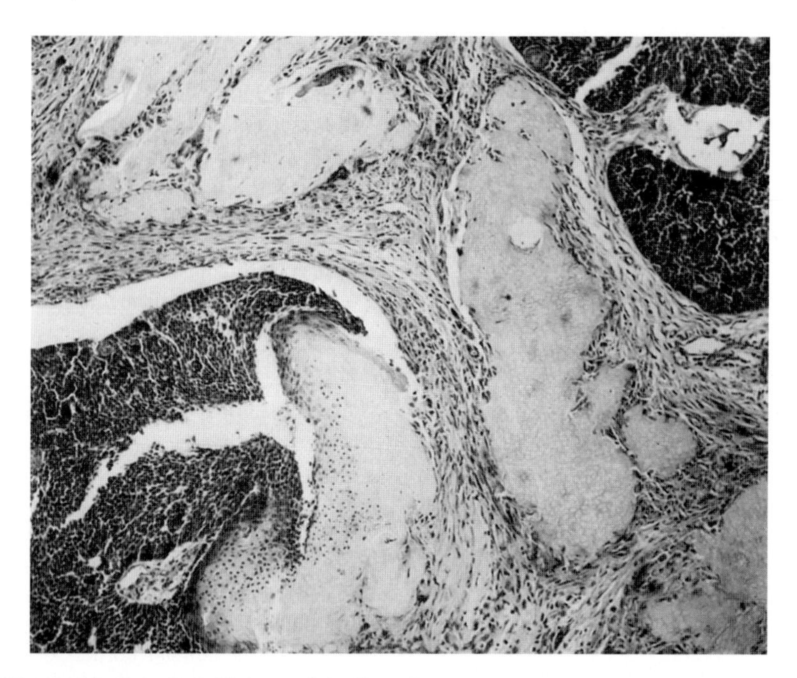

FIG. 31-13. Pilomatricoma (calcifying epithelioma)
The tumor consists of irregularly shaped islands embedded in a rather cellular stroma. Two types of cells comprise the islands: basophilic cells and shadow cells. The basophilic cells resemble hair matrix cells. The shadow cells show a central unstained shadow at the site of the lost nucleus. In the center of the field, one can see transformation of the basophilic cells into shadow cells. The stroma contains numerous multinucleated giant cells.

it was recognized in 1942 that the cells of the tumor differentiate in the direction of hair cortex cells,[76] a finding that was subsequently confirmed by electron microscopic studies. On this basis, the designation *pilomatricoma* was suggested.[73]

Histochemical studies have revealed in most tumor cells a strongly positive reaction with the periodic acid–Schiff stain for sulfhydryl or disulfide groups. This reaction is indicative of keratinization.[72,77] As further evidence of keratinization, the shadow cells show strong birefringence in polarized light.[78] A very similar birefringence is seen in the keratogenous zone of hair.[73]

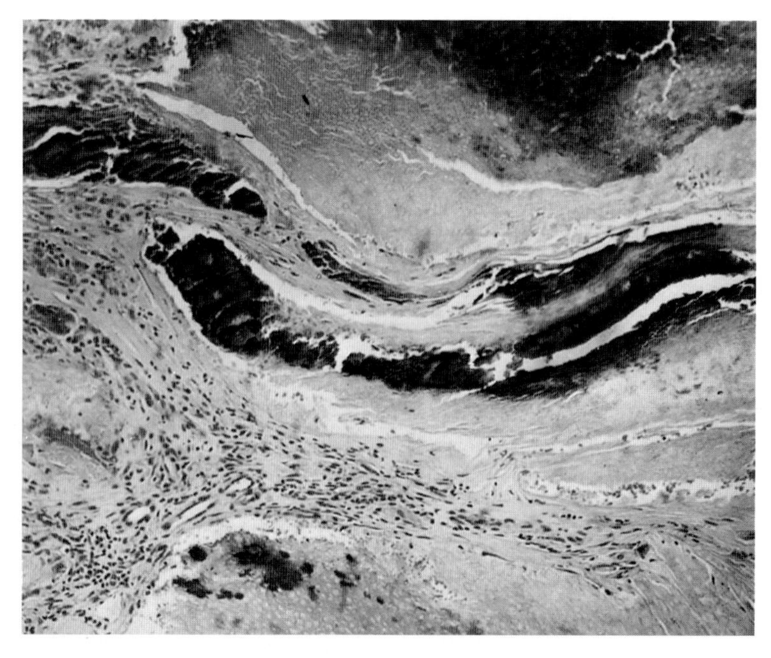

FIG. 31-14. Pilomatricoma (calcifying epithelioma)
Small and large areas of calcification are present within the lobules of shadow cells.

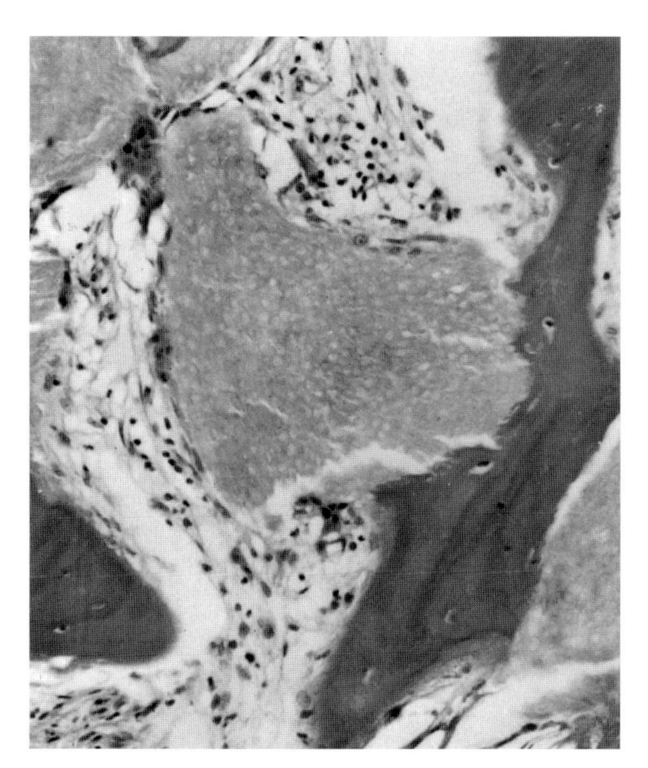

FIG. 31-15. Pilomatricoma (calcifying epithelioma) with ossification
Elongated, irregularly shaped areas of ossification are present in the stroma. In the center, an island of shadow cells is seen.

Electron microscopic examination has revealed a few desmosomes and a moderate number of tonofilaments in the areas of basophilic cells.[79] In cells that are in transition to shadow cells, numerous tonofilaments are seen aggregated into thick keratin fibrils. They form keratin without the appearance of keratohyaline granules. A striking resemblance exists between cells that are in transition to shadow cells and cells in the keratogenous zone of normal hair, because both types of cells show thick keratin fibrils concentrically arranged around a faintly visible nucleus. Fully developed shadow cells show numerous fused, electron-dense keratin fibrils surrounding the empty nuclear area.[77,80]

Differential Diagnosis. The wall of trichilemmal cysts also contains basophilic cells, which as they keratinize gradually lose their nuclei and often undergo calcification. The peripheral layer of basophilic cells in trichilemmal cysts, however, shows a palisading pattern, whereas the basophilic cells of pilomatricoma do not. Furthermore, shadow cells characterized by a central unstained area at the site of the disintegrated nucleus are seen only in pilomatricomas and, exceptionally, in basal cell epitheliomas with foci of matricial differentiation (see Chap. 30).[81]

Pilomatrix Carcinoma

On rare occasions, pilomatricomas show evidence of malignant transformation. Some cases show invasive growth upon recurrence.[82,83] Other cases are malignant from the beginning.[84,85] Pilomatrix carcinomas are not necessarily larger than benign pilomatricomas. Pulmonary metastases may occur.[67,86]

Histopathology. Many areas, especially at the periphery of the tumor, show proliferations of large, anaplastic, hyperchromatic basophilic cells with numerous mitoses.[82] Toward the center of the tumor, there may be transformation of basophilic cells into eosinophilic shadow cells of the type seen in benign pilomatricomas,[87] or there may be large cystic centers containing necrotic debris.[85]

Proliferating Trichilemmal Cyst

The proliferating trichilemmal cyst, also referred to as proliferating trichilemmal tumor,[88] is nearly always a single lesion; rarely, there are two proliferating trichilemmal cysts.[89] About 90% of the cases occur on the scalp, with the residual 10% occurring mainly on the back. More than 80% of the patients are women, most of them elderly.[90]

Starting as a subcutaneous nodule suggestive of a wen, the tumor may grow into a large, elevated, lobulated mass that may undergo ulceration and thus greatly resemble a squamous cell carcinoma.[90] The tumor may occur in association with one or even several trichilemmal cysts of the scalp (see Chap. 30).[91,92] There is evidence that a proliferating trichilemmal cyst may develop from an ordinary trichilemmal cyst.[90,93] However, the tumor may also give rise to one or several trichilemmal cysts, which ultimately may separate from it.[88] In several instances, rapid enlargement of nodular scalp lesions have indicated malignant transformation.[94] In such cases, metastases may arise (see Malignant Proliferating Trichilemmal Tumor).

Histopathology. The proliferating trichilemmal cyst, or proliferating trichilemmal tumor, usually is well demarcated from the surrounding tissue.[95] It is composed of variably sized lobules composed of squamous epithelium. Some of the lobules are surrounded by a vitreous layer and show palisading of their peripheral cell layer.[88] Characteristically, the epithelium in the center of the lobules abruptly changes into eosinophilic amorphous keratin (Fig. 31-16). This amorphous keratin is of the same type as that seen in the cavity of ordinary trichilemmal cysts (see Chap. 30).[96] In addition to showing trichilemmal keratinization, some proliferating trichilemmal cysts exhibit changes resembling the keratinization of the follicular infundibulum. These changes consist of epidermoid keratinization resulting in horn pearls, some of which resemble "squamous eddies."[90]

The tumor cells in many areas show some degree of nuclear atypia, as well as individual cell keratinization, which at first glance suggests a squamous cell carcinoma (see Fig. 31-16).[91,97] The tumor differs from a squamous cell carcinoma by its rather sharp demarcation from the surrounding stroma as well as by its abrupt mode of keratinization.[95] Foci of calcification, although generally small, are often present in the areas of amorphous keratin (Fig. 31-17).[92,95] Some tumors show vacuolization or clear cell formation of some of the tumor cells as a result of glycogen storage.[91,96]

Histogenesis. Keratinization in proliferating trichilemmal cysts is of the same type as in ordinary trichilemmal cysts (see Chap. 30). The "trichilemmal" keratinization in both is analogous to that of the outer root sheath as seen normally at the follicular isthmus above the zone of sloughing of the inner root

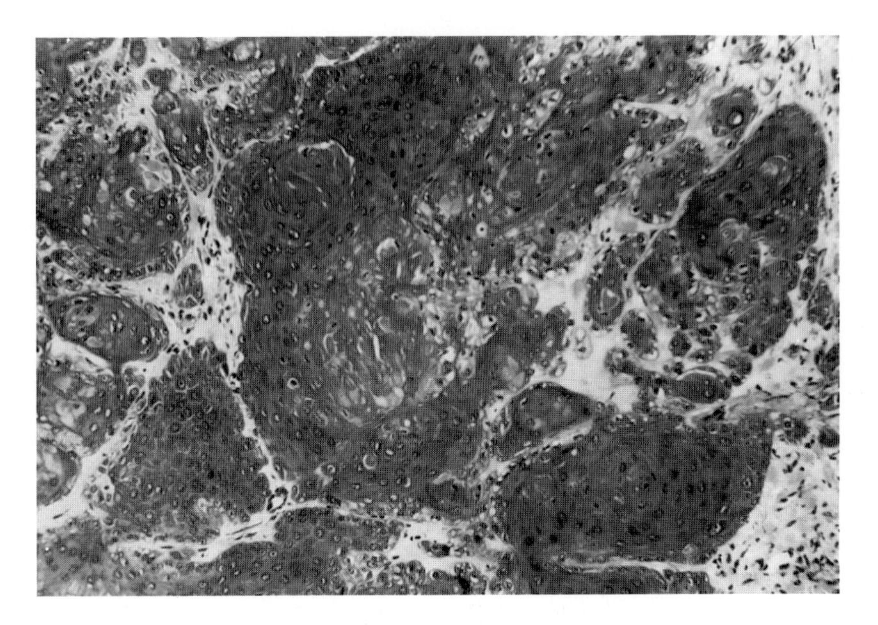

FIG. 31-16. Proliferating trichilemmal cyst
The tumor is composed of irregularly shaped lobules of squamous epithelium undergoing an abrupt change into amorphous keratin. A large area of amorphous keratin is present in the center.

sheath and in the sac surrounding the lower end of the telogen hair.[91,98] Analogous to the outer root sheath, proliferating trichilemmal cysts show (1) an abrupt change of squamous epithelium into amorphous keratin; (2) vacuolated cells containing glycogen, like the cells of the outer root sheath; and (3) a prominent glassy layer of collagen surrounding some tumor formations.[96] Focal calcification within the amorphous keratin is a feature that proliferating trichilemmal cysts and ordinary trichilemmal cysts have in common.

Differential Diagnosis. The presence of numerous sharply demarcated areas of amorphous eosinophilic keratin in the center of the tumor strands and lobules, and the absence of exten-

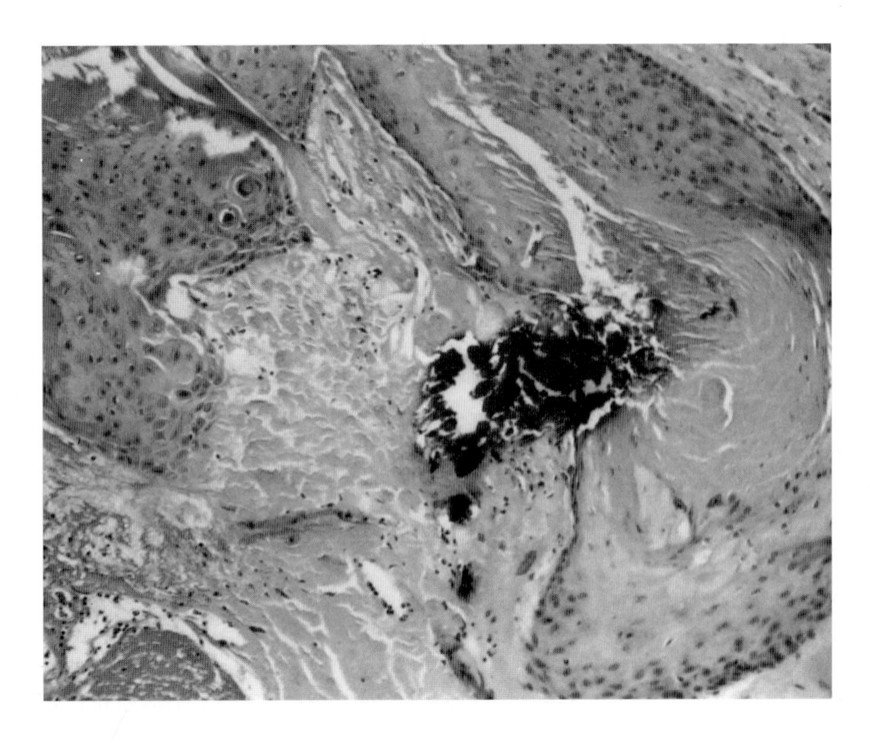

FIG. 31-17. Proliferating trichilemmal cyst
An area of calcification is present in the center. On the right side, an area of amorphous keratin is seen. On the left, two dyskeratotic cells are located in a lobule of squamous epithelium.

sive areas of severe atypia and of invasion of the surrounding tissue usually permit easy differentiation from squamous cell carcinoma.

Malignant Proliferating Trichilemmal Tumor

In rare instances malignant transformation of proliferating trichilemmal cysts takes place, indicated by rapid enlargement of the nodule.[94] There have been several reported instances of metastases, most of them regional.[91,99] In one instance, however, the metastases were generalized and fatal.[100] Penetration of the tumor into cerebral sinuses has occurred, causing death.[101]

Histopathology. Malignant proliferating trichilemmal tumors show extensive areas of severe atypia and invasion of the surrounding tissue.[94] Even though areas of trichilemmal keratinization are still in evidence, tissue invasion and the presence of nuclear atypia and giant nuclei indicate malignany.[100]

Trichilemmoma

Trichilemmoma is a fairly common solitary tumor. In addition, multiple facial trichilemmomas are specifically associated with Cowden's disease.

Solitary Trichilemmoma

Solitary trichilemmoma, first recognized as an entity in 1962,[102] generally is a small tumor, 3 to 8 mm in diameter, occuring usually on the face.[103] Occasionally, it measures several centimeters in diameter.[104] It has no characteristic clinical appearance. In some instances, it is found at the base of a cutaneous horn.[105]

Histopathology. One or several lobules are seen descending from the surface epidermis into the dermis. In some instances, the lobules are oriented about a central hair-containing follicle.[102] A variable number of tumor cells have the appearance of clear cells because of their content of glycogen (Fig. 31-18). The periphery of the tumor lobules usually shows palisading of columnar cells and a distinct, often thickened basement membrane zone resembling the vitreous layer surrounding the lower portion of normal hair follicles.[103] Paradoxically, trichilemmomas do not show the trichilemmal type of keratinization seen in trichilemmal cysts and proliferating trichilemmal cysts. Rather, at the surface, trichilemmomas display epidermoid keratinization, which is frequently pronounced and may even lead to the formation of an overlying cutaneous horn.[105]

In *desmoplastic trichilemmoma* there are irregular extensions of cells of the outer root sheath type that project into sclerotic collagen bundles and mimic invasive carcinoma.[106] Superficially, the lesion shows changes of a trichilemmoma, a finding which aids in the distinction from an invasive carcinoma (Figs. 31-19 and 31-20).

Differential Diagnosis. In instances with relatively few clear cells and marked hypergranulosis and hyperkeratosis, differentiation from a verruca vulgaris may be difficult. A PAS stain for the demonstration of glycogen may aid in the differentiation.

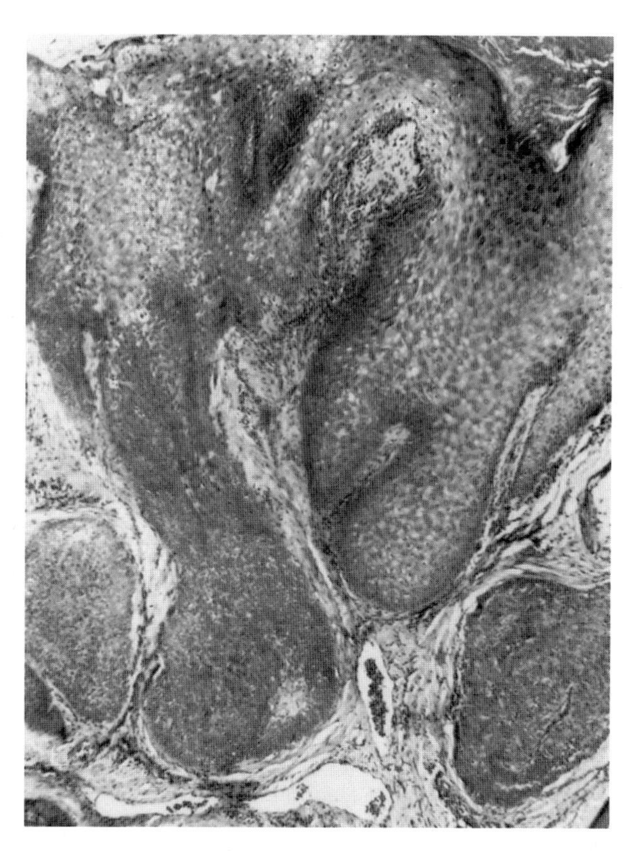

FIG. 31-18. Trichilemmoma
The tumor shows lobular formations extending into the dermis. As a result of their differentiation toward outer root sheath cells, many cells appear clear.

However, old verrucae, which often lack viral stigmata, may acquire cytoplasmic glycogen and mimic many features of trichilemmoma. Trichilemmomas differ from ordinary verrucae by their lobulated rather than papillary (verrucous) configuration, by their localization about follicular infundibula, by the presence of basaloid palisading at the periphery of tumor lobules, and by the presence of a thickened, hyalinized basement membrane. Molecular hybridization to detect the viral genome has not supported the notion that all trichilemmomas are the result of human papillomavirus infection.[107]

Multiple Trichilemmomas in Cowden's Disease

Cowden's disease, or multiple hamartoma syndrome, is an autosomal dominant genodermatosis with distinctive cutaneous findings. Recognition of Cowden's disease is important because of the high incidence of breast cancer in women with this disease. Multiple trichilemmomas precede the development of breast cancer and thus can identify women with a high risk of developing this cancer.[108] Other visceral malignancies also occasionally occur in Cowden's disease, but most of the internal lesions are fibrous hamartomas, especially of the breasts, thyroid, and gastrointestinal tract.[109]

Multiple trichilemmomas are found in all patients with Cowden's disease.[110] They are limited to the face, where they are

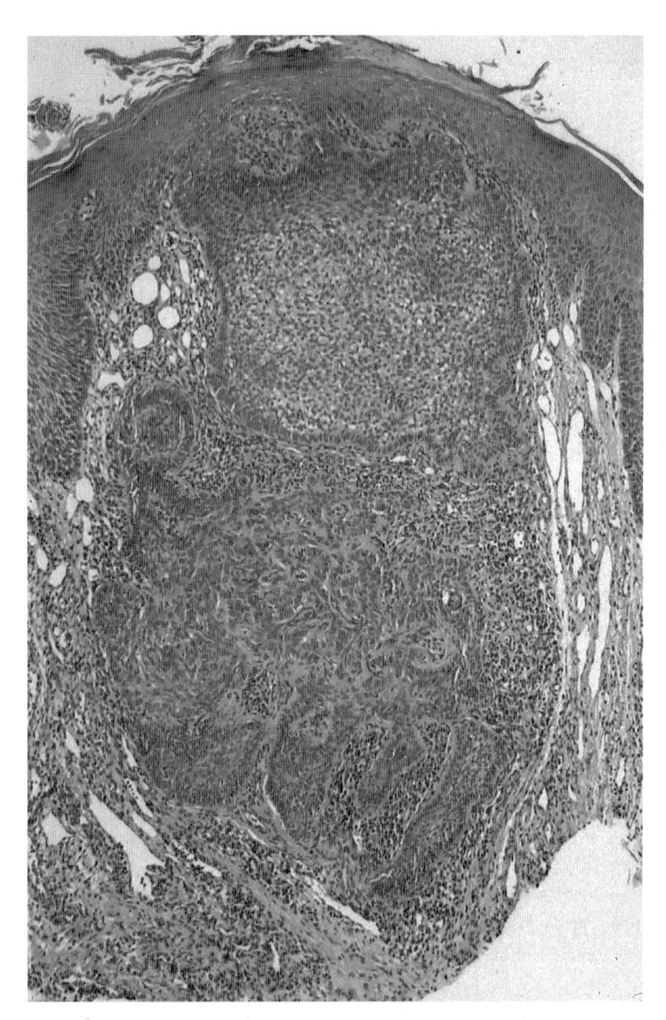

FIG. 31-19. Desmoplastic trichilemmoma
At the base of the lesion, there are irregular extensions of cells of the outer root sheath type that project into sclerotic collagen bundles and mimic invasive carcinoma.

found mainly about the mouth, nose, and ears. They consist of flesh colored, pink or brown papules that may resemble verrucae vulgares.[111] In addition, there may be closely set oral papules, giving the lips, gingiva, and tongue a characteristic "cobblestone" appearance, as well as multiple small acral keratoses. Small hyperkeratotic papillomas are commonly found on the distal portions of the extremities.[112]

Histopathology. Multiple biopsy specimens may be needed to find the diagnostic histologic picture of trichilemmoma in the facial lesions. Thus, in one series, only 29 of 53 facial lesions showed findings diagnostic of trichilemmoma.[110]

The oral lesions may show a fibromatous nodule composed of relatively acellular fibers patterned in whorls[113] or fibrovascular tissue with acanthosis.[110] The extrafacial cutaneous lesions may resemble verruca vulgaris or acrokeratosis verruciformis (see Chaps. 6 and 26). Only few specimens show mild follicular hyperplasia as seen in trichilemmoma.[112]

Differential Diagnosis. See Differential Diagnosis under Solitary Trichilemmoma.

Tumor of the Follicular Infundibulum

Besides the lobular type of trichilemmoma just described, there is a second type of trichilemmoma. This type, which shows platelike growth, was first described in 1961 as tumor of the follicular infundibulum.[114] It usually occurs as a solitary, flat, keratotic papule on the face.[115] Rarely, multiple papules are present.[116]

Histopathology. There is a platelike growth of epithelial cells in the upper dermis extending parallel to the epidermis and showing multiple connections with the lower margin of the epidermis (Fig. 31-21). The peripheral cell layer of the tumor plate shows palisading, and the centrally located cells show a pale-staining cytoplasm as a result of their content of glycogen. Small hair follicles enter the tumor plate from below and lose their identity and then are no longer recognizable.[115] Along the lower margin of the plate, there may be invaginations that resemble hair papillae.[116]

Differential Diagnosis. The platelike growth with multiple connections to the epidermis resembles superficial basal cell carcinoma, which may also show peripheral palisading. How-

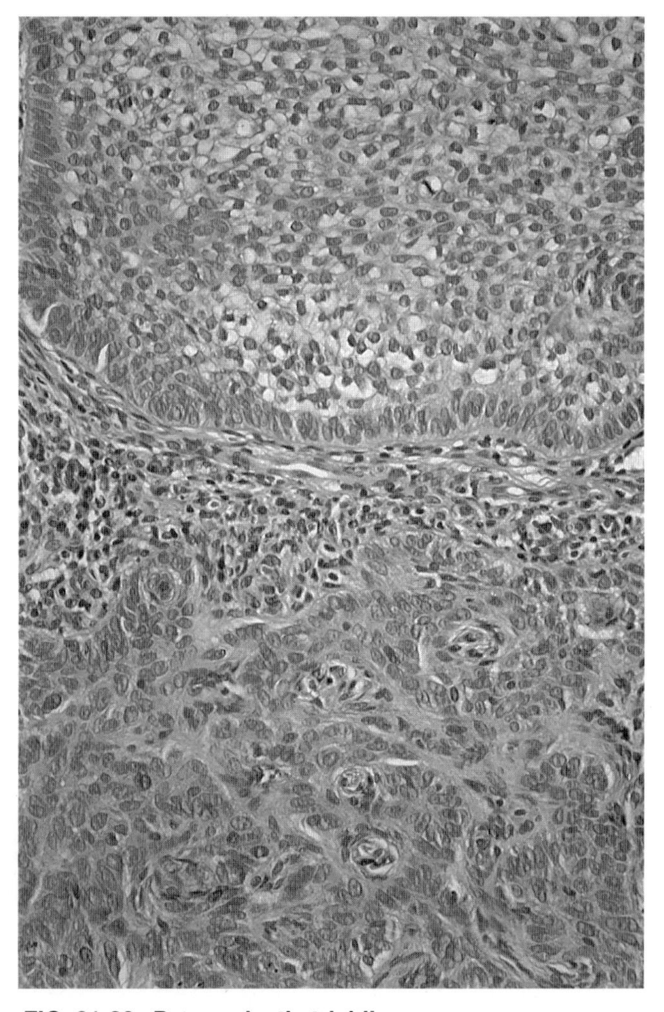

FIG. 31-20. Desmoplastic trichilemmoma
The superficial cells at the base exhibit clear cytoplasm and peripheral palisading, characteristic of trichilemmoma.

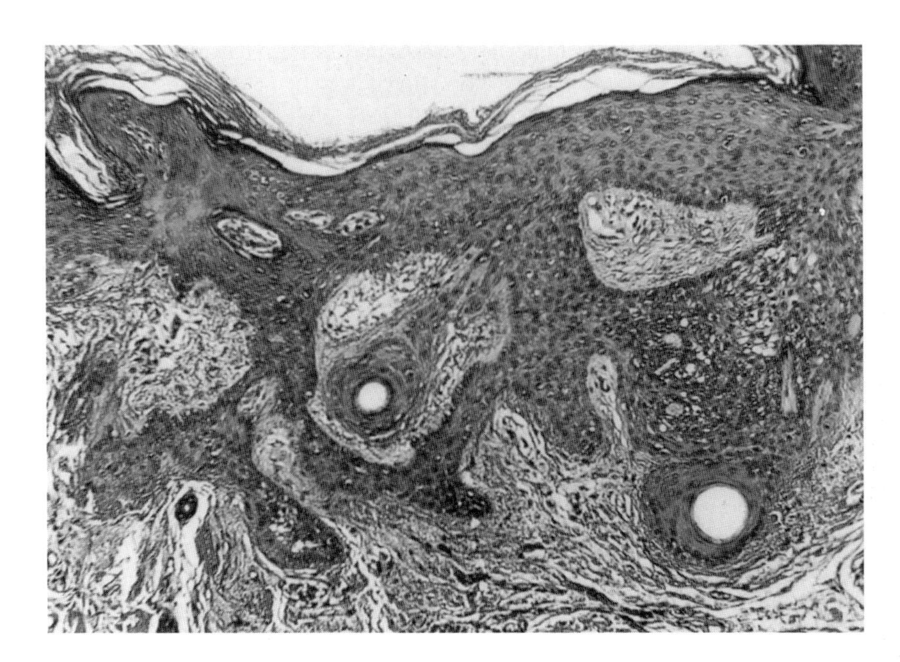

FIG. 31-21. Tumor of the follicular infundibulum
A platelike growth of pale-staining epithelial cells extends parallel to the epidermis in the upper dermis and shows multiple connections with the epidermis. The peripheral cell layer of the tumor plate shows palisading.

ever, the cells of the tumor of the follicular infundibulum possess a greater amount of cytoplasm, in which, furthermore, PAS-positive material is present.[117] Atypia, necrosis, and mitotic activity are generally lacking.

Trichilemmal Horn; Trichilemmomal Horn

Trichilemmal and trichilemmomal horns clinically have the appearance of a cutaneous horn, as seen in several other conditions (see Chap. 30). Both are solitary. The more common trichilemmal horn may be seen in many different areas[118]; the trichilemmomal horn occurs on the face or scalp.[119]

Histopathology. In a *trichilemmal horn,* trichilemmal keratinization occurs. At the base of the lesion there is a prominent basement membrane zone, with palisading of the basal cell layer and a tendency of the viable epithelial cells to become large and pale-staining. As trichilemmal cells, they keratinize without a granular layer.[118,120] Some nuclear atypicality analogous to a carcinoma in situ has been observed.[121]

In a *trichilemmomal horn,* a trichilemmoma is seen at the base of the lesion. At the surface, the trichilemmoma shows a cutaneous horn displaying epidermoid keratinization that is frequently pronounced, with a thick granular layer and massive hyperkeratosis.[119]

Trichilemmal Carcinoma

Trichilemmal carcinoma[122–125] occurs largely on the face or ears as a slow-growing epidermal papule, indurated plaque, or nodule that may ulcerate.[126] Mitoses and atypia may be prominent. However, recurrence and metastases are uncommon, and conservative surgical excision with clear margins is curative.[122,124,127]

Histopathology. This tumor is histologically invasive and consists of cytologically atypical clear cells resembling those of the outer root sheath.[128] The lesional cells have abundant glycogenated clear cytoplasm. They lie in solid, lobular, or trabecular growth patterns with foci of pilar-type keratinization and with peripheral palisading of cells with subnuclear vacuolization. Cytologic atypia is prominent, and there may be pagetoid spread of lesional cells into the epidermis, mimicking melanoma. The cells have hyperchromatic, pleomorphic, very large nuclei.[127] The cytoplasm contains glycogen, and this is PAS-positive and diastase-sensitive.[126] Areas of trichilemmal keratinization are frequently present.[129]

Histogenesis. A trichilemmal carcinoma may resemble a trichilemmoma by showing a lobular architecture[127] or may resemble a "tumor of the follicular infundibulum" by replacing the surface epidermis.[126] Differentiation from other clear cell carcinomas may be difficult.

TUMORS WITH SEBACEOUS DIFFERENTIATION

Nevus Sebaceus

Nevus sebaceus of Jadassohn is as a rule located on the scalp or the face as a single lesion and is present already at birth. In childhood, it consists of a cirumscribed, only slightly raised, hairless plaque that is often linear in configuration but may be round or irregularly shaped. In puberty, the lesion becomes verrucous and nodular.[130]

In rare instances, nevus sebaceus consists of multiple extensive plaques not limited to the head. Usually, at least some of the

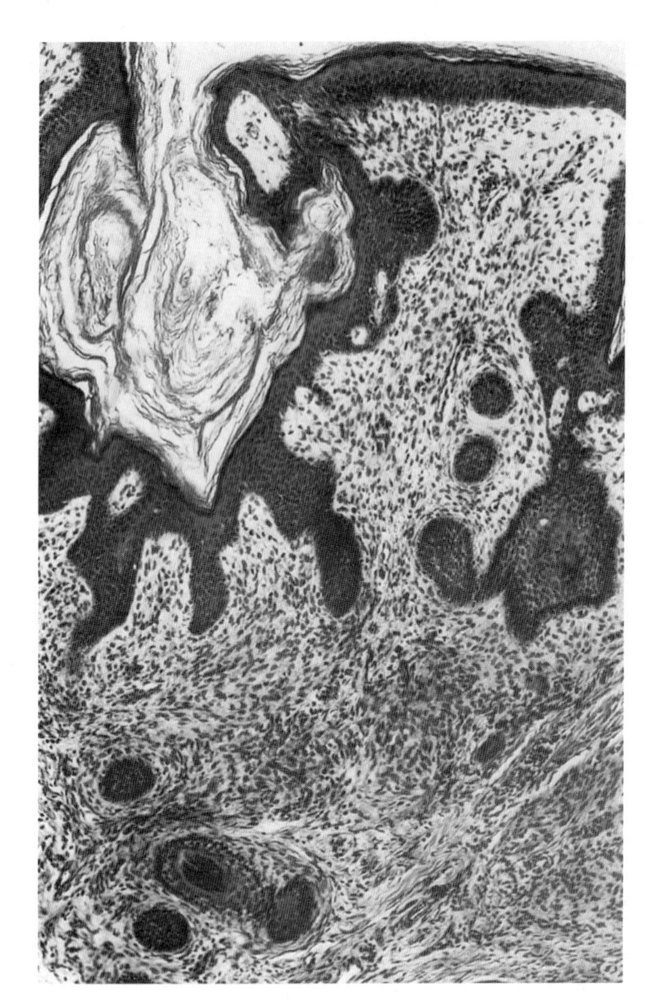

FIG. 31-22. Nevus sebaceus from the scalp of a child There are two dilated, keratin-filled infundibula showing multiple buds of undifferentiated cells representing malformed hair germs. The dermis contains many fibroblasts and one immature hair structure; sebaceous glands are absent in childhood. (Courtesy of Benjamin K. Fisher, MD.)

lesions have a linear configuration.[131] In addition, some patients with extensive nevus sebaceus show as evidence of a "neurocutaneous syndrome" epilepsy and mental retardation,[132,133] neurologic defects,[134] or skeletal deformities.[135] In some patients, the linear nevus is partially a linear nevus sebaceus and partially a linear epidermal nevus.[134,135] Thus the "neurocutaneous syndrome" that is associated with nevus sebaceus overlaps with the abnormalities associated with the epidermal nevus syndrome, in which skeletal deformities and central nervous system abnormalities may also occur (see Chap. 30).[136] The involvement of the central nervous system that may be seen in extensive cases of both linear nevus sebaceus and linear epidermal nevus closely resembles that of tuberous sclerosis by computed tomography and x-ray studies (see Chap. 33).[137]

Histopathology. The sebaceous glands in nevus sebaceus follow the pattern of normal sebaceous glands during infancy, childhood, and adolescence. In the first few months of life, they are well developed.[138] Thereafter, through childhood, the sebaceous glands in nevus sebaceus are underdeveloped and therefore greatly reduced in size and number (Fig. 31-22). Thus the diagnosis of nevus sebaceus may be missed. However, the presence of incompletely differentiated hair structures is typical of nevus sebaceus. There often are cords of undifferentiated cells resembling the embryonic stage of hair follicles.[130] Some hair structures consist of dilated, keratin-filled infundibula showing multiple buds of undifferentiated cells.

At puberty, the lesion assumes its diagnostic histologic appearance. This is brought on by the presence of large numbers of mature or nearly mature sebaceous glands and by papillomatous hyperplasia of the epidermis. The hair structures remain small except for occasional dilated infundibula. There are often buds of undifferentiated cells that resemble foci of basal cell carcinoma and represent malformed hair germs.[139] Ectopic aprocrine glands develop in about two thirds of the patients at puberty and sometimes at a younger age.[130,139] These glands are located deep in the dermis beneath the masses of sebaceous gland lobules (Fig. 31-23).

Quite commonly, in addition to the infantile and adolescent phases, there is a third stage in adulthood during which various types of appendage tumors develop secondarily within lesions of nevus sebaceus. A syringocystadenoma papilliferum has been found in 8% to 19% of the lesions of nevus sebaceus.[130,139] Less commonly found appendage tumors include nodular hidradenoma, syringoma, sebaceous epithelioma,[130] chondroid syringoma, trichilemmoma,[140] and proliferating trichilemmal cyst.[141]

A basal cell carcinoma that is clinically evident has been observed in 5% to 7% of the cases of nevus sebaceus (Fig.

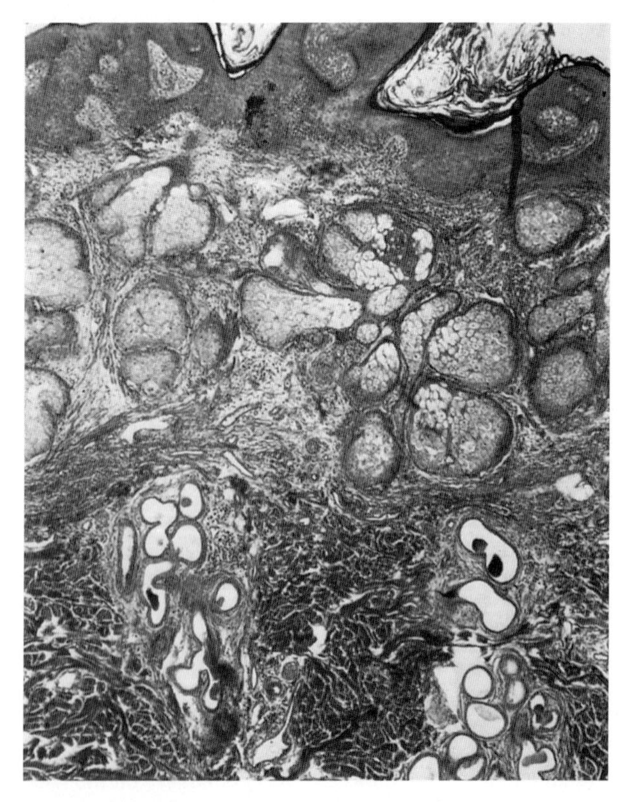

FIG. 31-23. Nevus sebaceus from the scalp of an adult Hyperkeratosis and papillomatosis are present. Numerous mature sebaceous glands lie in the upper dermis. Mature apocrine glands are located in the lower dermis.

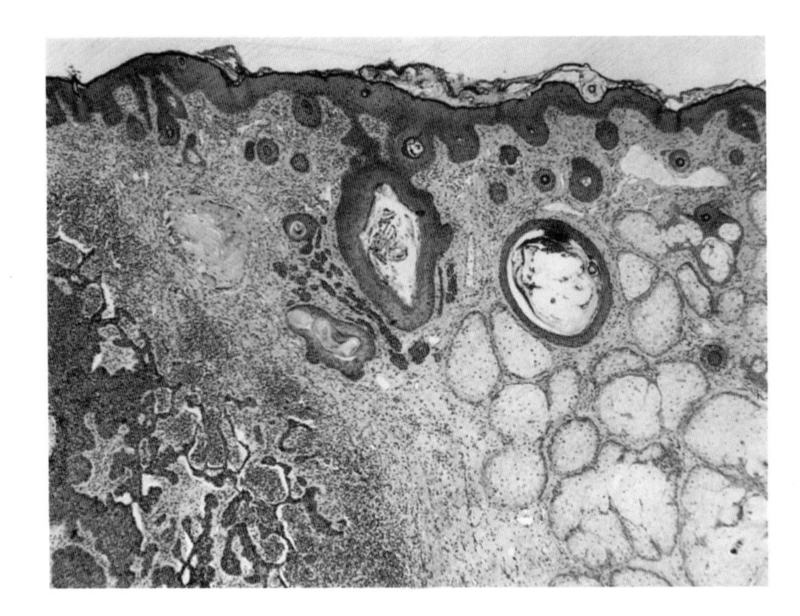

FIG. 31-24. Nevus sebaceus
A basal cell carcinoma has arisen within the lesion. The nevus sebaceus shows numerous tiny hair structures and two large, keratin-filled infundibula.

31-24).[139,142] In many instances, however, basal cell epitheliomas are found that are small and clinically not apparent and that show no aggressive growth pattern.[139] It is not always possible to differentiate histologically between a basal cell carcinoma and "basaloid proliferations" that arise in malformed hair germs and that are seen in as many as half of all cases of nevus sebaceus.[142] As evidence that the basal cell carcinoma–like proliferations in many instances are not true basal cell epitheliomas, these proliferations often contain Sudan-positive granules as an indication of sebaceous differentiation or glycogen as an indication of pilar differentiation.[143] Other proliferations show follicular differentiation with formation of hair papillae and hair bulbs.[144]

In only rare instances does a squamous cell carcinoma develop within a nevus sebaceus. This may be associated either with regional lymph node metastasis or with generalized metastases.[145] Apocrine carcinomas and, in one instance, a malignant eccrine poroma have developed in nevi sebacei, and they, too, may lead to regional or even generalized metastases.[145,146]

Histogenesis. The frequent association of nevus sebaceus with other appendage tumors and with apocrine glands suggests that nevus sebaceus is derived from the primary epithelial germ.[139]

Sebaceous Hyperplasia

The lesions of sebaceous hyperplasia occur on the face, chiefly on the forehead and cheeks, in persons past middle age. Rarely, the hyperplasia occurs in early adult life.[147] Either one or, more commonly, several elevated, small, soft, yellow, slightly umbilicated papules are present. Their usual size is 2 to 3 mm in diameter.

Histopathology. Most lesions consist of a single greatly enlarged sebaceous gland composed of numerous lobules grouped around a centrally located, wide sebaceous duct (Fig. 31-25). Its opening to the surface corresponds to the central umbilication of the lesion. Serial sections show that all sebaceous lobules grouped around the central duct are connected with that duct. Large lesions may consist of several enlarged sebaceous glands and contain several ducts, with sebaceous lobules grouped around each of them. Although some sebaceous gland lobules appear fully mature, others show more than one peripheral row of undifferentiated, generative cells in which there are few or no lipid droplets.[148]

Histogenesis. Labeling with tritiated thymidine has shown that the migration of sebocytes from the basal cell area to the center of the sebaceous lobules and into the sebaceous duct is distinctly slower in cases of sebaceous hyperplasia than in normal sebaceous glands.[148]

In sebaceous hyperplasia, in contrast to rhinophyma, only one sebaceous gland or, at the most, a few sebaceous glands are enlarged. This makes it appear likely that the lesions of sebaceous hyperplasia represent a hamartoma rather than a hypertrophy, as in rhinophyma.

Differential Diagnosis. In rhinophyma, which also shows large sebaceous glands and ducts, there is no grapelike grouping of the sebaceous lobules around the ducts, and the lesion is not sharply demarcated. In nevus sebaceus, ductal structures are less apparent than in sebaceous hyperplasia, and apocrine glands are often found beneath the sebaceous glands.

Fordyce's Condition

In Fordyce's condition, groups of minute, yellow, globoid lesions are observed on the vermilion border of the lips or on the oral mucosa. The incidence of the disorder increases with age, so that 70% to 80% of elderly persons show such lesions, which represents ectopic sebaceous glands.[149]

Histopathology. Each globoid lesion consists of a group of small but mature sebaceous lobules situated around a small

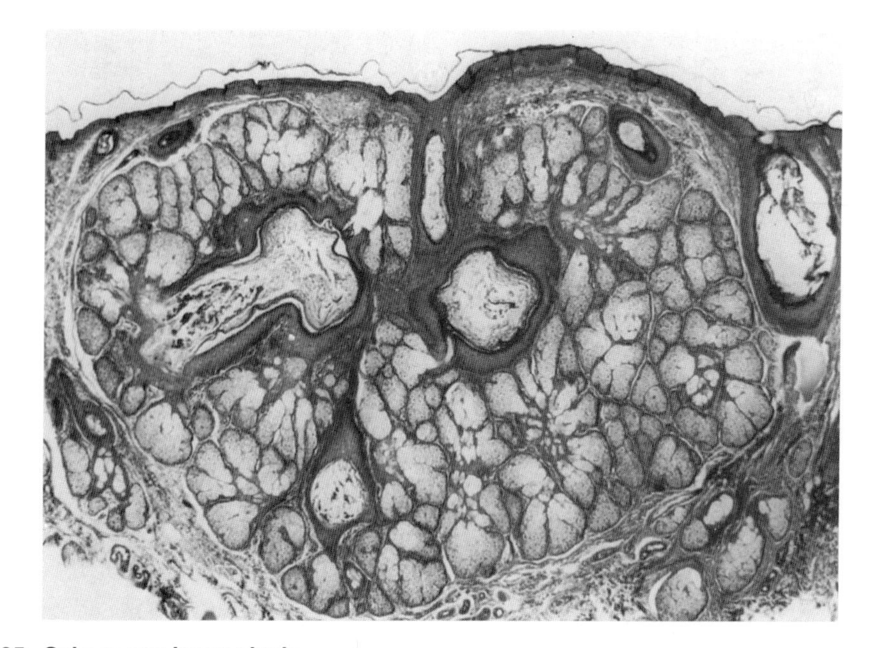

FIG. 31-25. Sebaceous hyperplasia
The lesion consists of a single greatly enlarged sebaceous gland with a wide, branching sebaceous duct in the center.

sebaceous duct leading to the surface epithelium.[149,150] Because of the small size of the sebaceous duct, serial sections may be required to demonstrate the duct.

Sebaceous Adenoma

Sebaceous adenoma represents a yellow, circumscribed nodule located on either the face or scalp. Up to 1968, sebaceous adenoma was regarded as a rare solitary tumor, and there were few publications about it.[151–153] Since then, however, its occurrence in many instances of the Muir-Torre snydrome has been described.

Histopathology. On histologic examination, sebaceous adenoma is sharply demarcated from the surrounding tissue. It is composed of incompletely differentiated sebaceous lobules that are irregular in size and shape (Fig. 31-26). Two types of cells are present in the lobules. The cells of the first type are identical to the cells present at the periphery of normal sebaceous glands and represent undifferentiated basaloid cells. The cells of the second type are mature sebaceous cells. In addition, there often are some cells in a transitional stage between these two types.[154] Distribution of the basaloid and sebaceous cells within the lobules varies. Some lobules contain predominantly basaloid cells. Other lobules contain mainly sebaceous cells and thereby resemble mature sebaceous lobules. In most lobules, however, the two types of cells occur in approximately equal proportions, often arranged in such a way that groups of sebaceous cells are surrounded by basaloid cells. Fat stains reveal the presence of lipid material in the sebaceous and transitional cells. Some large lobules contain cystic spaces in their center formed by the disintegration of mature sebaceous cells. Also, there may be foci of squamous epithelium with keratinization. These foci probably represent areas with differentiation toward cells of the infundibulum.

Differential Diagnosis. In degrees of differentiation, sebaceous adenoma stands between sebaceous hyperplasia, in which sebaceous lobules appear fully or nearly fully matured, and sebaceous epithelioma or sebaceoma (see text following), in which the tumor is composed predominantly or irregularly shaped cell masses and the percentage of tumor cells with sebaceous differentiation is far less than 50%. Sebaceous adenoma and sebaceous epithelioma lack nuclear atypia and invasive, asymmetric growth patterns, which are hallmarks of sebaceous carcinoma. Considerable mitotic activity in the basaloid regions may be present in either, however.

Sebaceoma (Sebaceous Epithelioma)

Clinically, sebaceoma, or sebaceous epithelioma, varies from a circumscribed nodule to that of an ill-defined plaque. Some of the lesions are yellow.[155] Most of the lesions are located on the face or scalp. In addition to occurring as a primary lesion, a sebaceous epithelioma occasionally arises within a nevus sebaceus.[130,139] Sebaceous epitheliomas may also be found among the multiple sebaceous neoplasms that occur in association with multiple visceral carcinomas and are referred to as Muir-Torre syndrome (see text following).

Histopathology. The histologic spectrum extends from that seen in sebaceous adenoma to lesions that may be difficult to distinguish from sebaceous carcinoma. Generally, a sebaceoma shows irregularly shaped cell masses in which more than half of the cells are undifferentiated basaloid cells but in which there are significant aggregates of sebaceous cells and of transitional cells.[156] Disintegration of sebaceous cells is seen

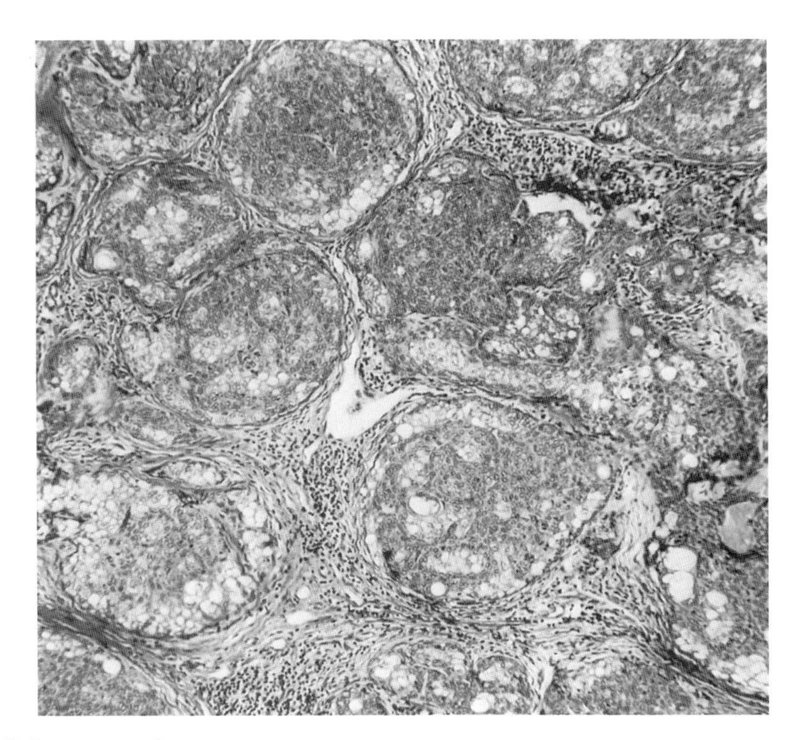

FIG. 31-26. Sebaceous adenoma
The tumor is composed of lobules of irregular size and shape. In the lobules, two types of cells can be recognized: generative and sebaceous.

in some areas.[155] Lesions verging on a sebaceous carcinoma show some degree of irregularity in the arrangement of the cell masses, and, although the majority of cells are basaloid cells, many cells show differentiation toward sebaceous cells (Fig. 31-27).[157]

Differential Diagnosis. Criteria listed by Steffen and Ackerman that may be of assistance in differentiating sebaceous adenoma from sebaceoma include the often greater size and depth of the latter, and the lack of structures resembling normal sebaceous lobules. Nuclear atypia is "rare," and mitoses may be numerous in sebaceomas, in contrast to adenomas, in which they are few or absent.[158] For a discussion of the more important differentiation of sebaceoma from sebaceous carcinoma, which may cause metastases, see p. 768.

Muir-Torre Syndrome

Since 1967, when the first publication by Muir appeared concerning the coexistence of frequently multiple sebaceous tumors and usually multiple visceral carcinomas,[159] scores of cases have been reported.[160] Keratoacanthomas also have occurred in these patients, in some cases without sebaceous lesions, in association with visceral malignancies.[161,162] A genetic predisposition exists in some cases of the Muir-Torre syndrome,[160] and the Muir-Torre syndrome has been found in association with the "cancer family syndrome."[163]

Among the internal malignancies, carcinoma of the colon is

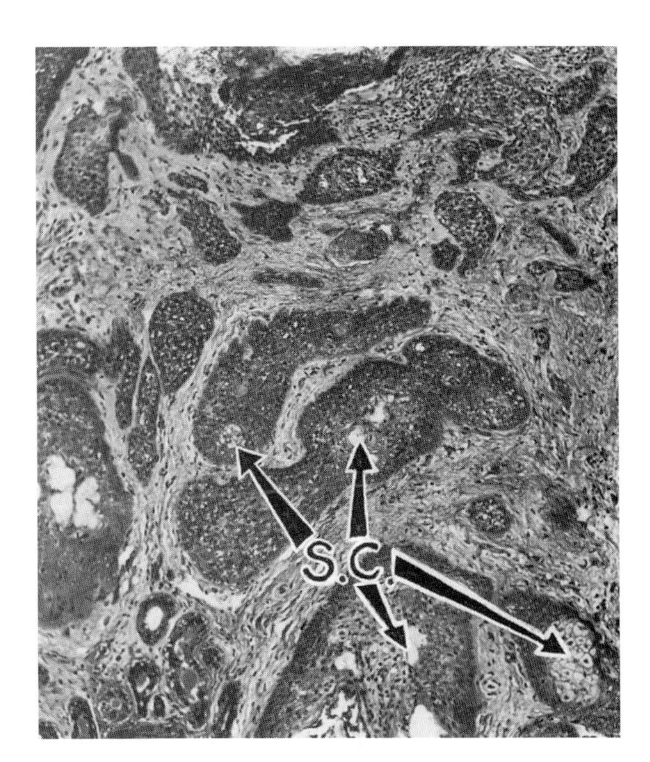

FIG. 31-27. Sebaceoma
The tumor is composed of irregularly shaped cell masses. The majority of cells are the same type as in basal cell carcinoma, but many cells show differentiation toward sebaceous cells (*S.C.*).

the most common malignancy, although a wide tumor spectrum exists, including hematologic malignancies.[160] Also common are adenomatous colonic polyps. Many of the malignant tumors are of relatively low malignancy, with only a slight tendency to metastasize.[164]

Cutaneous lesions vary from just 1 to more than 100 lesions.[165] Although the lesion in many instances is recognizable as a sebaceous tumor by its color or as a keratoacanthoma by its crater, histologic examination may be required to establish a diagnosis.

Histopathology. Sebaceous adenomas are the most distinctive cutaneous markers of the Muir-Torre syndrome. They may be solid, cystic, or keratoacanthoma-like.[154] Although ordinary keratoacanthomas occur in the Muir-Torre syndrome, often they have an accompanying sebaceous proliferation.[166] In addition to sebaceous adenomas, sebaceomas, and basal cell carcinomas with sebaceous differentiation, there are tumors with unusual appearance, so that a hard-to-classify sebaceous proliferation should be considered as a possible manifestation of the Muir-Torre syndrome.[166] Also, sebaceous carcinomas occur, but no metastases have been reported.[165,167]

Sebaceous Carcinoma

Carcinomas of the sebaceous glands occur most frequently on the eyelids, where they originate usually from the meibomian glands and less commonly from the glands of Zeis. However, they may occur elsewhere on the skin. On the eyelids, sebaceous carcinoma may be easily mistaken for chronic blepharoconjunctivitis or a chalazion.[168] On the skin, sebaceous carcinoma usually manifests itself as a nodule that may or may not be ulcerated.[169,170] Sebaceous carcinomas of the eyelids quite frequently cause regional metastases. Also, there may be orbital invasion, and in 22% of the cases reported in one study, death resulted from visceral metastases.[171] Sebaceous carcinomas arising on the skin away from the eyelids also may cause regional metastases.[172–174] However, visceral metastasis resulting in death is very rare, although it has been described.[170,175] The sebaceous carcinomas that may be found among the multiple sebaceous neoplasms occurring in association with multiple visceral carcinomas in the Muir-Torre syndrome do not metastasize, although the visceral malignant tumors may.[176] In some instances, a sebaceous carcinoma represents the only cutaneous manifestation of the syndrome.[177]

Histopathology. The irregular lobular formations show great variations in the size of the lobules (Fig. 31-28). Although many cells are undifferentiated, distinct sebaceous cells showing a foamy cytoplasm are present in the center of most lobules.[170] Many undifferentiated cells and sebaceous cells appear atypical, showing considerable variation in the shape and size of their nuclei.[172] Also, many of the undifferentiated cells have an eosinophilic cytoplasm, and when fat stains are used on frozen sections, the cells are found to contain fine lipid globules.[168] Some of the large lobules show areas composed of atypical keratinizing cells, as seen in squamous cell carcinoma.[169]

Sebaceous carcinomas of the eyelids in nearly half of the cases examined show a pagetoid spread of malignant cells in the conjunctival epithelium or the epidermis of the skin of the lid or both.[171] These changes are seen very rarely in extraocular sebaceous carcinoma.[175] The pagetoid cells contain no mucopolysaccharides but stain positively for fat with oil red O.[171] Recognition of the pagetoid growth pattern in biopsy material can be essential to recognition of the existence of an underlying sebaceous carcinoma.[178]

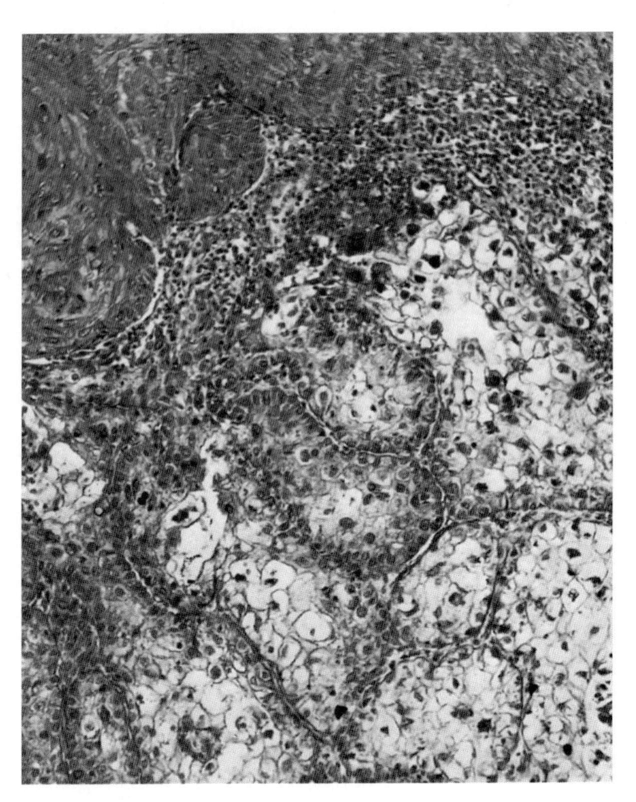

FIG. 31-28. Sebaceous carcinoma
Irregular lobular formations are composed of sebaceous and undifferentiated cells showing considerable variation in the shape and size of their nuclei. The undifferentiated cells differ from the undifferentiated cells of sebaceous epithelioma by showing greater atypicality of their nuclei and an eosinophilic rather than a basophilic cytoplasm.

Differential Diagnosis. Sebaceous carcinomas must be differentiated from basal cell carcinomas with sebaceous differentiation (see Chap. 30). Sebaceous carcinomas show no areas resembling basal cell carcinomas. Instead, the undifferentiated cells of sebaceous carcinoma show a more eosinophilic cytoplasm, greater cytologic atypia, and greater invasiveness (see Fig. 31-28).[179] The tumor cells are often large and squamoid in appearance, or show basaloid differentiation with only inconspicuous lipidization. In the latter case, the tumor must be distinguished from basal cell carcinomas with sebaceous differentiation,[180] and in the former case the differential diagnosis includes squamous cell carcinomas with hydropic changes.[181] When sebaceous carcinoma is suspected or found at frozen section, additional sections should be saved for fat stains. As in other malignant adnexal neoplasms, zones of necrosis, marked nuclear atypia, and abnormal mitotic figures are common. Pagetoid proliferation of tumor cells in the epidermis or conjunctiva may extend widely and confers a poorer prognosis. Other adverse prognostic attributes include multicentric involvement, poor differentiation (i.e., sparse lipid), necrosis, paucity of reactive lymphocytes,[182] extensive local invasion, and vascular or bony invasion. Metastases first involve regional lymph nodes of the periauricular, submaxillary, and cervical chains. Visceral spread may occur and lead to death. Steffen and Ackerman have listed the following criteria that may be of assistance in differentiating sebaceous carcinoma and sebaceoma: The carcinomas are larger, asymmetric, and poorly circumscribed, whereas sebaceomas may extend into the subcutis but are circumscribed and symmetrical. Carcinomas may ulcerate the epidermis, and there may be extensive necrosis ("necrosis en masse"). The relative percentage of differentiated (vacuolated) to undifferentiated (nonvacuolated) sebocytes varies but tends to be higher in sebaceomas. Nuclear atypia is often striking, and mitotic figures are numerous and sometimes atypical in carcinomas. Sebaceomas in contrast lack striking nuclear atypia, but may have few or many mitoses. According to these authors, basal cell carcinomas with sebaceous differentiation are exceedingly rare, and most putative examples are really benign sebaceomas.[158]

TUMORS WITH APOCRINE DIFFERENTIATION

Apocrine Nevus

Large numbers of mature apocrine secretory lumina are frequently present in scalp lesions of nevus sebaceus and syringocystadenoma papilliferum. Pure apocrine nevi, however, are very rare. The few reported cases presented as papules, a small nodule on the scalp, or as a soft mass found in each axilla.[183,184]

Histopathology. Numerous mature apocrine glands are seen, situated largely in the reticular layer of the dermis but extending into the subcutis.[184]

Apocrine Hidrocystoma

Apocrine hidrocystoma occurs usually as a solitary translucent nodule of cystic consistency. The diameter varies between 3 and 15 mm.[185] Quite frequently, instead of being skin-colored, the lesion has a blue hue and then resembles a blue nevus. The usual location of apocrine hidrocystoma is on the face, but it is occasionally seen on the ears, scalp, chest, or shoulders.[186,187] Multiple apocrine hidrocystomas are only rarely encountered.[186,188] Lesions described as occurring on the penis have been reclassified as median raphe cysts (see Chap. 30).[189]

Histopathology. The dermis contains one or several large cystic spaces into which papillary projections often extend. The inner surface of the wall and the papillary projections are lined by a row of secretory cells of variable height showing "decapitation" secretion indicative of apocrine secretion (Fig. 31-29). Peripheral to the layer of secretory cells are elongated myoepithelial cells, their long axes running parallel to the cyst wall.[186] In some cases, one finds superficially located lumina lined by a double layer of ductal epithelium in addition to the cysts lined by secretory cells.[185]

Histogenesis. The apocrine nature of the secretion of the luminal cells has been proved by the presence of numerous large PAS-positive, diastase-resistant granules in the secretory cells,[185] and by electron microscopy.

Electron microscopic examination shows abundant secretory

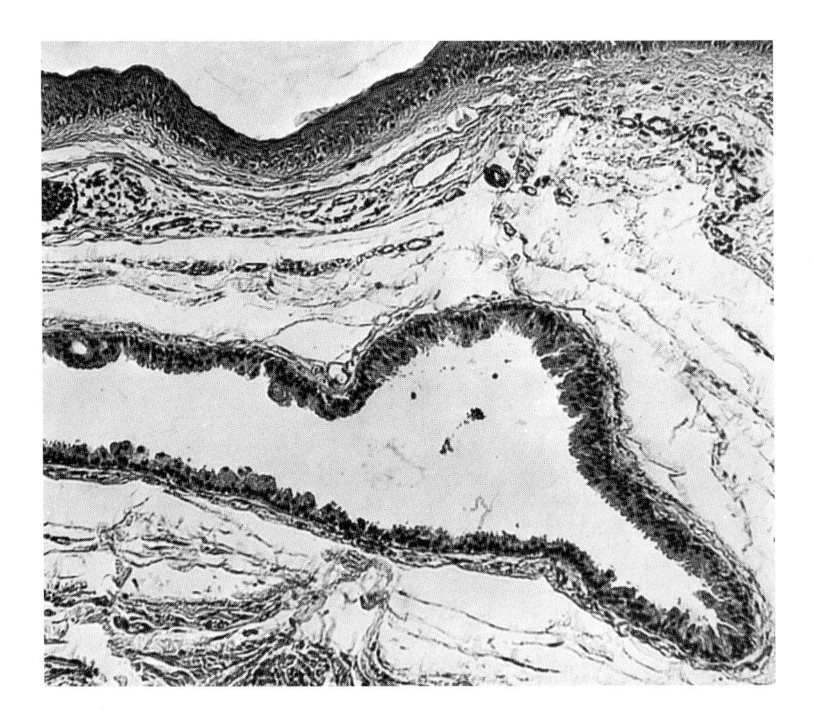

FIG. 31-29. Apocrine hidrocystoma
The dermis contains a cyst lined by a row of secretory cells showing secretion of the apocrine type, so-called *decapitation secretion.* Peripheral to the row of secretory cells are elongated myoepithelial cells.

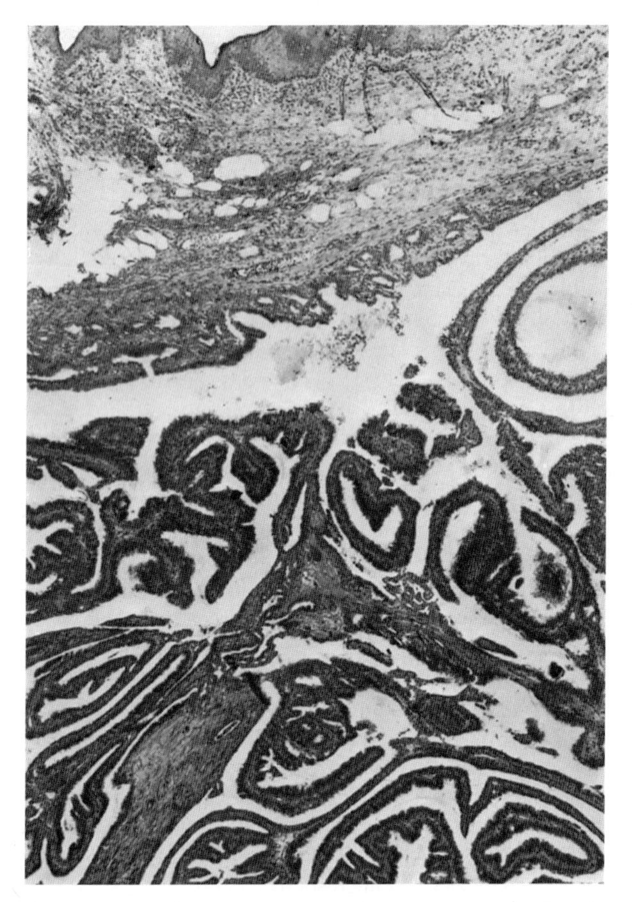

FIG. 31-30. Hidradenoma papilliferum, low magnification The tumor consists of a large cystic space. Numerous papillary folds project into the cystic lumen.

granules of moderate density and uniform internal structure in the secretory cells of apocrine hidrocystoma, particularly in their luminal portion, and evidence of apocrine secretion.[190–192]

The blue color in some of the cysts is not fully explained. According to most authors, it is a Tyndall effect caused by the scattering of light in a colloidal system and the resultant reflection of blue light.[186,188] The blue color has been attributed in a few cases to extravasated erythrocytes in the surrounding stroma.[193]

The apocrine hidrocystoma can be regarded as an adenoma rather than as a retention cyst because the secretory cells do not appear flattened, as they would be in a retention cyst, and because papillary projections extend into the lumen of the cystic spaces.[185]

Differential Diagnosis. Eccrine hidrocystomas, which are lined by ductal cells, differ from apocrine hidrocystomas by the absence of decapitation secretion, of PAS-positive granules, and of myoepithelial cells. However, those portions of an apocrine hidrocystoma in which the cystic spaces are lined by ductal epithelium have the same appearance as the cystic spaces in eccrine hidrocystomas, except that the latter usually are unilocular, and apocrine hidrocystomas are often multilocular. Median raphe cysts of the penis, which have been mistakenly reported as apocrine hidrocystomas, show a pseudostratified columnar cyst wall without evidence of decapitation secretion and without a row of myoepithelial cells.[189]

Hidradenoma Papilliferum

Hidradenoma papilliferum occurs only in women, usually on the labia majora or in the perineal or perianal region. One occurrence on an upper eyelid has been reported.[194] The tumor is covered by normal skin and measures only a few millimeters in diameter. Malignant changes have been reported in one pa-

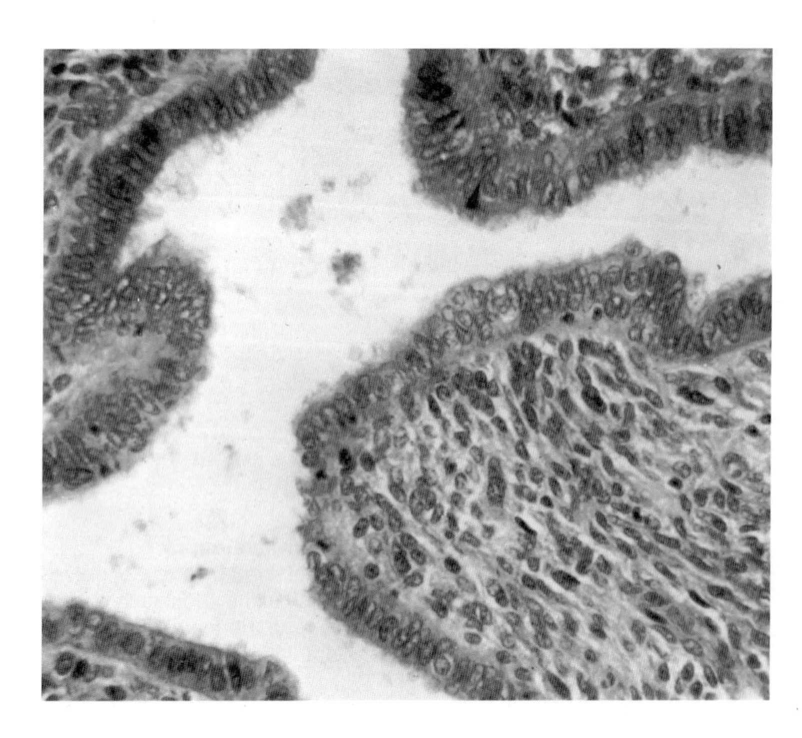

FIG. 31-31. Hidradenoma papilliferum High magnification of Fig. 31-30. The papillary folds are lined by one layer of high cylindric cells, which show evidence of active "decapitation" secretion like that seen in apocrine glands.

tient, in whom a metastasizing, fatal squamous cell carcinoma developed within a perianally located hidradenoma papilliferum.[195]

Histopathology. The tumor represents an adenoma with apocrine differentiation.[196] It is located in the dermis, is well circumscribed, is surrounded by a fibrous capsule, and shows no connection with the overlying epidermis. Some tumors have a peripheral epithelial wall showing areas of keratinization.[197] Within the tumor, one observes tubular and cystic structures (Fig. 31-30). Papillary folds project into the cystic spaces. The lumina are lined occasionally with only a single row of columnar cells, which show an oval, pale-staining nucleus located near the base, a faintly eosinophilic cytoplasm, and active decapitation secretion as seen in the secretory cells of apocrine glands (Fig. 31-31).[196] Usually, however, the lumina are surrounded by a double layer of cells consisting of a luminal layer of secretory cells and of an outer layer of small cuboidal cells with deeply basophilic nuclei. These are myoepithelial cells.[197]

Histogenesis. The apocrine nature of the secretion in hidradenoma papilliferum has been established by histochemical, enzyme histochemical, and electron microscopic examinations.

Histochemically, the luminal cells contain many large, PAS-positive, diastase-resistant granules as encountered in the secretory cells of apocrine glands. In addition, the luminal cells are positive for nonspecific esterase and acid phosphatase, the so-called apocrine enzymes, and negative for phosphorylase, a typical eccrine enzyme. Furthermore, the outer row of cells stains positive for alkaline phosphatase, as myoepithelial cells normally do.[196]

Electron microscopic examination shows in the luminal cells two features that are regarded as characteristic of the secretory cells of apocrine glands. First, numerous membrane-limited, secretory granules that are of varying size and density and that contain lipid droplets are present in the apical portion of these cells. Second, as evidence of decapitation secretion, portions of apical cytoplasm containing large secretory granules are released into the lumen.[197] The peripheral layer of cells contains numerous myofilaments.

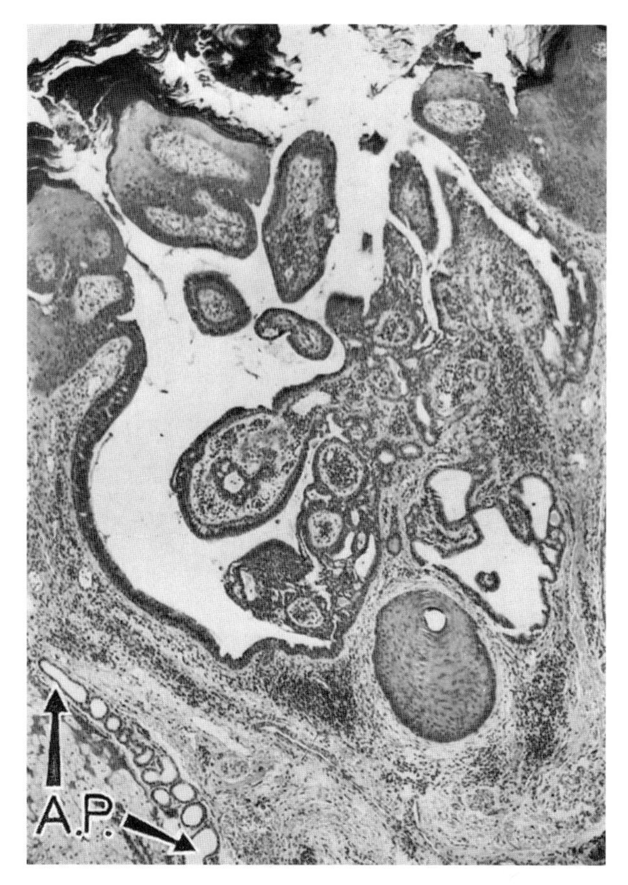

FIG. 31-32. Syringocystadenoma papilliferum, low magnification
A cystic invagination extends downward from the epidermis. Numerous papillary projections extend into the lumen of the cystic invagination. A group of apocrine glands (*A.P.*) is present in the left lower corner.

Syringocystadenoma Papilliferum

Syringocystadenoma papilliferum occurs most commonly on the scalp or the face. However, in about one fourth of the cases, it is seen elsewhere.[198] It is usually first noted at birth or in early childhood and consists of either one papule or several papules in a linear arrangement,[199] or of a solitary plaque. The lesion increases in size at puberty, becoming papillomatous and often crusted.[200] On the scalp, syringocystadenoma papilliferum frequently arises around puberty within a nevus sebaceus that has been present since birth.

Histopathology. The epidermis shows varying degrees of papillomatosis. One or several cystic invaginations extend downward from the epidermis (Fig. 31-32). The upper portion of the invaginations and, in some instances, large segments of the cystic invaginations are lined by squamous, keratinizing cells similar to those of the surface epidermis.[201] In the lower portion of the cystic invaginations, numerous papillary projections extend into the lumina of the invaginations. The papillary projections and the lower portion of the invaginations are lined by glandular epithelium often consisting of two rows of cells (Fig. 31-33). The luminal row of cells consists of high columnar cells with oval nuclei and faintly eosinophilic cytoplasm. Occasionally, some of these cells show active decapitation secretion, and cellular debris is found in the lumina.[8,202] The outer row of cells consists of small cuboidal cells with round nuclei and scanty cytoplasm. In some areas, the cells of the luminal layer are arranged in multiple layers and form a lacelike pattern resulting in multiple small, tubular lumina (Fig. 31-34).[198]

Beneath the cystic invaginations, deep in the dermis, one can find in many cases groups of tubular glands with large lumina (see Fig. 31-34). The cells lining the large lumina often show evidence of active decapitation secretion, indicating that they are apocrine glands (Fig. 31-35).[8,200] Connections of the apocrine glands deep in the dermis with the cystic invaginations in the upper dermis can be traced when step sections are carried out.[8]

A highly diagnostic feature is the almost invariable presence of a fairly dense cellular infiltrate composed nearly entirely of plasma cells in the stroma of this tumor, especially in the papillary projections. These are predominantly of the IgG and IgA classes.[203,204]

Frequently, there are malformed sebaceous glands and hair

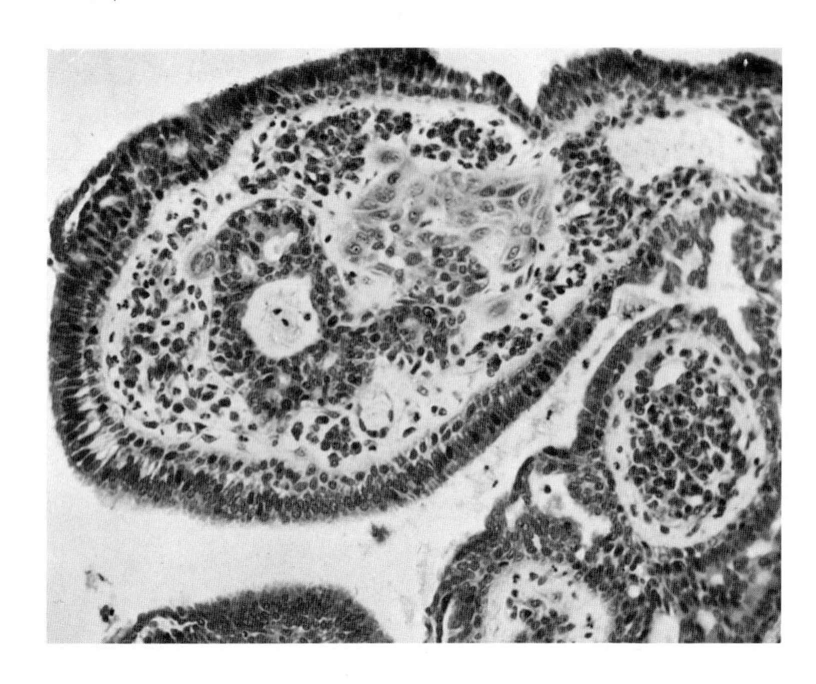

FIG. 31-33. Syringocystadenoma papilliferum
High magnification of Fig. 31-32. The papillary projections are lined by two rows of cells. The luminal row of cells consists of columnar cells with evidence of active "decapitation" secretion like that seen in apocrine glands. The outer row of cells consists of small cuboidal cells.

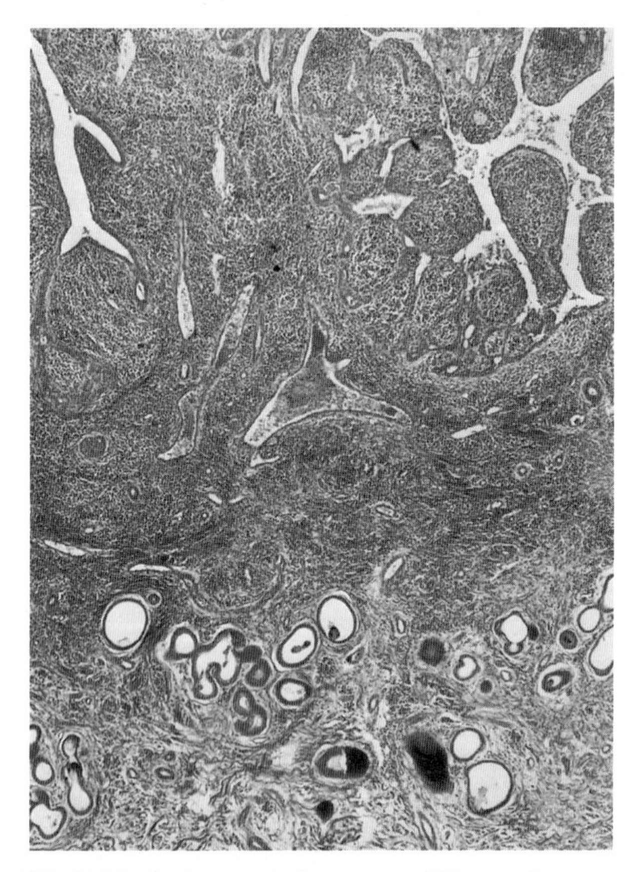

FIG. 31-34. Syringocystadenoma papilliferum, low magnification
In the upper dermis, numerous papillary projections extend into cystic spaces. A marked inflammatory infiltrate containing many plasma cells is present around the cystic invaginations. The lower dermis contains numerous apocrine glands.

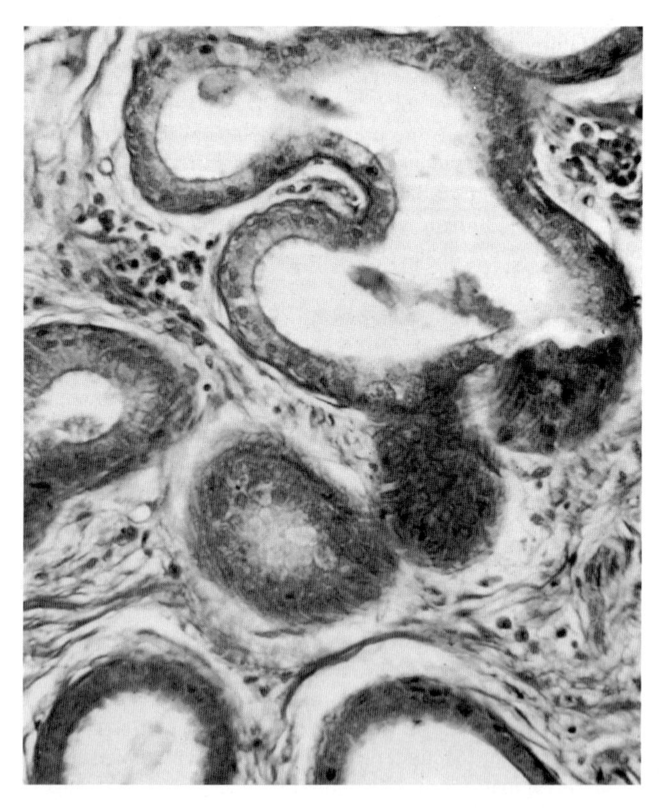

FIG. 31-35. Syringocystadenoma papilliferum
High magnification of Fig. 31-34. The secretory cells of the apocrine cells show evidence of active "decapitation" secretion.

structures in the lesions of syringocystadenoma papilliferum.[200] In about one third of the cases, syringocystadenoma papilliferum is associated with a nevus sebaceus. In about 10% of the cases, a basal cell carcinoma develops, but this is noted only in lesions that also exhibit a nevus sebaceus.[198] A few instances of transition of a syringocystadenoma papilliferum into an adenocarcinoma with regional lymph node metastases have been reported.[205,206]

Histogenesis. There is no unanimity about the direction of differentiation in syringocystadenoma papilliferum. Features of both apocrine and of eccrine differentiation can be seen in particular examples. For example, positive immunoreactivity for gross cystic disease fluid protein (GCDFP-15) in eight cases thus tested supports an apocrine genesis.[207] On the other hand, light and electron microscopic features of some lesions show evidence of eccrine differentiation.[208] It is likely that, rather than arising from mature structures, syringocystadenoma papilliferum arises from pluripotential cells with the potential to develop into primary epithelial germ structures of a variety of different types. In conclusion, the view expressed by Pinkus probably is correct: Although most lesions of syringocystadenoma papilliferum are apocrine in differentiation, some are eccrine.[200] The differentiation in either case may be predominantly ductal or secretory.

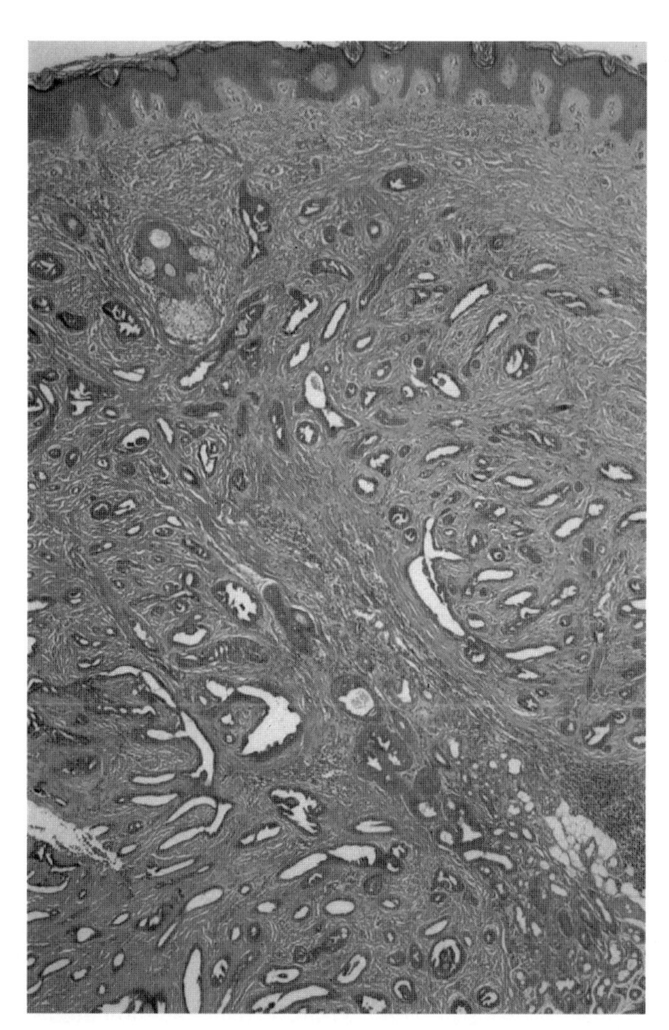

FIG. 31-36. Tubular apocrine adenoma
There are numerous irregularly shaped tubular structures in the dermis that are usually lined by two layers of epithelial cells, an indicator of benignancy. The peripheral layer consists of cuboidal or flattened cells, and the luminal layer is composed of columnar cells.

Tubular Apocrine Adenoma

First described in 1972,[209] several additional cases of tubular apocrine adenoma have been reported since.[210–215] This tumor consists of a well-defined nodule that is commonly located on the scalp. Most tumors have a smooth surface and are under 2 cm in diameter, although one reported lesion located on the scalp measured 7 by 4 cm.[209]

Histopathology. The characteristic feature of this tumor is the presence of numerous irregularly shaped tubular structures that are usually lined by two layers of epithelial cells (Fig. 31-36). The peripheral layer consists of cuboidal or flattened cells, and the luminal layer is composed of columnar cells.[209] Some of the tubules have a dilated lumen with papillary projections extending into it (Fig. 31-37). Decapitation secretion of the luminal cells is seen in many areas. In addition, cellular fragments are seen in some lumina. In two reported cases, the superficial portion of the tumor had the appearance of a syringocystadenoma papilliferum.[210,212]

Histogenesis. Electron microscopy has revealed secretory granules and evidence of apocrine-type decapitation secretion in the luminal cells.[209,211] In contrast to hidradenoma papilliferum, the peripheral cell layer contains no myofilaments. Enzyme histochemistry is also consistent with apocrine differentiation.[209]

Differential Diagnosis. In tubular apocrine adenomas with marked papillary proliferations, there may be some nuclear pleomorphism, which suggests sweat gland carcinoma or a metastatic adenocarcinoma. However, the presence of a peripheral layer of cuboidal or flattened cells is a feature favoring benignity.[213]

Tubular apocrine adenomas resemble papillary eccrine adenoma, and at one time these two tumors were regarded as identical.[212] Because of their differences in decapitation secretion, in enzyme histochemistry, and in electron microscopy, the suggestion was made that they be referred to as *tubulopapillary hidradenoma,* with apocrine or eccrine differentiation as the case may be.[216] For a description of papillary eccrine adenomas, see p. 785. The term *tubulopapillary hidradenoma* may be considered to conceptualize a spectrum of lesions that includes tubular apocrine adenoma and papillary eccrine adenoma,[217] and these are also closely related to syringocystadenoma papilliferum.[218]

Apocrine Adenoma; Apocrine Fibroadenoma

Rare variants of apocrine adenomas can occur in apocrine areas, such as in the axilla[219] and in the perianal region.[220]

Histopathology. Apocrine lumina are readily recognized by the presence of decapitation secretion. In addition, there may be cystically dilated spaces.

Erosive Adenomatosis of the Nipple

Erosive adenomatosis of the nipple represents an adenoma of the major nipple ducts. In the early stage, the nipple appears

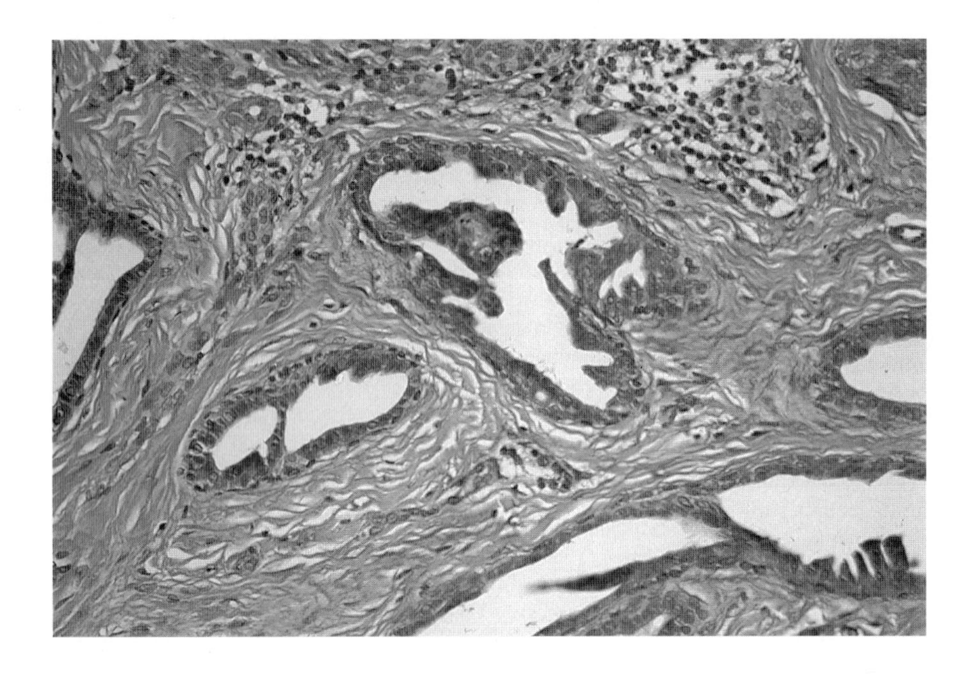

FIG. 31-37. Tubular apocrine adenoma
Some of the tubules have a dilated lumen with papillary projections. They are usually lined by two layers of epithelial cells, an indicator of benignancy.

eroded and inflamed and often shows a serous discharge. During this early erosive phase, clinical differentiation from Paget's disease of the breast may be impossible.[221,222] At a later stage, when the nipple shows nodular thickening, differentiation from Paget's disease is easy.[221]

Histopathology. Extending downward from the epidermis are irregular, dilated tubular structures greatly resembling those seen in tubular apocrine adenoma (Fig. 31-38). The tubules are lined by a peripheral layer of cuboidal cells and a luminal layer of columnar cells that in some areas show secretory projections at their luminal border (Fig. 31-39).[222] Within some of the tubules are papillary proliferations of the luminal cells into the lumen. This proliferation of cells may be so pronounced as to nearly fill the entire lumen. In other areas, detached, partially necrotic cells may be seen in the tubular lumina. In some lesions, considerable acanthosis of the epidermis is seen, with extension of squamous epithelium into some of the superficial ductal structures.

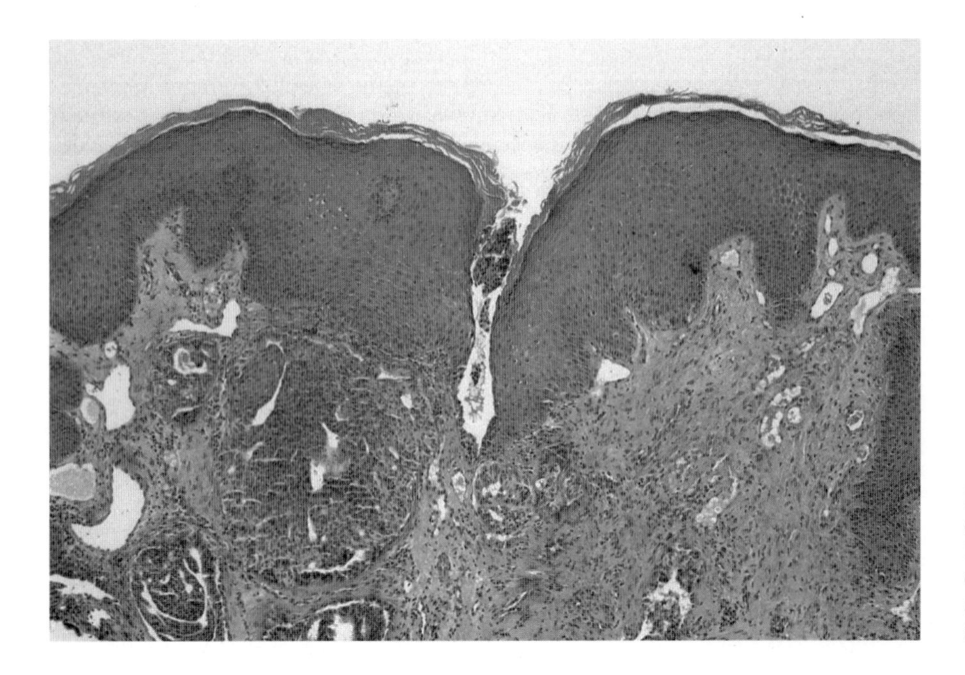

FIG. 31-38. Erosive adenomatosis of the nipple
Extending downward from the epidermis are irregular, dilated tubular structures greatly resembling those seen in tubular apocrine adenoma.

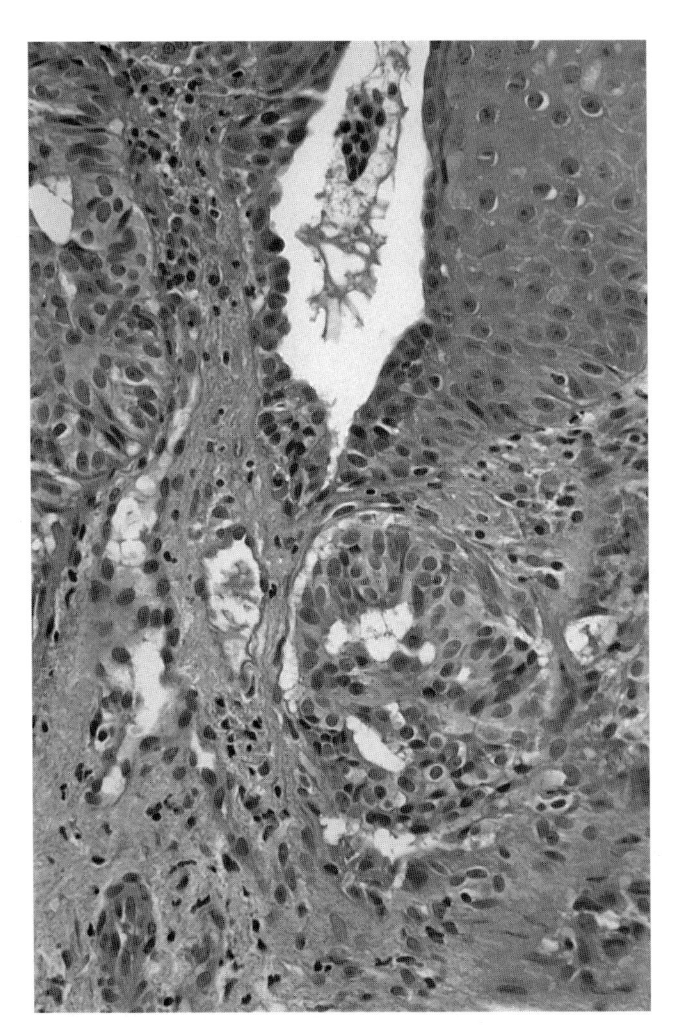

FIG. 31-39. Erosive adenomatosis of the nipple
The tubules are lined by a peripheral layer of cuboidal cells and a luminal layer of columnar cells that in some areas show secretory projections into the lumen.

Differential Diagnosis. Erosive adenomatosis of the nipple must be differentiated from intraductal carcinoma, which shows larger cuboidal cells and uniform atypicality of the nuclei, frequently with necrosis. Hidradenoma papilliferum, in contrast to erosive adenomatosis of the nipple, shows no connections of the tubular structures with the surface epidermis.[223]

Cylindroma

Cylindroma represents a tumor in which differentiation is probably in most cases in the direction of apocrine structures but is in some instances toward eccrine structures (see Histogenesis). It occurs more often as a solitary lesion than as multiple lesions.[224] Cases with multiple lesions are dominantly inherited and show numerous dome-shaped, smooth nodules of various sizes on the scalp. Occasionally, scattered nodules are also present on the face and, in rare instances, on the trunk and the extremities.[225] The lesions begin to appear in early adulthood and increase in number and size throughout life. They vary in size from a few millimeters to several centimeters. Nodules on the scalp may be present in such large numbers as to cover the entire scalp like a turban. For this reason, they are referred to occasionally as *turban tumors.*

The association of multiple lesions of cylindroma with multiple lesions of trichoepithelioma is quite common.[224,226–229] In these cases, the lesions of the scalp are cylindromas, and those elsewhere are partially cylindromas and partially trichoepitheliomas. The association of these two types of tumors, both of which are dominantly inherited, is also of interest in regard to their histogenesis.[230] In several instances, multiple cylindromas have been found in association with eccrine spiradenoma.[224,231,232]

Solitary cylindromas are not inherited; they appear in adulthood and occur either on the scalp or the face. Their histologic appearance is the same as that of multiple cylindromas.[224]

Histopathology. The tumors of cylindroma are composed of numerous islands of epithelial cells. Varying considerably in size and shape and lying close together, separated often only by their hyaline sheath and a narrow band of collagen, the islands of epithelial cells seem to fit together like pieces of a jigsaw puzzle (Figs. 31-40 and 31-41). The hyaline sheath surrounding the tumor islands, like a cylinder, is quite variable in thickness. In addition, droplets of hyalin are present in many islands, and some islands consist largely of hyalin and contain only a few cells. The hyalin is PAS-positive and diastase-resistant.[202]

Two types of cells constitute the islands: cells with small, dark-staining nuclei are present predominantly at the periphery of the islands, often in a palisade arrangement, and cells with large, light-staining nuclei lie in the center of the islands (see Fig. 31-41). In addition, tubular lumina are often present. In some cases, they are quite numerous, whereas, in others only a few are found after a thorough search. The lumina are lined by cells that usually have the appearance of ductal cells.[233] Occasionally, however, the luminal cells show active secretion, like the secretory cells of apocrine glands.[8] Often, amorphous material is found within the lumina; it contains both neutral and acid mucopolysaccharides, as shown by the fact that it stains positively both with the PAS reaction and with alcian blue.[202]

Histogenesis. The ultrastructural and immunohistochemical features best fit differentiation toward the intradermal coiled duct region of eccrine sweat glands,[234–236] with myoepithelial cell participation.[237]

Electron microscopic examination, similar to examination by light microscopy, has revealed two major types of cells; undifferentiated basal cells with small, dark nuclei, and differentiating cells with large, pale nuclei. Most of the differentiating cells still appear immature as "indeterminate cells," but some show a certain degree of differentiation toward secretory or ductal cells and are in part arranged around lumina.[80,233,238]

Interestingly, a study of two large pedigrees has led to the conclusion that cylindromas and trichoepitheliomas are different expressions of the same disorder and not merely examples of genetic linkage.[227] In contrast, the coexistence of cylindroma and eccrine spiradenoma in a few instances has been interpreted as evidence for the theory that cylindroma is of an eccrine nature.[224,231]

The thick hyaline band surrounding the tumor islands of cylindroma is composed mainly of an amorphous substance identical to the subepidermal lamina densa. It is connected with the tumor cells by half-desmosomes. Enmeshed in it are aggregated anchoring fibrils and thin collagen fibrils.[80] This thick

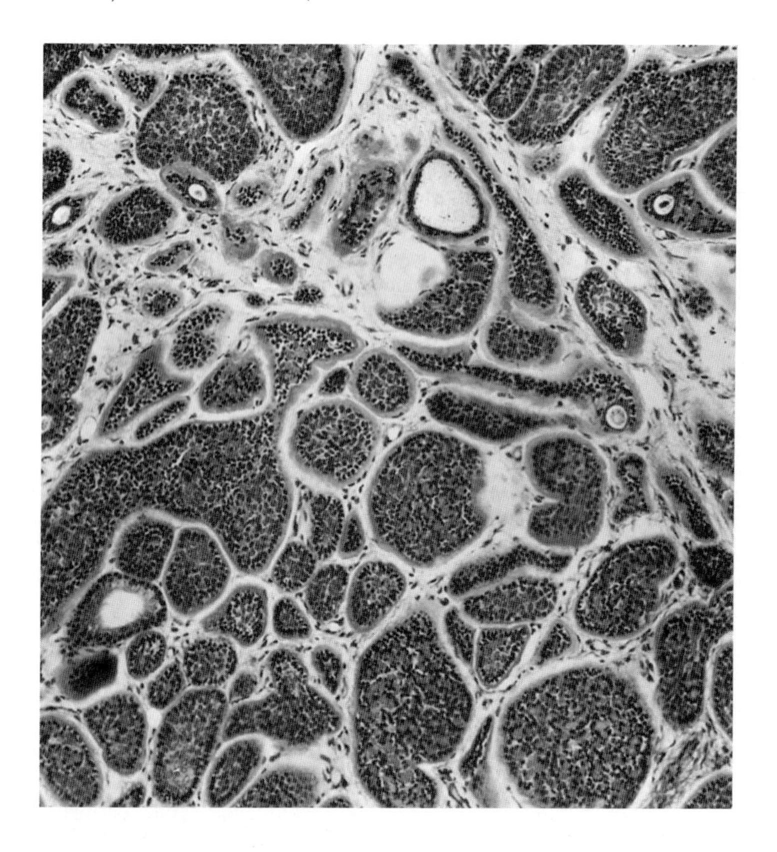

FIG. 31-40. Cylindroma, low magnification
The tumor is composed of irregularly shaped islands that fit together like pieces of a jigsaw puzzle. The islands are surrounded by a hyaline sheath. Several islands in the lower right quadrant contain droplets of hyalin.

hyaline membrane and also the particles of hyalin present between the cells of the tumor islands react positively to staining with antibodies against type IV collagen and laminin, analogous to the subepidermal lamina densa (see Chap. 3). This hyalin is synthesized by the tumor cells[239] and is similar to the deposits of basement membrane protein demonstrated in hyalinosis cutis et mucosae (see Chap. 17).

Malignant Cylindroma

Cylindromas rarely undergo malignant degeneration. Only about a score of cases are on record.[240,241] In most of these patients, there were multiple cylindromas of the scalp, but in several cases a single tumor was present.[242–244] Usually only one

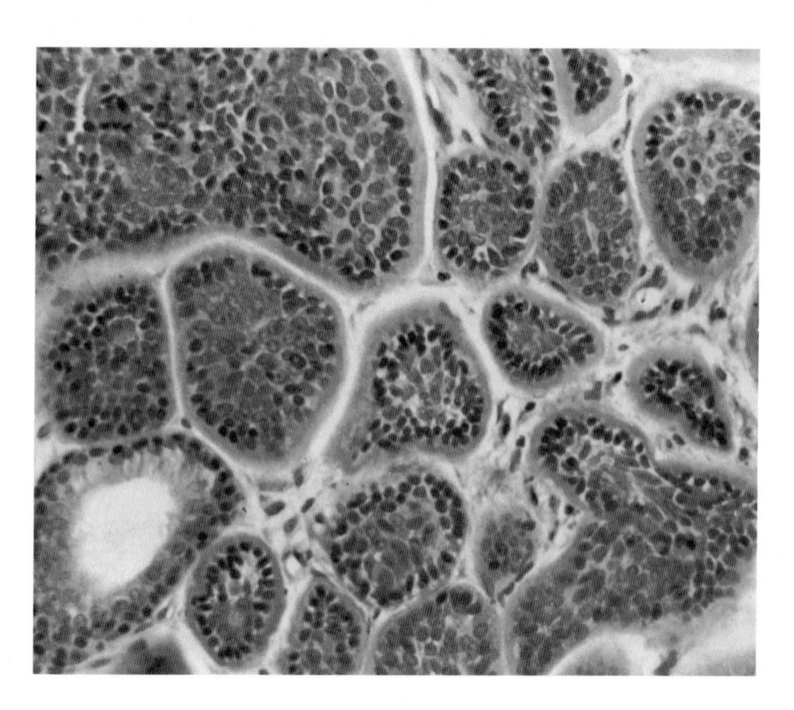

FIG. 31-41. Cylindroma
High magnification of Fig. 31-40. Two types of epithelial cells comprise the islands. There are cells with small dark nuclei representing undifferentiated cells, and cells with large pale nuclei, representing cells with a certain degree of differentiation toward ductal or secretory cells. In the lower left corner, a glandular lumen is lined by two rows of cells. The cells of the inner row show active secretion, like the secretory cells of apocrine glands.

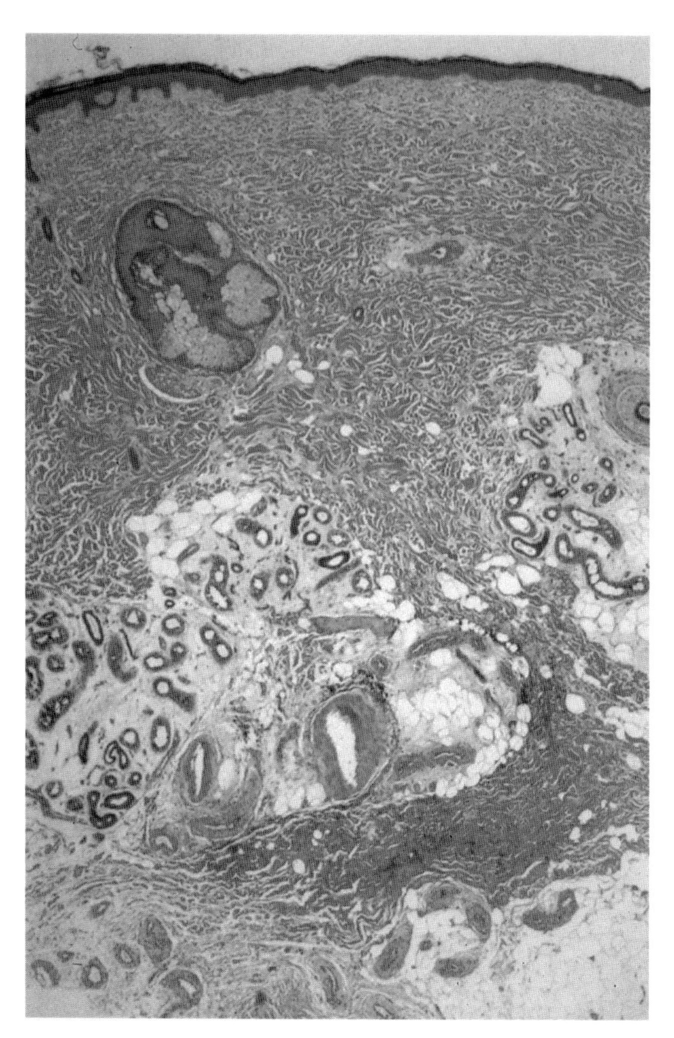

FIG. 31-42. Eccrine angiomatous hamartoma
There is an increased number of eccrine structures with intermingled capillary channels.

tumor was malignant, but in some cases malignant progression had occurred in several tumors.[245,246]

Death usually ensued through visceral metastases, but in a few patients it occurred as the result of invasion of the skull with ensuing hemorrhage or meningitis. Local excision of the tumors of the scalp may result in a cure.

Histopathology. Areas of malignant degeneration are characterized by islands of cells showing marked anaplasia and pleomorphism of the nuclei, many atypical mitotic figures, loss of the hyaline sheath, loss of palisading at the periphery, and invasion into the surrounding tissue.

TUMORS WITH ECCRINE DIFFERENTIATION

Eccrine Nevus

Eccrine nevi are very rare. They may show a circumscribed area of hyperhidrosis,[247,248] a solitary sweat-discharging pore,[249] or papular lesions in a linear arrangement.[250]

In the so-called eccrine angiomatous hamartoma, there may be one or several nodules[251] or a solitary large plaque.[252] The lesions are generally present on an extremity at birth. Hyperhidrosis and/or pain may be apparent.[253]

Histopathology. Eccrine nevi show an increase in the size of the eccrine coil or in both the size and the number of coils. In other cases there is ductal hyperplasia consisting of thickening of the walls and dilatation of the lumina.

Eccrine angiomatous hamartomas show increased numbers of eccrine structures and numerous capillary channels surrounding or intermingled with the eccrine structures.[254] These hamartomas may also contain fatty tissue and pilar structures (Figs. 31-42 and 31-43).[255,256]

Eccrine Hidrocystoma

In this condition, usually one lesion, but occasionally several, and rarely numerous lesions are present on the face.[257] As in apocrine hidrocystoma, the lesion consists of a small, translucent, cystic nodule 1 to 3 mm in diameter that often has a bluish

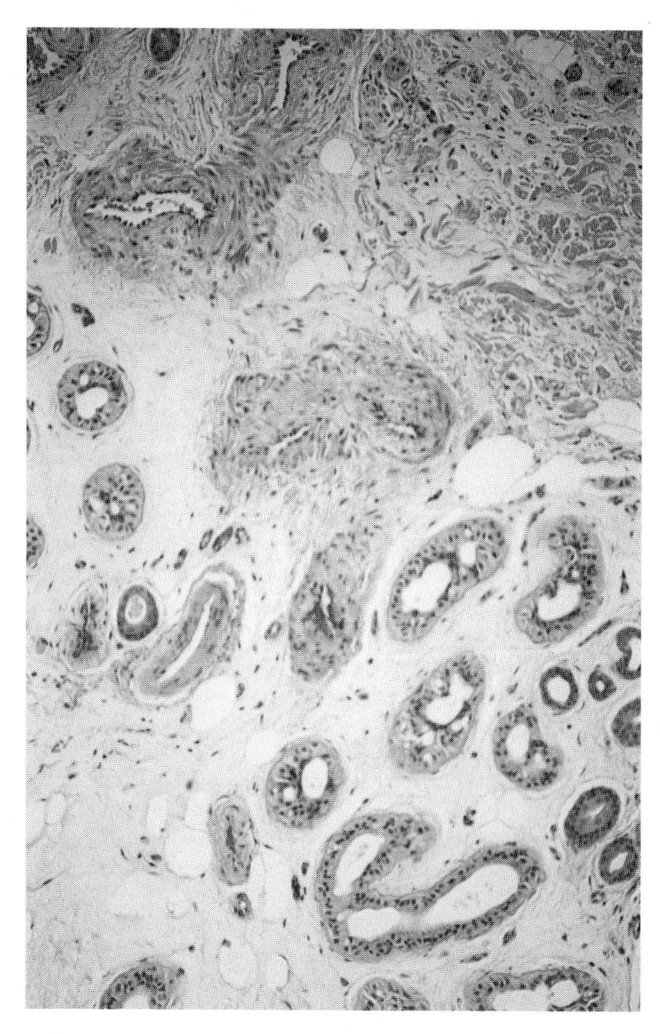

FIG. 31-43. Eccrine angiomatous hamartoma
The hamartoma also contains fatty tissue.

hue. In some patients with numerous lesions, the number of cysts increases in warm weather and decreases during winter.[258]

Histopathology. Eccrine hidrocystoma shows a single cystic cavity located in the dermis. The cyst wall usually shows two layers of small, cuboidal epithelial cells.[257] In some areas, only a single layer of flattened epithelial cells can be seen, their flattened nuclei extending parallel to the cyst wall. Small papillary projections extending into the cavity of the cyst are observed only rarely.[259] Eccrine secretory tubules and ducts are often located below the cyst and in close approximation to it, and, on serial sections, one may find an eccrine duct leading into the cyst from below.[80] However, no connection can be found between the cyst and the epidermis.

Histogenesis. Electron microscopy of eccrine hidrocystoma has established that the cyst wall is composed of ductal cells, since the luminal cell membrane shows numerous microvilli and no secretory granules.[260] Tonofilaments are seen in the luminal portion of the cells, and desmosomes connect the cells.[261]

Enzyme histochemistry in cases with numerous cysts has revealed phosphorylase[261] and succinic dehydrogenase,[260] which are eccrine enzymes, in the cyst walls.

It is likely that malformations of the eccrine ducts lead to either temporary or permanent retention of sweat.[261]

Differential Diagnosis. For a discussion of differentiation of eccrine from apocrine hidrocystoma, see p. 770.

Syringoma

According to histochemical and electron microscopic findings, syringoma represents an adenoma of intraepidermal eccrine ducts. It occurs predominantly in women at puberty or later in life. Although occasionally solitary, the lesions usually are multiple and may be present in great numbers. They are small, skin-colored or slightly yellow, soft papules usually only 1 or 2 mm in diameter. In many patients, the lesions are limited to the lower eyelids. Other sites of predilection are the cheeks, axillae, abdomen, and vulva.[262] In so-called eruptive hidradenoma or syringoma, the lesions arise in large numbers in successive crops on the anterior trunk of young persons.[263] Rarely, the lesions of syringoma show a unilateral, linear arrangement.[264] In rare instances, occult syringomas of the scalp are associated with diffuse thinning of the hair[265] or with cicatricial alopecia.[266,267] Inapparent syringoma has been found incidentally in close approximation to basal cell carcinoma.[268]

Histopathology. Embedded in a fibrous stroma are numerous small ducts (Fig. 31-44), the walls of which are lined usually by two rows of epithelial cells. In most instances, these cells are flat. Occasionally, the cells of the inner row appear vacuolated. The lumina of the ducts contain amorphous debris. Some of the ducts possess small, commalike tails of epithelial cells, giving them the appearance of tadpoles. In addition, there are solid strands of basophilic epithelial cells independent of the ducts.

Near the epidermis, there may be cystic ductal lumina filled with keratin and lined by cells containing keratohyaline granules (Fig. 31-45).[263] These keratin cysts resemble milia. Sometimes they rupture, producing a foreign-body reaction.[269]

In rare instances, many of the tumor cells appear as clear cells as a result of glycogen accumulation.[270] In such cases, one observes only a few ductal structures and epithelial cords but predominantly cell islands that are irregular in shape and size. With the occasional exception of the peripheral cell layer, these islands are composed entirely of clear cells (Fig. 31-46) and have more cell layers than are generally seen in ordinary syringomas.[271]

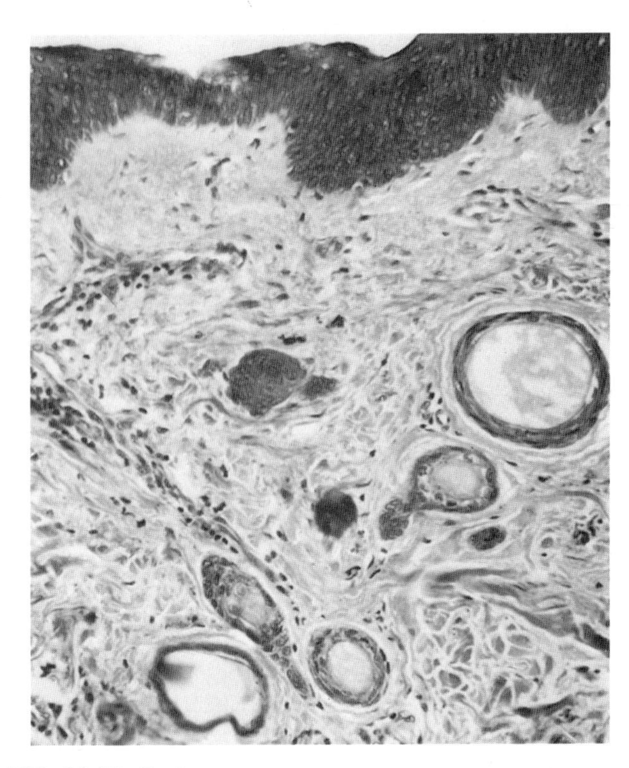

FIG. 31-44. Syringoma
The dermis contains several small ducts. The walls of the ducts are predominantly lined by two rows of epithelial cells. Two of the ducts have comma-like tails, giving them the appearance of tadpoles.

Histogenesis. Enzyme histochemical and electron microscopic studies have established syringoma as a tumor with differentiation toward intraepidermal eccrine sweat ducts.[272,273]

The enzyme pattern in the cells of syringoma shows a prevalence of eccrine enzymes such as succinic dehydrogenase,[274] as well as phosphorylase and leucine aminopeptidase.[275] In contrast to apocrine structures, syringomas react only weakly to lysosomal apocrine enzymes such as acid phosphatase and β-glucuronidase, except in a narrow, lysosome-rich periluminal zone.[263]

Electron microscopic examination reveals that the lumina of the ducts are lined not by secretory but by ductal cells showing numerous short microvilli, interconnecting desmosomes, a periluminal band of tonofilaments, and many lysosomes. In some tumor cells, intracytoplasmic cavities are formed by lysosomal action. Coalescence of several such intracytoplasmic cavities to form an intercellular lumen is the mode by which the ductal lumina are formed in syringoma; this is identical with the mode of formation of the embryonic and the regenerating intraepidermal eccrine ducts (see Chap. 3).[80,263]

The finding of cystic ductal lumina filled with keratin near the epidermis is compatible with the natural keratinizing propensity of the luminal cells of the intraepidermal eccrine sweat duct toward the upper strata of the epidermis.[263]

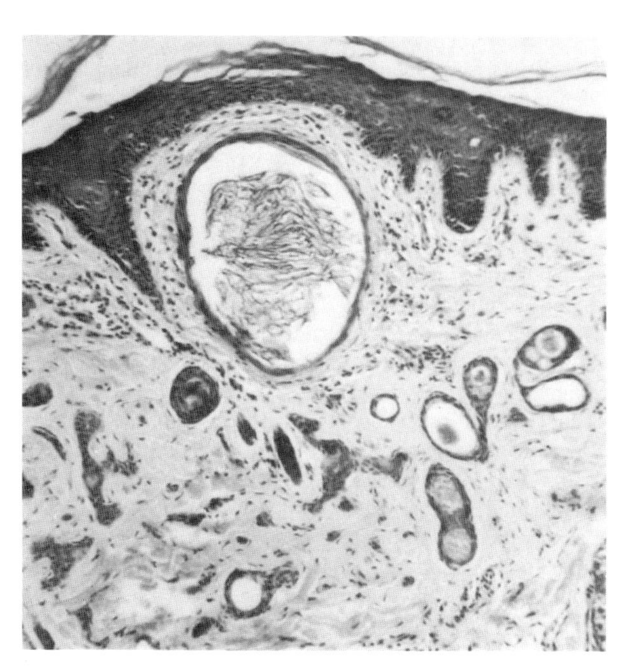

FIG. 31-45. Syringoma
Near the epidermis, the lumen of a cystic duct is filled with keratin.

The occasional presence of large amounts of glycogen in the cells of syringoma is analogous to that in nodular hidradenoma, a tumor that usually shows eccrine differentiation and often contains clear cells and then may be referred to as *clear cell hidradenoma.*[270]

Differential Diagnosis. The solid strands of basophilic epithelial cells embedded in a fibrous stroma seen in some cases of syringoma have an appearance similar to that of the strands seen in fibrosing basal cell carcinoma (see Chap. 30). The latter tumor, however, lacks ductal structures containing amorphous material. The horn cysts near the epidermis in syringoma resemble those occurring in trichoepithelioma, and their presence in syringoma was formerly misinterpreted as the occurrence of both types of tumors within the same lesion.[8] Although trichoepithelioma (including desmoplastic trichoepithelioma) shows solid strands of basophilic epithelial cells and horn cysts, it lacks ductal structures. Syringoma can be distinguished from microcystic adnexal carcinoma by its smaller size, its greater symmetry, and the lack of prominent horn cyst formation and infrequent single-file strand formation. Also, microcystic eccrine carcinoma, a much larger tumor than syringoma, extends into the subcutaneous tissue.[49] The diagnosis of microcystic eccrine carcinoma should always be considered in any apparently syringomatous or trichoepitheliomatous neoplasm that extends to the base of a superficial biopsy. For distinction from syringoid eccrine carcinoma, see p. 792.

Eccrine Poroma

Eccrine poroma, first described in 1956,[276] is a fairly common solitary tumor. In about two thirds of the cases, it is found on the sole or the sides of the foot,[277] occurring next in frequency on the hands and fingers. Eccrine poroma has also been observed in many other areas of the skin, such as the neck, chest, and nose.[278,279] Eccrine poroma generally arises in middle-aged persons. The tumor has a rather firm consistency, is raised and often slightly pedunculated, is asymptomatic, and usually measures less than 2 cm in diameter.

An unusual clinical variant is *eccrine poromatosis* in which more than 100 papules are observed on the palms and soles[280]; in one reported case, the papular poromas, in addition to involving the palms and soles, showed a widespread, diffuse distribution.[281]

Histopathology. In its typical form, eccrine poroma arises

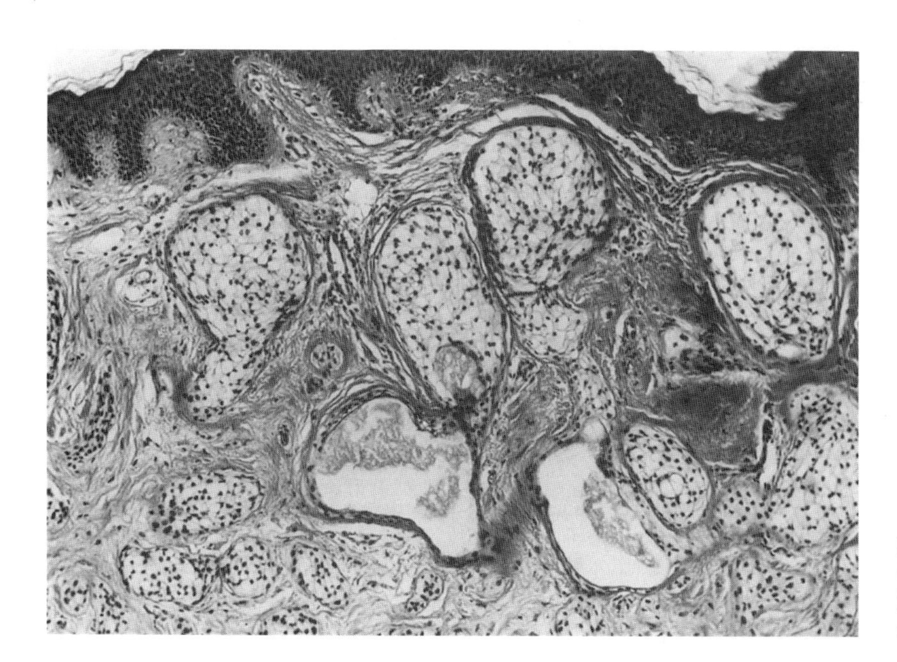

FIG. 31-46. Syringoma
In this rare variant, the tumor islands consist largely of clear cells as a result of glycogen accumulation.

within the lower portion of the epidermis, from where it extends downward into the dermis as tumor masses that often consist of broad, anastomosing bands. The border between epidermis and tumor is readily apparent because of the distinctive appearance of the tumor cells: they are smaller than squamous cells, have a uniform cuboidal appearance and a round, deeply basophilic nucleus, and are connected by intercellular bridges (Fig. 31-47). These cells show no tendency to keratinize within the tumor, but they are able to keratinize on the surface of the tumor in instances in which the tumor has replaced the overlying epidermis. Although the border between tumor formations and the stroma is sharp, tumor cells located at the periphery show no palisading.

As a characteristic feature, the tumor cells contain significant amounts of glycogen, usually in an uneven distribution.[282] Melanocytes and melanin often are absent,[276] although they may be present in tumors encountered in blacks,[283] Mongols,[284] and occasionally in whites.[285]

In most but not in all eccrine poromas, narrow ductal lumina and occasionally cystic spaces are found within the tumor bands.[282] They are lined by an eosinophilic, PAS-positive, diastase-resistant cuticle similar to that lining the lumina of eccrine sweat ducts and by a single row of luminal cells.

Poromas are occasionally located entirely within the epidermis, where they appear as discrete aggregates. Such intraepidermal poromas were first described under the designation *hidroacanthoma simplex* in 1956,[286] the same year in which poroma was first described.[276] These lesions represent one example of the so-called Borsst-Jadassohn phenomenon of intraepithelial epitheliomas, discussed in Chapter 30 (Figs. 31-48 and 31-49). A few ductal lumina lined by an eosinophilic cuticle can often be seen within the intraepidermal islands.[287] Eccrine poromas may also be located largely or entirely within the dermis, where they consist of variously shaped tumor islands containing ductal lumina. They are then referred to as *dermal duct tumors*.[288]

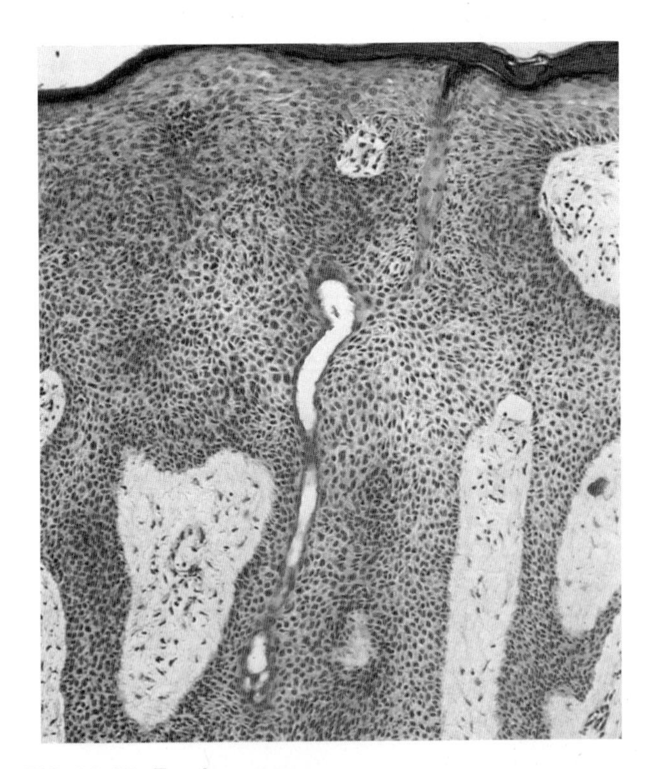

FIG. 31-47. Eccrine poroma
The tumor consists of broad anastomosing bands. The cells comprising the tumor have a uniformly small cuboidal appearance and are connected by intercellular bridges. A ductal lumen extends vertically through the tumor. It is lined by an eosinophilic cuticle and a single row of luminal cells.

Syringoacanthoma of Rahbari represents a clonal variant of eccrine poroma in which variously sized nests of small, deeply basophilic, ovoid or cuboidal sweat duct–like cells are embedded within an acanthotic epidermis.[289]

Histogenesis. Enzyme histochemical staining has shown the prevalence in eccrine poroma of eccrine enzymes, particularly phosphorylase and succine dehydrogenase.[288,290,291]

Electron microscopic examination reveals that the tumor cells, except for the luminal cells, contain a moderate number of tonofilaments, are connected with each other by desmosomes, and appear identical to the cells that compose the outer layer of the intraepidermal eccrine duct (poral epithelial cells).[291] The luminal cells show a periluminal filamentous zone and, extending into the lumen, numerous tortuous microvilli coated with amorphous material that forms the eosinophilic cuticle seen by light microscopy. Some of the tumor cells may also exhibit features considered indicative of dermal duct differentiation.[292,293]

Differential Diagnosis. Eccrine poroma must be differentiated from basal cell carcinoma and seborrheic keratosis. In basal cell carcinoma, the cells have no visible intercellular bridges, are more variable in size, often show peripheral palisading, and contain little or no glycogen. The cells of eccrine poroma greatly resemble the small basaloid cells of seborrheic keratosis, especially because they possess clearly visible intercellular bridges. However, seborrheic keratoses have an even demarcation at their lower border; moreover, their cells have the potential to keratinize, and when they keratinize, they form horn cysts. Also, both basal cell carcinoma and seborrheic keratosis lack lumina lined with an eosinophilic cuticle. Furthermore, these two types of tumors very rarely occur on the sole of the foot.

Eccrine Syringofibroadenoma

First described in 1963,[294] this usually is a solitary, hyperkeratotic, nodular plaque, several centimeters in diameter, on one extremity.[295,296] In one instance, a linear lesion extended along a lower extremity.[297]

Histopathology. Slender, anastomosing epithelial cords of acrosyringeal cells, with or without formation of lumina, are embedded in a fibrovascular stroma.[296] The netlike pattern of epithelial cells resembles that seen in fibroepithelioma (Figs. 31-50 and 31-51) (see Chap. 30).[297]

Malignant Eccrine Poroma (Porocarcinoma)

Malignant eccrine poroma, or porocarcinoma, may arise as such,[298,299] but usually it develops in an eccrine poroma of long standing.[285,300–302] The tumor favors extremities, particularly legs and feet, usually in adults of either sex. In some instances, the malignant eccrine poroma is still localized, manifesting

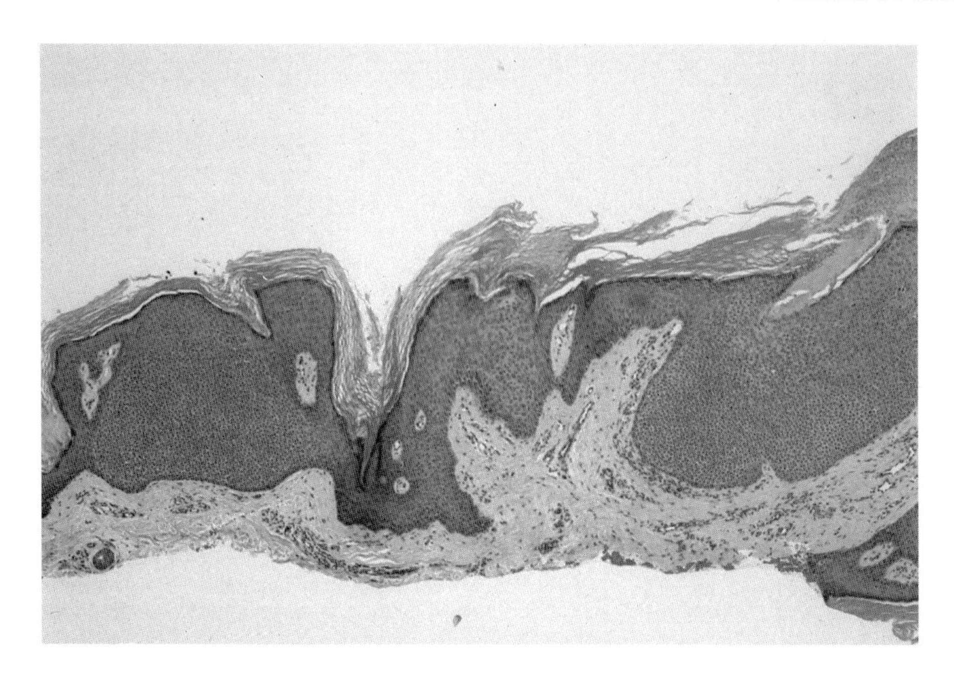

FIG. 31-48. Hidroacanthoma simplex
There are discrete aggregates of small cells in the epidermis, constituting one example of the so-called Borsst-Jadassohn phenomenon of intraepithelial epitheliomas.

itself as a nodule,[300] plaque,[299] or ulcerated tumor[302,303]; in other cases, there are multiple cutaneous metastases, which are usually associated with visceral metastases, resulting in death.[285,301,304,305] The propensity to form multiple cutaneous metastases is a unique feature of malignant eccrine poroma.

Histopathology. Malignant eccrine poroma may be seen adjoining a typical eccrine poroma[302] or a purely intraepidermal eccrine poroma.[300] In such cases, one observes areas composed of eccrine poroma cells with a benign appearance adjoining areas of anaplastic cells (Fig. 31-52). The malignant cells have large, hyperchromatic, irregularly shaped nuclei and may be multinucleated.[302] They are rich in glycogen.[304]

In the primary tumor, the malignant cells may be limited to the epidermis or may extend into the dermis. Some islands of tumor cells may lie free in the dermis. The epidermis often shows considerable acanthosis as a result of the proliferation of nu-

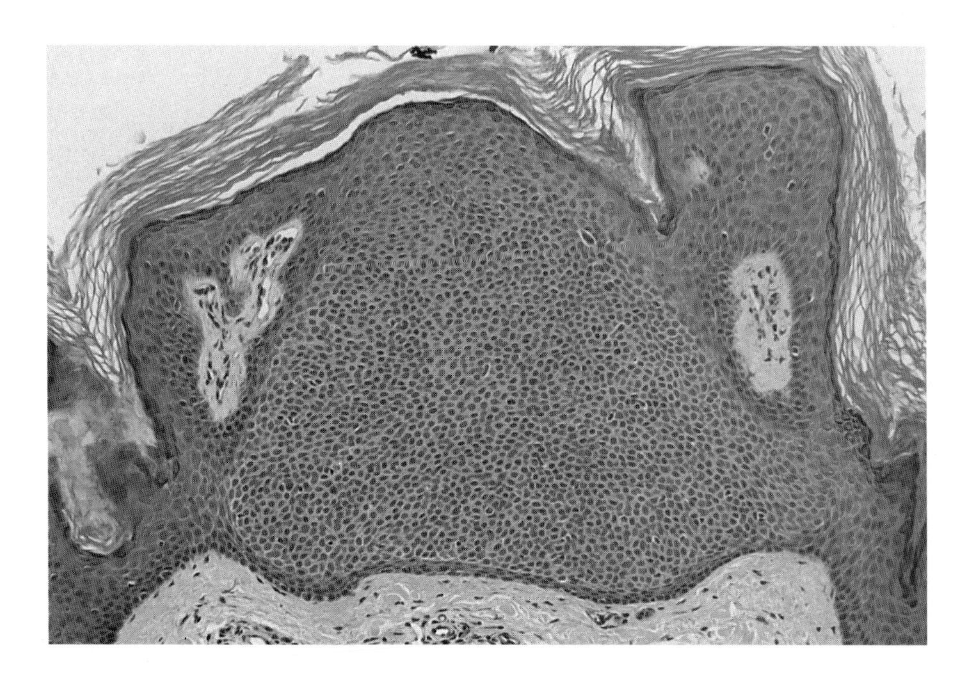

FIG. 31-49. Hidroacanthoma simplex
The cells are small and cytologically bland, distinguishing the lesion from Bowen's or Paget's disease. Some of these lesions contain small tubules, consistent with eccrine pore differentiation.

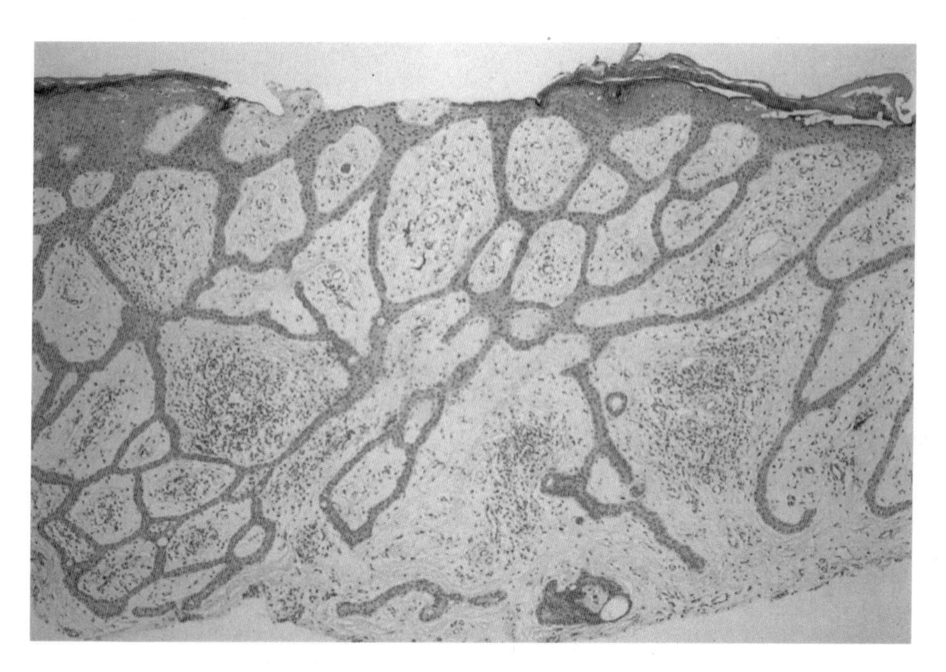

FIG. 31-50. Eccrine syringofibroadenoma
There is a hyperkeratotic, nodular plaque several centimeters in diameter.

merous well-defined tumor cell nests within it. Cystic lumina may be seen within the epidermal and dermal tumor nests. The tumors are asymmetrical, with cords and lobules of polygonal tumor cells, typically with a cribriform pattern. Nuclear atypia is evident, with frequent mitoses and necrosis. Useful clues to eccrine differentiation include spiraling ductular structures, ducts lined by cuticular material, zones of cytoplasmic glycogenation, and also intraepidermal cells in discrete aggregates, often centered on acrosyringial pores. Foci of squamous differentiation may have the histologic features of well-differentiated squamous cell carcinoma.[306] The stroma may be fibrotic, hyalinized, highly myxoid, or frankly mucinous. The distinction from metastatic adenocarcinoma, especially of breast and lung origin, can be difficult, especially for less differentiated tumors. Ductular differentiation with formation of a PAS-positive cuticle is strong evidence against a metastasis. An extracutaneous primary adenocarcinoma should be clinically ruled out.

The term *ductal eccrine carcinoma*[307] has been used to refer to tumors that may appear in the dermis as an infiltrative poroma (porocarcinoma) or as a moderately differentiated ade-

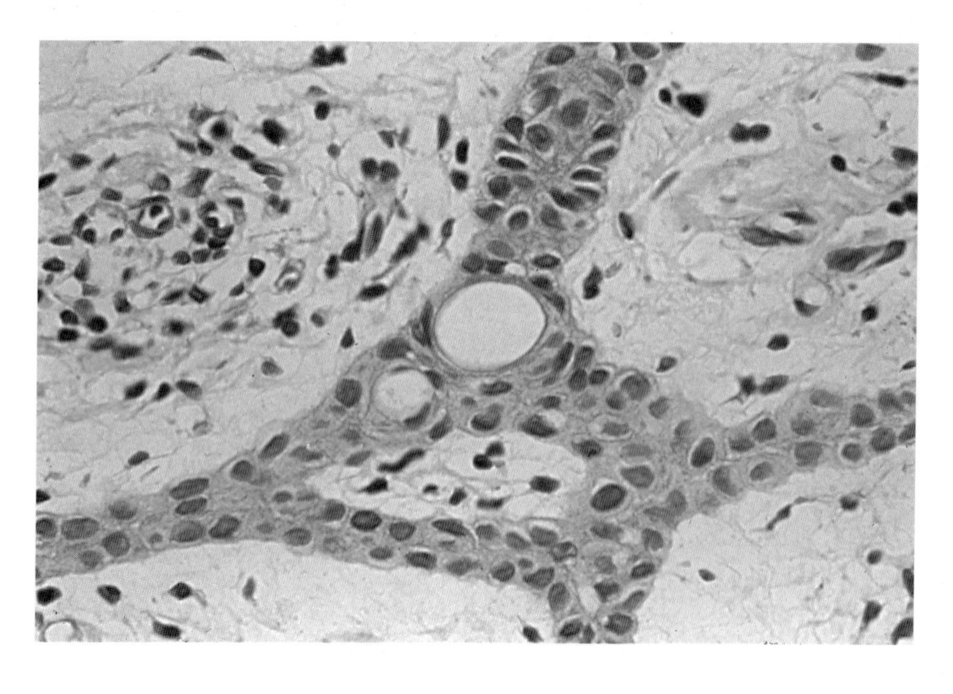

FIG. 31-51. Eccrine syringofibroadenoma
The tumor is composed of anastomosing epithelial cords of mature acrosyringeal cells, which may form lumina and are embedded in a fibrovascular stroma.

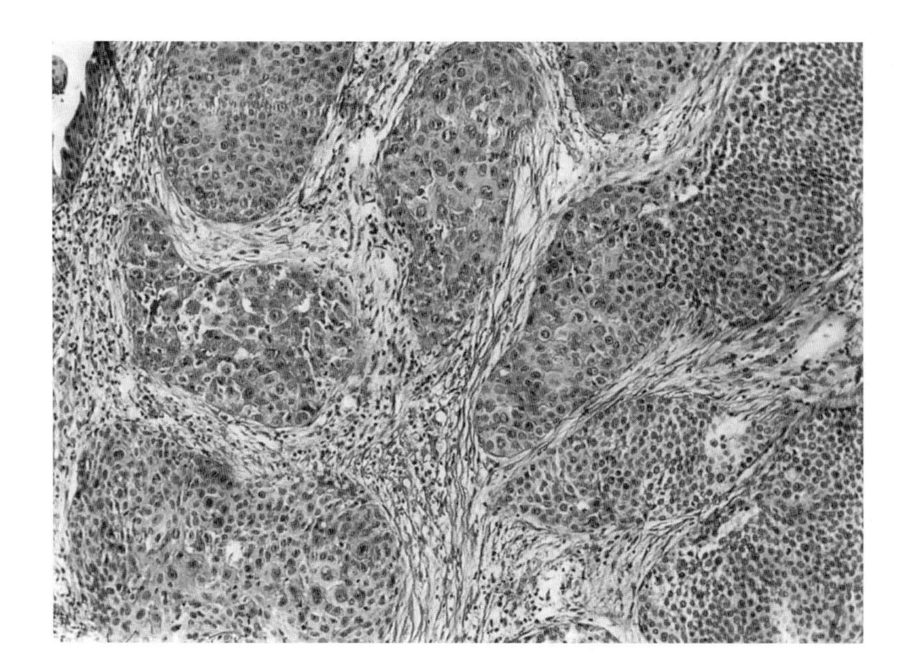

FIG. 31-52. Malignant eccrine poroma On the right side, the tumor has an appearance similar to that of an eccrine poroma; on the left side, the tumor lobules are composed of cells showing anaplastic nuclei and dyskeratosis.

nocarcinoma. About one third of ductal eccrine carcinomas are fatal, usually because of distant metastasis.[308]

Malignant eccrine poroma, analogous to its benign variant, can show a clonal ("intraepithelial epithelioma") pattern of its anaplastic acrosyringeal cells (see discussion in Chap. 30). The intraepidermal clones of such *malignant syringoacanthomas* may remain in situ or become invasive.[309]

In cutaneous metastases, numerous nests of tumor cells are present in both the epidermis and the dermis. In the epidermis, sharply defined small and large nests of tumor cells are seen surrounded by the squamous cells of the hyperplastic epidermis, resulting in a "pagetoid" pattern.[285,304] Some of the tumor nests in the dermis are located within dilated lymphatic vessels, suggesting spread of the tumor in the lymphatics of the skin.[304] From the lymphatics, the tumor cells invade the overlying epidermis because of the "epidermotropic" nature of the acrosyringeal tumor cells.

Mucinous Syringometaplasia

A rare condition first described in 1974,[310] mucinous syringometaplasia occurs as a solitary lesion in two different forms: as a verrucous lesion in an acral location on the sole of a foot[311] or a finger[312] and as a plaque resembling a basal cell carcinoma in a more central location.[312] With pressure, serous fluid can often be expressed.[311]

Histopathology. An invagination lined by squamous epithelium extends deeply into the dermis. One or several eccrine ducts lead into the invagination. They are lined in part by mucin-laden goblet cells.[311] In addition, there may be mucinous metaplasia in the underlying eccrine coils.[312,313] The epithelial mucin is PAS-positive and alcian-blue–reactive, suggesting that it is sialomucin.

Eccrine Spiradenoma

As a rule, eccrine spiradenoma occurs as a solitary intradermal nodule measuring 1 to 2 cm in diameter. Occasionally, there are several nodules,[314,315] and rarely, there are numerous small nodules in a zosteriform pattern[316] or large nodules, up to 5 cm, in a linear arrangement.[317] In most instances, eccrine spiradenoma arises in early adulthood. It has no characteristic location. The nodules are often tender and occasionally painful.

Histopathology. The tumor may consist of one large, sharply demarcated lobule, but more commonly there are several such lobules located in the dermis without connections to the epidermis. The lobules are evenly and sharply demarcated and may display a fibrous capsule.[318] On low magnification, the tumor lobules often appear deeply basophilic because of the close aggregation of the nuclei (Fig. 31-53).

On higher magnification, the epithelial cells within the tumor lobules are found to be arranged in intertwining cords.[319,320] These cords may enclose small, irregularly shaped islands of edematous connective tissue.[321] Two types of epithelial cells are present in the cords, both of which possess only scant amounts of cytoplasm. The cells of the first type possess small, dark nuclei; they are generally located at the periphery of the cellular aggregates. The cells of the second type have large, pale nuclei; they are located in the center of the aggregates and may be arranged partially around small lumina observed in about half of the tumors (Fig. 31-54).[318] The lumina frequently contain small amounts of a granular, eosinophilic material that is PAS-positive and diastase-resistant.[320] In the absence of lumina, the cells with pale nuclei may show a rosette arrangement. Glycogen is absent in the tumor cells or is present in insignificant amounts.

In some cases of eccrine spiradenoma, hyaline material is focally present in the stroma that surrounds the cords of tumor

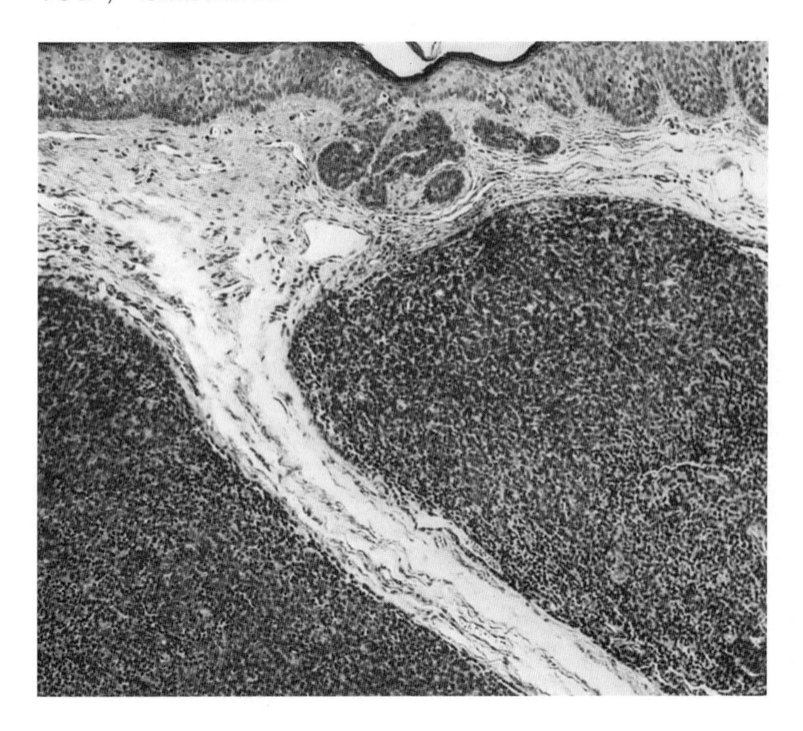

FIG. 31-53. Eccrine spiradenoma, low magnification
Two large masses of tumor cells composed of two types of cells are shown.

cells. In addition, hyalin may be seen within some of the cords among the tumor cells as hyaline droplets.[320] The stroma surrounding the tumor lobules occasionally shows lymphedema with greatly dilated blood or lymph capillaries.[320] A heavy diffuse lymphocytic infiltrate, mainly of T cells, may be present.[322] Malignant progression is rare.

Histogenesis. Enzyme histochemical staining has revealed a prevalence of eccrine enzymes in eccrine spiradenoma, but the reactions are not as strong as in syringoma or eccrine poroma.[315,321,323]

Electron microscopic examination, similar to light microscopic examination, has shown two types of cells: undifferentiated basal cells with small, dark nuclei, and differentiating cells with large, pale nuclei. Most of the differentiating cells are immature ("indeterminate cells") and, in some tumors, may show no further differentiation.[321] In most instances, however, there is some degree of differentiation toward intradermal eccrine ductal cells or toward eccrine secretory cells. Around the same lumen, some cells may show numerous microvilli and a well-developed periluminal zone of tonofilaments and thus resemble ductal cells, whereas other cells have only a few thin microvilli and thus resemble secretory cells.[80,315] All secretory cells have the appearance of serous cells (clear cells).[324] A few myoepithelial cells with typical myofilaments are present occasionally at the periphery of tubular structures.[315]

It can be concluded that differentiation in eccrine spirade-

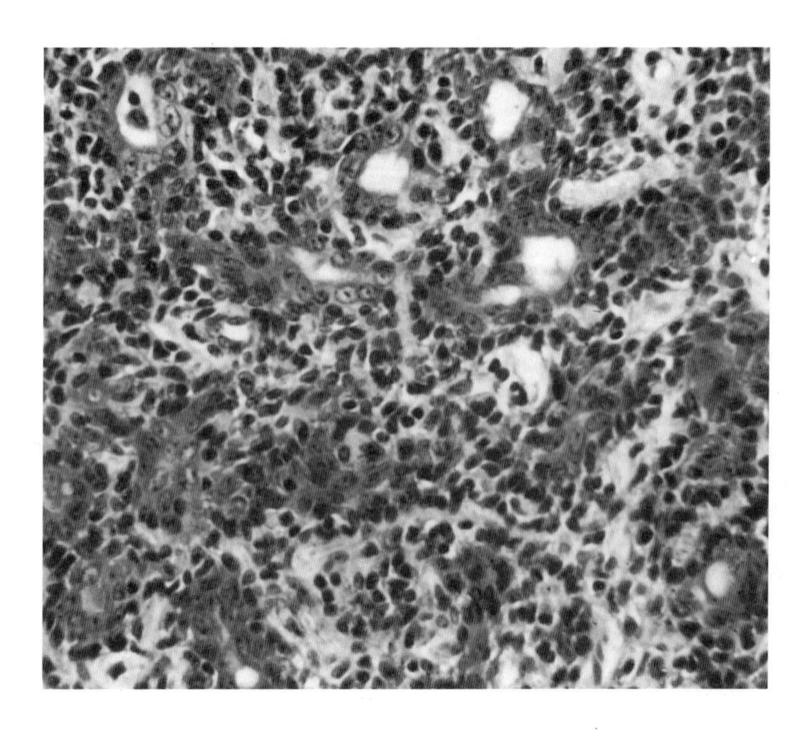

FIG. 31-54. Eccrine spiradenoma, high magnification
The epithelial cells are arranged in intertwining bands. Two types of cells can be seen. Cells with small dark nuclei lie at the periphery of the bands; they represent undifferentiated cells. Cells with large pale nuclei lie in the center of the bands and around small lumina.

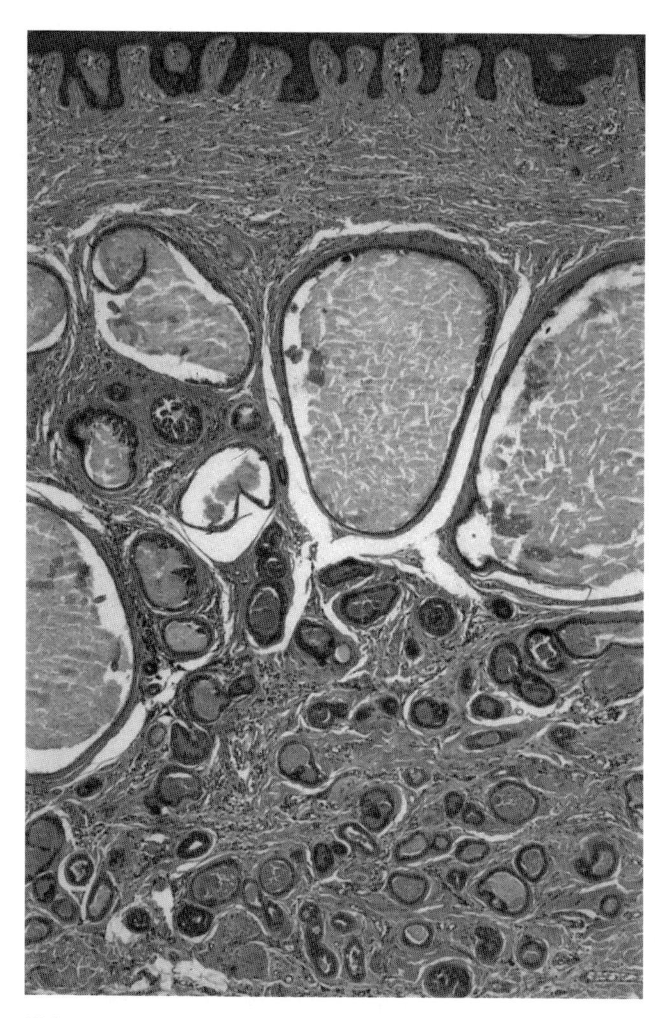

FIG. 31-55. Papillary eccrine adenoma
The tumor is well circumscribed and symmetrical and consists of dilated, occasionally branching tubular structures.

noma is in the direction of both the dermal duct and the secretory segment of the eccrine sweat gland. However, the weakness and inconsistency of the enzyme histochemical reactions, the presence largely of undifferentiated and indeterminate cells, and the absence of dark mucous cells indicate a rather low degree of differentiation.

Malignant Eccrine Spiradenoma

Occasionally, malignant degeneration takes place in longstanding solitary lesions of eccrine spiradenoma.[325–328] A few of these patients died of generalized metastases[327,329]; one had a regional lymph node metastasis.[330] Clinical features may include a history of enlargement in a previously stable lesion.

Histopathology. Two distinct components are seen: typical benign eccrine spiradenoma and carcinoma, with areas of transitions. The carcinoma may be undifferentiated or may show gland formation in some areas, squamous differentiation, or sarcomatous change.[328,330] Although mitoses may be seen in benign eccrine spiradenomas, malignant spiradenomas show a high mitotic rate (8–12 per hpf).[330] Because the malignant changes may be focal in a benign spiradenoma, the malignancy may be missed if the specimen is inadequately sampled.[331]

Papillary Eccrine Adenoma

This tumor represents the eccrine equivalent of tubular apocrine adenoma. First described in 1977,[332] it occurs most commonly on the distal portions of the extremities as a small, solitary nodule.

Histopathology. As in tubular apocrine adenoma, the tumor is well circumscribed and symmetrical and consists of dilated, occasionally branching tubular structures that are lined by usually two layers of epithelial cells (Fig. 31-55). Papillary projections extend into the lumina.[332] The ducts may contain amor-

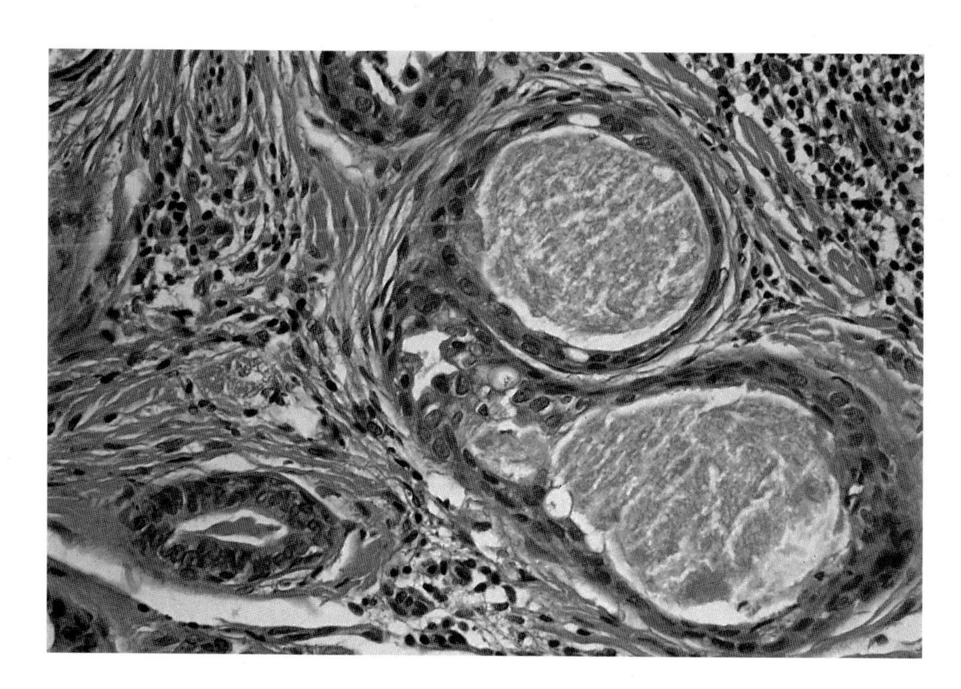

FIG. 31-56. Papillary eccrine adenoma
The dilated tubular structures are lined by two layers of cells, with papillary profections into the lumen.

'nophilic material (Fig. 31-56).[333] However, evidence ..pitation secretion is lacking.[334] Small microcysts representing dilated ducts may be present.[335–338] The low-power impression may suggest a benign breast lesion, such as intraductal hyperplasia, especially when, as is characteristic, the tumor is located within the superficial and deep dermis and is not continuous with the overlying epidermis. Amorphous and granular eosinophilic secretions are present in many of the duct lumens, and occasionally there are small, keratin-filled cysts. Adenomatous regions present variably spaced ducts and glands lined by one to several layers of cuboidal epithelium. The presence of a dense fibrovascular stromal tissue distinguishes this lesion from dermal endometriosis, which has a more cellular stroma. The tumor may recur locally but does not metastasize systemically.

A more aggressive variant that occurs primarily on the digits of the hand, called *aggressive digital papillary adenocarcinoma,* is discussed later as a variant of eccrine carcinoma.

Histogenesis. The amylophosphorylase reaction indicating eccrine differentiation is prominent, but the reaction with acid phosphatase, an apocrine enzyme, shows practically no staining in the tumor.[334] Immunoreactivity for S-100 protein, CEA, and EMA (see Chap. 4) is typically present, consistent with differentiation toward the secretory epithelium of sweat glands.[336,337]

Nodular Hidradenoma

Nodular hidradenoma,[339] referred to in the past as *clear cell myoepithelioma* (see Histogenesis), is presently also called *clear cell hidradenoma,*[340] *eccrine sweat gland adenoma of the clear cell type,*[341,342] *solid cystic hidradenoma,*[343,344] and *eccrine acrospiroma.*[345] It is a fairly common tumor without a preferred site.

Nodular hidradenoma, generally regarded as an ecccrine sweat gland tumor on the basis of its enzyme histochemical and electron microscopic features, occurs as a solitary tumor in most instances; rarely, several lesions are present.[346] The tumors present themselves as intradermal nodules and in most instances measure between 0.5 and 2.0 cm in diameter, although they may be larger. They are usually covered by intact skin, but some tumors show superficial ulceration[344] and discharge serous material. Although clinically the tumor only rarely gives the impression of being cystic, gross examination of the specimen often reveals the presence of cysts.[340,345]

Histopathology. The tumor is well circumscribed and may appear encapsulated. It is composed of lobulated masses located in the dermis and extending into the subcutaneous fat. Within the lobulated masses, tubular lumina of various sizes are often present (Fig. 31-57). However, such lumina may be absent or may be few in number, so that they are found only on step sectioning. The tubular lumina in some instances are branched. There are often cystic spaces, which may be of considerable size and contain a faintly eosinophilic, homogeneous material (Fig. 31-58).[344] The tubular lumina are lined by cuboidal ductal cells or by columnar secretory cells. Occasionally, the secretory cells show active secretion suggestive of decapitation secretion.[340,346] The wide cystic spaces are only rarely lined by a single row of luminal cells; more frequently, they are bordered by tumor cells that show no particular orientation and occasionally show degenerative changes.[340] This suggests that the cystic spaces form as a result of degeneration of tumor cells.

In solid portions of the tumor, two types of cells can be recognized.[340,344,347,348] The proportion of these two types of cells varies considerably in different tumors. One type of cell is usually polyhedral with a rounded nucleus and slightly basophilic cytoplasm. Some of these cells may appear fusiform and show an elongated nucleus (Fig. 31-59). The second type of cell is usually round and contains very clear cytoplasm, so that the cell

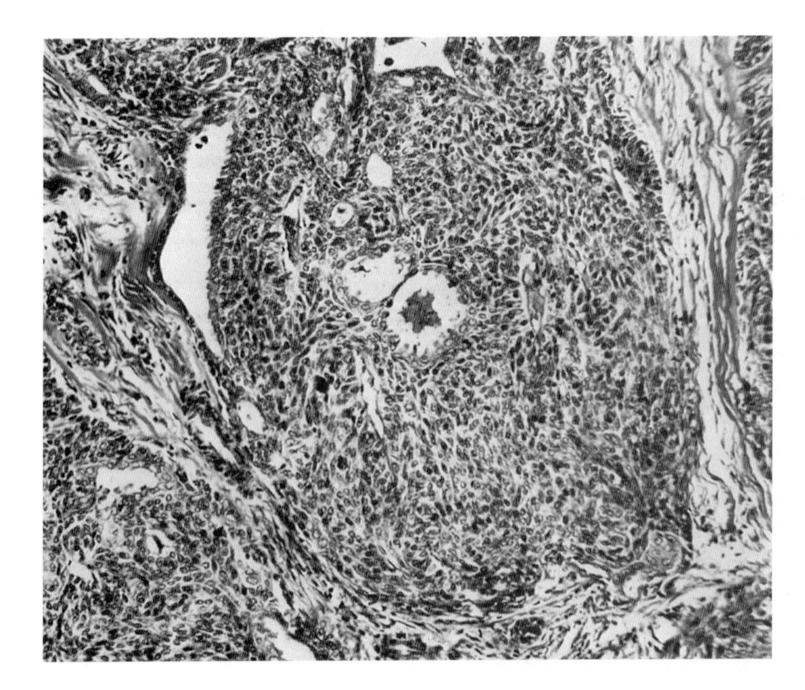

FIG. 31-57. Nodular hidradenoma
The tumor consists of lobular masses composed of cells with clear cytoplasm. Small and large lumina are present, lined either by cuboidal ductal cells or by columnar secretory cells.

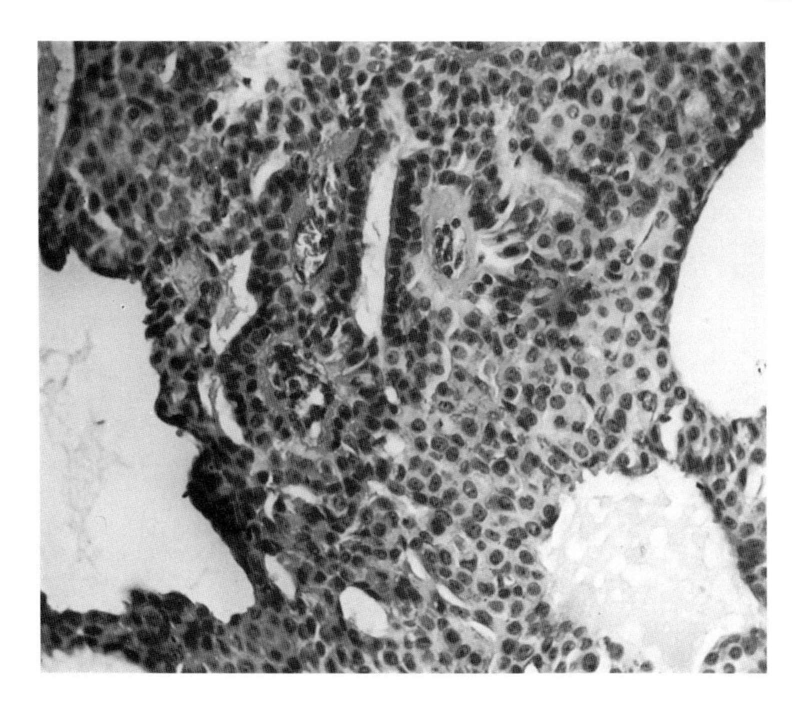

FIG. 31-58. Nodular hidradenoma
Tubular lumina and cystic spaces are present within the tumor. The cystic spaces seem to form as a result of degeneration of tumor cells.

membrane is distinctly visible. Its nucleus appears small and dark (Fig. 31-60). There also are cells transitional between these two varieties; these cells usually show a rather light, eosinophilic cytoplasm. The clear cells contain considerable amounts of glycogen, but they may show, in addition, significant amounts of PAS-positive, diastase-resistant material along their periphery.[347] In some tumors, epidermoid differentiation is seen, with the cells appearing large and polyhedral and showing eosinophilic cytoplasm.[349] There even may be keratinizing cells with formation of horn pearls.[340,341] In other tumors, groups of squamous cells are arranged around small lumina that are lined with a well-defined eosinophilic cuticle and thus resemble the intraepidermal portion of the eccrine duct.[345,347]

In most cases, no connections of the tumor lobules with the surface epidermis are noted; however, in some instances, the tumor replaces the epidermis centrally and merges with the acanthotic epidermis at the periphery of the tumor.[340,341,345] The tumor nodules are frequently associated with a characteristic eosinophilic hyalinized stroma (Fig. 31-61).

Histogenesis. The polyhedral and fusiform cells, because of

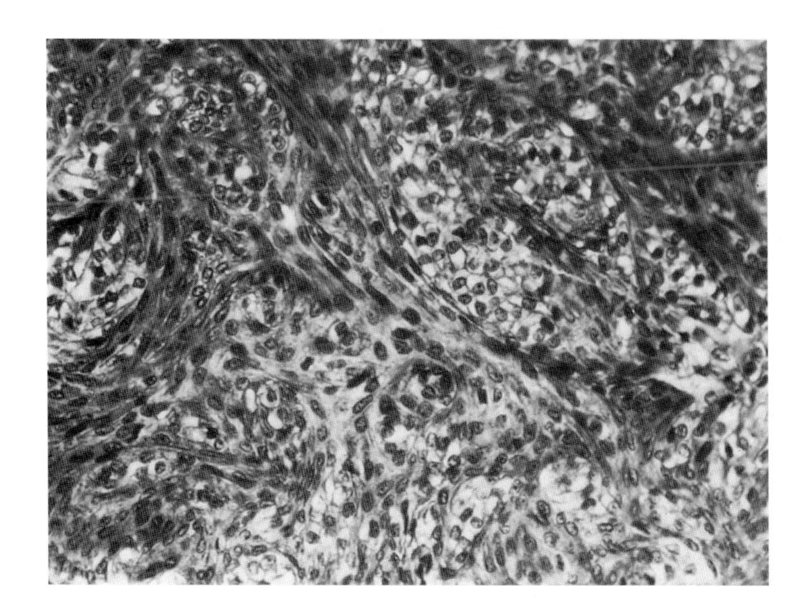

FIG. 31-59. Nodular hidradenoma
The tumor contains polyhedral cells, some of which appear fusiform. Others show a clear cytoplasm.

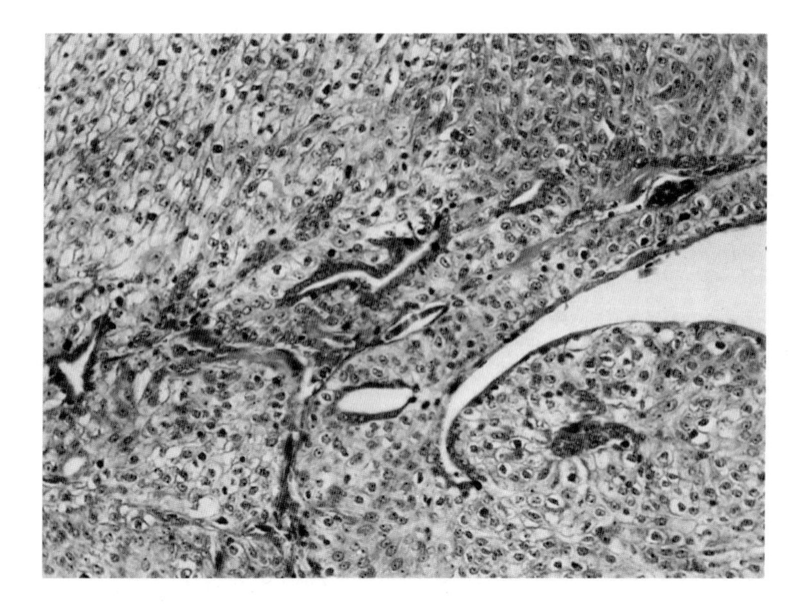

FIG. 31-60. Nodular hidradenoma
There are numerous clear cells and, in addition, tubular lumina lined by a single layer of cuboidal ductal cells.

their location peripheral to the luminal cells and because of their shape, were originally regarded as cells differentiating in the direction of myoepithelial cells.[340,346] However, the absence of alkaline phosphatase and, ultrastructurally, of myofilaments has disproved their relationship to myoepithelial cells.

Enzyme histochemical staining has established the presence in nodular hidradenoma of high concentrations of eccrine enzymes, particularly phosphorylase and respiratory enzymes, including succinic dehydrogenase and diphosphopyridine nucleotide (DPNH) diaphorase.[343,348] Immunohistochemical reactivity for keratin, EMA, CEA, S-100 protein, and vimentin is characteristic.[350]

Electron microscopic examination has shown a fair number of tonofilaments in the polyhedral and fusiform cells and an abundance of glycogen in the clear cells. These two types of tumor cells resemble the tumor cells of eccrine poroma and consequently also resemble the cells that compose the outer layers of the intraepidermal eccrine duct.[348] In addition, four types of luminal cells can be recognized: a secretory type, dermal-ductal and epidermal-ductal types, and an immature type.[348] It can be

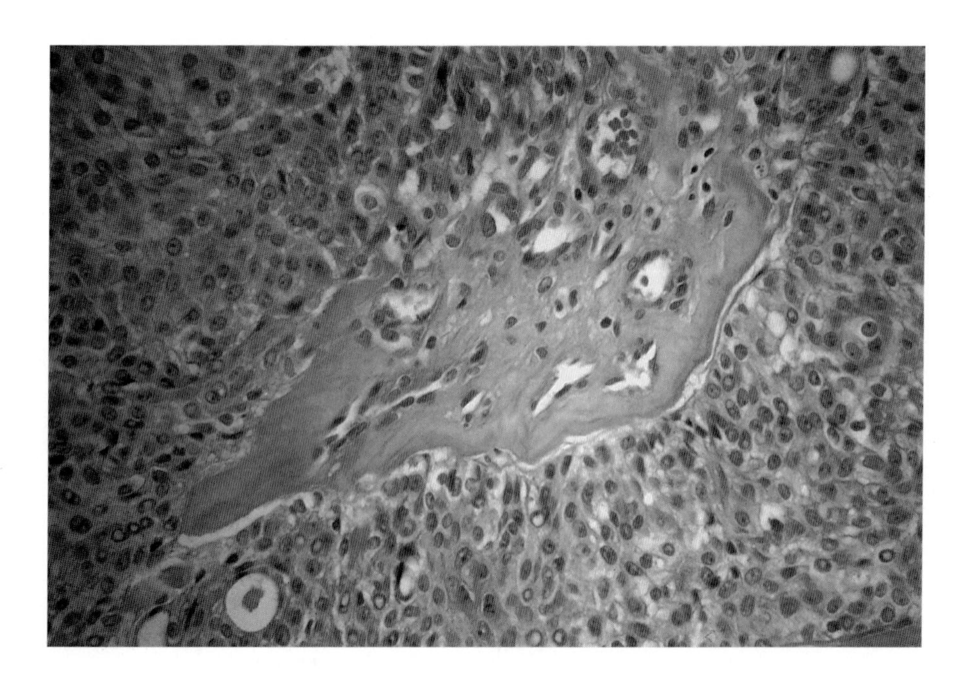

FIG. 31-61. Nodular hidradenoma
A characteristic eosinophilic hyalinized stroma is usually present.

concluded that nodular hidradenoma shows differentiation toward intraepidermal and intradermal eccrine structures ranging from the poral epithelium to the secretory segment.[342,348] Thus, ultrastructurally nodular hidradenoma seems to be intermediate between eccrine poroma, with its largely intraepidermal ductal differentiation, and eccrine spiradenoma, with is dermal-ductal and secretory differentiation. From this point of view, the clear cells represent immature poral epithelial cells, and the horn-pearl formation can be regarded as the keratinization of poral epithelial cells.

Differential Diagnosis. Nodular hidradenoma shares with trichilemmoma the presence of clear cells rich in glycogen. Foci of keratinization may also be found in both. However, only nodular hidradenoma usually shows the presence of large cystic spaces and of tubular lumina, and only trichilemmoma shows peripheral palisading of its tumor cells.

Although tumor nuclei may be hyperchromatic and there may be coarsely clumped chromatin, marked pleomorphism and frequent or atypical mitoses are not observed. If such changes are present, the tumor should be considered to have a potential for aggressive behavior. Zonal or diffuse patterns of necrosis also suggest malignancy, but the most important indicator of malignancy is an infiltrative, poorly circumscribed, and asymmetrical perimeter.

Nodular hidradenomas may occasionally reform after local excision. Associated distortion and fibrosis may impede the diagnostic interpretation when the histology of the primary lesion is unknown or unavailable. Lesions that have frequent mitoses or nuclear atypia but which lack clear evidence of asymmetric invasive growth may be termed atypical, and a reexcision to ensure their complete removal may be contemplated.

Malignant Nodular Hidradenoma

Malignant nodular hidradenomas are rare. Usually, they are malignant from their inception, but some develop from benign nodular hidradenomas.[351] These tumors present as a solitary nodule on the head, trunk, or distal extremity. Most reported cases are in patients over 50 years of age, though they may occur at any age. They tend to metastasize, and they may cause death. Although there is insufficient evidence in the literature, the recurrence rate may be estimated at about 50%, and the metastasis rate is about 60%, including regional nodes, bone, viscera, and skin.[351–355]

Histopathology. In contrast to benign nodular hidradenomas, which are well-demarcated, malignant nodular hidradenomas are larger, asymmetrical in their configuration, and show as a key feature evidence of invasion into the surrounding tissue (Fig. 31-62). There may be angiolymphatic invasion.[356] Mitoses are usually easily detected, and some may be atypical. Tumor necrosis, areas of high cellularity, and focal or diffuse areas of marked cytologic atypia in which differentiated elements are unrecognizable are present in some examples. In these, the diagnosis of malignancy may be evident, but the recognition of adnexal origin and the precise subclassification may be problematical. However, nuclear anaplasia may be only slight to moderate or even absent in both the primary tumor and the metastases. Nuclear anaplasia, if present, may be limited to the clear cells or affect both the polyhedral and the clear cells.

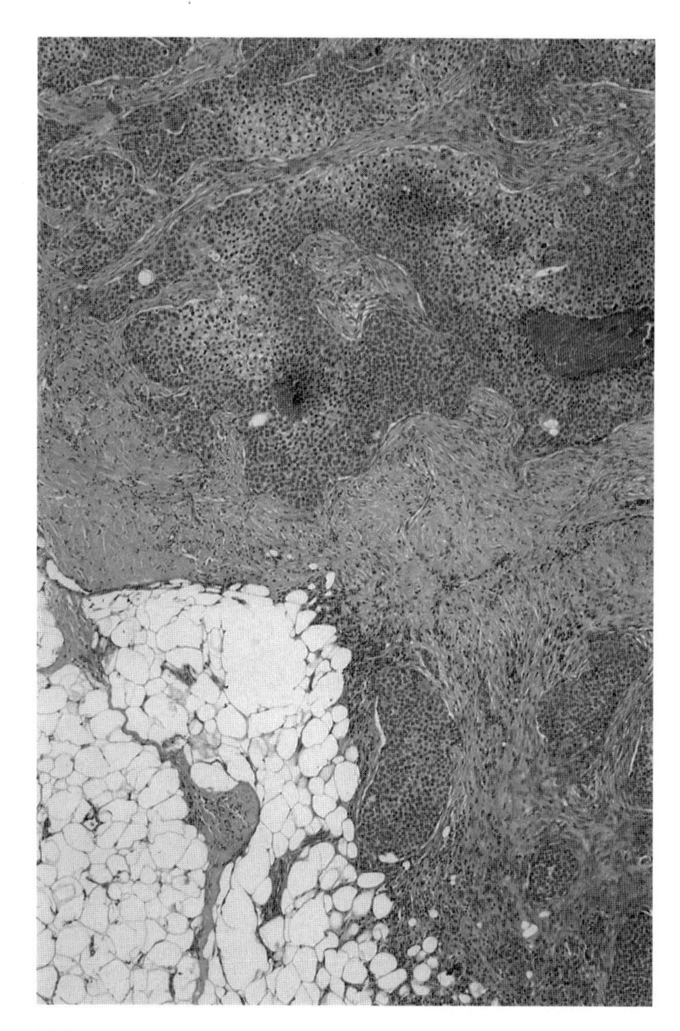

FIG. 31-62. Malignant nodular hidradenoma
A large, poorly circumscribed, and infiltrative tumor spans the dermis.

Chondroid Syringoma (Mixed Tumor of the Skin)

The term *chondroid syringoma,* introduced in 1961,[357] may be preferred to the alternative designation *mixed tumor of the skin* because of the recognition that the tumor is epithelial with merely secondary changes in the stroma. Chondroid syringomas are firm intradermal or subcutaneous nodules. Although the overlying skin may be attached to the tumor, it otherwise appears normal. Mixed tumors occur most commonly on the head and neck.[357] Their usual size is between 0.5 and 3.0 cm.

Histopathology. Histologically, two types of chondroid syringomas can be recognized: one with tubular and cystic, partially branching lumina, and the other with small, tubular lumina.[358] The former type is much more common than the latter.

Chondroid syringoma with tubular, branching lumina shows marked variation in the size and shape of the tubular lumina; it also shows cystic dilatation and branching (Fig. 31-63). Embedded in an abundant stroma, the tubular lumina are lined by two layers of epithelial cells: a luminal layer of cuboidal cells, and a peripheral layer of flattened cells. Furthermore, there are

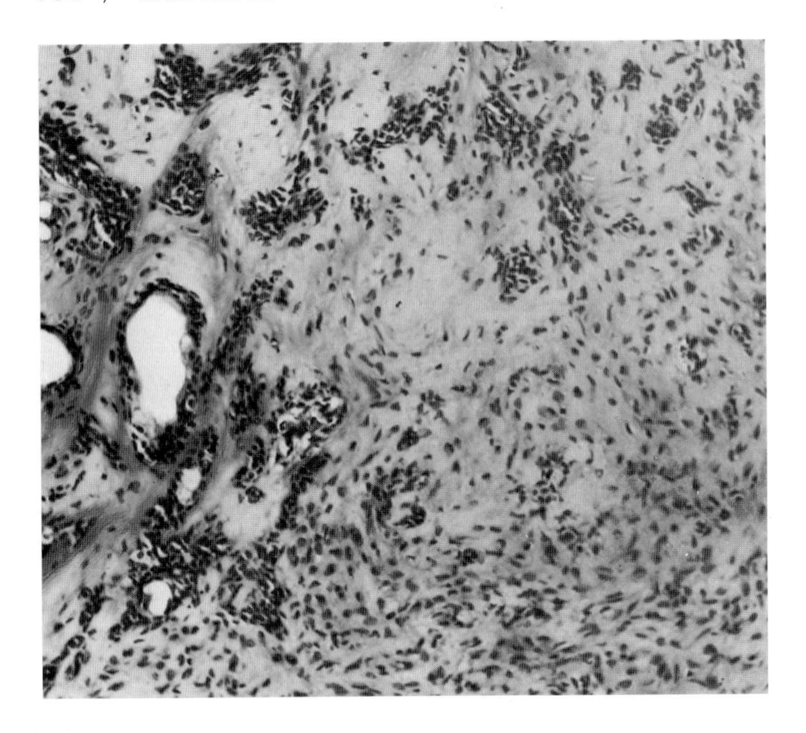

FIG. 31-63. Chondroid syringoma with tubular cystic lumina
Embedded in an abundant stroma, the tubular lumina are lined by two layers of cells: a luminal layer of cuboidal cells and a peripheral layer of flattened cells. Cells from the peripheral layer proliferate into the stroma, which has a mucoid, faintly basophilic appearance.

large and small aggregates of epithelial cells without lumina as well as single epithelial cells widely scattered through the stroma. It appears that cells from the peripheral cell layer of the tubular structures and from the solid aggregates proliferate into the stroma.[357] In most instances, the tubular lumina contain small amounts of amorphous, eosinophilic material that is PAS-positive and resistant to digestion with diastase. In general, the tubular structures are suggestive of eccrine differentiation.[357] Occasionally, the luminal cells show an apocrine type of decapitation secretion, at least in some areas.[358–361]

The abundant stroma in many areas has a mucoid, faintly basophilic appearance. As a result of shrinkage of the mucoid substance, the fibroblasts and epithelial cells that are scattered through it are surrounded by a halo, so that they resemble the cells of cartilage. The mucoid stroma stains with alcian blue, mucicarmine, and aldehyde-fuchsin. The alcian blue material is not appreciably decreased by predigestion with hyaluronidase.[357] Furthermore, on staining with toluidine blue or the Giemsa stain, there is distinct metachromasia.[362] Therefore, it can be concluded that the mucin consists largely of sulfated acid mucopolysaccharides, or chondroitin sulfate. The stroma is histochemically similar to normal cartilage.[357] In a few areas, the stroma may appear homogeneous and eosinophilic, like hyalin, and is then PAS-positive and diastase-resistant.[357,363]

Chondroid syringoma with small, tubular lumina shows numerous small ducts as well as small groups of epithelial cells and solitary epithelial cells scattered through a mucoid stroma (Fig. 31-64). The tubular lumina are lined by only a single layer of flat epithelial cells, from which small, comma-like proliferations often extend into the stroma, resembling a syringoma.[358] The mucoid stroma contains acid mucopolysaccharides that stain metachromatically with toluidine blue.

Histogenesis. By immunohistochemistry, the inner-layer cells express cytokeratin, CEA, and EMA. The outer cell layer is positive for vimentin, S-100 protein, NSE, and, occasionally, glial fibrillary acidic protein.[364–367] The tumor can show either eccrine or apocrine differentiation. In three cases examined by electron microscopy, eccrine differentiation was noted.[363,368] On the other hand, immunohistochemical examination with gross cystic disease fluid protein has indicated apocrine differentiation in both cases tested.[369] The stroma appears to evolve over time. Initially delicate stellate fibroblast-like cells possibly related to ductal myoepithelial cells are suspended in the alcian blue–positive, hyaluronidase-resistant myxoid stroma. Stromal cells may acquire cytoplasmic lipid, resulting in a scattering of mature signet ring fat cells within the myxoid background. In some lesions, there is complete synthesis and secretion of solid hyaline cartilage populated by cells in lacunae showing ultrastructural features of true chondrocytes and S-100 positivity.

Electron microscopic examination has shown that both ductal and secretory lumina are present, with the secretory lumina lined by clear and dark cells as in eccrine secretory lumina.[368] The cells of the outer layer of the tubuloalveolar and ductal structures, like myoepithelial cells, contain numerous filaments and extend into the chondroid matrix, which they apparently produce.[363] No chondrocytes were seen in the chondroid matrix in one study.[363] In another study, the stroma showed epithelial cells and fibroblasts embedded in a fibrocollagenous matrix and islands of cartilaginous tissue containing chondrocytes with ultrastructural features similar to mature cartilage.[368] In this particular case, foci of ossification were also observed, indicating that metaplasia into cartilage and bone had taken place.

Differential Diagnosis. Although most mixed tumors do not

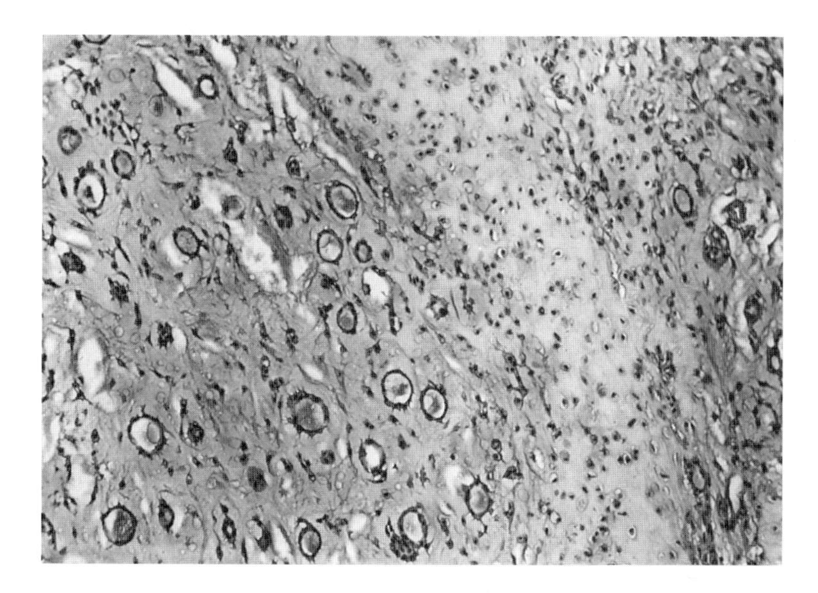

FIG. 31-64. Chondroid syringoma with small tubular lumina
There are numerous small tubular lumina lined with a single layer of epithelial cells. There also are small groups of epithelial cells and solitary epithelial cells. The epithelial structures are embedded in a mucoid stroma.

recur after surgical excision, seeding and regrowth of stromal and epithelial elements may occur, especially after an incomplete curettage. Lack of symmetry and an infiltrative pattern of growth are important features in distinguishing between benign mixed tumors and the rarely encountered malignant variant (see text following).[370]

Malignant Chondroid Syringoma

In most cases of malignant chondroid syringoma, anaplastic changes are present from the beginning.[371] Rarely, a chondroid syringoma of many years' duration suddenly undergoes malignant changes with widespread metastases.[372,373] The degree of malignancy varies. There may be only a local recurrence,[374] but some cases have shown regional lymph node metastases[375] or an osseous metastasis.[371] In several cases fatal visceral metastases have occurred.[376–379] When this tumor metastasizes, it generally does so as an adenocarcinoma, leaving behind any tendency to form chondroid stroma.

Histopathology. Histologically, malignant chondroid syringoma is composed of epithelial structures with glandular differentiation and carcinomatous features, embedded in a mucinous stroma with spindle mesenchymal cells and areas of chondroid differentiation. Unlike biphasic synovial sarcoma, in which both components express cytokeratins, only the epithelial structures of malignant chondroid syringoma are cytokeratin-positive. The malignant tumor and its metastases are recognizable as chondroid syringoma through their chondroid stroma and tubular structures. However, tubular differentiation is much less evident than in benign lesions.[376] Most of the epithelial cells in the malignant tumor are arranged in irregular cords.[374] The tumor cells appear atypical and hyperchromatic.[375] In addition, an increased mitotic rate, vascular invasion, infiltration into the surrounding tissue, and necrosis have been noted.[371]

MISCELLANEOUS CARCINOMAS OF ECCRINE GLANDS

Carcinomas of eccrine glands can be divided in several different ways.[380–383] For convenience of description, two groups can be established based on the relationship of the carcinoma to a benign sweat gland tumor. One group is related to benign eccrine tumors, in which they arise either through malignant degeneration by a process of tumor progression or de novo as malignant counterparts. These tumors have already been discussed along with their benign counterparts. In this group are malignant eccrine poroma, malignant eccrine spiradenoma, malignant nodular hidradenoma, and malignant chondroid syringoma. The second group comprises primary eccrine carcinomas that have no benign counterpart. In this group are the classic type of eccrine adenocarcinoma, syringoid eccrine carcinoma, microcystic adnexal carcinoma, mucinous (adenocystic) carcinoma, adenoid cystic carcinoma, and aggressive digital papillary adenocarcinoma.

Only few lesions of primary eccrine carcinoma possess a clinical appearance suggesting an eccrine malignancy. Although they may arise on the palms[10,384] or on the soles,[385] they more commonly arise elsewhere, particularly in the head and neck region.[386]

Classic Type of Eccrine Adenocarcinoma

The classic type of eccrine gland adenocarcinoma has a high incidence of metastases. Of 68 patients followed for 5 years or more, 29 had regional lymph node metastases, and visceral metastases were present in 26.[387]

The histologic configuration in the classic type of eccrine gland adenocarcinoma varies from fairly well differentiated tubular structures in some areas to anaplastic cells in other areas, not recognizable by themselves as eccrine sweat gland structures.[385] The tubular structures usually show only small lumina that are lined by either a single layer or a double layer of cells (Fig. 31-65).[385] In some areas, the lumina are lined by secretory cells, which appear large and vacuolated because of the presence of glycogen and which often contain also PAS-positive, diastase-resistant granules.[10,388]

It is often difficult to differentiate the classic type of eccrine sweat gland carcinoma from a metastatic adenocarcinoma. Therefore, the diagnosis of metastatic adenocarcinoma should always be given serious consideration before a diagnosis of eccrine sweat gland carcinoma is decided upon. Immunohistochemical techniques have been of no help.[386] So-called eccrine enzymes, such as amylophosphorylase and succinic dehydrogenase, may be present in moderate amounts, but their role in the recognition of the tumors as eccrine rather than as metastatic has not been well defined.[10,389]

Syringoid Eccrine Carcinoma

This tumor was originally referred to in 1969 as *basal cell tumor with eccrine differentiation*[390] and subsequently as *eccrine epithelioma*[391]; the term *syringoid eccrine carcinoma* is preferable because the tumor differs from basal cell carcinoma in its cytologic and enzymatic patterns. It represents a relatively well differentiated form of eccrine carcinoma.[392] Although first reported as a deeply invasive and destructive tumor of the scalp,[390] it also occurs in other locations.[392] Metastases rarely occur.[392]

Histologically, syringoid eccrine carcinoma resembles syringoma by showing ductal, cystic, and comma-like epithelial components and by containing eccrine enzymes such as phosphorylase and succinic dehydrogenase.[390] It differs from syringoma by its cellularity, anaplasia, and deep invasiveness. This uncommonly diagnosed tumor is probably related to the microcystic adnexal carcinoma described in text following.

Microcystic Adnexal Carcinoma

Microcystic adnexal carcinoma, or sclerosing sweat duct carcinoma,[393,394] may best be considered as a sclerosing variant of ductal eccrine carcinoma. This tumor, which is most commonly seen on the skin of the upper lip,[49] but occasionally also on the chin, nasolabial fold, or cheek,[394] is an aggressive neoplasm that invades deeply. Local recurrence is common; however, metastases have not been reported. Histologically, microcystic adnexal carcinoma is a poorly circumscribed dermal tumor that may extend into the subcutis and skeletal muscle. Continuity with the epidermis or follicular epithelium may be seen. Two components within a desmoplastic stroma may be evident. In some areas, basaloid keratinocytes are seen, some of which contain horn cysts and abortive hair follicles; in other areas, ducts and gland-like structures lined by a two-cell layer predominate (Figs. 31-66, 31-67, and 31-68).[49] The tumor islands typically reduce in size as the tumor extends deeper into the dermis. Cells with clear cytoplasm may be present, and sebaceous differentiation has been reported.[395] Cytologically, the cells are bland without significant atypia; mitoses are rare or absent. Perineural invasion may be seen, a feature that may account for the high recurrence rate.

Immunoperoxidase staining for carcinoembryonic antigen stains the glandular structures but not the pilar structures.[394] The presence of both pilar and eccrine structures allows differentiation from desmoplastic trichoepithelioma and syringoma. Lack of circumscription, deep dermal involvement, and perineural involvement all aid in diagnosis, since the cytology mimics benign adnexal neoplasms. This diagnosis should always be considered and complete excision contemplated when a syringo-

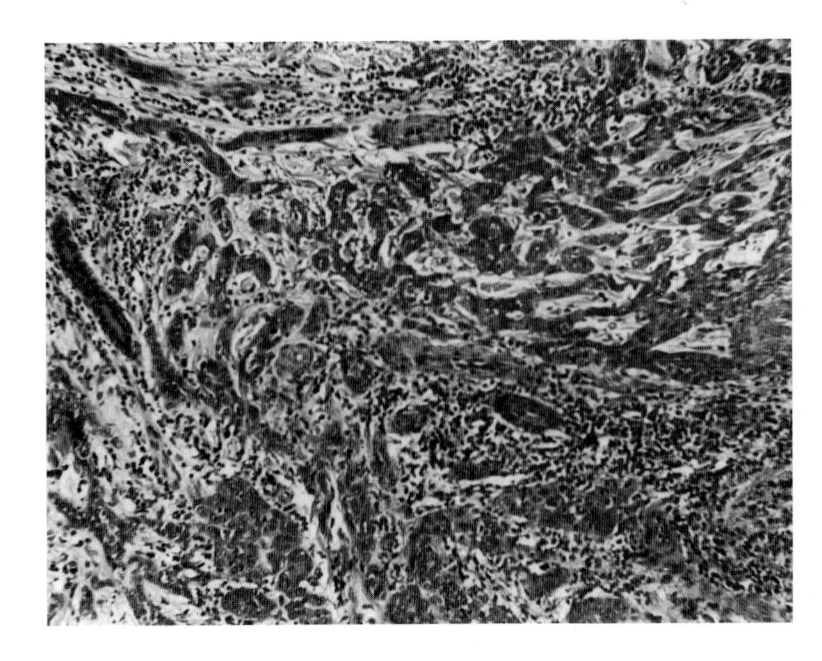

FIG. 31-65. Eccrine gland adenocarcinoma The tumor consists largely of tubular structures. Some of the tubules show a narrow lumen.

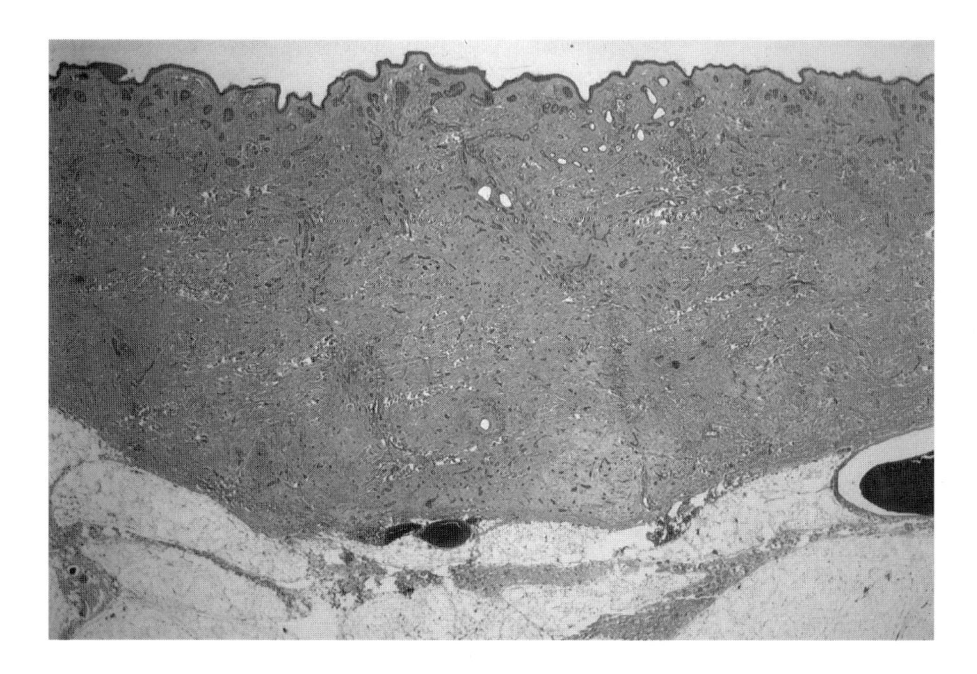

FIG. 31-66. Microcystic adnexal carcinoma
There is a large, poorly circumscribed tumor that invades deeply into the dermis and extends into the superficial subcutis.

matous or trichoepithelioma-like proliferation extends to the base of a biopsy, especially in an elderly patient.

Mucinous Eccrine Carcinoma

In this rather uncommon mucinous carcinoma of eccrine glands, first described in 1971,[396] regional lymph node metastases occur occasionally.[397] However, widespread metastases have been described very rarely.[398]

The histologic appearance is highly characteristic.[399] The tumor is divided into numerous compartments by strands of fibrous tissue. In each compartment, abundant amounts of pale-staining mucin surround nests or cords of moderately anaplastic epithelial cells, some of which show a tubular lumen (Fig. 31-69).[396,400] The mucin shows strongly positive reactions with both PAS and colloidal iron. The mucinous material is resistant to diastase and hyaluronidase but is sensitive to digestion with sialidase. The reaction with alcian blue is positive at pH 2.5 but negative at pH 1.0 and pH 0.4, which indicates that the mucin is

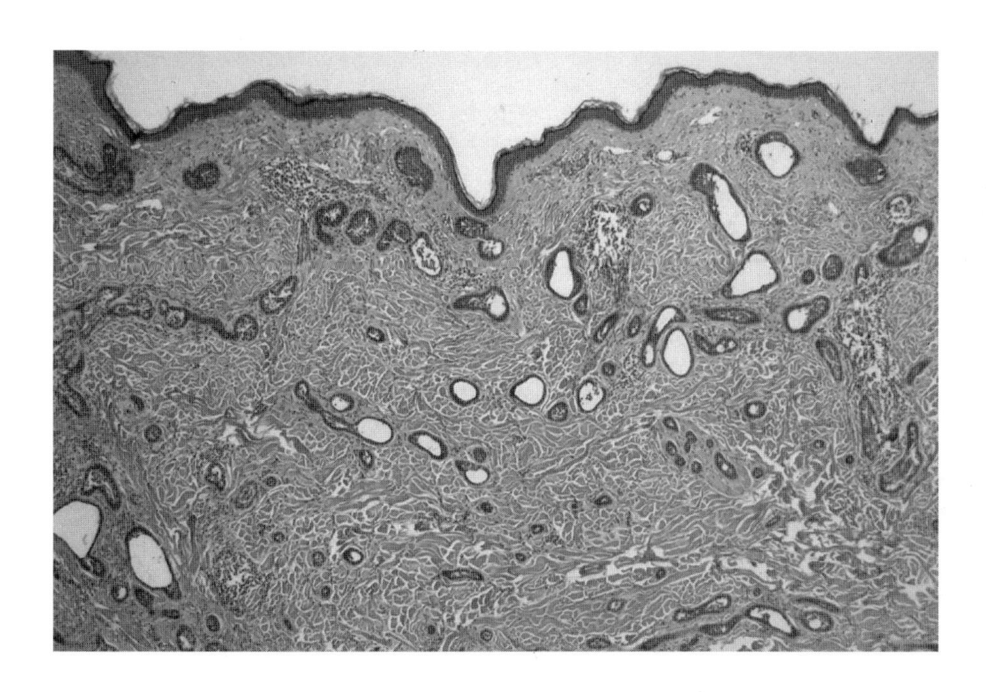

FIG. 31-67. Microcystic adnexal carcinoma
Superficial cystic glands may be mistaken for the cysts of a trichopithelioma or the glands of a benign syringoma, but the lesion invades deeply into the dermis (see also Fig. 31-68).

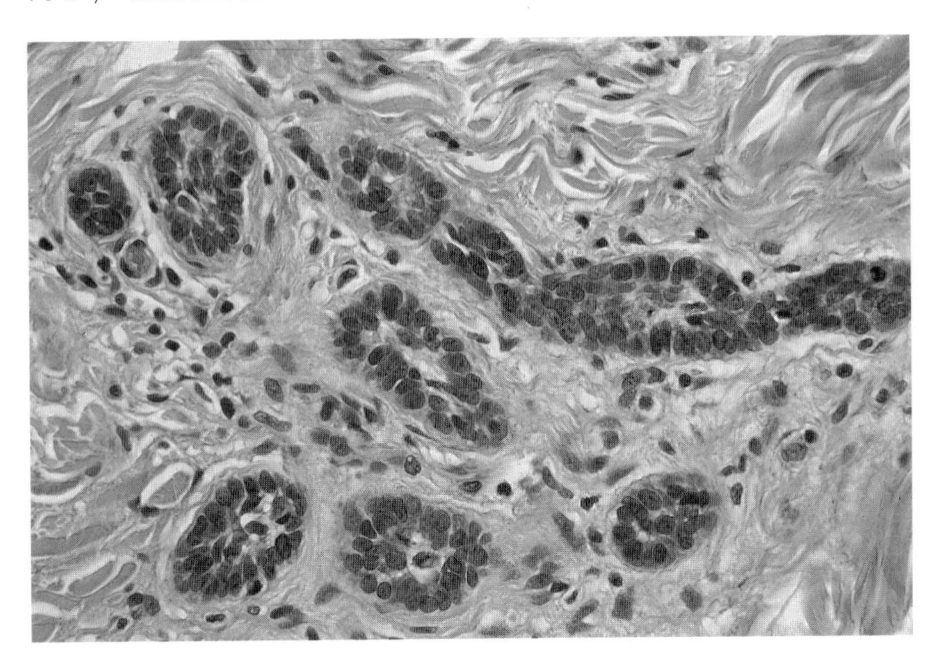

FIG. 31-68. Microcystic adnexal carcinoma
Low-grade nuclear atypia and occasional mitoses are present.

nonsulfated.[401] It can be concluded that the mucin represents sialomucin, an epithelial mucin.[396,400]

Enzyme histochemical examination has revealed a prevalence of enzymes of the eccrine type.[400] Electron microscopy has revealed two types of secretory cells in the tumor, dark and light, analogous to the two types normally encountered in eccrine coils. The sialomucin is secreted by the dark cells.[402] Immunohistochemical results also suggest differentiation toward eccrine secretory coil.[403]

It is important to differentiate this tumor from a metastatic mucinous adenocarcinoma, in which the primary lesion most commonly is located in the large intestines.[396] In both primary and metastatic mucinous adenocarcinoma, islands of tumor cells appear to be floating in lakes of mucin, but the tumor cells

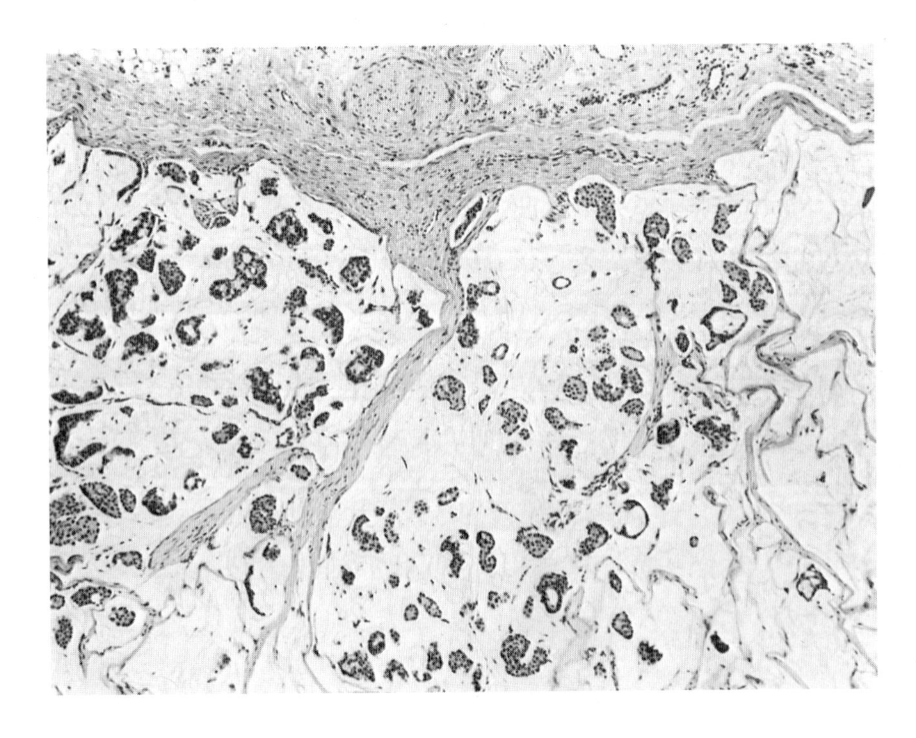

FIG. 31-69. Mucinous eccrine adenocarcinoma
The tumor is divided into numerous compartments. In each compartment, abundant amounts of mucin surround small islets of tumor cells, some of which show a lumen. (From Headington JT. Primary mucinous carcinoma of the skin. Cancer 1977;39:1055–1063.)

are more atypical in the metastatic type and the atypical cells invade between collagen bundles at the margin of the nodule.[404] Exclusion of primary visceral carcinomas is often impossible by histology alone.

Mucoepidermoid (Low-Grade Adenosquamous) Carcinoma

This tumor, which combines well-differentiated squamous and glandular epithelium, is histologically identical to that of salivary glands, and may occur as a primary cutaneous malignancy.[405,406]

Adenoid Cystic Carcinoma

The rarest type of eccrine sweat gland carcinomas is the adenoid cystic carcinoma, first described in 1975.[407] Metastases have been reported but are uncommon.[408] This indolent tumor, like its more aggressive counterpart in sweat glands, spreads in perineural spaces[408,409] and therefore recurs in 20% of cases.

Histologic examination reveals large cell masses with an adenoid or cribriform pattern and many small, solid epithelial islands (Fig. 31-70). Round spaces formed by malignant epithelial cells and containing amphophilic basement membrane–like material occur in the cribriform type and tubular variants.[410]

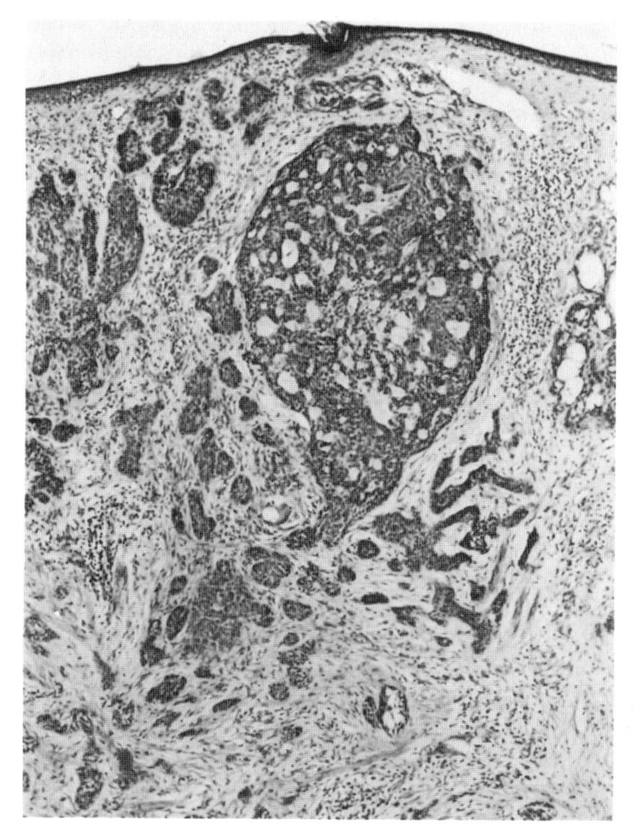

FIG. 31-70. Adenoid cystic carcinoma of eccrine glands A large cell mass shows an adenoid or cribriform pattern. In addition, many small, solid epithelial islands are present. (From Headington JT et al. Primary adenoid cystic carcinoma of the skin. Arch Dermatol 1978;114:421–424.)

Through the accumulation of mucin, the adenoid spaces may be transformed into multiple cystic spaces lined by a flattened cuboidal epithelium. The adenoid and cystic spaces contain pale-staining mucin that in some cases is hyaluronidase-sensitive[411] but in others was resistant to hyaluronidase digestion and reacted with the alcian blue stain at pH 2.5 and at pH 0.5.[412] In several instances there has been invasion of perineural spaces. The tumor is immunoreactive for carcinoembryonic antigen, amylase, and S-100 protein.[412]

Adenoid cystic carcinoma of eccrine glands must be distinguished from the adenoid type of basal cell carcinoma, from which it differs by lack of continuity with the epidermis or hair sheath and by the absence of palisading.[411] In addition, the adenoid type of basal cell carcinoma shows negative reactions to carcinoembryonic antigen, amylase, and S-100 protein.[412] Cutaneous extension from a parotid tumor or scar recurrence should be ruled out in adjacent body sites.

Aggressive Digital Papillary Adenoma/Adenocarcinoma

These tumors occur on the fingers, toes, and adjacent skin of the palms and soles, especially in adult males, as a single, often cystic mass that rarely ulcerates but often invades soft tissue.[413]

Histopathology. The tumor forms a spectrum with papillary eccrine adenoma. Characteristic histologic findings include tubuloalveolar and ductal structures with areas of papillary projections protruding into sometimes cystically dilated lumina. Macropapillae lined by atypical epithelial cells project into microcysts. These areas may merge with more cellular regions of moderately differentiated adenocarcinoma. Metastatic papillary carcinoma from breast, lung, thyroid, and ovary may be simulated. Low-grade ("aggressive digital papillary adenoma") and high-grade (adenocarcinoma) variants are distinguished by degree of pleomorphism, mitotic rate, and necrosis. As expected, the high-grade variants are more likely to recur and metastasize. About two thirds of these tumors can be classified as adenomas; but one third shows poor glandular differentiation, cellular atypia, areas of necrosis, and deep invasion, occasionally even of bone, and represent carcinomas.

Nearly half of the tumors regarded as carcinomas develop metastases, often involving the lung.

CARCINOMA OF APOCRINE GLANDS

Carcinomas of apocrine glands have been described only rarely.[414–419] They occur mainly in the axillae[415,416] and in other areas endowed with apocrine glands, such as the anogenital region, but occasionally elsewhere on the skin.[414,417] An occasional location of apocrine carcinomas is the external auditory meatus, where ceruminal glands are found as modified apocrine glands.[420,421] The tumor may extend to the ear and preauricular skin.[422]

Some cases of carcinoma of apocrine glands show only local invasiveness,[415,417] but others metastasize to regional lymph nodes,[416] and some patients have died from widespread metastases.[414,417]

Histopathology. The histologic picture is that of an adenocarcinoma that is fairly well, moderately, or poorly differentiated.[415]

In fairly well differentiated apocrine gland carcinomas, nuclear atypicality and invasiveness are limited in degree. Well-developed glandular lumina are present (Fig. 31-71). The lumina may be cystic and show branching.[415] The cytoplasm of the tumor cells is strongly eosinophilic. Evidence of decapitation secretion, typical of apocrine glands, is present at least in some areas. In addition, the cytoplasm of the tumor cells contains PAS-positive, diastase-resistant granules and often contains iron-positive granules.[415] Myoepithelial cells are seen rarely.[417]

In moderately or poorly differentiated apocrine gland carcinomas, recognition of an apocrine genesis may be difficult, although even poorly differentiated tumors often show fairly good differentiation in some areas.[415]

Histogenesis. Enzyme histochemical determinations are of value in establishing an apocrine genesis, because apocrine gland carcinomas show strong activity of apocrine enzymes, such as acid phosphatase, β-glucuronidase, and indoxyl acetate esterase, and low activity or absence of eccrine enzymes, such as phosphorylase and succinic dehydrogenase.[414,417]

Differential Diagnosis. Apocrine gland carcinoma of the axilla must be differentiated from a carcinoma arising in ectopic breast tissue. Features that favor the diagnosis of a carcinoma of apocrine glands are the presence of neoplastic glands high in the dermis, apocrine glands near the tumor, and intracytoplasmic granules of iron.[415]

CUTANEOUS ENDOMETRIOSIS

Cutaneous endometriosis is discussed here because it is composed of endometrial glands and stroma, which potentially could be confused with a skin appendage tumor. It is characterized by the presence of a solitary brown or blue nodule 0.5 to 6.0 cm in diameter. The lesion, which is quite rare, is seen only in adult women. Most commonly, it occurs in a surgical scar of the abdominal or genital region, especially following a cesarean section. However, the lesion may arise spontaneously in the umbilicus and, rarely, in the inguinal area.[423] Quite often, the lesion is slightly tender and painful. At the time of menstruation, these symptoms usually become more pronounced and may be associated with swelling and slight bleeding of the lesion. However, there are asymptomatic lesions, some of which are even unresponsive to menstruation.[424] It may, in rare cases, undergo malignant transformation, giving rise to endometrioid carcinoma.

Histopathology. Irregular glandular lumina are embedded in a highly cellular and vascular stroma resembling the stroma of the functioning endometrium.[425] The lining of the lumina may correspond to that of the uterine endometrium during the phases of the menstrual cycle. The proliferative phase is suggested by pseudostratification and epithelial mitotic activity; the secretory phase may be demonstrated by evidence of decapitation secretion within the glandular cells. Disintegration of the epithelium and the presence of erythrocytes in the lumina may resemble menstrual endometrium. However, no good correlation exists between the histologic appearance of the lumina in the cutaneous lesion and the menstrual stage.[426] The glandular component characteristic of genital endometriosis is often absent in extragenital lesions, which may be solely composed of stromal decidual nodules. Thus the absence of glands does not preclude a diagnosis of decidualized endometriosis. Evidence of stromal hemorrhage is usually also present.

Pathogenesis. In cases in which cutaneous endometriosis develops in surgical scars, implantation of viable endometrial cells is probably the cause. In contrast, in cases of spontaneously arising cutaneous endometriosis, it appears most likely that the endometrial tissue is transported to the area by way of lymphatic or vascular channels.[423]

Differential Diagnosis. Hypertrophic or myxoid decidual change during pregnancy may sometimes cause differential diagnostic difficulties with metastatic carcinoma or other malignancies, especially when large pools of sulfated mucopolysaccharides secreted by the decidual cells form pseudoalveoli.

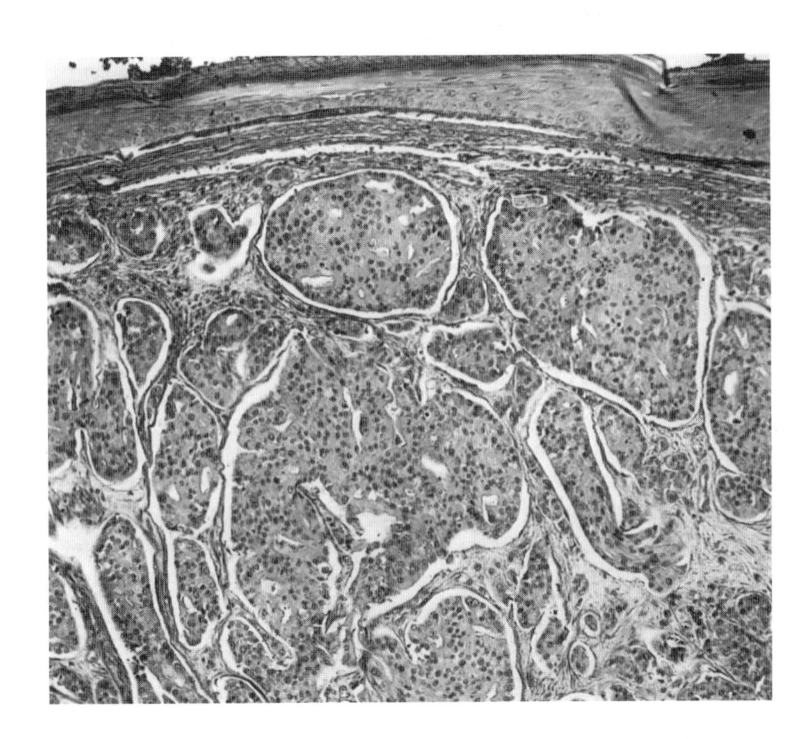

FIG. 31-71. Apocrine carcinoma of the vulva The tumor consists of atypical glandular cells with eosinophilic cytoplasm and active "decapitation" secretion.

Cutaneous Endosalpingiosis

On rare occasions, multiple brown papules averaging 5 mm in diameter develop after a salpingectomy around the umbilicus, but not necessarily within the laparotomy incision scar.

Histopathology. Each papule contains beneath an intact epidermis, a unilocular cyst with papillary projections into the lumen. The lining consists of epithelium as seen in the fallopian tube, that is, of columnar cells, some of them ciliated and others secretory.[427] The lining thus resembles that seen in cutaneous ciliated cysts (see Chap. 30).[428]

REFERENCES

1. Buchi ER, Peng Y, Eng AM et al. Eccrine acrospiroma of the eyelid with onocytic, apocrine and sebaceous differentiation: Further evidence for pluripotentiality of the adnexal epithelia. Eur J Ophthalmol 1991;1:187.
2. Sanchez Yus E, Requena L, Simon P, Sanchez M. Complex adnexal tumor of the primary epithelial germ with distinct patterns of superficial epithelioma with sebaceous differentiation, immature trichoepithelioma, and apocrine adenocarcinoma. Am J Dermatopathol 1992; 14:245.
3. Weyers W, Nilles M, Eckert F, Schill W-B. Spiradenomas in Brooke-Speigler syndrome. Am J Dermatopathol 1993;15:156.
4. Massa MC, Medenica M. Cutaneous adnexal tumors and cysts: A review. Part 1: Tumors with hair follicle differentiation and cysts related to different parts of the hair follicle. Pathol Annu 1985;20:189.
5. Wong T-Y, Suster S, Cheek RF, Mihm MC. Benign cutaneous adnexal tumors with combined folliculosebaceous, apocrine and eccrine differentiation: Clinicopathologic and immunohistochemical study of eight cases. Am J Dermatopathol 1996;18:124.
6. Penneys NS. Immunohistochemistry of adnexal neoplasma. J Cutan Pathol 1984;11:357.
7. Kligman AM, Pinkus H. The histogenesis of nevoid tumors of the skin. Arch Dermatol 1960;81:922.
8. Lever WF. Pathogenesis of benign tumors of cutaneous appendages and of basal cell epithelioma. Arch Dermatol Syph 1948;57:679.
9. Heenan PJ, Elder DE, Sobin LH. Histological typing of skin tumours. Berlin Heidelberg: Springer, 1996;3.
10. Hashimoto K, Lever WF. Appendage tumors of the skin. Springfield, IL: Charles C Thomas, 1968.
11. Wechsler HL, Fisher ER. A combined polymorphic and adnexal tumor in nevus unius lateris. Dermatologica 1964;130:158.
12. Pinkus H. Premalignant fibroepithelial tumors of the skin. Arch Dermatol Syph 1953;67:598.
13. Mehregan AH. The origin of the adnexal tumors of the skin: A viewpoint. J Cutan Pathol 1985;12:459.
14. Brownstein MH. The genodermatology of adnexal tumors. J Cutan Pathol 1984;11:457.
15. Albrecht E. Uber hamartome. Verh Dtsch Ges Pathol 1904;7:153.
16. Jadassohn J. Die benignen epitheliome. Arch Dermatol Syph 1914; 117:705, 833.
17. Murphy GF, Elder DE. Nomenclature, classification and staging. In: Murphy GF, Elder DE, eds. Non-melanocytic tumors of the skin. Washington, DC: Armed Forces Institute of Pathology, 1990;9.
18. Pippione M, Aloi F, Depaoli MA. Hair-follicule nevus. Am J Dermatopathol 1984;6:245.
19. Pinkus H, Sutton RL Jr. Trichofolliculoma. Arch Dermatol 1965;91: 46.
20. Gray HR, Helwig EB. Trichofolliculoma. Arch Dermatol 1962;86:619.
21. Hyman AB, Clayman SJ. Hair follicle nevus. Arch Dermatol 1957;75: 678.
22. Sanderson KV. Hair follicle naevus. Trans St Johns Hosp Dermatol Soc 1961;47:154.
23. Plewig G. Sebaceous trichofolliculoma. J Cutan Pathol 1980;7:394.
24. Winer L. The dilated pore, a trichoepithelioma. J Invest Dermatol 1954;23:181.
25. Mehregan AH, Brownstein MH. Pilar sheath acanthoma. Arch Dermatol 1978;114:1495.
26. Bhawan J. Pilar sheath acanthoma. J Cutan Pathol 1979;6:438.
27. Birt AR, Hogg GR, Dubé J. Hereditary multiple fibrofolliculomas with trichodiscomas and acrochordons. Arch Dermatol 1977;113: 1674.
28. Fujita WH, Barr RJ, Headley JL. Multiple fibrofolliculomas with trichodiscomas and acrochordons. Arch Dermatol 1981;117:32.
29. Weintraub R, Pinkus H. Multiple fibrofolliculomas (Birt-Hogg-Dubé associated with a large connective tissue nevus. J Cutan Pathol 1977; 4:289.
30. Pinkus H, Coskey R, Burgess GH. Trichodiscoma: A benign tumor related to the *Haarscheibe* (hair disk). J Invest Dermatol 1974;63:212.
31. Grosshans E, Dungler T, Hanau D. Le trichodiscome de Pinkus. Ann Dermatol Venereol 1981;108:837.
32. Scully K, Bargman H, Assaad D. Solitary fibrofolliculoma. J Am Acad Dermatol 1984;11:361.
33. Gaul LE. Heredity of multiple benign cystic epithelioma. Arch Dermatol Syph 1953;68:517.
34. Gray HR, Helwig EB. Epithelioma adenoides cysticum and solitary trichoepithelioma. Arch Dermatol 1963;87:102.
35. Pariser RJ. Multiple hereditary trichoepitheliomas and basal cell carcinomas. J Cutan Pathol 1986;13:111.
36. Howell JB, Anderson DE. Transformation of epithelioma adenoides cysticum into multiple rodent ulcers: Fact or fallacy? Br J Dermatol 1976;95:233.
37. Zeligman I. Solitary trichoepithelioma. Arch Dermatol 1960;82:35.
38. Müller-Hess S, Delacrétaz J. Trichoepitheliom mit strukturen eines apokrinen adenoms. Dermatologica 1973;146:170.
39. Tatnall FM, Wilson Jones E. Giant solitary trichoepitheliomas located in the perianal area: A report of three cases. Br J Dermatol 1986;115: 91.
40. Filho GB, Toppa NH, Miranda D et al. Giant solitary trichoepithelioma. Arch Dermatol 1984;120:797.
41. Headington JT. Tumors of the hair follicle: A review. Am J Pathol 1976;85:479.
42. Ackerman AB, de Viragh PA, Chonchitnant N. Trichoblastoma: Trichoepithelioma. In: Ackerman AB, de Viragh PA, Chonchitnant N, eds. Tumors with follicular differentation. Philadelphia: Lea & Febiger, 1993;359.
43. Gilks CB, Clement PB, Wood WS. Trichoblastic fibroma. Am J Dermatopathol 1989;11:397.
44. Kyllönen AP, Stenbäck F, Väänänen R. Trichoepitheliomatous tumors: Morphology and ultrastructure (abstr). J Cutan Pathol 1981;8: 167.
45. Kopf AW. The distribution of alkaline phosphatase in normal and pathologic human skin. Arch Dermatol 1957;75:1.
46. Brownstein MH, Shapiro L. Desmoplastic trichoepithelioma. Cancer 1977;40:2979.
47. MacDonald DM, Wilson Jones E, Marks R. Sclerosing epithelial hamartoma. Clin Exp Dermatol 1977;2:153.
48. Dupré A, Bonafé JL, Lassére J. Hamartome épithélial sclérosant: Forme clinique du trichoépithéliome. Ann Dermatol Venereol 1980; 107:649.
49. Goldstein DJ, Barr RJ, Santa Cruz DJ. Microcystic adnexal carcinoma: A distinct clinicopathologic entity. Cancer 1982;50:566.
50. Leppard BJ, Sanderson KV. The natural history of trichilemmal cysts. Br J Dermatol 1976;94:379.
51. Nikolowski W. Tricho-adenom. Arch Klin Exp Dermatol 1958;207:34.
52. Rahbari H, Mehregan A, Pinkus H. Trichoadenoma of Nikolowski: J Cutan Pathol 1977;4:90.
53. Nikolowski W. Trichoadenom. Z Hautkr 1977;53:87.
54. Undeutsch W, Rassner G. Das trichoadenom (Nikolowski). Hautarzt 1984;35:650.
55. Long SA, Hurt MA, Santa Cruz DJ. Immature trichoepithelioma: Report of six cases. J Cutan Pathol 1988;15:353.
56. Brown AC, Crounse RG, Winkelmann RK. Generalized hair-follicle hamartoma. Arch Dermatol 1969;99:478.
57. Ridley CM, Smith N. Generalized hair follicle hamartoma associated with alopecia and myasthenia gravis: Report of a second case. Clin Exp Dermatol 1981;6:283.
58. Starink TM, Lane EB, Meijer CJLM. Generalized trichoepithelioma with alopecia and myasthenia gravis (abstr). J Cutan Pathol 1986;13: 86.
59. Weltfriend S, David M, Ginzburg A et al. Generalized hair follicle hamartoma. Am J Dermatopathol 1987:9:428.

60. Mehregan AH, Baker S. Basaloid follicular hamartoma. J Cutan Pathol 1985;12:55.
61. Swerlick RA, Cooper PH, Mackel SE. Rapid enlargement of pilomatricoma. J Am Acad Dermatol 1982;7:54.
62. Uchiyama N, Shindo Y, Saida T. Perforating pilomatricomas. J Cutan Pathol 1986;13:312.
63. Moehlenbeck F. Pilomatrixoma: Calicifying epithelioma. Arch Dermatol 1973;108:532.
64. Chiaramonti A, Gilgor RS. Pilomatricomas associated with myotonic dystrophy. Arch Dermatol 1978;114:1363.
65. Panico L, Manivel JC, Pettinato G et al. Pilomatrix carcinoma: A case report with immunohistochemical findings, flow cytometric comparison with benign pilomatrixoma and review of the literature. Tumori 1994;80:308.
66. Sau P, Lupton GP, Graham JH. Pilomatrix carcinoma. Cancer 1993; 71:2491.
67. Gould E, Kurzon R, Kowalczyk P et al. Pilomatrix carcinoma with pulmonary metastases. Cancer 1984;54:370.
68. Hanly MG, Allsbrook WC, Pantazis CG et al. Pilomatrical carcinosarcoma of the cheek with subsequent pulmonary metatases: A case report. Am J Dermatopathol 1994;16:196.
69. Solanki P, Ramzy I, Durr N et al. Pilomatrixoma. Arch Pathol 1987; 111:294.
70. Lever WF, Griesemer RD. Calcifying epithelioma of Malherbe. Arch Dermatol Syph 1949;59:506.
71. Cazers JS, Okun MR, Pearson SH. Pigmented calcifying epithelioma. Arch Dermatol 1974;110:773.
72. Peterson WC Jr, Hult AM. Calcifying epithelioma of Malherbe. Arch Dermatol 1964;90:404.
73. Forbis R Jr, Helwig EB. Pilomatrixoma: Calcifying epithelioma. Arch Dermatol 1961;83:606.
74. Wiedersberg H. Das epithelioma calcificans Malherbe. Dermatol Monatsschr 1971;157:867.
75. Malherbe A, Chenantais J. Note sur l'épithéliome calcifié des glandes sebacées. Prog Med 1880;8:826.
76. Turhan B, Krainer L. Bemerkungen über die sogenannten verkalkenden epitheliome der haut und ihre genese. Dermatologica 1942;85:73.
77. Hashimoto K, Nelson RG, Lever WF. Calcifying epithelioma of Malherbe: Histochemical and electron microscopic studies. J Invest Dermatol 1966;46:391.
78. Lever WF, Hashimoto K. Die histogenese einiger hautanhangstumoren im lichte histochemischer und elektronenmikroskopischer befunde. Hautarzt 1966;17:161.
79. McGavran MH. Ultrastructure of pilomatrixoma: Calcifying epithelioma. Cancer 1965;18:1445.
80. Hashimoto K, Lever WF. Histogenesis of skin appendage tumors. Arch Dermatol 1969;100:356.
81. Aloi FG, Molinero A, Pippione M. Basal cell carcinoma with matricial differentiation. Ann J Dermatopathol 1988;10:509.
82. Lopansri S, Mihm MC Jr. Pilomatrix carcinoma or calcifying epitheliocarcinoma of Malherbe. Cancer 1980;45:2368.
83. Van der Walt JD, Rohlova B. Carcinomatous transformation in a pilomatrixoma. Am J Dermatopathol 1984;6:63.
84. Wood MG, Parhizzar B, Beerman H. Malignant pilomatricoma. Arch Dermatol 1984;120:770.
85. Green DE, Sanusi ID, Fowler MR. Pilomatrix carcinoma. J Am Acad Dermatol 1987;17:264.
86. Mir R, Cortes E, Papantoniou PA et al. Metastatic trichomatricial carcinoma. Arch Pathol 1986;110:660.
87. Weedon D, Bell J, Mayze J. Matrical carcinoma of the skin. J Cutan Pathol 1980;7:39.
88. Hanau D, Grosshans E. Trichilemmal tumor undergoing specific keratinization. J Cutan Pathol 1979;6:463.
89. Poiares Baptista A, Garcia E, Silva L, Born MC. Proliferating trichilemmal cyst. J Cutan Pathol 1983;10:178.
90. Brownstein MH, Arluk DJ. Proliferating trichilemmal cyst. Cancer 1981;48:1207.
91. Holmes EJ. Tumors of lower hair sheath: The common histogenesis of certain so-called "sebaceous cysts," adenomas, and "sebaceous carcinomas." Cancer 1968;21:234.
92. Korting GW, Hoede N. Zum sogenannten "pilar tumor of the scalp." Arch Klin Exp Dermatol 1969;234:409.
93. Leppard BJ, Sanderson KV. The natural history of trichilemmal cysts. Br J Dermatol 1976;94:379.
94. Mehregan AH, Lee KC. Malignant proliferating trichilemmal tumors: Report of three cases. J Dermatol Surg Oncol 1987;13:1339.
95. Wilson Jones E. Proliferating epidermoid cysts. Arch Dermatol 1966; 94:11.
96. Reed RJ, Lamar LM. Invasive hair matrix tumors of the scalp. Arch Dermatol 1966;94:310.
97. Dabska M. Giant hair matrix tumor. Cancer 1971;28:701.
98. Pinkus H. "Sebaceous cysts" are trichilemmal cysts. Arch Dermatol 1969;99:544.
99. Saida T, Oahara K, Hori Y et al. Development of a malignant proliferating trichilemmal cyst in a patient with multiple trichilemmal cysts. Dermatologica 1983;166:203.
100. Amaral ALM, Nascimento AG, Goellner Jr. Proliferating pilar (trichilemmal) cyst. Arch Pathol 1984;108:808.
101. Hödl S, Smolle J, Scharnagl E. Zur dignität der proliferierenden trichilemmalzyste. Hautarzt 1984;35:640.
102. Headington JT, French AJ. Primary neoplasms of the hair follicle. Arch Dermatol 1962;86:430.
103. Brownstein MH, Shapiro L. Trichilemmoma. Arch Dermatol 1973; 107:866.
104. Mehregan AH, Medenica M, Whitney D. A clear cell pilar sheath tumor of scalp: Case report. J Cutan Pathol 1988;15:380.
105. Brownstein MH, Shapiro EE. Trichilemmal horn: Cutaneous horn overlying trichilemmoma. Clin Exp Dermatol 1979;4:59.
106. Crowson AN, Magro CM. Basal cell carcinoma arising in association with desmoplastic trichilemmoma. Am J Dermatopathol 1966;18:43.
107. Leonardi CL, Zhu WY, Kinsey WH, Penneys NS. Trichilemmomas are not associated with human papillomavirus DNA. J Cutan Pathol 1991;18:193.
108. Brownstein MH, Wolf M, Bikowski JB. Cowden's disease: A cutaneous marker of breast cancer. Cancer 1978;41:2393.
109. Allen BS, Fitch MH, Smith JG Jr. Multiple hamartoma syndrome. J Am Acad Dermatol 1980;2:303.
110. Brownstein MH, Mehregan AH, Bikowski B et al. The dermatopathology of Cowden's syndrome. Br J Dermatol 1979;100:667.
111. Thyresson HN, Doyle JA. Cowden's disease: Multiple hamartoma syndrome (review). Mayo Clin Proc 1981;56:179.
112. Starink TM, Hausman R. The cutaneous pathology of extrafacial lesions in Cowden's disease. J Cutan Pathol 1984;11:338.
113. Weary PE, Gorlin RJ, Gentry WC Jr et al. Multiple hamartoma syndrome: Cowden's disease. Arch Dermatol 1972;106:682.
114. Mehregan AH, Buttler JD. A tumor of follicular infundibulum. Arch Dermatol 1961;83:924.
115. Mehregan AH. Tumor of follicular infundibulum. Dermatologica 1971;142:177.
116. Johnson WC, Hookerman BJ. Basal cell hamartoma with follicular differentiation. Arch Dermatol 1972;105:105.
117. Chan P, White SW, Pierson DL et al. Trichilemmoma. J Dermatol Surg Oncol 1979;5:58.
118. Brownstein MH. Trichilemmal horn: Cutaneous horn showing trichilemmal keratinization. Br J Dermatol 1979;100:303.
119. Brownstein MH. Shapiro EE. Trichilemmomal horn: Cutaneous horn overlying trichilemmoma. Clin Exp Dermatol 1979;4:59.
120. Nakamura K. Two cases of trichilemmal-like horn. Arch Dermatol 1984;120:386.
121. Grouls V. Tricholemmale keratose und tricholemmales karzinom. Hautarzt 1987;38:335.
122. Wong TY, Suster S. Tricholemmal carcinoma: A clinicopathologic study of 13 cases. Am J Dermatopathol 1994;16:463.
123. Hunt SJ, Abell E. Malignant hair matrix tumor ("malignant trichoepithelioma") arising in the setting of multiple hereditary trichoepithelioma. Am J Dermatopathol 1991;13:275.
124. Boscaino A, Terracciano LM, Donofrio V et al. Tricholemmal carcinoma: A study of seven cases. J Cutan Pathol 1992;19:94.
125. Reis JP, Tellechea O, Cunha MF, Baptista AP. Trichilemmal carcinoma: Review of 8 cases. J Cutan Pathol 1993;20:44.
126. Ten Seldam REJ. Tricholemmocarcinoma. Australas J Dermatol 1977;18:62.
127. Schell H, Haneke E. Tricholemmales karzinom: Bericht über 11 fälle. Hautarzt 1985;37:384.
128. Headington JT. Tumors of the hair follicle: A review. Am J Pathol 1976;85:480.
129. Swanson PE, Cherwitz DL, Wick MR. Trichilemmal carcinoma: A clincopathologic study of 6 cases (abstr). J Cutan Pathol 1988;14:374.

130. Mehregan AH, Pinkus H. Life history of organoid nevi. Arch Dermatol 1965;91:574.
131. Lentz CL, Altman J, Mopper C. Nevus sebaceus of Jadassohn. Arch Dermatol 1968;97:294.
132. Feuerstein R, Mims L. Linear nevus sebaceus with convulsions and mental retardation. Am J Dis Child 1962;104:675.
133. Marden PM, Venters HD. A new neurocutaneous syndrome. Am J Dis Child 1966;112:79.
134. Wauschkuhn J, Rohde B. Systematisierte talgdrüsen-, pigment-, und epitheliale naevi mit neurologischer symptomatik: Feuerstein-Mimssches neuroektodermales syndrom. Hautarzt 1971;22:10.
135. Hornstein OP, Knickenberg M. Zur kenntnis des Schimmelpenning-Feuerstein-Mims-syndroms. Arch Dermatol Forsch 1974;250:33.
136. Solomon LW, Fretzin DF, Dewald RL. The epidermal nevus syndrome. Arch Dermatol 1968;97:273.
137. Kuokkanen K, Koivikko M, Alavaikko M. Organoid nevus phakomatosis. Acta Derm Venereol (Stockh) 1980;60:534.
138. Lantis S, Leyden J, Thew M et al. Nevus sebaceus of Jadassohn: part of a new neurocutaneous syndrome. Arch Dermatol 1968;98:117.
139. Wilson Jones E, Heyl T. Naevus sebaceus. Br J Dermatol 1970;82:99.
140. Bonvalet D, Barrandon V, Foix C et al. Tumeurs annexielles bénignes de survenue tardive sur naevus verrucosébacé (Jadassohn). Ann Dermatol Venereol 1983;110:337.
141. Rahbari H, Mehregan AH. Development of proliferating trichilemmal cyst in organoid nevus. J Am Acad Dermatol 1986;14:123.
142. Brownstein MH, Shapiro L. The pilosebaceous tumors. Int J Dermatol 1977;16:340.
143. Morioka S. The natural history of *nevus sebaceus*. J Cutan Pathol 1985;12:200.
144. Allessi E, Wong SN, Advani HH et al. Nevus sebaceus is associated with unusual neoplasms. Am J Dermatopathol 1988;10:116.
145. Domingo J, Helwig EB. Malignant neoplasms associated with nevus sebaceus of Jadassohn. J Am Acad Dermatol 1979;1:545.
146. Tarkhan II, Domingo J. Metastasizing eccrine porocarcinoma developing in a sebaceous nevus of Jadassohn: Report of a case. Arch Dermatol 1985;121:413.
147. De Villez RL, Roberts LE. Premature sebaceous gland hyperplasia. J Am Acad Dermatol 1982;6:933.
148. Luderschmidt C, Plewig G. Circumscribed sebaceous gland hyperplasia: Autoradiographic and histoplanometric studies. J Invest Dermatol 1978;70:207.
149. Miles AEW. Sebaceous glands in the lip and cheek mucosa of man. Br Dent J 1958;105:235.
150. Chambers SO. The structure of Fordyce's disease as demonstrated by wax reconstruction. Arch Dermatol Syph 1928;18:666.
151. Woolhandler HW, Becker WS. Adenoma of sebaceous glands: Adenoma sebaceum. Arch Dermatol Syph 1942;45:734.
152. Lever WF. Sebaceous adenoma: Review of the literature and report of a case. Arch Dermatol Syph 1948;57:102.
153. Essenhigh DM, Jones D, Rack JH. A sebaceous adenoma. Br J Dermatol 1964;76:330.
154. Banse-Kupin L, Morales A, Barlow M. Torre's syndrome. J Am Acad Dermatol 1984;10:803.
155. Troy JL, Ackerman AB. Sebaceoma: A distinctive benign neoplasm of adnexal epithelium differentiating toward sebaceous cells. Am J Dermatopathol 1984;6:7.
156. Hori M, Egami K, Maejima K et al. Electron microscopic study of sebaceous epithelioma. J Dermatol 1978;5:139.
157 Urban FH, Winkelmann RK. Sebaceous malignancy. Arch Dermatol 1961;84:63.
158. Steffen C, Ackerman AB. Sebaceoma. In: Steffen C, Ackerman AB. Neoplasms with sebaceous differentiation. Philadelphia: Lea & Febiger, 1994;385.
159. Muir EG, Yates-Bell AJ, Barlow KA. Multiple primary carcinomata of the colon, duodenum and larynx associated with keratoacanthoma of the face. Br J Surg 1967;54:191.
160. Finan MC, Connolly SM. Sebaceous gland tumors and systemic disease: A clinicopathologic analysis. Medicine (Baltimore) 1984;63: 232.
161. Poleksic S. Keratoacanthoma and multiple carcinomas. Br J Dermatol 1974;91:461.
162. Fathizadeh A, Medenica MM, Soltani K et al. Aggressive keratoacanthoma and internal malignant neoplasm. Arch Dermatol 1982;118: 112.
163. Lynch HT, Fusaro RM, Roberts L et al. Muir-Torre syndrome in several members of a family with a variant of the Cancer Family syndrome. Br J Dermatol 1985;113:295.
164. Rulon DB, Helwig EB. Multiple sebaceous neoplasms of the skin: An association with multiple visceral carcinomas, especially of the colon. Am J Clin Pathol 1973;60:745.
165. Torre D. Multiple sebaceous tumors. Arch Dermatol 1968;98:549.
166. Burgdorf WHC, Pitha J, Fahmy A. Muir-Torre syndrome: Histologic spectrum of sebaceous proliferation. Am J Dermatopathol 1986;8: 202.
167. Worret WJ, Burgdorf WHC, Fahmi A et al. Torre-Muir syndrom. Hautarzt 1981;32:519.
168. Dixon RS, Mikhail GR, Slater HC. Sebaceous carcinoma of the eyelid. J Am Acad Dermatol 1980;3:241.
169. Urban FH, Winkelmann RK. Sebaceous malignancy. Arch Dermatol 1961;84:63.
170. King DT, Hirose FM, Gurevitch AW. Sebaceous carcinoma of the skin with visceral metastases. Arch Dermatol 1979;115:862.
171. Rao NA, Hidayat AA, McLeon IW. Sebaceous carcinomas of the ocular adnexa: A clinicopathologic study of 104 cases, with five-year follow-up data. Hum Pathol 1982;13:113.
172. Rulon DB, Helwig EB. Cutaneous sebaceous neoplasms. Cancer 1974;33:83.
173. Hernández-Pérez E, Baños E. Sebaceous carcinoma: Report of two cases with metastasis. Dermatologica 1978;156:184.
174. Mellette JR, Amonette RA, Gardner JH et al. Carcinoma of sebaceous glands on the head and neck. J Dermatol Surg Oncol 1981;7:404.
175. Wick MR, Goellner JR, Wolfe JT III et al. Adnexal carcinomas of the skin: II. Extraocular sebaceous carcinomas. Cancer 1985;56:1163.
176. Leonard DD, Deaton WR Jr. Multiple sebaceous gland tumors and visceral carcinomas. Arch Dermatol 1974;110:917.
177. Graham R, McKee P, McGibbon D. Torre-Muir syndrome: An association with isolated sebaceous carcinoma. Cancer 1985;55:2868.
178. Russell WG, Hough AG, Rogers LW. Sebaceous carcinoma of meibomian gland origin. Am J Clin Pathol 1980;73:504.
179. Prioleau PG, Santa Cruz DJ. Sebaceous gland neoplasia. J Cutan Pathol 1984;11:396.
180. Friedman KJ, Boudreau S, Farmer ER. Superficial epithelioma with sebaceous differentiation. J Cutan Pathol 1987;14:193.
181. Kuo T. Clear cell carcinoma of the skin. Am J Surg Pathol 1980;4:573.
182. Hasebe T, Mukai K, Yamaguchi N et al. Prognostic value of immunohistochemical staining for proliferating cell nuclear antigen, p53, and c-erbB-2 in sebaceous gland carcinoma and sweat gland carcinoma: Comparison with histopathological parameter. Mod Pathol 1994;7:37.
183. Civatte J, Tsoitis G, Préaux J. Le naevus apocrine. Ann Dermatol Syphiligr 1974;101:251.
184. Rabens SF, Naness JI, Gottlieb BF. Apocrine gland organic hamartoma: Apocrine nevus. Arch Dermatol 1976;112:520.
185. Mehregan AH. Apocrine cystadenoma. Arch Dermatol 1964;90:274.
186. Smith JD, Chernosky ME. Apocrine hidrocystoma (cystadenoma). Arch Dermatol 1974;109:700.
187. Benisch B, Peison B. Apocrine hidrocystoma of the shoulder. Arch Dermatol 1977;113:71.
188. Kruse TV, Khan MA, Hassan MO. Multiple apocrine cystadenomas. Br J Dermatol 1979;100:675.
189. Asarch RF, Golitz LE, Sausker WF et al. Median raphe cysts of the penis. Arch Dermatol 1979;115:1084.
190. Gross BG. The fine structure of apocrine hidrocystoma. Arch Dermatol 1965;92:706.
191. Hassan MO, Khan MA, Kruse TV. Apocrine cystadenoma. Arch Dermatol 1979;115:194.
192. Schaumburg-Lever G, Lever WF. Secretion from human apocrine glands. J Invest Dermatol 1975;64:38.
193. Hashimoto K, Lever WF. Appendage tumors of the skin. Springfield, IL: Charles C Thomas, 1968;52.
194. Santa Cruz DJ, Prioleau PG, Smith ME. Hidradenoma papilliferum of the eyelid. Arch Dermatol 1981;117:55.
195. Shenoy YMV. Malignant perianal papillary hidradenoma. Arch Dermatol 1961;83:965.
196. Meeker HJ, Neubecker RD, Helwig EG. Hidradenoma papilliferum. Am J Clin Pathol 1962;37:182.
197. Hashimoto K. Hidradenoma papilliferum: An electron microscopic study. Acta Derm Venereol (Stockh) 1973;53:22.

198. Helwig EB, Hackney VC. Syringadenoma papilliferum. Arch Dermatol 1955;71:361.
199. Rostan SE, Waller JD. Syringocystadenoma papilliferum in an unusual location. Arch Dermatol 1976;112:835.
200. Pinkus H. Life history of naevus syringadenomatosus papilliferus. Arch Dermatol Syph 1954;69:305.
201. Hashimoto K. Syringocystadenoma papilliferum: An electron microscopic study. Arch Dermatol Forsch 1972;245:353.
202. Fusaro RM, Goltz RW. Histochemically demonstrable carbohydrates of appendageal tumors of the skin: II. Benign apocrine gland tumors. J Invest Dermatol 1962;38:137.
203. Vanatta PR, Bangert JL, Freeman RG. Syringocystadenoma papilliferum: A plasmacytotropic tumor. Am J Surg Pathol 1985;9:678.
204. Mambo NC. Immunohistochemical study of the immunoglobulin classes of the plasma cells in papillary syringadenoma. Virchows Arch [A] 1982;397:1.
205. Seco Navado MA, Fresno Forcelledo M, Orduña Domingo A et al. Syringocystadénome papillifère à évolution maligne. Ann Dermatol Venereol 1982;109:685.
206. Numata M, Hosoe S, Itoh N et al. Syringadenocarcinoma papilliferum. J Cutan Pathol 1985;12:3.
207. Mazoujian G, Margolis R. Immunohistochemical gross cystic disease fluid protein (GCDFP-15) in 65 benign sweat gland tumors of the skin. Am J Dermatopathol 1988;10:28.
208. Hashimoto K, Lever WF. Appendage tumors of the skin. Springfield, IL: Charles C Thomas, 1968;47.
209. Landry M, Winkelmann RK. An unusual tubular apocrine adenoma. Arch Dermatol 1972;105:869.
210. Toribio J, Zulaica A, Peteiro C. Tubular apocrine adenoma. J Cutan Pathol 1987;14:114.
211. Umbert P, Winkelmann RK. Tubular apocrine adenoma. J Cutan Pathol 1976;3:75.
212. Civatte J, Belaich S, Lauret P. Adénome tubulaire apocrine. Ann Dermatol Venereol 1979;106:665.
213. Okun MR, Finn R, Blumental G. Apocrine adenoma versus apocrine carcinoma. J Am Acad Dermatol 1980;2:322.
214. Kanitakis J, Hermier C, Thivolet J. Adénome tubulaire apocrine. Dermatologica 1984;169:23.
215. Burket JM, Zelickson AS. Tubular apocrine adenoma with perineural invasion. J Am Acad Dermatol 1984;11:639.
216. Falck VG, Jordaan HF. Papillary eccrine adenoma. Am J Dermatopathol 1986;8:64.
217. Fox SB, Cotton DWK. Tubular apocrine adenoma and papillary eccrine adenoma: Entities or unity? Am J Dermatopathol 1992;14:149.
218. Ishiko A, Shimizu H, Inamoto N, Nakmura K. Is tubular apocrine adenoma a distinct clinical entity? Am J Dermatopathol 1993;15:482.
219. Warkel RL, Helwig EB. Apocrine gland adenoma and adenocarcinoma of the axilla. Arch Dermatol 1978;114:198.
220. Weigand DA, Burgdorf WHC. Perianal apocrine gland adenoma. Arch Dermatol 1980;116:1051.
221. Lewis HM, Ovitz ML, Golitz LE. Erosive adenomatosis of the nipple. Arch Dermatol 1976;112:1427.
222. Smith NP, Wilson Jones E. Erosive adenomatosis of the nipple. Clin Exp Dermatol 1977;2:79.
223. Brownstein MH, Phelps RG, Magnin PH. Papillary adenoma of the nipple. J Am Acad Dermatol 1985;12:707.
224. Crain RC, Helwig EB. Dermal cylindroma: Dermal eccrine cylindroma. Am J Clin Pathol 1961;35:504.
225. Baden H. Cylindromatosis simulating neurofibromatosis. N Engl J Med 1962;267:296.
226. Lausecker H. Beitrag zu den naevo-epitheliomen. Arch Dermatol Syph 1952;194:639.
227. Welch JP, Wells RS, Kerr CB. Ancell-Spiegler cylindromas (turban tumors) and Brooke-Fordyce trichoepitheliomas: Evidence for a single genetic entity. J Med Genet 1968;5:29.
228. Gottschalk HR, Graham JH, Aston EE IV. Dermal eccrine cylindroma, epithelioma adenoides cysticum, and eccrine spiradenoma. Arch Dermatol 1974;110:473.
229. Headington JT, Batsakis JG, Beals TF et al. Membranous basal cell adenoma of parotid gland, dermal cylindromas, and trichoepitheliomas. Cancer 1977;39:2460.
230. Guillot B, Buffière I, Barnéon G et al. Trichoépitheliomas multiples, cylindromes, grain de milium. Ann Dermatol Venereol 1987;114:175.
231. Goette DK, McConnell MA, Fowler VR. Cylindroma and eccrine spiradenoma coexistent in the same lesion. Arch Dermatol 1982;118:273.
232. Ferrándiz C, Campo E, Baumann E. Dermal cylindromas (turban tumours) and eccrine spiradenomas in a patient. J Cutan Pathol 1985;12:72.
233. Urbach F, Graham JH, Goldstein J et al. Dermal eccrine cylindroma. Arch Dermatol 1963;88:880.
234. Penneys N, Kaiser M. Cylindroma expresses immunohistochemical markers linking it to eccrine coil. J Cutan Pathol 1993;20:40.
235. Cotton DWK, Braye SG. Dermal cylindromas originate from the eccrine sweat gland. Br J Dermatol 1984;111:53.
236. Kallioinen M. Immunoelectron microscope demonstration of the basement membrane components laminin and type IV collagen in the dermal cylindroma. J Pathol 1985;147:97.
237. Tellechea O, Reis JP, Ilheu O, Poiares Baptista A. Dermal cylindroma: An immunohistochemical study of thirteen cases. Am J Dermatopathol 1995;17:260.
238. Munger BL, Graham JH, Helwig EB. Ultrastructure and histochemical characteristics of dermal eccrine cylindroma: Turban tumor. J Invest Dermatol 1962;39:577.
239. Weber L, Wick G, Gebhart W et al. Basement membrane components outline the tumour islands in cylindroma. Br J Dermatol 1984;111:45.
240. Gerretsen AL, van der Putte SC, Deenstra W. Cutaneous cylindroma with malignant transformation. Cancer 1993;72:1618.
241. Lo JS, Peschen M, Snow SN et al. Malignant cylindroma of the scalp. J Dermatol Surg Oncol 1991;17:897.
242. Bourlond A, Clerens A, Sigart H. Cylindrome malin. Dermatologica 1979;158:203.
243. Urbanski SJ, From L, Abramowicz A et al. Metamorphosis or dermal cylindroma: Possible relation to malignant transformation. J Am Acad Dermatol 1985;12:188.
244. Galadari E, Mehregan AH, Lee KC. Malignant transformation of eccrine tumors. J Cutan Pathol 1987;14:15.
245. Luger A. Das cylindrom der haut und seine maligne degeneration. Arch Dermatol Syph 1949;188:155.
246. Beideck M, Kuhn A. Maligne entartung bei kutanen zylindromen. Z Hautkr 1985;60:73.
247. Arnold HL. Nevus seborrheicus et sudoriferus. Arch Dermatol 1945;51:370.
248. Goldstein N. Ephidrosis (local hyperhidrosis): Nevus sudoriferus. Arch Dermatol 1967;96:67.
249. Herzberg JJ. Ekkrines syringocystadenom. Arch Klin Exp Dermatol 1962;214:600.
250. Imai S, Nitto H. Eccrine nevus with epidermal changes. Dermatologica 1983;166:84.
251. Hyman AB, Harris H, Brownstein MH. Eccrine angiomatous hamartoma. NY State J Med 1968;68:2803.
252. Zeller DJ. Goldman RL. Eccrine-pilar angiomatous hamartoma. Dermatologica 1971;143:100.
253. Challa VR, Jona J. Eccrine angiomatous hamartoma: A rare skin lesion with diverse histological features. Dermatologica 1977;155:206.
254. Sanmartin O, Botella R, Alegre V et al. Congenital eccrine angiomatous hamartoma. Am J Dermatopathol 1992;14:161.
255. Velasco J, Almeida V. Eccrine pilar angiomatous nevus. Dermatologica 1988;177:317.
256. Donati P, Amantea A, Balus L. Eccrine angiomatous hamartoma: A lipomatous variant. J Cutan Pathol 1989;16:227.
257. Smith JD, Chernosky ME. Hidrocystomas. Arch Dermatol 1973;108:676.
258. Cordero AA, Montes LF. Eccrine hidrocystoma. J Cutan Pathol 1976;3:292.
259. Hassan MO, Khan MA. Ultrastructure of eccrine cystadenoma. Arch Dermatol 1979;115:1217.
260. Sperling LC, Sakas EL. Eccrine hidrocystomas. J Am Acad Dermatol 1982;7:763.
261. Ebner J, Erlach E. Ekkrine hidrozystome. Dermatol Monatsschr 1975;161:739.
262. Thomas J, Majmudar B, Gorelkin L. Syringoma localized to the vulva. Arch Dermatol 1979;115:95.
263. Hashimoto K, Dibella, Borsuk GM et al. Eruptive hidradenoma and syringoma. Arch Dermatol 1967;96:500.
264. Yung CW, Soltani K, Bernstein JE et al. Unilateral linear nevoidal syringoma. J Am Acad Dermatol 1981;4:412.

265. Shelley WB, Wood MG. Occult syringomas of scalp associated with progressive hair loss. Arch Dermatol 1980;116:843.
266. Dupré A, Bonafe JL, Christol B. Syringomas as a causative factor for cicatricial alopecia (letter). Arch Dermatol 1981;117:315.
267. Pujol R, Moreno A, Gonzalez MJ et al. Syringoma du cuir chevelu. Ann Dermatol Venereol 1986;113:693.
268. Spitz DF, Stadecker MJ, Grande DJ. Subclinical syringoma coexisting with basal cell carcinoma. J Dermatol Surg Oncol 1987;13:793.
269. Friedman SJ, Butler DF. Syringoma presenting as milia. J Am Acad Dermatol 1987;16:310.
270. Headington JT, Koski J, Murphy PJ. Clear cell glycogenosis in multiple syringomas. Arch Dermatol 1972;106:353.
271. Feibelman CE, Maize JC. Clear-cell syringoma. Am J Dermatopathol 1984;6:139.
272. Asai Y, Ishii M, Hamada T. Acral syringoma: Electron microscopic studies on its origin. Acta Derm Venereol (Stockh) 1982;62:64.
273. Hashimoto K, Lever WF. Histogenesis of skin appendage tumors. Arch Dermatol 1969;100:356.
274. Mustakallio KK. Succinic dehydrogenase activity of syringomas. Acta Dermatol 1964;89:827.
275. Winkelmann RK, Muller SA. Sweat gland tumors. Arch Dermatol 1964;89:827.
276. Pinkus H, Rogin JR, Goldman P. Eccrine poroma. Arch Dermatol 1956;74:511.
277. Hyman AB, Brownstein MH. Eccrine poroma: An analysis of 45 new cases. Dermatologica 1969;138:29.
278. Okun MR, Ansell HB. Eccrine poroma. Arch Dermatol 1963;88:561.
279. Penneys NS, Ackerman AB, Indgin SN et al. Eccrine poroma. Br J Dermatol 1970;82:613.
280. Goldner R. Eccrine poromatosis. Arch Dermatol 1970;101:606.
281. Wilkinson RD, Schopflocher P, Rozenfeld M. Hidrotic ectodermal dysplasia with diffuse eccrine poromatosis. Arch Dermatol 1977;113:472.
282. Freeman RG, Knox JM, Spiller WF. Eccrine poroma. Am J Clin Pathol 1961;36:444.
283. Knox JM, Spiller WF. Eccrine poroma. Arch Dermatol 1958;77:726.
284. Yasuda T, Kawada A, Yoshida K. Eccrine poroma. Arch Dermatol 1964;90:428.
285. Krinitz K. Malignes intraepidermales ekkrines porom. Z Hautkr 1972; 47:9.
286. Smith JLS, Coburn JG. Hidroacanthoma simplex. Br J Dermatol 1956;68:400.
287. Mehregan AH, Levson DN: Hidroacanthoma simplex. Arch Dermatol 1969;100:303.
288. Winkelmann RK, McLeod WA. The dermal duct tumor. Arch Dermatol 1966;94:50.
289. Rahbari H. Syringoacanthoma: Acanthotic lesion of the acrosyringium. Arch Dermatol 1984;120:751.
290. Sanderson KV, Ryan EA. The histochemistry of eccrine poroma. Br J Dermatol 1963;75:86.
291. Hashimoto K, Lever WF. Eccrine poroma: Histochemical and electron microscopic studies. J Invest Dermatol 1964;43:237.
292. Hashimoto K, Lever WF. Histogenesis of skin appendage tumors. Arch Dermatol 1969;100:356.
293. Hu CH, Marques AS, Winkelmann RK. Dermal duct tumor. Arch Dermatol 1978;114:1659.
294. Mascaro JM. Considérations sur les tumeurs fibroépithéliales: Le syringofibroadénome eccrine. Ann Dermatol Syphilgr 1963;90:143.
295. Weedon D, Lewis J. Acrosyringeal nevus. J Cutan Pathol 1977;4:166.
296. Mehregan AH, Marufi M, Medenica M. Eccrine syringofibroadenoma (Mascaro). J Am Acad Dermatol 1985;13:433.
297. Ogino A. Linear eccrine poroma. Arch Dermatol 1976;112:841.
298. Pinkus H, Mehregan AH. Epidermotropic eccrine carcinoma. Arch Dermatol 1963;88:597.
299. Mishima Y, Morioka S. Oncogenic differentiation of the intraepidermal eccrine sweat duct: Eccrine poroma, poroepithelioma and porocarcinoma. Dermatologica 1969;138:238.
300. Bardach H. Hidroacanthoma simplex with in situ porocarcinoma. J Cutan Pathol 1978;5:236.
301. Gschnait F, Horn F, Lindlbauer R et al. Eccrine porocarcinoma. J Cutan Pathol 1980;7:349.
302. Mohri S, Chika K, Saito I et al. A case of porocarcinoma. J Dermatol 1980;7:431.
303. Ishikawa K. Malignant hidroacanthoma simplex. Arch Dermatol 1971;104:529.
304. Pinkus H, Mehregan AH. Epidermotropic eccrine carcinoma. Arch Dermatol 1963;88:597.
305. Miura Y. Epidermotropic eccrine carcinoma. Jpn J Dermatol [B] 1968;78:226.
306. Peña J, Suster S. Squamous differentiation in malignant eccrine poroma. Am J Dermatopathol 1993;15:492.
307. Urso C, Paglierani M, Bondi R. Histologic spectrum of carcinomas with eccrine ductal differentiation: Sweat-gland ductal carcinomas. Am J Dermatopathol 1993;15:435.
308. Kolde G, Macher E, Grundmann E. Metastasizing eccrine porocarcinoma: Report of two cases with fatal outcome. Pathol Res Pract 1991; 187:477.
309. Rahbari H. Syringoacanthoma: Acanthotic lesion of the acrosyringium. Arch Dermatol 1984;120:751.
310. Kwittken J. Muciparous epidermal tumors. Arch Dermatol 1974;109: 554.
311. King DT, Barr RJ. Syringometaplasia: Mucinous and squamous variants. J Cutan Pathol 1979;6:284.
312. Scully K, Assaad D. Mucinous syringometaplasia. J Am Acad Dermatol 1984;11:503.
313. Mehregan AH. Mucinous syringometaplasia. Arch Dermatol 1980; 116:988.
314. Munger BL, Berghorn BM, Helwig EB. A light and electron-microscopic study of a case of multiple eccrine spiradenoma. J Invest Dermatol 1962;38:289.
315. Hashimoto K, Gross BG, Nelson RG et al. Eccrine spiradenoma: Histochemical and electron microscopic studies. J Invest Dermatol 1966; 46:347.
316. Shelley WB, Wood MG. A zosteriform network of spiradenoma. J Am Acad Dermatol 1980;2:59.
317. Tsur H, Lipskier E, Fisher BK. Multiple linear spiradenomas. Plast Reconstr Surg 1981;68:100.
318. Mambo NC. Eccrine spiradenoma: Clinical and pathologic study of 49 tumors. J Cutan Pathol 1983;10:312.
319. Lever WF. Myoepithelial sweat gland tumor: Myoepithelioma. Arch Dermatol Syph 1948;57:332.
320. Kersting DW, Helwig EB. Eccrine spiradenoma. Arch Dermatol 1956;73:199.
321. Castro C, Winkelmann RK. Spiradenoma: Histochemical and electron microscopic study. Arch Dermatol 1974;109:40.
322. van den Oord JJ, De Wolf-Peeters C. Perivascular spaces in eccrine spiradenoma: A clue to its histological diagnosis. Am J Dermatopathol 1995;17:266.
323. Winkelmann RK, Wolff K. Histochemistry of hidradenoma and eccrine spiradenoma. J Invest Dermatol 1967;49:173.
324. Hashimoto K, Kanzaki T. Appendage tumors of the skin: Histogenesis and ultrastructure. J Cutan Pathol 1984;11:365.
325. Cooper PH, Frierson HF Jr. Morrison G. Malignant transformation of eccrine spiradenoma. Arch Dermatol 1985;121:1445.
326. Galadari C, Mehregan AH, Lee KC. Malignant transformation of eccrine tumors. J Cutan Pathol 1987;14:15.
327. Wick MR, Swanson PE, Kaye VN et al. Sweat gland carcinoma ex eccrine spiradenoma. Am J Dermatopathol 1987;9:90.
328. Herzberg AJ, Elenitsas R, Strohmeyer CR. Unusual case of early malignant transformation of spiradenoma. Dermatol Surg Oncol 1995; 21:1.
329. Dabska M. Malignant transformation of eccrine spiradenoma. Pol Med J 1972;11:388.
330. Evans HL, Su WPD, Smith JL et al. Carcinoma arising in eccrine spiradenoma. Cancer 1979;43:1881.
331. Argenyi ZB, Nguyen AV, Balogh K et al. Malignant eccrine spiradenoma: A clinicopathologic study. Am J Dermatopathol 1992;14:381.
332. Rulon DB, Helwig EB. Papillary eccrine adenoma. Arch Dermatol 1977;113:596.
333. Urmacher C, Lieberman PH. Papillary eccrine adenoma. Am J Dermatopathol 1987;9:243.
334. Falck VG, Jordaan HF. Papillary eccrine adenoma. Am J Dermatopathol 1986;8:64.
335. Sexton M, Maize JC. Papillary eccrine adenoma. J Am Acad Dermatol 1988;18:1114.
336. Magahed M, Hölzle E. Papillary eccrine adenoma: A case report with immunohistochemical examination. Am J Dermatopathol 1993;15:150.
337. Aloi F, Pich A. Papillary eccrine adenoma: A histopathological and immunohistochemical study. Dermatologica 1991;182:47.

338. Nova MP, Kress Y, Jennings TA et al. Papillary eccrine adenoma and low-grade eccrine carcinoma: A comparative histologic, ultrastructural, and immunohistochemical study. Surg Pathol 1990;3:179.
339. Lund HZ. Tumors of the skin. In: Atlas of tumor pathology. Section I, Fascicle 2. Washington, DC: Armed Forces Institute of Pathology, 1957.
340. Lever WF, Castleman B. Clear cell myoepithelioma of the skin. Am J Pathol 1952;28:691.
341. O'Hara JM, Bensch K, Ioannides G et al. Eccrine sweat gland adenoma, clear cell type. Cancer 1966;19:1438.
342. O'Hara JM, Bensch KG. Fine structure of eccrine sweat gland adenoma, clear cell type. J Invest Dermatol 1967;49:261.
343. Winkelmann RK, Wolff K. Histochemistry of hidradenoma and eccrine spiradenoma. J Invest Dermatol 1967;49:173.
344. Winkelmann RK, Wolff K. Solid-cystic hidradenoma of the skin. Arch Dermatol 1968;97:651.
345. Johnson BL Jr., Helwig EB. Eccrine acrospiroma. Cancer 1969;23:641.
346. Efskind J, Eker R. Myo-epitheliomas of the skin. Acta Derm Venereol (Stockh) 1954;34:279.
347. Kersting DW. Clear cell hidradenoma and hidradenocarcinoma. Arch Dermatol 1963;87:323.
348. Hashimoto K, Di Bella RJ, Lever WF. Clear cell hidradenoma: Histologic, histochemical, and electron microscopic study. Arch Dermatol 1967;96:18.
349. Stanley RJ, Sanchez NP, Massa MC et al. Epidermoid hidradenoma. J Cutan Pathol 1982;9:293.
350. Haupt HM, Stern JB, Berlin SJ. Immunohistochemistry in the differential diagnosis of nodular hidradenoma and glomus tumor. Am J Dermatopathol 1992;14:310.
351. Mambo NC. The significance of atypical nuclear changes in benign eccrine acrospiromas: A clinical and pathological study of 18 cases. J Cutan Pathol 1984;11:35.
352. Keasbey LE, Hadley GC. Clear-cell hidradenoma: Report of three cases with widespread metastases. Cancer 1954;7:934.
353. Santler R, Everhartinger C. Malignes klarzellen-myoepitheliom. Dermatologica 1965;130:340.
354. Hernändez-Pérez E, Cestoni-Parducci R. Nodular hidradenoma and hidradenocarcinoma. J Am Acad Dermatol 1985;12:15.
355. Mehregan AH, Hashimoto K, Rahbari H. Eccrine adenocarcinoma: A clinicopathologic study of 35 cases. Arch Dermatol 1983;119:104.
356. Headington JT, Niederhuber JE, Beals TF. Malignant clear cell acrospiroma. Cancer 1978;41:641.
357. Hirsch P, Helwig EB. Chondroid syringoma. Arch Dermatol 1961;84:835.
358. Headington JT. Mixed tumors of the skin: Eccrine and apocrine types. Arch Dermatol 1961;84:989.
359. Tsoitis G, Brisou B, Destombes. Mummified cutaneous mixed tumor. Arch Dermatol 1975;111:194.
360. Gartmann H, Pullmann H. Apokriner und ekkriner mischtumor der kopfhaut. Z Hautkr 1979b;54:952.
361. Welke S, Goos M. Das chondroide syringom. Hautarzt 1982;33:15.
362. Gartmann H, Pullmann H. Chondroides syringom. Z Hautkr 1979a; 54:908.
363. Varela-Duran J, Diaz-Flores L, Varela-Nuñez R. Ultrastructure of chondroid syringoma. Cancer 1979;44:148.
364. Banerjee SS, Harris M, Eyden BP et al. Chondroid syringoma with hyaline cell change. Histopathology 1993;22:235.
365. Hasseb-el-Naby HM, Tam S, White WL, Ackerman AB. Mixed tumors of the skin: A histological and immunohistochemical study. Am J Dermatopathol 1989;11:413.
366. Iglesias FD, Forcelledo FF, Sanchez TS et al. Chondroid syringoma: A histological and immunohistochemical study of 15 cases. Histopathology 1990;17:311.
367. Kanitakis J, Zambruno G, Viac J et al. Expression of neural-tissue markers (S-100 protein and Leu-7 antigen) by sweat gland tumors of the skin. J Am Acad Dermatol 1987;17:187.
368. Hernandez FJ. Mixed tumors of the skin of the salivary gland type: A light and electron microscopic study. J Invest Dermatol 1976;66:49.
369. Mazoujian G, Margolis R. Immunohistochemistry of gross cystic disease fluid protein (GCDFP-15) in 65 benign sweat gland tumors of the skin. Am J Dermatopathol 1988;10:28.
370. Trown K, Heenan PJ. Malignant mixed tumor of the skin: Malignant chondroid syringoma. Pathology 1994;26:237.
371. Harrist TJ. Aretz TH, Mihm MC Jr et al. Malignant chondroid syringoma. Arch Dermatol 1981;117:719.
372. Shvili D, Rothem A. Fulminant metastasizing chondroid syringoma of the skin. Am J Dermatopathol 1986;8:321.
373. Metzler G, Schaumburg-Lever G, Hornstin O, Rassner G. Malignant chondroid syringoma: Immunohistopathology. Am J Dermatopathol 1996;18:83.
374. Botha JBC, Kahn LB. Aggressive chondroid syringoma. Arch Dermatol 1978;114:954.
375. Hilton JMN, Blackwell JB. Metastasizing chondroid syringoma. J Pathol 1973;109:167.
376. Matz LR. McCully DJ, Stokes BAR. Metastasizing chondroid syringoma: Case report. Pathology 1969;1:77.
377. Redono C, Rocamora A, Villoria F et al. Malignant mixed tumor of the skin, malignant chondroid syringoma. Cancer 1982;49:1690.
378. Ishimura E, Iwamoto H, Kobashi Y et al. Malignant chondroid syringoma. Cancer 1983;52:1966.
379. Devine P, Sarno RC, Ucci AA. Malignant cutaneous mixed tumor (letter). Arch Dermatol 1984;120:576.
380. Cooper PH. Carcinomas of sweat glands. Pathol Annu 1987;22:83.
381. Santa Cruz DJ. Sweat gland carcinomas. A comprehensive review. Semin Diagn Pathol 1987;4:38.
382. Alessi E, Caputo R. Syringomatous carcinoma of the scalp presenting as a slowly enlarging patch of alopecia. Am J Dermatopathol 1993;15:503.
383. Urso C, Paglierani M, Bondi R. Histologic spectrum of carcinomas with eccrine ductal differentiation: Sweat-gland ductal carcinomas. Am J Dermatopathol 1993;15:435.
384. Grant RA. Sweat gland carcinoma with metastases. JAMA 1960;173:490.
385. Teloh HA, Balkin RB, Grier JP. Metastasizing sweat gland carcinoma. Arch Dermatol 1957;76:80.
386. Swanson PE, Cherwitz DL, Neumann MP et al. Eccrine sweat gland carcinoma. J Cutan Pathol 1987;14:65.
387. El-Domeiri AA, Brasfield RD, Huvos AG et al. Sweat gland carcinoma. Ann Surg 1971;173:270.
388. Dave VK. Eccrine sweat gland carcinoma with metastases. Br J Dermatol 1972;86:95.
389. Orbaneja JG, Yus ES, Diaz-Flores L et al. Adenocarcinom der ekkrinen schweissdrüsen. Hautarzt 1973;24:197.
390. Freeman RG, Winkelmann RK. Basal cell tumor with eccrine differentiation. Arch Dermatol 1969;100:234.
391. Sanchez NP, Winkelmann RK. Basal cell tumor with eccrine differentiation: Eccrine epithelioma. J Am Acad Dermatol 1982;6:514.
392. Mehregan AH, Hashimoto K, Rahbari H. Eccrine adenocarcinoma. Arch Dermatol 1983;119:104.
393. Cooper PH. Sclerosing carcinomas of sweat ducts: Microcystic adnexal carcinoma. Arch Dermatol 1986;122:261.
394. Nickoloff BJ, Fleischmann HE, Carmel J et al. Microcystic adnexal carcinoma: Immunohistologic observations suggesting dual (pilar and eccrine) differentiation. Arch Dermatol 1986;122:290.
395. Leboit P, Sexton M. Microcystic adnexal carcinoma of the skin: A reappraisal of the differentiation and differential diagnosis of an under-recognized neoplasm. J Am Acad Dermatol 1993;29:609.
396. Mendoza S, Helwig EB. Mucinous (adenocystic) carcinoma of the skin. Arch Dermatol 1971;103:68.
397. Santa Cruz DJ, Meyers JH, Gnepp DR et al. Primary mucinous carcinoma of the skin. Br J Dermatol 1978;98:645.
398. Yeung KY, Stinson JC. Mucinous (adenocystic) carcinoma of sweat glands with widespread metastases. Cancer 1977;39:2556.
399. Snow SN, Reizner GT. Mucinous eccrine carcinoma of the eyelid. Cancer 1992;70:2099.
400. Headington JT. Primary mucinous carcinoma of the skin. Cancer 1977;39:1055.
401. Baandrup U, Leftarr, Gaard H. Mucinous (adenocystic) carcinoma of the skin. Dermatologica 1982;164:338.
402. Wright JD, Font RL. Mucinous sweat gland adenocarcinoma of the eyelid. Cancer 1979;44:1757.
403. Eckert F, Schmid U, Hardmeier T, Altmannsberger M. Cytokeratin expression in mucinous sweat gland carcinomas: An immunohistochemical analysis of four cases. Histopathology 1992;21:161.
404. Balin AK, Fine RM, Golitz LE. Mucinous carcinoma. J Dermatol Surg Oncol 1988;14:521.
405. Landman G, Farmer ER. Primary cutaneous mucoepidermoid carcinoma: Report of a case. J Cutan Pathol 1991;18:56.

406. Friedman KJ. Low-grade primary cutaneous adenosquamous (mucoepidermoid) carcinoma: Report of a case and review of the literature. Am J Dermatology 1989;11:43.
407. Boggio R. Adenoid cystic carcinoma of the scalp. Arch Dermatol 1975;111:793.
408. Seab JA, Graham JH. Primary cutaneous adenoid cystic carcinoma. J Am Acad Dermatol 1987;17:113.
409. Cooper PH, Adelson GL, Holthaus WH. Primary cutaneous adenoid cystic carcinoma. Arch Dermatol 1984;120:774.
410. Fukai K, Ishii M, Kobayashi H et al. Primary cutaneous adenoid cystic carcinoma: Ultrastructural study and immunolocalization of types I, III, IV, and V collagens and laminin. J Cutan Pathol 1990; 17:374.
411. Headington JT, Tesars R, Niederhuber JE et al. Primary adenoid cystic carcinoma of the skin. Arch Dermatol 1978;114:421.
412. Wick MR, Swanson PE. Primary adenoid cystic carcinoma of the skin. Am J Dermatopathol 1986;8:2.
413. Kao GF, Helwig EB, Graham JH. Aggressive digital papillary adenoma and adenocarcinoma. J Cutan Pathol 1987;14:129.
414. Baes H, Suurmond D. Apocrine sweat gland carcinoma. Br J Dermatol 1970;83:483.
415. Warkel RL, Helwig EB. Apocrine gland adenoma and adenocarcinoma of the axilla. Arch Dermatol 1978;114:198.
416. Futrell JW, Krueger GR, Chretien PB et al. Multiple primary sweat gland carcinoma. Cancer 1971;28:686.
417. Sakamoto F, Ito M, Sato S et al. Basal cell tumor with apocrine differentiation: apocrine epithelioma. J Am Acad Dermatol 1985;13:355.
418. Paties C, Taccagni GL, Papotti M et al. Apocrine carcinoma of the skin: A clinicopathologic, immunocytochemical, and ultrastructural study. Cancer 1993;71:375.
419. Nishikawa Y, Tokusashi Y, Saito Y et al. A case of apocrine adenocarcinoma associated with hamartomatous apocrine gland hyperplasia of both axillae. Am J Surg Pathol 1994;18:832.
420. Neldner KH. Ceruminoma. Arch Dermatol 1968;98:344.
421. Michel RG, Woodard BH, Shelburne JD et al. Ceruminous gland adenocarcinoma. Cancer 1978;41:545.
422. Lynde CW, McLean DI, Wood WS. Tumors of ceruminal glands. J Am Acad Dermatol 1984;11:841.
423. Steck WD, Helwig EB. Cutaneous endometriosis. JAMA 1965;191: 167.
424. Williams HE, Barsky S, Storino W. Umbilical endometrioma: Silent type. Arch Dermatol 1976;112:1435.
425. Popoff L, Raitchev R, Andreev VC. Endometriosis of the skin. Arch Dermatol 1962;85:186.
426. Tidman MJ, MacDonald DM. Cutaneous endometriosis: A histopathologic study. J Am Acad Dermatol 1988;18:373.
427. Doré N, Landry M, Cadotte M et al. Cutaneous endosalpingiosis. Arch Dermatol 1980;116:909.
428. Farmer ER, Helwig EB. Cutaneous ciliated cysts. Arch Dermatol 1978;114:70.

Lever's Histopathology of the Skin, eighth edition,
edited by David Elder et al. Lippincott–
Raven Publishers, Philadelphia © 1997.

CHAPTER 32

Cutaneous Lymphomas and Leukemias

Philip E. LeBoit and Timothy H. McCalmont

The explosion of knowlege about the human immune system witnessed in the last two decades has led to profound changes in the way that histopathologists look at lymphoproliferative disorders and lymphomas. As workers correlate clinical, histologic, cytomorphologic, immunologic, and genetic information, several distinct entities, each with a definable natural history, have come into focus.

There have been several attempts to classify lymphomas so as to permit microscopists and clinicians to be certain that they are speaking about the same disease, and to permit students of the subject to organize their thoughts about a group of diseases that is as heterogeneous as the cells that comprise the immune system. The classifications of Rappaport, Lukes and Collins, and the Kiel group were based primarily on cytomorphology. The "Working Formulation" was not intended to be a classification, but rather as a schema so that workers using different classifications could find equivalent terms for the same disease in each of the commonly used classifications, and so that clinicians could plan appropriate therapies based on grade, irrespective of the terminology of the interpreting pathologist. The recent REAL (Revised European American Lymphoma) classification is the first major structure to take advances in immunopathology into account, and its categories represent distinct clinicopathologic entities rather than merely morphologic ones.[1]

This chapter follows the spirit of the REAL classification, dividing lymphoproliferative disorders into those of B-cell and T-cell lineage and then discussing Hodgkin's lymphoma and proliferations of hematopoietic cells. In considering the large variety of lymphoproliferative diseases in this chapter, it is worth remembering that in many respects the most important determination to be made microscopically is simply that one is indeed dealing with a lymphoma. In general, lymphomas primary to the skin have favorable prognoses, whereas those that are disseminated at presentation have unfavorable ones.

P. E. LeBoit: Departments of Pathology and Dermatology, University of California Medical Center, San Francisco, CA

T. H. McCalmont: Departments of Pathology and Dermatology, University of California Medical Center, San Francisco, CA

PROLIFERATIONS OF B CELLS

B-Cell Cutaneous Lymphoid Hyperplasia (B-Cell Pseudolymphoma, or B-CLH)

The term "pseudolymphoma" loosely refers to a group of conditions in which the microscopic appearance of lymphocytic infiltrates in the skin resembles that of one of the cutaneous lymphomas. The growing appreciation of the diversity of cutaneous lymphomas has similarly led to the recognition that there are many cutaneous pseudolymphomas, including lymphoid proliferations of B-cell or T-cell composition. B-CLH is often referred simply to as pseudolymphoma, because it was the first simulant of cutaneous lymphoma to be studied comprehensively. "Lymphadenosis benigna cutis," "cutaneous lymphoplasia," "lymphocytoma cutis," and other even more arcane and archaic terms are also synonymous with B-CLH. In reviewing the literature on B-CLH, it should be kept in mind that many older cases might be reclassified as low grade B-cell lymphomas using current methods. Cutaneous immunocytoma, marginal zone lymphoma, and follicular lymphoma all contain either reactive or neoplastic follicles, and can simulate B-CLH microscopically. Until recently, criteria for distinguishing these conditions from B-CLH did not exist.

In B-CLH, nodules or plaques result from the recapitulation in the skin of the elements found in the cortices of reactive lymph nodes (Fig. 32-1).[2] Clinically, B-CLH generally presents with red to purple nodules or plaques, usually on the face or scalp. Lesions are usually solitary but may be multiple. Patients with multiple lesions often have only a few lesions affecting a circumscribed area (most often the skin of the head or neck), but rare patients have generalized lesions.[3] Most lesions persist for months or years, sometimes to resolve spontaneously.

Histopathology. The infiltrates of B-CLH are nodular or diffuse, and involve the dermis and/or the subcutis. A "top-heavy" pattern is often observed at scanning magnification—i.e., the infiltrate is denser in the dermis than in the subcutis (Fig. 32-2). Depending on the degree to which the reaction resembles the cortex of a reactive lymph node, follicles may be distinct or inconspicuous. In the follicular pattern of B-CLH, distinct germinal centers, identical in composition to secondary follicles in

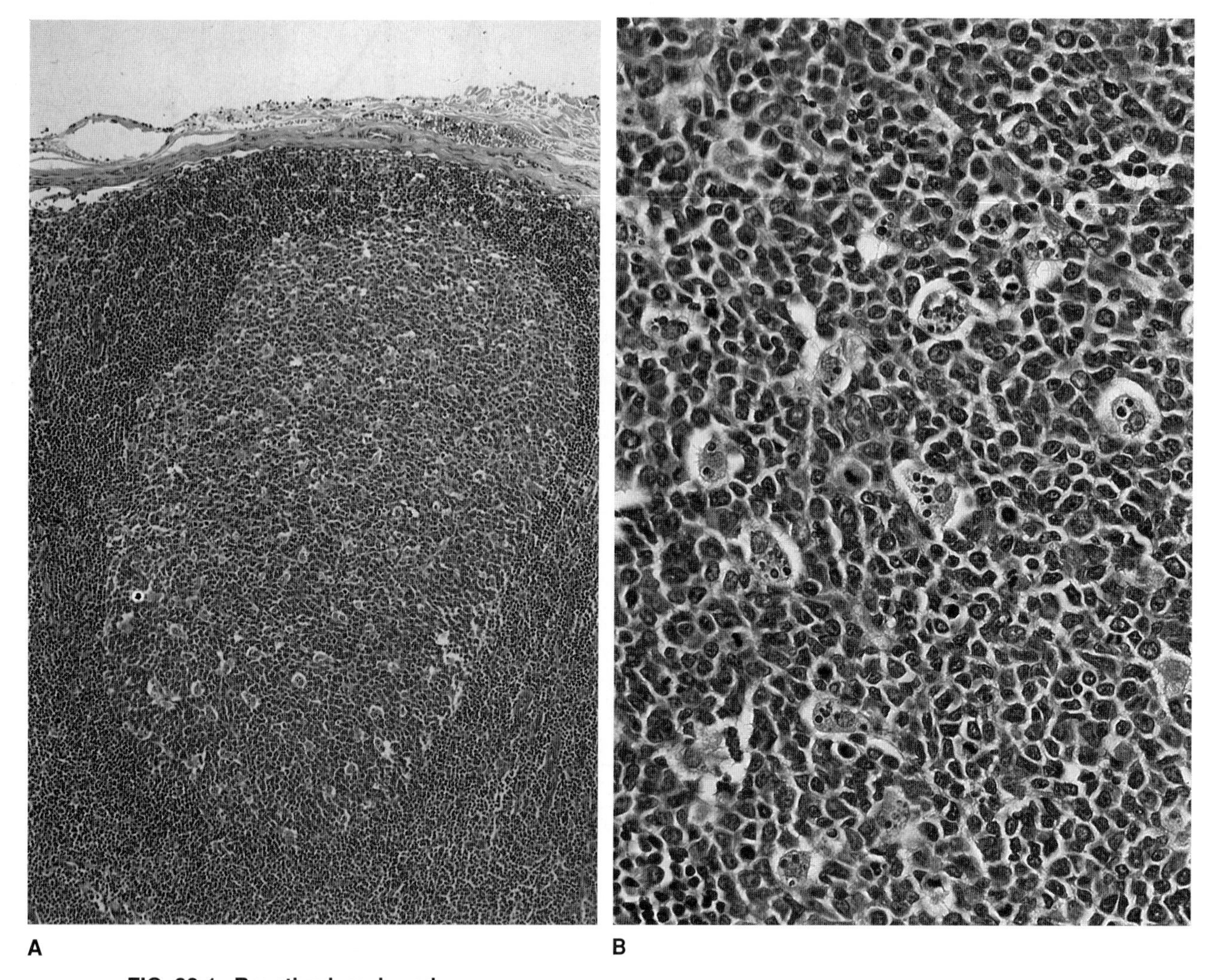

FIG. 32-1. Reactive lymph node
(**A**) The outermost cortex of a reactive lymph node shows elements that are also identifiable within skin infiltrates of B-cell cutaneous lymphoid hyperplasia. (**B**) There are germinal centers composed of follicular center cells and immunoblastic lymphocytes, stippled by tingible body macrophages, and blanketed by thick mantles.

reactive lymph nodes, are present. As lymph nodes develop, B cells aggregate in primary follicles as collections of small lymphocytes. Antigen stimulation produces secondary follicles, with a more complex composition. Secondary follicles consist of follicular center cells surrounded by a mantle of small lymphocytes that resemble those observed in primary follicles. The follicular center cells include small cleaved and large lymphocytes (centrocytes and centroblasts), follicular dendritic cells (which present antigen to immunologically naive B cells), and tingible body macrophages, whose cytoplasm contains the debris of small lymphocytes that have undergone apoptosis (programmed cell death), the result of failure to bind avidly with antigens presented by dendritic cells. Mitotic figures are commonly found in reactive follicles. The follicles in reactive lymph nodes are polarized, with dark areas rich in centroblasts and tingible body macrophages at one end and light areas populated by many centrocytes. This polarization is not evident in most examples of B-CLH. The mantle zone, as noted earlier, is composed of small lymphocytes. Whereas in reactive nodes it is thickened on the side adjacent to the capsule, in B-CLH no such orientation is evident. However, there are usually complete mantles around the follicles. Peripheral to the follicles and their mantles is an admixture of cells that consist of T cells with small but irregularly shaped nuclei, immunoblasts (antigen-stimulated cells of either B or T lineage that have large vesicular nuclei and prominent, central nucleoli), histiocytes, and rarely histiocytic giant cells, eosinophils, polytypic plasma cells (i.e., both κ- and λ-expressing cells), and plasmacytoid monocytes.[4] The venules found in these interfollicular areas resemble the "high endothelial venules" of lymph nodes in that their endothelial cells have protuberant nuclei.

The nonfollicular pattern of B-CLH can present as a nodular or diffuse infiltrate with a mixture of cell types. A *sine qua non* is the presence of follicular center cells (centrocytes and centroblasts) as described earlier, but there are often eosinophils, macrophages, and plasma cells. Hints of follicles are sometimes apparent at scanning magnification as zones of pale-staining cells; the presence of follicular elements in such areas can be

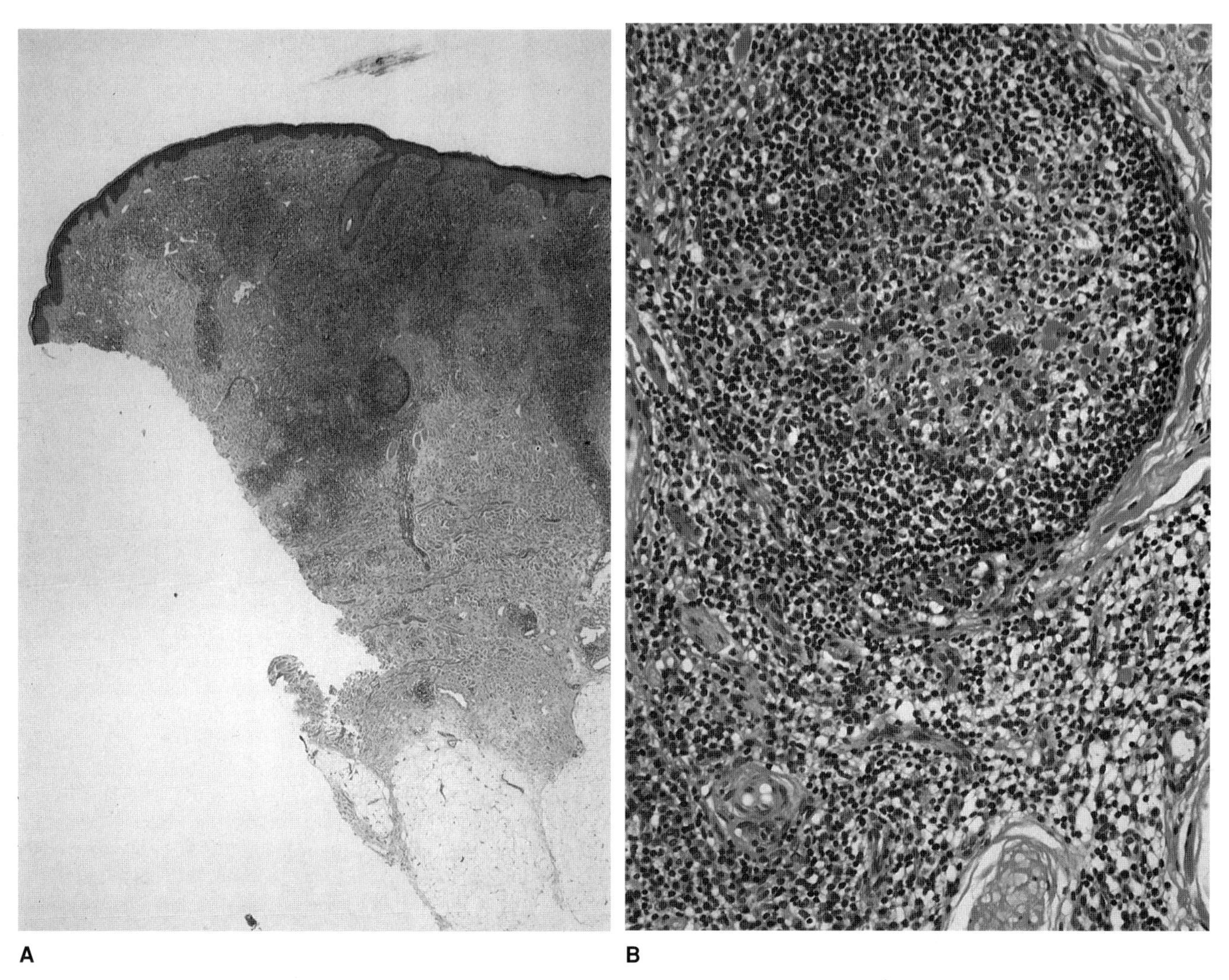

FIG. 32-2. B-cell cutaneous lymphoid hyperplasia
(**A**) Scanning magnification. There is a wedge-shaped, heterogeneous infiltrate. (**B**) Eosinophils, plasma cells, and a germinal center are identifiable at high magnification.

confirmed by immunostaining for antigens such as CD35 that recognize follicular dendritic cells, whose processes form a meshwork in lymphoid follicles.

Other immunophenotypic aspects of B-CLH also resemble those of reactive follicles. The follicular center and mantle zones consist of polyclonal populations of B lymphocytes. Helper T cells are present within follicles, and comprise some of the small lymphocytes therein that have irregular nuclei. The dendrites of antigen-presenting cells are coated with polyclonal immunoglobulin. Cell-membrane-bound immunoglobulin is present in follicular center cells and in those of the mantle zone. At this time, only a few laboratories are able to demonstrate it in routinely processed tissue, using antigen-retrieval techniques. Cytoplasmic immunoglobulin is present in plasma cells, plasmacytoid lymphocytes, and some B immunoblasts. It can be stained by routine immunoperoxidase methods, and the cells that produce it can also be demonstrated by in situ hybridization for messenger RNA. In reactive follicles, κ or λ light-chain-bearing cells can each be present in both follicular and interfollicular zones, in a ratio of approximately 2:1. Because this can vary, most laboratories require ratios of κ:λ expression greater than 5:1 or less than 1:1 as evidence of clonality. The demonstration of clonality is presumptive evidence of neoplasia and is not consistent with a diagnosis of mere B-CLH, but one must be cognizant of the fact that clonality is not necessarily an indicator of biological aggressiveness.

Differential Diagnosis. Follicular B-CLH needs to be distinguished from other processes that contain reactive follicles, as well as from lymphomas that have a follicular pattern or feature reactive follicles. Follicular lymphomas can spread from nodes to the skin, and there are cutaneous lymphomas that have a follicular pattern as well, their immunophenotypic differences from nodal follicular lymphomas notwithstanding (see discussion of cutaneous follicular lymphoma). A "bottom-heavy" (deep dermis and subcutaneous) pattern and close apposition of follicles are clues to follicular lymphoma that are evident at low magnification. In follicular lymphoma, there are nodules nearly entirely composed of small cleaved cells (centrocytes) or small cleaved and large lymphocytes (centrocytes and centroblasts), rather than the mixture of cell types observed in reactive follicles. There are few mitoses in follicular lymphoma when centrocytes predominate, and they become more frequent as the number of large cells (centroblasts) increases. Mitotic figures are numerous in reactive follicles. Thus the finding of but a few mitoses within follicles composed largely of small cells favors lymphoma. Attenuated or absent mantle zones around follicles favor lymphoma over B-CLH. In cases in which a diagnosis is unattainable by routine methods, immunoperoxidase staining can be used to show whether or not there is light chain restriction. In some follicular lymphomas, the interstitial polyclonal immunoglobulins that coat follicular dendritic cells are absent (resulting in so-called immunoglobulin-negative follicular lymphoma). Molecular studies using probes to the immunoglobulin heavy and light chain genes can also be studied to assay clonality. An important caveat is that B-CLH can seem polyclonal by immunophenotypic studies, but its infiltrates can harbor a clone that can be detected only by genotypic analysis.[5]

A variety of other conditions can have conspicuous lymphoid follicles, including angiolymphoid hyperplasia with eosinophilia, Kimura's disease (which is distinct from the former), morphea, dermatofibroma, necrobiosis lipoidica, and necrobiotic xanthogranuloma with paraproteinemia. These conditions are usually readily distinguishable from B-CLH by virtue of their other microscopic attributes.

In the diffuse pattern of B-CLH, centrocytes, centroblasts, and immunoblasts are distributed throughout the infiltrate but cells with striking cytologic atypia are usually absent. There are usually many admixed small T lymphocytes, and varying numbers of eosinophils, plasma cells, and histiocytes. These features overlap with those of low-grade B-cell lymphomas (extranodal marginal cell lymphoma or immunocytoma, the distinction between which is unsettled at this time; see text following). In cases in which several cutaneous sites are involved, or the process recurs over several years, rebiopsy for frozen section immunohistochemistry to test for light chain restriction and hence clonality, or assessment seeking evidence of clonal rearrangement of immunoglobulin genes, can help resolve the differential diagnosis.

Histogenesis. Most cases of B-CLH are unexplained. The putative causes are many, and most texts list hypersensitivity reactions to tattoos, gold earrings, insect bites, infections, folliculitis, trauma, or infection with the spirochete *Borrelia burgdorferi*.[6–8] B-CLH is a late complication of borreliosis, and it occurs in patients with borreliosis more frequently in Europe than in North America, where it appears to be a reaction to *B. burgdorferi afzelius*, a local strain of the spirochete. A distinctive presentation of *Borrelia*-induced B-CLH is bilateral earlobe lesions.

B-Lymphoblastic Lymphoma

Lymphoblastic lymphomas are proliferations of cells with many of the characteristics of primitive lymphocytes, similar to those in the thymic cortex. Peripheral blood involvement by similar cells is termed acute lymphocytic (lymphoblastic) leukemia (ALL). There are both B- and T-cell forms of lymphoblastic lymphoma and of ALL. Most systemic lymphoblastic lymphomas are of T-cell lineage, with T-cell neoplasms comprising roughly 85% of all cases. In contrast, the small numbers of cutaneous lymphoblastic lymphomas analyzed to date have been disproportionately of B-cell lineage.

Systemic T-lymphoblastic lymphoma is a malignancy of high grade that is prone to dissemination. In contrast to this often dire picture, B-lymphoblastic lymphoma usually presents in the skin of children with papules and nodules on the head and neck. Although the outlook is unfavorable for children with disseminated disease, those who present with cutaneous involvement only (stage IE) often do well.[9]

Histopathology. B-lymphoblastic lymphoma most often presents as a nodular or diffuse, monomorphous proliferation of small to medium-sized lymphocytes sparing the epidermis (Fig. 32-3). The cells have scant cytoplasm, which is often undetectable in routinely processed sections. The nuclei are slightly to moderately convoluted with thin but well-defined nuclear membranes and finely dispersed chromatin. Some cases have a subpopulation of cells with multilobated nuclei. Touch preparations can be helpful in demonstrating the cytologic features.

Histogenesis. Although B-cell lymphoblastic lymphomas do not bear cell surface immunoglobulin, the cells often contain intracytoplasmic immunoglobulin and can be considered pre-B cells. Other B-cell associated antigens such as CD20 are present, and most cases express CD10, known also as CALLA (common ALL antigen). The enzyme terminal deoxynucleotidyl transferase (TdT) can be detected by immunoperoxidase staining in the cells of both B- and T-cell lymphoblastic lymphoma, in fresh or routinely processed tissues. TdT is not present in the cells of other lymphomas. T-cell determinants such as CD3 and CD45RO point to the diagnosis of T-lymphoblastic lymphoma if other attributes are present.

Differential Diagnosis. Small, noncleaved cell (or "undifferentiated") lymphoma, either of the Burkitt's or so-called non-Burkitt's type, can be difficult to distinguish from lymphoblastic lymphoma. The differential diagnosis between them is seldom decided on skin biopsy, and a solitary cutaneous lesion in a child in whom this choice arises is far more likely to have lymphoblastic lymphoma. Small, noncleaved cell lymphoma is more apt to present with a "starry sky" pattern resulting from interspersed macrophages, and mitotic figures are more conspicuous. The nuclei of the cells of small noncleaved lymphomas differ by being larger, with a more coarse chromatin pattern, and often have multiple nucleoli. The cytoplasms of small noncleaved lymphoma cells stain more deeply with methyl green pyronine, and contain vacuoles that are best seen on touch imprints. Small cleaved (centrocytic) and mantle zone lymphoma can also resemble lymphoblastic lymphoma, and differentiation is important in that the chemotherapies appropriate for these conditions are different. The so-called "small round cell tumors" may enter the diagnosis of small noncleaved cell and lymphoblastic lymphoma. Immunohistochemistry is of great assistance in this differential diagnosis.

Small B-Lymphocytic Lymphoma (SLL)

Small lymphocytic lymphoma (SLL) is a proliferation of cells resembling those comprising primary lymphoid follicles—i.e., the collections of immunologically naive B cells seen in lymph nodes prior to antigenic challenge. Its cells are indistinguishable from those of B-cell chronic lymphocytic leukemia (B-CLL), and the dividing line between the two conditions, based on the degree of peripheral blood lymphocytosis, is arbitrary, with cutoff points ranging from 4 to 15,000 cells per cubic millimeter. SLL was referred to as well-differentiated lym-

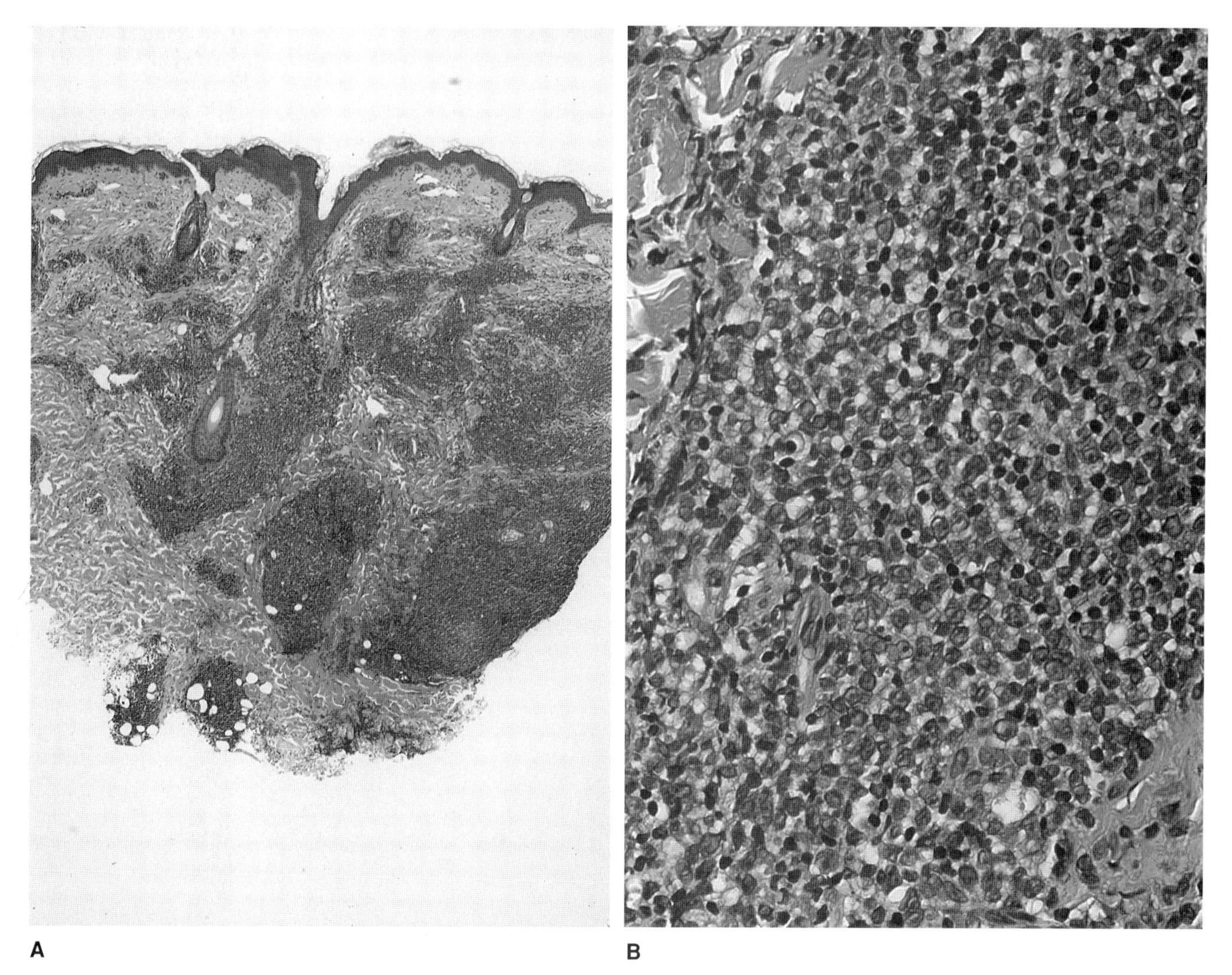

A B

FIG. 32-3. B-lymphoblastic lymphoma, scanning magnification
(**A**) A diffuse infiltrate of lymphocytes permeates the reticular dermis. (**B**) The neoplastic nuclei have delicate nuclear membranes that enclose finely distributed chromatin. Nucleoli are inconspicuous, as is cytoplasm.

phocytic lymphoma in the Rappaport classification of lymphoma and in previous editions of this text.

Cutaneous nodules or tumors or diffuse infiltrates that can cause a leonine facies are among the presentations of SLL/CLL that have been noted.[10] Some patients with CLL have had vesicles and bullae above plaques. Whether the vesiculation is a result of the infiltrates or marks the sites of insect bites to which neoplastic cells have homed is uncertain.

Histopathology. There are three main histologic patterns that the infiltrates of SLL/CLL can demonstrate.[11] One is a superficial and deep perivascular pattern, which spares the epidermis but can involve venules in the subcutaneous fat. Another is an interstitial pattern, in which the cells are arranged perivascularly and as strands between reticular dermal collagen bundles, in a fashion similar to that observed in many forms of leukemia (Fig. 32-4). In the third pattern, there is a nodular or diffuse infiltrate, which spares the epidermis. The cytologic features of small lymphocytic lymphoma include scant cytoplasm; a small, round to oval nucleus with small aggregates of chromatin in apposition to the nuclear membrane; and a small nucleolus. In some examples with a diffuse pattern of cutaneous infiltration, "proliferation centers" or "pseudofollicles" are present (Fig. 32-5). These are pale-staining zones containing slightly larger cells, termed prolymphocytes and paraimmunoblasts, whose nuclei tend to be more pale-staining.

Histogenesis. The cells of small lymphocytic lymphoma are B lymphocytes that have a single type of immunoglobulin light chain on their membranes, a finding that can be exploited in fresh material, but not yet in routinely processed sections. The cells also express a variety of B-cell determinants, such as CD20 and CD79a. CD23 is an antigen that is found on the cells of the mantles of secondary lymphoid follicles, and also on those of SLL/CLL. CD23 is infrequently found in other B-cell neoplasms. SLL/CLL can aberrantly coexpress the T-cell-associated antigens CD43 and CD5 in addition to B-cell determinants.[11] These T-cell antigens are present in normal B cells early in their development. CD43 is preserved in formalin-fixed, paraffin-embedded tissue, and demonstration of its coexpression by a cutaneous infiltrate of B lymphocytes with small round nuclei can clinch the diagnosis of SLL/CLL. Although

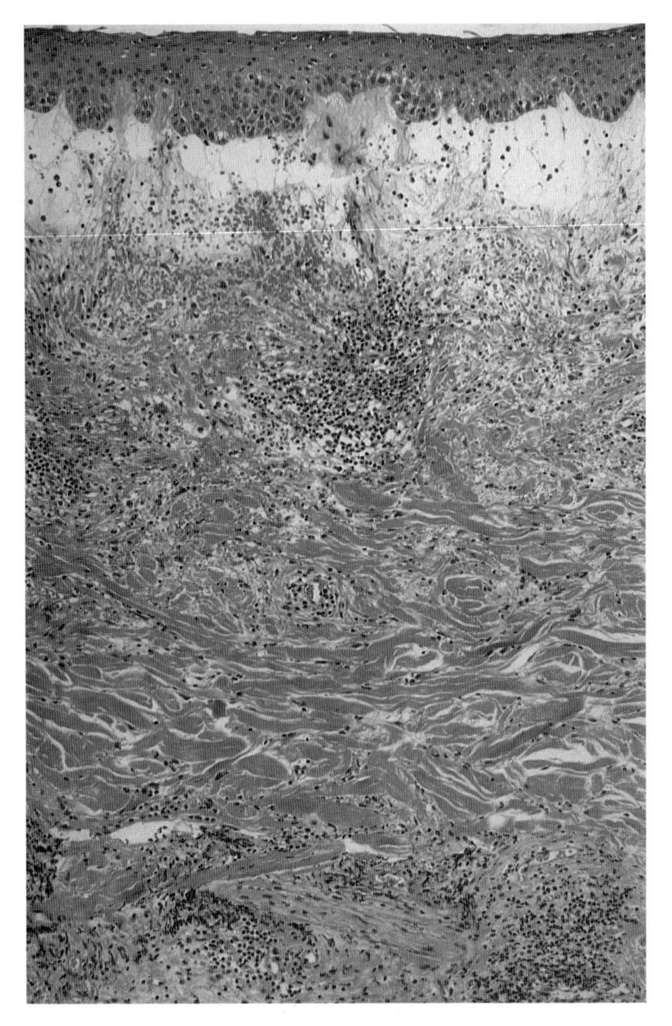

FIG. 32-4. SLL/CLL
This specific infiltrate of SLL/CLL consists of lymphocytes distributed interstitially. Expression of both CD20 and CD43 was detected immunohistochemically. The presence of papillary dermal edema is an unusual feature.

coexpression of CD5 is diagnostically useful in fresh material, the epitope that is preserved in paraffin-embedded sections is frequently not detectable. Ki-67, a marker of cell proliferation, is expressed at a higher rate in the proliferation centers of SLL/CLL than in the surrounding smaller cells.[11] Other T-cell antigens such as CD3 and CD45RO are expressed by small reactive cells (marked by slightly irregular nuclei) rather than by neoplastic lymphocytes.

The cells of SLL/CLL often have trisomy of chromosome 12 and a t(11;14) translocation that results in rearrangement of the *bcl*-1 oncogene. This gene encodes a cell cycle regulatory protein. Rearrangements of *bcl*-1 can be detected by the polymerase chain reaction.

Differential Diagnosis. Inflammatory skin diseases with superficial and deep perivascular, or perivascular and interstitial, infiltrates, in which small lymphocytes predominate but spare the epidermis, can resemble SLL/CLL. Polymorphous light eruption, "tumid" lesions of lupus erythematosus (a variant of discoid lupus erythematosus in which the epidermis is largely spared), reactions to some arthropod bites, the deep form of gyrate erythema, and early inflammatory lesions of morphea in which sclerosis has not supervened all share this pattern and enter the differential diagnosis. The cells of SLL/CLL have round nuclei, whereas most reactive infiltrates are composed of T cells with slightly convoluted nuclei. Other microscopic clues include mucin and a perifollicular distribution of cells in tumid lupus erythematosus and plasma cells in lupus and in morphea, especially around the deep vascular plexus. Immunohistochemical staining can be quite helpful in difficult cases (see preceding text for the characteristic features). The lymphocytes of virtually all inflammatory skin diseases are T cells; for practical purposes, a predominant population of B cells is evident only in B-cell lymphoma or leukemia and B-CLH.

Marginal zone cell lymphoma also is composed of small lymphocytes resembling the cells of both primary follicles and follicular mantles (further discussion following). Its cutaneous infiltrates frequently have the remnants of reactive follicles scattered within them, and do not demonstrate the proliferation centers observed in SLL/CLL.

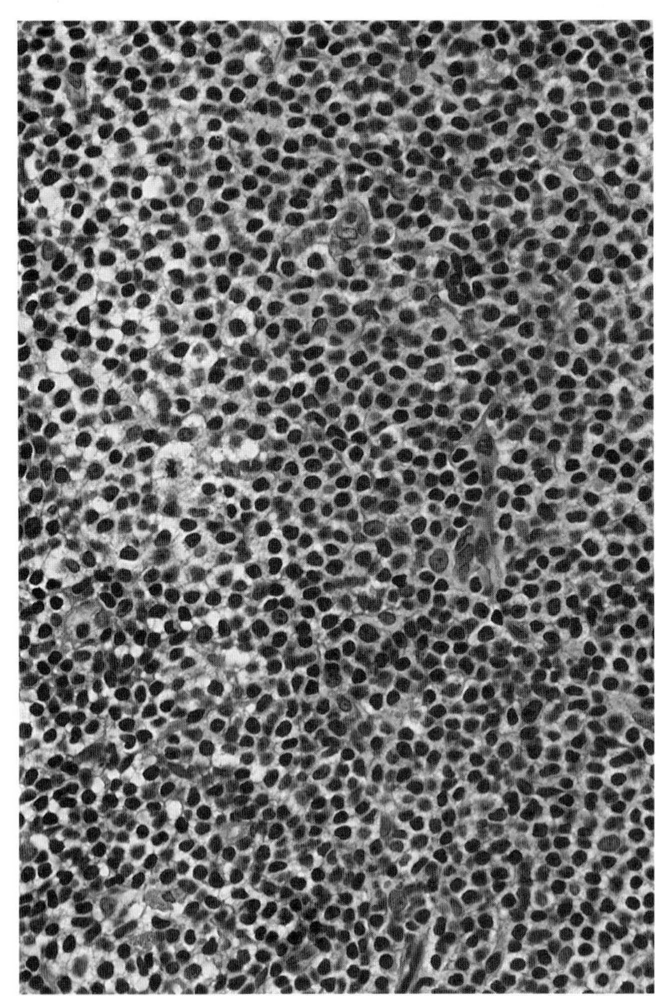

FIG. 32-5. SLL/CLL
A diffuse infiltrate of SLL/CLL is punctuated by poorly defined nodular zones of larger "prolymphocytic" cells, a configuration known as proliferation centers.

Immunocytoma (Lymphoplasmacytoid or Lymphoplasmacellular Lymphoma)

Immunocytoma is a low-grade B-cell lymphoma in which some of the neoplastic cells include plasmacytoid lymphocytes, sometimes termed immunocytes, which is a confusing designation that has been largely abandoned because so many other types of lymphocytes also play a role in immunity. Plasmacytoid lymphocytes have the eccentric nuclei and cytoplasms, but not the coarse chromatin distributed in a "clock-face" pattern, typical of plasma cells. Immunocytoma is thought to be a distinct neoplasm by some, whereas others believe that it lies within the spectrum of mucosal and marginal zone lymphomas. In the spleen, the marginal zone is a ring of pale-staining cells peripheral to the mantle zone that encircles secondary lymphoid follicles both in the spleen and at other sites. Marginal zone lymphomas of the spleen, and many of those arising in mucosal associated lymphoid tissue (MALT), are composed in part of centrocyte-like lymphocytes. These cells are small lymphocytes with indented nuclei and varying amounts of pale cytoplasm. The plasma cells and plasmacytoid lymphocytes found in marginal zone and MALT lymphomas express the same immunoglobulin types as the centrocyte-like cells.[12]

Primary cutaneous immunocytoma usually presents with a single nodule or plaque on the trunk or an extremity. Lesions are less frequently found on the skin of the head and neck, in contast to primary cutaneous follicular lymphomas. Nodules of immunocytoma have reportedly occurred in patches of acrodermatitis chronica atrophicans.[10,13] In secondary cutaneous immunocytoma, cutaneous lesions are often multiple and widely distributed.

The course of patients with primary cutaneous immunocytoma is favorable, and that of secondary disease is less so.[14] Immunoblastic lymphoma and leukemia are rare complications. IgM κ, or less frequently IgG κ or λ, are produced by the neoplastic cells.[15] If there is abundant secretion of IgM, Waldenstrom's macroglobulinemia can result. Autoimmune diseases such as autoimmune hemolytic anemia, Sjögren's syndrome, or Hashimoto's thyroiditis can accompany systemic immunocytoma.

Histopathology. Primary cutaneous immunocytoma violates many of the traditional rules for differentiating lymphoma from "pseudolymphoma." There is usually a "top-heavy" rather than a "bottom-heavy" pattern—that is, the superficial dermis is more densely infiltrated than the deep dermis, and the subcutis is often spared. Its infiltrates are heterogeneous rather than monomorphous (Fig. 32-6). Eosinophils can be plentiful. Nonneoplastic lymphoid follicles are characteristically present.[16,18] For these reasons, many cases have been misinterpreted as B-CLH, and undoubtedly some of the cases in which lymphoma purportedly arose in B-CLH were immunocytomas from the outset.

Several details regarding this histologically deceptive lymphoma are pertinent. There are often vertically oriented pillars of cells that follow the courses of hair follicles. The heterogeneous composition includes plasmacytoid lymphocytes, immunoblasts, and plasma cells, as well as the above-mentioned centrocyte-like lymphocytes. Rarely, the plasmacytoid lymphocytes of an immunocytoma have convoluted nuclei.[16] Cells with features intermediate between any of the earlier types can also be present. There is a tendency for plasmacytoid cells or plasma cells to be present at the peripheries of aggregations in primary cutaneous, but not in secondary cutaneous, infiltrates. The reactive elements in immunocytomas, both primary and secondary, can include lymphoid follicles, eosinophils, T cells, and histiocytes (sometimes comprising small granulomas). Colonization of secondary lymphoid follicles by centrocyte-like cells can occur, a finding previously noted in MALTomas and marginal zone lymphomas.

In both lesions resulting from relapse of primary cutaneous immunocytoma and lesions of secondary disease, sheets of plasmacytoid or immunoblastic lymphocytes can be encountered.

Histogenesis. The cells of immunocytoma do not represent mature plasma cells, but rather represent B lymphocytes that display varying degrees of plasmacytic differentiation. Although the plasmacytoid cells of immunocytoma are of B lineage, they sometimes do not express CD20 and can aberrantly express the T-cell determinant CD43, findings that can lead to misinterpretation as a T-cell lymphoma. Cytoplasmic immunoglobulin is well preserved in routinely processed tissue, in contrast to cell-membrane-bound immunoglobulin. Light chain restriction can therefore be used to confirm the clonality of immunocytoma. Although immunoperoxidase staining often gives clear-cut results, any cell with plasmacytic differentiation can nonspecifically absorb immunoglobulin; therefore, excellent technique and careful interpretation are necessary. Nonspecific absorption results in pale diffuse cytoplasmic deposition of the chromagen, in contrast to the more intense, granular staining of a specific reaction. In situ hybridization for light chain messenger RNA (mRNA) does not suffer from this limitation and often yields superior results.

Differential Diagnosis. As noted earlier, immunocytoma shares many features with B-CLH. Key features in its identification are vertically oriented perifollicular infiltrates and the presence of cells with plasmacytoid or centrocyte-like features. Because immunocytoma is monoclonal and B-CLH is polyclonal, light chain restriction can be the key to distinguishing these conditions.

Although myeloma also shows plasmacytic differentiation, in myeloma there are monomorphous nodules of plasma cells, some of which show aberrant nuclei.

Cutaneous Follicular Lymphoma (FL)

Cutaneous lymphomas with a follicular pattern comprise a heterogeneous group. The skin can be involved by follicular lymphoma (FL) of nodal origin, and sometimes a follicular pattern is evident in these secondary ("metastatic") infiltrates.[18] The existence of primary cutaneous lymphomas with a follicular pattern has only recently been recognized, as the morphologic criteria used to distinguish reactive from neoplastic follicles in lymph nodes began to be applied to the skin.[19] Primary cutaneous FL was at first regarded as the cutaneous counterpart of nodal follicular center lymphoma. More recently, it has become apparent that primary cutaneous lymphomas with a follicular pattern show closer resemblance to mucosal lymphomas (MALTomas) and marginal zone lymphoma of the spleen than to true follicular center lymphomas of lymph nodes, and share the more favorable prognosis of these extranodal neo-

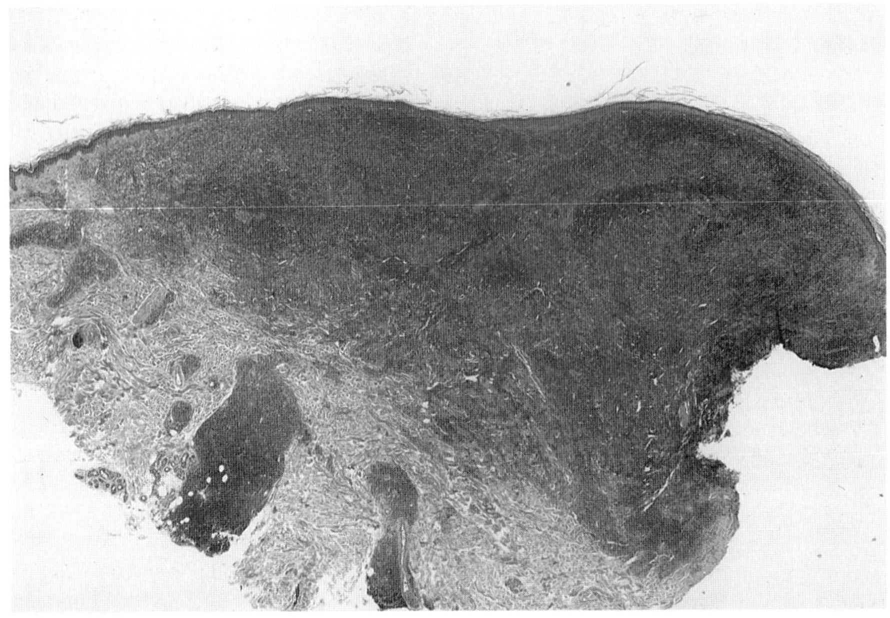

A

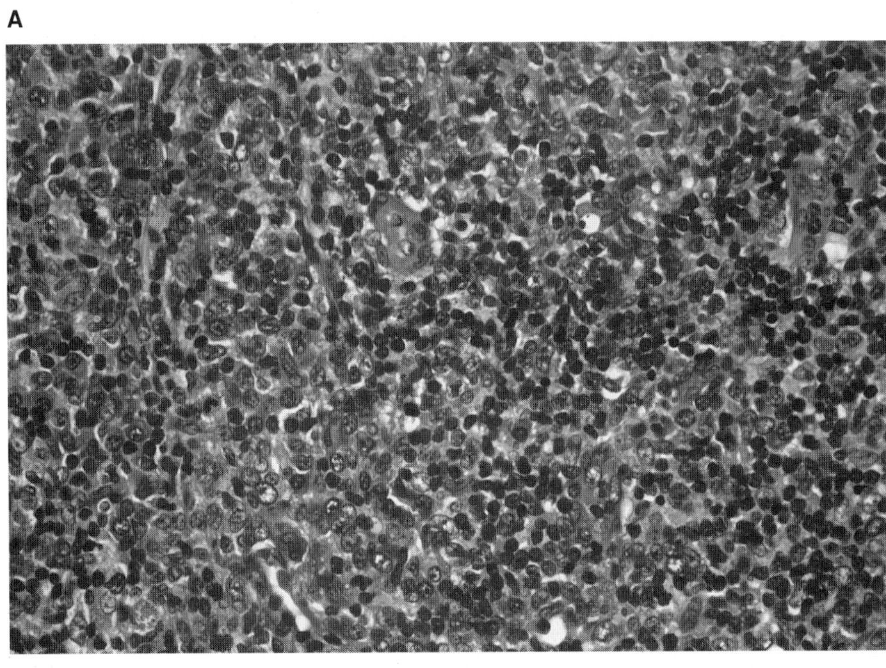

B

FIG. 32-6. Immunocytoma (lymphoplasmacellular lymphoma)
(**A**) There is a vaguely wedge-shaped infiltrate that is denser in the upper half of the reticular dermis. Although the pattern is "top-heavy," there is a vertically oriented column of lymphoid elements surrounding adnexa in the deep reticular dermis, a pattern characteristic of this small B-cell lymphoma. (**B**) The infiltrate is heterogeneous but includes both plasmacytoid lymphocytes and many mature plasma cells, particularly at the periphery of the infiltrate. Eosinophils are often present in large numbers, although they are lacking in this example.

plasms.[12,20] Cutaneous lymphoma with a follicular pattern and MALToma-like features may overlap with primary cutaneous immunocytoma, as noted earlier. The follicular pattern in both lymphomas may result from colonization of reactive follicles. A third form of cutaneous lymphoma in which a follicular pattern is evident is mantle zone lymphoma, in which reactive follicles can be compressed or overrun.

Because the prognosis of cutaneous B-cell lymphomas, in which a follicular pattern is evident, is favorable if the disease is primary and unfavorable if the skin is secondarily involved, distinction among these subtypes of primary cutaneous lymphoma is mostly of academic interest. For the purpose of this discussion we will lump these conditions together under the rubric of primary cutaneous FL.

The clinical presentation of primary cutaneous FL stereotypically comprises one or several nodules situated in a single area, most often the skin of the scalp or forehead. The lesions are red to purple and can have intact or ulcerated surfaces.

Secondary spread to the skin is observed in about 4% of the cases of nodal FL. A lymphoma in which small cleaved cells predominate in lymph nodes can feature large noncleaved ones in secondary skin lesions. This "dedifferentiation" or transformation is an unfavorable prognostic sign.

Histopathology. The infiltrates of cutaneous follicular lymphoma are most easily diagnosed when they are bottom-heavy, but top-heavy patterns also occur. In cases that resemble follicular center lymphomas of lymph nodes, or in secondary spread to the skin of nodal follicular lymphoma, many of the same criteria that apply to the diagnosis of follicular center lymphoma in nodes can be applied to the skin.[22] The neoplastic follicles can be of uniform size, with mantles that are thin or absent, resulting in coalescence of follicles (Fig. 32-7). Tingible body macrophages, which represent cells engulfing the remnants of apoptotic lymphocytes, are rare.[20] The mitotic rate is low in cases in which small cleaved cells (centrocytes) predominate, and higher as the proportion of large noncleaved cells or centroblasts increases. Most of the many variations of FL that occur in lymph nodes, such as irregularly shaped follicles, follicles with serrated outlines, follicles with thick mantles, conspicuous follicular dendritic cells, many tingible body macrophages, and follicles with extracellular amorphous material, can also occur in cutaneous lesions. In lesions with an immunophenotype resembling MALToma, the cells can be more centrocyte-like (see section on Immunocytoma) or monocytoid.

Histogenesis. Cutaneous FL is a proliferation of B cells that expresses monotypic cell surface immunoglobulin, or fails to express immunoglobulin at all (in so-called "immunoglobulin-negative" FL). The cells of the neoplasms that share this pattern express CD20 and CD79a.

In North America, about 85% of patients with node-based FL display the t(14;18) translocation, an event that results in the apposition of an oncogene on the long arm of chromosome 14, *bcl*-2, with the heavy chain joining gene (J_H) on the long arm of chromosome 14 (for unexplained reasons, this translocation

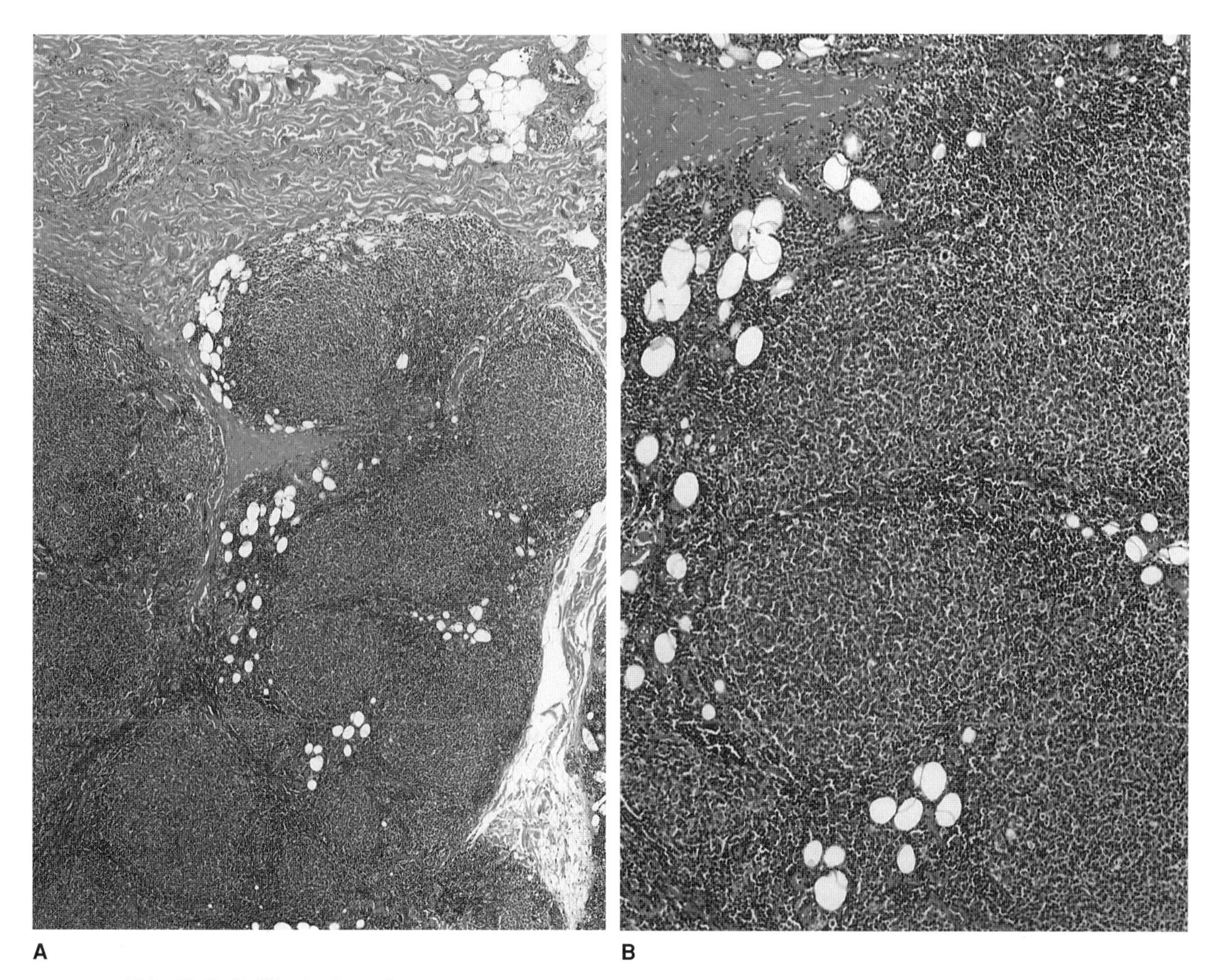

FIG. 32-7. Follicular lymphoma
(**A**) A multinodular pattern is clearly evident in this lymphomatous infiltrate situated at the dermal-subcutaneous junction, composed of small, cleaved, follicular center cells arrayed as coalescing follicles. (**B**) Note the absence of tingible body macrophages.

occurs less frequently in FL patients from Europe and Asia). As a result, there is increased production of the protein *bcl*-2. The *bcl*-2 protein is present on the membranes of mitochondria. It is one of many molecules that regulate apoptosis. B lymphocytes that contain high levels of *bcl*-2 are resistant to apoptosis, and tend to accumulate as a result of their longevity. Immunoperoxidase staining can detect *bcl*-2 in the cells of most examples of FL that have the t(14;18) translocation. In studies from Europe, the t(14;18) translocation is rare in primary cutaneous FL, and *bcl*-2 protein is not expressed immunohistochemically by the follicular B cells. Additional genetic defects beyond *bcl*-2 rearrangement appear to occur in aggressive subtypes of follicular lymphoma.

Along with a *bcl*-2-negative phenotype, the cells of marginal-zone-like or MALToma-like FL lack CD10, or CALLA, in contrast to those of authentic nodal FL.[20]

Differential Diagnosis. The principal simulant of cutaneous FL is follicular B-CLH. The heterogeneous composition of follicles, with many tingible body macrophages and well-formed mantles of small lymphocytes around them, are findings that favor a benign interpretation. Although cytologically normal follicular center cells can predominate in lymphoma, some examples of FL contain cytologically aberrant cells, such as "dysplastic" small cleaved cells that have remarkably attenuated nuclei.

Light chain restriction can be used to demonstrate clonality in problematic cases. In immunoglobulin-negative FL, the polyclonal immunoglobulin that permeates reactive follicles is absent.[21] Genotypic studies can detect clonal rearrangement of the immunoglobulin heavy or light chain genes, or both.

Mantle Cell Lymphoma (MCL)

Mantle cell lymphoma (MCL) is a neoplasm whose normal cellular counterparts are the cells that comprise the mantles that surround secondary follicles in lymph nodes and extranodal sites. Originally termed "intermediate lymphocytic lymphoma," MCL has emerged as a distinct clinicopathologic entity with unique molecular and immunohistochemical features.

Most patients with MCL have disseminated disease at the outset, with lymph node disease accompanied by involvement of other organs. A leukemic phase can ensue in up to one-third of all patients.

Only a few well-characterized patients with cutaneous disease have been reported, but it seems likely that this is largely a result of the fact that the salient characteristics have only recently been described. In some cases, cutaneous lesions preceded visceral, nodal, or leukemic disease by years, suggesting that although the disease can be primary in the skin, it is not as indolent as cutaneous immunocytoma or FL.[22,23]

Histopathology. The neoplastic cells of MCL range from small lymphocytes that resemble the cells of SLL/CLL to larger cells that resemble small, cleaved cells or centrocytes but are more apt to have a clumped chromatin pattern. The microscopic hallmark, which is best seen in lymph nodes but can also be observed in cutaneous infiltrates, is the tendency of the neoplastic lymphocytes to surround and seemingly compress nonneoplastic lymphoid follicles, which are visible as small, round collections of pale-staining cells in a sea of dark-staining lymphocytes. Cases with this pattern are referred to as mantle zone, as opposed to merely mantle cell, lymphoma. There are often foci of plasmacytic differentiation in cutaneous lesions. In many cases, the infiltrates are patchy and "top-heavy."

MCL cells express pan-B-cell markers, such as CD19, CD20, and CD21, and also are IgM- and often IgD-positive. Lambda light chains are often expressed, in contrast to the k predominance of some other lymphomas. Mantle cell lymphoma cells express CD5, and anomalously express the T-cell determinant CD43, as do the cells of SLL/CLL. Unlike SLL/CLL cells, MCL cells lack CD23.

Histogenesis. MCL is a B-cell neoplasm that is characteristically associated with a t(11;14)q(13;32) translocation that results in the apposition of *bcl*-1 to the immunoglobulin heavy chain gene. The resulant overexpressed protein, also known as PRAD1 or cyclin D1, can be detected immunohistochemically.

Differential Diagnosis. MCL can present in the skin with or without a so-called mantle zone pattern. When a mantle zone pattern is present, the differential diagnosis includes other lymphoproliferative diseases in which follicles are present—namely, B-CLH, FL, and immunocytoma/extranodal marginal zone lymphoma. The small, compressed follicles of MCL within a sea of small lymphocytes make a distinctive pattern not seen in these other conditions. Thick follicular mantles can sometimes be present in B-CLH, and follicles can be inconspicuous, but the B-CLH differs from those of MCL in that they are not small, sharply circumscribed and round. The follicles in mantle cell lymphoma are not neoplastic, unlike those in follicular lymphoma. Infiltration of follicles by centrocytoid cells occurs in immunocytoma or marginal zone lymphoma, so that follicles can have irregular outlines (so-called colonization of follicles by neoplastic lymphocytes). The resultant follicles have irregular outlines. The interfollicular infiltrates in immunocytoma or marginal zone lymphoma are often markedly heterogeneous in composition, with small lymphocytes, plasmacytoid lymphocytes, plasma cells, immunoblasts, eosinophils, and histiocytes, whereas most examples of mantle cell lymphoma feature monomorphous infiltrates (rare cases can demonstrate blastic cells or ones with plasmacytoid differentiation). The follicles of the mantle zone pattern must also be distinguished from proliferation centers in SLL/CLL (see earlier discussion). These pale-staining foci contain cells with large central nucleoli, rather than typical follicular center cells. If a mantle zone pattern is absent, the principal differential diagnosis is SLL/CLL. In the absence of proliferation centers, immunohistochemical studies can be helpful, because the infiltrates of these conditions express CD23 and lack cyclin D1, in contrast to MCL.

Cutaneous Plasmacytoma and Multiple Myeloma (MM)

Plasmacytomas are localized collections of monoclonal plasma cells. Cutaneous plasmacytomas either arise in the skin or spread secondarily to it from internal (usually osseous) foci of myeloma. There is a broad range of disease. Cutaneous plasmacytoma can occur in patients with no evidence of myeloma, or can be a harbinger of future myeloma. In some patients with solitary cutaneous plasmacytoma, there is laboratory evidence of myeloma at the time of presentation. In others, the process appears to be localized, because ablation of the lesion effects a cure. Systemic spread has apparently occurred in some patients with plasmacytomas either of the skin or of internal organs.[24]

Multiple myeloma (MM) is an often rapidly fatal, disseminated malignant neoplasm of plasma cells. The diagnosis of MM is based on clinical, laboratory, and microscopic findings. These findings include not only the presence of a pathologically established plasmacytoma but also the spread of plasma cells to the bone marrow, paraproteinemia or a monoclonal immunoglobulin or light chain protein in the urine, lytic bone lesions, or plasma cell leukemia. Bone pain, pathologic fractures, systemic amyloidosis, and renal failure are important consequences of plasma cell infiltration or secretion. The frequency of extraosseous infiltration by plasma cells is related to the type of immunoglobulin produced by the neoplastic plasma cells. Only 1% to 3% of patients having IgA or IgG-producing cells exhibit extraosseous deposits of myeloma, whereas in 10% of patients who produce only light chains and in 63% of those with IgD-producing tumors, the lesions spread to other sites.[25]

Cutaneous lesions of MM or plasmacytoma are usually circumscribed, violaceous papules or nodules. Diffusely infiltrated plaques are occasionally observed.[26] Cutaneous deposits of myeloma are rare, occurring in only about 2% of myeloma patients.[27] Patients with myeloma can also develop a variety of nonspecific cutaneous complications, including deposits of light-chain derived amyloid (primary systemic amyloidosis), purpuric lesions resulting from monoclonal cryoglobulinemia, diffuse normolipemic plane xanthoma, pyoderma gangrenosum, Sweet's syndrome, leukocytoclastic vasculitis, and erythema elevatum diutinum.

Monoclonal gammopathies can complicate a variety of other cutaneous diseases, such as scleromyxedema, necrobiotic xanthogranuloma with paraproteinemia, POEMS syndrome (polyneuropathy, organomegaly, endocrinopathy, M protein, and skin lesions), and scleredema. Myeloma supervenes in a small minority of patients with any of these disorders.

Histopathology. In cutaneous lesions of MM and in plasmacytomas, there are monomorphous infiltrates of plasma cells, arrayed as densely cellular nodules or interstitially between collagen bundles (Fig. 32-8).[28] In the nodular pattern, clusters of macrophages are sometimes present. Multinucleate plasmal cells, plasmacytes with large atypical nuclei, and mitotic figures can be observed. Plasma cell bodies, round eosinophilic fragments of plasma cell cytoplasm, can be present in the background between intact cells, but are not specific for MM because they can be present in any plasmacyte-rich infiltrate. Intranuclear inclusions of immunoglobulin, known as Dutcher bodies, which can be mistaken for eosinophilic nucleoli, are rare in MM. Infiltrates that are composed of nuclei with a "clock-face" clumping of chromatin typical of mature, or Marshalko-type, plasma cells have been referred to as the plasmacytic variant. Infiltrates that are composed of cells with nuclei that resemble those of immunoblasts are sometimes referred to as plasmablastic plasmacytoma, whereas an even greater degree of nuclear atypia is observed in the anaplastic variant. Ultrastructurally, the cells of MM and plasmacytoma have prominent cisternae lined by rough endoplasmic reticulum, as do normal plasma cells.

Histogenesis. Plasmacytomas and myelomas are composed of neoplastic plasma cells whose cytoplasms contain immunoglobulin, which can be demonstrated in paraffin-embedded tissue. Light chain restriction is generally easily shown, although nonspecific absorption of immunoglobulin can lead to difficulties in interpretation of clonality. Accentuation of staining in the Golgi region is specific evidence of clonal immunoglobulin synthesis by the cells in question. Like normal plasma cells, neoplastic cells do not express leukocyte common antigen (CD45) or the most common B-lymphocyte marker, CD20. A further pitfall is that neoplastic plasma cells can express epithelial membrane antigen, leading to the erroneous diagnosis of carcinoma in rare cases.

Differential Diagnosis. Infiltrates in which mature plasma cells predominate can be confused with MM or plasmacytomas.

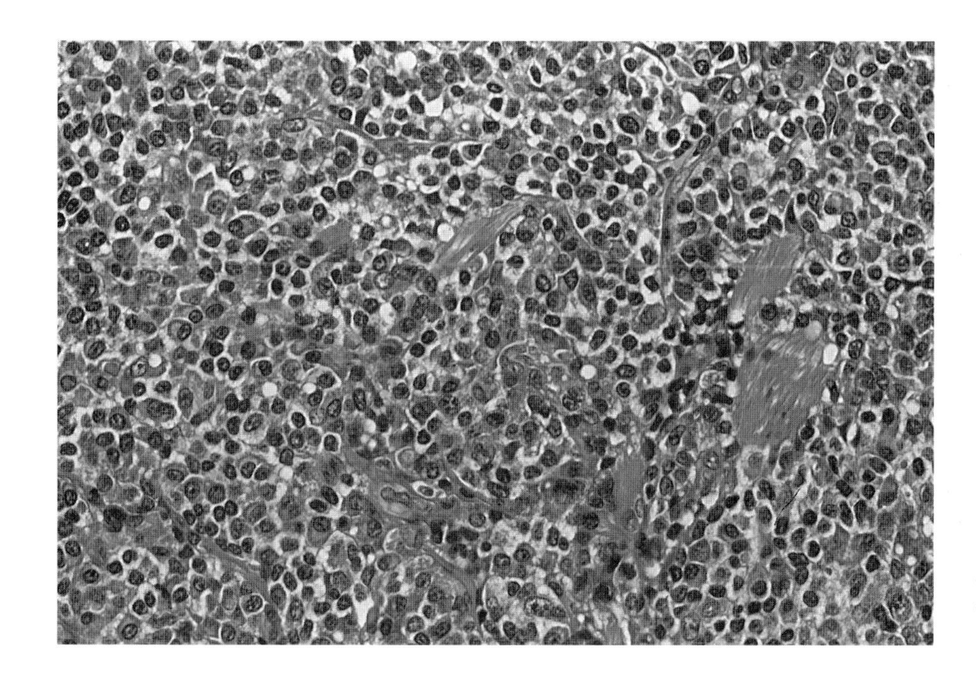

FIG. 32-8. Plasmacytes
Atypical, vesicular nuclei are distributed in a nodular configuration in this cutaneous infiltrate of IgM+ plasmacytoma.

Inflammatory reactions involving the scalp or mucous membranes are frequently replete with plasma cells, a finding known as circumorificial plasmacytosis.[29] Systemic plasmacytosis is an apparently nonneoplastic proliferation of plasma cells that has been observed in Japanese patients, manifested as cutaneous plaques accompanied by lymphadenopathy and polyclonal hypergammaglobulinemia.[30] Histologically, there are perivascular or dermal nodules of well-differentiated plasma cells. Cutaneous inflammatory pseudotumors present as fibrotic nodules, situated in the dermis or subcutis, with patterned sclerosis, thickened vessels, lymphoid follicles, and dense plasma-cell-rich but heterogeneous infiltrates.[31]

Immunoperoxidase staining using antisera to κ and λ light chains is helpful in discerning clonality. Light chain expression can also help in confirming a diagnosis of MM, if the neoplastic cells are not morphologically recognizable as plasma cells. Large-cell lymphomas, especially B-cell immunoblastic lymphoma and immunocytoma, can be confused with myeloma and plasmacytoma. The nuclei of the cells of immunoblastic lymphoma are larger and more vesicular than those of neoplastic plasma cells. Although chromatin is marginated along nuclear membranes, it does not occur in blocks large enough to impart the "clock-face" pattern observed in plasma cells. Plasma cells have more cytoplasm than do the cells of immunoblastic lymphoma cells, and their nuclei are more centrally situated. The cytoplasm of myeloma cells is intensely pyroninophilic, staining dark red with pyronine. Cutaneous immunocytoma (see discussion earlier) is an indolent disease, in contrast to the fulminant course characteristic of myeloma. The cells of immunocytoma can vary considerably, and centrocyte-like, small plasmacytoid, and immunoblast-like forms can be present. A key finding in many immunocytomas is the presence of a spectrum of differentiation in contrast to the monomorphous differentiation within a single lesion of myeloma. Heterologous elements, such as eosinophils, lymphoid follicles, and granulomata, are much more common in immunocytoma than in myeloma.

Diffuse Large B-Cell Lymphoma (Centroblastic and Immunoblastic Lymphoma, B-Cell Type)

Large-cell types of B-cell lymphoma of nodal origin are aggressive neoplasms when a diffuse rather than a follicular pattern is evident. They can spread secondarily to the skin, and some forms can arise within the skin. The distinction between different morphologic forms of diffuse large-cell B-cell lymphoma may not be possible. Large noncleaved B cells with small nucleoli are thought to correspond to similar cells in follicles, and proliferations with similar features have been termed centroblastic lymphoma in the Kiel classification. Immunoblastic lymphomas have been said to be neoplasms of cells that resemble immunoblasts—reactive B cells that have large, vesicular nuclei, prominent central nucleoli, distinct nuclear membranes, and moderate amounts of amphophilic cytoplasm. Immunoblasts are believed to be precursors of plasma cells, and hence their cytoplasms can contain immunoglobulin. Both T- and B-cell immunoblastic lymphomas can occur. The distinction between centroblastic and immunoblastic types of large-cell lymphoma rests on the size and position of nucleoli (larger and more centrally placed in immunoblasts than in centroblasts) and the amounts of cytoplasm (more abundant and basophilic in immunoblastic lymphoma). The authors of the REAL classification recognized the unreliability of making this differential diagnosis and established a category titled simply "diffuse large B-cell lymphoma."[1] The distinction between immunoblasts and immunocytes should also be mentioned here. Although the terms are similar, the cells differ greatly in appearance. Immunocytes (plasmacytoid lymphocytes) have some features of small lymphocytes and others of plasma cells. Immunoblasts, on the other hand, are large lymphocytes with far larger nuclei and nucleoli. Immunocytoma is a low-grade lymphoma, whereas immunoblastic lymphoma is a high-grade neoplasm.

Diffuse B-cell lymphomas of the large-cell type appear on the skin as red to purplish papules, nodules, or plaques. Primary cutaneous diffuse large-cell lymphoma can be diagnosed if lesions are solitary, or few and confined to a single area, and if a staging work-up is negative. Secondary large-cell lymphoma metastatic to skin often presents with disseminated lesions.

Many patients with diffuse large B-cell lymphoma primary in the skin, whose lesions are localized to one area, can be cured or put into long remissions with local modalities. An exception may be patients with localized lesions involving the lower legs, who seem to undergo a more aggressive course.[32] Another localization of large-cell lymphoma worthy of comment is involvement of the skin of the back. The term "reticulohistiocytoma of the dorsum (of Crosti)" has been used in the European literature for this condition, which is simply large-cell lymphoma of B-cell lineage presenting as plaques on the back.[33]

Histopathology. Diffuse large-cell lymphoma of the B-cell type often fulfills the expectations of students as to what to expect of a cutaneous lymphoma: there are "bottom-heavy" dermal and subcutaneous infiltrates that often are composed of cells with monomorphous, large nuclei, accompanied by numerous mitotic figures, necrosis of adnexa, and ulceration (Fig. 32-9). The amount of cytoplasm is often difficult to appreciate in any but the best hematoxylin-eosin–stained preparations. In Europe and Asia, many hematopathologists also evaluate Giemsa-stained sections, in which immunoblastic lymphomas exhibit distinct basophilic cytoplasms. Pseudocarcinomatous epidermal hyperplasia and infiltration of the epidermis by neoplastic cells are unusual findings. Variable cytologic features include marked nuclear pleomorphism, plasmacytoid differentiation, and folded or indented nuclei.

Histogenesis. Diffuse large-cell lymphomas of B lineage comprise a histogenetically heterogeneous group. Some appear to begin as follicular center-cell lymphomas, which can have varying proportions of large cells. Rearrangements of *bcl* are present in a proportion of cases of nodal diffuse large-cell lymphoma and may indicate a follicular center-cell origin. It seems likely that other genetic findings will define clinicopathologic subsets among these neoplasms.

Differential Diagnosis. The differential diagnosis of diffuse large-cell B-cell lymphoma versus cutaneous lymphoid hyperplasia is usually easy. A rare variant that can pose difficulties is so-called T-cell-rich B-cell lymphoma. The neoplastic cells of this condition are large B lymphocytes, but their presence is obscured by an infiltrate of small, reactive T cells. Various criteria for the diagnosis of this variant include a composition ranging

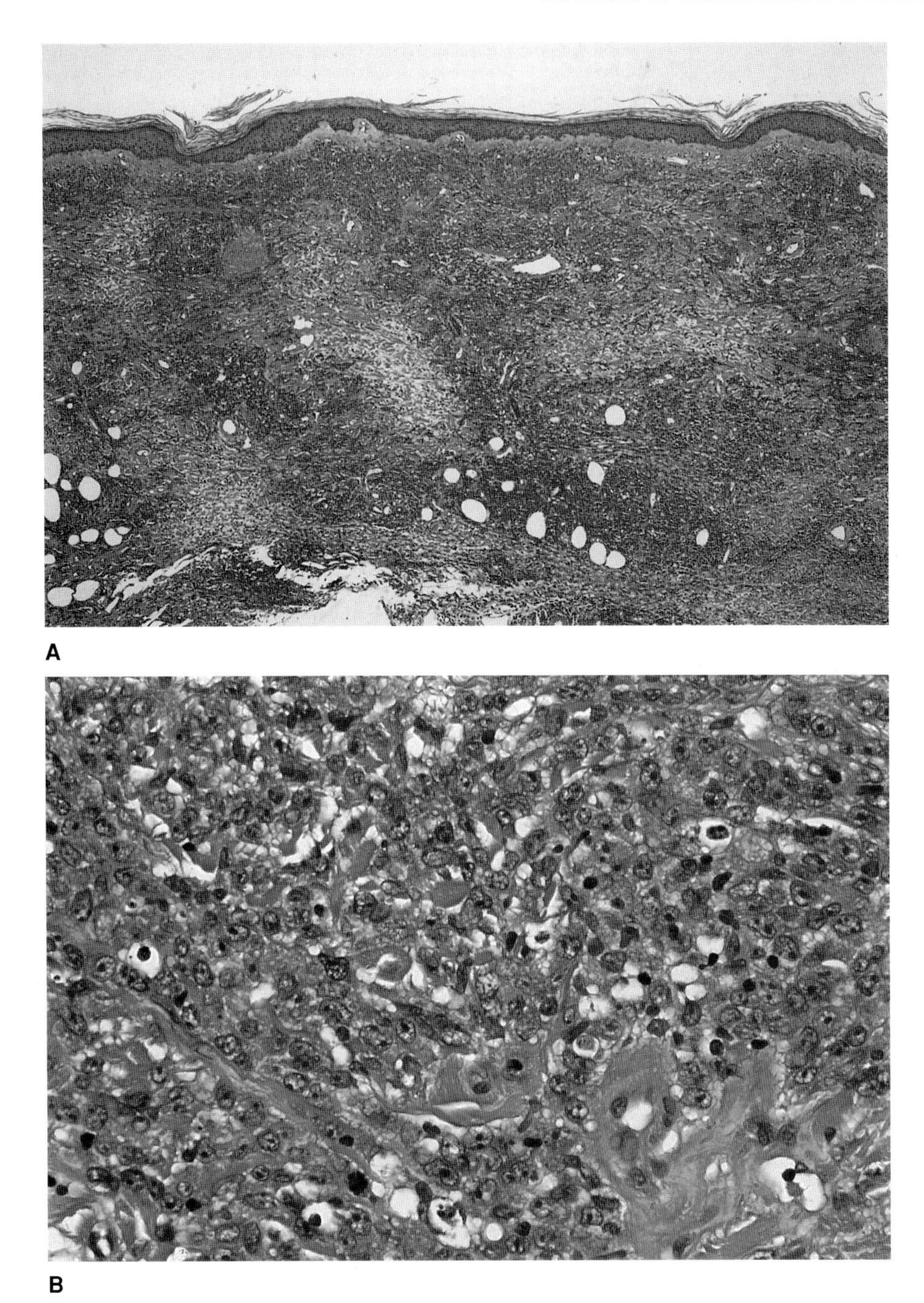

FIG. 32-9. Large B-cell lymphoma
(**A**) Large neoplastic lymphocytes diffusely infiltrate the reticular dermis in this large-cell B-cell lymphoma. Necrosis was manifest in the underlying subcutaneous fat. (**B**) High magnification reveals neoplastic B cells with vesicular nuclei, and one or more prominent nucleoli.

from more than 50% to more than 90% reactive T cells, with a predominance of T cells throughout the infiltrate. Light chain restriction and the finding of clonal rearrangement of the immunoglobulin genes, along with a germline configuration of the T-cell receptor genes, can help in differential diagnosis. Nonlymphoid malignancies also need to be considered. Immunoblastic lymphomas, like plasmacytomas, sometimes do not express leukocyte common antigen (CD45), illustrating how important it is not to use single markers in immunohistochemical differential diagnosis. The distinction between large-cell T- or B-cell lymphomas may not be of clinical importance. Most large-cell lymphomas will be readily typable, expressing either the T-cell antigen CD3 or such B-cell markers as L26 (CD20) and/or CD79a. Some routinely processed B-cell lymphomas are composed of cells with sufficient cytoplasmic immunoglobulin so that sections can be stained successfully with light chain reagents by immunoperoxidase methods. Frozen section immunohistochemistry, flow cytometry, or gene-rearrangement studies may be needed to arrive at a precise phenotype in reticent cases.

Intravascular Lymphoma

The cells of intravascular lymphoma lodge in the lumina of small blood vessels in the skin and many other organs. Archaic terms for intravascular lymphoma include "malignant angioendotheliomatosis," "angioendotheliomatosis proliferans systemisata," "intravascular lymphomatosis," and "intravascular endothelioma," most of which date to a time when the nature of the condition was debated and some believed that it was a proliferation of endothelial cells. Because most intravascular lymphomas are proliferations of B cells, we will present the condition in this section, although intravascular T-cell lymphoma can also be encountered.

The skin and brain are the organs most commonly affected by intravascular lymphoma, although any small vessel in the body can be occluded by the cells of this malignancy. Fever, dementia, and aberrations in vision, speech, and sensation are common and often present confusing signs, because lymphadenopathy, a mass lesion, or marrow involvement often cannot be found. Cutaneous lesions produced by intravascular lymphoma are often hemorrhagic plaques, with or without telangiectasia, scale, or ulceration, on the trunk or extremities. Nonspecific laboratory abnormalities that have been recorded include positive antinuclear antibody (ANA) and rheumatoid factor tests, and an elevated erythrocyte sedimentation rate.

Histopathology. The cells of intravascular lymphoma lodge in the lumens of small vessels throughout the dermis and subcutis (Fig. 32-10). Although they sometimes infiltrate beneath endothelial cells, they seldom permeate vessel walls or exit them. They are frequently enmeshed in fibrin. In some cases the lumens of vessels are indented by papillations lined by prominent endothelial cells, and sometimes a glomeruloid configuration results.[34] The neoplastic cells often have large vesicular nuclei, irregular nuclear membranes, prominent multiple nucleoli, and moderate amounts of cytoplasm.

Differential Diagnosis. Conditions other than intravascular lymphoma can feature the accumulation of neoplastic cells in the lumens of blood vessels. In so-called "inflammatory carcinoma" of the breast, patients present with erythematous, indurated plaques, biopsy of which reveals adenocarcinomatous cells in vascular lumens. Other "inflammatory" carcinomas and even "inflammatory melanoma" have been noted. Immunoperoxidase staining can readily distinguish these neoplasms. The cells of intravascular lymphoma express leukocyte common antigen (LCA, CD45) and CD20 in most instances, whereas intravascular carcinoma cells contain keratin filaments and melanoma cells express S-100 protein.

Reactive angioendotheliomatosis is a hyperplasia of endothelial cells and pericytes, usually with associated luminal occlusion and recanalization. As for intravascular lymphoma, this proliferation can result in the formation of glomeruloid structures.[34] Its bruiselike clinical lesions resemble those of intravascular lymphoma, and thus the two conditions were confused for many years.[35] Luminal occlusion by fibrin or cryoproteins appears to be pathogenetically important, although there are some cases in which a hypersensitivity vasculitis may be the initial event. In well-prepared sections, the cells of reactive angioendotheliomatosis are clearly endothelial and pericytic, and not lymphoid. They express such endothelial molecules as von Willebrand's factor and L-fucose (recognized by *Ulex europeus* agglutinin), and they do not express lymphocytic antigens.

Histogenesis. Defective lymphocyte–endothelial cell interaction can complicate both B- and T-cell lymphomas, with a few cases of the latter having recently been described. The Hermes-3 homing receptor is present on high endothelial venules, by means of which lymphocytes commonly exit the blood vascular system. The receptor is present on endothelial cells in intravascular lymphoma. However, CD11a/CD18, which binds to endothelial cell membranes, is absent from the surfaces of the neoplastic lymphocytes.[36,37]

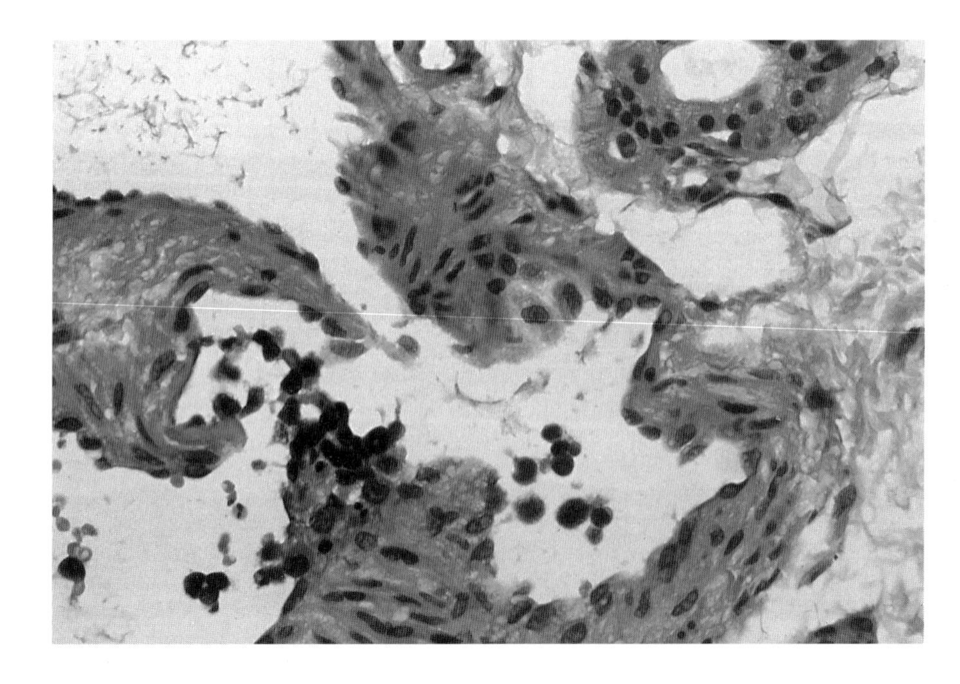

FIG. 32-10. Intravascular lymphoma
Hyperchromatic lymphocytes and fibrin hug the endothelial lining of a small dermal vessel. Strong CD20 expression was confirmed immunohistochemically.

PROLIFERATIONS OF T CELLS

T-Cell Cutaneous Lymphoid Hyperplasia (T-Cell Pseudolymphoma or T-CLH)

Although benign lymphoid infiltrates are often thought of as aberrations of B lymphocytes, benign infiltrates of T-cells that simulate lymphoma clinically and microscopically also occur. As is the case for B-CLH, T-CLH does not comprise a single entity but is a heterogeneous grouping of disorders. There is diversity in the clinical manifestations of T-CLH, which undoubtedly reflects etiologic diversity, but most of the clinical lesions are plaques or nodules Unilesional or oligolesional presentations are typical, but extensive or generalized eruptions can also be observed.[2,38,39] Most reported cases involve adults. Although the causes of many reactive infiltrates cannot be discerned, established causes include medications (so-called lymphomatoid drug eruptions), including anticonvulsant drugs; contactants (lymphomatoid contact dermatitis); and arthropod venom reactions.[2,38] Even within a given group there is diversity: lymphomatoid drug eruptions that mimic mycosis fungoides, lymphomatoid papulosis, or nodular lymphoma can be observed. Although some T-cell lymphomas of the skin (such as lymphomatoid papulosis) exhibit indolent clinical behavior and have thus been considered pseudolymphomatous by some observers, the terms "T-CLH" and "T-cell pseudolymphoma" are strictly reserved for nonlymphomatous T-cell infiltrates in this chapter.

Histopathology. T-CLH is characterized microscopically by either a bandlike or nodular pattern under scanning magnification.[2,38] In the bandlike pattern, medium-sized to large lymphocytes are arrayed within an expanded papillary dermis (Fig. 32-11). Cells with convoluted nuclear membranes can be observed at higher magnifications. Most examples also show extension of the infiltrate around the deep vascular plexus. Small lymphocytes, macrophages, eosinophils, and plasma cells can be found in the infiltrate, with the first two cell types being the most common.[38,39] Overt granuloma formation is only occasionally encountered.[38] Lymphocytes are also arrayed intraepidermally, with associated spongiosis that varies from negligible to near vesiculation (Fig. 32-12). Lymphocytes tend to be dispersed singly among keratinocytes within the epidermis, and intraepidermal lymphocyte collections are rare.

Nodular T-cell CLH is manifested as a diffuse infiltrate of lymphocytes arrayed throughout the reticular dermis, with extension into the subcutis in a minority of cases. In most examples, a T-cell pattern is evident, with lymphocytes arrayed within the papillary dermis and epidermis, but on occasion the entire infiltrate is confined to the reticular dermis with a subepidermal grenz zone.[2,38] Medium-sized convoluted lymphocytes comprise the bulk of the lymphoid component of the infiltrate, but scattered large convoluted lymphocytes and small lymphocytes can also be observed. The nonlymphoid component is highly variable and can include plasma cells, eosinophils, and macrophages, with the last two cell types being present in vast numbers in exceptional cases.

Histogenesis. Most examples of T-CLH express a mature helper T-cell phenotype (CD4+), and expression of other T-cell determinants (CD3, CD45RO+) is also common.[2,38] CD30 expression can also be observed, albeit only rarely. In addition to expressing an immunophenotype similar to that of mycosis fungoides, the cells of T-CLH are cytomorphologically indistinguishable from those of mycosis fungoides, because a similar degree of nuclear convolution can be seen in both entities using standard techniques.[38] Insufficient numbers of cases have been studied to ascertain if clonal aberrations of the T-cell receptor (TCR) gene or CD7 deletions are common in this disorder, or if the presence of these alterations has any diagnostic significance.

Differential Diagnosis. Although B lymphocytes can be de-

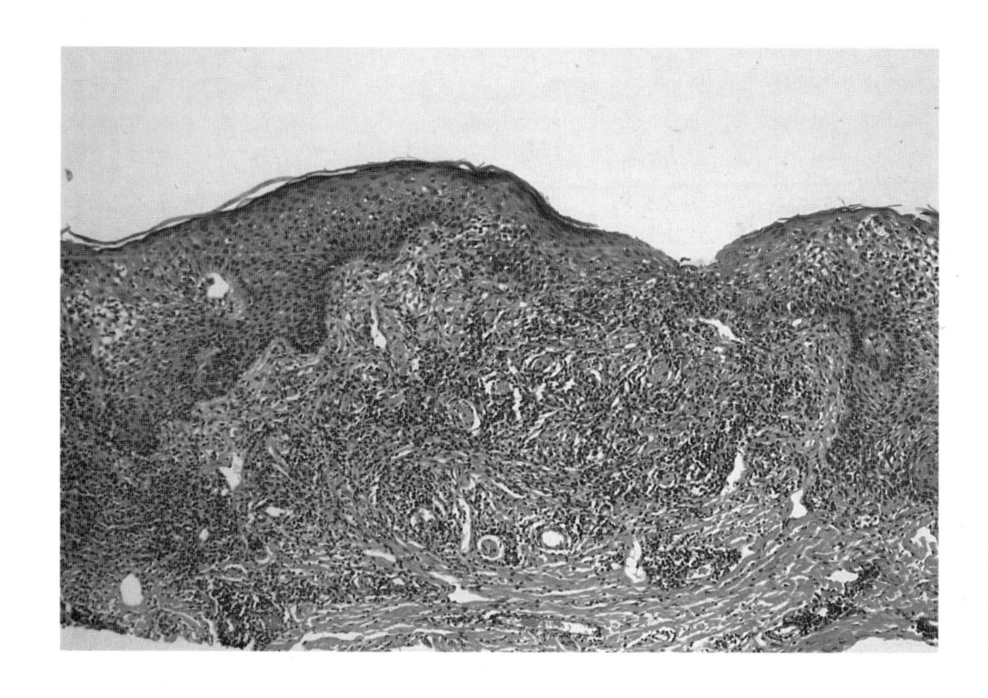

FIG. 32-11. T-cell pseudolymphoma, scanning magnification A bandlike array of lymphocytes fills the papillary dermis and many lymphocytes are present intraepidermally, in association with variable spongiosis.

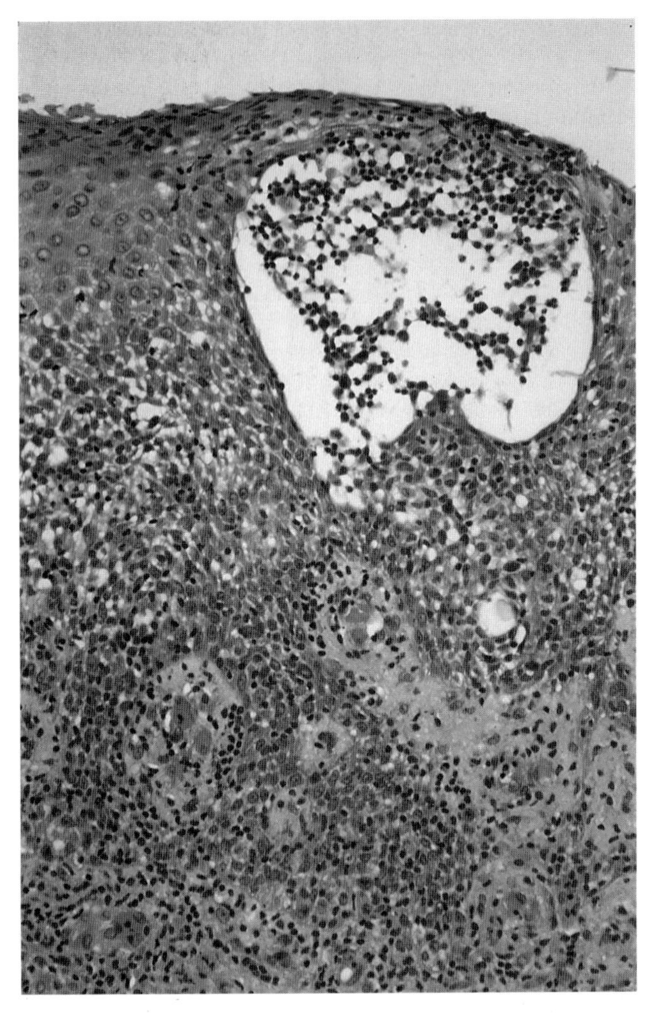

FIG. 32-12. T-cell pseudolymphoma
A heterogeneous infiltrate, with numerous admixed eosinophils and macrophages, is appreciable at high magnification of T-cell pseudolymphoma. The intraepidermal collection of mononuclear cells does not constitute a Pautrier collection, because the aggregate is composed of cells of disparate lineage (lymphocytes, macrophages, Langerhans' cells, acantholytic keratinocytes) rather than convoluted T lymphocytes.

tected immunohistochemically in T-cell CLH, the B cells typically comprise less than 10% of the total lymphoid component, without the formation of clusters or germinal centers, a pattern helpful in excluding B-cell CLH or B-cell lymphoma from the differential diagnosis.[3,40] Furthermore, the B lymphocytes are small, in contrast to the medium-sized or large B cells observed in most T-cell-rich B-cell lymphomas.

Distinction of the bandlike pattern of T-CLH from mycosis fungoides can be impossible on histopathologic grounds, although a greater degree of epidermotropism and the presence of intraepidermal lymphocyte collections are held to be more common in the lymphoma.[40] The clinical context can be of value in making the distinction, because T-CLH is prone to be oligolesional and recently acquired. However, because mycosis fungoides can present as a solitary lesion, definitive classification based on the clinical presentation is clearly not possible.[42]

In contrast, the nodular pattern of T-CLH is more readily distinguished from nonepidermotropic T lymphomas such as pleomorphic T-cell lymphoma, based on the heterogeneity of the infiltrate, the heterogeneity of the lymphoid component, a greater tendency to display granulomatous features, and a lack of sheetlike arrays of atypical lymphocytes in large numbers.[38]

T-Lymphoblastic Lymphoma

T-lymphoblastic lymphomas display differentiation toward pre- and intrathymic T lymphocytes. These neoplasms account for the majority of noncutaneous (usually nodal) lymphoblastic lymphomas. The presentation typically occurs in childhood, adolescence, or young adulthood as a mediastinal mass, often with involvement of the marrow and peripheral blood. In contrast to the systemic form, T-lymphoblastic lymphoma seems to comprise a smaller percentage of cases of cutaneous lymphoblastic lymphoma. Cutaneous lesions are generally red to purple papules and nodules, and involvement of the head and neck area is common.[9]

Histopathology. The infiltrate is dermal and nonepidermotropic. The neoplastic cells have scant cytoplasm and slightly to moderately convoluted nuclei with finely dispersed chromatin.[9,41] Nuclear grooves can be seen in some instances.[41] Nucleoli are typically inconspicuous. Touch preparations are often the best venue for the appreciation of the delicate nuclear characteristics of this neoplasm. Some T-lymphoblastic lymphomas are accompanied by eosinophils.

Differential Diagnosis. T- and B-lymphoblastic lymphomas cannot be distinguished by routine microscopy. Although the nuclei of lymphoblastic lymphomas are medium-sized to large, the nucleoli are typically small. Neuroendocrine (Merkel cell) carcinoma of the skin is the chief nonlymphoid simulant, but differs from lymphoblastic lymphoma in that the neoplastic aggregations are typically cohesive and are sometimes arrayed in nodular or trabecular configurations. Furthermore, neuroendocrine carcinomas tend to display prominent nuclear molding, which is usually not conspicuous in lymphoblastic lymphomas. Immunohistochemical phenotyping is useful to confirm T-cell lineage and to exclude nonlymphoid neoplasms from the differential diagnosis.

Mycosis Fungoides (MF)

Mycosis fungoides (MF) is a form of T-cell lymphoma that initially involves the epidermis and papillary dermis, comprising the *patch stage* of the disease. With time, the neoplastic lymphocytes often acquire the capacity to proliferate within the reticular dermis, and plaques, nodules, and tumors *(plaque* and *tumor stages)* are manifest clinically. In some patients, generally after extended periods of time, the neoplasm disseminates to extracutaneous sites such as lymph nodes and viscera. MF is usually thought of as a disease of older adults, but the neoplasm can develop at any age, including early childhood.[28] The term MF is a descriptive misnomer, coined by Alibert after observing mushroomlike nodules in the tumor stage of the disease. Morphologic descriptions that refer to MF pervade the dermatologic lexicon, including such terms as "parapsoriasis en plaques," "large plaque parapsoriasis," "poikiloderma vasculare atrophicans," "prereticulotic poikiloderma," "chronic superficial dermatitis," "xanthoerythrodermia perstans," and "parapsoriasis variegata."[43] Although some authors still regard these terms as valid diagnostic categories for an early, preneoplastic stage of MF, most present investigators contend that the disorders described historically in association with these terms would be reclassified by present criteria as MF. These designations are unlikely to disappear in the forseeable future, because of the fondness for morphologic nomenclature among dermatologists.

Patches of MF are technically very thin, virtually macular plaques. Patches are usually pinkish red and slightly scaly, typically distributed on the trunk and proximal extremities. The buttocks and breasts are often involved, probably reflecting the multilayered photoprotection by clothing that exists at these sites, because the neoplastic infiltrates of early disease are easily suppressed by radiation in the ultraviolet spectrum.[43] At least some of the patches exceed 10 cm in diameter in most patients, corresponding to the morphologic pattern of "large plaque parapsoriasis." Large, garment-sized patches are not uncommon. In some individuals, patches become "poikilodermatous," as epidermal atrophy, dyspigmentation, and telangiectasia develop secondary to the chronic neoplastic infiltrate. This appearance corresponds to the morphologic pattern of "poikiloderma vasculare atrophicans," a nonspecific term that is potentially misleading because it is also used in reference to atrophic, dyschromic lesions of lupus erythematosus and dermatomyositis. Some patches of MF develop a reticulated appearance, which comprises the morphologic pattern known as "parapsoriasis variegata." The proportion of patients with patch stage MF that will progress to develop plaques is not precisely known but is thought to be low.[43,44]

Plaques of MF are sharply marginated and are usually red to reddish brown. The centers of plaques can involute, yielding annular or serpiginous morphology. Plaques and patches of MF often coexist in a given patient.

Nodules and tumors are the least common, most advanced, and biologically most ominous cutaneous lesions of MF. Tumors of MF are morphologically indistinguishable from tumors of other cutaneous lymphomas, except for the clinical context from which they sprout: residual patch and plaque stages of the disease are virtually always evident.[43,44] MF tumors are reddish-brown or violaceous and firm, and ulceration can occur. The form of cutaneous lymphoma known historically as "d'emblee MF," characterized by the abrupt onset of tumors in the absence of patches and plaques, was probably not a variant of MF at all, but rather pleomorphic T-cell lymphoma.

In some patients, macular lesions become generalized, either transiently or persistently. If generalized cutaneous involvement develops without seeding of the peripheral blood, the process is classified as erythrodermic MF. If significant numbers of atypical lymphocytes are present in the peripheral vasculature, the process is known as Sézary syndrome (SS), which some investigators consider to be a leukemic phase of MF.[43,45] Although the histologic features of SS are indistinguishable from those of conventional MF, there are differences in its clinical presentation, including a greater degree of pruritus and conspicuous involvement of the head, neck, and acral sites (including the palms and soles), as well as a less favorable prognosis.

In addition to conventional patches, plaques, and tumors, MF can assume a wide variety of other clinical patterns.[46] At times, the neoplastic infiltrate of MF is associated with varying degrees of epidermal hyperplasia and hyperkeratosis. If the degree of epidermal thickening is pronounced, with thick, scaly plaques or nodules manifested clinically, the term "verrucous hyperkeratotic MF" has been forwarded.[46] Similar morphology can also be seen in Woringer-Kolopp lymphoma (pagetoid reticulosis). In other patients, a lesser degree of acanthosis and hyperkeratosis is evident, and clinical lesions can resemble acanthosis nigricans.[47] The epidermal infiltrate of MF can also induce dyspigmentation, eliciting a clinical pattern known as hypopigmented MF.[48,49] Relatively common, hypopigmentation is a manifestion of MF with onset in childhood, and hypopigmented lesions have commonly been observed in dark-skinned patients—probably because the lesions are conspicuous in that context. If neoplastic lymphocytes are folliculotropic, follicular papules can be observed on the head, trunk, or extremities, and comedones and acquired follicular cysts can ensue.[46]

Uncommon clinical variants include bullous and pustular MF.[46] If an unusual morphologic pattern is encountered in a patient with an established diagnosis of mycosis fungoides, the possibility of a second, concurrent skin disease should be thoroughly considered. In some reports of unusual patterns of MF, neoplastic cells have not been documented in the area of unique morphology, raising the possibility that a coincidental skin condition was also present.

Staging of MF is most commonly based on a TNM ("tissue-node-metastasis") system. The T value represents the extent of cutaneous disease (T1 denotes less than 10% body surface involvement; T2, more than 10% body surface involvement; T3, tumors; T4, erythroderma), the N value reflects the presence or absence of lymph node disease, and the M value reflects the presence or absence of visceral disease.[43,50] Based on a patient's TNM values, a specific stage can be assigned. A sophisticated scheme for lymph node staging has been forwarded in the hope of enhancing the prognostic import of lymph node biopsy. Lymph nodes are assigned a score from LN1 to LN4, with LN1 and LN2 representing nodes with noneffaced architecture, LN3 representing nodes containing clusters of atypical lymphocytes, and LN4 representing nodes with architectural effacement resulting from lymphomatous infiltration.[51,52] In addition to microscopic examination, genotypic analysis of nodal tissue is of diagnostic and prognostic value in the staging of MF.[53,54] LN1 and LN2 nodes do not typically contain clonal lymphocyte populations, whereas LN3 nodes commonly do and LN4 nodes virtually always do. The identification of a clonal lymphoid population within a node is highly associated with the presence of adenopathy and a shorter survival, irrespective of the histologic pattern of nodal involvement.[54]

Although strides have been made, the natural history of MF remains somewhat enigmatic. The long-term prognosis associated with the early patch stage of the disease remains a key question, and why some patients bear the limited morbidity of patches for decades, whereas others suffer from systemic lymphoma after a brief course of macular disease, is still a mystery. The refinement of criteria for patch lesions has resulted in an increase in diagnosis, which has been interpreted by some as an indicator of an increase in incidence.[55,56] However, there are no data that confirm that a sizable increase in the incidence of MF has occurred. Despite the need for further prognostic investigation, it is clear that the median survival for patients in the patch or plaque stage of the disease is a decade or longer. In contrast, the prognosis for patients with cutaneous or extracutaneous tumors is grim, with 5-year survival rates below 50%.[43,44]

Histopathology of Patch Stage MF. The microscopic findings in the earliest patches of MF are subtle, consisting of a sparse intraepidermal and papillary dermal infiltrate of lymphocytes, arrayed within a fibrotic papillary dermis below an epidermis that shows slight psoriasiform hyperplasia (Fig. 32-13). Because of the sparse infiltrate, multiple biopsies and close clinicopathologic correlation are often needed for diagnosis. Despite the paucity of neoplastic cells, however, characteristic features sufficient for specific diagnosis can be identified when carefully sought. Small numbers of lymphocytes, with relatively small but irregular nuclei, are arrayed within the epidermis with minimal associated spongiosis.[57] The lymphocytes are often distributed in a linear fashion on the epidermal side of the basement membrane zone, but the pattern differs from that of an interface dermatitis by virtue of the fact that there is little vacuolar change and there are few if any necrotic keratinocytes.[58] This linear array of lymphocytes has been likened to a string of pearls (Fig. 32-14). Although clusters of intraepidermal lymphocytes, so-called Pautrier collections, are often sought as the key to a diagnosis of MF, a pattern in which lymphocytes are dispersed among keratinocytes is more common in biopsies of macular lesions.

It is vital to remember that patch mycosis fungoides is largely an architectural diagnosis and not a cytologic one. The architectural alterations involve both the papillary dermis and the epidermis. Even in developing lesions, the papillary dermis is expanded by fibrosis. The degree of fibrosis and collagen bundle thickening increases in rough proportion to lesional age. Thus, in the earliest patches, fibrosis is noticeable but subtle, whereas the papillary dermis is coarsely fibrotic late in the patch stage or in fully developed plaques. Thickened collagen bundles often lie roughly parallel to the epidermal surface, in contrast to the vertically oriented collagen bundles that develop secondary to lichenification. The overlying epidermis is nearly normal in the earliest patch lesions, but typically shows slight, regular psoriasiform hyperplasia and hyperkeratosis, although atrophy can be seen in poikilodermatous patches.

Readily discernible nuclear atypia of lymphocytes is the exception rather than the rule in conventional histologic sections of patch stage disease.[57] At high magnification, some degree of nuclear convolution is usually appreciable, but because of the thickness of ordinary sections, it is difficult to distinguish neoplastic lymphocytes from nonneoplastic ones, although the neoplastic lymphocytes are typically slightly larger and display some degree of nuclear hyperchromatism. Although it is difficult to appreciate nuclear atypism in any given individual cell, sometimes nuclear enlargement can be detected in the entire epidermal infiltrate, even in relatively early lesions. This is possible because virtually all the intraepidermal lymphocytes are neoplastic ones, whereas the lymphocytes in the papillary dermis consist of both neoplastic and smaller nonneoplastic cells. Thus, when taken as a whole, the lymphocytes within the epidermis are slightly larger and more darkly staining than the ones within the papillary dermis (Fig. 32-15). In some cases, this difference in size can be striking and can serve as a valuable diagnostic clue.[59]

Poikilodermatous mycosis fungoides differs from conventional patch style disease in that the fibrotic expansion of the papillary dermis is marked, in conjunction with a diminishment of the rete ridge pattern and the deposition of melanophages (Fig. 32-16). The diagnosis still rests on identification of lymphocytes with convoluted nuclei, in clusters or in a linear array along the dermalepidermal junction. Because the specific histologic features of MF are attenuated in poikilodermatous disease, multiple biopsies may be necessary for unequivocal diagnosis. The microscopic appearance of poikilodermatous MF shares features with other cell-mediated immune reactions directed against native or neoplastic elements of the junctional zone, including cutaneous lupus erythematosus, atrophic lichen planus, and regression of melanoma. Thus, poikilodermatous MF could represent incomplete regression of patch stage MF, in which reactive lymphocytes are suppressing neoplastic ones.

Histopathology of Plaque Stage MF. Not surprisingly, the architectural features of patch stage MF are preserved in plaques of the disease. The papillary dermis is similarly

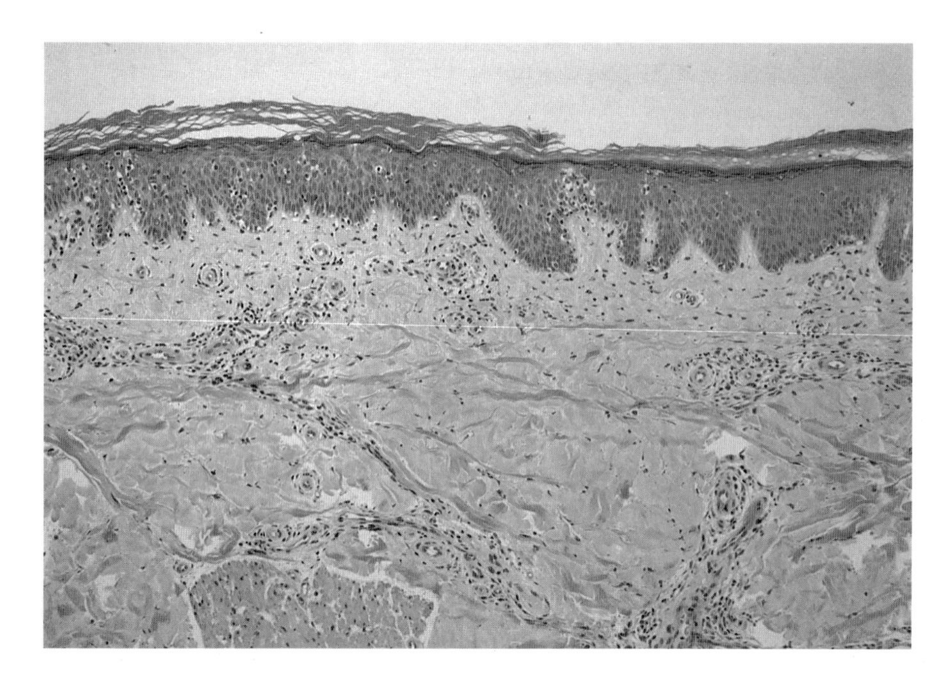

FIG. 32-13. Mycosis fungoides, patch stage
A sparse infiltrate of lymphocytes is present along the junction of an epidermis that shows slight hyperplasia, above a papillary dermis exhibiting fibrosis.

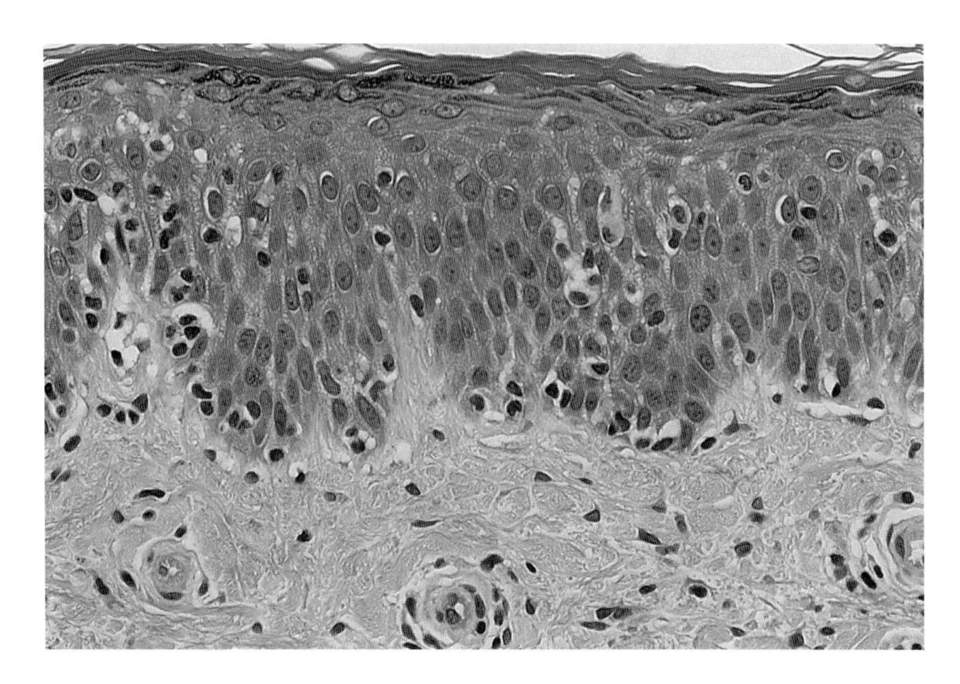

FIG. 32-14. Mycosis fungoides, patch stage
A linear array of convoluted lymphocytes is present along the epidermal side of the epidermal basement membrane zone.

expanded by coarse fibrosis but contains denser, bandlike infiltrates of lymphocytes, which, in combination with slight, regular epidermal thickening, account for the "lichenoid-psoriasiform" pattern that is characteristic of the late patch stage and the plaque stage (Fig. 32-17). In addition to a papillary dermal infiltrate, the reticular dermis holds superficial and deep perivascular or nearly diffuse infiltrates of lymphocytes. Cytologic atypism, particularly of intraepidermal lymphocytes, is often conspicuous in biopsies from plaques, in contrast to the subtle cytologic changes evident in macular lesions. Follicular mucinosis (FM) is an epithelial reaction pattern that can be seen in a benign, nonneoplastic condition, alopecia mucinosa, but can also be seen sporadically in a variety of other contexts, including a close association with plaque stage MF.[60–62] In FM, epithelial mucin is aberrantly produced by hair follicle epithelium, yielding a spongiosis-like pattern as spaces between keratinocytes are widened by accumulations of mucopolysaccharide. In FM associated with MF, atypical lymphocytes can be present within follicular epithelium, but it is difficult or impossible to distinguish follicular mucinosis associated with MF from so-called benign follicular mucinosis by conventional microscopy.[61] As a rule, a diagnosis of MF should be based only on histologic findings away from the involved follicle or follicles.

Histopathology of Tumor Stage MF. Histologic sections from nodules or tumors of MF display neoplastic cells in a dense array in the reticular dermis, and the degree of epider-

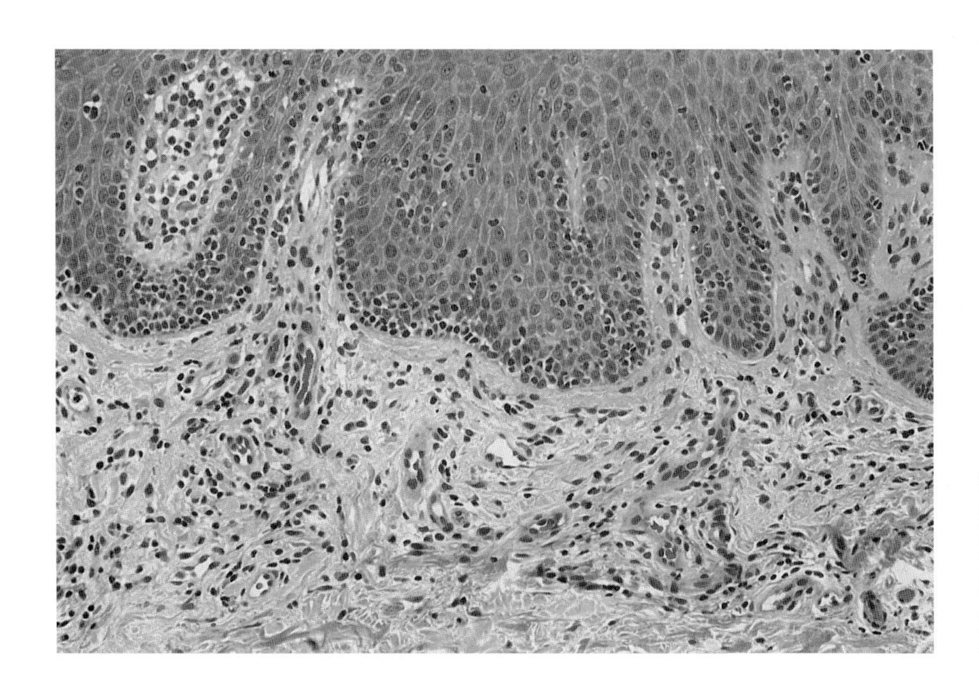

FIG. 32-15. Mycosis fungoides, patch stage
In this area of prominent epidermotropism, intraepidermal lymphocytes have slightly larger nuclei than those of the cells arrayed within the papillary dermis.

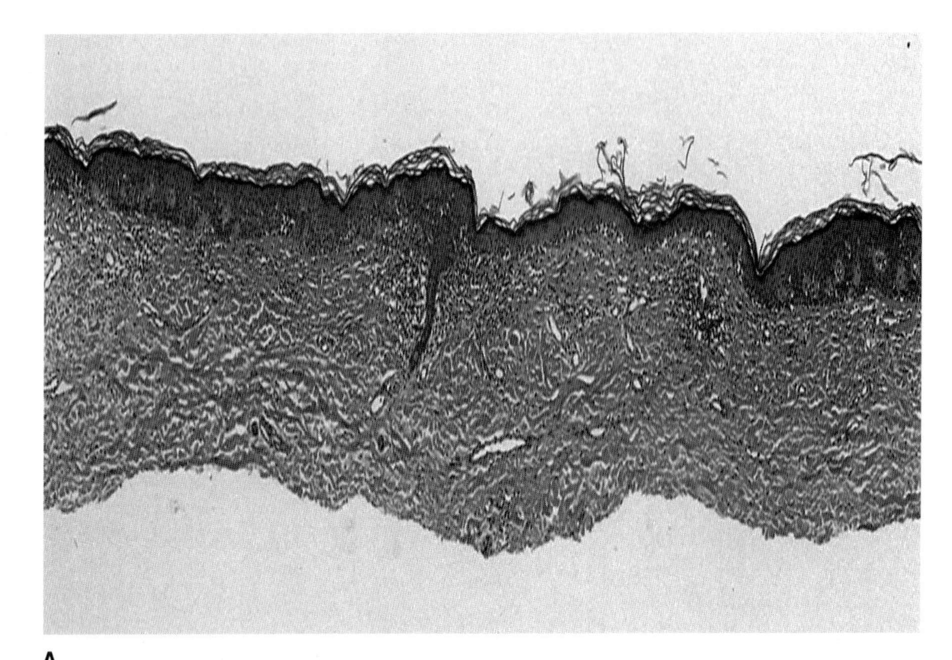

A

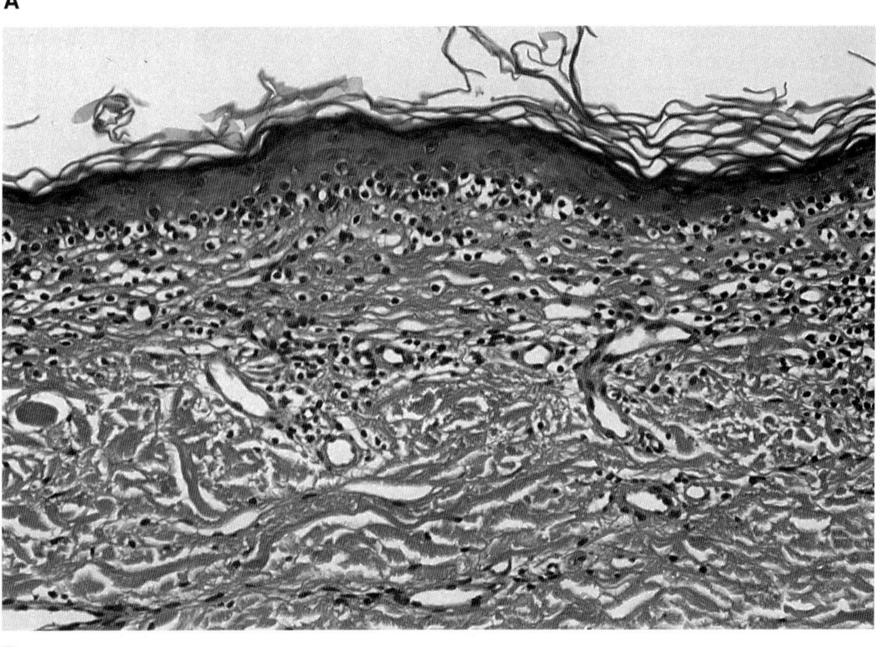

B

FIG. 32-16. Mycosis fungoides, atrophic patch stage
(**A**) Scanning magnification. The rete ridge pattern is attenuated, in contrast to the psoriasiform pattern of conventional patch stage disease. (**B**) At high magnification, a linear array of lymphocytes is disposed on the epidermal side of the basement membrane zone.

motropism often diminishes (Fig. 32-18). Tumors are either composed virtually entirely of small to medium-sized cells with cerebriform nuclei, or are composed of both convoluted and large lymphocytes (with large cells comprising 25% or more of the infiltrate), a pattern known as "transformed MF."[63] Scattered eosinophils, plasma cells, and macrophages can be found in most tumors.[64]

It has been proposed that MF tumors with histologic evidence of transformation be classified under the modified Kiel classification.[63] In this scheme, MF tumors are classified as medium-sized or large-cell pleomorphic T-cell lymphoma, characterized by medium to large cells with markedly irregular or folded nuclei; immunoblastic T-cell lymphoma, characterized by relatively monomorphous large cells with vesicular nuclei and prominent central nucleoli; large-cell anaplastic T-cell lymphoma, characterized by large cells, sometimes multinucleate, with abundant cytoplasm, vesicular nuclei, and one or several large nucleoli; or unclassifiable large-cell T-cell lymphoma.

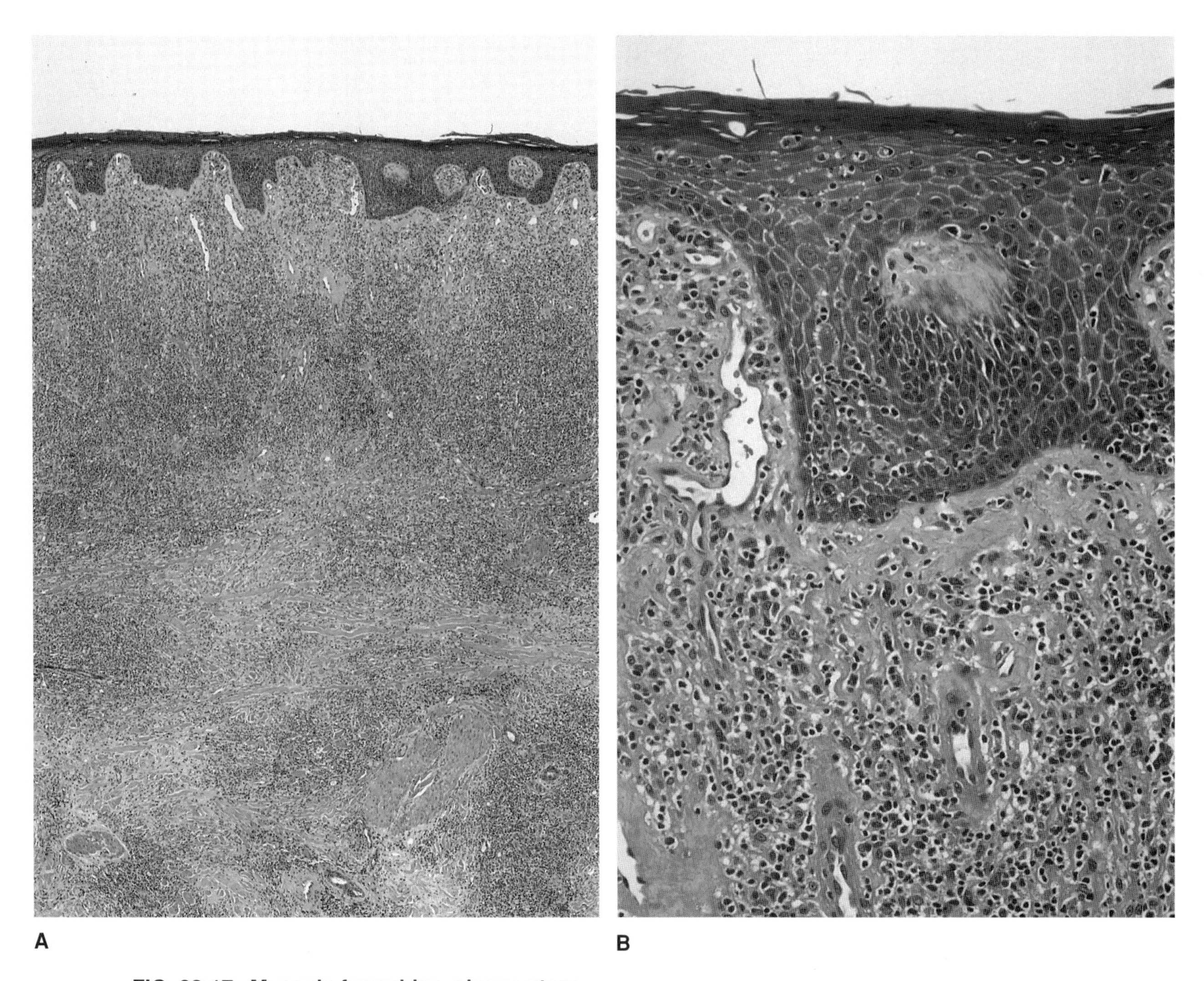

FIG. 32-17. Mycosis fungoides, plaque stage
(**A**) A diffuse infiltrate of lymphocytes permeates the reticular dermis. (**B**) At high magnification, an epidermis riddled with convoluted lymphocytes overlies massive fibrotic expansion of the papillary dermis.

The prognostic significance of this classification relative to tumor stage MF is not established. In the pilot study, the mortality rate was similar for patients with transformed and nontransformed tumors, but the rate of neoplastic progression was accelerated in patients with transformed disease.[63]

Histopathologic Variations. Biopsies from some patients with clinically stereotypical patches, plaques, or tumors of MF display unusual microscopic features, with granulomatous MF constituting the foremost variant pattern. In granulomatous MF, nodular, interstitial, or palisaded collections of macrophages occur in concert with the epidermotropic infiltrate that is requisite for diagnosis (Fig. 32-19).[65] It now appears that granulomatous inflammation is not of prognostic significance.[65] Angiocentric MF constitutes another variant histologic pattern.[46] In angiocentric MF, changes of lymphocytic vasculitis are observed, often within an otherwise typical MF lesion. The lymphocytes noted within vessel walls are not reactive cells, but are identifiable as neoplastic lymphoctyes on the basis of their nuclear characteristics.[46]

Histogenesis. Currently it is generally accepted that MF represents a clonal neoplastic disorder of T helper cell lineage. There are several adjunctive techniques that were developed in the hope of improving diagnostic accuracy in early MF. Fresh tissue immunophenotyping, assessment of nuclear contour (convolution) by plastic sectioning or electron microscopy, and measurement of nuclear DNA content by image analysis cytometry have all been forwarded with the hope of enhancing the diagnosis and biologic understanding of MF.

Immunophenotyping is the most readily accessible and the most commonly used adjunctive technique. In light of the T helper (CD4+) lineage of MF, early studies held out hope that an elevated helper-to-suppressor (CD4:CD8) ratio might be specific for MF, but it is apparent that rare examples of MF are of suppressor cell lineage (CD8+) whereas many inflammatory skin diseases consist largely of T helper cells, thus rendering the ratio irrelevant to the diagnosis. The simultaneous aberrant expression of CD4 and CD8 by the same T cells, although rare, suggests a neoplastic infiltrate. Claims have been made that the cells of MF fail to express CD7, an antigen expressed on most mature T helper cells, but other workers have not found the

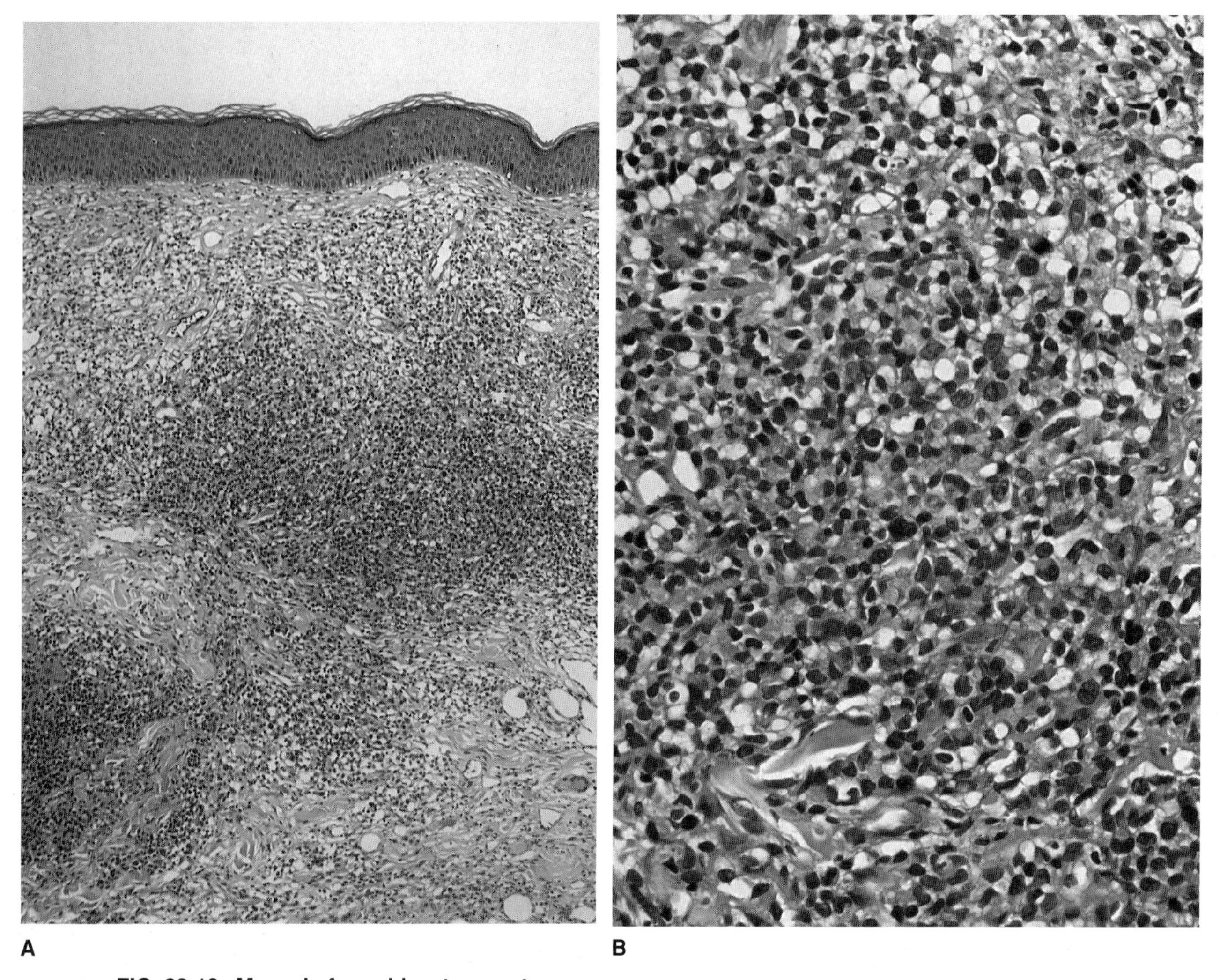

FIG. 32-18. Mycosis fungoides, tumor stage
(**A**) Scanning magnification. Epidermotropism is inconspicuous. (**B**) At high magnification, large convoluted lymphocytes predominate in the dermal neoplastic infiltrate.

absence of CD7 to be a reliable marker for MF.[66] Plaques and tumors of MF, which are easier to diagnose with certainty by routine methods, often have lymphocytes with abnormal immunophenotypes, lacking common T-cell determinants such as CD2, CD3, and CD5.

Analysis of the genetic sequences that code for the T-cell receptor (TCR) is proving to be a major advance in the study of the biology of MF as well as an adjunctive diagnostic test of considerable utility. Studies of the TCR genetic configuration have shown that densely infiltrated patches, plaques, and tumors of MF are produced by single clones of neoplastic T cells.[67] Because early patches of MF contain relatively small numbers of neoplastic lymphocytes, it has been difficult to use conventional methods of DNA extraction from lesional tissue to assess clonality. The polymerase chain reaction (PCR) should make it possible to detect clonal populations of lymphocytes in early macular lesions. Because even minor clones can be amplified by PCR, quantification of clonal populations will likely be important for the reliable use of this technique as an ancillary test.

Differential Diagnosis. The main simulants of patch stage MF include skin conditions that display spongiotic and/or lichenoid microscopic patterns. Spongiotic dermatitides display papillary dermal infiltrates of lymphocytes as well as a few lymphocytes in the epidermis, and can simulate patch stage MF—particularly chronic patch stage MF, in which papillary dermal fibrosis and hyperkeratosis are also present. Distinguishing features include a lichenoid lymphocytic infiltrate, slight but regular psoriasiform epidermal hyperplasia, and intraepidermal lymphocytes arrayed with negligible spongiosis—features that are not observed in the so-called spongiotic simulants. A "psoriasiform-lichenoid" or "spongiotic-psoriasiform-lichenoid" pattern in which lymphocytes predominate favors MF over any primary spongiotic dermatitis.[68] Slight spongiosis often is present in MF in areas infiltrated by lymphocytes, but in spongiotic dermatitis the degree of spongiosis is greater and is identifiable in the absence of intraepidermal lymphocytes in some foci. Spongiotic vesiculation is uncommon in MF. When present, lymphocytes with unequivocal nuclear atypia are requisite for diagnosis.

The intraepidermal collections of mononuclear cells that develop in spongiotic dermatitis can simulate so-called Pautrier collections.[69] Spongiotic collections exhibit a flask-shaped con-

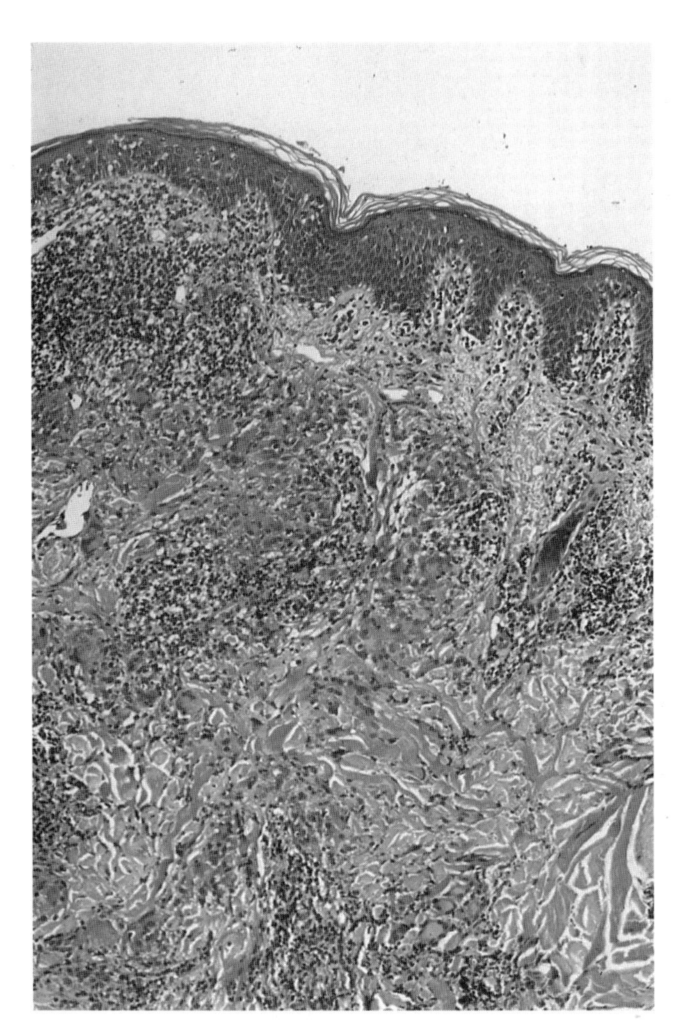

FIG. 32-19. Granulomatous mycosis fungoides
An interstitial infiltrate of macrophages involves the dermis beneath an epidermotropic infiltrate.

figuration and are heterogeneous in composition, comprising lymphocytes, macrophages, Langerhans' cells, and degenerating keratinocytes, in contrast to the rounded collections observed in MF, which are composed largely of convoluted lymphocytes.

Lichenoid interface dermatitides can also simulate patch stage MF. Although lichen planus and lichenoid drug eruptions show lymphocytes in bandlike arrays, sometimes in association with papillary dermal fibrosis, the associated destruction of basilar keratinocytes yields a jagged rete ridge pattern and loss of the basal layer, changes that are only rarely present in MF. Lichenoid purpura and lichen aureus, two of the persistent pigmented purpuric dermatitides, can produce lesions with a psoriasiform-lichenoid pattern and numerous lymphocytes in a nearly normal or slightly spongiotic epidermis.[70] Deep papillary dermal collections of siderophages, edema of the papillary dermis, numerous intraepidermal and papillary dermal erythrocytes, and an absence of lymphocytes with cytologically atypical nuclei are all features that favor pigmented purpuric dermatitis over MF. Some lichenoid simulants of MF presenting as solitary lesions defy specific classification, but can generally be separated histologically from MF.[38] Some of these solitary lesions could represent lichenoid keratoses (lichen planus-like keratoses) that simulate MF rather than lichen planus, a pattern that has humorously been referred to as mycosis fungoides-like keratosis (MFLK). Others represent true T-CLH. Total reliance cannot be placed on the clinical context as a criterion for diagnosis, however, because unilesional presentations of MF have been clearly documented.[40]

Despite the difficulty in diagnosis that can be posed by an unusual presentation of MF, it is fortifying to remember that there is little risk of harm from a delay in diagnosis, in light of the generally indolent clinical course.

Sézary Syndrome (SS)

Sézary syndrome (SS) is a form of epidermotropic lymphoma characterized by erythroderma resulting from a cutaneous infiltrate of neoplastic T lymphocytes, with neoplastic cells also present in the peripheral blood. Because of features shared with mycosis fungoides (MF), including epidermotropism, nuclear hyperconvolution, and a similar immunophenotype, some investigators consider SS and MF to be different clinical expressions of a single disorder.[43,45] Although there is considerable overlap with the findings of MF, as there are significant differences in clinical presentation and prognostic significance, SS is considered separately from MF in this chapter.

Clinical Features. SS is uncommon as strictly defined. As this time, a confident diagnosis of SS can be based on the constellation of erythroderma, increased numbers of convoluted lymphocytes in the peripheral blood, and either a skin biopsy diagnostic of epidermotropic T-cell lymphoma or a skin or blood sample that confirms the presence of clonal rearrangement of the TCR gene. Any sense of commonness of SS is probably attributable to inclusion of examples of erythrodermic MF or misdiagnosed nonneoplastic erythrodermas. The age of onset is similar to that of MF, with a peak in the seventh decade.[45] The disorder is spectacularly rare in childhood or early adulthood.

In addition to erythroderma, common cutaneous manifestations include alopecia and palmoplantar keratoderma, and "leonine facies" can complicate advanced disease.[43] Systemic involvement is present by definition, and lymphadenopathy and hepatomegaly are typically evident in addition to the seeding of the peripheral blood.

The prognosis of SS is poor, with less than 50% survival at 5 years.[43,45] Disease progression is similar to but more rapid than that in MF, with plaques and tumors developing from macular lesions. Morbidity is generally attributable to infection.

Histopathology. Under the microscope, the erythrodermic skin of SS patients resembles patch stage MF, with a bandlike lymphocytic infiltrate, intraepidermal lymphocytes with disproportionately little spongiosis, and papillary dermal fibrosis (Fig. 32-20). Eosinophils and plasma cells can be present in small numbers. Most examples include at least a few lymphocytes with enlarged and hyperconvoluted nuclei, although nuclear contour is sometimes difficult to appreciate in all but the thinnest of conventional microscopic sections. Plaques and tumors of SS are indistinguishable from those of MF. The diagnosis can be exceedingly difficult in some instances. Some patients with clinical and hematologic evidence of SS have histopathologic findings, even after the examination of repeated biopsies, that suggest spongiotic dermatitis rather than epidermotropic T-cell lymphoma.[71]

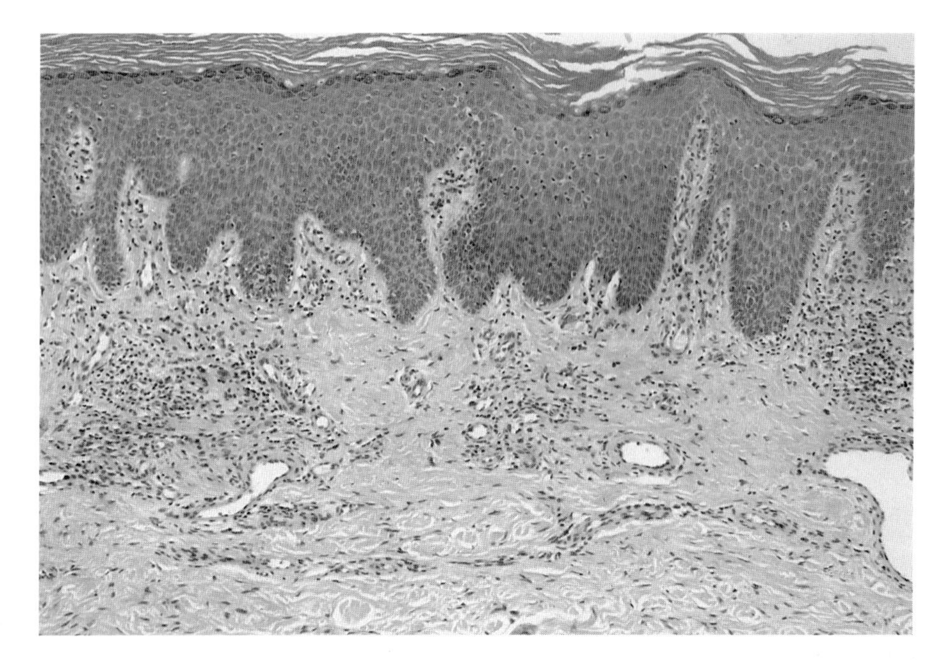

FIG. 32-20. Sézary syndrome
This palmar biopsy from an erythrodermic patient yielded specific diagnostic features, with medium-sized lymphocytes arrayed among keratinocytes, in association with only scant spongiosis.

The peripheral blood of patients with SS contains an increased number of abnormal lymphocytes with convoluted nuclei (Sézary cells). Sézary cells were at first thought to be unique to MF and SS; however, a similar cytologic configuration has been detected in the blood of some patients with a variety of inflammatory skin diseases.[45] Several methods have been proposed to assess the degree of convolution, including the nuclear contour index, comprising the ratio of the perimeter measurement of the nucleus to the nuclear radius. Irrespective of the method of identification, the number of circulating Sézary cells required for diagnosis is controversial. The most commonly forwarded criteria have been an absolute Sézary lymphocytosis of more than 1000 cells per cubic millimeter and the presence of more than 10% Sézary lymphocytes in the peripheral blood.[45,71] Because considerable variation in Sézary lymphocyte counts can occur among different observers, diagnosis of SS should not be based solely on peripheral blood lymphocyte counts.

Histogenesis. SS lymphocytes express a mature T helper cell (CD4+) phenotype. Similar to MF, the neoplastic lymphocytes sometimes fail to express CD7.

Clonal TCR gene rearrangements have been detected in most cases of SS.[45,72] A limited number of samples from patients with erythrodermic inflammatory skin diseases have been analyzed as controls without identification of clonality.

Differential Diagnosis. The cutaneous infiltrate observed in SS so closely resembles MF that many consider the two conditions to be variants of the same disorder, and refer to both collectively by the overly generic term "cutaneous T-cell lymphoma."[43] Several studies have compared the cutaneous histopathologies of SS and MF.[73,74] Based on these studies, Pautrier collections are held to be more common in SS, and papillary dermal edema can be seen in SS whereas patch stage MF usually exhibits wiry papillary dermal fibrosis. Eosinophils and plasma cells are also more common in MF than in SS.

Patients with erythroderma resulting from an underlying inflammatory skin disease such as psoriasis, pityriasis rubra pilaris, or allergic contact dermatitis pose a greater diagnostic challenge. In the absence of definitively diagnostic microscopic findings, genotypic analysis of the TCR gene, using DNA from skin biopsies or peripheral blood as a substrate, may prove useful in such cases.[45] It is important to remember that sufficient DNA for analysis cannot be extracted from sparsely infiltrated skin specimens.

Strikingly convoluted nuclei are not unique to SS. Convoluted, multilobate, cloverleaf-like, and pedunculated nuclear segments are often present in the neoplastic lymphocytes of patients with adult T-cell leukemia/lymphoma (ATLL, discussed later). Circulating Sézary cells can also be found in erythrodermic follicular mucinosis, a rare condition involving widespread cutaneous lesions of alopecia mucinosa and peripheral blood eosinophilia.[75]

Pagetoid Reticulosis (PR)

Pagetoid reticulosis (PR) is an indolent form of T-cell lymphoma in which lesions prototypically present on acral skin and microscopically show pronounced epidermotropism.[76] If localized, the disorder is termed Woringer-Kolopp lymphoma, in attribution to the original describers. If microscopically similar lesions are present in a disseminated fashion, the disorder is known as the Ketron-Goodman variant.[77] Clinically, localized PR is characterized by verrucous, scaling plaques that often display an annular or polycyclic configuration.[76] The clinical presentation of localized PR overlaps with that of unilesional mycosis fungoides (MF), with localized PR having a greater tendency to exhibit an acral distribution and associated hyperkeratosis.[40,78] Localized PR responds well to localized therapy, comprising surgical extirpation or irradiation, in most instances. Lifelong follow-up is warranted, however, because dissemination or the development of systemic lymphoma has been occasionally documented in patients with localized disease.[79,80]

Lesions of disseminated PR resemble those of conventional MF and consist of slightly scaly patches or plaques.[77] The existence of the Ketron-Goodman variant has been questioned, because some cases follow a clinical course indistinguishable from that of MF.[81] Although it has not yet been proven that distinction of disseminated PR from MF is warranted biologically, the entity is included in this discussion for completeness.

Histopathology. In microscopic sections, the neoplastic lymphocytes display striking infiltration of the epidermis and pericellular halos, imparting an appearance that reminded early observers of Paget's disease (Fig. 32-21). The neoplastic cells have intermediate-sized, convoluted nuclei and scant cytoplasm. The epidermis generally is thickened and hyperkeratotic, and a pseudocarcinomatous pattern is not uncommon.[76] Eosinophils and plasma cells are usually not present in PR.

Histogenesis. Although there has been a historical debate regarding the lineage of PR, immunophenotypic studies have demonstrated that PR is a T-cell neoplasm.[77,78,82] Rearrangements of the T-cell receptor gene have been documented, confirming the clonal nature of the proliferation.[83] A summation of reported cases reveals a heterogeneous immunophenotype.[77,78,82] Most cases express CD4, although some are CD8+ proliferations of suppressor cells. Diminished or absent expression of CD7 is common. In contrast to MF and SS, there has been documentation of a lack of expression of CD45 (leukocyte common antigen) and CD45RO (UCHL1, the T-cell-associated epitope of the same molecular complex) by the cells of localized PR.[77] Interestingly, the cells of some examples of disseminated PR have been demonstrated to be CD45+ and CD45RO−.[77] Because CD45 interacts with lymphocyte-specific kinases that are important in regulating lymphocyte turnover, the absence of CD45 has been forwarded as a possible explanation for the indolent clinical behavior of this lymphoma.

Differential Diagnosis. Some cases with the clinical presentation of PR may not display striking epidermotropism, and such cases could alternatively be classified as solitary MF. Marked epidermotropism is present by definition in the Ketron-Goodman variant and serves as a criterion for distinction from conventional MF.

Granulomatous Slack Skin

Granulomatous slack skin (GSS) is an extraordinarily rare, clinically unique form of epidermotropic T-cell lymphoma that displays microscopic features in common with mycosis fungoides. Fewer than 50 patients with this condition have been documented in the literature.

Clinical Features. Like MF, GSS begins as patches, thin papules, and plaques.[84] Over time, distinctive plaques that manifest as pendulous skin folds evolve, and the lesions are most commonly distributed in the axillae and groin, although involvement of the trunk or extremities has been noted.[84]

Histopathology. The earliest lesions of GSS show the same microscopic features as patches of MF, with a sparse epidermotropic infiltrate within a slightly fibrotic papillary dermis.[84] In contrast, biopsies of lax skin show a pathognomonic constellation of features, with a papillary dermal and epidermal array of small convoluted lymphocytes above a massively expanded reticular dermis that contains a diffuse infiltrate of lymphocytes and multinucleate macrophages.[84–86] The multinucleate cells are memorable because they contain extraordinary numbers of nuclei in clusters or a wreath-like configuration, and some show lymphophagocytosis.[84] Evidence of elastolysis is detectable by elastic fragments within macrophage cytoplasm, and elastic tissue stains demonstrate near absence of elastic fibers throughout the dermis.

Histogenesis. The neoplastic cells of GSS have T-helper cell lineage and express CD3 and CD4. Absence or diminution of CD7 expression is common.[84] Clonal rearrangements of the T-cell receptor β-chain gene have been confirmed by a number of different investigators.[84–86]

Differential Diagnosis. The clinical differential diagnosis of GSS includes cutis laxa and anetoderma, both of which can usually be readily excluded based on clinical and histopathologic features. The distinction of GSS and granulomatous MF poses the greatest challenge because both are clonal, epidermotropic, T-helper cell proliferations. In addition to the clinical context, the most distinguishing microscopic attributes include fewer nuclei within multinucleate cells and a greater tendency to show an interstitial pattern in granulomatous MF. In addition, the degree of lymphocyte convolution and hyperchromatism tends to be greater in early MF than GSS.[84]

Adult T-Cell Leukemia/Lymphoma (ATLL)

Adult T-cell leukemia/lymphoma (ATLL) is a high-grade T-cell lymphoma induced by genomic integration of the retrovirus HTLV-1. The highest incidence of ATLL is in areas endemic for HTLV-1 infection, including southern Japan, Southeast Asia, and the Caribbean.[87] HTLV-1 seropositivity and ATLL have also been documented in African-Americans in the southeastern United States. HTLV-1 is transmissible through bodily fluids. Serologic testing reveals that HTLV-1 seropositivity is much more common than overt ATLL.

Clinical Features. ATLL often has an abrupt onset and an aggressive clinical course. *H*ypercalcemia, *o*steolytic bone lesions, *T*-cell leukemia, and *s*kin lesions (HOTS) describes a clinical constellation that is manifested in some cases, along with lymphadenopathy.[87] Cutaneous lesions of ATLL consist of papules, plaques, and nodules/tumors. Patches, commonplace in MF, are extraordinary in ATLL. Unusual clinical presentations include purpuric plaques, subcutaneous nodules, and acral papulovesicles.

Histopathology. Small papules of ATLL display a dense dermal infiltrate of lymphocytes with medum-sized convoluted nuclei. A bandlike array of lymphocytes in the papillary dermis, with some convoluted lymphocytes within the epidermis, can also be seen, similar to the changes of MF (Fig. 32-22). Nodules and tumors of ATLL contain lymphocytes with large, vesicular nuclei and clumped chromatin, similar to anaplastic large-cell lymphoma.[87,88] Angiocentricity can be seen in nodules or tumors.[88] The peripheral blood commonly contains lymphocytes with multilobated nuclei.[87] Peripheral eosinophilia is also frequently observed.[89]

Histogenesis. The lymphocytes of ATLL are of T helper lineage and express CD3 and CD4. Paradoxically, the cells may exert suppressor activity in vitro. Southern blot analysis of the T-cell receptor gene reveals a clonal patten in most cases. The

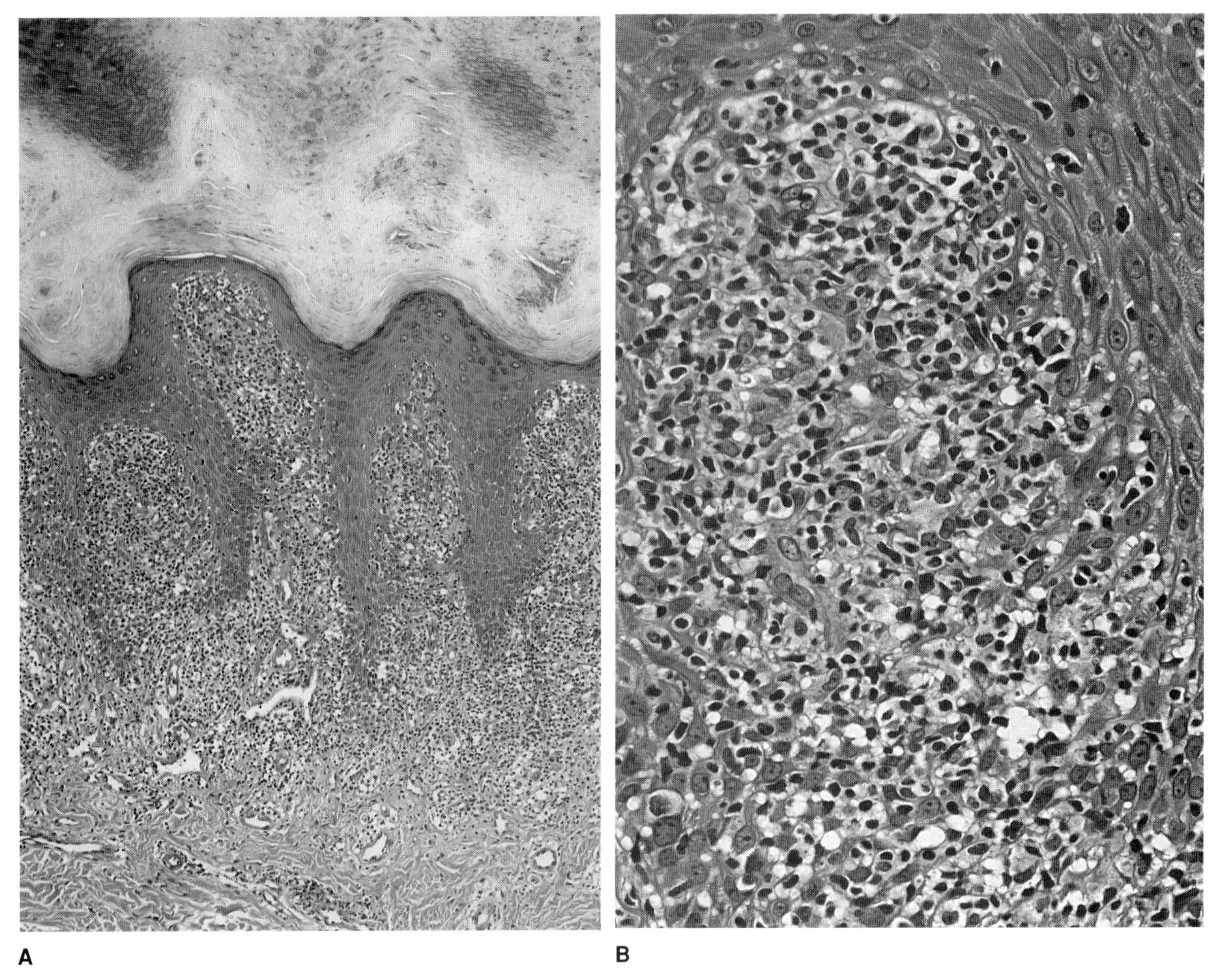

FIG. 32-21. Localized pagetoid reticulosis (Woringer-Kolopp lymphoma) (**A**) Low magnification. There is a dense, bandlike array of lymphocytes in concert with massive hyperkeratosis. (**B**) High magnification reveals many convoluted lymphocytes in array within the epidermis, and many lymphocytes display pericellular halos.

circulating cells of ATLL express CD25, the interleukin-2 (IL-2) receptor, in higher percentages than do the cells of Sézary syndrome.[90] Indeed, IL-2 may drive the proliferation of T cells in ATLL, and antireceptor antibodies have been utilized to block IL-2 binding, resulting in remission.

Differenial Diagnosis. ATLL is most easily confused with MF and SS. It is important to recognize ATLL in light of its morbid course and the transmissibility of HTLV-1. The clinical course is helpful in distinguishing MF from ATLL, because the course of MF is typically indolent and the disease presents as patches rather than papules or nodules. Histologic features alone do not allow differentiation between plaques or tumors of MF and ATLL in all instances. The changes observed in patches of MF are histologically distinctive, however, because the earliest reported lesions of ATLL are papules with involvement of the reticular dermis.

Distinction between ATLL and SS can also be difficult. Seropositivity for HTLV-1 does not always indicate ATLL, because the prevalence of such antibodies in endemic populations is high.[45] Peripheral blood smears may be useful, because the multilobated nuclei of ATLL are not encountered in SS. The "gold standard" for diagnosis of ATLL is the demonstration of clonal integration of the HTLV-1 genome within the neoplastic cells.[91] Testing for clonal integration can be perfomed on either lesional skin or blood from ATLL patients, using the Southern blot method.

Peripheral T-Cell Lymphoma

Histologic, immunophenotypic, and genotypic data have made it possible to recognize a variety of T-cell lymphomas unrelated to MF and SS. The term "nonepidermotropic T-cell lymphoma" is inadequate, because some degree of infiltration of the epidermis can occur in any of these conditions, and the lumping of these conditions does not acknowledge differences in biological behavior. Although the revised Kiel classification recognizes several types, the diagnosis of some of these categories is not reproducible, and therefore several are recognized as provisional categories within the REAL classification.[1]

Lennert's (lymphoepithelioid) lymphoma (LL) is a low-grade T-cell neoplasm with numerous associated epithelioid

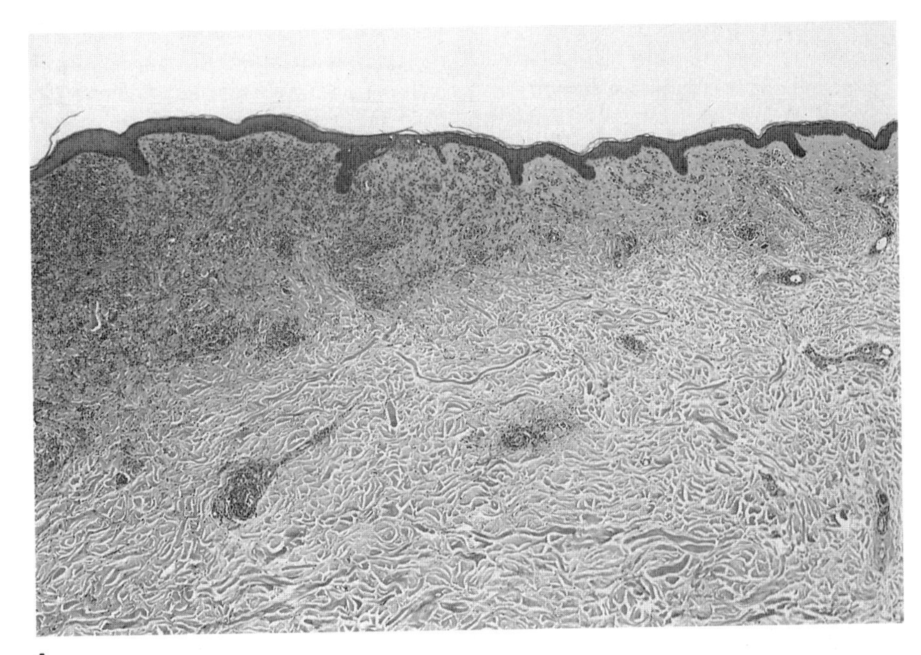

A

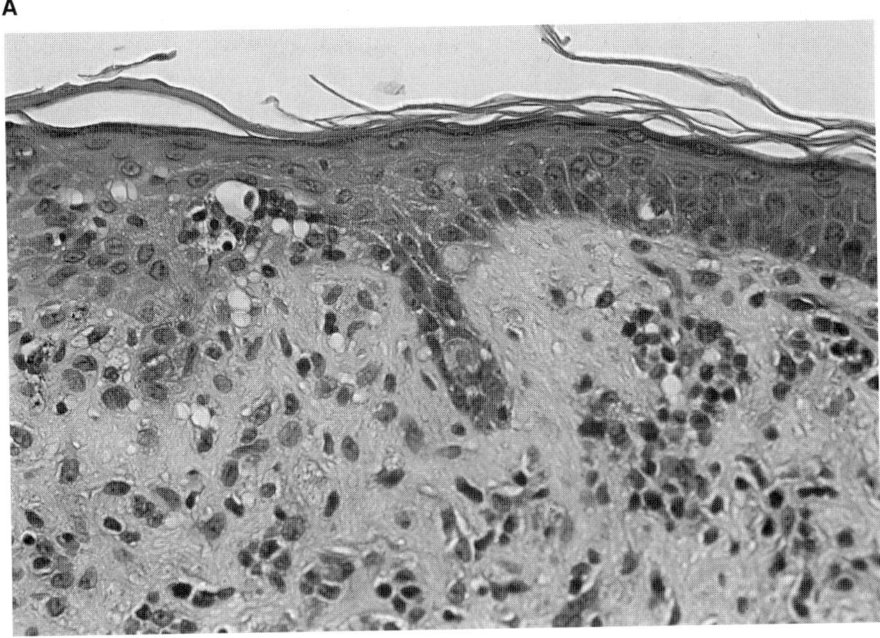

B

FIG. 32-22. Adult T-cell leukemia/lymphoma
(**A**) Scanning magnification. The infiltrate assumes a T-cell pattern, with a bandlike array of lymphocytes that also involve the superficial reticular dermis. (**B**) At high magnification, small numbers of convoluted epidermotropic lymphocytes are identifiable. Lymphocytes with multilobate nuclei were identifiable in a peripheral blood smear.

macrophages. Systemic manifestations include cervical lymphadenopathy, hepatosplenomegaly, bone marrow involvement, and fever. The skin is involved in less than 10% of the cases.[92] There are no distinctive clinical features. Dense nodular and diffuse infiltrates of neoplastic lymphocytes with convoluted or twisted nuclei, with clusters of epithelioid macrophages and rare plasma cells, typify LL. Large lymphocytes are often directly adjacent to the clusters of macrophages. In addition to nodular or diffuse dermal infiltrates, there can be bandlike infiltrates in the papillary dermis, and lymphocytes may occasionally infiltrate the epidermis.[43] LL can resemble granulomatous MF histologically, but the patches observed in the latter are never found clinically. Immunophenotyping is not useful for differentiating these conditions, because both are of T-helper lineage. The clusters of macrophages are smaller than those found in sarcoidosis or other sarcoidal granulomatous dermatitides.

Angioimmunoblastic lymphadenopathy (AILD) is a condition characterized by fever, lymphadenopathy, and dysproteinemia. Infiltrates in lymph nodes are heterogeneous and feature immunoblasts, plasma cells, and small lymphocytes, with a background in which there are increased numbers of small blood vessels with extravascular accumulations of glycoprotein. Overt T-cell lymphomas evolve in some patients. Large, atypical lympocytes with clear cytoplasm are found next to small vessels in AILD-like T-cell lymphoma. It is conceivable that early examples of AILD have minor clonal populations and are already low-grade lymphomas. Roughly 40% of patients develop cutaneous macules and papules, but the histopathologic findings are not specific. A pattern of lymphocytic vasculitis has been reported.

Pleomorphic T-cell lymphoma (PTL) was first described in Japanese patients infected with HTLV-1, but it is now known that PTL also develops in seronegative individuals. The disease is defined by cytologic features, with irregularly shaped, variably sized hyperchromatic nuclei, with small nucleoli (Fig. 32-23). In the modified Kiel classification, the small-cell (3 to 7 μm) variant of pleomorphic T-cell lymphoma is a low-grade lymphoma and the medium-sized (7 to 11 μm) and large-cell (more than 11 μm) variants are high-grade lymphomas.[61] The REAL classification recognizes the difficulty that many pathologists have in classifying these lesions and consolidates them into a group termed "peripheral T-cell lymphoma, unspecified."[1]

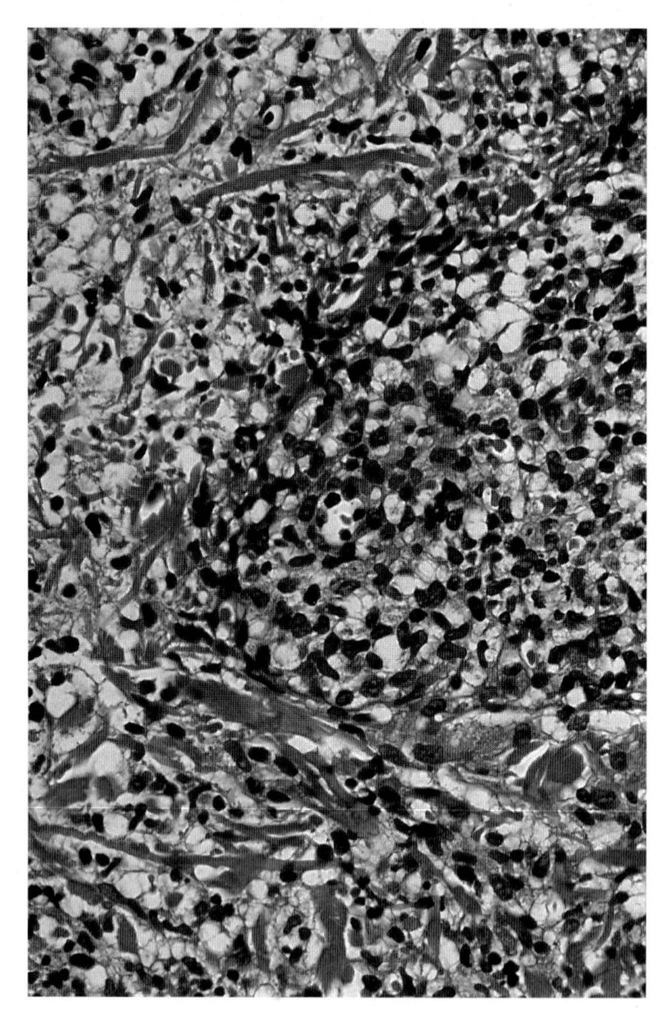

FIG. 32-23. Pleomorphic T-cell lymphoma
A nodular infiltrate of small to medium-sized lymphocytes, with convoluted nuclei and small nucleoli, involves the reticular dermis. Epidermotropism was not pronounced, and only nodular lesions were present clinically.

The clinical lesions of PTL do not have a distinctive appearance. Patches do not occur. The infiltrates display a T-cell pattern, with focal infiltration of the epidermis and hair follicle epithelium. Multilobated T-cell lymphoma is a variant of PTL with a propensity to involve the skin and bones of elderly patients.[94,95]

Subcutaneous panniculitic or lipotropic T-cell lymphoma presents with subcutaneous nodules, usually on the extremities. Some patients with this condition have associated hemophagocytic syndrome, which can prove fatal.[96] The morphologic pattern overlaps with angiocentric lymphoma, as infiltration of vessel walls often accompanies subcutaneous infiltrates. Histopathologic features include a dense, subcutaneous infiltrate with a mixed septal and lobular distribution (Fig. 32-24). The neoplastic cells have cytologic features similar to those of medium-sized or large-cell PTL; rarely, anaplastic large cells are prominent. Foci of karyorrhexis and fat necrosis can occur and can be associated with a granulomatous inflammatory reaction. Phagocytosis of erythrocytes by nonneoplastic macrophages is present in the subcutaneous infiltrate or the bone marrow. The neoplastic cells express a mature helper T-cell phenotype but can show loss of CD5 and CD7 antigens, and a natural killer cell phenotype (CD16+, CD56+) with evidence of Epstein-Barr virus (EBV) genomic integration has also been documented. Subcutaneous T-cell lymphomas resemble panniculitis at scanning magnification, and in the cases in which small pleomorphic T cells predominate, their infiltrates may not be obviously malignant, even under close scrutiny. Careful attention to cytologic detail, a search for morphologic and laboratory evidence of erythrophagocytosis, and prudent utilization of molecular studies such as genotypic analysis can be of help with this challenging diagnosis.

Cutaneous CD30+ (Ki-1) Anaplastic Large-Cell Lymphoma (ALCL) and Lymphomatoid Papulosis (LyP)

The entity historically described as "Ki-1+ lymphoma" was first recognized as a neoplasm manifested as cutaneous nodules composed of lymphocytes with large, strikingly atypical nuclei. The neoplastic cells, usually of T-cell lineage, by definition expressed the Ki-1 (now known as CD30) antigen. It is now established that CD30+ lymphoma is not a single entity but comprises a spectrum of disorders linked by the presence of a common neoplastic cell type. Within the spectrum, a striking range of clinical behavior can be seen. The spectrum includes CD30+ ALCL, so-called regressing atypical histiocytosis (RAH), and LyP.[97,98] It is worth remembering that CD30+ expression can be observed in tumor stage MF, some pleomorphic T-cell lymphomas, and some nonneoplastic eruptions, and thus the mere identification of CD30+ expression does not constitute grounds for the diagnosis of a CD30+ lymphoproliferative process. The CD30 antigen is an inducible marker of lymphocyte activation that can be identified on either B or T cells. Because the atypical cells of LyP, RAH, and ALCL all share similar cellular morphology, CD30 expression, and clonal rear-

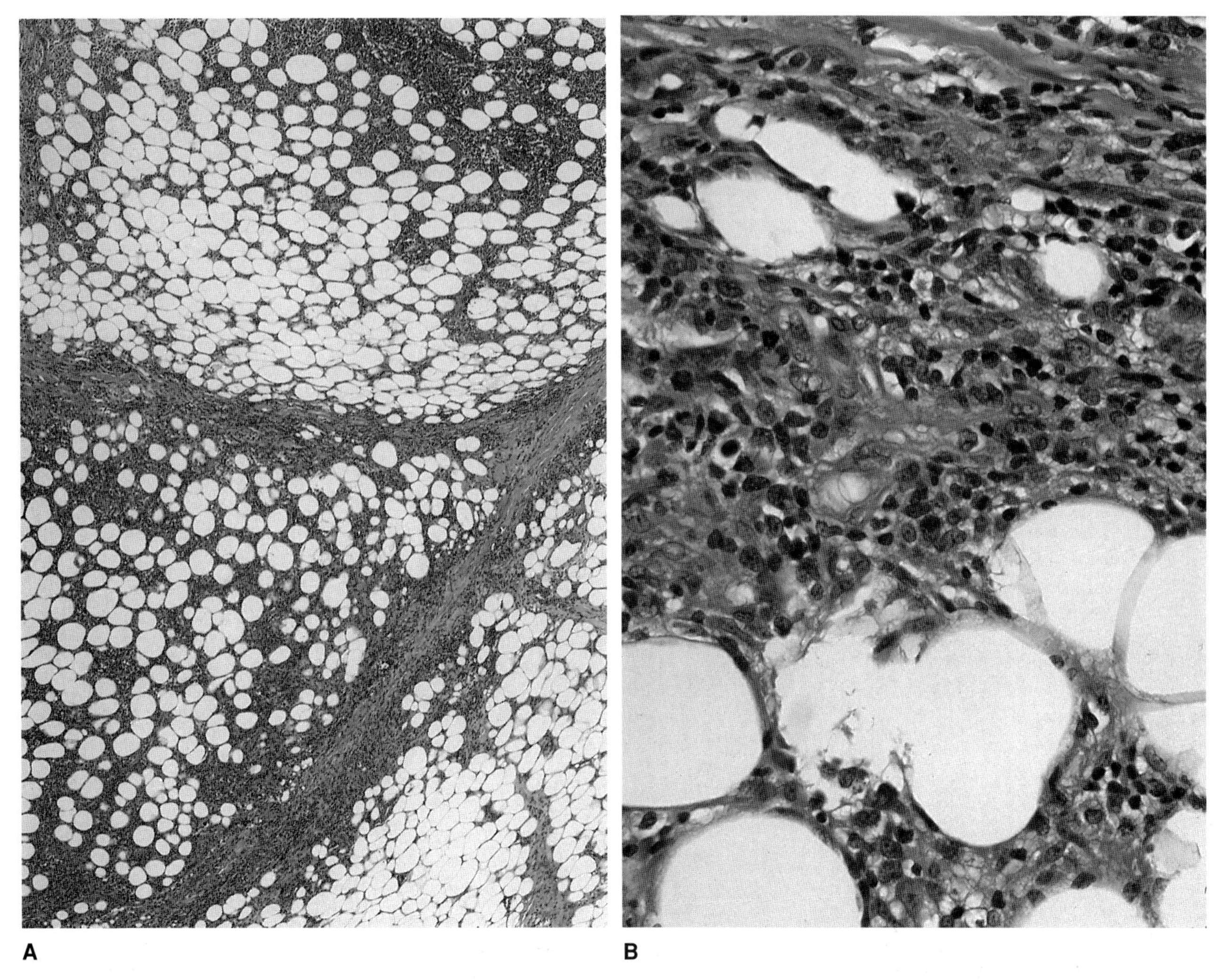

FIG. 32-24. Subcutaneous T-cell lymphoma, scanning magnification
(**A**) A septal and lobular pattern is punctuated by foci of necrosis. (**B**) Neoplastic lymphocytes are often inconspicuous in a heterogeneous infiltrate of macrophages, lymphocytes of varying size, and eosinophils. Genotypic analysis can be useful as an adjunctive diagnostic tool in such instances.

rangement of the T-cell receptor gene, a strong case can be made that the three conditions comprise a disease spectrum.[97,98] Within this spectrum, the overall number of clinical lesions is roughly inversely proportional to the durability of the lesions. Thus, lesions of LyP tend to be numerous, short-lived, and recurrent in most instances, whereas ALCL lesions tend to be few in number and persistent.

Clinical Features. CD30+ ALCL and RAH lesions typically present as large nodules or tumors located on the extremities, and ulceration and crusting are common. ALCL and RAH are oligolesional disorders, and often only one cutaneous lesion is present at a time in ALCL. The lymphoma can present at any age.[97–99] Many examples of systemic CD30+ ALCL develop in children, whereas primary cutaneous ALCL is more common in adults. Patients with RAH or cutaneous ALCL do not usually develop systemic symptoms, in contrast to patients with nodal involvement at presentation.[100] The clinicopathologic features observed in patients with RAH support the conclusion that RAH and CD30+ ALCL are two expressions of the same entity. The two patients who were described in the initial report of RAH went on to die from systemic lymphoma.[101,102] Some patients with cutaneous CD30+ lymphoma secondarily involving lymph nodes exhibit spontaneous regression and relapse of the cutaneous lesions but persistence of nodal disease. CD30+ ALCL appears to be the most common cutaneous lymphoma in patients with HIV.[99,103] In contrast to immunocompetent individuals, HIV-seropositive patients with CD30+ ALCL have a dismal prognosis.

Histopathology. Both RAH and CD30+ ALCL are characterized by a nodular dermal and subcutaneous infiltrate of large lymphocytes with abundant, faintly basophilic cytoplasm; large, irregularly shaped vesicular nuclei with coarsely clumped chromatin along nuclear membranes; and large, irregularly shaped nucleoli (Fig. 32-25). Wreath-shaped multinucleated cells are often present, as are "embryo"-shaped nuclei. Sarcomatoid (spindled) cellular morphology is encountered in rare cases.[100] Epidermal hyperplasia or ulceration and an inflammatory infiltrate rich in neutrophils are commonly observed.

Lesions of LyP are usually separable histologically in that atypical lymphocytes are arrayed in small numbers or in small clusters rather than sheets, within a heterogeneous infiltrate in which neutrophils and/or eosinophils are usually conspicuous

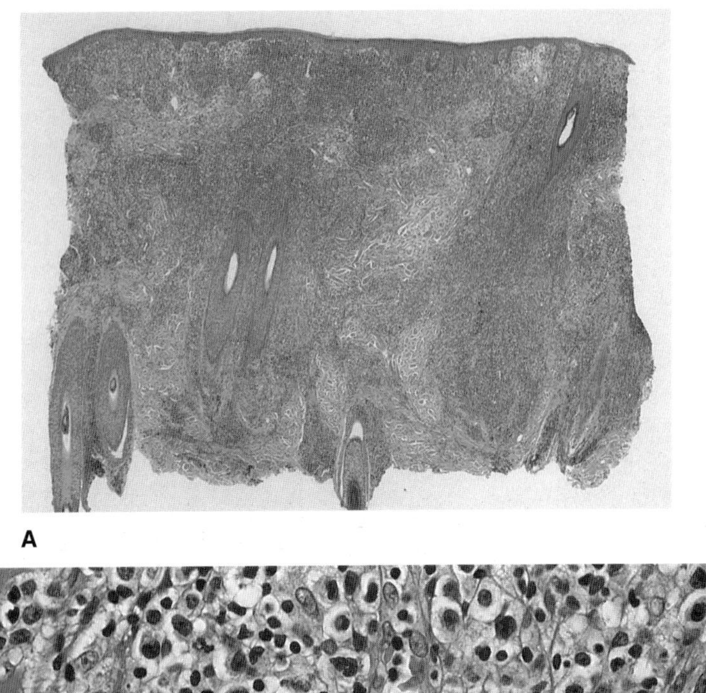

A

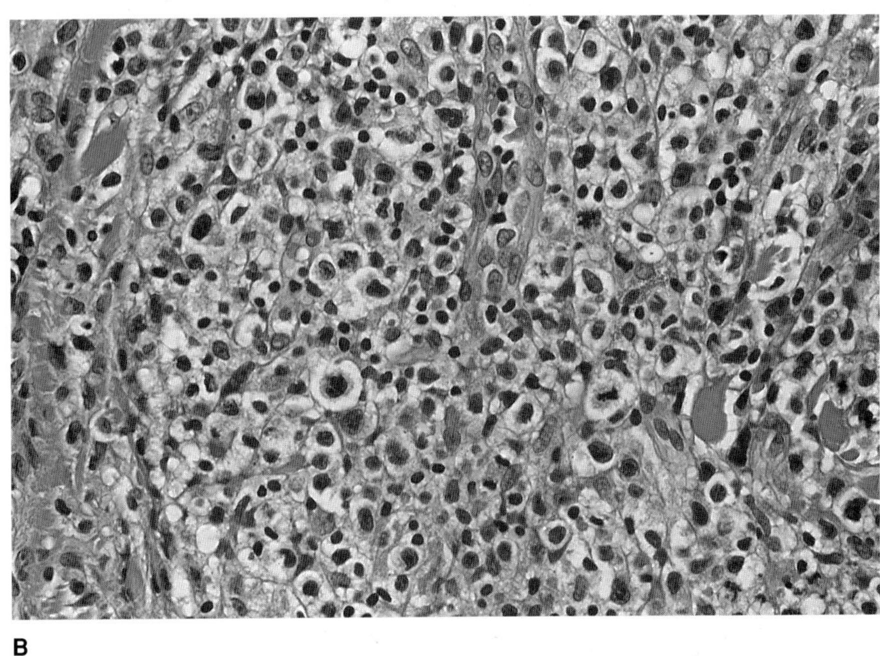

B

FIG. 32-25. CD30+ anaplastic large-cell lymphoma, scanning magnification
(**A**) The view of this lesion from the scalp shows a diffuse infiltrate of large lymphocytes in conjunction with epidermotropism. (**B**) Lymphocytes with large (and often multilobate) nuclei, prominent and multiple nucleoli, and ample cytoplasm comprise the infiltrate. Mitotic figures are often conspicuous.

(Fig. 32-26). The epidermis can show a variety of patterns in LyP biopsies, including infiltration by small to medium-sized convoluted lymphocytes, an interface reaction with necrotic keratinocytes, or necrosis and ulceration.

Histogenesis. Immunophenotypic and genotypic studies indicate T-cell lineage for LyP and RAH, in most instances for CD30+ ALCL.[97,98] Even though RAH cells sometimes display abundant cytoplasm and erythrophagocytosis, which lead to the erroneous initial notion that the process represents a histiocytic disorder on morphologic grounds, genotypic analysis has unequivocally demonstrated the T-cell lineage of the proliferation.[101,105] Surprisingly (and perhaps aberrantly), expression of CD1 has been documented in some examples of RAH/ALCL.[91] HTLV-1 genomic segments have been documented in ALCL cells from patients who reside in areas in which the virus is not endemic.[107] EBV genomic DNA is also identifiable in the cells of CD30+ ALCL in immunosuppressed, but not in immunocompetent, patients.[108] Because in situ hybridization demonstrates viral genome in most of the cells of such infiltrates, it seems likely that there is clonal integration of viral DNA in the

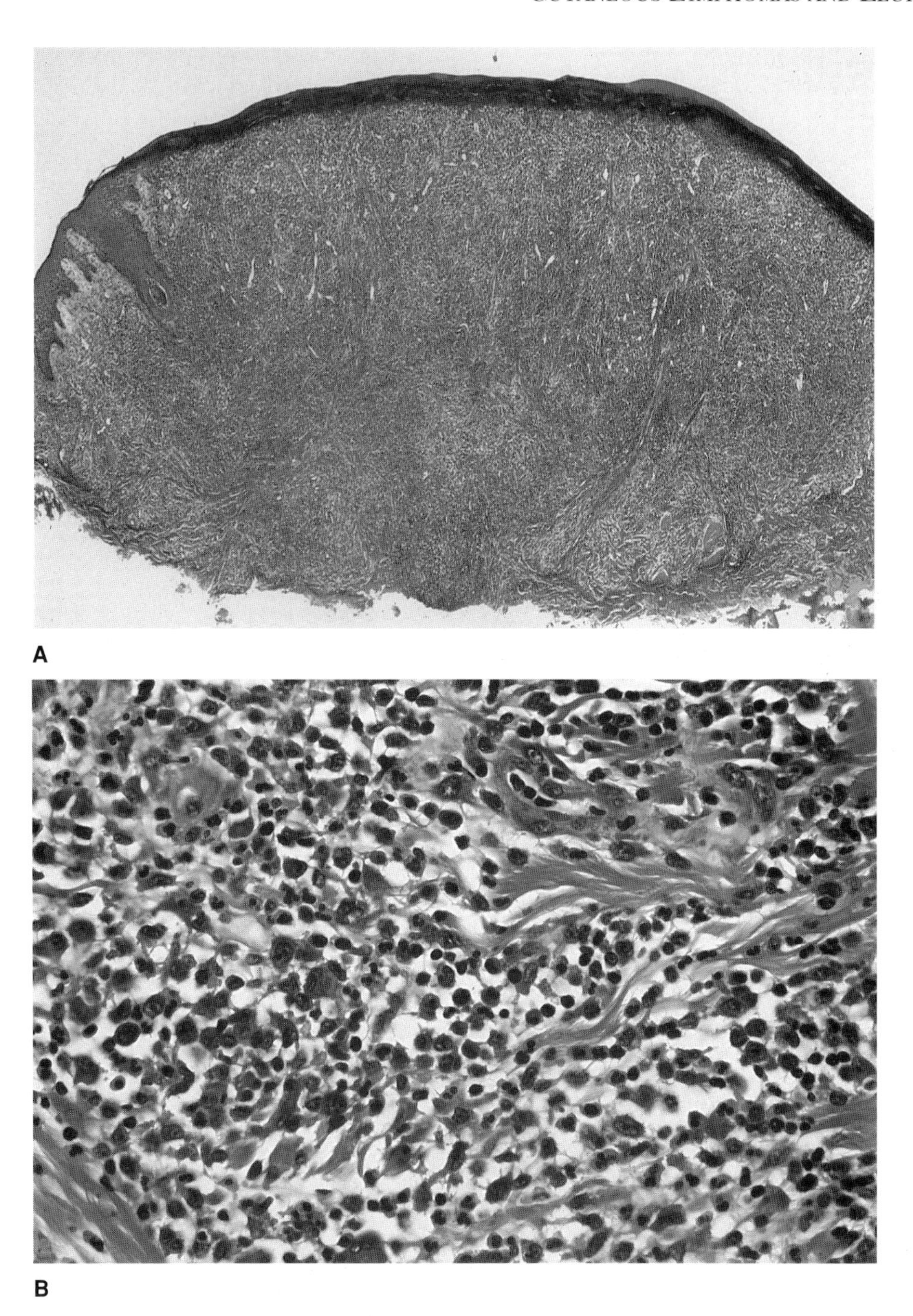

FIG. 32-26. Lymphomatoid papulosis, ulcerated lesion, scanning magnification
(**A**) There is a diffuse and vaguely wedge-shaped infiltrate in the reticular dermis. (**B** and **C**) The infiltrate is heterogeneous and includes many neutrophils and eosinophils, and contains relatively small numbers of neoplastic lymphocytes, as demonstrated in a CD30 immunostain. (*continued on next page*)

neoplastic cells in at least some patients. Nevertheless, viral integration is insufficient to explain the pathogenesis of all CD30+ lymphoproliferative disorders, because most if not all examples of LyP do not contain EBV genome.[99]

Progression from LyP to CD30+ ALCL has occurred in some patients and is marked clinically by the advent of larger, persistent lesions. The lack of lesional involution may reflect loss of the receptor for transforming growth factor (TGF)-b, which has an inhibitory effect on the cells of LyP.[109]

Differential Diagnosis. Although LyP is morphologically and biologically related to RAH and CD30+ ALCL, its course (unless complicated by another lymphoproliferative disease) is indolent, and thus it is important to make a specific diagnosis of LyP or CD30+ ALCL, if possible. The fact that LyP presents as numerous small lesions containing small numbers of atypical lymphocytes is usually helpful in making the distinction. In CD30+ ALCL, the atypical lymphocytes usually comprise the majority of the infiltrate and are often arrayed as sheets. Multinucleate, wreathlike cells are more often found in CD30+ ALCL than in LyP.

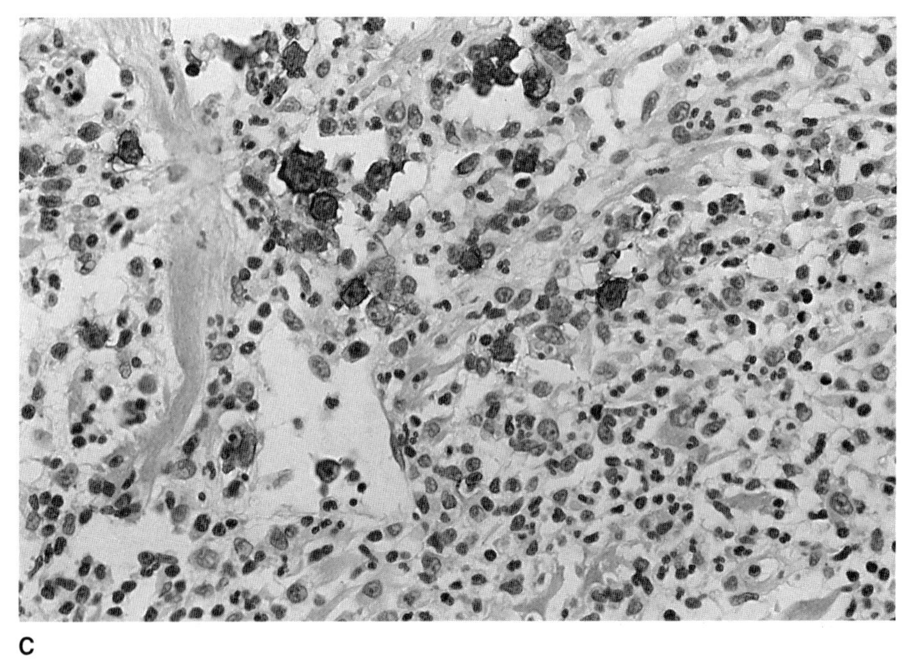

C

FIG. 32-26. *Continued*

Cutaneous lesions of Hodgkin's lymphoma (HL) may also pose considerable difficulty in the differential diagnosis of CD30+ lymphoproliferative disorders. It is vital to remember that HL most often involves the skin by direct extension from involved lymph nodes, and that disseminated cutaneous lesions of HL are extraordinary. The fact that HL and LyP often coexist in the same patient serves as a further caution against the assumption that an atypical infiltrate in an HL patient represents cutaneous HL. Reed-Sternberg (RS) cells are nearly always found in infiltrates of HL but are not present in CD30+ lymphoma. RS cells common express CD15, a determinant usually not expressed by CD30+ ALCL or LyP. If there is lymphadenopathy, a node biopsy can prove helpful, because nodes involved by CD30+ lymphoma often display a sinusoidal pattern distinct from the interfollicular or diffuse pattern commonly observed in HL.

Overinterpretation of the significance of CD30 expression is to be avoided. CD30 can be expressed by a variety of carcinomas, including embryonal carcinoma.[110] Thus, a diagnosis of carcinoma should be considered before concluding that a cutaneous infiltrate of anaplastic CD30+ cells is large-cell lymphoma. Other cutaneous lymphomas can also express CD30, making it imperative that a panel of lymphoid and nonlymphoid markers be evaluated as part of the diagnostic evaluation, in addition to careful conventional microscopic assessment.

Angiocentric Lymphoma

The neoplastic lymphocytes of angiocentric lymphoma display a tendency to infiltrate blood vessel walls and also involve other structures. Systemic disease is usually present. The terms "lymphomatoid granulomatosis" and "angiocentric immunoproliferative lesion" have been used to refer to a spectrum of diseases with similar histopathologic patterns, ranging from heterogeneous infiltrates, in which the neoplastic cells are inconspicuous, to frank lymphoma. Despite the heterogeneity, the observation of clonal integration of EBV genome in a distinct subset of patients suggests that some angiocentric lymphoproliferative disorders constitute lymphoma from the outset. Angiocentricity seems to be a pattern expressed by several distinct entities that involve the skin, including conventional T-cell neoplasms and proliferations of natural killer (NK) and NK-like cells.

Clinical Features. Subcutaneous or dermal nodules are the most common clinical morphologies, but great morphologic heterogeneity, from papules to ulcerated tumors, has been noted.[111] Concurrent pulmonary and central nervous system diseases are common and can precede or follow cutaneous lesions.[111] In light of the systemic presentation of the malignancy, it is not surprising that the prognosis is grim in some variants of angiocentric lymphoma, with 5-year survival rates of less than 50%.[111]

Histopathology. The proportion of neoplastic cells in the infiltrate is highly variable.[112] Some infiltrates are virtually nondiagnosable histologically, because the cytologic aberrancies in the neoplastic cells are subtle. Most commonly, the neoplastic lymphocytes display medium-sized nuclei with rounded or irregularly shaped borders. Nuclear clefts and grooves can be seen, but true cerebriform morphology is exceptional.[113] In most cases, medium-sized and small vessels contain lymphocytes within their walls, although this finding can be subtle (Fig. 32-27). Concentric perivascular fibrosis, fibrin deposition in vessel walls or lumens, and intimal fibrosis are clues to the presence of vascular damage from the neoplastic infiltrate.[113] The compromise of the vasculature can lead to anoxic cutaneous necrosis and can potentially obscure the microscopic picture. Epidermotropism can be seen in some instances. Some cases in which there is a prominent pagetoid pattern have been reported as disseminated pagetoid reticulosis, and could represent MF or

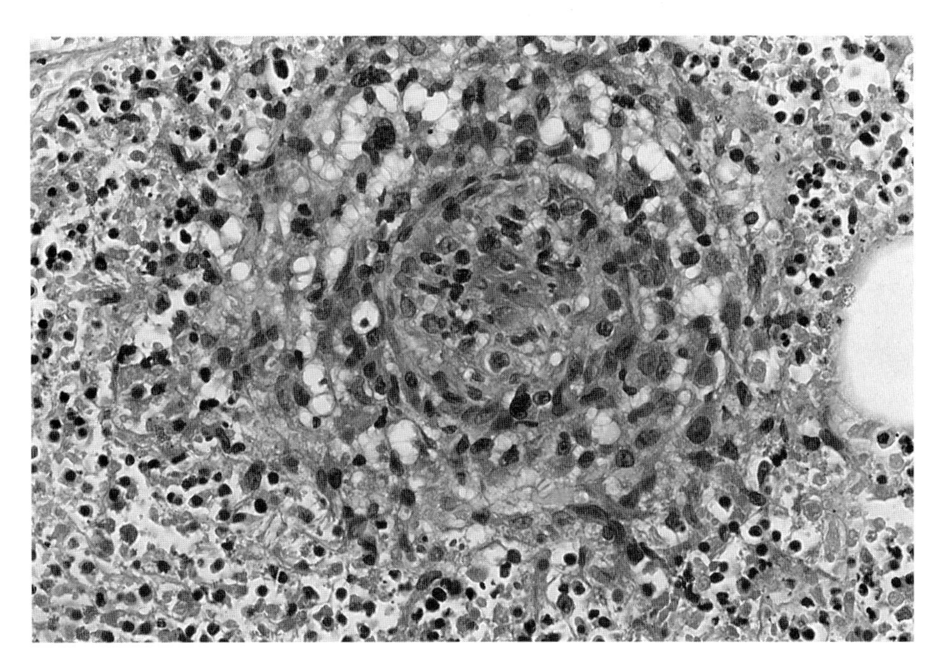

FIG. 32-27. Angiocentric lymphoma
The wall of a medium-sized vessel is obliterated by an infiltrate of neoplastic T lymphocytes. There are adjacent foci of necrosis.

an MF-like lymphoma with angiocentricity.[114] The clinical and pathologic features also overlap with those of subcutaneous lymphoma. In short, the microscopic pattern of angiocentric lymphoma is heterogeneous in that it does not constitute a single clinicopathologic entity, but rather comprises a group of lymphoproliferative disorders that are linked by angiocentricity.

Histogenesis. Immunophenotypic studies reveal aberrant T-cell phenotypes in many cases of angiocentric lymphoma, with loss of the CD3, CD5, and CD7 antigens.[113] Other examples are of natural killer (NK) cell or NK-cell-like lineage, because they fail to express T-cell markers but express CD16 and CD56.[115] Touch imprints of some of these infiltrates show large granular lymphocytes when stained by the Wright-Giemsa method.[115] Although the cells do not express CD3 on their surfaces, cytoplasmic CD3 can be detected. Despite the enduring name "lymphomatoid granulomatosis," neither granulomatous inflammation nor macrophages are usually conspicuous.

Clonal EBV genomic integration appears to play an important role in the pathogenesis of some angiocentric lymphomas, especially those of NK-cell or NK-cell-like lineage. In situ hybridization or immunoperoxidase staining for EBV genome or proteins can be employed to seek evidence of EBV integration in routine specimens.[101]

Differential Diagnosis. The differential diagnosis includes both nonneoplastic and neoplastic disorders. If the cells of angiocentric lymphoma are few in number, the infiltrate can be mistaken for a mere perivascular infiltrate or dermatitis. If vascular changes are prominent, the lymphocytic vasculitis associated with perniosis and pityriasis lichenoides enters the differential diagnosis. Careful examination of the infiltrate for atypical lymphocytes remains the best approach to the differential diagnosis, and the clinical context and molecular studies should also be heavily relied upon.

Among neoplastic disorders, LyP most commonly displays angiocentricity that simulates angiocentric lymphoma. LyP can usually be distinguished by the presence of a wedge-shaped infiltrate, involvement of the superficial dermis and epidermis, and CD30 immunopositivity. Angiocentricity can also be rarely encountered in patients with various forms of epidermotropic cutaneous T-cell lymphoma, including MF. The epidermotropism of angiocentric MF tends to be the predominant pattern, in contrast to angiocentric lymphoma, in which epidermotropism is usually no more than spotty.

Angiocentric lymphoma is often confused with angiotropic lymphoma, historically known as malignant angioendotheliomatosis. Angiotropic lymphoma or intravascular lymphomatosis is distinguishable in that the neoplastic cells are within vessel lumens rather than vessel walls, and furthermore most angiotropic lymphomas are of B-cell lineage.

PROLIFERATIONS OF OTHER HEMATOLYMPHOID CELLS

Hodgkin's Lymphoma (HL)

Hodgkin's lymphoma (HL) is manifest histologically as a heterogeneous infiltrate containing scattered, strikingly atypical mononuclear cells of uncertain lineage, known as Reed-Sternberg (RS) cells. Whereas most lymphomas spread in the patient in a haphazard fashion, HL generally extends through contiguous sites. HL typically develops within a single lymph node, disseminates through lymphatics to involve adjacent nodes, and in some cases then invades vessel walls and spreads hematogenously. The classical Rye scheme recognizes four histologic patterns: lymphocyte-predominant, nodular sclerosing, mixed-cellularity, and lymphocyte-depleted. Whether HL is a single disease entity or a group of lymphoproliferative diseases with shared histologic and immunophenotypic features is currently debatable. The distinctions between nodular lymphocyte-predominant HL and B-cell lymphoma and between lymphocyte-depleted HL and ALCL are ambiguous. Although the lineage of the malignancy remains unestablished (at least in some instances), HL is considered as a lymphoma in this chapter.

HL comprises 20 to 30% of all lymphomas but only a minute fraction of cutaneous lymphomas. There are different clinicopathologic groups of patients with HL. In developing countries, many children are affected, whereas in developed nations there are age peaks among young adults and in late middle age. There is a variety of clinical presentations of HL. Lymphadenopathy alone is observed in early cases, whereas disseminated disease results in hepatosplenomegaly, abdominal or thoracic tumors, and systemic or "B" symptoms. Skin involvement by HL is almost always secondary to visceral or nodal involvement. Secondary cutaneous HL is rare, occurring in 0.5 to 3.4% of the cases.[116,117] The most common source of secondary cutaneous HL is distal retrograde spread from involved lymph nodes. Papules, plaques, or subcutaneous nodules arise in the skin of an arm or leg following HL in the axillary or inguinal nodes. Less commonly, HL spreads by direct extension from lymph nodes. Even more rarely, hematogenous spread disseminates papules or nodules throughout the skin. Cutaneous involvement in HL portends a poor prognosis.

Primary cutaneous HL appears to be an exceedingly rare but authentic entity. Most older reports purporting to describe cutaneous HL were really depictions of lymphomatoid papulosis or CD30+ ALCL. Some patients with primary cutaneous HL have developed mixed-cellularity HL in their lymph nodes, but the disease has been limited to the skin in others.[118]

HL in its early stages spreads in a predictable fashion from node group to node group through lymphatics, and even viscera are involved in sequence. Staging of the disease by lymphangiography and exploratory laparotomy (splenectomy, liver biopsy, and biopsy of iliac and para-aortic lymph nodes) was performed for many years, but imaging studies and the risk of damage to the immune system from splenectomy have made classical staging obsolete in many centers. The commonly used staging system for HL is the modified Ann Arbor Staging Classification. Four stages are recognized:[119]

Stage I: Involvement of a single lymph node region (I) or of a single extralymphatic organ or site (I_E).

Stage II: Involvement of two or more lymph node regions on the same side of the diaphragm (II) or localized involvement of an extralymphatic organ or site (II_E).

Stage III: Involvement of lymph node regions on both sides of the diaphragm (III) or localized involvement of an extralymphatic organ or site (III_E) or spleen (III_S), or both (III_{SE}).

Stage IV: Diffuse or disseminated involvement of one or more extralymphatic organs with or without associated lymph node involvement.

The presence or absence of systemic symptoms, such as fever and weight loss, is another staging criterion, denoted by the suffix letters B and A, respectively. Biopsy-proven HL of the liver or bone marrow implies stage IV disease. Involvement of other extralymphatic organs, such as the lung, pleura, or bone, may represent either E lesions, if localized, or stage IV disease, if multiple or disseminated.

Histopathology. HL has a vast range of microscopic appearances, but a common feature is the presence of RS cells or their variants. Classic RS cells range up to 50 μm in diameter, are binucleate, and have large vesicular nuclei, clumped chromatin, and irregular nuclear membranes (Fig. 32-28). In addition, true RS cells have brightly eosinophilic nucleoli that measure more than one-third of the diameter of the nucleus. Immunoblasts in histopathologic simulants of HL, such as infectious mononucleosis, often have smaller nucleoli. The term "Hodgkin's cell" is used for large lymphocytes that have the other features of RS

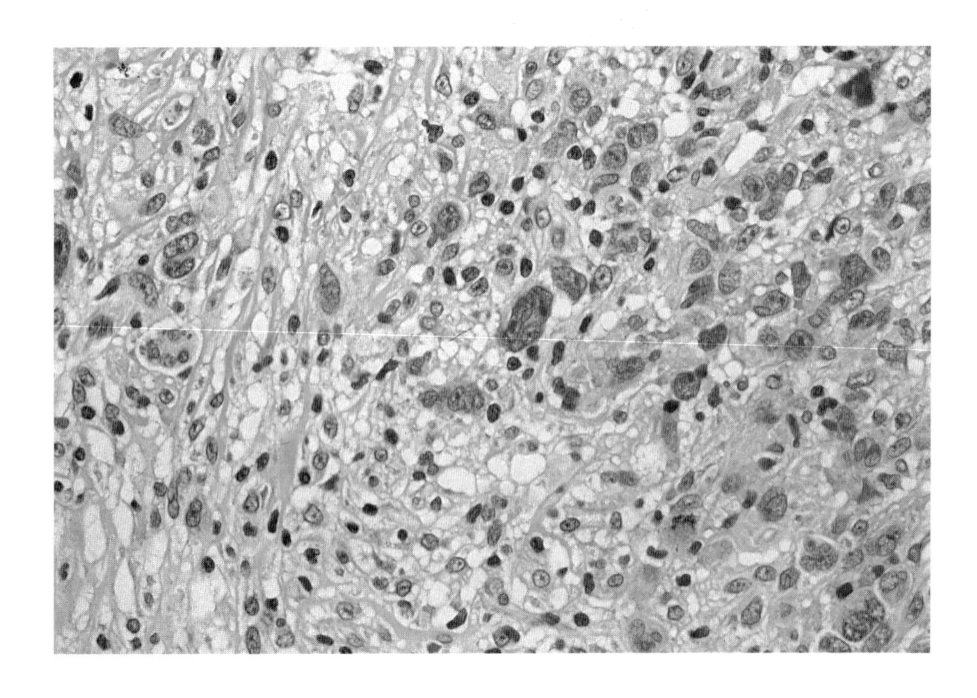

FIG. 32-28. Hodgkin's lymphoma, Reed-Sternberg cell There is a binucleate form with prominent nucleoli in the center of the field. Variant Reed-Sternberg forms are also evident.

cells but are not binucleate. Three variants of Hodgkin's cells occur in cutaneous infiltrates of HL. Lymphocytic-histiocytic (L&H) cells, observed in lymphocyte-predominant HL, have large, multilobate, vesicular nuclei with minute nucleoli and moderate amounts of pale cytoplasm. The lacunar cell of nodular sclerosing HL is so named because it has clear cytoplasm that often appears retracted from a sharply defined peripheral margin. In the reticular type of lymphocyte-depleted HL, Hodgkin's cells can appear "sarcomatoid"—i.e., spindled and pleomorphic. Extreme variation in nuclear appearance typifies the pleomorphic variant of lymphocyte-depleted HL.

Cutaneous HL histologically resembles nodal disease in most patients. In occasional cases, the skin harbors an infiltrate of higher histologic grade. As is the case with nodal HL, the majority of cells are inflammatory and usually consist of small lymphocytes, eosinophils, neutrophils, and plasma cells.

A few generalizations apply to the infiltrates of various types of HL in the skin. The infiltrates are generally nodular or diffuse, and spare the epidermis (Fig. 32-29). In cases with large numbers of RS cells, areas of necrosis can be present.

Lymphocyte-predominant HL only rarely involves the skin. It appears as sheets of small, convoluted lymphocytes and scattered RS cells.

In nodes affected by nodular sclerosing HL, there are bands of polarizable collagen that replace nodal parenchyma. This feature is not usually evident in cutaneous infiltrates. One hallmark of nodular sclerosing HL that can be seen in cutaneous involvement is the lacunar type of the RS cell. Lacunar cells are surrounded by a retraction space in formalin-fixed tissues and often have multilobulated nuclei with small nucleoli.

Mixed-cellularity HL features an infiltrate with a balance between small lymphocytes and RS cells that is intermediate between the lymphocyte-predominant and lymphocyte-depleted forms of HL. More macrophages and eosinophils are present than in lymphocyte predominant HL.

Lymphocyte-depleted HL presents in the skin as relatively monomorphous infiltrates of RS or Hodgkin's cells. Necrosis is often present.

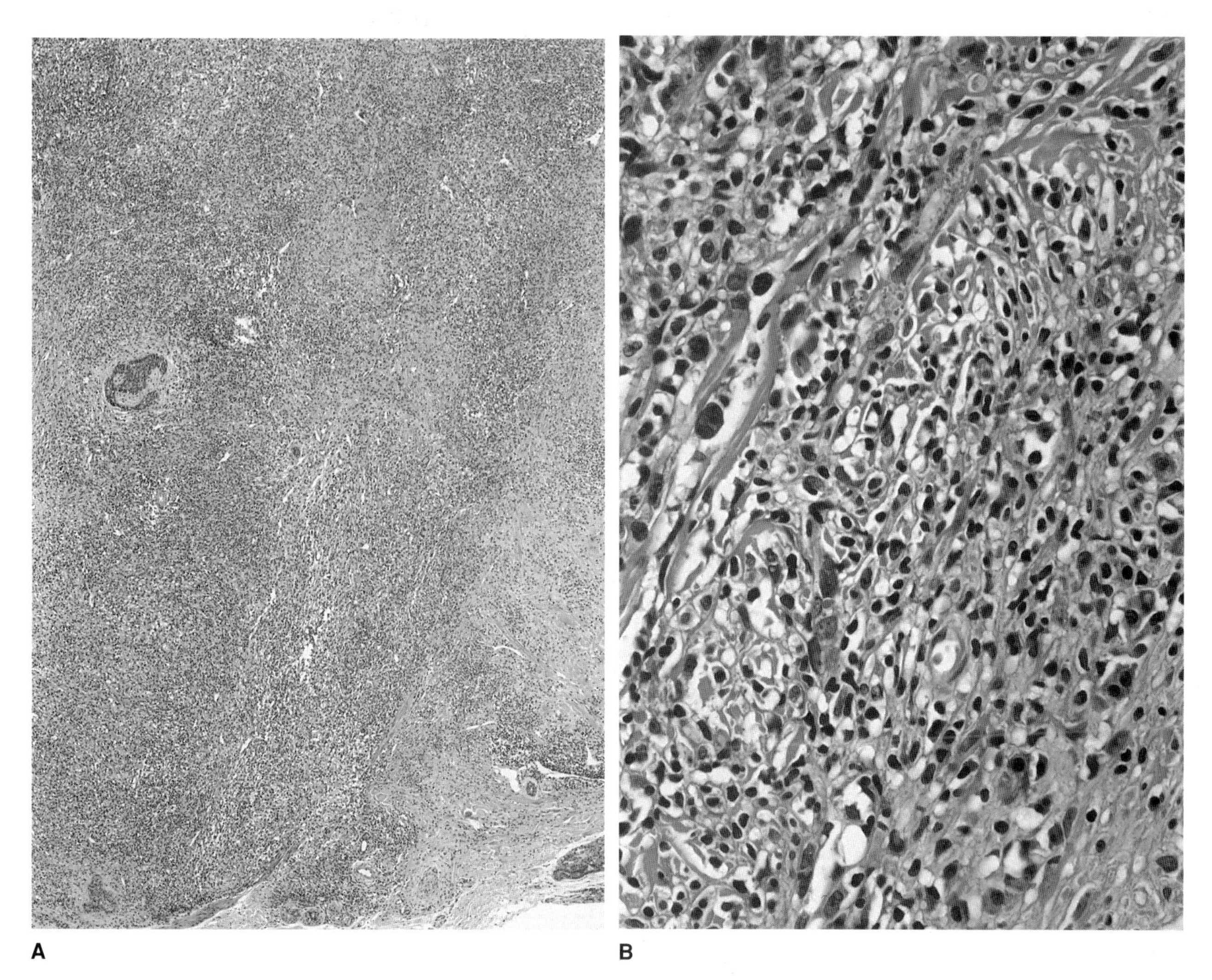

FIG. 32-29. Hodgkin's lymphoma
(**A**) Scanning magnification. There is a dense, diffuse infiltrate arrayed throughout the reticular dermis, to the level of the eccrine glands. (**B**) High magnification reveals variant Reed-Sternberg forms and admixed eosinophils. There was confirmation of nodal Hodgkin's lymphoma involving an adjacent lymph node chain.

Despite the fact that the lineage of HL has not been confirmed, the cells do display a consistent immunophenotype. RS cells in most cases of HL of all types express CD30, a receptor found on cell membranes whose ligands are homologous to nerve growth factor, and on activated lymphocytes.[120] Another activation antigen, CD15, is also present on RS cells in all types of HL except for the nodular lymphocyte-predominent variety.[121] There is inconsistent expression of T- and B-cell determinants by RS cells, which lack these molecules in most cases but clearly bear them in others. Clonal rearrangements of T-cell receptor or immunoglobulin genes are generally absent.

Histogenesis. The cells in normal lymph nodes that most resemble RS cells appear in the paracortex as solitary CD30 + dendritic cells. The role of these cells in the immune system is unknown. It is unknown whether these cells proliferate in HL, or whether HL arises from other undifferentiated lymphocytes.

Epidemiologic, immunophenotypic, and genotypic studies point to EBV as a major factor or cofactor in the genesis of HL. Patients with HL report a history of infectious mononucleosis more commonly than the population at large. There are aberrant serologic responses to EBV among HL patients. In roughly half of HL patients there is EBV genomic DNA in the nuclei of RS cells. EBV is even more commonly found in RS cells of immunosuppressed patients or those in the third world. If EBV is causative, it may infect and transform lymphocytes, which then proliferate and induce a polyclonal lymphocytic reaction and recruit other cell types by means of cytokine secretion.[122] Speaking against a global pathogenetic role for EBV is its seeming absence from roughly one-half of all cases.

Differential Diagnosis. Cutaneous infiltrates of HL are usually found in the context of known nodal disease, facilitating its identification. Cutaneous HL most commonly presents in an extremity in which proximally situated lymph nodes are involved, or by direct extension from prominently involved nodes. More problematic is the situation in which randomly distributed or disseminated cutaneous lesions are present. Among cutaneous lymphoproliferative disorders, the main simulants of HL include CD30+ disorders such as LyP and ALCL. The distinction is sometimes challenging, because CD30+ lymphoproliferative disorders have been documented to coexist with HL. Patients can have LyP, CD30+ ALCL, MF, and HL, in any combination, and lesions of LyP can precede, occur in synchrony with, or follow HL.[99] The distinctions among these disorders are not merely academic, because the prognosis of patients with miliary cutaneous HL is far worse than that of patients with HL and coexistent LyP. Additional information regarding this differential diagnosis is contained in the discussion of CD30+ lymphoproliferative disorders.

Tumor stage MF can also simulate HL. The distinction between these diseases is important, because both can occur in the same patient but require different therapies.[123] Nodules of MF can contain cells that resemble RS cells, but the infiltrate usually contains a range of large lymphocytes with hyperchromatic, irregularly shaped nuclei, whereas the reactive T cells in the infiltrate of HL are smaller and are all of fairly uniform size. Distinctive RS variants such as L&H or lacunar cells can occur in cutaneous lesions of HL but are not found in MF.

Immunophenotypic studies can assist or obscure the correct diagnosis. Whereas MF is usually a disease of CD4+ helper T lymphocytes, CD8+ (suppressor/cytotoxic) T cells can sometimes compose the majority of cells in HL involving the skin. The large cells of MF can express CD30 or (rarely) CD15, whereas these antigens can be absent in roughly 10% of HL cases. Strong CD3 immunopositivity favors a diagnosis of MF, but weak or absent CD3 staining does not exclude MF, because antigen expression can diminish with disease progression.[124]

Leukemia Cutis

Leukemias are neoplasms of hematolymphoid cells that usually present with prominent involvement of the peripheral blood. In some instances, the malignant cells essentially completely replace the bone marrow whereas only a few cells are detectable in the blood, but most leukemias display an associated leukocytosis. In contrast, most lymphomas show very few cells in the peripheral compartment compared with the number that infiltrate tissues, but a leukemic phase can sometimes supervene, especially in small B-cell lymphoma (SLL/CLL), mantle-cell lymphoma, and epidermotropic T-cell lymphoma (MF/SS).

The leukemias can be broadly grouped into acute and chronic forms of either lymphoid or myeloid lineage. The distinction of myeloid from lymphoid lineage is established on the basis of immunohistochemical and histochemical attributes of the leukemic cells. Myeloid lineage encompasses proliferations with myelocytic, myelomonocytic, strict monocytic, and megakaryocytic differentiation. Acute leukemias are neoplasms of immature cells or blasts, whereas chronic leukemias are composed of mature cells, often with a range of differentiation. Acute leukemias are typically proliferations with considerable malignant potential that often exhibit near-total replacement of the marrow by neoplastic cells, whereas in chronic leukemias portions of the marrow are spared, resulting in greater preservation of normal hematopoietic elements and a slower progression of disease.

Acute myeloid leukemia (AML) can be further classified into eight subtypes (M0 to M7), depending on the predominant pattern of differentiation in the leukemic cells. "Undifferentiated" examples of AML are included in the M0 and M1 classes. AML with myeloblastic differentiation, detectable on the basis of myeloperoxidase content or cytoplasmic Sudan black B reactivity, falls within the M2 class. Promyelocytic AML, in which promyelocytic differentiation is recognizable microscopically on the basis of specific cytoplasmic granules and Auer rods, is included in the M3 class. Myelomonocytic and monocytic AML, in which monocytic differentiation is identifiable by the presence of nonspecific esterase (butyrate esterase or a-naphthyl esterase) activity, belong to the M4 and M5 classes, respectively. Acute erythroleukemia is included in the M6 class, and acute megakaryocytic (megakaryoblastic) leukemia falls within the M7 class.

Acute lymphocytic (lymphoblastic) leukemia (ALL) can also be subcategorized on the basis of blast morphology into L1, L2, and L3 classes. The morphologic differences among these lymphoid classes are recognizable only in smears and touch preparations and are not appreciable in conventional histologic sections.

Clinical Features. Specific infiltrates of leukemia, in which neoplastic cells are present within tissue, can be seen in any leukemia but are especially common in the M4 and M5 variants of AML. Cutaneous leukemic infiltrates present as macules, papules, plaques, nodules, and ulcers.[125] Lesions can be erythematous or purpuric. Certain types of mucocutaneous lesions are specifically associated with certain types of leukemia. Gingival hypertrophy can be observed in association with AML. Vesicles and bullae, which may represent an unusual hypersensitivity reaction, are found in patients with CLL.[11] Extramedullary deposits of myeloblastic AML are commonly referred to as granulocytic sarcomas or chloromas. Extramedullary deposits may precede the appearance of blasts in the peripheral blood or marrow of a previously healthy patient (so-called "aleukemic" leukemia cutis), occur in a patient with myelodysplastic syndrome as the first sign of blastic transformation (conversion of myelodysplastic syndrome to myelogenous leukemia), or complicate known (AML) or herald its relapse. Patients with aleukemic leukemia cutis usually develop systemic disease within a year. In addition to these specific infiltrates of leukemia, there is a variety of inflammatory skin diseases that occur in conjunction with leukemia, sometimes referred to as nonspecific infiltrates or leukemids. These disorders include leukocytoclastic vasculitis, pyoderma gangrenosum, Sweet's syndrome, urticaria, erythroderma, erythema nodosum, and erythema multiforme.

Histopathology. Cutaneous leukemic infiltrates display several characteristic patterns, irrespective of lineage. The most common pattern consists of an interstitial infiltrate, constituting the so-called reticular pattern, marked by diffuse permeation of the reticular dermis by leukemic cells in horizontal strands between collagen bundles (Fig. 32-30). Nodular infiltrates of leukemic cells can also occur, but are less distinctive. Dense, bandlike infiltrates in the superficial dermis and sparse superficial and deep perivascular infiltrates are occasionally observed.

AML can assume either an interstitial (reticular) or a nodular pattern. The epidermis is spared, but the subcutis is often involved. The diagnosis hinges in large part on the recognition of myeloblasts, which can be a tricky business. Myeloblasts are most readily identified in touch imprints. Toward that end, Wright-Giemsa-stained touch preparations obtained from the fresh surfaces of cut biopsy specimens can delineate fine azurophilic granules, or, in the case of the M3 type of AML, Auer rods, thus facilitating the recognition of myeloblastic differentiation. In tissue sections, myeloblasts have scant cytoplasm, large vesicular nuclei, and nucleoli of variable size. Unusual appearances include the presence of cells with anaplastic or signet-ring nuclei. Eosinophilic myelocytes or metamyelocytes are not pathognomonic of AML, but strongly favor that diagnosis in the proper context. These immature cells have the granules of mature eosinophils with monolobed nuclei.

Cutaneous infiltrates of chronic myeloid leukemia (CML) are less common than those of AML. Similar diffuse or nodular patterns occur. The infiltrates contain a range of myelocytic differentiation from myeloblasts to segmented neutrophils.

Acute lymphocytic (lymphoblastic) leukemia (ALL) shares features with lymphoblastic lymphoma, as CLL does with SLL. SLL/CLL is discussed comprehensively in a previous section.

Hairy cell leukemia (HCL) is a B-cell neoplasm named for the delicate cytoplasmic processes that its cells exhibit in peripheral blood or in body fluids. There are only a few reports of cutaneous involvement by HCL. In most organs, such as the spleen, lymph nodes, and bone marrow, there are sheets of cells with voluminous clear cytoplasm and evenly distributed, centrally situated monomorphous vesicular nuclei. The villous projections that are so distinctive in the peripheral blood cannot be discerned in tissue sections. The cutaneous infiltrates of HCL described to date have not had this stereotypic appearance but have resembled those in other forms of leukemia.[126]

Differential Diagnosis. Malignant lymphoma can form interstitial (reticular), nodular, or bandlike infiltrates in the skin, and can be quite difficult to distinguish from leukemia cutis. A nearly perfect reticular pattern throughout a lesion is usually found only in leukemic infiltrates. The most problematic lymphomas include the large-cell types of B-cell lymphoma, immunoblastic lymphoma, the blastic variant of MCL, and several of the subtypes of peripheral T-cell lymphoma. The presence of eosinophilic myelocytes favors acute myelogenous leukemia, that of segmented neutrophils favors chronic myelocytic leukemia, and pale-staining, reniform nuclei can indicate monocytic leukemia.

Both histochemical and immunophenotypic studies can help in the identification of leukemic infiltrates. Unfortunately, some classic techniques available to hematopathologists are not applicable to fixed tissue sections, but can be applied only to blood smears, marrow aspirates, frozen sections, or touch imprints. Histochemical reactions include those for myeloperoxidase and Sudan black B stains, which can be used to identify myeloblastic differentiation. The chloroacetate esterase or Leder stain also labels cells with myeloid or myelomonocytic differentiation. Immunoperoxidase stains have recently been applied to leukemic infiltrates. Mac-387, useful as a marker of a subset of tissue macrophages, also labels cells of myeloid lineage. Other antibodies that can prove useful in the differential diagnosis include lysozyme, myeloperoxidase, CD33 (My-9), and neutrophil-specific elastase. A panel of at least three antisera has been recommended because no single reagent is sufficiently sensitive and specific.[127] The human progenitor cell antigen, CD34, is expressed by the blasts of several forms of leukemia, but not by the cells of most malignant lymphomas. It is preserved in routinely processed tissue.[128] CD68, normally expressed by macrophages, is found on the cells of myeloid and myelomonocytic leukemias. An important caveat is that myeloblasts react with a variety of reagents that also identify lymphoid cells, including CD43, CD45RO, and CD20.

The infiltrates of HCL were at first identified by histochemical staining for tartrate-resistant acid phosphatase. This enzyme is not well preserved in routinely processed tissue, but such B-cell determinants as CD20 are identifiable.[129] An antibody known as B-ly7 can also be used to identify specifically the infiltrates of HCL.

A reticular pattern can also be observed in metastatic adenocarcinomas, such as ductal carcinomas of the breast and prostate. A few small nests of cells are generally present in metastatic adenocarcinoma, and glandular lumens are often discernible and should be carefully sought. Mucin can be detected with either the periodic acid-Schiff method or the mucicarmine stain. The differential diagnosis can readily be resolved using immunohistochemistry, because hematolymphoid cells fail to express keratin filaments and other adenocarcinomatous markers.

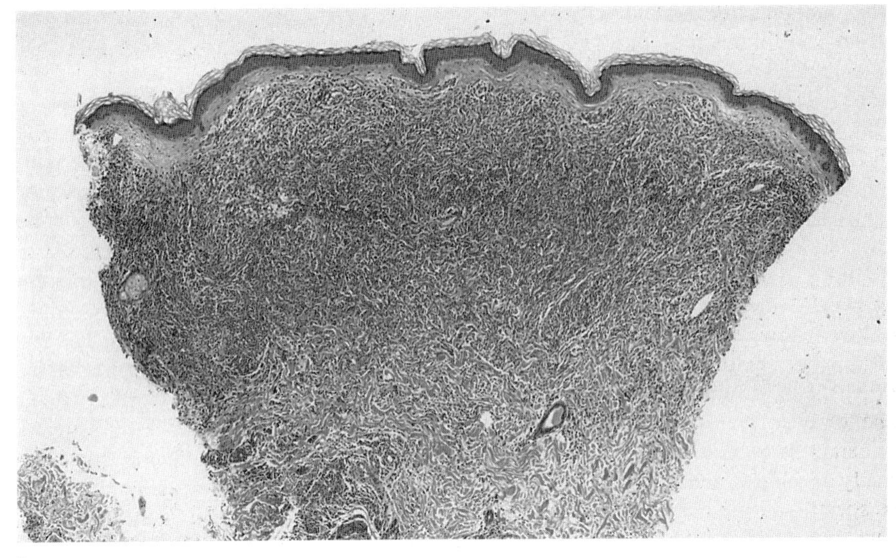

A

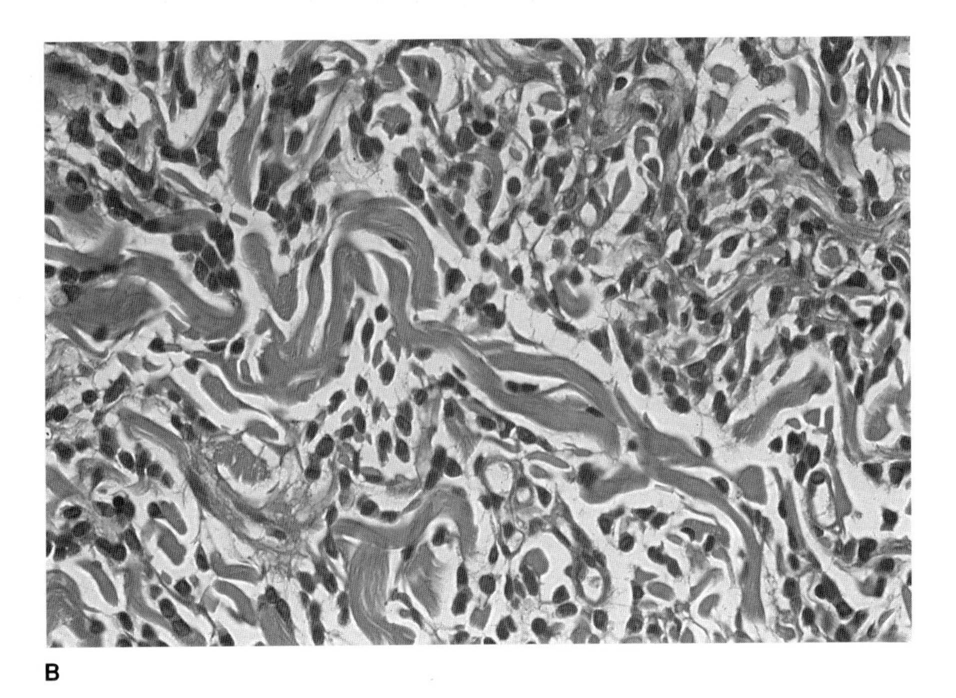

B

FIG. 32-30. Myeloid leukemia cutis
(**A**) Scanning magnification. There is an interstitial infiltrate of mononuclear cells within the upper reticular dermis. (**B**) High magnification reveals cells with ample cytoplasm arrayed between collagen bundles, and myeloperoxidase immunostaining confirmed myeloid lineage.

Dermal Erythropoiesis and Dermal Hematopoiesis

The term *dermal erythropoiesis* refers to the presence in the dermis of red blood cell precursors. When these cells are accompanied by myeloid cells, megakaryocytes, or both, the appropriate term is *dermal hematopoiesis*. The rationale for distinguishing these processes is that there are differences in the clinical settings in which they occur. Extramedullary hematopoiesis is a broad term that encompasses both conditions.

The most frequent setting of dermal erythropoiesis is in newborns, in whom it seems to occur as a reaction to stress. Congenital viral infections such as those caused by rubella, coxsackie, or cytomegalovirus, or hematologic disease (e.g., hemolysis resulting from ABO or Rh incompatibility, twin transfusion syndrome, or hereditary spherocytosis), are common precipitating events.

Dermal hematopoiesis occurs chiefly in adults with myelofibrosis. It occasionally occurs in neonates in the setting mentioned above.

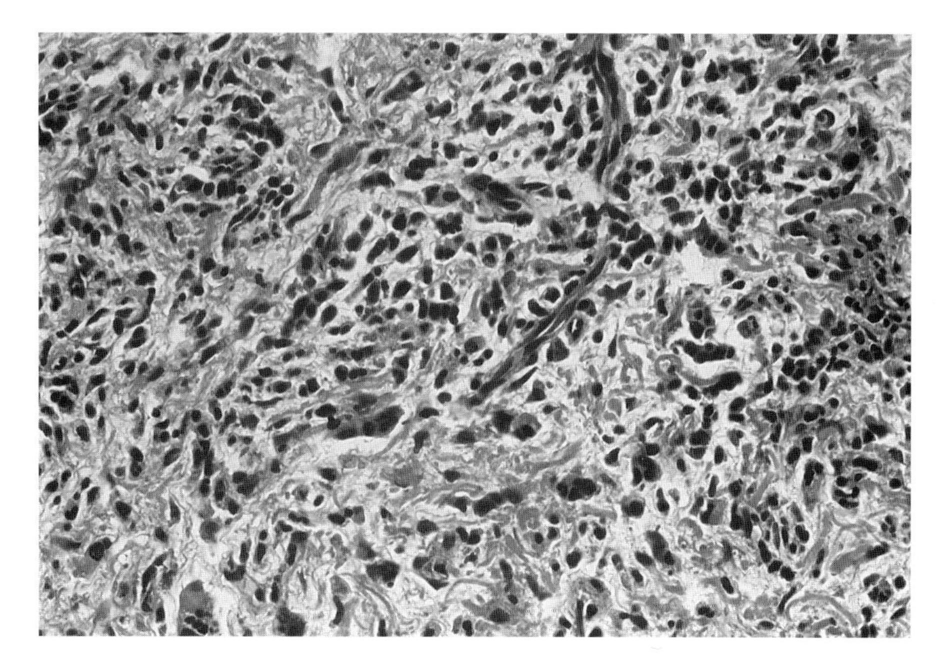

FIG. 32-31. Dermal hematopoiesis
A heterogeneous infiltrate contains both erythroid precursors, evident microscopically as cells with dark round nuclei, and megakaryocytic precursors, evident as large multinucleate cells with ample granular cytoplasm.

Clinical Features. Dermal erythropoiesis and dermal hematopoiesis present with reddish-blue macules, papules, and nodules. The lesions of dermal erythropoiesis in neonates are mainly macules that occur on the head and neck, a clinical pattern memorialized in the picturesque description "blueberry muffin baby." Lesions of dermal hematopoiesis in adults often present on the trunk. Splenectomy may accelerate the spread of hematopoietic cells to the skin, and lesions of hematopoiesis are often found in postsplenectomy scars.

Histopathology. The reticular (interstitial) pattern of infiltration, similar to the pattern observed in leukemia cutis, is also typical of dermal erythropoiesis (Fig. 32-31). Erythroblasts, which have scant cytoplasm and round nuclei, are difficult to recognize and can resemble the cells of lymphoma or leukemia. Fortunately, nucleated erythrocytes are quite distinctive and mark the presence of the erythroid cell line. These cells have deeply eosinophilic cytoplasms and small, round, deeply basophilic nuclei. Extramedullary hematopoiesis in neonates can sometimes feature a few myeloblasts and metamyelocytes, but megakaryocytes are usually absent.[130]

Dermal hematopoiesis resulting from myelofibrosis can result in cutaneous infiltrates containing all three cell lines. In addition to myeloid and erythroid cells, there are megakaryocytes, which are identifiable by their huge size, copious cytoplasm, and multilobulated nuclei. If atypical-appearing megakaryocytes are present, the appropriate diagnosis may well be megakaryocytic leukemia.[131]

Differential Diagnosis. Leukemia cutis usually assumes a reticular pattern similar to that of extramedullary hematopoiesis. Leukemia cutis does not contain nucleated erythrocytes, and thus the confirmation of the presence of the erythroid line can serve as a diagnostic key. *Ulex europeus* lectin binds to L-fucose, which is found in all of the blood group antigens present on the membranes of erythroid precursors. If there is any doubt about the presence of megakaryocytes, they can be specifically identified with CD61 (platelet glycoprotein IIB/IIIA).

CONCLUSION

If anything is clear about the course of future developments in the realm of cutaneous lymphomas and leukemias, it is that changes in this field will come with extraordinary rapidity. Whereas correlations of immunologic data with traditional clinicopathologic findings have led to many of the advances of the last 20 years, the next decade will doubtless be one in which advances in molecular biology will revise our concepts regarding many issues.

Among the subjects that are unclear or controversial at this time, there are several that are likely to be clarified by the time of the next edition of this book, including the following:

- Are many cases of cutaneous lymphoid hyperplasia (B-cell pseudolymphoma) diagnosed by traditional methods actually low-grade B-cell lymphomas?
- Are there primary cutaneous lymphomas of follicular center cell type, or are all such lesions of extracutaneous origin?
- Is cutaneous immunocytoma simply a variant of extranodal marginal zone lymphoma?
- Do primary cutaneous lymphomas with a follicular pattern, which differ from nodal follicular lymphomas in so many ways, constitute one group? Do they more closely resemble marginal zone or mantle cell lymphoma?
- Is small plaque parapsoriasis simply an indolent form of patch stage mycosis fungoides?
- Are there ways to recognize which patients with patch stage

mycosis fungoides will progress to develop plaques and tumors?

- Does HTLV-1 play a significant role in the development of mycosis fungoides and Sézary's syndrome?
- What is Hodgkin's lymphoma? Is it a collection of morphologically and immunophenotypically similar lesions, or is it a cohesive biologic entity?

Finally, readers should be aware that information regarding these and many other aspects, of cutaneous lymphoproliferative diseases will change rapidly. We look forward to learning the answers to these and other questions.

REFERENCES

1. Harris NL, Jaffe ES, Stein H et al. A revised European-American classification of lymphoid neoplasms: A proposal from the International Lymphoma Study Group. Blood 1994;84:1361.
2. Smolle J, Torne R, Soyer HP, Kerl H. Immunohistochemical classification of cutaneous pseudolymphomas: Delineation of distinct patterns. J Cutan Pathol 1990;17:149.
3. Torne R, Roura M, Umbert P. Generalized cutaneous B-cell pseudolymphoma: Report of a case studied by immunohistochemistry. Am J Dermatopathol 1989;11:544.
4. Eckert F, Schmid U. Identification of plasmacytoid T cells in lymphoid hyperplasia of the skin. Arch Dermatol 1989;125:1518.
5. Wood GS, Ngan BY, Tung R et al. Clonal rearrangements of immunoglobulin genes and progression to B cell lymphoma in cutaneous lymphoid hyperplasia. Am J Pathol 1989;135:13.
6. Iwatsuki K, Yamada M, Takigawa M et al. Benign lymphoplasia of the earlobes induced by gold earrings: Immunohistologic study on the cellular infiltrates. J Am Acad Dermatol 1987;16:83.
7. Hovmark A, Asbrink E, Olsson I. The spirochetal etiology of lymphadenosis benigna cutis solitaria. Acta Derm Venereol 1986;66:479.
8. Blumental G, Okun MR, Ponitch JA. Pseudolymphomatous reaction to tattoos: Report of three cases. J Am Acad Dermatol 1982;6:485.
9. Sander CA, Medeiros LJ, Abruzzo LV et al. Lymphoblastic lymphoma presenting in cutaneous sites: A clinicopathologic analysis of six cases. J Am Acad Dermatol 1991;25:1023.
10. Burg G, Braun-Falco O. Cutaneous lymphomas, pseudolymphomas, and related disorders. New York: Springer-Verlag 1983;236.
11. Cerroni L, Zenahlik P, Hofler G et al. Specific cutaneous infiltrates of B-cell chronic lymphocytic leukemia: A clinicopathologic and prognostic study of 42 patients. Am J Surg Pathol 1996;20:1000.
12. Isaacson PG. Gastrointestinal lymphoma. Hum Pathol 1994;25:1020.
13. Frithz A, Lagerholm B. Acrodermatitis chronica atrophicans, erythema chronicum migrans and lymphadenosis benigna cutis: Spirochetal diseases? Acta Derm Venereol 1983;63:432.
14. Rijlaarsdam JU, van der Putte SC, Berti E et al. Cutaneous immunocytomas: A clinicopathologic study of 26 cases. Histopathology 1993;23:117.
15. Marti RM, Estrach T, Palou J et al. Primary cutaneous lymphoplasmacytic lymphoma. J Am Acad Dermatol 1987;16:1106.
16. van der Putte SC, Toonstra J, Schuurman HJ, van Unnik JA. Immunocytoma of the skin simulating lymphadenosis benigna cutis. Arch Dermatol Res 1985;277:36.
17. LeBoit PE, McNutt NS, Reed JA et al. Primary cutaneous immunocytoma: A B-cell lymphoma that can easily be mistaken for cutaneous lymphoid hyperplasia. Am J Surg Pathol 1994;18:969.
18. Dabski K, Banks PM, Winkelmann RK. Clinicopathologic spectrum of cutaneous manifestations in systemic follicular lymphoma: A study of 11 patients. Cancer 1989;64:1480.
19. Garcia CF, Weiss LM, Warnke RA, Wood GS. Cutaneous follicular lymphoma. Am J Surg Pathol 1986;10:454.
20. Giannotti B, Santucci M. Skin-associated lymphoid tissue (SALT)–related B-cell lymphoma (primary cutaneous B-cell lymphoma): A concept and a clinicopathologic entity. Arch Dermatol 1993;129(Editorial):353.
21. Ngan B, Warnke A, Cleary ML. Variability of immunoglobulin expression in follicular lymphoma: An immunohistologic and molecular genetic study. Am J Pathol 1989;135:1139.
22. Bertero M, Novelli M, Fierro MT, Bernengo MG. Mantle zone lymphoma: An immunohistologic study of skin lesions. J Am Acad Dermatol 1994;30:23.
23. Geerts ML, Busschots AM. Mantle-cell lymphomas of the skin. Dermatol Clin 1994;12:409.
24. Wong KF, Chan JK, Li LP et al. Primary cutaneous plasmacytoma: Report of two cases and review of the literature. Am J Dermatopathol 1994;16:392.
25. Gomez EC, Margulies M, Rywlin A et al. Cutaneous involvement by IgD myeloma. Arch Dermatol 1978;114:1700.
26. Kois JM, Sexton FM, Lookingbill DP. Cutaneous manifestations of multiple myeloma. Arch Dermatol 1991;127:69.
27. Edwards GA, Zawadzki ZA. Extraosseous lesions in plasma cell myeloma: A report of six cases. Am J Med 1967;43:194.
28. Patterson JW, Parsons JM, White RM et al. Cutaneous involvement of multiple myeloma and extramedullary plasmacytoma. J Am Acad Dermatol 1988;19:879.
29. White JW Jr, Olsen KD, Banks PM. Plasma cell orificial mucositis: Report of a case and review of the literature. Arch Dermatol 1986;122:1321.
30. Watanabe S, Ohara K, Kukita A, Mori S. Systemic plasmacytosis: A syndrome of peculiar multiple skin eruptions, generalized lymphadenopathy, and polyclonal hypergammaglobulinemia. Arch Dermatol 1986;122:1314.
31. Hurt MA, Santa Cruz DJ. Cutaneous inflammatory pseudotumor: Lesions resembling "inflammatory pseudotumors" or "plasma cell granulomas" of extracutaneous sites. Am J Surg Pathol 1990;14:764.
32. Willemze R, Meijer CJ, Sentis HJ et al. Primary cutaneous large cell lymphomas of follicular center cell origin: A clinical follow-up study of nineteen patients. J Am Acad Dermatol 1987;16:518.
33. Pimpinelli N, Santucci M, Bosi A et al. Primary cutaneous follicular centre-cell lymphoma: A lymphoproliferative disease with favourable prognosis. Clin Exp Dermatol 1989;14:12.
34. Bhawan J. Angioendotheliomatosis proliferans systemisata: An angiotropic neoplasm of lymphoid origin. Semin Diagn Pathol 1987;4:18.
35. Wick MR, Mills SE, Scheithauer BW et al. Reassessment of malignant "angioendotheliomatosis": Evidence in favor of its reclassification as "intravascular lymphomatosis." Am J Surg Pathol 1986;10:112.
36. Ferry JA, Harris NL, Picker LJ et al. Intravascular lymphomatosis (malignant angioendotheliomatosis): A B-cell neoplasm expressing surface homing receptors. Mod Pathol 1988;1:444.
37. Jalkanen S, Aho R, Kallajoki M et al. Lymphocyte homing receptors and adhesion molecules in intravascular malignant lymphomatosis. Int J Cancer 1989;44:777.
38. Rijlaarsdam JU, Scheffer E, Meijer CJ, Willemze R. Cutaneous pseudo-T-cell lymphomas: A clinicopathologic study of 20 patients. Cancer 1992;69:717.
39. van der Putte SC, Toonstra J, Felten PC, van Vloten WA. Solitary nonepidermotropic T cell pseudolymphoma of the skin. J Am Acad Dermatol 1986;14:444.
40. Oliver GF, Winkelmann RK. Unilesional mycosis fungoides: A distinct entity. J Am Acad Dermatol 1989;20:63.
41. Quintanilla-Martinez L, Zukerberg LR, Harris NL. Prethymic adult lymphoblastic lymphoma: A clinicopathologic and immunohistochemical analysis. Am J Surg Pathol 1992;16:1075.
42. Koch SE, Zackheim HS, Williams ML et al. Mycosis fungoides beginning in childhood and adolescence. J Am Acad Dermatol 1987;17:563.
43. Braverman IM. Cutaneous T-cell lymphoma. Curr Probl Dermatol 1991;3:184.
44. Epstein EH Jr, Levin DL, Croft JD Jr, Lutzner MA. Mycosis fungoides: Survival, prognostic features, response to therapy, and autopsy findings. Medicine (Baltimore) 1972;51:61.
45. Wieselthier JS, Koh HK. Sézary syndrome: Diagnosis, prognosis, and critical review of treatment options. J Am Acad Dermatol 1990;22:381.
46. LeBoit PE. Variants of mycosis fungoides and related cutaneous T-cell lymphomas. Semin Diagn Pathol 1991;8:73.
47. Willemze R, Scheffer E, Van Vloten WA. Mycosis fungoides simulating acanthosis nigricans. Am J Dermatopathol 1985;7:367.
48. Zackheim HS, Epstein EH Jr, Grekin DA, McNutt NS. Mycosis fungoides presenting as areas of hypopigmentation: A report of three cases. J Am Acad Dermatol 1982;6:340.

49. Lambroza E, Cohen SR, Phelps R et al. Hypopigmented variant of mycosis fungoides: Demography, histopathology, and treatment of seven cases. J Am Acad Dermatol 1995;32:987.
50. Bunn PA Jr, Lamberg SI. Report of the Committee on Staging and Classification of Cutaneous T-Cell Lymphomas. Cancer Treat Rep 1979;63:725.
51. Sausville EA, Worsham GF, Matthews MJ et al. Histologic assessment of lymph nodes in mycosis fungoides/Sézary syndrome: (cutaneous T-cell lymphoma): Clinical correlations and prognostic import of a new classification system. Hum Pathol 1985;16:1098.
52. Sausville EA, Eddy JL, Makuch RW et al. Histopathologic staging at initial diagnosis of mycosis fungoides and the Sézary syndrome: Definition of three distinctive prognostic groups. Ann Intern Med 1988;109:372.
53. Bakels V, Van Oostveen JW, Geerts ML et al. Diagnostic and prognostic significance of clonal T-cell receptor beta gene rearrangements in lymph nodes of patients with mycosis fungoides. J Pathol 1993;170: 249.
54. Lynch JW Jr, Linoilla I, Sausville EA et al. Prognostic implications of evaluation for lymph node involvement by T-cell antigen receptor gene rearrangement in mycosis fungoides. Blood 1992;79:3293.
55. Weinstock MA, Horm JW. Mycosis fungoides in the United States: Increasing incidence and descriptive epidemiology. JAMA 1988;260: 42.
56. Weinstock MA, Horm JW. Population-based estimate of survival and determinants of prognosis in patients with mycosis fungoides. Cancer 1988;62:1658.
57. Sanchez JL, Ackerman AB. The patch stage of mycosis fungoides: Criteria for histologic diagnosis. Am J Dermatopathol 1979;1:5.
58. Nickoloff BJ. Light-microscopic assessment of 100 patients with patch/plaque-stage mycosis fungoides. Am J Dermatopathol 1988;10: 469.
59. Ackerman AB, Jacobson M, Vitale P. Clues to diagnosis in dermatopathology. Vol. 1. Chicago: ASCP Press 1991;414.
60. Hempstead RW, Ackerman AB. Follicular mucinosis: A reaction pattern in follicular epithelium. Am J Dermatopathol 1985;7:245.
61. Mehregan DA, Gibson LE, Muller SA. Follicular mucinosis: Histopathologic review of 33 cases. Mayo Clin Proc 1991;66:387.
62. Nickoloff BJ, Wood C. Benign idiopathic versus mycosis fungoides–associated follicular mucinosis. Pediatr Dermatol 1985;2:201.
63. Cerroni L, Rieger E, Hodl S, Kerl H. Clinicopathologic and immunologic features associated with transformation of mycosis fungoides to large-cell lymphoma. Am J Surg Pathol 1992;16:543.
64. Shapiro PE, Pinto FJ. The histologic spectrum of mycosis fungoides/Sézary syndrome (cutaneous T-cell lymphoma): A review of 222 biopsies, including newly described patterns and the earliest pathologic changes. Am J Surg Pathol 1994;18:645.
65. LeBoit PE, Zackheim HS, White CR Jr. Granulomatous variants of cutaneous T-cell lymphoma: The histopathology of granulomatous mycosis fungoides and granulomatous slack skin. Am J Surg Pathol 1988;12:83.
66. Ralfkiaer E. Immunohistological markers for the diagnosis of cutaneous lymphomas. Semin Diagn Pathol 1991;8:62.
67. Weiss LM, Hu E, Wood GS et al. Clonal rearrangements of T-cell receptor genes in mycosis fungoides and dermatopathic lymphadenopathy. N Engl J Med 1985;313:539.
68. Ackerman AB, Guo Y, Vitale P. Clues to diagnosis in dermatopathology. Vol. 2. Chicago: ASCP Press 1992;423.
69. LeBoit PE, Epstein BA. A vase-like shape characterizes the epidermal-mononuclear cell collections seen in spongiotic dermatitis. Am J Dermatopathol 1990;12:612.
70. Toro JR, Sander CA, LeBoit PE. Persistent pigmented purpuric dermatitis and mycosis fungoides: Simulant, precursor, or both? A study by light microscopy and molecular methods. Am J Dermatopathol (in press).
71. Buechner SA, Winkelmann RK. Sézary syndrome: A clinicopathologic study of 39 cases. Arch Dermatol 1983;119:979.
72. Weiss LM, Wood GS, Hu E et al. Detection of clonal T-cell receptor gene rearrangements in the peripheral blood of patients with mycosis fungoides/Sézary syndrome. J Invest Dermatol 1989;92:601.
73. Sentis HJ, Willemze R, Scheffer E. Histopathologic studies in Sézary syndrome and erythrodermic mycosis fungoides: A comparison with benign forms of erythroderma. J Am Acad Dermatol 1986;15:1217.
74. Imai S, Burg G, Braun-Falco O. Mycosis fungoides and Sézary's syndrome show distinct histomorphological features. Dermatologica 1986;173:131.
75. LeBoit PE, Abel EA, Cleary ML et al. Clonal rearrangement of the T cell receptor beta gene in the circulating lymphocytes of erythrodermic follicular mucinosis. Blood 1988;71:1329.
76. Mandojana RM, Helwig EB. Localized epidermotropic reticulosis (Woringer-Kolopp disease). J Am Acad Dermatol 1983;8:813.
77. Sterry W, Hauschild A. Loss of leukocyte common antigen (CD45) on atypical lymphocytes in the localized but not disseminated type of pagetoid reticulosis. Br J Dermatol 1991;125:238.
78. Burns MK, Chan LS, Cooper KD. Woringer-Kolopp disease (localized pagetoid reticulosis) or unilesional mycosis fungoides? An analysis of eight cases with benign disease. Arch Dermatol 1995;131:325.
79. Yagi H, Hagiwara T, Shirahama S et al. Disseminated pagetoid reticulosis: Need for long-term follow-up. J Am Acad Dermatol 1994;30: 345.
80. Ralfkiaer E, Thomsen K, Agdal N et al. The development of a Ki-1–positive large cell non-Hodgkin's lymphoma in pagetoid reticulosis. Acta Derm Venereol 1989;69:206.
81. Lacour JP, Juhlin L, el Baze P et al. Disseminated pagetoid reticulosis associated with mycosis fungoides: Immunomorphologic study. J Am Acad Dermatol 1986;14:898.
82. Mielke V, Wolff HH, Winzer M, Sterry W. Localized and disseminated pagetoid reticulosis: Diagnostic immunophenotypical findings. Arch Dermatol 1989;125:402.
83. Wood GS, Weiss LM, Hu CH et al. T-cell antigen deficiencies and clonal rearrangements of T-cell receptor genes in pagetoid reticulosis (Woringer-Kolopp disease). N Engl J Med 1988;318:164.
84. LeBoit PE. Granulomatous slack skin. Dermatol Clin 1994;12:375.
85. LeBoit PE, Beckstead JH, Bond B et al. Granulomatous slack skin: Clonal rearrangement of the T-cell receptor beta gene is evidence for the lymphoproliferative nature of a cutaneous elastolytic disorder. J Invest Dermatol 1987;89:183.
86. Grammatico P, Balus L, Scarpa S et al. Granulomatous slack skin: Cytogenetic and molecular analyses. Cancer Genet Cytogenet 1994;72: 96.
87. Broder S, Bunn PA Jr, Jaffe ES et al. NIH conference. T-cell lymphoproliferative syndrome associated with human T-cell leukemia/lymphoma virus. Ann Intern Med 1984;100:543.
88. Manabe T, Hirokawa M, Sugihara K et al. Angiocentric and angiodestructive infiltration of adult T-cell leukemia/lymphoma (ATLL) in the skin: Report of two cases. Am J Dermatopathol 1988;10:487.
89. Murata K, Yamada Y, Kamihira S et al. Frequency of eosinophilia in adult T-cell leukemia/lymphoma. Cancer 1992;69:966.
90. Waldmann TA, Greene WC, Sarin PS et al. Functional and phenotypic comparison of human T cell leukemia/lymphoma virus positive adult T cell leukemia with human T cell leukemia/lymphoma virus negative Sézary leukemia, and their distinction using anti-Tac: Monoclonal antibody identifying the human receptor for T cell growth factor. J Clin Invest 1984;73:1711.
91. Gessain A, Moulonguet I, Flageul B et al. Cutaneous type of adult T cell leukemia/lymphoma in a French West Indian woman: Clonal rearrangement of T-cell receptor beta and gamma genes and monoclonal integration of HTLV-I proviral DNA in the skin infiltrate. J Am Acad Dermatol 1990;23:994.
92. Roundtree JM, Burgdorf W, Harkey MR. Cutaneous involvement in Lennert's lymphoma. Arch Dermatol 1980;116:1291.
93. Kiesewetter F, Haneke E, Lennert K et al. Cutaneous lymphoepithelioid lymphoma (Lennert's lymphoma): Combined immunohistological, ultrastructural, and DNA-flow-cytometric analysis. Am J Dermatopathol 1989;11:549.
94. Van der Putte SC, Toonstra J, De Weger RA, Van Unnik JA. Cutaneous T-cell lymphoma, multilobated type. Histopathology 1982;6: 35.
95. Goldman BD, Bari M, Kantor GR et al. Cutaneous multilobated T-cell lymphoma with aggressive course. J Am Acad Dermatol 1991;25:345.
96. Gonzalez CL, Medeiros LJ, Braziel RM, Jaffe ES. T-cell lymphoma involving subcutaneous tissue. A clinicopathologic entity commonly associated with hemophagocytic syndrome. Am J Surg Pathol 1991;15:17.
97. Paulli M, Berti E, Rosso R et al. CD30/Ki-1–positive lymphoproliferative disorders of the skin: Clinicopathologic correlation and statistical analysis of 86 cases. A multicentric study from the European Organization for Research and Treatment of Cancer Cutaneous Lymphoma Project Group. J Clin Oncol 1995;13:1343.
98. Karp DL, Horn TD. Lymphomatoid papulosis. J Am Acad Dermatol 1994;30:379.

99. LeBoit PE. Lymphomatoid papulosis and cutaneous CD30+ lymphoma. Am J Dermatopathol 1996;18:221.
100. Pileri S, Falini B, Delsol G et al. Lymphohistiocytic T-cell lymphoma (anaplastic large cell lymphoma CD30+/Ki-1+ with a high content of reactive histiocytes). Histopathology 1990;16:383.
101. Headington JT, Roth MS, Schnitzer B. Regressing atypical histiocytosis: A review and critical appraisal. Semin Diagn Pathol 1987;4:28.
102. Flynn KJ, Dehner LP, Gajl-Peczalska KJ et al. Regressing atypical histiocytosis: A cutaneous proliferation of atypical neoplastic histiocytes with unexpectedly indolent biologic behavior. Cancer 1982;49: 959.
103. Kerschmann RL, Berger TG, Weiss LM et al. Cutaneous presentations of lymphoma in human immunodeficiency virus disease: Predominance of T cell lineage. Arch Dermatol 1995;131:1281.
104. Chan JK, Buchanan R, Fletcher CD. Sarcomatoid variant of anaplastic large-cell Ki-1 lymphoma. Am J Surg Pathol 1990;14:983.
105. Headington JT, Roth MS, Ginsburg D et al. T-cell receptor gene rearrangement in regressing atypical histiocytosis. Arch Dermatol 1987;123:1183.
106. Jaworsky C, Cirillo-Hyland V, Petrozzi JW et al. Regressing atypical histiocytosis: Aberrant prothymocyte differentiation, T-cell receptor gene rearrangements, and nodal involvement. Arch Dermatol 1990;126:1609.
107. Anagnostopoulos I, Hummel M, Kaudewitz P et al. Detection of HTLV-I proviral sequences in CD30-positive large cell cutaneous T-cell lymphomas. Am J Pathol 1990;137:1317.
108. Chadburn A, Cesarman E, Jagirdar J et al. CD30 (Ki-1) positive anaplastic large cell lymphomas in individuals infected with the human immunodeficiency virus. Cancer 1993;72:3078.
109. Kadin ME, Cavaille-Coll MW, Gertz R et al. Loss of receptors for transforming growth factor beta in human T-cell malignancies. Proc Natl Acad Sci USA 1994;91:6002.
110. Pallesen G. The diagnostic significance of the CD30 (Ki-1) antigen. Histopathology 1990;16:409.
111. James WD, Odom RB, Katzenstein AL. Cutaneous manifestations of lymphomatoid granulomatosis: Report of 44 cases and a review of the literature. Arch Dermatol 1981;117:196.
112. Jambrosic J, From L, Assaad DA et al. Lymphomatoid granulomatosis. J Am Acad Dermatol 1987;17:621.
113. Chan JK, Ng CS, Ngan KC et al. Angiocentric T-cell lymphoma of the skin: An aggressive lymphoma distinct from mycosis fungoides. Am J Surg Pathol 1988;12:861.
114. Fujiwara Y, Abe Y, Kuyama M et al. CD8+ cutaneous T-cell lymphoma with pagetoid epidermotropism and angiocentric and angiodestructive infiltration. Arch Dermatol 1990;126:801.
115. Wong KF, Chan JK, Ng CS et al. CD56 (NKH1)-positive hematolymphoid malignancies: An aggressive neoplasm featuring frequent cutaneous/mucosal involvement, cytoplasmic azurophilic granules, and angiocentricity. Hum Pathol 1992;23:798.
116. White RM, Patterson JW. Cutaneous involvement in Hodgkin's disease. Cancer 1985;55:1136.
117. Smith JL Jr, Butler JJ. Skin involvement in Hodgkin's disease. Cancer 1980;45:354.
118. Sioutos N, Kerl H, Murphy SB, Kadin ME. Primary cutaneous Hodgkin's disease: Unique clinical, morphologic, and immunophenotypic findings. Am J Dermatopathol 1994;16:2.
119. Lister TA, Crowther D, Sutcliffe SB et al. Report of a committee convened to discuss the evaluation and staging of patients with Hodgkin's disease: Cotswolds meeting (published erratum appears in J Clin Ocol 1990;8:1602) J Clin Oncol 1989;7:1630.
120. Moretti S, Pimpinelli N, Di Lollo S et al. In situ immunologic characterization of cutaneous involvement in Hodgkin's disease. Cancer 1989;63:661.
121. Timens W, Visser L, Poppema S. Nodular lymphocyte predominance type of Hodgkin's disease is a germinal center lymphoma. Lab Invest 1986;54:457.
122. Harris NL. Epstein-Barr virus in lymphoma: Protagonist or passenger? Am J Clin Pathol 1992;98:278.
123. Simrell CR, Boccia RV, Longo DL, Jaffe ES. Coexisting Hodgkin's disease and mycosis fungoides: Immunohistochemical proof of its existence. Arch Pathol Lab Med 1986;110:1029.
124. Salhany KE, Cousar JB, Greer JP et al. Transformation of cutaneous T cell lymphoma to large cell lymphoma: A clinicopathologic and immunologic study. Am J Pathol 1988;132:265.
125. Su WP, Buechner SA, Li CY. Clinicopathologic correlations in leukemia cutis. J Am Acad Dermatol 1984;11:121.
126. Arai E, Ikeda S, Itoh S, Katayama I. Specific skin lesions as the presenting symptom of hairy cell leukemia. Am J Clin Pathol 1988;90: 459.
127. Davey FR, Olson S, Kurec AS et al. The immunophenotyping of extramedullary myeloid cell tumors in paraffin-embedded tissue sections. Am J Surg Pathol 1988;12:699.
128. Hanson CA, Ross CW, Schnitzer B. Anti-CD34 immunoperoxidase staining in paraffin sections of acute leukemia: Comparison with flow cytometric immunophenotyping. Hum Pathol 1992;23:26.
129. Stroup R, Sheibani K. Antigenic phenotypes of hairy cell leukemia and monocytoid B-cell lymphoma: An immunohistochemical evaluation of 66 cases. Hum Pathol 1992;23:172.
130. Bowden JB, Hebert AA, Rapini RP. Dermal hematopoiesis in neonates: Report of five cases. J Am Acad Dermatol 1989;20:1104.
131. Schofield JK, Shun JL, Cerio R, Grice K. Cutaneous extramedullary hematopoiesis with a preponderance of atypical megakaryocytes in myelofibrosis. J Am Acad Dermatol 1990;22:334.

Lever's Histopathology of the Skin, eighth edition,
edited by David Elder et al. Lippincott–
Raven Publishers, Philadelphia © 1997.

CHAPTER 33

Tumors of the Fibrous Tissue Involving the Skin

Peter J. Heenan

BENIGN FIBROUS HISTIOCYTOMA (DERMATOFIBROMA)

Benign fibrous histiocytoma has also been known as dermatofibroma, histiocytoma, and sclerosing hemangioma. These tumors occur in the skin as firm, indolent single or multiple nodules, usually on the extremities of adults, although they may arise elsewhere. They are seen only rarely on the palms and soles.[1] Although they are as a rule only a few millimeters in diameter, they occasionally measure 2 to 3 cm. Rarely, as a result of hemorrhage into the tumor, they may attain a larger size.[2] Most lesions have a red color, but they may be red-brown because of hyperpigmentation of the overlying skin or, rarely, blue-black because of large amounts of hemosiderin within the tumor. In the latter case, the clinical appearance resembles that of a malignant melanoma. The cut surface of the lesions varies in color from white to yellowish brown, depending on the proportions of fibrous tissue, lipid, and hemosiderin present (Fig. 33-1A). Benign fibrous histiocytomas usually persist indefinitely, although spontaneous involution has been observed.[3]

Histopathology. The epidermis is usually hyperplastic, with hyperpigmentation of the basal layer and elongation of the rete ridges, separated by a clear (Grenz) zone from the spindle cell tumor in the dermis (see Fig. 33-1B), which is composed of fibroblastlike spindle cells, histiocytes, and blood vessels in varying proportions (see Fig. 33-1C). Foamy histiocytes and multinucleated giant cells containing lipid or hemosiderin may be present, sometimes in large numbers, forming xanthomatous aggregates. Capillaries may be plentiful in the stroma, giving the lesion an angiomatous component; when associated with a sclerotic stroma, such lesions have been referred to as "sclerosing hemangioma." In some small lesions the spindle cells are distributed singly between the collagen bundles, forming a zone of subtly increased cellularity, whereas in larger tumors there is much denser cellularity and the spindle cells are arranged in sheets or interlocking strands in storiform pattern. The dermal tumor is poorly demarcated on both sides, so that the fibroblasts and thc young basophilic collagen extend between the mature, eosinophilic collagen bundles of the dermis and surround them, thus trapping normal collagen bundles at the periphery of the tumor nodule.

Pronounced hyperplasia of the overlying epidermis in the center of the lesion occurs in more than 80% of benign fibrous histiocytomas.[4] The presence of this hyperplasia often has considerable value in the diagnosis of benign fibrous histiocytoma and in distinguishing the atypical variant from atypical fibroxanthoma.[5] Most commonly the hyperplasia consists of regular elongation of the rete ridges, which may be associated with hyperpigmentation of the basal layer. In some cases the epidermal hyperplasia is reminiscent of seborrheic keratosis through the interlacing of thickened rete ridges. Occasionally, downward proliferations are present that imitate the hair matrix to the point of having a connective tissue papilla.[6] In 2% to 5% of the lesions the downward proliferations are indistinguishable from those of superficial basal cell carcinoma.[7] Even though the proliferations in most of these instances are to be regarded as similar to basal cell carcinoma, in rare instances a truly invasive basal cell carcinoma associated with ulceration develops.[8,9]

Variants of Benign Fibrous Histiocytoma

Cellular Benign Fibrous Histiocytoma[10]

This is a very densely cellular tumor with fascicular and storiform growth patterns and frequent extension into the subcutis (Fig. 33-2A). The neoplasm shares some features, therefore, with dermatofibrosarcoma protuberans, from which it is distinguished by the overlying epidermal hyperplasia, polymorphism of the tumor cell population, extension of tumor cells at the edge of the lesion to surround individual hyalinized collagen bundles (see Fig. 33-2B), and the absence of immunostaining for CD34 (human hemopoietic progenitor cell antigen).[11] The cellular benign fibrous histiocytoma also extends into the subcutis along the septa or in a bulging, expansile pattern, rather than in the more diffusely infiltrative pattern of dermatofibrosarcoma protuberans, which produces a typical honeycomblike pattern.[12]

P. J. Heenan: Cutaneous Pathology, Nedlands, WA, Australia

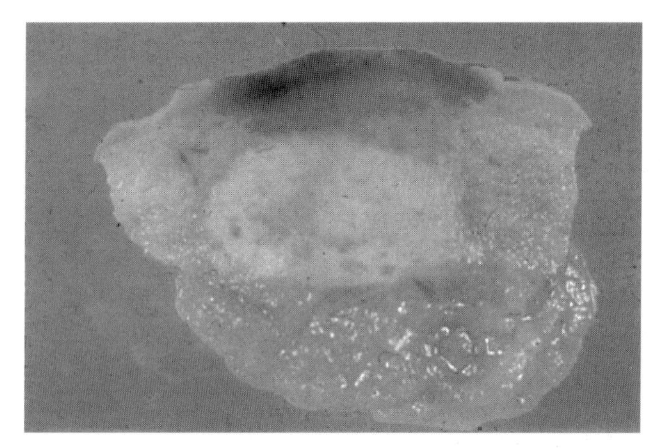

A

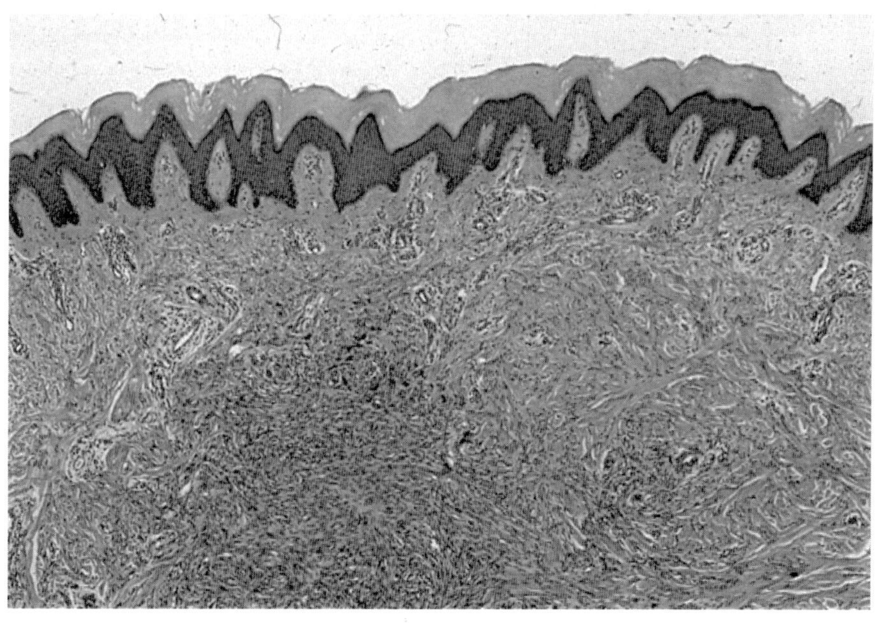

B

FIG. 33-1. Benign fibrous histiocytoma (dermatofibroma)
(**A**) Gross specimen. A circumscribed nodular lesion with a yellow cut surface is present in the dermis. The epidermis shows brownish pigmentation and is separated from the underlying tumor by a clear zone. (**B**) The epidermis is hyperplastic and separated by a narrow clear zone from a moderately cellular spindle cell tumor extending into the deep dermis.

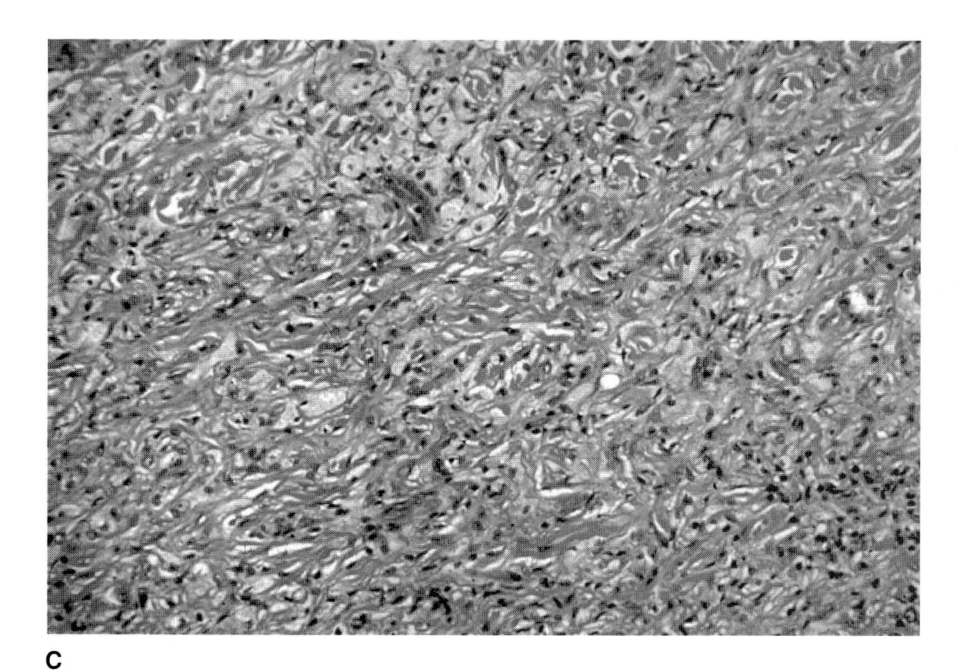

FIG. 33-1. *Continued*
(**C**) The tumor is composed of plump spindle cells with pale eosinophilic cytoplasm in a collagenous stroma, as well as groups of histiocytes with pale cytoplasm.

Aneurysmal Benign Fibrous Histiocytoma

In these tumors, collections of capillaries, foci of hemorrhage, siderophages, and foamy macrophages surround cleft-like and cavernous blood-filled spaces in the center of the tumor, which otherwise shows typical features of benign fibrous histiocytoma (Fig. 33-3A and B).[13]

Atypical (Pseudosarcomatous) Benign Fibrous Histiocytoma

Atypical cells are occasionally present in benign fibrous histiocytomas and may lead to misdiagnosis as atypical fibroxanthoma, which may represent a superficial variant of malignant fibrous histiocytoma. Such lesions are best referred to as "atypical benign fibrous histiocytoma."[5,14,15] They usually are less than 1.2 cm in diameter but occasionally are as large as 2.5 cm.[16] The pseudomalignant changes may consist of scattered, strikingly atypical cells with an extremely large nucleus, referred to as monster cells,[16] or there may be marked focal cellular atypia without mitoses or with only a few normal mitoses. The atypical cells may also consist of multinucleated giant cells that possess bizarre, large, hyperchromatic nuclei with little cytoplasm or irregular, vesiculated nuclei with abundant foamy cytoplasm. (Fig. 33-4A and B).[5]

Epithelioid Benign Fibrous Histiocytoma

This variant was originally described as epithelioid cell histiocytoma.[17] This is a distinctive form, composed of epithelioid cells with abundant eosinophilic cytoplasm, binucleate cells, foamy macrophages, and spindle cells forming a polypoid tumor with an epidermal collarette.[18]

Neoplasm Versus Fibrosis

The view has been expressed that benign fibrous histiocytomas are not true neoplasms but reactive fibroblastic proliferation subsequent to trauma, including arthropod bites. These tumors have been referred to as "nodular subepidermal fibrosis"[19] and have been regarded as fibrosing inflammatory lesions, even in the presence of "monster cells."[16] However, the fact that the lesions with very few exceptions show no tendency to regress but persist indefinitely speaks in favor of a neoplastic rather than a reactive inflammatory genesis.[20]

Hyperplasia of the Epidermis

The hyperplasia of the epidermis overlying benign fibrous histiocytomas can be explained by the presence of young collagen and of abundant amounts of metachromatic ground substance in the subepidermal region. This material stimulates the epidermis in a fashion similar to that of embryonic mesenchyme, causing the formation of immature hair structures and even of primary epithelial germs. Because the benign fibrous histiocytoma prevents their downward growth, the immature hair structures, including the primary epithelial germ formations, proliferate in the narrow space between the epidermis and the tumor.[21] The primary epithelial germ proliferations resemble the proliferations of a basal cell carcinoma and in rare instances even give rise to a true basal cell carcinoma. The view has been expressed that the basal cell carcinoma–like masses represent regressed adnexal structures pushed up against the overlying epidermis by the tumor.[22]

Histogenesis. Dermatofibroma was originally described as fibroma simplex by Unna in 1894.[23] In 1932, Woringer and Kviatkowski showed that some dermatofibromas contain

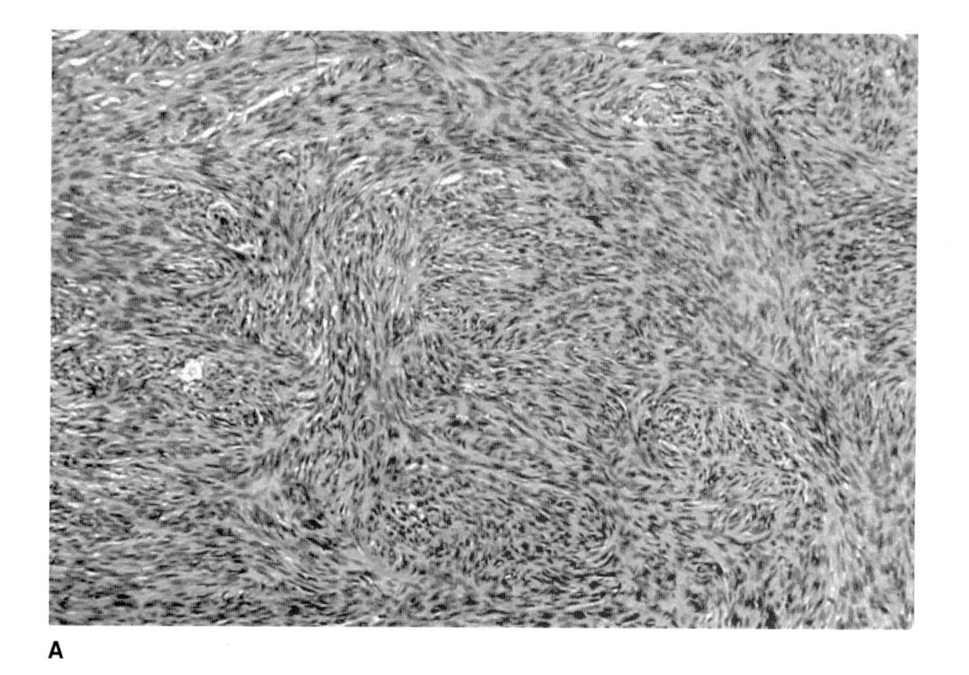

A

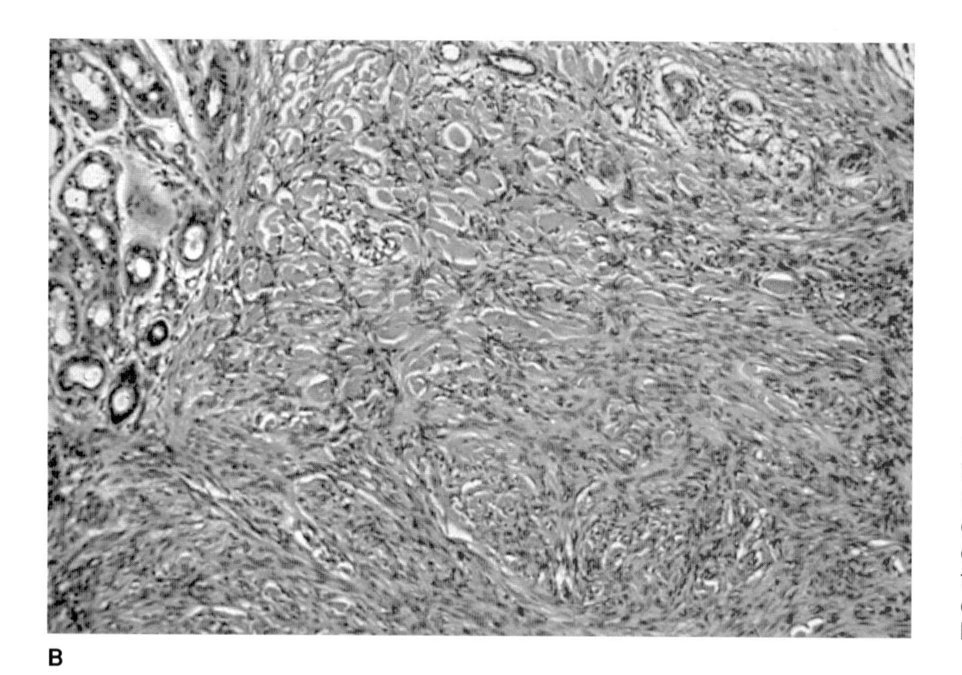

B

FIG. 33-2. Cellular benigh fibrous histiocytoma (dermatofibroma) (**A**) The tumor consists of spindle cells arranged in densely cellular fascicular and storiform patterns. (**B**) At the border of the lesion the spindle cells surround individual collagen bundles.

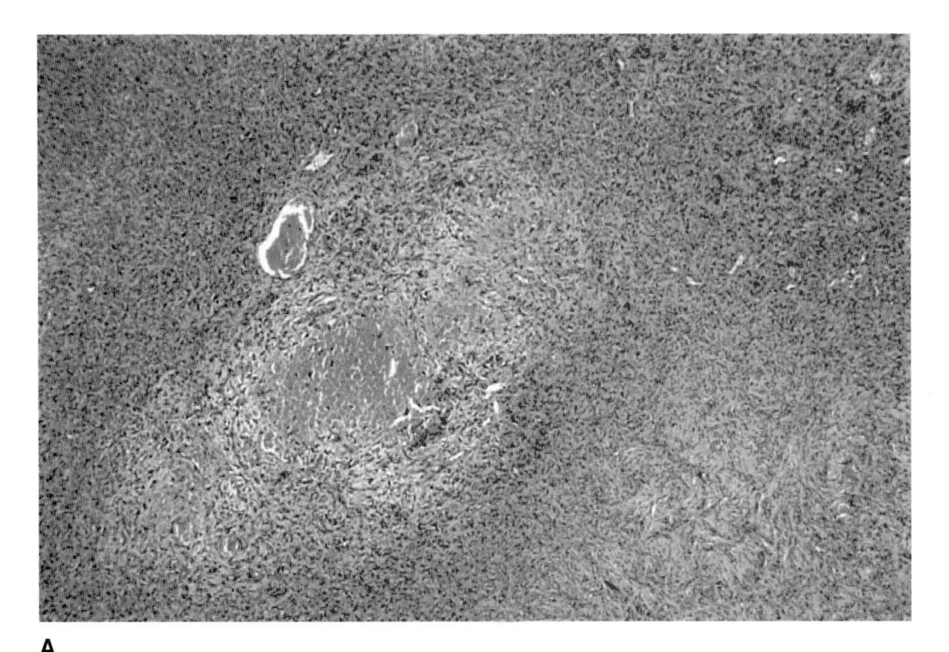

A

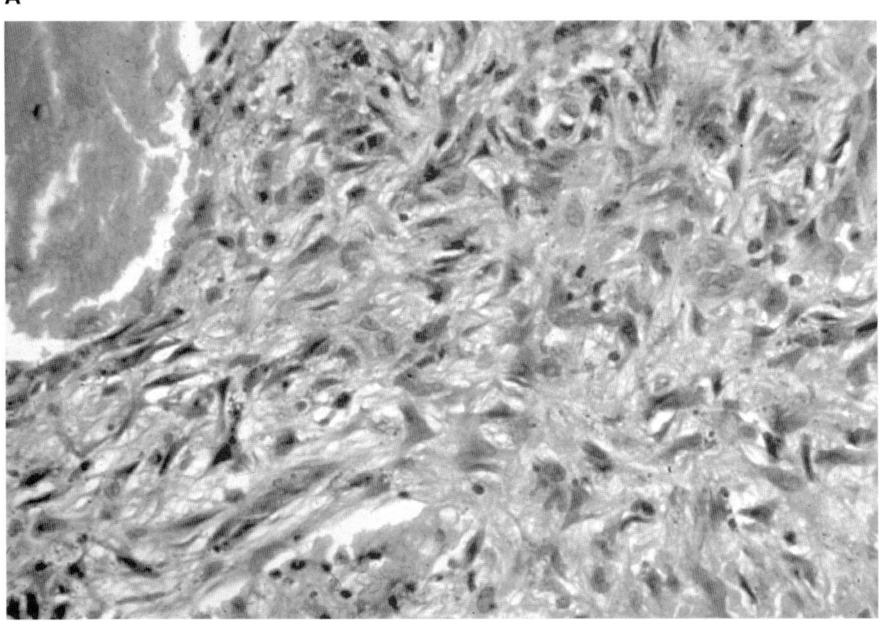

B

FIG. 33-3. Aneurysmal benign fibrous histiocytoma (dermatofibroma)
(**A**) Central congested, dilated blood vessels and hemorrhage are surrounded by plump spindle cells. (**B**) Spindle cells and siderophages are adjacent to blood-filled spaces.

phagocytizing cells, which they regarded as histiocytes, and therefore they proposed the term *histiocytoma*.[24] In 1936, Senear and Caro injected colloidal iron under six dermatofibromas before excision and found that all tumors phagocytized iron; they therefore concluded that all dermatofibromas are histiocytomas.[25] It became common practice, however, to refer to those tumors composed predominantly of collagen fibers and fibroblastlike spindle cells as "dermatofibromas," and to tumors containing a larger component of histiocytelike cells as "histiocytomas."

More recent enzyme histochemical, electron microscopic, and immunohistochemical studies have indicated variously that these tumors demonstrate histiocytic, myofibroblastic, and fibroblastic differentiation[26–30] and are probably of primitive mesenchymal origin.[31] The term *benign fibrous histiocytoma* is now used as a general designation for this varied group of spindle cell neoplasms.[31]

The alternative term *dermal dendrocytoma* has also been suggested for benign fibrous histiocytoma on the basis of immunohistochemical studies using antibodies to factor XIIIa and MAC387.[32] Most cells in these tumors were found to react with factor XIIIa, whereas only a few were MAC387-positive. Factor XIIIa labels the normal dermal population of fixed connective tissue cells, or fibroblasts, also termed "dermal dendro-

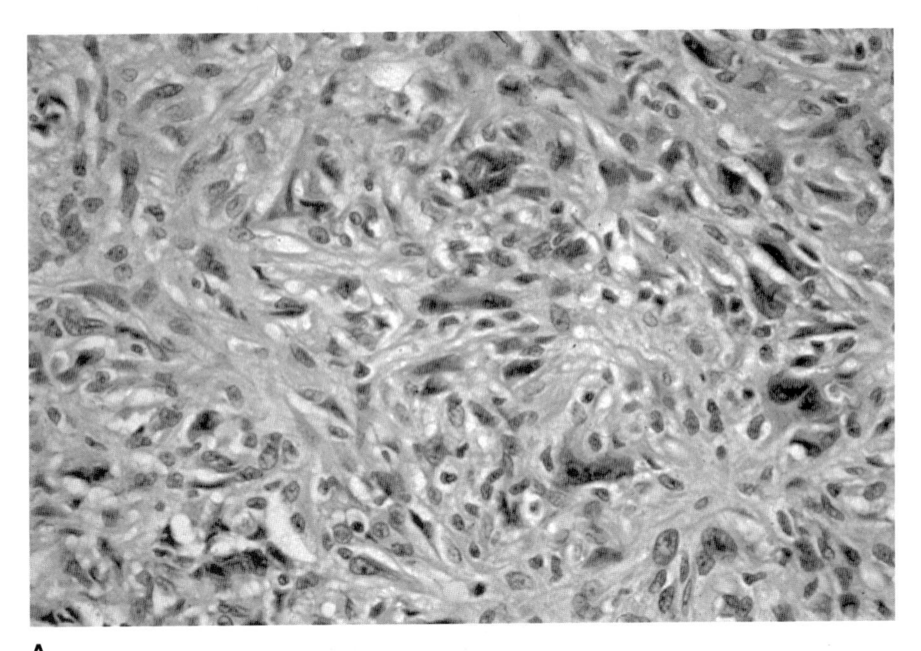

A

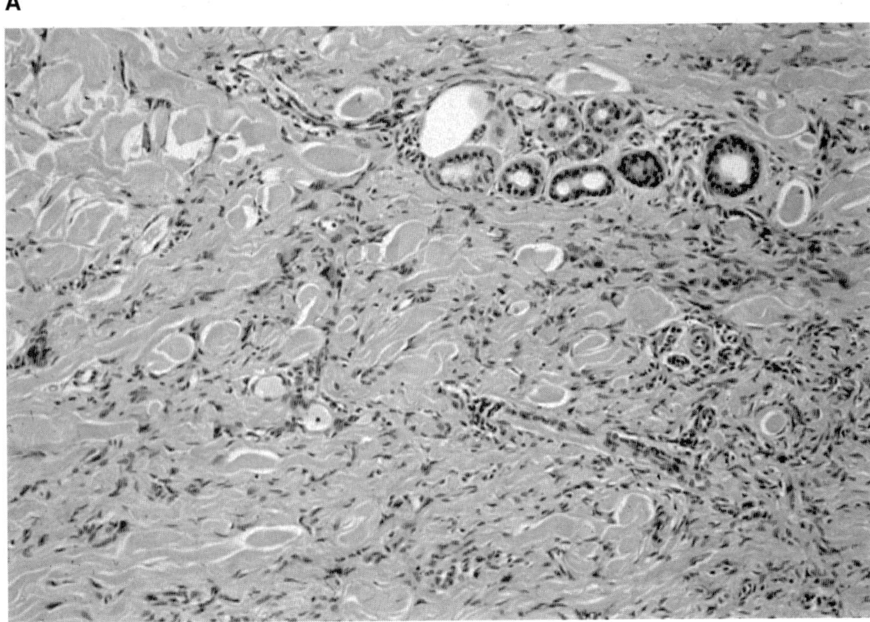

B

FIG. 33-4. Atypical benign fibrous histiocytoma (dermatofibroma) (**A**) This variant includes spindle cells, epithelioid cells, and giant cells with large, pleomorphic nuclei. (**B**) At the border of this tumor the cells are arranged around individual collagen bundles in the pattern typical of benign fibrous histiocytoma.

cytes" because of their characteristic dendritic processes.[33] MAC387, on the other hand, is expressed by monocyte-derived macrophages. Other investigators, however, believe that the factor XIIIa–positive cells seen in benign fibrous histiocytoma represent reactive stromal cells rather than true tumor cells.[31]

Electron Microscopy. Reports of electron microscopic studies have variously described the cells of benign fibrous histiocytoma as fibroblasts,[34] histiocytes,[35] and myofibroblasts.[36]

Enzyme Histochemistry. The results of enzymic studies on benign fibrous histiocytoma have also yielded varied results. Positive staining for lysozyme and α_1-antitrypsin have been interpreted as indicating histiocytic differentiation,[37] whereas negative results for these enzymes have led to the speculation that both the fibroblastic and histiocytelike cells in these tumors arise from primitive mesenchymal cells.[38,39] The presence of HLA-DR antigens in the majority of cells in benign fibrous histiocytoma has also been regarded as evidence in favor of histiocytic origin.[40]

Differential Diagnosis. The cellular variant of benign fibrous histiocytoma, frequently showing a storiform growth pattern and extending into the subcutis, shares these features with dermatofibrosarcoma protuberans, from which it is distinguished by the overlying epidermal hyperplasia, polymorphism of the tumor cells, extension of tumor cells at the edge of the lesion to surround individual hyalinized collagen bundles, and the absence of immunostaining for CD34.[41] Cellular benign fibrous histiocytoma also extends into the cutis along the interlobular septa or in a bulging, expansile pattern, rather than in the characteristic infiltrating honeycomblike pattern of dermatofibrosarcoma protuberans.[12] Dermatofibrosarcoma protuberans also is usually a much larger lesion at the time of diagnosis, often consisting of multiple nodules. Cellular benign fibrous histiocytoma may also be confused with leiomyosarcoma, which, however, has plumper spindle cells with eosinophilic cytoplasm and nuclei with rounded extremities, and shows positive staining for desmin and alpha smooth muscle actin.[31]

Aneurysmal benign fibrous histiocytoma may be confused with neoplasms of vascular origin and angiomatoid malignant fibrous histiocytoma. Benign and malignant angiomatous tumors are characterized by the formation of vascular structures lined by endothelial cells that stain positively for factor VIII and CD34. Nodular Kaposi sarcoma, in particular, demonstrates slitlike spaces containing erythrocytes and a monomorphic CD34 positive spindle cell population.[31]

Aneurysmal benign fibrous histiocytoma is distinguished from angiomatoid malignant fibrous histiocytoma by the presence in the latter tumor of monomorphic histiocytelike cells with a prominent lymphocytic infiltrate,[42] and its presentation in a younger age group, occasionally with systemic symptoms, usually in a subcutaneous location.[43]

The cells of epithelioid benign fibrous histiocytoma may resemble those of intradermal Spitz nevus, but the latter tumor is characterized by a nested pattern in the superficial layers, spindle cells as well as epithelioid cells, intranuclear cytoplasmic invaginations, desmoplastic stroma, maturation of cells in the deeper layers, and immunostaining for S-100 protein. Reticulohistiocytoma, which may also bear some resemblance to the epithelioid benign fibrous histiocytoma, is composed of characteristic multinucleated giant cells with glassy cytoplasm.

Atypical fibroxanthoma differs from atypical benign fibrous histiocytoma in its location on the sun-exposed skin of elderly patients, usually the head and neck, frequent ulceration, severe cellular pleomorphism, and frequent mitoses, including bizarre forms.

DERMATOFIBROSARCOMA PROTUBERANS

Dermatofibrosarcoma protuberans (DFSP) is a slowly growing dermal spindle cell neoplasm of intermediate malignancy that usually forms an indurated plaque on which multiple reddish purple, firm nodules subsequently arise, sometimes with ulceration (Fig. 33-5A). The tumors occur most frequently on the trunk or the proximal extremities of young adults and only rarely in the head and neck.[44,45] A small proportion of cases have been reported in childhood and, rarely, as congenital lesions.[46] Local recurrence is common but metastasis is rare.[47,48]

Histopathology. DFSP is composed of densely packed, monomorphous, plump spindle cells arranged in a storiform (matlike) pattern in the central areas of tumor nodules, whereas at the periphery there is diffuse infiltration of the dermal stroma, frequently extending into the subcutis and producing a characteristic honeycomb pattern (see Fig. 33-5B–D).[12] Infiltration into the underlying fascia and muscle is a late event.[49] Lateral extension of irregular strands of spindle cells into the dermal stroma is often pronounced, where the peripheral elements of the tumor may have a deceptively bland appearance, approaching that of normal collagen. This can cause difficulties in determining the true extent of the tumor and may result in recurrence after presumed adequate resection.[47]

Myxoid areas, sometimes resembling liposarcoma, include a characteristic vascular component of slitlike anastomosing thin-walled blood vessels presenting a crow's foot or chicken wire appearance (Fig. 33-6A and B).[50] Melanin-containing cells may be present in a small proportion of tumors, so-called Bednar tumor (pigmented DFSP, storiform neurofibroma).[51,52]

Fibrosarcomatous areas are seen in a small proportion of DFSP, characterized by a fascicular or herringbone growth pattern of the spindle cells.[53] This variant does not appear to have any greater propensity for local recurrence, which is related to the adequacy of primary surgical excision.

Giant cells are seen in a small proportion of otherwise typical DFSP. The histologic resemblance between giant cell fibroblastoma and DFSP, and recurrences of DFSP showing features of giant cell fibroblastoma, and vice versa, suggests that giant cell fibroblastoma is a juvenile variant of DFSP.[54–59]

Histogenesis. On the basis of electron microscopic findings, the tumor cells have been regarded as fibroblasts, because they show active synthesis of collagen in a well-developed endoplasmic reticulum.[35,60,61] In some tumors the presence of interrupted basement membrane–like material along the cell membrane has indicated that the cells are modified fibroblasts possessing features of perineural and endoneural cells.[62] Immunohistochemical studies have suggested fibroblastic[63] or myofibroblastic[64] differentiation, but the expression of CD34 (human progenitor cell antigen) by DFSP has also been interpreted as supporting the view that these neoplasms are variants of nerve sheath tumors.[65]

Differential Diagnosis. DFSP shares common features with other dermal spindle cell neoplasms, but it is characterized by the uniformity of the spindle cells and the more prominent storiform pattern than is associated with benign or malignant fibrous histiocytoma. Superficial biopsies contribute to the difficulty in distinguishing between DFSP, benign fibrous histiocytoma, and diffuse neurofibroma. In contrast with cellular benign fibrous histiocytoma, the epidermis overlying DFSP is usually attenuated or ulcerated rather than hyperplastic, and a clear zone between the epidermis and tumor may not be present (Fig. 33-7). DFSP is more densely cellular and monomorphic, with a more prominent storiform pattern, and the extension into the subcutis presents either the classic honeycomblike pattern or a multilayered pattern, in contrast with the well-demarcated bulging deep margin of cellular benign fibrous histiocytoma, which may also extend into the subcutis but is predominantly along the septa.[12,41] Immunostaining for CD34 is usually positive in DFSP and negative in cellular benign fibrous histiocytoma (Fig. 33-8).[12,65–67] Neurofibroma expresses S-100 protein, which is absent in DFSP, and it also has other histologic features of neural differentiation, without the dense, uniform cellularity of DFSP.

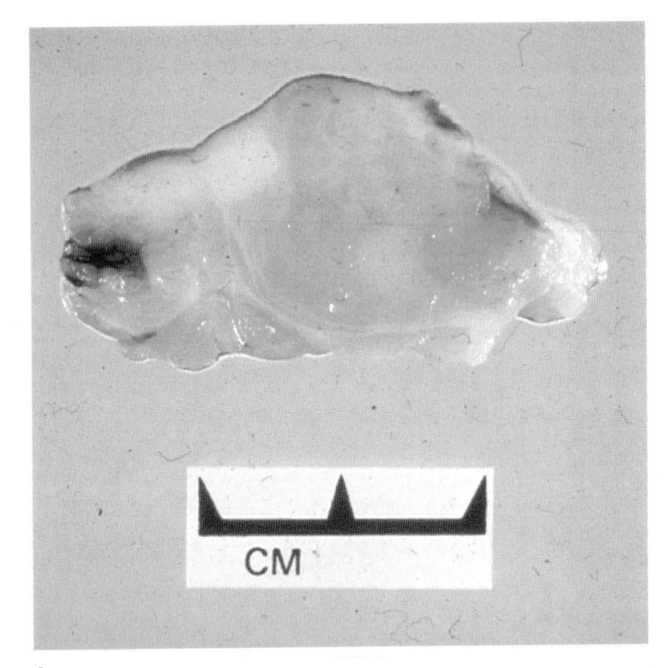

A

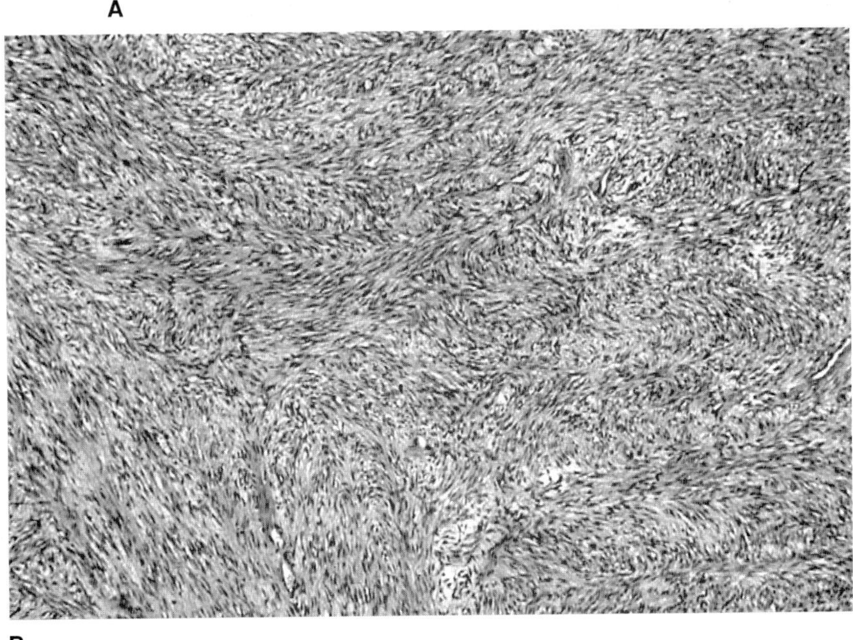

B

FIG. 33-5. Dermatofibrosarcoma protuberans
(**A**) Gross specimen of a myxoid variant of dermatofibrosarcoma protuberans forming a central nodule extending into the subcutis, with lateral extension in the dermis of a component of firmer white tissue. (**B**) Densely packed spindle cells arranged in a storiform pattern.

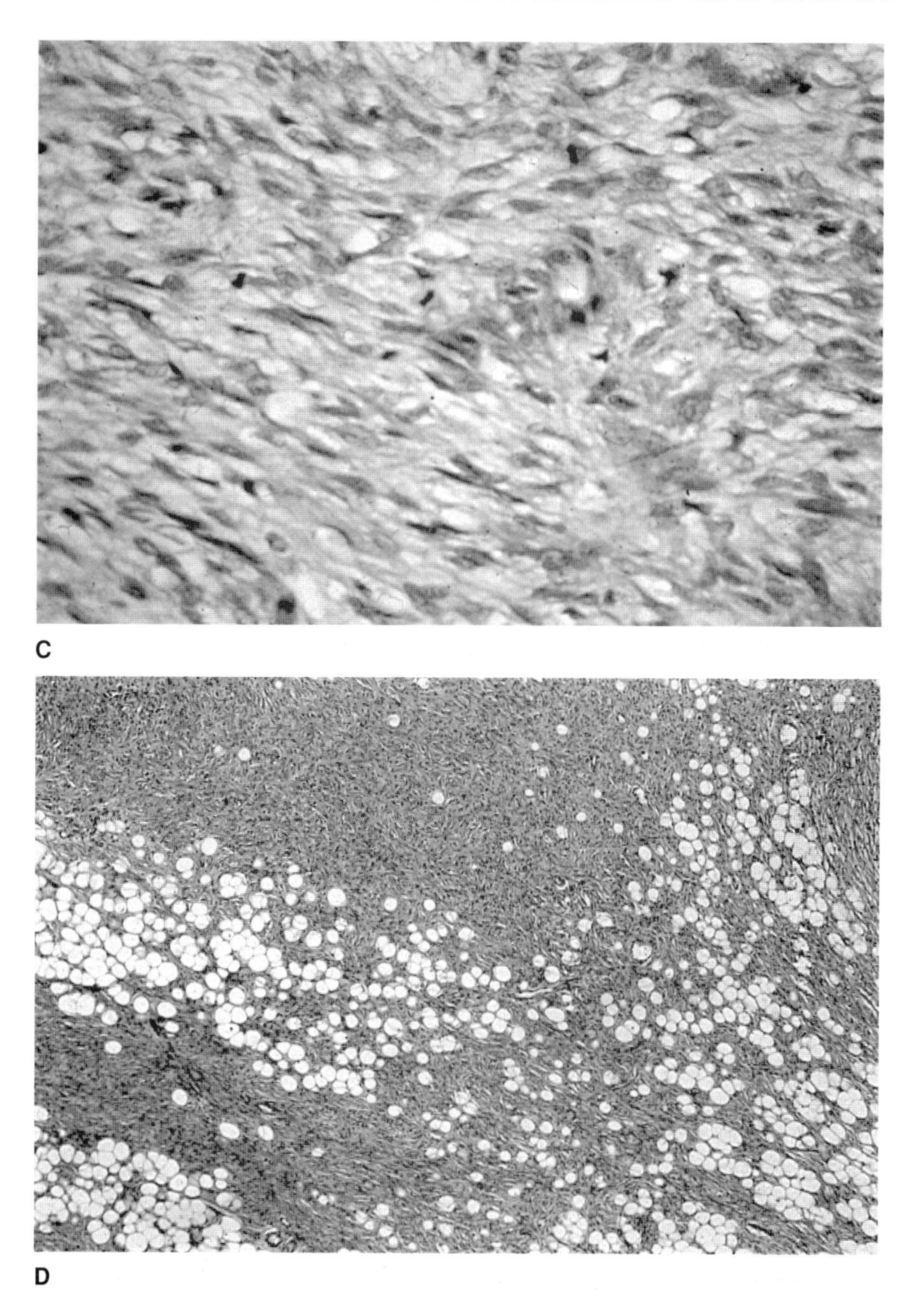

FIG. 33-5. ***Continued***
(**C**) Uniform, plump spindle cells with scattered mitoses. (**D**) Diffuse infiltration of the subcutis producing a honeycomblike pattern.

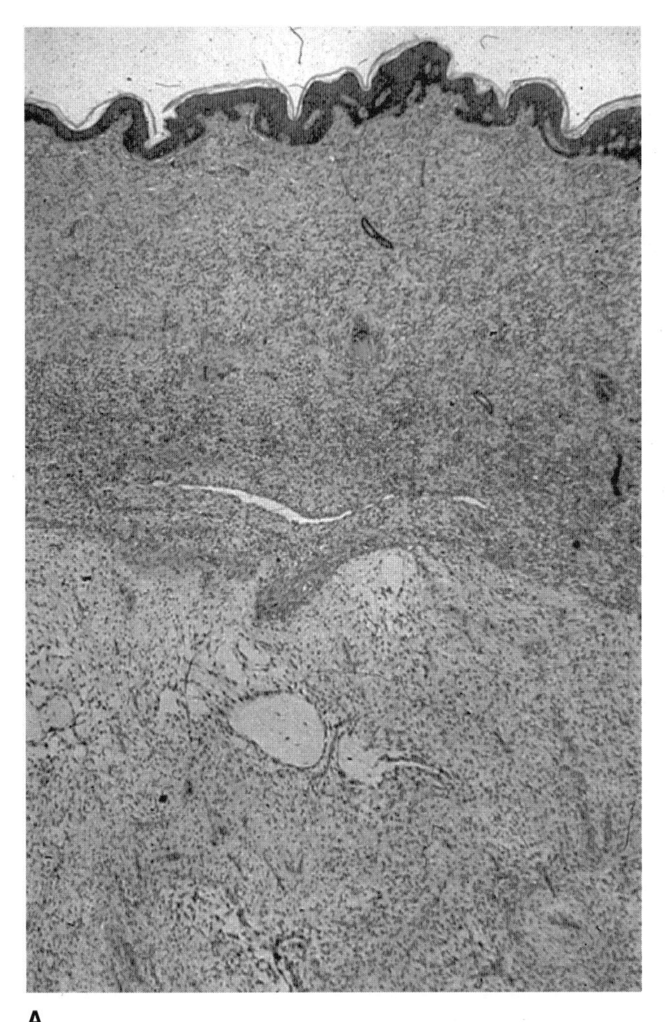

A

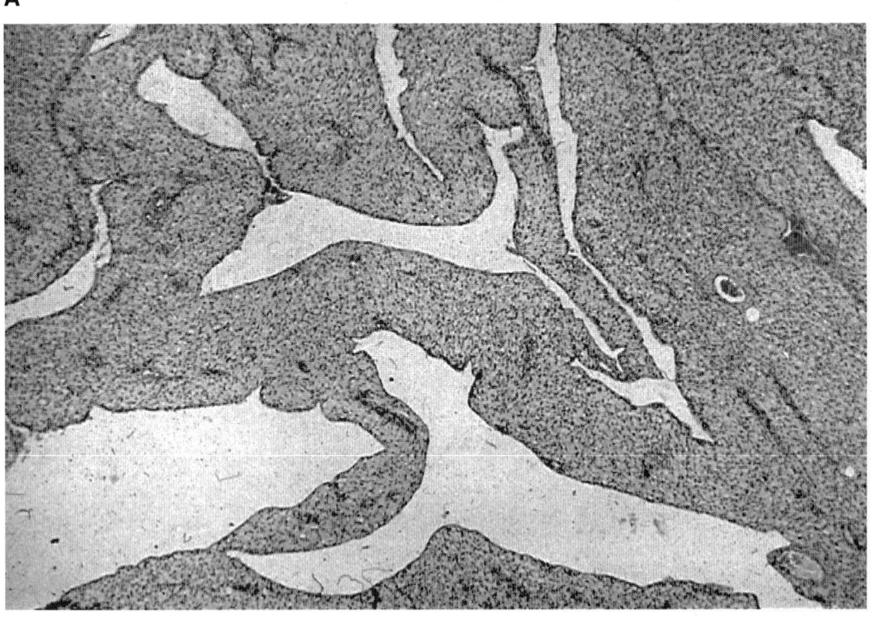

B

FIG. 33-6. Myxoid dermatofibrosarcoma protuberans
(**A**) This example of dermatofibrosarcoma protuberans has a myxoid component in the deeper dermis. (**B**) Blood vessels in myxoid dermatofibrosarcoma protuberans producing a characteristic "crow's foot" or "chicken wire" pattern.

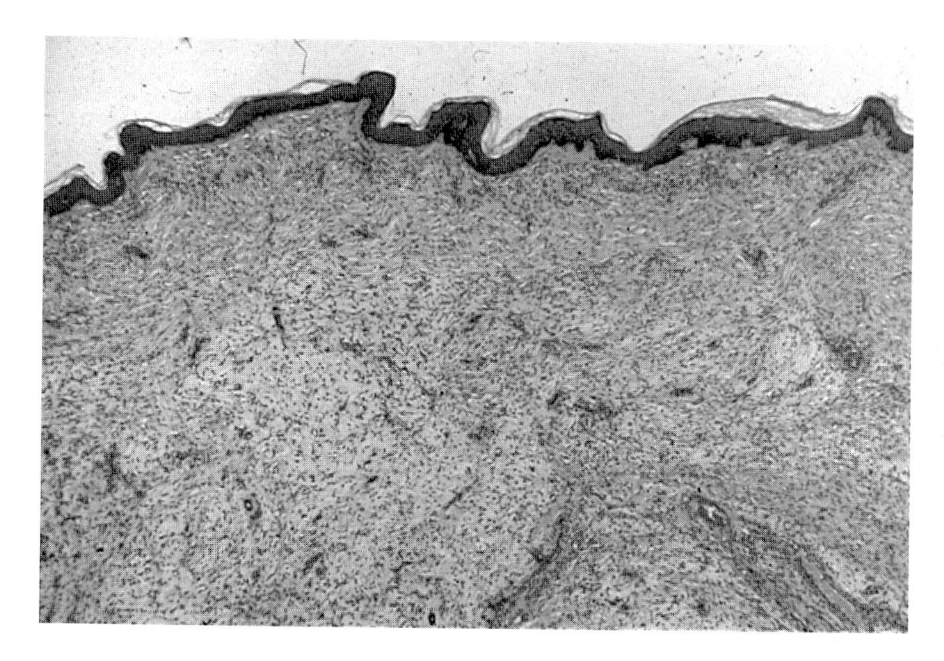

FIG. 33-7. Dermatofibrosarcoma protuberans
The epidermis is not hyperplastic, and there is no Grenz zone between the epidermis and the underlying dermatofibrosarcoma protuberans.

GIANT CELL FIBROBLASTOMA

Giant cell fibroblastoma, first described by Shmookler and Enzinger in 1982,[68] is a rare benign tumor occurring almost exclusively in children as a solitary dermal or subcutaneous nodule, most often on the back, thigh, or chest wall. Local recurrence following incomplete excision is common,[69] but no metastases have been reported.[70]

Histopathology. The dermal and subcutaneous nodules are composed of poorly circumscribed, loosely structured collections of pleomorphic spindle cells in a collagenous or myxoid stroma (Fig. 33-9A). Distinctive multinucleated giant cells line cleftlike, angiectoid spaces (see Fig. 33-9B). The apparently multiple nuclei of the giant cells have been shown by electron microscopy to represent multiple sausagelike lobations of a single nucleus.[54] In the more solid, spindle cell areas of the tumor the appearances resemble DFSP.

Histogenesis. Ultrastructurally the cells resemble fibroblasts. Immunohistochemical studies have shown that the tumors express vimentin but not S-100 protein or vascular mark-

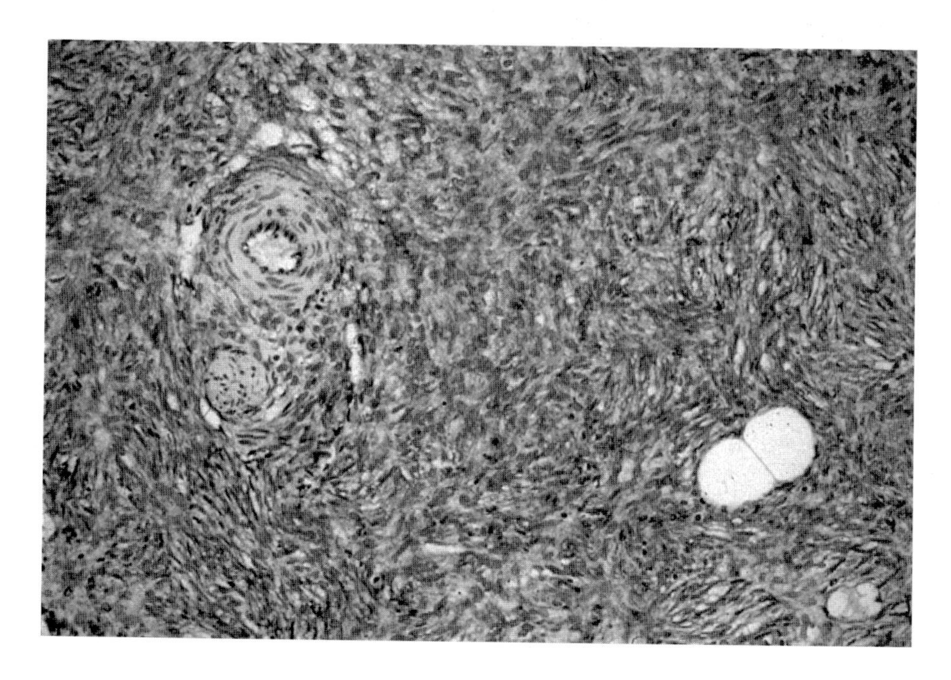

FIG. 33-8. Dermatofibrosarcoma protuberans
Positive immunostaining for CD34 in dermatofibrosarcoma protuberans and in the endothelium of blood vessels.

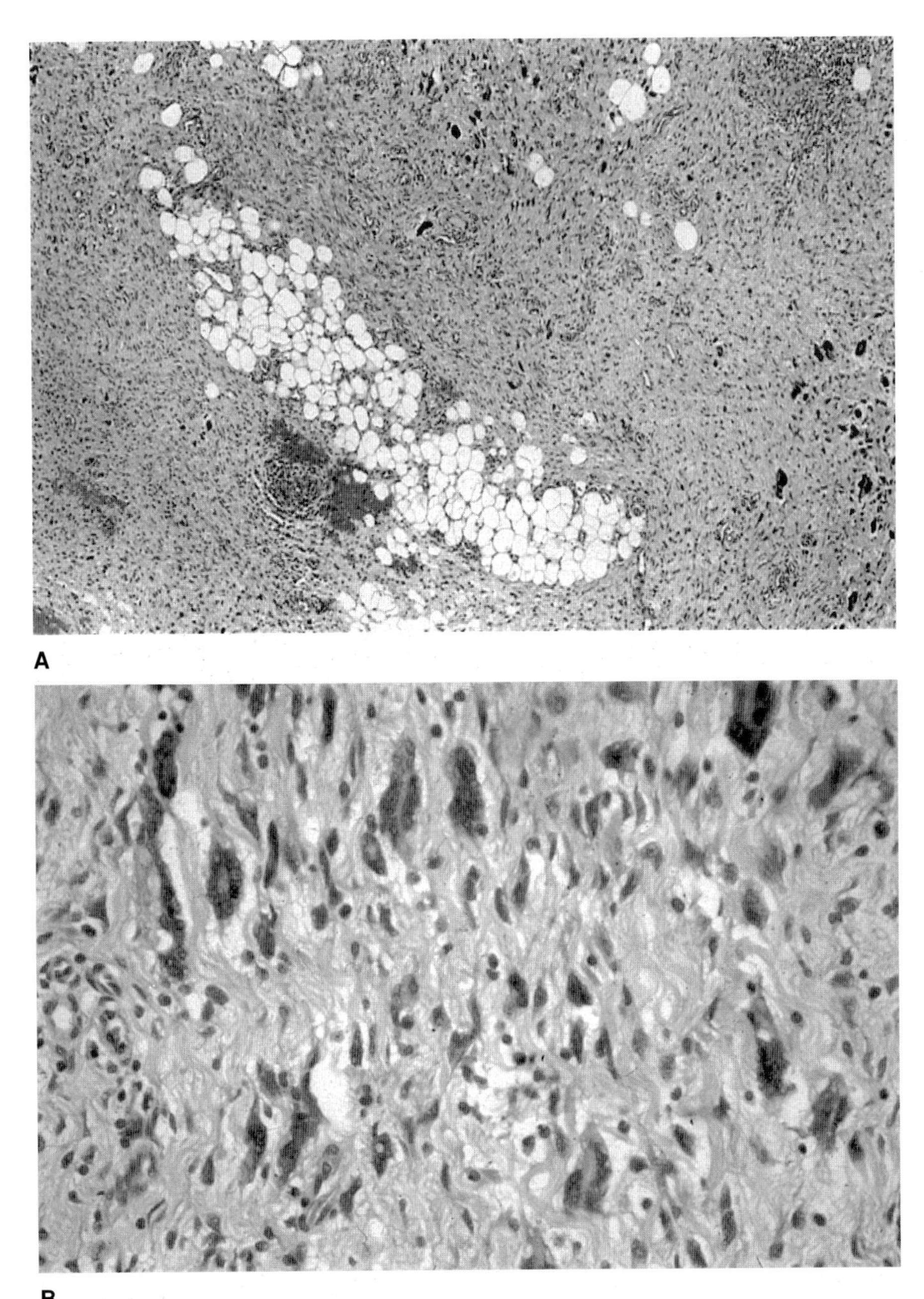

FIG. 33-9. Giant cell fibroblastoma
(**A**) The growth pattern resembles that of dermatofibrosarcoma protuberans with infiltration of subcutaneous fat by uniform spindle cells, with the additional feature of scattered giant cells. (Courtesy of Dr. Inara Strungs, Adelaide Children's Hospital, and Dr. P. W. Allen.) (**B**) Spindle cells and numerous giant cells with mainly single, pleomorphic, multilobated nuclei.

ers,[71] and positive immunostaining for CD34 has recently been demonstrated in some cases.[65] The histologic similarity to dermatofibrosarcoma protuberans, emphasized by reports of tumors sharing common features of both types and recorded cases in which recurrence of either DFSP or giant cell fibroblastoma has presented features of the other tumor, all suggest that giant cell fibroblastoma may be the juvenile counterpart of DFSP.[54–59] Giant cell fibroblastoma with a Bednar tumor (pigmented dermatofibrosarcoma protuberans) component has also been reported.[72,73]

DESMOID TUMOR (MUSCULOAPONEUROTIC FIBROMATOSIS)

Desmoid tumors are benign fibrous neoplasms that arise as firm nontender masses from a muscular aponeurosis and tend to invade the muscle. Although their rate of growth is slow, they may attain considerable size, as large as 25 cm in diameter.[74] Although usually solitary, they may be multiple.[75]

Desmoid tumors may occur in children, but they are seen mainly in young adults, particularly in women. The most common type of desmoid tumor arises in women from the rectus abdominis muscle following pregnancy. In some instances, desmoid tumors develop in scars resulting from abdominal operations. However, they may arise as extraabdominal desmoid tumors within any skeletal muscle.[74]

In addition, desmoid tumors occur in the rare, dominantly transmitted *Gardner's syndrome*. This syndrome consists of (1) intestinal polyposis, which is usually limited to the large intestine and which, in about half of the cases, results in a malignant transformation of one or several adenomatous polyps into adenocarcinoma; (2) epidermal cysts, especially on the face and scalp; (3) osteomatosis with a predilection for the membranous bones of the head; and (4) fibrous tissue tumors consisting either of well-demarcated fibromas in the skin, the subcutaneous tissue, or the abdominal cavity or of desmoid tumors that invade adjacent muscles. The latter arise either in an abdominal scar following colectomy or spontaneously at other sites.[76]

Histopathology. Desmoid tumors are composed of poorly circumscribed bundles of spindle cells surrounded by abundant collagen (Fig. 33-10A). Although most desmoid tumors are quite cellular, at least in some areas, and show arrangement of their spindle cells in interlacing bundles, the nuclei are regular

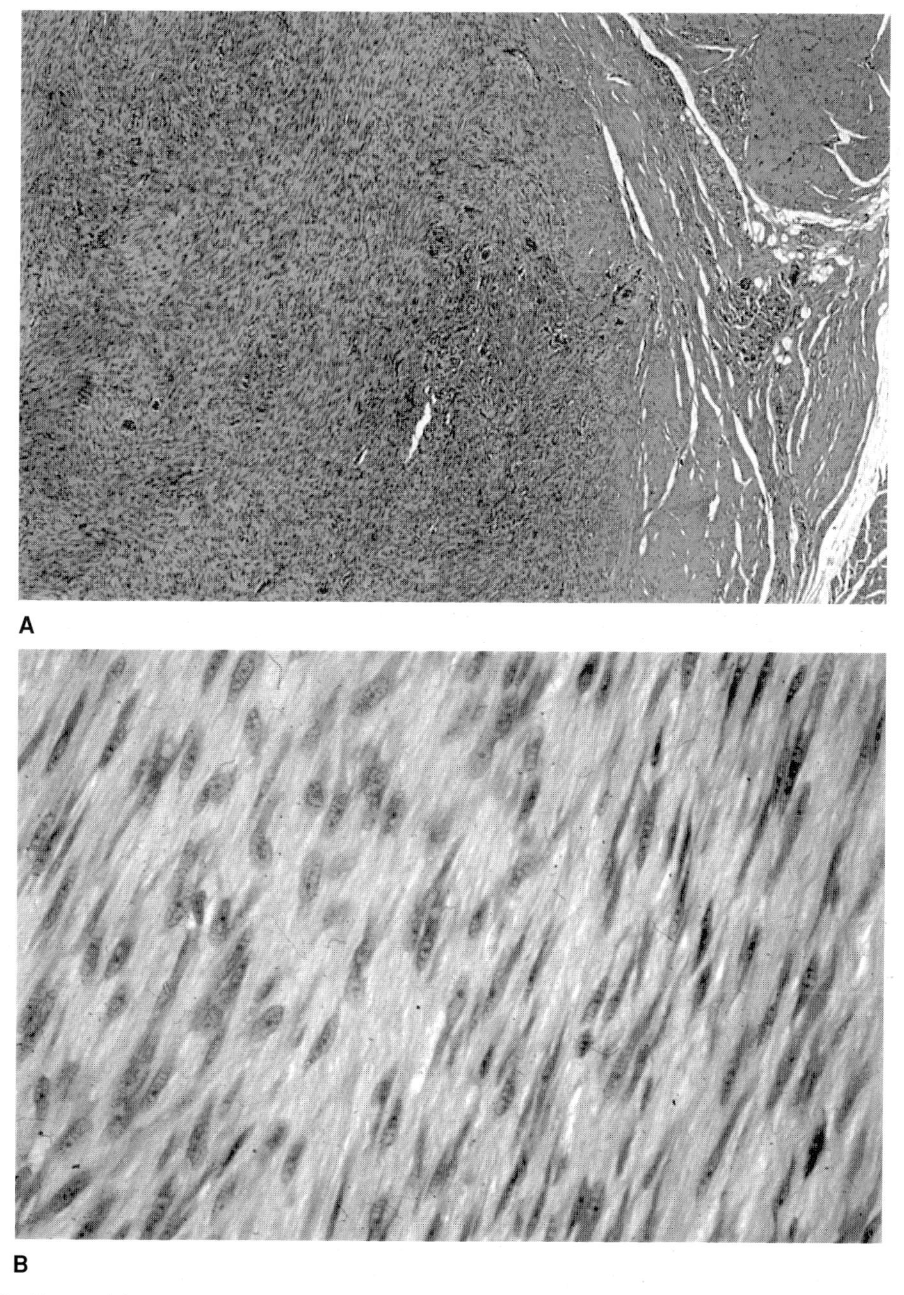

FIG. 33-10. Desmoid tumor
(**A**) A mass composed of dense bundles of eosinophilic spindle cells is present within striated muscle.
(**B**) The tumor cells are monomorphous, with regular nuclei and pale cytoplasm; there are no mitoses or giant cells. *(continued on next page)*

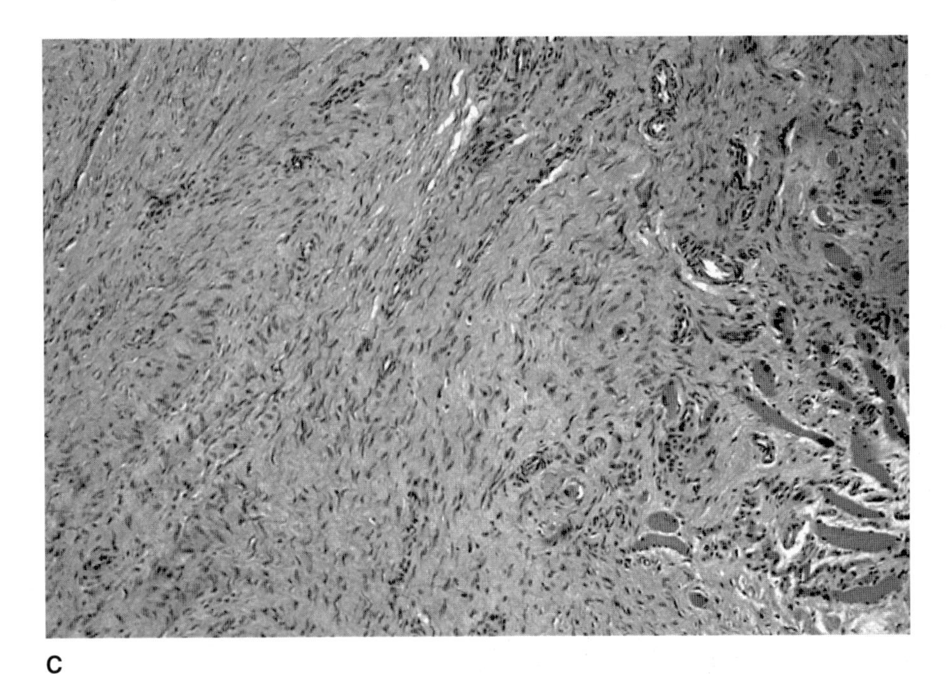

C

FIG. 33-10. *Continued*
(**C**) In this area the spindle cells are more dispersed and infiltrate the striated muscle, isolating degenerate segments of muscle fibers.

and pale staining, mitoses are infrequent, and giant cells are absent (Fig. 33-10B).[75] Desmoid tumors show a great tendency to infiltrate adjacent striated muscle bundles. Isolated degenerating and sometimes multinucleated muscle fibers are frequently found entrapped in the tumors (Fig. 33-10C).[74]

Histogenesis. Desmoid tumors are generally regarded as neoplasms, although some investigators believe that they represent a hyperplasia of connective tissue analogous to keloids.[74] They differ from keloids in their location, their invasive tendency, their potential to occur without trauma, and their histopathologic appearance.

On electron microscopic examination, the spindle cells of desmoid tumors show the features of myofibroblasts.[75,77,78] This may reflect an abnormal persistence and proliferation of myofibroblasts, which normally disappear gradually in the late stages of wound healing.[75] Immunostaining for vimentin, alpha smooth muscle actin, and muscle actin with only rare positivity for desmin, is also typical of myofibroblasts.[79]

PLEXIFORM FIBROHISTIOCYTIC TUMOR

Plexiform fibrohistiocytic tumor is a multinodular neoplasm of the dermis and subcutis, composed of histiocytelike cells, fi-

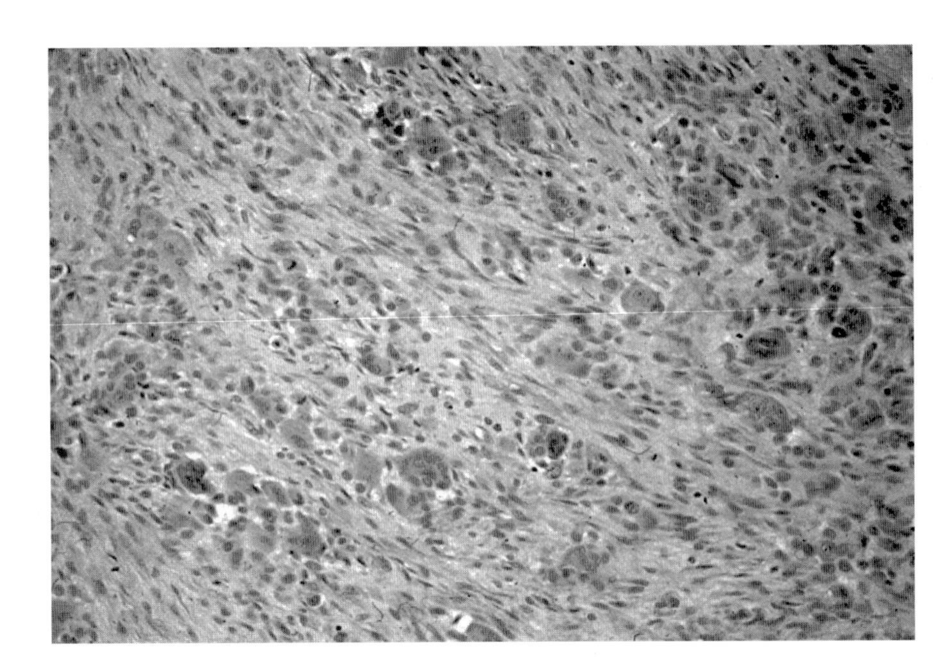

FIG. 33-11. Plexiform fibrohistiocytic tumor
Small groups of epithelioid and osteoclastlike giant cells are surrounded by fascicles of spindle cells in a plexiform pattern.

broblasts, and multinucleated giant cells in a plexiform pattern.[79] This distinctive lesion is a slowly growing mass, occurring usually in the extremities of children and young adults. Local recurrence is common and regional lymph node metastasis has been described, but visceral metastasis has not been recorded.

Histopathology. Nodules of histiocytic and osteoclastlike giant cells are surrounded by fascicles of fibroblastlike spindle cells intersecting the stroma in a plexiform pattern (Fig. 33-11).

Histogenesis. Ultrastructural and immunocytochemical studies have indicated histiocytic and myofibroblastic differentiation.[80]

Differential Diagnosis. Cellular benign fibrous histiocytoma and dermatomyofibroma do not have the distinctive nodules of histiocytelike cells of plexiform fibrohistiocytic tumor, whereas fibromatosis and nodular fasciitis are usually more deeply situated and lack the characteristic plexiform growth pattern. Fibrous hamartoma of infancy has no histiocytic nodules.

DERMATOMYOFIBROMA

Dermatomyofibroma[81] (also termed "plaquelike dermal fibromatosis"[82]) is a benign dermal plaquelike proliferation of fibro-

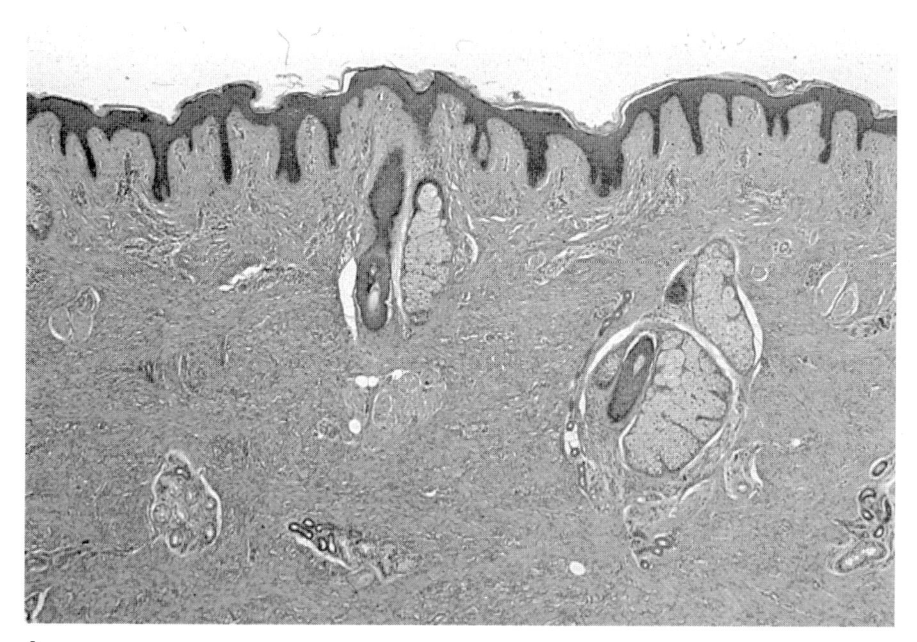

A

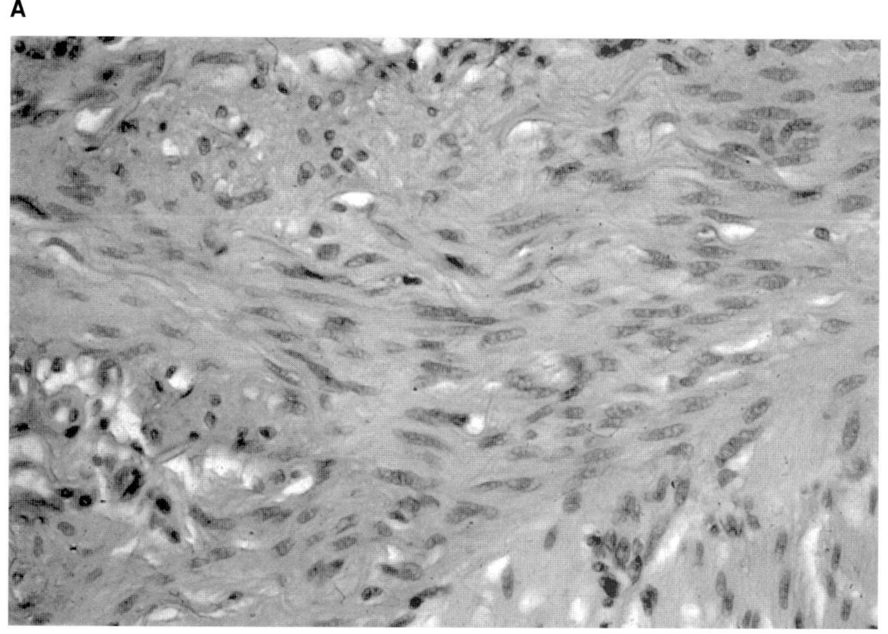

B

FIG. 33-12. Dermatomyofibroma (**A**) The epidermis shows elongation of the rete ridges, which overlie a plaque of increased cellularity extending into the reticular dermis, surrounding but not replacing appendages. (Courtesy of Hideko Kamino, MD, New York University Medical Center.) (**B**) The plaque is composed of uniform spindle cells with eosinophilic cytoplasm arranged parallel to the epidermal surface.

blasts and myofibroblasts, occurring mainly in young adults, more commonly in females, and most frequently in the shoulder region.

Histopathology. Uniform spindle cells in elongated and intersecting fascicles mainly arranged parallel to the epidermis surface form a well-circumscribed plaque in the reticular dermis and may extend into the upper subcutis (Fig. 33-12A and B).[81,83]

Histogenesis. Immunohistochemical reactivity for vimentin and nonspecific muscle actin and the ultrastructural features suggest myofibroblastic differentiation in this recently described neoplasm.[81,83]

Differential Diagnosis. The orientation parallel to the epidermis of monomorphic spindle cells and their location in the reticular dermis and upper subcutis have been suggested as points of distinction from benign fibrous histiocytoma, whereas the immunohistochemical features of these two lesions are similar. Dermatomyofibroma may also resemble DFSP, but the former lesion does not express CD34.[83]

MALIGNANT FIBROUS HISTIOCYTOMA

Malignant fibrous histiocytoma is a pleomorphic sarcoma that represents the most common soft tissue sarcoma of middle

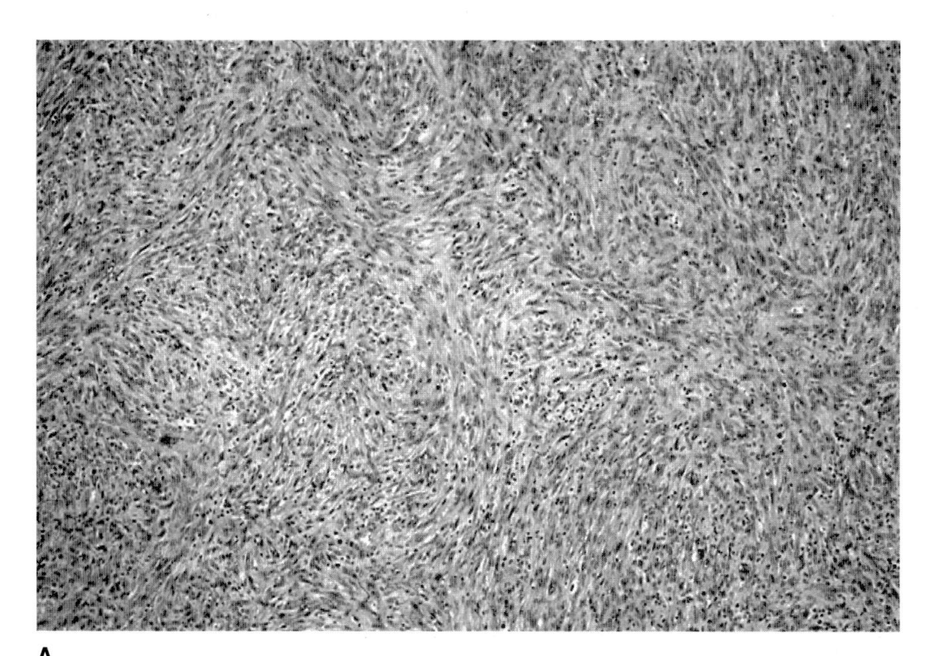

A

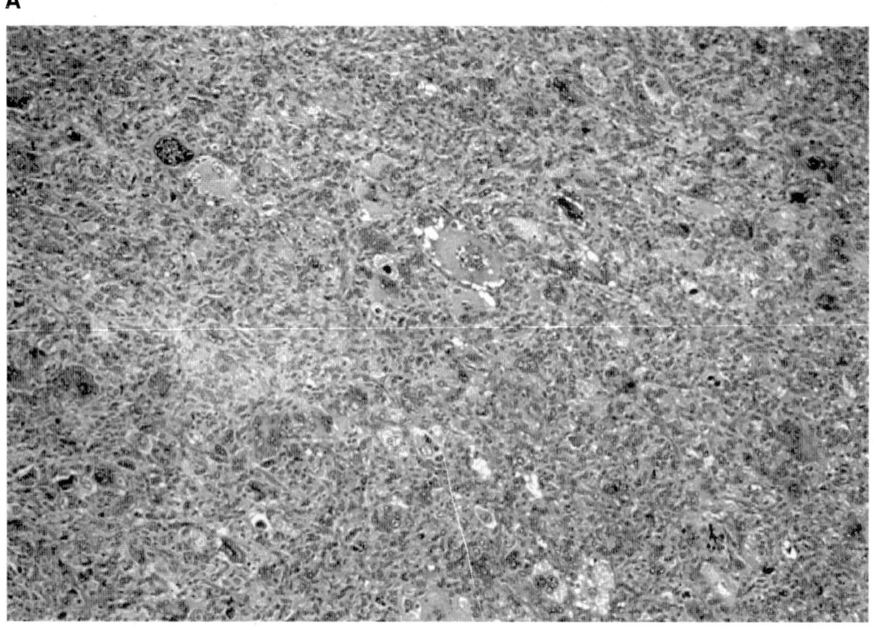

B

FIG. 33-13. Malignant fibrous histiocytoma
(**A**) The tumor is composed of densely cellular, pleomorphic spindle cells arranged in a storiform pattern. (**B**) Spindle cells are intermingled with numerous giant cells with markedly pleomorphic single and multiple nuclei.

and late adulthood.[84] The most common sites of origin are the proximal extremities, particularly the thigh and buttock.[84] The tumors are multilobular fleshy masses, often apparently circumscribed on gross examination, although the microscopic growth pattern is frequently infiltrative along fascial planes and between muscle fibers, accounting for the high rate of local recurrence.[70] Involvement of the dermis, occasionally with ulceration, is rare;[85] most tumors occur in striated muscle, less than 10% being confined to the subcutis.[70] Metastasis is related to tumor size, depth, and grade.[70] The rates of local recurrence and metastasis have improved in recent studies, probably because of more effective primary surgical therapy. A recent study of prognostic factors reported a local recurrence rate of 25%, a metastatic rate of 34%, and an overall survival rate of 50%.[86]

Histopathology. Malignant fibrous histiocytoma is a highly cellular, pleomorphic tumor composed of fibroblastlike spindle cells, histiocytelike cells, foam cells, and giant cells. Mitotic figures, including atypical forms, are plentiful.[26, 87] Four subtypes are recognized:

1. Storiform-pleomorphic[84,88]
2. Myxoid (myxofibrosarcoma)[89,90]
3. Giant cell (malignant giant cell tumor of soft parts)[91]
4. Inflammatory (xanthosarcoma, malignant xanthogranuloma)[92]

Angiomatoid fibrous histiocytoma, formerly regarded as another subtype of malignant fibrous histiocytoma,[93] has been reclassified as a fibrohistiocytic tumor of intermediate grade[94] on the basis of its excellent prognosis.[43]

The most common variant is the storiform-pleomorphic type, composed of spindle cells, plump histiocytelike cells, and pleomorphic multinucleate giant cells. The spindle cells are arranged in whorled or storiform pattern, with a delicate collagenous stroma (Fig. 33-13A and B). Those tumors composed of a high proportion of relatively uniform spindle cells in a storiform pattern may resemble DFSP, whereas other tumors are anaplastic. The myxoid variant shows marked myxoid change in the stroma and more cellular foci of pleomorphic type. The giant cell variant contains osteoclastlike giant cells with abundant cytoplasm and numerous vesicular nuclei of uniform size.[12] The inflammatory variant is characterized by a dense infiltrate of neutrophils and numerous xanthoma cells, as seen in fibroxanthosarcoma.[92]

Histogenesis. It was originally assumed that malignant fibrous histiocytoma was composed of malignant histiocytes capable of acting as facultative fibroblasts.[95,96] Electron microscopic studies, however, indicate that the progenitor cell in malignant fibrous histiocytoma is a mesenchymal cell capable of showing both histiocytic and fibroblastic differentiation.[26,97] It has recently been shown that some tumors demonstrating the light microscopic criteria for malignant fibrous histiocytoma also express intermediate filaments including keratin.[98–100] It has also been suggested that pleomorphic malignant fibrous histiocytoma may not be a distinct entity, but rather a collection of mesenchymal and nonmesenchymal tumors in which a large proportion could be reclassified more specifically on the basis of careful examination of extensively sampled material, immunohistochemistry, and electron microscopy.[101] Atypical fibroxanthoma is histologically indistinguishable from pleomorphic malignant fibrous histiocytoma, its almost invariably benign course being attributed to its superficial location in the dermis.[102] Lesions reported as metastasizing atypical fibroxanthoma are regarded by other authorities as malignant fibrous histiocytomas on the basis of their deep invasion, necrosis, or vascular invasion.[102]

ANGIOMATOID FIBROUS HISTIOCYTOMA

This tumor was previously termed "angiomatoid malignant fibrous histiocytoma."[93] In recognition of the relatively good prognosis of this distinctive neoplasm of children and young adults,[43] however, the term *malignant* has been deleted from the title.[94] The tumor occurs most often on the extremities as a slowly growing nodular or cystic mass of the dermis or subcutis, sometimes associated with systemic systems, including anemia, pyrexia, and weight loss, and less often with local pain and tenderness.

Histopathology. The tumors characteristically include hemorrhagic cystic spaces, sheets of histiocytelike cells, and an infiltrate of lymphocytes and plasma cells. The lymphoid tissue may include follicles with germinal centers and a thick pseudocapsule, thus resembling lymph node architecture. The hemorrhagic cystic structures are lined by flattened tumor cells rather than endothelium.

Histogenesis. Immunohistochemical studies have produced conflicting results with regard to histiocytic differentiation.[42,103] The expression of desmin in some cases has been interpreted as evidence of myoid or myofibroblastic differentiation.[42]

ATYPICAL FIBROXANTHOMA (PSEUDOSARCOMA, PARADOXICAL FIBROSARCOMA)

Atypical fibroxanthoma is a pleomorphic spindle cell neoplasm of the dermis that, despite apparently malignant histologic features, usually follows an indolent or locally aggressive course. It is a fairly common tumor, first described in 1963[104] and interpreted as a benign reactive lesion.[105,106] Because a small number of metastases have been reported, atypical fibroxanthoma has become regarded as a neoplasm of low-grade malignancy related to malignant fibrous histiocytoma, from which it is indistinguishable histologically.[107,108] According to this view, the more favorable prognosis of atypical fibroxanthoma is related to its small size and superficial location.[108] The specificity of pleomorphic malignant fibrous histiocytoma as an entity, its relationship with atypical fibroxanthoma, and the precise nature of cases of atypical fibroxanthoma reported to have metastasized[109,110] have recently been questioned.[31] Atypical fibroxanthoma usually presents as a solitary nodule less than 2 cm in diameter on the exposed skin of the head and neck or dorsum of the hand of elderly patients, often with a short history of rapid growth. The lesions are usually associated with severe actinic damage, and a few have arisen in areas treated by radiation. Several cases described on the trunk and extremities of younger persons[111,112] may have represented cases of atypical benign fibrous histiocytoma.[113]

Histopathology. Atypical fibroxanthoma is an exophytic, densely cellular neoplasm, unencapsulated but with only lim-

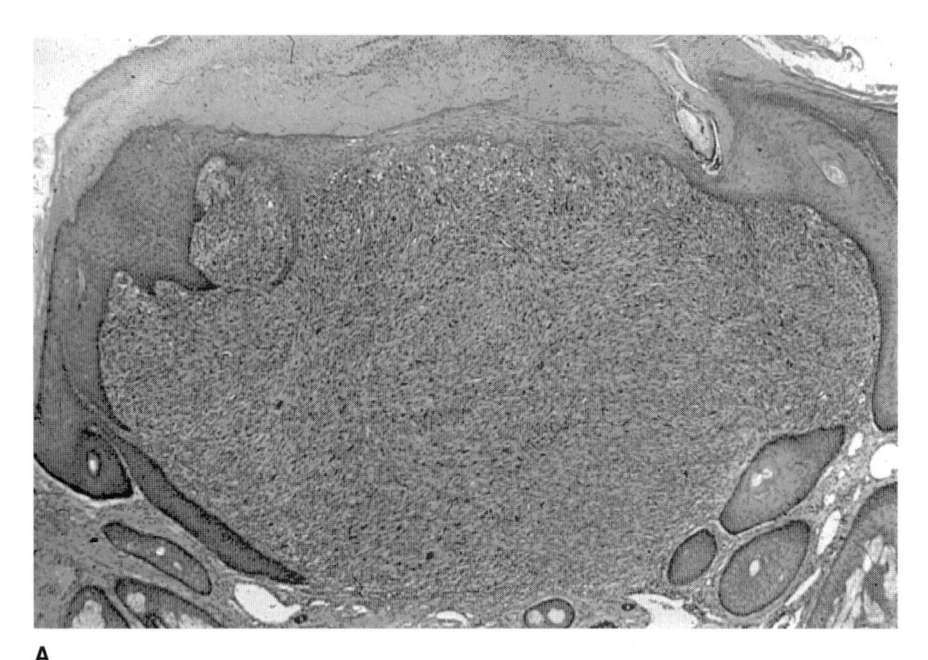

A

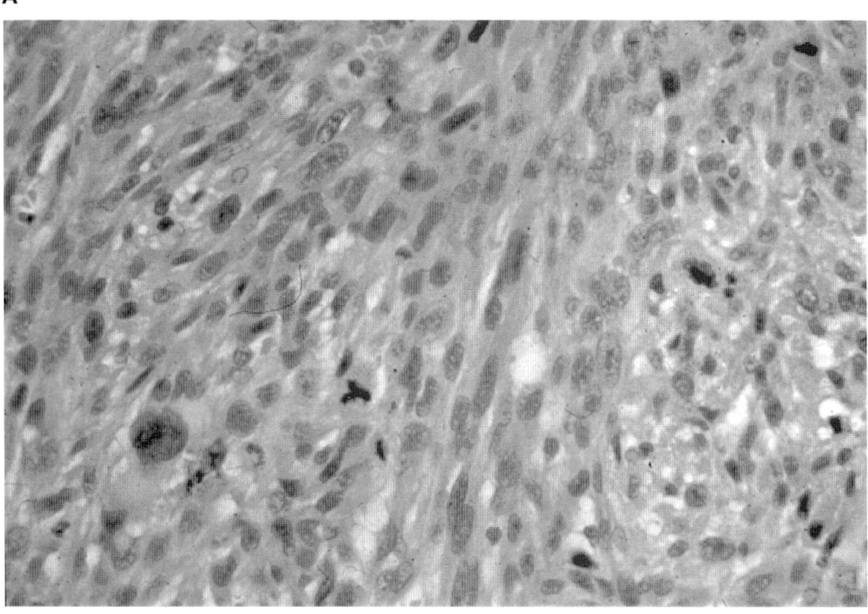

B

FIG. 33-14. Atypical fibroxanthoma
(**A**) The tumor is an exophytic densely cellular nodule, with a collarette of epidermis. (**B**) The cytologic characteristics are very similar to those of malignant fibrous histiocytoma, with pleomorphic spindle cells and giant cells with scattered mitoses, including atypical forms.

ited infiltration of the stroma, frequently with an epidermal collarette (Fig. 33-14A). The tumor may extend to the dermoepidermal junction, but there is no direct continuity with the squamous epithelium, although ulceration is often present. Severe solar elastosis is present in the adjacent dermis. The classical tumor is composed of pleomorphic histiocytelike cells and atypical giant cells, often with bizarre nuclei[106,111] and numerous mitotic figures, including abnormal forms (see Fig. 33-14B).[108] The cells are arranged in compact, although disorderly pattern, surrounding but not destroying adnexal structures. Fibroblastlike spindle cells are present in variable numbers; cells of morphology intermediate between these spindle cells and histiocytelike cells are also present.[107,114] Scattered inflammatory cells and numerous small blood vessels are present, commonly with focal hemorrhage.

The spindle cell variant of atypical fibroxanthoma consists of eosinophilic spindle cells with vesicular nuclei and eosinophilic nucleoli arranged in fascicular pattern.[115]

Histogenesis. Electron microscopic[107,116] and immunohistochemical[64,117] studies indicate that, as for malignant fibrous histiocytoma, the progenitor cell is an undifferentiated mesenchymal cell, capable of showing histiocytic, fibroblastic, and myofibroblastic differentiation.

Differential Diagnosis. The histologic features of most cases

TABLE 33-1. *Suggested immunohistochemical reactions as an aid to the differential diagnosis of cutaneous spindle cell tumors*

	Epithelioid sarcoma	Atypical fibroxanthoma	Dermato-fibrosarcoma protuberans	Cellular benign fibrous histiocytoma	Spindle cell squamous cell carcinoma	Desmoplastic melanoma	Leiomyo-sarcoma
Cytokeratin	+	−	−	−	+	−	−
Vimentin	+	+	+	+	−	+	+
S-100	−	−	−	−	−	+	−
Desmin	−	R	−	−	−	−	+
CD34	V	V	+	V	−	−	−
Factor XIIIa	U	V	V	+	U	U	U
Epithelial membrane antigen	+	−	−	−	−	−	−

This table is limited to reagents in common use. It is emphasized that the immunohistochemical reactions should be regarded as adjuncts to routine histological methods.
V = variable; R = rare; U = unknown.

of atypical fibroxanthoma are diagnostic. In some cases, especially the less pleomorphic tumors, immunohistochemical staining is helpful in distinguishing atypical fibroxanthoma from other spindle cell neoplasms. Atypical fibroxanthoma expresses vimentin and is nonreactive for cytokeratin, S-100 protein, and usually desmin, thereby excluding spindle cell squamous cell carcinoma, spindle cell melanoma, and most cases of leiomyosarcoma (Table 33-1).[64]

EPITHELIOID SARCOMA

Epithelioid sarcoma, thus designated by Enzinger[118] in 1970, is a distinctive rare malignant soft tissue neoplasm of uncertain origin, occurring most commonly in the distal extremities of young adult males as a slowly growing dermal or subcutaneous nodule (Color Fig. 33-1).[119] However, the tumor has been reported in a wide range of anatomic sites, including the head and neck region and the pelvis in children,[120,121] the penis,[122,123] and the vulva.[124,125] This aggressive neoplasm is characterized by multiple recurrences, often producing ulcerated nodules and plaques in the dermis and subcutis. In the study of Chase and Enzinger,[119] 77% of cases developed one or more recurrences, and metastases occurred in 45% of the patients. The most important prognostic factors are sex of the patient and size of the tumor.[126,127] The more favorable prognosis for females is emphasized by the study of Bos et al.,[126] in which the 5-year survival rate was 80% for females, as against 40% for males.

Histopathology. The tumors are composed of irregular nodules of atypical epithelioid cells with abundant eosinophilic cytoplasm and pleomorphic nuclei, merging with spindle cells. These aggregates are embedded in collagenous fibrous tissue in which there may be focal hemorrhage, hemosiderin, and mucin deposition with a patchy lymphocytic infiltrate. Mitoses are present in varied frequency, vascular invasion is a common feature, and foci of necrosis are present in the centers of tumor nodules. Ulceration follows epidermal involvement by the larger tumor nodules, and invasion extends diffusely into the subcutis and deeper soft tissues (Fig. 33-15A–C).

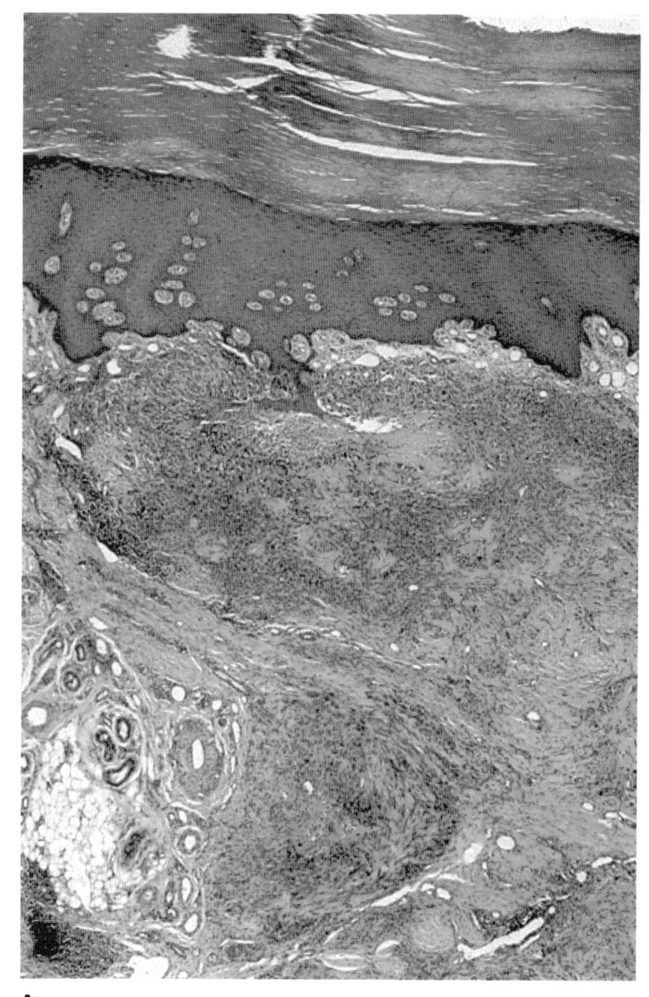

A

FIG. 33-15. Epithelioid sarcoma
(**A**) The epidermis is hyperplastic and overlies several poorly defined nodules in the dermis with central foci of necrosis. *(continued on next page)*

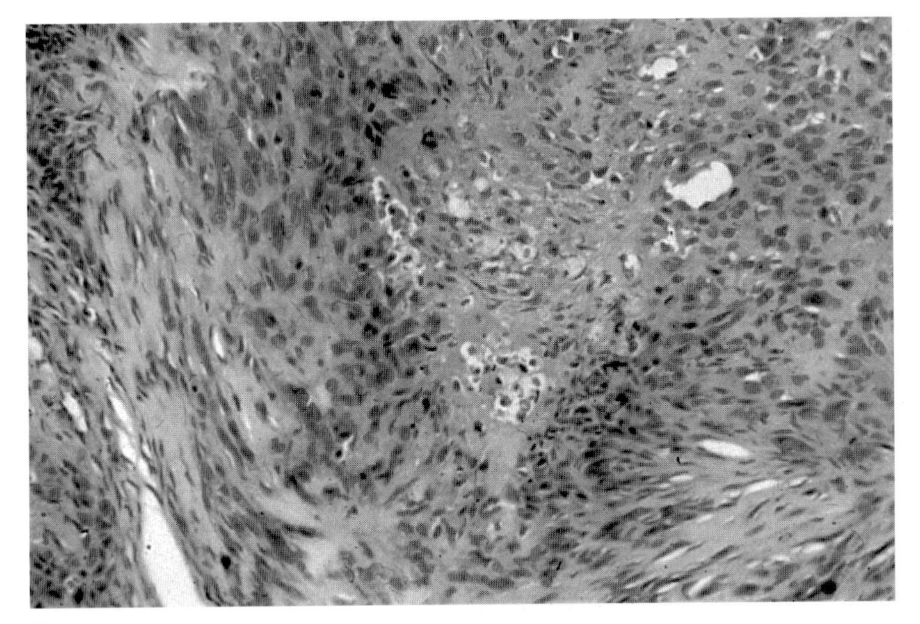

B

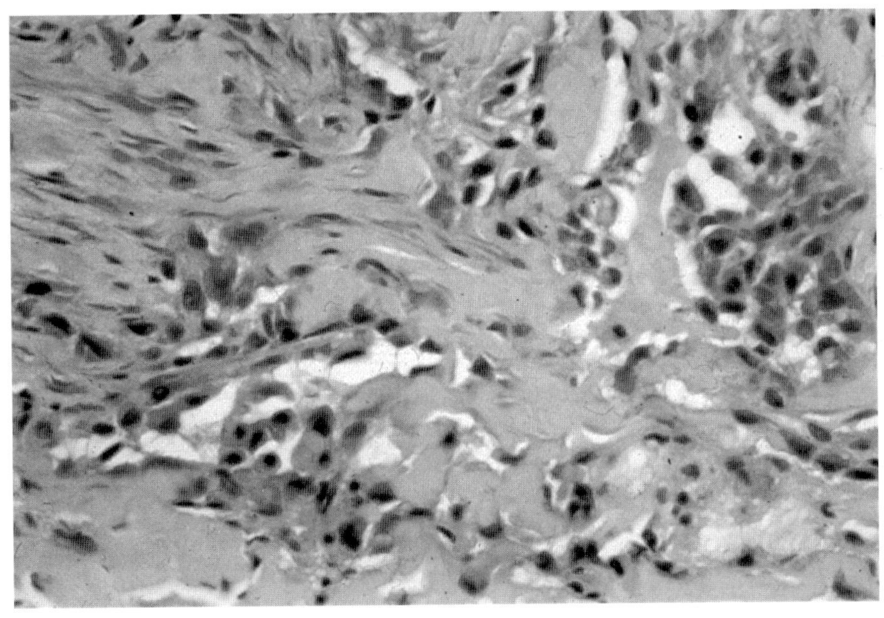

C

FIG. 33-15. ***Continued***
(**B**) Epithelioid cells with eosinophilic cytoplasm and pleomorphic nuclei surround a central zone of necrosis. (**C**) Atypical epithelioid cells line irregular spaces, producing an angiosarcomalike pattern, with spindle cells in the intervening stroma.

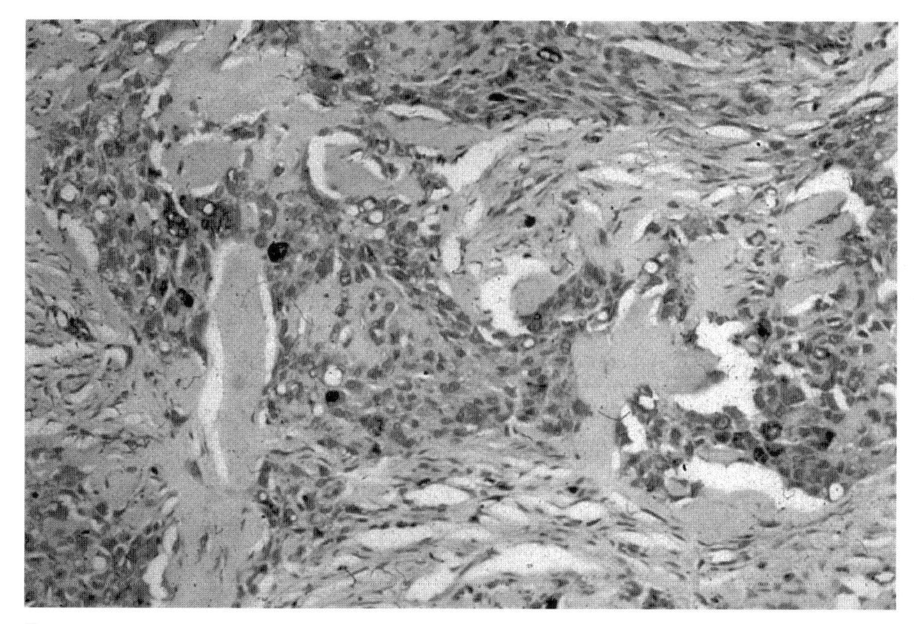

D

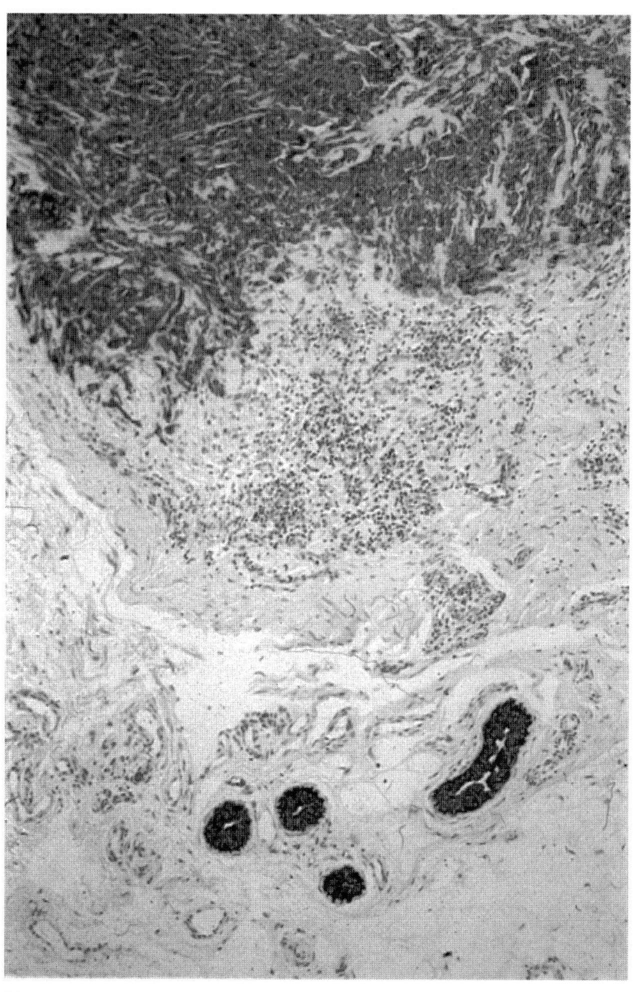

E

FIG. 33-15. ***Continued***
(**D**) Positive immunostaining for vimentin in the tumor cells. (**E**) Intensely positive immunostaining for cytokeratins AE1 and AE3.

A fibromalike variant of epithelioid sarcoma has also been reported, in which the spindle cell pattern predominates without the characteristic epithelioid cells and nodularity.[128]

Histogenesis. The histogenesis of epithelioid sarcoma is still uncertain, but the ultrastructural features of desmosomelike intercellular junctions, numerous microvilli, and whorled arrangements of intermediate filaments,[120,129,130] together with positive immunostaining for epithelial membrane antigen, cytokeratin, and vimentin,[121,130] suggest an origin from primitive mesenchymal cells with the capacity for epithelial differentiation.[130] A recent report, however, described three cases of epithelioid sarcoma showing strong positivity for cytokeratin and epithelial membrane antigen while failing to react for vimentin. Staining for CD34 was positive in these cases, possibly representing a unique immunophenotypic variant (see Table 33-1).[131]

Differential Diagnosis. At low power, the neoplasm may suggest a granulomatous process such as granuloma annulare, necrobiosis lipoidica, or rheumatoid nodule. The cellular atypia, diffuse stromal invasion, and foci of necrosis involving tumor cells and not only stroma, as in the necrobiotic granulomatous processes,[129] identify the process as malignant, and the diagnosis is supported by positive immunostaining for cytokeratin and vimentin (Fig. 33-15D and E).[119,130,132] and negativity for leucocyte common antigen.[133] Epithelioid sarcoma may also be confused with other neoplasms, including malignant fibrous histiocytoma, synovial sarcoma, fibrosarcoma, angiosarcoma, epithelioid hemangioendothelioma, malignant extrarenal rhabdoid tumor, and amelanotic melanoma; the characteristic clinical, morphologic, and immunocytochemical features usually permit the distinction from these tumors, although the diagnosis may present difficulty. Although epithelioid sarcoma, like synovial sarcoma, shows both mesenchymal and epithelial differentiation, it lacks the characteristic biphasic pattern of synovial sarcoma.[133]

SYNOVIAL SARCOMA

Synovial sarcoma most commonly occurs on the extremities, particularly the thigh. Superficial lesions adjacent to joints of the foot or hand sometimes present with dermal involvement.[134]

Histopathology. The tumor typically presents a biphasic pattern including an epithelioid cell component forming pseudoglandular spaces, and a spindle cell component resembling fibrosarcoma (Fig. 33-16). One of the two patterns, however, may predominate.[134] Immunostaining demonstrates reactivity for low- and high-molecular-weight cytokeratins in both the epithelioid and spindle cells, with less intense positivity for epithelial membrane antigen; vimentin is present in the spindle cells but not in the epithelioid cells.[135–137] According to one report, the expression of cytokeratins 7 and 19 and desmoplakin is specific for synovial sarcoma, whereas the presence of cytokeratins 8 and 18 is shared with some other spindle cell neoplasms, including epithelioid sarcoma.[136] The epithelioid cells and pseudoglandular spaces contain mucin of the epithelial type, whereas the spindle cells produce mesenchymal mucin.

Histogenesis. Immunohistochemical and ultrastructural differences between normal synovial cells and the cells of synovial sarcoma indicate that the tumor may not be derived from synovium, leading to suggestions of alternative terms, including connective tissue carcinosarcoma and soft tissue carcinoma.[138,139] An immunohistochemical study of the distribution of collagens, fibronectin, laminin, and tenascin in synovial sarcoma has produced results suggesting resemblances between synovial sarcoma and the embryonic development of epithelia

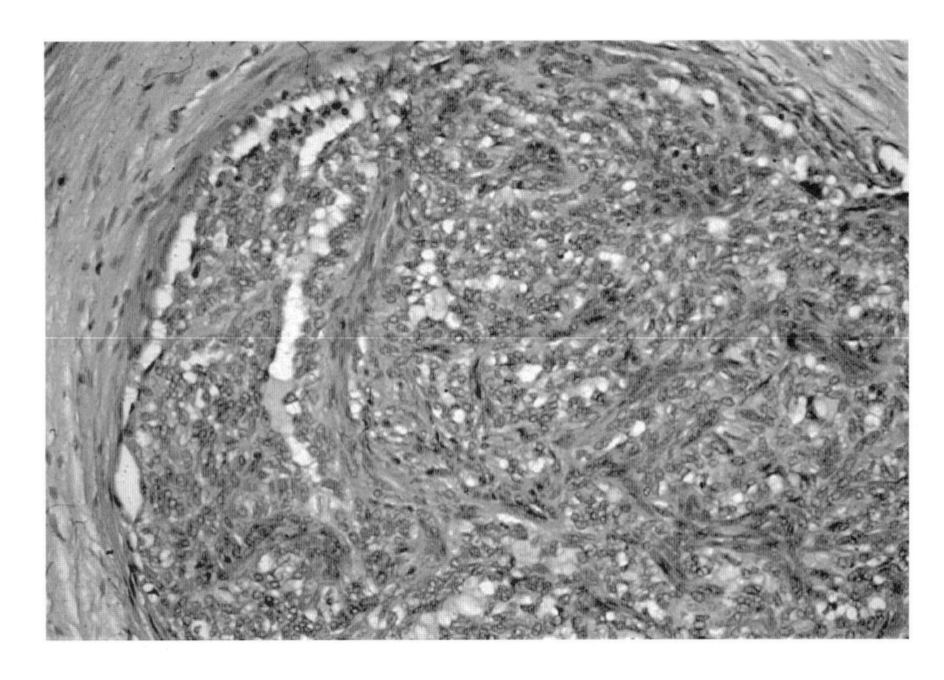

FIG. 33-16. Synovial sarcoma The classical biphasic pattern of epithelioid cells forming pseudoglandular spaces surrounded by spindle cells.

from mesenchymal cells, supporting the concept that synovial sarcomas are soft tissue carcinosarcomas.[140]

INFANTILE DIGITAL FIBROMATOSIS (RECURRING DIGITAL FIBROUS TUMOR OF CHILDHOOD, INCLUSION BODY FIBROMATOSIS)

In infantile digital fibromatosis, single or multiple nodules are present on the fingers or toes, excluding the great toe and the thumb. They may be present at birth, but they usually appear during the first year of life or, less commonly, later in childhood. The nodules rarely exceed 2 cm in diameter and involute spontaneously. In about 75% of the cases, recurrences are observed during early childhood.[141]

Histopathology. The dermis is infiltrated by uniform spindle cells and collagen bundles arranged in interlacing fascicles, extending from just below the epidermis into the subcutis (Fig. 33-17A). A characteristic diagnostic feature is the presence of eosinophilic cytoplasmic inclusion bodies, often indenting the

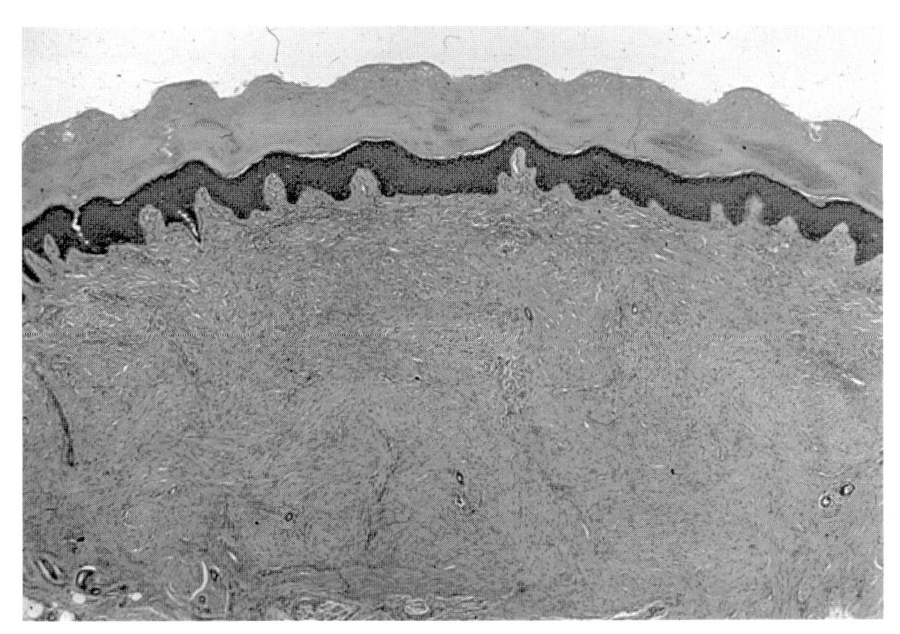

A

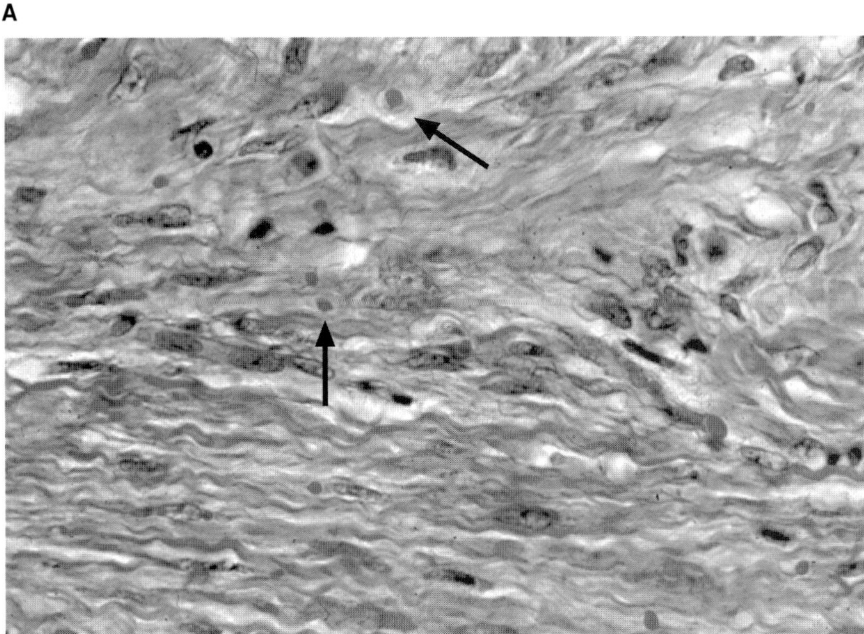

B

FIG. 33-17. Infantile digital fibromatosis
(**A**) Interlacing fascicles extend from the papillary dermis into the subcutis. (**B**) Fascicles of spindle cells, some of which contain small, round, eosinophilic, cytoplasmic inclusions (*arrows*).

nucleus (see Fig. 33-17B). These bodies measure from 3 to 10 μm in diameter.[142] In hematoxylin-eosin sections they resemble erythrocytes; these inclusions stain deep red with Masson trichome and purple with phosphotungstic acid–hematoxylin.

Histogenesis. Ultrastructurally, the spindle cells contain narrow bundles of filaments arranged longitudinally within the cell. Dense bodies of the type seen in the contractile apparatus of smooth muscle cells are distributed along each bundle, some of which are attached to the cell membrane. These features suggest that the tumor cells are myofibroblasts and that the bundles are composed of myofilaments.[143] The inclusion bodies are non-membrane-bound, granular-filamentous structures with elongated processes of 5 to 12 nm-filaments[143] containing condensations (dense bodies).[144] The cytoplasmic bodies are composed, at least partially, of actin. Immunocytochemical staining for vimentin and actin in the tumor cells supports their myofibroblastic nature.[145,146]

ACQUIRED DIGITAL FIBROKERATOMA

A solitary rounded, firm, more or less hyperkeratotic projection is seen most commonly on a finger or toe, and occasionally on the palms or soles.[147] Some fibrokeratomas appear to originate from the proximal nail fold.[148] The outgrowth is either elongated or dome-shaped, and if dome-shaped, often slightly pedunculated. It protrudes from a collarette of slightly raised skin. In contrast to infantile digital fibromatosis, acquired fibrokeratoma occurs in adults.

Histopathology. The epidermis shows marked hyperkeratosis and acanthosis with thickened, often branching rete ridges. The core of the lesion is formed by thick, interwoven bundles of collagen predominantly oriented in the direction of the vertical axis of the lesion (Fig. 33-18).[149] Elastic fibers are usually present but are apt to be thin and scanty.[150] Many tumors are highly vascular.[147]

Differential Diagnosis. Although acquired digital fibrokeratoma may resemble a rudimentary supernumerary digit in its clinical and histologic appearance, rudimentary polydactyly almost always occurs at the base of the fifth finger, is present from birth, and is often bilateral. Histologically, rudimentary polydactyly differs from digital fibrokeratoma by the presence of numerous nerve bundles, especially at the base of the lesion.[149]

FOLLICULAR FIBROMA (TRICHODISCOMA, FIBROFOLLICULOMA, PERIFOLLICULAR FIBROMA)

Perifollicular fibroma, fibrofolliculoma, and trichodiscoma are distinct, rare tumors of the pilosebaceous mesenchyme, probably hamartomas. Their clinical features are similar; they occur as small, flat, or dome-shaped lesions, usually multiple, on the face, trunk, and extremities.[73,151–156] Multiple fibrofolliculomas and trichodiscomas may occur in association with fibroepithelial polyps as a triad known as the Birt-Hogg-Dubé syndrome, which is inherited as an autosomal dominant trait.[152,157,158] Perifollicular fibromas may be solitary[159] or multiple[160] and may be associated with fibrofolliculomas, trichodiscomas,[161] and colonic polyps.[155]

Histopathology. Trichodiscoma is a sharply defined fibrovascular lesion of the superficial dermis, sometimes associated with an adjacent hair follicle. The overlying epidermis is flattened, and the fibrillar collagen of the elliptical parafollicular lesion contains abundant connective tissue mucin. Fibrofolliculoma consists of a circumscribed proliferation of compact collagen and fibroblasts surrounding one or more distorted keratin-plugged hair follicles from which interlocking strands of basaloid cells protrude into the surrounding stroma. Perifollicular fibroma comprises concentric layers of cellular fibrous tis-

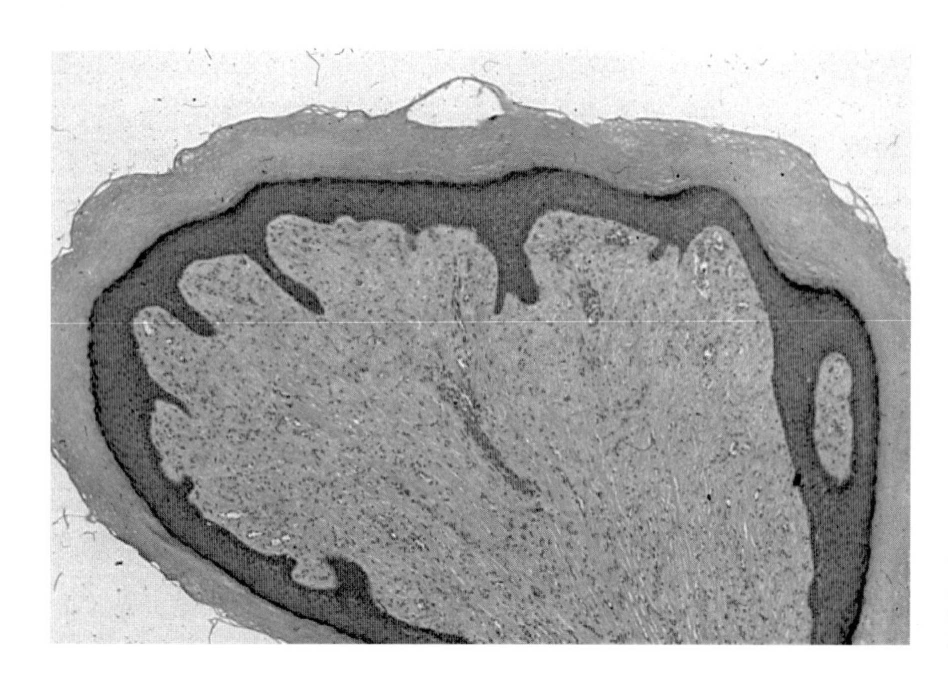

FIG. 33-18. Digital fibrokeratoma A polypoid lesion with acanthotic epidermis overlying collagen bundles oriented mainly in the vertical plane.

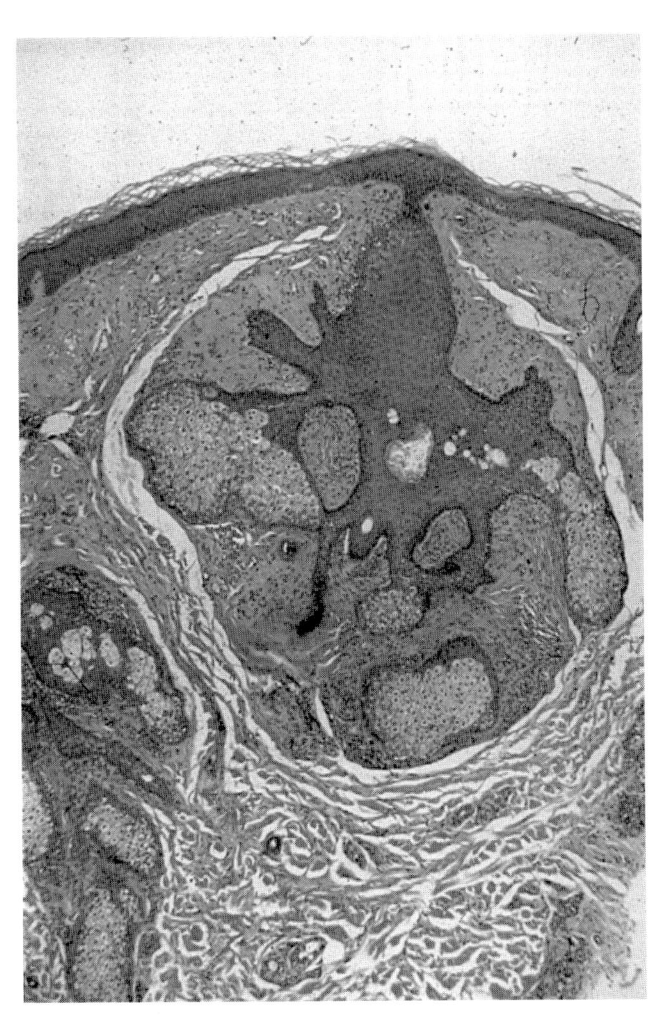

FIG. 33-19. Perifollicular fibroma
A circumscribed zone of compact cellular fibrous tissue surrounds a central pilosebaceous complex.

sue in perifollicular arrangement, without the interlocking strands of proliferating epithelium seen in fibrofolliculoma (Fig. 33-19).

Histogenesis. Trichodiscoma is believed to arise from the hair disk, which is a specialized component of the perifollicular mesenchyme, overlying which the epidermis contains Merkel cells.[151]

FIBROUS PAPULE OF THE FACE

Fibrous papule of the face, a common lesion, occurs in mature persons nearly always as a solitary lesion on the lower portion of the nose or on the adjacent skin of the face. It is usually dome-shaped, firm, and small, not exceeding 5 mm in diameter. In most cases it is skin-colored, but it may be red or slightly pigmented. Originally described as an involuting melanocytic nevus,[162,163] subsequent reports suggest that this lesion represents an angiofibroma.[164,165]

Histopathology. The epidermis is raised, overlying a localized area of fibroplasia and vascular proliferation in the upper dermis. In nearly all cases, there are scattered, large triangular and stellate cells, some of which may be multinucleated.[165,166] In some cases, an increased number of melanocytes is seen at the dermoepidermal junction (Fig. 33-20).

Histogenesis. The prevalence of melanocytes at the dermoepidermal junction and the resemblance of the large triangular and stellate cells in the dermis to nevus giant cells explain why authors in the past have regarded fibrous papules of the face as involuting melanocytic nevi. However, electron microscopic studies[167,168] have identified the triangular or stellate cells as fibroblasts rather than melanocytes. Several studies have shown that the spindle and stellate cells of fibrous papule express factor XIIIa but not S-100 protein, indicating that the tumors are composed of dermal dendritic cells or dermal fibroblasts rather than melanocytic nevus cells.[169–173]

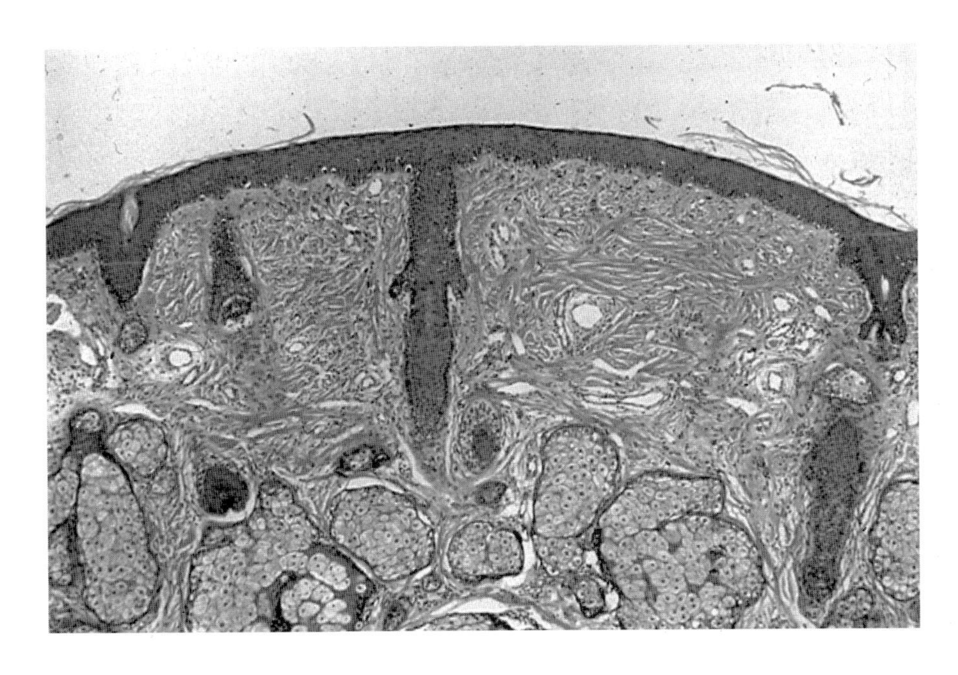

FIG. 33-20. Fibrous papule of the face
The epidermis is slightly raised and overlies a zone of vascular fibroplasia in the superficial dermis, with scattered spindle and stellate cells in the upper layers.

Differential Diagnosis. Because the facial lesions of tuberous sclerosis also show angiofibrosis and may contain stellate cells, differentiation from fibrous papule of the face may require clinical data.[174]

TUBEROUS SCLEROSIS

Tuberous sclerosis, a dominantly inherited disorder, is characterized by the triad of mental deficiency, epilepsy, and angiofibromas of the face. The triad is not necessarily complete. The angiofibromas consist of numerous small, red, smooth papules in symmetric distribution in the nasolabial folds, on the cheeks, and on the chin. Other organs are frequently involved.[175]

Additional cutaneous manifestations may include asymmetrically arranged, large, raised, soft, brown fibromas on the face and the scalp, subungual and periungual fibromas, and so-called shagreen patches, usually found in the lumbosacral region and consisting of slightly raised and thickened areas of the skin. Scattered hypopigmented, leaf-shaped areas are present in more than half of the patients with tuberous sclerosis, and best visualized with the aid of a Wood light. Their diagnostic significance lies in the fact that they are present at birth or appear very early in life and thus are the earliest cutaneous sign of tuberous sclerosis.[176]

Systemic Lesions. Multiple tumors are commonly found in the brain (gliomas, often calcified),[177] retina (gliomas),[178] heart (rhabdomyomas),[179] and kidneys (angiomyolipomas).[180]

Histopathology. In the past, the symmetrically distributed, small, red angiofibromas of the face were mistakenly called adenoma sebaceum of Pringle. However, the sebaceous glands are generally atrophic, and the main findings are dermal fibrosis and dilatation of some of the capillaries. In some lesions, the fibrosis has a "glial" appearance because of the large size and stellate shape of the fibroblasts. Occasionally, multinucleated giant cells are also present. In some cases, one observes vascular proliferation and perivascular proliferation of fibroblasts in addition to vascular dilatation.[174] In old lesions, there may be perifollicular proliferation of collagen, leading to the compression of atrophic hair follicles by concentric layers of collagen. Elastic tissue is absent in the angiofibromas (Fig. 33-21A and B).

The larger, asymmetric fibromas on the face and scalp show markedly sclerotic collagen arranged in thick, concentric layers around atrophic pilosebaceous follicles. In contrast to the smaller lesions, dilated capillaries usually are absent. Giant angiofibroma[181] and a cluster growth of large nodules[182] have also been reported.

The ungual fibromas show fibrosis, usually without but occasionally with capillary dilatation. The areas of fibrosis may have a glial appearance because of the presence of large stellate fibroblasts.[174,183]

The shagreen patches show two somewhat different types of changes in the collagen. In the more common variety, a dense, sclerotic mass of very broad collagenous bundles is seen in the lower dermis, mimicking the appearance of morphea. In the other type, normal collagen bundles throughout the dermis are seen in an interwoven pattern, so that some bundles are cut transversely and others longitudinally. The elastic tissue in some instances shows fragmentation and clumping[174] but generally is reduced in amount.[184]

The hypopigmented, leaf-shaped areas show a normal number of melanocytes with decreased pigmentation. On electron microscopy, the melanosomes within the melanocytes and keratinocytes are smaller and show less melanization than normal melanosomes.[176,184]

Differential Diagnosis. The angiofibromas of tuberous sclerosis are histologically indistinguishable from the solitary angiofibroma or fibrous papule of the face or nose. The shagreen patches of tuberous sclerosis differ from other connective tissue nevi by the regular absence of any increase in elastic tissue.

ELASTOFIBROMA

A deep-seated, firm mass, usually several centimeters in diameter, is observed most commonly in the lower subscapular area in elderly individuals. Since elastofibroma occurs rarely at sites other than the back, this term is preferred to the original title of *elastofibroma dorsi.*[185]

Histopathology. The mass consists of dense bundles of collagen interspersed with many thick, deeply eosinophilic, homogeneous elastic fibers, some of which have a beaded appearance.[186] In the course of further degeneration, the thick elastic fibers may become wavy and disintegrate into numerous small eosinophilic globules.[187]

Histogenesis. Elastofibroma appears to be the result of excessive formation of collagen and abnormal elastic fibers secondary to repeated injury. It has also been suggested that the lesion may be the result of disturbed elastic fibrillogenesis by periosteal-derived cells.[188]

SOFT FIBROMA

Soft fibromas, also called "fibroepithelial polyps," "acrochordons" or "cutaneous tags," occur as three types: (1) multiple small, furrowed papules, especially on the neck and in the axillae, generally only 1 to 2 mm long; (2) single or multiple filiform, smooth growths in varying locations, about 2 mm wide and 5 mm long; and (3) solitary baglike, pedunculated growths, usually about 1 cm in diameter but occasionally much larger, seen most commonly on the lower trunk.[189,190]

Several reports have suggested an association between the presence of soft fibroma and colonic polyps,[191–194] diabetes,[195–197] and acromegaly.[198] The association with colonic polyps, however, has not been confirmed by subsequent reports.[199–201]

Histopathology. The multiple small furrowed papules usually show papillomatosis, hyperkeratosis, and regular acanthosis and occasionally also horn cysts within their acanthotic epidermis. Thus there is often considerable resemblance to a pedunculated seborrheic keratosis.

The filiform, smooth growths show slight to moderate acanthosis and occasionally mild papillomatosis. The connective tissue stalk is composed of loose collagen fibers and often contains numerous dilated capillaries filled with erythrocytes.[189] Nevus cells are found in as many as 30% of the filiform growths, indicating that some of them represent involuting melanocytic nevi.[202]

The baglike, soft fibromas generally show a flattened epidermis overlying loosely arranged collagen fibers and mature fat cells in the center.[190] In some instances, the dermis is quite thin, so that the fat cells compose a significant portion of the tumor, which may then be regarded as a lipofibroma.[203]

Other Histologic Variants

Sclerotic Fibroma

This is composed of interwoven fascicles of collagen bundles with a laminated or tortuous appearance, occurring as a solitary tumor[204] or as multiple papules in patients with Cowden disease.[205]

Pleomorphic Fibroma

Grossly indistinguishable from a fibroepithelial polyp, this variant shows severe nuclear atypia, occasional mitoses, and sparse cellularity. Positive immunostaining for vimentin and actin support a fibroblastic or myofibroblastic origin of these cells.[206]

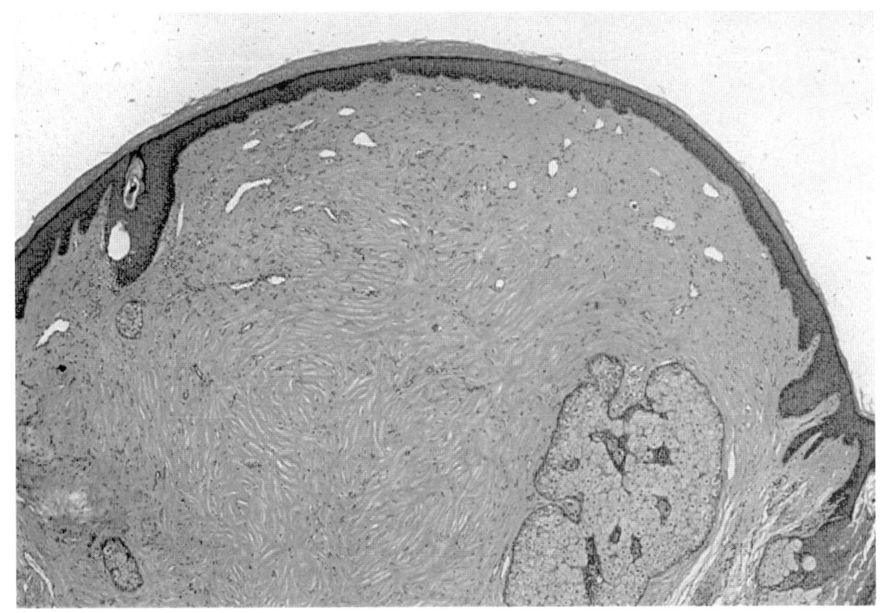

A

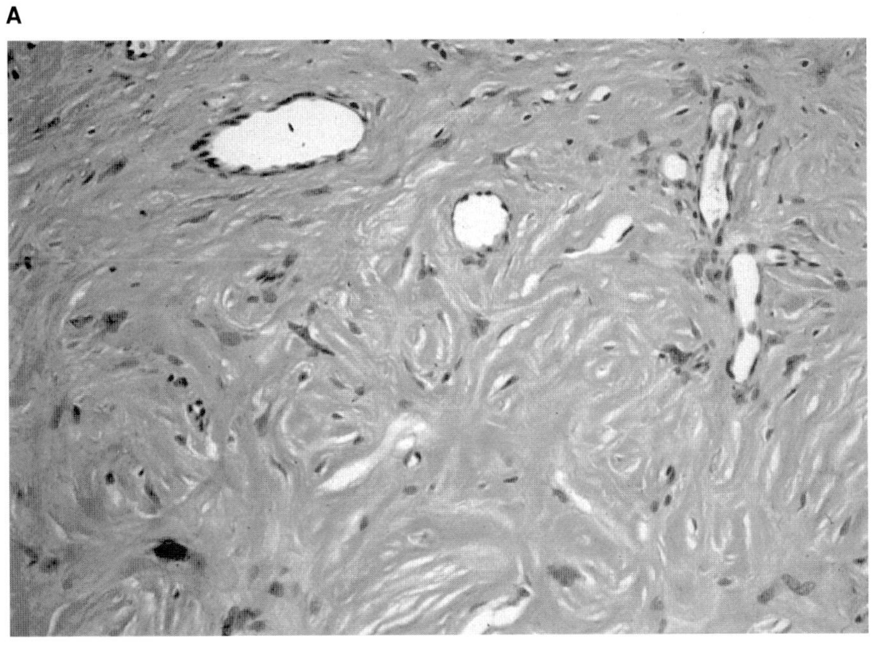

B

FIG. 33-21. Angiofibroma of tuberous sclerosis
(**A**) The epidermis is raised in a dome-shaped pattern overlying a zone of compact fibroplasia with prominent blood vessels in the upper half. (**B**) Sclerotic, hyalinized collagenous stroma, with scattered spindle and stellate cells and telangiectatic blood vessels.

Myoid Fibroma

Occurring in adolescence, this variant forms papules or plaques of cells resembling smooth muscle cells arranged in lobules or fascicles. The immunohistochemical and ultrastructural features support fibroblastic origin.[207]

GIANT CELL TUMOR OF TENDON SHEATH

The giant cell tumor of tendon sheath occurs most commonly on the fingers, hands, and wrists, where it is attached to a tendon sheath. It is firm in consistency with a yellowish tan cut surface and measures from 1 to 3 cm in diameter. There is no tendency toward spontaneous involution. The tumor may extend to the synovium of an adjacent joint space and, on rare occasions, may even extend into the overlying skin.[208]

Histopathology. The tumor consists of lobules of varied cellularity surrounded by dense collagen (Fig. 33-22A). In cellular areas, most cells are plump histiocytelike cells with vesicular nuclei. Often they contain hemosiderin or lipid. Some of the lipid-laden cells have the appearance of foam cells. Less cellular areas consist of spindle cells within a fibrous or hyalinized stroma.[208,209] The characteristic giant cells, often of consider-

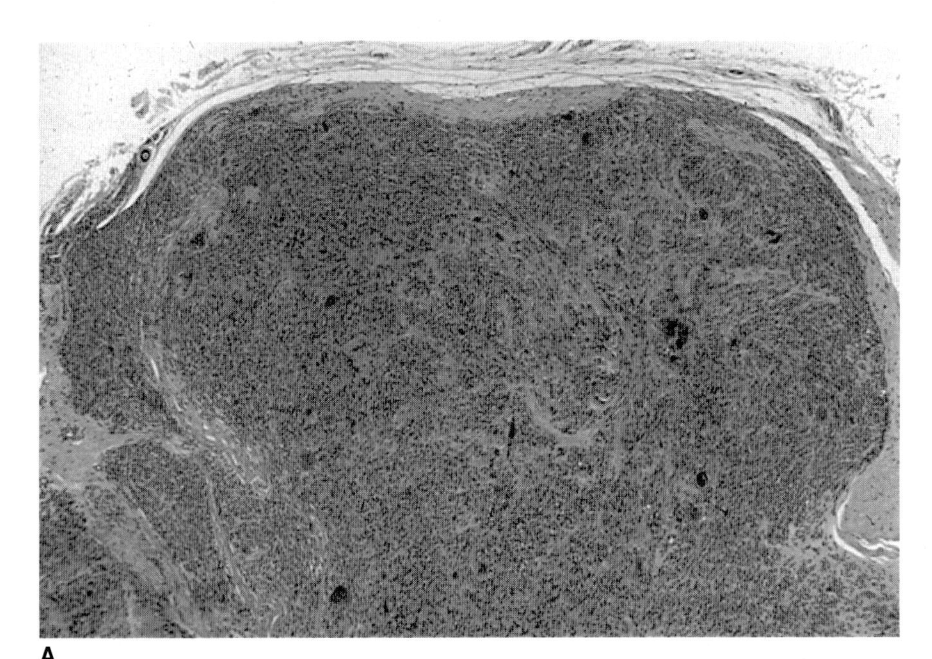

A

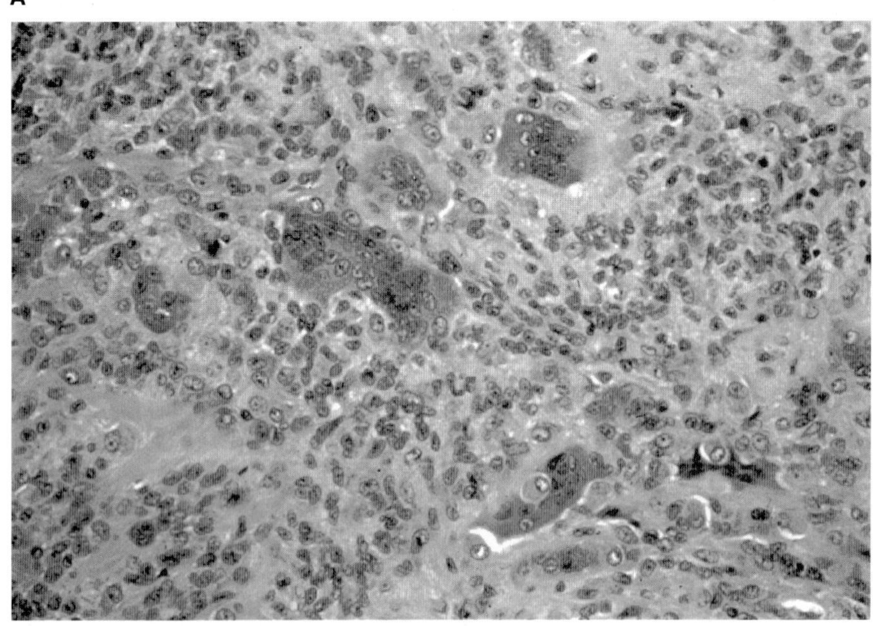

B

FIG. 33-22. Giant cell tumor of tendon sheath
(**A**) The tumor is composed of sharply circumscribed, densely cellular lobules surrounded by fibrofatty tissue. (**B**) Giant cells with multiple nuclei, resembling osteoclasts, are scattered among plump epithelioid and spindle cells.

able size and resembling osteoclasts,[210] are scattered through both the cellular and fibrous areas; their cytoplasm is deeply eosinophilic and they contain a variable number of haphazardly distributed nuclei (see Fig. 33-22B). Although mitotic figures are seen in a large proportion of cases and may be frequent,[211] there is no evidence that mitotic activity is related to metastasis, which is an extremely rare event in these tumors.[212]

Histogenesis. Ultrastructural,[210,213] enzymatic,[214,215] and immunohistochemical studies[214–216] have indicated variously that the cells of this tumor may be related to synovial cells, monocytes, and osteoclasts.

FIBROMA OF TENDON SHEATH

Fibroma of tendon sheath was first described in 1979[217] as a distinct clinicopathologic entity. Its clinical characteristics resemble those of giant cell tumor of tendon sheath.[218]

Histopathology. The lesion is largely composed of interlacing bundles of hyalinized, hypocellular fibrous tissue with occasional more cellular areas.[219] A characteristic feature is the presence of slitlike vascular channels.[218] No foam cells are seen, and multinucleated giant cells are very rare.[219]

Histogenesis. The cells of fibroma of tendon sheath show myofibroblastic differentiation.[220]

NODULAR FASCIITIS (PSEUDOSARCOMATOUS FASCIITIS)

Although nodular fasciitis is a relatively common soft tissue lesion, it was not recognized as an entity until 1955.[221] The lesion is usually a solitary, rapidly developing subcutaneous nodule that reaches its ultimate size of 1 to 5 cm within a few weeks. The lesion is self-limited in duration and thus, even if it is incompletely excised, regresses, usually within a few months.[222] The longest known duration of a nodule is 26 months.[223] Often the lesion is slightly tender. Although the arm is the most common site, the lesion may occur in any subcutaneous area. The overlying skin is freely movable over the nodule. Although most patients are middle-aged, about 5% are infants or children.[224]

The cause is unknown. Although trauma does not seem to play a role, the general view is that nodular fasciitis represents a reactive fibroblastic and vascular proliferation.

Histopathology. Nodular fasciitis occurs as three types according to the plane of soft tissue involved: subcutaneous, intramuscular, and fascial. An outstanding feature of the lesion is the infiltrative manner of growth along several of the thin fibrous septa of the subcutaneous fat, resulting in poor demarcation. The nodule consists of numerous large, pleomorphic fibroblasts growing haphazardly in a vascular stroma containing varying amounts of mucoid ground substance, argyrophilic reticulum fibers, and collagen fibers (Fig. 33-23A).[225,226] The vascular component includes well-formed capillaries and slitlike spaces. Erythrocytes are present, not only in the capillaries and slitlike spaces but also free in the tissue.[225] The fibroblasts show a moderate number of mitoses, which are not atypical. In about half of the cases, small spindle-shaped giant cells are found containing two to six centrally placed nuclei (see Fig. 33-23B).[223] In some instances, degenerate muscle fibers have the appearance of multinucleated giant cells.[227] A scattered chronic inflammatory infiltrate is often present, particularly at the periphery of the nodule.[228] In older lesions, the fibroblasts appear more mature, showing a more compact arrangement of spindle cells with increased production of collagen.[223]

Dermal fasciitis is a rare variant arising within the dermis,[229–231] and another variant, intravascular fasciitis,[231,232] occurs in intimate association with blood vessels, forming small nodules of myofibroblasts, apparently originating from the vessel walls and protruding into the lumen. Proliferative fasciitis appears to be related to nodular fasciitis, but it includes giant cells resembling ganglion cells, similar to those of proliferative myositis and showing an abundant, irregularly outlined, basophilic cytoplasm with one or two large vesicular nuclei.[233,234]

Histogenesis. The spindle cells in lesions of nodular fasciitis on electron microscopy appear to be myofibroblasts.[235] As in other myofibroblastic lesions, the cells show immunoreactivity for vimentin, smooth muscle actin, and muscle-specific actin, but not for desmin.[236]

Differential Diagnosis. The presence of numerous large, pleomorphic fibroblasts and the infiltrative type of growth may be suggestive of fibrosarcoma. In addition to rapid growth and tenderness, however, the combination of fibroblastic and vascular proliferation is the most helpful diagnostic feature of nodular fasciitis. Other findings suggesting the diagnosis of nodular fasciitis are the presence of a mucoid ground substance and of an inflammatory infiltrate, especially near the margin of the lesion. Because nodular fasciitis as a reactive lesion does not recur, the recurrence of a lesion originally diagnosed as such should spur a careful reappraisal of the histologic findings.[227]

CRANIAL FASCIITIS OF CHILDHOOD

Cranial fasciitis of childhood is an unusual variant of nodular fasciitis that occurs in infants and children as a rapidly growing mass in the subcutaneous tissue of the scalp that extends into the underlying cranium. No recurrence has been reported after excision of the mass with resection or curettage of the underlying bone.[237]

Histopathology. The histologic features closely resemble those of nodular fasciitis. An origin in one of the deep fascial layers of the scalp appears likely.[237]

Histogenesis. The lesion contains fibroblasts and myofibroblasts.[238]

INFANTILE MYOFIBROMATOSIS

This rare disorder, formerly called congenital fibromatosis, affects two subgroups of patients. In patients with *superficial myofibromatosis*, the nodules are confined to the skin, subcutaneous tissue, skeletal muscle, and bone, and the prognosis is good; in patients with *generalized myofibromatosis*, visceral lesions are also present and the mortality rate is as high as 80% because visceral nodules can obstruct and compress vital organs, most commonly the lungs.[239,240] In both the superficial and the generalized types, dermal and subcutaneous nodules usually are present at birth. Additional nodules may subse-

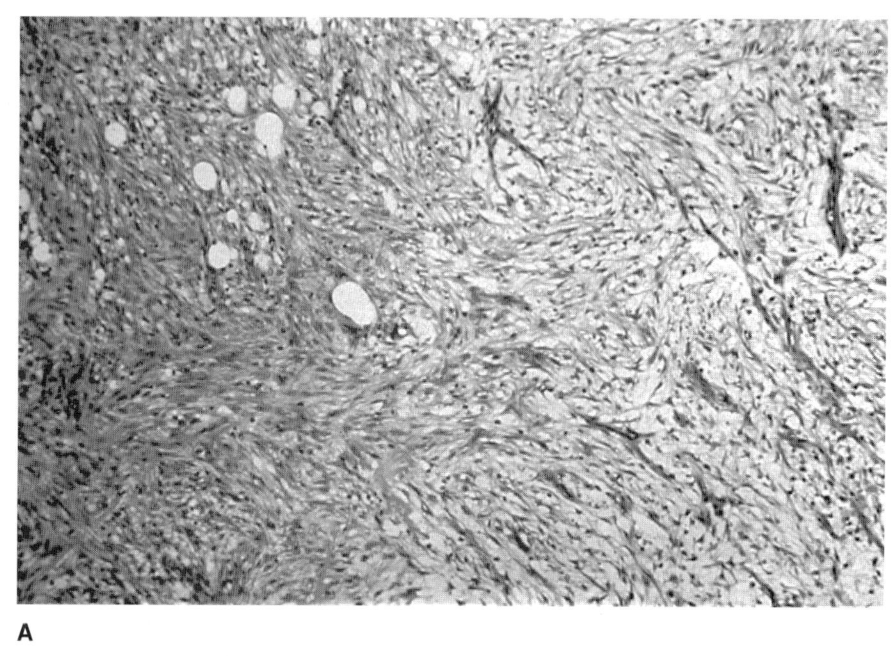

A

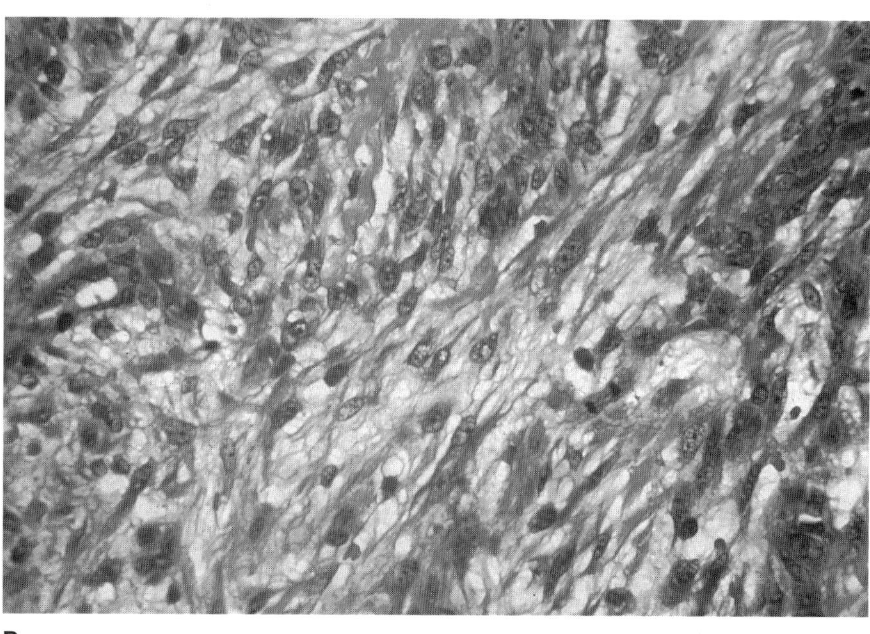

B

FIG. 33-23. Nodular fasciitis
(**A**) Plump spindle cells are arranged in varied cellularity in a loosely structured, vascular stroma. (**B**) Plump spindle cells with ovoid, vesicular nuclei and scattered mitoses are embedded in a loosely structured stroma with capillaries, slitlike spaces, and scattered erythrocytes.

quently appear. In some cases only a solitary cutaneous nodule is present.[241,242]

In infants with visceral involvement, death, if it occurs, takes place in the first few months of life. In infants with the generalized form who survive and in those with superficial myofibromatosis, spontaneous involution of the lesions takes place, often within the first year of life,[2] possibly mediated by apoptosis.[243]

Histopathology. The cutaneous lesions consist of nodular dermal aggregates of plump spindle cells resembling smooth muscle cells arranged in short fascicles, sometimes with areas of central hyalinization (Fig. 33-24A).[241] Most tumors present a characteristic biphasic growth pattern. A peripheral component of leiomyomalike fascicles of plump spindle cells surrounds a central hemangiopericytomalike component where more rounded cells are arranged around the blood vessels (see Fig. 33-24B). Collagen is present, but it is not abundant, and in less cellular areas the stroma may appear mucoid.[244] A monophasic cellular variant has also been described recently; in these lesions

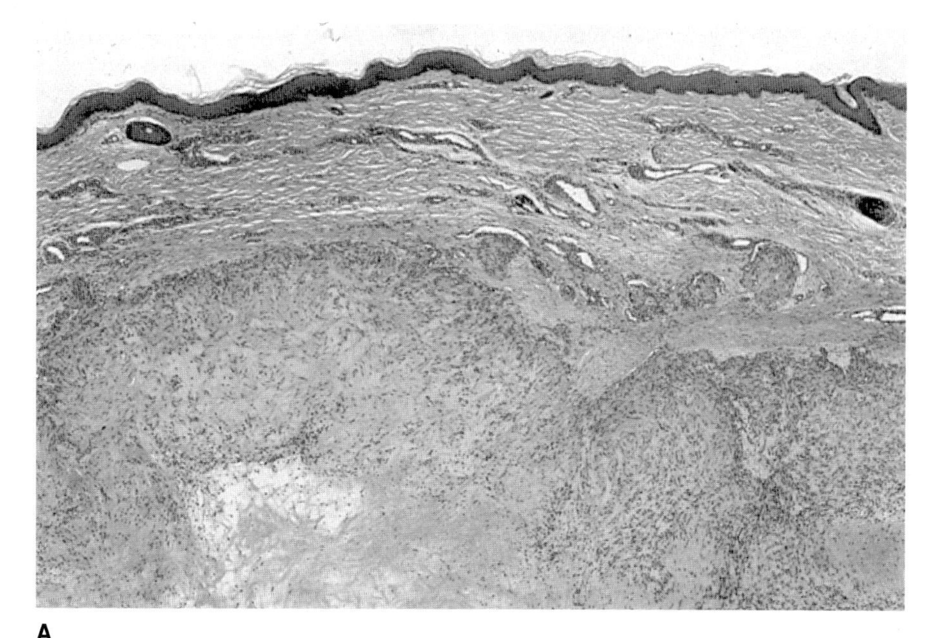

A

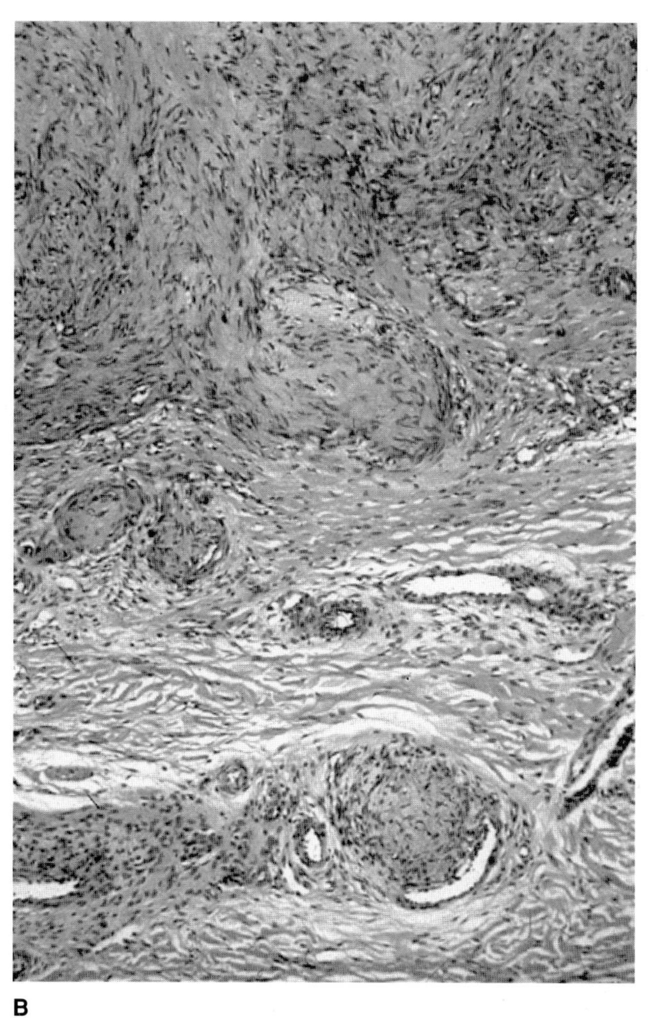

B

FIG. 33-24. Infantile myofibromatosis
(**A**) Circumscribed dermal nodules of varied size, with hyalinization in the center of the largest nodule. (**B**) The nodules consist of fascicles of plump spindle cells with pale eosinophilic cytoplasm, some of which indent the walls of blood vessels.

the more characteristic biphasic pattern developed during the course of the disease.[245]

Histogenesis. Ultrastructural evidence and immunoreactivity for vimentin and actin, with negative staining for desmin,[246,247] have indicated that the spindle cells are myofibroblasts, but it has also been suggested that the spindle cells show true smooth muscle differentiation.[248]

SOLITARY MYOFIBROMA

Solitary myofibroma is the adult counterpart of infantile myofibromatosis, presenting as a painless nodule of the skin or oral cavity.[239–241]

Histopathology. The lesions are composed of spindle cells in a biphasic pattern similar to that of infantile myofibromatosis, with peripheral leiomyomalike and central hemangiopericytomalike areas.

Histogenesis. Ultrastructural and immunohistochemical studies suggest that the spindle cells are myofibroblasts or fibroblasts.[241]

FIBROUS HAMARTOMA OF INFANCY

In fibrous hamartoma of infancy, usually one and rarely two subcutaneous nodules are present at birth or develop before the end of the first year of life.[249] After an initial period of growth, there is no further increase in the size of the nodule. In a recent study of 40 cases, 29 patients were males and 11 were females, and the lesions were distributed in a wide range of anatomic sites.[250]

Histopathology. The nodule consists of three different tissue components: rather cell-poor fibrous trabeculae, whorls of immature appearing spindle cells in a mucoid matrix, and mature adipose tissue (Fig. 33-25A,B).[249,251] In addition, capillary proliferations may be present.[252] The fibrous component may vary in cellularity, pattern, and amount, resembling granulation tissue, deep fibrous histiocytoma, or fibromatosis in some areas.[250]

JUVENILE HYALINE FIBROMATOSIS

A rare, recessively inherited disorder, juvenile hyaline fibromatosis starts in early infancy with flexural contractures, innumerable skin nodules that gradually increase in size, and a hypertrophic gingiva. The largest nodes are usually seen on the scalp.[253] Juvenile hyaline fibromatosis has been reported in association with skull and encephalic abnormalities[254] and in the hand of an adult.[255] The uncommon occurrence of widespread visceral involvement is known as infantile systemic hyalinosis.[256]

Histopathology. The nodules are composed to varying degrees of fibroblasts and ground substance. Small, newly developed tumors are more cellular, whereas larger tumors contain much more ground substance.[257] In paraffin-embedded, formalin-fixed material, empty spaces are seen around the fibroblasts as a shrinkage artifact, giving these cells a chondroid appearance.[258]

Histogenesis. The fibroblasts, in tissue culture, show an increased synthesis of chondroitin sulfate.[259] The progressive enlargement of the lesions is due to an increase in the amount of intercellular hyalin produced by the cells.[260]

CUTANEOUS EXTRASKELETAL EWING'S SARCOMA

Cutaneous extraskeletal Ewing's sarcoma is a highly malignant primary soft tissue neoplasm, rarely involving the skin,[261] as distinct from extension of Ewing's sarcoma of bone into adjacent tissue.

Histopathology. Multiple tumor lobules in the subcutis may infiltrate the dermis. The lobules are composed of masses of uniform, round, or oval cells with round or ovoid vesicular nuclei and scanty pale cytoplasm containing glycogen.

Histogenesis. Although the cells of Ewing's sarcoma have been regarded as primitive, noncommitted mesenchymal cells,[262] a recent immunocytochemical and ultrastructural study has indicated that Ewing's sarcoma of bone and peripheral neuroepithelioma are both peripheral primitive neuroectodermal neoplasms.[263] It has also been suggested, on the basis of a tissue culture–associated differentiation assay study, that extraosseous Ewing's sarcoma comprises a heterogeneous group of tumors showing differentiation arrested at more advanced stages of neural crest development than Ewing's sarcoma of bone.[264]

CUTANEOUS MYXOMA

Cutaneous myxomas are sharply demarcated nodules of the dermis or subcutis, occurring as multiple lesions in association with cardiac and mammary myxomas, spotty pigmentation, and endocrine overactivity in Carney complex[265] (NAME[266] or LAMB[267] syndrome) or, rarely, as a solitary lesion.[268]

Histopathology. Cutaneous myxomas are sharply circumscribed lesions composed of a vascular, mucinous matrix with a network of fine collagen and reticulin fibers and containing stellate and spindle-shaped fibroblasts (Fig. 33-26). An epithelial component, possibly derived from outer root sheath epithelium, is sometimes present, taking the form of strands of epithelium with trichoblastic features or small keratinous cysts.[265,268] Fibromyxoma has been described as a lesion containing histiocytes and more fibroblasts than cutaneous myxoma in addition to the mucinous matrix. These lesions may occur as multiple tumors, clinically resembling dermatofibroma.[269]

Differential Diagnosis. Cutaneous myxoma is more sharply circumscribed and more vascular than cutaneous focal mucinosis.[270]

DIGITAL MUCOUS CYST

Two types of digital mucous cysts exist.[271,272] One type is analogous to focal mucinosis. It differs from focal mucinosis only by its location near the proximal nail fold and by its greater tendency to fluctuation. The other type is located on the dorsum of a finger near the distal interphalangeal joint and is due to a herniation of the joint lining, thus representing a ganglion.[271]

Histopathology. The *myxomatous* type of digital mucous cyst in its early stage has the same histologic appearance as that

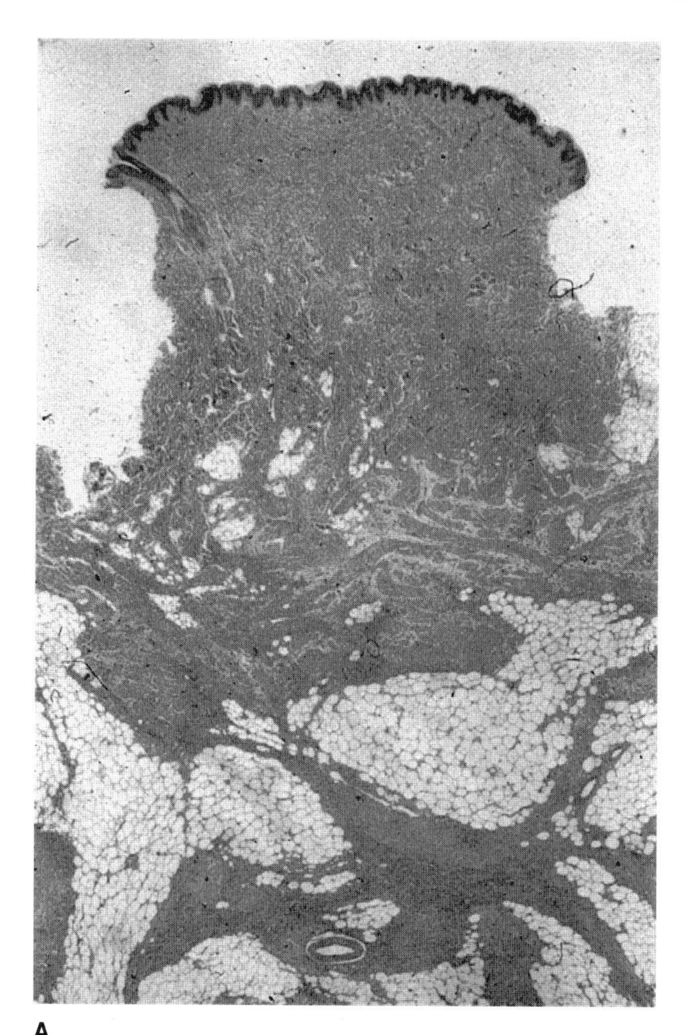

A

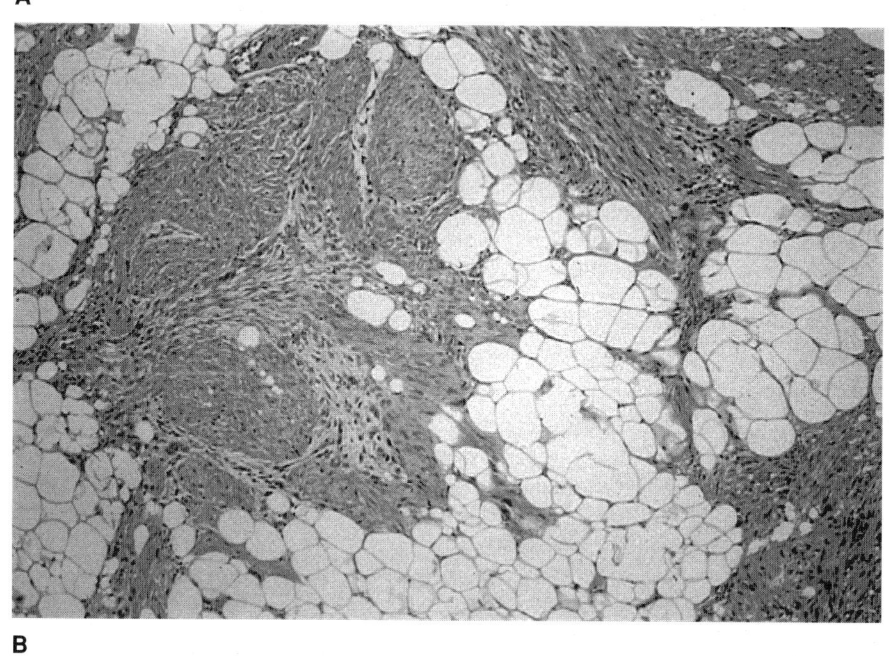

B

FIG. 33-25. Fibrous hamartoma of infancy
(**A**) Trabeculae of varied thickness intersect lobules of fat in the subcutis. (**B**) The trabeculae are composed of spindle cells arranged in loosely structured myxoid areas and more densely collagenous foci.

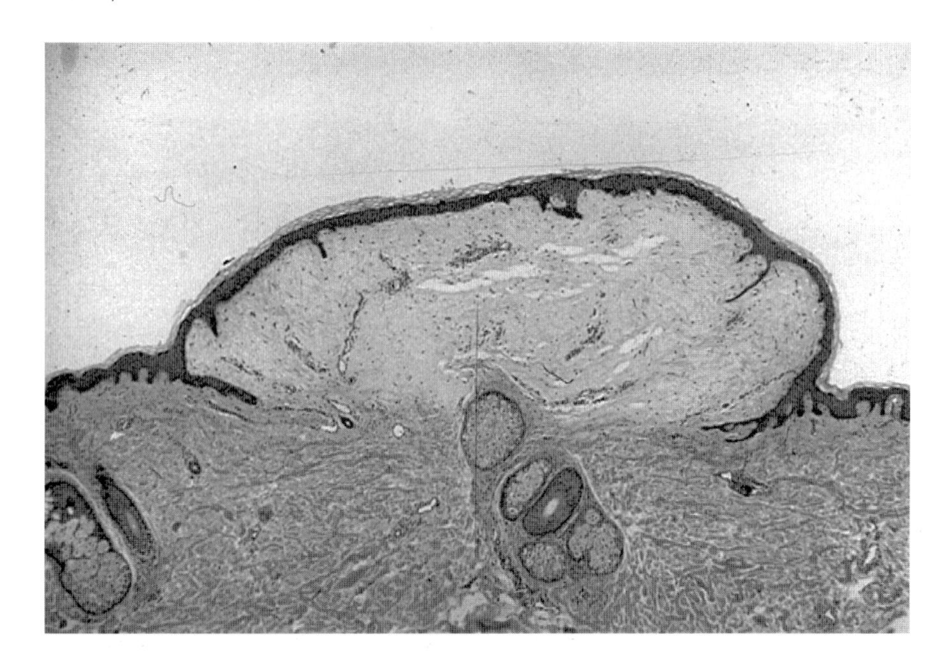

FIG. 33-26. Cutaneous myxoma The lesion is a sharply circumscribed nodule composed of a vascular mucinous matrix in which are scattered spindle cells.

seen in focal mucinosis, namely, an ill-defined area of mucinous material. Subsequently, multiple clefts form and then coalesce into one large cystic space containing mucin composed largely of hyaluronic acid, which stains with alcian blue and colloidal iron.[273] The cystic space in early lesions is separated from the epidermis by mucinous stroma but in older lesions is found in a subepidermal location with thinning of the overlying epidermis. The collagen at the periphery of the cyst appears compressed. No lining of the cyst wall is apparent (Fig. 33-27).[273–275]

In the *ganglion type* of digital mucous cyst, on surgical exploration the cyst shows an epithelial lining and evidence of a pedicle leading to the joint spaces.[272]

Histogenesis. The type of digital mucous cyst that is analogous to focal mucinosis results from an overproduction of hyaluronic acid by fibroblasts. The overproduction is associated with a decrease in or absence of collagen formation.[273,274]

In the ganglion type of digital mucous cyst, the hyaluronic acid is derived from the joint fluid of the distal interphalangeal joint. The origin of the mucous material from the joint fluid is supported by the observation that, after the injection of methy-

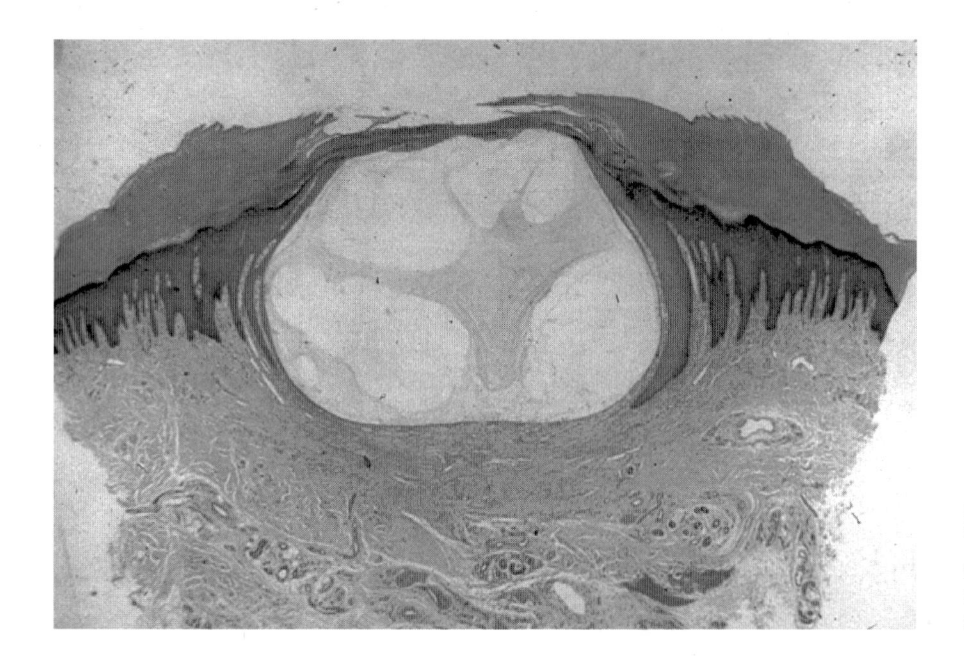

FIG. 33-27. Digital mucous cyst The epidermis is raised and attenuated and overlies a circumscribed mucinous cystic nodule, with an epidermal collarette.

lene blue into the volar aspect of the distal interphalangeal joint space, the cyst regularly contains the dye.[275,276]

MUCOUS CYST OF THE ORAL MUCOSA

Mucous cysts of the oral mucosa, also known as mucoceles, occur as solitary asymptomatic lesions, usually on the mucous surface of the lower lip and only rarely elsewhere on the oral mucosa, such as the buccal mucosa[277] or the tongue.[278] The cysts usually measure less than 1 cm in diameter, appear dome-shaped, are translucent, and contain a clear, viscous fluid. The cysts may disappear spontaneously, with or without evacuating their mucous content.[279]

Mucous cysts of the oral mucosa usually are the result of minor trauma causing rupture of a mucous duct and an outpouring of sialomucin into the tissue. Although most patients with an oral mucous cyst have no preexisting abnormality, mucous cysts of the lower lip may occur in patients with *cheilitis glandularis*, a condition in which the labial mucous glands and ducts are hyperplastic.[280]

Histopathology. In early lesions, one finds multiple small spaces filled with sialomucin and surrounded by or intermixed with granulation tissue. Older lesions show either a solitary large cystic space or several large spaces lined by a thick layer of granulation tissue composed of neutrophils, lymphocytes, fibroblasts, macrophages, and capillaries.[277,278,281] The macrophages contain prominent[277,278,281] vacuoles representing phagocytized sialomucin.[278] The wall of some cysts shows a ruptured salivary duct opening into the cavity (Fig. 33-28).[281] The sialomucin within the cysts appears as amorphous, slightly eosinophilic material in routinely stained sections. It is periodic acid–Schiff positive and diastase-resistant, and also stains with alcian blue and colloidal iron. Superficial mucoceles are small, subepithelial, vesicular lesions. Minor salivary gland ducts in the underlying stroma provide a clue to the diagnosis.[282]

HYPERTROPHIC SCAR AND KELOID

Hypertrophic scars and keloids initially have the same clinical appearance: they are red, raised, and firm and possess a

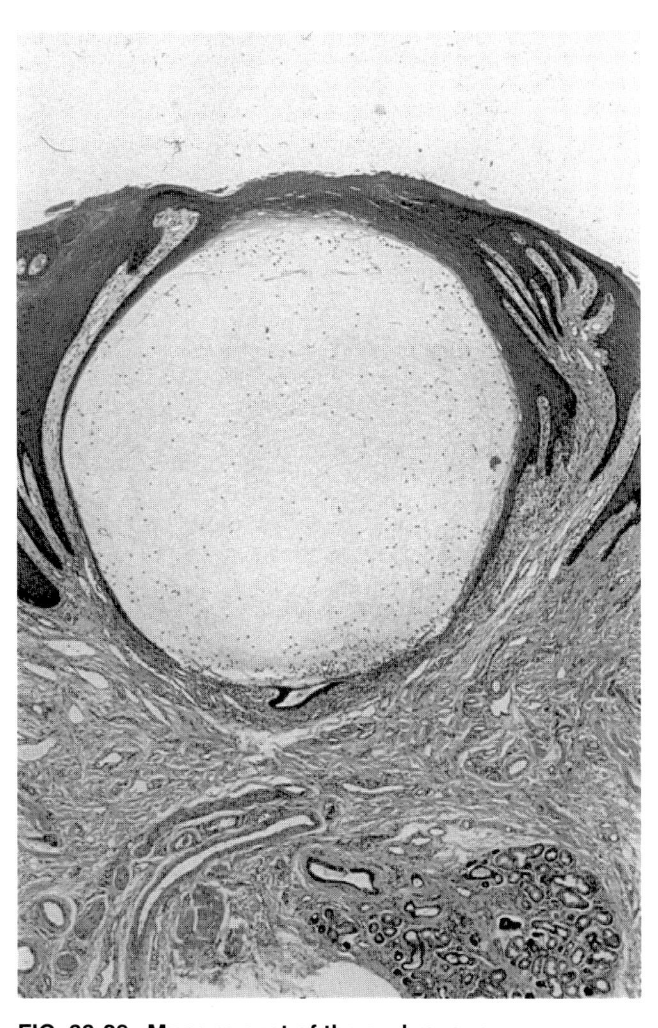

FIG. 33-28. Mucous cyst of the oral mucosa
The squamous epithelium is raised with a collarette formation and overlies a circumscribed mucinous nodule. A segment of salivary gland duct opens into the base of the cyst.

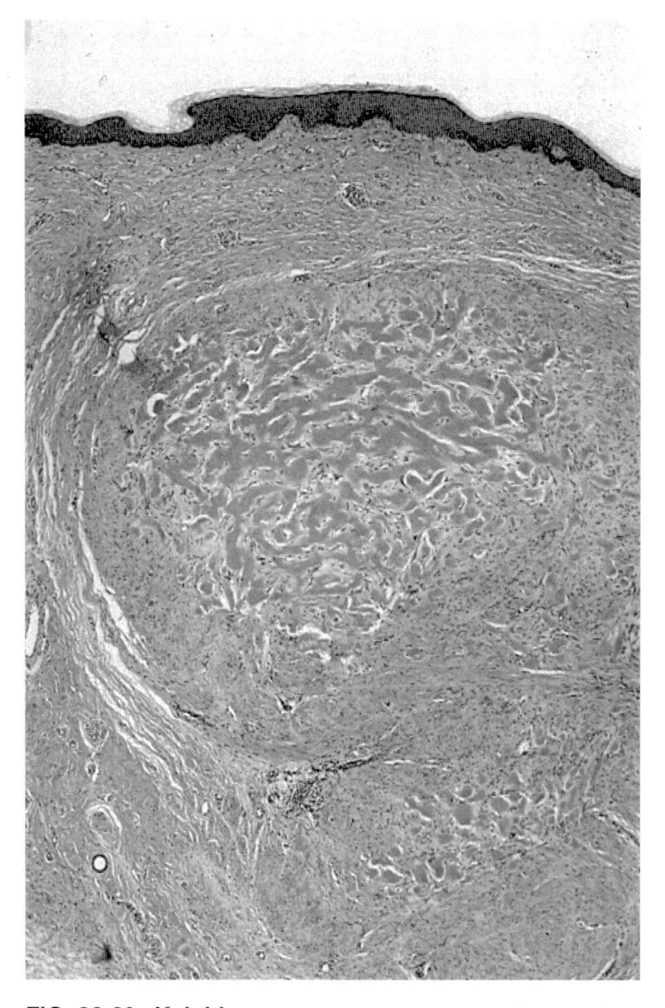

FIG. 33-29. Keloid
Large nodules of cellular collagenous tissue extend into the deep dermis, with central collections of broad hyalinized collagen bundles.

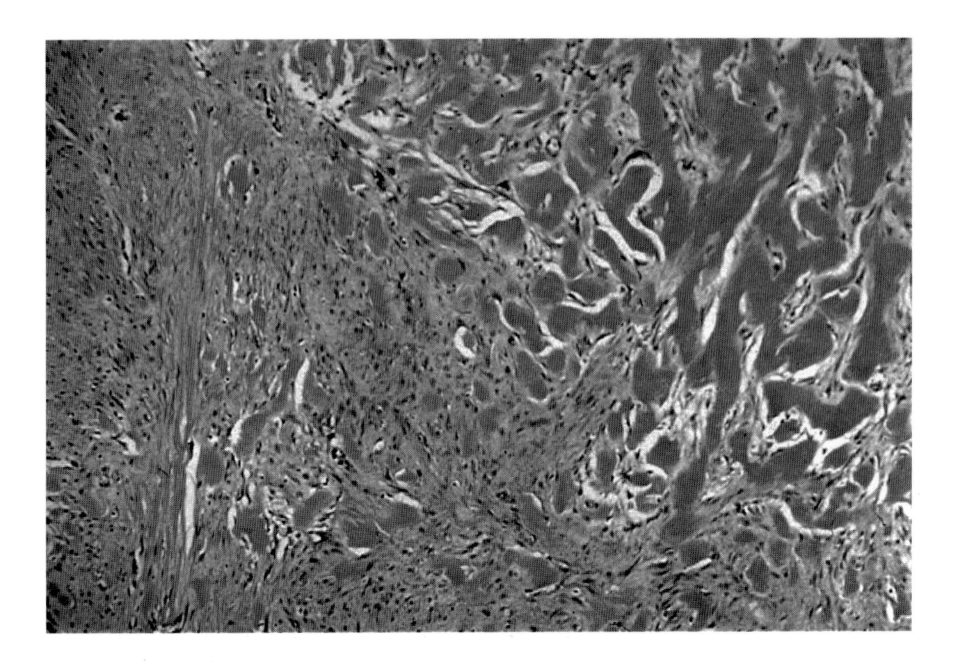

FIG. 33-30. Keloid
Irregular broad segments of hypereosinophilic, hyalinized collagen and adjacent strands of cellular collagen with plump fibroblasts.

smooth, shiny surface. Whereas hypertrophic scars flatten spontaneously in the course of one or several years, keloids persist and may even extend beyond the site of the original injury.

Keloids usually follow an injury, but patients sometimes have no recollection of prior injury. This is particularly true in the case of presternal keloids. Occasionally, there is a familial predilection for keloid formation.[283] Also, keloids are much more common in blacks than in whites.[284] In the rare Rubinstein-Taybi syndrome, keloids are apt to develop spontaneously in adolescence or early adulthood. This syndrome is characterized by microcephaly, mental retardation, beaking of the nose, and characteristic broadening of the terminal phalanges of the thumbs and first toes.[285]

Histopathology. The difference between normal wound healing and healing with a hypertrophic scar or keloid lies not only in the rate at which new collagen is formed but also in the arrangement of the newly formed collagen. Normal wound healing proceeds through an early inflammatory stage to a "fibroblastic" stage in which one finds granulation tissue composed of numerous capillaries, fibroblasts, and collagen fibers. The collagen fibers in the reticular dermis show a parallel, wavy orientation.[286] Usually after 5 weeks, the number of capillaries and fibroblasts has decreased, and the collagen lies as thick hyalinelike bundles in parallel arrangement.[287]

In hypertrophic scars and keloids, the formation of new collagen following the inflammatory stage is slower than in normally healing wounds. Even in the early period of the fibroblastic stage, the collagen fibers in the granulation tissue are arranged in a whorl or nodular pattern.[286] The nodules gradually grow and ultimately show thick, highly compacted, hyalinized bands of collagen lying in a concentric arrangement.[288]

Depending upon whether the nodule condensation of the collagen encroaches upon the papillary dermis, the epidermis appears either flattened or normal.[289]

Keloids differ from hypertrophic scars by extending beyond the confines of the original wound and usually protruding prominently above the surrounding skin, whereas hypertrophic scars remain within the boundaries of the wound and are flat or only slightly elevated.[290] The mature keloid also contains more markedly thickened and hypereosinophilic collagen bundles, with few adnexal structures and elastic fibers.

In keloids, the nodular condensation of the collagen persists indefinitely; in contrast, in hypertrophic scars, the thick and hyalinized collagen bundles in the nodules gradually become thinner and straighten, so that the orientation of the collagen bundles begins to parallel the free surface of the skin.

Histogenesis. Myofibroblasts were first observed in granulation tissue,[287,291] and it has been assumed that they aid in the gradual contraction of granulation tissue. Because early keloids contain granulation tissue, it is not surprising that many fibroblasts in them have the appearance of myofibroblasts.[292] Occasional myofilament bundles are seen in fibroblasts of maturing keloids.[293] In mature keloids myofibroblasts are absent (Figs. 33-29 and 33-30).[294]

REFERENCES

1. Bedi TR, Pandhi RK, Bhutani LK. Multiple palmoplantar histiocytomas. Arch Dermatol 1976;112:1001.
2. Hairston MAJ, Reed RJ. Aneurysmal sclerosing hemangioma of skin. Arch Dermatol 1966;93:439.
3. Niemi KM. The benign fibrohistiocytic tumours of the skin (review). Acta Derm Venereol (Stockh) 1970;50:1.
4. Schoenfeld RJ. Epidermal proliferations overlying histiocytomas. Arch Dermatol 1964;90:266.
5. Leyva WH, Santa Cruz DJ. Atypical cutaneous fibrous histiocytoma. Am J Dermatopathol 1986;8:467.
6. Dalziel K, Marks R. Hair follicle-like changes over histiocytomas. Am J Dermatopathol 1986;8:462.
7. Bryant J. Basal cell carcinoma overlying longstanding dermatofibromas. Arch Dermatol 1977;113:1445.
8. Goette DK, Helwig EB. Basal cell carcinomas and basal cell carci-

noma-like changes overlying dermatofibroma. Arch Dermatol 1975; 111:589.

9. Buselmeier TJ, Uecker JH. Invasive basal cell carcinoma with metaplastic bone formation associated with a long-standing dermatofibroma. J Cutan Pathol 1979;6:496.
10. Calonje E, Mentzel T, Fletcher CDM. Cellular benign fibrous histiocytoma: Clinicopathologic analysis of 74 cases of a distinctive variant of cutaneous fibrous histiocytoma with frequent recurrence. Am J Surg Pathol 1994;18:668.
11. Cohen PR, Rapini RP, Farhood AI. Expression of the human hemopoietic progenitor cell antigen CD34 in vascular and spindle cell tumors. J Cutan Pathol 1993;20:15.
12. Kamino H, Jacobson M. Dermatofibroma extending into the subcutaneous tissue: Differential diagnosis from dermatofibrosarcoma protuberans. Am J Surg Pathol 1990;14:1156.
13. Santa Cruz DJ, Kyriakos M. Aneurysmal ("angiomatoid") fibrous histiocytoma of the skin. Cancer 1981;47:2053.
14. Reed RJ. New concepts in surgical pathology of the skin. New York: Wiley, 1976;68.
15. Fukamizu H, Oku T, Inoue K et al. Atypical ("pseudocarcinomatous") cutaneous histiocytoma. J Cutan Pathol 1983;10:327.
16. Tamada S, Ackerman AB. Dermatofibroma with monster cells. Am J Dermatopathol 1987;9:380.
17. Wilson Jones E, Cerio R, Smith NP. Epithelioid cell histiocytoma: A new entity. Br J Dermatol 1989;120:185.
18. Singh Gomez C, Calonje E, Fletcher CDM. Epithelioid benign fibrous histiocytoma of skin: Clinico-pathological analysis of 20 cases of a poorly known variant. Histopathology 1994;24:123.
19. Klaus SN, Winkelman RK. The enzyme histochemistry of nodular subepidermal fibrosis. Br J Dermatol 1966;78:398.
20. Bandmann HJ. Ein beitrag zur morphologischen pathologie des dermatofibroma lenticulare bzw. des histiocytoms. Arch Klin Exp Dermatol 1957;204:584.
21. Pinkus H. Pathobiology of the pilary complex. Jpn J Dermatol [B] 1967;77:304.
22. Rahbari H, Mehregan AH. Adnexal displacement and regression in association with histiocytoma (dermatofibroma). J Cutan Pathol 1985; 12:94.
23. Unna PG. Histopathologic de hautkrankheiten. Berlin: August Hirschwald, 1894;839.
24. Woringer F, Kviatkowski S. L'histiocytome de la peau. Ann Dermatol Syphiligr 1932;3:998.
25. Senear FE, Caro MR. Histiocytoma cutis. Arch Dermatol Syph 1936; 33:209.
26. Fu Y-S, Gabbiani G, Kaye GI, Lattes R. Malignant soft tissue tumors of probable histiocytic origin (malignant fibrous histiocytomas): General considerations and electron microscopy and tissue culture studies. Cancer 1975;35:176.
27. Fletcher CDM. Malignant fibrous histiocytoma? Histopathology 1987;11:433.
28. Soini Y, Miettinen M. Widespread immunoreactivity for alpha-1-antichymotrypsin in different types of tumors. Am J Clin Pathol 1988; 89:131.
29. Soini Y, Meittinen M. Alpha-1-antitrypsin and lysozyme: Their limited significance in fibrohistiocytic tumors. Am J Clin Pathol 1989;91: 515.
30. Kempson RL, Hendrickson MR. What is a fibrohistiocytic tumour? In: Fletcher C, McKee PH, eds. Pathobiology of soft tissue tumours. Edinburgh: Churchill Livingstone, 1990;105.
31. Calonje E, Fletcher CDM. Cutaneous fibrohistiocytic tumors: An update. Adv Anat Pathol 1994;1:2.
32. Cerio R, Spaull J, Wilson Jones E. Histiocytoma cutis: A tumour of dermal dendrocytes (dermal dendrocytoma). Br J Dermatol 1989;120: 197.
33. Headington JT. The dermal dendrocyte. In: Callen JP, Dahl MV, Golitz LE, eds. Advances in dermatology. Vol. 1. Chicago: Year Book Medical Pub, 1986;157.
34. Mihatsch-Konz B, Schaumburg-Lever G, Lever WF. Ultrastructure of dermatofibroma. Arch Dermatol Forsch 1973;246:181.
35. Aubock L. Zur Ultrastruktur fibroser und histiocytarer hauttumoren. Virchows Arch [A] 1975;368:253.
36. Katenkamo D, Stiller D. Cellular composition of the so-called dermatofibroma (histiocytoma cutis). Virchows Arch 1975;367:325.
37. Kindblom LG, Jacobsen GK, Jacobsen M. Immunohistochemical investigations of tumors of supposed fibroblastic-histiocytic origin. Hum Pathol 1982;13:834.
38. Burgdorf W, Moreland A, Wasik R. Negative immunoperoxidase staining for lysozyme in nodular subepidermal fibrosis. Arch Dermatol 1982;118:241.
39. Kerdel FA, Morgan EW, Holden CA. Demonstration of alpha-1-antitrypsin and alpha-1-antichymotrypsin in cutaneous histiocytic infiltrates. J Am Acad Dermatol 1982;7:177.
40. Kanitakis J, Schmitt D, Thivolet J. Immunohistologic study of cellular populations of histiocytofibromas ("dermatofibromas"). J Cutan Pathol 1984;11:88.
41. Zelger B, Sidoroff A, Stanzl U et al. Deep penetrating dermatofibroma versus dermatofibrosarcoma protuberans. Am J Surg Pathol 1994;18: 677.
42. Fletcher CDM. Angiomatoid "malignant fibrous histiocytoma": An immunohistochemical study indicative of myoid differentiation. Hum Pathol 1991;22:563.
43. Costa MJ, Weiss SW. Angiomatoid malignant fibrous histiocytoma: A follow-up study of 108 cases with evaluation of possible histologic predictors of outcome. Am J Surg Pathol 1990;14:1126.
44. Peters CW, Hanke CW, Pasarell HA et al. Dermatofibrosarcoma protuberans of the face. J Dermatol Surg Oncol 1982;8:823.
45. Gutierrez G, Ospina JE, De Baez NE et al. Dermatofibrosarcoma protuberans. Int J Dermatol 1984;23:396.
46. McKee PH, Fletcher CDM. Dermatofibrosarcoma protuberans presenting in infancy and childhood. J Cutan Pathol 1991;18:241.
47. Kahn LB, Saxe N, Gordon W. Dermatofibrosarcoma protuberans with lymph node and pulmonary metastases. Arch Dermatol 1978;114:599.
48. Berbis P, Devant O, Echinard C et al. Dermatofibrosarcome de Darier-Ferrand métastasé. Ann Dermatol Venereol 1987;114:1217.
49. Taylor HB, Helwig EB. Dermatofibrosarcoma protuberans. Cancer 1961;15:717.
50. Fletcher CDM, Evans BJ, MacArtney JC et al. Dermatofibrosarcoma protuberans: A clinicopathological and immunohistochemical study with a review of the literature. Histopathology 1985;9:921.
51. Bednar F. Storiform neurofibromas of the skin, pigmented and nonpigmented. Cancer 1957;10:368.
52. Ding JA, Hashimoto H, Sugimoto T et al. Bednar tumor (pigmented dermatofibrosarcoma protuberans): An analysis of six cases. Acta Pathol Jpn 1990;40:744.
53. Connelly JH, Evans HL. Dermatofibrosarcoma protuberans: A clinicopathologic review with emphasis on fibrosarcomatous areas. Am J Surg Pathol 1992;16:921.
54. Shmookler BM, Enzinger FM, Weiss SW. Giant cell fibroblastoma: A juvenile form of dermatofibrosarcoma protuberans. Cancer 1989;64: 2154.
55. Beham A, Fletcher DC. Dermatofibrosarcoma protuberans with areas resembling giant cell fibroblastoma: Report of two cases. Histopathology 1990;17:165.
56. Alguacil-Garcia A. Giant cell fibroblastoma recurring as dermatofibrosarcoma protuberans. Am J Surg Pathol 1991;15:798.
57. Allen PW, Zwi J. Giant cell fibroblastoma transforming into dermatofibrosarcoma protuberans (letter). Am J Surg Pathol 1992;15: 1127.
58. Coyne J, Kaftan SM, Craig RD. Dermatofibrosarcoma protuberans recurring as a giant cell fibroblastoma. Histopathology 1992; 21:184.
59. Michael M, Zamecnik M. Giant cell fibroblastoma with a dermatofibrosarcoma protuberans component. Am J Dermatopathol 1992;14: 549.
60. Alguacil-Garcia A, Unni KH, Goellner JR. Histogenesis of dermatofibrosarcoma protuberans: An ultrastructural study. Am J Clin Pathol 1978;69:427.
61. Zina AM, Bundino S. Dermatofibrosarcoma protuberans: An ultrastructural study of five cases. J Cutan Pathol 1979;6:265.
62. Hashimoto K, Brownstein MH, Jacobiec FA. Dermatofibrosarcoma protuberans. Arch Dermatol 1974;110:874.
63. Lautier R, Wolff HH, Jones RE. An immunohistochemical study of dermatofibrosarcoma protuberans supports its fibroblastic character and contradicts neuroectodermal or histiocytic components. Am J Dermatopathol 1990;12:25.
64. Ma CK, Zarbo RJ, Gown AM. Immunohistochemical characterization of atypical fibroxanthoma and dermatofibrosarcoma protuberans. Am J Clin Pathol 1992;97:478.
65. Weiss SW, Nickoloff BJ. Cd-34 is expressed by a distinctive cell pop-

ulation in peripheral nerve, nerve sheath tumors, and related lesions. Am J Surg Pathol 1993;17:1039.
66. Aiba S, Tabata N, Ishil H et al. Dermatofibrosarcoma protuberans is a unique fibrohistiocytic tumour expressing CD34. Br J Dermatol 1992; 127:79.
67. Altman DA, Nickoloff BJ, Fivenson DP. Differential expression of factor XIIIa and CD34 in cutaneous mesenchymal tumors. J Cutan Pathol 1993;20:154.
68. Shmookler BM, Enzinger FM. Giant cell fibroblastoma: A peculiar childhood tumor (abstr). Lab Invest 1982;46:76A.
69. Dymock RB, Allen PW, Stirling JW et al. Giant cell fibroblastoma: A distinctive, recurrent tumor of childhood. Am J Surg Pathol 1987;11: 263.
70. Enzinger FM, Weiss SW. Soft tissue tumors. 3rd ed. St Louis: Mosby, 1995;337.
71. Fletcher CDM. Giant cell fibroblastoma of soft tissue: A clinicopathological and immunohistochemical study. Histopathology 1988; 13:499.
72. De Chadarevian JP, Coppola D, Billmure DF. Bednar tumor pattern in recurring giant cell fibroblastoma. Am J Clin Pathol 1993;100:164.
73. Zamecnik M, Michael M. Giant cell fibroblastoma with pigmented dermatofibrosarcoma protuberans component. Am J Surg Pathol 1994;18:736.
74. Gonatas K. Extra-abdominal desmoid tumors: Report of six cases. Arch Pathol 1961;71:214.
75. Goellner JR, Soule EH. Desmoid tumors: An ultrastructural study of eight cases. Hum Pathol 1980;11:43.
76. Weary PR, Linthicum A, Cawley EP et al. Gardner's syndrome. Arch Dermatol 1964;90:20.
77. Stiller D, Katenkamp D. Cellular features in desmoid fibromatosis and well differentiated fibrosarcomas: An electron microscopic study. Virchows Arch [A] Pathol Anat 1975;369:155.
78. Hasegawa T, Hirose T, Kudo E et al. Cytoskeletal characteristics of myofibroblasts in benign neoplastic and reactive fibroblastic lesions. Virchows Arch [A] Pathol Anat 1990;416:375.
79. Enzinger FM, Zhang R. Plexiform fibrohistiocytic tumor presenting in children and young adults: An analysis of 65 cases. Am J Surg Pathol 1988;12:818.
80. Hollowood K, Holley MP, Fletcher CDM. Plexiform fibrohistiocytic tumor: Clinicopathological, immunohistochemical and ultrastructural analysis in favour of a myofibroblastic lesion. Histopathology 1991; 19:503.
81. Kamino H, Reddy VB, Guo M, Greco MA. Dermatomyofibroma. J Cutan Pathol 1992;19:85.
82. Hugel H. Plaque-like dermal fibromatosis/dermatomyofibroma. J Cutan Pathol 1993;20:94.
83. Colome MI, Sanchez RL. Dermatomyofibroma: Report of two cases. J Cutan Pathol 1994;21:371.
84. Weiss SW, Enzinger FM. Malignant fibrous histiocytoma: An analysis of 200 cases. Cancer 1978;41:2250.
85. Kempson RL, Kyriakos M. Fibroxanthosarcoma of the soft tissues: A type of malignant fibrous histiocytoma. Cancer 1972;29:961.
86. Pezzi CM, Rawlings MS Jr, Esgro JJ et al. Prognostic factors in 227 patients with malignant fibrous histiocytoma. Cancer 1992;69:2098.
87. Hardy TJ, An T, Brown PW et al. Postirradiation sarcoma (malignant fibrous histiocytoma) of axilla. Cancer 1978;42:118.
88. Weiss SW. Malignant fibrous histiocytoma. Am J Surg Pathol 1982; 6:773.
89. Weiss SW, Enzinger FM. Myxoid variant of malignant fibrous histiocytoma. Cancer 1977;39:1672.
90. Lillemoe T, Steeper T, Manivel JC, Wick MR. Myxoid malignant fibrous histiocytoma (MMFH) of the skin (abstr). J Cutan Pathol 1988; 15:324.
91. Guccion JG, Enzinger FM. Malignant giant cell tumor of soft parts: An analysis of 32 cases. Cancer 1972;29:1518.
92. Kyriakos M, Kempson RL. Inflammatory fibrous histiocytoma. Cancer 1976;37:1584.
93. Enzinger FM. Angiomatoid malignant fibrous histiocytoma: A distinct fibrohistiocytic tumor of children and young adults simulating a vascular neoplasm. Cancer 1979;44:2147.
94. Weiss SW. Histological typing of soft tissue tumours. International histological classification of tumours. 2nd ed. Berlin and New York: Springer-Verlag, 1994;21.
95. Angervall L, Hagmar B, Kindblom LG et al. Malignant giant cell tumor of soft tissue. Cancer 1981;47:736.
96. Soule EH, Enriquez P. Atypical fibrous histiocytoma, malignant fibrous histiocytoma, malignant histiocytoma, and epithelioid sarcoma: A comparative study of 65 tumors. Cancer 1974;30:128.
97. McCarthy EF, Matsuno T, Dorfman HD. Malignant fibrous histiocytoma of bone. Hum Pathol 1979;10:57.
98. Roholl PJ, Prinsen I, Rademakers LP et al. Two cell lines with epithelial cell-like characteristics established from malignant fibrous histiocytomas. Cancer 1991;68:1963.
99. Litzky LA, Brooks JJ. Cytokeratin immunoreactivity in malignant fibrous histiocytoma and spindle cell tumors: Comparison between frozen and paraffin-embedded tissues. Mod Pathol 1992;5:30.
100. Rosenberg AE, O'Connell JX, Dickerson GR, Bhan AK. Expression of epithelial markers in malignant fibrous histiocytoma of the musculoskeletal system: An immunohistochemical and electron microscopic study. Hum Pathol 1993;24:284.
101. Fletcher CDM. Pleomorphic malignant fibrous histiocytoma: Fact or fiction? A critical reappraisal based on 159 tumors diagnosed as pleomorphic sarcoma. Am J Surg Pathol 1992;16:213.
102. Enzinger FM, Weiss SW. Soft tissue tumors. 3rd ed. St Louis: Mosby, 1995;355.
103. Smith ME, Costa MJ, Weiss SW. Evaluation of CD68 and other histiocytic antigens in angiomatoid malignant fibrous histiocytoma. Am J Surg Pathol 1991;15:757.
104. Helwig EB. Atypical fibroxanthoma. Tex State J Med 1963;59:664.
105. Fretzin DFJ, Helwig EB. Atypical fibroxanthoma of the skin. Cancer 1973;31:1541.
106. Kroe OJ, Pitcock JA. Atypical fibroxanthoma of the skin. Am J Clin Pathol 1969;51:487.
107. Barr RJ, Wuerker RB, Graham JH. Ultrastructure of atypical fibroxanthoma. Cancer 1977;40:1471.
108. Enzinger FM. Atypical fibroxanthoma and malignant fibrous histiocytoma. Am J Dermatopathol 1979;1:185.
109. Jacobs DS, Edwards WD, Ye RC. Metastatic atypical fibroxanthoma of the skin. Cancer 1975;35:457.
110. Helwig EB, May D. Atypical fibroxanthoma of the skin with metastasis. Cancer 1986;57:368.
111. Vargas-Cortes F, Winkelmann RK, Soule EH. Atypical fibroxanthoma of the skin. Mayo Clin Proc 1973;48:211.
112. Dahl I. Atypical fibroxanthoma of the skin. Acta Pathol Microbiol Immunol Scand [A] 1976;84:183.
113. Beham A, Fletcher CDM. Atypical "pseudosarcomatous" variant of cutaneous benign fibrous histiocytoma: A report of eight cases. Histopathology 1990;17:165.
114. Kemp JD, Stenn KS, Arons M et al. Metastasizing atypical fibroxanthoma. Arch Dermatol 1978;14:1533.
115. Calonje E, Wadden C, Wilson Jones E, Fletcher CDM. Spindle-cell non-pleomorphic atypical fibroxanthoma: Analysis of a series and delineation of a distinctive variant. Histopathology 1992;22:247.
116. Alguacil-Garcia A, Unni KK, Goellner JR et al. Atypical fibroxanthoma of the skin: An ultrastructural study of two cases. Cancer 1977; 40:1471.
117. Longacre TA, Smoller BR, Rouse RU. Atypical fibroxanthoma: Multiple immunohistologic profiles. Am J Surg Pathol 1993;17:1199.
118. Enzinger FM. Epithelioid sarcoma: A sarcoma simulating a granuloma or a carcinoma. Cancer 1970;26:1029.
119. Chase DR, Enzinger FM. Epithelioid Sarcoma: Diagnosis, prognostic indicators and treatment. Am J Surg Pathol 1985;9:241.
120. Kodet R, Smelhais V, Newton WA et al. Epithelioid sarcoma in childhood. Pediatr Pathol 1994;14:433.
121. Schmidt D, Harms D. Epithelioid sarcoma in children and adolescents: An immunohistochemical study. Virchows Arch [A] Pathol Anat 1987;410:423.
122. Moore SW, Wheeler JE, Hefter LG. Epithelioid sarcoma masquerading as Peyronie's disease. Cancer 1975;35:1706.
123. Huang DJ, Stanisic TH, Hansen KK. Epithelioid sarcoma of the penis. J Urol 1992;147:1370.
124. Weismann D, Amenta PS, Kantor GR. Vulvar epithelioid sarcoma metastatic to scalp: A case report and review of the literature. Am J Dermatopathol 1990;12:462.
125. Kudo E, Hirose E, Fuji Y et al. Undifferentiated carcinoma of the vulva mimicking epithelioid sarcoma. Am J Surg Pathol 1991;15:990.

126. Bos GD, Pritchard DJ, Reiman HM et al. Epithelioid sarcoma: An analysis of fifty-one cases. J Bone Joint Surg [Am] 1988;70:862.
127. Evans HL, Baer SC. Epithelioid Sarcoma: A clinicopathologic and prognostic study of 26 cases. Semin Diagn Pathol 1993;10:286.
128. Mirra JM, Kessler S, Bhuta S, Eckardt J. The fibroma-like variant of epithelioid sarcoma: A fibrohistiocytic/myoid cell lesion often confused with benign and malignant spindle cell tumors. Cancer 1992;15: 1382.
129. Heenan PJ, Quirk CJ, Papadimitriou JM. Epithelioid Sarcoma: A diagnostic problem. Am J Dermatopathol 1986;8:95.
130. Ishida T, Oka T, Matsushita H, Machinami R. Epithelioid sarcoma: An electron-microscopic, immunohistochemical and DNA flow cytometric analysis. Virchows Arch A Pathol Anat Histopathol 1992;421: 401.
131. Arber DA, Kandalaft PL, Mehta P, Battifora H. Vimentin-negative epithelioid sarcoma: The value of an immunohistochemical panel that includes CD34. Am J Surg Pathol 1993;17:302.
132. Manivel JC, Wick MR, Dehner LP et al. Epithelioid sarcoma: An immunohistochemical study. Am J Clin Pathol 1987;87:319.
133. Fisher C. Epithelioid sarcoma. Hum Pathol 1988;19:265.
134. Fletcher CDM, McKee PH. Sarcomas: III. Synovial sarcoma. Clin Exp Dermatol 1985;10:332.
135. Abenoza P, Manivel JC, Swanson PE. Synovial sarcoma: Ultrastructural study and immunohistochemical analysis by a combined peroxidase-antiperoxidase/avidin-biotin-peroxidase complex procedure. Hum Pathol 1986;17:1107.
136. Miettinen M. Keratin subsets in spindle cell sarcomas: Keratins are widespread but synovial sarcoma contains a distinctive keratin polypeptide pattern and desmoplakins. Am J Pathol 1991;138:505.
137. Fisher C. Synovial sarcoma: Ultrastructural and immunohistochemical features of epithelial differentiation in monophasic and biphasic tumors. Hum Pathol 1986;17:996.
138. Miettinen M, Virtanen I. Synovial sarcoma: A misnomer. Am J Pathol 1984;117:18.
139. Ghadially FN. Is synovial sarcoma a carcinosarcoma of connective tissue? Ultrastruct Pathol 1987;11:147.
140. Guarino M, Christensen L. Immunohistochemical analysis of extracellular matrix components in synovial sarcoma. J Pathol 1994;172: 279.
141. Santa Cruz DJ, Reiner CB. Recurrent digital fibroma of childhood. J Cutan Pathol 1978;5:339.
142. Shapiro L. Infantile digital fibromatosis and aponeurotic fibroma. Arch Dermatol 1969;99:37.
143. Bhawan J, Bacchetta C, Joris I. A myofibroblastic tumor: Infantile digital fibroma. Am J Pathol 1979;94:19.
144. Iwasaki H, Kiruchi M, Mori R et al. Infantile digital fibromatosis. Cancer 1980;46:2238.
145. Choi KC, Hashimoto K, Setoyama M et al. Infantile digital fibromatosis: Immunohistochemical and immunoelectron microscopic studies. J Cutan Pathol 1990;17:225.
146. Mukai M, Torikata C, Iri H et al. Immunohistochemical identification of aggregated actin filaments in formalin-fixed, paraffin-embedded sections. Am J Surg Pathol 1992;16:110.
147. Verallo VVM. Acquired digital fibrokeratomas. Br J Dermatol 1968; 80:730.
148. Kint A, Baran R. Histopathologic study of Koenen tumors: Are they different from acquired digital fibrokeratoma? J Am Acad Dermatol 1988,18:369.
149. Bart RS, Andrade R, Kopf AW et al. Acquired digital fibrokeratomas. Arch Dermatol 1968;97:120.
150. Hare PJ, Smith PAJ. Acquired (digital) keratoma. Br J Dermatol 1969; 81:667.
151. Pinkus H, Coskey R, Burgess GH. Trichodiscoma: A benign tumor related to Haarscheibe (hair disk). J Invest Dermatol 1974;63:212.
152. Birt AR, Hogg GR, Dubé WJ. Hereditary multiple fibrofolliculomas with trichodiscomas and acrochordons. Arch Dermatol 1977;113: 1674.
153. Fujita WH, Barr RJ, Headley JL. Multiple fibrofolliculomas with trichodiscomas and acrochordons. Arch Dermatol 1981;117:32.
154. Foucar K, Rosen T, Foucar E, Cochran RJ. Fibrofolliculoma: A clinicopathologic study. Cutis 1981;28:429.
155. Hornstein OP, Knickenberg M. Perifollicular fibromatosis cutis with polyps of the colon: A cutaneointestinal syndrome sui generis. Arch Dermatol Res 1975;253:161.
156. Starink TM, Kisch LS, Meijer CJLM. Familial multiple trichodiscomas: A clinicopathologic study. Arch Dermatol 1985;121:888.
157. Ubogy-Rainey Z, James WD, Lupton GP, Rodman OG. Fibrofolliculomas, trichodiscomas, and acrochordons: The Birt-Hogg-Dubé syndrome. J Am Acad Dermatol 1987;16:452.
158. Rongioletti F, Hazini R, Gianotti G, Rebora A. Fibrofolliculomas, trichodiscomas and achrocordons (Birt-Hogg-Dubé) associated with intestinal polyposis. Clin Exp Dermatol 1989;14:72.
159. Freeman RG, Chernosky ME. Perifollicular fibroma. Arch Dermatol 1969;100:66.
160. Smith LR, Heaton CL. Perifollicular fibroma. Cutis 1979;23:354.
161. Chemaly PH, Cavelier B, Civatte J. Syndrome de Birt, Hogg et Dubé. Ann Dermatol Venereol 1983;110:699.
162. Graham JH, Saunders JB, Johnson WC, Helwig EB. Fibrous papule of the nose: A clinicopathological study. J Invest Dermatol 1965;45:194.
163. Saylan T, Marks R, Wilson Jones E. Fibrous papule of the nose. Br J Dermatol 1971;85:111.
164. Reed RJ, Hairston MA, Palomeque FE. The histologic identity of adenoma sebaceum and solitary melanocytic angiofibroma. Dermatol Int 1966;5:3.
165. Meigel WN, Ackerman AB. Fibrous papule of the face. Am J Dermatopathol 1979;1:329.
166. McGibbon DH, Wilson Jones E. Fibrous papule of the nose. Am J Dermatopathol 1979;1:345.
167. Ragaz A, Berezowsky V. Fibrous papule of the face: A study of five cases by electron microscopy. Am J Dermatopathol 1979;1:353.
168. Kimura S, Yamasaki Y. Ultrastructure of fibrous papule of the nose. J Dermatol 1983;10:571.
169. Spiegel J, Nadji M, Penneys NS. Fibrous papule: An immunohistochemical study with antibody to S100 protein. J Am Acad Dermatol 1983;9:360.
170. Nemeth AJ, Penneys NS, Bernstein HB. Fibrous papule: A tumor of fibrohistiocytic cells that contain factor XIIIa. J Am Acad Dermatol 1988;19:1192.
171. Cerio R, Rao BK, Spaull J, Wilson Jones E. An immunohistochemical study of fibrous papule of the nose: 25 cases. J Cutan Pathol 1989;16: 194.
172. Nemeth AJ, Penneys NS. Factor XIIIa is expressed by fibroblasts in fibrovascular tumors. J Cutan Pathol 1989;16:266.
173. Cerio R, Wilson Jones E. Factor XIIIa positivity in fibrous papule. J Am Acad Dermatol 1990;20:138.
174. Nickel WR, Reed WB. Tuberous sclerosis: Special reference to the microscopic alterations in the cutaneous hamartomas. Arch Dermatol 1962;85:209.
175. Sanchez NP, Wick MR, Perry HO. Adenoma sebaceum of Pringle: A clinicopathologic review, with a discussion of related pathologic entities. J Cutan Pathol 1981;8:395.
176. Fitzpatrick TB, Szabo G, Hori Y et al. White leaf-shaped macules. Arch Dermatol 1968;98:1.
177. Reed WB, Nickel WR, Campion G. Internal manifestations of tuberous sclerosis (review). Arch Dermatol 1963;87:715.
178. Scheig RL, Bornstein P. Tuberous sclerosis in the adult. Arch Intern Med 1961;108:789.
179. Moreles JB. Congenital rhabdomyoma, tuberous sclerosis, and splenic histiocytosis. Arch Pathol 1961;71:485.
180. Price EB Jr, Mostofi FK. Symptomatic angiomyolipoma of the kidney. Cancer 1965;18:761.
181. Willis WF, Garcia RL. Giant angiofibroma in tuberous sclerosis. Arch Dermatol 1978;114:1843.
182. Park YK, Hann SK. Cluster growths in adenoma sebaceum associated with tuberous sclerosis. J Am Acad Dermatol 1989;20:918.
183. Yasuki Y. Acquired periungual fibrokeratoma. J Dermatol 1985;12: 349.
184. Kobayasi RT, Wolf-Jurgensen P, Danielsen L. Ultrastructure of shagreen patch. Acta Derm Venereol (Stockh) 1973;53:275.
185. Enzinger FM, Weiss SW. Soft tissue tumors. 3rd ed. St Louis: Mosby, 1995;187.
186. Dixon AY, Lee SH. An ultrastructural study of elastofibromas. Hum Pathol 1980;11:257.
187. Gartmann H, Groth W, Kuhn A. Elastofibroma dorsi. Z Hautkr 1988; 63:525.
188. Kumaratilake JS, Krishnan R, Lomax-Smith J et al. Elastofibroma: Disturbed elastic fibrillogenesis by periosteal-derived cells? An immunoelectron microscopic and in situ hybridization study. Hum Pathol 1991;22:1017.

189. Flegel H, Tessmann K. Gibt es ein weiches fibrom der haut? Hautarzt 1967;18:251.
190. Field LM. A giant pendulous fibrolipoma. J Dermatol Surg Oncol 1982;8:54.
191. Chobanian SJ, Van Ness MM, Winters C, Cattau EL. Skin tags as a marker for adenomatous polyps of the colon. Ann Intern Med 1985; 103:892.
192. Beitler M, Eng A, Kilgour M, Lebwohl M. Association between acrochordons and colonic polyps. J Am Acad Dermatol 1986;14:1042.
193. Chobanian SJ, Van Ness MM, Winters C. Skin tags as a screening marker for colonic neoplasia. Gastrointest Endosc 1986;32:162.
194. Chobanian SJ. Skin tags and colonic polyps: A gastroenterologist's perspective. J Am Acad Dermatol 1987;16:407.
195. Margolis J, Margolis LS. Skin tags: A frequent sign of diabetes mellitus. N Engl J Med 1976;294:1184.
196. Kahana M, Grossman E, Feinstein A et al. Skin tags: A cutaneous marker for diabetes mellitus. Acta Derm Venereol (Stockh) 1987;67: 175.
197. Agarwal JK, Nigam PK. Acrochordon: A cutaneous sign of carbohydrate intolerance. Australas J Dermatol 1987;28:132.
198. Lawrence JH, Tobias CA, Linfoot JA et al. Successful treatment of acromegaly: Metabolic and clinical studies in 145 patients. J Clin Endocrinol Metab 1970;31:180.
199. Dalton AD, Coghill SB. No association between skin tags and colorectal adenomas. Lancet 1985;1:1332.
200. Luk GD. Colonic polyps and acrochordons (skin tags) do not correlate in familial colonic polyposis kindreds. Ann Intern Med 1986;104:209.
201. Graffeo M, Cesari P, Buffoli F et al. Skin tags: Markers for colonic polyps? J Am Acad Dermatol 1989;21:1029.
202. Stegmaier OC. Natural regression of the melanocytic nevus. J Invest Dermatol 1959;32:413.
203. Huntley AC. Eruptive lipofibromata. Arch Dermatol 1983;119:612.
204. Rapini RP, Golitz LE. Sclerotic fibromas of the skin. J Am Acad Dermatol 1989;20:266.
205. Starink TM, Meijer CJLM, Brownstein MH. The cutaneous pathology of Cowden's disease: New findings. J Cutan Pathol 1985;12:83.
206. Kamino H, Lee JY-Y, Berke A. Pleomorphic fibroma of the skin; a benign neoplasm with cytologic atypia: A clinicopathologic study of eight cases. Am J Surg Pathol 1989;13:107.
207. Poomeechaiwong S, Bonelli JE, DeSpain JD et al. Myoid fibroma: Piloleiomyoma-like fibroma of the skin (abstr). J Cutan Pathol 1989;16: 320.
208. King DT, Millman AJ, Gurevitch AW. Giant cell tumor of the tendon sheath involving the skin. Arch Dermatol 1978;114:944.
209. Ushijima M, Hashimoto H, Tsuneyoshi M. Giant cell tumor of the tendon sheath (nodular tenosynovitis). Cancer 1986;57:875.
210. Carstens P. Giant cell tumors of tendon sheath. Arch Pathol 1978;102: 99.
211. Rao AS, Vigorita VJ. Pigmented villonodular synovitis (giant cell tumor of the tendon sheath and synovial membrane): A review of 81 cases. J Bone Joint Surg 1984;66a:76.
212. Enzinger FM, Weiss SW. Soft tissue tumors. 3rd ed. St Louis: Mosby, 1995;736.
213. Alguacil-Garcia A, Unni KK, Goellner JR. Giant cell tumor of tendon sheath and pigmented villonodular synovitis: An ultrastructural study. Am J Clin Pathol 1978;69:6.
214. Ushijima M, Hashimoto H, Tsuneyoshi M et al. Giant cell tumor of the tendon sheath (nodular tenosynovitis): A study of 207 cases to compare the large joint group with the common digit group. Cancer 1985; 57:875.
215. Wood GS, Beckstead JH, Medeiros LJ et al. The cells of giant cell tumor of tendon sheath resemble osteoclasts. Am J Surg Pathol 1988;12: 444.
216. Medeiros LJ, Beckstead JH, Rosenberg AE et al. Giant cells and mononuclear cells of giant cell tumor of bone resemble histiocytes. Appl Immunohistochem 1993;1:115.
217. Chung EB, Enzinger FM. Fibroma of tendon sheath. Cancer 1979;44: 1945.
218. Cooper PH. Fibroma of tendon sheath. J Am Acad Dermatol 1984;11: 625.
219. Humphreys S, McKee PH, Fletcher CDM. Fibroma of tendon sheath. J Cutan Pathol 1986;13:331.
220. Hashimoto H, Tsuneyoshi M, Daimaru Y et al. Fibroma of tendon sheath: A tumor of myofibroblasts. A clinicopathologic study of 18 cases. Acta Pathol Jpn 1985;35:1099.
221. Konwaler BE, Keasbey L, Kaplan L. Subcutaneous pseudosarcomatous fibromatosis (fasciitis). Am J Clin Pathol 1955;25:241.
222. Hutter RVP, Stewart FW, Foote FW Jr. Fasciitis. Cancer 1962;15:992.
223. Soule EH. Proliferative (nodular) fasciitis. Arch Pathol 1962;73:437.
224. Stout AP. Pseudosarcomatous fasciitis in children. Cancer 1961;14: 1216.
225. Price EP Jr, Siliphant WM, Shuman R. Nodular fasciitis: A clinicopathologic analysis of 65 cases. Am J Clin Pathol 1961;35:122.
226. Rockl H, Schubert E. Fasciitis nodularis pseudocarcinomatosa. Hautarzt 1971;22:150.
227. Bernstein KE, Lattes R. Nodular (pseudosarcomatous) fasciitis: A nonrecurrent lesion. Cancer 1982;49:1668.
228. Mehregan AH. Nodular fasciitis. Arch Dermatol 1966;93:204.
229. Lai FM-M, Lam WY. Nodular fasciitis of the dermis. J Cutan Pathol 1993;20:66.
230. Goodland JR, Fletcher CDM. Intradermal variant of nodular "fasciitis." Histopathology 1990;17:569.
231. Price S, Kahn LB, Saxe N. Dermal and intravascular fasciitis: Unusual variants of nodular fasciitis. Am J Dermatopathol 1993;15:539.
232. Patchefsky AS, Enzinger FM. Intravascular fasciitis: A report of 17 cases. Am J Surg Pathol 1982;5:29.
233. Chung EB, Enzinger FM. Proliferative fasciitis. Cancer 1975;36: 1450.
234. Diaz-Flores L, Martin Herrera AI, Garcia Montelongo R, Gutierrez Garcia R. Proliferative fasciitis: Ultrastructure and histogenesis. J Cutan Pathol 1989;16:85.
235. Wirman JA. Nodular fasciitis: A lesion of myofibroblasts. Cancer 1976;38:2378.
236. Montgomery EA, Meis JM. Nodular fasciitis: Its morphologic spectrum and immunohistochemical profile. Am J Surg Pathol 1991;15: 942.
237. Laver DH, Enzinger FM. Cranial fasciitis of childhood. Cancer 1980; 45:401.
238. Patterson JW, Moran SL, Konerding H. Cranial fasciitis. Arch Dermatol 1989;125:674.
239. Venencie PV, Bigel P, Desgruelles C et al. Infantile myofibromatosis. Br J Dermatol 1987;117:255.
240. Spraker MK, Stack C, Esterly NB. Congenital generalized fibromatosis. J Am Acad Dermatol 1984;10:365.
241. Chung EB, Enzinger FM. Infantile myofibromatosis. Cancer 1981;48: 1807.
242. Barnes L, Mimouni F, Lucky AW. Solitary nodule on the arm of an infant. Arch Dermatol 1986;122:89.
243. Fukasawa Y, Ishikura H, Takada A et al. Massive apoptosis in infantile myofibromatosis: A putative mechanism of tumor regression. Am J Pathol 1994;144:480.
244. Benjamin SP, Mercer RD, Hawk WA. Myofibroblastic contraction in spontaneous regression of multiple congenital mesenchymal hamartoma. Cancer 1977;40:2343.
245. Zelger BWH, Calonje E, Sepp N et al. Monophasic cellular variant of infantile myofibromatosis: An unusual histopathologic pattern in two siblings. Am J Dermatopathol 1995;17:131.
246. Smith KJ, Skelton HG, Barrett TL et al. Cutaneous myofibroma. Mod Pathol 1989;2:603.
247. Daimaru Y, Hashimoto H, Enjoji M. Myofibromatosis in adults: Adult counterpart of infantile myofibromatosis. Am J Surg Pathol 1989;13:859.
248. Fletcher CDM, Achu P, Van Noorden S, McKee PH. Infantile myofibromatosis: A light microscopic, histochemical and immunohistochemical study suggesting true smooth muscle differentiation. Histopathology 1987;11:245.
249. Enzinger FM. Fibrous hamartoma of infancy. Cancer 1965;18:241.
250. Sotelo-Avila C, Bale PM. Subdermal fibrous hamartoma of infancy: Pathology of 40 cases and differential diagnosis. Pediatr Pathol 1994; 14:39.
251. King DF, Barr RJ, Hirose FM. Fibrous hamartoma of infancy. J Dermatol Surg Oncol 1979;5:482.
252. Aberer E, Mainitz M, Entacher U et al. Fibrous hamartoma of infancy. Dermatologica 1988;176:46.
253. Kitano Y. Juvenile hyalin fibromatosis. Arch Dermatol 1976;112:86.
254. Gilaberte Y, Gonzalez Mediero I, Lopez Barrantes V, Zambrano A.

Juvenile hyaline fibromatosis with skull-encephalic anomalies: A case report and review of the literature. Dermatology 1993;187:114.
255. Hallock GG. Juvenile hyaline fibromatosis of the hand in an adult. J Hand Surg [Am] 1993;18:614.
256. Kan AE, Rogers M. Juvenile hyaline fibromatosis: An expanded clinicopathologic spectrum. Pediatr Dermatol 1989;6:68.
257. Kitano Y, Horiki M, Aoki T et al. Two cases of juvenile hyalin fibromatosis. Arch Dermatol 1972;106:877.
258. Remberger K, Krieg T, Kunze D et al. Fibromatosis hyalinica multiplex (juvenile hyalin fibromatosis). Cancer 1985;56:614.
259. Iwata S, Horiuchi R, Haeda H et al. Systemic hyalinosis or juvenile hyalin fibromatosis. Arch Dermatol Res 1980;267:115.
260. Mayer-Da-Silva A, Polares-Baptista A, Rodrigo FG et al. Juvenile hyalin fibromatosis. Arch Pathol 1988;112:928.
261. Patterson JW, Maygarden SJ. Extraskeletal Ewing's sarcoma with cutaneous involvement. J Cutan Pathol 1986;13:46.
262. Peters MS, Reiman HM, Muller SA. Cutaneous extraskeletal Ewing's sarcoma. J Cutan Pathol 1985;12:476.
263. Navarro S, Cavazzana AO, Llombart-Bosch A, Truche TJ. Comparison of Ewing's sarcoma of bone and peripheral neuroepithelioma: An immunocytochemical and ultrastructural analysis of two primitive neuroectodermal neoplasms. Arch Pathol Lab Med 1994;118:608.
264. Noguera R, Navarro S, Peydro-Olaya A, Llombar-Bosch A. Patterns of differentiation in extraosseous Ewing's sarcoma cells: An in vitro study. Cancer 1994;74:616.
265. Carney JA, Headington JT, Su WPD. Cutaneous myxomas: A major component of the complex of myxomas, spotty pigmentation, and endocrine overactivity. Arch Dermatol 1986;122:790.
266. Atherton DJ, Pitcher DW, Wells RS, MacDonald DM. A syndrome of various cutaneous pigmented lesions, myxoid neurofibromata and atrial myxoma: The NAME syndrome. Br J Dermatol 1980;103:421.
267. Rhodes AR, Silverman RA, Harrist TJ, Perez-Atayde AR. Mucocutaneous lentigines, cardiomucocutaneous myxomas, and multiple blue nevi: The "LAMB" syndrome. J Am Acad Dermatol 1984;10:72.
268. Allen PW, Dymock RB, MacCormac LB. Superficial angiomyxomas with and without epithelial components. Am J Surg Pathol 1988;12: 519.
269. Zina AM, Bundino S. Multiple cutaneous fibromyxomas: A light and electron microscopic study. J Cutan Pathol 1980;7:335.
270. Wilk M, Schmoekel C. Cutaneous focal mucinosis: A histopathological and immunohistochemical analysis of 11 cases. J Cutan Pathol 1994;21:446.
271. Armijo M. Mucoid cysts of the fingers. J Dermatol Surg Oncol 1981; 7:317.
272. Salasche SJ. Myxoid cysts of the proximal nail fold. J Dermatol Surg Oncol 1984;10:35.
273. Johnson WC, Graham JH, Helwig EB. Cutaneous myxoid cyst. JAMA 1965;191:15.
274. Gotz H, Koch R. Zur klinik, pathogenese und therapie der sogenannten "dorsalcysten." Haurtarzt 1956;7:533.
275. Goldman JA, Goldman L, Jaffe MS et al. Digital mucinous pseudocysts. Arthritis Rheum 1977;20:997.
276. Newmeyer WL, kilgore ES Jr, Graham WP. Mucous cysts: The dorsal distal interphalangeal joint ganglion. Plast Reconstr Surg 1974;53: 313.
277. Lattanand A, Johnson WC, Graham JH. Mucous cyst (mucocele). Arch Dermatol 1970;101:673.
278. Braun-Falco O. Uber ein schleimgranuloma der zunge. Hautarzt 1960; 11:131.
279. Nikolowski W. Schleimcysten und sogenanntes schleimgranulom der unterlippe. Arch Klin Exp Dermatol 1956;203:246.
280. Weir TW, Johnson WC. Cheilitis glandularis. Arch Dermatol 1971; 103:433.
281. Ehlers G. Zur histogenese der lippenschleimcysten. Z Hautkr 1963; 34:77.
282. Jensen JL. Superficial mucoceles of the oral mucosa. Am J Dermatopathol 1990;12:88.
283. Murray JC, Pollack SV, Pinnel SR. Keloids: A review. J Am Acad Dermatol 1981;4:461.
284. Onwukwe MF. Classification of keloids. J Dermatol Surg Oncol 1978; 4:534.
285. Kurwa AR. Rubinstein-Taybi syndrome and spontaneous keloid. Clin Exp Dermatol 1978;4:251.
286. Linares HA, Larson DL. Early differential diagnosis between hypertrophic and nonhypertrophic healing. J Invest Dermatol 1974;62:514.
287. Mancini RE, Quaife JV. Histogenesis of experimentally produced keloids. J Invest Dermatol 1962;38:143.
288. Linares HA, Kischer CW, Dobrkovsky M et al. The histiotypic organization of the hypertrophic scans in humans. J Invest Dermatol 1972; 59:323.
289. Nikolowski W. Pathogenese, klinik und therapie des keloids. Arch Klin Exp Dermatol 1961;212:550.
290. Ketchum LD, Cohen IK, Masters FW. Hypertrophic scars and keloids: A collective review. Plast Reconstr Surg 1974;53:140.
291. Ryan GB, Cliff WJ, Gabbiani G et al. Myofibroblasts in human granulation tissue. Hum Pathol 1974;5:55.
292. James WD, Besanceney CD, Odom RB. The ultrastructure of a keloid. J Am Acad Dermatol 1980;3:50.
293. Katenkamp D, Stiller D. Untersuchungen zur ultrastruktur des keloids. Zentralbl Allg Pathol 1978;122:312.
294. Matsuoka LV, Uitto J, Wortsman J et al. Ultrastructural characteristics of keloid fibroblasts. Am J Dermatopathol 1988;10:505.

Lever's Histopathology of the Skin, eighth edition,
edited by David Elder et al. Lippincott–
Raven Publishers, Philadelphia © 1997.

CHAPTER 34

Vascular Tumors

Tumors and Tumor-Like Conditions of Blood Vessels and Lymphatics

Eduardo Calonje and Edward Wilson-Jones

The classification of vascular lesions and in particular benign vascular tumors is far from satisfactory. The division between developmental, reactive, benign (neoplastic), and occasionally malignant vascular tumors is often blurred, and many conditions cannot be neatly classified into a specific category. This often reflects either limited knowledge about the pathogenesis or the presence of overlapping features among different entities. While advances in knowledge and research have undoubtedly led to the improvement of this situation, the classification of many vascular tumors still remains controversial. A few examples include pyogenic granuloma and angiolymphoid hyperplasia with eosinophilia (reactive vs. neoplastic), and more importantly Kaposi's sarcoma (neoplastic vs. infectious). The classification of vascular tumors proposed in this chapter and in Table 34-1 intends only to provide a framework to define and present different vascular tumors in a coherent manner based on recent developments. It does not intend to be definitive because future changes in our understanding of vascular tumors will give way to further modifications.

REACTIVE CONDITIONS

Intravascular Papillary Endothelial Hyperplasia (Masson's Hemangio-Endotheliome Vegetant Intravasculaire)

This not uncommon condition probably represents an unusual endothelial proliferation in an organizing thrombus that can be misdiagnosed as angiosarcoma.[1] Intravascular papillary endothelial hyperplasia arises primarily within a venous channel or secondarily within a preceding angioma or some type of vascular anomaly, including hemorrhoids, as in Masson's original description.[2] An exceptional case of an extravascular location in association with a hematoma has been reported.[3] The lesions are almost always solitary, arising in the skin, subcutaneous tissue, or even muscle with the head and neck region, and the upper extremities, especially the fingers, are the most common sites. A rare instance of multiple lesions of the lower extremities simulating Kaposi's sarcoma has been described.[4] All ages can be affected, although there is a slight predominance of females.[5] Primary lesions are usually tender nodules less than 2 cm in size, whereas secondary lesions occur because some preceding vascular abnormality increases in size.

Histopathology. Often, low-power examination allows recognition of the intravascular nature of the process in a single thin-walled vein (Fig. 34-1) or as part of a preceding angiomatous condition. Extravascular lesions fail to reveal a blood vessel wall despite serial sectioning. The main lesion consists of a mass of anastomosing vascular channels with a variable degree of intraluminal papillary projections (Fig. 34-2). The stroma consists of hyalinized eosinophilic material that may merge with uncanalized thrombus remnants. The infiltrating vascular channels show enlarged and prominent endothelial cells that may be "heaped up" to give rise to intraluminal prominences, but atypia and mitotic activity are slight. Factor VIII–related antigen positivity of endothelial cells in the lesion may be related to vessel maturity.[6]

Differential Diagnosis. The occurrence of areas of somewhat atypical endothelial-lined channels apparently showing a "dissection of collagen" appearance can closely simulate a well-differentiated angiosarcoma. However, the stroma is not collagen and thus is not refractile on polarization and the changes are localized and occur within a preceding vessel or a vascular anomaly. Usually angiosarcoma shows a much greater degree of nuclear atypia and mitotic activity.

Angioendotheliomatosis

Until the last decade two distinctive forms of angioendotheliomatosis were recognized: an aggressive variant with systemic involvement and poor prognosis, and a reactive self-limited

E. Calonje: Consultant Dermatopathologist and Honorary Senior Lecturer, St. John's Institute of Dermatology, St. Thomas' Hospital, London, United Kingdom

E. Wilson-Jones: Emeritus Professor of Dermatology, St. John's Institute of Dermatology, St. Thomas' Hospital, London, United Kingdom

TABLE 34-1. *A classification of vascular tumors*

Reactive conditions
- Intravascular papillary endothelial hyperplasia
- Reactive angioendotheliomatosis
- Glomeruloid hemangioma
- Angiolymphoid hyperplasia with eosinophilia (epithelioid hemangioma)
- Pyogenic granuloma (lobular capillary hemangioma)
- Bacillary angiomatosis
- Verruca peruana (not discussed)

Developmental abnormalities
- Nevus flammeus (salmon patch, port-wine stain)
- Angiokeratoma
- Generalized essential telangiectasia
- Unilateral nevoid telangiectasia
- Angioma serpiginosum
- Hereditary hemorrhagic telangiectasia (Osler-Rendu-Weber disease)
- Nevus araneus (spider nevus)
- Nevus lake

Benign tumors
- Capillary hemangioma
  - Strawberry nevus
  - Cherry angioma (Campbell de Morgan spot, senile angioma)
  - Tufted angioma (angioblastoma)
- Cavernous hemangioma
  - Sinusoidal hemangioma
- Verrucous hemangioma
- Microvenular hemangioma
- Targetoid hemosiderotic hemangioma (hobnail hemangioma)
- Arteriovenous (venous) hemangioma (cirsoid aneurysm)
- Angiomatosis
- Spindle cell hemangioendothelioma

Low-grade malignant vascular tumors
- Kaposi's sarcoma
- Epithelioid hemangioendothelioma
- Retiform hemangioendothelioma
- Malignant endovascular papillary angioendothelioma (Dabska's tumor)
- Kaposi-like infantile hemangioendothelioma

Malignant vascular tumors
- Angiosarcoma
  - Idiopathic (head and neck)
  - Associated with lymphoedema
  - Postradiotherapy
  - Epithelioid

Lymph vessel tumors
- Lymphangioma circumscriptum
- Cystic hygroma/cavernous lymphangioma
- Progressive lymphangioma (benign lymphangioendothelioma)

Tumors of perithelial and glomus cells
- Glomus tumor
  - Solid
  - Glomangioma
  - Glomangiomyoma
  - Infiltrating glomus tumor
  - Glomangiosarcoma
- Hemangiopericytoma (adult and infantile)

form with a benign course restricted to the skin. However, with the advent of immunohistochemistry, many studies in recent years have demonstrated that malignant angioendotheliomatosis shows no endothelial differentiation but represents a form of angiotropic lymphoma that has been renamed *intravascular lymphomatosis* (see Chap. 32).

Reactive Angioendotheliomatosis

This is an uncommon condition that exclusively affects the skin and presents in patients of either gender with a wide anatomic distribution. Clinical presentation varies from erythematous or brown macules to papules and/or plaques that can be associated with purpura. Most cases are idiopathic, but some cases are associated with cryoglobulinemia,[7] paraproteinemia and systemic infections, especially bacterial endocarditis.[8] Recently a variant associated with peripheral vascular atherosclerotic disease has been described as diffuse dermal angiomatosis.[9]

Histopathology. Lesions are predominantly dermal and composed of closely packed, variably dilated vascular spaces (mainly capillaries) (Fig. 34-3) lined by bland but plump endothelial cells surrounded by pericytes. Small lumina might be apparent, but some are obliterated by endothelial cells or fibrin thrombi. Often the capillaries appear to proliferate in the lumina of dilated preexisting blood vessels. Hyaline refractile eosinophilic thrombi representing immunoglobulins are present in cases associated with cryoglobulinemia (Fig. 34-4).

Histogenesis. Reactive angioendotheliomatosis, in contrast to malignant angioendotheliomatosis, displays universal reactivity for endothelial markers and negativity for leukocyte common antigen, proving that the proliferating cells are endothelial cells.[8] It has been proposed that the endothelial cell proliferation is induced by a circulating angiogenic factor or alternatively, especially in cases associated to cryoglobulinemia, by occlusion of vascular spaces.[7]

Glomeruloid Hemangioma

This is a highly distinctive, rare, recently described reactive vascular proliferation that presents in patients with POEMS syndrome (**P**olyneuropathy, **O**rganomegaly, **E**ndocrinopathy, **M**-protein, and **S**kin changes), usually but not always in association with multicentric Castleman's disease.[10,11] The skin changes in POEMS syndrome include hypertrichosis, hyperpigmentation, hyperhidrosis, sclerodermoid features, and multiple small vascular papules on the trunk and limbs.

Histopathology. Most vascular lesions in POEMS syndrome show the features of cherry angiomas, and only a very small percentage have the appearance of a glomeruloid hemangioma. In the latter there are numerous ectatic vascular spaces throughout the dermis that contain in their lumina clusters of small congested capillaries surrounded by pericytes bearing a striking resemblance to renal glomeruli (Fig. 34-5). Although the endothelial cells are flat, a few scattered cells appear vacuolated and can show PAS-positive hyaline globules that correspond to deposition of immunoglobulins.[11]

Histogenesis. Glomeruloid hemangioma probably represents a

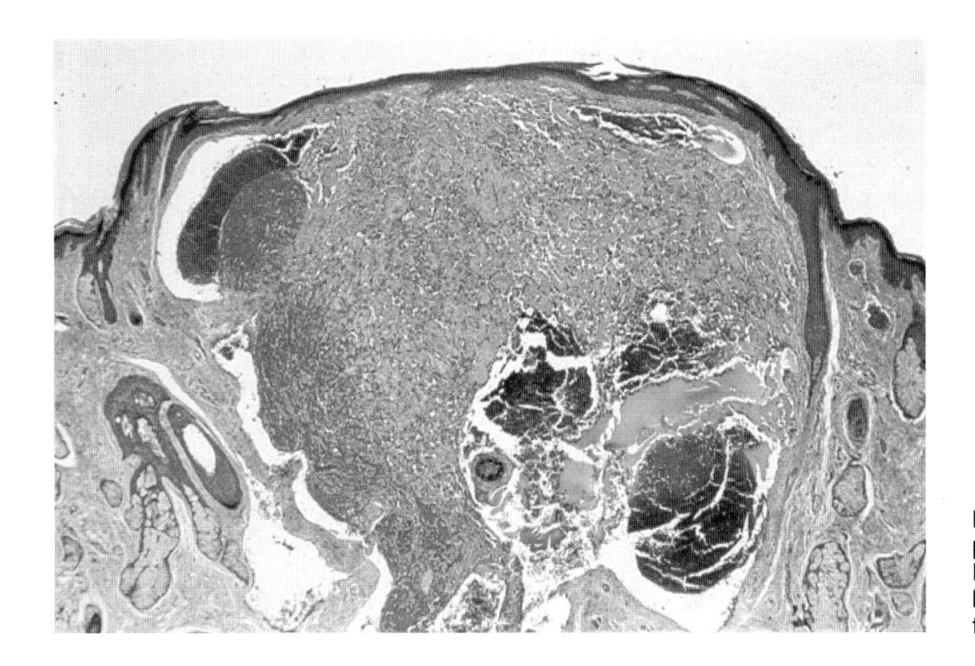

FIG. 34-1. Primary intravascular papillary endothelial hyperplasia
Note a markedly dilated thin-walled blood vessel appearing to contain a thrombus.

variant of reactive angioendotheliomatosis. It has not been established what causes the vascular proliferation in POEMS syndrome, but it may be induced by an angiogenic factor, possibly the abnormal immunoglobulin in the vascular spaces.

Angiolymphoid Hyperplasia with Eosinophilia: Epithelioid Hemangioma

The two parts of the title of this section highlight the controversy about whether this entity represents a vascular neoplasm or a reactive process consequent to trauma or some other stimulus. The term *epithelioid hemangioma* has been used by some authors to encompass vascular lesions at the benign end of the spectrum of conditions characterized by transformed endothelial cells that have an epithelioid or histiocytoid morphology.[12–15] It seems apparent in lesions of angiolymphoid hyperplasia that an inflammatory component is an integral part of the pathology and that not all the vascular endothelial cells show an epithelioid appearance. These histological features taken in conjunction with the fluctuating clinical course and the frequent

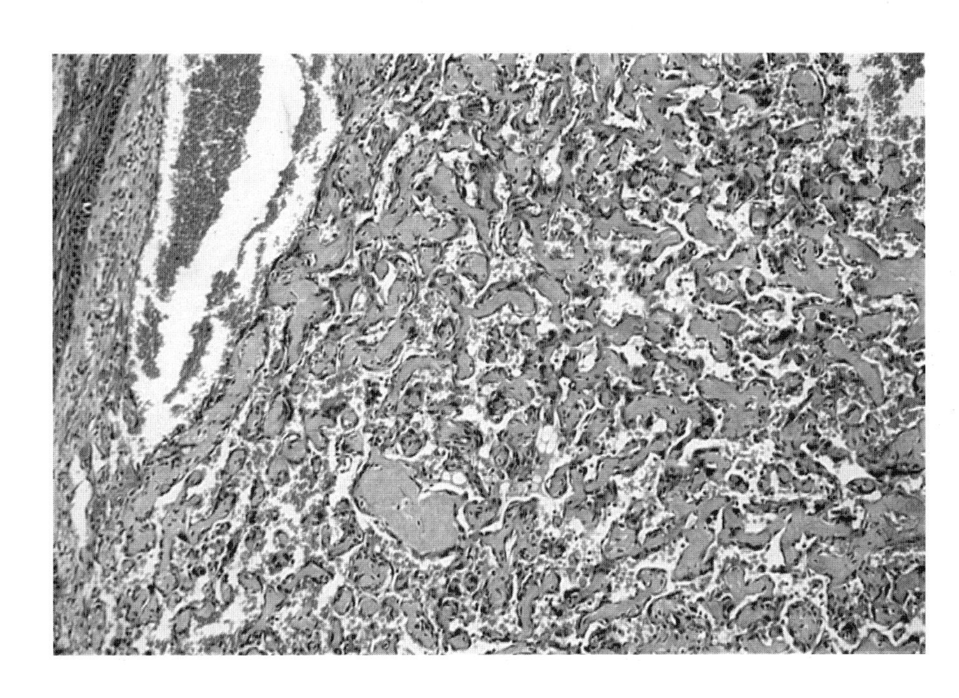

FIG. 34-2. Intravascular papillary endothelial hyperplasia
Typical hyaline papillary projections lined by endothelial cells focally mimicking a dissection of collagen pattern.

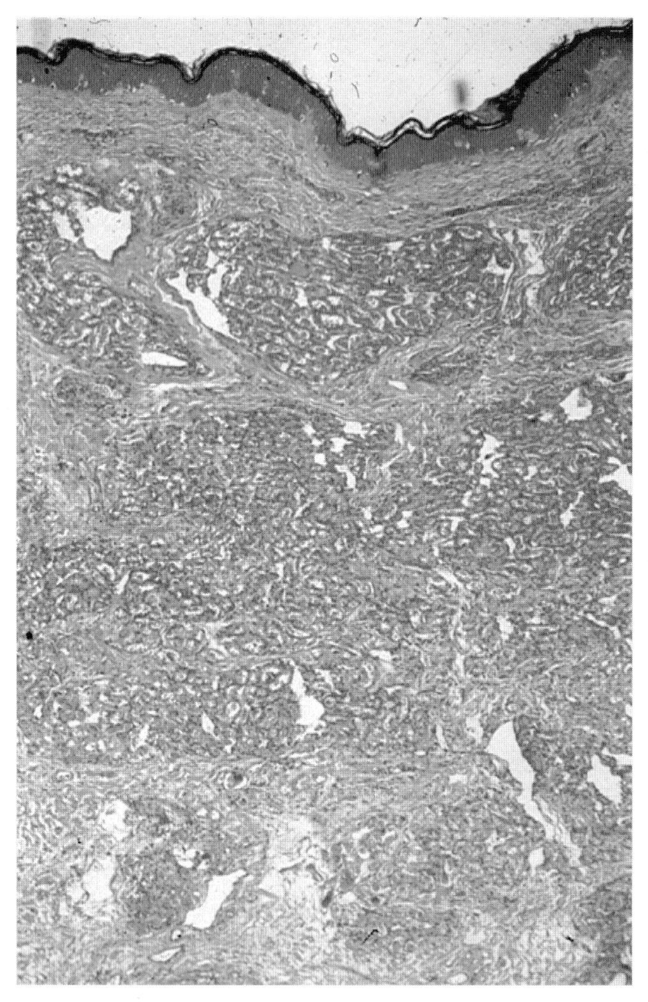

FIG. 34-3. Reactive angioendotheliomatosis
Numerous closely packed capillaries within preexisting dilated blood vessels are seen throughout the dermis.

multifocality of the disease seem to point to an inflammatory or reactive pathogenesis rather than a neoplasm.[16]

Clinical Features. Most lesions arise either superficially in the dermis, or in the subcutaneous tissue or deeper tissues, although occasionally both superficial and deep tissues are affected together.[17,18]

Superficial lesions. Young to middle-aged women are mainly affected with the development of pruritic papules and plaques at or around the external ear. The lesions can be numerous but are limited to one side. Typically the clinical course is chronic over several years despite excision and other treatment modalities. Such superficial lesions were originally referred to as pseudopyogenic granuloma.[19] Occlusion of the external auditory canal can bring patients to the attention of ear, nose and throat specialists.[20] Sometimes other areas in the head and neck region, especially the occipital region and the vicinity of the temporal artery, are affected.

Lesions of subcutaneous and deeper tissues. Adults are mainly affected, and there is no gender predilection. The typical lesion is a solitary, slowly growing, firm, subcutaneous swelling 2 to 10 cm in size in the head and neck region with some predilection for the pre- or postauricular sites. Sometimes more than one lesion arises. Most lesions are asymptomatic except for occasional pruritus. Blood eosinophilia and modest enlargement of neighboring lymph nodes and salivary tissue may occur. Occasionally other body sites are affected, such as the arm, axillae, or inguinal region.[17,21,22] An exceptional case has been described in association with a traumatically induced arteriovenous fistula involving the popliteal artery.[23] The condition can persist for years, but serious complications or lymphomatous transformation does not occur. It is problematic to consider inflammatory vascular proliferative lesions of the tongue[24] or internal sites as part of angiolymphoid hyperplasia.

Histopathology. The main components of the pathology are:

1. Proliferation of small to medium-sized blood vessels often showing a lobular architecture (Fig. 34-6). Many of these

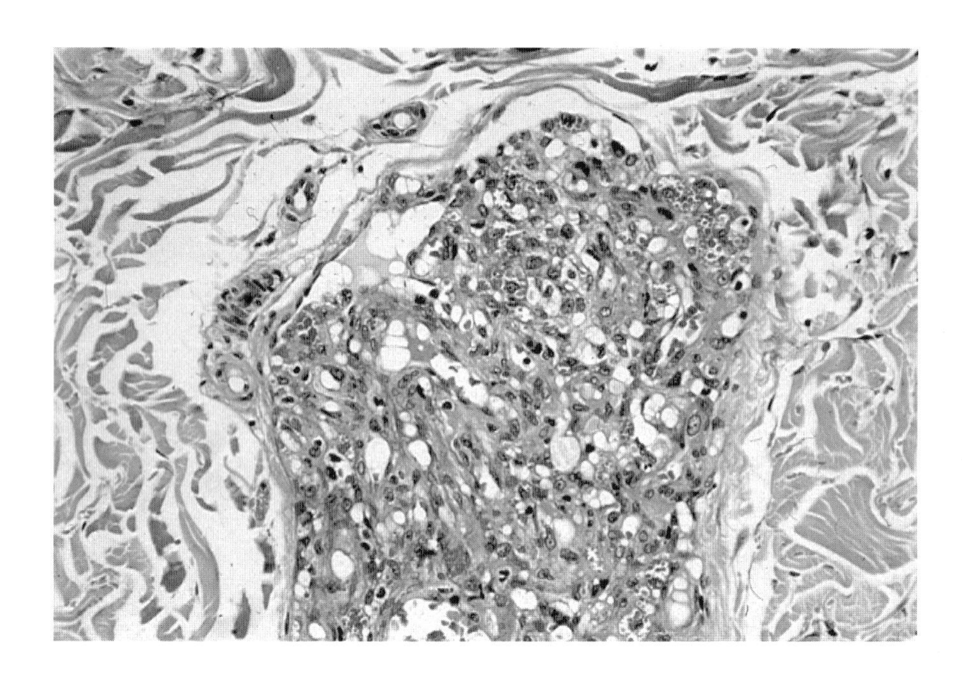

FIG. 34-4. Reactive angioendotheliomatosis
Plump endothelial cells and intraluminal eosinophilic globules in a case associated with cryoglobulinemia.

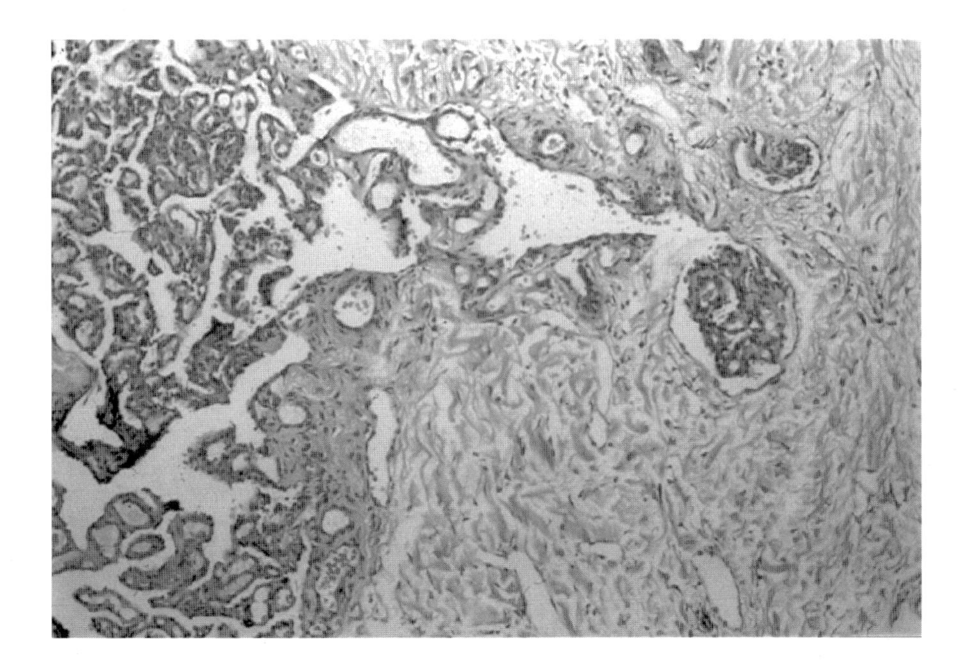

FIG. 34-5. Glomeruloid hemangioma
Note resemblance to reactive angioendotheliomatosis and two glomerular-like structures to the right. (Courtesy of Dr. F. Rongioletti, Genoa, Italy.)

vascular channels are lined by greatly enlarged (epithelioid) endothelial cells (Fig. 34-7).
2. A perivascular inflammatory cell infiltrate composed mainly of lymphocytes and eosinophils.
3. Nodular areas of lymphocytic infiltrate occurring with or without follicle formation.
4. Inflammatory vascular occlusive changes in medium-sized arteries (Fig. 34-8) associated with endothelial cell proliferation through the vessel walls.

In superficial lesions there is variable degree of vascular hyperplasia that can include areas in which the proliferation is almost angiomatous. A distinctive feature is the "cobblestone" appearance of enlarged endothelial cells that project into the lumina of some vessels. The nucleus of these cells is ovoid and orthochromatic without atypia or evidence of mitotic activity. Affected vessels often show endothelial cells with intracytoplasmic vacuoles, a prominent feature of some diagnostic value (Fig. 34-9).[19] The most abnormal blood vessels are usually sur-

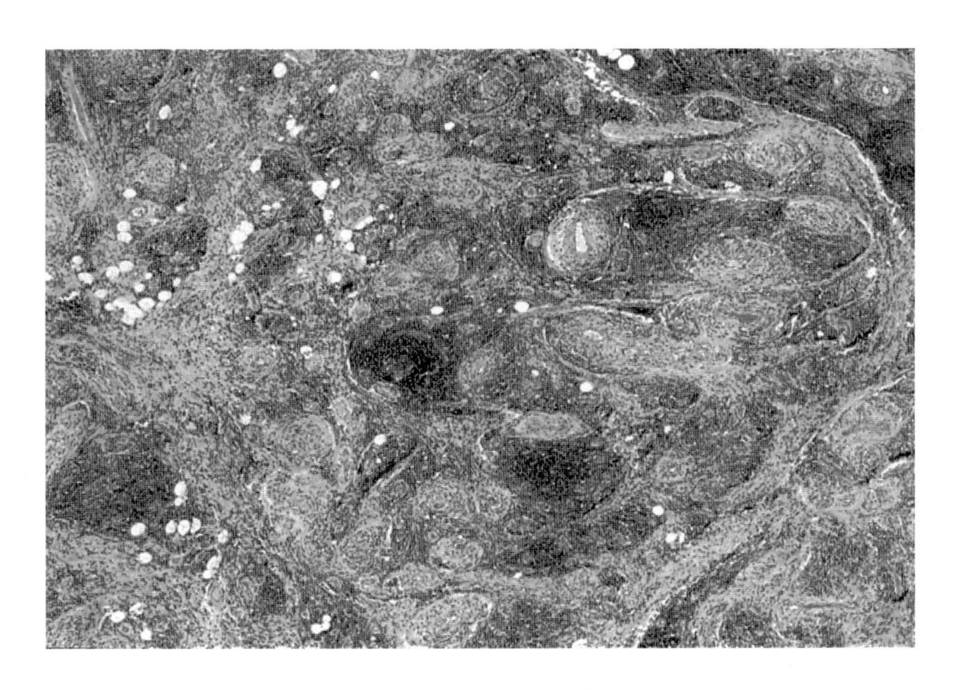

FIG. 34-6. Angiolymphoid hyperplasia with eosinophilia
Subcutaneous lesion with lobular architecture and prominent lymphoid infiltrate.

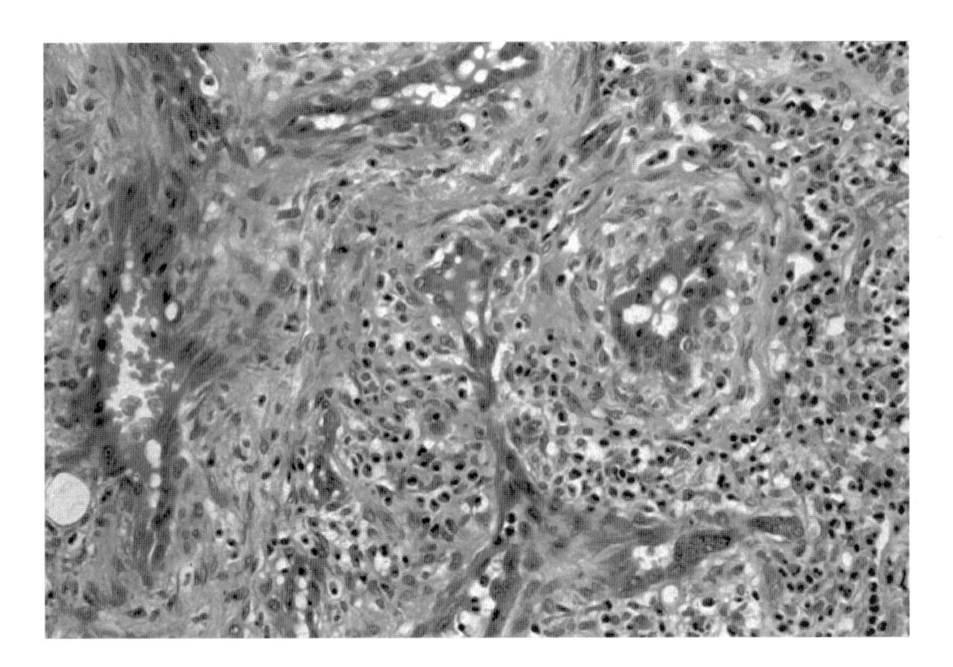

FIG. 34-7. Angiolymphoid hyperplasia with eosinophilia
Prominent endothelial cells with abundant eosinophilic cytoplasm and numerous eosinophils in the surrounding stroma.

rounded by stellate and spindle-shaped cells in a mucoid stroma. The associated perivascular inflammatory cell infiltrate is usually loosely scattered around the affected vessel, but in places it may be almost completely absent. Generally eosinophils make up 5% to 15% of the cells. A complete absence of eosinophils should cast doubt on the diagnosis. Occasionally more extensive areas of lymphoid infiltrate develop in the lower dermis, but lymphoid follicle formation is rare compared with subcutaneous lesions.

The epidermis above the lesions may show acanthosis or erosions due to superficial trauma. The skin appendages are usually unaffected except for the occasional finding of follicular mucinosis.[25]

In subcutaneous lesions the inflammatory cell infiltrate is usually more massive, with a central, poorly circumscribed nodule that replaces the fat. The nodule is composed of confluent sheets of small lymphocytes and eosinophils in which a network of poorly canalized thick-walled capillaries is embedded. Satellite smaller islands of

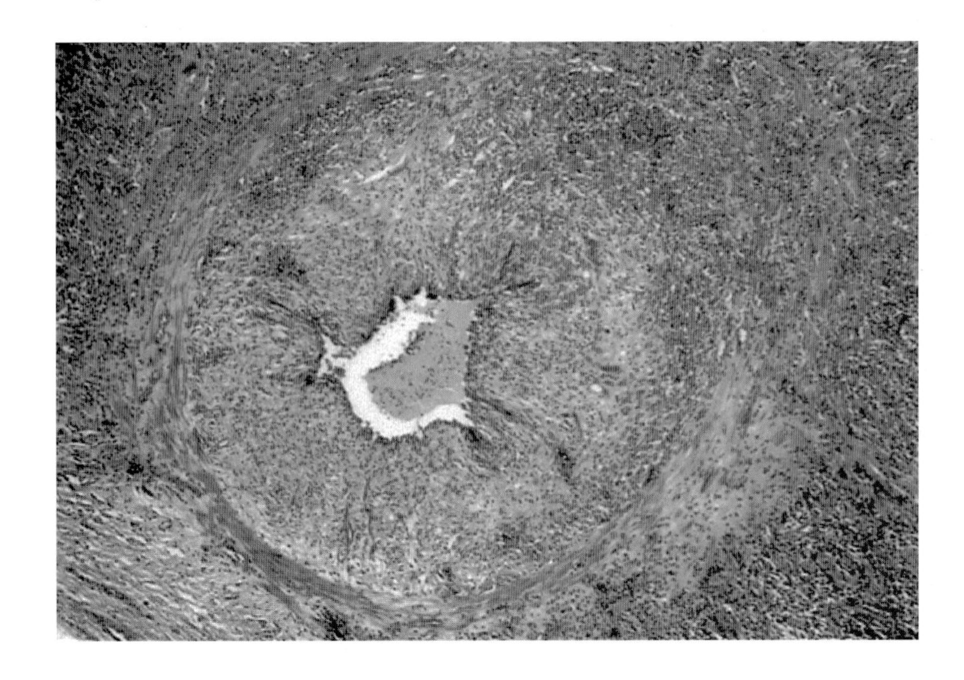

FIG. 34-8. Angiolymphoid hyperplasia with eosinophilia
Involvement of a medium-sized artery.

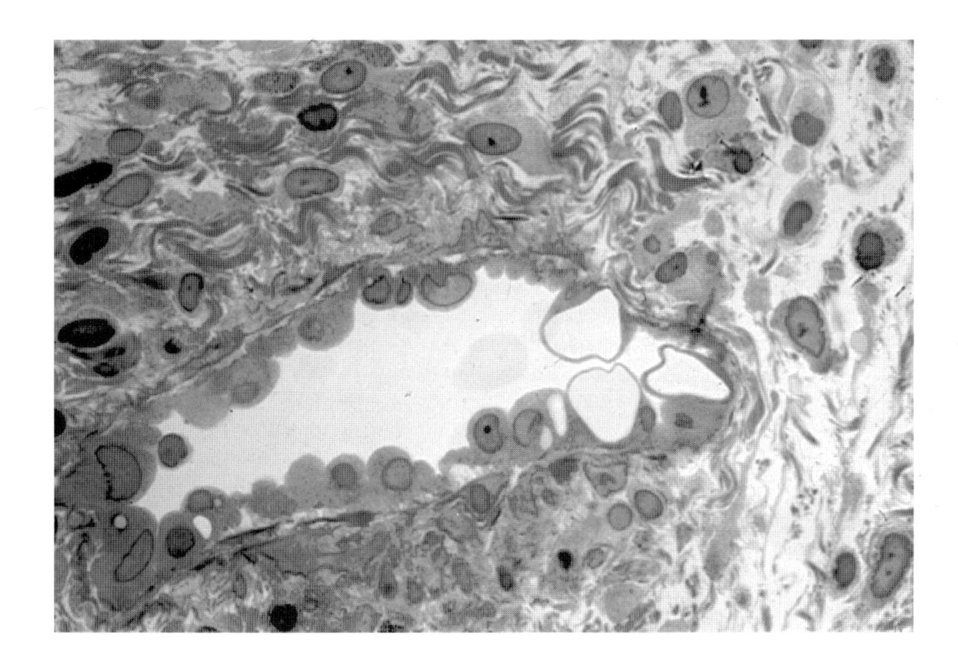

FIG. 34-9. Angiolymphoid hyperplasia with eosinophilia
Thin epon-embedded section highlighting the epithelioid cells and the cytoplasmic vacuoles.

lymphoid cells with lymphoid follicles usually surround the central nodule. Eosinophils can form up to 50% of the cell population.

In about 50% of cases, evidence of involvement of medium to large-sized arteries can be found.[17] A variable degree of blood-vessel damage occurs, with infiltration of the vessel wall by inflammatory cells and occlusion of the lumen. Partial loss of the internal elastic lamina is often seen.

Pathogenesis. The etiology and pathogenesis of angiolymphoid hyperplasia is at present uncertain. Occasionally trauma[16] or external otitis can precede the onset of the disease. Many of the histologic features suggest chronic allergic inflammation in which certain aspects, such as vessel changes, are exaggerated. Ultrastructural studies have not confirmed that the enlarged endothelial cells are developing histiocytic properties, as has been suggested.[13,14,19]

Differential Diagnosis. The proliferation of endothelial-lined channels with large irregular cells in angiolymphoid hyperplasia can be misinterpreted as angiosarcoma. The latter can be accompanied by a lymphocytic infiltrate, but eosinophils are rarely present. The main distinguishing feature is the presence of nuclear atypia with hyperchromatism, mitotic activity, and dissection of collagen pattern in angiosarcoma, but not in angiolymphoid hyperplasia. Distinction from the recently described retiform hemangioendothelioma is easy: angiolymphoid hyperplasia lacks a retiform growth pattern and does not show tall, narrow endothelial cells with a typical hobnail appearance, as is the case in retiform hemangioendothelioma.

Angiolymphoid hyperplasia can be distinguished from most benign angiomas or ectasias by the absence of an intrinsic inflammatory cell infiltrate in the latter. Greatly enlarged endothelial cells with an eosinophilic cytoplasm rarely feature in benign angiomas, although they can be seen focally in lobular capillary hemangioma (pyogenic granuloma).

Persistent insect bite reactions can show overlapping histologic features with angiolymphoid hyperplasia, but the vascular proliferation is rarely as exuberant. A somewhat similar pathology can also arise as a reaction to injected vaccines.[26–28] The histology is characterized by a deep lymphoid infiltrate with lymphoid follicles, tissue eosinophilia, and fibrosis. Vascular hyperplasia is, however, less marked than in angiolymphoid hyperplasia, and epithelioid endothelial cells are not a feature. A diagnostic feature is the presence of aluminium-containing crystals as demonstrated by solochrome-azurin when aluminium-adsorbed vaccines have been used.[26]

When angiolymphoid hyperplasia with eosinophilia was first described in Western Europe, similarities to *Kimura's disease* as reported in the Far East were noted. Indeed, many authors thought that both conditions might be part of one disease spectrum.[17] However, more recently most authorities emphasize differences between the two entities.[12,15,21,22,29–31] Subcutaneous angiolymphoid hyperplasia and Kimura's disease occur most commonly in the head and neck region in adults and both share the histological features of extensive lymphoid proliferation, tissue eosinophilia, and evidence of vascular hyperplasia. Kimura's disease, however, demonstrates a wider age span with male predominance and a tendency for more extensive lesions to occur, often with involvement of salivary tissue and lymph nodes and at sites distant from the head and neck region.[32] Authors from the Far East have stressed the histologic differences, the most important of which are the lesser degree of exuberant vascular hyperplasia lacking prominent eosinophilic endothelial cells and the absence of uncanalized blood vessels in Kimura's disease. Other points of difference are eosinophilic abscesses and marked fibrosis around the lesions in Kimura's disease and the absence of lesions centered around damaged arteries. There is an important association between Kimura's disease and renal disease, particularly nephrotic syndrome.[33]

Pyogenic Granuloma (Lobular Capillary Hemangioma)

Pyogenic granuloma is a common proliferative lesion that often occurs shortly after a minor injury or infection of the skin. Typically the lesion grows rapidly for a few weeks before stabilizing as an elevated, bright red papule, usually not more than 1 to 2 cm in size; it then may persist indefinitely unless destroyed. Recurrence after surgery or cautery is not rare. Pyogenic granuloma most often affects children or young adults of either gender, but the age range is wide; the hands, fingers, and face, especially the lips and gums, are the most common sites.[34,35] Pyogenic granuloma of the gingiva in pregnancy (epulis of pregnancy) is a special subgroup.

A rare and alarming event is the development of multiple satellite angiomatous lesions at and around the site of a previously destroyed pyogenic granuloma.[36,37] This usually occurs following lesions on the shoulder or upper trunk in children. Histologically lesions that are similar to pyogenic granuloma can occur in the deep dermis, the subcutaneous tissue,[38] and even within dilated venous channels.[39] Widely scattered angiomatous lesions resembling pyogenic granulomas have also been described,[40–43] sometimes in association with visceral disease.

Histopathology. The typical lesion presents as a polypoid mass of angiomatous tissue protruding above the surrounding skin. It is often constricted at its base by a collarette of acanthotic epidermis (Fig. 34-10). An intact flattened epidermis may cover the entire lesion, but surface erosions are common. In ulcerated lesions a superficial inflammatory cell reaction can give rise to an appearance suggestive of granulation tissue, but inflammation does not appear to be an intrinsic feature. Inflammation is usually slight in the deeper part of the lesion and may be absent when the epidermis is intact. The angiomatous tissue tends to occur in discrete masses or lobules, resembling a capillary hemangioma, hence the preference by Mills et al[34] for the term "lobular capillary hemangioma" to describe this condition (Fig. 34-11). The angiomatous tissue is surrounded by myxoid stroma (Fig. 34-12) containing scattered spindle- and stellate-shaped connective tissue cells and occasional mast cells. The angiomatous tissue is composed of a variably dilated network of blood-filled capillary vessels and groups of poorly canalized vascular tufts. Mitotic activity varies and can be prominent. Feeding vessels often extend into the adjacent dermis and rare lesions show a deep component in the reticular dermis. Occasionally foci of intravascular papillary endothelial hyperplasia occur within the larger deep vessels. Focal epithelioid endothelial cells sometimes can be seen. The histology of recurrent or satellite lesions is similar, but the angiomatous proliferation can extend more deeply into the dermis. Pyogenic granulomas of the subcutaneous tissue or in veins show similar histologic features but lack an inflammatory component. Intravascular lesions can so distend the veins that the surrounding muscle coat can be thinned and difficult to detect.

Pathogenesis. It was once assumed that granuloma pyogenicum was caused by pyogenic infection. However, the histologic picture of early lesions suggests a capillary hemangioma, and even in eroded lesions that show inflammation, the appearance mimics that of a capillary hemangioma in its deeper portions. Therefore, terms like eruptive hemangioma[44] and lobular capillary hemangioma[34] have been suggested.

Immunohistochemical studies have demonstrated positive labeling of endothelial cells for factor VIII–related antigen, Ulex europaeus agglutinin-1 and vimentin, and also of perithelial cells for muscle-specific actin and type IV collagen. Antibodies to estrogen and progesterone-receptor proteins were negative.[45] These studies tend to support a reactive rather then neoplastic etiology of pyogenic granuloma.

Differential Diagnosis. Both Kaposi's sarcoma and angiosarcoma should be considered as part of the differential diagnosis, especially when multiple lesions are present. Elevated polypoid lesions are rare in Kaposi's sarcoma; most show obvious spindle cells woven between delicate vascular spaces, unlike in pyogenic granuloma. A much greater degree of cell atypia with intraluminal spreading of malignant cells characterizes well-differentiated angiosarcomas. Focal areas of intravascular papillary endothelial hyperplasia within a pyogenic gran-

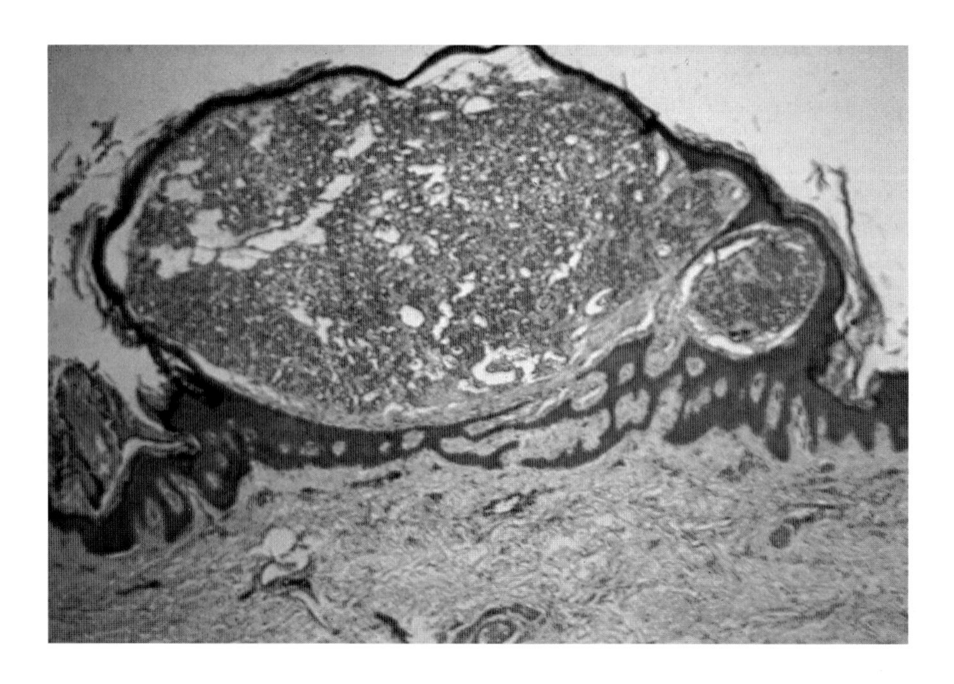

FIG. 34-10. Pyogenic granuloma Early, nonulcerated lesion with the typical epithelial collarette.

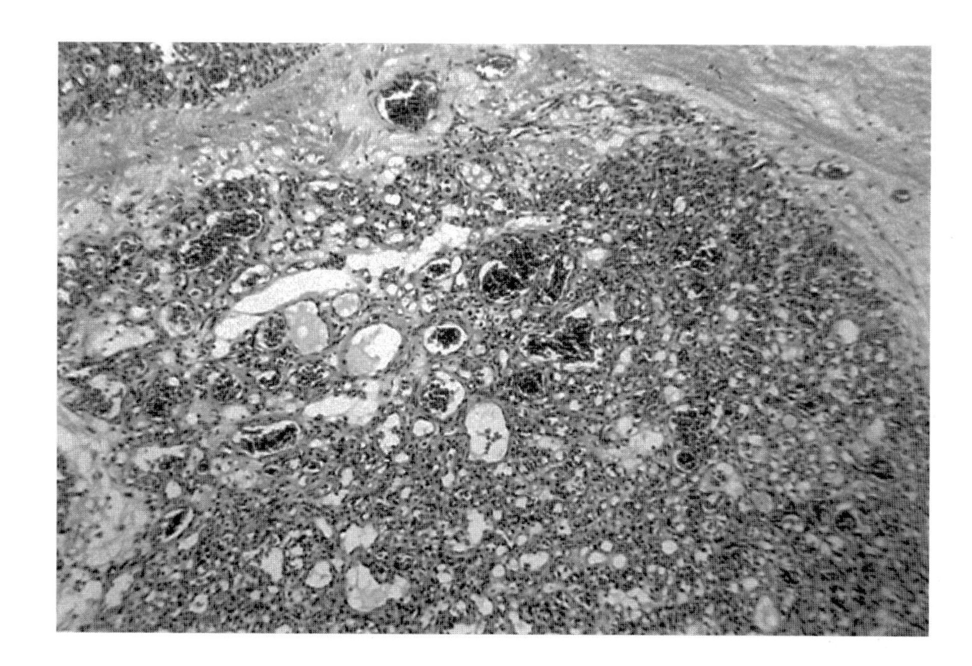

FIG. 34-11. Pyogenic granuloma Note lobules of dilated and congested capillaries.

uloma occasionally can simulate angiosarcoma, but, even so, nuclear atypia is slight.

In recent years further differential diagnosis of pyogenic granuloma is with bacillary angiomatosis, a recently described infectious vascular proliferation common in HIV-infected patients and caused by *Rochalimaea henselae,* a small, gram-negative rod belonging to the family Bartonellaceae[46] (see Chap. 21). Clinically, and especially histologically, lesions of bacillary angiomatosis can look remarkably similar to a pyogenic granuloma. In the former, however, a lobular architecture is not apparent, the endothelial cells often have abundant pale cytoplasm (Fig. 34-13), and aggregates of neutrophils are present throughout the lesion, often in relation to clumps of granular basophilic material. This basophilic material shows bacilli when stained with Warthin-Starry (Fig. 34-14) or Giemsa stains.

Vascular granulomatous lesions mimicking pyogenic granulomas occasionally arise as a complication of retinoid therapy, but the histology is that of nonspecific vascular granulation tissue lacking a lobular architecture.[47,48]

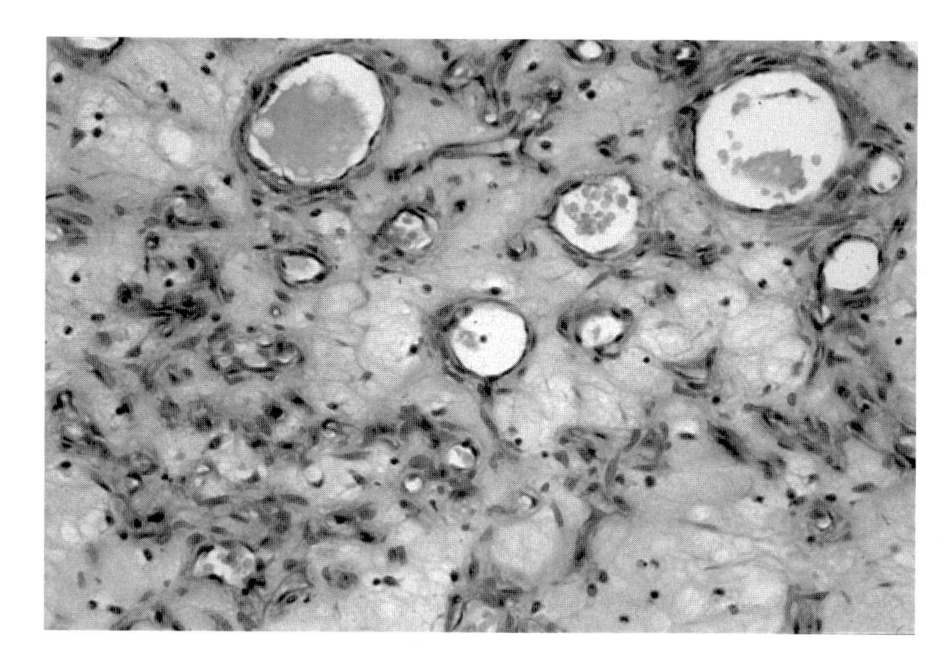

FIG. 34-12. Pyogenic granuloma Myxoid stroma and bland endothelial cells.

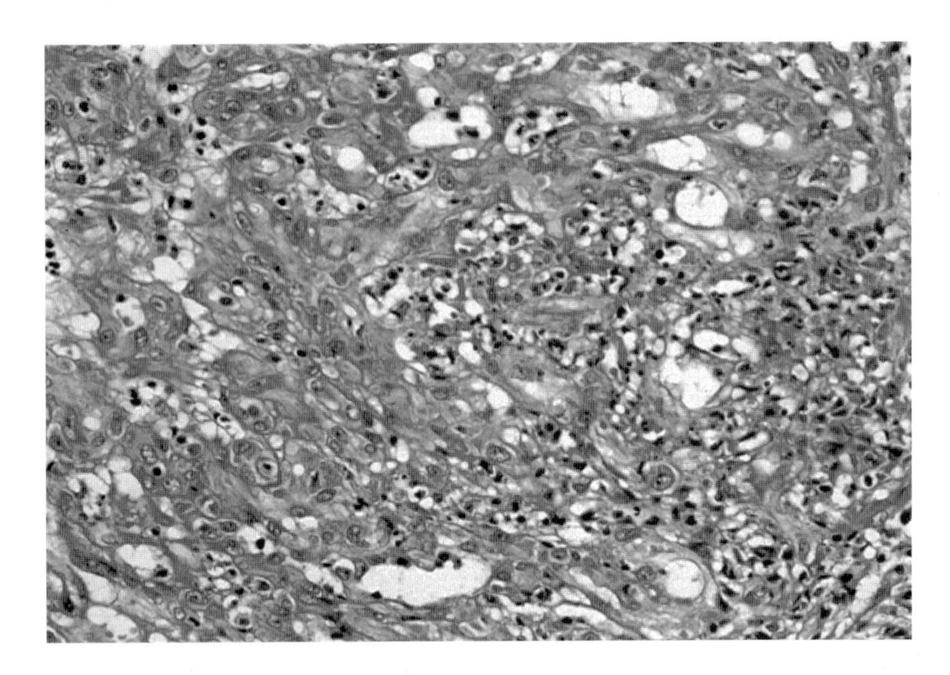

FIG. 34-13. Bacillary angiomatosis Note the pale epithelioid endothelial cells and numerous neutrophils with nuclear dust.

DEVELOPMENTAL ABNORMALITIES

Nevus Flammeus

The term nevus flammeus is often used to refer to two different lesions: the *salmon patch* and the *port-wine stain*. Although both lesions are congenital, the former tends to involute in the first years of life and usually has no association with other types of anomalies, while the latter tends to be persistent and is often related to other malformations. The salmon patch is present in up to 50% of newborns of either gender as an ill-defined, red to pale pink macule mainly in the nape of the neck, the glabella, or the eyelids.[49,50] The port-wine stain occurs in about 0.3% of newborns as a macular, usually unilateral, red-pink lesion with predilection for the face.[50] Later in life the lesion becomes darker and raised.

Sturge-Weber syndrome (encephalotrigeminal angiomatosis) is characterized by the presence of a facial port-wine stain, often in the distribution of the trigeminal nerve associated with an ipsilateral leptomeningeal venous malformation, atrophy and calcification of the underlying cerebral cortex, epilepsy, mental retardation, ocular vascular malformations, glaucoma, and contralateral hemiparesis.

In *Klippel-Trenaunay syndrome* (osteohypertrophic nevus flammeus), one observes hypertrophy of the soft tissues and bones of one or several extremities affected with a nevus flammeus. Associated with this are varicosities or arteriovenous fistulas or both and, less commonly, spindle-cell hemangioendotheliomas. Cases presenting with arteriovenous fistulas

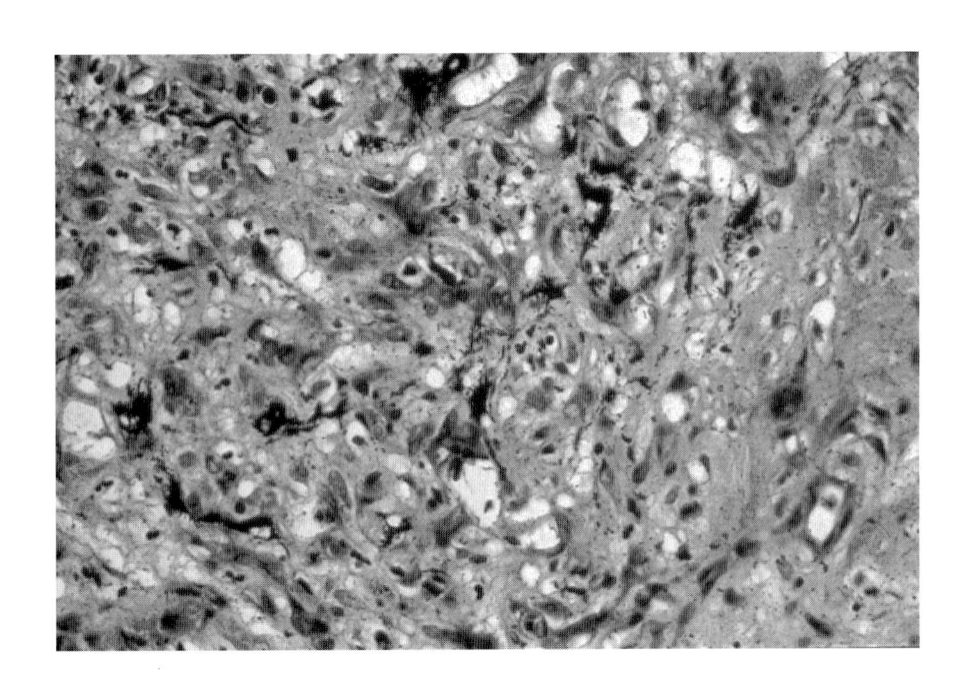

FIG. 34-14. Bacillary angiomatosis Warthin-Starry stain showing numerous clumps of bacilli.

are sometimes known as Parkes-Weber syndrome. Complications of note are cutaneous ulcers and high-output cardiac failure.

Histopathology. In the *salmon patch,* dilated capillaries are seen in the papillary dermis. In the *port-wine stain,* no telangiectases are apparent histologically until the patient has reached about 10 years of age.[51] The capillary ectasias thereafter gradually increase with age. Ultimately, when the lesion is raised or nodular, not only the superficial capillaries but also some of the blood vessels in the deeper layers of the dermis and in the subcutaneous layer are dilated. Many ectatic vessels are filled with red blood cells. Lesions with a deep component can be associated with a cavernous hemangioma or an arteriovenous malformation.[51]

Histogenesis. Because no histologic abnormalities are present early in life with port-wine stain, it appears likely that this malformation is the result of a congenital weakness of the capillary walls.[51] Thus, the port-wine stain represents a progressive telangiectasia. Antibodies directed against components of the blood vessel wall, collagenous basement membrane protein (type IV collagen), fibronectin, and factor VIII–related antigen have an equivalent distribution and intensity in normal skin and nevus flammeus. Although this does not rule out a structural abnormality of these components, it has been suggested that the alteration may be related to the supporting dermal elements rather than to an intrinsic abnormality in the vessel wall.[52] An abnormality in neuromodulation has been proposed as an alternate theory.[53]

Angiokeratoma

Four types of angiokeratoma have been described that represent true ectasias of blood vessels of the superficial dermis:[54]

1. *Angiokeratoma corporis diffusum.* Patients present with numerous clusters of tiny red papules in a symmetrical distribution usually in the "bathing-trunk" area. Although often considered synonymous with Fabry's disease, which is an X-linked genetic disorder associated with deficiency of the lysosomal enzyme A-galactosidase, identical clinical appearances have been described in patients with other enzymatic deficiencies including B-galactosidase, neuraminidase, and L-fucosidase.[55,56] An exceptional case was reported in an individual with no detectable biochemical abnormalities.[57]
2. *Angiokeratoma of Mibelli.* Several dark red papules with a slightly verrucous surface are seen on the dorsa of the fingers and toes. Usually the lesions appear during childhood or adolescence and measure from 3 to 5 mm in diameter.[58]
3. *Angiokeratoma of Fordyce.* Multiple vascular papules 2 to 4 mm in diameter are seen on the scrotum. Similar lesions have been described on the vulva.[59] They arise in middle or later life. Early lesions are red, soft, and compressible; later, they become blue, keratotic, and noncompressible.[60]
4. *Solitary or multiple angiokeratomas.* Usually one and occasionally several papular lesions arise in young adults, most commonly on the lower extremities. The lesions range from 2 to 10 mm in diameter. Early lesions appear bright red and soft, but they later become blue to black, firm, and hyperkeratotic.[54] Thrombosed lesions are not uncommonly misdisgnosed clinically as malignant melanomas.

Histopathology. The histologic findings are essentially the same in all four above-mentioned types of angiokeratoma and consist of numerous, dilated, thin-walled, congested capillaries mainly in the papillary dermis underlying an epidermis that shows variable degrees of acanthosis with elongation of the rete ridges and hyperkeratosis (Fig. 34-15).[54] In cutaneous lesions of Fabry's disease, cytoplasmic vacuoles representing lipids can sometimes be detected in endothelial cells, fibroblasts, and pericytes.[61]

Generalized Essential Telangiectasia

Widespread linear telangiectases, mainly on the extremities, may develop gradually in adults, predominantly in women.[62]

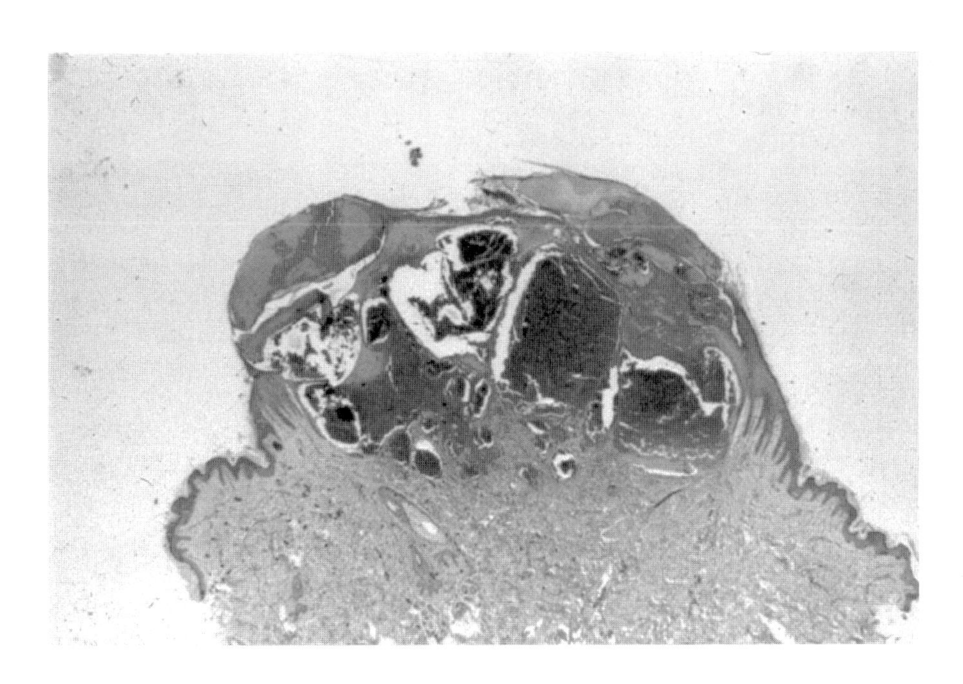

FIG. 34-15. Angiokeratoma
Note ectatic blood vessels in the papillary dermis with overlying epidermal hyperplasia.

Histopathology. Dilated, often congested, vessels are seen in the papillary dermis. The walls of the vessels are composed only of endothelium. The absence of alkaline phosphatase activity suggests that it is the venous portion of the capillary loop that participates in the disease process.[62]

Unilateral Nevoid Telangiectasia

Although unilateral nevoid telangiectasia may be congenital, in most instances its onset is related to high estrogen levels because they occur in pregnancy, during puberty, and in chronic hepatic disease associated with alcoholism.[63] The telangiectases, which are largely punctate and stellate rather than linear, follow a dermatomal distribution, particularly those associated with the trigeminal nerve and cranial nerves III and IV. Rare cases are associated with gastric involvement.[64]

Histopathology. Numerous dilated vessels are seen in the upper and middle dermis and, to a lesser extent, in the deeper part of the dermis.

Histogenesis. It has been proposed that the changes seen in this condition are induced by an increase in estrogen receptors in a dermatomal distribution.[65]

Angioma Serpiginosum

Angioma serpiginosum is a rare acquired vascular lesion that usually presents in the first two decades of life with predilection for females.[66] Anatomic distribution is wide, but lesions often present in the lower extremities. The disorder is asymptomatic, and there is slow progression over the years. Focal spontaneous regression rarely occurs. Most cases are sporadic but inherited cases have been reported.[67] A typical lesion is characterized by deeply red nonpalpable puncta that are grouped closely together in a macular or netlike pattern. Irregular extension at the periphery of the macules may cause them to have serpiginous borders. The deeply red puncta represent dilated capillaries.

Histopathology. Dilated, thin-walled capillaries are seen in some of the dermal papillae and the superficial reticular dermis (Fig. 34-16). Epidermal changes and extravasation of red blood cells are absent.

Histogenesis. On electron microscopic examination, it is apparent that the thickening of the capillary walls is caused by a heavy precipitate of basement membrane–like material mixed with thin collagen fibers and an increased number of concentrically arranged pericytes.[68] In addition, some of the dilated capillaries show slit-like protrusions of their lumina and endothelial lining into the surrounding thickened vessel walls. These findings indicate that angioma serpiginosum is not just a simple telangiectasia but represents a vascular malformation.[68]

Hereditary Hemorrhagic Telangiectasia (Osler-Weber-Rendu Disease)

Osler-Weber-Rendu disease is inherited as an autosomal dominant trait. Although epistaxis may already begin in childhood, the characteristic telangiectases on the mucous membranes do not begin to appear until adolescence, and the cutaneous lesions often appear much later in life, involving particularly the upper part of the body. Typical lesions are small bright red nonpulsating papules.

Concomitant involvement of other organs including the gastrointestinal tract, liver, brain, lungs, spleen, kidneys, and adrenal glands is common. Associated vascular malformations are often a feature.[69] Morbidity and mortality are mainly related to bleeding from internal organs.

Histopathology. Irregularly dilated capillaries and venules

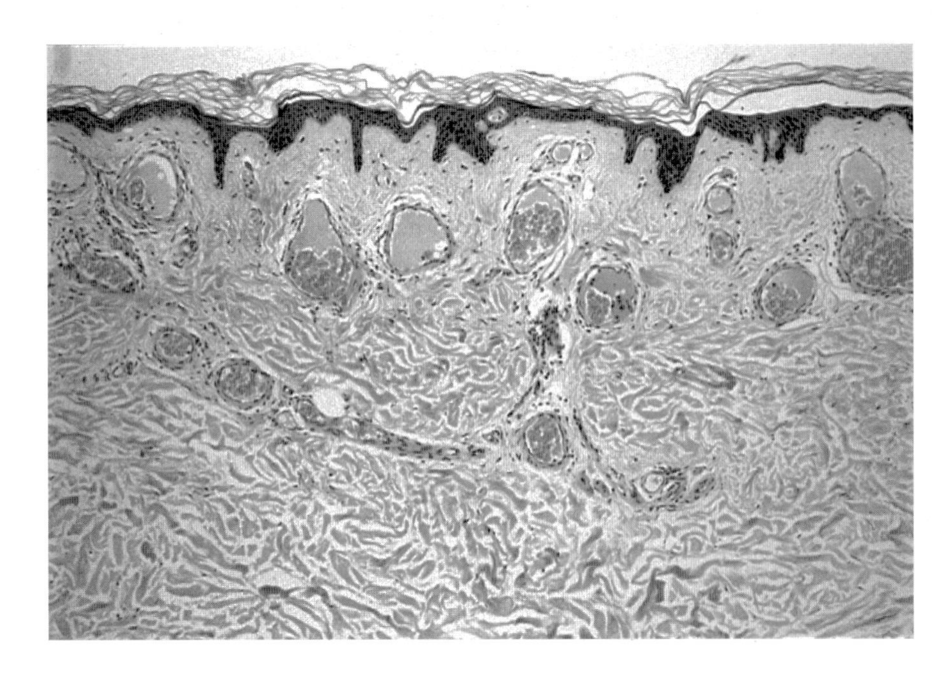

FIG. 34-16. Angioma serpiginosum
Dilated and congested capillaries in the superficial dermis. (Courtesy of Dr. Michele Clement, Farnborough, United Kingdom.)

lined by flat endothelial cells are seen in the papillary and subpapillary dermis.

Histogenesis. On electron microscopy, the dilated vessels in the skin and oral mucosa are seen to be small postcapillary venules that normally do not possess pericytes. A defect in the perivascular supportive tissue has been found responsible for the breakdown of the junctions between endothelial cells and the resultant hemorrhage.[70] The presence of a mild perivascular lymphocytic infiltrate has been regarded as important in inducing the pathologic changes.[71]

Nevus Araneus (Spider Nevus)

Nevus araneus, or spider nevus, considered the most common form of telangiectasia, presents at any age, especially in children, with predilection for the face and upper limbs.[69,72] It is characterized by a central, slightly elevated, red punctum from which blood vessels radiate. Occasionally pulsation can be observed. Although spider nevi often arise spontaneously, pregnancy, the use of oral contraceptives, and liver disease are factors predisposing their appearance.[69] Spontaneous regression is common as children grow older and after pregnancy.

Histopathology. In the center of the lesion is an ascending artery that branches and communicates with multiple dilated capillaries.

Venous Lakes

Venous lakes are small, dark blue, slightly raised, soft lesions occurring on the exposed skin of elderly persons. They can usually be emptied of most of their blood using sustained pressure. Usually several lesions are present. The face, ears, and lips are the most common sites.

Histopathology. Venous lakes represent telangiectasias. In the upper dermis, close to the epidermis, they show either one greatly dilated space or several interconnected dilated spaces filled with erythrocytes and lined by a single layer of flattened endothelial cells and a thin wall of fibrous tissue.[73] In some instances, there is, in place of fibrous tissue, a thin irregular noncontinuous smooth muscle layer.[74]

BENIGN TUMORS

Capillary Hemangioma Variants

Strawberry Nevus (Juvenile Hemangioendothelioma)

Capillary hemangioma, mostly represented by strawberry nevus, constitutes the most common vascular tumor of infancy, affecting as many as one of every 100 live births. Overall, it comprises between 32% and 42% of all vascular tumors.[75,76] Lesions usually first appear between the third and fifth week of life, increase in size for several months to one year, and then start to regress. A typical lesion consists of one or several bright red, soft, lobulated tumors that vary greatly in size and have a wide anatomic distribution with predilection for the head and neck area. Females are slightly more affected than males. On occasion lesions can involve deeper soft tissues or even internal organs and can be associated with high morbidity, especially if located near vital structures. Complete spontaneous resolution is common, occurring in about 70% of capillary hemangiomas by the time the patient has reached the age of 7 years.

Kasabach-Merritt syndrome. The association of extensive capillary hemangiomas in infants with thrombocytopenia and purpura is known as Kasabach-Merritt syndrome. However, this syndrome is seen occasionally in adults with numerous or very large cavernous hemangiomas. The purpura is not just a result of thrombocytopenia, as first assumed, but represents a consumption coagulopathy within the hemangioma.[77]

Histopathology. All tumors have a lobular architecture (Fig. 34-17), but microscopic features change as the lesion evolves. During their period of growth in early infancy, capillary hemangiomas show considerable proliferation of their endothelial cells. The endothelial cells are large, mitotically active, and aggregated predominantly in solid strands and masses in which there are only a few small capillary lumina. Not uncommonly crystalline intracytoplasmic inclusions can be seen in the endothelial cells. The lumina can be highlighted with the use of a reticulin stain. In maturing lesions, the capillary lumina are wider and the lining endothelial cells then appear flatter (Fig. 34-18). In mature lesions, some of the lumina may be greatly dilated, resembling focally a cavernous hemangioma. In the invo-

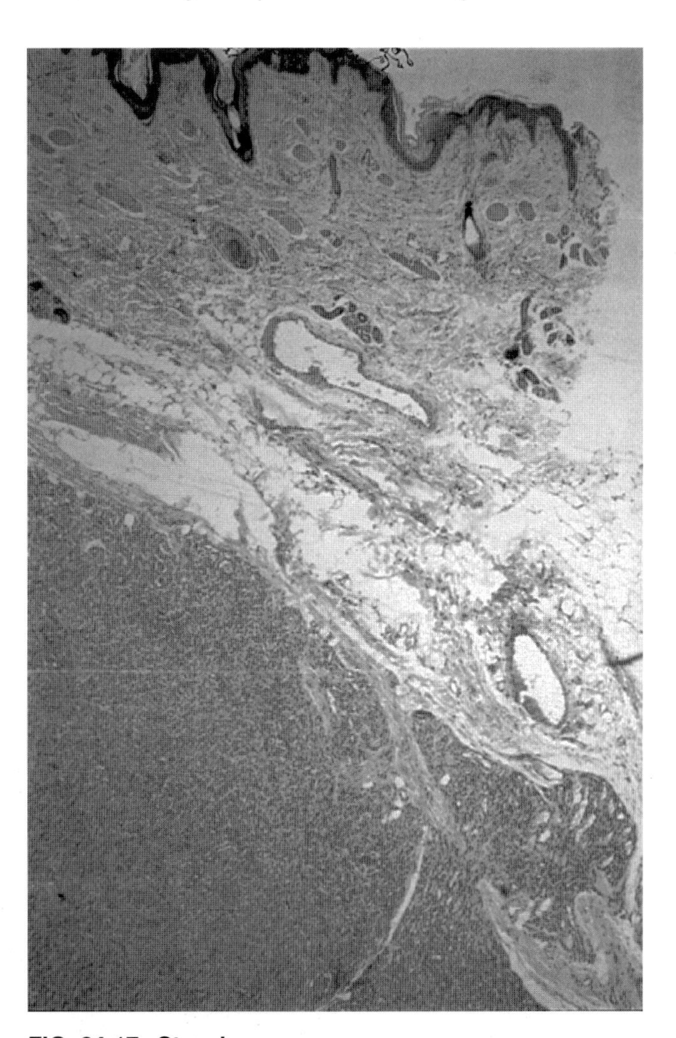

FIG. 34-17. Strawberry nevus
Note lobular architecture in an early lesion.

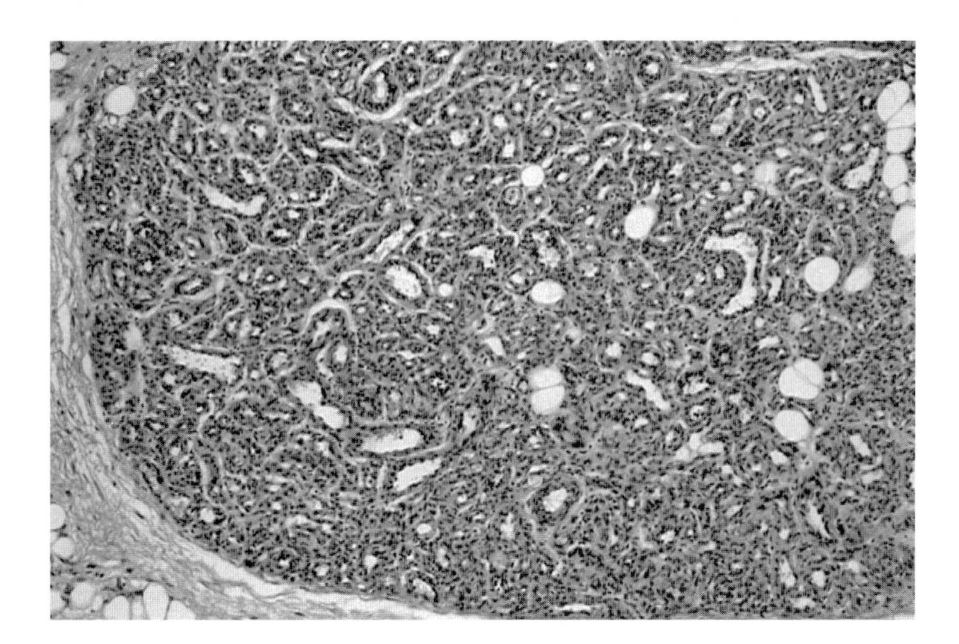

FIG. 34-18. Strawberry nevus More mature lesion with a number of canalized capillaries.

luting phase, there is progressive fibrosis with disappearance of the blood vessels and the vascular nature of the tumor might be difficult to establish. However, the lobular pattern is often preserved. A worrying but entirely benign feature seen in a number of capillary hemangiomas is the presence of perineural invasion.[78,79]

Pathogenesis. Ultrastructural and immunohistochemical studies of capillary hemangiomas have demonstrated that tumors show remarkable cellular heterogeneity. A large proportion of the cells in a given tumor are endothelial cells and pericytes, but fibroblasts, mast cells, and a population of as yet unidentified factor XIIIa–positive cells have been described.[80–82] A complex interaction among these cell populations may modulate the progression and latter evolution of capillary hemangiomas.[81]

Cherry Hemangioma (Senile Angioma, Campbell de Morgan Spot)

Cherry hemangiomas are bright red lesions varying in size from a hardly visible punctum to a soft, raised, dome-shaped lesion measuring several millimeters in diameter. This very common lesion, often present in large numbers, may start appearing in early adulthood and the number of lesions increases with age. Cherry hemangiomas may occur anywhere on the skin, but the trunk and the upper limbs are the most common sites.

Histopathology. In the early stage of development, cherry hemangiomas have the appearance of true capillary hemangiomas, being composed of numerous newly formed capillaries with narrow lumina and prominent endothelial cells arranged in a lobular fashion in the subpapillary region.[83] As the lesion ages the capillaries become dilated. In a fully mature cherry hemangioma, one observes numerous moderately dilated capillaries lined by flattened endothelial cells. The intercapillary stroma shows edema and homogenization of the collagen. The epidermis is thinned and often surrounds most of the angioma as a collarette.[84]

Differential Diagnosis. In its early stage, cherry hemangioma, like granuloma pyogenicum, shows capillary proliferation; however, endothelial proliferation is much less pronounced than in granuloma pyogenicum, so that solid aggregates of endothelial cells are not seen.

Tufted Angioma (Angioblastoma)

This benign angiomatous condition can be regarded as identical to the angioblastoma reported by Japanese authors.[85,86] The angiomas affect the genders equally, usually arising between the age of 1 to 5 years[87]; occasionally the lesions are present at birth, but they may develop in adults or even in old age.[88] There are exceptional instances of angiomas arising in pregnancy with regression after parturition,[89] the occurrence in several members of a family[90] and the development of lesions after liver transplantation.[91] The most common sites for the angiomatous papules and plaques are the upper trunk, neck, and the proximal part of the limbs. The lesions usually slowly progress for several years and can come to cover wide segments of the body; some are tender on palpation. Some lesions can regress.[92]

Histopathology. Circumscribed foci of closely set capillaries are found scatttered through the dermis and occasionally reach the subcutis. At lower magnification these discrete, ovoid angiomatous lobules or tufts have been alluded to as giving rise to a "cannonball" appearance (Fig. 34-19).[87] The vascular nature of the tufts may not be immediately apparent as vascular lumina are compressed by enlarged endothelial cells and contain few red blood cells. Some of the vascular tufts appear to indent lymphatic-like channels (Fig. 34-20). Mitotic activity and cell atypia are insignificant.

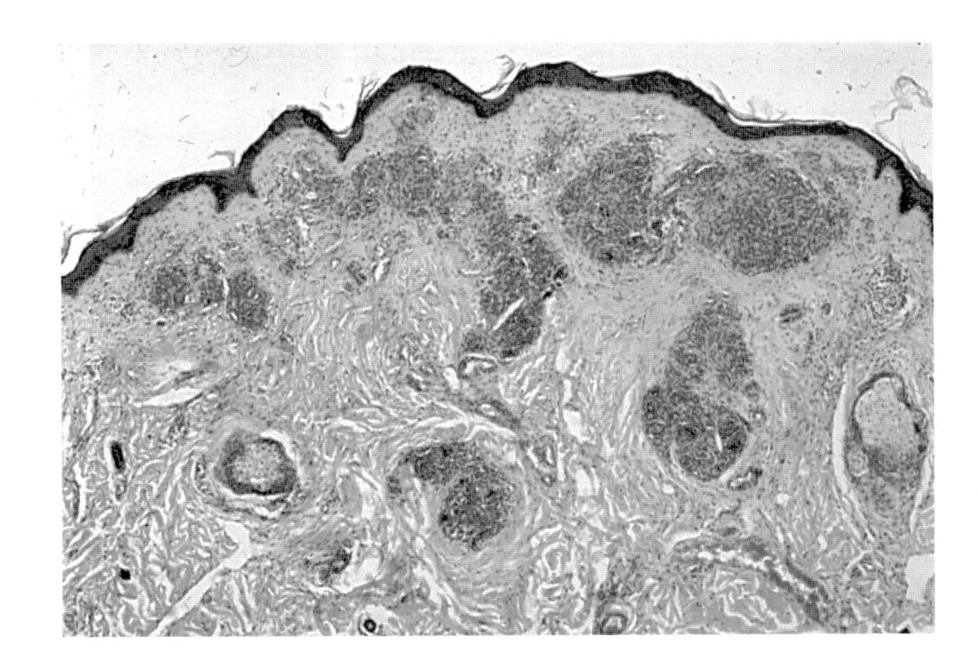

FIG. 34-19. Tufted angioma
Scattered round or ovoid dermal lobules in a typical "cannonball" distribution.

Positivity for FVIII-RA is usually limited to few vessels.[87,93] The presence of strong labeling for actin has been interpreted as indicating a prominent perithelial component among the tumor capillaries.[93]

The main importance of this uncommon angioma, especially if it develops in adults, is the differential diagnosis from *Kaposi's sarcoma* or possibly a low-grade *angiosarcoma*. Endothelial cells in tufted angioma may show slight spindling but not the elongated spindle cells of Kaposi's sarcoma. The discrete focal arrangement of vascular tufts having few red blood cells also differs greatly from the mature lesions of Kaposi's sarcoma. The absence of cell atypia is the main distinguishing feature from angiosarcoma.

The hypertrophic cellular appearance of the tufts is similar to the angiomatous tissue in strawberry nevi, but the angiomatous aggregates are far more massive in the latter, where they tend to replace wide segments of the dermis and fat. It seems likely that tufted angioma is a variant of capillary hemangioma; this is supported by the finding of characteristic cytoplasmic crystalline lamellae in both disorders.[94]

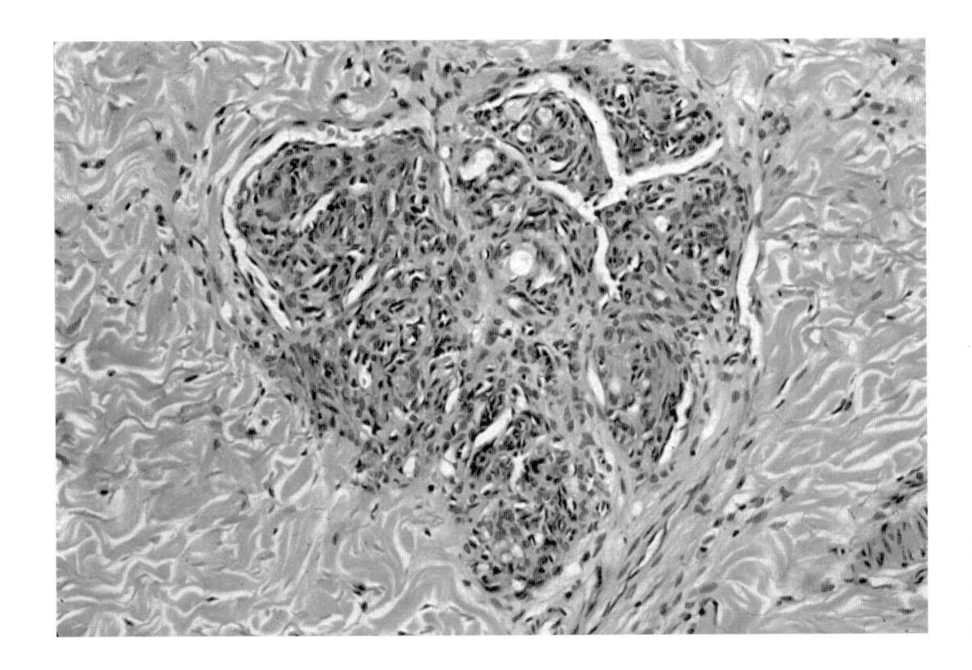

FIG. 34-20. Tufted angioma
Lobule composed of bloodless capillaries surrounded by dilated crescent-shaped vascular channels.

Cavernous Hemangioma

Sharing with strawberry nevus the same age, gender, and anatomic distribution, cavernous hemangioma still is less common and tends to be larger, deeper and less well-defined than the former and shows no tendency for spontaneous regression.[75,76] Rare cavernous hemangiomas may be associated with an overlying capillary hemangioma. There are two rare conditions in which numerous cavernous hemangiomas occur: Maffucci's syndrome and the blue rubber bleb nevus.

Maffucci's Syndrome

The outstanding features of Maffucci's syndrome are dyschondroplasia resulting in defects in ossification; fragility of the bones, causing severe deformities; and osteochondromas, which may develop into chondrosarcomas.[50] In addition, large, compressible subcutaneous cavernous hemangiomas may be present at birth or appear in childhood or early adulthood.

Blue Rubber Bleb Nevus

In the blue rubber bleb nevus, cavernous hemangiomas are present at birth but may subsequently increase in size and number. The hemangiomas have a distinct appearance, and most of them are protuberant, dark blue, soft, and compressible, and some are pedunculated. They vary from a few millimeters to 3 cm in diameter. In addition, subcutaneous hemangiomas are felt on palpation. There also are hemangiomas in the oral mucosa, the gastrointestinal tract, and less commonly in other organs.[50] Some blue rubber bleb nevi are probably telangiectatic glomus tumors in which the glomus cells are sparse.

Histopathology. Cavernous hemangiomas appear in the lower dermis and the subcutaneous tissue with large, irregular spaces containing red blood cells and fibrinous material (Fig. 34-21). The spaces are lined by a single layer of thin endothelial cells. Not uncommonly, a capillary component is present, especially in the superficial portion of a tumor. Dystrophic calcification is often present.

Variant Sinusoidal Hemangioma

Sinusoidal hemangioma is a relatively rare, recently described variant of cavernous hemangioma.[95] The lesion presents as a bluish subcutaneous mass, especially in middle-aged adults, and has predilection for females. Although the anatomic distribution is wide, tumors often present in the breast and in this setting angiosarcoma is considered in the differential diagnosis.

Histopathology. Sinusoidal hemangioma is lobular and focally ill-defined with partial or total replacement of subcutaneous fat lobules. The typical feature is the presence of gaping, markedly dilated and congested, thin walled, back-to-back vascular spaces in a sieve-like or sinusoidal arrangement (Fig. 34-22). Pseudopapillary structures due to cross-sectioning of these spaces focally resemble intravascular papillary endothelial hyperplasia. The blood vessels are lined by bland, flat endothelial cells, which can be focally prominent and mildly pleomorphic. Thrombosis, hyalinization, dystrophic calcification, and even areas of infarction can be seen in older lesions. Distinction from a well-differentiated angiosarcoma is based on the presence in the latter of an infiltrative growth pattern, cytologic atypia, and multilayering. In breast lesions it is worth remembering that mammary angiosarcomas are always intraparenchymal.

Verrucous Hemangioma

Verrucous hemangioma is a rare form of vascular malformation that is usually congenital and only rarely presents later in

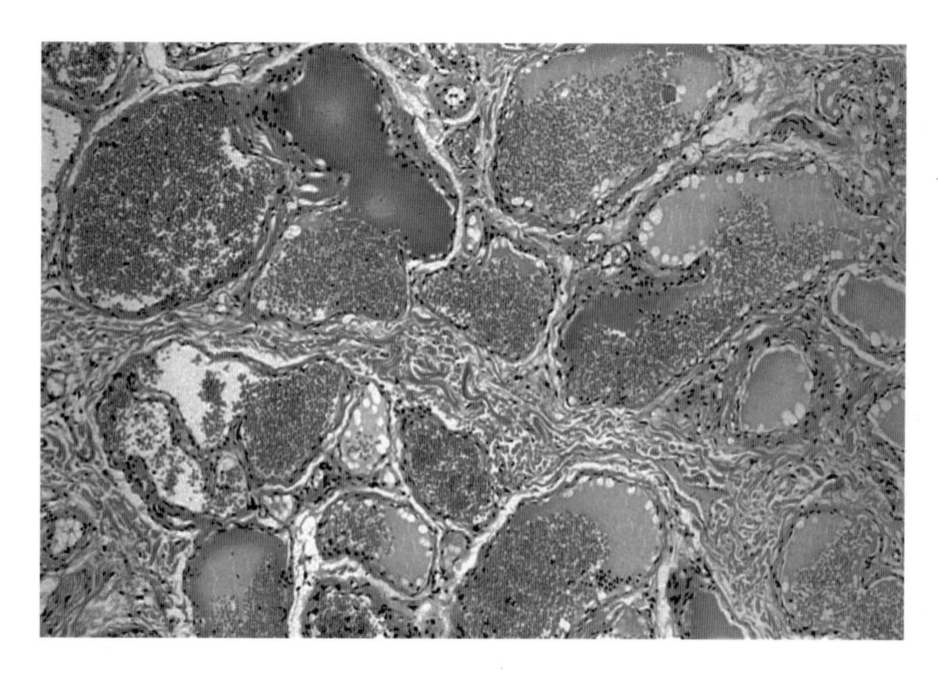

FIG. 34-21. Cavernous hemangioma
Markedly dilated and congested vascular spaces.

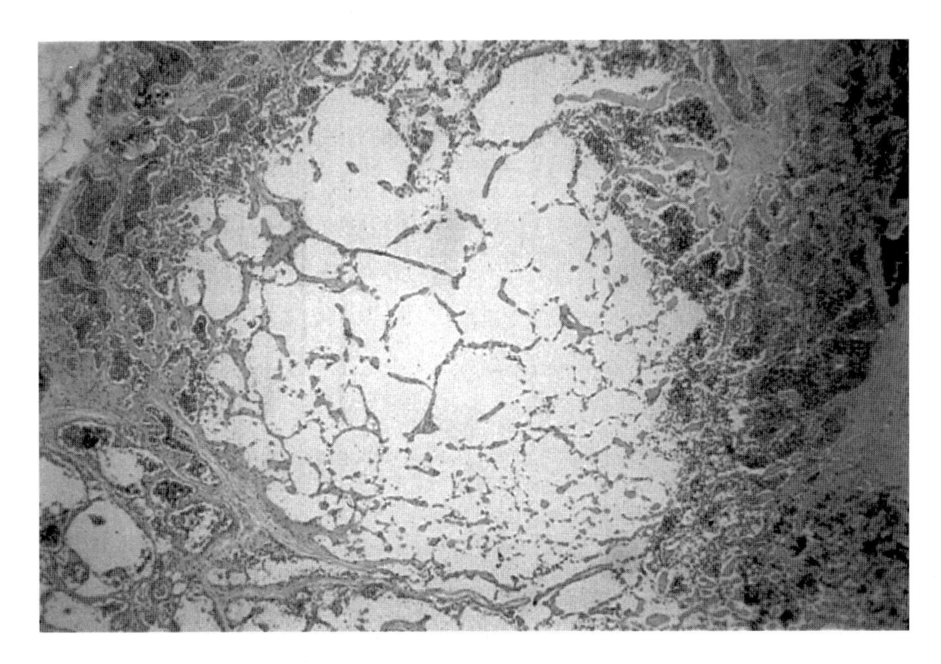

FIG. 34-22. Sinusoidal hemangioma
Anastomosing vascular spaces with a typical sieve-like appearance.

life. Most cases present as wart-like, dark blue papules or nodules with special predilection for the distal lower limbs. Although the majority of cases are solitary, an exceptional case with multiple lesions on different parts of the body has been reported.[96] Often cases are confused clinically and histologically with angiokeratomas, but verrucous hemangiomas always have a deep component and recurrence after incomplete excision occurs in up to one third of cases.[97,98]

In *Cobb syndrome*, a lesion identical to a verrucous hemangioma presents on the trunk with a dermatomal distribution and in association with an underlying meningospinal hemangioma.[99]

Histopathology. The superficial portion of a verrucous hemangioma is indistinguishable from an angiokeratoma. However, a combination of congested capillaries and cavernlike vascular spaces is seen extending into the deep dermis and subcutaneous tissue (Fig. 34-23). These vascular spaces are lined by flattened endothelial cells and are usually surrounded by a layer of pericytes. A lobular growth pattern is often apparent in the deep component.

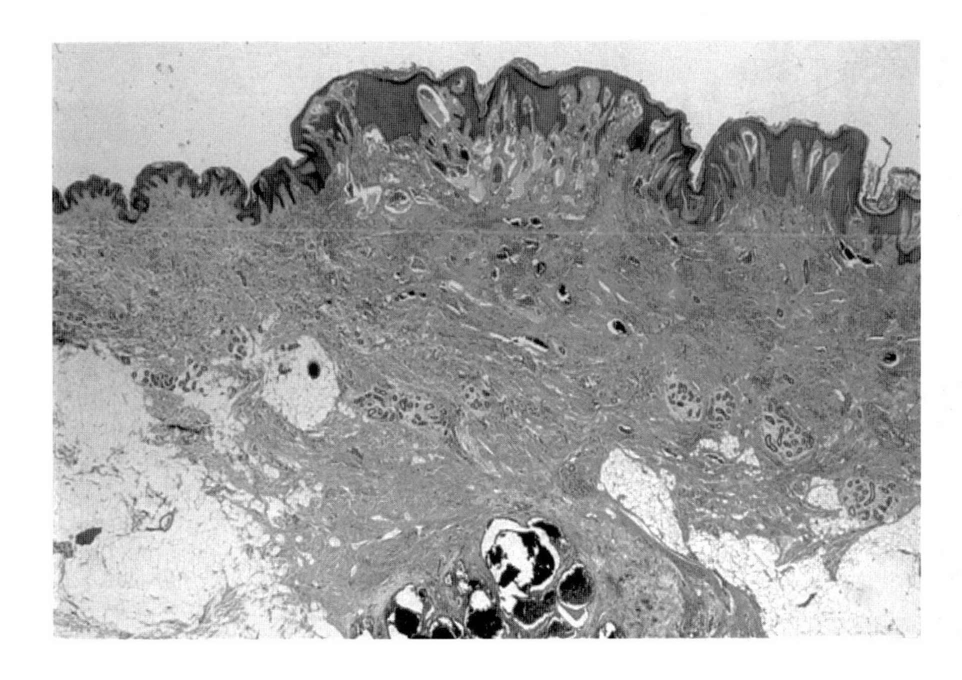

FIG. 34-23. Verrucous hemangioma
Note the superficial component similar to angiokeratoma but with a deep component similar extending to the subcutaneous tissue.

Microvenular Hemangioma

This is a recently described uncommon acquired vascular lesion that usually arises as a small reddish lesion in young to middle-aged individuals of either gender.[100,101] The arms, trunk, and legs are favored sites. The development of lesions in relationship to pregnancy or a change in the use of oral contraception may suggest a hormonal influence on the disease in women.[102]

Histopathology. Histologically thin branching capillaries and small venules with narrow or slightly dilated lumina are found widely throughout the dermis (Fig. 34-24). There is no obvious endothelial cell atypia or accompanying inflammation, but slight dermal sclerosis is often present (Fig. 34-25). The vessels are strongly positive for factor VIII–related antigen and with CD34 and Ulex europaeus agglutinin-I. In two cases, angiomatous tufts in the deeper part of the lesion could indicate a possible relationship to tufted angioma.[101]

Differential Diagnosis. The importance of microvenular hemangioma as an acquired vascular anomaly in young persons lies in the differential diagnosis from an early or macular lesion of Kaposi's sarcoma. The lymphangioma-like channels of Kaposi's sarcoma are more delicate, do not contain erythrocytes, show angulated outlines, and tend to wrap around collagen bundles. Furthermore, plasma cells and other inflammatory cells are common in Kaposi's sarcoma but not in microvenular hemangioma.

Targetoid Hemosiderotic Hemangioma (Hobnail Hemangioma)

This is an uncommon, recently described vascular tumor that usually presents in the trunk or extremities of young or middle-aged adults with a slight male predominance.[103–105] Rare cases occur in the oral mucosa. The descriptive name given to this tumor reflects a typical clinical appearance characterized by a small solitary lesion consisting of a brown to violaceous papule, 2 to 3 mm in diameter, surrounded by a thin, pale area and a peripheral ecchymotic ring. However, these features are only present in 20% of cases,[105] and most often the clinical appearance is that of a red-blue or brown papule. An alternative name of *hobnail hemangioma*, which emphasizes a special histologic feature, has been proposed (see text following).[106]

Histopathology. In the superficial reticular dermis there are a number of thin-walled, dilated, and irregular vascular spaces often lined by bland endothelial cells with scanty cytoplasm and rounded nuclei that protrude into the lumina and closely resemble hobnails (Fig. 34-26). Focally, epithelioid cells are rarely present. Intraluminal papillary projections and fibrin thrombi can be seen in the superficial blood vessels. The vascular channels in the deeper dermis become less conspicuous, irregular, and angulated, are lined by flattened endothelial cells, and dissect between collagen bundles. Extensive red blood cell extravasation, inflammatory aggregates predominantly of lymphocytes, and, in a later stage, extensive stromal hemosiderin deposition are commonly seen.

Pathogenesis. Because there is a family of vascular tumors characterized by epithelioid endothelial cells, it has been proposed that this tumor represents the benign end of the spectrum of a group of vascular tumors characterized by hobnail endothelial cells that includes *Dabska's tumor* and the recently described *retiform hemangioendothelioma.*[106]

Differential Diagnosis. These include patch-stage Kaposi's sarcoma, retiform hemangioendothelioma, and benign lymphangioendothelioma.

Arteriovenous (Venous) Hemangioma (Cirsoid Aneurysm)

Arteriovenous (venous) hemangioma, or cirsoid aneurysm, usually occurs as a solitary dark-red papule or nodule on the

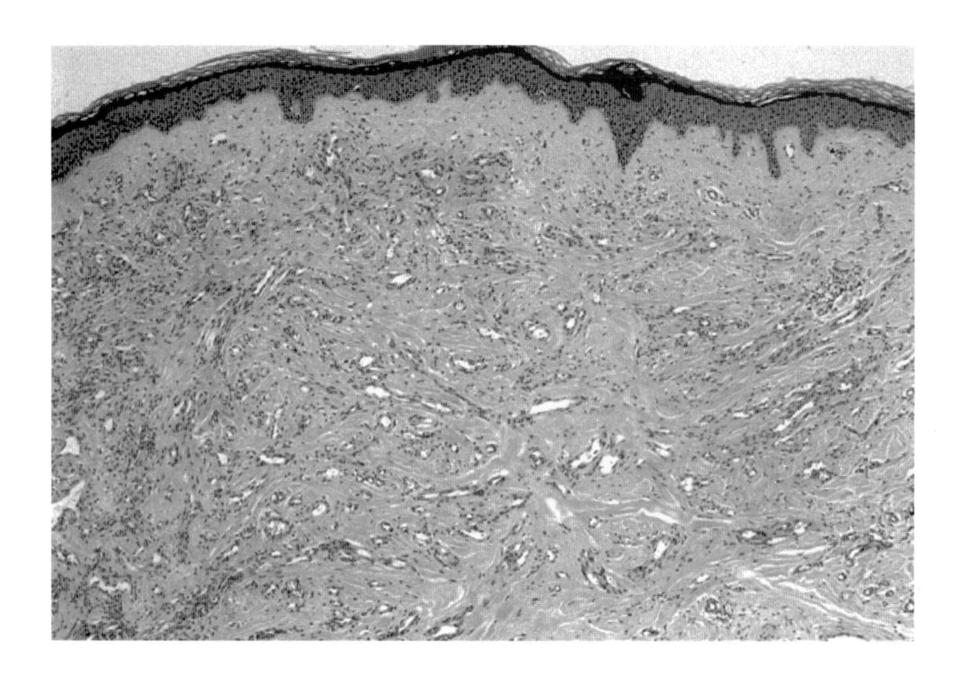

FIG. 34-24. Microvenular hemangioma
Irregular, branching, thin-walled venules throughout the dermis.

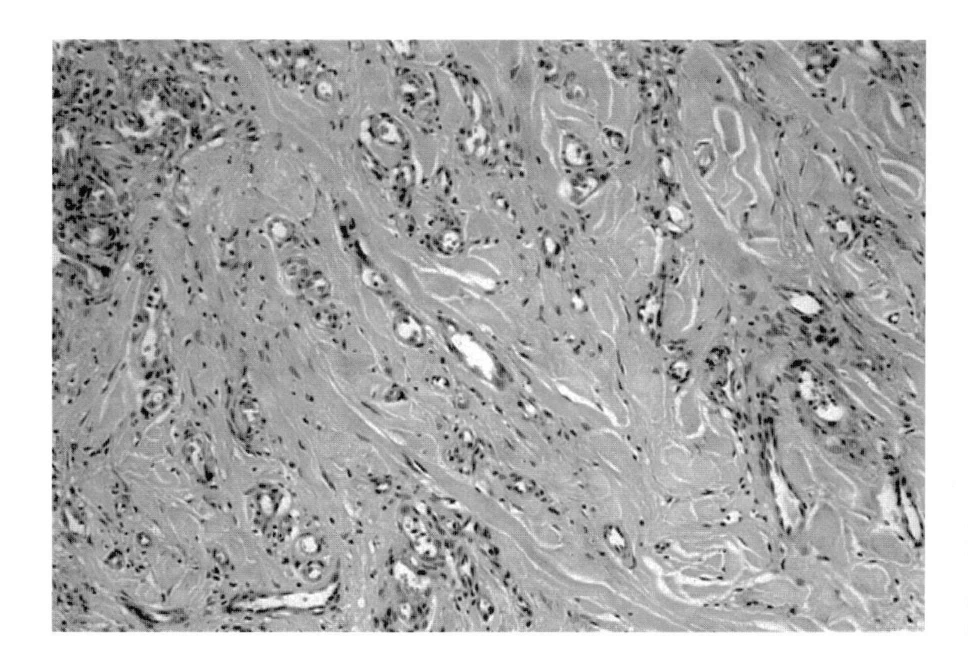

FIG. 34-25. Microvenular hemangioma
Note small venules surrounded by somewhat hyalinized collagen bundles.

face (especially the lip) or, less commonly, on the extremities of adults, with equal gender incidence.[107,108] Rare cases present in the oral cavity.[109] Most of the lesions measure less than 1 cm in diameter.

Histopathology. Within a circumscribed area, usually restricted to the dermis, one observes densely aggregated, thick-walled and thin-walled vessels lined by a single layer of endothelial cells (Fig. 34-27). The walls of the thick-walled vessels consist mainly of fibrous tissue but in most instances also contain some smooth muscle. Internal elastic lamina is found in very few vessels, indicating that most of the blood vessels are veins. Many vessels contain red blood cells, and thrombi are occasionally seen.[108] Lesions with similar histologic appearances can be seen in the deeper soft tissues of younger patients and can be associated with hemodynamic complications due to shunting.

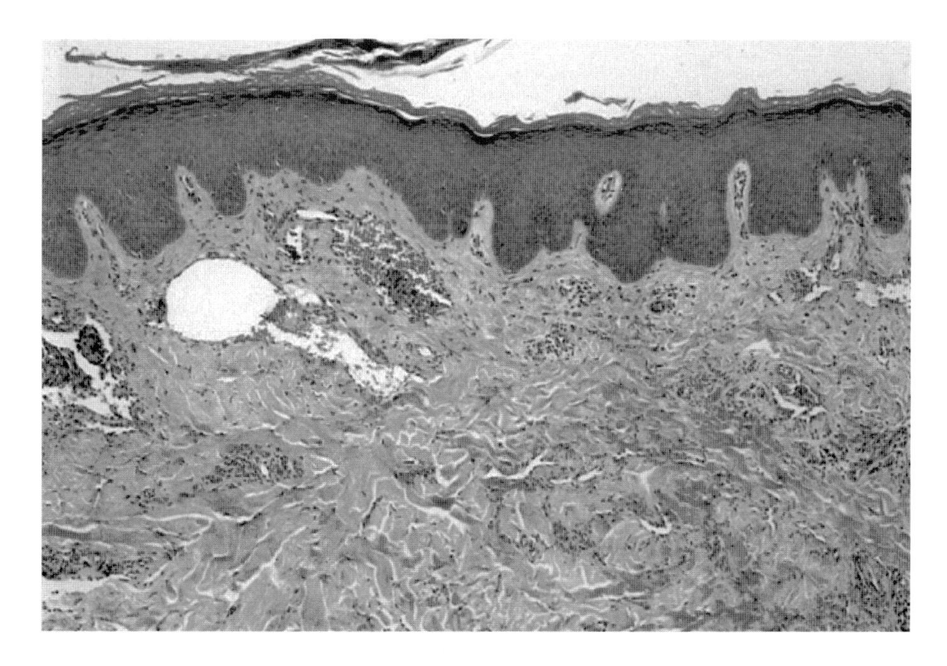

FIG. 34-26. Targetoid hemosiderotic hemangioma
Note irregular, thin-walled vascular spaces with focal papillary projections and prominent stromal hemorrhage.

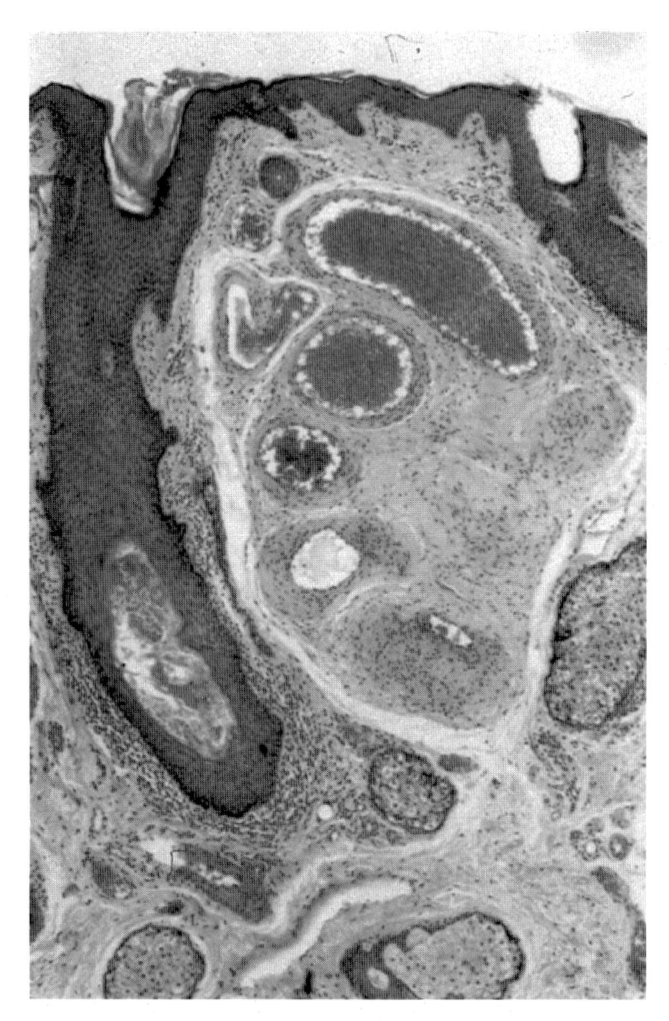

FIG. 34-27. Cirsoid aneurysm
Thick- and thin-walled vascular channels in the superficial dermis.

Histogenesis. It seems likely that many of these lesions represent pure venous hemangiomas, some of which have arterialized veins.[109]

Angiomatosis

Angiomatosis is an uncommon condition that presents exclusively in children and adolescents and is defined as a diffuse proliferation of blood vessels affecting a large contiguous area of the body.[110,111] Anatomic distribution is wide, but there is a preference for limb involvement. A typical case presents with involvement of the skin, underlying soft tissues, and even bone. Associated limb hypertrophy is common. Involvement of parenchymal organs and the central nervous system can be present. Due to extensive involvement, surgical treatment is difficult and recurrences are common.

Histopathology. Most tumors are composed of abundant mature fat intermixed with blood vessels in two histologic patterns.[111] The most common pattern is a mixture of veins with irregular walls, cavernous vascular spaces, and capillaries. The veins often show an incomplete muscular layer, and smaller blood vessels can be seen in the walls of larger vessels. The second pattern is composed mainly of capillaries with a focal lobular architecture. Perineural invasion can be a feature in both patterns.

Spindle-Cell Hemangioendothelioma

This tumor was first described in 1986[112] as a form of low-grade angiosarcoma, although mounting evidence in recent years widely favors a nonneoplastic process most likely related to a vascular malformation (see pathogenesis). Gender incidence is equal, and most lesions arise in the second or third decade of life. It presents as multiple red-blue nodules in the dermis and subcutaneous tissue, most commonly involving the distal aspects of the extremities with predilection for the hands. Visceral lesions do not occur, and involvement of deeper soft tissues is rare.[113] The clinical course is indolent with multiple new lesions appearing over the years. Spontaneous regression is exceptional. In aproximately 10% of cases, associated anomalies include lymphoedema, Maffucci's syndrome, Klippel–Trenaunay syndrome, and early onset varicose veins.[112,114,115]

Histopathology. Tumors tend to be poorly circumscribed and may present totally or partially in an intravascular location especially involving medium-sized veins. A typical lesion is composed of two elements: irregularly dilated, thin-walled congested cavernous spaces often with organizing thrombi and phleboliths intermixed with more solid areas composed of spindle-shaped cells (Fig. 34-28) generally bland in appearance, although rare cases might show focal degenerative cytological atypia. Mitotic figures are rare. Commonly in the solid areas focal aggregates of epithelioid cells with eosinophilic cytoplasm and bundles of smooth muscle are seen. The epithelioid cells may show vacuolation or intracytoplasmic lumina (Fig. 34-29). Slit-like vascular spaces are common in the solid areas and are accompanied by scattered extravasated red blood cells and hemosiderin-laden macrophages. Focal areas with changes resembling Masson's tumor can be a feature. Irregular, thick-walled vascular spaces reminiscent of those seen in vascular malformations are often seen in the periphery of many lesions. Occasionally cases show combined features of epithelioid and spindle-cell hemangioendothelioma.[116,117]

Pathogenesis. Original classification of this tumor as a form of low-grade angiosarcoma was based on the development of lymph node metastasis in one of the patients reported.[112] However, the patient had been treated with radiotherapy, and it is very likely that the metastasis was from a radiation-induced sarcoma. Further series of cases in recent years have provided evidence favoring the theory that spindle-cell hemangioendothelioma represents a reactive condition or a form of vascular malformation.[114,118–120]

By immunohistochemistry, the endothelial cells lining the vascular spaces and the epithelioid cells in the solid areas stain variably with endothelial markers. The spindle cells stain focally with actin and less commonly with desmin.

Differential Diagnosis. The main differential diagnosis is with nodular stage Kaposi's sarcoma, as discussed next.

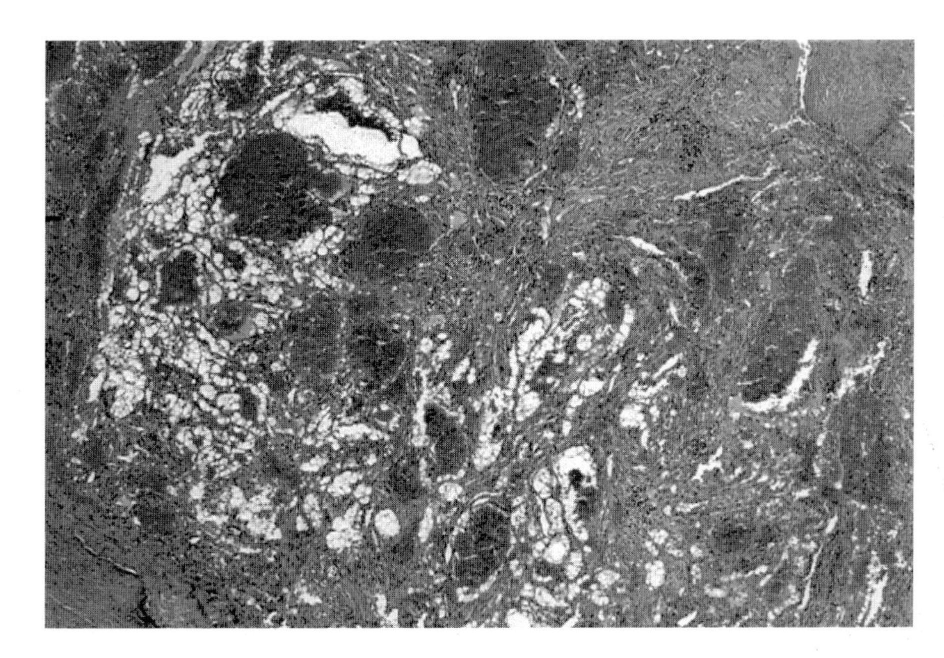

FIG. 34-28. Spindle-cell hemangioendothelioma
Cavernous vascular spaces combined with solid areas representing spindle cells.

LOW-GRADE MALIGNANT TUMORS

Kaposi's Sarcoma

Until the late 1960s, Kaposi's sarcoma was described as an uncommon, slowly progressive, multifocal tumor arising mostly in elderly male patients of Eastern and Southern European descent, a clinical pattern now referred to as the "classic" form of the disease. The current intense interest in the disease stems from the recognition that Kaposi's sarcoma is an extremely common tumor in tropical Africa and that it is also a prime marker of acquired immunodeficiency syndrome (AIDS). In addition, the sarcoma can arise in association with other causes of immunodeficiency, especially when drug induced. There remain many unusual facets about the disease, the genetic and epidemiologic aspects, the clinical course, the histopathologic features, the transmission, and the pathogenesis that as yet defy adequate scientific explanation.

Clinical Features. Nearly all cases of Kaposi's sarcoma can be classified in four groups:[121–124]

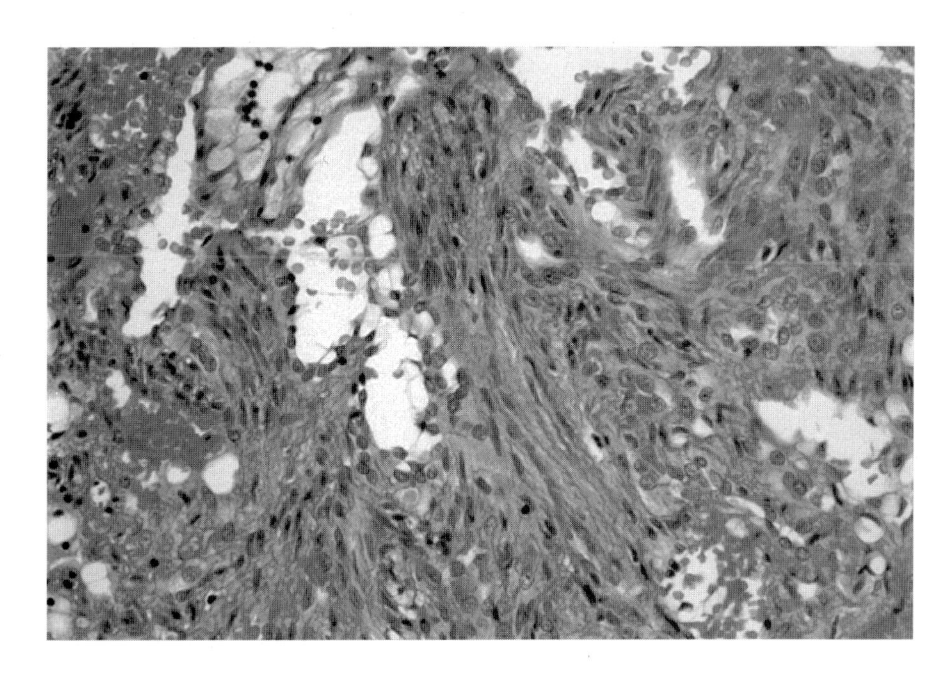

FIG. 34-29. Spindle-cell hemangioendothelioma
Spindle-shaped cells and focal epithelioid and vacuolated cells.

1. *Classic Kaposi's sarcoma.* This arises 10 to 15 times more commonly in men than women, affecting mainly patients of Eastern European, Jewish and Mediterranean origin. Studies of clusters of cases in the Peloponnese may suggest the role of an infectious agent in the etiology of the disease.[125] The disease mainly arises in patients over the age of 50 with the slow development of angiomatous nodules and plaques on the lower extremities. Affected patients may survive 10 to 20 years; even at late stages with widespread skin nodules, visceral disease is unusual, although asymptomatic involvement of lymph nodes, lungs, or gastrointestinal tract can often be found at necropsy.[123] Occasionally before the advent of AIDS, an aggressive type of Kaposi's sarcoma occurred in young adults or children with early lymph node involvement.[122] Various types of lymphoma have been reported to occur in the classic type of Kaposi's sarcoma with an incidence of 10% or more.

2. *Kaposi's sarcoma in Africa.* In the 1960s it was realized that Kaposi's sarcoma was very common among native blacks in Central Africa, representing the most common tumor in pathology departments in Uganda and parts of Zaire. In South Africa it has been estimated that Kaposi's sarcoma is 10 times more common in blacks than whites. In Africans the disease can run a similar indolent course as in classic Kaposi's sarcoma, but a higher proportion of young people are affected, with a more aggressive disease manifested by widespread tumors, deep infiltrative or elevated fungating lesions, and bone involvement. A distinctive childhood type of Kaposi's sarcoma occurs with massive lymph node involvement and early death. Mucocutaneous lesions are usually a late or minor clinical feature in this lymphadenopathic form.[122] The male to female ratio in these children is approximately 3:1.

3. *AIDS-associated Kaposi's sarcoma.* In the early 1980s reports of groups of young homosexual males in New York and California who were developing Kaposi's sarcoma[126] was one of the keys in establishing the existence of AIDS. Originally about 40% of patients with AIDS had concomitant Kaposi's sarcoma, but this high percentage has gradually fallen to around 20% in the United States[121,124,127] and Europe.[128] Collected data from the Centers for Disease Control in the United States suggest that Kaposi's sarcoma is at least 201,000 times more common with AIDS than in the general population.[121] The risk of Kaposi's sarcoma occurring with AIDS is much greater in active homosexuals than in heterosexual males or females, such as hemophiliacs who receive contaminated blood products or drug abusers who share needles. These epidemiologic peculiarities call into question whether the human immunodeficiency virus (HIV) is the sole or main transmissible agent causing Kaposi's sarcoma.

The clinical features of AIDS-related Kaposi's sarcoma differ from the classic disease in the rapid evolution of the lesions, their atypical distribution affecting the trunk, and the mucosal involvement.[123] Visceral involvement is very common at autopsy[129–132] but such internal lesions are often unapparent clinically during life. Visceral involvement may be present without any skin lesions. Most patients die as a result of infections due to immunodeficiency rather than from the direct effect of the sarcoma.

4. *Kaposi's sarcoma and iatrogenic immunosuppression.* Drug-induced immunosuppression to prevent rejection of transplanted organs greatly increases the risk of developing lymphomas and other tumors, including Kaposi's sarcoma. In one study, 13 cases of Kaposi's sarcoma arose in 820 kidney transplant recipients.[133] A peculiarity of this type of Kaposi's sarcoma is the frequent regression or apparent cure on discontinuation of immunosuppressive therapy. The male-dominant gender ratio is much smaller in this group.

Histopathology. The histopathology of fully developed nodules of Kaposi's sarcoma in all types of the disease is distinctive and should rarely cause problems for pathologists. The diagnostic pitfalls lie mainly in the early macular lesions where misinterpretation as banal inflammation or some form of minor angiomatous or lymphatic anomaly is easy to make.[134] A further difficulty is that in some late lesions cytologic atypia increases and the vascular component of the nodules becomes effaced, giving rise to the differential diagnosis of other spindle-cell sarcomas.

For descriptive convenience, the histologic spectrum can be divided into stages roughly corresponding to the clinical type of lesion: early and late macules, plaques, nodules, and aggressive late lesions. In reality there is overlap between stages, and multiple biopsies taken at the same time or even a single biopsy may show features of different histologic stages. There are no differences in the pathology of the disease in the different risk groups.

1. *Macular (patch stage).* In early macules there is usually a patchy, sparse, upper dermal perivascular infiltrate consisting of lymphocytes and plasma cells. Narrow cords of cells, insinuated between collagen bundles, may at first suggest histiocytes or connective tissue cells, but close inspection should reveal evidence of luminal differentiation or connection with discernable small vessels. Usually a few dilated irregular or angulated lymphatic-like spaces lined by delicate endothelial cells are also present. Vessels with "jagged" outlines tending to separate collagen bundles are especially characteristic (Fig. 34-30).[126,135] Normal adnexal structures and preexisting blood vessels often protrude into newly formed blood vessels (Fig. 34-31). This finding, known as the "promontory sign," is commonly present but is not specific to Kaposi's sarcoma. In late macular lesions there is a more extensive infiltrate of vessels in the dermis: "jagged" vessels and cords of thicker-walled vessels similar to those in granulation tissue. Some of these vessels may in part be reactive rather than an intrinsic part of the tumor. At this stage, red blood cell extravasation and the presence of siderophages may be encountered. In some lesions, ramifying variably dilated bloodless lymphatic-like spaces dissect out collagen to give an appearance that suggests a well-differentiated angiosarcoma or progressive lymphangioma.[136] This exaggerated lymphangioma-like appearance has led some authors to designate this as a special variant of the disease.[135] Occasional fascicles of spindle-shaped cells may occur independent of blood vessels.

2. *Plaque stage.* In this stage a diffuse infiltrate of small blood vessels extends through most parts of the dermis and tends to displace collagen. The vessels show variable morphology, some occurring as poorly canalized cords, some as blood containing ovoid vessels, and some showing lymphatic-like features. Loosely distributed spindle cells, arranged in short fascicles, are also encountered (Fig. 34-32). Intracytoplasmic hyaline globules[137,138] may be found in areas of denser infiltrate. These hyaline globules are seen more often in lesions from patients with AIDS.

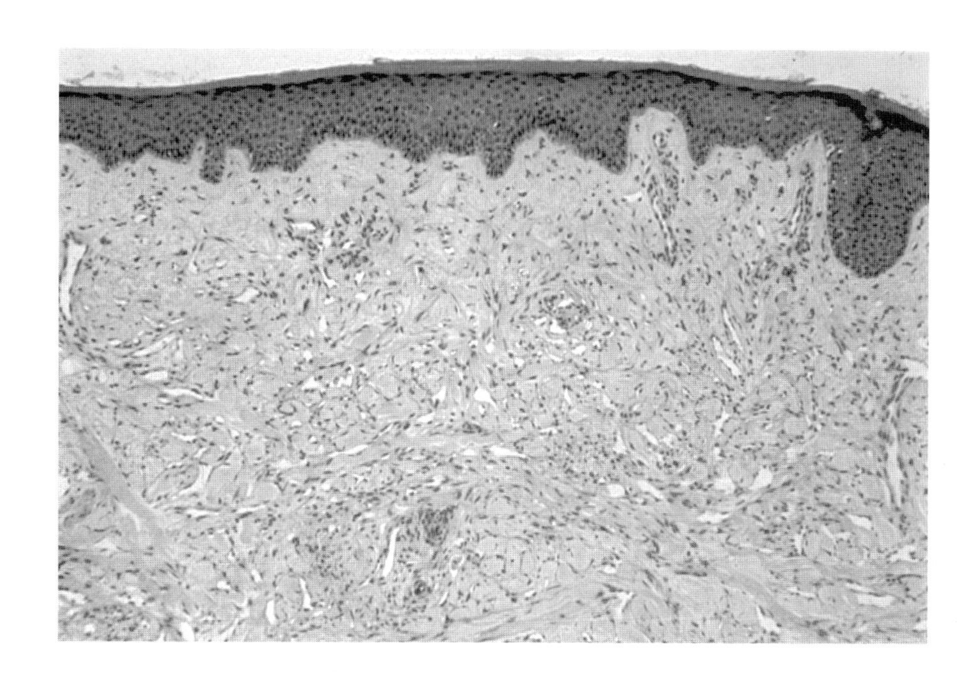

FIG. 34-30. Patch-stage Kaposi's sarcoma
Numerous, small jagged vascular spaces throughout the dermis.

3. *Nodular stage*. In the tumor stage, well-defined nodules composed of vascular spaces and spindle cells replace dermal collagen. These tumor nodules tend to be compartmentalized by dense bands of fibrocollagenous tissue. Dilated lymphatic spaces can also be seen between tumor aggregates. The characteristic feature is a honeycomb-like network of blood-filled spaces or slits, closely associated with interweaving spindle cells (Fig. 34-33). Although generally vascular spaces and fascicles of spindle cells are present, either element can predominate focally. The vascular lumina in the angiomatous tissue are so closely set that they lie next to each other in a "back-to-back" arrangement. Delicate flattened endothelial cells lining the vascular clefts are hardly discernable with routine stains but are easily seen with the newer immunocytochemical markers CD31 and CD34.[139] The vascular slits in the nodules appear to be in direct contact with spindle cells, leading to the suggestion that they are pseudovascular spaces.[138] The presence of a closely set honeycomb-like pattern of vascular spaces is perhaps the single most important diagnostic feature of Kaposi's sarcoma. In the vascular spaces of pyogenic granuloma and most angiomas, the

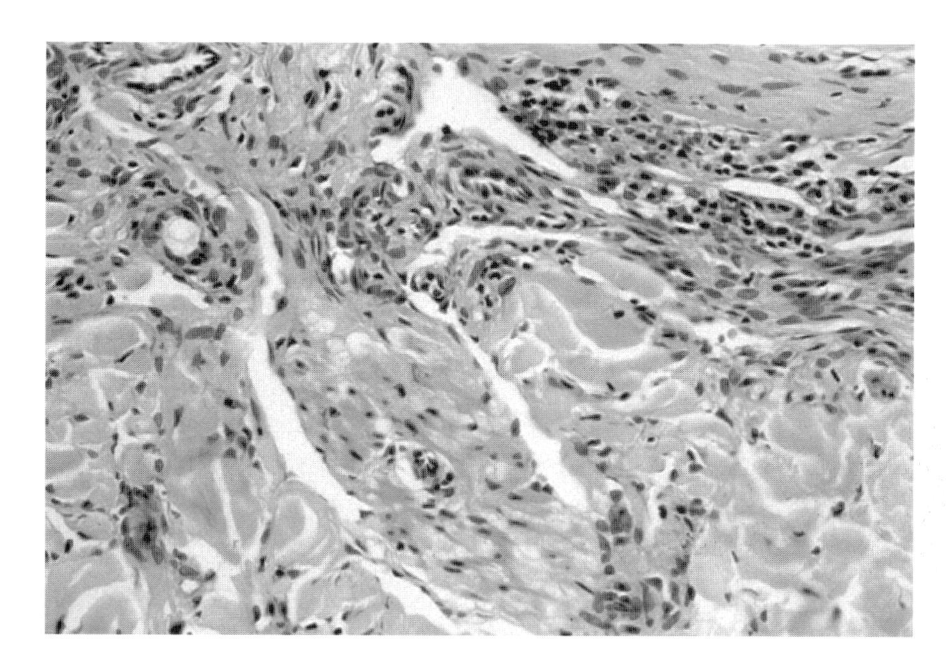

Fig. 34-31. Patch-stage Kaposi's sarcoma
Normal blood vessels and an arrector pili muscle protruding into newly formed blood vessels ("promontory sign"). Also note focal hemorrhage and plasma cells.

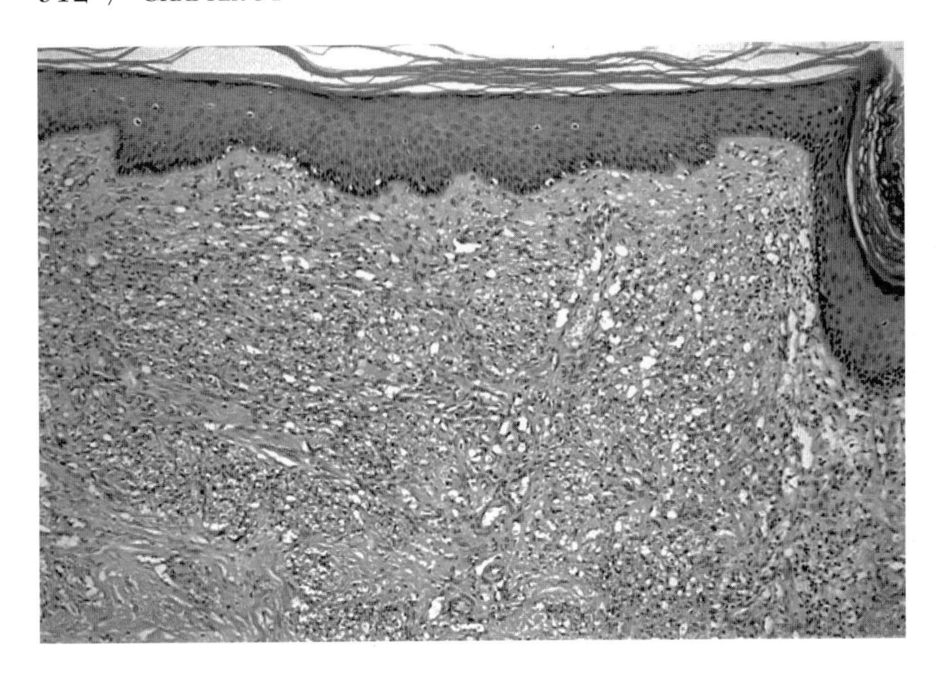

FIG. 34-32. Plaque-stage Kaposi's sarcoma
Numerous irregular blood vessels and the appearance of spindle-shaped cells in the background.

endothelial cells of the capillary walls are more prominent and the vessels are set farther apart by intervening stroma. Around the nodules varying numbers of thicker-walled vessels are encountered that may represent reactive or "feeder" vessels, not a basic component of the tumor. Blood pigment–containing macrophages are nearly always prominent adjacent to the nodules, especially in lesions at dependent sites.

The spindle cells in the nodules are elongated and fusiform with a well-defined cytoplasm. The nuclei are ovoid and somewhat flattened with finely granular chromatin in the long axis of the cells. The nucleoli are generally inconspicuous and nuclear atypia is absent or slight. Mitosis is infrequent. Prominent and consistent positivity for CD34 is seen in the spindle cell population (Fig. 34-34).

Intra- and extracellular hyaline globules occur more frequently than in plaque-stage lesions (Fig. 34-35). They present in groups as faintly eosinophilic spheres 1 to 7 μm in size and are PAS positive and diastase resistant.[135] The globules probably represent partially digested erythrocytes.[138] Although characteristic and of some diagnostic significance, hyaline globules are not entirely specific for Kaposi's sarcoma because they can

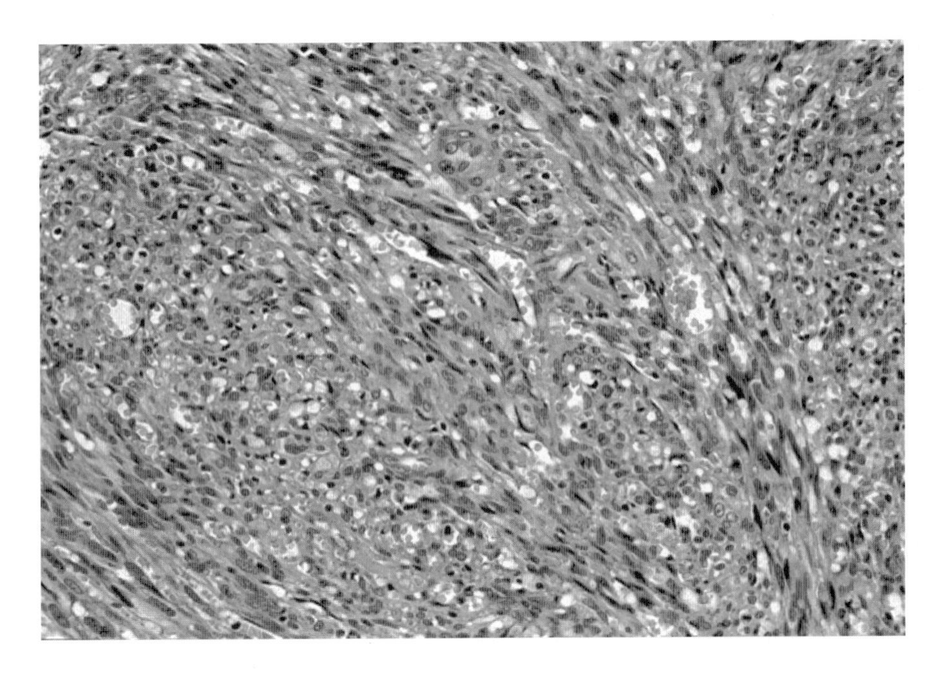

FIG. 34-33. Nodular Kaposi's sarcoma
Bland spindle cells forming slit-like spaces occupied by red blood cells.

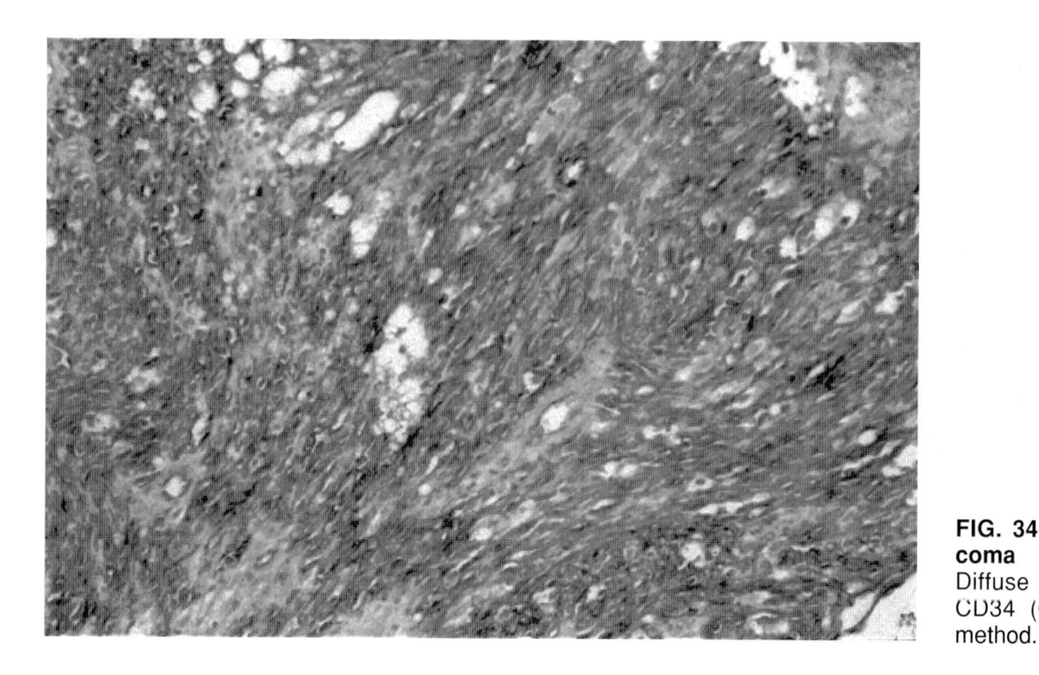

FIG. 34-34. Nodular Kaposi's sarcoma
Diffuse staining of spindle cells with CD34 (QBEND/10) using the ABC method.

be found occasionally in other connective tissue conditions with interstitial hemorrhage. Usually the epidermis and skin appendages remain intact.

4. *Aggressive late stage lesions.* Mostly in Africans, but sometimes with other types of Kaposi's sarcoma, "infiltrating" lesions show a more obviously sarcomatous character with reduction or loss of the vascular component. The spindle cells demonstrate a greater degree of cytologic atypia with regard to size, shape, and nuclear features, with mitosis becoming frequent. In such lesions, phagocytozed erythrocytes and the presence of hyaline globules may provide clues about the tumor's origin. Very rarely angiosarcoma is mimicked by the development of vascular spaces lined by grossly atypical endothelial cells.

It has been questioned whether the histologic features of Kaposi's sarcoma can be used as a guide to the prognosis. It seems reasonable to suggest that as the disease progresses from the macular to plaque and nodular stages, the presence of histologic characteristics of the polar macular and nodular stages might be a guide to the clinical evolution. Surprisingly this does not seem

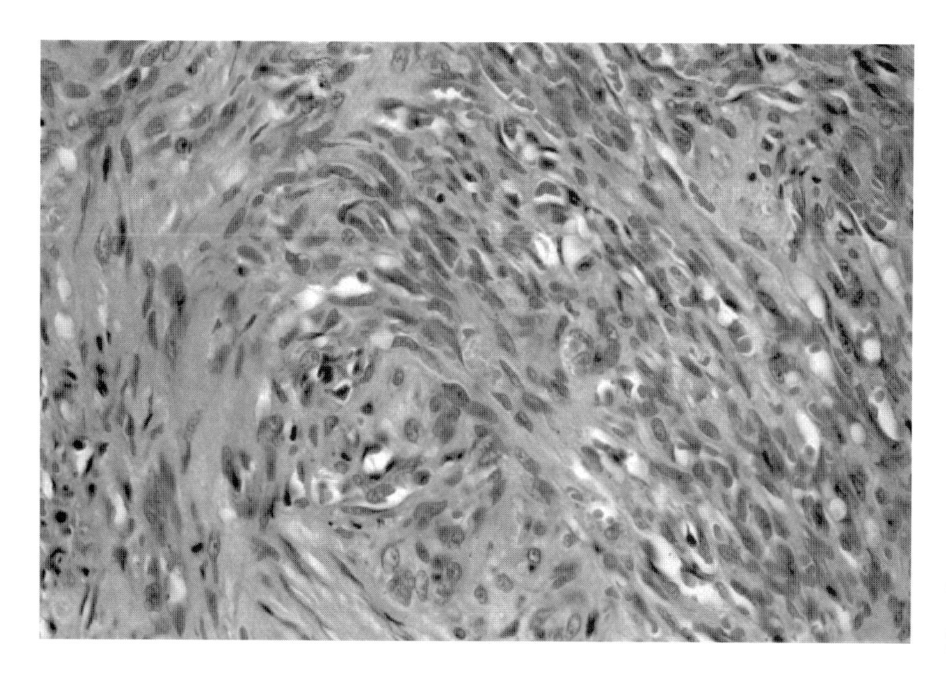

FIG. 34-35. Nodular Kaposi's sarcoma
Note numerous eosinophilic intracytoplasmic globules.

to be the case as a recent study[140] has indicated that lesions histologically indicative of nodular Kaposi's sarcoma carry a better prognosis than that of macular lesions.

Differential Diagnosis. The differential diagnosis is wide,[134] with the most difficulties encountered with either early macular or late aggressive lesions. Vascular proliferations in stasis and multinucleate-cell angiohistiocytoma are discussed here in more detail because they are not described elsewhere in this chapter.

In *early macular lesions* an inflammatory condition or a cell-poor (atrophic) histiocytoma may be suspected since the vascular nature of vessels with collapsed lumina may not be apparent. Appropiate cell markers may clarify the vascular nature of the underlying lesion. The cryptic vessels are universally positive with CD31 and CD34, variably positive with Ulex europaeus agglutinin-I, but negative with factor XIIIa. Factor VIII–related antigen is negative in lymphangioma-like channels of Kaposi's sarcoma with positive labeling limited to thicker-walled vessels. In later macular lesions, differential diagnosis includes well-differentiated angiosarcoma, progressive lymphangioma, targetoid hemosiderotic hemangioma, and microvenular hemangioma. Angiosarcoma shows a "dissection" of collagen's infiltrative pattern, but endothelial cell atypia with hyperchromatism and intraluminal shedding of malignant cells occurs unlike in Kaposi's sarcoma. Histologically, progressive lymphangioma is almost indistinguishable from Kaposi's sarcoma with prominent lymphangioma-like features, but inflammatory cells, especially plasma cells, tend to be absent in the former. When the clinical features are taken into account, distinction is not difficult. In targetoid hemosiderotic hemangioma, lymphangioma-like channels are mainly confined to the upper dermis; in places plump "hobnail" endothelial cells invaginate vascular spaces, inflammatory cells are rare, and hemosiderin deposition is prominent, unlike in early Kaposi's sarcoma. Microvenular hemangioma differs in showing blood containing vessels, many of which are surrounded by pericytes or smooth-muscle cells (positive for smooth-muscle actin) suggestive of venular differentiation.

Spindle-cell hemangioendothelima, the rare recently described kaposiform hemangioendothelioma of childhood, and moderately differentiated angiosarcomas with spindle-cell differentiation are the most important histologic simulants of *nodular Kaposi's lesions.*

Spindle cell hemangioendothelioma differs by showing cavernous or widely dilated vascular spaces and collections of epithelioid cells with or without intracytoplasmic lumina.

Kaposiform hemangioendothelioma is mainly a disease of children that usually affects deep soft tissues although the skin can be affected.[141,142] Histologically, the tumor shows intermediate features of capillary hemangioma and Kaposi's sarcoma and has a lobular growth pattern that is absent in Kaposi's sarcoma.

Sometimes spindle-cell differentiation is prominent in angiosarcoma, but usually markedly atypical cells are present, allowing differentiation from Kaposi's sarcoma.

Other acquired vascular conditions that can cause problems from the clinical and histologic point of view are bacillary angiomatosis, and pyogenic granuloma, especially if complicated by satellite lesions and tufted angioma. Spindle-cell fascicles with a bland cytologic appearance do not feature as a prominent component of any of these entities.

Aneurysmal benign fibrous histiocytoma is a nonvascular, highly cellular spindle-cell lesion with pseudovascular spaces and hemosiderin deposition that can be confused with nodular Kaposi's sarcoma.[143] The variability of pathology, the presence of peripheral areas similar to common dermal fibrous histiocytoma, and immunohistochemistry should prevent error in diagnosis.

In *aggressive late-stage lesions,* many malignant spindle cell tumors can come into the differential diagnosis especially if clinical details are unavailable. The most important differential diagnoses are fibrosarcoma, leiomyosarcoma, monophasic synovial sarcoma, malignant cellular blue nevus with sparse melanin deposition, and desmoplastic malignant melanoma. Accurate diagnosis may be impossible unless reliable immunohistochemistry is available. The newer markers CD31 and CD34 are particularly helpful in suggesting a vascular derivation even in poorly diffentiated Kaposi's lesions.

Hypostasis and high venous pressure gives rise to vascular proliferation (pseudo-Kaposi's sarcoma and acroangiodermatits). Angiomatous papules and plaques near the ankles that are secondary to high venous pressure result from incompetent veins and are common causes of Kaposi-like lesions.[134,135] Less commonly, high venous pressure can arise due to congenital or acquired arteriovenous anomalies.[144,145] Histologically there is expansion of the whole capillary bed throughout the dermis. In the papillary dermis there is reduplication and corkscrewing of thick-walled capillaries, which increase in size and become angiomatous in appearance. Similarly, venules and deeper, vertically small veins become hypertrophied and tortuous. Erythocyte extravasation, fibrosis with horizontally oriented spindle cells, and numerous siderophages are additional features. The angiomatous capillaries appear separated from each other by an edematous matrix, and they do *not* lie "back-to-back" as in Kaposi's sarcoma. To complicate matters, hypostatic vascular proliferation can coexist with Kaposi's sarcoma. A key difference between Kaposi's sarcoma and pseudo-Kaposi's sarcoma is that in the latter vascular hyperplasia results from hyperplasia of the preexisting vasculature, whereas in the former the vascular proliferation is mainly independent.

Multinucleate-cell angiohistiocytoma, a recently described reactive vascular condition, arises as slowly developing grouped vascular papules usually on the legs[146] but also at other sites including the face and hands.[147] Most patients are older women. Histologically, an increased number of capillaries and venules with few inflammatory cells are found throughout the dermis, but the extent of the proliferation does achieve angiomatous proportions. Increased numbers of histiocytes and scattered multinucleate cells are usually found but not in every biopsy. Blood-pigment deposition is generally insignificant.

Pathogenesis. The multifocal development, slow evolution of the classic form of the disease, occasional regression, and histology of inflammation which lacks cytologic atypia, has led many to suggest that at least initially Kaposi's sarcoma is a reactive condition and not a sarcoma in the neoplastic sense.[122,125,148,149] The morphogenesis of the differing tumor elements—in particular the derivation of the spindle-cell component of plaque and nodular lesions—used to be controversial. Ultrastructural studies tend to indicate that the spindle cells represent transformed endothelial cells and have received strong support from recent immunohistochemical studies. The spindle cells label with newer endothelial cell markers CD31 and CD34.[139,150–152] CD34 is a less specific label for endothelial cells than CD31 since labeling of other mesenchymal cells also occurs. The possibility of deriving spindle cells from dermal dendrocytes has not been supported by studies using markers against factor XIIIa, although reactive hyperplasia of dendrocytes occurs around Kaposi nodules.[153] Nevertheless, Nickoloff suggests that activated dendrocytes may have an important role in the initiation of Kaposi lesions. Earlier cell-marker studies also provide evidence suggesting that the spindle cells of Kaposi's sarcoma are endothelial-cell derived.[137,154–157]

Dorfmann's earlier morphologic observations led him to suggest that Kaposi's sarcoma may originate from lymphatic rather than vascular endothelial cells.[122] This would account for lymphangioma-like instances of Kaposi's sarcoma.[136] This suggestion has been supported by cell markers used by some authors [154,155] but not others.[156] Dictor and Anderson[158] suggest, because of the close association between veins and lymphatics, that endothelium with hybrid characteristics could give rise to the lymphatic and blood-vascular aspects of the pathology. The role of growth-promoting factors causing angiogenesis and recruitment of other cells in Kaposi's sarcoma has also been studied using molecular biologic techniques.[124,127]

The peculiar epidemiologic aspects of Kaposi's sarcoma have stimulated research on whether viruses other than HIV or some other transmissible agent helps induce the disease. There is much evidence of the association of cytomegalic virus with Kaposi's sarcoma, but the relevance of this association is uncertain.[149] The fine structure of tumor cells in Kaposi's sarcoma reveals tuboreticular structures and cylindrical-confronting cisternae, which may suggest a cellular reaction to a viral infection. Retrovirus-like structures have also been identified.[125] Recently herpesvirus-like DNA sequences have been detected not only in AIDS-related Kaposi's sarcoma[159] but also in African endemic[160] and Mediterranean[161] Kaposi's sarcoma. This novel herpesvirus has been named *human herpesvirus 8*.[162]

Epithelioid Hemangioendothelioma

This is a low-grade tumor of vascular endothelial origin that was originally described as mainly arising in the superficial and deep soft tissue and muscle of the extremities.[163] However, it soon became apparent that the tumor can arise at internal sites and in the viscera (especially the liver, lungs, and bone) and that such tumors were described previously by different names.[15,164] Middle-aged patients, with an equal gender distribution, are mainly affected, but the tumor has a wide age distribution. In about half the cases, the tumor apparently arises from a medium-sized vein or, less often, an artery. Multicentricity is common in visceral lesions, particularly those affecting the lungs, liver, and bones. Skin involvement is rare and usually associated with an underlying soft-tissue or bone lesion or with multicentric disease.[164–166] Exceptional cases present with pure cutaneous involvement.[167] Local recurrences or metastases after surgery develop in about one third of cases involving superficial soft tissues, but the prognosis is worse for internal sites.

Histopathology. Typically, epithelioid hemangioendothelioma shows an infiltrative growth pattern of ovoid, cuboidal, or short spindle cells with a prominent eosinophilic cytoplasm. The nucleus is vesicular showing slight or no atypia, and the nucleolus lacks prominence. Cells tend to be arranged in short fascicles, small nests, or in an "indian-file" pattern, often set in a distinctive hyalinized or mucoid stroma rich in sulphated acid mucoplysaccharides (Figs. 34-36 and 34-37). There is often a chondroid appearance. Obvious vascular channels are generally lacking, but intracytoplasmic vacuoles, sometimes containing erythrocytes, are usually present. Infiltration through large-ves-

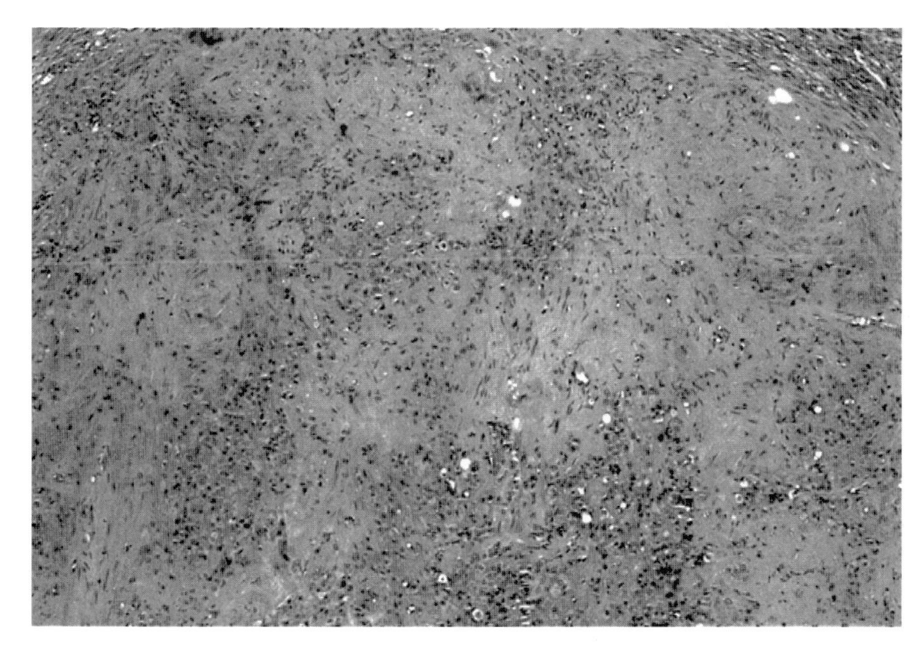

FIG. 34-36. Epithelioid hemangioendothelioma
Note hyaline stroma and trabecular growth pattern.

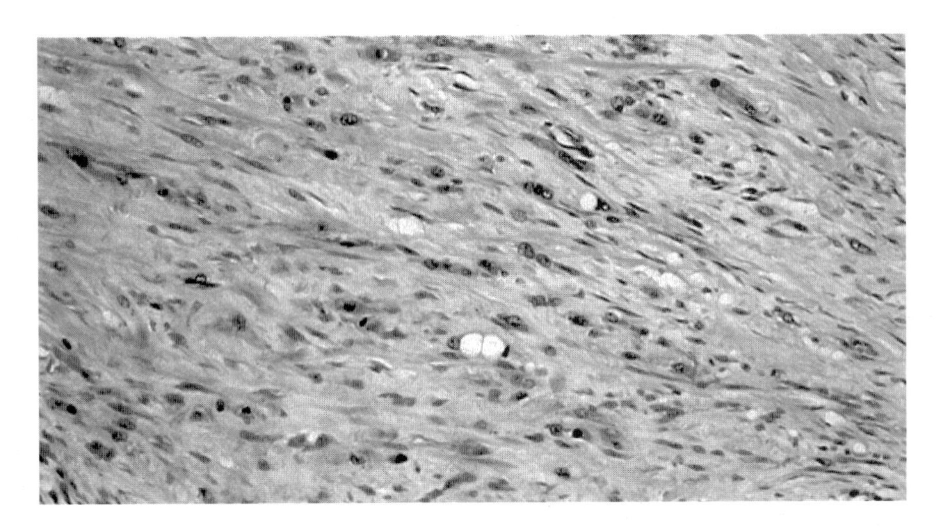

FIG. 34-37. Epithelioid hemangioendothelioma
Strands of of epithelioid cells, some of which show prominent cytoplasmic vacuoles.

sel walls and evidence of endothelial origin may be found. A subset of the tumor with a more aggressive clinical course shows prominent cytologic atypia and a high mitotic rate, overlapping histologically with epithelioid angiosarcoma.[168] Although lesions with cytologic atypia and mitoses are associated with a poorer prognosis, behavior of tumors with bland morphology is difficult to predict.

Tumor cells often stain for endothelial markers including CD31, CD34, and FVIII-RA. Positivity for pan-keratin can be focally found[169] and in our experience this is present in up to 15% of cases.

Differential Diagnosis. The differential diagnosis includes angiolymphoid hyperplasia with eosinophilia, which often has a lobular architecture, prominent inflammation, and numerous well-formed blood vessels; metastatic adenocarcinoma, which is negative for endothelial markers and positive for mucin stains; and myxoid chondrosarcoma, which has a lobular growth pattern, S-100 positive cells, and absence of intracytoplasmic lumina.

Retiform Hemangioendothelioma

Retiform hemangioendothelioma is a rare, recently described variant of low-grade angiosarcoma characterized by indolent clinical behavior and closely related to Dabska's tumor (see text following).[106] There is predilection for young adults, and it presents as a slowly growing nondistinct tumor with equal gender incidence and predilection for the extremities, especially the distal lower limbs. Rare cases can be associated with radiotherapy or chronic lymphedema. Multiple recurrences are common, but metastases has so far been reported in only one case. Retiform hemangioendothelioma appears to be part of the spectrum of a family of vascular tumors that are characterized by endothelial cells with a distinctive hobnail appearance. This includes a benign tumor originally described as targetoid hemosiderotic hemangioma (hobnail hemangioma) and another low-grade malignant lesion, Dabska's tumor.

Histopathology. Tumors are ill-defined and involve the reticular dermis with frequent extension into the subcutis. In most cases, there is a striking low-power resemblance to the normal rete testis conferred by the presence of elongated, arborizing blood vessels (Fig. 34-38) lined by monomorphic bland endothelial cells with prominent apical nuclei and scanty cytoplasm. These cells have been described as having a "matchstick" or hobnail appearance (Fig. 34-39). A lymphocytic inflammatory cell infiltrate is often not only in the stroma but also in the vascular lumina (though not invariably present). The intravascular lymphocytes commonly appear in close contact with the hobnail endothelial cells. Occasional intravascular papillae with hyaline cores can be seen. In most tumors there are solid areas composed of bland spindle cells that stain for endothelial markers.

Differential Diagnosis. Retiform hemangioendothelioma shares clinical and histologic features with Dabska's tumor, and it has been proposed that the former is the adult variant of the latter. However, in Dabska's tumor, cavernous vascular spaces resembling lymphatics predominate, there is no retiform architecture, and intravascular papillae with collagenous cores are a striking feature. Targetoid hemosiderotic hemangioma (hobnail hemangioma) is more superficial, lacks a retiform architecture, and has hobnail endothelial cells that are mainly seen in vessels near the surface. Angiosarcoma often presents in a different clinical setting and shows cytologic atypia, mitosis, and absence of hobnail endothelial cells.

Malignant Endovascular Papillary Angioendothelioma (Dabska's Tumor)

Malignant endovascular papillary angioendothelioma is a very rare tumor that was first described in 1969.[170] Since its original description, very few additonal cases have been reported in the literature, and there seems to be a lack of consensus regarding its specific histologic features. Tumors present mainly in infants and children with a wide anatomic distribution but show predilection for the head and neck area. Regional lymph-node metastasis can occur.

Histopathology. Low-power examination reveals a dermal and often subcutaneous tumor composed of markedly dilated,

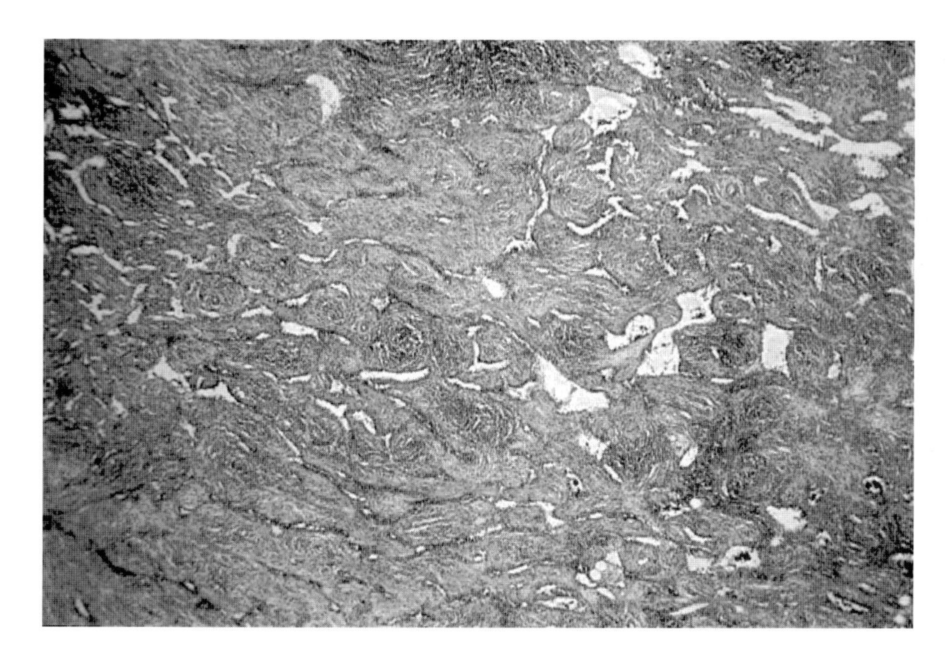

FIG. 34-38. Retiform hemangioendothelioma
Branching blood vessels and a prominent lymphocytic inflammatory cell infiltrate.

thin-walled vascular channels resembling a cavernous lymphangioma. These vascular channels are lined by bland hobnail endothelial cells with protruding nuclei and very scanty cytoplasm. A prominent intra- and extravascular lymphocytic inflammatory cell infiltrate is often present, and intravascular papillae with collagenous cores are a frequent finding (Fig. 34-40). Commonly, the lymphocytes appear to be in close apposition to the endothelial cells.

Pathogenesis. Based on the close interaction between lymphocytes and endothelial cells in Dabska's tumor, it has been proposed that the hobnail endothelial cells differentiate towards high endothelial cells, which are normally responsible for the selective homing of lymphocytes in lymphoid organs.[171] A similar theory can be proposed for retiform hemangioendothelioma, which shares some histologic features with Dabska's tumor.

Differential Diagnosis. See Differential Diagnosis for retiform hemangioendothelioma.

Kaposi-like Infantile Hemangioendothelioma

Although this tumor has only been described recently, individual cases of the same condition were reported in the past us-

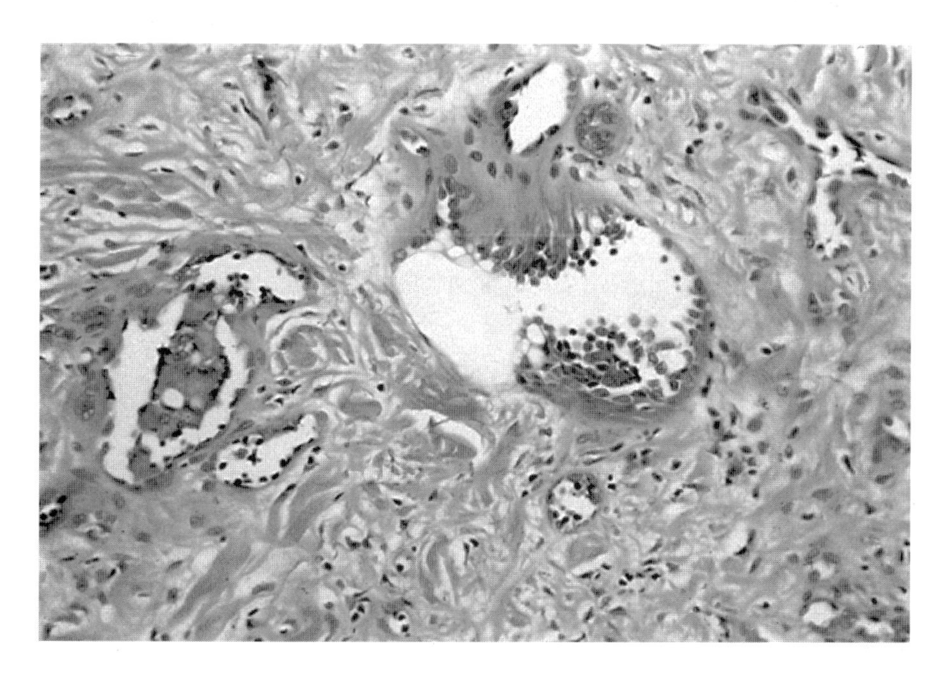

FIG. 34-39. Retiform hemangioendothelioma
Typical hobnail endothelial cells and focal papillary projections.

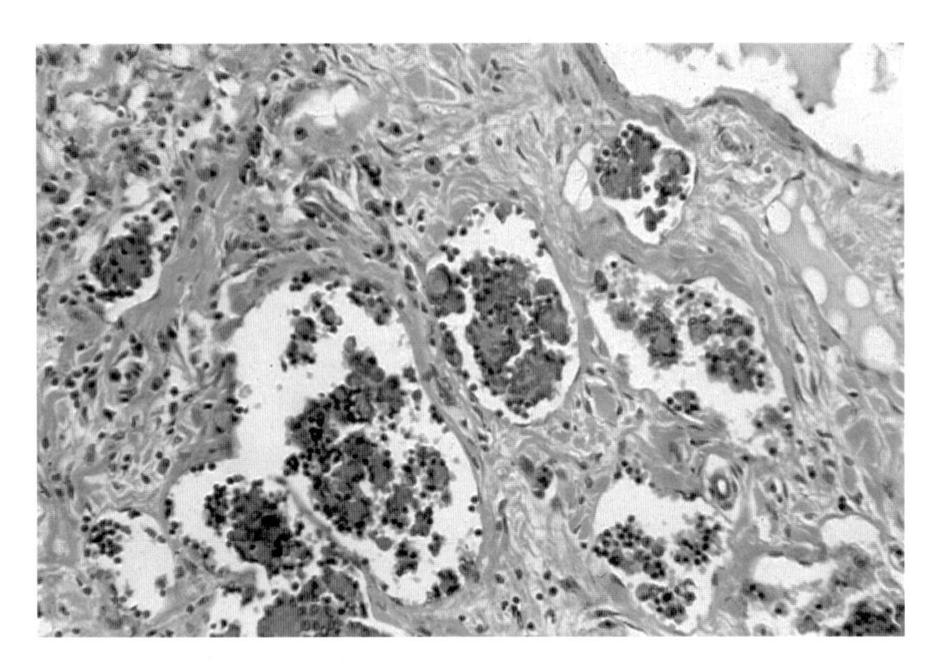

FIG. 34-40. Malignant endovascular papillary angioendothelioma Cavernous lymphangioma–like vascular spaces and intravascular papillae with collagenous cores.

ing different names.[141,142,172,173] It is a rare vascular tumor that usually presents in the retroperitoneum or deep soft tissues of infants. It is classified as a low-grade malignant vascular tumor because of its locally aggressive growth, yet metastases have not been reported. Cases presenting in the skin are exceptional but have been described.[142] A number of cases are associated with Kasabach-Merritt syndrome or lymphangiomatosis.[141]

Histopathology. A typical lesion combines a lobular and infiltrative growth pattern with fascicles of bland spindle-shaped endothelial cells intermixed with engorged capillaries and scattered epithelioid cells. Slit-like vascular spaces are often a feature.

Distinction from Kaposi's sarcoma is discussed on page 909.

MALIGNANT TUMORS

Angiosarcoma

Malignant tumors of endothelial cell origin can be broadly divided into those of high- or low-grade malignancy (see Table 31-1); high-grade tumors mainly arise in the elderly, whereas the low-grade malignancies may affect younger age groups. There is a tendency to designate high-grade malignant vascular tumors as angiosarcomas and low-grade tumors as hemangioendotheliomas, but some authors use the terms interchangeably. It must also be remembered that the term hemangioendothelioma was used in the past to refer to some benign vascular tumors, especially strawberry nevus in children.

It is doubtful whether sarcomas of probable lymphatic origin can be distinguished histologically from those of presumptive vascular endothelial origin; hence there is a tendency to disregard the term lymphangiosarcoma in favor of angiosarcoma. In fact, there is some evidence to suggest that not only angiosarcoma but also Kaposi's sarcoma could be of lymphatic endothelial cell origin.

Most angiosarcomas of the skin arise in the following clinical settings: (1) angiosarcoma of the face and scalp in the elderly, (2) angiosarcoma (lymphangiosarcoma) secondary to chronic lymphoedema, and (3) angiosarcoma as a complication of chronic radiodermatitis or arising from the effects of severe skin trauma or ulceration.[174]

Recently an aggressive variant known as epithelioid angiosarcoma[175] has been described, which is difficult to diagnose histologically because of undifferentiated cytomorphology without the help of immunohistochemistry (see text following).

Apart from these circumstances, cutaneous angiosarcomas are extremely rare. Exceptional case reports include angiosarcoma arising in preceding vascular nevi,[176,177] in association with neural tumors[178,179] and xeroderma pigmentosum.[180] With the exception of epithelioid angiosarcoma, the histopathologies of angiosarcomas are similar regardless of the clinical setting.

1. *Angiosarcoma of the scalp and face of the elderly.* This is almost invariably a fatal tumor that usually arises innocuously as erythematous or bruise-like lesions on the scalp or middle and upper face with predilection for men.[181–184] Subsequent plaques, nodules, or ulcerations develop; metastasis to nodes or internal organs usually arises only as a late complication with many patients dying as a result of extensive local disease. This sarcoma has only rarely been reported in black patients; the disease mainly affects whites and sometimes Asians.[185] Only a very small percentage of patients, usually those with lesions less than 10 cm in diameter at presentation, can be successfully treated with radical widefield radiotherapy and surgery.[181,186]

2. *Angiosarcoma following lymphedema (postmastectomy lymphangiosarcoma or the Stewart-Treves syndrome).* Typically the tumor presents in women who have had severe long-

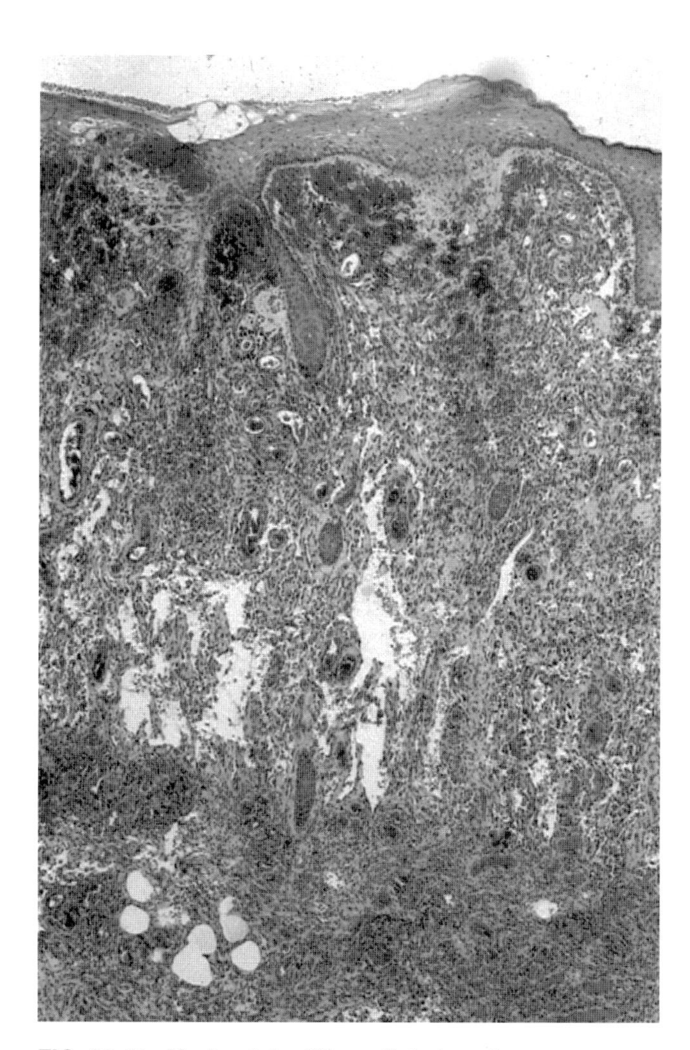

FIG. 34-41. Moderately differentiated angiosarcoma
Note numerous irregular vascular channels, more solid areas, and extensive hemorrhage.

standing lymphedema of the arm following breast surgery.[186–188] In most cases, lymphedema is present for about 10 years before the tumor arises, usually in the inner portion of the upper arm. Radiotherapy can usually be excluded as an etiologic factor because the sarcoma nearly always develops beyond the areas of chronic radiodermatitis. Lymphedema-induced angiosarcoma has also been described in men[189] and in a lower extremity[190] from causes other than cancer surgery, including congenital lymphedema[191] and tropical lymphedema due to filaria.[192] The prognosis despite radical surgery is extremely poor.[187] Exceptionally, a low-grade angiosarcoma with lesions simulating lymphangioma circumscriptum has been described as complicating chronic lymphedema after surgery.[193]

3. *Post-irradiation angiosarcoma.* There are many reports of angiosarcoma arising in the skin after radiotherapy for internal cancer. The most common sites are the breast or chest wall[194–196] and the lower abdomen[197,198] after therapy for breast or gynecologic cancer. There are also rare reports of previous radiotherapy being a factor in the etiology of angiosarcoma of the head and neck region.[181]

Histopathology. Usually the tumor extends well beyond the limits of the apparent clinical lesion.[184] As a rule, the tumor shows varied differentiation in different biopsies, even within different fields in a single biopsy (Fig. 34-41). In well-differentiated areas, irregular anastomosing vascular channels lined by a single layer of somewhat enlarged endothelial cells permeate between collagen bundles. Isolation and enclosure of collagen bundles, figuratively referred to as "dissection of collagen" by Rosai et al.[199] is a characteristic feature (Fig. 34-42). Nuclear atypia is always present and may be slight to moderate, but occasional large hyperchromatic cells may be encountered (Fig. 34-43). At this stage the vascular lumens are generally bloodless, but they may contain free-lying shed malignant cells.

In less well-differentiated areas endothelial cells increase in size and number, forming intraluminal papillary projections where there is enhanced mitotic activity. In poorly differentiated areas, solid sheets of large pleomorphic cells with little or no evidence of luminal differentiation, can resemble metastatic carcinoma or melanoma.[199] Focally, areas showing epithelioid cells are not uncommon. Other areas may simulate a poorly differentiated spindle cell sarcoma. Interstitial hemorrhage and widely dilated blood-filled spaces may sometimes develop.

The histopathology of angiosarcomas secondary to lymphedema and radiotherapy shows a similar range of well differentiated to poorly differentiated neoplasms as idiopathic

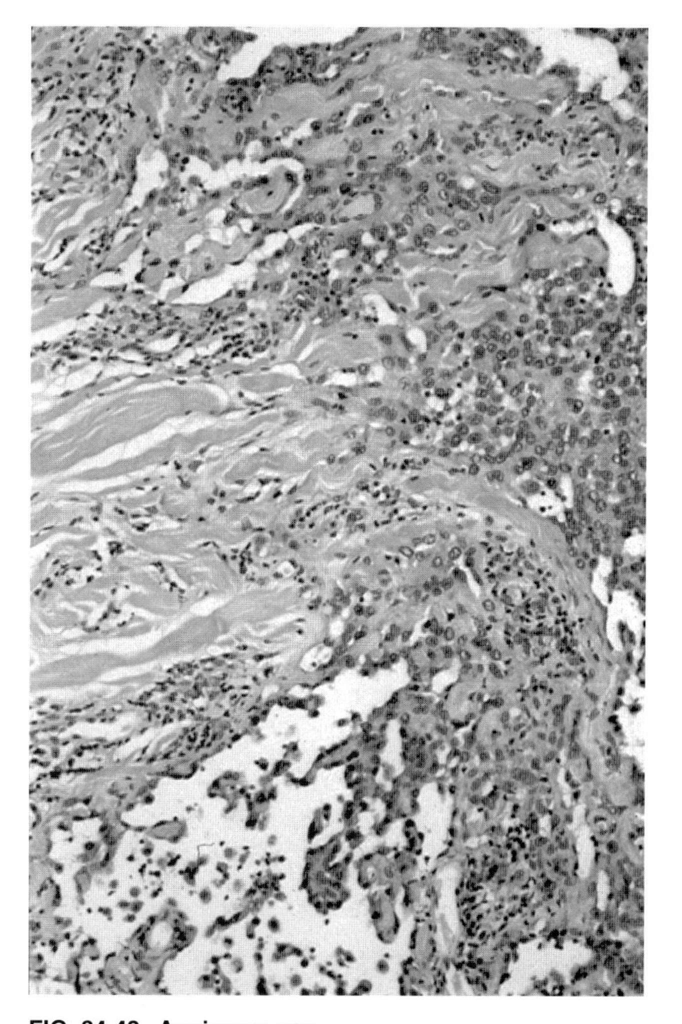

FIG. 34-42. Angiosarcoma
Typical dissection of collagen pattern and poorly formed vascular channels with papillary projections.

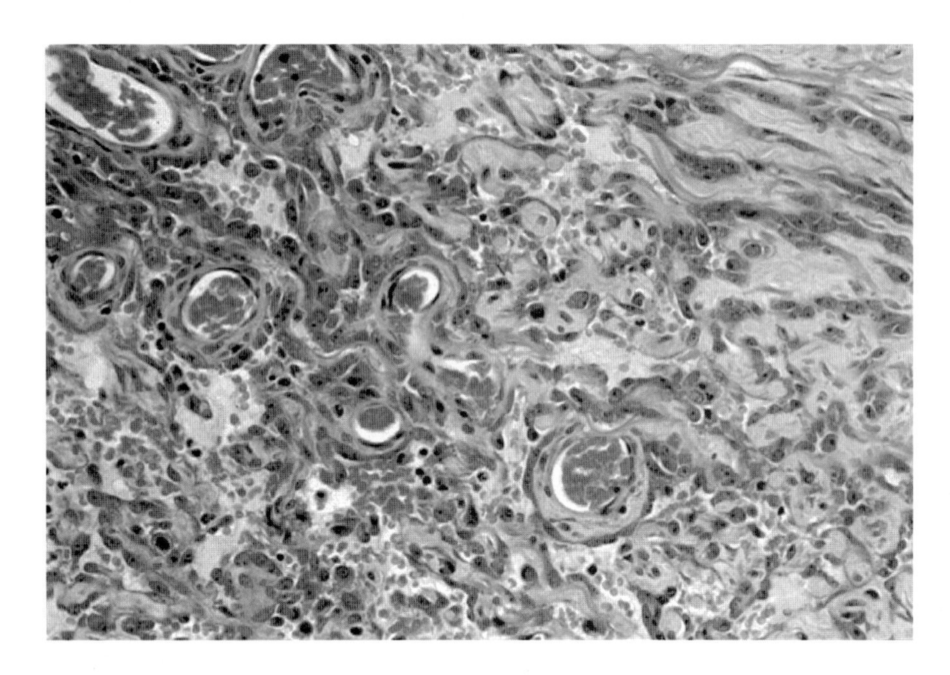

FIG. 34-43. Angiosarcoma
Marked cytologic atypia and mitotic figures.

angiosarcoma of the face and scalp. There are no reliable histologic differentiating features, although sometimes evidence of chronic lymphedema or chronic radiation dermatitis may be apparent in the tissue adjacent to the sarcoma.

Histogenesis. Earlier immunohistochemical markers for factor VIII–related antigen (FVIII-RA) and Ulex europaeus agglutinin-I (UEA-1) are of little value as an aid to diagnosis of this type of angiosarcoma. FVIII-RA is generally negative even in well differentiated tumors[181] but patchy, weak, diffuse staining may be found focally in less well-differentiated tumors that require caution in interpretation. Also faulty technique can give rise to FVIII-RA false positivity in squamous cell carcinoma that sometimes simulates angiosarcoma. UEA-1 is usually strongly positive in moderately and well-differentiated angiosarcomas, but UEA-1 has a very low specificity. The newer markers CD34 and especially the more specific CD31 are much more reliable as sensitive markers of tumors of endothelial cell origin for use in routine biopsies (Fig. 34-44).[139] On electron microscopic examination well-differentiated tumors may show the ovoid laminated organelle-like Weibel-Palade bodies char-

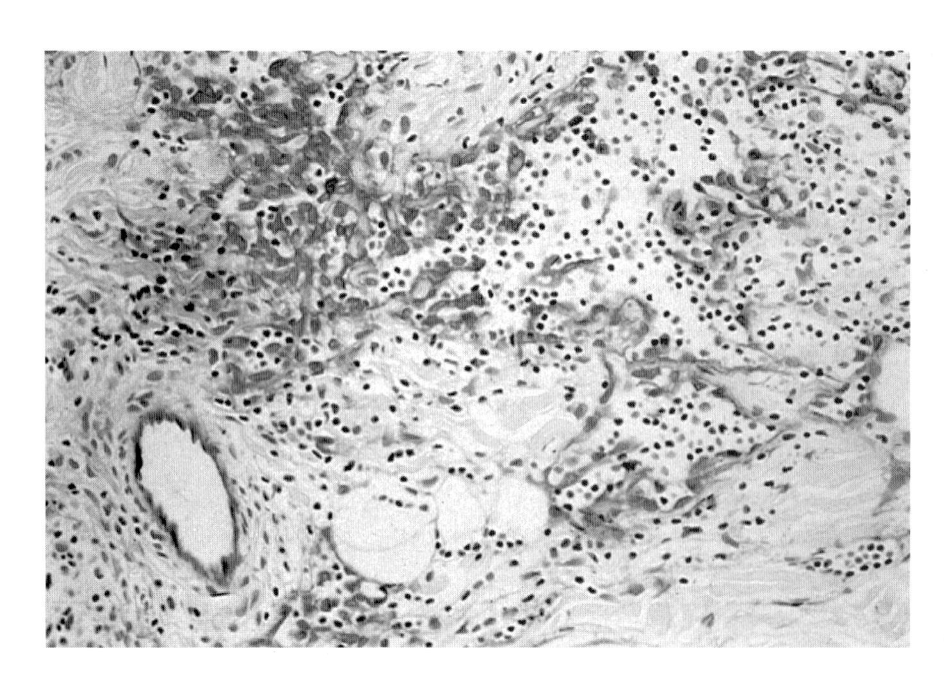

FIG. 34-44. Angiosarcoma
Uniform staining of tumor cells for CD31 using the ABC method.

acteristic of vascular endothelial cells, but they are absent in most tumors.[200] The absence of FVIII-RA labeling and the paucity of Weibel-Palade bodies can be said to favor a lymphatic endothelial origin of this type of angiosarcoma.[181]

Differential Diagnosis. Well-differentiated angiosarcomas, if cell atypia is slight, may closely resemble early macular lesions of Kaposi's sarcoma and benign lymphangioendothelioma because all these conditions can demonstrate to a greater or lesser extent a "dissection of collagen" pattern. The major differences in clinical presentation of the disorders, (absence of mitosis and the bland appearances of the endothelial cells in macular lesions of Kaposi's sarcoma and benign lymphangioendothelioma) should prevent any difficulties. Focal dissection of collagen pattern is also mimicked in intravascular papillary endothelial hyperplasia by new vessels invading thrombotic material. In poorly differentiated angiosarcomas it is usually possible to find evidence of channel formation in peripheral areas that allows diagnosis. However, the recent use of endothelial markers, especially CD31, is an important aid in diagnosis. Finally, occasionally adenoid squamous carcinomas, with intratumor hemorrhage, can simulate angiosarcoma.[201–203] Immunohistochemistry is useful in these cases since only angiosarcomas with epithelioid morphology are positive for cytokeratin,[175,204] but these also show staining for CD31 and CD34.

Epithelioid Angiosarcoma

This is a rare form of angiosarcoma that usually arises in deep soft tissues[175] but may also occur in the skin and internal organs, including the thyroid and adrenal gland.[204,205] Personal experience indicates that cutaneous lesions are more common than previously thought, and it is likely that such lesions were diagnosed in the past as epithelial or melanocytic neoplasms. There is wide anatomic distribution, and cases present in adults with slight predilection for males. Rare examples have been associated with radiation therapy,[175] an arteriovenous fistula,[206] and a foreign body.[207] The outlook is extremely poor, although a slow course has been described for some skin tumors.[205]

Histopathology. Tumors are composed of sheets of pleomorphic large cells with prominent eosinophilic cytoplasm, a large nucleus, and an eosinophilic nucleolus, usually with little evidence of vascular differentiation other than the occasional presence of intracytoplasmic vacuoles sometimes containing red blood cells (Fig. 34-45). This angiosarcoma can easily be mistaken for a carcinoma deposit or even malignant melanoma. Usually the tumor cells demonstrate consistent positivity for FVIII–related antigen and CD31 (Fig. 34-46). However, cytokeratin positivity is present in up to 50% of cases, and rare cases are focally positive for EMA; this might be a source of confusion with metastatic carcinoma and epithelioid sarcoma which are negative for endothelial markers.

TUMORS OF LYMPHATIC VESSELS

Lymphangiomas constitute only about 4% of all vascular tumors[208] and about 26% of benign vascular tumors in children.[76] They can be classified as four types: (1) cavernous lymphangioma, (2) cystic hygroma, (3) lymphangioma circumscriptum,[209] and (4) acquired progressive lymphangioma or benign lymphangioendothelioma.[210] In addition, lesions of lymphangiectasia, which are indistinguishable from classic lymphangioma circumscriptum, may occur, though rarely, in association with congenital or acquired lymphedema.[211] Although traditionally cavernous lymphangioma and cystic hygroma have been considered independent entities, it is likely that the latter is an ectatic variant of the former, which arises in areas of loose connective tissues; therefore, they will be discussed under the same heading.[212] The existence of capillary lymphangioma is doubtful, and will not be considered further.

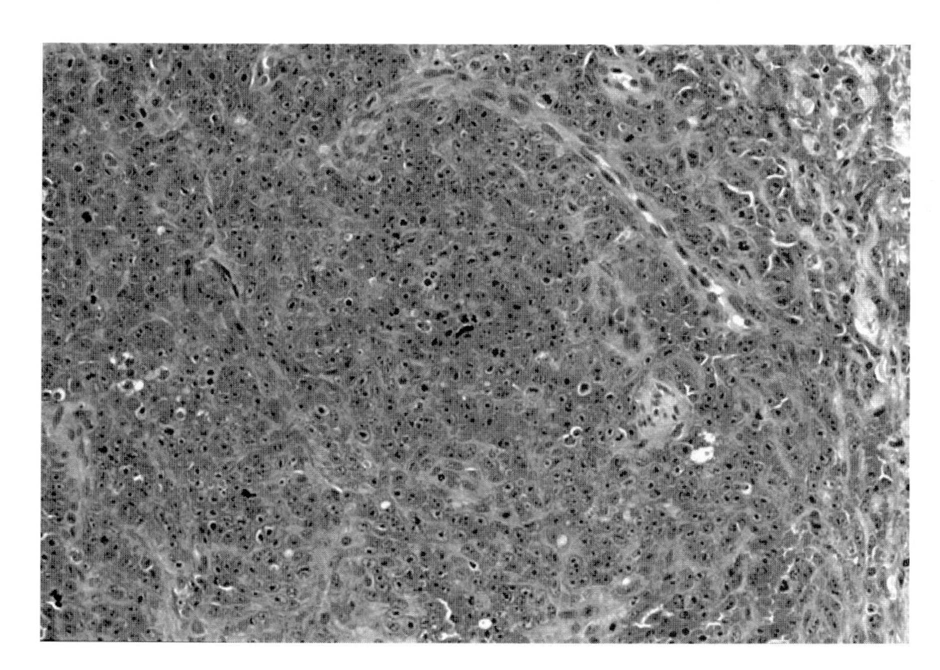

FIG. 34-45. Epithelioid angiosarcoma
Solid proliferation of atypical epithelioid cells with occasional cytoplasmic vacuoles. Note the melanoma-like nuclei with eosinophilic nucleoli.

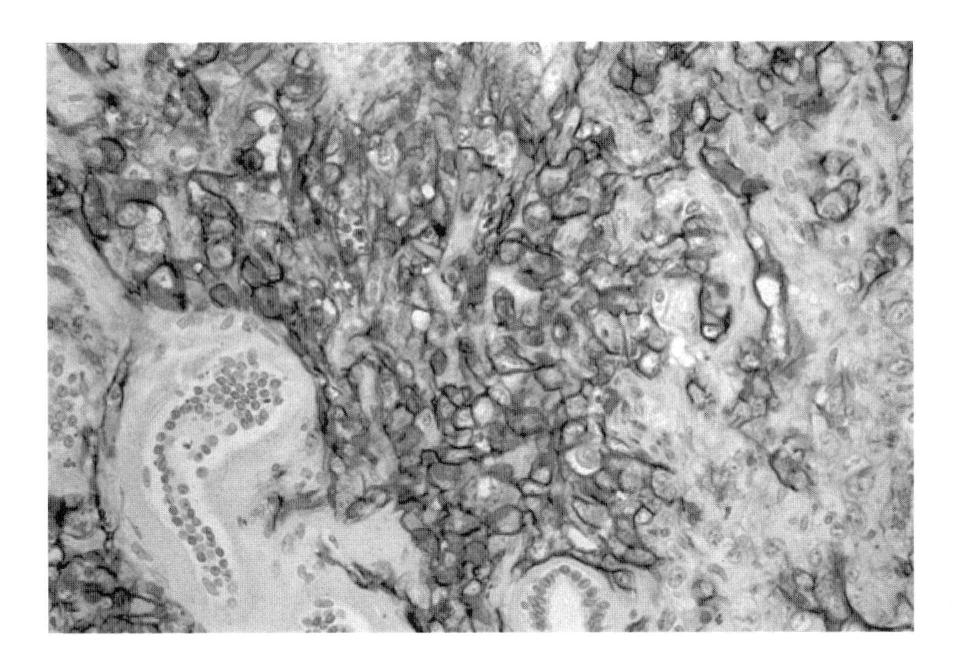

FIG. 34-46. Epithelioid angiosarcoma
The epithelioid cells are positive for CD31 in contrast to the neighboring negative sweat ducts (ABC method).

Histogenesis. The great majority of tumors of lymphatic vessels are benign, and most of them appear to represent developmental abnormalities rather than true neoplasms. Although in hemangiomas the endothelial cells stain positively for factor VIII–related antigen, the endothelial cells in lymphangiomas are for the most part negative for factor VIII–related antigen.[213] This is in contrast with Ulex europaeus agglutinin-I, which is positive in the endothelial cells of both hemangiomas and lymphangiomas. The presence of fragmented basal lamina and anchoring filaments in hemangiomas is a more reliable ultrastructural feature to use to distinguish lymphatics and blood vessels. However, distinction between angiomas and lymphangiomas is not always clear even when light microscopy is combined with immunohistochemistry and electron microscopy.[214]

Cavernous Lymphangioma and Cystic Hygroma

Cavernous lymphangioma usually presents at birth or during the first two years of life with an equal gender incidence.[215,216] The most common locations are the head and neck area (particularly the oral cavity) and, less often, the extremities. It presents as a large, diffuse, subcutaneous, often fluctuant soft mass. Recurrences are common after limited excision.

Cystic hygroma has a similar age and gender distribution, and lesions tend to affect the neck, axillae, and groin.[216] Tumors tend to be better circumscribed than cavernous lymphangiomas, but there is also a tendency for local recurrence unless a wide excision is performed.

Histopathology. Cavernous lymphangioma shows large, irregularly shaped spaces in the dermis and subcutaneous tissue lined by a single layer of bland endothelial cells (Fig. 34-47). The surrounding stroma can be loose or fibrotic and shows a lymphocytic inflammatory cell infiltrate with scattered lymphoid follicles. An incomplete layer of smooth muscle can be seen in the walls of some vessels. The vascular lumina show pink proteinaceous fluid with lymphocytes, but erythrocytes can also be seen. Large cavernous lymphangiomas, particularly in areas of the lip or tongue, may extend between the muscle bundles, separating them from one another.[209]

In cystic hygroma microscopic features are similar to those of cavernous lymphangioma except for the presence of numerous cystically dilated thin-walled lymphatic spaces.

Differential Diagnosis. Distinction from cavernous hemangioma can be impossible since the vascular channels in both conditions can show red blood cells in their lumina. The presence of lymphoid aggregates in the stroma tends to favor the diagnosis of lymphangioma.

Lymphangioma Circumscriptum

Lymphangioma circumscriptum is predominantly a developmental malformation of infancy with an equal gender incidence, but it may arise at any age.[209,217] Similar acquired lesions arising in adults in relation to chronic lymphedema or radiotherapy are best regarded as *lymphangiectasia.*[211] The anatomic distribution is wide, but the proximal portions of the limbs and limb girdle are most frequently affected. Association with cavernous lymphangioma, cystic hygroma, and even lymphangiomatosis is common. A typical lesion consists of collections of numerous vesicles containing clear fluid and less commonly, blood. Due to the presence of a deep component (see text following), lesions arising in infancy tend to recur after simple excision.

Histopathology. Lymphangioma circumscriptum is composed of numerous dilated lymphatics in the superfical and papillary dermis (Fig. 34-48). There is clear fluid (Fig. 34-49) and, less frequently, red blood cells in their lumina. In the overlying epidermis there is some degree of acanthosis and hyperkeratosis. The surrounding stroma shows scattered lymphocytes. Le-

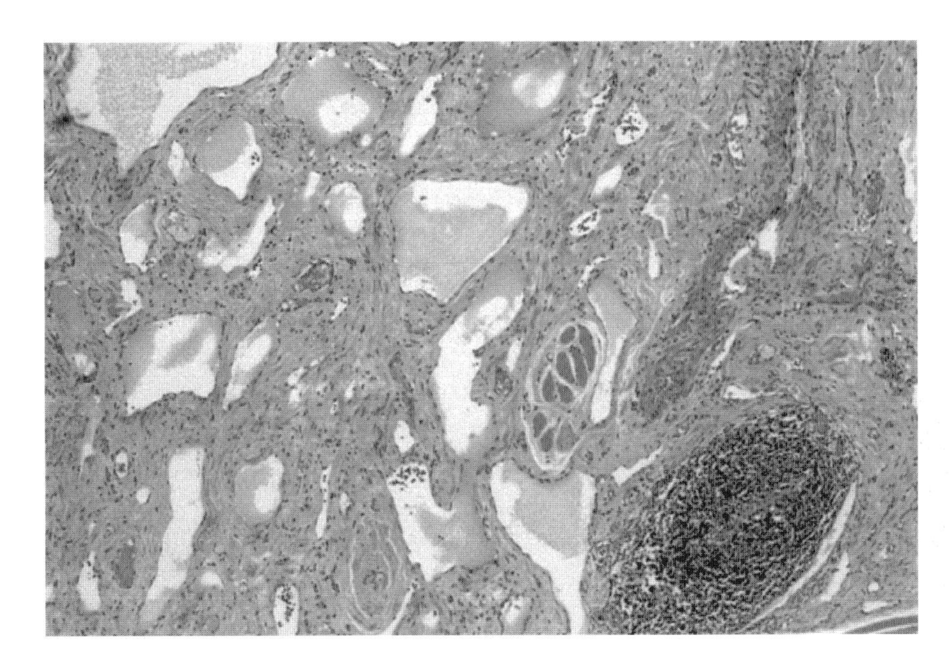

FIG. 34-47. Cavernous lymphangioma
Dilated lymphatic channels lined by flat endothelial cells with aggregates of lymphocytes in the stroma.

sions developing in infancy often show a large-caliber, muscular lymphatic space in the subcutaneous tissue, which has to be ligated at the time of excision to avoid recurrence.

Progressive Lymphangioma (Benign Lymphangioendothelioma)

Progressive lymphangioma (benign lymphangioendothelioma) is a benign rare tumor that has a tendency to present in children and to evolve slowly over the years. Males and females are equally affected, and although the anatomic distribution is wide, there is preferential involvement of the limbs.[210,218] Clinically, a typical lesion is a solitary well-circumscribed erythematous macule or plaque. Recurrence after simple excision has not been described, and occasional lesions can show focal or complete spontaneous regression.[219]

Histopathology. Most lesions involve predominantly the superficial dermis but extension into the dermis and subcutis can be present.[219] Irregular, horizontal, thin-walled vascular channels lined by a single layer of bland endothelial cells are seen dissecting collagen bundles (Fig. 34-50).[210,218] Endothelial cell

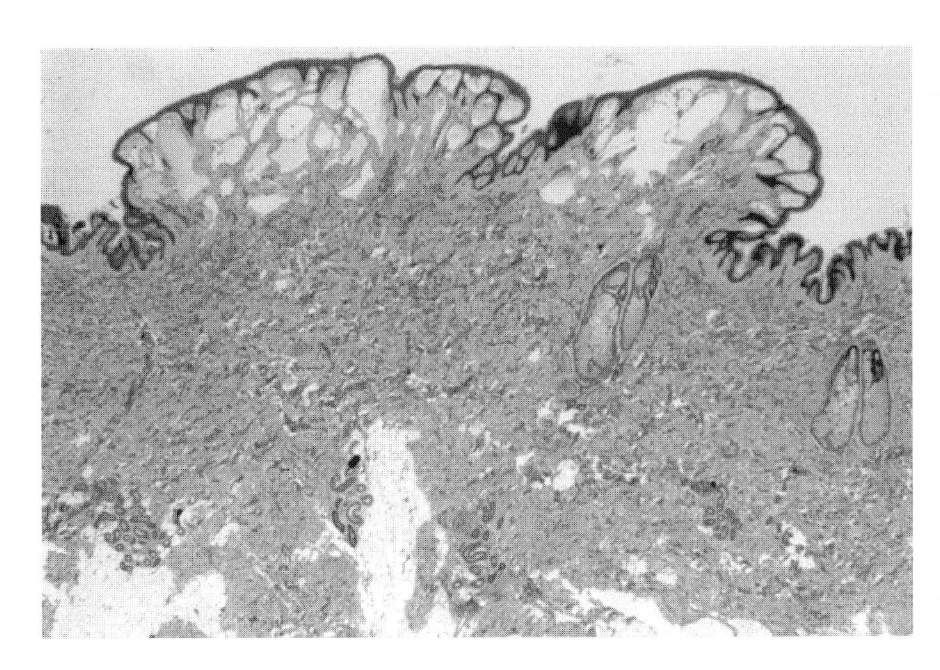

FIG. 34-48. Lymphangioma circumscriptum
Numerous dilated lymphatic channels expand the papillary dermis.

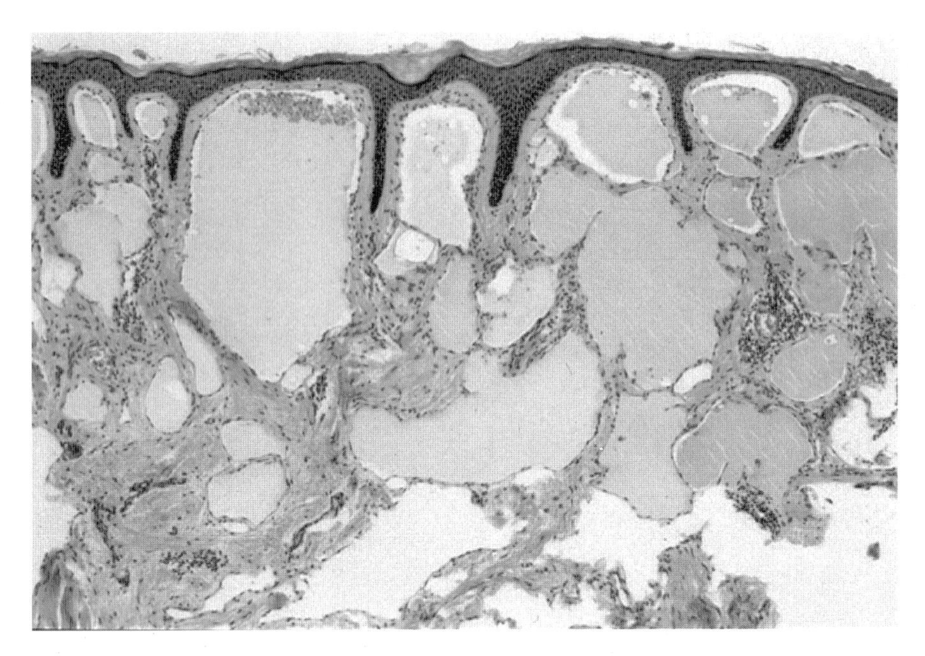

FIG. 34-49. Lymphangioma circumscriptum
Note intraluminal lymph and scattered lymphocytes in the surrounding dermis.

atypia and mitotic figures are absent. The vascular channels appear empty or have scanty proteinaceous material and/or a few red blood cells.

Differential Diagnosis. The main differential diagnosis is with well-differentiated angiosarcoma and patch-stage Kaposi's sarcoma. Although sharing with angiosarcoma the presence of extensive dissection of collagen bundles, the latter conditions occur in completely different settings and in angiosarcoma there is usually, at least focally, cytologic atypia and mitotic figures. Patch-stage Kaposi's sarcoma often presents clinically with multiple lesions, and histologically the abnormal blood vessels tend to cluster around normal preexisting blood vessels. There is hemosiderin deposition with an inflammatory cell infiltrate with lymphocytes and plasma cells.

Lymphangiomatosis

Lymphangiomatosis is a rare developmental abnormality that affects children with an equal gender incidence. Although most

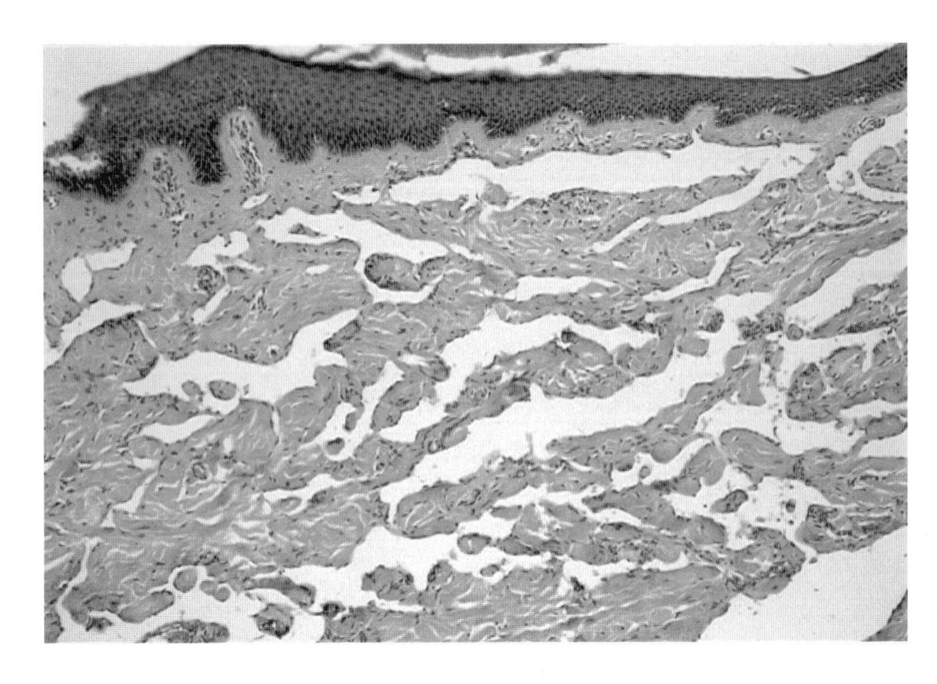

FIG. 34-50. Progressive lymphangioma
Extensive dissection of collagen bundles by irregular vascular channels lined by bland flat endothelial cells.

cases appear to be congenital the disease is often not diagnosed until childhood. The majority of cases involve soft tissues, skin, bone and parenchymal organs. When vital organs are affected the prognosis is very poor.[220,221] Cases with involvement limited to skin and soft tissues of a limb (with or without bone involvement) have been described and are associated with a better prognosis.[221] Rare cases can present in association with kaposiform hemangioendothelioma of infancy and childhood.[141] Lymphangiomatosis is the lymphatic counterpart of angiomatosis. In some instances distinction between them can be difficult, although lymphangiographic studies can be very helpful in establishing the difference.

Histopathology. The appearance of lymphangiomatosis is very similar to that of progressive lymphangioma, but the changes in lymphangiomatosis are more extensive and diffuse with involvement of deeper soft tissues, fibrosis in long-standing cases, and stromal hemosiderin deposition.

TUMORS OF PERIVASCULAR CELLS

Glomus Tumor

Glomus tumors are relatively common lesions that usually present in young adults between the third and fourth decade of life with no gender predilection except for subungual tumors which have a marked female predilection.[222] The hand (particularly subungual region and palm) is the most commonly affected site, followed by the foot and forearm. Lesions, however, can occur with a wide anatomic distribution not only in the skin but also rarely in mucosae and internal organs. Most tumors classically present as solitary, small (less than 1 cm), blue-red nodules that are characteristically associated with paroxysmal pain often elicited by changes in temperature (especially cold) or pressure.

A very small proportion of glomus tumors are multiple. As opposed to solitary glomus tumors, the latter usually arise in children, tend to be asymptomatic, are rarely subungual, and are thought to be inherited in an autosomal dominant fashion.[223] Clinically, these lesions can be confused with those of the blue rubber bleb nevus syndrome, and it is likely that cases of this condition reported in the past represented examples of multiple glomus tumors. Histologically, multiple glomus tumors are predominantly glomangiomas (see text following).

Local recurrence is very uncommon, and when seen, is usually in deep-seated tumors with an infiltrative growth pattern (so-called infiltrating glomus tumor, see text following).[224] Exceptionally, glomus tumors originate within a blood vessel[225,226] or nerve.[227] Malignant glomus tumor or glomangiosarcoma is rare to the point of vanishing.

Histopathology. Glomus tumors show varying proportions of glomus cells, blood vessels, and smooth muscle and are classified accordingly into *solid glomus tumor* (25% of cases), *glomangioma* (60% of cases), and *glomangiomyoma* (15% of cases). Most cases of glomus tumor are well circumscribed, and a classic solid lesion is composed of sheets of uniform cells with pale or eosinophilic cytoplasm, well-defined cell margins (highlighted distinctively by a PAS stain), and round or ovoid punched-out central nuclei (Fig. 34-51). Small blood vessels are uniformly distributed in the tumor but may not be apparent without the use of special stains. The stroma is often edematous, and extensive myxoid change may be present. Normal mitotic figures may be conspicuous in some cases, but cytologic atypia is usually absent. Numerous stromal nerve fibers may be highlighted with special stains. Exceptional cases show extensive oncocytic change.[228] In glomangioma there are numerous dilated, cavernous-like, thin-walled vascular spaces surrounded by one or a few layers of glomus cells (Fig. 34-52). In glomangiomyoma there is an important number of spindle-shaped smooth-muscle cells, which tend to be distributed near the vascular spaces and blend with the adjacent collections of glomus cells (Fig. 34-53).

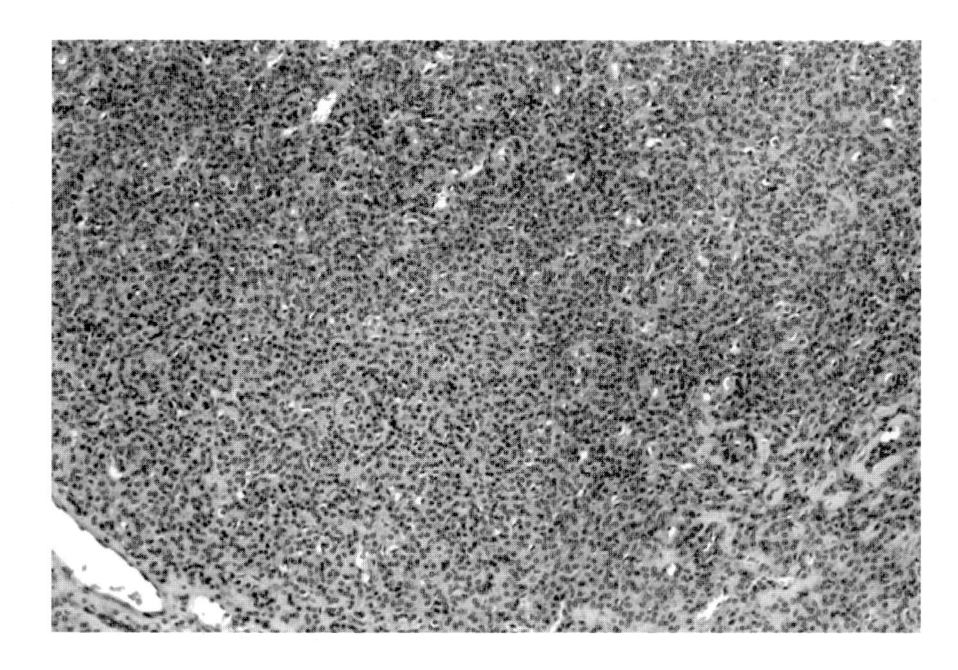

FIG. 34-51. Solid glomus tumor Monomorphic round cells with eosinophilic cytoplasm and central nuclei.

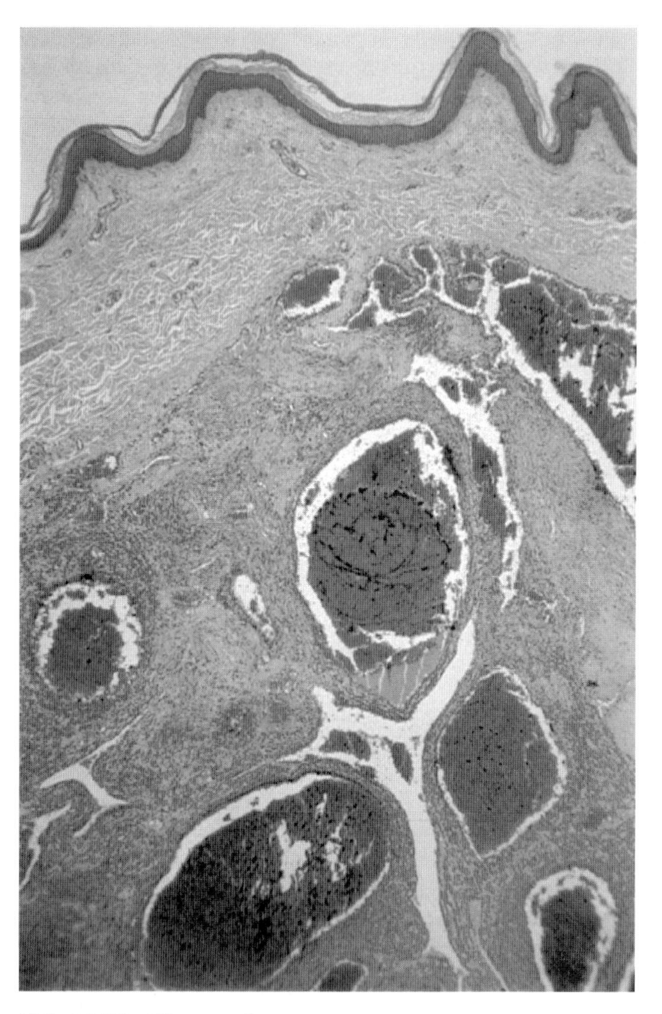

FIG. 34-52. Glomangioma
Cavernous vascular spaces surrounded by layers of glomus cells.

Infiltrating glomus tumor is a very rare variant that occurs in deep soft tissues and is characterized by solid nests of glomus cells with an infiltrative growth pattern.[224] It is associated with a high recurrence rate.

The histologic diagnosis of glomangiosarcoma is made when an otherwise typical glomus tumor coexists with a frankly sarcomatous component.[224,229] Metastasis, however, appears to be an exception.

Histogenesis. Glomus tumors closely resemble the modified smooth muscle cells of a segment of a specialized arteriovenous anastomoses (Sucquet–Hoyer canal) that is involved in the regulation of temperature, the *glomus body*. Glomus bodies are usually found in acral skin, particularly on the hands. However, many glomus tumors arise from sites where glomus bodies are not known to exist. In view of this it is likely that some glomus tumors arise from differentiation of pluripotential mesenchymal cells or ordinary smooth-muscle cells. On immunohistochemical examination, glomus tumor cells stain for smooth muscle actin (Fig. 34-54), muscle-specific actin, and myosin.[230,231] Staining for desmin is only focally positive.

Differential Diagnosis. Solid glomus tumor can be distinguished from eccrine spiradenoma by the presence in eccrine spiradenoma of two populations of cells, focal ductal differentiation, and positivity for epithelial markers. Occasionally intradermal nevus with pseudovascular spaces resembles a glomus tumor, but in the former there is always evidence of nesting, maturation, and positivity of lesional cells for S-100.[232]

Multiple glomus tumors differ from lesions of the blue rubber bleb nevus by the presence of glomus cells in nearly all tumors. It is likely that some previously reported cases of blue rubber bleb nevus actually represented examples of multiple glomus tumors.

Hemangiopericytoma

Traditionally, hemangiopericytoma is divided into two main categories: an infantile and an adult variant.[233] Both variants,

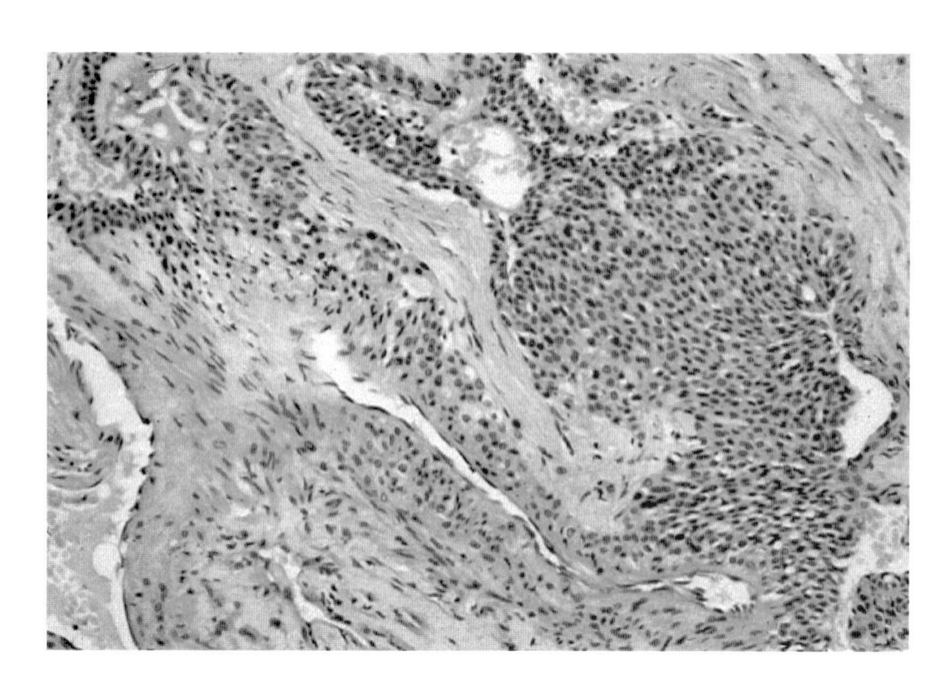

FIG. 34-53. Glomangiomyoma
Spindle-shaped cells with pink cytoplasm combined with glomus cells.

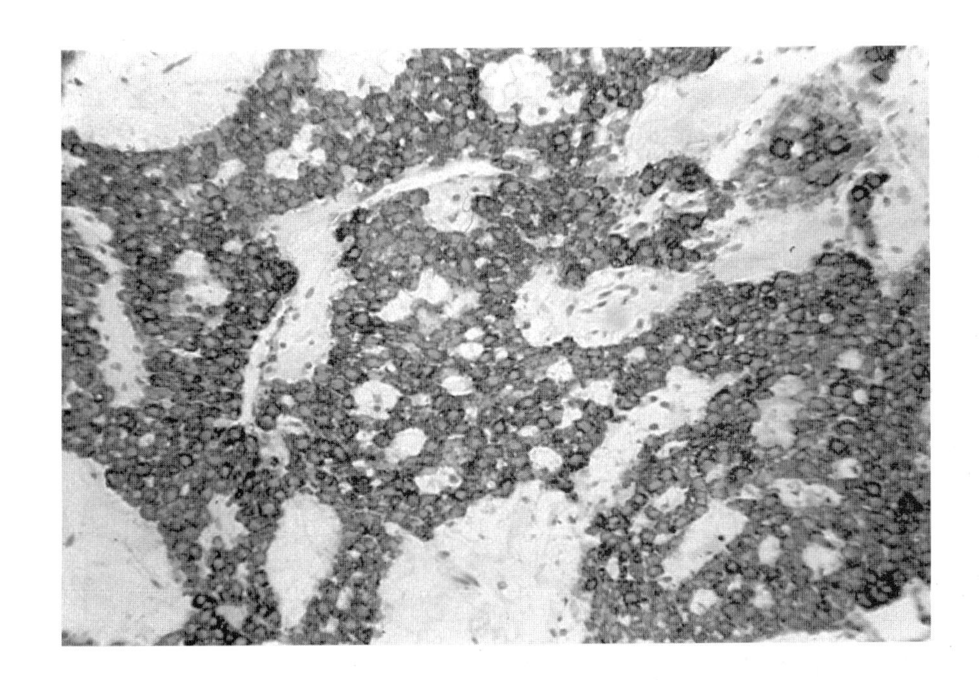

FIG. 34-54. Glomus tumor
Strong positivity of tumor cells for smooth muscle actin (ABC method).

however, appear to have very little in common except for the histologic presence of a pericytomatous vascular pattern (see text following).

Adult hemangiopericytoma presents in middle-aged to elderly adults as a deep-seated mass in the retroperitoneum, lower limbs, orbit or sinonasal area. Involvement of the skin is increasingly rare.

Infantile hemangiopericytoma usually presents at birth or in the first years of life as single or multiple dermal or subcutaneous nodules. Local recurrence is common, and distant spread has been described, but it is likely that spread represents multicentricity rather than true metastasis. Clinical and histologic features are remarkably similar to those of infantile myofibromatosis (see Chap. 33), and it has been proposed that both entities represent different maturation stages of the same condition.[234,235]

Histopathology. Adult hemangiopericytomas are well circumscribed, often multinodular, and composed of short spindle-shaped cells with oval nuclei and scanty cytoplasm. Tumor cells are typically disposed around numerous thin-walled ramifying blood vessels, often arranged in a staghorn configuration (pericytomatous vascular pattern) (Fig. 34-55). Increased cellularity,

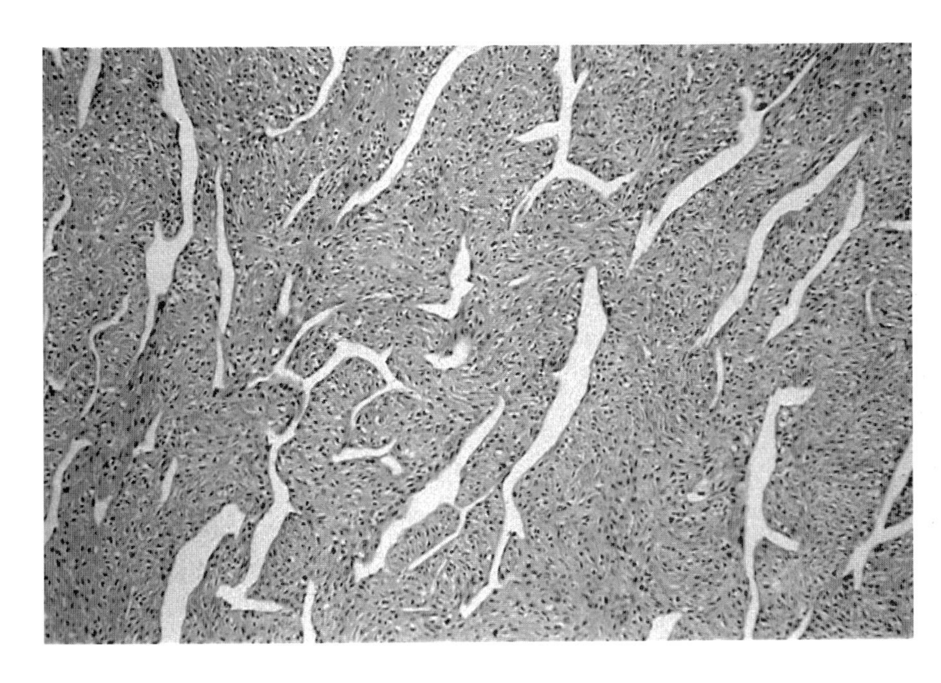

FIG. 34-55. Adult hemangiopericytoma
Short spindle-shaped cells arranged around numerous, branching elongated blood vessels.

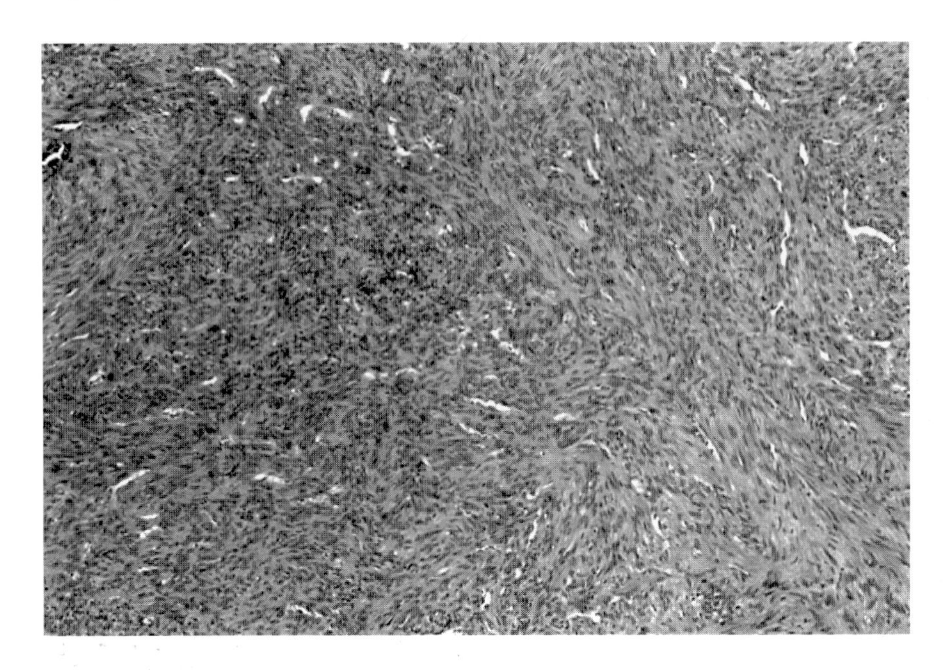

FIG. 34-56. Infantile hemangiopericytoma
Typical biphasic pattern showing immature round cells with scanty cytoplasm (*left*) alternating with bundles of spindle cells with a myofibroblastic appearance (*right*).

necrosis, hemorrhage, and, especially, more than four mitotic figures per 10 high-power fields are indicative of malignancy.[233]

Infantile hemangiopericytomas are multinodular and, as opposed to the adult counterpart, show at least focally a biphasic growth pattern. Hemangiopericytomatous areas composed of small round hyperchromatic cells blend with areas of bundles and nodules of more mature spindle-shaped cells with eosinophilic cytoplasm resembling myofibroblasts (Fig. 34-56). This zoning phenomenon is identical to, although less pronounced than, that seen in infantile myofibromatosis (see Chap. 33). Mitosis, necrosis, and vascular invasion are common features.

Pathogenesis. Since its original description hemangiopericytoma has been described as a tumor derived from the pericyte, a modified smooth muscle cell that normally surrounds small blood vessels.[233,236] This theory, initially based on light microscopy appearances (i.e., pericytomatous vascular pattern), was later partially supported by ultrastructural studies.[237–239] However, with the introduction of immunohistochemistry, it became apparent that most cases classified as adult hemangiopericytoma do not stain for actin or other myoid markers.[240,241] Moreover, with the combination of immunohistochemistry and electron microscopy, most tumors classified as adult hemangiopericytoma on light microscopy show other lines of differentiation.[242] These include synovial sarcoma, mesenchymal chondrosarcoma, solitary fibrous tumor, and deep benign fibrous histiocytoma. The few cases for which the line of differentiation remains obscure are the "true" adult hemangiopericytomas, but it is likely that they arise from an undifferentiated mesenchymal cell.

In infantile hemangiopericytoma the darker, less mature cells in the pericytomatous areas usually do not stain for any markers whereas the more mature spindle-shaped cells resembling myofibroblasts stain for alpha-smooth muscle actin. Identical features are seen in infantile myofibromatosis, and it is believed that the two entities are part of the same spectrum.[234,235]

REFERENCES

1. Clearkin KP, Enzinger FM. Intravascular papillary endothelial hyperplasia. Arch Pathol Lab Med 1976;100:441.
2. Hashimoto H, Daimaru Y, Enjoji M. Intravascular papillary endothelial hyperplasia. A clinicopathologic study of 91 cases. Am J Dermatopathol 1983;5:539.
3. Pins MR, Rosenthal DI, Springfield DS et al. Florid extravascular papillary endothelial hyperplasia (Masson's pseudosarcoma) presenting as a soft tissue sarcoma. Arch Pathol Lab Med 1993;117:259.
4. Reed CN, Cooper PH, Swerlick RA. Intravascular papillary endothelial hyperplasia: Multiple lesions simulating Kaposi's sarcoma. J Am Acad Dermatol 1984;10:110.
5. Miyamoto H, Nagatami T, Mohri S et al. Intravascular papillary endothelial hyperplasia. Clin Exp Dermatol 1988;13:411.
6. Albretch S, Khan HJ. Immunohistochemistry of intravascular papillary endothelial hyperplasia. J Cutan Pathol 1990;17:16.
7. LeBoit PE, Solomon AR, Santa Cruz DJ et al. Angiomatosis with luminal cryoprotein deposition. J Am Acad Dermatol 1992;27:969.
8. Wick MR, Rocamora A. Reactive and malignant "angioendotheliomatosis:" A discriminant clinicopathological study. J Cutan Pathol 1988;15:260.
9. Krell JM, Sanchez RL, Solomon AR. Diffuse dermal angiomatosis: A variant of reactive cutaneous angioendotheliomatosis. J Cutan Pathol 1994;21:363.
10. Chan JKC, Fletcher CDM, Hicklin GA et al. Glomeruloid hemangioma: A distinctive cutaneous lesion of multicentric Castleman's disease associated with POEMS syndrome. Am J Surg Pathol 1990;14:1036.
11. Rongioletti F, Gambini C, Lerza R. Glomeruloid hemangioma: A cutaneous marker of POEMS syndrome. Am J Dermatopathol 1994;16:175.
12. Allen PW, Ramakrishna B, MacCormac LB. The histiocytoid hemangiomas and other controversies. Pathol Ann 1992;27:51.
13. Rosai J. Angiolymphoid hyperplasia with eosinophilia of the skin: Its nosological position in the spectrum of histiocytoid hemangioma. Am J Dermatopathol 1982;4:175.

14. Rosai J, Gold J, Landy R. The histiocytoid hemangiomas: A unifying concept embracing several previously described entities of skin, soft tissue, large vessels, bone and heart. Hum Pathol 1979;10:707.
15. Tsang WYW, Chan JKC. The family of epithelioid vascular tumors. Histol Histopathol 1993;8:187.
16. Fetsch JF, Weiss SW. Observations concerning the pathogenesis of epithelioid hemangioma (angiolymphoid hyperplasia). Mod Pathol 1991;4:449.
17. Olsen TG, Helwig EB. Angiolymphoid hyperplasia with eosinophilia: A clinicopathologic study of 116 patients. J Am Acad Dermatol 1985; 12:781.
18. Mehregan AH, Shapiro L. Angiolymphoid hyperplasia with eosinophilia. Arch Dermatol 1971;103:50.
19. Eady RAJ, Wilson-Jones E. Pseudopyogenic granuloma: Enzyme, histochemical and ultrastructural study. Hum Pathol 1977;8:653.
20. DelGaudio JM, Myers MW, Telian SA. Angiolymphoid hyperplasia with eosinophilia involving the external auditory canal. Otolaryngol Head Neck Surg 1994;111:669.
21. Chan JKC, Hui PK, Ng CS et al. Epithelioid hemangioma (angiolymphoid hyperplasia with eosinophilia) and Kimura's disease in Chinese. Histopathology 1989;15:557.
22. Kuo TT, Shih LY, Chan HL. Kimura's disease: Involvement of regional lymph nodes and distinction from angiolymphoid hyperplasia with eosinophilia. Am J Surg Pathol 1988;12:843.
23. Moesner J, Pallesen R, Sorensen B. Angiolymphoid hyperplasia with eosinophilia (Kimura's disease): A case with dermal lesions in the knee region and a popliteal arteriovenous fistula. Arch Dermatol 1981;117:650.
24. Razquin S, Mayayo E, Citores MA et al. Angiolymphoid hyperplasia with eosinophilia of the tongue: Report of a case and review of the literature. Hum Pathol 1991;22:837.
25. Wolff HH, Kinney J, Ackerman AB. Angiolymphoid hyperplasia with follicular mucinosis. Arch Dermatol 1978;114:229.
26. Fawcett HA, Smith NP. Injection site granuloma due to aluminium. Arch Dermatol 1984;120:1318.
27. Hallam LA, Mackinlay GA, Wright AMA. Angiolymphoid hyperplasia with eosinophilia: Possible aetiological role for immunisation. J Clin Pathol 1989;42:944.
28. Miliauskas JR, Mukherjee T, Dixon B. Postimmunization (vaccination) injection-site reactions: A report of four cases and review of the literature. Am J Surg Pathol 1993;17:516.
29. Googe PB, Harris NL, Mihm MC Jr. Kimura's disease and angiolymphoid hyperplasia with eosinophilia: Two distinct histopathological entities. J Cutan Pathol 1987;14:263.
30. Kung IT, Gibson JB, Bannatyne PM. Kimura's disease: A clinicopathological study of 21 cases and its distinction from angiolymphoid hyperplasia with eosinophilia. Pathology 1984;16:39.
31. Urabe A, Tsuneyoshi M, Enjoji M. Epithelioid hemangioma versus Kimura's disease: A comparative clinicopathologic study. Am J Surg Pathol 1987;10:758.
32. Kawada A. Morbus Kimura: Darstellung der erkrankung und ihre differential diagnose. Hautarzt 1976;27:309.
33. Yamada A, Mitsuhashi K, Miyakawa Y. Membranous glomerulonephritis associated with eosinophilic lymphfolliculosis of the skin (Kimura's disease): Report of a case and review of the literature. Clin Nephrol 1982;18:211.
34. Mills SE, Cooper PH, Fechner RE. Lobular capillary hemangioma: the underlying lesion of pyogenic granuloma. A study of 73 cases from the oral and nasal mucous membranes. Am J Surg Pathol 1980;4:471.
35. Patrice SJ, Wiss K, Mulliken JB. Pyogenic granuloma (lobular capillary hemangioma): A clinicopathologic study of 178 cases. Pediatr Dermatol 1994;8:267.
36. Blickenstaff RD, Roeningk RK, Peters MS et al. Recurrent pyogenic granuloma with satellitosis. J Am Acad Dermatol 1989;21:1241.
37. Vicente MA, Estrach T, Zamora E et al. Granuloma piogenico recidivante con lesiones satelites multiples: Presentacion de dos casos. Med Cutan Ibero Lat Am 1990;18:331.
38. Cooper PH, Mills SE. Subcutaneous granuloma pyogenicum: Lobular capillary hemangioma. Arch Dermatol 1982;118:30.
39. Saad RW, Sau P, Mulvaney MP et al. Intravenous pyogenic granuloma. Int J Dermatol 1993;32:130.
40. Braunstein B, Greer KE, Cooper PH. Eruptive disseminated lobular capillary hemangioma (pyogenic granuloma). J Am Acad Dermatol 1989;21:391.
41. Nappi O, Wick MR. Disseminated lobular capillary hemangioma (pyogenic granuloma). Am J Dermatopathol 1986;8:379.
42. Torres JE, Sanchez JL. Disseminated pyogenic granuloma after an exfoliative dermatitis. J Am Acad Dermatol 1995;32:280.
43. Wilson BB, Greer KE, Cooper PH. Eruptive disseminated lobular capillary hemangioma (pyogenic granuloma). J Am Acad Dermatol 1989; 21:391.
44. Marsch WC. The ultrastructure of eruptive hemangioma ("pyogenic granuloma")(abstr). J Cutan Pathol 1981;8:144.
45. Nichols GE, Gaffey MJ, Mills SE et al. Lobular capillary hemangioma: An immunohistochemical study including steroid hormone status. Am J Clin Pathol 1992;97:770.
46. Cockerell CJ. Bacillary angiomatosis and related diseases caused by *Rochalimaea*. J Am Acad Dermatol 1995;32:783.
47. Exner JH, Dahod S, Pochi PE. Pyogenic granuloma-like acne lesions during isotretinoin therapy. Arch Dermatol 1983;119:808.
48. Valentic JP, Barr RJ, Weinstein GD. Inflammatory neovascular nodules associated with oral isotretinoin treatment of severe acne. Arch Dermatol 1983;119:871.
49. Leung AKC, Telmesani AMA. Salmon patches in caucasian children. Pediatr Dermatol 1989;6:185.
50. Esterly NB. Cutaneous hemangiomas, vascular stains and malformations, and associated syndromes. Curr Probl Dermatol 1995;7:67.
51. Finley JL, Noe JM, Arndt KA et al. Port-wine stains: Morphologic variations and developmental lesions. Arch Dermatol 1984;120:1453.
52. Finley JL, Clark RAF, Colvin RB et al. Immunofluorescent staining with antibodies to factor VIII, fibronectin, and collagenous basement membrane in normal human skin and port wine stains. Arch Dermatol 1982;118:971.
53. Smoller BP, Rosen S. Port-wine stains: A decrease of altered neural modulation of blood vessels? Arch Dermatol 1986;122:177.
54. Imperial R, Helwig EB. Angiokeratoma. Arch Dermatol 1967;95:166.
55. Epinette WW, Norins AL, Drew AL et al. Angiokeratoma corporis diffusum with a L-fucosidase deficiency. Arch Dermatol 1973; 107:754.
56. Ishibashi A, Tsuboi R, Shinmei M. B-galactosidase and neuraminidase deficiency associated with angiokeratoma corporis diffusum. Arch Dermatol 1984;120:1344.
57. Holmes RC, Fensom AH, McKee P et al. Angiokeratoma corporis diffusum in a patient with normal enzyme activities. J Am Acad Dermatol 1984;10:384.
58. Hayes KR, Rebello DJA. Angiokeratoma of Mibelli. Acta Derm Venereol (Stockh) 1961;41:56.
59. Imperial R, Helwig EB. Angiokeratoma of the vulva. Obstet Gynecol 1967;29:307.
60. Agger P, Osmundsen PE. Angiokeratoma of the scrotum (Fordyce). Acta Dermatol Venereol (Stockh) 1970;50:221.
61. Tarnowski WM, Hashimoto K. New light microscopic findings in Fabry's disease. Acta Derm Venereol (Stockh) 1969;49:386.
62. McGrae JD Jr, Winkelmann RK. Generalized essential telangiectasia. JAMA 1963;185:909.
63. Wilken JK. Unilateral dermatomal superficial telangiectasia. Arch Dermatol 1984;120:579.
64. Anderson RL, Smith JG Jr. Unilateral nevoid telangiectasia with gastric involvement. Arch Dermatol 1975;111:617.
65. Uhlin SR, McCarty KS Jr. Unilateral nevoid telangiectatic syndrome: The role of estrogen and progesterone receptors. Arch Dermatol 1983; 119:226.
66. Hunt SJ, Santa Cruz DJ. Acquired benign and "borderline" vascular lesions. Dermatol Clin 1992;10:97.
67. Marriott PJ, Munro O, Ryan T. Angioma serpiginosum: Familial incidence. Br J Dermatol 1975;93:701.
68. Chavaz P, Laugier P. Angiome serpigineux de Hutchinson. Ann Dermatol Venereol 1981;108:429.
69. Abahamian LM, Rothe MJ, Grant-Kels JM. Primary telangiectasia of childhood. Int J Dermatol 1992;31:307.
70. Hashimoto K, Pritzker MS. Hereditary hemorrhagic telangiectasia: An electron microscopic study. Oral Surg 1972;34:751.
71. Braverman IM. Ultrastructure and organization of the cutaneous microvasculature in normal and pathological states. J Invest Dermatol 1989; 93 (Suppl):25.
72. Johnson WC. Pathology of cutaneous vascular tumors. Int J Dermatol 1976;15:239.

73. Bean WB, Walsh JR. Venous lakes. Arch Dermatol 1956;74:459.
74. Alcalay J, Sandbank M. The ultrastructure of cutaneous venous lakes. Int J Dermatol 1987;26:645.
75. Edgerton MT, Hiebert JM. Vascular and lymphatic tumors in infancy, childhood and adulthood: Challenge of diagnosis and treatment. Curr Probl Cancer 1978;2:4.
76. Coffin CM, Dehner LP. Vascular tumors in children and adolescents: A clinicopathologic study of 228 tumors in 222 patients. Pathol Annu 1993;28:97.
77. Esterly NB. Kasabach-Merritt syndrome in infants. J Am Acad Dermatol 1983;8:504.
78. Perrone T. Vessel-nerve intermingling in benign infantile hemangioendothelioma. Hum Pathol 1985;16:198.
79. Calonje E, Mentzel T, Fletcher CDM. Pseudosarcomatous neural invasion in capillary hemangiomas. Histopathology 1995;26:159.
80. Taxy JB, Gray SR. Cellular angiomas of infancy: An ultrastructural study of two cases. Cancer 1979;43:2322.
81. Gonzales-Crussi F, Reyes-Mugica M. Cellular hemangiomas ("hemangioendotheliomas") in infants: Light microscopic, immunohistochemical and ultrastructural observations. Am J Surg Pathol 1991;15:769.
82. Smoller BR, Apfelberg DB. Infantile (juvenile) capillary hemangioma: A tumor of heterogeneous cellular elements. J Cutan Pathol 1993;20:330.
83. Schnyder UW, Keller R. Zur klinik und histologie der angiome: III. Mitteilung. Zur histologie und pathogenese der senilen angiome. Arch Dermatol Syph (Berlin) 1954;198:333.
84. Salamon T, Lazovic O, Milicecic M. Uber einige histologische befunde bei dem sogenannten angioma senile. Dermatol Monatsschr 1973;159:1021.
85. Cho KH, Kim SH, Park KC et al. Angioblastoma (Nakagawa): Is it the same as tufted angioma? Clin Exp Dermatol 1991;16:110.
86. Kimura S. Ultrastructure of so-called angioblastoma of the skin before and after soft x-ray therapy. J Dermatol 1981;8:235.
87. Wilson Jones E, Orkin M. Tufted angioma (angioblastoma): A benign progressive angioma, not to be confused with Kaposi's sarcoma or low-grade angiosarcoma. J Am Acad Dermatol 1989;20:214.
88. Alessi E, Bertoni E, Sala F. Acquired tufted angioma. Am J Dermatopathol 1986;8:426.
89. Kim YK, Kim HJ, Lee KG. Acquired tufted angioma associated with pregnancy. Clin Exp Dermatol 1992;17:458.
90. Heagerty AHM, Rubin A, Robinson TWE. Familial tufted angioma. Clin Exp Dermatol 1992;17:344.
91. Chu P, LeBoit PE. An eruptive vascular proliferation resembling acquired tufted angioma in the recipient of a liver transplant. J Am Acad Dermatol 1992;26:322.
92. Lam WY, Lai Mac-Moune F, Look CN et al. Tufted angioma with complete regression. J Cutan Pathol 1994;21:461.
93. Padilla RS, Orkin M, Rosai J. Acquired "tufted" angioma (progressive capillary hemangioma). Am J Dermatopathol 1987;9:292.
94. Kumakiri M, Muramoto F, Tsukniaga I. Crystalline lamellae in the endothelial cells of a type of hemangioma characterized by the proliferation of immature endothelial cells and pericytes: Angioblastoma (Nakagawa). J Am Acad Dermatol 1983;8:68.
95. Calonje E, Fletcher CDM. Sinusoidal hemangioma: A distinctive benign vascular neoplasm within the group of cavernous hemangiomas. Am J Surg Pathol 1991;15:1130.
96. Cruces MJ, De La Torre C. Multiple eruptive verrucous hemangiomas: A variant of multiple hemangiomatosis. Dermatologica 1985; 171:106.
97. Imperial R, Helwig EB. Verrucous hemangioma. Arch Dermatol 1967;96:247.
98. Chan JKC, Tsang WYW, Calonje E et al. Verrucous hemangioma: A distinct but neglected variant of cutaneous hemangioma. Intl J Surg Pathol 1995;2:171.
99. Jessen RT, Thompson S, Smith EB. Cobb syndrome. Arch Dermatol 1977;113:1587.
100. Hunt SJ, Santa Cruz DJ, Barr RJ. Microvenular hemangioma. J Cutan Pathol 1991;18:235.
101. Aloi F, Tomasini C, Pippione M. Microvenular hemangioma. Am J Dermatopathol 1993;15:534.
102. Satge D, Grande-Goburdhun J, Grosshans E. Hemangiome microcapillaire. Ann Dermatol Venereol 1993;120:297.
103. Santa Cruz DJ, Aronberg J. Targetoid hemosiderotic hemangioma. J Am Acad Dermatol 1988;19:550.
104. Rapini RP, Golitz LE. Targetoid hemosiderotic hemangioma. J Cutan Pathol 1990;17:233.
105. Ho C, McCalmont TH. Targetoid hemosiderotic hemangioma: Report of 24 cases, with emphasis on unusual features and comparison to early Kaposi's sarcoma (abstr). J Cutan Pathol 1995;22:67.
106. Calonje E, Fletcher CDM, Wilson Jones E et al. Retiform hemangioendothelioma: A distinctive form of low-grade angiosarcoma delineated in a series of 15 cases. Am J Surg Pathol 1994;18:115.
107. Connelly MG, Winkelmann RK. Acral arteriovenous tumor: A clinicopathologic review. Am J Surg Pathol 1985;9:15.
108. Girard C, Graham JH, Johnson WC. Arteriovenous hemangioma (arteriovenous shunt). J Cutan Pathol 1974;1:73.
109. Koutlas IG, Jessurun J. Arteriovenous hemangioma: A clinicopathological and immunohistochemical study. J Cutan Pathol 1994;21: 343.
110. Howat AJ, Campbell PE. Angiomatosis: A vascular malformation of infancy and childhood. Report of 17 cases. Pathology 1987;19:377.
111. Rao VK, Weiss SW. Angiomatosis of soft tissue: An analysis of the histologic features and clinical outcome in 51 cases. Am J Surg Pathol 1992;16:764.
112. Weiss SW, Enzinger FM. Spindle cell hemangioendothelioma: A low-grade angiosarcoma resembling cavernous hemangioma and Kaposi's sarcoma. Am J Surg Pathol 1986;10:521.
113. Ono CM, Mitsunaga MM, Lockett LJ. Intragluteal spindle cell hemangioendothelioma: An unusual presentation of a recently described vascular neoplasm. Clin Orthop 1992;281:224.
114. Fletcher CDM, Beham A, Schmid C. Spindle cell haemangioendothelioma: A clinicopathological and immunohistochemical study indicative of a non-neoplastic lesion. Histopathology 1991;18:291.
115. Scott GA, Rosai J. Spindle cell hemangioendothelioma: Report of seven additional cases of a recently described vascular neoplasm. Am J Dermatopathol 1988;10:281.
116. Zoltie N, Roberts PF. Spindle cell haemangioendothelioma in association with epithelioid haemangioendothelioma. Histopathology1989; 15:544.
117. Azadeh B, Attallah MF, Ejeckam GC. Spindle cell hemangioendothelioma in association with epithelioid hemangioendothelioma. Cutis 1994;53:134.
118. Ding J, Hashimoto H, Imayama S et al. Spindle cell hemangioendothelioma: Probably a benign vascular lesion not a low-grade angiosarcoma. A clinicopathological, ultrastructural and immunohistochemical study. Virchows Arch A 1992;420:77.
119. Perkins P, Weiss SW. Spindle cell hemangioendothelioma: A clinicopathologic study of 78 cases. Mod Pathol 1994;7:9A.
120. Imayama S, Murakamai Y, Hashimoto H et al. Spindle cell hemangioendothelioma exhibits the ultrastructural features of reactive vascular proliferation rather than of angiosarcoma. Am J Clin Pathol 1992;97:279.
121. Beral V, Peterman TA, Berkelman R et al. Kaposi's sarcoma among persons with AIDS: A sexually transmitted infection. Lancet 1990; 335:123.
122. Dorfmann RF. Kaposi's sarcoma with special reference to its manifestations in infants and children and to the concepts of Arthur Purdy Stout. Am J Surg Pathol 1986;10(Suppl):68.
123. Friedman-Kien AE, Saltzman BR. Clinical manifestations of classical, endemic African, and epidemic AIDS-associated Kaposi's sarcoma. J Am Acad Dermatol 1990;22:1237.
124. Tappero JW, Conant MA, Wolfe SF et al. Kaposi's sarcoma: Epidemiology, pathogenesis, histology, clinical spectrum, staging criteria and therapy. J Am Acad Dermatol 1993;28:371.
125. Wolff K. The enigma of Kaposi's sarcoma: An answer at last? Clin Exp Dermatol 1992;17:146.
126. Gottlieb GJ, Ackerman AB. Kaposi's sarcoma: An extensively disseminated form in young homosexual men. Hum Pathol 1982;13:882.
127. Roth WK. HIV-associated Kaposi's sarcoma: New developments in epidemiology and molecular pathology. J Cancer Res Clin Oncol 1991;117:186.
128. Casabona J, Melbye M, Biggar RJ et al. Kaposi's sarcoma and non-Hodgkin's lymphoma in European AIDS cases: No excess risk of Kaposi's sarcoma in Mediterranean countries. Int J Cancer 1991;47:49.
129. Lee WA, Hutckins GM. Cluster analysis of the metastatic patterns of human immunodeficiency virus-associated Kaposi's sarcoma. Hum Pathol 1992;23:306.
130. Lemlich G, Scham L, Lebwokl M. Kaposi's sarcoma and acquired im-

munodeficiency syndrome: Postmortem findings in twenty-four cases. J Am Acad Dermatol 1987;16:319.
131. McKenzie R, Travis WD, Dolan SA et al. The causes of death in patients with human immunodeficiency virus infection: A clinical and pathologic study with emphasis on the role of pulmonary diseases. Medicine (Baltimore) 1991;70:326.
132. Moskowitz LB, Hensley GT, Gould EW. Frequency and anatomic distribution of lymphadenopathic Kaposi's sarcoma in the acquired immunodeficiency syndrome: An autopsy series. Hum Pathol 1985;16: 447.
133. Montagnimo G, Bencini PL, Tarantino A et al. Clinical features and course of Kaposi's sarcoma in kidney transplant patients: Report of 13 cases. Am J Nephrol 1994;14:121.
134. Blumenfield W, Egbert BM, Sagebiel RW. Differential diagnosis of Kaposi's sarcoma. Arch Pathol Lab Med 1985;109:123.
135. Chor PJ, Santa Cruz DJ. Kaposi's sarcoma: A clinicopathologic review and differential diagnosis. J Cutan Pathol 1992;19:6.
136. Gange RW, Wilson Jones E. Lymphangioma-like Kaposi's sarcoma: A report of three cases. Br J Dermatol 1979;100:327.
137. Facchetti F, Lucini L, Gavazzoni R et al. Immunomorphological analysis of the role of blood vessel endothelium in the morphogenesis of cutaneous Kaposi's sarcoma: A study of 57 cases. Histopathology 1988;12:581.
138. Kao GF, Johnson FB, Sulica VI. The nature of hyaline (eosinophilic) globules and vascular slits of Kaposi's sarcoma. Am J Dermatopathol 1990;12:256.
139. Orchard GE, Wilson Jones E, Russel Jones R. Immunocytochemistry in the diagnosis of Kaposi's sarcoma and angiosarcoma. Br J Biomed Sci 1995;52:35.
140. Niedt GW, Myskowski PL, Urmacher C. Histologic predictors of survival in acquired immunodeficiency syndrome-associated Kaposi's sarcoma. Hum Pathol 1992;23:1419.
141. Zukerberg LR, Nickoloff BJ, Weiss SW. Kaposiform hemangioendothelioma of infancy and childhood: An aggressive neoplasm associated with Kasabach-Merritt syndrome and lymphangiomatosis. Am J Surg Pathol 1993;17:321.
142. Lam WY, Lai FMM, To KF et al. Cutaneous lesions of kaposiform hemangioendothelioma: Report of two cases. Int J Surg Pathol 1995; 2(Suppl):521.
143. Calonje E, Fletcher CDM. Aneurysmal benign fibrous histiocytoma: Clinicopathological analysis of 40 cases of a tumour frequently misdiagnosed as a vascular neoplasm. Histopathology 1995;26:323.
144. Del-Rio E, Aguilar A, Ambrojo P et al. Pseudo-Kaposi's sarcoma induced by minor trauma in a patient with Klippel-Trenaunay-Weber syndrome. Clin Exp Dermatol 1993;18:151.
145. Strutton G, Weedon D. Acro-angiodermatitis: A simulant of Kaposi's sarcoma. Am J Dermatopathol 1987;9:85.
146. Wilson Jones E, Cerio R, Smith NP. Multinucleate cell angiohistiocytoma: An acquired vascular anomaly to be distinguished from Kaposi's sarcoma. Br J Dermatol 1990;122:651.
147. Smolle J, Auboeck L, Gogg-Retzer I et al. Multinucleate cell angiohistiocytoma: A clinicopathological, immunohistochemical and ultrastructural study. Br J Dermatol 1989;121:113.
148. Brooks JJ. Kaposi's sarcoma: A reversible hyperplasia. Lancet 1986; 2:1309.
149. Ioachim HL, Dorsett B, Melamed J et al. Cytomegalovirus, angiomatosis, and Kaposi's sarcoma: New observations of a debated relationship. Mod Pathol 1992;5:169.
150. Nickoloff BJ. PECAM-1(CD31) is expressed on proliferating endothelial cells, stromal-shaped cells, and dermal dendrocytes in Kaposi's sarcoma. Arch Dermatol 1993;129:250.
151. Nickoloff BJ. The human progenitor cell antigen (CD34) is localized on endothelial cells, dermal dendritic cells, and perifollicular cells in formalin-fixed normal skin, and on proliferating endothelial cells and stromal spindle-shaped cells in Kaposi's sarcoma. Arch Dermatol 1991;127:523.
152. Regezi JA, MacPhail LA, Daniels TE et al. Human immunodeficiency virus-associated oral Kaposi's sarcoma: A heterogeneous cell population dominated by spindle-shaped endothelial cells. Am J Pathol 1993; 143:240.
153. Gray MH, Trimble CL, Zirn J. Relationship of Factor XIIIa-positive dermal dendrocytes to Kaposi's sarcoma. Arch Pathol Lab Med 1991; 115:791.
154. Beckstead JH, Wood GS, Fletcher V. Evidence for the origin of Kaposi's sarcoma from lymphatic endothelium. Am J Pathol 1985; 119:294.
155. Russel Jones R, Spaull J, Wilson Jones E. Histogenesis of Kaposi's sarcoma in patients with and without acquired immune deficiency syndrome (AIDS). J Clin Pathol 1986;39:742.
156. Rutgers JL, Wieczoreck R, Bonetti F et al. The expression of endothelial cell surface antigens by AIDS-associated Kaposi's sarcoma. Am J Pathol 1986;122:493.
157. Scully PA, Steinman HK, Kennedy C et al. AIDS-related Kaposi's sarcoma displays differential expression of endothelial surface antigens. Am J Pathol 1988;130:244.
158. Dictor M, Andersson C. Lymphaticovenous differentiation in Kaposi's sarcoma: Cellular phenotypes by stage. Am J Pathol 1988;130: 411.
159. Chang Y, Cesarman E, Pessin MS. Identification of herpesvirus-like DNA sequences in AIDS-associated Kaposi's sarcoma. Science 1994; 266:1865.
160. Huang YQ, Li JJ, Kaplan MH et al. Human herpesvirus-like nucleic acid in various forms of Kaposi's sarcoma. Lancet 1995;345:759.
161. Dupin N, Grandadam M, Calvez V et al. Herpesvirus-like DNA sequences in patients with Mediterranean Kaposi's sarcoma. Lancet 1995;345:761.
162. Levy JA. A new human herpesvirus KSHV or HHV8? Lancet 1995; 346:786.
163. Weiss SW, Enzinger FM. Epithelioid hemangioendothelioma: A vascular lesion often mistaken for a carcinoma. Cancer 1982;50:970.
164. Weiss SW, Ishak KG, Dail DH et al. Epithelioid hemangioendothelioma and related lesions. Semin Diagn Pathol 1986;3:259.
165. Tyring S, Guest P, Lee P et al. Epithelioid hemangioendothelioma of the skin and femur. J Am Acad Dermatol 1989;20:362.
166. Malane SL, Sau P, Benson PM. Epithelioid hemangioendothelioma associated with reflex sympathetic dystrophy. J Am Acad Dermatol 1992;26:325.
167. Resnik KS, Kantor GR, Spielvogel RL et al. Cutaneous epithelioid hemangioendothelioma without systemic involvement. Am J Dermatopathol 1993;15:272.
168. Suster S, Moran CA, Koss MN. Epithelioid hemangioendothelioma of the anterior mediastinum: Clinicopathologic, immunohistochemical, and ultrastructural analysis of 12 cases. Am J Surg Pathol 1994;18: 871.
169. Gray MF, Rosenberg AE, Dickersin GR, et al. Cytokeratin expression in epithelioid vascular neoplasms. Hum Pathol 1990;21:211.
170. Dabska M. Malignant endovascular papillary angioendothelioma of the skin in childhood: Clinicopathologic study of 6 cases. Cancer 1969;24:503.
171. Manivel JC, Wick MR, Swanson PE et al. Endovascular papillary angioendothelioma of childhood: A vascular lesion possibly characterized by "high" endothelial cell diferentiation. Hum Pathol 1986;17: 1240.
172. Tsang WYW, Chan JCK. Kaposi-like infantile hemangioendothelioma: A distinctive vascular neoplasm of the retroperitoneum. Am J Surg Pathol 1991;15:982.
173. Tsang WYW, Chan JCK, Fletcher CDM. Recently characterized vascular tumors of skin and soft tissues. Histopathology 1991;19:489.
174. Calixto MMP, Pacheco FA. Angiosarcoma of the leg in a patient with chronic osteomyelitis. Skin Cancer 1986;1:77.
175. Fletcher CDM, Beham A, Bekir S et al. Epithelioid angiosarcoma of deep soft tissue: A distinctive tumor readily mistaken for an epithelial neoplasm. Am J Surg Pathol 1991;15:915.
176. Gloor M, Adler D, Bersch A et al. Hamangiosarkom in einem naevus telangiectaticus lateralis. Hautarzt 1983;34:182.
177. Nagata M, Semba I, Ooya K et al. Malignant endothelial neoplasm arising in the area of lymphangioma: Immunohistochemical and ultrastructural observation. J Oral Pathol 1984;13:560.
178. Chadhuri B, Ronan SG, Manahgod JR. Angiosarcoma arising in a plexiform neurofibroma. Cancer 1980;46:605.
179. Brown RW, Tornos C, Evans HL. Angiosarcoma arising from malignant Schwannoma in a patient with neurofibromatosis. Cancer 1992; 70:1141.
180. Leake J, Sheehan MP, Rampling D et al. Angiosarcoma complicating xeroderma pigmentosum. Histopathology 1992;21:179.
181. Holden CA, Spittle MF, Wilson Jones E. Angiosarcoma of the face and scalp: prognosis and treatment. Cancer 1987;59:1046.
182. Mark RJ, Tron LM, Sercarz J et al. Angiosarcoma of the head and

neck: The UCLA experience 1955 through 1990. Arch Otolaryngol Head Neck Surg 1993;119:973.
183. Wilson Jones E. Malignant vascular tumours. Clin Exp Dermatol 1976;1:287.
184. Haustein U-F. Angiosarcoma of the face and scalp. Int J Dermatol 1991;30:851.
185. Matsumoto K, Inoue K, Fukamizu H et al. Prognosis of cutaneous angiosarcoma in Japan: A statistical study of sixty-nine cases. Chir Plastica 1986;8:151.
186. Maddox JC, Evans HL. Angiosarcoma of the skin and soft tissue: A study of forty-four cases. Cancer 1981;48:1907.
187. Woodward AH, Ivins JC, Soule EH Jr. Lymphangiosarcoma arising in chronic lymphedematous extremities. Cancer 1972;20:562.
188. Alessi E, Sala F, Berti E. Angiosarcomas in lymphedematous limbs. Am J Dermatopathol 1986;8:371.
189. Chen KTK, Bauer V, Flam MS. Angiosarcoma in postsurgical lymphedema: An unusual occurrence in a man. Am J Dermatopathol 1991;13:488.
190. Hultberg BM. Angiosarcomas in chronically lymphedematous extremities: Two cases of Stewart-Treves syndrome. Am J Dermatopathol 1987;9:406.
191. Offori TW, Platt CC, Stephens M et al. Angiosarcoma in congenital hereditary lymphedema (Milroy's disease): Diagnostic beacons and a review of the literature. Clin Exp Dermatol 1993;18:174.
192. Muller R, Hajdu SI, Brennan MF. Lymphangiosarcoma associated with chronically lymphedematous extremities: Two cases of Stewart-Treves syndrome. Cancer 1987;59:179.
193. Drachman D, Rosen L, Sharaf D et al. Postmastectomy low-grade angiosarcoma: An unusual case resembling a lymphangioma circumscriptum. Am J Dermatopathol 1988;10:247.
194. Davies JD, Rees GJG, Mera SL. Angiosarcoma in irradiated post-mastectomy chest wall. Histopathology 1983;7:947.
195. Edeiken S, Russo DP, Knecht J et al. Angiosarcoma after tylectomy and radiation therapy for carcinoma of the breast. Cancer 1992;70:644.
196. Moskaluk CA, Merino MJ, Danforth DN et al. Low-grade angiosarcoma of the skin of the breast: A complication of lumpectomy and radiation therapy for breast carcinoma. Hum Pathol 1992;23:710.
197. Goette DK, Detlefs RL. Postirradiation angiosarcoma. J Am Acad Dermatol 1985;12:922.
198. Laaff H, Vibrans U. Cutaneous angiosarcoma after telecobalt irradiation. Hautarzt 1992;43:654.
199. Rosai J, Summer HW, Major MC et al. Angiosarcoma of the skin: A clinicopathologic and fine structural study. Hum Pathol 1976;7:83.
200. Matejka M, Konrad K. Cutaneous angiosarcoma of the face and scalp. Clin Exp Dermatol 1984;9:232.
201. Banerjee SS, Eyden BP, Wells S et al. Pseudoangiosarcomatous carcinoma: A clinicopathological study of seven cases. Histopathology 1992;21:13.
202. Nappi O, Wick MR, Pettinato G et al. Pseudovascular adenoid squamous cell carcinoma of the skin: A neoplasm that may be mistaken for angiosarcoma. Am J Surg Pathol 1992;16:429.
203. McGrath JA, Schofield OM, Mayou BJ et al. Metastatic squamous cell carcinoma resembling angiosarcoma complicating dystrophic epidermolysis bullosa. Dermatologica 1991;182:235.
204. Prescott RJ, Banerjee SS, Eyden BP et al. Cutaneous epithelioid angiosarcoma: A clinicopathological study of four cases. Histopathology 1994;25:421.
205. Marrogi AJ, Hunt SJ, Santa Cruz DJ. Cutaneous epithelioid angiosarcoma. Am J Dermatopathol 1990;12:350.
206. Byers RJ, McMahon RFT, Freemont AJ et al. Epithelioid angiosarcoma arising in an arteriovenous fistula. Histopathology 1992;21:87.
207. Jennings TA, Peterson L, Axiotis CA et al. Angiosarcoma associated with foreign body material. Cancer 1988;62:2436.
208. Watson WL, McCarthy WB. Blood and lymph vessel tumors: A report of 1056 cases. Surg Gynecol Obstet 1940;71:569.
209. Peachey RDG, Lim CC, Whimster IW. Lymphangioma of the skin. Br J Dermatol 1970;83:519.
210. Wilson Jones E, Winkelmann RK, Zacharay CB et al. Benign lymphangioendothelioma. J Am Acad Dermatol 1990;23:229.
211. Prioleav PG, Santa Cruz DJ. Lymphangioma circumscription following radical mastectomy and radiation therapy. Cancer 1978;42:1989.
212. Zadvinskis DP, Benson MT, Kerr HH et al. Congenital malformations of the cervicothoracic lymphatic system: Embriology and pathogenesis. Radiographics 1992;12:1175.
213. Burgdorf WHC, Mukai K, Rosai J. Immunohistochemical identification of factor VIII-related antigen in endothelial cells of cutaneous lesions of alleged vascular nature. Am J Clin Pathol 1981;75:167.
214. Pearson JM, McWilliam LJ. A light microscopical, immunohistochemical, and ultrastructural comparison of hemangiomata and lymphangiomata. Ultrastruct Pathol 1990;14:497.
215. Harkins GA, Sabiston DC. Lymphangioma in infancy and childhood. Surgery 1960;47:811.
216. Chervenak FA, Isaacson G, Blakemore KJ et al. Fetal cystic hygroma: Cause and natural history. N Engl J Med 1983;309:822.
217. Flanagan BP, Helwig EB. Cutaneous lymphangioma. Arch Dermatol 1977;113:24.
218. Herron GS, Rouse RV, Kosek JC et al. Benign lymphangioendothelioma. J Am Acad Dermatol 1994;31:362.
219. Mehregan DR, Mehregan AH, Mehregan DA. Benign lymphangioendothelioma: Report of 2 cases. J Cutan Pathol 1992;19:502.
220. Ramani P, Shah A. Lymphangiomatosis: Histologic and immunohistochemical analysis of four cases. Am J Surg Pathol 1993;17:329.
221. Singh Gomez C, Calonje E, Ferrar DW et al. Lymphangiomatosis of the limbs: Clinicopathologic analysis of a series. Am J Surg Pathol 1995;19:125.
222. Tsuneyoshi M, Enjoji M. Glomus tumor: A clinicopathologic and electron microscopic study. Cancer 1982;50:1601.
223. Tran LP, Velanovich V, Kaufmann CR. Familial multiple glomus tumors: Report of a pedigree and literature review. Ann Plast Surg 1994;32:89.
224. Gould EW, Manivel JC, Albores-Saavedra J et al. Locally infiltrative glomus tumors and glomangiosarcoma: A clinical, ultrastructural and immunohistochemical study. Cancer 1990;65:310.
225. Beham A, Fletcher CDM. Intravascular glomus tumor: A previously undescribed phenomenon. Virchows Arch (A) 1991;418:175.
226. Googe PB, Griffin WC. Intravenous glomus tumor of the forearm. J Cutan Pathol 1993;20:359.
227. Calonje E, Fletcher CDM. Cutaneous intraneural glomus tumor: Report of a case. Am J Dermatopathol 1995;15:395.
228. Slater DN, Cotton DWK, Azzopardi JG. Oncocytic glomus tumor: A new variant. Histopathology 1987;11:523.
229. Aiba M, Hirayama A, Kuramochi S. Glomangiosarcoma in a glomus tumor. Cancer 1988;61:1467.
230. Dervan PA, Tobbin IN, Casey M et al. Glomus tumour: An immunohistochemical profile of 11 cases. Histopathology 1989;14:483.
231. Porter PL, Bigler SA, McNutt M et al. The immunophenotype of hemangiopericytomas and glomus tumors with special reference to muscle protein expression: An immunohistochemical study and review of the literature. Mod Pathol 1991;4:46.
232. Kaye VM, Dehner LP. Cutaneous glomus tumor: A comparative immunohistochemical study with pseudoangiomatous intradermal melanocytic nevi. Am J Dermatopathol 1991;13:2.
233. Enzinger FM, Smith BH. Hemangiopericytoma: An analysis of 106 cases. Hum Pathol 1976;7:61.
234. Coffin CM, Dehner LP. Fibroblastic-myofibroblastic tumors in children and adolescents: A clinicopathologic study of 108 examples in 103 patients. Pediatr Pathol 1991;11:569.
235. Mentzel T, Calonje E, Nascimiento AG, Fletcher CDM. Infantile hemangiopericytoma versus infantile myofibromatosis: A study of a series suggesting a spectrum of infantile myofibroblastic lesions. Am J Surg Pathol 1994;18:922.
236. McMaster MJ, Soule EH, Ivins JC. Hemangiopericytoma: A clinicopathologic study and long-term follow-up of 60 patients. Cancer 1975; 36:2232.
237. Battifora H. Hemangiopericytoma: Ultrastructural study of five cases. Cancer 1973;31:1418.
238. Hahn MJ, Dawson R, Esterly JA et al. Hemangiopericytoma: An ultrastructural study. Cancer 1973;31:255.
239. Nunnery EW, Kahn LB, Reddick RL et al. Hemangiopericytoma: A light microscopic and ultrastructural study. Cancer 1981;47:906.
240. Schurch W, Skalli O, Lagace R et al. Intermediate filament proteins and actin isoforms as markers of soft tissue tumor differentiation and origin: III. Hemangiopericytomas and glomus tumors. Am J Pathol 1990;136:771.
241. Dardick I, Hammar SP, Scheithauer BW. Ultrastructural spectrum of hemangiopericytoma: A comparative study of fetal, adult, and neoplastic pericytes. Ultrastruct Pathol 1989;13:111.
242. Fletcher CDM. Haemangiopericytoma: A dying breed? Reappraisal of an entity and its variants. Curr Diagn Pathol 1994;1:19.

Lever's Histopathology of the Skin, eighth edition,
edited by David Elder et al. Lippincott–
Raven Publishers, Philadelphia © 1997.

CHAPTER 35

Tumors of Fatty, Muscular, and Osseous Tissue

Fat as a Tissue, an Organ, and a Source of Tumors

Bruce D. Ragsdale

THE BASIC SCIENCE OF FAT RELEVANT TO TUMORS

Adipose tissue can be divided into two types, brown and white. In adult humans, most fat is of the white, univesicular variety. White fat serves as the depot for stored lipid, which is an efficient energy reserve, and protects against external trauma.

The red-brown to tan color of brown adipose tissue results from cytochrome pigment in the numerous mitochondria of its cells. Brown fat has been considered an immature or fetal stage in the development of white fat, but most evidence now substantiates the unique identity of brown fat and its role in basal metabolism and thermoregulation. In humans, brown fat is more prevalent in the newborn period than later in life, but it persists throughout adulthood in the neck, axilla, and mediastinum, as well as elsewhere, embedded within the common white fat.[1]

Most investigators agree that perivascular cells resembling pericytes and fibroblasts play an important transition role in the development of benign and malignant lipoblasts. Both white and brown fat cells modulate from these primitive fat organ precursors through multivesicular stages easily mistaken for histiocytes, to preadipocytes in which lipid inclusions coalesce and glycogen decreases, and finally to univacuolar adipocytes (Fig. 35-1).[2] The multivacuolar stage is observed in various tumors and is likely to reappear with involution following injury. In these settings, the cells with foamy cytoplasm are commonly mistaken for histiocytes—e.g., the CD68-negative foam cells in subcutis following biopsy. This is the source of much nosologic confusion, particularly with regard to some of the lesions popularly regarded as "histiocytomas."[3]

Fatty tumors of dermatologic interest are common and are generally situated in subcutaneous position.[4]

B. D. Ragsdale: Department of Dermatology, University of Alabama, Birmingham, AL; Central Coast Pathology Consultants, San Luis Obispo, CA

NEVUS LIPOMATOSUS SUPERFICIALIS

Nevus lipomatosus superficialis is a fairly uncommon lesion showing groups of soft, flattened papules or nodules that have smooth or wrinkled surfaces and are skin-colored or pale yellow. Characteristically, the lesions are linearly distributed on one hip or buttock (nevus lipomatosus superficialis of Hoffman and Zurhelle) (Fig. 35-2),[5] from where they may overlap onto the adjacent skin of the back or the upper thigh.[6] Other areas, such as the thorax or the abdomen, are only rarely affected. The lesions may be present at birth or may begin in infancy (nevus angiolipomatosus of Howell),[7] in which case the replacement of hypoplastic dermis may cause pseudotumorous yellow protrusions and be associated with skeletal and other malformations, but they develop most commonly during the first two decades of life and occasionally later. Multiple lesions may coalesce.

Solitary lesions have been diagnosed as nevus lipomatosus superficialis,[6] but it seems preferable to regard them instead as solitary, baglike, soft fibromas[5] (Chap. 33) or polypoid fibrolipomas. The rather common presence of fat cells within long-standing intradermal melanocytic nevi represents an involutionary phenomenon rather than an association of a nevus lipomatosus with a melanocytic nevus[8] (Chap. 29).

Histopathology. Groups and strands of fat cells are found embedded among the collagen bundles of the dermis, often as high as the papillary dermis (Fig. 35-2B). The proportion of fatty tissue varies greatly, from more than 50% of the dermis to less than 10%. In cases with only small deposits, the fat cells are apt to be situated in small foci around the subpapillary vessels. In instances with relatively large amounts of fat, the fat lobules are irregularly distributed throughout the dermis, and the boundary between the dermis and the hypoderm is ill-defined or lost. The fat cells may all be mature, but in some instances an occasional small, incompletely lipidized cell may be observed.[6]

Aside from the presence of fat cells, the dermis may be entirely normal, but in some instances the density of the collagen bundles, the number of fibroblasts, and the vascularity are greater than in normal skin.[5]

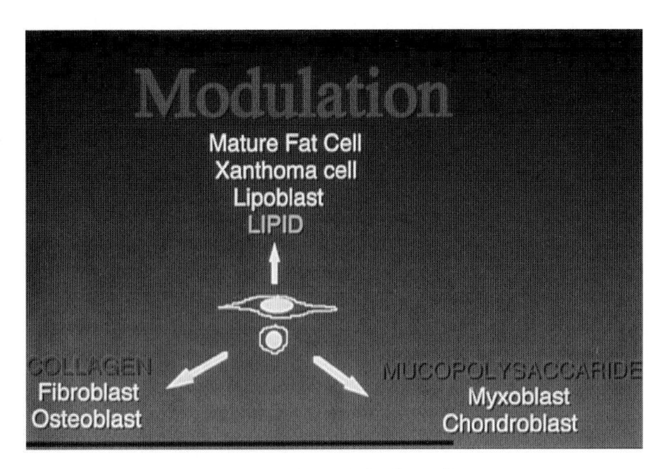

FIG. 35-1. Mesenchymal modulation diagram
Uncommitted mesenchyme is the product of differentiation. Further adoption of specific function and corresponding cell structure can be distinguished as modulation. Matrix products can be collagen-dominant (fibrous or osseous) or mucopolysaccharide-dominant (chondroid or myxoid). A signet-ring fat cell represents the end product of storage of cytoplasmic fat that begins as multiple small vacuoles. The structure and function of some fully modulated mesenchymal cells can change with altered systemic or local influences in the realms of metabolic, mechanical (e.g., trauma, friction), and/or circulatory (increased arterial flow vs. venous congestion) factors. Initially in this process, regression leads to spindle or round cells that can be easily mistaken for fibroblasts or lymphocytes. This is followed by cytoplasmic reorganization and acquisition, making possible new functions. Also, more than one modulational potential may be seen in mesenchymal tumors as they grow (e.g., Figs. 35-7 and 35-8). (After Lent C. Johnson, AFIP, Washington, DC.)

Pathogenesis. It is generally agreed that nevus lipomatosus represents, as the name implies, a nevoid anomaly. The ectopic fat cells in the dermis are derived from the perivascular mesenchymal tissue.[6] This view has found support in electron microscopic studies of nevus lipomatosus superficialis, which in some instances showed, in the vicinity of capillaries, immature lipocytes containing numerous small lipid droplets and a centrally located nucleus.[9,10]

Differential Diagnosis. In focal dermal hypoplasia, fat cells are also present in the dermis, often in close proximity to the epidermis. However, this disorder differs from nevus lipomatosus by the extreme attenuation of the collagen (Chap. 6).

FOLDED SKIN WITH LIPOMATOUS NEVUS

Newborn babies showing generalized folding of the skin[11–13] have an appearance that has given rise to the term *Michelin-tire baby*. The folding diminishes gradually during childhood.[13]

Histopathology. In some areas, fat lobules extend close to the epidermis, as in nevus lipomatosus superficialis, and surround adnexal structures. In other areas, the dermis is of normal thickness, but excessive amounts of adipose tissue are beneath the dermis and around adnexal structures. Several bands of fibrous tissue penetrate the subcutaneous fat.[11]

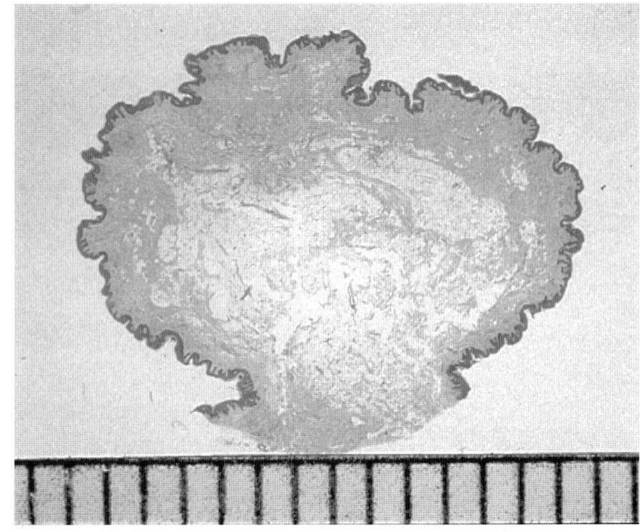

A

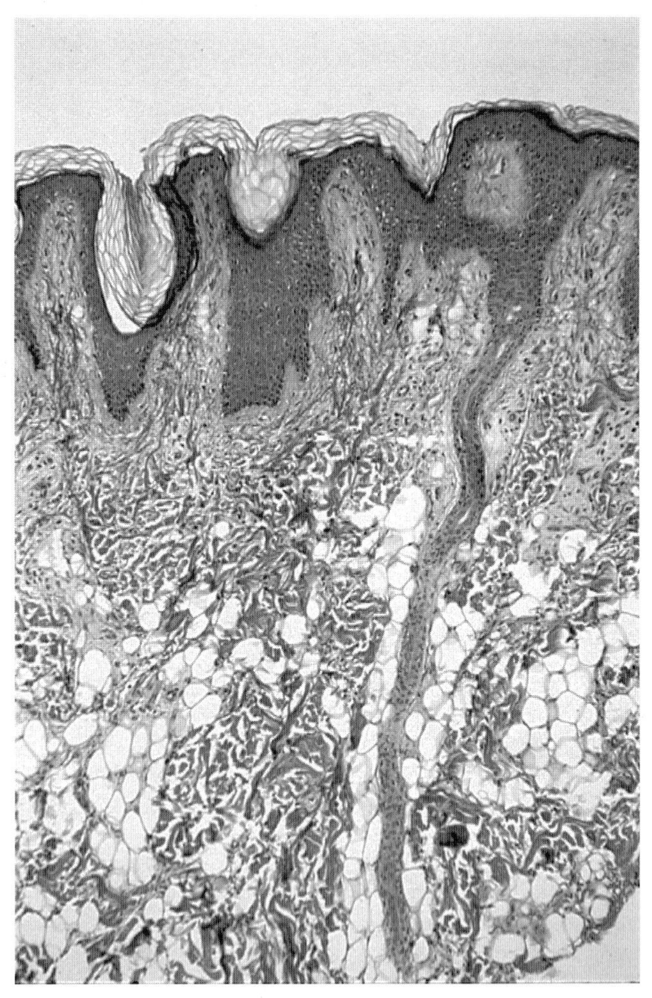

B

FIG. 35-2. Nevus lipomatosus (45-year-old male; 2-cm lesion from buttock)
(**A**) A polypoidal projection of crenated epidermis has a fatty core. (**B**) Mature signet-ring fat cells displace dermal collagen. A sweat gland duct runs vertically through the field.

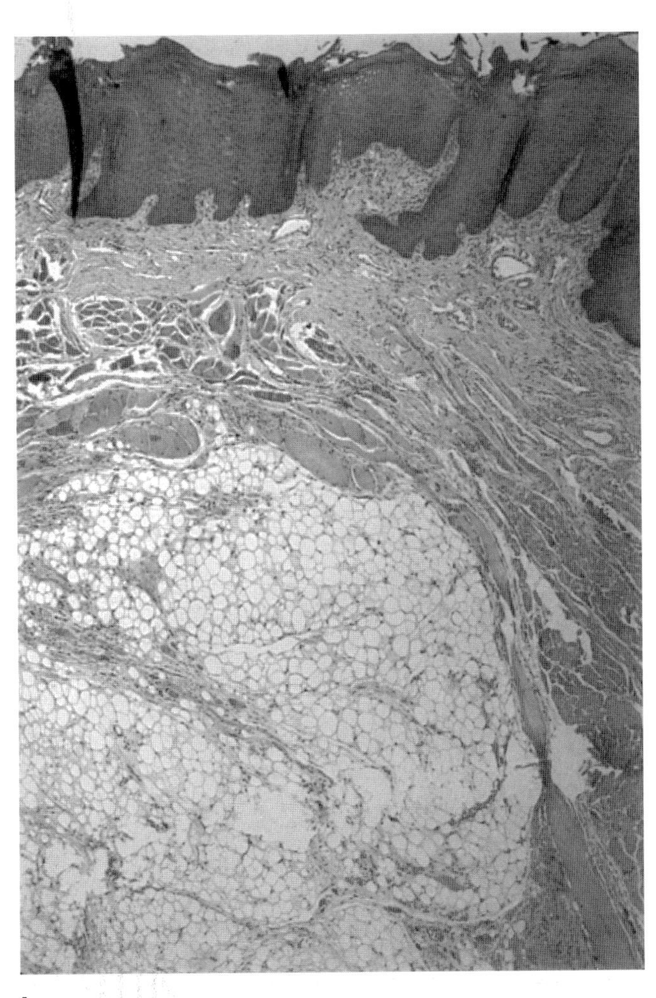

A

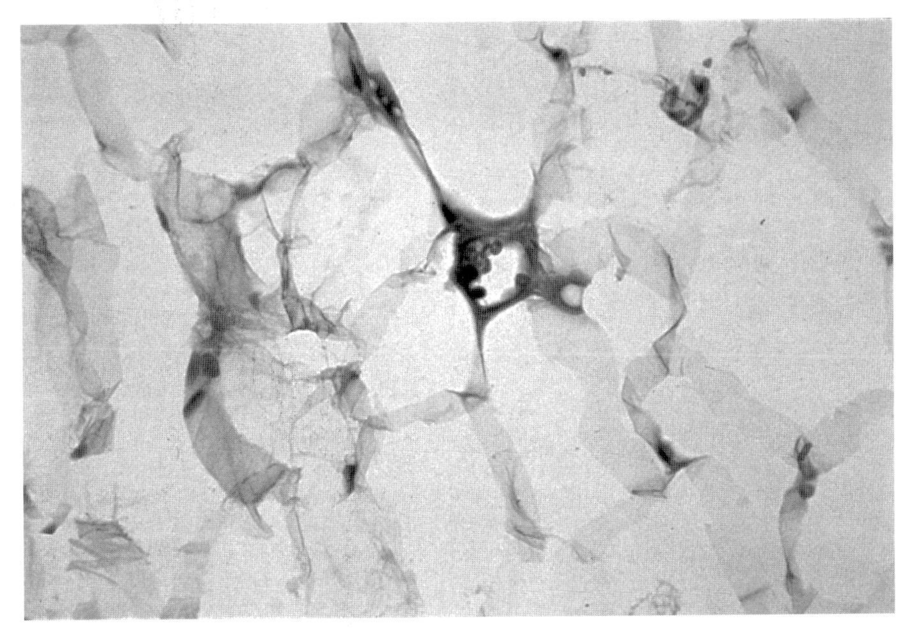

B

FIG. 35-3. Lipoma, tongue (36-year-old male)
(**A**) A lobulated, well-circumscribed collection of mature-appearing signet-ring fat cells occurs within skeletal muscle and connective tissue beneath tongue mucosa. (**B**) The delicate cell membranes of adipocytes create a "chicken-wire" pattern. A nuclear pseudoinclusion (Lochkern), as shown in the nucleus to the right of the central blood vessel, is not to be mistaken for the nucleus of a lipoblast.

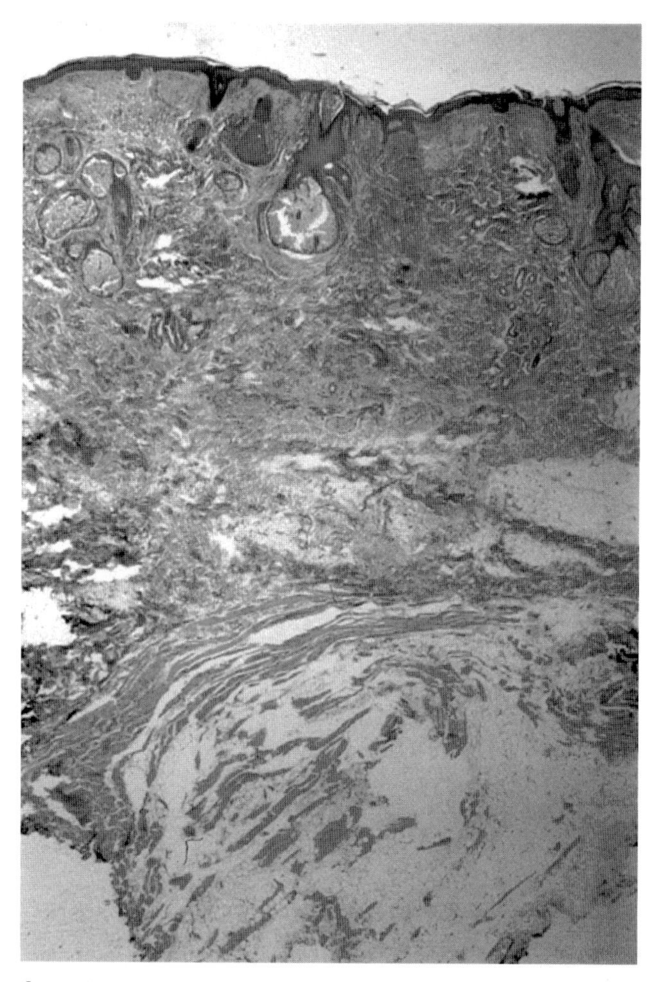

A

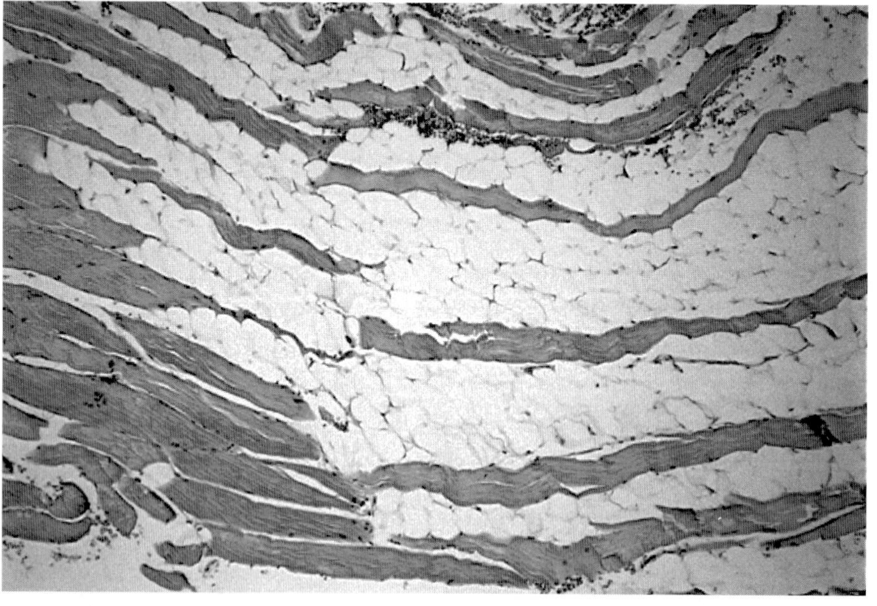

B

FIG. 35-4. Intramuscular (infiltrating) lipoma (adult male with clinically recurrent nodule on forehead) (**A**) Skeletal muscle beneath hair-bearing skin shows separation of myocytes by pale-staining lipoma tissue. (**B**) At higher magnification, signet-ring fat cells with inconspicuous nuclei splay skeletal muscle fibers.

Differential Diagnosis. Folded skin has also been reported overlying smooth muscle hamartoma.[14]

LIPOMAS

Common lipomas consist of mature fat cells throughout (Fig. 35-3) and are the most common neoplasms of mesenchyme. Most lipomas (98%) occur as single or multiple subcutaneous growths that are soft, rounded or lobulated, and movable against the overlying skin. They often grow insidiously, displaying an initial growth phase followed by a period of quiescence. They come to clinical attention only if they reach inordinate size or are perceived as blemishes in need of cosmetic removal. Approximately 6% of all cases are multifocal. The patient commonly presents with an asymptomatic, slowly growing round mass having a gelatinous or cystic consistency. Well-circumscribed lipomas are easily "shelled out" and only rarely reform, generally when initially incompletely encapsulated or infiltrative. Deep-seated variants of ordinary lipomas tend to be less well-circumscribed than their superficial counterparts, often sending out pseudopod-like processes within fascial planes, engulfing aponeuroses, and potentially compressing local structures. Large size, rapid growth, deep location, fixation, pain, and thigh or retroperitoneal location are features that suggest the wisdom of preoperative radiographic characterization and a cautious surgical approach to exclude a more significant lesion.

Some lipomas are characterized by specific clinical presentation and location. *Perineural lipoma* involves the median nerve in 9 out of 10 cases, and may be associated with macrodactyly. *Lumbosacral lipomas* frequently occur in conjunction with spina bifida and intraspinal lipoma. *Lipomas of tendon sheath and joint synovium* are centered on the named structures. *Lipoma arboresens of synovium* is papillomatous with a tendency for repeated regrowth. *Inter- and intramuscular lipomas* infiltrate muscle and tend to recur unless completely excised.[15] *Myolipomas of soft tissue* are rarely subcutaneous.[16] *Angiomyolipomas* are best known in the kidney. *Cutaneous angiomyolipoma* is rare, occurs in men of mean age 53 years, and presents as a single, painless, subcutaneous nodule on an extremity.[17] Here they are independent of tuberous sclerosis, as of pulmonary lymphangiomyomatosis that can accompany the renal lesion. The *adenolipoma* is a dermal or subcutaneous variant of the common lipoma that does not deviate appreciably in presentation or gross appearance but microscopically has inclusions of sweat gland apparatus.[18] *Atypical lipoma* is discussed in the section Liposarcoma.

In two rare conditions, multiple lipomas composed of mature fat cells arise in adult life. These conditions are *adiposis dolorosa*, or Dercum's disease, in which there are tender, circumscribed or diffuse fatty deposits,[19] and *benign symmetric lipomatosis*, which is characterized by the gradual development of many large, coalescent, asymptomatic lipomas, mainly on the trunk and arms and beginning in early adulthood.[20] In some instances, referred to as *Madelung's disease*, the lipomas are present especially in the region of the neck in a "horse-collar" distribution.[21] Occasionally, benign symmetric lipomatosis is inherited as an autosomal dominant trait. The *Bannayan-Zonana syndrome* is the congenital combination of multiple lipomas, including lipomas in body cavities in some instances, hemangiomas, and macrocephaly. Multiple lipomas and hemangiomas occur in *Cowden's syndrome*. *Fröhlich's syndrome* exhibits multiple lipomas, obesity, and sexual infantilism. The *Proteus syndrome* features multiple lipomatous lesions, including pelvic lipomatosis and fibroplasia of the feet and hands, skeletal hypertrophy, exostoses and scoliosis, and pigmented skin lesions.

Histopathology. By definition, lipomas contain mature adipocytes as a principal component. They tend to be sur-

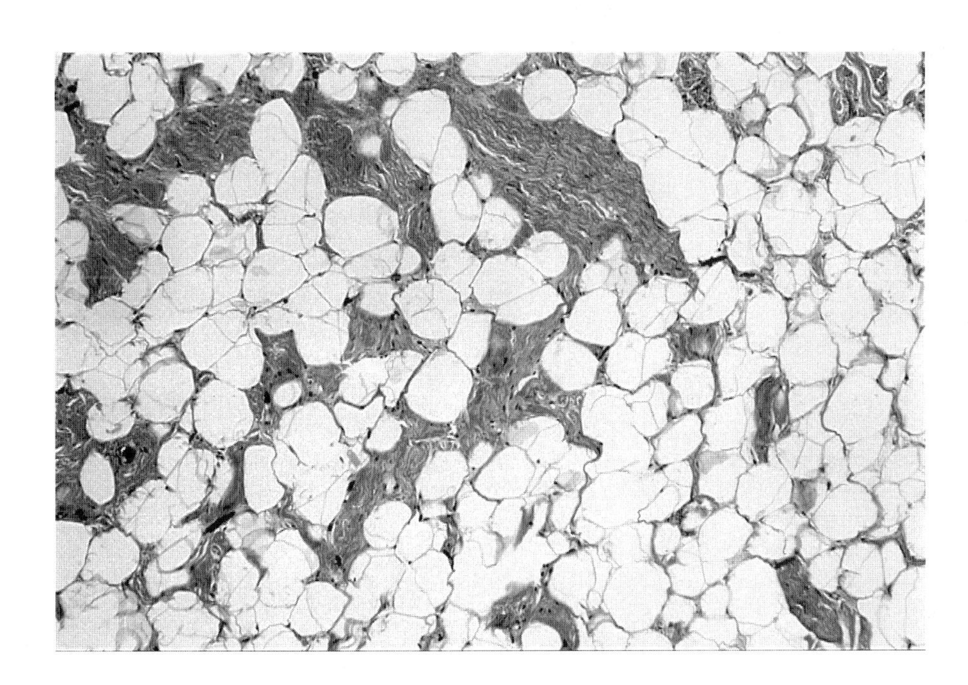

FIG. 35-5. Fibrolipoma
Strands of collagenous, fibrous connective tissue can be seen within a tumor composed of mature adipocytes. In other cases, the nodule may be predominantly fibrous with little fat.

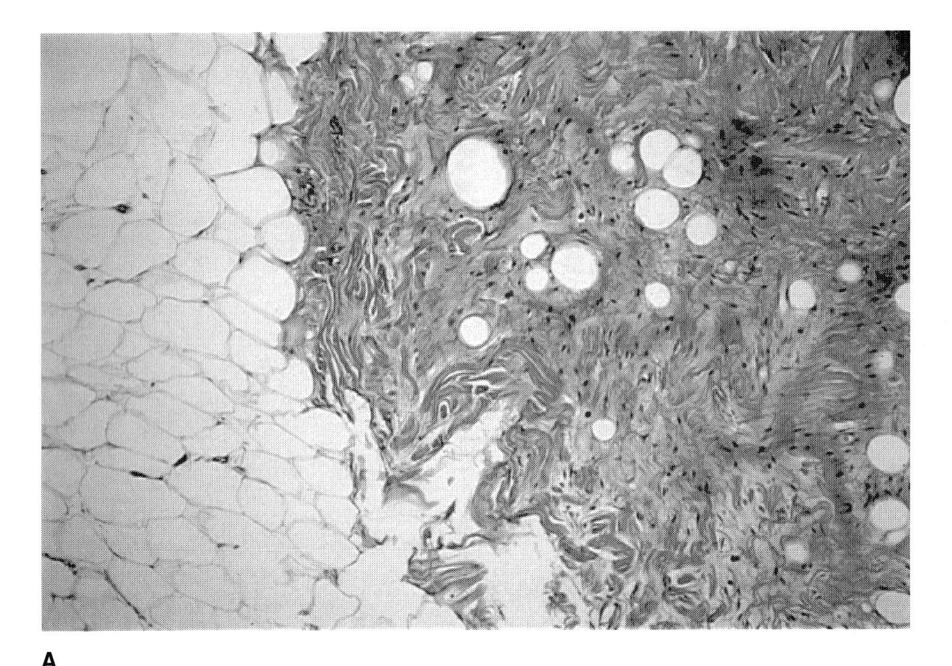

A

B

FIG. 35-6. Myxolipoma (48-year-old female, left shoulder region)
(**A**) A medium-magnification view shows a fibromyxoid area within a fatty tumor containing isolated mature signet-ring fat cells. (**B**) At higher magnification, cells within the myxoid background are stellate and spindle-shaped without accumulation of cytoplasmic lipid or nuclear atypia, features permitting distinction from myxoid liposarcoma despite focal similarity resulting from capillary vessel prominence.

rounded by a thin connective tissue capsule and are composed, often entirely, of normal fat cells that are indistinguishable from the fat cells in the subcutaneous tissue. Occasional "hibernoma-like" cells or multivesicular cells around foci of necrosis should not be misinterpreted as lipoblasts, which differ in having coarse vacuoles and irregular nuclei. *Intramuscular (infiltrating) lipomas* consist of mature fat cells that infiltrate muscle, splaying fibers but showing no nuclear atypia (Fig. 35-4). In some lipomas, one finds more or less of a connective tissue framework than in the normal subcutaneous fat. Those containing considerable proportions of fibrous connective tissue are called *fibrolipomas* (Fig. 35-5). Substantial basophilic mucopolysaccharide may fill regions of the tumor and recommends the term *myxolipoma* (Fig. 35-6). Focal chondroid (Fig. 35-7) and/or osteoid production (Fig. 35-8) have no significance other than underscoring the common ancestry of functional mesenchymal cells.

Myolipomas are comprised of variable amounts of benign

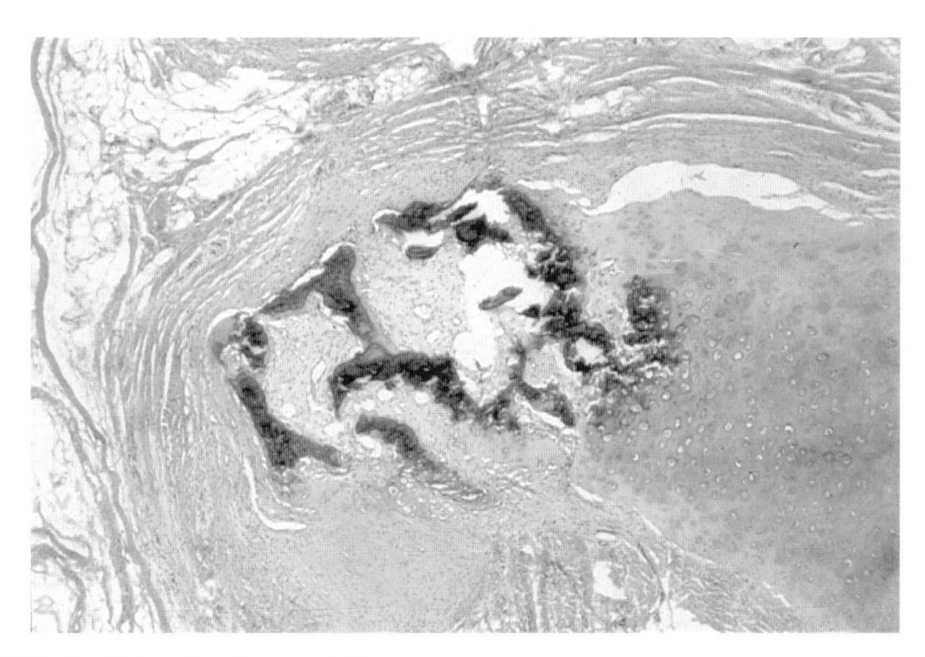

FIG. 35-7. Ossifying chondromyxoid lipoma
Within a fatty and myxoid background are areas of chondrification (*right*) and ossification (*center*). The contact between the bone and cartilage to the right of center suggests that part of the bone was formed through the enchondral mechanism, analogous to longitudinal bone growth at the growth plate. A portion of the bone has formed directly from the fibrous background (intramembranous ossification). This lesion manifests all three directions of modulation outlined in Fig. 35-1.

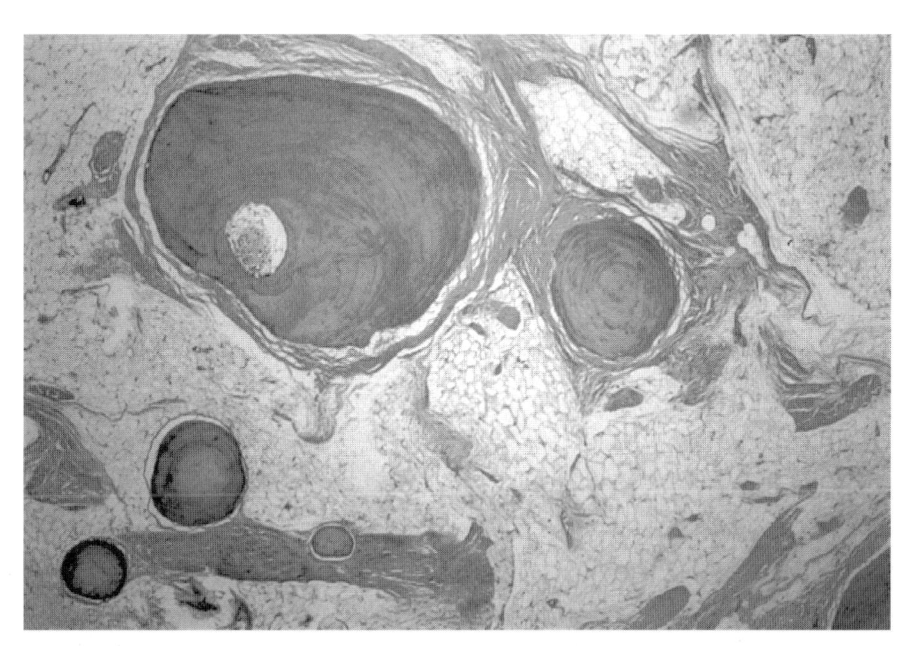

FIG. 35-8. Osteolipoma (63-year-old male with "cyst" on forehead for many years)
Rounded islands of bone are visible within a fibrofatty background in this mass. The largest ossicle (upper left) has undergone central haversianization.

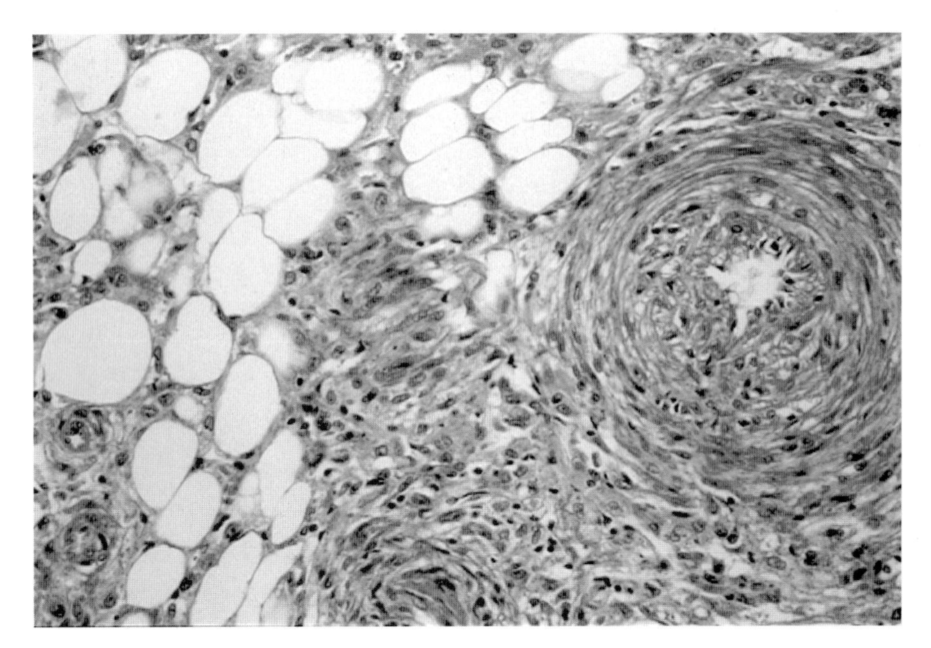

FIG. 35-9. Angiomyolipoma
Plump cells with features of smooth muscle appear to derive from the wall of a vessel within a fatty background. The basic components of the tumor are mature adipose tissue, and thick-walled, medium-sized vascular channels from which sheets of plump, smooth muscle cells appear to be derived. Moderate pleomorphism of the fatty and smooth muscle components is expected and does not connote malignancy.

smooth muscle and mature adipose tissue. The smooth muscle component of a cutaneous *angiomyolipoma* (Fig. 35-9) may show pronounced cellular and nuclear pleomorphism and hyperchromatism, as is common in the renal tumor of the same name.[22] The distinctive feature of an *adenolipoma* (Fig. 35-10) is an admixture of displaced and distorted sweat glands within the fatty background.[18] In *adiposis dolorosa* (Dercum's disease), most authors have found the lipomas to be indistinguishable histologically from ordinary lipomas. In some cases, the histologic appearance is that of an angiolipoma, a tumor that is

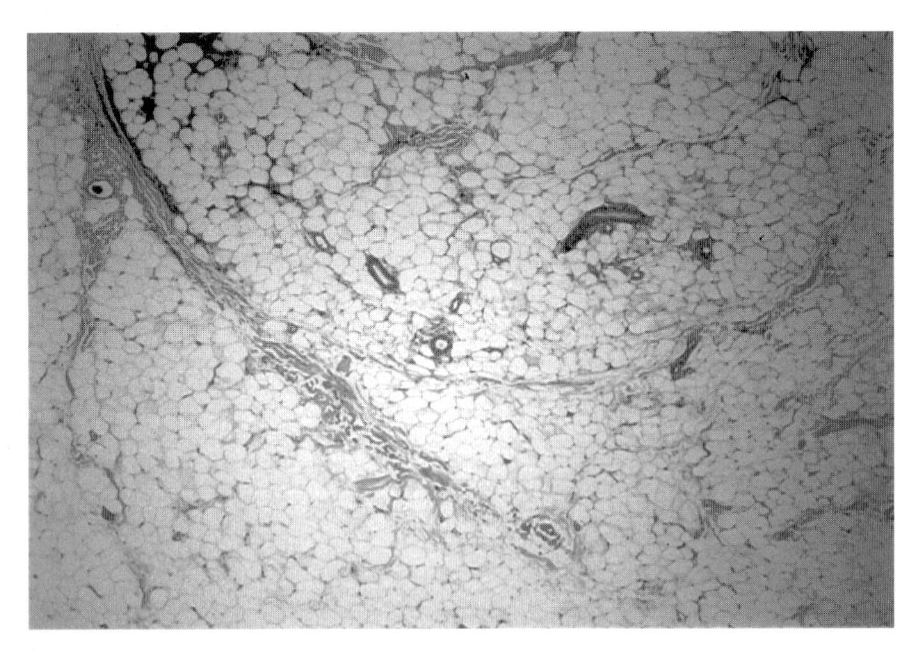

A

FIG. 35-10. Adenolipoma
(**A**) Low-magnification view shows lobulated fat within which are isolated tubular eccrine structures (59-year-old female with 1.5-cm nodule on left shoulder).

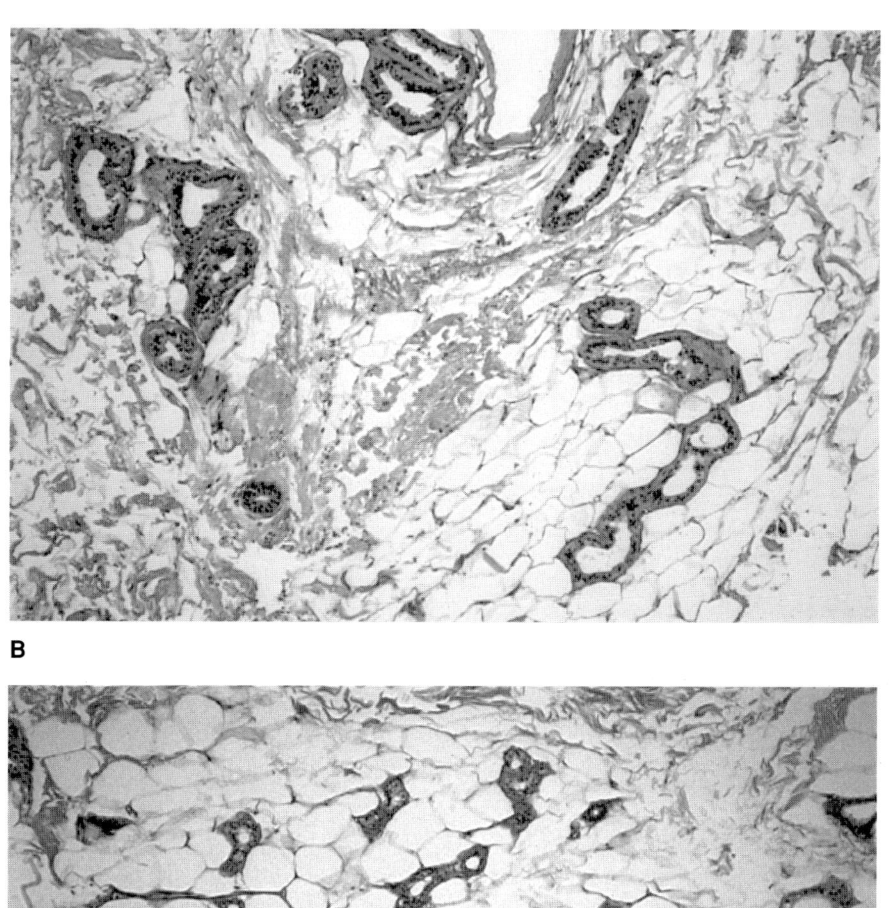

B

C

FIG. 35-10. *Continued*
(**B**) Excess mature fat in this medium-magnification view surrounds sweat gland coils and tubules (52-year-old male with 2-cm left neck nodule). (**C**) Apocrine glandular elements (*bottom*) can be seen with sweat gland elements in a background of mature fat (62-year-old female with small axillary mass).

often painful (see text following). In other cases, granulomas of the foreign-body type have been noted within the fatty tissue.[19] In *benign symmetric lipomatosis* (Madelung's disease), the lipomas have the histologic appearance characteristic of ordinary lipomas.[21] Hundreds of slowly growing subcutaneous and deep or visceral lipomas may be acquired in the autosomal dominant condition, *familial multiple lipomatosis*.

Efforts to distinguish true adipocyte neoplasms from lipomatous hamartomas and localized overgrowth of fat have been limited by the lack of reproducible markers for adipose neoplasms. Identification of a (12:16) (q13p11) translocation in myxoid liposarcomas, and of a similar translocation in lipomas with breakpoints at 12q14,[23] makes future prospects of resolving these issues of pathogenesis seem bright. For the present, lipomatous tumors are still classified morphologically (Table 35-1).

Differential Diagnosis. Growth pattern and size may suggest well-differentiated liposarcoma, but superficial (dermal or subcutaneous) liposarcomas are extremely rare. Lipomas do not contain diagnostic lipoblasts. This fact and the absence of the characteristic delicate capillary network distinguish lipomas with focal or substantial basophilic mucopolysaccharide from myxoid liposarcomas. Instances of malignant transformation of ordinary lipomas are anecdotal at best.

Deeply situated myolipomas can be confused with well-differentiated liposarcomas.[16]

TABLE 35-1. *Benign lipomatous tumors of skin and soft tissue*

Hamartomas
Nevus lipomatosus cutaneous superficialis
Folded skin with lipomatous nevus
Congenital lipomatosis
Proteus syndrome
Benign neoplasms of white fat
Homogeneous
Mature lipoma
With heterogeneous mesenchymal elements:
Fibrolipoma
Myxolipoma
Ossifying lipoma
Angiolipoma
Myolipoma
Angiomyolipoma
With specific clinicopathogenic settings:
Perineural lipoma
Lipoma of tendon sheath and joints
Multiple lipoma syndromes
Adiposis dolorosa (Dercum's disease)
Benign symmetric lipomatosis
Familial multiple lipomatosis
Pseudosarcomatous benign adipose tumors
Spindle cell lipoma
Pleomorphic lipoma
Chondroid lipoma
Lipoblastoma and lipoblastomatosis
Inter- and intramuscular lipoma
Cervical symmetrical lipomatosis
Pelvic lipomatosis
Diffuse lipomatosis
Benign neoplasm of brown fat
Hibernoma

ANGIOLIPOMA

Angiolipomas usually occur as encapsulated subcutaneous lesions. As a rule, they arise in young adults. The forearm is the single most common location for this tumor, which is more often multifocal than solitary. Clinically, angiolipomas resemble lipomas, although they have a greater tendency to be multiple. They are often tender or painful.[24] Some, it is alleged, can be moved for considerable distances under the skin,[25] although it is argued that these are actually areas of nodular-cystic fat necrosis in which dead fat lobules undergo fibrous encapsulation.[26]

Histopathology. Inapparent at the gross level, angiolipomas microscopically show sharp encapsulation, numerous small-caliber vascular channels containing characteristic microthrombi, and variable amounts of mature adipose tissue (Fig. 35-11). These thrombi are well demonstrated by phosphotungstic acid–hematoxylin staining[27] and are likely artifacts of removal because they show no organization. The degree of vascularity is quite variable, ranging from only a few small angiomatous foci to lesions with a predominance of dense vascular and stromal tissue.[24] The angiomatous foci are composed in part of well-formed, dilated capillaries engorged with erythrocytes. Other capillaries appear tortuous and have poorly formed lumina and prominent proliferation of pericytes. Perivascular fibrosis may be prominent.

Differential Diagnosis. Lesions with prominent perithelial fibrocytes may bring to mind spindle cell lipoma, which, however, lacks the conspicuous capillary channels with fibrin thrombi. Nearly all angiolipomas contain fibrin thrombi within their capillaries, often to a considerable degree. Cellular angiolipomas composed almost entirely of vascular channels and prominent spindle cells are sometimes confused with Kaposi's sarcoma or angiosarcoma. Subcutaneous position, encapsulation, septation, small size, diminutive nonatypical endothelial cells, microthrombi, and clinical presentation in healthy individuals help to exclude a malignant diagnosis.[28] The term *infiltrating angiolipoma*, as used by Dionne and Seemayer[29] and by Puig et al.,[30] is synonymous with *intramuscular angioma* (Fig. 35-12),[31] a soft tissue tumor with copious mature fat that is not acknowledged in its name. Its vessels are larger, and this lesion has a significant recurrence rate.

SPINDLE CELL LIPOMA

A solitary, slowly growing subcutaneous tumor, spindle cell lipoma exhibits a predilection for the posterior neck and shoulder girdle region in men in their sixth decade. Clinically, the tumor is a slowly growing, painless nodule centered in the dermis or subcutis and measuring from 1.0 to 13.0 cm. in diameter. This tumor does not recur or metastasize.

Histopathology. Although the lesion is well circumscribed, it is seldom encapsulated. It is comprised of mature fat cells and uniform, slender spindle cells within a mucinous matrix.[32] Spindle cell lipoma is polymorphous as a result of variations in cellularity, collagen content, and the ratio of spindle cells to mature adipocytes. In some areas, the neoplasm consists of a pure spindle cell population, often arranged in thick bundles, without fat

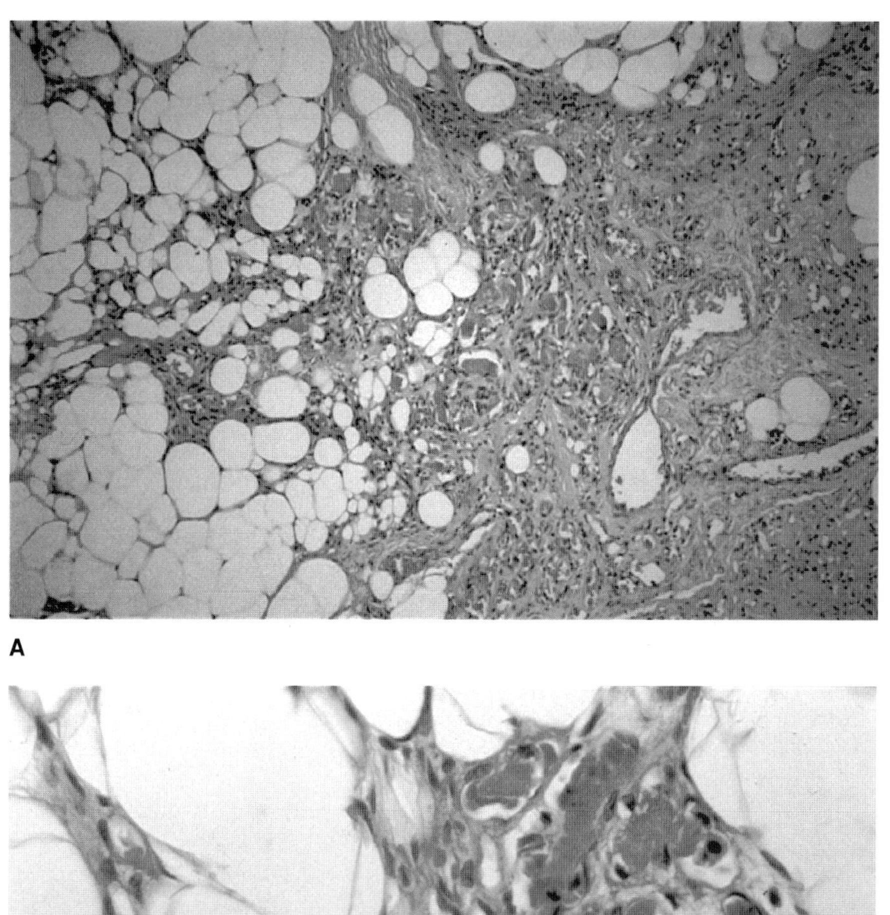

A

B

FIG. 35-11. Angiolipoma
(**A**) Prominent vessels radiate through a fibrous background into mature fat. Prominent vascularity can impersonate a primary vascular neoplasm. (**B**) At higher magnification, fibrin thrombi without organization occur in capillary lumina.

cells. In other areas, the spindle cells are intermingled with scattered groups of mature fat cells (Fig. 35-13).[33] The spindle cells, functioning as fibroblasts, produce varying amounts of collagen. A unique feature is the presence of numerous mast cells throughout the tumor.[33] Some tumors also show a prominent admixture of blood vessels ranging from capillaries to thick-walled vessels containing smooth muscle bundles[34] to prominent sinusoidal channels dividing the tumor into irregular lobules.

Differential Diagnosis. The diagnosis of liposarcoma or fibrosarcoma can usually be excluded without difficulty because of the uniformity of the proliferated spindle cells and the absence of lipoblasts and atypical mitotic figures in spindle cell lipoma.[32]

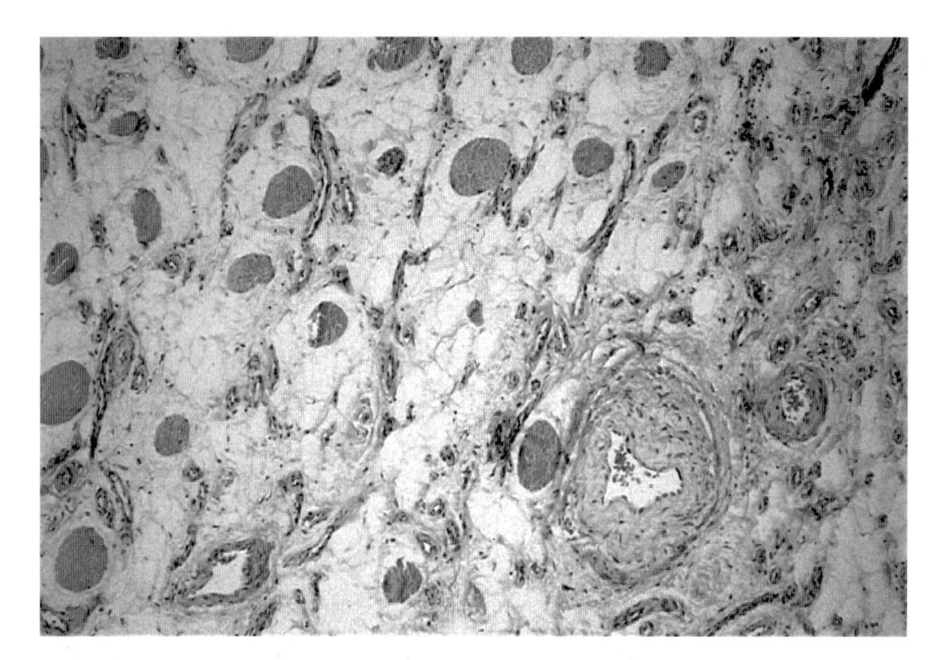

FIG. 35-12. Intramuscular hemangioma (43-year-old male with 8-cm mass in deltoid muscle) Mature skeletal muscle fibers cut end-on, resulting in circular profiles, are separated by abundant blood vessels and mature fat cells. This soft tissue tumor has in the past been reported under the term *cellular* or *infiltrating angiolipoma.* This lesion has a significant propensity for local regrowth if incompletely excised.

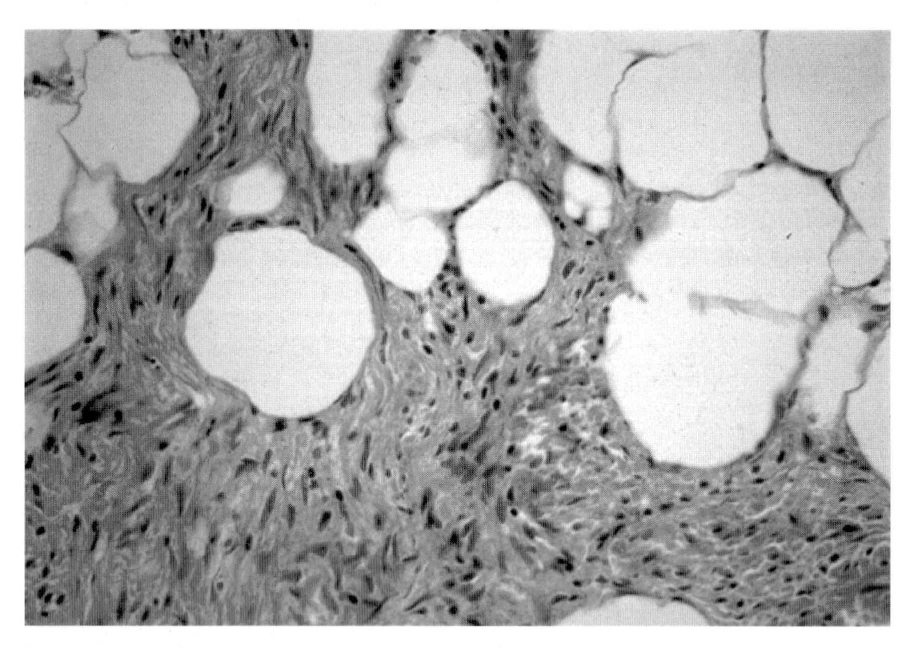

FIG. 35-13. Spindle cell lipoma (60-year-old male with small neck nodule) Uniform collagen-forming spindle cells expand the space between mature fat cells. (Courtesy of William B. Dupree.)

PLEOMORPHIC LIPOMA

Like spindle cell lipomas, the great majority of pleomorphic lipomas are solitary tumors of the shoulder girdle and neck in men in the fifth to seventh decade. The lesion presents as a slowly growing, well-circumscribed dermal or subcutaneous mass grossly resembling an ordinary lipoma.[35] Despite occasional lipoblast-like cells and atypical mitotic figures, local excision should be curative.

Histopathology. The well-circumscribed tumor displays a wide morphologic spectrum. Although areas of mature fat cells are present, some of them show enlarged, hyperchromatic nuclei.[36] In addition, most fat cells show marked variation in size. About half of the tumors contain occasional multivacuolated cells that have the appearance of lipoblasts.[35] The mature and immature fat cells are situated singly and in groups in a mucinous stroma traversed by dense collagen bundles (Fig. 35-14A).

A very helpful feature in the diagnosis of pleomorphic

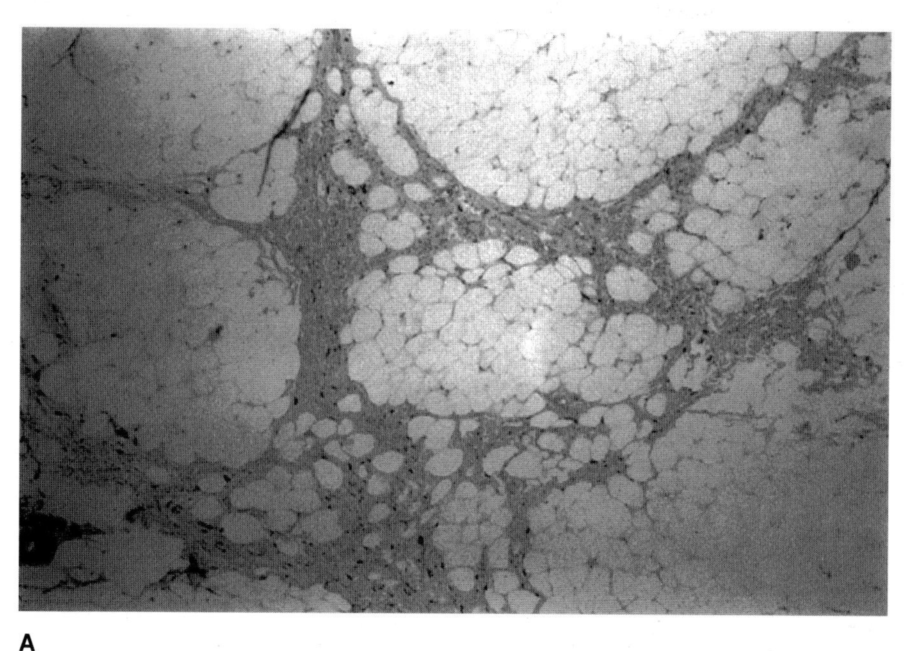

A

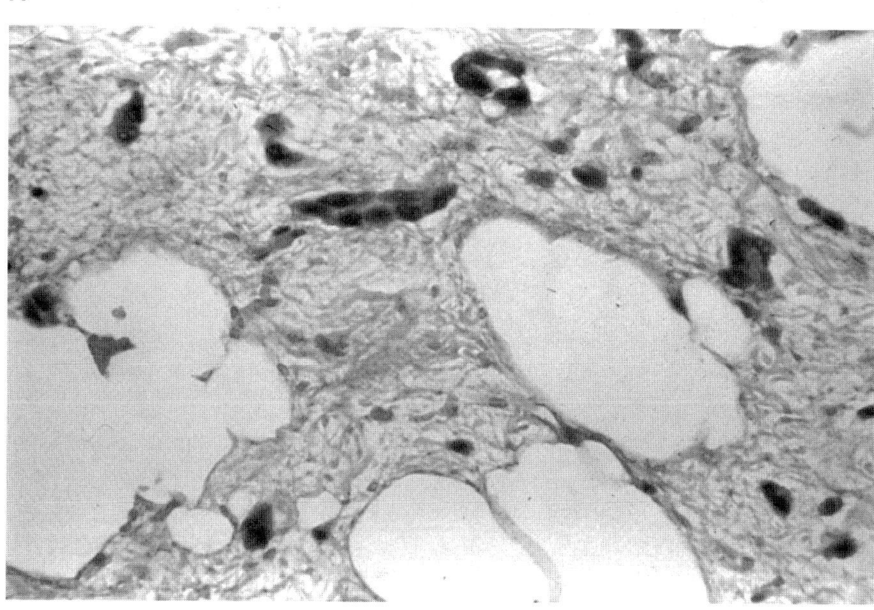

B

FIG. 35-14. Pleomorphic lipoma with local regrowth (59-year-old male)
(**A**) Most of a 9-cm mass at the posterior base of the patient's neck was initially excised. Lobulation is created by hypercellular fibrous bands. (**B**) Characteristic floret-type giant cells with multiple peripherally placed nuclei and deeply eosinophilic cytoplasm are visible in the fibrous regions. This view comes from a local regrowth that had regained a size of 9 cm 8 years after initial surgery.

lipoma is the presence of characteristic multinucleated giant cells, which are found in most but not all cases.[36] These giant cells exhibit, within an eosinophilic cytoplasm, multiple, marginally placed, and often overlapping hyperchromatic nuclei. This peculiar arrangement is not unlike that of the petals of a small flower, and these giant cells are therefore referred to as *floret-type giant cells* (Fig. 35-14B).[35,37] Rarely, pleomorphic lipoma histology comprises a sharply demarcated nodule within an otherwise ordinary lipoma. Also, small foci of spindle cell lipoma may be encountered in some pleomorphic lipomas.[35] Some pleomorphic lipomas have inflammatory cells, including lymphocytes, plasma cells, mast cells, and occasional histiocytes in a perivascular or diffuse stromal distribution.

Differential Diagnosis. No single feature confirms the diagnosis of pleomorphic lipoma and excludes liposarcoma. Only a multivariate analysis leads to the correct diagnosis, and such an analysis should consider (1) the age and sex of the patient, (2) anatomic location, (3) size, (4) epicenter of growth (deep or su-

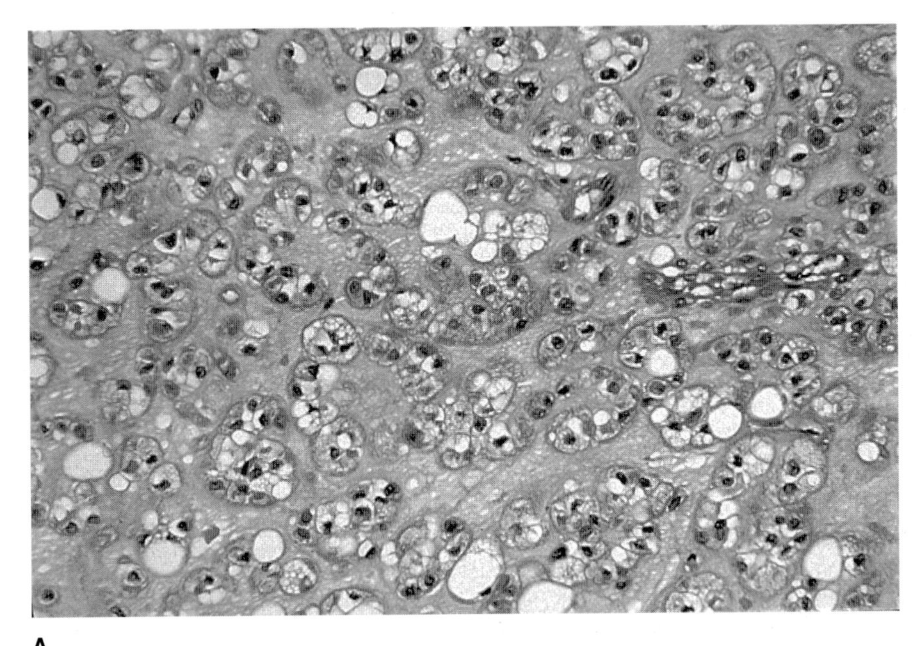

A

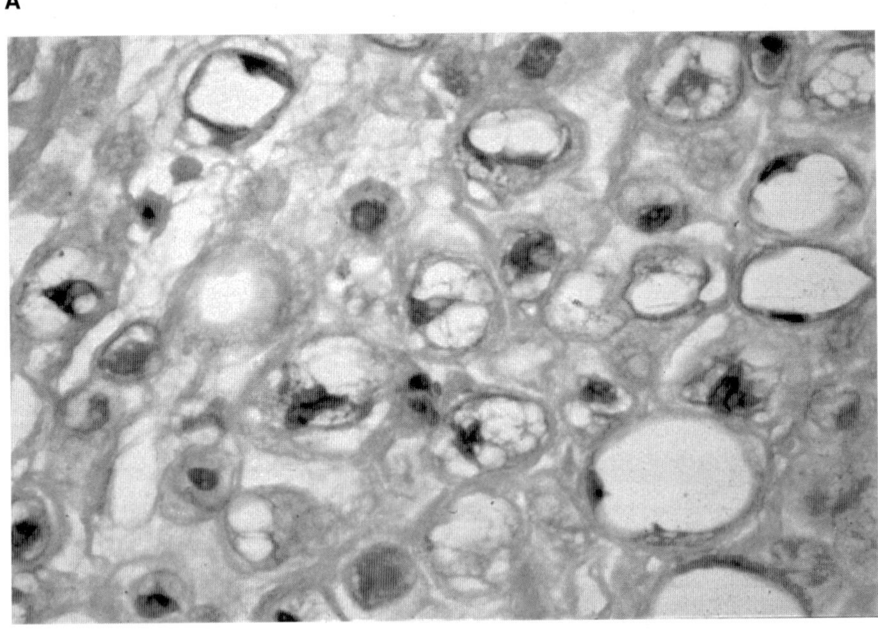

B

FIG. 35-15. Chondroid lipoma
(**A**) Chondroid lipoma has a lobular pattern consisting of strands and nests of rounded or polygonal eosinophilic cells in a stroma of mature fat, myxoid and chondroid material, and partly hyalinized fibrous tissue. (**B**) The polygonal eosinophilic tumor cells have lipid vacuoles and grossly simulate lipoblasts. They contain neutral fat and glycogen and stain positively with oil red O and PAS stains. They are positive for vimentin and S-100 protein. (Courtesy of Andrew E. Rosenberg.)

perficial), (5) degree of local invasion, and (6) histologic appearance. Liposarcomas differ from pleomorphic lipomas by their infiltrative growth, greater cellularity, more nuclear atypicality including atypical mitoses, more numerous multivacuolated lipoblasts, prominent necrosis, and absence of thick collagen bundles. Floret-type giant cells are rarely seen in liposarcomas, and then only in small numbers.[35]

CHONDROID LIPOMA

Chondroid lipoma must be added to the list of lipoma variants that are at risk of being misdiagnosed as sarcomas. Based on 20 cases,[38] the age range is 14 to 70 years with a 4:1 female predominance and predilection for the limbs and limb girdles. These nonpainful masses of weeks' or years' duration ranged from 1.5 to 11 cm in diameter, with a median of 4 cm. Perhaps half of these well-demarcated, encapsulated, yellow-to-white or gray-tan masses are in the subcutis or involve the superficial fascia of the skeletal muscle. The remainder are more deeply situated, possibly within muscles.

Histopathology. In chondroid lipoma, a variable background of mature adipose tissue is associated with a predominant, partially fibrinous to hyalinized myxoid matrix (Fig. 35-15A). Within this matrix are nests, strands, and sheets of eosinophilic and vacuolated cells, which contain glycogen and fat droplets, resembling brown fat cells, lipoblasts, and chondroblasts. These S-100-positive cells lack pleomorphism and mitoses and adopt a lacunar appearance when surrounded by the prominent myxoid or hyalin matrix (Fig. 35-15B). This lesion, almost invariably mistaken for a sarcoma, especially myxoid liposarcoma or myxoid chondrosarcoma, is nonaggressive and has a benign clinical course without local regrowth or metastases in the original 12 cases with follow-up.[38]

Pathogenesis. Electron microscopy reveals that the tumor cells have abundant intracytoplasmic lipid and glycogen, and also numerous pinocytotic vesicles characteristic of adipocytes rather than chondroblasts. This favors the view that chondroid lipoma is a tumor of pure white adipocytes with a hyalinized extracellular matrix that resembles cartilage under light microscopy.[39]

HIBERNOMA

Hibernoma[40] is a benign, moderately firm, solitary, subcutaneous, tan or red-brown tumor generally from 3 to 12 cm in diameter, but occasionally larger. Although usually asymptomatic, it is occasionally tender.[41] Hibernomas may appear in childhood and slowly increase in size,[42] but they more commonly arise in adulthood. This rare tumor arises most frequently in the subcutis of the shoulder girdle, posterior neck, and axilla, but some hibernomas occur at sites where brown fat is not normally located, such as the abdomen.[41] Clinically, hibernomas are indistinguishable from lipomas and, like lipomas, have no tendency to recur locally.

Histopathology. Histologic examination reveals that the tumor is divided into numerous lobules by well-vascularized connective tissue (Fig. 35-16A). In contrast to ordinary lipoma of white fat, the highly vascular nature of the tumor is readily apparent in most sections. The tumor cells are round or polygonal and are closely apposed to one another within the lobules (Fig. 35-16B).[42] Three principal types of cells can be recognized: (1) a small cell (average, 37 μm) with granular, eosinophilic cytoplasm and with or without rare, small lipid vacuoles; (2) a larger, multivacuolated fat cell (average, 54 μm) with scanty granular, eosinophilic cytoplasm, referred to as a mulberry cell; and (3) a still larger, univacuolated fat cell (average, 64 μm).[43] The nuclei of the granular and multivacuolated cells are usually centrally located; and the nuclei of the univacuolated fat cells are peripheral. Cells of the three principal types, with transitional forms, usually are dispersed randomly throughout the lobules. In most tumors, multivacuolated mulberry cells predominate. Some tumors, however, contain a few lobules, particularly at their peripheries, that are composed entirely of univacuolated cells.[41] The vacuoles in both the multivacuolated and univacuolated cells stain positively with Sudan black.[44]

Pathogenesis. The term *hibernoma* reflects the fact that these tumors are composed of cells that resemble the brown fat of hibernating animals. The incomplete modulation of the mulberry cells may be attributable to underdevelopment of enzyme systems.[45]

Differential Diagnosis. Hibernomas are to be distinguished from granular cell tumors, which have no lipid vacuoles, and also from certain forms of round cell liposarcoma, which usually contain diagnostic multivacuolar lipoblasts.

BENIGN LIPOBLASTOMA

Lipoblastoma is an uncommon, solitary, circumscribed variant of lipoma arising in the subcutaneous fat between the time of birth and 7 years of age.[46] The slowly growing tumor may reach considerable size. About 70% occur in limbs, mostly in the lower extremities.[47]

Two basic forms of benign lipoblastoma occur. One, which is a variant called lipoblastomatosis, is deeply situated and poorly circumscribed and tends to grow into the surrounding tissue spaces and musculature.[45] The other is relatively superficial and encapsulated.[46] Each form commonly presents as a painless nodule or mass, affecting boys twice as frequently as girls.

A breakpoint in the long arm of chromosome 8q11-13 appears to be emerging as a consistent finding.[48]

Despite the cellular immaturity, prognosis is excellent after simple excision for lipoblastoma and after wide local excision for diffuse lipoblastomatosis. Cellular maturation has been reported in serial biopsies over time.

Histopathology. Peripheral immature lipoblasts with fat vacuoles of various sizes and central mature fat cells containing single, large, fat vacuoles are characteristic whether the tumor is deeply or superficially situated (Fig. 35-17). The lipoblasts vary in size. Most of them contain single vacuoles that are variable in size but smaller than those found in mature fat cells. These vacuoles displace the nuclei against the cytoplasmic membrane.[45] A few small lipoblasts contain two, three, or occasionally more vacuoles. Some benign lipoblastomas also show lipoblasts with finely vacuolar cytoplasm and centrally placed nuclei resembling hibernoma cells.[49] Nonvacuolated cells that are spindle-shaped or stellate are observed in the mucinous stroma. Fibrous septae partition lobules in the circumscribed form.

Differential Diagnosis. Only the age of the patient, the abundance of lipoblasts, the absence of atypical mitoses,[49] and a

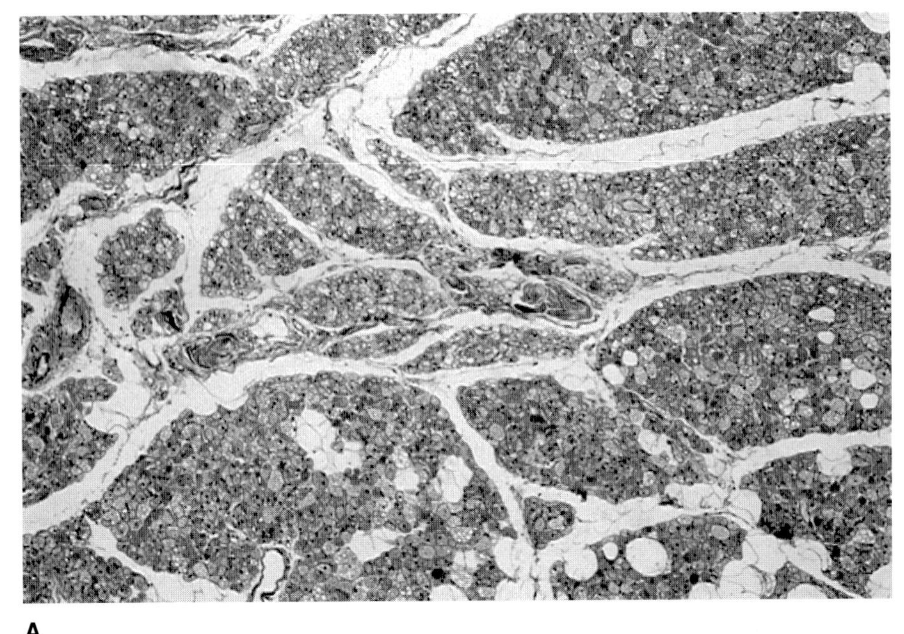

A

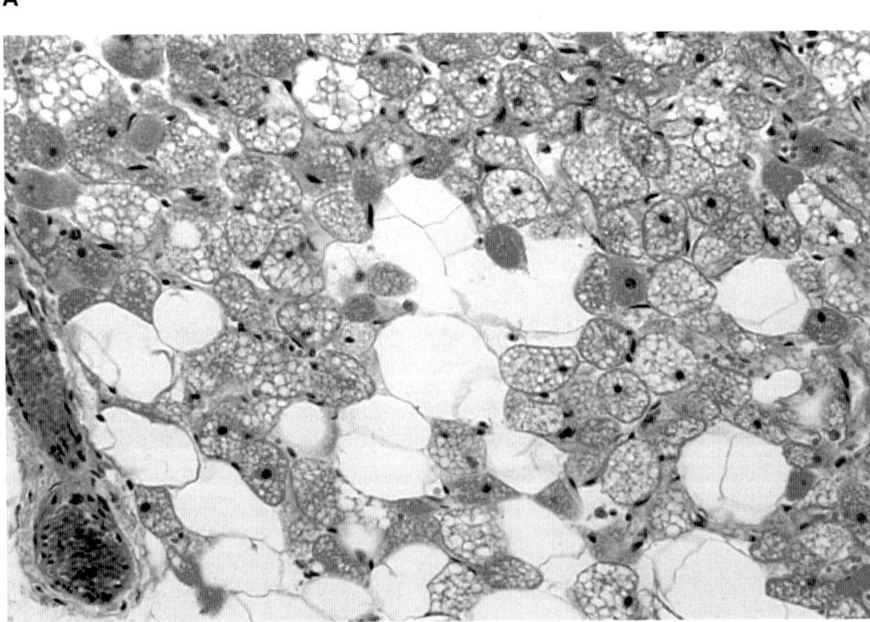

B

FIG. 35-16. Hibernoma
(**A**) A low-magnification view displays the distinct lobular pattern characteristic of hibernoma. (**B**) At higher magnification, hibernoma cells show varying degrees of complete modulation to signet-ring fat cells. These cells range from uniform round to oval granular eosinophilic cells to multivacuolated cells with multiple small oil-red-O–positive lipid droplets and centrally placed nuclei, to intermixed univacuolar cells with one or more large lipid droplets and peripherally placed nuclei (lipocytes). The gross brown color of hibernoma results from the prominent vascularity and many mitochondria in tumor cells.

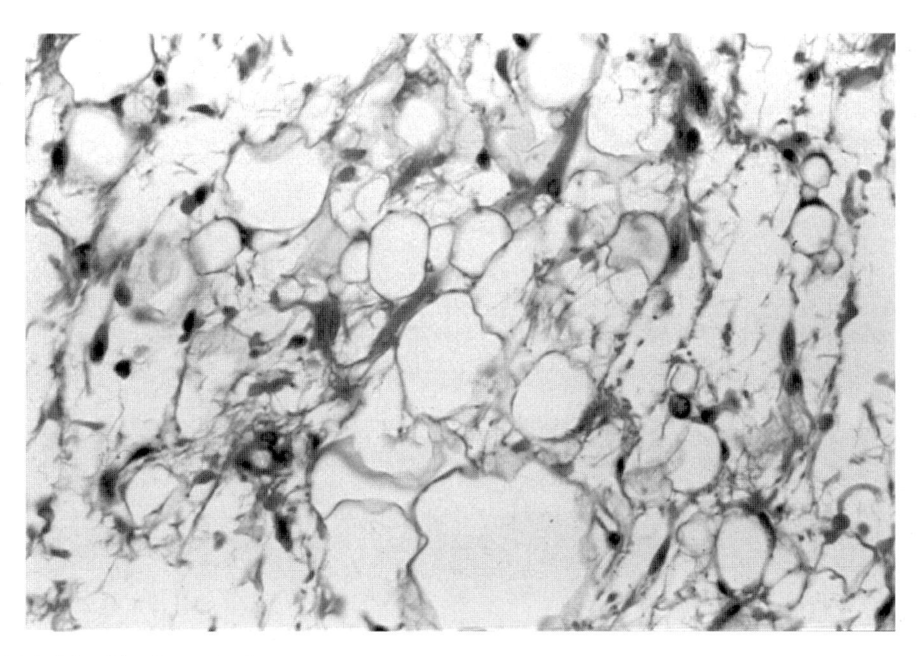

FIG. 35-17. Lipoblastomatosis
The tumor is comprised of partly differentiated lipoblasts and has a prominent capillary vascular pattern with areas of mucoid matrix. Cells with large hyperchromatic nuclei are absent.

sometimes subtle lobularity distinguish it from liposarcoma—especially the myxoid type.[50] Liposarcomas occur very rarely in infants and young children.

LIPOSARCOMA

Although liposarcomas constitute 15% to 20% of all soft tissue sarcomas, they rarely arise in the subcutaneous fat. Most commonly, they originate in the intermuscular fascial planes, with a special predilection for the thighs.[51] From a fascial plane, they can extend to the subcutaneous tissue. Liposarcomas arise as such and for practical purposes do not develop from lipomas. The average age of onset is 50 years. Occasionally, liposarcomas arise in children from 10 to 15 years of age, comprising 4% of childhood soft tissue sarcomas,[52] but are exceedingly rare, if not nonexistent, in children younger than 10 years.[53] Liposarcomas are slightly more prevalent in males and tend to occur on the right side of the body more commonly than on the left. Infrequently, liposarcomas may be multicentric.

Four major types of liposarcomas are generally recognized and have epidemiologic and prognostic differences: (1) well-differentiated, (2) myxoid, (3) round cell, and (4) pleomorphic.[51,54] In some tumors, more than one type can be recognized. Myxoid variants are more common in the young, whereas well-differentiated and pleomorphic subtypes are more often encountered in older patients. The well-differentiated and myxoid types have better prognoses than the round cell and pleomorphic types.[55]

Well-differentiated liposarcomas are further divided into three closely related subtypes: (1) "lipoma-like," (2) inflammatory, and (3) sclerosing. Well-differentiated liposarcomas are low grade and may regrow locally but do not metastasize. The clinical outcome of well-differentiated lipoma-like liposarcoma is best predicted by anatomic location.[56] In the subcutis they are usually cured by local excision, rarely regrow, and do not metastasize. Therefore the term *atypical lipoma* has been introduced for the subcutaneous form of well-differentiated liposarcoma.[57] This is the form of liposarcoma most likely to be biopsied by the dermatologist. Because of this benign course, Evans[58] has suggested an even less commital designation for this neoplasm, *atypical lipomatous tumor*. It has been recommended that this term be restricted to the subcutaneous tumors, especially those of small size with minimal atypical changes.[59]

For the more aggressive liposarcomas, circumscription of the lesion may offer false hope of eradication by simply shelling out the tumor. In reality, liposarcomas extend microscopic pseudopod-like extensions that commonly insinuate between fascial planes. Occasionally, small satellite nodules become separated from the lobulated sarcomatous mass, leading to an erroneous impression of multicentricity. Biopsy and resection should be carefully planned, guided by MR and radiographic findings in a manner that eliminates prior biopsy tracts and any plane potentially contaminated by surgical exposure or spreading hematoma.

Metastases are common, especially in poorly differentiated liposarcomas, the lungs and liver being the most common sites.

Histopathology. The diagnosis of liposarcoma depends on recognition of lipoblasts. For a cell to be designated as a lipoblast, it must show the ability to synthesize and accumulate non-membrane-bound lipid in the cytoplasmic matrix. Acceptable malignant lipoblasts are quite variable because they may recapitulate any stage in the normal maturation sequence. Their common morphologic denominator is well-demarcated cytoplasmic lipid that displaces or indents one or more irregular hyperchromatic nuclei. The nucleus conforms to the contours of the lipid droplet, creating an apparent delicate scalloping of the nuclear membrane. Hyperchromaticity and variability from lipoblast to lipoblast support a malignant diagnosis. Despite these criteria, the distinction between malignant lipoblast and "atypical lipocyte" is at times subjective, especially in the more well-differentiated lipoma-like variants of liposarcoma. Benign fat necrosis, myxoid changes in structural fat, lipogranulomas, lymphomas with signet-ring changes, and carcinomas can contain vacuolated cells that mimic lipoblasts. Lesions such as pleomorphic lipomas and lipoblastomas illustrate that even unequivocal lipoblasts do not always signal malignancy.

The cells of liposarcoma bear a close resemblance to different stages in the development of fat and are found in variable proportions as a function of histologic subtype, but show a much greater individual variability.

In *well-differentiated lipoma-like liposarcoma*, the tumor is composed predominantly of univacuolated fat cells of various sizes. The nuclei of the fat cells are slightly pleomorphic, and some of them are hyperchromatic. *Atypical lipoma* (Fig. 35-18) histologically features distended fat cells that vary slightly in size and shape, with occasional interspersed lipoblasts. Broad, fibrous septa containing cells with enlarged hyperchromatic atypical nuclei are a characteristic feature (Fig. 35-18A). Foci of well-differentiated smooth muscle may be found but do not in-

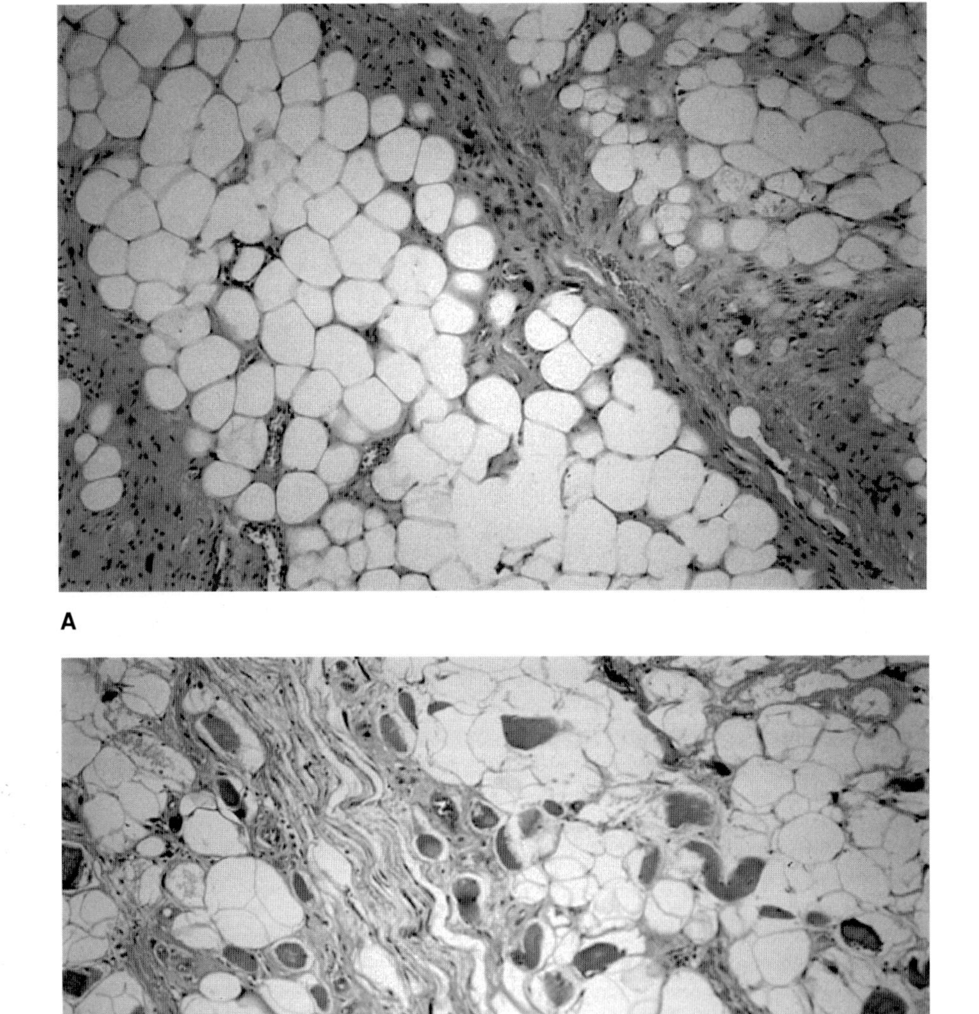

FIG. 35-18. Well-differentiated liposarcoma (atypical lipoma)
(**A**) Broad, fibrous septa containing cells with atypical hyperchromatic nuclei partition a tumor of fat-filled rounded cells, some of which are lipoblasts. (**B**) At a similar magnification, an atypical lipoma with hypercellular fibrous bands infiltrates skeletal muscle (compare Fig. 35-4B).

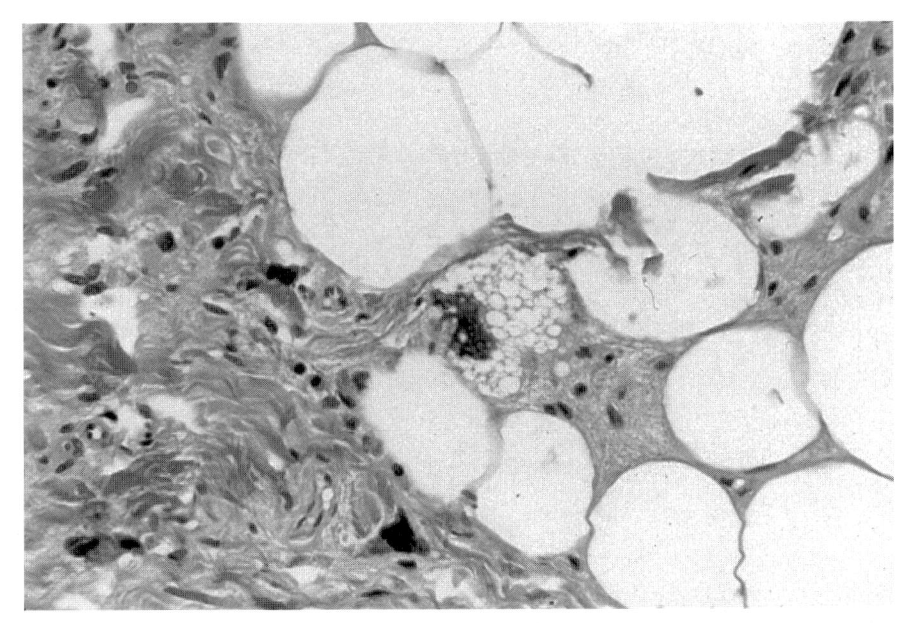

C

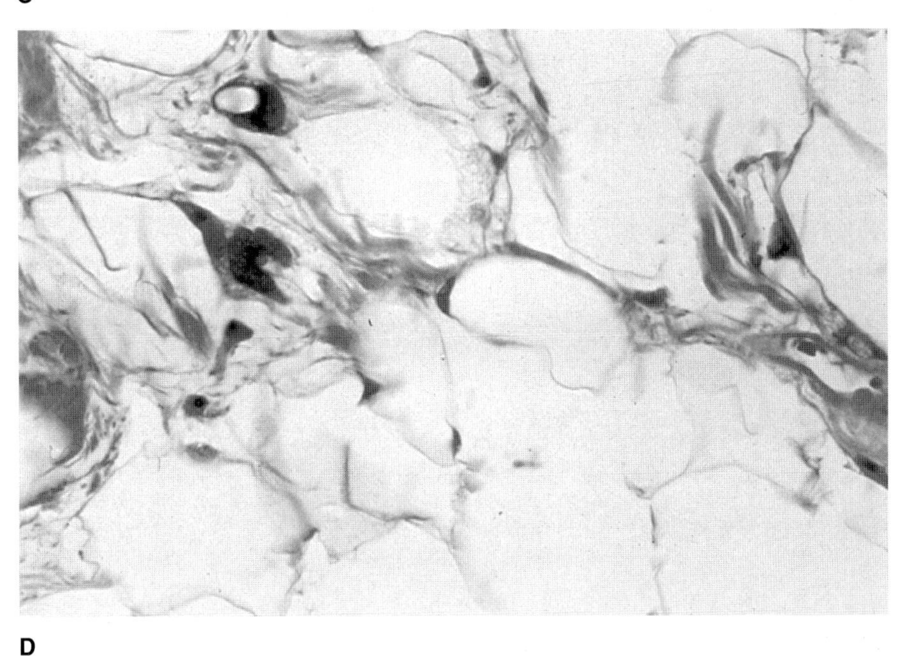

D

FIG. 35-18. ***Continued***
(**C**) In addition to atypical and large hyperchromatic nuclei in the fibrous bands (*left*), lipoblasts with hyperchromatic nuclei indented by lipid vacuoles (*center*) should be sought. (Courtesy of Andrew E. Rosenberg.) (**D**) Prolonged searching may be required to find enlarged, irregular, hyperchromatic nuclei, some indented by clear lipid vacuoles (*upper left*), in atypical lipoma.

fluence the behavior.[60] The emergence of a high-grade sarcoma pattern within a well-differentiated liposarcoma or in recurrence is known by the biologically imprecise term "dedifferentiation" and is limited for practical purposes to these tumors when they are located in body spaces, especially retroperitoneum.[61]

Myxoid liposarcomas (Fig. 35-19) are the most common type of liposarcoma and display various quantities of four elements: (1) proliferating lipoblasts, (2) delicate plexiform capillaries, (3) myxoid matrix, and (4) acid mucopolysaccharide lakes (Fig. 35-19A). Mitotic figures are conspicuously absent. These tumors have been subdivided into a well-differentiated type with little tendency to metastasize and a poorly differentiated type that commonly metastasizes.[51] A well-differentiated myxoid liposarcoma contains, in addition to lipoblasts with spindle-shaped nuclei and several lipid vacuoles, more highly differentiated fat cells, such as so-called *signet-ring* cells (Fig. 35-19C), which have single large vacuoles occupying a major portion of the cytoplasm, and even mature fat cells. The tumor cells are arranged loosely in a myxoid stroma. In a poorly differentiated myxoid liposarcoma, the spindle-shaped lipoblasts have large, atypical nuclei and usually only small numbers of lipid droplets. Depending on the amount of myxoid stroma, there is consider-

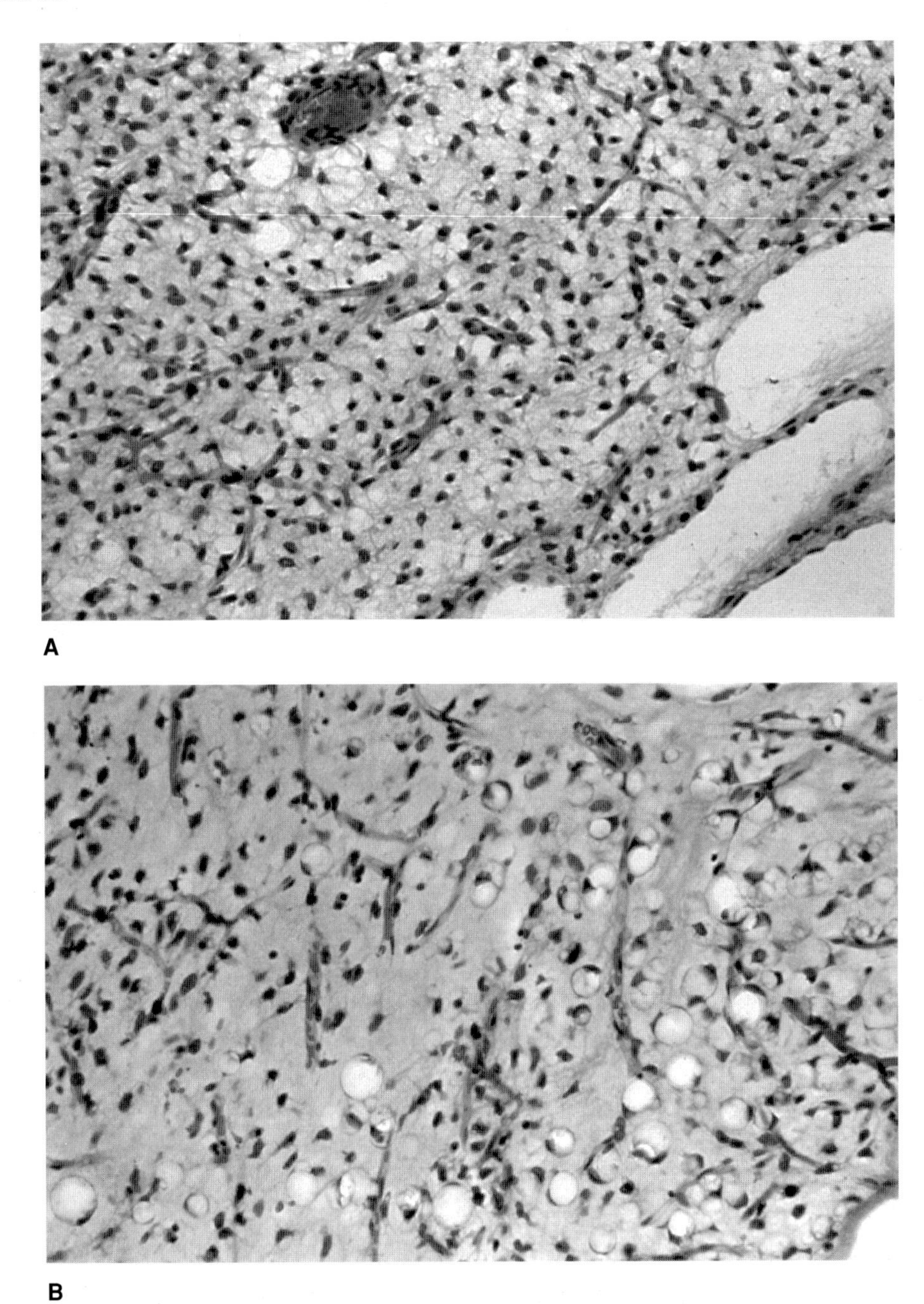

FIG. 35-19. Myxoid liposarcoma
(**A**) Angular hyperchromatic nuclei of densely packed lipoblasts might be mistaken for stellate cells of a myxoma. Pooling of myxoid material may result in a cribriform or lacelike pattern (lower right). (**B**) Another case presents lipoblasts in varying stages of cytoplasmic lipid accumulation, a prominent plexiform capillary pattern, and an abundance of myxoid material between vessels and tumor cells.

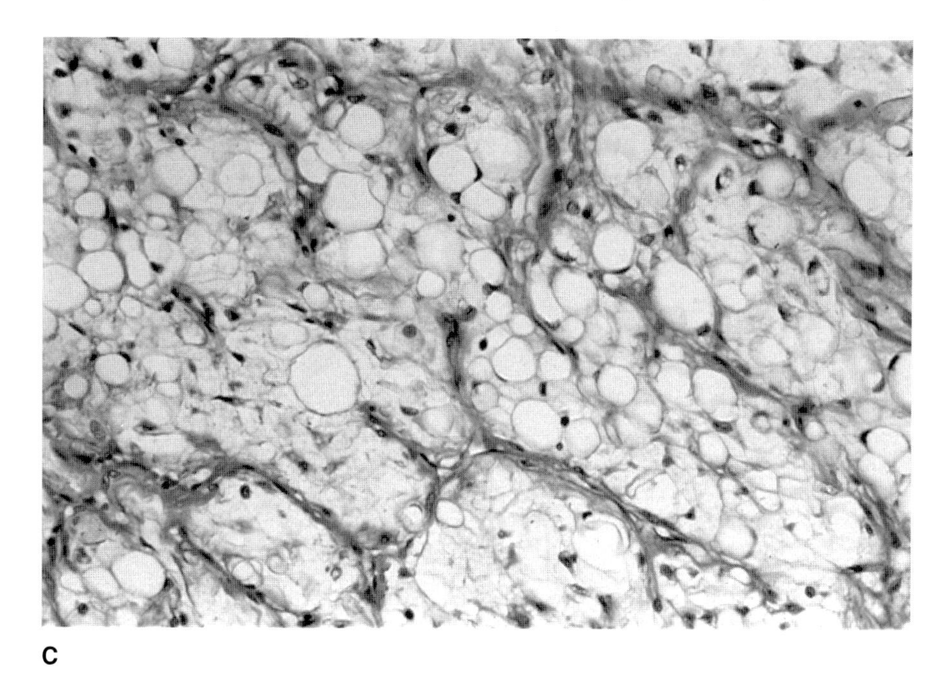

C

FIG. 35-19. *Continued*
(**C**) This example exhibits lipoblasts well-distended with fat, a prominent vascular pattern, and a minimal intercellular mucoid background.

able resemblance to either a myxosarcoma or an undifferentiated fibrosarcoma, because the latter may also have a certain amount of myxoid stroma.

Because of the more aggressive behavior of *round cell liposarcoma*, accurate diagnosis is important. As indicated by its name, round cell liposarcoma is characterized by an excessive proliferation of uniform, closely packed, rounded or oval cells, some of which contain no lipid. Others contain only small cytoplasmic vacuoles (Fig. 35-20). These cells are vaguely reminiscent of Ewing's sarcoma (and, similarly, may contain glycogen), malignant lymphoma, or small cell anaplastic carcinoma. Their association with other patterns of liposarcoma points to their liposarcomatous nature. Multivacuolated lipoblasts are few in number. Most tumor cells have hyperchromatic and atypical nuclei, with frequent mitoses. This tumor can be thought of as a less differentiated modification of liposarcoma in which the

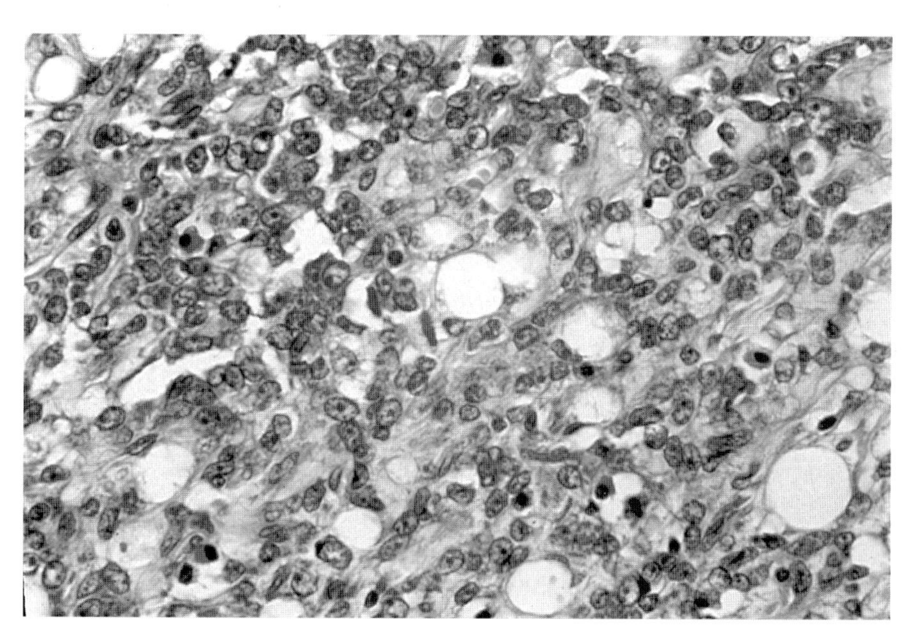

FIG. 35-20. Round cell liposarcoma
Numerous undifferentiated tumor cells can be seen with rare univacuolar lipoblasts. Because glycogen is involved in lipogenesis, these cells are PAS-positive, and this should not be taken as evidence for Ewing's sarcoma.

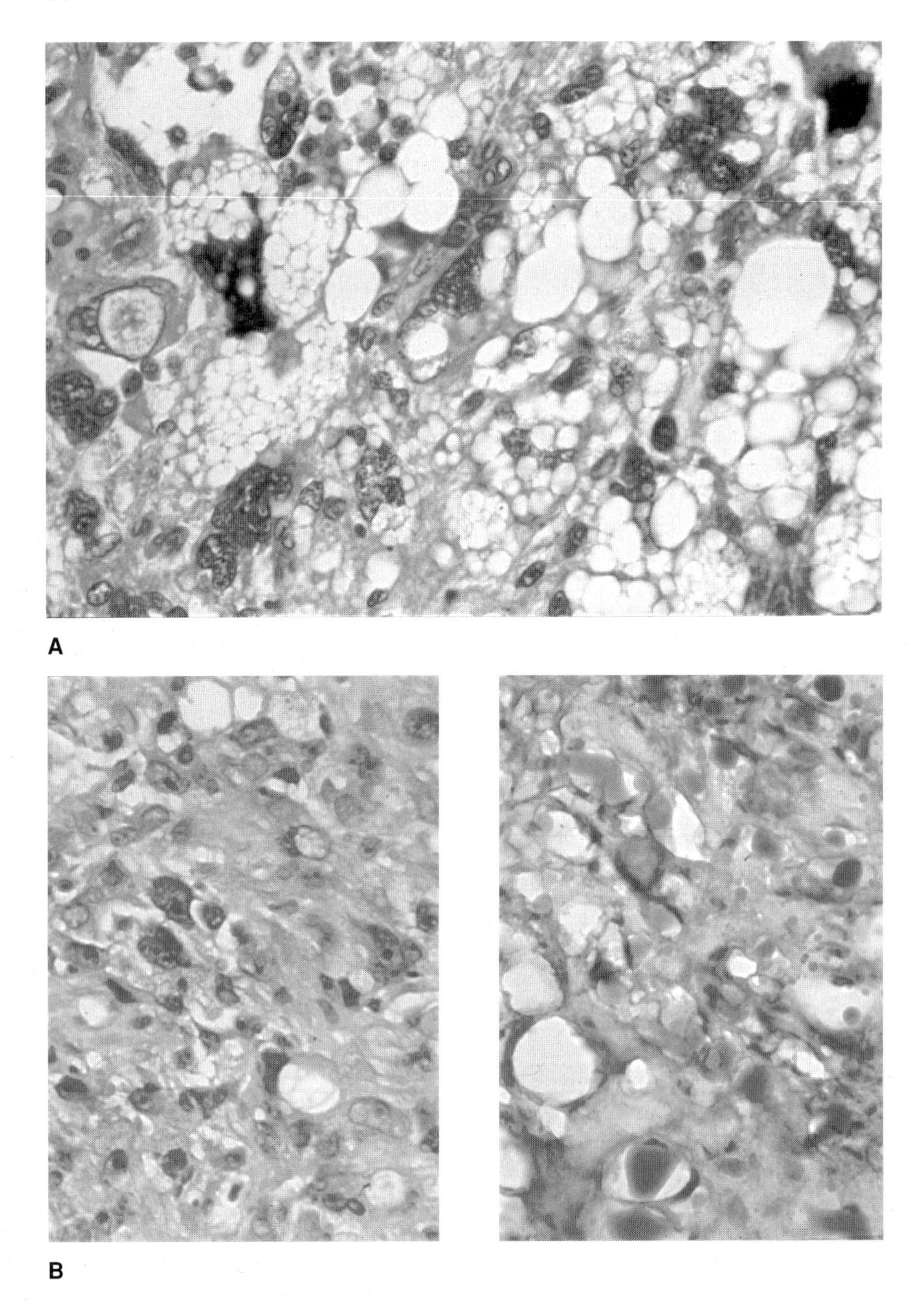

FIG. 35-21. Pleomorphic liposarcoma
(**A**) Multivacuolar lipoblasts with large, irregular hyperchromatic nuclei predominate in this example. (**B**) Univacuolar lipoblasts (*left*) have a cytoplasmic lipid content that can be revealed in a frozen section stained with oil red O (*right*).

cells are largely incapable of lipid accumulation. At least focal transition toward the myxoid variant, or, less frequently, a well-differentiated or pleomorphic subtype, is always present. As previously indicated, these transitions are central to the correct diagnosis of round cell liposarcoma. In general, when more than 25% of the cellular elements are round cells, the diagnosis of round cell liposarcoma should be made. However, any more than 5% round cell component in a myxoid liposarcoma portends a higher risk of metastasis or death from disease.[62]

Pleomorphic liposarcoma is characterized by a disorderly growth pattern, an extreme degree of cellular pleomorphism, and bizarre giant cells. Two histologic variants of pleomorphic liposarcoma have been described. The majority of pleomorphic liposarcomas display limited numbers of lipoblasts admixed with smaller, polygonal, round or spindle-shaped cells with eosinophilic cytoplasm. Mitotic figures are usually rare. In any given microscopic field lacking a lipoblast, the separation of this entity from the pleomorphic storiform variant of malignant fibrous histiocytoma is difficult if not impossible. The less common variant contains giant lipoblasts. These extremely large cells have numerous cytoplasmic lipid droplets of variable size (Fig. 35-21). Multinucleation and amphophilia of the cytoplasm causes these cells to have the appearance of atypical mulberry cells, so that the tumor is suggestive of a malignant hibernoma. No myogenic (skeletal and smooth) ultrastructural features, and expressed vimentin but not desmin or alpha-smooth muscle actin, are expected.[63] The histologic subgroups of pleomorphic liposarcoma have not been shown to have prognostic value, perhaps because of the limited number of cases available for study.

DNA flow analysis shows benign and low grade tumors to be diploid, and high-grade tumors to be generally aneuploid, regardless of histogenetic type.[64]

Differential Diagnosis. A poorly differentiated myxoid liposarcoma may contain very little lipid material. A lipid stain then often aids in the diagnosis. The demonstration of neutral lipid in cells with special stains (e.g., Sudan black, oil red O) on frozen sections of tumor tissue is insufficient for a diagnosis of liposarcoma unless lipoblasts are also found (Fig. 35-21B). Many other mesenchymal tumors and some carcinomas (e.g., of kidney and adrenal) routinely contain fat, as do tumors injured by ischemia or radiation.

The main utility of immunohistochemistry in the diagnosis of liposarcoma is one of exclusion, because no specific or useful immunohistochemical marker has been found for malignant fatty tumors. Immunohistochemistry can be quite helpful in revealing the true identities of various sarcomas that may contain vacuolated bizarre cells, such as malignant schwannoma (S-100 protein), rhabdomyosarcoma (myoglobin), and leiomyosarcoma (desmin). Alpha-1-antitrypsin and alpha-1-antichymotrypsin can be demonstrated in malignant fibrous histiocytoma regardless of subtype, and are constant and diagnostically useful characteristics. However, these markers may also be present in other spindle cell malignant tumors. For differentiation from benign lipoblastoma, a tumor that occurs in infancy and early childhood, see the section on Benign Lipoblastoma.

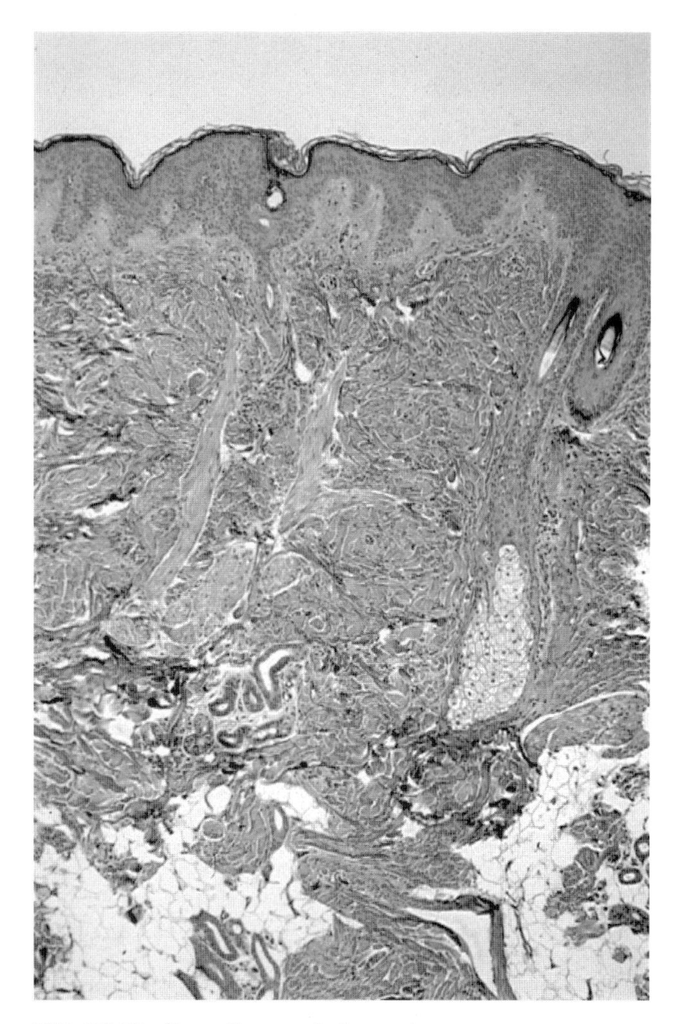

FIG. 35-22. Smooth muscle hamartoma
This lesion consists microscopically of numerous thick, long, straight, well-defined bundles of smooth muscle fibers extending in various directions throughout the dermis.

SMOOTH MUSCLE HAMARTOMA

Smooth muscle hamartoma usually presents as a single patch several centimeters in diameter, most commonly in the lumbar region. It may be present at birth or may arise in childhood or early adulthood.[65] Usually, there are small, follicular papules throughout the patch, although the entire lesion may be slightly elevated. The patch shows hyperpigmentation and hypertrichosis in some patients[66,67] but not in others.[68] If hyperpigmentation and hypertrichosis are present, an association with Becker's melanosis (Chap. 29) exists.[69] These two entities represent different poles of the same developmental spectrum of hamartomatous change.[67] There is no known associated systemic involvement or malignant transformation.[65]

Histopathology. Numerous thick, long, straight, well-defined bundles of smooth muscle fibers are scattered throughout the dermis and extend in various directions (Fig. 35-22). Smooth muscle bundles can be readily distinguished from collagen bundles by the trichrome stain, which stains smooth muscle red and collagen green or blue. In patients with hypertrichosis, some of the smooth muscle bundles show connections with large hair follicles.[66,69]

Differential Diagnosis. The arrangement of the smooth muscle bundles in the dermis differs from that observed in piloleiomyoma, in which the smooth muscle bundles form a large aggregate.

Pathogenesis. In fetal life, hair muscles originate in a diffuse metachromatic zone of the mesoderm, near but not part of the fibroepithelial hair germ. Overproduction in these pilar fields may lead to stable hamartomatous overgrowths or progressive neoplasms.[70]

LEIOMYOMA

Five types of leiomyomas of the skin are: (1) multiple piloleiomyomas and (2) solitary piloleiomyomas, both arising from arrectores pilorum muscles; (3) solitary genital leiomyomas, arising from the dartoic, vulvar, or mammillary muscles; (4) solitary angioleiomyomas, arising from the muscles of veins; and (5) leiomyomas with additional mesenchymal elements.

Multiple piloleiomyomas, by far the most common type of leiomyoma, are small, firm, red or brown intradermal nodules arranged in a group or in a linear pattern. Often, two or more areas are affected. Usually, but not always, the lesions are tender and give rise spontaneously to occasional attacks of pain.[70]

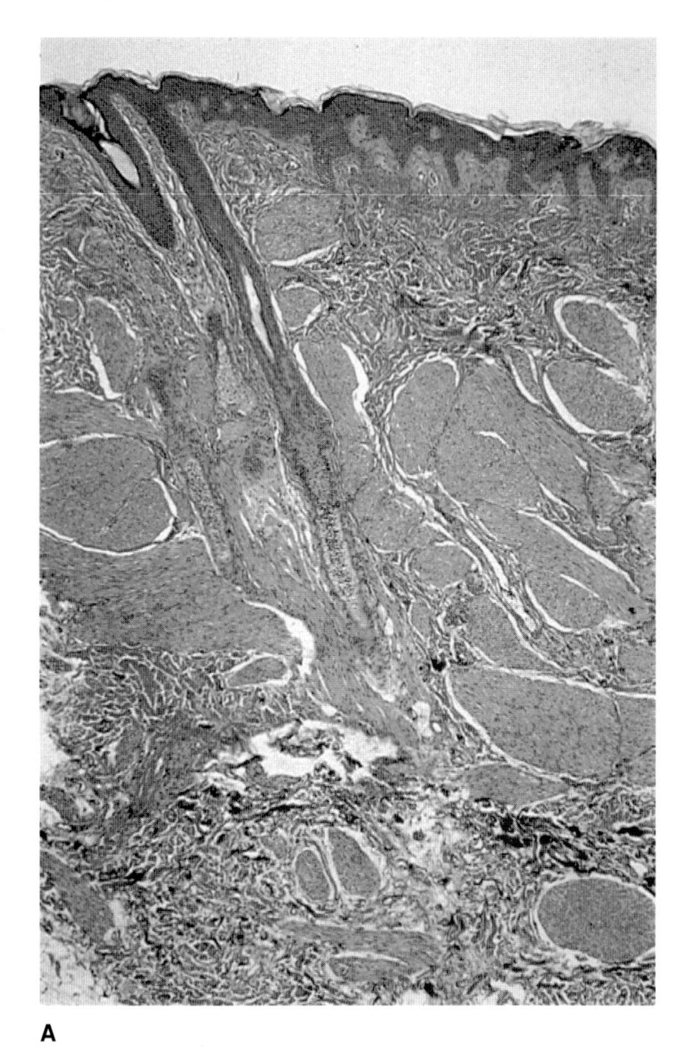

A

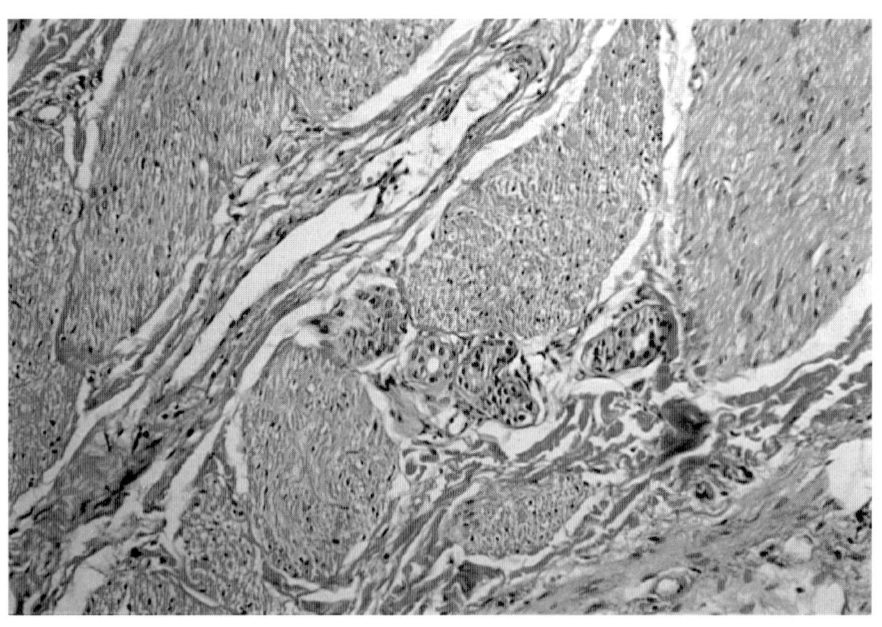

B

FIG. 35-23. Piloleiomyoma
(**A**) Bundles of smooth muscle interlace around follicular structures in the dermis. (**B**) Well-defined smooth muscle bundles resembling pilar muscles surround sweat gland coils.

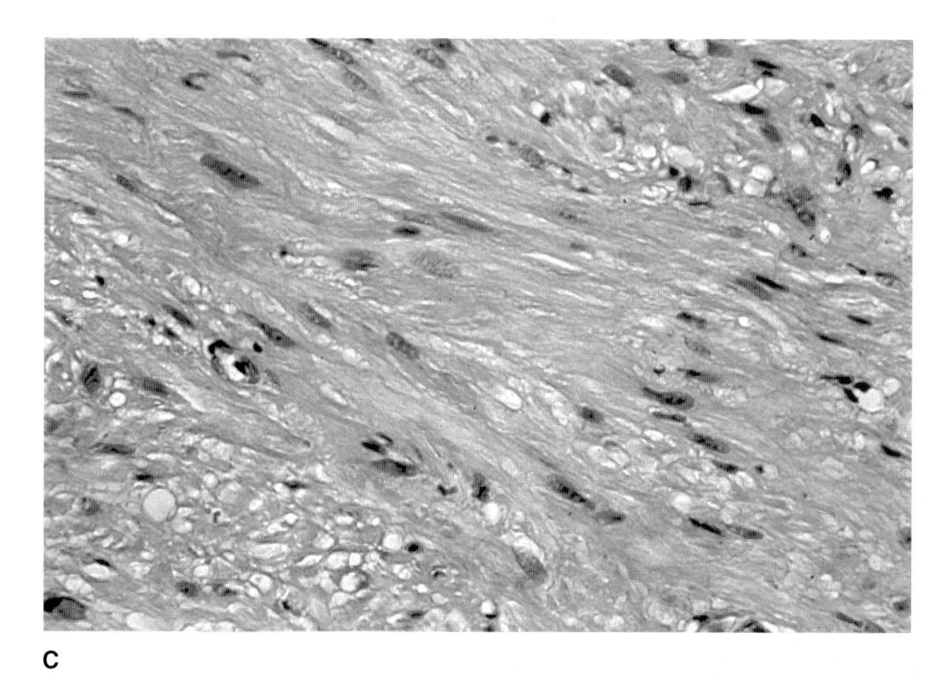

C

FIG. 35-23. *Continued*
(**C**) Benign smooth muscle cells have some variation in nuclear size and chromaticity, blunt nuclear ends, and no conspicuous mitotic activity.

Solitary piloleiomyomas are intradermal nodules that are usually larger than those of multiple piloleiomyomas, measuring up to 2 cm in diameter. Most of them are tender and also occasionally painful.[71]

Solitary genital leiomyomas are located on the scrotum, the labia majora, or, rarely, the nipples. Their location is intradermal. In contrast to the other leiomyomas, most genital leiomyomas are asymptomatic.[71]

Solitary angioleiomyomas are usually subcutaneous and only rarely intracutaneous in location. As a rule, they do not exceed 4 cm in diameter. The lower extremities are the most common site. Pain and tenderness are evoked by most, but not all, angioleiomyomas.[70]

Histopathology. Piloleiomyomas, whether multiple or solitary, and genital leiomyomas are similar in histologic appearance.[71] They are poorly demarcated and are composed of interlacing bundles of smooth muscle fibers with which varying amounts of collagen bundles are intermingled (Fig. 35-23). The muscle fibers composing the smooth muscle bundles are generally straight, with little or no waviness; they contain centrally located, thin, very long, blunt-edged, "eel-like" nuclei.

The muscle bundles stain pink with hematoxylin-eosin, just as collagen does, but can be distinguished from collagen bundles by the following differences in the appearance. The nuclei of the fibroblasts located in the collagen are shorter than the nuclei located in the smooth muscle fibers and show tapering at their ends whereas smooth muscle nuclei tend to have blunt ends; the cytoplasm of the smooth muscle cell is more conspicuous than in quiescent fibroblasts. In contrast to collagen bundles, smooth muscle bundles usually show slight vacuolization, especially in cross sections, as a result of a perinuclear clear zone.[71] Reliable differentiation between muscle and collagen bundles is possible with the aid of one of the collagen stains, such as the aniline blue stain or the trichrome stain. With the aniline blue stain, muscle stains red and collagen blue; with the trichrome stain, muscle stains dark red and collagen green or blue. Longitudinal intracytoplasmic myofibrils often can be visualized as striations in H&E sections and can be more easily resolved if stained with phosphotungstic acid–hematoxylin, where they appear as purple threads.

Angioleiomyomas differ from the other types of leiomyomas in that they are encapsulated and contain numerous vessels (Fig. 35-24A). As a rule, they contain only small amounts of collagen. The numerous veins that are present vary in size and have muscular walls of varying thickness. On this basis, angioleiomyomas have been subdivided into a capillary or solid type, a cavernous type, and a venous type.[72] In the capillary type, the vascular channels are numerous but small. Tumors of the cavernous type are composed of dilated vascular channels with small amounts of smooth muscle. Tumors of the venous type exhibit veins with thick muscular walls. In venous tumors, smooth muscle cells extend tangentially from the peripheries of the veins and merge with the intervascular tumor substance (Fig. 35-24B). The veins usually have a rounded or slitlike lumen, but some, because of contraction of their muscular tissue, have a stellate lumen. The veins have no elastic lamina. Areas of mucinous alteration are often present, especially in large angioleiomyomas.

Lipoleiomyomas comprise long, intersecting bundles of bland, smooth muscle mixed with the additional mesenchymal element of nests of mature fat cells.[73]

Cutaneous angiolipoleiomyoma could arguably be considered an angioleiomyoma with fat cell modulation. However, elastic lamina completely or partially rim the vascular channels, and the lesion has a strong male rather than female predilection.[74] It is a rare acquired asymptomatic tumor, always acral, and independent of signs of tuberous sclerosis or renal angiomyolipoma. These subcutaneous, well-circumscribed tu-

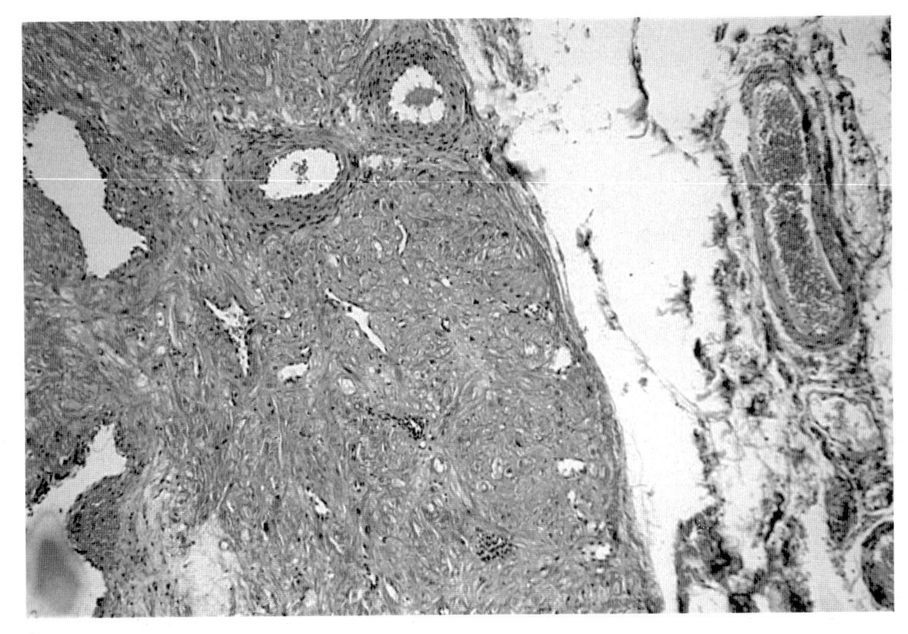

A

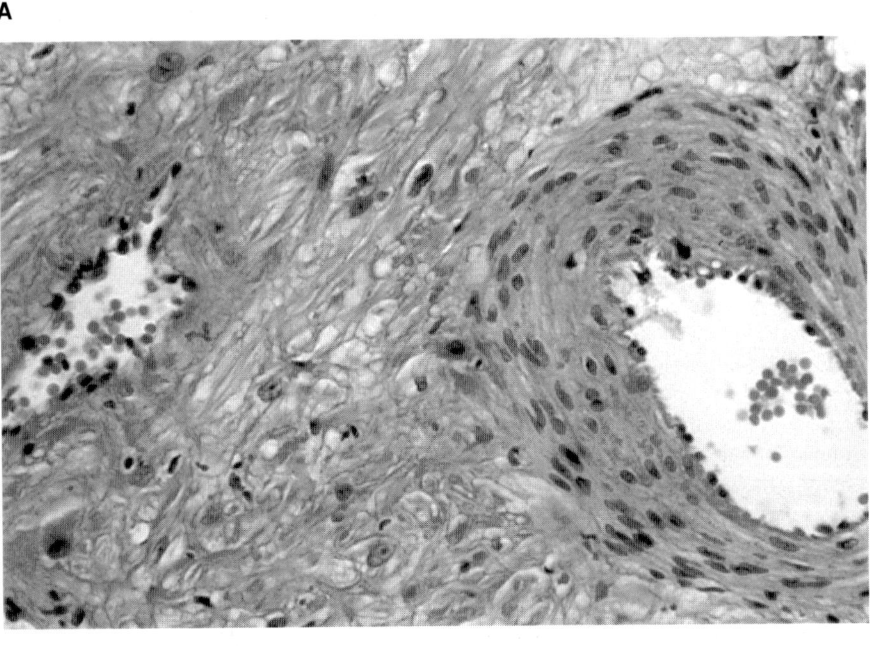

B

FIG. 35-24. Angioleiomyoma
(**A**) A medium-magnification view shows the well-circumscribed border of a subcutaneous nodule containing prominent blood vessels and comprised of cells with copious eosinophilic cytoplasm. (**B**) At higher magnification, the blood vessel walls seem continuous with the benign smooth muscle cells comprising the tumor substance.

mors are composed of smooth muscle, vascular spaces, connective tissue, and mature fat.

Differential Diagnosis. A trichrome stain is useful in differentiating angiolipoleiomyomas from angiolipomas with increased fibrous tissue. Arteriovenous hemangiomas in the subcutaneous tissues may have vascular spaces of both arterial and venous types associated with areas that resemble capillary or cavernous hemangioma. Arteriovenous hemangioma can be excluded because it is not circumscribed, lacks a fibrous pseudocapsule, and lacks fascicles of smooth muscle intermixed with lipocytes. Subcutaneous cavernous hemangiomas may also occur, but the vascular spaces are larger, the vessel walls are thinner, the tissue surrounding the vessels lacks fascicles of smooth muscle, and the tumor lacks a fibrous pseudocapsule.

Pathogenesis. Electron microscopic examination has shown that piloleiomyomas are composed of normal-appearing smooth muscle cells. Each of these cells has a central nucleus surrounded by an area containing endoplasmic reticulum and mitochondria and, peripheral to this area, numerous myofilaments arranged in bundles. Both cytoplasmic and marginal dense bodies are present.

The cause of the frequent pain or tenderness has not been satisfactorily determined. Some authors have observed, by electron microscopy, damage to nerve fibers through distortion and disruption of the myelin sheath and regard this damage as the cause.[75] Others, however, have observed only scanty unmyelinated nerve fibers.[76] It is probable, therefore, that the pain is a result of muscular contractions.

LEIOMYOSARCOMA

Cutaneous leiomyosarcomas are believed to derive from the erector pili muscles, which are smooth muscles that surround sweat glands in the nearby adipose tissue at or below the junction of the cutis and subcutis, and also from vascular tissue.[77] They are most common in the fifth and sixth decades and are two to three times more likely to occur in males than in females.[78] These tumors account for 2% to 3% of all soft tissue sarcomas. In 1992, less than 125 cases of cutaneous and subcutaneous leiomyosarcoma could be found in the English literature.[79] Because of their different prognoses, it is important to distinguish between cutaneous and subcutaneous leiomyosarcomas and superficial leiomyosarcomas of the genital areas.[80]

Cutaneous leiomyosarcomas exhibit a predilection for extremity extensor surface location,[81] which coincide with the areas of greatest hair distribution. There is usually a solitary red-pink nodule that may be painful or tender[70] but only rarely ulcerates. In some cases, several nodules are present,[77] but this should arouse suspicion of metastases—for example, from a retroperitoneal, uterine, or alimentary tract primary.[82] Origination in an ectopic areola has been reported.[83] Cutaneous leiomyosarcomas have a good prognosis. Metastases to regional lymph nodes may occur, but they are not usually fatal.[79] In at least one reported instance, however, distant metastases ultimately led to the death of the patient.[82]

Subcutaneous leiomyosarcomas have a guarded prognosis. They manifest themselves as subcutaneous nodules or diffuse swellings over which the nondiscolored skin usually is freely movable. They cause pain of a local or radiating nature in only a few patients. They may cause hematogenous metastases, especially to the lungs, and lead to death in about one-third of the patients.[78] Purely subcutaneous leiomyosarcomas must be differentiated from leiomyosarcomas involving skeletal muscle or fascia, which are nearly always fatal.[84,85]

Vulvar and scrotal leiomyosarcomas tend to be larger and better circumscribed than those in skin or subcutaneous locations. Their traditional inclusion under the general heading of cutaneous leiomyosarcoma has been challenged.[80,84]

Histopathology. Cutaneous leiomyosarcomas (Fig. 35-25) vary from moderately well to poorly delimited intradermal tumors that may extend into the subcutaneous tissue. In the center, the tumor shows nodular aggregates and densely packed, interlacing bundles of smooth muscle cells. At the margin of the tumor, strands of smooth muscle cells extend between collagen bundles. Cutaneous leiomyosarcomas, with their fascicular, infiltrative, peripheral growth pattern, presumably are derived from arrectores pilorum muscles.[78] Minimal criteria for malignancy in a well-differentiated lesion include crowded cellularity, some plump and hyperchromatic nuclei constituting cellular atypia, and a few mitoses (Fig. 35-25B). Areas of lesser differentiation are present in all tumors, although to varying degrees. They show numerous irregularly shaped, anaplastic nuclei and usually also atypical giant cells with bizarre nuclei (Fig. 35-25C).[78] Still, the nature of the sarcoma usually can be established even in rather anaplastic tumors, because in some areas there are bundles of fairly well-differentiated smooth muscle cells in which delicate myofibrils can be revealed by staining with phosphotungstic acid–hematoxylin[78] or trichrome. The number of mitoses may be high in anaplastic areas even when there will be no metastases.[85] When confined to the dermis, the sarcoma may recur in up to half of all cases.

Subcutaneous leiomyosarcomas[86] are deemed to be vascular in origin and analogous to angioleiomyomas. Radiation dermatitis may be a substrate.[87] The de novo tumor may be well-circumscribed and partially surrounded by a compressed rim of connective tissue. Irregular aggregates of more or less atypical smooth muscle cells can be seen intertwining haphazardly without the fascicular pattern characteristic of cutaneous leiomyosarcomas. Subcutaneous leiomyosarcomas show endothelium-lined, thin-walled blood vessels with variously shaped but often large lumina surrounded by smooth muscle cells.[78] Mitoses should be easily found.[85] No correlation seems to exist between the degree of histologic malignancy of the tumor and metastases, which occur in up to 40% of the cases.[84] DNA content, as determined by flow cytometry, was a strong predictor of metastatic potential in one study.[88] Involvement of underlying muscular fasciae or skeletal muscle is a likely harbinger of metastases.[84]

Pathogenesis. Immunohistochemical staining of deparaffinized sections shows expression of desmin in all cutaneous leiomyosarcomas and of muscle-specific actin in the great majority.[82] Only about half of the subcutaneous leiomyosarcomas show significant numbers of tumor cells that are positive for desmin and actin.[84] These smooth muscle markers may be demonstrated in "myofibroblastic" lesions and therefore are not absolute diagnostic criteria. Some hold that ultrastructural study is a more reliable means for definite identification. Positivity for cytokeratin may be found and is attributed to "phenotypic shift" in terms of vimentin and cytokeratin expression for the supposed muscle of origin.[89]

Electron microscopic examination has shown that the tumor cells have the characteristics of smooth muscle cells even when there is marked nuclear atypicality.[85] Thus, the tumor cells show skeins of intermediate filaments punctuated by dense bodies, subplasmalemmal plaques, pinocytotic vesicles, and external pericellular lamina.[81,85] However, in some instances the basal lamina is discontinuous.[82]

Differential Diagnosis. The presence of bizarre giant cells in cutaneous leiomyosarcomas may cause a resemblance to malignant fibrous histiocytoma.[85] However, at least in some areas, there are greatly elongated, thin, blunt-ended nuclei characteristic of smooth muscle cells. Also, demonstration of the enhancement of longitudinal striation due to myofibrils by staining with trichrome or phosphotungstic acid–hematoxylin will aid in the differentiation. The same holds true for subcutaneous leiomyosarcomas, in which the presence of endothelial-lined vessels may suggest a hemangiopericytoma.

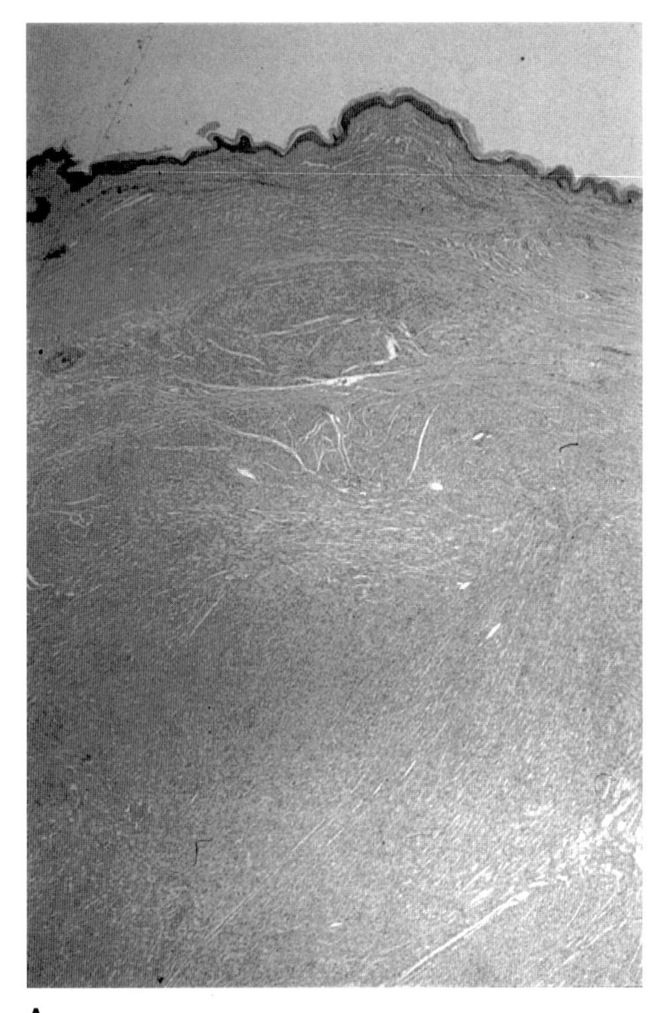

A

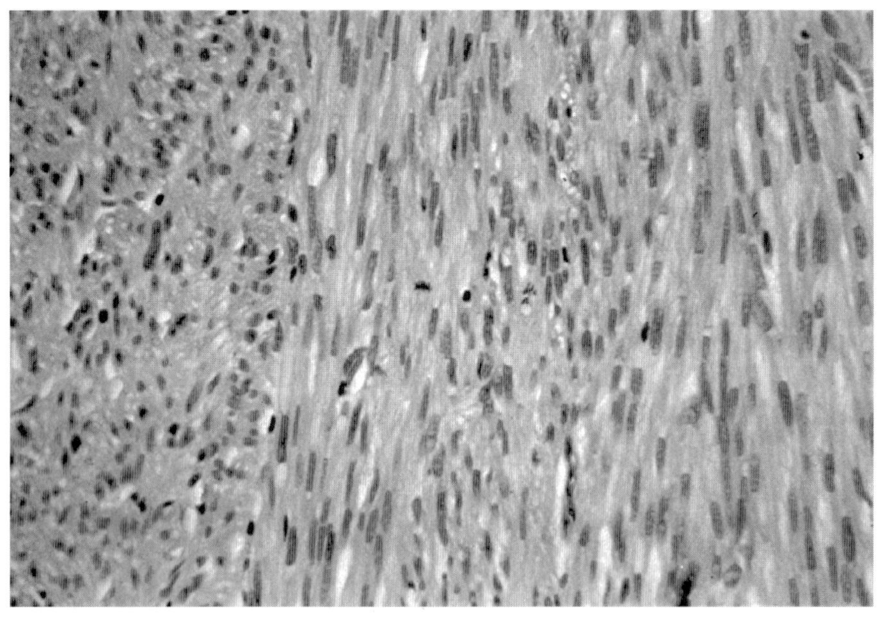

B

FIG. 35-25. Leiomyosarcoma (**A**) A low-magnification view presents a poorly circumscribed lobulated dermal tumor. (**B**) A higher-magnification view of the well-differentiated leiomyosarcoma shown in part A indicates that it is comprised of minimally atypical smooth muscle cells with elongate blunt nuclei but a high mitotic rate.

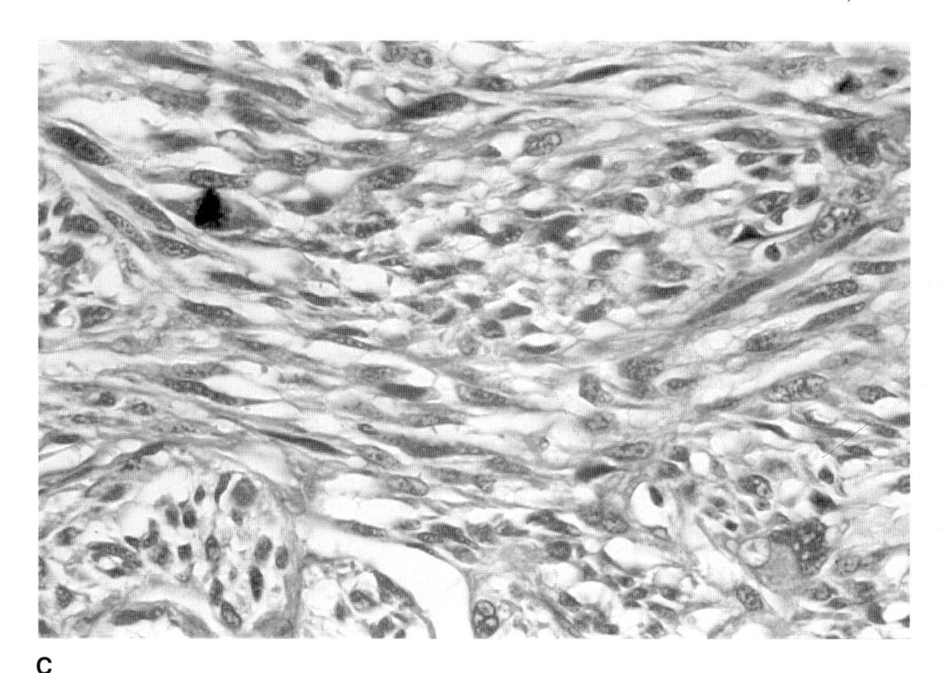
C

FIG. 35-25. *Continued*
(**C**) Another case presents considerable cellular pleomorphism and abnormal mitotic activity. The longitudinally striated eosinophilic cytoplasm characteristic of smooth muscle cells is retained. (Courtesy of Jeffrey C. Warner.)

RHABDOMYOMA

Rhabdomyomas are extremely rare benign tumors of striated muscle[90] that can be subtyped on the basis of clinical and morphologic differences. *Adult-type rhabdomyomas* are slowly growing lesions that nearly always occur in the head and neck areas of older persons (Fig. 35-26). *Fetal-type rhabdomyomas* occur in the head and neck areas of children and adults. *Genital-type rhabdomyomas* are polypoidal tumor masses in the vaginas and vulva of middle-aged women. *Rhabdomyomatous mesenchymal hamartomas* present as polypoid striated muscle proliferation in the periorbital and perioral regions of infants and young children.

RHABDOMYOSARCOMA

Although rare in adults, rhabdomyosarcomas are the most common soft tissue sarcomas in children. Most of these tumors are located in intramuscular locations, and involvement of the skin is rare. Skeletal muscle in skin occurs only in the face. Only a few rhabdomyosarcomas presenting as dermal nodules[91] or subcutaneous indurations have been reported.

Histopathology. Rhabdomyosarcomas often exhibit a low degree of differentiation so that their identification requires immunohistochemical studies (Fig. 35-27). Only some of these tumors contain cells recognizable as rhabdomyoblasts by virtue of their cytoplasm exhibiting cross-striation that is best revealed by phosphotungstic acid–hematoxylin staining.[91] Round cells of the embryonal variant, unlike those of lymphoma, neuroblastoma, trabecular carcinoma, and Ewing's sarcoma, tend to have cytoplasmic rims that are stained red by trichrome. Some tumors show alveolar spaces lined with small, round, neoplastic cells and with tumor cells floating within these spaces (alveolar rhabdomyosarcoma) (Fig. 35-28A).[91,92] Cells with elongated eosinophilic cytoplasm, so-called "strap cells," are suggestive but not diagnostic of rhabdomyosarcoma[92] and may be found in the pleomorphic type (Fig. 35-28B).

Histogenesis. Immunohistochemical studies of deparaffinized tissue may show undifferentiated cells to be positive only for vimentin, indicating a mesenchymal origin. More-differentiated cells may be positive for desmin and myoglobin, which is indicative of muscular differentiation.[91,92]

CUTANEOUS OSSIFICATION

Cutaneous bone formation may be primary or secondary. If it is primary, there is no preceding cutaneous lesion; if it is secondary, bone forms through metaplasia within a preexisting lesion. Primary cutaneous ossification can occur in Albright's hereditary osteodystrophy and as osteoma cutis.

Albright's Hereditary Osteodystrophy

In Albright's hereditary osteodystrophy (AHO), first described in 1952,[93] multiple areas of subcutaneous or intracutaneous ossification are often encountered (Fig. 35-29). These areas may be present at birth or may arise later in life. No definite area of predilection seems to exist; areas of ossification have been described on the trunk,[94] on the extremities,[95] and on the scalp.[96] The areas of ossification may be so small as to be hardly perceptible or as large as 5 cm in diameter.[97] Those located in the skin may cause ulceration, and bony spicules may be extruded through the ulcer.[95] In addition to cutaneous and subcutaneous osteomas, bone formation may be observed in some cases along fascial planes.[97]

AHO includes the syndromes of pseudohypoparathyroidism and pseudopseudohypoparathryoidism. Patients with the former

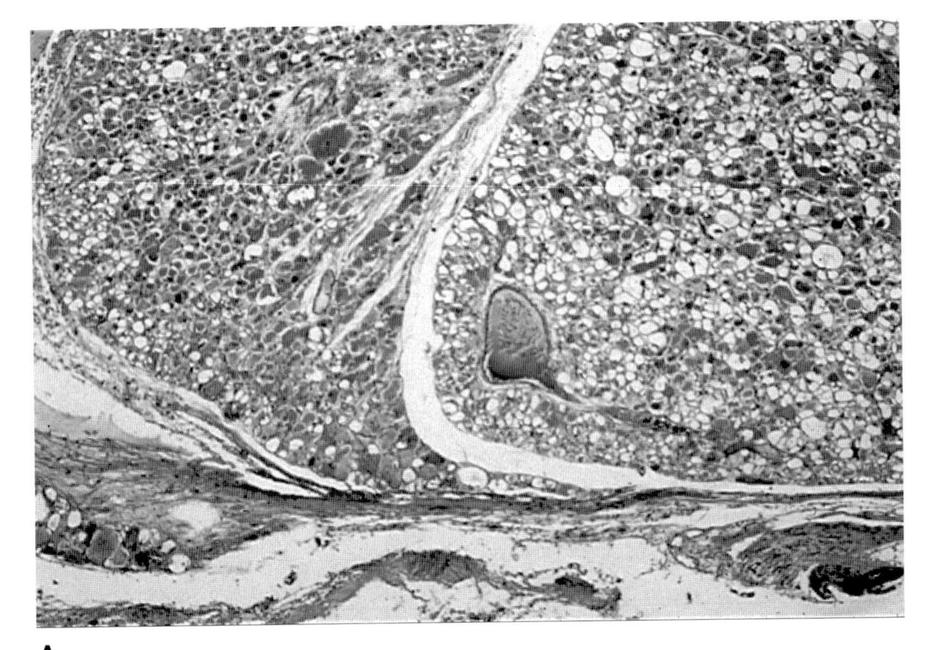

A

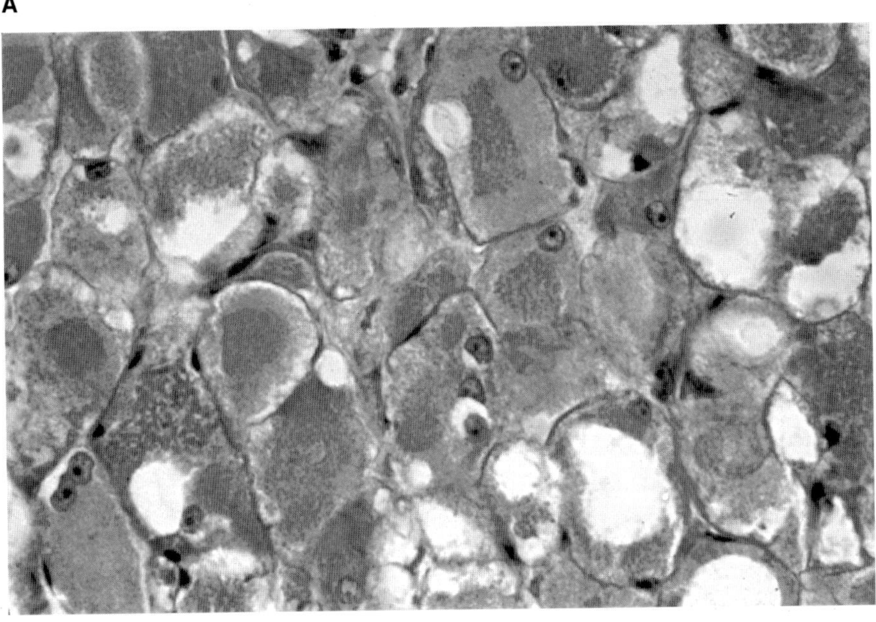

B

FIG. 35-26. Adult-type rhabdomyoma (55-year-old male with 4-cm lateral neck mass)
(**A**) This lobulated tumor resembles hibernoma under low-magnification examination. (**B**) Variably sized, deeply eosinophilic polygonal cells comprising this tumor have peripherally situated nuclei and occasional intracellular vacuoles. Cytoplasmic cross- striations may be seen. Removal of intracellular glycogen results in the pronounced vacuolated appearance of many of the cells. This lesion should not be mistaken for a granular cell tumor (myoblastoma).

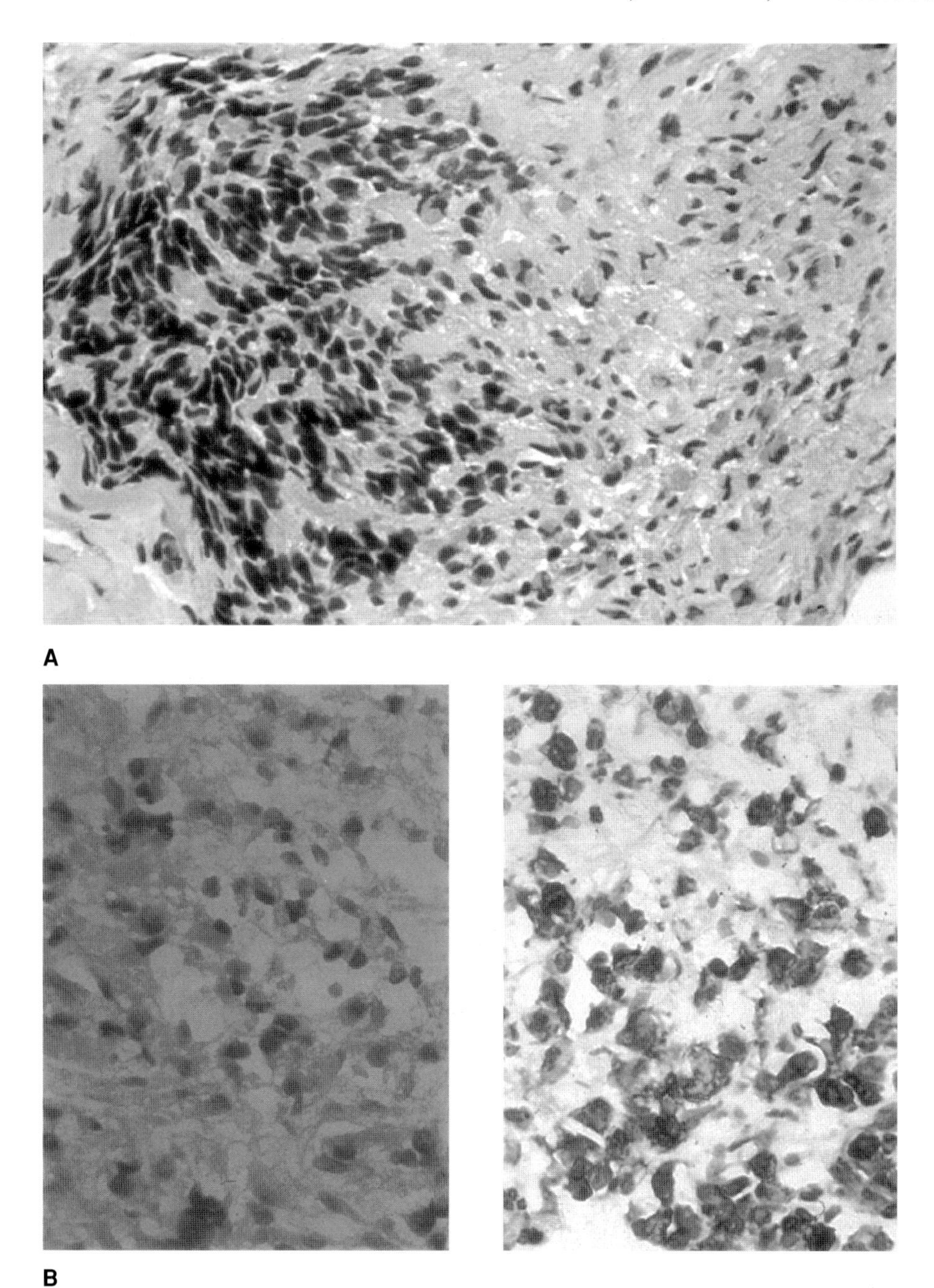

FIG. 35-27. Embryonal rhabdomyosarcoma (49-year-old male with 3-cm mass in foot)
(**A**) An undifferentiated round cell pattern (*left*) grades into a region where tumor cells acquire a small amount of eosinophilic cytoplasm (*right*). (**B**) An H&E view (left) of a tumor cell region where cells have acquired myoplasm is compared with a positive immunoperoxidase reaction for desmin in the same region (*right*).

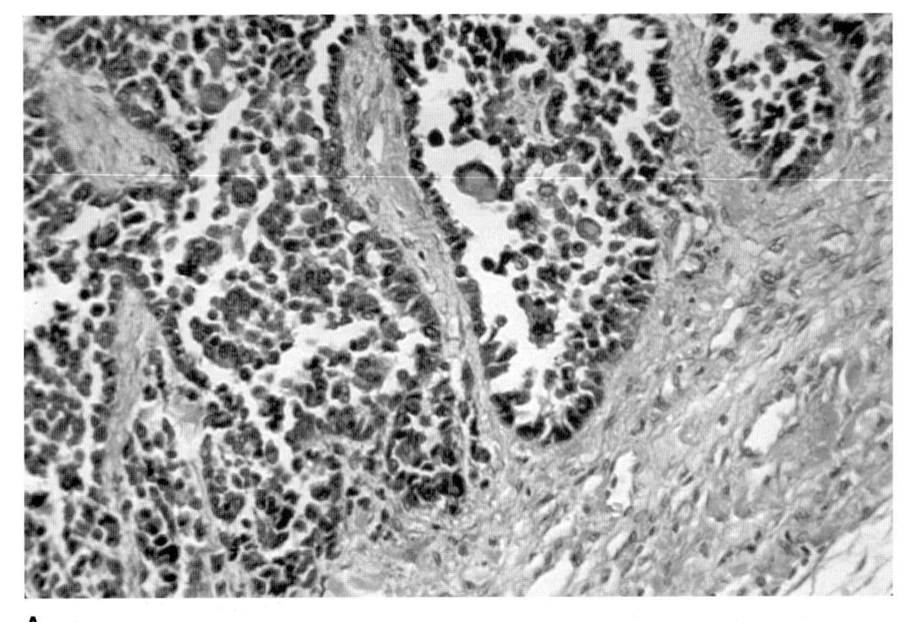

A

B

FIG. 35-28. Other rhabdomyosarcoma variants
(**A**) Alveolar rhabdomyosarcoma is comprised of rounded cells with eosinophilic cytoplasmic rims, lining spaces that contain similar or larger tumor cells. (**B**) Round, "tadpole," and strap-shaped rhabdomyoblasts occur with atypical mitoses in pleomorphic rhabdomyosarcoma. The differential diagnosis would include liposarcoma and malignant fibrous histiocytoma.

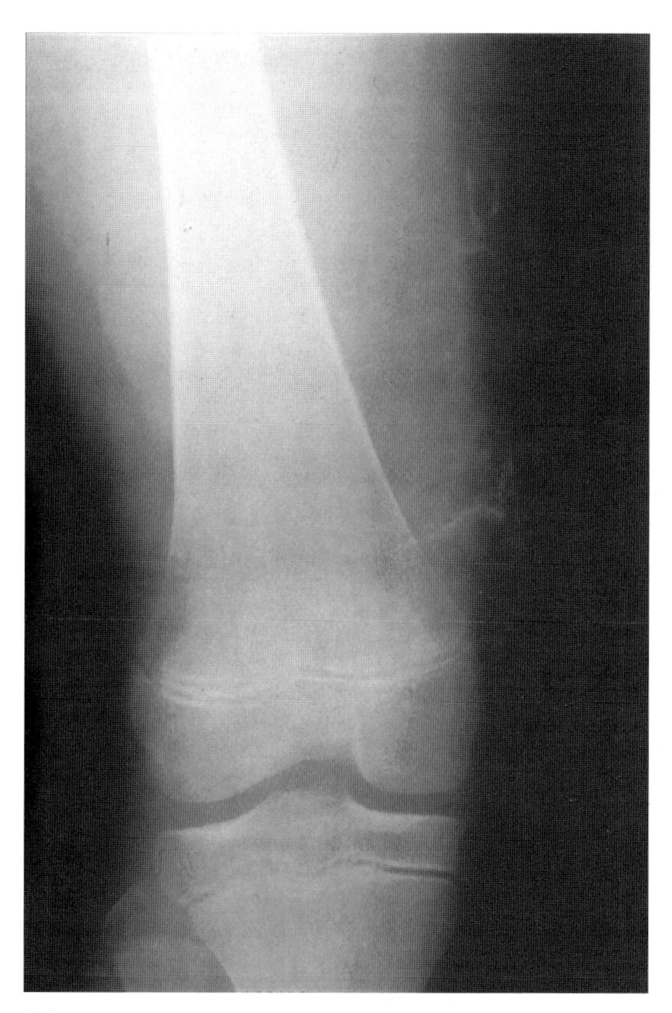

FIG. 35-29. Heterotopic ossification in pseudohypoparathyroidism
A plain film radiograph of a juvenile's thigh features irregular branching spicules and cords of bone in dermis and subcutaneous tissue medial to the femur.

condition have hypocalcemia with a failure to respond to parathyroid hormone, whereas patients with the latter syndrome fail to respond to parathyroid hormone but have normal serum calcium values.[97] Patients with AHO have short stature, round facies, and multiple skeletal abnormalities, such as curvature of the radius and shortening of some of the metacarpal bones.[97] As a result of this shortening, some knuckles are absent when the fists are clenched, and depressions or dimples are apparent there instead. This important diagnostic sign is referred to as the Albright dimpling sign.

Additional manifestations include basal ganglia calcification and mental retardation. The mode of inheritance is dominant, possibly X-linked dominant.[97]

Histopathology. Spicules of bone of various sizes may be found within the dermis[96] or in the subcutaneous tissue.[97,98] The bone contains fairly numerous osteocytes as well as cement lines that are best revealed with a strong (e.g., Harris) hematoxylin or in polarized light. In addition, osteoblasts with elongated nuclei can usually be seen along the margins of the bone where new bone is being laid down. Osteoclasts, if present, are cells with multiple large nuclei resembling multinucleated foreign-body giant cells but are distinguished by their attachment to a bone surface. They excavate surface pits called Howship's lacunae into the bone substance as the initial step in remodeling. Osteons with haversian canals containing blood vessels and connective tissue are produced through internal remodeling and indicate the passage of significant time.

The spicules of bone may enclose, either partially or completely, areas of mature fat cells,[97] which represents the maturation of the lesion with establishment of a medullary cavity. Hematopoietic elements, however, are observed only rarely among the fat cells.

Pathogenesis. The osteoblasts that form bone in primary cutaneous ossification originate in preexisting fibrous connective tissue, and thus their product is termed *intramembranous* rather than *enchondral* bone.

The incidence of cutaneous ossification in AHO is fairly high. It has been estimated that cutaneous ossification is found in 42% of the patients with pseudohypoparathyroidism and in 27% of those with pseudopseudohypoparathyroidism.[99] However, the reason for the bone formation is not clear.

Because the association of AHO with cutaneous ossification was not recognized until 1965,[100] the question arises as to how many cases of primary cutaneous ossification reported before then occurred in association with AHO. In a review examining this question,[98] several cases originally reported as primary osteoma of the skin were recognized as showing evidence of AHO.[95] Although the conclusion that most cases of primary osteoma cutis are associated with AHO seems somewhat exaggerated, it is nevertheless apparent that patients with extensive foci of ossification usually have AHO.

Differential Diagnosis. Progressive osseous heteroplasia (POH)[101] is a disease of females that is clinically distinguishable from AHO and fibrodysplasia (myositis) ossificans progressiva (FOP). The initial skin involvement tends to be plaque-like or papulovesicular rash or reddened in duration,with dermal ossification. Unlike in AHO, deeper connective tissues become ossified. Also, the endocrine disturbances are lacking. Unlike in FOP, the disturbance is asymmetrical and random. In FOP, cartilage production precedes ossification of deeper tissues (enchondral ossification), whereas the predominant pathway of bone formation in POH and AHO is intramembranous.

Osteoma Cutis

The term *osteoma cutis* is applied to cases of primary cutaneous ossification in which there is no evidence of AHO in either the patients or their families.

Apparently, there are four groups of patients with osteoma cutis, with the osteomas limited in extent in all but the first group. The four groups are (1) patients with *widespread osteomas* since birth or early life but without evidence of Albright's hereditary osteodystrophy[102]; (2) patients with *single, large, plaquelike osteomas* present since birth either in the skin of the scalp[103,104] or in the skin or subcutaneous tissue of an extremity[105]; (3) patients with *single small osteomas* arising in later life in various locations[105] and in some instances showing transepidermal elimination of bony fragments; and (4) patients with *multiple miliary osteomas of the face.* In (all of them women) some instances, the osteomas do not appear until late in life.[106] In others, they are observed in young women in association with longstanding acne

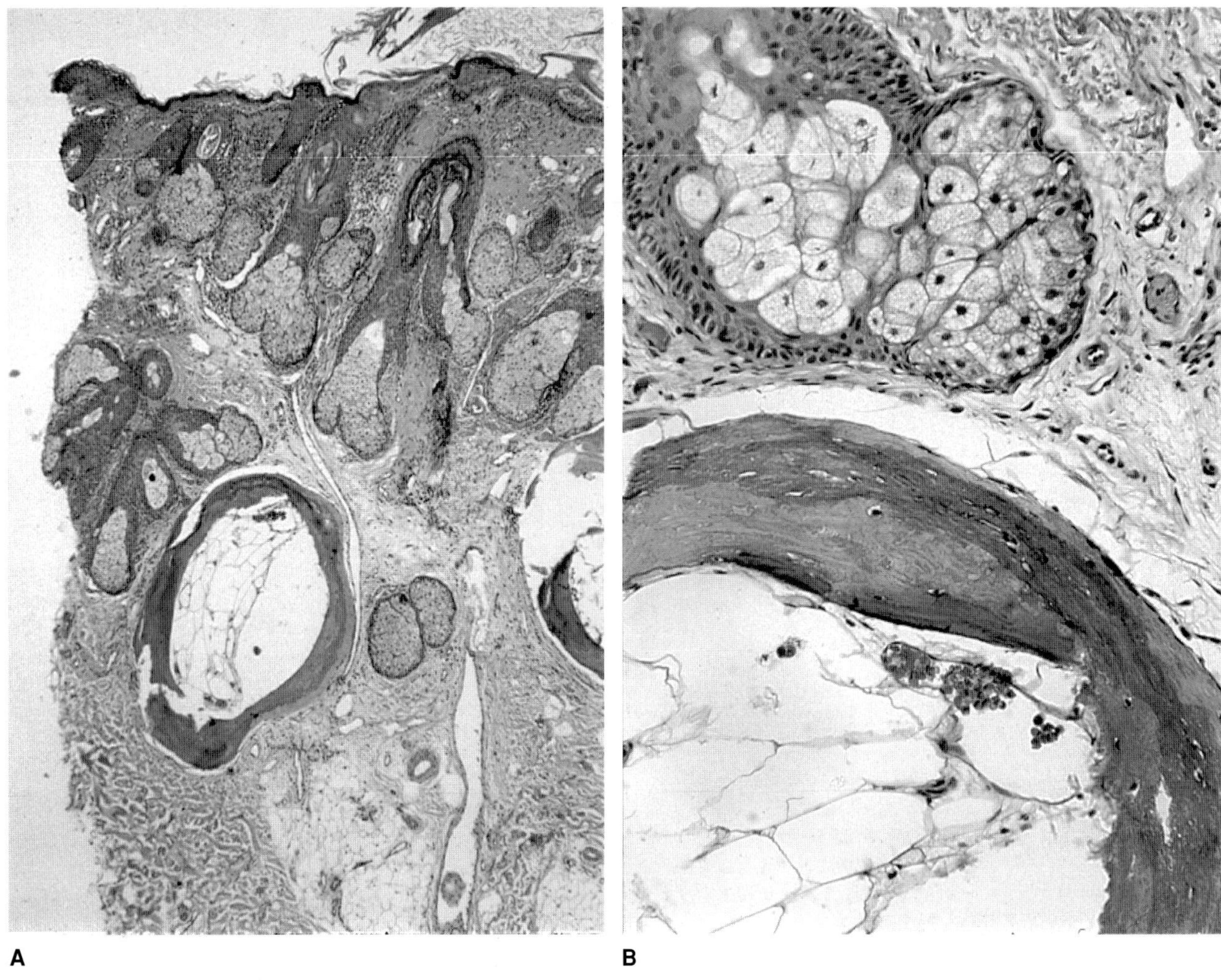

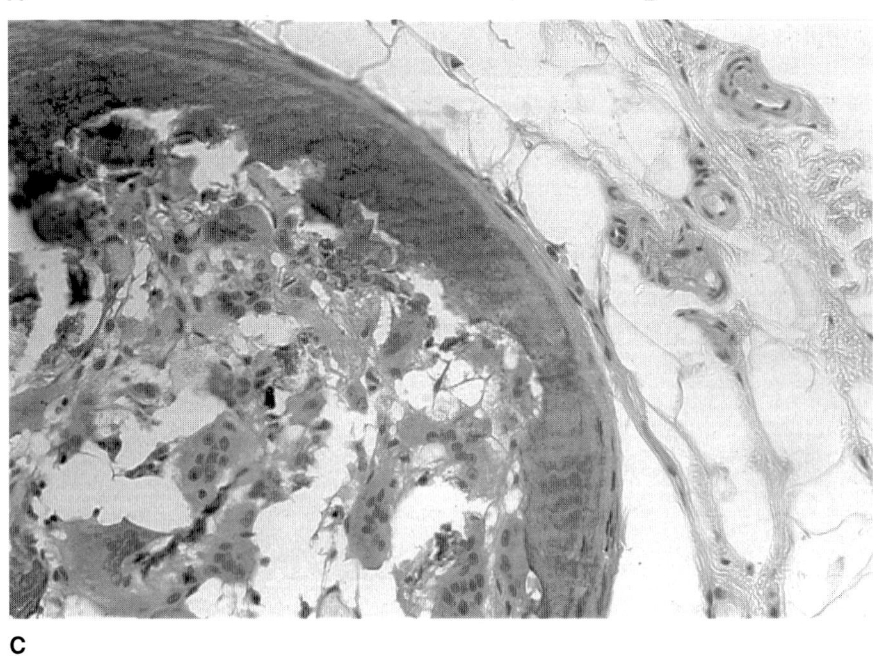

FIG. 35-30. Osteoma cutis
(**A**) Beneath an actinic keratosis is a rounded ossicle with fatty marrow in lower dermis. The edge of a second ossicle is shown at the right. (**B**) Higher-magnification view of field in part A shows the rounded cortex of compact bone and a vascularized fatty marrow. (**C**) Small, incidentally found dermal ossicles generally start out as solid, rounded particles that enlarge by slow peripheral apposition of lamellar bone. Osteoclastic remodeling activity may appear in the center, as indicated in this view, hollowing it out and making room for fatty marrow.

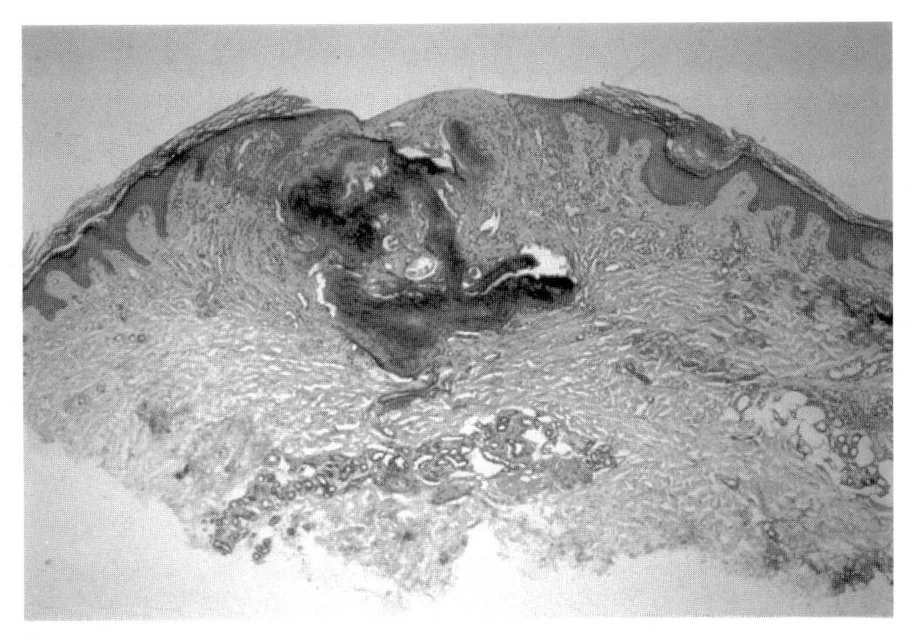

D

FIG. 35-30. ***Continued***
(**D**) Dermal ossicles may be eliminated like foreign bodies through surface ulceration (49-year-old male with focal leg ulceration).

vulgaris.[107–109] In the latter cases, the miliary osteomas have been interpreted as metaplastic ossification within acne scars. However, the absence of acne vulgaris among the patients in the older age group and the presence in one case of miliary osteomas also in the scalp, where acne does not occur,[106] raise the possibility that the acne vulgaris is coincidental.

Histopathology. The histologic findings in osteoma cutis are the same as in primary cutaneous ossification occurring in conjunction with Albright's hereditary osteodystrophy. Small foci of ossification within the dermis or stroma in other lesions, such as melanocytic nevi, are formed by the activities of flattened osteoblasts that appear to be derived through modulation from dermal fibroblasts (Fig. 35-30). A minority of the formative cells persist to be included in the osseous product as indigenous osteocytes. Continued bone application at the surface creates an enlarging dermal ossicle that eventually incurs central remodeling, beginning with osteoclast erosion (Fig. 35-30C). A circular outline is commonly achieved, and central hollowing creates a space for fatty marrow. In cases with transepidermal elimination, some patients show fragments of bone within channels lined by epidermis and leading to the surface, and others show such fragments within breaks in the epidermis (Fig. 35-30D). A sinus tract draining an osteomyelitis or septic joint should enter the differential.

Pathogenesis. In situ hybridization techniques indicate that, given appropriate stimulation, indigenous fibroblasts have the ability to modulate into osteoblastic cells (see Fig. 35-1) that have the same properties as those of osteoblasts, such as high alkaline phosphatase activity and a high expression of osteonectin.[110] In multiple miliary osteoma cutis, a dynamic bone study using a tetracycline double-labeling technique demonstrated a high rate of internal remodeling.[111]

METAPLASTIC OSSIFICATION

Metaplastic or secondary ossification occurs within a preexisting lesion. It may be observed in association with cutaneous tumors, scars, or inflammatory processes.

Histopathology. The tumor that most commonly shows metaplastic ossification is pilomatricoma, or calcifying epithelioma (Chap. 31). Calcification of shadow cells is followed by the attraction of osteoclastic giant cells. Osteoclastic erosion of mineralized epithelium is followed by ("coupled to") osteoblastic deposition of osteoid against remnants of the shadow cell islands. The process is therefore similar to the normal process of enchondral ossification wherein mineralized cartilage is the inducing factor. Ossification is found in 14% to 20% of pilomatricomas.[105] It also occurs on rare occasions in basal cell carcinomas, where it takes place usually in the stroma but sometimes in calcifying areas of keratinization. Some basal cell carcinomas with ossification are cases of the nevoid basal cell carcinoma syndrome.[112] In intradermal nevi, ossification usually is secondary to a folliculitis. In desmoplastic malignant melanoma, fibroplasia may be accompanied by cement production resulting in bone formation.[113,114] Rare melanomas in which there is osteoid synthesis by S-100-positive tumor cells have been termed "osteogenic melanomas."[115] Ossification may also occur in chondroid syringomas or mixed tumors of the skin by means of the enchondral mechanism.

In contrast to metaplastic ossification in association with tumors, metaplastic ossification in scars and in inflammatory processes of the skin, such as morphea, systemic scleroderma, and dermatomyositis[116] or venous stasis (Fig. 35-31), is rare.

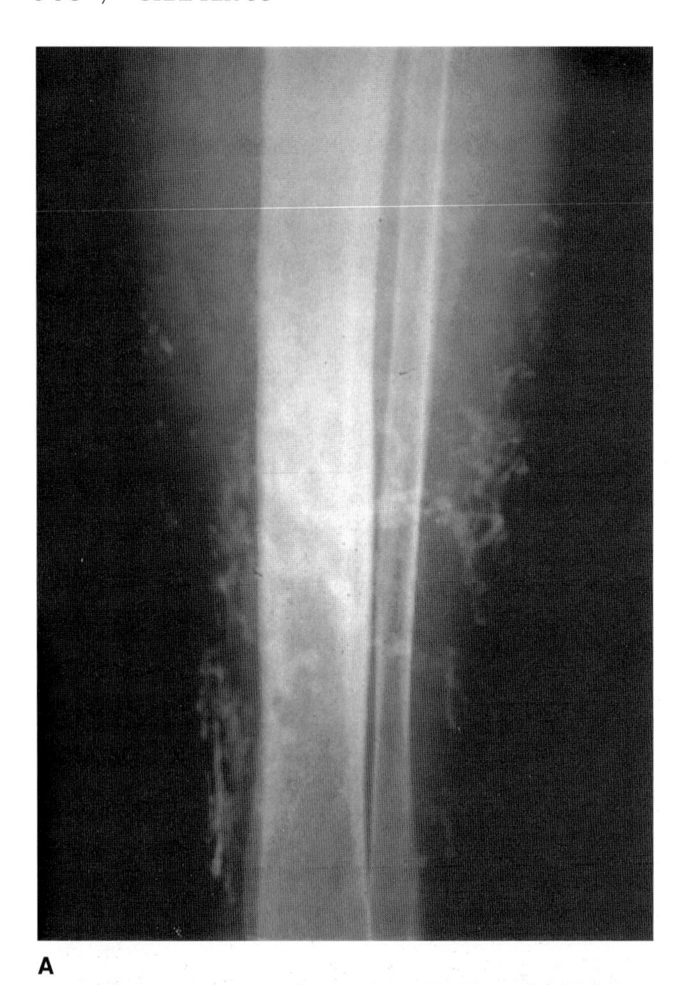

A

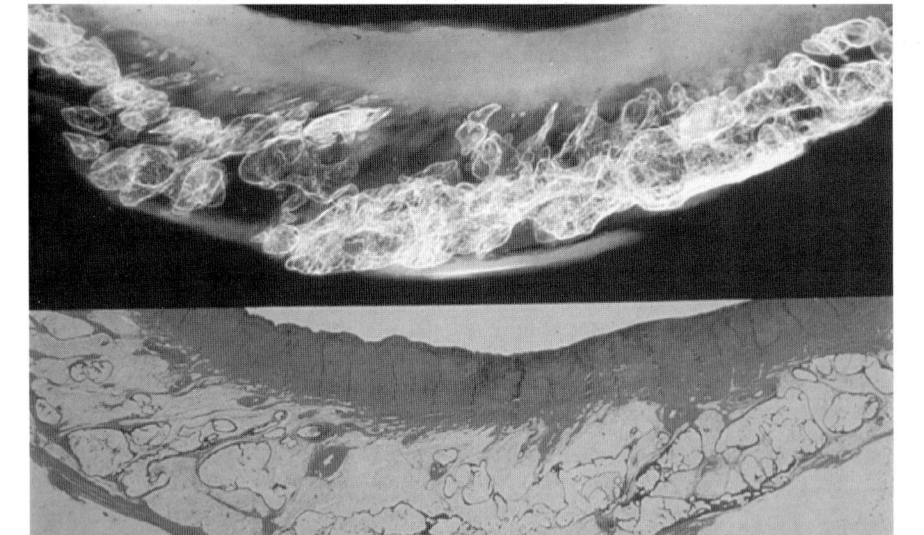

B

FIG. 35-31. Heterotopic subcutaneous ossification associated with chronic venous stasis (60-year-old female with chronic venous stasis of lower legs)
(**A**) In this plain film radiograph, irregular bony deposits unrelated to veins can be seen in the absence of fat necrosis or abnormal serum calcium or phosphorus. (**B**) A specimen radiograph (*top*) correlates well with the large format histologic section (*bottom*) in showing the distribution of irregular lobulated ossific plates in and around subcutaneous fat. The ossification seems to have taken place in interlobular septa. In the histologic view, fibrosis markedly thickens dermis. Thick-walled veins are present in subcutaneous fat (e.g., left of center).

SUBUNGUAL EXOSTOSIS

Subungual exostosis is a fairly common condition that exhibits a solitary tender nodule beneath the free edge of a nail, most commonly beneath the nail of the great toe. Although the nodule usually measures only a few millimeters in diameter,[117] it can be larger and cause swelling of the entire distal phalanx, possibly with ulceration that is treated for a time as an ingrown nail with infection. Less than half of all patients with this lesion will relate its onset to a specific traumatic event, but these anecdotes argue persuasively for traumatic induction of aberrant modulation.

Radiologic examination reveals a bony projection from the edge of the terminal phalangeal tuft (Fig. 35-32A). Its length and radiologic density are proportional to its duration.[118]

Histopathology. In an exostosis (Fig. 35-32B), the earliest

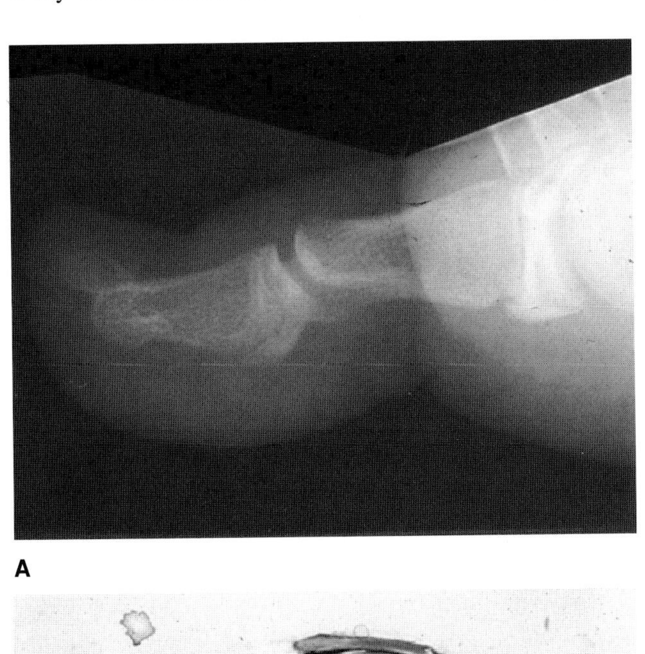

A

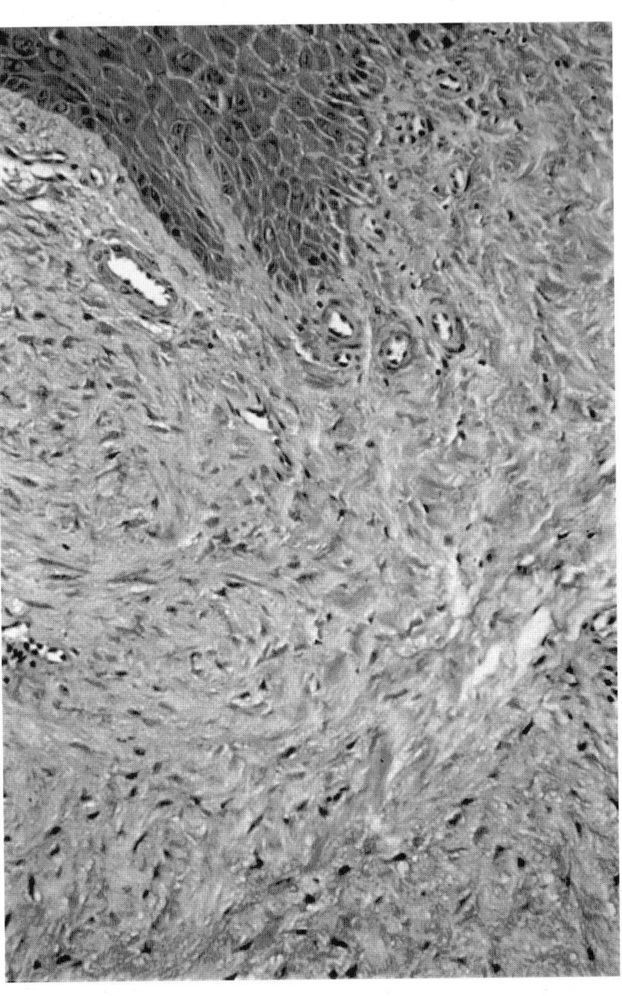

C

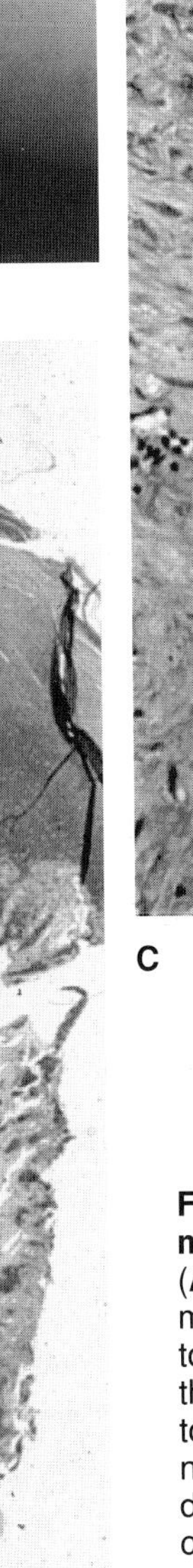

B

FIG. 35-32. Subungual exostosis (14-year-old female; 4 months previously, a horse stepped on her great toe) (**A**) A polypoid bony projection extends from the tuft of terminal phalanx beneath the nail. An osteocartilaginous exostosis (osteochondroma) would be expected to be attached to the metaphyseal (more proximal) region of the phalanx, not to the tip. (**B**) The excised exostosis consists of a cartilaginous cap (*top*) emerging from dermis beneath stretched epidermis and nail bed epithelium. This cartilage overlies a cancellous bony stalk built largely through the process of enchondral ossification. (**C**) The earliest stage in the progressive enlargement of a subungual exostosis is the elaboration of myxoid material between dermal fibroblasts (*bottom*). (continued on next page)

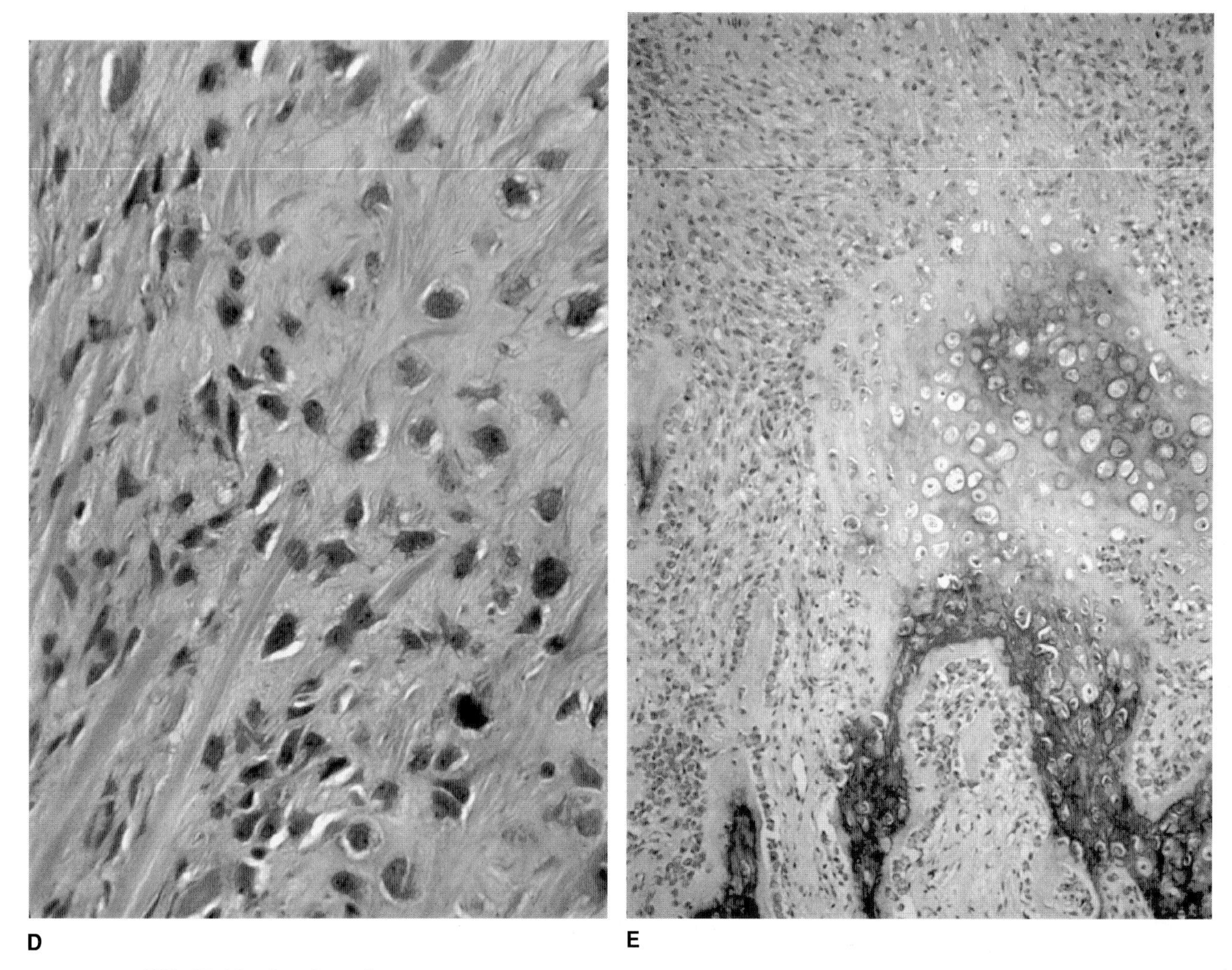

FIG. 35-32. *Continued*
(**D**) With time, the myxoid material assumes the solidity of hyaline cartilage and the intervening cells occupy lacunae within it. Deletion by osteoclastic erosion and substitution of bone tends to follow. (**E**) Exuberant and reactive/reparative chondro-osseous tissue, as illustrated from another case, can be histologically disconcerting.

change is mucopolysaccharide and osteoid elaboration by periosteum and contiguous dermal fibroblasts, eventuating in a gradational continuum of chondroid and osteoid that can be alarmingly cellular (Fig. 35-32E). As the cartilage achieves solid hyalin qualities, it becomes focally eroded along its deep surface by osteoclastic giant cells, followed immediately by enchondral bone deposition on any chondroid matrix remnant. In this way, a cancellous bony stalk is built out from original cortex. The process continues, perhaps from ongoing irritation by footwear, as long as dermal fibroblasts continue to modulate into matrix-producing cells.[119]

CHONDROMAS OF SKIN AND SOFT TISSUE

Benign cartilage nodules and masses independent of bone, including cutaneous cartilage tumors, are variously regarded as neoplastic, metaplastic, or anomalous. Generically referred to as soft part or extraskeletal chondromas, most of these nodules are located in the hands and feet, especially in the fingers of middle-aged adults. These slowly enlarging nodules are seldom painful or tender and rarely exceed 3 cm in diameter. Most are solitary and may attach to tendons, tendon sheaths, or joint capsules (Fig. 35-33A).[120,121] Tenosynovial chondromatosis is a metaplastic process that may create a mass around a joint or along a tendon. Because of their location, these tumors come to the attention of the dermatopathologist only rarely.

Histopathology. Soft tissue chondromas consist of lobules of aggregates of plump chondrocytes (Fig. 35-33B). The lesions appear to develop and grow at their edges by the enlargement of fibroblasts into plump cells that inflate the preexisting structural fibrous tissue with mucopolysaccharides, creating hyalin cartilage (Fig. 35-33C). A minority exhibit secondary stippled (Fig. 35-33D) or heavy calcification. The well-circumscribed, solid-appearing cartilage may exhibit focal fibrosis, enchondral ossification (soft tissue osteochondroma), myxoid change (myxochondroma), cystification, and/or hemorrhage. There may be a granulomatous reaction ("chondrogranuloma") with multinucleated giant cells along the margins and interlobular vascular channels. Biopsy interpretation should ignore substantial atypia

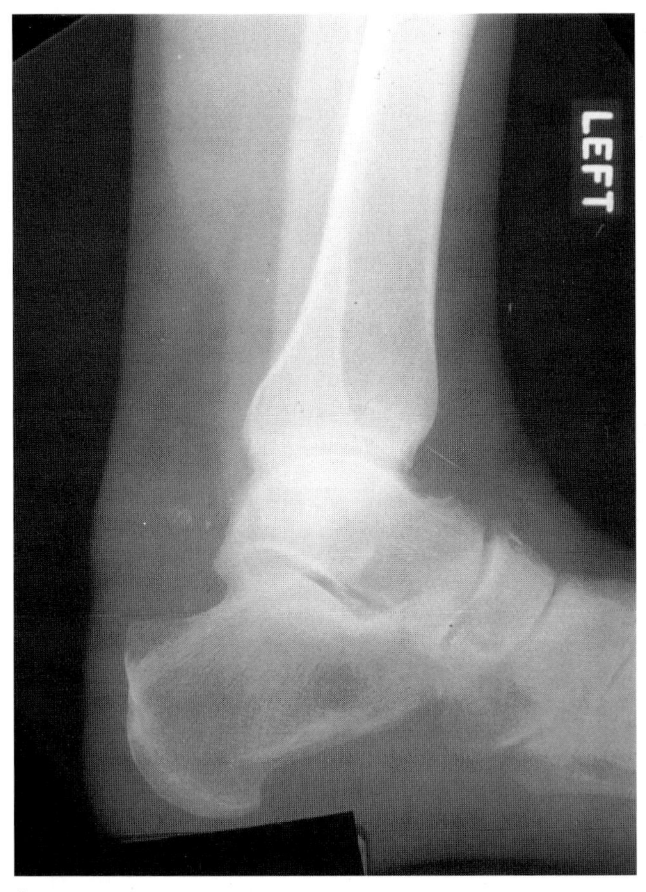

A

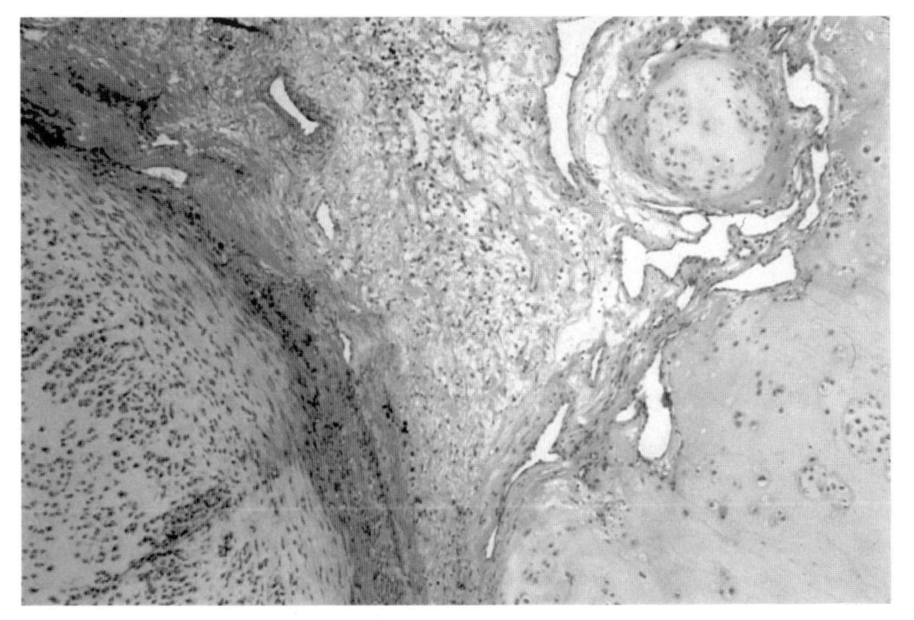

B

FIG. 35-33. Extraskeletal (soft tissue) chondroma
(**A**) An adult male presented with a focally mineralized 4-cm mass posterior to the ankle joint, as shown in this plain film radiograph. (**B**) The tumor consists of rounded masses of variably cellular hyaline cartilage that appear to have emerged from surrounding fibrovascular tissue. *(continued on next page)*

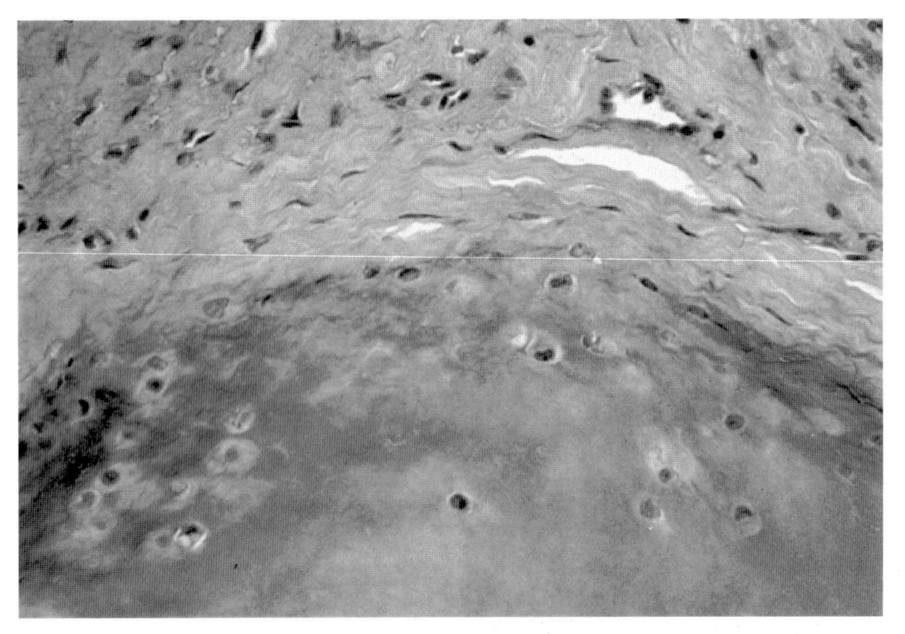

C

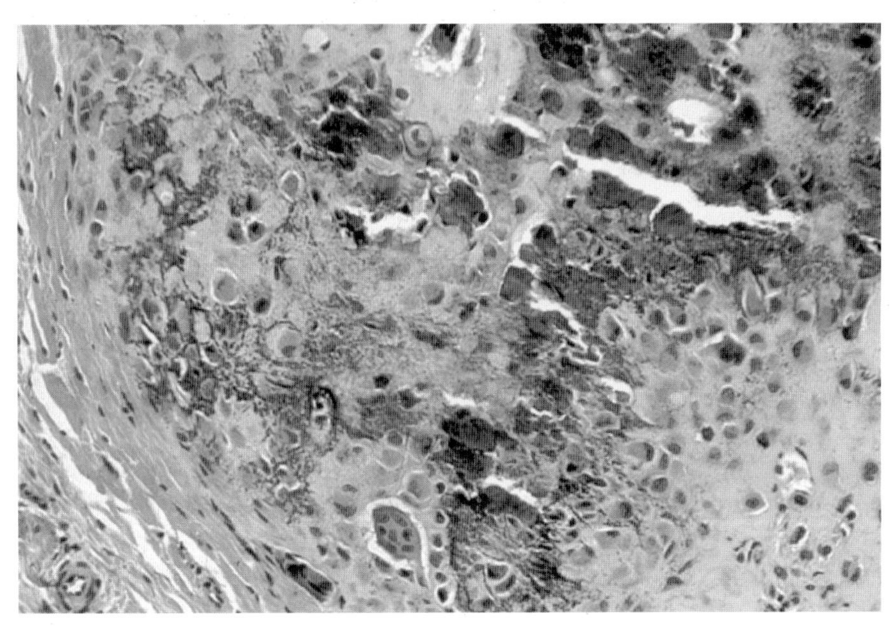

D

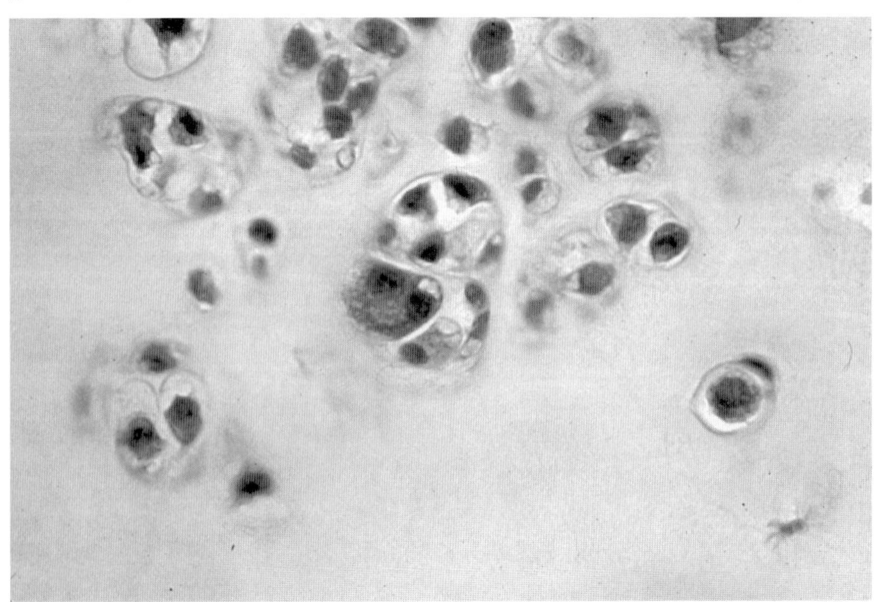

E

FIG. 35-33. ***Continued***
(**C**) The gradual emergence of lesional chrondroid tissue from surrounding fibrous tissue suggests an in situ transformation of "fibroblasts," through the stage of chondroblasts, to become chondrocytes in lacunae within lesional cartilage. (**D**) Particulate mineralizations and basophilic mineral outlining in matrix around tumor cells correlate with the speckled radiographic densities in part A. (**E**) Binucleation and moderate variations in size, shape, and staining do not necessarily connote malignancy in soft tissue cartilage lesions.

in what is radiologically or clinically a small lesion to avoid unnecessarily disfiguring surgery. Plump, immature-appearing chondrocytes that are bi- or multinucleated are not uncommon and, as in bone lesions, do not necessarily connote malignancy (Fig. 35-33E); lesions associated with them behave no differently from the well-differentiated forms. Few recur locally.

Differential Diagnosis. Several soft tissue processes may contain histologically disconcerting cartilage. Extraskeletal chondromas are to be distinguished from developmental cartilagenous rests of branchial origin (usually in the lateral neck in children or infants). Tumorous masses that may be in part cartilagenous to be considered include juvenile aponeurotic fibroma, giant-cell tumor of tendon sheath, fibromatosis, metaplastic cartilage in occasional lipoma varieties, tenosynovial chondromatosis, and cartilage produced in myositis ossificans and fracture callus. Heavily calcified chondromas show granular areas with giant-cell reaction resembling tumoral calcinosis or tenosynovial giant-cell tumors. Radiographs distinguish tumors extending from bone, such as osteochondroma or subungual exostosis.[122]

REFERENCES

1. Seemayer TA, Knaack J, Wang N, Ahmed MN. On the ultrastructure of hibernoma. Cancer 1975;36:1785.
2. Napolitano L. The differentiation of white adipose cells: An electron microscope study. Anat Rec 1963;147:273.
3. Headington JT. The histiocyte in memoriam. Arch Dermatol 1986; 122:532.
4. Ragsdale BD, Dupree WB. Fatty neoplasms. In: Bogumill GP, Fleegler EJ, eds. Tumors of the hand and upper limb. Edinburgh: Churchill Livingstone, 1993;254.
5. Mehregan AH, Tavafoghi V, Ghandchi A. Nevus lipomatosus cutaneus superficialis (Hoffmann-Zurhelle). J Cutan Pathol 1975;2:307.
6. Wilson-Jones E, Marks R, Pongsehirun D. Naevus superficialis lipomatosus. Br J Dermatol 1975;93:121.
7. Howell JB. Nevus lipomatosus vs focal dermal hypoplasia. Arch Dermatol 1965;92:238.
8. Maize JC, Foster G. Age-related changes in melanocytic nevi. Clin Exp Dermatol 1979;4:49.
9. Reymond JL, Stoebner P, Amblard P. Nevus lipomatosus cutaneus superficialis: An electron microscopic study of four cases. J Cutan Pathol 1980;7:295.
10. Dotz W, Prioleau PG. Nevus lipomatosus cutaneus superficialis: A light and electron microscopic study. Arch Dermatol 1984;120:376.
11. Gardner EW, Miller HM, Lowney ED. Folded skin associated with underlying nevus lipomatosus. Arch Dermatol 1979;115:978.
12. Burgdorf WHC, Doran CK, Worret WI. Folded skin with scarring: Michelin tire baby syndrome? J Am Acad Dermatol 1982;7:90.
13. Ross CM. Generalized folded skin with underlying lipomatosus nevus: The Michelin tire baby (letter). Arch Dermatol 1972;106:766.
14. Oku T, Iwasaki K, and Fujita H. Folded skin with an underlying cutaneous smooth muscle hamartoma. Br J Dermatol 1993;129:606.
15. Kashima M, Saito K. A case of atypical inter-muscular lipoma (Evans). J Dermatol 1991;18:532.
16. Meis JM, Enzinger FM. Myolipoma of soft tissue. Am J Surg Pathol 1991;15:121.
17. Mehregan DA, Mehregan DR, Mehregan AH. Angiomyolipoma. J Am Acad Dermatol 1992;27:331.
18. Hitchcock MG, Hurt MA, Santa Cruz DJ. Adenolipoma of the skin. A report of nine cases. J Am Acad Dermatol 1993;29:82.
19. Blomstrand R, Juhlin L, Nordenstam H et al. Adiposis dolorosa associated with defects of lipid metabolism. Acta Derm Venereol (Stockh) 1971;51:243.
20. Enzi G. Multiple symmetric lipomatosis. An update clinical report. Medicine (Baltimore) 1984;63:56.
21. Uhlin SR. Benign symmetric lipomatosis. Arch Dermatol 1979;115: 94.
22. Rodriguez-Fernández A, Caro-Manilla A. Cutaneous angiomyolipoma with pleomorphic changes. J Am Acad Dermatol 1993;29: 115.
23. Mrozek K, Karakousis CP, Bloomfield CD. Chromosome 12 breakpoints are cytogenetically different in benign and malignant lipogenic tumors. Localization of breakpoints in lipoma to 12q15 and in myxoid liposarcoma to 12q13.3. Cancer Res 1993;53:1670.
24. Howard WR, Helwig EB. Angiolipoma. Arch Dermatol 1960;82:924.
25. Sahl WJ Jr. Mobile encapsulated lipomas: Formerly called angiolipomas. Arch Dermatol 1978;114:1684.
26. Hurt MA, Santa Cruz DJ. Nodular cystic fat necrosis: A reevaluation of the so-called mobile encapsulated lipoma. J Am Acad Dermatol 1989;21:493.
27. Dixon AY, McGregor DH, Lee SH. Angiolipomas: An ultrastructural and clinicopathological study. Hum Pathol 1981;12:737.
28. Hunt SJ, Santa Cruz DJ, Barr RJ. Cellular angiolipoma. Am J Surg Pathol 1990;14:75.
29. Dionne GP, Seemayer TA, Infiltrating lipomas and angiolipomas revisited. Cancer 1974;33:732.
30. Puig L, Moreno S, DeMoragas JM. Infiltrating angiolipoma. J Dermatol Surg Oncol 1986;12:617.
31. Allen PW, Enzinger FM. Hemangiomas of skeletal muscle: An analysis of 89 cases. Cancer 1972;29:8.
32. Enzinger FM, Harvey DA. Spindle cell lipoma. Cancer 1975;36:1852.
33. Brody HJ, Meltzer HD, Someren A. Spindle cell lipoma. Arch Dermatol 1978;114:1065.
34. Warkel RL, Rehme CG, Thompson WH. Vascular spindle cell lipoma. J Cutan Pathol 1982;9:113.
35. Shmookler BM, Enzinger FM. Pleomorphic lipoma. A benign tumor simulating liposarcoma. Cancer 1981;47:126.
36. Evans HL, Soule EH, Inkelmann RK. Atypical lipoma, atypical intramuscular lipoma, and well differentiated retroperitoneal liposarcoma. Cancer 1979;43:574.
37. Bryant J. A pleomorphic lipoma in the scalp. J Dermatol Surg Oncol 1981;7:323.
38. Meis JM, Enzinger FM. Chondroid lipoma: A unique tumor simulating liposarcoma and myxoid chondrosarcoma. Am J Surg Pathol 1993;17:1103.
39. Nielsen GP, O' Connell JX, Dickersin GR, Rosenberg AE. Chondroid lipoma, a tumor of white fat cells: A brief report of two cases with ultrastructural analysis. Am J Surg Pathol 1995;19: 1272.
40. Rigor VU, Goldstone SE, Jones J, Bernstein J. Hibernoma: A case report and a discussion of a rare tumor. Cancer 1986;57:2207.
41. Dardick I. Hibernoma: A possible model of brown fat histogenesis. Hum Pathol 1978;9:321.
42. Novy FG Jr, Wilson JW. Hibernomas: brown fat tumors. Arch Dermatol 1956;73:149.
43. Gaffney EF, Hargreaves HK, Semple E et al. Hibernoma: Distinctive light and electron microscopic features and relationship to brown adipose tissue. Hum Pathol 1983;14:677.
44. Levine GD. Hibernoma: An electron microscopic study. Hum Pathol 1972;3:351.
45. Vellios F, Baez J, Shumacker HB. Lipoblastomatosis: A tumor of fetal fat different from hibernoma. Am J Pathol 1958;34:1149.
46. Chung EB, Enzinger FM. Benign lipoblastomatosis: An analysis of 35 cases. Cancer 1973;32:483.
47. Coffin CM, Williams RA. Congenital lipoblastoma of the hand. Pediatr Pathol 1992;12:857.
48. Sawyer JR, Parsons EA, Crowson ML et al. Potential diagnostic implications of breakpoints in the long arm of chromosome 8 in the lipoblastoma. Cancer Genet Cytogenet 1994;76:39.
49. Chaudhuri B, Ronan SG, Ghosh L. Benign lipoblastoma. Cancer 1980;46:611.
50. Mentzel T, Calonje E, Fletcher CD. Lipoblastoma and lipoblastomatosis: A clinicopathological study of 14 cases. Histopathology 1993; 23:527.
51. Enterline HT, Culberson JD, Rochlin DB et al. Liposarcoma. Cancer 1960;13:932.
52. Miser JS, Pizzo PA. Soft tissue sarcomas in childhood. Pediatr Clin North Am 1985;32:779.
53. Shmookler BM, Enzinger FM. Liposarcoma occurring in children: An analysis of 17 cases and review of the literature. Cancer 1983;52:567.
54. Enzinger FM, Winslow DJ. Liposarcoma: A study of 103 cases. Virchows Arch Pathol Anat 1962;335:367.
55. Reitan JB, Kaalhus O, Brennhovd IO et al. Prognostic factors in liposarcoma. Cancer 1985;55:2482.

56. Azumi N, Curtis J, Kempson RL, Hendrickson MR. Atypical and malignant neoplasms showing lipomatous differentiation: A study of 111 cases. Am J Surg Pathol 1987;11:161.
57. Evans HL, Soule EH, Winkelman RK. Atypical lipoma, atypical intramuscular lipoma, well-differentiated retroperitoneal liposarcoma. Cancer 1979;43:574.
58. Evans HL. Liposarcomas and atypical lipomatous tumors. A study of 66 cases followed for a minimum of 10 years. Surg Pathol 1988;1:41.
59. Enzinger FM, Weiss SW. Soft tissue tumors. 3rd ed. St Louis: Mosby, 1995;450.
60. Evans HL. Smooth muscle in atypical lipomatous tumors. Ann J Surg Pathol 1990;14:714.
61. Kransdorf MJ, Meis JM, Jelinek JS. Dedifferentiated liposarcoma of the extremities. Imaging and findings in four patients. Am J Radiol 1993;161:127.
62. Smith TA, Easley KA, Goldblum JR. Myxoid/round cell liposarcoma of the extremities: A clinicopathologic study of 29 cases with particular attention to extent of round cell liposarcoma. Am J Surg Pathol 1996;20:171.
63. Sühurch W, Bégin LR, Seemayer TA et al. Pleomorphic soft tissue myogenic sarcomas of adulthood: A reappraisal in the mid-1990's. Am J Surg Pathol 1996;20:131.
64. Kreichbergs A, Tribukait B, Willems J, Bauer HCF. DNA flow analysis of soft tissue tumors. Cancer 1987;59:128.
65. Gagne, EJ, Su WPD. Congenital smooth muscle hamartoma of the skin. Pediatr Dermatol 1993;10:142.
66. Bronson DM, Fretzin DF, Farrell LN. Congenital pilar and smooth muscle nevus. J Am Acad Dermatol 1983;8:111.
67. Slifman NR, Harrist TJ, Rhodes AR. Congenital arrector pili hamartoma. Arch Dermatol 1985;121:1034.
68. Darling TN, Kamino H, Murray JC. Acquired cutaneous smooth muscle hamartoma. J Am Acad Dermatol 1993;28:844.
69. Urbanek RW, Johnson WC. Smooth muscle hamartoma associated with Becker's nevus. Arch Dermatol 1978;114:104.
70. Montgomery H, Winkelmann RK. Smooth-muscle tumors of the skin. Arch Dermatol 1959;79:32.
71. Fisher WC, Helwig EB. Leiomyomas of the skin. Arch Dermatol 1963;88:510.
72. Hachisuga T, Hashimoto H, Enjoji M. Angioleiomyoma: A clinicopathologic reappraisal of 562 cases. Cancer 1984;54:126.
73. Scurry JP, Carey MP, Targett CS, Dowling JP. Soft tissue lipoleiomyoma. Pathology 1991;23:360.
74. Fitzpatrick JE, Mellette JR, Hwang RJ et al. Cutaneous angiolipoleiomyoma. J Am Acad Dermatol 1990;23:1093.
75. Mann PR. Leiomyoma cutis: An electron microscope study. Br J Dermatol 1970;82:463.
76. Seifert HW. Ultrastructural investigation on cutaneous angioleiomyoma. Arch Dermatol Res 1981;271:91.
77. Jegasothy BV, Gilgor RS, Hull DM. Leiomyosarcoma of the skin and subcutaneous tissue. Arch Dermatol 1981;117:478.
78. Fields JP, Helwig EB. Leiomyosarcoma of the skin and subcutaneous tissue. Cancer 1981;47:156.
79. Wascher RA, Lee MY. Recurrent cutaneous leiomyosarcoma. Cancer 1992;70:490.
80. Newman PL, Fletcher CD. Smooth muscle tumors of the external genitalia: Clinicopathologic analysis of a series. Histopathology 1991;18: 523.
81. Manivel JC, Wick MR, Dehner LP. Non-vascular sarcomas of the skin. In: Wick MR, ed. Pathology of unusual malignant cutaneous tumors. New York: Marcel Dekker, 1985;211.
82. Swanson PE, Stanley MW, Scheithauer BW et al. Primary cutaneous leiomyosarcoma. J Cutan Pathol 1988;15:129.
83. Alessi E, Sala F. Leiomyosarcoma in ectopic areola. Am J Dermatopathol 1992;14:165.
84. Hashimoto H, Daimaru Y, Tsuneyoshi M, Enjoji M. Leiomyosarcoma of the external soft tissue. Cancer 1986;57:2077.
85. Headington JT, Beals TF, Niederhuber JE. Primary leiomyosarcoma of skin: A report and critical appraisal. J Cutan Pathol 1977;4:308.
86. Yamamura T, Takada A, Higashiyama M, Yoshikawa K. Subcutaneous leiomyosarcoma. Br J Dermatol 1991;124:252.
87. Yamamura T, Takada A, Higashiyama M, Yoshikawa K. Subcutaneous leiomyosarcoma developing in radiation dermatitis. Dermatologica 1991;183:154.
88. Oliver GF, Reiman HM, Gonchoroff NJ et al. Cutaneous and subcutaneous leipmysarcoma. Br J Dermatol 1991;124:252.
89. Lundgren L, Kindblom LG, Seidal T, Angervall L. Intermediate and fine cytofilaments in cutaneous and subcutaneous leiomyosarcomas. APMIS 1991;99:820.
90. Kapadia SB, Meis JM, Frisman DM et al. Adult rhabdomyoma of the head and neck: A clinicopathologic and immunophenotypic study. Hum Pathol 1993;24:608.
91. Wiss K, Solomon AR, Raimer SS. Rhabdomyosarcoma presenting as a cutaneous nodule. Arch Dermatol 1988;124:1687.
92. Agamanolis DP, Dasu S, Krill CE Jr. Tumors of skeletal muscle. Hum Pathol 1986;17:778.
93. Albright F, Forbes AP, Henneman PH. Pseudohypoparathyroidism. Trans Assoc Am Physicians 1952;65:337.
94. Peterson WC Jr, Mandel SL. Primary osteomas of skin. Arch Dermatol 1963;87:626.
95. Donaldson EM, Summerly R. Primary osteoma cutis and diaphyseal aclasis. Arch Dermatol 1962;85:261.
96. Barranco VP. Cutaneous ossification in pseudohypoparathyroidism. Arch Dermatol 1971;104:643.
97. Eyre WG, Reed WB. Albright's hereditary osteodystrophy with cutaneous bone formation. Arch Dermatol 1971;104:636.
98. Brook CGD, Valman HG. Osteoma cutis and Albright's hereditary osteodystrophy. Br J Dermatol 1971;85:471.
99. Spranger J. Skeletal dysplasia: Albright's hereditary osteodystrophy. In: Bergsma D, ed. The first conference on the clinical delineation of birth defects. New York: National Foundation March of Dimes, 1968; 122.
100. Piesowicz AT. Pseudohypoparathyroidism with osteoma cutis. Proc R Soc Med 1965;58:126.
101. Kaplan FS, Craver R, MacEwen GD et al. Progressive osseus hetroplasia: A distinct developmental disorder of heterotopic ossification. J Bone Joint Surg [Am] 1994;76A:425.
102. O'Donnell TF Jr, Geller SA. Primary osteoma cutis. Arch Dermatol 1971;104:325.
103. Sanmartin O, Alegre V, Martinez-Aparicio A et al. Congenital platelike osteoma cutis. Case report and review literature. Pediatric Dermatol 1993;10:182.
104. Monroe AB, Burgdorf WHC, Sheward S. Platelike cutaneous osteoma. J Am Acad Dermatol 1987;16:481.
105. Burgdorf W, Nasemann T. Cutaneous osteomas. A clinical and histopathologic review. Arch Dermatol Res 1977;260:121.
106. Helm F, De La Pava S, Klein E. Multiple miliary osteomas of the skin. Arch Dermatol 1967;96:681.
107. Basler RSW, Taylor WB, Peacor DR. Postacne osteoma cutis. Arch Dermatol 1974;110:113.
108. Walter JF, Macknet KD. Pigmentation of osteoma cutis caused by tetracycline. Arch Dermatol 1979;115:1087.
109. Moritz DL, Elewski B. Pigmented post acne osteoma cutis in a patient treated with minocycline: Report and review of the literature. J Am Acad Dermatol 1991;24:851.
110. Oikarinen A, Tuomi M-L, Kallionen M et al. A study of bone formation in osteoma cutis employing biochemical, histochemical and in situ hybridization techniques. Acta Derm Venereol (Stockh) 1992;72: 172.
111. Goldminz D, Greenberg RD. Multiple miliary osteoma cutis. J Am Acad Dermatol 1991;24:878.
112. Mason JK, Helwig EB, Graham JH. Pathology of the nevoid basal cell carcinoma syndrome. Arch Pathol 1965;79:401.
113. Urmacher C. Unusual stromal pattern in truly recurrent and satellite metastatic lesions of malignant melanoma. Am J Dermatopathol 1984; 1(Suppl):331.
114. Moreno A, Lamarca J, Martinez R et al. Osteoid and bone formation in desmoplastic malignant melanoma. J Cutan Pathol 1986;13:128.
115. Lucas DR, Tazelaar HD, Unni KK, Wold LE. Osteogenic melanoma: A rare varient of malignant melanoma. Am J Surg Pathol 1993;17: 400.
116. Roth SI, Stowell RE, Helwig EB. Cutaneous ossification. Arch Pathol 1963;76:44.

117. Woo TY, Rasmussen JE. Subungual osteocartilaginous exostosis. J Dermatol Surg Oncol 1985;11:534.
118. Cohen HJ, Frank SB, Minkin W et al. Subungual exostoses. Arch Dermatol 1973;107:431.
119. Ragsdale, BD. Morphologic analysis of skeletal lesions: Correlation of imaging studies and pathologic findings. In: Reynaldo A, Weinstein RS, eds. Advances in pathology and laboratory medicine. St. Louis: Mosby–Year Book, 1993;445.
120. Chung EB, Enzinger FM. Chondroma of soft parts. Cancer 1978;41:1414.
121. DelSignore JL, Torre BA, Miller RJ. Extraskeletal chondroma of the hand: Case report and review of the literature. Clin Orthop 1990;254:147.
122. Ragsdale BD, Vihn TN, Sweet DE. Radiology as gross pathology in evaluating chondroid lesions. Hum Pathol 1989;20:930.

Lever's Histopathology of the Skin, eighth edition, edited by David Elder et al. Lippincott–Raven Publishers, Philadelphia © 1997.

CHAPTER 36

Tumors of Neural Tissue

Richard J. Reed and Zsolt Argenyi

GENERAL ANATOMIC RELATIONSHIPS

Structural Components

A *nerve*, an anatomic unit, is composed of nerve fibers, endoneurium, and perineurium. *Nerve fibers*, the functioning element, are aggregated to form axial bundles (parallel arrays of nerve fibers with longitudinal symmetry). Individually, each fiber consists of an axon or axons and related *Schwann cells*.[1–3] *Axons* are cytoplasmic extensions from the perikaryon of *neurons* in the central nervous system or in sympathetic ganglia. From origin to terminus, the entire length of the peripheral portion of an axon is enclosed by enveloping Schwann cells. Along nonmyelinated nerve fibers, a single Schwann cell encloses segments of several axons in cytoplasmic invaginations. Along myelinated nerve fibers, a single Schwann cell encloses a segment of an axon in concentric layers of its cytoplasmic membrane, and where neighboring Schwann cells abut end to end, a node of Ranvier is formed. In sympathetic ganglia, neurons are rimmed by satellite cells. Ultrastructurally, microfilaments, specialized intermediate (neural) filaments, and microtubules are components of axons. Schwann cells have complex cytoplasmic processes, are surrounded by continuous basal lamina, and contain densely packed intermediate filaments.

The *perineurium*, a tubular fibrous sheath, delimits each nerve. It extends from the pia-arachnoid of the central nervous system to the terminus of each nerve or to specialized sensory receptors. Slender bipolar or tripolar cells (*perineurial cells*) are isolated among its concentric fibrous lamellae. Ultrastructurally, discontinuous basal lamina, numerous pinocytotic vesicles, and tight intercellular junctions are features. The perineurium is a relatively impervious barrier.

The *endoneurium* is a delicate, mucinous matrix between the perineurium and the axial collection of nerve fibers. Fibroblasts, mast cells, collagen, mucin, and capillaries are its components.

In proximal locations, several large nerves, in bundles, are encased in a dense fibrous matrix, the *epineurium* (a fibrous sheath that is continuous with the dura mater at the junction of the spinal nerves with the central nervous system). Individual nerves, in their course, leave the bundles and continue without an epineurium. Near the terminus of each nerve, nerve fibers extend beyond an open-ended perineurium into the mesenchyme, and naked axons even extend into the epithelium. Ensheathed receptors of the skin include mucocutaneous corpuscles and the corpuscles of Vater-Pacini, Meissner, and Merkel. Meissner corpuscles are ovoid structures in which an axon is sinuously enclosed in stacks of distinctive cells. Pacinian corpuscles are spherical structures in soft tissue. In them, concentrically laminated, distinctive cells and fibrous lamellae are arranged around a centrally located axon. The ultrastructural features of the laminated cells of both Meissner and pacinian corpuscles are perineurial cell-like.[4]

ONTOGENY AND REACTIONS TO INJURY AS RELATED TO THE INTERPRETATION OF PHENOTYPIC EXPRESSIONS OR PATTERNS IN NEOPLASIA

Neurosustentacular cells of peripheral nerves, related cells of the peripheral ganglia, melanocytes, and even cells of some cranial mesenchyme are all of neurocristic origin.

In reactions of peripheral nerves to injury, reserve cells of neural origin proliferate and subsequently express either a schwannian or perineurial phenotype. Expressions of phenotype are fortuitous: the environs in which uncommitted reserve cells find themselves influence the expressions. The available options probably include a capacity to function facultatively as endoneurial fibroblasts.[5]

Once incorporated into a microscopist's store of virtual images, various patterns, some relating to the structural components of peripheral nerves, some to the embryologic development of their neurocristic precursors, and some to the reactions of normal nerves to injury, provide clues to the interpretation of the puzzling histologic patterns of nerve sheath tumors and, in turn, for the structuring of a correct histologic diagnosis. For example, the structure of Meissner corpuscles is recapitulated in the tactile corpuscle–like structures (tactoid bodies) of diffuse neurofibromas. The features of wallerian degeneration are recapitulated in a most distorted manner in granular cell nerve sheath

R. J. Reed: Reed Laboratory of Skin Pathology, New Orleans, LA
Z. Argenyi: University of Iowa College of Medicine, Iowa City, IA

tumor. The intravaginal hyaline nodules of Renaut[3] may provide a model for the patterns manifested in nerve sheath myxomas.

When damaged, axons form multiple sproutlike extensions. In the ensuing reparative process, newly formed axons are accompanied by newly formed Schwann cells. These patterns are incompletely recapitulated in spontaneous, intraneural neuromas. The distorted patterns that are manifested in intraneural neurofibromas and even in some small schwannomas may relate to a local excess of thin, nonmyelinated axons.

PHENOTYPES AND HISTOCHEMICAL AND IMMUNOHISTOCHEMICAL REACTIONS

Neurosustentacular cells, melanocytes, and even some mesenchymal cells are intermutable. In tumors of peripheral nerves, the structural qualities of either Schwann cells or perineurial cells are commonly expressed, but either cell type may in turn express an immunohistochemical marker of a conflicting type. For example, the cells of tactoid bodies mark with antibodies for S-100 protein (as do Schwann cells) but have the ultrastructural features of perineurial cells.

S-100 protein is a cytoplasmic antigen of glial cells but is expressed in a variety of other cells, including melanocytes, lipocytes, chondrocytes, some cells of sweat glands, and Schwann cells. *Neuron-specific enolase* (NSE) is a cytoplasmic product common to a variety of cells including Schwann cells, and both neurons and their axons. An immunoreaction for the demonstration of neural filaments provides a pure demonstration of the reaction of axons. Silver impregnation techniques are the time-honored method of demonstrating axons but are less sensitive than immunohistochemical reactions: fewer axons are demonstrated. The luxol-fast blue stain and antibodies for myelin-basic protein (MBP) and CD57 (Leu-7) antigen demonstrate myelin products. An immunoreaction for glial fibrillary acidic protein (GFAP) is positive in glial cells and even in some of the cells in some tumors of salivary glands. In some large schwannomas of soft tissue, neoplastic Schwann cells are immunoreactive for GFAP. *Epithelial membrane antigen* (EMA) is a cytoplasmic antigen commonly expressed in a variety of normal and neoplastic tissue, including cells of the perineurium and sebaceous cells.

NEUROFIBROMAS (HAMARTOMAS WITH PHENOTYPIC DIVERSITY)

Extraneural sporadic cutaneous neurofibromas (ESCNs) (the common sporadic neurofibromas) are soft, polypoid, skin-colored or slightly tan, and small (rarely larger than a centimeter in diameter). They usually arise in adulthood. The identification of as many as four, small, cutaneous neurofibromas in a single patient, in the absence of other confirmatory findings, would not qualify as stigmata of neurofibromatosis.

Histopathology. Most examples of ESCN are faintly eosinophilic, and are circumscribed but not encapsulated: they are extraneural. Thin spindle cells with elongated, wavy nuclei are regularly spaced among thin, wavy collagenous strands (Fig. 36-1). The strands are either closely spaced (homogeneous pattern) or loosely spaced in a clear matrix (loose pattern) (see Fig. 36-1).[1] The two patterns are often intermixed in a single lesion. Rarely, ESCNs are composed of widely spaced spindle and stellate cells in a myxoid matrix. The regular spacing of adnexae is preserved in cutaneous neurofibromas. Entrapped small nerves occasionally are enlarged and hypercellular. Tactoid (tactile corpusclelike) bodies and pigmented dendritic melanocytes are most uncommon.

Histogenesis. With silver impregnations (Bodian or Bielschowsky stain), only a few axons, mostly in small, entrapped nerves, are demonstrable. Immunohistochemically, axons are more uniformly and generously represented. With monoclonal antibodies for NSE, an intense punctate and fiberlike cytoplasmic reaction, in a background of diffuse cytoplasmic staining, identifies the axons of a cutaneous neurofibroma. A similar response without diffuse cytoplasmic staining characterizes the reaction for neural filaments. Immunoreactions and ultrastructural features identify the schwannian (neurosustentacular) nature of the tumor cells in ESCN.

Differential Diagnosis. A schwannoma is intraneural (encapsulated) and usually does not contain axons as demonstrated by antibodies to neurofilaments.

In a neurotized nevus, nests and fascicles of nevocytic cells usually can be identified in scattered foci. Tactoid bodies are common in neurotized nevi but rare in ESCN.

In the absence of an intraneural plexiform component, a cutaneous neurofibroma of neurofibromatosis may be histologically indistinguishable from ESCN.

Some sporadic cutaneous neurofibromas, including subcutaneous variants, differ in patterns from ESCN. Confined by the perineurium of the nerve of origin, they are circumscribed and intraneural.[1–3] Their internal patterns are indistinguishable from the patterns variously manifested in the intraneural components of plexiform neurofibromas.

On rare occasions, dermatofibromas and subcutaneous spindle cell lipomas may be mistaken for a nerve sheath tumor.

NEUROFIBROMATOSIS (PHENOTYPIC DIVERSITY EXPRESSED IN GENETICALLY DETERMINED HAMARTOMAS AND NEOPLASMS)

Multiple cutaneous neurofibromas are characteristic of most, but not all, examples of neurofibromatosis (von Recklinghausen's disease). Other important stigmata include plexiform (intraneural) and deep, diffuse (extraneural) neurofibromas, multiple periareolar neurofibromas, intraocular Lisch nodules, and macular cutaneous hyperpigmentations (e.g., café-au-lait spots and bilateral axillary freckling).[6,7]

Neurofibromatosis type I (NF1) can arise as an autosomal dominant condition, but in nearly half of the patients, it arises by spontaneous mutation.[8] In it, cutaneous neurofibromas usually appear first in late childhood or in adolescence and gradually increase in size and number.

For NF1, the gene, which is huge, has been localized to the pericentromeric region of the long arm of chromosome 17. A high spontaneous mutation rate,[9] an attribute of huge genes, would account for the high incidence of sporadic cases. The gene shows functional and structural homology with guanosine triphosphatase–activating protein, which controls the ras oncogene. In turn, the role of the ras oncogene in growth, development, and differentiation may be aberrantly expressed in the NF1 phenotype.[9] The protein product of the gene is called *neurofibromin.*[10]

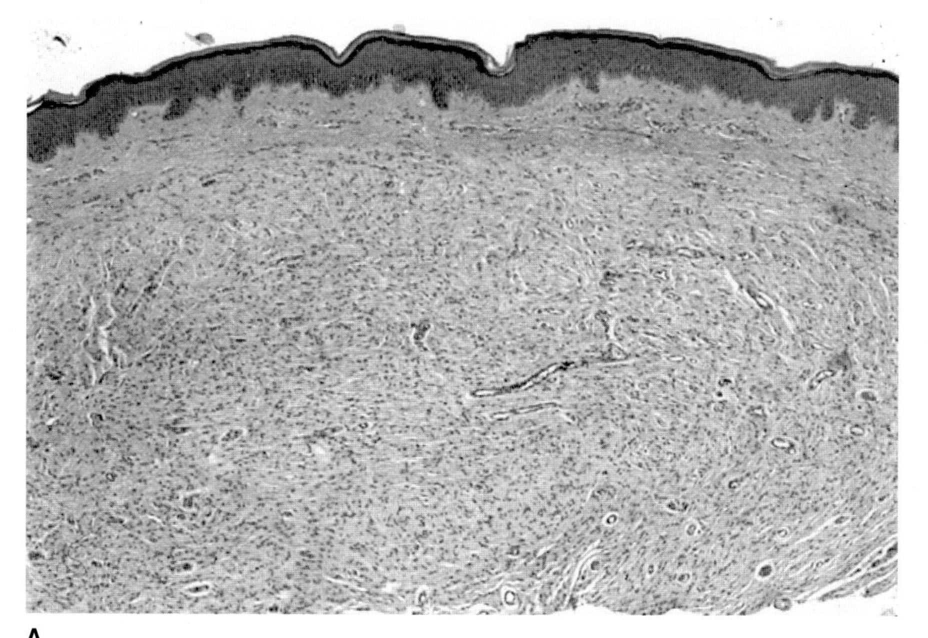

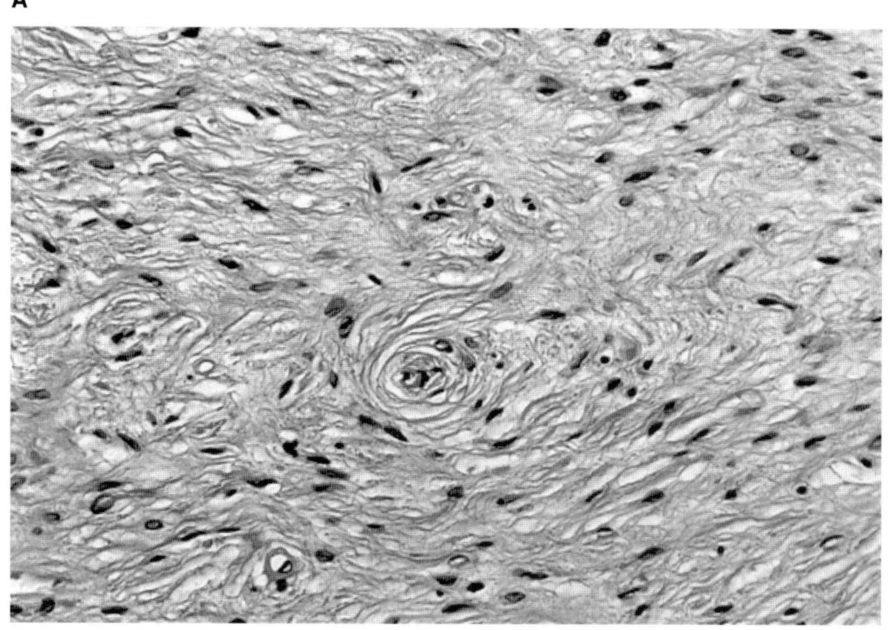

FIG. 36-1. Extraneural sporadic cutaneous neurofibroma
(**A**) A circumscribed nonencapsulated tumor of the dermis is composed of loosely spaced spindle cells and wavy collagenous strands. (**B**) Thin spindle cells are associated with thin, wavy collagen bundles. The cells and collagen bundles are loosely spaced in a clear matrix.

In NF1, superficial peripheral nerves, deep peripheral nerves, nerve roots, and the autonomic nerves of viscera and blood vessels may be affected. Large, pendulous plexiform neurofibromas have the flabby texture of a "bag of worms." Deep, diffuse neurofibromas are poorly defined at their limits with the adjacent soft tissue.[3] Elephantiasic changes may be associated with large neurofibromas of the skin and subcutaneous fat. Spinal nerve root tumors may cause compression of the spinal cord.[8] Tumors of the central nervous system occur in 5% to 10% of the patients.[6] The pressure of an adjacent or intraosseous neurofibroma may result in erosive defects in bones. Nonspecific lesions, such as kyphoscoliosis or an increase in the length of long bones, may occur. NF1, diffuse intestinal ganglioneuromatosis, and multiple endocrine neoplasia, type 2b, are unpredictably associated.[11,12] An association between juvenile xanthogranuloma, juvenile chronic myelogenous leukemia, and NF1 has been observed.[13]

In localized or segmental neurofibromatosis, cutaneous neurofibromas are few in number and the family history is negative.[14]

In *neurofibromatosis type 2* (NF2) (a genetically distinct variant), café-au-lait spots, neurofibromas, schwannomas, and a variety of intracranial tumors, including bilateral schwannomas of the acoustic nerves, are manifestations.[10] The gene locus has been linked to chromosome 22q11-q13. The protein gene product, called *merlin*, is similar to a group of cytoskeleton-linked proteins.[10]

The syndrome of *multiple schwannomas* (schwannomatosis

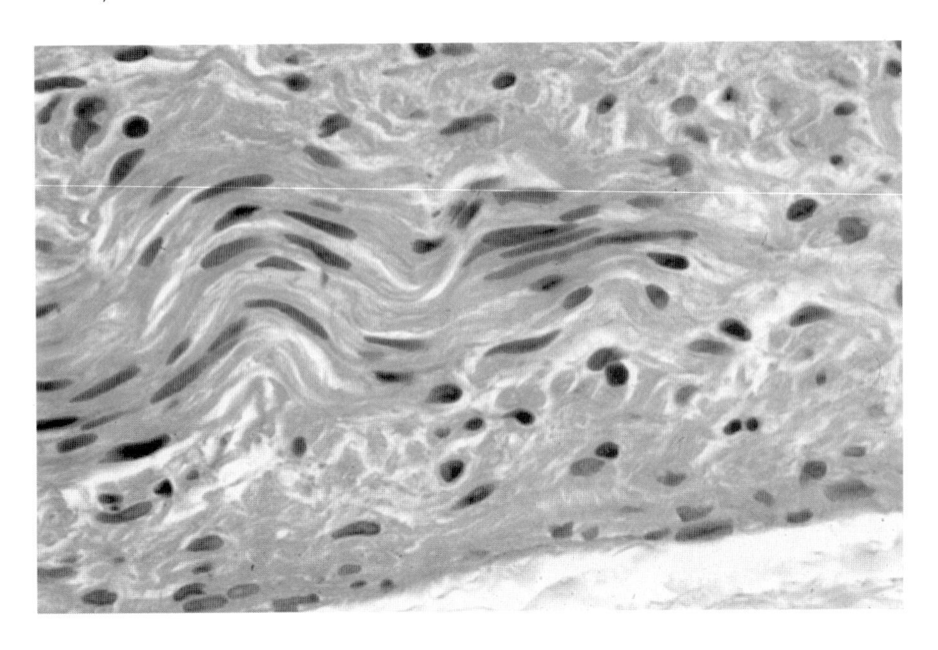

FIG. 36-2. Small component of a plexiform, intraneural neurofibroma
The symmetrical axial bundle of the nerve of origin is preserved centrally.

or neurilemmomatosis) [15] is characterized by multiple schwannomas and plexiform schwannomas.

Café-au-lait spots occur in nearly all patients with neurofibromatosis and usually precede cutaneous tumors.[6] Although a few café-au-lait spots are occasionally seen in patients without neurofibromatosis, the presence of more than six spots, each exceeding 1.5 cm in diameter, is indicative of neurofibromatosis.[6,8]

Histopathology. The histologic spectrum of neurofibromas in NF1 is broad. Cutaneous, extraneural variants (as manifested in ESCN); cutaneous or deep, circumscribed (intraneural) variants; plexiform (intraneural) variants; deep, diffuse (extraneural) variants; and various combinations of the above are manifested in an array of histologic patterns.

In many deep, circumscribed neurofibromas and in most plexiform neurofibromas, axial bundles of symmetrically arranged nerve fibers are remnants of the axial bundle of the nerve of origin (Fig. 36-2).[3,16] They appear to have a role in the histogenesis of NF. They retain their symmetry in a field of distorted and asymmetrical patterns. In some axial bundles, Schwann cells are hyperplastic and tightly packed. In cross sections of the involved nerve, these hypercellular bundles appear as micronodules and qualify as *microscopic schwannomatosis* (Fig. 36-3).[3] From the periphery of these nidi, which function as growth centers, cells and collagenous strands, streaming asymmetrically into the expanded endoneurium, contribute to the expansion of the intraneural component. Many of the cellular nidi may be independent of a true axial bundle (see Fig. 36-3), but all function as growth centers.

In the evolution of a neurofibroma, the contributions from each anatomic component of a peripheral nerve are variable. *Perineurial variants* are rather uniformly and densely fibrous, and their cells are bipolar or tripolar with rigid processes (Fig. 36-4). *Endoneurial variants* are characterized by a thickened perineurium, one or several axial bundles, and isolated cells in an expanded, mucinous endoneurial component (Fig. 36-5). Some of the cells in the mucinous matrix resemble the "cellules godronné" of Renaut (round cells with complexly interconnected cytoplasmic processes that enclose a mucinous ma-

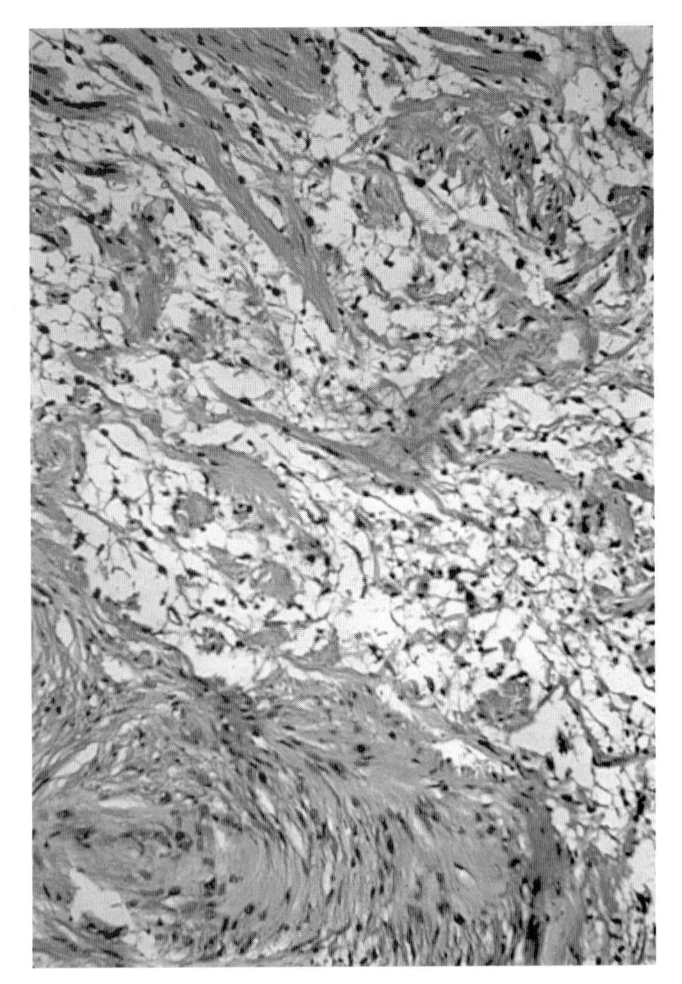

FIG. 36-3. Intraneural neurofibroma, schwannian type, showing focal schwannomatosis
Coarse collagen bundles that vary in size are interconnected and are spaced in a myxoid matrix. Near the left-hand margin of the field, Schwann cells are tightly clustered and focally are arranged in ill-defined palisades (microscopic schwannomatosis).

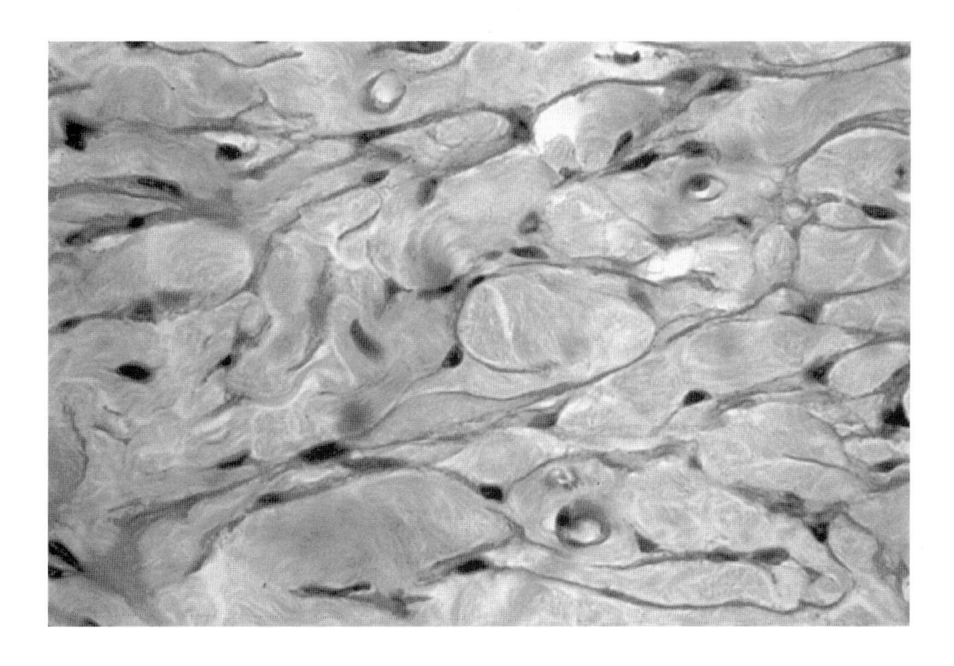

FIG. 36-4. Intraneural neurofibroma, perineurial pattern of differentiation
Thin cells with polar cytoplasmic extensions are spaced among and outline coarse collagen bundles. The cells are joined to their neighbors by cytoplasmic extensions. The cells have features of perineurial cells.

trix).[1,3] *Schwannian variants* are characterized by a thickened perineurium, one or several axial bundles, and an expanded mucinous endoneurial component in which spindle cells are spaced among asymmetrical collagen bundles (Fig. 36-6).

In the expanded endoneurial component of endoneurial and schwannian variants, the matrix is myxoid (see Figs. 36-5 and 36-6) and rich in hyaluronic acid.[1]

In a lesion in which the patterns of neurofibroma are otherwise preserved and in the absence of mitotic activity, a spotty representation of scattered cells with enlarged, hyperchromatic, and irregular nuclei is not a significant finding (see Fig. 36-6).[1]

At the interface of *extraneural (diffuse) neurofibromas* with soft tissue, margins are poorly defined (Fig. 36-7) and lipocytes are often entrapped. The matrix of extraneural neurofibroma is either delicately fibrous and faintly acidophilic or more coarsely fibrous and brightly acidophilic. Nerves within the lesion usually are small, internally symmetrical, and hypercellular, and the perineuria are hyperplastic. In cross section, these nerves

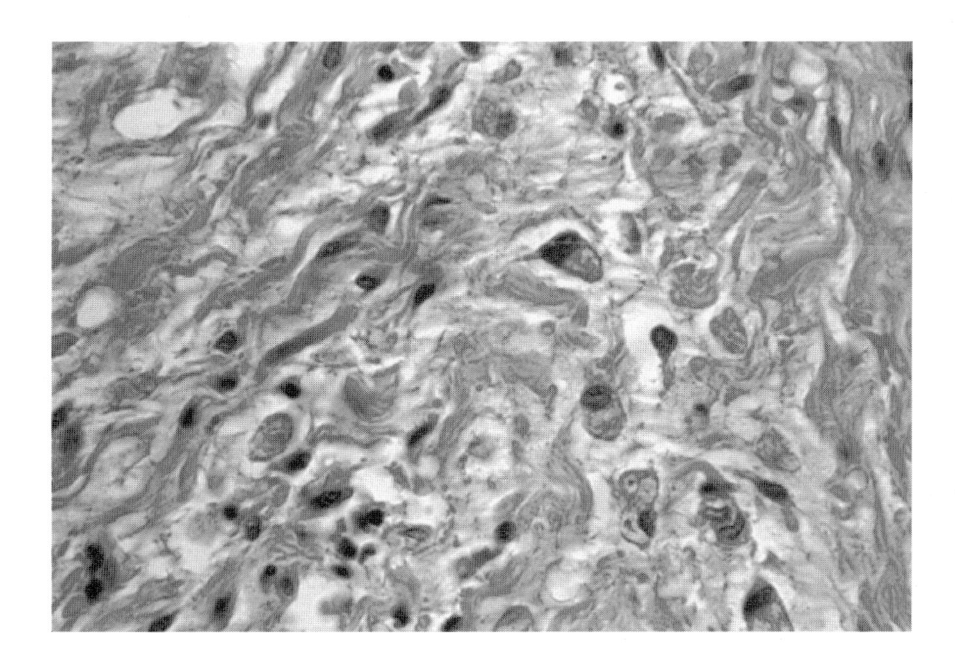

FIG. 36-5. Intraneural neurofibro-993ma, endoneurial pattern of differentiation
Rounded cells are spaced among wavy collagen bundles in a basophilic, myxoid matrix. The cells have rounded nuclei with dense chromatin patterns and contain intracytoplasmic mucin. They resemble the "cellules godronné" as seen in the intravaginal hyaline system of Renaut.

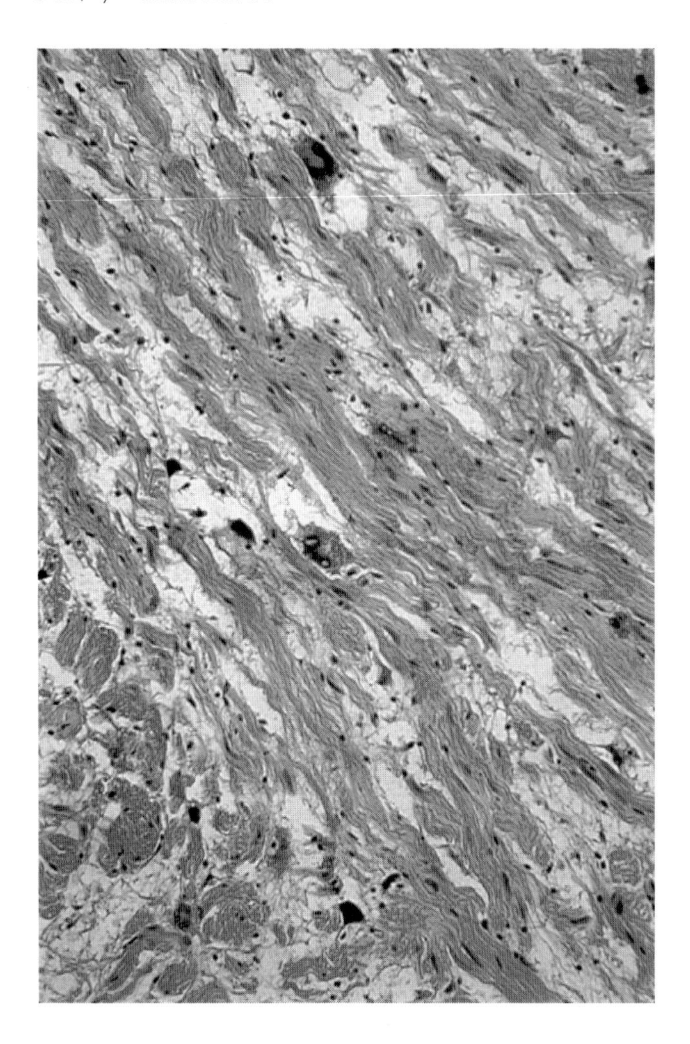

FIG. 36-6. Intraneural neurofibroma, cytologic atypia Delicate spindle cells are associated with coarse collagen bundles. The bundles are interconnected and loosely spaced in a myxoid matrix. Bizarre giant cells are irregularly spaced among the bundles. The pattern is schwannian in type.

might be mistaken as evidence of pacinian corpuscle–like differentiation.[26] The patterns of a plexiform (intraneural) neurofibroma and a diffuse (extraneural) neurofibroma are combined[3] in *paraneurofibroma*. Focal collections of tactoid bodies (see Fig. 36-7) and pigmented dendritic melanocytes, a common feature of deep extraneural neurofibromas,[3] are rare in the intraneural components of plexiform, or circumscribed, intraneural neurofibromas.

Ultrastructurally, the cells of neurofibromas (including those of tactoid bodies) mostly resemble those of perineurial cells,[17] but cells with the characteristics of Schwann cells, as well as endoneurial fibroblasts, also have been identified: a morphologic continuum of neurosustentacular cells is manifested.[3,18] Endoneurial fibroblasts, like common mesenchymal fibroblasts, do not have basal lamina. The average diameter of their collagen fibrils lies well below that of dermal collagen fibrils, which is about 100 nm.[19]

Histogenesis. The immunohistochemical profile of neurofibroma is as follows: S-100 protein (+), CD57 (Leu-7) antigen (+), and myelin basic protein (+). In extraneural cutaneous neurofibromas, axons, as demonstrated with NSE, are fairly uniform in distribution among collagen bundles. This finding is less consistent in deep intraneural neurofibromas.

The ultrastructural features of neurofibromas (a preponderance of cells that resemble perineurial cells[17]) and the respective immunohistochemical findings (e.g., S-100 [+] and EMA [−]) are discordant qualities.

Schwann cells with enclosed axons, as demonstrated with monoclonal antibodies for NSE or neural filaments, have been characterized as an integral part of neurofibromas, or simply as a consequence of the entrapment of uninvolved nerve fibers.[17] Nonplexiform but circumscribed neurofibromas in von Recklinghausen disease contain abundant, peptide-rich nerves.[20] Undoubtedly, similar associations exist in plexiform variants. The innervation of neurofibromas of NF1 apparently is much richer than has been appreciated in the past, when one relied on the results of silver impregnation techniques.

The extraneural distribution of the common dermal neurofibroma may be a manifestation of the extension of tumor through

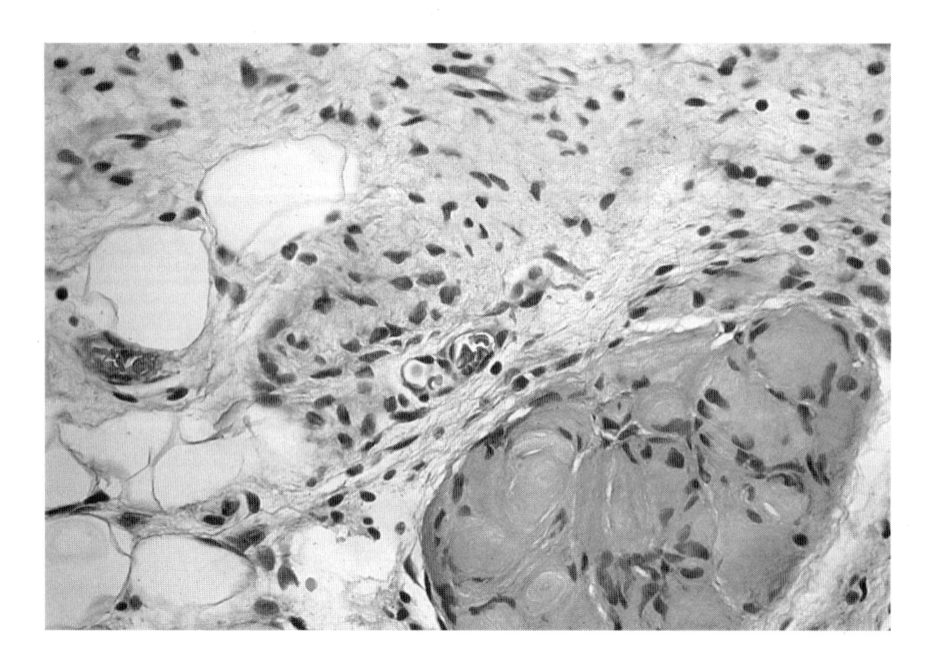

FIG. 36-7. Extraneural (diffuse) neurofibroma with cluster of tactoid bodies Small cells that appear as naked nuclei are loosely spaced in a delicate, faintly acidophilic matrix. Near the lower, right-hand corner, acidophilic spindle cells are clustered in tactile corpuscle–like patterns (tactoid bodies).

the open-ended terminal of perineurial sheaths or through the thin perineurium of small dermal nerves.[16] Deep extraneural neurofibroma may represent a diffuse, neurocristic dysplasia that is expressed in mesenchymal patterns.[3,21]

Differential Diagnosis. Plexiform and pseudoplexiform lesions of the skin and subcutaneous tissue include plexiform schwannoma,[3] plexiform neuroma,[22] the neuromas of the mucosal neuroma syndrome,[23] nerve sheath myxoma,[1,24] and plexiform fibrous histiocytoma.[25]

Subcutaneous extraneural (diffuse) neurofibromas may be confused with the deep component of *dermatofibrosarcoma protuberans*. The confounding patterns account for the characterization of pigmented dermatofibrosarcoma protuberans as *pigmented storiform neurofibroma*.[26,27]

In infancy, fibrous hamartoma also might be considered in the differential diagnosis of an extraneural neurofibroma.

The nodular myxoid components of a low-grade *malignant myxoid fibrous histocytoma* might be misinterpreted as the pattern of a plexiform nerve sheath tumor.

In NF1, mucinous and proliferative endarteritis and aneurysms affect mainly muscular renal vessels, but similar changes may be manifested in other sites.[3,28,29] Aneurysmal changes have been a prominent feature of muscular vessels in some examples of extraneural neurofibromas of the skin and soft tissue, particularly in the distribution of the trigeminal nerve.[3] Such lesions may be mistaken for *hemangioma*.

TRUE NEOPLASMS OF SCHWANN CELLS

Schwannomas (neurilemmomas) are benign, Schwann cell neoplasms.[1,17,30] As solitary, skin-colored tumors along the course of peripheral or cranial nerves, their usual size is between 2 and 4 cm and their usual location is the head or the flexor aspect of the extremities. Superficial schwannomas are rare in the subcutaneous tissue (Fig. 36-8) and even less common in the dermis. In deep soft tissue, they may be large.[31] Internal viscera[32] and bones may be involved. When small, most schwannomas are asymptomatic, but pain, localized to the tumor or radiating along the nerve of origin, can be a complaint.

Histopathology. Schwannomas, with the exception of infiltrating fascicular variants, are intraneural and symmetrically expansile. They are confined by the perineurium of the nerve of origin (see Fig. 36-8) and displace and compress the endoneurial matrix. Most of the symmetrically bundled nerve fibers of the nerve of origin are displaced eccentrically and, if identified, usually are to be found between the tumor and the perineurium (see Fig. 36-8).[3,30] Some of the nerve fibers may extend from the axial bundle into the tumor at the interface with the nerve of origin (see Fig. 36-8). The observations of Russell and Rubinstein[33] contradict the dictum that schwannomas are universally devoid of axons. Loosely and randomly spaced, nonmyelinated axons have been observed in small peripheral schwannomas and in small and medium-sized acoustic nerve schwannomas.[33]

Two variant patterns, namely *Antoni A* and *Antoni B* types, have been described.[34] In the Antoni type A tissue, uniform spindle cells are arranged back to back (Fig. 36-9), and each cell is outlined by delicate, rigid reticular fibers (basement membranes). The cells tend to cluster in stacks, and the respective nuclei tend to form palisades. Two neighboring palisades, the intervening cytoplasms of Schwann cells, and associated reticular fibers, all constitute a *Verocay body* (see Fig. 36-9).

In Antoni type B tissue, files of elongated Schwann cells, arranged end to end, and individual Schwann cells are loosely spaced in a clear, watery matrix (Fig. 36-10).[1,35]

Clusters of dilated, congested vessels with hyalinized walls, thrombi, and subendothelial collections of foam cells[35] are rep-

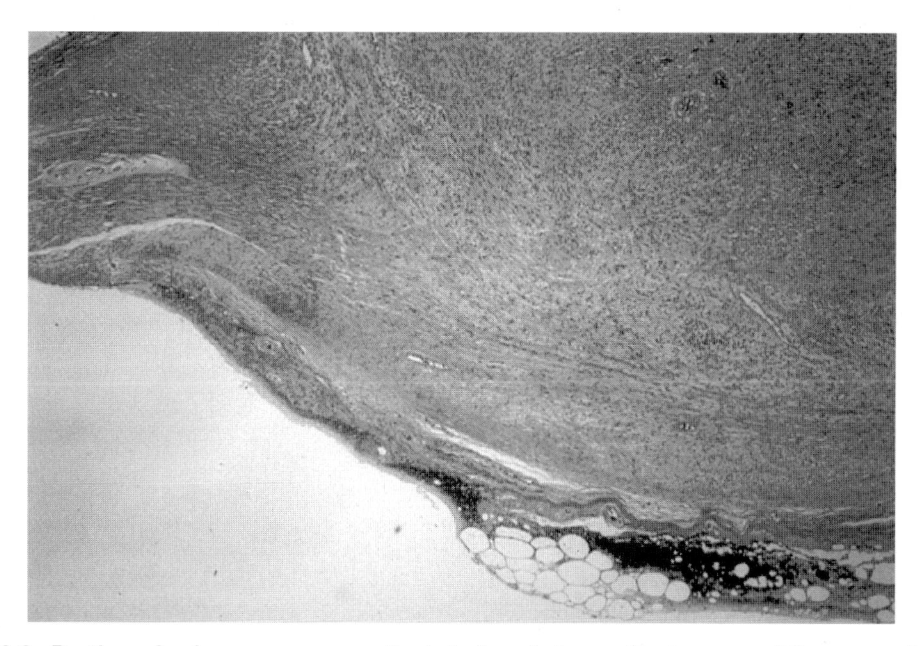

FIG. 36-8. Portion of schwannoma, near the interface between the tumor and the nerve of origin The perineurium is represented as a zone of condensed fibrous tissue between the tumor and the adipose tissue. The nerve of origin is represented at the left-hand side of the field, and the symmetrical axial bundle of nerve fibers extends between the tumor and the perineurium. Some of the nerve fibers extend from the axial bundle into the substance of the schwannoma.

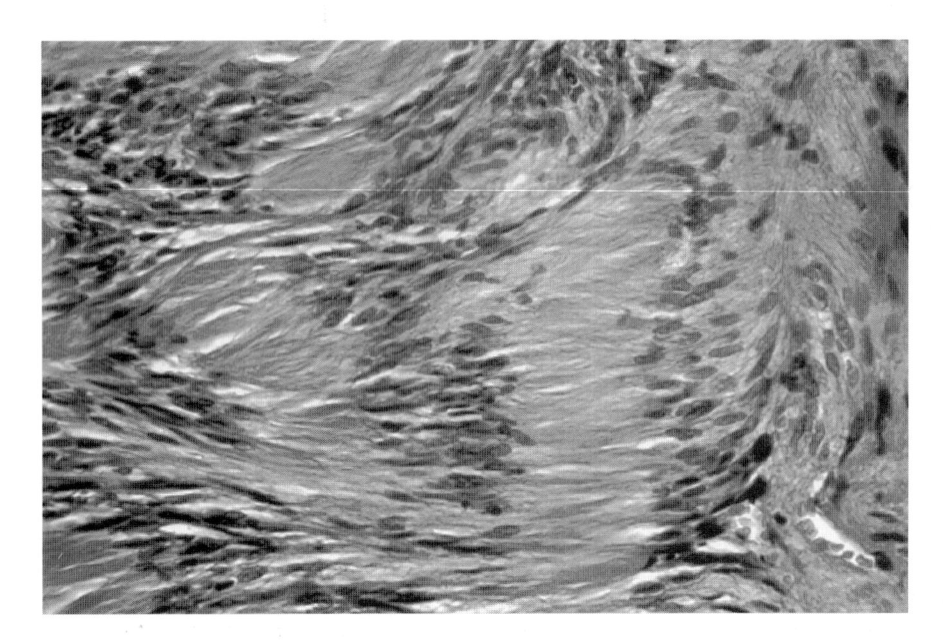

FIG. 36-9. Schwannoma, Verocay body
Schwann cells are arranged in regularly spaced palisades. In aggregate the collections of palisades of nuclei with intervening collections of cytoplasm constitute a Verocay body (variation of patterns in Antoni A tissue).

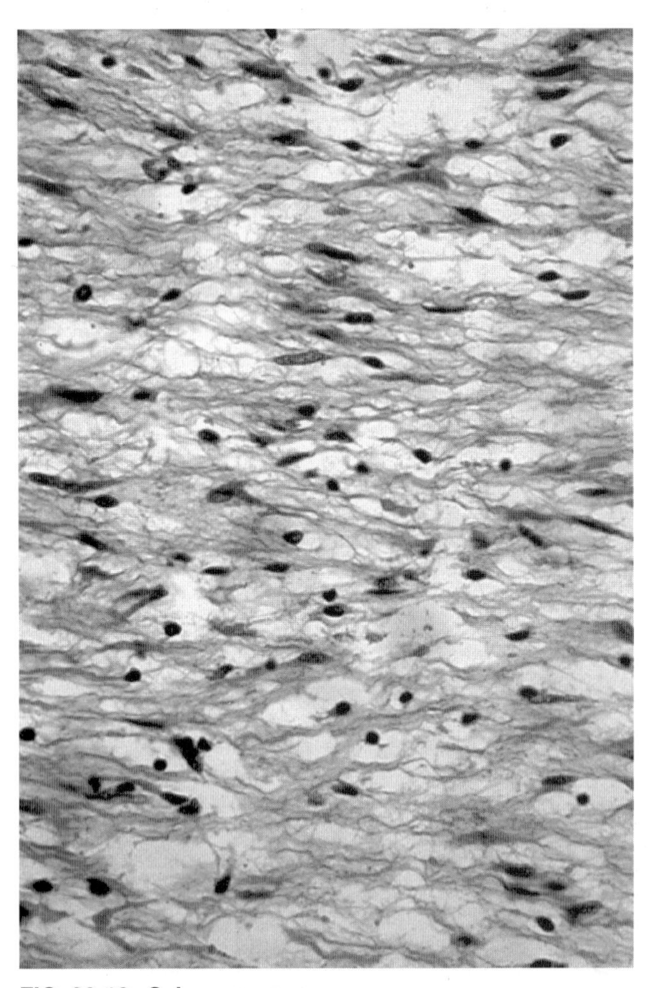

FIG. 36-10. Schwannoma
Thin spindle cells are associated with thin wavy collagen bundles in a clear matrix (Antoni B tissue). A few lymphoid cells are also represented.

resented in both Antoni A and Antoni B tissue. Cystic changes,[3,34] extravasated erythrocytes, and hemosiderin deposits are variable features.

If other common features are preserved, scattered cells having large, hyperchromatic nuclei are of no significance. A low mitotic rate (<10/10 hpf) in association with areas of cytologic atypia in a schwannoma is, in part, a requisite for the diagnosis of a variant of "cellular schwannoma."

Ultrastructurally, the tumor cells manifest the features of Schwann cells.[17] Axons usually are not a significant component. Long-spacing collagen may be represented.[33]

The patterns in Antoni type B tissue are degenerative in nature and at the level of the light microscope have been characterized as "ancient change."[35] Ultrastructurally, tumor cells are widely separated by an electron-lucid, homogeneous matrix containing strands of fibrin and detached segments of basement membrane. Autophagic lysosomes, some containing myelin figures, are seen in many cells. The cells show extensive loss of their basement membrane, disruption of their cell membrane, and degenerative changes in their nuclei.[36]

Histogenesis. The immunohistochemical profile is S-100 protein (+) and collagen type IV (+). In the capsule, cells are EMA (+). A Bodian stain and an immunoreaction for the demonstration of neural filaments reveal few or no axons, except in the peripherally displaced axial bundle.

Apoptosis is a deletion of selected cells in both physiologic and pathologic processes.[37,38] A modification of this process may be the operative phenomema promoting the expression of Antoni B patterns in a schwannoma.

Differential Diagnosis. For a nerve sheath tumor involving a significant sensory or motor nerve, the distinctions between intraneural neurofibroma and schwannoma are important. The intact, but displaced, symmetrical axial bundle of a schwannoma often can be preserved during surgical dissections. On the other hand, excision of an intraneural neurofibroma requires sacrifice of the nerve of origin (including the axial bundle).

Variant Types of Schwannomas

Cellular Schwannoma (CS)

The generic designation of cellular schwannoma, which embraces a variety of histologic patterns, has found a degree of legitimacy in the documentation of a favorable prognosis in several retrospective studies. Classes 1 and 2 (CS1 and CS2) are defined here.

In *CS1*, or atypical schwannoma (a restricted application of the designation in the manner of Harkin and Reed[1]), most examples are large tumors of the retroperitoneum and mediastinum (and may incidentally show immunoreactivity for glial fibrillary acidic protein (GFAP).[39,40] The lesions of CS1 are mostly cellular with solid sheets and interlacing fascicles of spindle cells (Fig. 36-11).[1,3] The basic patterns of a variant of schwannoma, such as a common schwannoma or an epithelioid schwannoma, are preserved, but in some examples most of the cells are cytologically atypical (see Fig. 36-11). Cellular pleomorphism is acceptable. In some examples, nuclear atypia is uniform and extensive. By definition, mitoses are infrequent (<2/10 hpf). A background population of small lymphocytes also may contribute to the cellularity.[1] Nuclear palisades, Verocay bodies, and Antoni type B components may be inconspicuous.[1,3]

In *CS2* (cellular schwannoma of Woodruff[41]; transformed schwannoma of Reed and Harkin[3]), increased cell density, storiform patterns, mitotic activity (even up to 20 or more mitoses per 10 hpf), zones of necrosis, and cytologic atypia are features.[40–45] Although some have argued that these lesions are unequivocally benign, the prospective studies that would certify CS2 as something other than a low-grade, intraneural malignant schwannoma (transformed schwannoma of Reed and Harkin[3]), are not available. The patterns are of a type that in other organ systems would be consistent with a transition from benignancy to low-grade malignancy. In practice, most of these lesions are amenable to local surgery. Confinement of such lesions by the perineurium of the nerve of origin may be prognostically and therapeutically important in providing a distinction between these lesions and infiltrating low-grade malignant schwannomas.[46]

Differential Diagnosis. The differential diagnosis of CS1 includes *leiomyoma*, low-grade *leiomyosarcoma*, and *gastrointestinal stromal tumor*. In a problematic lesion, an intense reaction for S-100 protein would offer support for a diagnosis of schwannoma. Smooth muscle cells, in turn, react with antibodies to smooth muscle actin and desmin. In gastrointestinal stromal tumors, divergent phenotypes may be expressed. Variants of soft tissue sarcoma must be included in the differential diagnosis of CS1 and CS2.

In the rare *epithelioid schwannoma* (with or without radial sclerosis),[3] spindle and round cells are clustered in epithelioid patterns and often have round nuclei (Fig. 36-12). Nuclear atypia and dense nuclear chromatin are common features. In some examples, the cells have acidophilic cytoplasm. In one variation, the cells have round nuclei and scanty cytoplasm, and some of the cells are radially arranged in palisades around distinctive zones of sclerosis.[3,47–49] In the zones of sclerosis, fibrous lamellae are radially oriented and interdigitate with cytoplasmic projections of the surrounding tumor cells.[49] Such lesions have been characterized as epithelioid schwannoma with radial sclerosis,[3] collagenous spherulosis in a schwannoma,[49] and neuroblastomalike epithelioid schwannoma.[47,48] Neither the patterns nor the clinical behavior of these lesions justifies the last-mentioned characterization. Collagenous spherulosis, as originally defined for breast lesions, is distinct from the patterns of radial sclerosis as manifested in nerve sheath tumors. Some examples of epithelioid schwannoma have been characterized as cellular. Some epithelioid schwannomas are also plexiform (see Fig. 36-12).

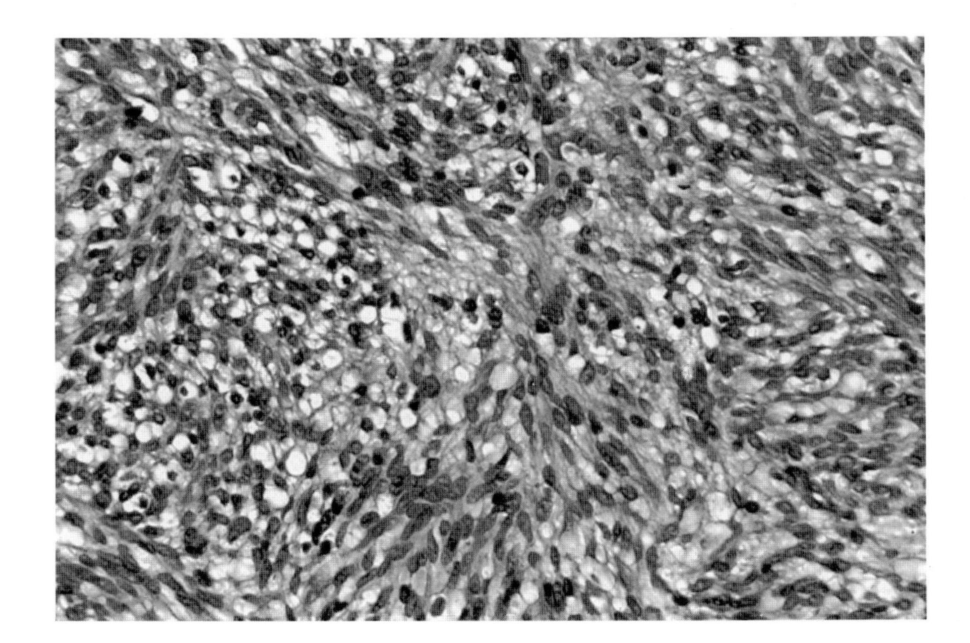

FIG. 36-11. Cellular schwannoma This schwannoma is both cellular and cytologically atypical. The nuclei are uniform but hyperchromatic. Ill-defined storiform patterns are represented (CS, class I).

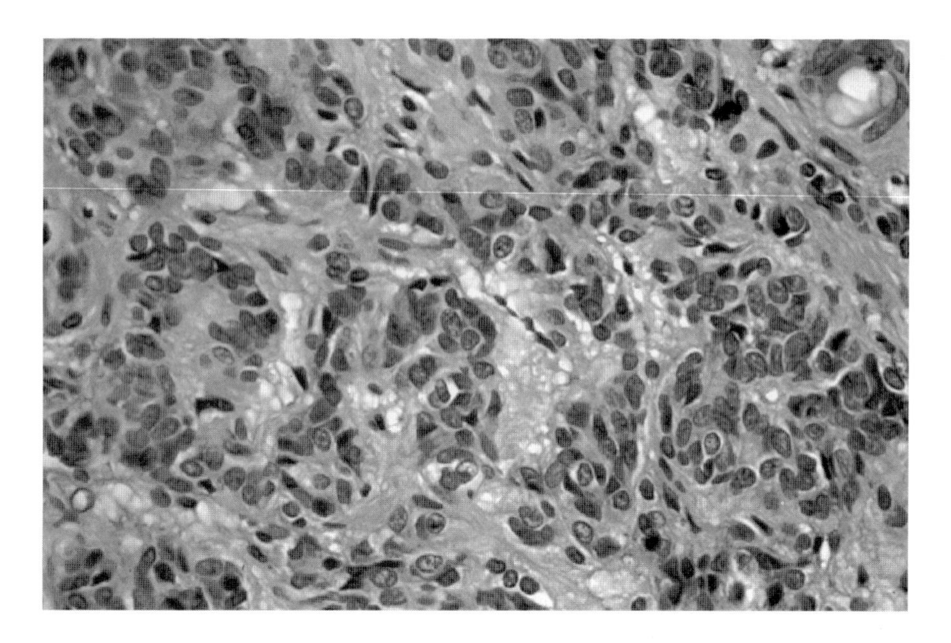

FIG. 36-12. Plexiform, epithelioid schwannoma
In this schwannoma, the cells are polygonal and are closely spaced in epithelioid and fascicular patterns in a delicate fibrous matrix. At low magnification, the overall pattern of this lesion was plexiform.

Glandular Schwannoma

Glands, with the features of sweat glands, are occasionally found within subcutaneous schwannomas.[50–52] Woodruff and Christensen,[51] having demonstrated a component of myoepithelial cells, proposed that the glands are nothing more than entrapped sweat glands. Yoshida and Toot[52] proposed *divergent differentiation* as an alternate explanation for the glandular inclusions. Glandular patterns of a different (entodermal) type are a feature of some malignant schwannomas and also have been observed in a benign neurofibroma.[51]

Plexiform Schwannoma

These occur mostly in the subcutaneous tissue (Fig. 36-13) and rarely are confined to the dermis.[3,16,51–58] They may be a feature of the syndrome of *multiple schwannomas* (schwannomatosis or neurilemmomatosis) [55,59] or they may be solitary.[57] The gene of NF2 and that of multiple schwannomas may be identical.[60,61]

Histopathology. Plexiform schwannoma is intraneural. Spindle cells in solid Antoni A patterns fill the expanded endoneurial space of a limited segment of a nerve plexus. The

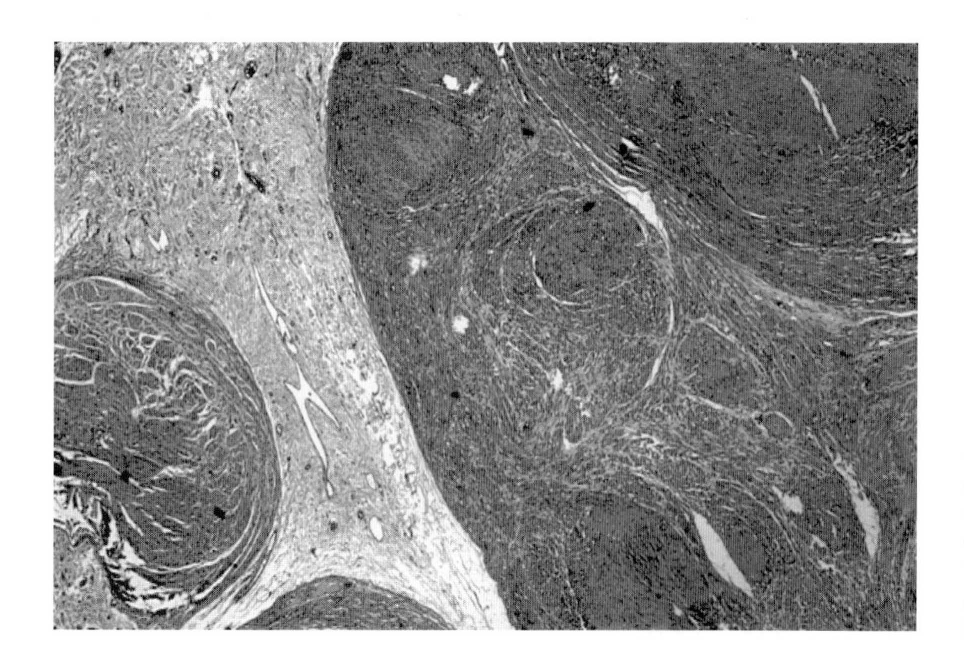

FIG. 36-13. Plexiform schwannoma of dermis and subcutis
The components of the plexus are defined by a peripheral condensation of fibrous tissue that is an extension of the perineurium of the nerve of origin. This example is cellular and purely Antoni A in type. Cytologic atypia is not a feature (CS, class I).

sampled portions present as columns and nodules that are surrounded by perineuria. The vascular changes and Antoni type B tissue of a common schwannoma are variable features. Cystic changes are uncommon. In some examples, fascicles of Schwann cells extend beyond the confines of the perineurium into the neighboring mesenchyme. The limited patterns in the adjacent soft tissue resemble those of a small, circumferential, extraneural neuroma.[53] Some examples of plexiform schwannoma are "cellular."

The category of plexiform schwannoma may be heterogeneous. Kao et al.[57] have documented a relationship between neurofibroma and plexiform schwannoma in one case. In our experience, plexiform schwannoma is commonly associated with a background of diffuse neurofibroma. Examples of plexiform schwannoma that focally are rich in axons may be plexiform schwannoma ex plexiform neurofibroma or ex plexiform neuroma.

Schwannoma Arising in Neurofibroma (with Emphasis on Relationships with Intraneural Microscopic Schwannomatosis)

Schwannomas in continuity with neurofibromas have been documented. *Intraneural microscopic schwannomatosis* (see Fig. 36-3),[3] a proliferative change affecting axial bundles of nerve fibers in intraneural neurofibromas, may, with progression, become a *schwannoma ex neurofibroma*.[16] The phenomena of microscopic intraneural schwannomatosis may be operative in the evolution of some plexiform schwannomas. Rarely, remnants of an intraneural neurofibroma are found at the periphery of a cellular schwannoma (CS1).

Borderline Variants

Infiltrating (Extraneural) Fascicular Schwannoma (IFS) of Infancy and Childhood

Also called plexiform malignant peripheral nerve sheath tumor of infancy and childhood[62] or fascicular schwannoma or congenital hamartoma of nerve,[63] this is a rare Schwann cell neoplasm most often affecting an extremity. In contrast to all other variants of schwannoma, IFS is chiefly extraneural. True plexiform patterns (intraneural by definition) are not a prominent feature.

Histopathology. Uniform spindle cells are arranged in tortuous, interlacing fascicles that vary in size. In some of the thin fascicles, spindle cells tend to cluster in palisades with anuclear collections of cytoplasm separating neighboring palisades. IFS infiltrates skin and soft tissue and, in some examples, erodes bone. In one example, a richly cellular and mitotically active intraneural component was identified.[63] In it, components of the original axial bundle were displaced peripherally.

In the only published collection,[62] four of the six patients with follow-up had local recurrences. In addition, one patient with an invasive lesion of the orbit died.

The malignant nature of IFS has not been convincingly demonstrated. The histologic patterns overlap with those of both infiltrating and fascicular epithelioid malignant schwannoma (IFEMS) and neurotropic melanoma.

Histogenesis. The most characteristic feature of IFS is its extraneural invasion of soft tissue. The tumor cells of IFS, both immunohistochemically and ultrastructurally, are clearly identifiable as Schwann cells.

The nature of IFS is controversial. To assign IFS to the category of malignant nerve sheath tumor would only mask its undefined biologic nature. A malignant nerve sheath tumor unequivocally behaves in a malignant fashion, with a predictable capacity for local recurrence and metastasis. To include IFS in the category of cellular or plexiform schwannoma[64] would be an unwarranted extension of what is already too broadly defined.[64] Cellular schwannoma, as defined by Woodruff, shares the histologic features of malignant schwannoma, but in the available retrospective studies all examples, *by definition*, have been biologically benign. IFS should be characterized as a borderline lesion of indeterminant malignant potential until its nature is better documented.

Psammomatous Melanotic Schwannoma (PMS)

This may be either sporadic or a stigma of a complex (*Carney complex*) that includes myxomas (including trichogenic and cardiac variants),[65] spotty pigmentation, pigmented adrenal cortical hyperplasia, large-cell calcifying Sertoli cell tumor,[66] and endocrine overactivity (including Cushing syndrome).[67,68] Some examples of PMS have behaved in a malignant fashion.

Histologically, psammoma bodies and pigmented, dendritic melanocytes are features. Most examples of PMS are quite distinct, but some show nuclear palisades and Verocay bodies.[67]

Transformed (Borderline) Schwannoma (TBS) (CS2)

This borderline lesion of uncertain malignant potential,[3] like benign schwannoma, is intraneural (confined by an expanded perineurium).[3] Its internal patterns, but not its setting, are reminiscent of patterns seen in minimal-deviation (low-grade) malignant schwannomas of neurofibromatosis (a lesion that is not confined by the perineurium of the nerve of origin). Some examples of TBS contain scattered globular deposits of melanotic pigment.[3]

TBS, as defined by Reed and Harkin,[3] shares many features with cellular schwannoma as defined by Woodruff et al.[41] The overlaps in patterns are given recognition here in the characterization of TBS as cellular schwannoma, class 2 (CS2).

Malignant transformation of benign schwannoma has been a rarely documented event.[69] In the most recent report,[70] only histologically "high-grade" variants were represented. "High-grade," transformed malignant schwannomas,[70] in contrast to TBS, show a greater degree of cellular atypia and pleomorphism and a higher mitotic rate. They may show infiltrative growth beyond the confines of the perineurium,[70] a quality that excludes TBS.

MALIGNANT SCHWANNOMA

Malignant schwannoma (neurofibrosarcoma; malignant peripheral nerve sheath tumor [MPNST]) is the characteristic malignancy arising in neurofibromatosis. Related malignancies may be de novo or may be transformations in other neurocristic neoplasms, such as schwannoma or ganglioneuroma. The criteria for the diagnosis of malignant schwannoma include some, or all, of the following: (1) origin from, or continuity with, a major nerve or neurofibroma; (2) association with classic stigmata of neurofibromatosis; (3) identification of characteristic histologic patterns; and (4) demonstration of immunohistochemical or ultrastructural features of Schwann cells.[74] It has been argued that since most malignant schwannomas arise in association with neurofibromas of neurofibromatosis and since malignant schwannoma ex schwannoma is rare, the designation, malignant schwannoma, is inaccurate. The designation "malignant peripheral nerve sheath tumor," an alternative lacking discrimination, provides no distinctions between the common malignancy of neurofibromatosis and a lesion such as peripheral neuroepithelioma (primitive neuroectodermal tumor). If schwannomas (including "cellular" variants) arising in intraneural neurofibromas are acceptable as "schwannomas," and if the demonstration of both immunoreactivity for S-100 protein (an acceptable marker for Schwann cell differentiation) and ultrastructural features of Schwann cell differentiation are important as evidence favoring nerve sheath differentiation in the common malignancy arising in neurofibromatosis, then the generic designation, malignant schwannoma, retains validity. In it, the schwannian character of the tumor cells is emphasized.

Malignant schwannoma is the common malignant tumor of peripheral nerves.[1,3,21,71–73] Its association with neurofibromatosis is established, but even in this setting it is uncommon. In a series of 678 patients with neurofibromatosis, a malignant schwannoma was observed in only 21 (3.1%) of the patients.[72] In only 2 of the 678 patients did a malignant schwannoma primarily involve the skin and subcutis.

Malignant schwannomas usually arise contiguous with either an extra- or intraneural component of a neurofibroma: in turn, they may be intraneural or extraneural. In the deep soft tissue, involvement of a large nerve trunk, such as a femoral, tibial, or intercostal nerve, is characteristic, but in some instances no such connections are apparent. Malignant schwannomas may also arise as sporadic or de novo lesions (i.e., not associated with neurofibromatosis).[73] An origin in a benign schwannoma, as a documented phenomenon, has been rarely reported.[70]

Histopathology. The variable patterns of differentiation in malignant schwannomas include (1) mesenchymal (fibrosarcomatous, osteo-, and chondrosarcomatous,[3] rhabdomyosarcomatous,[1,71,75] and even liposarcomatous patterns), (2) glandular (entodermal) patterns,[51,76] (3) epithelioid patterns in which individual spindle and round cells often have acidophilic cytoplasm[3,77,78] and are closely spaced in nests, fascicles, and sheets, and (4) neuroepitheliomalike patterns.[79]

Histologically, *mesenchymal patterns* are preponderant in the setting of neurofibromatosis. Thin, rigid spindle cells are arranged in interlacing fascicles in a fibromyxoid matrix. The fascicles are rigid and are alternatingly light (pale) and dark (more intensely stained) (Fig. 36-14). Often the spindle cells are remarkably uniform. Around vessels, neoplastic cells tend to be concentrically or radially arranged. Having identified these basic features, an additional search for and the identification of specific expressions of mesenchymal differentiation provide strong support for a diagnosis of malignant schwannoma. Patterns of specific mesenchymal differentiation, when found, usually are spotty in distribution. Having identified one specific pattern of mesenchymal differentiation, it is often possible for the observer to then find another. The mitotic rate provides a correlate for the diagnosis of malignant schwannoma. It is not a prime determinant of biologic potential. In the setting of neurofibromatosis, rates may be low (<10/10 hpf) or high (>50/10 hpf),

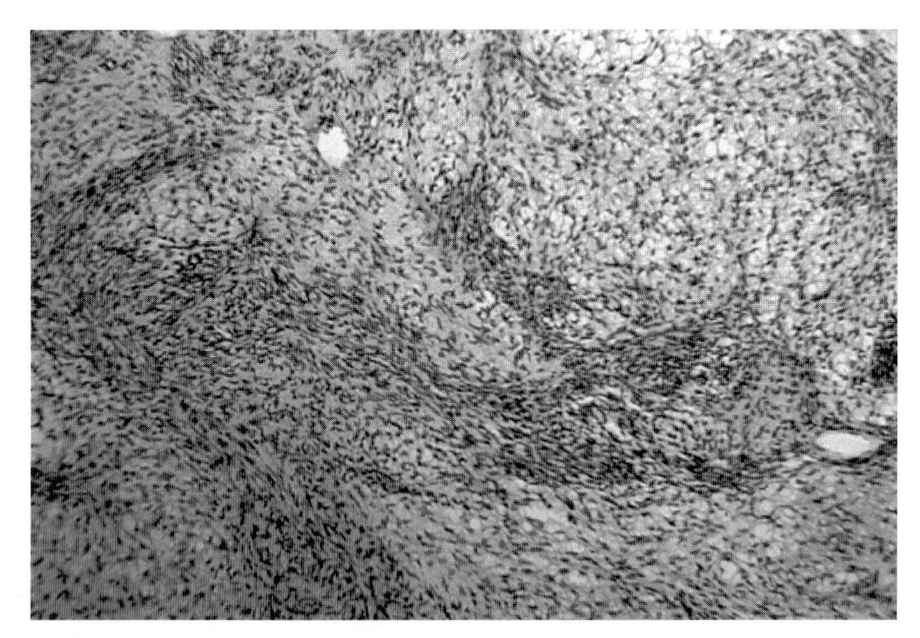

FIG. 36-14. Malignant schwannoma, mesenchymal type
In this large, mitotically active lesion, uniform spindle cells form fascicles that are alternately light and dark. In the light fascicles, the cells are spaced in a clear or myxoid matrix. In the dark fascicles, the matrix is condensed and delicately fibrous. Lesions with similar patterns may also show specific differentiation, such as patterns of rhabdomyoblastic or osteochrondrosarcomatous differentiation.

and the outcome for either category may be poor, depending on other factors, such as the size and location of the lesions and the age of the patient.

Epithelioid patterns are a variant expression of malignant schwannomas in the setting of neurofibromatosis. De novo malignant schwannomas[73] and "high-grade" malignant schwannomas arising in benign schwannomas (*malignant transformed schwannoma*) [70] tend to be intraneural in origin and are manifested in "epithelioid" patterns.[77,78] The study of Hruban et al.[79] does not support this generalization but is compromised by including, as de novo variants, examples of both neuroepithelioma and malignant schwannoma arising in neurofibroma.[79]

Histologically, in epithelioid variants, plump tumor cells in nests and sheets are closely spaced with scanty intercellular matrix (Fig. 36-15).[3,77,78] Nuclei are large and often rounded. In pleomorphic variants, tumor giant cells are common. Specific patterns of mesenchymal differentiation are variant features. In some examples, the cells form nests and cords in a sparsely cellular mucinous, or hyaline, matrix. The "purely epithelioid" (epithelial) malignant schwannoma, a lesion with no "sarcomatous" component, is rare.[3,76,80] In some "epithelial" examples, plump, acidophilic tumor cells manifest a striking cytoplasmic argyrophilia.[3]

Malignant epithelioid schwannomas, some of which appear to have had their origin from, and are in continuity with, a peripheral nerve, may manifest extraneural, infiltrating, and fascicular patterns[26,77] in the skin and subcutaneous tissue. They qualify as *infiltrating fascicular epithelioid malignant schwannomas* (IFEMSs) (Fig. 36-16).

Zones of necrosis with peripheral palisades of tumor cells, a feature of both mesenchymal and epithelioid variants, are reminiscent of patterns in high-grade gliomas of the central nervous system.

Attempts to predict an association of malignant schwannoma with neurofibromatosis simply on the basis of histologic findings usually are defeated by common expressions of overlap in patterns of differentiation.

Ultrastructure. Features supporting a light microscopic diagnosis of malignant schwannoma include (1) slender, overlapping cytoplasmic processes enveloping other processes or cell bodies that may be connected by intercellular junctions; (2) granular, flocculent material preferably coursing parallel to the plasma membrane and occasionally assuming the linear form of basal lamina; and (3) the absence or relative paucity of fine intracytoplasmic filaments.[74]

Histogenesis. In 40% to 80% of cases of malignant schwannoma,[26,77,80–82] the tumor cells are immunoreactive for S-100 protein. CD57 can be detected in over half the cases.[81] MBP is less commonly detected.[81]

Of the many peripheral stigmata in neurofibromatosis, only neurofibromas are predisposed to malignant transformations.

Differential Diagnosis. In the absence of discernible stigmata of neurofibromatosis, differentiation of malignant schwannoma from fibrosarcoma is difficult. Patterns of interlacing fascicles that are alternately light and dark are characteristic of malignant schwannoma. In a mesenchymal variant of malignant schwannoma with patterns of specific differentiation, but with no history or stigmata of neurofibromatosis, a diagnosis of malignant mesenchymoma would be a consideration.

For deep epithelioid variants of malignant schwannoma, malignant fibrous histiocytoma,[83] rhabdomyosarcoma, leiomyosarcoma, and malignant melanoma are considerations.

If confronted with infiltrating and fascicular patterns in a tumor of the skin, a distinction between neurotropic melanoma[3,84] and cutaneous primary infiltrating and fascicular epithelioid malignant schwannoma may be impossible in the absence of melanocytic lentiginous and junctional patterns in the overlying or adjacent epidermis. Fortunately, the distinction as to whether such a lesion is one or the other has no major therapeutic or prognostic implications: for both lesions the management

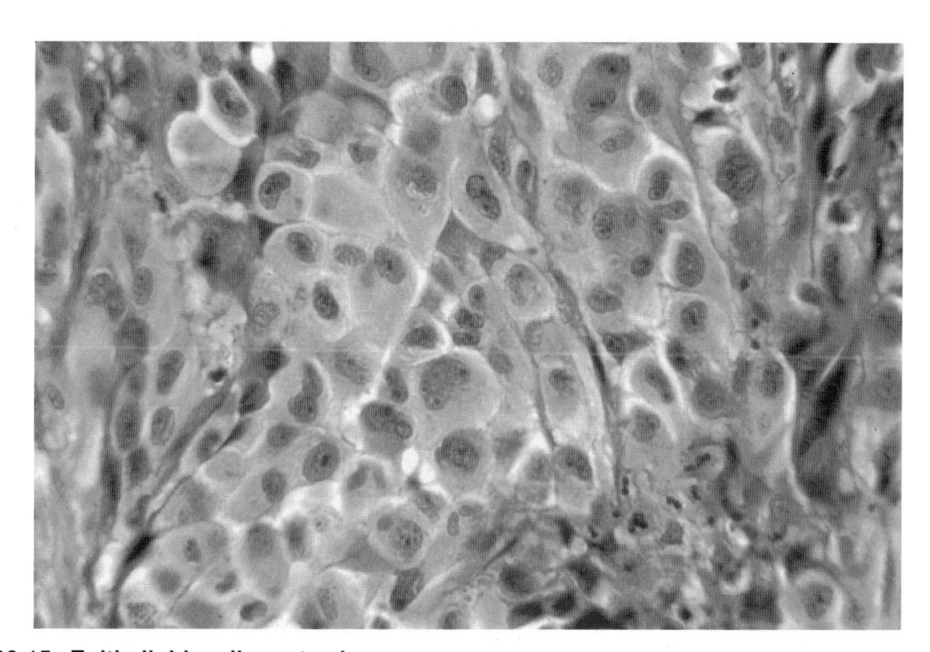

FIG. 36-15. Epithelioid malignant schwannoma
In this example, plump, round, and polygonal cells are clustered in epithelioid patterns. The cells have plump, hyperchromatic nuclei and acidophilic cytoplasm. Some show condensation of the cytoplasm and have rigid, polar cytoplasmic processes. With a Bodian stain, the cells were remarkably argyrophilic.

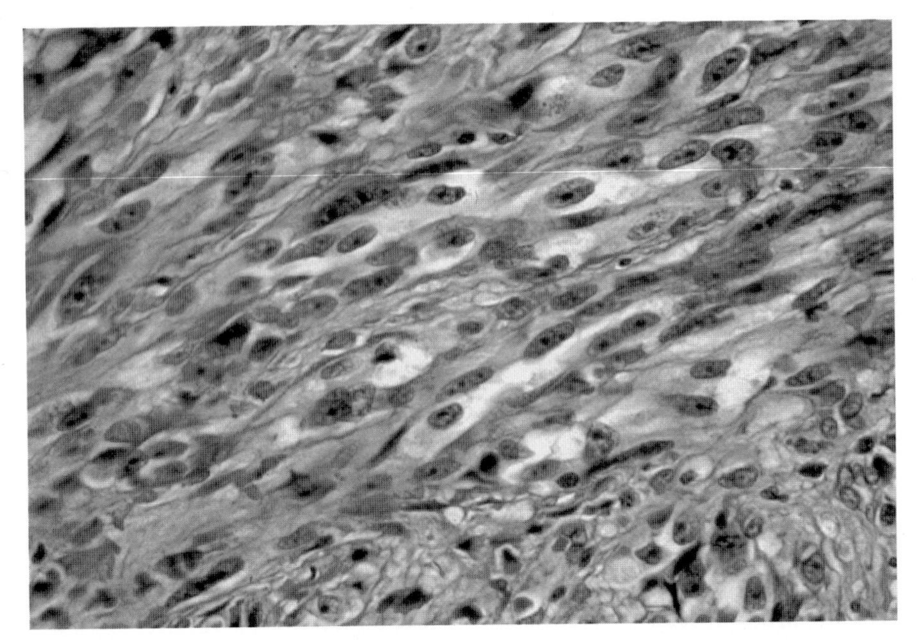

FIG. 36-16. Malignant epithelioid schwannoma: analogue of neurotropic melanoma Plump spindle cells are arranged in ill-defined fascicles. The cells show variations in nuclear size, staining, and outlines. They have pale or clear cytoplasm. This lesion had its origin from a deep peripheral nerve, but the pattern is indistinguishable from patterns commonly manifested in neurotropic melanomas of the skin.

would be similar. Patterns of radial sclerosis, as seen in rare epithelioid schwannomas, occasionally are a feature of dermal lesions in this overlap category of malignant fascicular epithelioid schwannoma and neurotropic melanoma.

Infiltrating fascicular schwannoma of infancy (*IFS*), in its histologic, but not its cytologic, patterns, shows overlaps with the patterns of both infiltrating fascicular epithelioid malignant schwannoma (IFEMS) and neurotropic melanoma.

Glandular, entodermal patterns may be more commonly associated with epithelioid than with mesenchymal variants of malignant schwannoma (Fig. 36-17). If glandular patterns are represented in a problem lesion, then carcinosarcoma might be a consideration. Rarely, entodermal glandular patterns, in the absence of sarcomatous components, characterize a malignant schwannoma.[76]

Ganglioneuroma of the deep soft tissue has been the rare site of origin for a malignant schwannoma.[21,85,86]

Prognostication and Treatment. A moderate increase in cel-

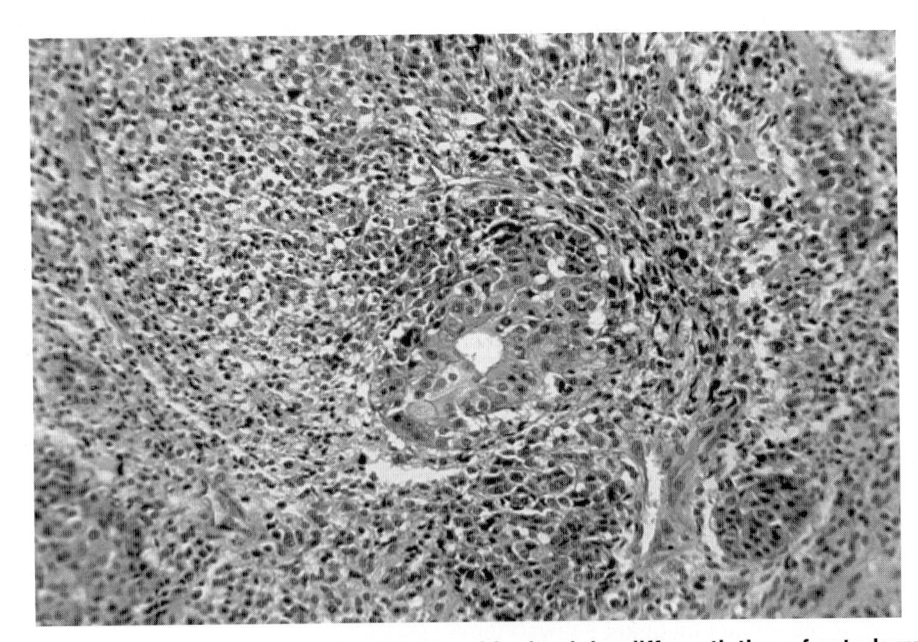

FIG. 36-17. Epithelioid malignant schwannoma with glandular differentiation of entodermal type The lesional tissue in the background is composed of atypical spindle and polygonal cells that are arranged in epithelioid patterns. In the center of the field, epithelial cells are arranged in glandular patterns.

lularity, focal storiform patterns, mild nuclear atypia, and the presence of mitoses (<10/10 hpf) may be the only features that distinguish low-grade malignant schwannoma from neurofibroma.[3,43] Such examples qualify as *minimal deviation variants of indeterminant malignant potential* and may be controlled with local surgery.

In the setting of neurofibromatosis, malignant schwannoma generally has a poor prognosis. High-grade tumors show high mitotic rates (as many as 50/10 hpf), dense cellularity, scanty stroma, marked nuclear atypia, pleomorphism, and palisaded zones of necrosis. For intraneural, high-grade malignant schwannoma ex schwannoma (confined by the perineurium of the nerve of origin), confinement favorably modifies the significance of the "high grade." In one series of epithelioid malignant schwannoma, superficial location (skin and subcutis) and small size were favorable prognostic parameters.[77] In general, adverse prognostic factors include large tumor size; age greater than, or equal to, 7 years; tumor necrosis greater than, or equal to, 25%; and von Recklinghausen disease.[87,88] A high mitotic rate and the need for resection by amputation have also been cited as factors related to a poor prognosis.[79] Aggressive surgical treatment is required for high-grade tumors with extensive spread along the involved nerve.[89]

TUMORS OF UNCERTAIN NATURE WITH NERVE SHEATH–LIKE FEATURES

Nerve sheath myxoma (*NSM; neurothekeoma*) was originally defined by Harkin and Reed [1] and was reintroduced by Gallager and Helwig[90] under the designation *neurothekeoma*. Additional designations include pacinian neurofibroma,[91] bizarre cutaneous neurofibroma,[92] cutaneous lobular neuromyxoma,[93] perineurial myxoma,[94] and myxoma of nerve sheath.[95] In the accumulated studies, the patterns are divisible into a pure myxoid category, a pure "cellular" category, and an overlap category.[96–98] Herein, in the fashion of Argenyi, LeBoit, et al.,[24] the category of nerve sheath myxoma will be divided into a small group, designated *mature nerve sheath myxoma* (*NSM1*) (a myxoid and loosely cellular lesion that mostly appears micronodular), and a larger group (*NSM2*) that includes both immature nerve sheath myxoma (cellular, or epithelioid and fascicular, neurothekeoma) and differentiating immature nerve sheath myxoma, in which immature (epithelioid) and mature (myxoid) patterns are mixed. In all variations, NSM is a rare neoplasm of the dermis. To encounter somewhat similar lesions in the soft tissue is even more infrequent. NSM, in all its expressions, has been benign, although in cases of incomplete removal, rare examples, probably of the NSM2 type, have recurred. Axons are not a component of any of the variants. Neither neurofibromatosis nor multiple mucosal neuroma syndrome has been a documented association.

Mature Nerve Sheath Myxoma (Myxoid Neurothekeoma: NSM1)

Mature (micronodular) NSM ("classical" type of Argenyi et al.[24]) is most common in middle-aged adults (mean age 48 years) with a male-female ratio of approximately 1:2.[24] Asymptomatic, soft, skin-colored or translucent papules or nodules ranging from 0.5 to 1.0 cm in diameter are typically located on the face and the upper extremities, but can occur anywhere on the body.[98]

Histopathology. Symmetrically expansile, myxoid micronodules that vary in size are loosely clustered in a fibrous matrix in the reticular dermis to form a multilobulated mass that is often poorly circumscribed and not always symmetrical (Fig. 36-18). The myxoid matrix is rich in acid mucopolysaccharides (sulfated glycosaminoglycans). In it, bipolar and tripolar cells

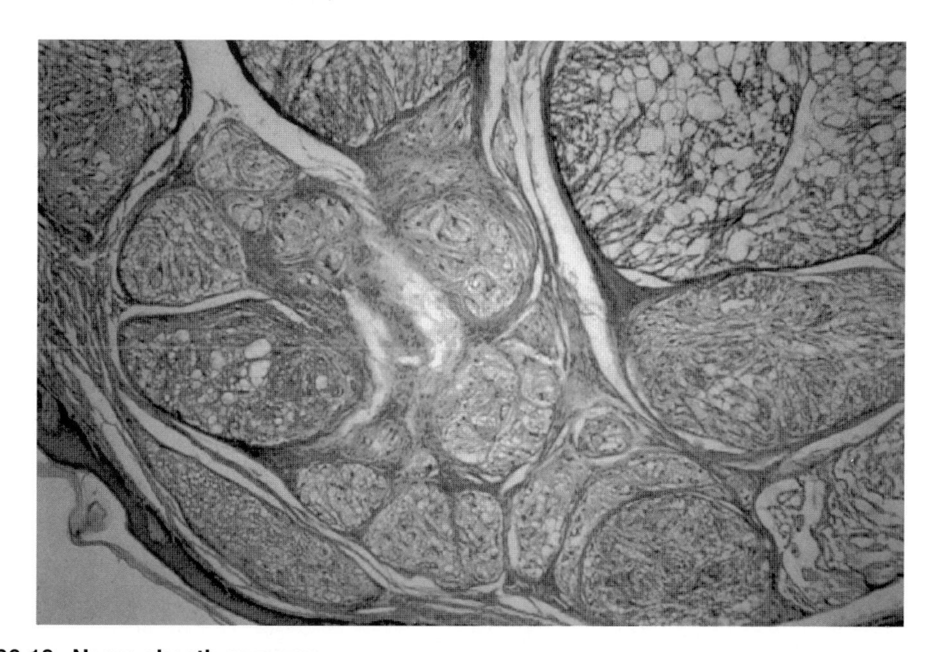

FIG. 36-18. Nerve sheath myxoma
Myxoid cords and nests are closely spaced in the dermis, and each is outlined by a condensation of fibrous tissue. The patterns are plexiform. Within the myxoid matrix, cells with prominent cytoplasmic processes are loosely spaced.

are widely and fairly regularly spaced. Nuclei are elongated and often angulated with inconspicuous nucleoli and uniformly distributed, dense chromatin. Cytoplasms are pale, and cell membranes are sharply defined. Centrally in the micronodules, cells tend to be arranged in loose whorls. Each micronodule is partially or completely outlined, in perineuriumlike patterns, by a thin condensation of fibrous tissue. Continuity with adjacent nerves is rarely identified.[1,90,94,95,98]

Ultrastructurally in lesions of NSM1, a continuous basal lamina outlines most cells, but in some reports discontinuous basal lamina and pinocytotic vesicles have been features.[98] Engulfment of collagen fibers in the manner of Schwann cells has been observed. Fibroblasts and mast cells are also represented.[99]

Histogenesis. The immunohistochemical profile is S-100 protein (+), collagen type IV (+), and vimentin (+).[24,98] A smaller number of cells are EMA (+).[24,95,99]

Immature Nerve Sheath Myxoma (Cellular or Epithelioid and Fascicular Nerve Sheath Myxoma: NSM2)

The second and larger group (NSM2; *cellular neurothekeoma)* includes both immature (NSM2 A) and differentiating immature (NSM2 B) variants. In NSM2, the mean age is 24 years, but examples have been reported in children. Women are more commonly affected, and the head is the favored site. The lesions are firm, pink, red-brown papules or nodules measuring 0.5 to 3.0 cm, and some may produce symptoms.[98]

Histopathology. In immature *NSM2 A*, fascicles of cells tend to be rather uniform in diameter, and their margins are poorly defined. They are arranged in infiltrating (dissecting) patterns among collagen bundles of the reticular dermis (Fig. 36-19) and often extend into the subcutis. Exclusive of the fascicular component, individual tumor cells and small, irregular clusters of tumor cells may infiltrate the reticular dermis and may even extend into arrector muscles. In the fascicles, the cells are closely spaced and tend to be polygonal, but in rare examples they are plump and spindle-shaped. Their cytoplasm is conspicuous and acidophilic. Rigid cytoplasmic processes are prominent. The nuclei are plump, rounded, or elongated, and somewhat irregular in outline. The chromatin is stippled, and the nuclear membranes are heavy.

In *NSM2 B*, some of the aggregates become locally expanded to form broad fascicles and nodules in which both immature (cellular) and mature (myxoid) patterns are represented (Fig. 36-20). In the myxoid zones, stellate cells are loosely spaced: their cytoplasmic processes are broader and more irregular in diameter than those of the cells of mature (NSM1) variants. The mature components tend to be focal, with a preference for the periphery of broad fascicles and nodules. Compact whorls of cells are focally prominent in all variations of NSM2. Spotty, incomplete condensations of fibrous tissue are observed at the periphery of the broad fascicles and nodules.

In some examples of NSM2, the stroma consists of a sclerotic fibrous matrix with no preservation of the interwoven fiber patterns of the reticular dermis.

Mitoses are not a prominent feature in most examples of both variants of NSM2, but atypical variants are characterized by nuclear atypia and pleomorphism with scattered mitoses, some of which may be atypical.[94]

In some examples of NSM2, histocytelike, multinucleated giant cells are represented among the tumor cells.

Rarely in lesions of NSM2, tumor cells extend within the perineurium or in the endoneurial space of small nerves into the adjacent dermis.

Ultrastructurally, NSM2 A and B are composed preponderantly of undistinguished cells. Focal densities of the cell membranes that are suggestive of attachment plaques and focal, poorly formed, basal lamina–like material have been described. Some of the cells contain phagolyosomelike structures, irregularly arranged microfilaments, and rare microfilament-attached dense bodies.[99] Mature fibroblasts are common. In a single case, perineurial cell–like features have been described.[98]

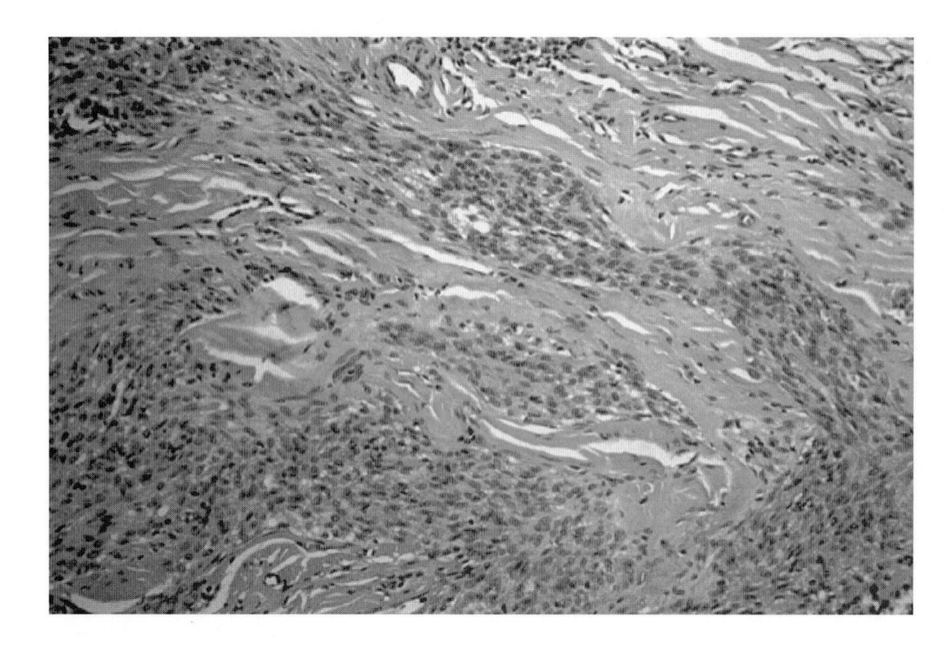

FIG. 36-19. Immature nerve sheath myxoma
Uniform, closely spaced cells form thin, rigid fascicles among collagen bundles of the reticular dermis.

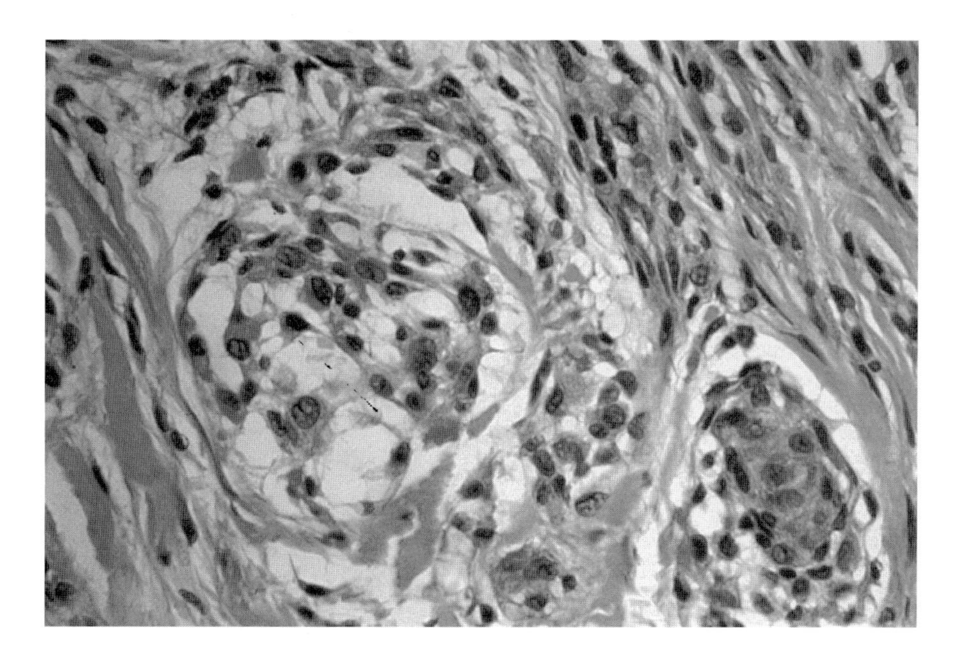

FIG. 36-20. Differentiating immature nerve sheath myxoma
In this differentiating portion, the cells are loosely spaced in a myxoid matrix. Some of the cells are arranged in whorls. In areas showing the most abundant matrix, the cells have rigid, cytoplasmic processes.

Histogenesis. Immunohistochemically, the cells of NSM2 exhibit a variable and inconsistent phenotype. They are positive for vimentin but do not stain convincingly for S-100 protein or epithelial membrane antigen. Weak and variable expression of smooth muscle–specific actin, collagen type IV, NK1/C3, and CD57 have been reported.[24,97–101] The immunohistochemical distinctions seem to contradict the position that NSM1 and NSM2 are related. They may provide evidence that the expressions of phenotype and the respective histologic patterns are dependent on the degree of differentiation.

Differential Diagnosis. Intraneural neurofibromas are rare in the dermis and only slightly more common in the subcutis. Immunoreactive axons may be a feature of intraneural neurofibroma but are not a feature of NSM1.

Cellular myxomas of the skin, including *angiomyxomas* [102] and *trichogenic myxomas,*[65] are rare, and some are poorly documented. They are solid, uniform lesions: neither the micronodular qualities of NSM1 nor the fascicular and nodular qualities of NSM2 A and B are represented. In cellular myxomas, immunoreactions for S-100 protein are negative.[24] Examples of cellular myxoma appear to have been included in some reports of NSM.

Spindle cell nevus of the Spitz type, particularly dermal variants, might be confused with NSM2. A strong and uniform reaction for S-100 protein would favor a variant of Spitz nevus or some other variant of nevus, such as a cellular blue nevus with prominent fascicular components. The pigmentation of deep penetrating nevus is not a feature of NSM2.

In rare examples, minimal deviation *neurotropic melanoma* would be a consideration. Most spindle cell melanomas are S-100 protein positive. Not all desmoplastic and neurotropic melanomas are immunoreactive for HMB45, but a positive reaction excludes NSM2. NSM2 A may be mistaken for a metastatic malignant melanoma (a lesion lacking a primary configuration). A positive reaction for S-100 protein and HMB45 would strongly favor a diagnosis of malignant melanoma.

Some examples of NSM2 B with involvement of the subcutis, and with numerous giant cells, would be difficult to distinguish from plexiform fibrous histiocytoma of children and young adults.[25] In the nodular portions of plexiform fibrous histiocytoma, the cells are closely spaced and often are admixed with multinucleated giant cells. Plexiform fibrous histiocytoma has a close association with fascia. A myxoid matrix is not prominent but focally may be a feature.

Rare sclerosing myofibroblastomas as well as rare myxoid or epithelioid pilar leiomyomas of the skin should be considered in the differential diagnosis. In the cellular portions of myxoid leiomyomas, the cells clearly are smooth muscle in type. In NSM2 A, in which some of the cells are immunoreactive for smooth muscle actin, the tumor cells are consistently negative for desmin.[24]

Epithelioid fibrous histiocytoma (*EFH*) (epithelioid cell histiocytoma, adventitial cellular myxofibroblastoma)[103,104] tends to be polypoid and is mostly confined to a widened papillary dermis. Some examples are mostly myxoid. Large, vacuolated cells with muciparous qualities are occasionally a feature. Many of the dendritic histiocytes among tumor cells of EFH are reactive for factor XIIIa, and some are reactive for S-100 protein. Examples of EFH can be identified in some reports of NSM.

Granular Cell Tumors

Granular Cell Nerve Sheath Tumor (GCNST)

These tumors have been characterized as granular cell myoblastomas, granular cell schwannomas, and granular cell tumors. They usually are solitary but in about 10% of the cases are multiple and may be multifocal. Forty percent of the cases involve the tongue,[105] but the skin and the subcutaneous tissue also are a common site. Other reported sites include the esophagus, stomach, appendix, larynx, bronchus, pituitary gland, uvea, and skeletal muscle.[106]

GCNSTs of the skin are well-circumscribed, raised, firm, and nodular. Some examples are verrucoid at the surface. Generally, lesions range from 0.5 to 3.0 cm in diameter. The cut surface often is faintly yellow and homogeneous. Tenderness or pruritus has been an occasional complaint.

Histopathology. Most GCNSTs are extraneural: rare examples have been intraneural, at least in part. Broad fascicles of tumor cells infiltrate the dermis among the collagen bundles (Fig. 36-21). Rarely, they are entrapped in a dense fibrous matrix (sclerosing variant). Extension of fascicles of tumor into the subcutis is common. The tumor cells are large and polygonal (see Fig. 36-21), and cell membranes are distinct. Faintly eosinophilic, uniform, small granules that are PAS (+) and diastase-resistant fill the cytoplasms. Scattered, laminated cytoplasmic globules with peripheral halos (residual bodies) are also represented. Nuclei usually are small, round to oval, and centrally located (see Fig. 36-21), but in some examples are plump, irregular, and hyperchromatic. Mitoses are uncommon. Some clusters of tumor cells are surrounded by PAS (+), diastase-resistant membranes, strands of collagen fibers, and occasional flattened, satellite cells.[105] Interstitial spindle cells have fibroblastlike qualities.[26]

Neurotropic spread along peripheral nerves, both within and at the advancing margins, is often a feature. Rarely, deep GCNSTs have an intraneural component that expands the involved nerve.

Mitoses are an acceptable feature and are not a marker for malignant transformation. GCNST is a locally infiltrative lesion and should be completely excised. Recurrences are common after incomplete excision.

Infiltration of skeletal muscle and regenerating and degenerating muscle fibers are common features of GCNST involving the squamous mucosae. *Plexiform GCNST* is characterized by perineurial extensions of tumor along the neural plexus of the dermis in the absence of a discrete mass.[107]

Ultrastructurally, tumor cells are outlined by basal lamina.[108] The preponderant cytoplasmic granules are largely phagolysosomes. They appear as membrane-bound vacuoles measuring 200 to 900 nm in diameter. Some of the larger cytoplasmic bodies have the appearance of residual bodies or myelin figures.[106,108,109] The peripheral satellite cells of the fascicles are outlined by discontinous lamina.[110] Interstitial cells of the tumor contain angulate bodies.[26]

Histogenesis. The immunohistochemical profile is S-100 protein (+), peripheral nerve myelin proteins, such as P2 protein and PO protein (+),[111] NSE (+), and vimentin (+).

Differential Diagnosis. A *xanthoma* is excluded by the identification of cytoplasmic granules rather than vacuoles, and by the fascicular arrangement of cells.

Angulated, elongated columns of bland squamous cells occasionally extend from the epidermis into GCNST among the fascicles of tumor cells (*pseudoepitheliomatous hyperplasia).* On biopsy specimens from tumoral lesions of the tongue, genitalia, or the mucous membranes of the upper respiratory tract, esophagus, or anus, such patterns should be interpreted with caution. If confronted with such patterns, a careful search for a component of granular cells may avoid a mistaken diagnosis of carcinoma and, in turn, needless aggressive surgery.

Tumor cells with granular qualities are occasionally a feature of *lesions of diverse lineage*, such as basal cell carcinoma[112] and dermatofibroma. The granules of rare granular squamous cell carcinomas, in contrast to those of other benign and malignant granular cell tumors, are PAS (−), and desmosomes are seen on electron microscopy.[113] In the jawbones, a granular cell variant of ameloblastoma has been described. Granular cell change has been noted in smooth muscle tumors.[114]

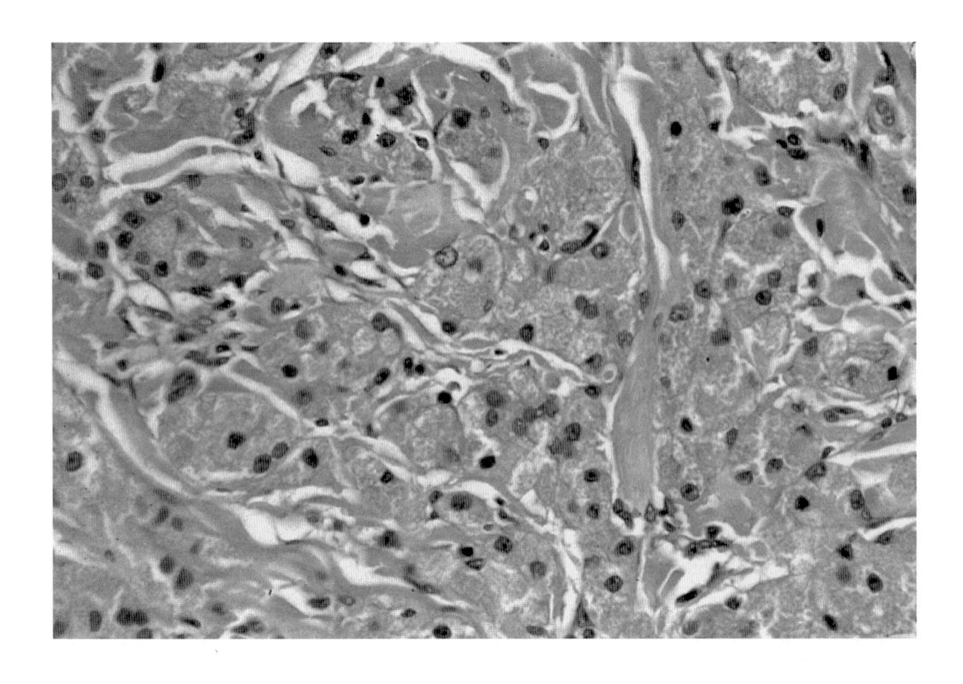

FIG. 36-21. Granular cell tumor Plump, polygonal cells are arranged in nests and fascicles. They have uniform nuclear characteristics and granular cytoplasm.

Granular Cell Epulis of Infancy

This is a polypoid tumor of the gingiva of the newborn, with a predilection for girls.[115] It shares the basic histologic features of *GCNST* but is immunohistochemically distinctive. The immunohistochemical profile is NSE (+), vimentin (+), S-100 protein (−), GFAP (−), CD57 (−), MBP (−), lysozyme (−), a1-ACT (−), and laminin (−). Interstitial cells are positive for S-100 protein. They do not contain angulate bodies.[116]

Malignant Granular Cell Tumor (MGCT)

This tumor is uncommon. Most of the reported cases have occurred on the skin or in the subcutaneous tissue, but, as in benign GCNST, a few cases have been reported from other areas, such as the sciatic nerve[117] and the viscera. A variety of malignant tumors may masquerade in granular cell patterns. In all instances, an acceptance of the diagnosis, MGCT, is predicated on circumspection.

In the skin and subcutaneous tissue, MGCT, a rapidly growing, poorly defined nodule or mass, may reach considerable size and undergo ulceration.[118] Extensive metastases to viscera, skin, and skeletal musculature occur, either with or without regional lymph node metastases. Some lesions, even in the absence of demonstrable metastases, have been characterized as MGCT.[119]

Histopathology. There are two types of MGCT.[120] In one type, in spite of the clinically malignant course, the histologic appearance of the primary lesion, and even of the metastases, is that of a benign GCNST, except for occasional mitotic figures and mild pleomorphism with nuclei that are slightly larger than those seen in most benign GCNSTs.[118,120,121] In the general category of GCNST, these cytologic features are too common to provide a reliable identification of lesions with the potential for metastases. In evaluating the malignant potential of histologically benign or indeterminant granular cell tumors, clinical data, such as the large size of the tumor, rapid growth, ulceration, and invasion into adjacent tissue, are of greater diagnostic value than the histologic features.[122] The average diameter of "histologically benign, clinically malignant," granular cell tumors has been found to be 9 cm, as compared with 1.85 cm for the benign variety.[120,122]

In the second type of MGCT, both the primary lesion and the metastases are histologically malignant: they show transitions from typical granular cells through pleomorphic granular cells to pleomorphic, nongranular spindle and giant cells with numerous mitotic figures.[123,124]

In benign GCNST, immunohistochemical tests for S-100 protein, NSE, and vimentin are regularly positive. In MGCT, the same tests often are negative.[125]

Fibrolamellar Nerve Sheath Tumor

Fibrolamellar nerve sheath tumor (FNST) ("pacinian neurofibroma"[126]) is a solitary tumor of the dermis.

Histopathology. FNST is nonencapsulated but sharply defined in the dermis. Coarse, rigid, brightly eosinophilic lamellae are arranged in parallel arrays in stacks of four or more (Fig. 36-22). Neighboring stacks are random in orientation, one to the other, but in some areas the patterns that result from the abutment of neighboring stacks are storiform. Some examples are mostly myxoid, and in them the fibrous lamellae are more delicate and widely spaced. Tumor cells, each with a small nucleus, scanty perikaryon, and rigid, thin, polar extensions of cytoplasm, resemble perineurial cells. They are isolated in clear or mucinous matrix among the fibrous lamellae. Rarely, a few loosely clustered, pigmented dendritic melanocytes have been a feature.

FNST is histologically distinctive but may be simply an exaggeration of perineurial-like patterns that are occasionally manifested in cutaneous neurofibromas.

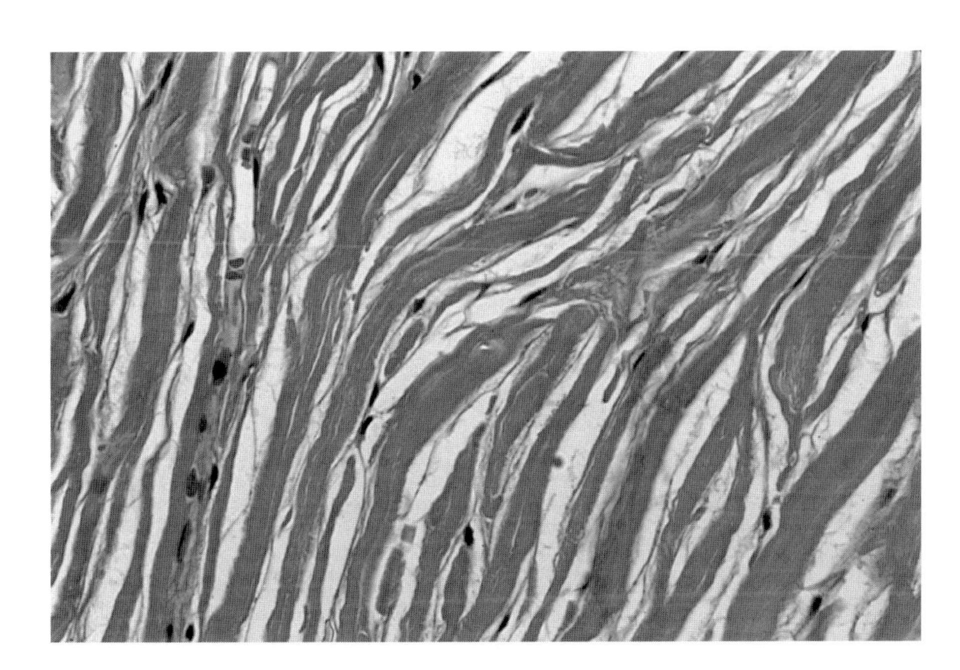

FIG. 36-22. Fibrolamellar nerve sheath tumor
Thin, wavy fibrous lamellae are regularly spaced in a delicate, mucinous matrix and are stacked. The cells among the lamellae have thin, elongated polar processes (perineurial cell–like).

FNST shares features with *sclerosing fibroma* as manifested either sporadically or in the setting of *Cowden* disease.[126] An appreciation of subtle cytologic differences and a demonstration of immunoreactivity by some of the tumor cells for S-100 protein strongly favor the diagnosis of FNST.

Storiform Nerve Sheath Tumor

Storiform nerve sheath tumor (SNST) (storiform perineurial fibroma; "perineurioma") is a solitary, symmetrically expansile, and well-circumscribed tumor[3,127,128] of the subcutis, but the deep soft tissue and even viscera may be involved. The clinical features are not well established.

Histopathology. SNST is circumscribed. At its periphery, the interface with soft tissue is defined by a thin capsule consisting of several loosely spaced, delicate fibrous lamellae. Beneath the capsule, thin, rigid, fibrous lamellae are regularly spaced in a delicate matrix. Cells with plump, angulated nuclei and rigid, polar, cytoplasmic extensions are loosely spaced among the fibrous lamellae. Fascicles in storiform patterns are variably represented. In most examples, small nerves are embedded in, or may be traced into, the tumor. The tumor cells tend to form thin, concentric layers around entrapped small nerves, blood vessels, and collagen bundles. Onion skin patterns occasionally are a focal variation in such lesions.

Histogenesis. The cytologic features are perineurial cell–like. In some examples, tumor cells are immunoreactive for vimentin and EMA, although the latter reaction may be weak or patchy[129] and best developed in cells in or near the capsule. In other examples, scattered aggregates of tumor cells in more central locations are reactive for S-100 protein.

Storiform patterns appear to be variations that are expressed in a variety of nerve sheath tumors, and perhaps variants of both schwannomas and neurofibromas may be included in this category. The evidence that the category is purely perineurial in character is unconvincing. Some examples would also qualify as "cellular" schwannoma.

Differential Diagnosis. Dermatofibrosarcoma protuberans, in its nodular, well-differentiated components, may be confused with SNST. Fibrous histiocytoma of the subcutis and dermatofibroma also are considerations in the differential diagnosis.

Dermatofibrosarcoma Protuberans

Dermatofibrosarcoma protuberans (DFSP) has been variously classified as a fibroblastic, fibrohistiocytic, or neurocristic tumor. The pigmented variant of DFSP (*Bednar tumor*) has been characterized as pigmented storiform neurofibroma. The nature of pigmented dermatofibrosarcoma is controversial, but in one study perineurial cell–like qualities were observed.[130] The cells of DFSP, like those of nerve sheath tumors, are immunoreactive for CD34.[131] DFSP is described in detail elsewhere (Chap. 33).

Pacinian Neurofibroma

The designation *pacinian neurofibroma* has been assigned to a variety of lesions. The list includes the lesion characterized herein as dermal fibrolamellar nerve sheath tumor (FNST);[126] cellular blue nevus;[132] a lesion of uncertain nature with perivascular concentric lamellar fibrosis;[133] diffuse neurofibroma with tactoid bodies;[4] a giant pacinian corpuscle with an increased number of coarse fibrous lamellae;[3] and nerve sheath myxoma.[91]

PERINEURIAL TUMORS

Perineurioma

Perineurioma (hypertrophic interstitial neuritis; hypertrophic mononeuropathy)[134–136] is an intraneural, solitary, segmental, and cylindrical enlargement of a nerve. Sensorimotor defects are characteristic.

Histopathology. Cells with both the structural qualities and the immunoreactivity of perineurial cells form concentric sheaths (pseudo–onion bulbs) around affected nerve fibers (Fig. 36-23) and even around small clusters of pseudo–onion

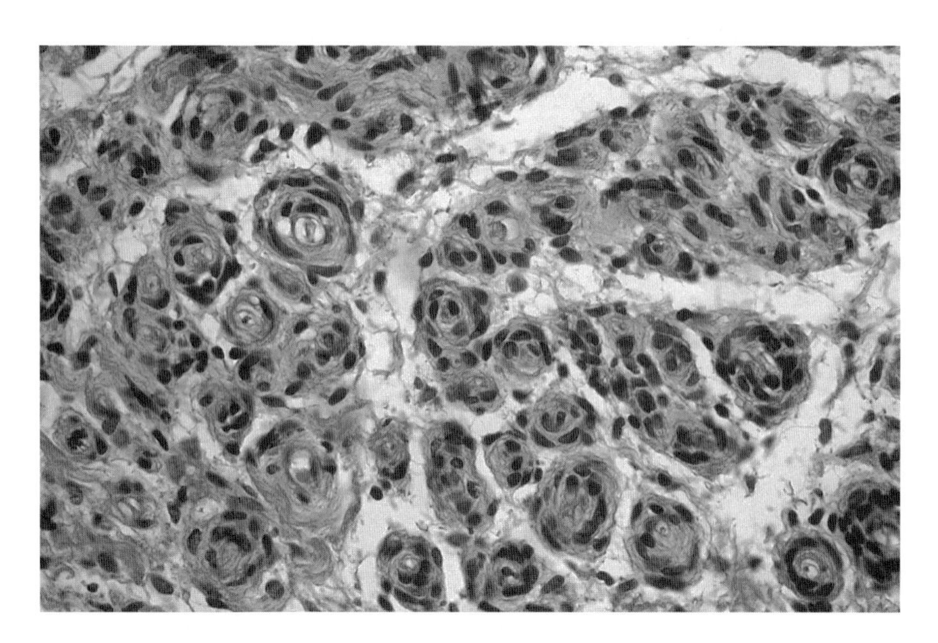

FIG. 36-23. Mononeural neuropathy; intraneural symmetrical neurofibroma; hypertrophic interstitial neuritis
In this tumor of a spinal nerve root, perineurial cells are concentrically layered around preexisting nerve fibers (pseudo–onion skin patterns).

bulbs.[134] Collagen bundles and vessels may be similarly embraced. Demyelination and degeneration of axons are associated phenomena.

Histogenesis. The concentrically arranged cells immunoreact with antibodies for EMA and have the ultrastructural features of perineurial cells.

A defect in the integrity of the perineurial barrier has been proposed as the primary alteration. Delamination of the perineurium and migration of perineurial cells into the endoneurium have been offered as an explanation for the origin of pseudo–onion bulbs.[135]

In common with descriptions of the clonal chromosomal abnormalities in benign and malignant schwannomas, neurofibromas, meningiomas, and gliomas, deletion of 22q11.2-qter has been described in perineurioma,[134] and is a finding favoring neoplasia.

Differential Diagnosis. The *hereditary degenerative neuropathies* are not localized and segmental.[135] They are characterized by concentric hyperplasia of Schwann cells (onion bulbs).

NEUROMAS

Neuromas are hyperplasias of axons and associated nerve sheath cells. In most but not all cutaneous neuromas, Schwann cells and axons are arranged in broad, interlacing (tortuous) fascicles, and axons are easily demonstrated with silver impregnation techniques. Axons are also easily demonstrated with monoclonal antibodies, such as those for neurofilaments, but such reactions, in themselves, do not distinguish between the innervated fascicles of a neuroma and those of cutaneous neurofibroma.

Neuromas can be divided into four types: (1) extraneural (traumatic or acquired) neuromas, (2) intraneural (isolated and spontaneous, solitary or multiple) neuromas, (3) intraneural (multiple mucosal) neuromas occurring in multiple endocrine neoplasia, type 2b, and (4) abnormalities of sensory receptors.

Extraneural Neuromas

Acquired (Traumatic) Neuroma

Traumatic neuromas are usually solitary, skin-colored or pink, firm papules or nodules at the sites of scars following local trauma. In mature neuromas a lancinating type of pain may be elicited in response to local pressure.

Histopathology. Interlacing fascicles of regenerating nerve fibers extend from the proximal end of a damaged nerve through an acquired defect in the perineurium into the neighboring mesenchyme. They insinuate in asymmetrical patterns among collagen bundles. With maturation, perineuria form around the extraneural fascicles (Fig. 36-24). Tangled fascicles in a scar form the tumor. The distal end of a severed nerve does not contribute to the neuroma. In pretumorous stages, nerve fibers of both the proximal and distal segments of the disrupted nerve show wallerian degeneration.

Rudimentary Supernumerary Digits

These usually are asymptomatic, smooth or verrucous papules. Like intact supernumerary digits, they occur at the base of the ulnar side of the fifth finger. They are assumed to represent the residua of either autoamputation in utero, or postnatal destruction, of a supernumerary digit.[138]

Histopathology. Much of what comprises a rudimentary digit shows the histologic pattern of an acquired neuroma. Nerve fibers of the neuroma that are located close to the epi-

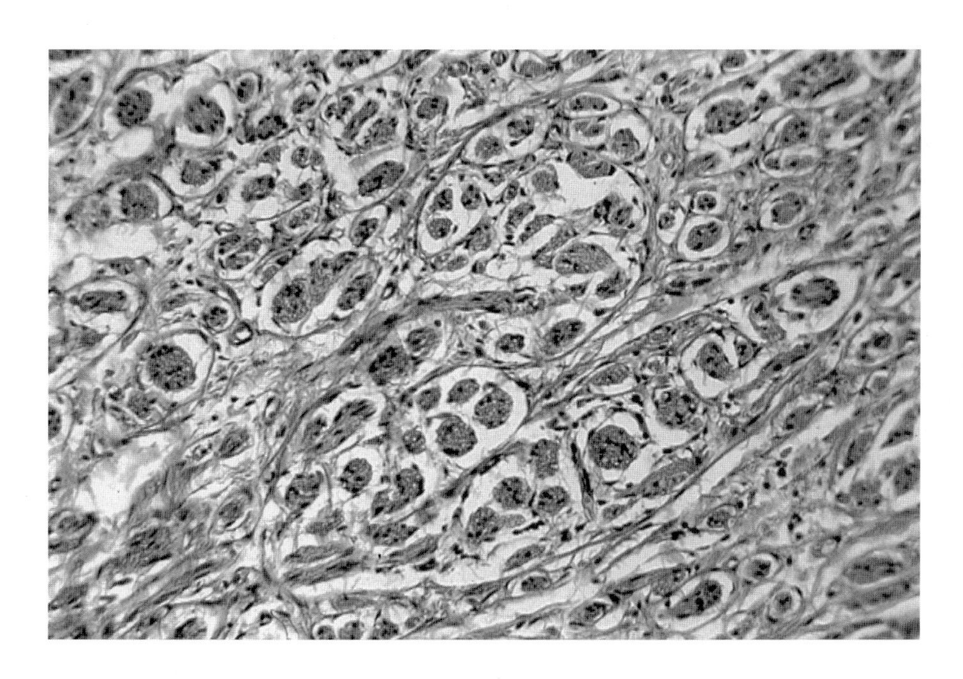

FIG. 36-24. Acquired (traumatic) extraneural neuroma
Innervated fascicles are mostly cut in cross sections. They are supported by a space containing myxoid matrix, and each fascicle and its supporting matrix are confined by a thin condensation of fibrous tissue (regenerated perineurium). All are supported by a background fibrous matrix (mature neuroma).

dermis may terminate in closely spaced Meissner corpuscles.[138]

Intraneural Neuromas

Palisaded and Encapsulated (Sporadic and Spontaneous) Neuroma (PEN)

This neuroma is uncommon. Solitary examples may arise in either early childhood or adulthood (mean age, 45.5 years). Multiple neuromas arise in adulthood. Both solitary and multiple cutaneous intraneural neuromas usually are asymptomatic. In neither presentation are the lesions associated with the stigmata of *multiple endocrine neoplasia* (MEN).

PEN is a firm, rubbery, skin-colored or pink papule or nodule[139–142] that commonly affects the "butterfly area" of the face. During biopsy, it often is ennucleated from its dermal bed and then submitted to the pathologist without any surrounding skin.

Histopathology. PEN is a bulbous expansion of a peripheral nerve, appearing as a well-circumscribed, ovoid or rounded nodule in the dermis (Fig. 36-25). Intraneurally, Schwann cells form uniform, broad (4–5+ cell layers), interlacing fascicles that are closely spaced in a clear matrix (Fig. 36-26). Nuclear palisades are ill defined. Nuclear pleomorphism and mitoses are not features. PEN is confined by a thin, expanded perineurial sheath. In many examples, the sheath is attenuated along the surface that approximates the epidermis. This variation is a consequence of the anatomy of a nerve: the perineurial sheath is open-ended in this site. At some site along the periphery, it is usually possible to identify in continuity extensions into the endoneurial space of small neighboring nerves.

The fascicles are rich in axons with silver stains (Fig. 36-27)[141,142] and with immunoreactions for neural filaments. A weak, sometimes discontinuous reaction for EMA is a feature in the capsule of PEN.[141]

Intraneural Plexiform Neuroma

Plexiform neuroma is an uncommon intraneural tumor of the dermis and subcutis. It has been characterized as a variant of PEN,[22] but some examples may represent incipient plexiform schwannoma.

Histopathology. Nodules and broad cords are circumscribed by the perineurium of the involved segment of nerve. The internal patterns of all the nodules and broad cords are basically those of PEN.

Clustered, dilated vessels with sclerotic walls and subendothelial collections of foam cells are features in common with schwannoma.

In contrast to fully developed plexiform schwannoma, plexiform neuroma, with both silver stains and immunoreactions for neural filaments, is rich in axons.

Mucosal Neuroma Syndrome

Multiple endocrine neoplasia (MEN), type 2b, first described in 1968,[23] is the only one of three types (i.e., types 1, 2, and 2b) to show mucosal and cutaneous neuromas (*mucosal neuroma syndrome, MNS*). *Multiple* (*intraneural*) *neuromas*, many of which are periorificial, are often its earliest manifestation. First appearing in early childhood, they are seen as small nodules, often in large numbers, on the mucosa of the lips, tongue, and oral cavity[143,144] and on the conjunctiva and sclera. Some patients show small, nodular neuromas on the skin of the face, usually only in small numbers[144] but occasionally in large numbers on and around the nose and on the eyelids. Quite frequently, the

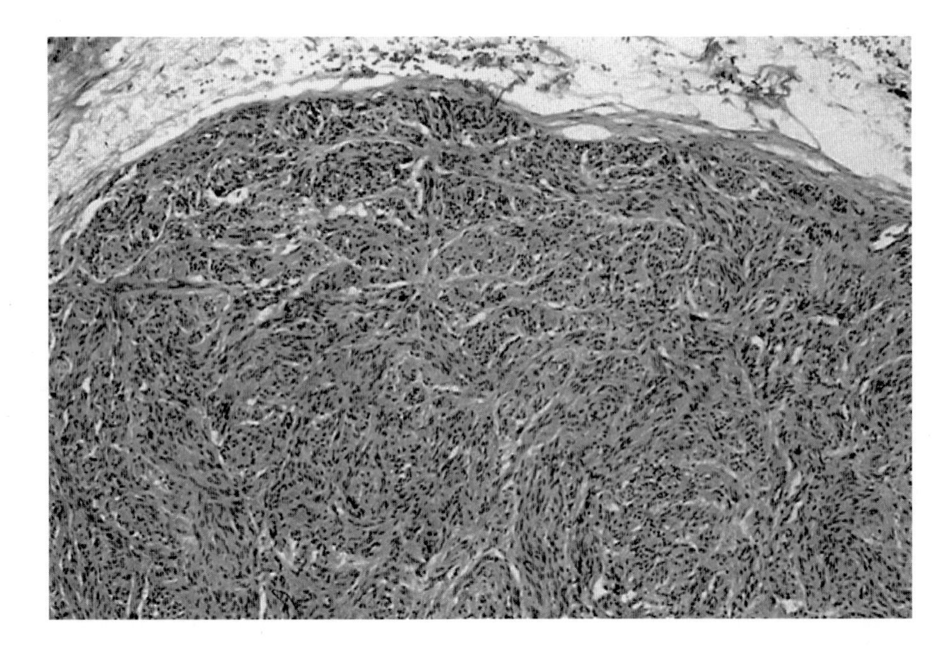

FIG. 36-25. Palisaded encapsulated neuroma
An expansile tumor is outlined by a condensation of fibrous tissue (expanded perineurium). Broad fascicles of axons and Schwann cells are interlaced in a scanty, clear matrix.

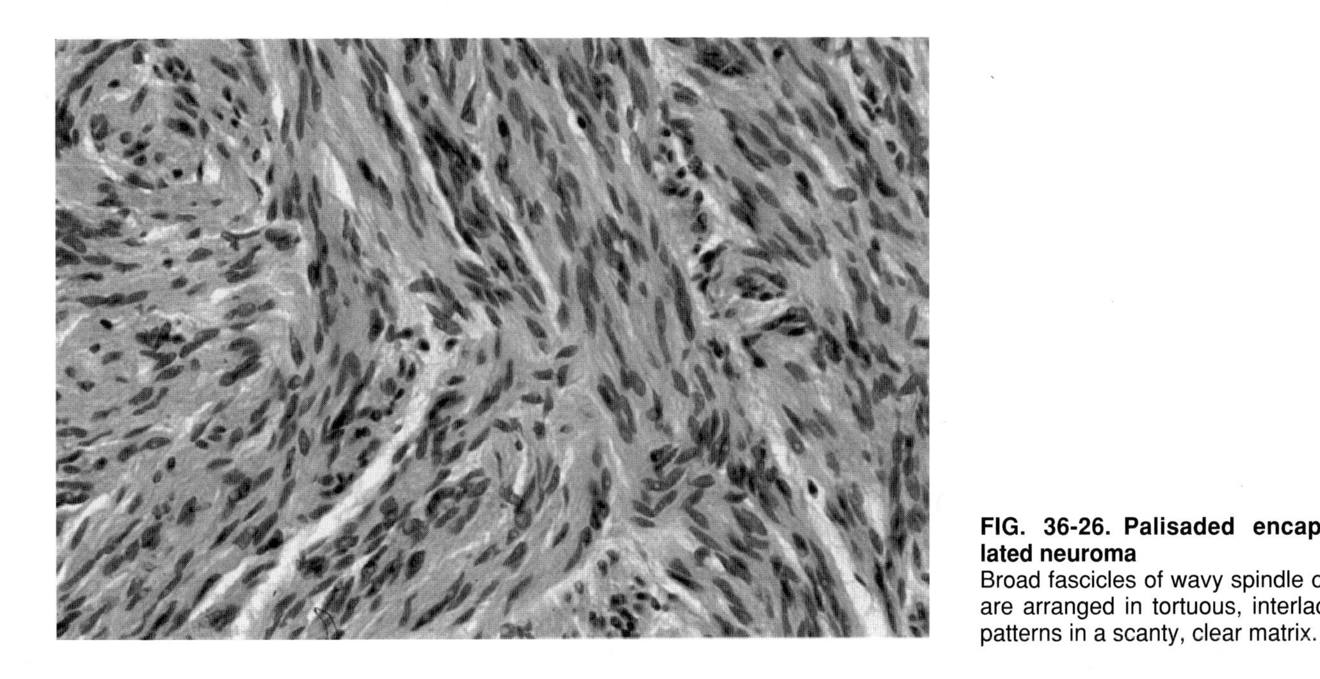

FIG. 36-26. Palisaded encapsulated neuroma
Broad fascicles of wavy spindle cells are arranged in tortuous, interlacing patterns in a scanty, clear matrix.

lips are thick, fleshy, and protruding.[145] Marfanoid features and skeletal abnormalities may be present.[145]

MEN, type 2b, may be inherited as an autosomal dominant trait,[143] and *medullary thyroid carcinoma, bilateral pheochromocytoma,*[144] and *diffuse alimentary tract ganglioneuromatosis* are associated disorders of variable frequency.[146]

Histopathology. The neuromas of the MNS are intraneural and plexiform. Characteristically, the involved nerves are slender. Many are uniform in diameter, but bulbous expansions also are a feature. Within the confines of the perineurium, fascicles that are fairly uniform in diameter and composed of two or more nerve fibers are interlaced in asymmetrical patterns and are closely spaced, back to back, in a clear (endoneurial) matrix. The fascicles of nerve fibers in the mucosal and cutaneous lesions are richly innervated.

Linear cutaneous neuroma (dermatoneurie en strie), a sporadic variant of an intraneural neuroma, is manifested clinically as a group of raised linearities. It differs from the mucosal neuroma syndrome in clinical presentation and in the size of the altered nerves in the dermis.

Histologically, nerves of the dermis and subcutis are slightly enlarged and hypercellular. Internally, Schwann cells are in-

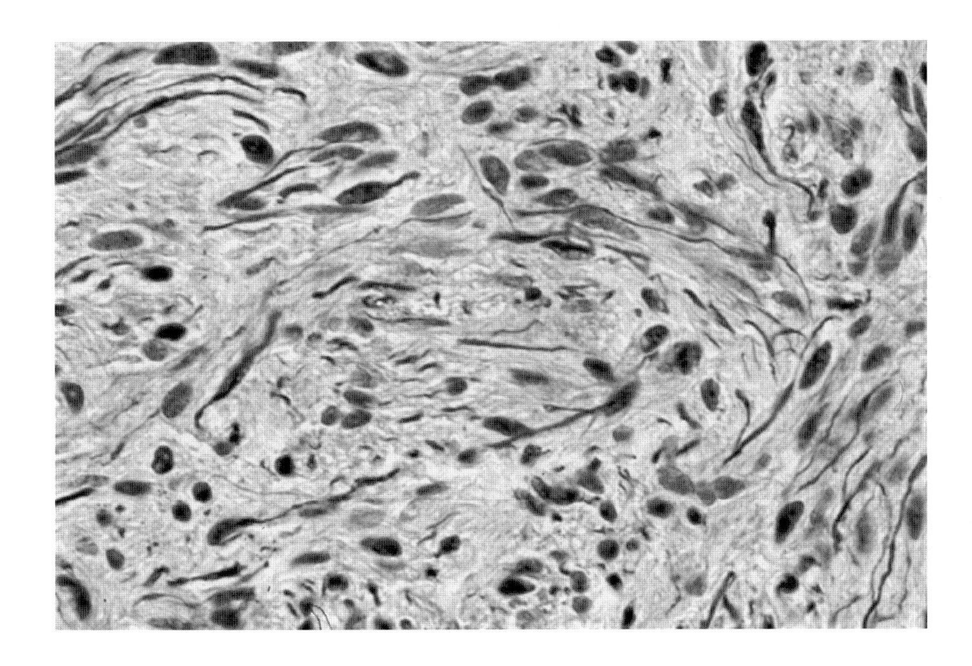

FIG. 36-27. Palisaded encapsulated neuroma
Bodian stain. Argyrophilic axons are numerous among the Schwann cells.

creased in number and nerve fibers are tortuous; this combination of features results in loss of axial symmetry in the affected segments.

It has been proposed that linear cutaneous neuromas are a manifestation of multiple endocrine neoplasia, type 2b.[147]

Special Stains (Applicable to All Neuromas). With luxol-fast blue stain, some of the fibers in all forms of neuroma may be myelinated.

Electron Microscopy (Applicable to All Neuromas). Ultrastructurally, fascicles that are composed of myelinated and nonmyelinated nerve fibers are the chief feature of both extraneural[148] and intraneural neuromas. Those of a mature, extraneural neuroma are ensheathed by multiple lamina of perineurial cells.[148] Generally, perineuria do not outline the individual, asymmetrical fascicles of intraneural neuromas.

Histogenesis (Applicable to All Neuromas). The immunohistochemical profile is S-100 protein (+), collagen type IV (+), vimentin (+), and NSE and neural filaments (+).

In mature traumatic neuroma, the majority of the individual nerve fascicles are surrounded by cells that are immunoreactive for EMA, indicating perineurial differentiation.[140] Collagens type I and III are deposited among the fascicles. The nerve fibers of the newly formed fascicles are supported by matrix that is rich in acid mucopolysaccharides.[140]

In spontaneous intraneural neuromas, such as PEN and those of the mucosal neuroma syndrome, the local proliferation of axons within the confines of the perineurium has not been adequately explained.

Pacinian Neuroma

Pacinian neuroma is found in the same anatomic sites as pacinian corpuscles[149] and is an occult, painful lesion.

Histopathology. Pacinian corpuscles form a localized cluster but are otherwise unremarkable. The corpuscles may vary in size.

If a cluster of corpuscles is continuous with an extraneural neuroma, it would be difficult to attribute the symptomatology to the cluster of corpuscles.

Patterns in which cells and fibers are concentrically layered are common in the setting of nerve sheath tumors. Some examples of nerve sheath tumors with such patterns have been characterized as "pacinian neurofibroma."

SMALL ROUND CELL TUMORS

This category includes primary, cutaneous, small-cell undifferentiated carcinoma (Merkel cell tumor); primitive neuroectodermal tumors (PNET) such as Ewing sarcoma, neuroblastoma, and neuroepithelioma; primitive mesenchymal tumors such as small-cell osteosarcoma and embryonal and alveolar rhabdomyosarcoma; rare melanomas of infancy that arise in the setting of giant congenital nevus (melanoblastoma of infancy);[150] and melanotic neuroectodermal tumor of infancy.[151] In all of these lesions on hematoxylin-eosin–stained sections, cells with few distinguishing characteristics other than scanty cytoplasm, and with closely spaced, "dark" nuclei, provide a challenge in differential diagnosis. In this category, some of the lesions that have been grouped as "primitive neuroectodermal tumors" share certain features but may also be distinguished by patterns of divergent differentiation.[152] Small round cell tumors are more common in the soft tissue or bone.[153,154] In the skin, cutaneous small (Merkel) cell undifferentiated carcinoma is most frequent.

Cutaneous Small (Merkel) Cell Undifferentiated Carcinoma

Cutaneous small-cell undifferentiated carcinoma (CSCUC) (Merkel cell, neuroendocrine, or trabecular carcinoma[155–157]), an uncommon tumor, mostly occurs as a solitary nodule, usually on the head or on the extremities.[158] Multiple lesions have been observed, either localized to one area or widely distributed. The tumors are usually few in number but occasionally are multitudinous.

The lesions of CSCUC are firm, nodular, and red-pink. They usually are nonulcerated and range in size from 0.8 to 4.0 cm in diameter.

Histopathology. Tumor cells with scanty cytoplasm and plump, round or irregular nuclei are closely spaced in sheets and trabecular patterns (Fig. 36-28),[159,160] and less commonly in ribbons and festoons. Pseudorosettes are an occasional feature.[160] The nuclear chromatin often is dense and uniformly distributed. In some examples, nuclei focally or uniformly show margination of chromatin. Nucleoli generally are inconspicuous. Nuclear molding may be a feature. Mitoses and nuclear fragments are regular features.[155] In some CSCUC, the nests of cells are supported by scant, delicate, and paucicellular stroma. Lymphoid infiltrates are common at the margin and focally in the stroma. Contact with the epidermis is rare, but if a lesion invades the epidermis, the patterns may include rounded defects in which tumor cells are collected.[161,162] Patterns of keratinocytic dysplasia in the overlying epidermis and even islands of squamous cell differentiation in the dermal nests are uncommon features. At the interface between the tumor and the epidermis and at the margins of the tumor, dilated, thin-walled vessels commonly contain tumor cells.

The immunohistochemical profile is NSE (+),[163] protein gene product (+), chromogranins (+), Ber-EP4 (+),[161] and CD57 (+).[164] A single punctate zone of cytoplasmic immunoreactivity for cytokeratins, especially CK20, or neurofilaments is most characteristic.[165] EMA is expressed in 75% to 80% of CSCUC.[166] A reaction for cytokeratin 20 has been offered as a finding against the diagnosis of metastatic small-cell carcinoma of the lung.

Ultrastructurally, cytoplasmic, membrane-bound, round, dense-core granules of neuroendocrine type measure 100 to 200 nm in diameter.[157,160] Perinuclear bundles or whorls of intermediate filaments 7 to 10 nm wide[167] and small desmosomes are regularly present. Tonofilaments attached to the desmosomes have been found in only a few cases.[168]

Histogenesis. The origin of the CSCUC is controversial. Divergent differentiation is expressed in neuroendocrine, squamous (see Fig. 36-28), adnexal,[165,169] and melanocytic phenotypes.[170]

Differential Diagnosis. Cutaneous metastases from atypical carcinoids or small-cell undifferentiated carcinoma (oat cell carcinoma) of the lung may be confused with primary CSCUC.[171]

The nuclear characteristics of the cells of CSCUC differ from those of most lymphomas.[172] Immunoreactions are an aid in the

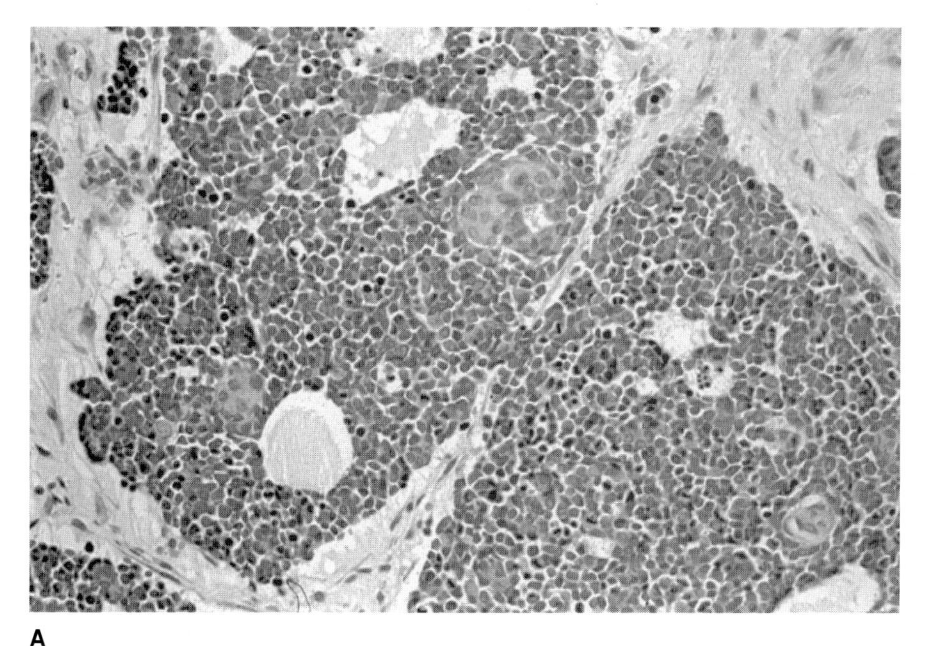

A

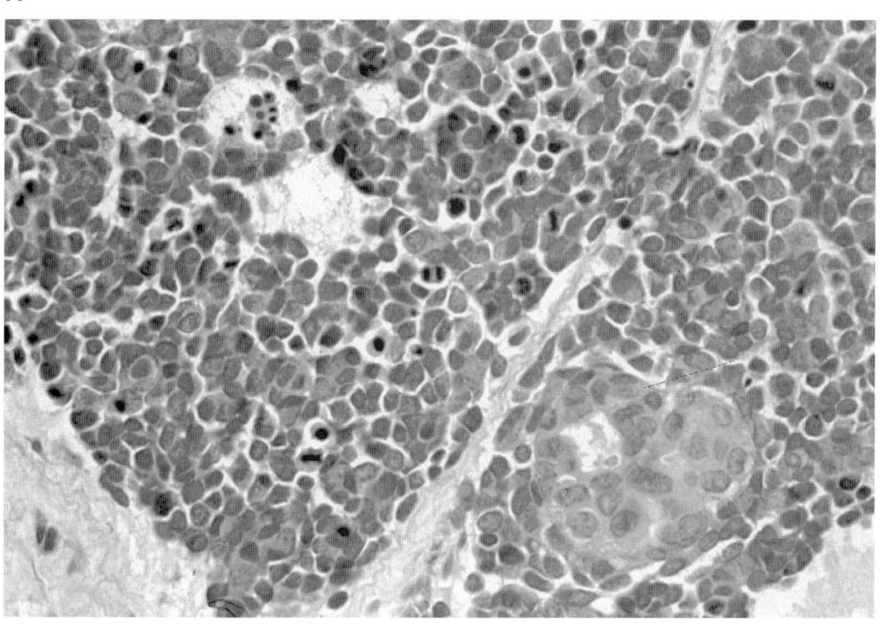

B

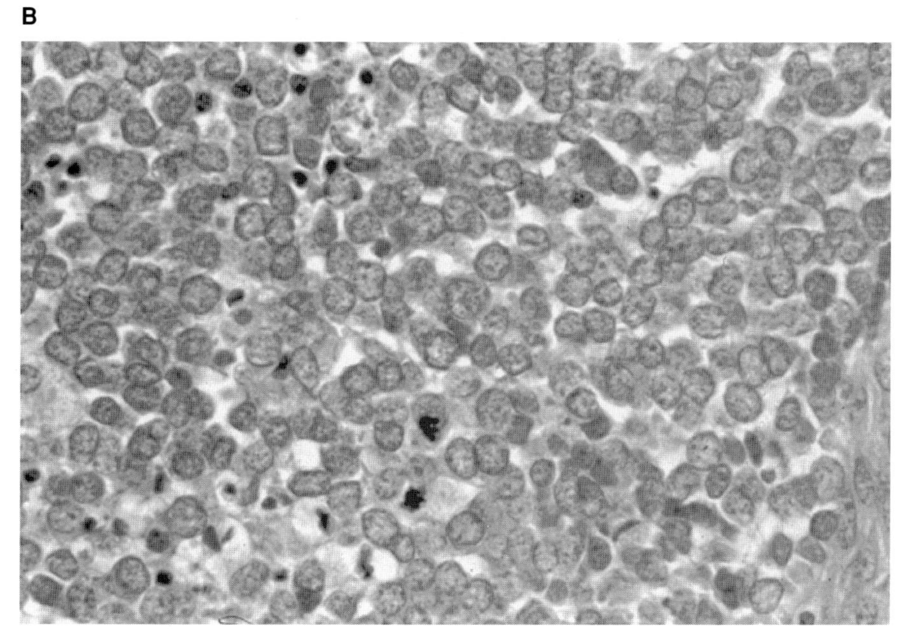

C

FIG. 36-28. Cutaneous small-cell undifferentiated carcinoma, Merkel cell type
(**A**) Small undifferentiated cells with scanty cytoplasm and uniformly dense nuclear chromatin are arranged in trabecular patterns in a delicate fibrous matrix. (**B**) In the lower right-hand corner, squamoid cells form a cluster (divergent differentiation). (**C**) Nucleoli are small or inconspicuous. Pynotic nuclei and fragments of nuclear debris, as represented in this field, are correlated with a high apoptotic index.

differential diagnosis.[171] If lymphoma remains a problem, even in the face of a negative reaction for leukocyte common antigen, reactions for the antigens L-26 and CD-3 may provide more definitive information.

Primary small-cell undifferentiated carcinomas have been observed in most organ systems. They are not peculiar to the skin, but those in the skin often have distinguishing characteristics. Small-cell undifferentiated carcinomas of both the skin and lung are neuroendocrine carcinomas, but the former designation has a greater degree of specificity and gives recognition to basic patterns that are expressed in distinctive primary neoplasms in a variety of organ systems. The nuclei of pulmonary small-cell undifferentiated carcinomas (PSCUC) are irregular and often have a pointed extremity. Patterns of squamous cell and glandular differentiation are variable features of PSCUC. Unlike the primary cutaneous variant, the cells of a PSCUC may stain for bombesin and leucine enkephalin.[171] Clinicopathologic correlations are an aid in the differential diagnosis.

The primary basaloid and undifferentiated carcinomas of the skin appendages, including lymphoepithelial variants, also must be considered in the differential diagnosis.

Tumors that are similar to CSCUC have been observed as isolated lesions in lymph nodes.[173]

Primitive Neuroectodermal Tumors (PNETs)

Peripheral Neuroblastoma

Neuroblastoma, as a primary soft tissue tumor, is a diagnosis of exclusion. The skin is a most unlikely site. In infancy, the differential diagnosis of undifferentiated, small-cell malignancies of the skin and soft tissue includes metastatic neuroblastoma. A thorough workup to rule out a metastasis from an occult site such as the adrenal gland or paravertebral ganglia is required. Metastatic neuroblastoma of infancy may present the picture of blueberry muffin baby[174] or as blanching subcutaneous nodules.[175] Adult neuroblastomas have been documented.[176,177]

Histopathology. Neuroblastomas are undifferentiated, small-cell malignancies. Solid sheets of undifferentiated cells often are the preponderant patterns, but septation, neuropil, differentiation, and pseudorosettes (Homer Wright), if identified, are an aid in diagnosis. Neuroblasts are distinguished by the formation of cell processes. The designation *neuropil* gives recognition to a matrix of cytoplasmic processes, including those of neurons, Schwann cells, and glial cells. It gives recognition to patterns of matrical differentiation in neuroectodermal tumors. A sprinkling of larger, neuronlike cells with slightly eccentric nuclei, prominent central nucleoli, and marginated chromatin are features of neuroblastic differentiation.

Depending on the degree of differentiation, the immunohistochemical profile is as follows: neural filaments (+), NSE (+), S-100 protein (+), synaptophysin (+), and even other neuroendocrine markers.[178]

Metastatic neuroblastoma possesses an innate tendency for maturation (differentiation). As a consequence, metastases from a neuroblastoma may present as immature or mature ganglioneuroma.[179] The problems are complicated by the rare example in which a primary neuroblastoma of the adrenal gland with distant metastases undergoes complete regression in the primary site.

Ganglioneuroma

Ganglioneuroma is exceedingly uncommon in the skin. Rare examples appear to be in the nature of heterotopias. Some may represent divergent differentiation of phenotypically pluripotent neurocristic cells. Others may represent metastatic neuroblastoma that has matured into a ganglioneuroma.

Histopathology. The basic pattern of a ganglioneuroma is that of a neuroma in which characteristic ganglion cells are clustered and individually isolated.[180] Small, primary ganglioneuromas of the skin may be characterized by numerous, mature ganglion cells and an inconspicuous background of neurosustentacular cells.[181]

Histogenesis. With immunoperoxidase stain for S-100 protein, ganglion cells are not, and Schwann cells are, reactive.[182] Like all neuromas, Schwann cell fascicles of a ganglioneuroma are innervated. Ganglion cells are reactive for NSE and chromogranins. Immaturity, as manifested by foci of small, dark cells, spongy neuropil, and lymphoid infiltrates, signals the need for additional studies to rule out a differentiating metastatic neuroblastoma. In immature ganglioneuroma, the neurons may not be associated with satellite cells.

Ewing Sarcoma (EWS) and Peripheral Neuroepithelioma (PNE)

These are examples of *primitive neuroectodermal tumors* (*PNET*). EWS, including an atypical variant,[183] is a rare malignant neoplasm of bone and soft tissue. *Peripheral neuroepithelioma* (PNE) (the "primitive neuroectodermal tumor"; peripheral neuroblastoma) generally is a tumor of the deep soft tissue. Some examples have had their origin in a peripheral nerve[184] or have been a component of malignant schwannoma.[79]

Histogenesis. Immunoreactions are variable in the category of PNET, and the useful positive reactions include NSE, CD57, and synaptophysin. In some examples of EWS and peripheral neuroepithelioma, tumor cells have been immunoreactive for HBA71 (MIC2).[185–186]

Both EWS and PNE are characterized by the presence of a recurrent chromosomal translocation t(11;22)(q24;q12), and the EWS gene has recently been identified at the breakpoint on chromosome 22.[187]

Differential Diagnosis. Neuroepitheliomalike patterns may be encountered as a regional variation in malignant schwannoma[79] and in the setting of cutaneous small-cell undifferentiated carcinoma.[159,188]

The distinctions between neuroblastoma and PNE have been a source of confusion. PNET cannot always be assigned to a specific category as either neuroblastoma or PNE. In practice, evidence of maturation, in the form of neuronlike cells, favors a diagnosis of neuroblastoma, although maturation has been documented in recurrent PNE.[189]

Melanotic Neuroectodermal Tumor of Infancy

This tumor[190–192] affects the tissues of the oral cavity but also may be found in other sites. In it, polyphenotypic expressions of neural and epithelial markers, melanogenesis, and occasional glial and rhabdomyoblastic differentiation are variably represented. Its patterns have been compared to those of the retina at 5 weeks' gestation.[193]

HETEROTOPIAS

Cephalic brain–like heterotopias (*CBHs*) (nasal gliomas) are found most commonly on the skin near the root of the nose, but they may be intranasal (40%) or extranasal (60%). Extranasal CBHs are smooth, firm, noncompressible, and skin-colored, ranging in size from 1 to 5 cm. They do not pulsate or transilluminate. On the external surface of the nose, they usually are not midline. Intranasally, CBHs present as a firm, smooth, red to purple protrusion, and usually measure 2 to 3 cm in diameter. They may resemble a hemangioma. Those that are both intranasal and extranasal are connected through a defect in the nasal bone.[194] The other most commonly associated bony defects involve the fonticulus frontalis, the cribriform plate, and the space between nasal bone and cartilage.[194] Some examples are connected by a fibrous cord to the dura. Other sites include the scalp, oropharynx, nasopharynx, and tongue.

Histopathology. CBHs are not encapsulated. They are disorganized and commonly show admixtures of glial tissue (Fig. 36-29), randomly distributed, mature neurons, increased vascularity, focal calcification, and fibrous tissue.[195] Strands of neural and fibrous tissue are interwoven.[196] Fibrillary and gemistocytic astrocytes, activated oligodendrocytes, and giant astrocytes are variably represented. Astrocytes are the most conspicuous cellular component. In some examples, the astrocytic component may resemble a low-grade astrocytoma. Neurons usually are small and may be absent.[197] Occasionally, they are focally prominent. Ependymal[198] and retinal epithelium, and even choroid plexus–like components have been observed. Focal areas of oligodendroglial differentiation may be prominent, and in these areas the neuropil may be immunoreactive for both NSE and synaptophysin. The degree of differentiation in these heterotopias may reflect the age of the patient at the time of excision. Some examples are remarkable for the diversity of cell types, all representative of neuroectodermal differentiation. An oligodendroglioma arising in ectopic brain tissue of the nasopharynx has been reported.

Immunohistochemically, neurons react for NSE and neural filaments. Astrocytes and ependymal cells are, and oligodendroglial cells are not, immunoreactive for GFAP. The latter share immunoreactions with Schwann cells.

Differential Diagnosis. Encephaloceles (extracranial protrusions of brainlike tissue that are in continuity with the subarachnoid space) may show a high degree of organization.[198] CBH and encephaloceles of the same anatomic sites have similar clinical features. A distinction between CBH and encephalocele is not always possible, but encephaloceles are connected to the subarachnoid space by a sinus tract, thus making an ordinary biopsy inadvisable. A rhinorrhea with leakage of spinal fluid and septic encephalitis may ensue. Computerized tomography[199] and neurosurgical consultation should precede any operative intervention of either CBH or encephalocele.[196]

CUTANEOUS MENINGIOMAS AND MENINGOTHELIAL HETEROTOPIAS

Cells with the features of meningothelial cells may be encountered in skin and soft tissue beyond the confines of the central nervous system.[200] They may be represented either in patterns of a neoplasm and properly characterized as *ectopic* meningioma, or in patterns similar to those manifested in the coverings of *meningoceles*, *meningomyeloceles*, and *meningoencephaloceles* and properly characterized as heterotopia or dysplasia.

A definition of various pathways and phenomena provides an explanation for the presence of meningothelial cells in the skin and soft tissue:

1. Precursors of meningothelial cells may be displaced into the dermis and subcutis during embryogenesis. Such remnants,

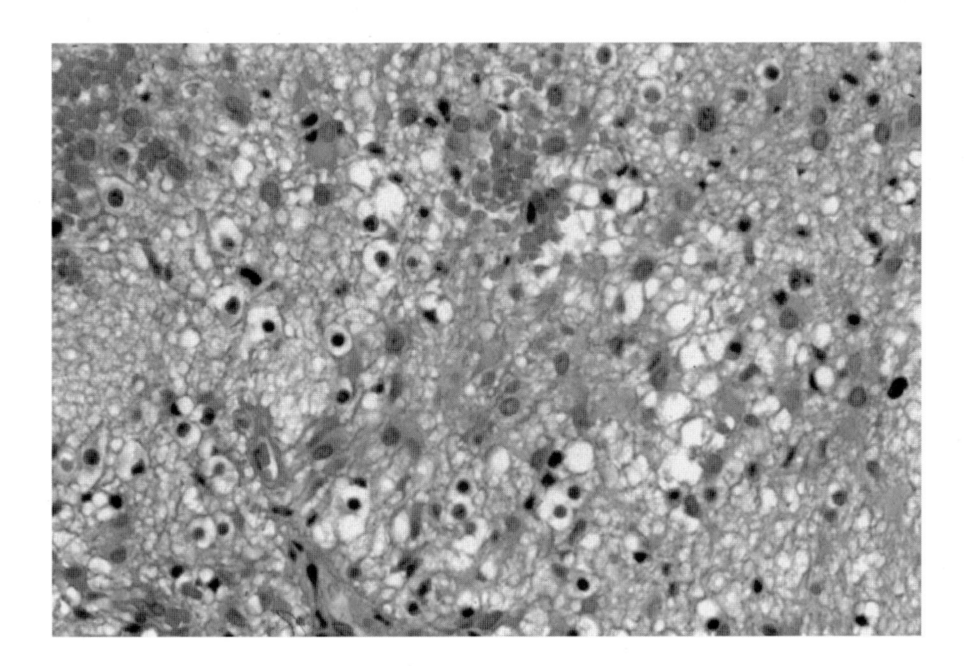

FIG. 36-29. Parapharyngeal cephalic brain–like heterotopia Astrocytes and oligodendroglial cells are supported by neuropil.

located mainly in subcutaneous tissue of the scalp, forehead, and paravertebral regions of children and young adults,[200] may develop into congenital meningeal heterotopias. They are relatively restricted in distribution along the lines of closure of the developing neural tube. Some of these lesions qualify as acelic meningeal heterotopias (rudimentary meningoceles).[201] They have occult connections with the central nervous system that may become apparent only at the time of surgery with the leakage of spinal fluid into the surgical defect. Histologic patterns include those of both the dura and the leptomeninges.

2. True ectopic meningomas, distributed along the course of cranial nerves of the sensory organs of the face and head, tend to occur in adults and arise from extensions of arachnoidal lining cells along peripheral nerves.[202] Some ectopic meningiomas arise in sites that are far from the axial skeleton. The histologic patterns of benign ectopic meningiomas recapitulate those of the meningiomas of the central nervous system.

3. Large, intracranial meningiomas may extend in direct continuity through foramina [33] or old operative defects into the neighboring soft tissue. They qualify as *perforating* meningiomas. Their histology corresponds to that of the primary intracranial lesion and, once defined, is predictive of their behavior.

4. *Anaplastic (malignant) meningiomas*, including sarcomatous as well as papillary and hemangiopericytomatous variants, may aggressively invade bone, soft tissue, and scalp. They also may be associated with intracranial seeding and with extracranial, mostly pulmonary, metastases.[33] Rarely, histologically benign meningiomas have seeded the brain surface or metastasized.

Histopathology. Heterotopias are not well circumscribed.[202] The cells are cytologically bland and loosely attached to their neighbors. They commonly outline thin, angulated clefts, a feature that may be mistaken as evidence of vascular differentiation (Fig. 36-30).[201,203] Whorls of cells and psammoma bodies, if identified, are an aid in diagnosis. The supporting matrix is fibrous and loosely fissured.

The histopathology and classification of true meningiomas, whether intracranial, ectopic, or metastatic, are complex. The basic features include sheets and nests of polygonal or spindle cells, whorls of cells, psammoma bodies, intranuclear inclusions of cytoplasm, immunoreactivity for EMA, and scanty, condensed stroma or thin clefts at the interface between nests.

Anaplastic (malignant) meningiomas are characterized by dense cellularity, nuclear atypia, mitoses, necrosis, and invasion of the brain and even soft tissue. The basic patterns of common meningiomas usually are preserved, but some examples are frankly sarcomatous.

Ultrastructurally, meningothelial cells are characterized by poorly formed basal lamina, rare desmosomes, abundant mitochondria, and elaborate interdigitating cytoplasmic processes.

Histogenesis. Like intracranial meningiomas, the cells of ectopic meningiomas and meningeal heterotopias react immunohistochemically for vimentin and EMA.[204,205] Depending on the histologic subtypes, the expression of certain antigens, especially of cytokeratins and to S-100 protein, is variable.[201,207] The clonal nature of the antibody to S-100 protein may also influence the results of the tests.

Differential Diagnosis. Meningoceles, meningomyeloceles, and meningoencephaloceles, like meningeal heterotopias, present along the lines of closure of the neural tube. They consist of both dense and loosely laminated, vascularized fibrous tissue, some of which is arachnoidal in quality. If there is an associated encephalocele (or myelocele), then tissue of the central nervous system will also be represented.

Ependymal rests also may be found in the sacrococcygeal region. Some are organized in patterns that resemble microscopic myxopapillary ependymomas.[208] They may provide an explanation for the origin of rare *ectopic ependymomas* in the sacrococcygeal region.[209]

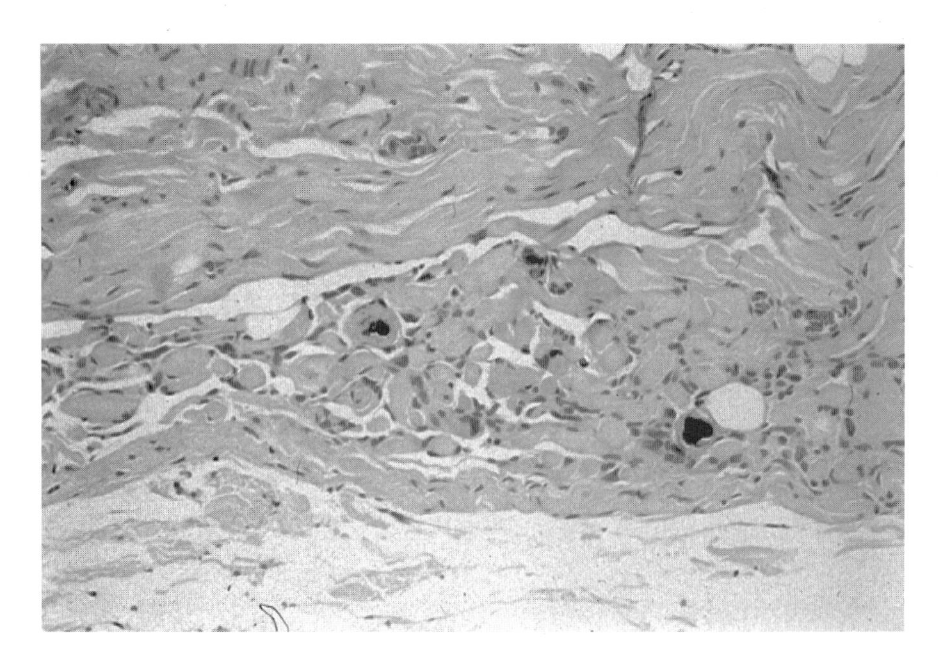

FIG. 36-30. Meningothelial heterotopia
Thin spindle and stellate cells incompletely outline the spaces between coarse collagen bundles. Small psammoma bodies are also represented.

NEURAL TUMORS OF A DEGENERATIVE NATURE

In *impingement neurofasciitis (Morton or interdigital "neuroma")*, the compression of nerves and soft tissue between bony surfaces may induce degenerative changes. The responses include demyelination and endoneurial fibrosis, mucinous and fibrinous degeneration of soft tissue (fascia), deposition of pre-elastin over the surfaces of elastic fibers (in patterns resembling those seen in lesions of elastofibroma dorsi), and fibrinous bursitis.[210] All of these phenomena, manifested in the interdigital area of so-called Morton neuroma, have nothing in common with the neuromas. In the altered nerves, localized, oval zones of mucinous or fibrous matrix may focally displace the nerve fibers. In them, spindle and stellate cells are loosely arranged in whorls. Similar epiphenomena, found incidentally in normal nerves, were characterized by Renaut as an "intravaginal hyaline system."

Ganglion cyst of nerve is an uncommon tumor of a degenerative nature. In preferential sites, a superficial nerve impinges upon a bony protuberance.

Initially, the perineurium and endoneurium are mucinous, expanded, and paucicellular. In one or more sites, cystic changes ensue. The end result is a mucinous cyst that expands the endoneurial space, compresses the axial bundle, and balloons the perineurial sheath. A condensation of fibrous tissue forms the wall of the cyst.[1]

Ganglion cyst of nerve is distinguished from periarticular ganglion cyst by location.

NEUROTROPIC GROWTH (GENERAL COMMENTS)

Neurotropic growth of tumor is common in the skin. Generally, the identification of this phenomenon is sufficient to characterize any related primary neoplasm of the skin as aggressive (e.g., microcystic adenexal carcinoma,[211] neurotropic melanoma,[84] epidermoid carcinoma,[212] and keratoacanthoma). Rarely, benign invasion of nerve sheaths by squamous epithelium has been noted in reexcision specimens after a biopsy.[213]

REFERENCES

1. Harkin JC, Reed RJ. Tumors of the peripheral nervous system. 2nd series, Fasc. 3. Washington, DC: Armed Forces Institute of Pathology, 1969.
2. Ortiz-Hidalgo C, Weller RO. Peripheral nervous system. In: Sternberg SS, ed. Histology for pathologists. New York: Raven Press, 1992;169.
3. Reed RJ, Harkin JC. Supplement: Tumors of the peripheral nervous system. 2nd series, Fasc. 3. Washington, DC: Armed Forces Institute of Pathology, 1983.
4. Weiser G. An electron microscopic study of "pacinian neurofibroma." Virchows Arch A 1975;366:331.
5. Morris JH, Hudson AR, Weddell G. A study of degeneration and regeneration in the divided rat sciatic nerve based on electron microscopy. Part 1. Z Zellforsch Mikrosk Anat 1972;124:76.
6. Riccardi VM. Von Recklinghausen neurofibromatosis (review). N Engl J Med 1981;305:1617.
7. Crowe FW. Axillary freckling as a diagnostic aid in neurofibromatosis. Ann Intern Med 1964;61:1142.
8. Crowe FW, Schull WJ, Neel JV, eds. Clinical, pathological, and genetic study of multiple neurofibromatosis. Springfield, IL. Charles C Thomas, 1956.
9. Goldberg NS, Collins FS. The hunt for the neurofibromatosis gene. Arch Dermatol 1991;127:1705.
10. Zvulunov A, Easterly NB. Neurocutaneous syndromes associated with pigmentary skin lesions. J Am Acad Dermatol 1995;32:915.
11. Shekitka KM, Sobin LH. Ganglioneuromas of the gastrointestinal tract: Relation to von Recklinghausen disease and other multiple tumor syndromes. Am J Surg Pathol 1994;18:250.
12. DeLellis RA. Biology of disease: Multiple endocrine neoplasia syndromes revisited. Clinical, morphologic, and molecular features. Lab Invest 1995;72:494.
13. Zvulunov A, Barak Y, Metzker A. Juvenile xanthogranuloma, neurofibromatosis, and juvenile chronic myelogenous leukemia: World statistical analysis. Arch Dermatol 1995;131:904.
14. Jaakkola S, Muona P, James WD et al. Segmental neurofibromatosis: Immunocytochemical analysis of cutaneous lesions. J Am Acad Dermatol 1990;22:617.
15. Honda M, Arai E, Sawade S et al. Neurofibromatosis 2 and neurilemmomatosis gene are identical. J Invest Dermatol 1995;104:74.
16. Masson P. Human tumors: Histology, diagnosis and technique. 2nd ed. Detroit: Wayne State Univ Press, 1970.
17. Erlandson RA, Woodruff JM. Peripheral nerve sheath tumors. Cancer 1982;49:273.
18. Friede RL. The organization of endoneurial collagen in peripheral nerves as revealed with the scanning electron microscope. J Neurol Sci 1978;38:83.
19. Lassmann H, Jurecka W, Lassmann G et al. Different types of benign nerve sheath tumors. Virchows Arch Pathol Anat 1977;375:197.
20. Vaalasti A, Suomalainen H, Kuokkanen K, Rechardt L. Neuropeptides in cutaneous neurofibromas of von Recklinghausen's disease. J Cutan Pathol 1990;17:377.
21. Reed RJ. The neural crest, its migrants, and cutaneous malignant neoplasms related to neurocristic derivatives. In: Lynch HT, Fusaro RM, eds. Cancer-associated genodermatoses. New York: Van Nostrand Reinhold, 1982;177.
22. Argenyi ZB, Cooper PH, Santa Cruz D. Plexiform and other unusual variants of palisaded encapsulated neuroma. J Cutan Pathol 1993;20:34.
23. Gorlin RJ, Sedano HO, Vickers RA et al. Multiple mucosal neuromas, pheochromocytoma and medullary carcinoma of the thyroid: A syndrome. Cancer 1968;22:293.
24. Argeny ZB, LeBoit PE, Santa Cruz D et al. Nerve sheath myxoma (neurothekeoma) of the skin: Light microscopic and immunohistochemical reappraisal of the cellular variant. J Cutan Pathol 1993;20:294.
25. Enzinger F, Zhang R. Plexiform fibrohistiocytic tumor presenting in children and young adults: An analysis of 65 cases. Am J Surg Pathol 1988;12:818.
26. Enzinger FM, Weiss SW. Soft tissue tumors. 3rd ed. St Louis: Mosby-Year Book, 1995;335.
27. Dupree WB, Langloss JM, Weiss SH. Pigmented dermatofibrosarcoma protuberans (Bednar tumor): A pathologic, ultrastructural, and immunohistochemical study. Am J Surg Pathol 1985;9:630.
28. Greene JF, Fitzwater JE, Burgess J. Arterial lesions associated with neurofibromatosis. Am J Clin Pathol 1974;62:481.
29. Salyer WR, Salyer DC. The vascular lesions of neurofibromatosis. Angiology 1974;25:510.
30. Masson P. Experimental and spontaneous schwannomas (peripheral gliomas). Am J Pathol 1932;8:367.
31. Ackerman LV, Taylor FH. Neurogenous tumors within the thorax: A clinicopathologic evaluation of forty-eight cases. Cancer 1951;4:669.
32. Stout AP. The peripheral manifestations of the specific nerve sheath tumor (neurilemmoma). Am J Cancer 1935;24:751.
33. Russell DS, Rubinstein LJ. Pathology of tumours of the nervous system. 5th ed. Baltimore: Williams & Wilkins, 1989;544.
34. Stout AP. Tumors of the peripheral nervous system. 1st series, Fasc. 6. Washington, DC: Armed Forces Institute of Pathology, 1949.
35. Argenyi ZB, Balogh K, Abraham AA. Degenerative ("ancient") changes in benign cutaneous schwannoma: A light microscopic, histochemical, and immunohistochemical study. J Cutan Pathol 1993;20:148.
36. Sian CS, Ryan SF. The ultrastructure of neurilemmoma with emphasis on Antoni B tissue. Hum Pathol 1981;12:145.
37. Kerr JFR, Winterford CM, Harmon BV. Apoptosis: Its significance in cancer and cancer therapy. Cancer 1994;73:2013.

38. Farber EM. Programmed cell death: Necrosis versus apoptosis. Mod Pathol 1994;7:605.
39. Kawahara E, Oda Y, Ooi A et al. Expression of glial fibrillary acidic protein (GFAP) in peripheral nerve sheath tumors. Am J Surg Pathol 1988;12:115.
40. Lodding P, Kindblom LG, Angerval L, Stenman G. Cellular schwannoma: A clinicopathologic study of 29 cases. Virchows Arch [A] Pathol Anat 1990;416:237m.
41. Woodruff JM, Godwin TA, Erlandson RA et al. Cellular schwannoma: A variety of schwannoma sometimes mistaken for a malignant tumor. Am J Surg Pathol 1981;5:733.
42. Fletcher CDM, Davis SE, McKee PH. Cellular schwannoma: A distinct pseudosarcomatous entity. Histopathology 1987;11:21.
43. Hajdu SI. Schwannomas. Mod Pathol 1995;8:109.
44. Casadei GP, Scheithauer BW, Hirose T et al. Cellular schwannoma. Cancer 1995;75:1109.
45. White W, Shiu MH, Rosenblum MK et al. Cellular schwannoma: A clinicopathologic study of 57 patients and 58 tumors. Cancer 1990;66: 1266.
46. George E, Swanson PE, Wick MR. Malignant peripheral nerve sheath tumor of the skin. Am J Dermatopathol 1989;11:213.
47. Fisher C, Chappell ME, Weiss SW. Neuroblastoma-like epithelioid schwannoma. Histopathology 1995;26:193.
48. Goldblum JR, Beals TF, Weiss SW. Neuroblastoma-like neurilemmoma. Am J Surg Pathol 1994;18:266.
49. Skelton HG, Smith KJ, Lupton GP. Collagenous spherulosis in a schwannoma. Am J Dermatopathol 1994;16:549.
50. Elston DM, Bergfeld WF, Biscotti CV, McMahon JT. Schwannoma with sweat duct differentiation. J Cutan Pathol 1993;20:254.
51. Woodruff JM, Christensen WN. Glandular peripheral nerve sheath tumors. Cancer 1993;72:3618.
52. Yoshida SO, Toot BV. Benign glandular schwannoma. Am J Clin Pathol 1993;100:167.
53. Iwashita T, Enjoji M. Plexiform neurilemmoma: A clinicopathological and immunohistochemical analysis of 23 tumors from 20 patients. Virchows Arch A Pathol Anat Histopathol 1987;411:305.
54. Rongioletti F, Drago F, Rebora A. Multiple cutaneous plexiform schwannomas with tumors of the central nervous system. Arch Dermatol 1989;125:431.
55. Sasaki T, Nakajima H. Congenital neurilemmomatosis. J Am Acad Dermatol 1992;26:786.
56. Woodruff JM, Marshall MI, Godwin TA et al. Plexiform (multinodular) schwannoma: A tumor simulating the plexiform neurofibroma. Am J Surg Pathol 1983;7:691.
57. Kao GF, Laskin WB, Olsen TG. Solitary cutaneous plexiform neurilemmoma (schwannoma): A clinicopathologic, immunohistochemical, and ultrastructural study of 11 cases. Mod Pathol 1989;2:20.
58. Shishiba T, Niimura M, Ohtsuka F et al. Multiple cutaneous neurilemmomas as a skin manifestation of neurilemmomatosis. J Am Acad Dermatol 1984;10:744.
59. Murata Y, Kumano K, Ugai K et al. Neurilemmomatosis. Br J Dermatol 1991;125:466.
60. Rouleau GA, Merel P, Lutchman M et al. Alteration in a new gene encoding a putative membrane-organizing protein causes neurofibromatosis type 2. Nature 1993;363:515.
61. Honda M, Arai E, Sawada S et al. Neurofibromatosis 2 and neurilemmomatosis gene are identical. J Invest Dermatol 1995;104:74.
62. Meis-Kindblom JM, Enzinger FM. Plexiform malignant peripheral nerve sheath tumor of infancy and childhood. Am J Surg Pathol 1994; 18:479.
63. Argenyi ZB, Goodenberger ME, Strauss JS. Congenital neural hamartoma ("fascicular schwannoma"): A light microscopic, immunohistochemical, and ultrastructural study. Am J Dermatopathol 1990;12: 283.
64. Woodruff JM, Erlandson RA, Scheithauer BW. Nerve sheath tumors: Letter to editor. Am J Surg Pathol 1995;19:608.
65. Cohen C, Davis TS. Multiple trichogenic adnexal tumors. Am J Dermatopathol 1986;8:241.
66. Proppe KH, Scully RE. Large cell calcifying Sertoli cell tumor of the testis. Am J Clin Pathol 1980;74:607.
67. Carney JA. Psammomatous melanotic schwannoma: A distinctive, heritable tumor with special associations, including cardiac myxoma and the Cushing syndrome. Am J Surg Pathol 1990;14:206.
68. Carney JA, Hruska LS, Beauchamp GD, Gordon H. Dominant inheritance of the complex of myxomas, spotty pigmentation, and endocrine overactivity. Mayo Clin Proc 1986;61:165.
69. Carstens PHB, Schrodt GR. Malignant transformation of a benign encapsulated neurilemmoma. Am J Clin Pathol 1969;51:144.
70. Woodruff JM, Selig AM, Crowley K, Allen PW. Schwannoma (neurilemmoma) with malignant transformation: A rare, distinctive peripheral nerve tumor. Am J Surg Pathol 1994;18:882.
71. Guccion JG, Enzinger FM. Malignant schwannoma associated with von Recklinghausen's neurofibromatosis. Virchows Arch Anat Pathol 1979;39:43.
72. D'Agostino AN, Soule EH, Miller RH. Sarcomas of the peripheral nerves and somatic soft tissues associated with multiple neurofibromatosis (von Recklinghausen's disease). Cancer 1963;16:1015.
73. D'Agostino AN, Soule EH, Miller RH. Primary malignant neoplasms of nerves (malignant neurilemmomas) in patients without manifestations of multiple neurofibromatosis (von Recklinghausen's disease). Cancer 1963;16:1003.
74. Taxy JB, Battifora H, Trujillo Y et al. Electron microscopy in the diagnosis of malignant schwannoma. Cancer 1981;48:1381.
75. Woodruff JM, Perino G. Non-germ-cell or teratomatous malignant tumors showing additional rhabdomyoblastic differentiation, with emphasis on malignant triton tumor. Semin Diagn Pathol 1994;11:69.
76. Reed RJ. Case 13, proceedings of the 49th annual anatomic pathology slide seminar, American Society of Clinical Pathologists. Chicago: American Society of Clinical Pathologists Press, 1983;97.
77. Laskin WB, Weiss SW, Bratthauer GL. Epithelioid variant of malignant peripheral nerve sheath tumor (malignant epithelioid schwannoma). Am J Surg Pathol 1991;15:1136.
78. Lodding P, Kindblom L-G, Angervall L. Epithelioid malignant schwannoma: A study of 14 cases. Virchows Arch A 1986;409:437.
79. Hruban RH, Shiu MH, Senie RT, Woodruff JM. Malignant peripheral nerve sheath tumors of the buttocks and lower extremity: A study of 43 cases. Cancer 1990;66:1253.
80. Dicarlo EF, Woodruff JM, Bansal M, Erlandson RA. The purely epithelioid malignant peripheral nerve sheath tumor. Am J Surg Pathol 1986;10:478.
81. Wick MR, Swanson PE, Scheithauer BW, Manivel JC. Malignant peripheral nerve sheath tumor: An immunohistochemical study of 62 cases. Am J Clin Pathol 1987;87:425.
82. Daimaru Y, Hashimoto H, Enjoji M. Malignant peripheral nerve sheath tumors (malignant schwannomas): An immunohistochemical study of 29 cases. Am J Surg Pathol 1983;9:434.
83. Fletcher CDM. Pleomorphic malignant fibrous histiocytoma: Fact or fiction? Am J Surg Pathol 1992;16:213.
84. Reed RJ, Leonard DD. Neurotropic melanoma: A variant of desmoplastic melanoma. Am J Surg Pathol 1979;3:301.
85. Ricci A, Parham DM, Woodruff JM et al. Malignant peripheral nerve sheath tumor arising from ganglioneuroma. Am J Surg Pathol 1984; 8:19.
86. Ghali VS, Gold JE, Vincent RA et al. Malignant peripheral nerve sheath tumor arising spontaneously from retroperitoneal ganglioneuroma: A case report, review of the literature, and immunohistochemical study. Hum Pathol 1992;23:72.
87. Meis JM, Enzinger FM, Martz KL, Neal JA. Malignant peripheral nerve sheath tumors (malignant schwannomas) in children. Am J Surg Pathol 1992;16:694.
88. Wanebo JE, Malik JM, Vandenberg SR et al. Malignant peripheral nerve sheath tumors: A clinicopathologic study of 28 cases. Cancer 1993;71:1247.
89. Sordillo PP, Helson L, Hajdu SI et al. Malignant schwannoma: Clinical characteristics, survival, and response to therapy. Cancer 1981;47: 2503.
90. Gallager RL, Helwig EB. Neurothekeoma: a benign cutaneous tumor of neural origin. Am J Clin Pathol 1980;74:759.
91. MacDonald DM, Wilson-Jones E. Pacinian neurofibroma. Histopathology 1977;1:247.
92. King DT, Barr RJ. Bizarre cutaneous neurofibromas. J Cutan Pathol 1980;7:21.
93. Holden CA, Wilson-Jones E, MacDonald DM. Cutaneous lobular neuromyxoma. Br J Dermatol 1982;106:211.
94. Pulitzer DR, Reed RJ. Nerve-sheath myxoma (perineurial myxoma). Am J Dermatopathol 1985;7:409.
95. Goldstein J, Lifshitz T. Myxoma of the nerve sheath: Report of three cases, observations by light and electron microscopy and histochemical analysis. Am J Dermatopathol 1985;7:423.
96. Rosati LA, Fratamico FCM, Eusebi V. Cellular neurothekeoma. Appl Pathol 1986;4:186.

97. Barnhill RL, Mihm MC. Cellular neurothekeoma: A distinctive variant of neurothekeoma mimicking nevomelanocytic tumors. Am J Surg Pathol 1990;14:113.
98. Barnhill RL, Dickerson GR, Nickeleit V et al. Studies on cellular origin of neurothekeoma: Clinical, light microscopic, immunohistochemical, and ultrastructural observations. J Am Acad Dermatol 1991;25:80.
99. Aronson PJ, Fretzin DF, Potter BS. Neurothekeoma of Gallager and Helwig: Dermal nerve sheath myxoma variant. J Cutan Pathol 1985; 12:506.
100. Argenyi ZB, Kutzner H, Seaba MM. Ultrastructural spectrum of cutaneous nerve sheath myxoma/cellular neurothekeoma. J Cutan Pathol 1995;22:137.
101. Calonje E, Wilson-Jones E, Smith NP, Fletcher CDM. Cellular "neurothekeoma:" An epithelioid variant of pilar leiomyoma? Morphological and immunohistochemical analysis of a series. Histopathology 1992;20:397.
102. Allen PW, Dymock RB, MacCormac LB. Superficial angiomyxomas with and without epithelial components: Report of 30 tumors in 28 patients. Am J Surg Pathol 1988;12:519.
103. Wilson-Jones E, Cerio R, Smith NP. Epithelioid cell histiocytoma: A new entity. Br J Dermatol 1989;120:185.
104. Gomez CS, Calonje E, Fletcher CDM. Epithelioid benign fibrous histiocytoma of skin: Clinicopathological analysis of 20 cases of a poorly known variant. Histopathology 1994;24:123.
105. Aparicio SR, Lumsden CE. Light and electron microscopic studies on the granular cell myoblastoma of the tongue. J Pathol 1969;97:339.
106. Sobel HJ, Marquet E. Granular cells and granular cell lesions. Pathol Annu 1974;9:43.
107. Lee J, Bhawan J, Wax F, Farber J. Plexiform granular cell tumor: A report of two cases. Am J Dermatopathol 1994;16:537.
108. Garancis JC, Komorowski RA, Kuzma JF. Granular cell myoblastoma. Cancer 1970;25:542.
109. Weiser G. Granularzelltumor (granulares neurom feyrter) und schwannsche Phagen: Elektronenoptische untersuchung von 3 fallen. Virchows Arch A 1987;380:49
110. Tamaki K, Ishibashi Y, Kukita A. A granular cell tumor. J Dermatol 1978;5:127.
111. Mukai M. Immunohistochemical localization of S-100 protein and peripheral nerve myelin (P2 protein, PO protein) in granular cell tumors. Am J Pathol 1983;112:139.
112. LeBoit PE, Barr RJ, Burall S et al. Primitive polypoid granular-cell tumor and other cutaneous granular-cell neoplasms of apparent nonneural origin. Am J Surg Pathol 1991;15:48.
113. Gilliet F, MacGee W, Stoian M et al. Zur histogenese granuliertzelliger tumoren. Hautarzt 1973;24:52.
114. Mentzel T, Wadden C, Fletcher CDM. Granular cell change in smooth muscle tumours of skin and soft tissue. Histopathology 1994;24:223.
115. Takahashi H, Fujita S, Satoh H, Okabe H. Immunohistochemical study of congenital gingival granular cell tumor (congenital epulis). J Oral Pathol Med 1990;19:492.
116. Lack EE, Perez-Atayde AR, McGill TJ, Vawter CF. Gingival granular cell tumor of the newborn (congenital "epulis"): Ultrastructural observations relating to histogenesis. Hum Pathol 1982;13:686.
117. Shimamura K, Osamura RY. Malignant granular cell tumor of the right sciatic nerve: Report of an autopsy case with electron microscopic, immunohistochemical, and enzyme histochemical studies. Cancer 1984;53:524.
118. Klima M, Peters J. Malignant granular cell tumor. Arch Pathol 1987; 111:1070.
119. Gokasian ST, Terzakis JA, Santagada EA. Malignant granular cell tumor. J Cutan Pathol 1994;21:263.
120. Gamboa LG. Malignant granular-cell myoblastoma. Arch Pathol 1955;60:663.
121. Uzoaru I, Firfer B, Ray V et al. Malignant granular cell tumor. Arch Pathol Lab Med 1992;116:206.
122. Strong EW, McDivitt RW, Brasfield RD. Granular cell myoblastoma. Cancer 1970;25:415.
123. Al-Sarraf M, Loud AV, Vaitkevicius VK. Malignant granular cell tumor: Histochemical and electron microscopic study. Arch Pathol 1971;91:550.
124. Gartmann H. Malignant granular cell tumor. Hautarzt 1977;28:40.
125. Kuhn A, Mahrle G, Steigleder GK. Benigne und maligne granularzelltumoren. Z Hautkr 1987;62:952.
126. Requena L, Sangueza OP. Benign neoplasms with neural differentiation: A review. Am J Dermatopathol 1995;17:75.
127. Lazarus SS, Trombetta LD. Ultrastructural identification of a benign perineurial cell tumor. Cancer 1978;41:1823.
128. Tsang WYW, Chan JKC, Chow LTC, Tse CCH. Perineurioma: An uncommon soft tissue neoplasm distinct from localized hypertrophic neuropathy and neurofibroma. Am J Surg Pathol 1992;16:756.
129. Mentzel T, Dei Tos AP, Fletcher CDM. Perineurioma (storiform perineurial fibroma): Clinico-pathological analysis of four cases. Histopathology 1994;25:261.
130. Dupree WB, Langloss JM, Weiss SW. Pigmented dermatofibrosarcoma protuberans (Bednar tumor): A pathologic, ultrastructural, and immunohistochemical study. Am J Surg Pathol 1985;9:630.
131. Weiss SW, Nickoloff BJ. CD-34 is expressed by a distinctive cell population in peripheral nerve, nerve sheath tumors, and related lesions. Am J Surg Pathol 1993;17:1039.
132. Pritchard KW, Custer RP. Pacinian neurofibroma. Cancer 1952; 5:297.
133. Prose PH, Gherardi GJ, Coblenz A. Pacinian neurofibroma. Arch Dermatol 1957;76:65.
134. Emory TS, Scheithauer BW, Hirose T et al. Intraneural perineurioma: A clonal neoplasm associated with abnormalities of chromosome 22. Am J Clin Pathol 1995;103:696.
135. Stanton C, Perentes E, Phillips L, VandenBerg SR. The immunohistochemical demonstration of early perineurial change in the development of localized hypertrophic neuropathy: Case studies. Hum Pathol 1988;19:1455.
136. Mitsumoto H, Wilbourn AJ, Goren H. Perineurioma as the cause of localized hypertrophic neuropathy. Muscle Nerve 1980;3:403.
137. Anthony DC, Hevner RF. Advances in the genetics of hereditary peripheral neuropathies. Adv Anat Pathol 1995;2:283.
138. Shapiro L, Juhlin EA, Brownstein HM. Rudimentary polydactyly. Arch Dermatol 1973;108:223.
139. Fletcher CDM. Solitary circumscribed neuroma of the skin (so-called palisaded, encapsulated neuroma): A clinicopathologic and immunohistochemical study. Am J Surg Pathol 1989;13:574.
140. Argenyi ZB, Santa-Cruz D, Bromley C. Comparative light-microscopic and immunohistochemical study of traumatic and palisaded and encapsulated neuromas of the skin. Am J Dermatopathol 1992;14: 504.
141. Argenyi ZB. Immunohistochemical characterization of palisaded, encapsulated neuroma. J Cutan Pathol 1990;17:329.
142. Reed RJ, Fine RM, Meltzer HD. Palisaded, encapsulated neuromas of the skin. Arch Dermatol 1972;106:865.
143. Hurwitz S. Sipple syndrome. Arch Dermatol 1974;110:139.
144. Khairi MRA, Dexter RN, Burzynski NJ et al. Mucosal neuroma, pheochromocytoma and medullary thyroid carcinoma: Multiple endocrine neoplasia type 3 (review). Medicine (Baltimore) 1975;54:89.
145. Ayala F, Derosa G, Scippa L et al. Multiple endocrine neoplasia, type IIb. Dermatologica 1981;162:292.
146. Carney JA, Go VLW, Sizemore GW et al. Alimentary-tract ganglioneuromatosis: A major component of the syndrome of multiple endocrine neoplasia, type 2b. N Engl J Med 1976;295:1287.
147. Guillet G, Gauthier Y, Tamisier JM et al. Linear cutaneous neuromas (dermatoneurie en stries): A limited phakomatosis with striated pigmentation corresponding to cutaneous hyperrneury (featuring multiple endocrine neoplasia syndrome?). J Cutan Pathol 1987;14:43.
148. Waggener JD. Ultrastructure of benign peripheral nerve sheath tumors. Cancer 1966;19:699.
149. Fletcher CDM, Theaker JM. Digital pacinian neuroma: A distinctive hyperplastic lesion. Histopathology 1989;15:249.
150. Reed RJ. Giant congenital nevi: A conceptualization of patterns. J Invest Dermatol 1993;100:300s.
151. Pettinato G, Manivel JC, d'Amore ESG et al. Melanotic neuroectodermal tumor of infancy: A reexamination of a histogenetic problem based on immunohistochemical, flow cytometric, and ultrastructural study of 10 cases. Am J Surg Pathol 1991;15:233.
152. Pearson JM, Harris M, Eyden BP, Banerjee SS. Divergent differentiation in small round-cell tumours of the soft tissues with neural features: An analysis of 10 cases. Histopathology 1993;23:1.
153. Navarro S, Cavazzana AO, Llombart-Bosch A, Triche TJ. Comparison of Ewing's sarcoma of bone and peripheral neuroepithelioma: An immunocytochemical and ultrastructural analysis of two primitive neuroectodermal neoplasms. Arch Pathol Lab Med 1994;118:608.
154. Kushner BH, Hajdu SI, Gulati SC et al. Extracranial primitive neuroectodermal tumors: The Memorial Sloan-Kettering Cancer Center experience. Cancer 1991;67:1825.

155. Toker C. Trabecular carcinoma of the skin. Arch Dermatol 1972;105: 107.
156. Tang CK, Toker C. Trabecular carcinoma of the skin. Cancer 1978;42: 2311.
157. Ratner D, Nelson BR, Brown MD, Johnson TM. Merkel cell carcinoma. J Am Acad Dermatol 1993;29:143.
158. Raaf JH, Urmacher C, Knapper WK et al. Trabecular (Merkel cell) carcinoma of the skin. Cancer 1986;57:178.
159a. Sibley RK, Dehner LP, Rosai J. Primary neurocrine (Merkel cell?) carcinoma of the skin. Am J Surg Pathol 1985;9:95.
159b. Sibley RK, Dahl D. Primary neuroendocrine (Merkel cell?) carcinoma of the skin: An immunocytochemical study of 21 cases. Am J Surg Pathol 1985;9:109.
160. Silva EG, MacKay B, Goepfert H et al. Endocrine carcinoma of the skin: Merkel cell carcinoma. Pathol Annu 1984;19:1.
161. Smith KJ, Skelton HG III, Holland TT et al. Neuroendocrine (Merkel cell) carcinoma with an intraepidermal component. Am J Dermatopathol 1993;15:528.
162. LeBoit PE, Crutcher WA, Shapiro PE. Pagetoid intraepidermal spread in Merkel cell (primary neuroendocrine) carcinoma of the skin. Am J Surg Pathol 1992;16:584.
163. Wick MR, Scheithauer BW, Kovacs K. Neuron-specific enolase in neuroendocrine tumors of the thymus, bronchus, and skin. Am J Clin Pathol 1983;79:703.
164. Michels S, Swanson PE, Robb JA, Wick MR. Leu-7 in small cell neoplasms: An immunohistochemical study with ultrastructural correlations. Cancer 1987;60:2958.
165. Merot Y, Margolis RJ, Dahl D et al. Coexpression of neurofilament and keratin proteins in cutaneous neuroendocrine carcinoma cells. J Invest Dermatol 1986;86:74.
166. Wick MR, Goellner JR, Scheithauer BW et al. Primary neuroendocrine carcinomas of the skin: Merkel cell tumors. Am J Clin Pathol 1983;79:6.
167. Haneke E. Electron microscopy of Merkel cell carcinoma from formalin-fixed tissue. J Am Acad Dermatol 1985;12:487.
168. van Muijen GNP, Ruiter DJ, Warnaar SO. Intermediate filaments in Merkel cell tumors. Hum Pathol 1985;16:590.
169. Gould E, Albores-Saavedra J, Dubner B et al. Eccrine and squamous differentiation in Merkel cell carcinoma: An immunohistochemical study. Am J Surg Pathol 1988;12:768.
170. Isimbaldi G, Sironi M, Taccagni GL et al. Tripartite differentiation (squamous, glandular, and melanocytic) of a primary cutaneous neurocrine carcinoma. Am J Dermatopathol 1993;15:260.
171. Wick MR, Millns JL, Sibley RK. Secondary neuroendocrine carcinomas of the skin. J Am Acad Dermatol 1985;13:134.
172. Wick MR, Kaye VN, Sibley RK et al. Primary neuroendocrine carcinoma and small-cell malignant lymphoma of the skin. J Cutan Pathol 1986;13:347.
173. Eusebi V, Capella C, Cossu A, and Rosai J. Neuroendocrine carcinoma within lymph nodes in the absence of a primary tumor, with special reference to Merkel cell carcinoma. Am J Surg Pathol 1992;16: 658.
174. Aleshire SL, Glick AD, Cruz VE et al. Neuroblastoma in adults: Pathologic findings and clinical outcome. Arch Pathol Lab Med 1985; 109:352.
175. Mackay B, Luna MA, Butler JJ. Adult neuroblastoma: Electron microscopic observations in nine cases. Cancer 1976;37:1334.
176. Shown TE, Durfee ME. Blueberry muffin baby: Neonatal neuroblastoma with subcutaneous metastases. J Urol 1970;104:193.
177. Hawthorne HC, Nelson JS, Witzleben CL, Giangiacomo J. Blanching subcutaneous nodules in neonatal neuroblastoma. J Pediatr 1970;77: 297.
178. Osborn M, Dirk T, Kaser H et al. Immunohistochemical localization of neurofilaments and neuron-specific enolase in 29 cases of neuroblastoma. Am J Pathol 1986;122:433.
179. Joshi VV, Silverman JF. Pathology of neuroblastic tumors. Semin Diagn Pathol 1994;11:107.
180. Collins JP, Johnson WC, Burgoon LF Jr. Ganglioneuroma of the skin. Arch Dermatol 1972;105:256.
181. Rios JJ, Diaz-Cano SJ, Rivera-Hueto F, Villar JL. Cutaneous ganglion cell choristoma. J Cutan Pathol 1991;18:469.
182. Lee JY, Martinez AJ, Abell E. Ganglioneuromatous tumor of the skin: A combined heterotopia of ganglion cells and hamartomatous neuroma. Report of a case. J Cutan Pathol 1988;15:58.
183. Hartman KR, Triche TJ, Kinsella TJ, Miser JS. Prognostic value of histopathology in Ewing's sarcoma: Long-term follow-up of distal extremity primary tumors. Cancer 1991;67:163.
184. Hashimoto H, Enjoji M, Nakajima T et al. Malignant neuroepithelioma (peripheral neuroblastoma): A clinicopathologic study of 15 cases. Am J Surg Pathol 1983;7:309.
185. Fellinger EJ, Garin-Chesa P, Glasser DB et al. Comparison of cell surface antigen HBA71 (p30/32 mic2), neuron specific enolase, and vimentin in the immunohistochemical analysis of Ewing's sarcoma of bone. Am J Surg Pathol 1992;16:746.
186. Perlman EJ, Dickman PS, Askin FB et al. Ewing's sarcoma—routine diagnostic utilization of MIC2 analysis: A pediatric oncology group/children's cancer group intergroup study. Hum Pathol 1994;25: 304.
187. Ladanyi M, Garin-Chesa P, Rettig WJ et al. EWS rearrangement in Ewing's sarcoma and peripheral neuroectodermal tumor: Molecular detection and correlation with cytogenetic analysis and MIC2 expression. Diag Mol Pathol 1993;2:141.
188. Argenyi ZB, Bergfeld WF, McMahon JT et al. Primitive neuroectodermal tumor in the skin with features of neuroblastoma in an adult patient. J Cutan Pathol 1986;13:420.
189. Argenyi ZB, Schelper RL, Balogh K. Pigmented neuroectodermal tumor of infancy: A light microscopic and immunohistochemical study. J Cutan Pathol 1991;18:40.
190. Kapadia SB, Frisman DM, Hitchcock CL, Popek EJ. Melanotic neuroectodermal tumor of infancy: Clinicopathological, immunohistochemical, and flow cytometric study. Am J Surg Pathol 1993;17: 566.
191. Raju U, Zarbo RJ, Regezi JA et al. Melanotic neuroectodermal tumors of infancy: Intermediate filament-, neuroendocrine-, and melanoma-associated antigen profiles. Appl Immunohistochem 1993;1:69.
192. Pettinato G, Manivel JC, d'Amore ESG et al. Melanotic neuroectodermal tumor of infancy: A reexamination of a histogenetic problem based on immunohistochemical, flow cytometric, and ultrastructural study of 10 cases. Am J Surg Pathol 1991;15:233.
193. Baran R, Kopf A, Schnitzler L. Le gliome nasal. Ann Dermatol Syphiligr 1973;100:395.
194. Christianson HB. Nasal glioma. Arch Dermatol 1966;93:68.
195. Kopf AW, Bart RS. Nasal glioma. J Dermatol Surg Oncol 1978;4:128.
196. Fletcher CDM, Carpenter G, McKee PH. Nasal glioma: A rarity. Am J Dermatopathol 1986;8:341.
197. Yeoh GPS, Bale PM, de Silva M. Nasal cerebral heterotopia: The so-called nasal glioma or sequestered encephalocele and its variants. Pediatr Pathol 1989;9:531.
198. Mirra SS, Pearl GS, Hoffman JC et al. Nasal "glioma" with prominent neuronal component. Arch Pathol 1981;105:540.
199. Berry AD, Patterson JW. Meningoceles, meningomyeloceles, and encephaloceles: A neuro-dermatopathologic study of 132 cases. J Cutan Pathol 1990;18:164.
200. Sibley DA, Cooper PH. Rudimentary meningocele: A variant of "primary cutaneous meningioma." J Cutan Pathol 1989;16:72.
201. Lopez DA, Silvers DN, Helwig EB. Cutaneous meningioma: A clinicopathologic study. Cancer 1974;34:728.
202. Laymon CW, Becker FT. Massive metastasizing meningioma involving the scalp. Arch Dermatol Syph 1949;59:626.
203. Suster S, Rosai J. Hamartoma of the scalp with ectopic meningothelial elements: A distinctive benign soft tissue lesion that may simulate angiosarcoma. Am J Surg Pathol 1990;14:1.
204. Theaker JM, Fleming KA. Meningioma of the scalp: A case report with immunohistochemical features. J Cutan Pathol 1987;14:49.
205. Gelli MC, Pasquinelli G, Martinelli G et al. Cutaneous meningiomas: Histochemical, immunohistochemical, and ultrastructural investigation. Histopathology 1993;23:576.
206. Argenyi ZB, Theiberg MD, Hayes CM, Whitaker DC. Primary cutaneous meningioma associated with von Recklinghausen's disease. J Cutan Pathol 1994;21:549.
207. Theaker JM, Gatter KC, Puddle J. Epithelial membrane antigen expression by the perineurium of peripheral nerve and in peripheral nerve tumors. Histopathology 1988;13:171.
208. Pultizer DR, Martin PC, Collins PC, Ralph DR. Subcutaneous sacro-

coccygeal ("myxopapillary") ependymal rests. Am J Surg Pathol 1988;12:672.
209. Anderson MS. Myxopapillary ependymomas presenting in the soft tissue over the sacrococcygeal region. 1966;19:585.
210. Reed RJ, Bliss BO. Morton's neuroma: Regressive and productive intermetatarsal elastofibrositis. Arch Pathol 1973;95:123.
211. Martin PC, Smith JL, Pultizer DR, Reed RJ. Compound (primordial) adnexal carcinoma arising in a systematized compound epithelial nevus. Am J Surg Pathol 1992;16:417.
212. Lawrence N, Cottel WI. Squamous cell carcinoma of the skin with perineural invasion. J Am Acad Dermatol 1994;31:30.
213. Stern JB, Haupt HM. Reexcision perineural invasion: Not a sign of malignancy. Am J Dermatopathol 1990;14:183.

Lever's Histopathology of the Skin, eighth edition,
edited by David Elder et al. Lippincott–
Raven Publishers, Philadelphia © 1997.

CHAPTER 37

Metastatic Carcinoma of the Skin

Incidence and Dissemination

Waine C. Johnson

Cutaneous metastases are of diagnostic importance because they may be the first manifestation of an undiscovered internal malignancy or the first indication of metastasis of a supposedly adequately treated malignancy. Cutaneous metastases are generally uncommon but have been reported more frequently in recent years. In a study of 7316 patients with internal cancer, Lookingbill et al.[1] found 367 (5%) to have skin involvement. Of 4020 patients with metastatic disease, Lookingbill et al.[2] reported that 420 (10%) had cutaneous metastases. Nine percent of 7518 patients with internal cancer who were autopsied at Roswell Park Memorial Institute had skin metastases.[3] The incidence of various tumors that are metastatic to the skin correlates well with the frequency of occurrence of the primary malignant tumor in each gender.

Review of 724 patients with cutaneous metastases in 1972 by Brownstein and Helwig[4] showed that, in women, commensurate with the greater frequency of carcinoma of the breast, 69% of all cutaneous metastases originated in the breast. Carcinoma of the large intestine accounted for 9% of cutaneous metastases, and carcinoma of the lungs and ovaries accounted for 4%. In recent years, the incidence of cutaneous metastasis from carcinoma of the lungs in women has significantly increased, and carcinoma of the lungs has become the most frequent cause of cancer deaths in women (as it is in men).[5] The study by Brownstein and Helwig,[4] of cutaneous metastases in men revealed the following incidences of primary carcinoma: lungs = 24%, large intestine = 19%, oral cavity = 12%, kidney and stomach each = 6%. Metastatic melanoma (13%) is discussed in Chap. 29.

Due to the relative rarity of carcinomas of the thyroid gland, pancreas, liver, gall bladder, urinary bladder, endometrium, prostate, testes, and neuroendocrine system, cutaneous metastases of these tumors are also relatively rare. A recent review by Schwartz[6] reported cutaneous metastatic disease as the first sign of internal cancer most commonly seen with cancer of the lung, kidney, and ovary.

Dissemination may take place through the lymphatics or the blood stream. In carcinomas of the breast and the oral cavity, metastases reach the skin largely through lymphatic channels and are often located in the overlying skin. In contrast, cutaneous metastatic lesions in other carcinomas are often the result of hematogenous dissemination and may appear in any area of the skin.[7]

W. C. Johnson: Johnson & Griffin Dermatopathology Associates, Glenside, PA

CARCINOMA OF THE BREAST

Cutaneous metastases that occur predominantly by lymphatic dissemination include inflammatory carcinoma, carcinoma en cuirasse, telangiectatic and nodular carcinoma, and carcinoma of the inframammary crease. Alopecia neoplastica and mammary carcinoma of the eyelid are probably caused by hematogenous spread.[6]

Inflammatory breast carcinoma is characterized by an erythematous patch or plaque with an active spreading border that resembles erysipelas and usually affects the breast and nearby skin.[6] Rarely, inflammatory metastatic carcinoma may arise from primary involvement of other organs. The inflammatory appearance and warmth are attributed to capillary congestion.

En cuirasse metastatic carcinoma is characterized by a diffuse morphea-like induration of the skin and rarely involves skin from other primary carcinomas. It usually begins as scattered papular lesions coalescing into a sclerodermoid plaque without inflammatory changes.

Telangiectatic metastatic breast carcinoma is characterized by violaceous papulovesicles resembling lymphangioma circumscriptum.[6] A violaceous hue, which is often present, is caused by blood in dilated vascular channels.

The nodular form appears as multiple firm nodules that may show ulceration. An exophytic nodule may occur in the infra-

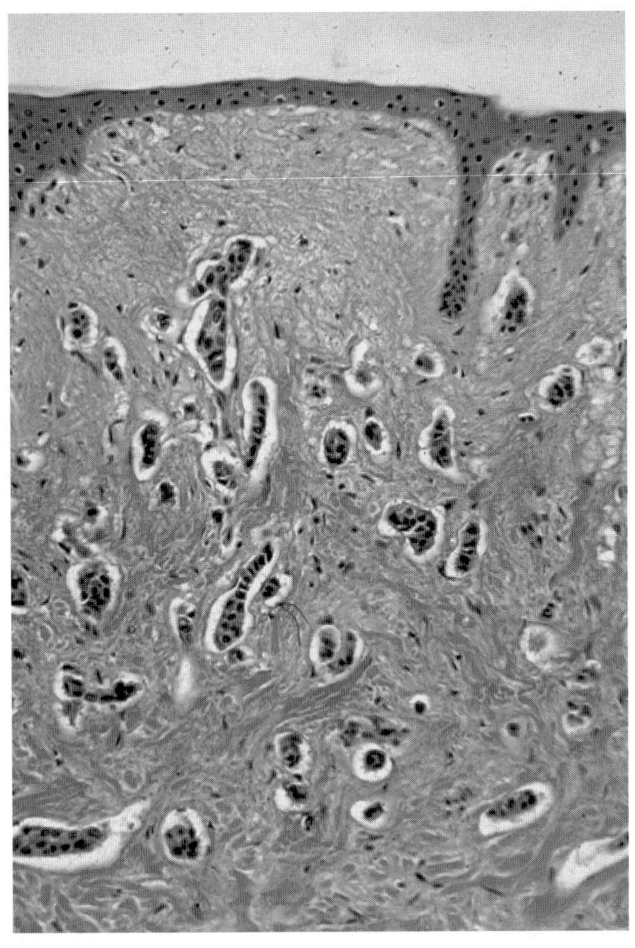

FIG. 37-1. Inflammatory breast carcinoma metastatic to skin
Dilated lymphatics contain groups and cords of tumor cells.

mammary crease resembling a primary squamous cell or basal cell carcinoma and occurs more frequently in women with large breasts.

Alopecia neoplastica occurs as oval plaques or patches of the scalp and may be confused clinically with alopecia areata or a scarring alopecia. Metastatic mammary carcinoma in the eyelid clinically presents as a painless swelling with induration or as a discrete nodule.[6]

Histopathology. In inflammatory carcinoma histologic examination of the skin reveals extensive invasion of the dermis and often the subcutaneous lymphatics by groups and cords of tumor cells (Fig. 37-1). The tumor cells are similar to those in the primary growth and atypical in character with large, pleomorphic, hyperchromatic nuclei. There is marked capillary congestion, which is the reason for the clinical appearance of erythema and warmth.[6] Often there is interstitial edema and a slight perivascular lymphoid infiltrate. The extensive lymphatic dissemination is caused by retrograde lymphatic spread into the skin secondary to blockage of the deep lymphatics and lymph nodes.[8] Fibrosis is not a significant feature. Some studies indicate only 1% to 4% of patients with metastatic breast carcinoma present with the inflammatory or erysipeloid type and that most of these patients have intraductal breast carcinoma.[9]

In en cuirasse carcinoma, also referred to as scirrhous carcinoma, the indurated areas show fibrosis and may contain only a few tumor cells. The tumor cells may be confused with fibroblasts. The tumor cells have elongated nuclei similar to fibroblasts, but the nuclei are larger, more angular, and more deeply basophilic. The tumor cells often lie singly, but in some areas they may form small groups or single rows between fibrotic and thickened collagen bundles (Fig. 37-2). This latter feature of "Indian filing" is of particular diagnostic importance (Fig. 37-3) and may be seen in any histologic variety.

In telangiectatic carcinoma the tumor cells tend to be located more superficially in the dermis within dilated lymphatic vessels than those in inflammatory carcinoma. The blood vessels

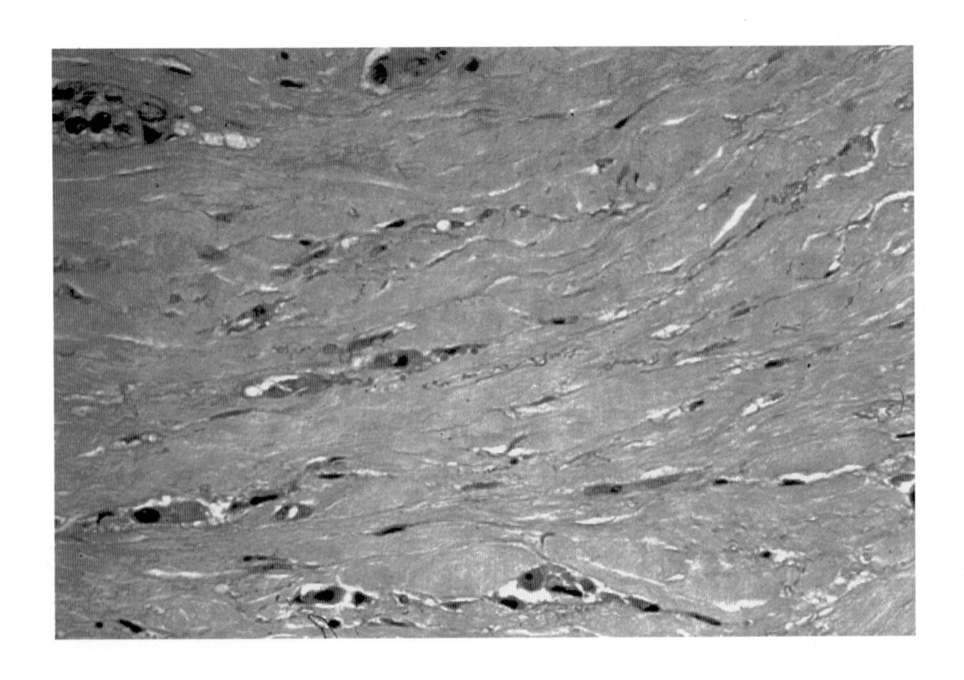

FIG. 37-2. En cuirasse carcinoma of the breast metastatic to skin
There are strands and groups of tumor cells between fibrotic collagen bundles.

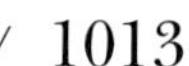

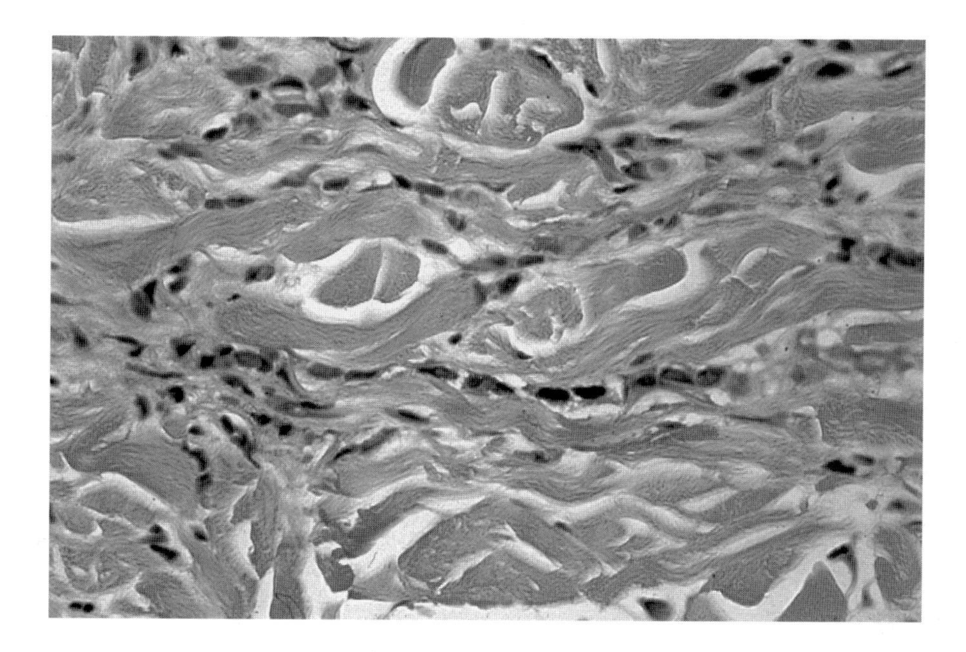

FIG. 37-3. Breast carcinoma metastatic to skin
The tumor cells show a linear arrangement, referred to as "Indian Filing," highly suggestive of metastatic carcinoma.

are congested with red blood cells, as in inflammatory carcinoma, but usually also contain aggregates of neoplastic cells.[10] The presence of many dilated blood vessels immediately beneath the epidermis gives rise to the clinical appearance of hemorrhagic vesicles.

In nodular carcinoma there are variably-sized groups of tumor cells in the dermis, and these nodular areas are surrounded by fibrosis. Depending on the tumor type, some cells may show glandular arrangement. Sometimes a nodule may be pigmented and clinically suggestive of a melanoma or pigmented basal cell carcinoma. The pigment results from melanin accumulation within the cytoplasm of neoplastic cells and in the stroma.[11]

In carcinoma of the inframammary crease islands of epithelial cells with hyperchromatic nuclei extend contiguously with the epidermis into the dermis.[12]

In hematogenous metastases the histologic picture varies with clinical presentation. In alopecia neoplastica, the features resemble those of en cuirasse type with single files of tumor cells between thickened collagen bundles.[13] Metastatic mammary carcinoma involving the eyelid has been described in 13 patients,[6] and in 8 of them the microscopic features had a prominent histiocytoid appearance.[14]

Immunoperoxidase. Cutaneous metastases are positive with keratin and often are positive with epithelial membrane antigen (EMA) and carcinoembryonic antigen (CEA). Reactivity with S-100 protein has been reported in as many as 84% of cases of primary and metastatic breast carcinoma.[15] The presence of melanin granules and melanosomes within tumor cells that give a positive HMB-45 is rare and probably occurs secondarily to phagocytosis or melanocyte colonization of the tumor cells.[11] In lesions in which there are cells positive with S-100 or HMB-45, reactivity with keratins, EMA, and/or CEA would rule out melanoma.

CARCINOMA OF THE LUNG

Metastasis to skin is more common in men, but the incidence of lung carcinoma in women is increasing.[5] In 56 patients reported with skin metastasis from lung carcinoma, 7% had a skin nodule before the diagnosis of the primary tumor and 16% had a nodule at the same time.[16] In 11 of 21 patients with cutaneous metastasis, the skin was the first extranodal site.[1] Metastases may occur on any cutaneous surface, but the most common sites are the chest wall and posterior abdomen.[6] Oat cell carcinoma shows predilection for the skin of the back.[2] Most lesions present as a localized cluster of cutaneous papules or nodules or as a solitary nodule.

Histopathology. Cutaneous metastases were undifferentiated in approximately 40% and adenocarcinoma and squamous cell carcinoma in approximately 30% each.[4] The undifferentiated tumors were often of the small cell type (Fig. 37-4) with hyperchromatic nuclei and scant cytoplasm.[4] The closely packed tumor cells may suggest a malignant lymphoma. Immunoperoxidase studies are extremely helpful im making this distinction. Larger cells require consideration of metastatic amelanotic melanoma and, again, immunoperoxidase studies may be required for distinction.

Squamous cell carcinomas metastatic to skin are usually poorly or moderately differentiated.[4] They can usually be distinguished from primary squamous cell carcinoma by the absence of proliferation from the surface epidermis and seldom show an orderly pattern of differentiation from basaloid to prickle cells with centers of keratinization. They show occasional whorls of squamoid cells with imperfect keratinization and individually keratinized cells, and sometimes have large, bizarre forms with frequent mitotic figures.[4] In larger tumors areas of central necrosis are often present. Most cutaneous metastatic squamous cell carcinomas arise in the lung, oral cavity, or esophagus (Fig. 37-5). Tumors from the oral cavity tend to be more differentiated and nearly always appear on the head or neck. Squamous carcinoma metastatic from the esophagus shows essentially similar features to that from the lung.[4]

Adenocarcinomas metastatic to skin from lung are often moderately differentiated, but some show well-formed, mucin-secreting, glandular structures (Fig. 37-6). Individual tumor cells sometimes contain abundant cytoplasmic mucin, but usually lack large pools of mucin, which is more characteristically seen from gastrointestinal metastatic adenocarcinomas.[4]

Immunoperoxidase. In addition to keratins that are positive

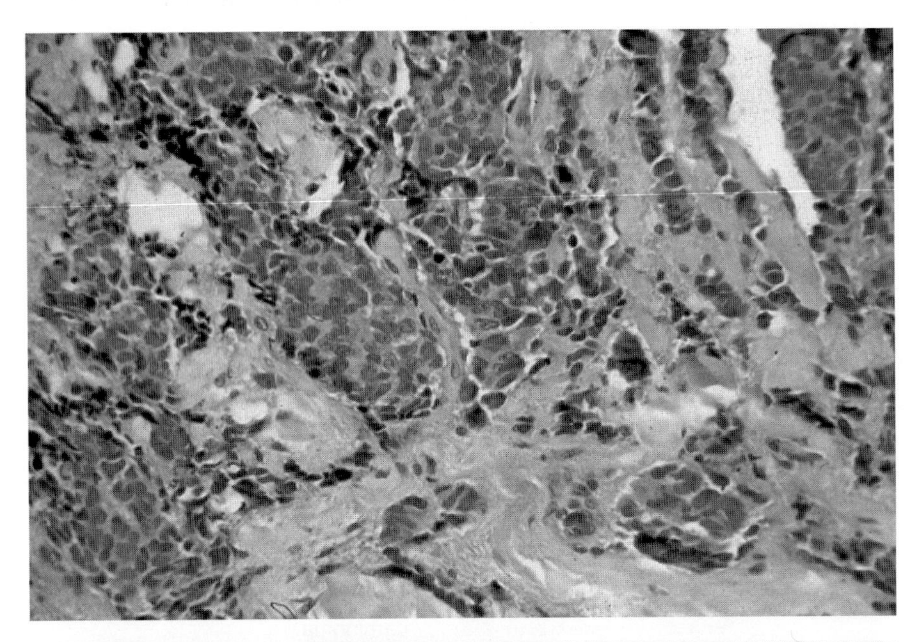

FIG. 37-4. Small cell carcinoma of lung metastatic to skin
Histologically indistinguishable from Merkel cell carcinoma.

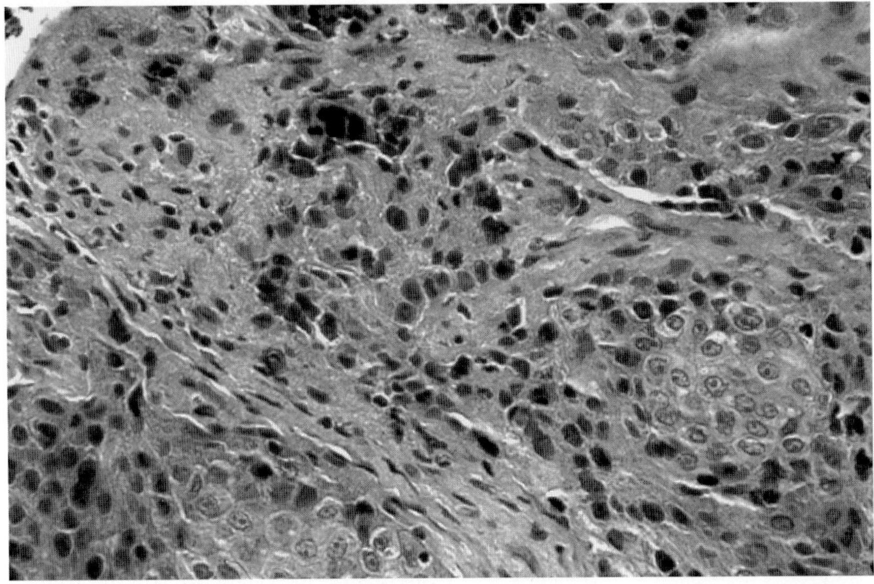

FIG. 37-5. Bronchogenic squamous cell carcinoma metastatic to skin

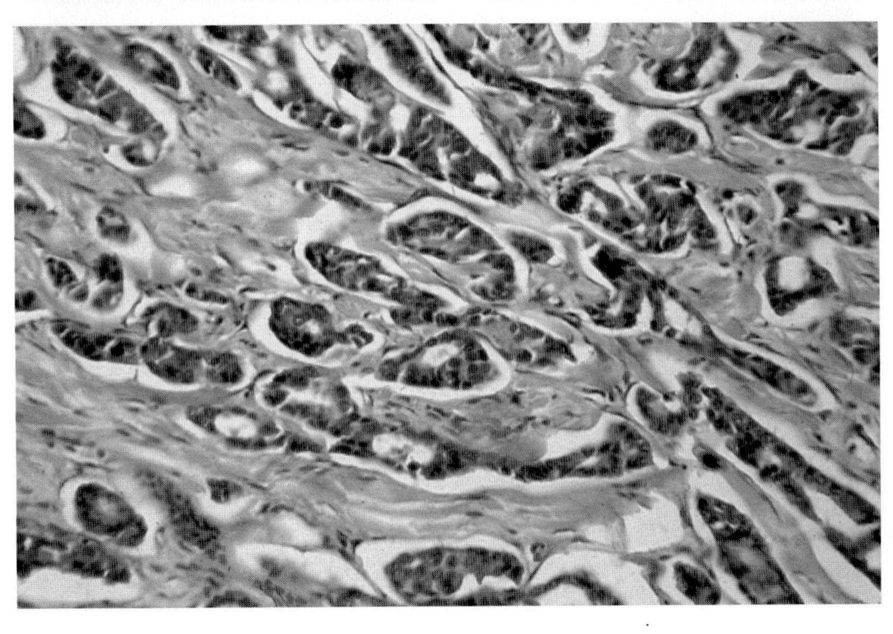

FIG. 37-6. Adenocarcinoma of lung metastatic to skin

in most metastatic carcinomas, most metastatic adenocarcinomas are positive with EMA and CEA. Metastatic small cell or neuroendocrine carcinoma characteristically shows a "dot-like" paranuclear reaction for cytokeratin that is also seen in primary Merkel's cell carcinomas of skin.[17–19] It has been stated that a positive reaction with CEA (seen in 50% of secondary neuroendocrine carcinomas) may be most helpful in differentiating between primary and secondary lesions.[17] A rare exception to this consideration is the presence of duct-like structures in two instances of Merkel cell carcinoma, and these were CEA-positive.[18] This was assumed to be eccrine differentiation. Either primary or secondary neuroendocrine carcinoma, in addition to the dot-like paranuclear or diffuse cytoplasmic reactivity to keratin, are almost always positive with neuron-specific enolase (NSE) and EMA. They may show reactivity to one or more of the following: protein gene product (PCP), chromogranin-A, CD56 antigen (Leu-7), and Synaptophysin.[17] Negative reactions with lymphocyte common antigen (LCA) and other lymphoid markers are most helpful in ruling out malignant lymphomas.[19]

GASTROINTESTINAL CARCINOMA

Carcinoma of the colon and rectum is the second most common type of primary cancer in both men and women.[6] Cutaneous lesions usually appear after the primary tumor has been recognized and occur more commonly on the abdomen or perineal areas, although the head and neck areas are sometimes involved. Metastases from gastric carcinoma may occur at any distant site, but the umbilical region is perhaps most common.

Histopathology. Most cutaneous metastases from the large intestine and all from the stomach as reported by Brownstein and Helwig[20] were adenocarcinomas. A mucinous carcinoma pattern with small groups of tumor cells that lie in large pools of mucin is common in lesions from the large intestine (Fig. 37-7). Signet-ring cell differentiation is not usually seen in lesions from the large intestine but may be present in lesions from the stomach.[4] The stomach metastases are usually anaplastic, infiltrating carcinomas with variable cellularity, a loose stroma, and varying proportions of signet-ring cells. The mucin present in metastatic carcinoma from the gastrointestinal tract as well as in mucinous carcinomas from the breast and lung is a nonsulfated, hyaluronidase-resistant, sialic acid–type of mucosubstance.[21–23] Histochemical procedures show this mucin to be positive with colloidal iron, hyaluronidase resistant, alcian blue positive at pH 2.5 and negative at pH 0.4, and aldehyde-fuchsin positive at pH 1.7 and negative at pH 1.0. It shows metachromasia with toluidine blue at pH 3.0, and is negative at pH 2.0, is is PAS positive and diastase resistant, and is mucicarmine positive.[24] In contrast, histochemical studies of adenoid squamous cell carcinoma show the mucin to be predominantly hyaluronic acid. Also, distinction from adenoid basal cell carcinoma and adenocystic carcinoma from lacrimal and salivary glands can be made based on the fact that these latter tumors contain a predominance of sulfated acid mucosaccharides.[24] The differential diagnosis for metastatic carcinoma includes carcinomas of cutaneous adnexae such as sweat gland carcinomas.

ORAL CAVITY CARCINOMA

Most lesions metastasizing from carcinomas of the oral cavity are spread by lymphatic invasion and are located on the face or neck.[4] They usually appear as multiple or solitary nodules and sometimes are ulcerated.

Histopathology. The lesions are almost always squamous cell in type and are usually moderately or well differentiated.[4] They are located usually in the deeper dermis and subcutaneous tissue with sparing of the superficial cutis. In examples with ulceration and involvement of the upper corium, distinction from primary squamous cell carcinoma of skin may not be possible.[4]

RENAL CELL CARCINOMA

The tumors are most common in the head and neck area, although any site may be involved.[6,25] They often present as soli-

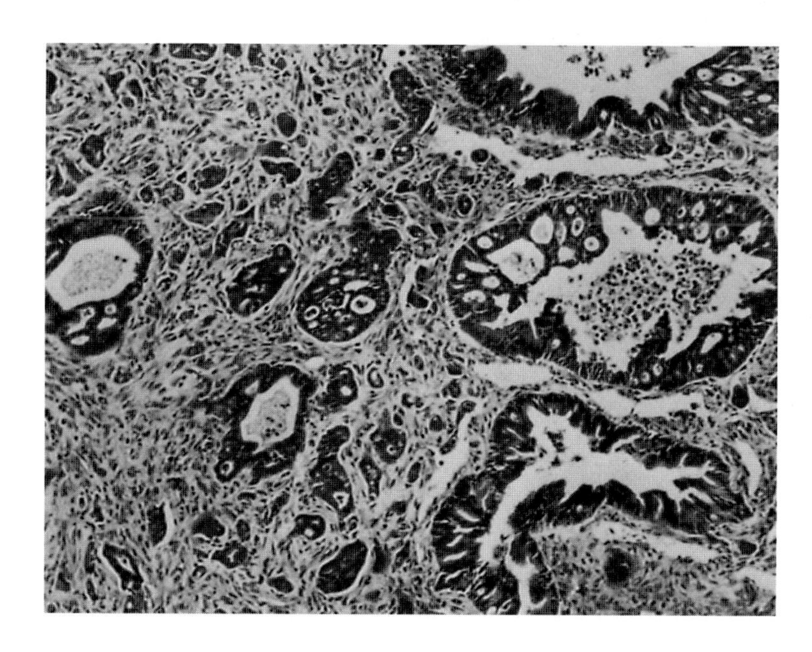

FIG. 37-7. Cutaneous metastasis from an adenocarcinoma of the colon
Numerous glandular lumina are present.

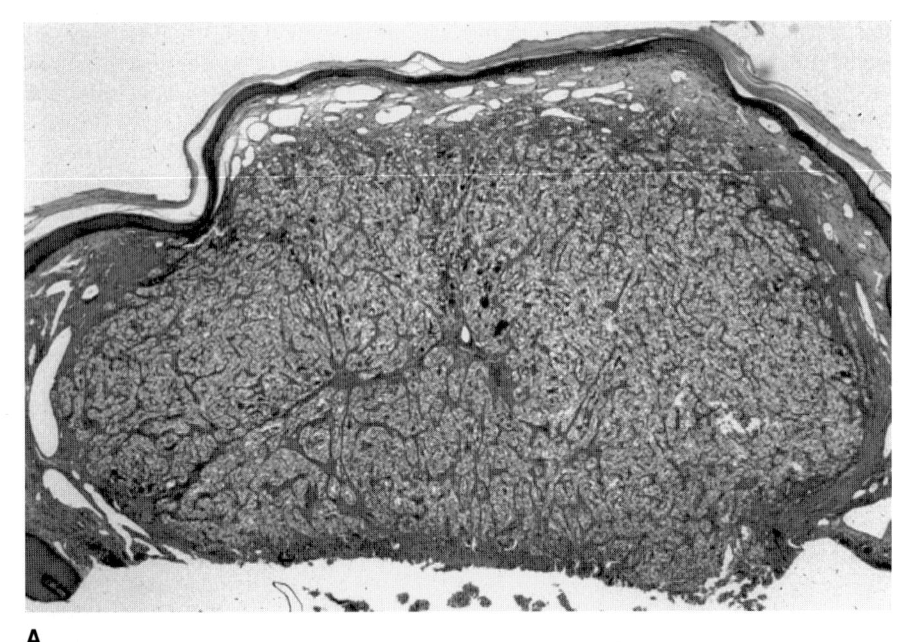

A

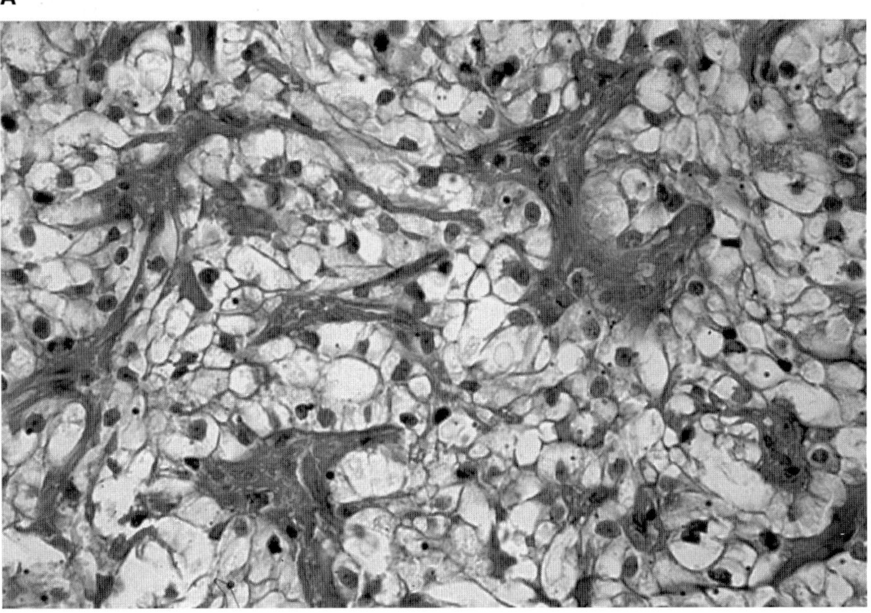

B

FIG. 37-8. Renal cell carcinoma metastatic to skin
There are thick-walled capillaries between clear cells.

tary or a few nodules and may be skin colored, reddish, or violaceous. They may occur as the first sign of internal cancer or as late as ten years after diagnosis of the primary. They occur almost always in men.

Histopathology. The histologic features are usually those of a clear cell adenocarcinoma. They are often localized intradermal nodules and may stretch the overlying epidermis.[4] The tumor cells show oval nuclei with abundant, clear cytoplasm and often are in a glandular configuration (Fig. 37-8). The stroma is vascular, and extravasated red blood cells are frequent. Intracytoplasmic glycogen is uniformly present as demonstrated by staining with PAS stain and diastase-labile intracytoplasmic material. Frozen sections stained with oil-red–O show the presence of lipid droplets in many tumor cells.[25] The histologic differential diagnosis includes adnexal tumors and especially eccrine acrospiroma. In contrast to the usual unilobular and hemorrhagic renal cell carcinoma, the eccrine acrospiroma tends to be multilobular and nonhemorrhagic, and often distinct ductal structures are present. Sebaceous cell tumors also may be confused, but the markedly vascular stroma and hemorrhagic nature of the renal cell cancer is fairly distinctive.

Immunoperoxidase. In most cases the tumor cells are reactive with cytokeratin and EMA and negative with CEA. One rare example was positive with S-100, and 25% of examples are reported to be positive with Vimentin.[26]

CARCINOMA OF THE OVARY

The most frequent sites involved are the abdomen including the umbilicus, the vulva, or the back.[6] Lesions of the abdomen may be in the scar sites from surgery or diagnostic procedures.[2]

Histopathology. The features are usually of a moderately or well-differentiated adenocarcinoma, often having a papillary configuration and containing psammoma bodies.[4] Psammoma bodies in cutaneous metastases in 724 patients studied by these authors were found only in metastases from the ovary (but might also be seen in papillary carcinomas from other sites including, for example, the thyroid).

CARCINOID AND NEUROENDOCRINE CARCINOMAS

These tumors are assumed to be derived from the neural crest tissues and are classified as amine precursor uptake and decarboxylase (APUD) system.[18] Lesions appear as solitary or multiple cutaneous papules or nodules and may occur at any site. Primary carcinoids giving rise to cutaneous metastases occur most frequently in the bronchi but have been reported in various sites, including the small intestines, sigmoid, colon, pancreas, stomach, thymus, and thyroid.[27] In addition to carcinoid tumors, cutaneous metastases from neuroendocrine carcinomas of a variety of sites including the uterus, vulva, gall bladder, and fallopian tubes have been reported.[6,28] Neuroblastoma, which is the most common cancer identified at birth, has been reported to metastasize to the subcutaneous tissue in 32% of patients with congenital neuroblastoma.[6] Clinically, they have a fairly specific appearance, which has been described as like a "blueberry muffin." This term has also been used to describe some cases of congenital leukemia. Cutaneous neuroblastoma is very rare in adults, and it is impossible to distinguish between primary and metastatic lesions except for finding an internal primary tumor.[29]

Histopathology. Carcinoid metastases in the skin and subcutaneous tissue consist of solid islands, nests, and cords of tumor cells. As a rule, the cells appear quite uniform in size and shape, have small, rounded nuclei, and abundant, clear, or eosinophilic cytoplasm occasionally containing numerous eosinophilic granules.[30] However, in some instances the nuclei are hyperchromatic and there may be areas in which the nuclei show anaplasia by being irregularly shaped, large, and hyperchromatic. Carcinoids of the bronchus usually contain argyrophil granules in contrast to those of the small intestine, which usually contain argentaffin granules, which can be demonstrated by the Fontana-Masson stain.[31] Cutaneous metastases of bronchial carcinoids may have either argyrophil or argentaffin granules.[32] The histologic differential diagnosis may include sweat gland carcinoma or glomus tumor because of their arrangement in well-defined islands, as well as metastases from noncarcinoid neuroendocrine tumors, and primary Merkel cell carcinoma. The latter usually show more immature cells or greater cellular atypism, a greater number of mitotic figures, and a "trabecular" pattern. The presence of an intraepidermal component would also favor a primary Merkel cell carcinoma.[18] Involvement of the deep dermis and multiple skin sites favor a metastatic lesion.[28] Primary or metastatic neuroblastomas (peripheral neuroectodermal tumor) show identical features of undifferentiated, small, hyperchromatic cells with frequent rosettes of the Homer Wright type and numerous mitoses.[29] Some examples of undifferentiated lesions may not show rosettes. The histologic differential diagnosis includes other small cell carcinomas that sometimes show rosette-like structures, extraskeletal Ewing's sarcoma, lymphoma, and leukemia. Merkel cell carcinoma tends to display a trabecular arrangement, but this is not always specific.

Immunoperoxidase and Electron Microscopy. Immunoperoxidase studies are of limited value in distinguishing a primary Merkel cell carcinoma of the skin from a metastatic neuroendocrine carcinoma. If the lesion is positive for CEA in nonductal or nonglandular sites, this would strongly favor a metastatic lesion.[17,18] The presence of a positive reaction with NSE and EMA is not necessarily helpful, since these can be reactive in primary or secondary neuroendocrine carcinomas as well as sweat gland carcinomas. Reactivity with CK20 favors a Merkel cell tumor. If the tumor is positive with S-100, this favors an eccrine sweat gland carcinoma, a metastatic breast carcinoma, or a malignant melanoma. If the tumor is positive with LCA, this identifies the lesion as a malignant lymphoma. Calcitonin has been demonstrated in cutaneous metastasis of medullary carcinoma of the thyroid.[33] Electron microscopic studies of carcinoid, neuroendocrine carcinomas, and primary Merkel cell carcinomas show "neurosecretory" membrane-bound, dense-core granules measuring 100 to 250 nm in diameter.[27,28,32,34] These granules do not distinguish among members of this group. Immunoelectron microscopic studies confirm the presence of cytokeratin (AE1/AE3) arranged in paranuclear areas, while cytoplasmic synaptophysin and chromogranin positivity over dense-core granules tend to confirm light microscopic immunohistochemical studies.[34] Neuroblastoma has been reported to be positive with NSE but often is negative with other commonly reactive antigens of neuroendocrine tumors such as EMA, chromagranin-A, and synaptophysin.[29] Electron microscopy shows membrane-bound, dense-core granules concentrated in the cytoplasmic processes. Desmosomes and microtubules are usually seen in more differentiated tumors.

MISCELLANEOUS CARCINOMAS

In metastatic carcinoma from the liver the arrangement of malignant hepatocytes in irregular columns are fairly distinctive[30] and, if there are acinar structures containing bile, the diagnosis is definite.[35]

In choriocarcinoma the cutaneous metastases show the two types of cells that arise from the fetal trophoblast: cytotrophoblasts and syncytiotrophoblasts. The cytotrophoblasts usually grow in clusters, and the cells appear cuboidal with large, vesicular nuclei and a pale cytoplasm. The syncytiotrophoblasts, which have large and irregular nuclei and a basophilic cytoplasm, grow around the clusters of cytotrophoblasts in a plexiform pattern resembling chorionic villi.[36] The syncytiotrophoblasts have been reported to be strongly positive for human chorionic gonadotropin antigen.[37]

Metastatic carcinoma of the prostate to skin is rare and usually occurs in the inguinal area, lower abdomen, or thighs, but distant sites of the scalp and face have been reported.[6] Reactivity with prostate-specific antigen establishes the diagnosis.[38]

Pancreatic cancer metastatic to skin is rare, and the most common site is the umbilical area.[6,39] Histologically it usually represents an adenocarcinoma. Immunoperoxidase with a carbohydrate antigen (CA19-9) is found to be positive.[39] This antigen is commonly present in adenocarcinoma of the pancreas but is not specific. It is usually negative in adenocarcinomas of the breast.

Cutaneous metastases from thyroid carcinoma tend to involve the abdominal skin or the head area.[6] Medullary, follicular, and papillary thyroid carcinomas may retain their histologic patterns in the cutaneous metastases. Immunoperoxidase studies often show a positive reaction to antithyroglobulin antibody.[40]

REFERENCES

1. Lookingbill DP, Spangler N, Sexton FM. Skin involvement as the presenting sign of internal carcinoma. J Am Acad Dermatol 1990;22:19.
2. Lookingbill DP, Spangler N, Helm KF. Cutaneous metastases in patients with metastatic carcinoma: A retrospective study of 4020 patients. J Am Acad Dermatol 1993;29:228.
3. Spencer PS, Helm TN. Skin metastases in cancer patients. Cutis 1987; 39:119.
4. Brownstein MH, Helwig EB. Metastatic tumors of the skin. Cancer 1972;29:1298.
5. Fielding JE. Smoking and women. N Engl J Med 1987;317:1343.
6. Schwartz RA. Cutaneous metastatic disease. J Am Acad Dermatol 1995;33:161.
7. Brownstein MH, Helwig EB. Patterns of cutaneous metastasis. Arch Dermatol 1972;105:862.
8. Zala L, Jenni C. Das carcinoma erysipelatodes. Dermatologica 1980; 160:80.
9. Cox SE, Cruz PD. A spectrum of inflammatory metastasis to skin via lymphatics: Three cases of carcinoma erysipeloides. J Am Acad Dermatol 1994;30:304.
10. Ingram JT. Carcinoma erysipelatodes and carcinoma telangiectaticum. Arch Dermatol 1958;77:227.
11. Shamai-Lubovitz O, Rothem A, Ben-David E et al. Cutaneous metastatic carcinoma of the breast mimicking malignant melanoma clinically and histologically. J Am Acad Dermatol 1994;31:1058.
12. Waisman M. Carcinoma of the inframammary crease. Arch Dermatol 1978;114:1520.
13. Carson HJ, Pellettiere EV, Lack E. Alopecia neoplastica simulating alopecia areata and antedating the detection of primary breast carcinoma. J Cutan Pathol 1994;21:67.
14. Hood CI, Font RL, Zimmerman LE. Metastatic mammary carcinoma in the eyelid with histiocytoid appearance. Cancer 1973;31:793.
15. Stroup RM, Pinkus GS. S-100 immunoreactivity in primary and metastatic carcinoma of the breast: A potential source of error in immunodiagnosis. Hum Pathol 1988;19:949.
16. Brady LW, O'Neill EA, Farber SH. Unusual sites of metastases. Semin Oncol 1977;4:59.
17. Wick MR, Swanson PE, Ritter JH, Fitzgibbon JF. The immunohistology of cutaneous neoplasia: A practical perspective. J Cutan Pathol 1993;20:481.
18. Smith KJ, Skelton HG III, Holland TT et al. Neuroendocrine (Merkel cell) carcinoma with an intraepidermal component. Am J Dermatopathol 1993;15:528.
19. Guinee DG Jr, Fishback NF, Koss MN et al. The spectrum of immunohistochemical staining of small-cell lung carcinoma in specimens from transbronchial and open-lung biopsies. Am J Clin Pathol 1994;102:406.
20. Brownstein MH, Helwig EB. Spread of tumors to the skin. Arch Dermatol 1973;107:80.
21. Johnson WC, Helwig EB. Histochemistry of primary and metastatic mucus-secreting tumors. Ann NY Acad Sci 1963;106:794.
22. Johnson WC, Helwig EB. Histochemistry of the acid mucopolysaccharides of skin in normal and in certain pathologic conditions. Am J Clin Pathol 1963;40:123.
23. Werner I. Studies on glycoproteins from mucous epithelium and epithelial secretions. Acta Soc Med Ups 1953;58:1.
24. Johnson WC. Histochemistry of the skin. In: Graham JH, Johnson WC, Helwig EB, eds. Dermal pathology. Hagerstown: Harper & Row, 1972; 75.
25. Connor DH, Taylor HB, Helwig EB. Cutaneous metastasis of renal cell carcinoma. Arch Pathol 1963;76:339.
26. Coffin CM, Swanson PE, Wick MR, Dehner LP. An Immunohistochemical comparison of chordoma with renal cell carcinoma, colorectal adenocarcinoma, and myxopapillary ependymoma: A potential diagnostic dilemma in the diminutive biopsy. Mod Pathol 1993;6:531.
27. Rodriquez G, Villamizar R. Carcinoid tumor with skin metastasis. Am J Dermatopathol 1992;14:263.
28. Fogaca MF, Fedorciw BJ, Tahan SR et al. Cutaneous metastasis of neuroendocrine carcinoma of uterine origin. J Cutan Pathol 1993;20:455.
29. Van Nguyen A, Argenyi ZB. Cutaneous neuroblastoma. Am J Dermatopathol 1993;15:7.
30. Reingold IM, Escovitz WE. Metastatic cutaneous carcinoid. Arch Dermatol 1960;82:971.
31. Brody HJ, Stallings WP, Fine RM, Someren A. Carcinoid in an umbilical nodule. Arch Dermatol 1978;114:570.
32. Keane J, Fretzin DV, Wellington J, Shapiro CM. Bronchial carcinoid metastatic to skin: Light and electron microscopic findings. J Cutan Pathol 1980;7:43.
33. Ordonez NG, Samaan NA. Medulary carcinoma of the thyroid metastatic to the skin: Report of two cases. J Cutan Pathol 1987;14:251.
34. Mount SL, Taatjes DJ. Neuroendocrine carcinoma of the skin (Merkel cell carcinoma): An immunoelectron-microscopic case study. Am J Dermatopathol 1994;16:60.
35. Kahn JA, Sinhamohapatra SB, Schneider AF. Hepatoma presenting as a skin metastasis. Arch Dermatol 1971;104:299.
36. Cosnow I, Fretzin DF. Choriocarcinoma metastatic to skin. Arch Dermatol 1974;109:551.
37. Chhieng DC, Jennings TA, Slominski A, Mihm MC Jr. Choriocarcinoma presenting as a cutaneous metastasis. J Cutan Pathol 1995;22:374.
38. Segal R, Penneys NS, Nahass G. Metastatic prostatic carcinoma histologically mimicking malignant melanoma. J Cutan Pathol 1994;21: 280.
39. Taniguchi S, Hisa T, Hamada T. Cutaneous metastases of pancreatic carcinoma with unusual clinical features. J Am Acad Dermatol 1994; 31:877.
40. Toyota N, Asaga H, Hirokawa M, Iizuka H. A case of skin metastasis from follicular thyroid carcinoma. Dermatology 1994;188:69.

APPENDIX

Electron Micrographs

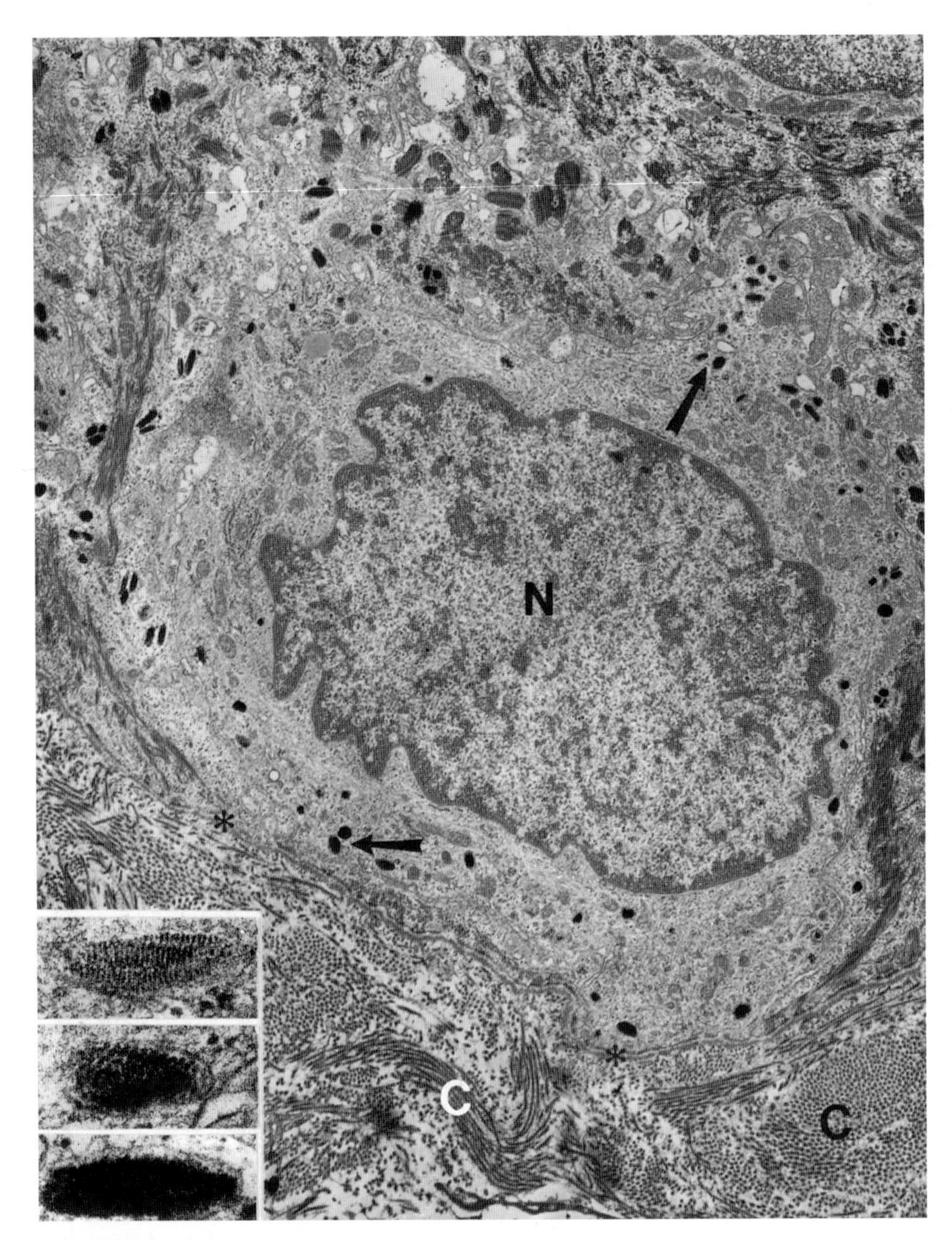

EM 1. Melanocyte, (Inset) Melanosomes
N, nucleus of melanocyte; *arrows,* melanosomes; *C,* collagen in the dermis; *asterisk,* basal lamina. *(Insets)* Melanosomes in different stages of development: Stage II (*upper inset*), Stage III (*middle inset*), and Stage IV (*lower inset*).

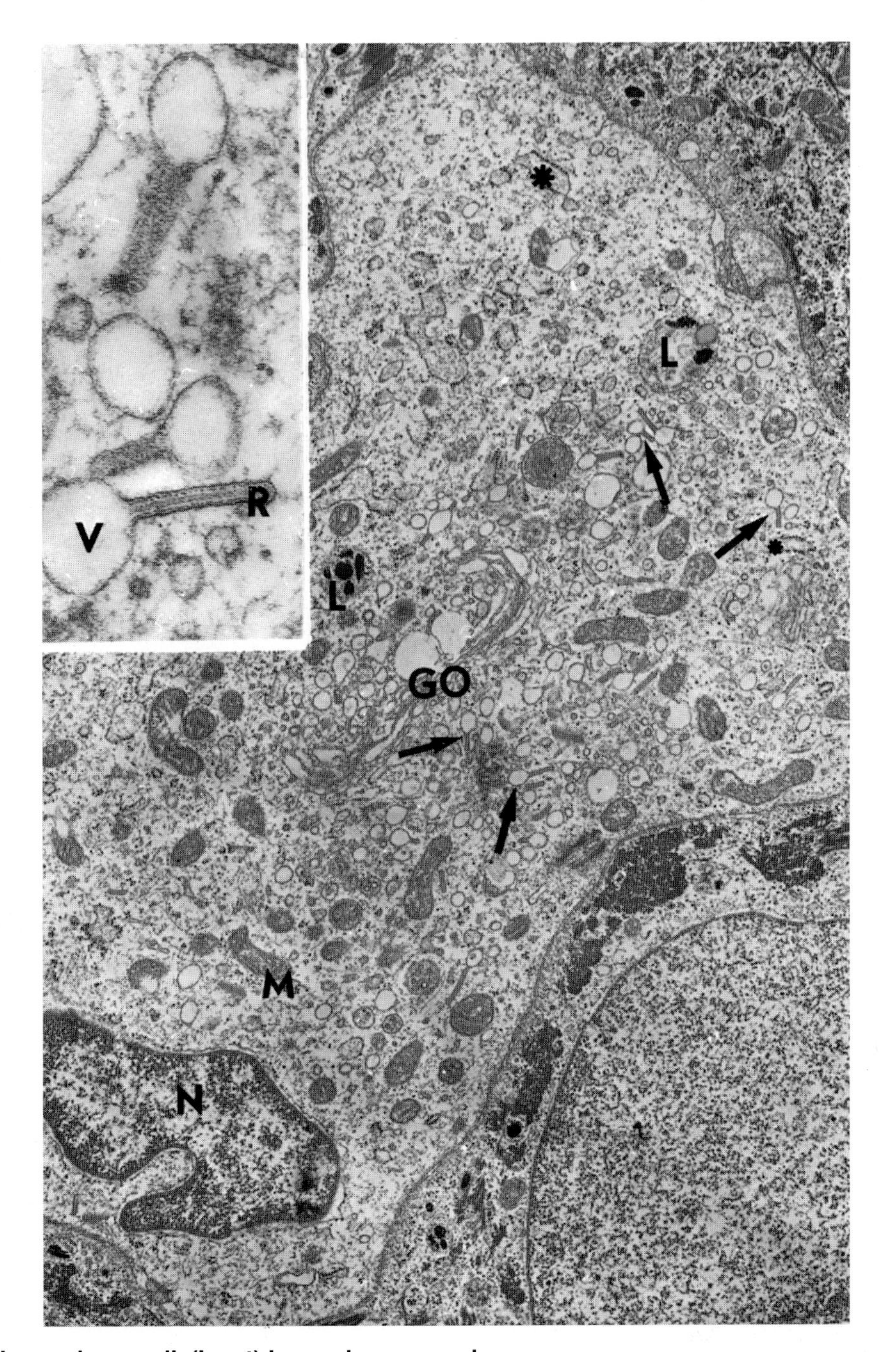

EM 2. Langerhans cell, (Inset) Langerhans granules

N, nucleus of Langerhans cell; *L,* lysosomes containing melanosomes; *GO,* Golgi complex; *M,* mitochondrium; *asterisk,* rough endoplasmic reticulum; *arrows,* Langerhans granules. (*Inset*) Langerhans granules at higher magnification consisting of a vesicle (*V*) and a rod (*R*), both giving the appearance of a tennis racquet.

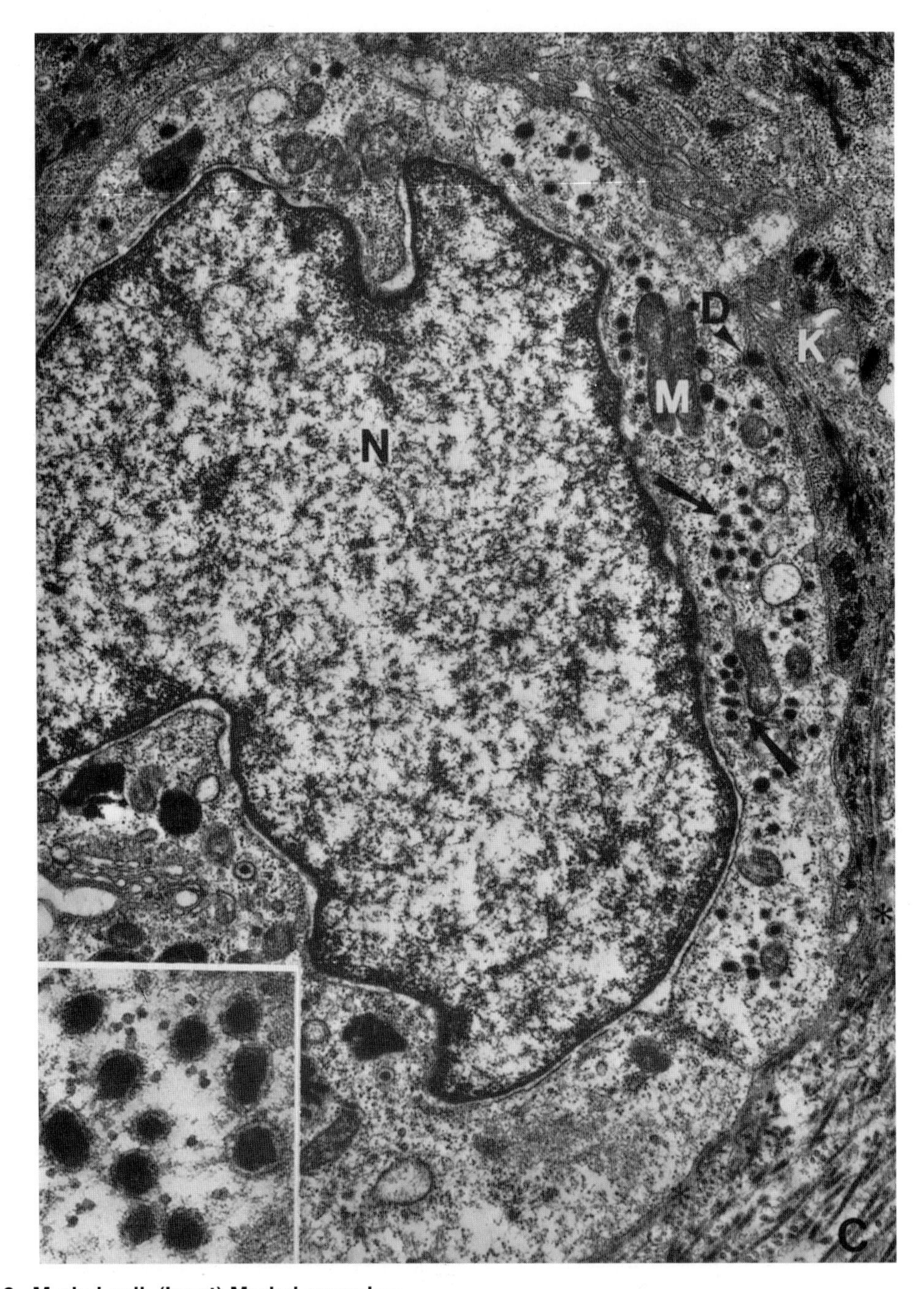

EM 3. Merkel cell, (Inset) Merkel granules
N, nucleus of Merkel cell; *asterisk,* on basal lamina; *M,* mitochondria; *arrows,* specific granules of the Merkel cell; *D with pointer,* desmosome between Merkel cell and keratinocyte (*K*); *C,* collagen with cross striation. (*Inset*) Specific membrane-bound granules at higher magnification.

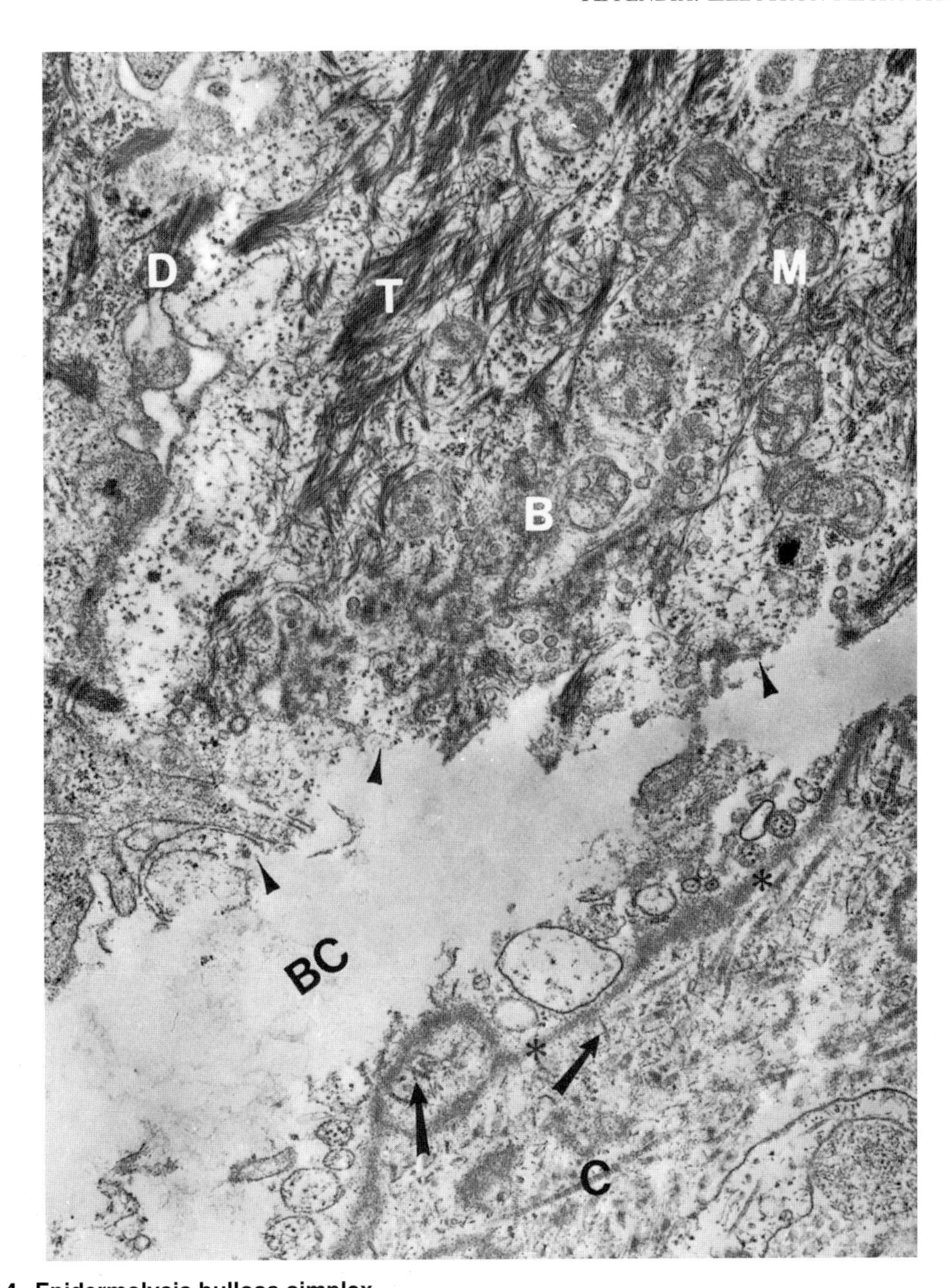

EM 4. Epidermolysis bullosa simplex
The blister formed as the result of degenerative, cytolytic changes in the basal cells (*B*). The bulla cavity (*BC*) is situated above the basement membrane (*asterisk*). The basal cells are severely damaged, lacking a plasma membrae (*pointers*). *T,* tonofilaments; *M,* mitochondria; *D,* desmosome.

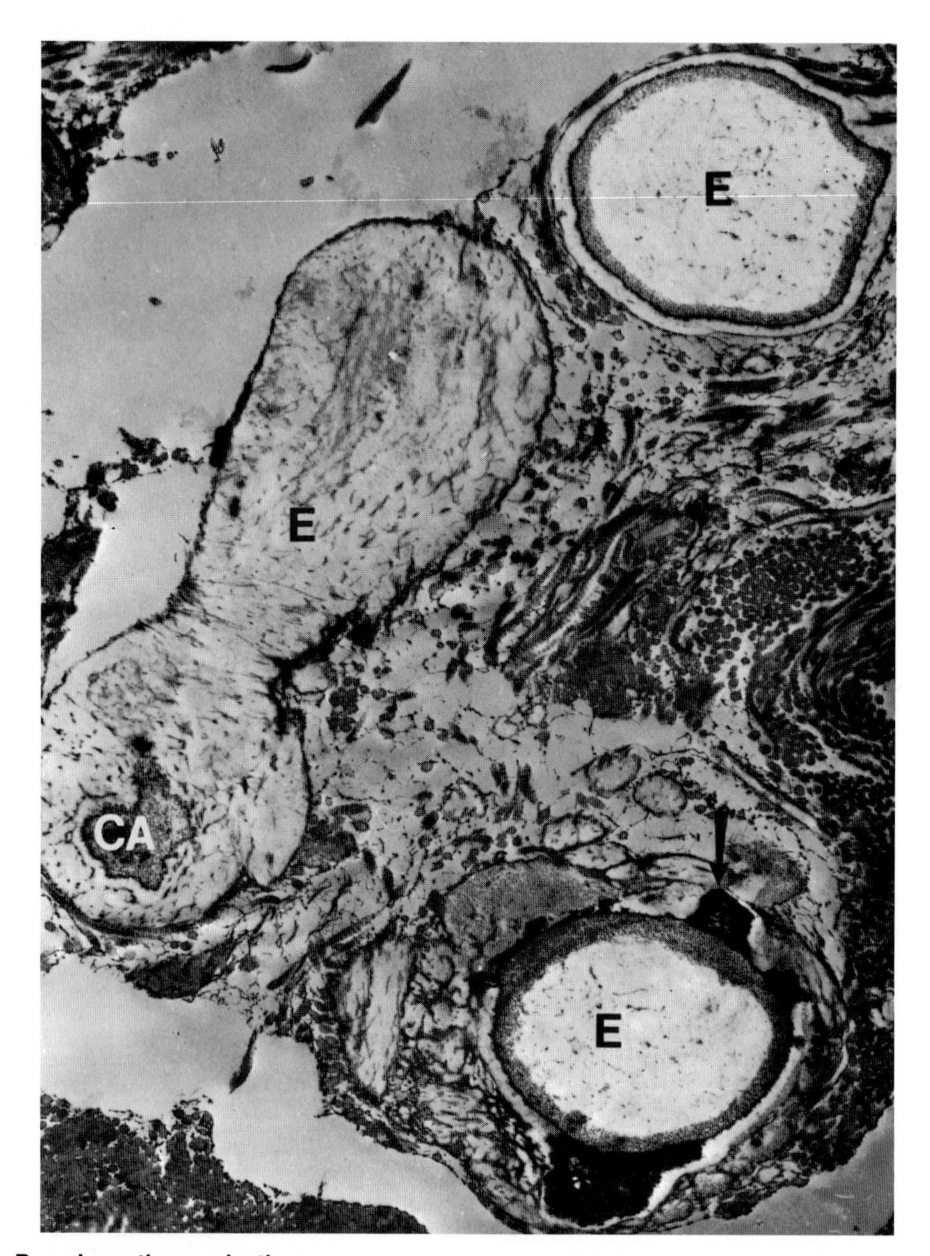

EM 5. Pseudoxanthoma elasticum
The elastic fibers (*E*) are bizarrely shaped. Calcium (*CA; arrows*) is deposited on or around elastic fibers.

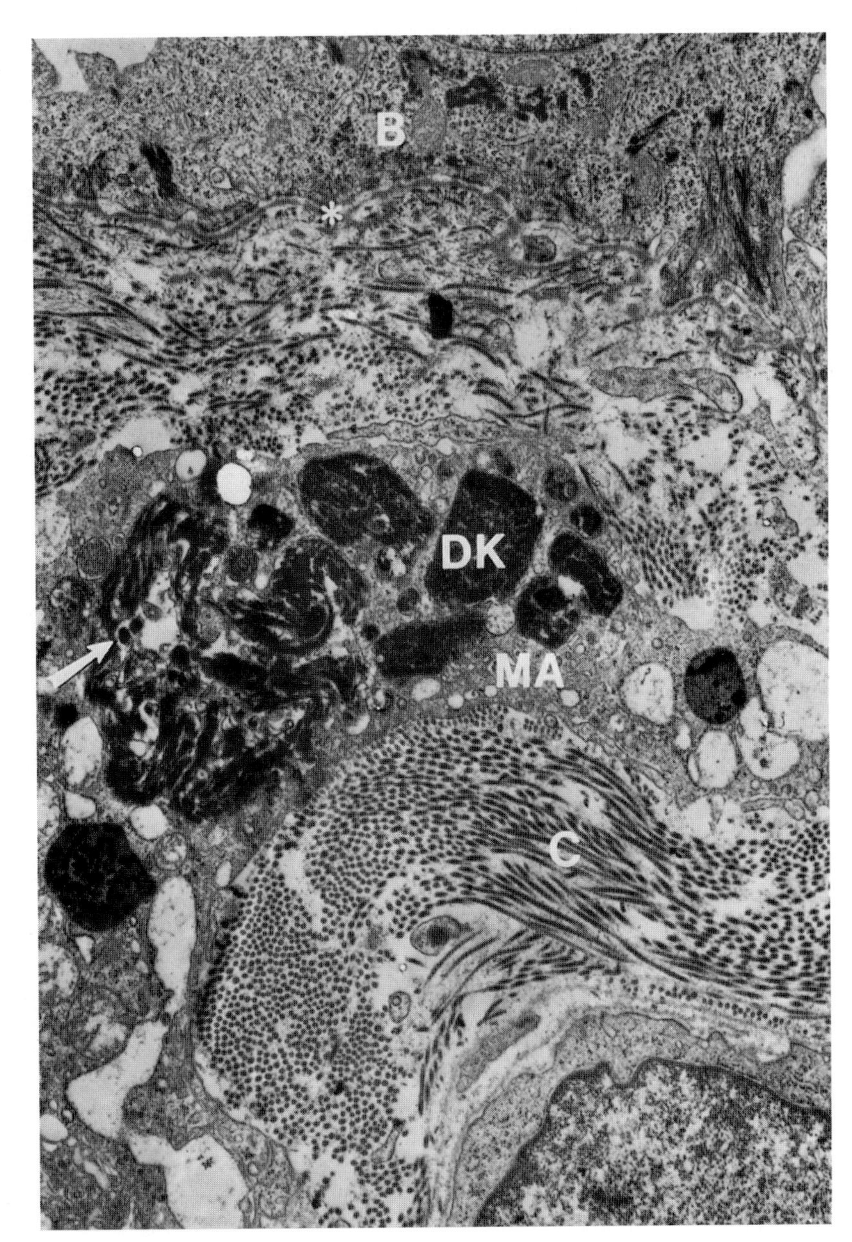

EM 6. Incontinentia pigmenti
In this disease, dyskeratotic cells are found in the epidermis. Macrophages migrate into the epidermis, phagocytize these dyskeratotic cells as well as melanosomes, and subsequently return to the dermis. *MA,* macrophage containing dyskeratotic material (*DK*) and melanosomes (*arrow*); *B,* basal cell; *asterisk,* basal lamina; *C,* collagen.

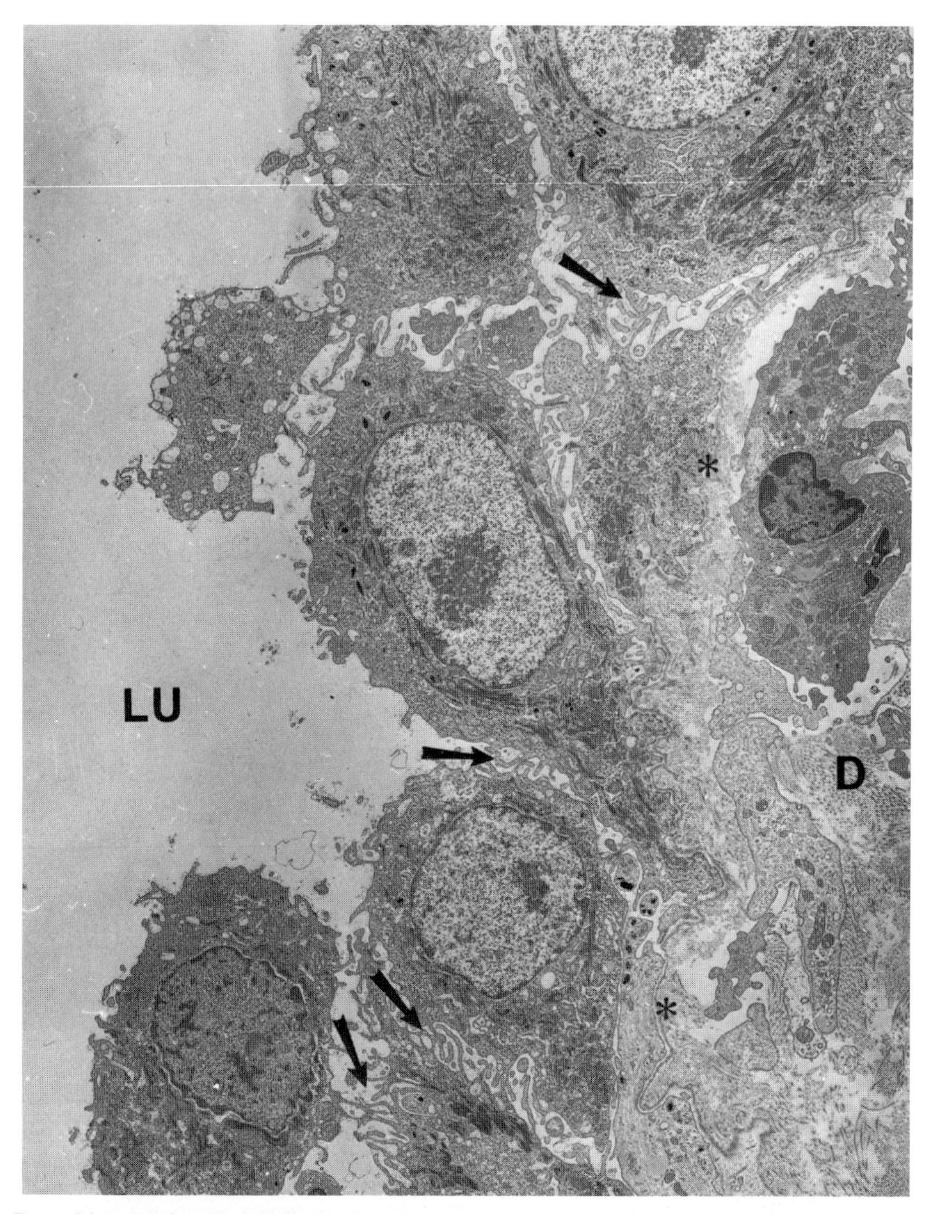

EM 7. Pemphigus vulgaris, tombstone row
The dissolution of the intercellular cement led to the formation of a blister. At the base of the blister, one or two rows of keratinocytes are left. The cohesion of the basal cells with the dermis is well preserved. *LU,* blister lumen; *asterisks,* basement membrane; *arrows,* microvilli of keratinocytes; *D,* dermis.

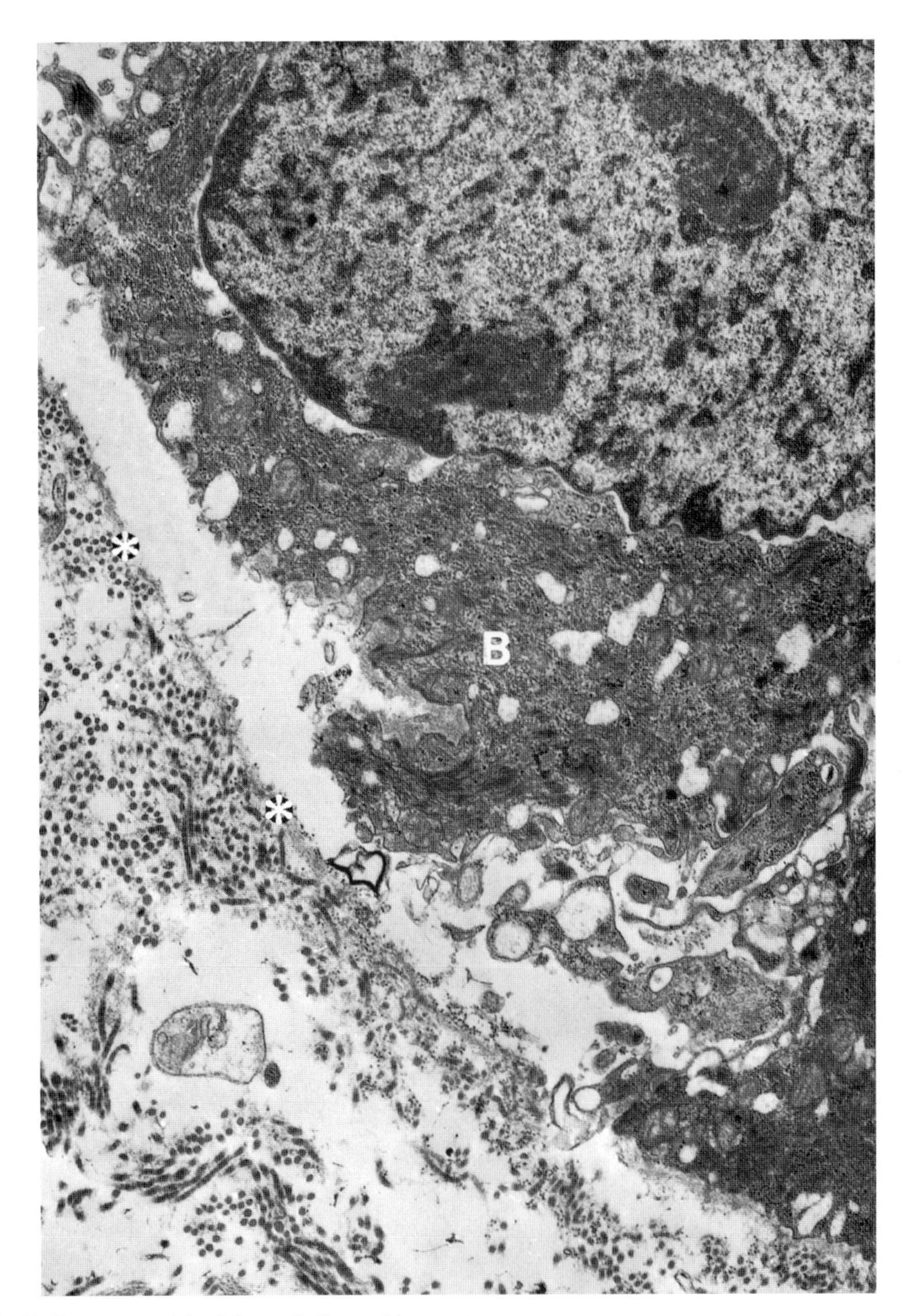

EM 8. Bullous pemphigoid, noninflamed type
In this type of bullous pemphigoid, the blister forms between the basal cell (*B*) and the basement membrane (*asterisks*).

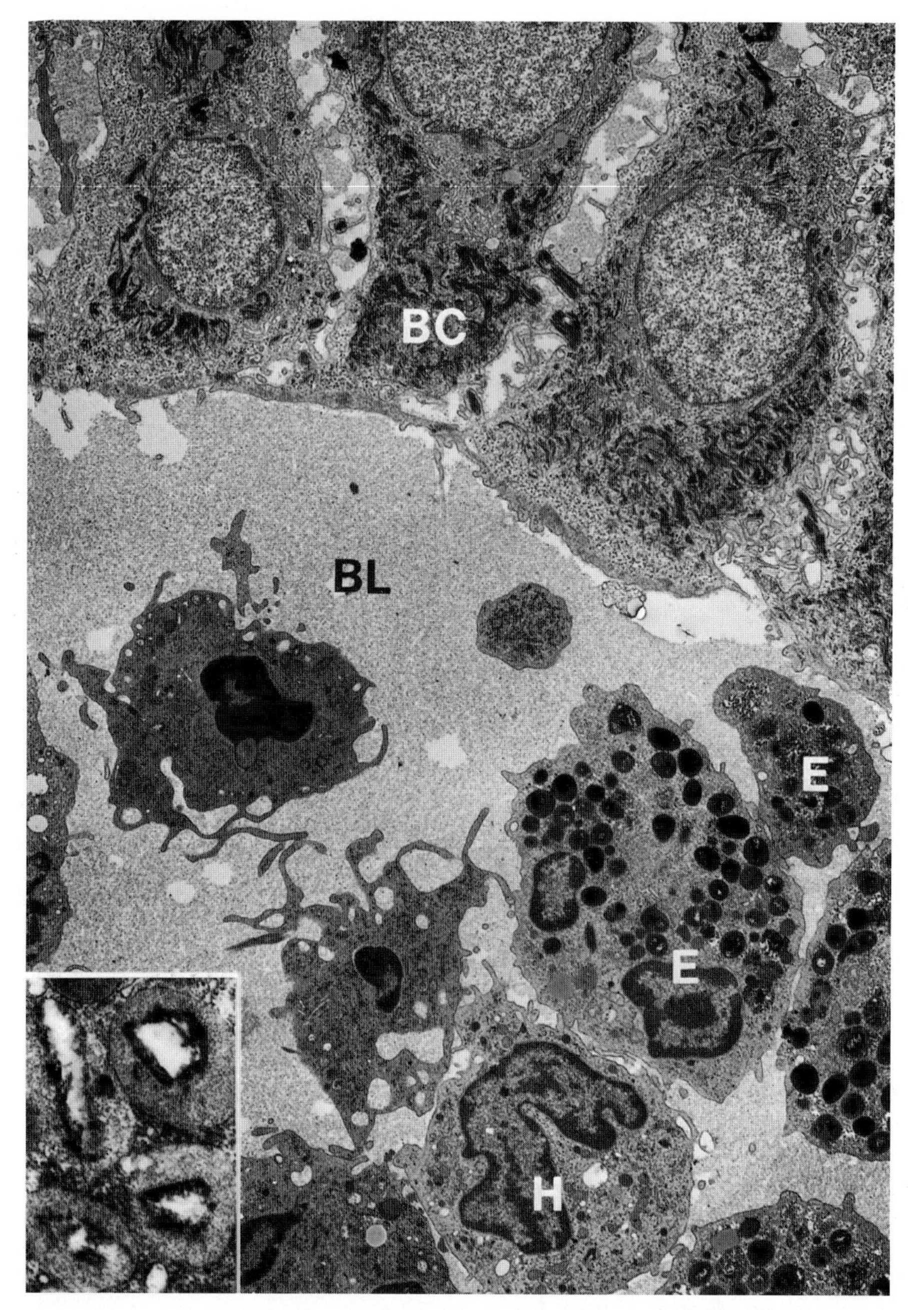

EM 9. Bullous pemphigoid inflamed type, (Inset) Granules of eosinophils
The blister (*BL*) contains several histiocytes (*H*) and eosinophils (*E*). The basement membrane has disappeared. The basal cells (*BC*) at the top of the blister are well preserved. (*Inset*) Eosinophilic granules at higher magnification show a "crystal" at their center.

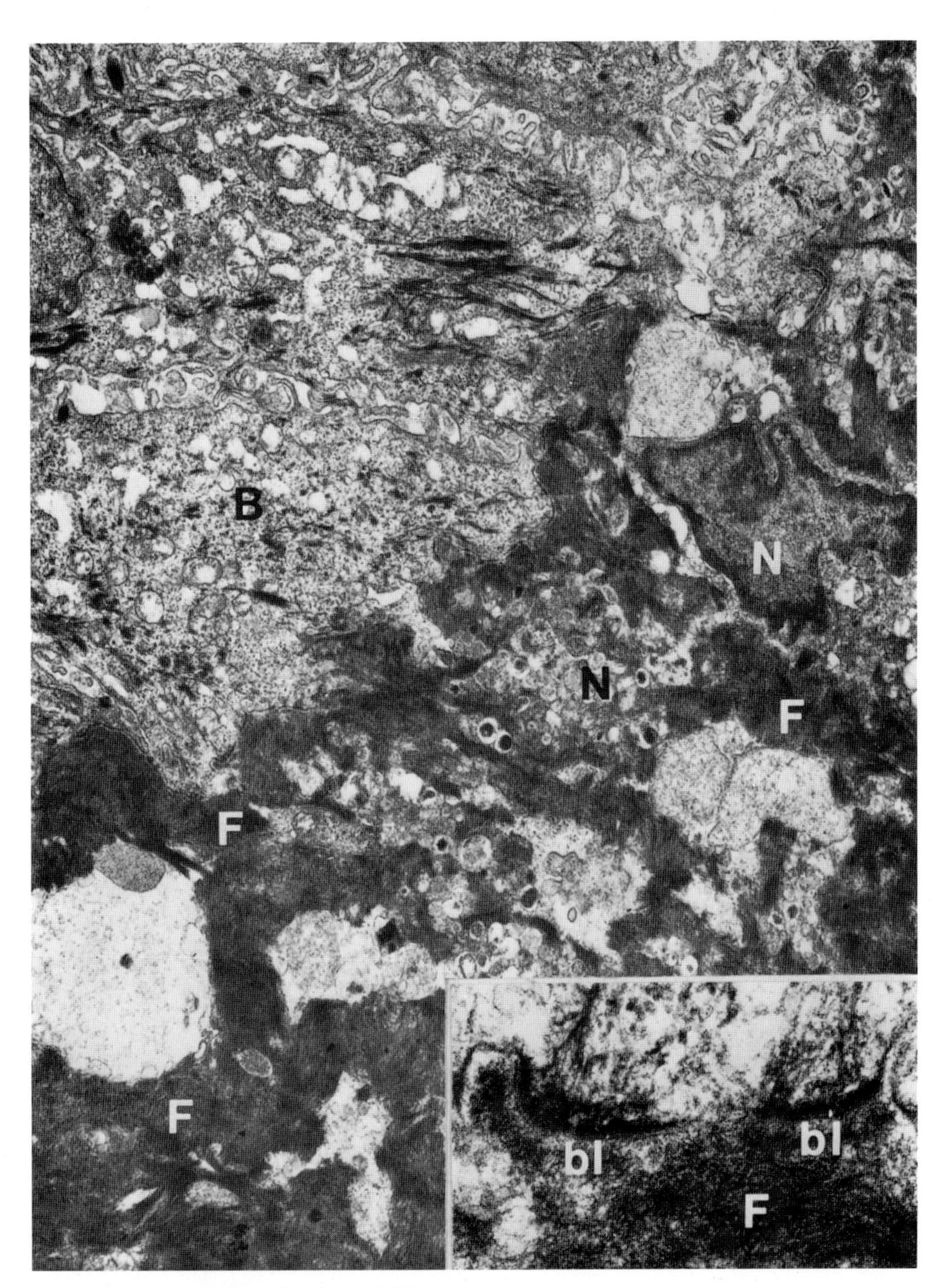

EM 10. Dermatitis herpetiformis, (Inset) Fibrin
The dermal papillae contain abundant amounts of fibrin (*F*). Between the meshes of fibrin, fragments of neutrophilic leukocytes (*N*) can be seen. *B,* basal cell. (*Inset*) The fibrin (*F*) is attached to the dermal side of the basement membrane or basal lamina (*bl*). The basement membrane shows discontinuities.

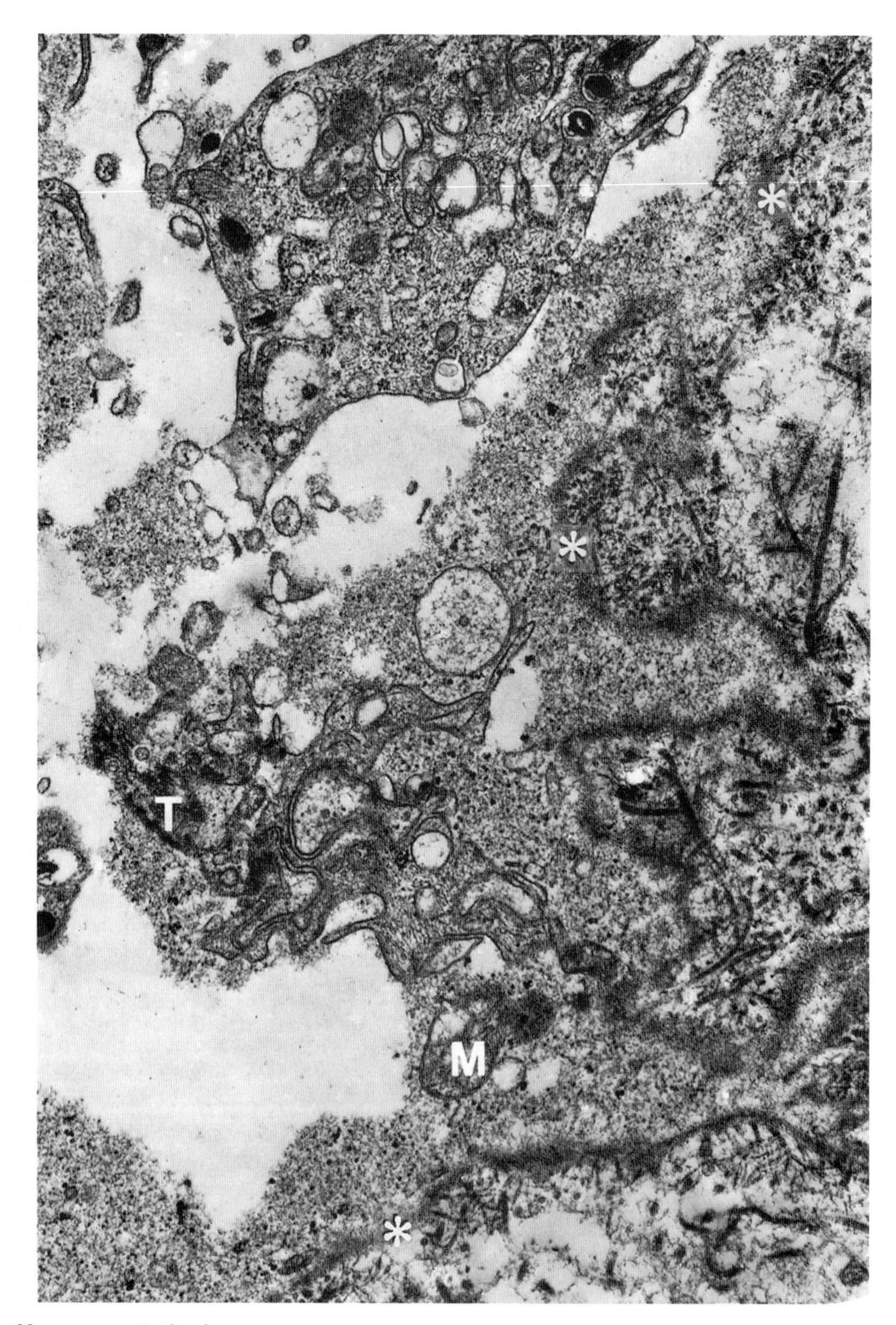

EM 11. Herpes gestationis
In this disease, the blister forms either between basal cells and the basement membrane or, subsequent to dissolution of basal cells, between squamous cells and the basement membrane. A disintegrated basal cell containing tonofilaments (*T*) and mitochondria (*M*) and the basement membrane (*asterisks*) form the floor of the blister.

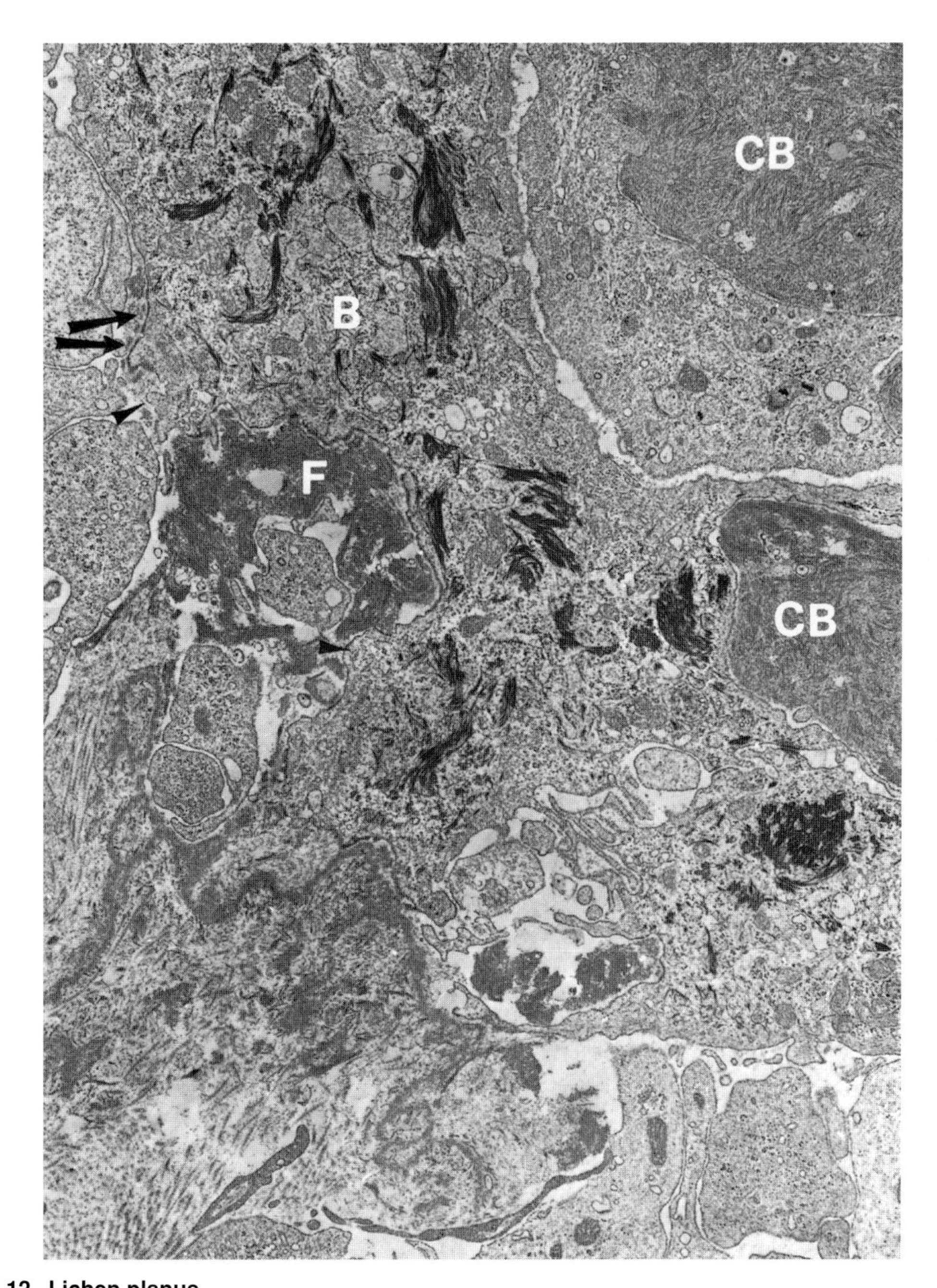

EM 12. Lichen planus
The basement membrane is split up in some areas (*arrows*) and has disappeared in other (*pointers*). The lower epidermis contains colloid bodies (*CB*) consisting of numerous filaments and remnants of organelles. *F,* fibrin beneath the basal cell (*B*).

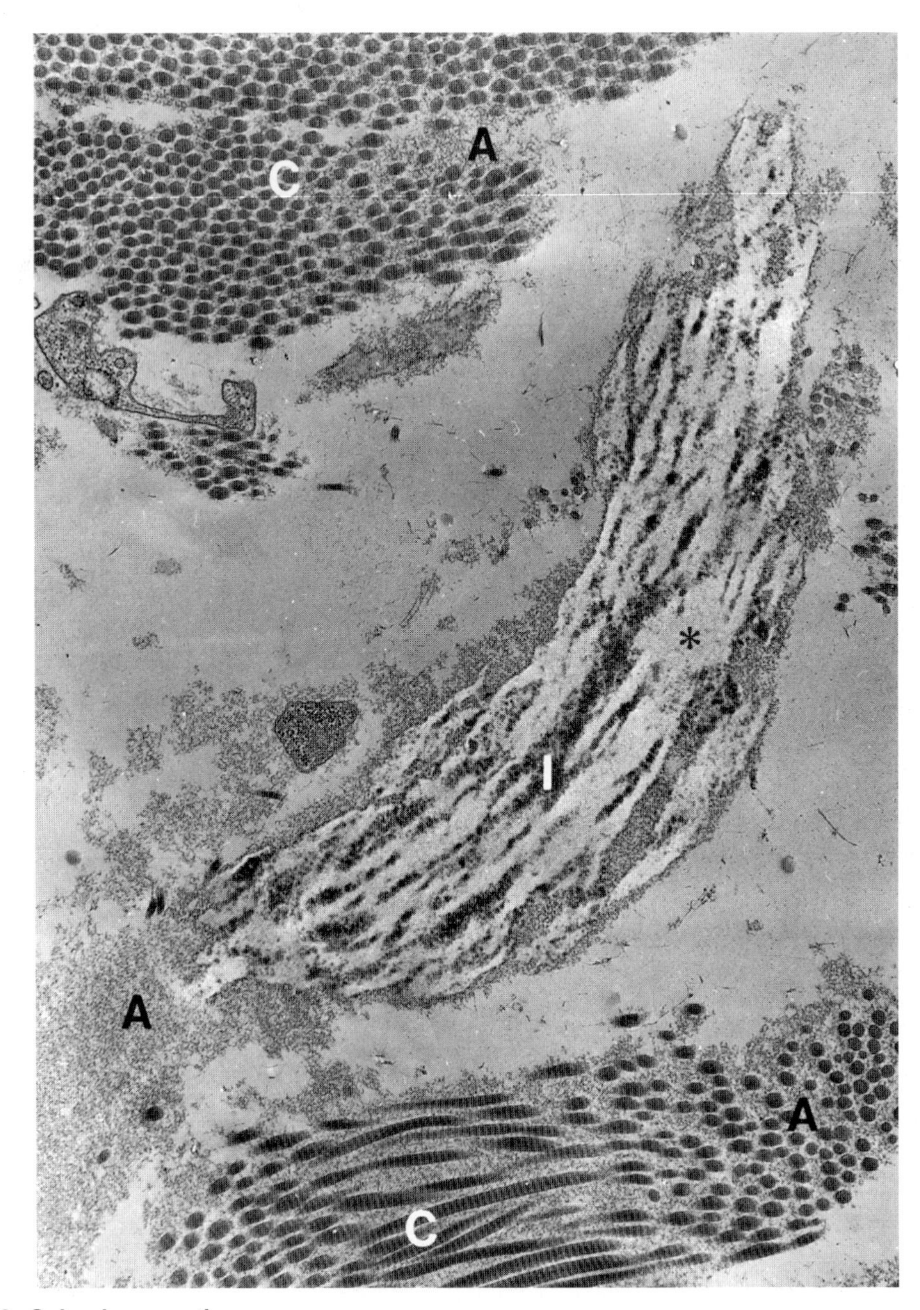

EM 13. Solar degeneration

The elastic fiber contains in its amorphous matrix (*asterisk*) numerous electron-dense inclusions (*I*). Extensive amorphous material (*A*) can be seen around the elastotic fiber and among the collagen fibrils (*C*).

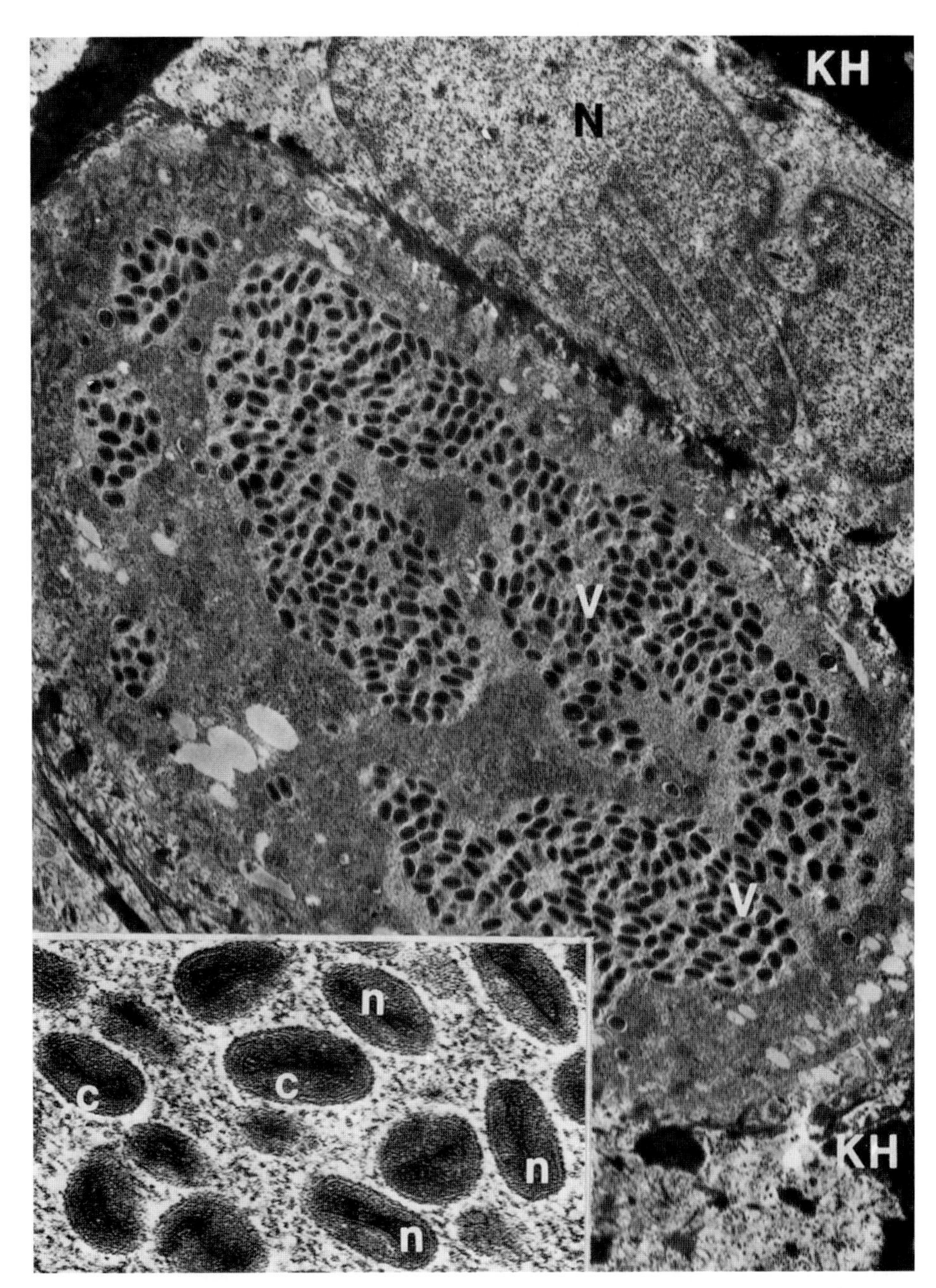

EM 14. Molluscum contagiosum, (Inset) High magnification of viruses
The granular cell contains an inclusion body consisting of numerous molluscum contagiosum viruses (*V*). The nucleus (*N*) of the cell has been displaced to the periphery of the cell. *KH,* keratohyaline granules. (*Inset*) The virus consists of the dumbbell-shaped nucleoid (*n*) surrounded by the capsid (*c*).

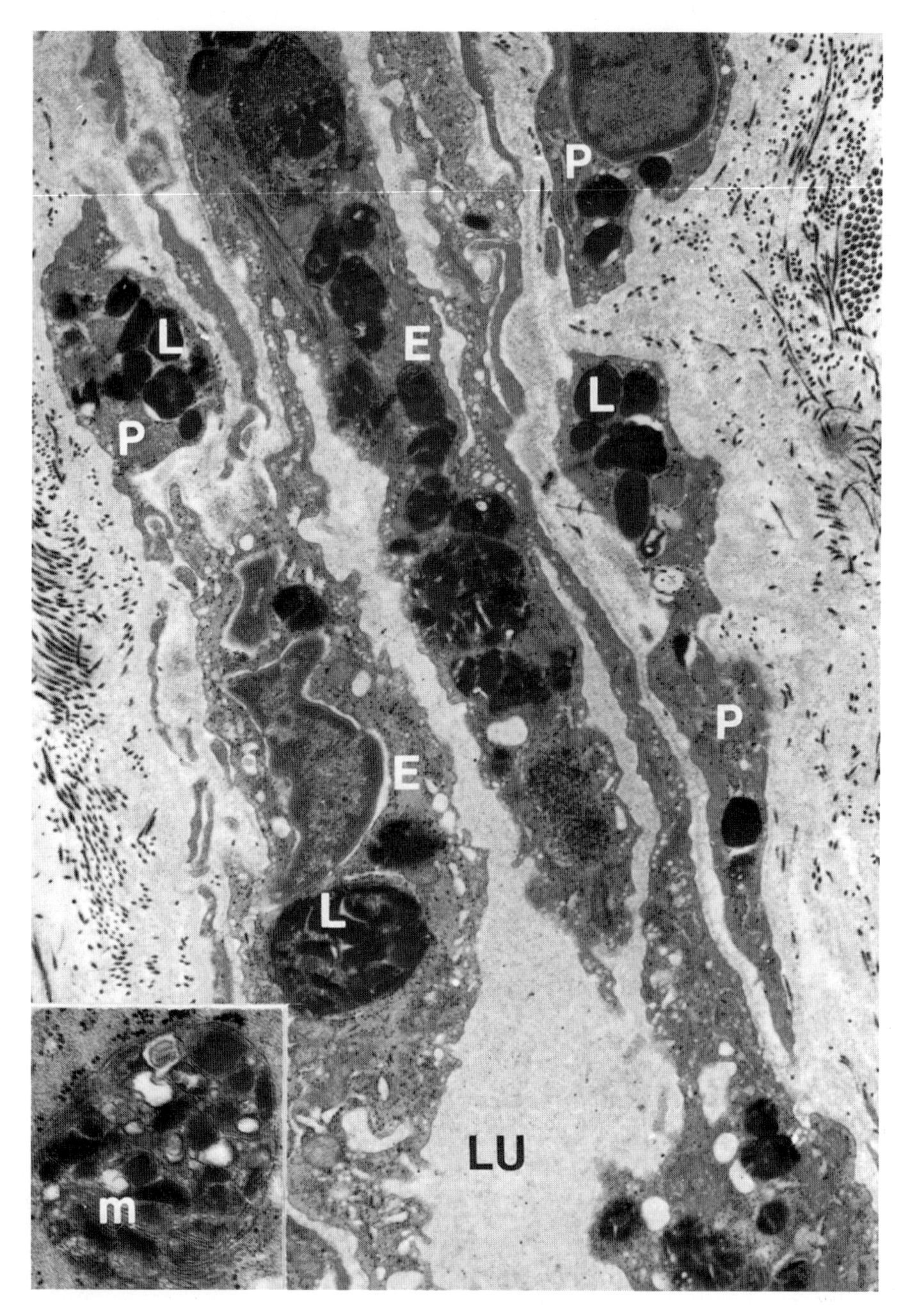

EM 15. Angiokeratoma corporis diffusum (Fabry's disease), (Inset) Lysosomal residual body Endothelial cells (*E*) and pericytes (*P*) contain lipid deposits (*L*) within greatly enlarged lysosomes. *LU,* lumen of capillary. (*Inset*) A large matured lysosome as a residual body shows laminated myelin figures (*m*).

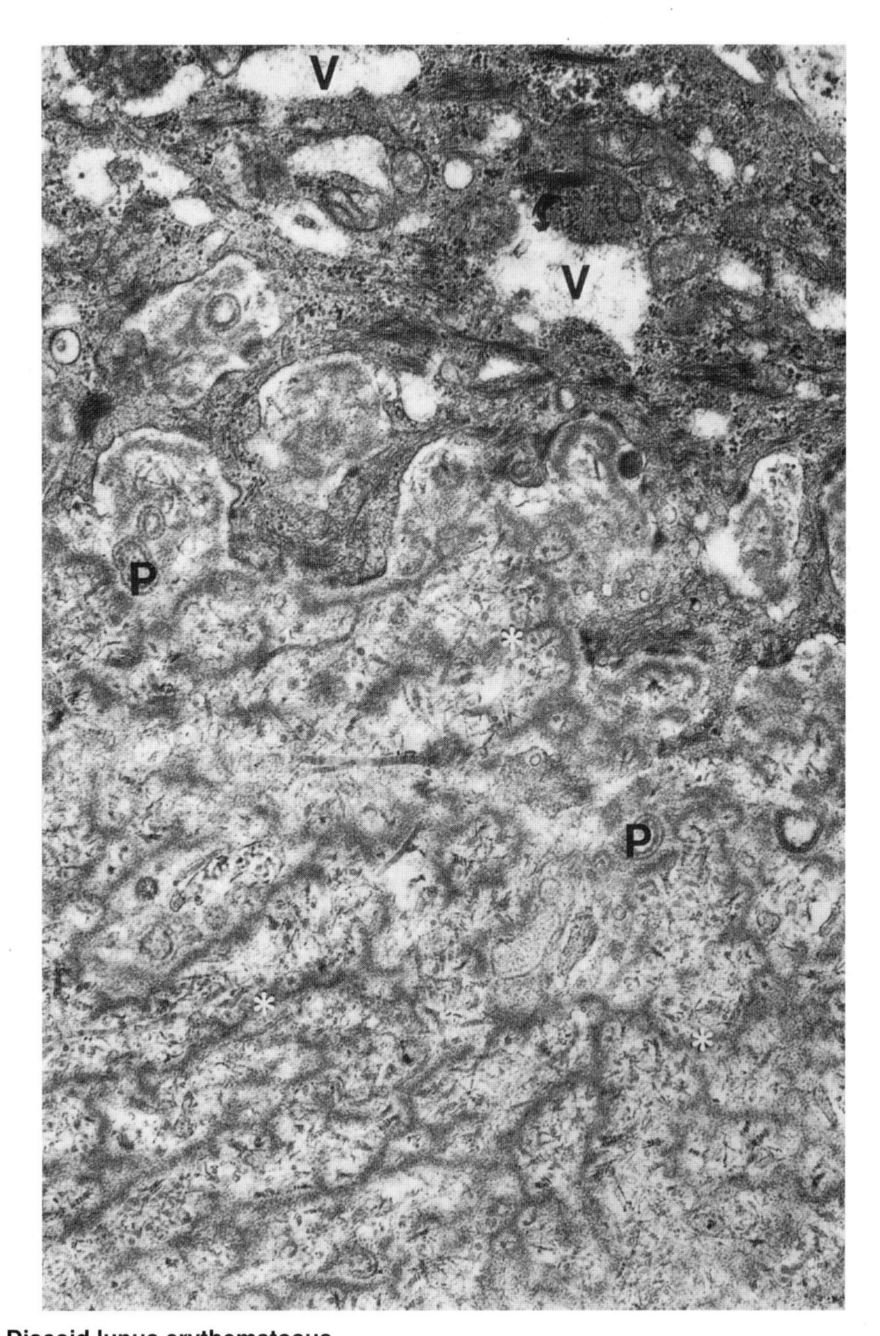

EM 16. Discoid lupus erythematosus

The basal cell contains several vacuoles (*V*), which ultimately may cause disintegration of the cell. Many cross-sectioned projections (*P*) of the basal cell into the dermis can be seen, as can a greatly increased amount of basal lamina material (*asterisks*).

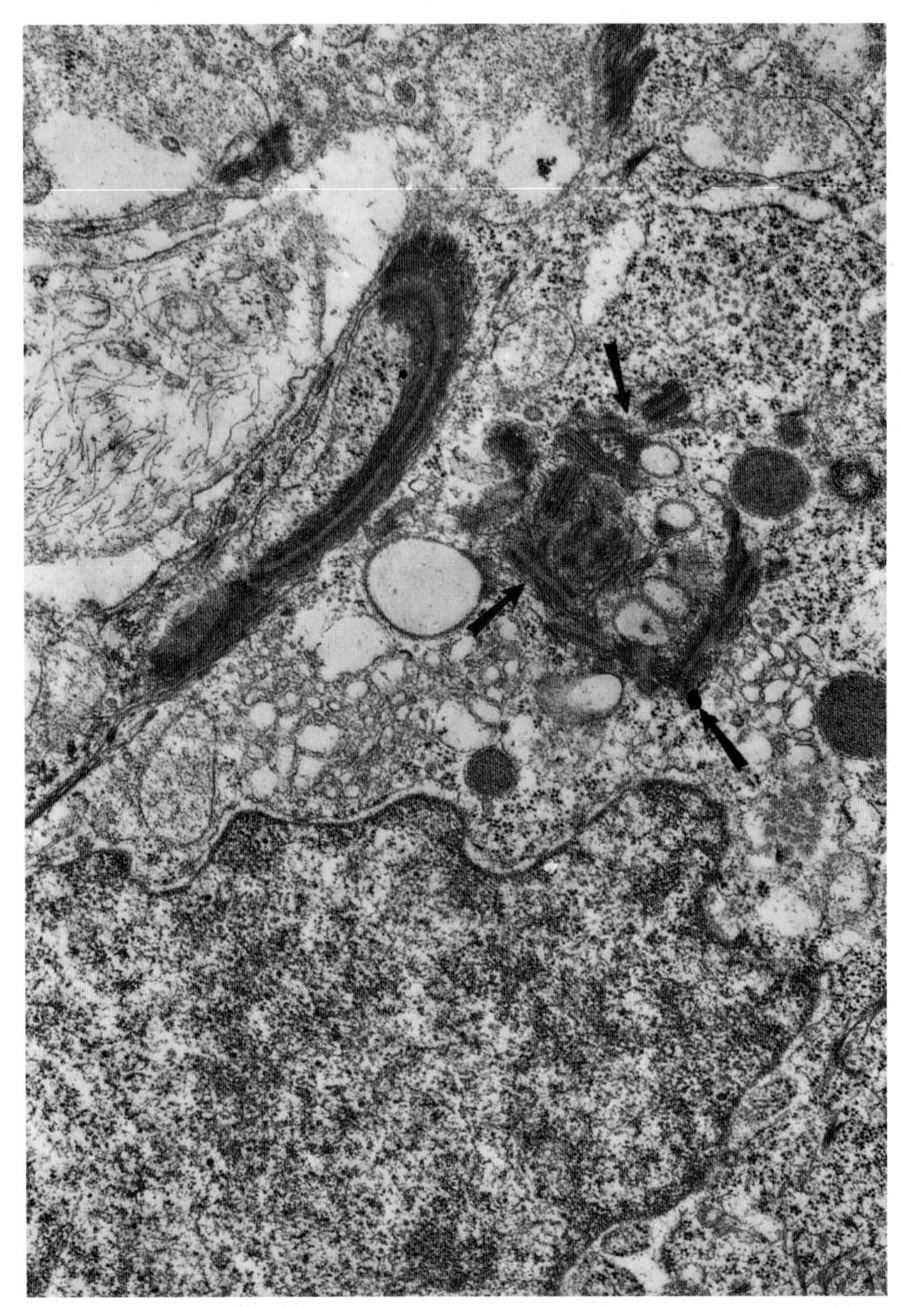

EM 17. Squamous cell carcinoma
Desmosomes attached to tonofilaments (*arrows*) can be seen within the cytoplasm of the tumor cell.

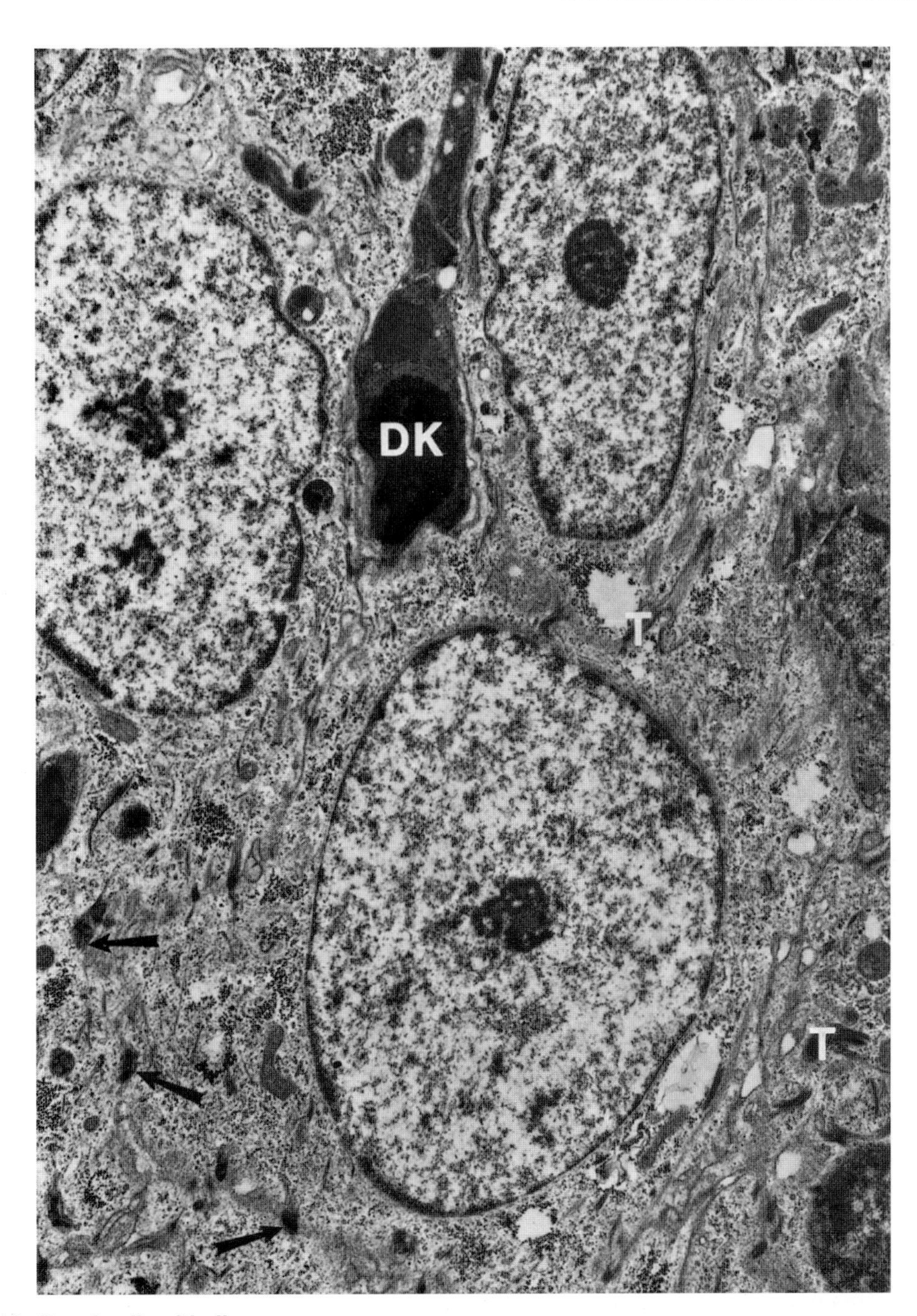

EM 18. Basal cell epithelioma

The cells show evidence of keratinization. In addition to tonofilaments (*T*) and desmosomes (*arrows*), some dyskeratotic material (*DK*) is present.

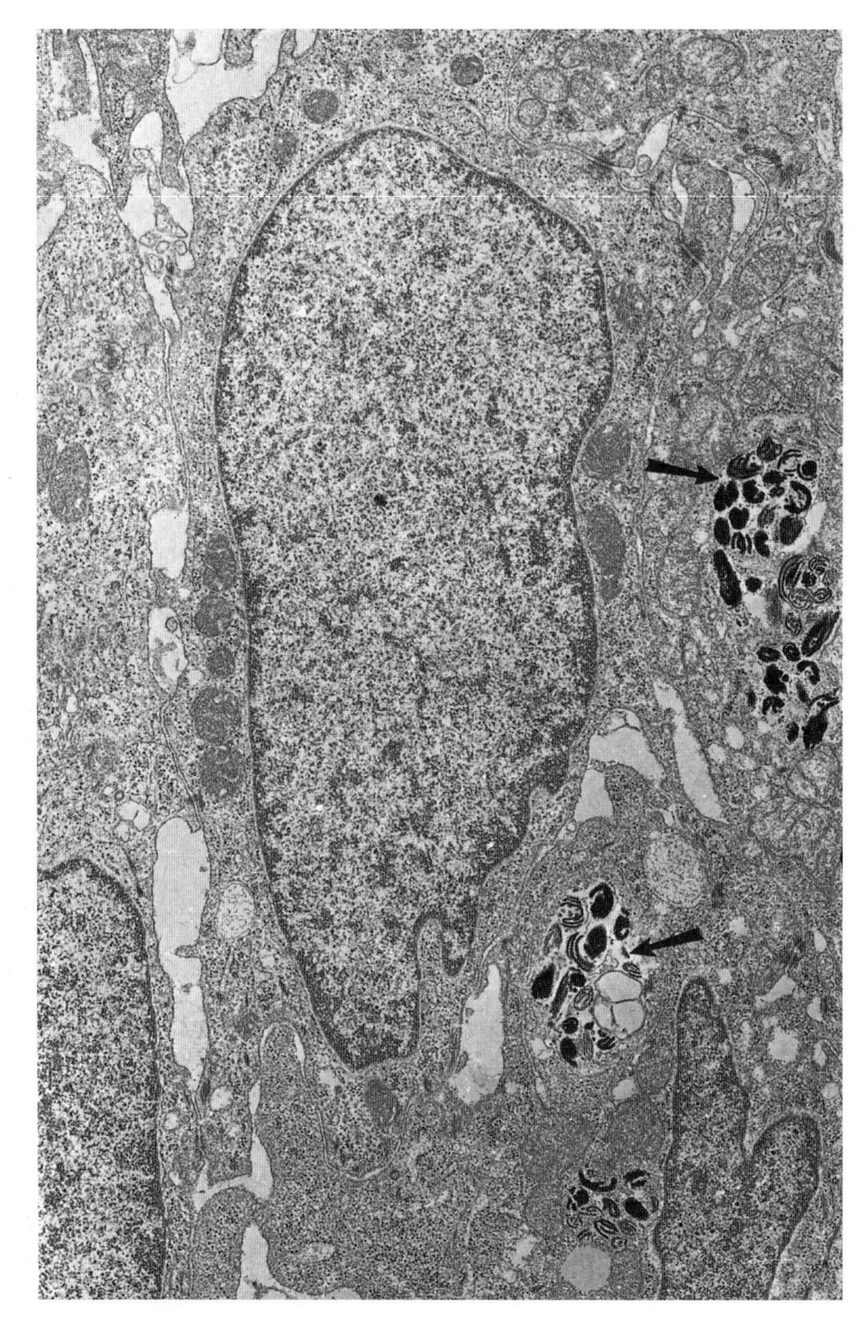

EM 19. Pigmented basal cell carcinoma
Some of the tumor cells contain melanosome complexes located within lysosomes (*arrows*).

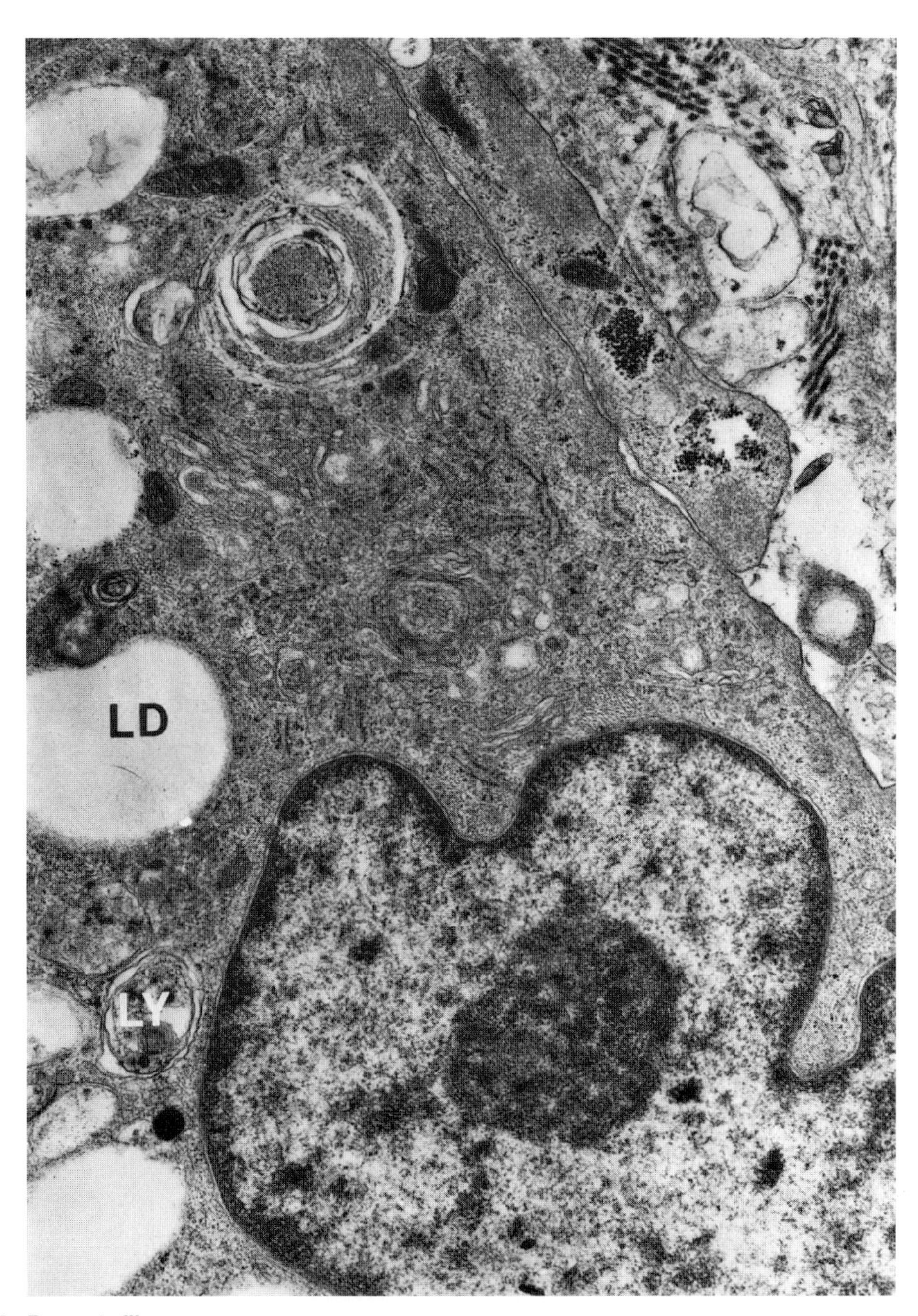

EM 20. Dermatofibroma
The essential cells are fibroblasts, which, in addition to producing collagen, are engaged in phagocytosis and storage of lipid. *LY,* lysosome; *LD,* lipid droplets. (Courtesy of Dr. B. Mihatsch-Konz.)

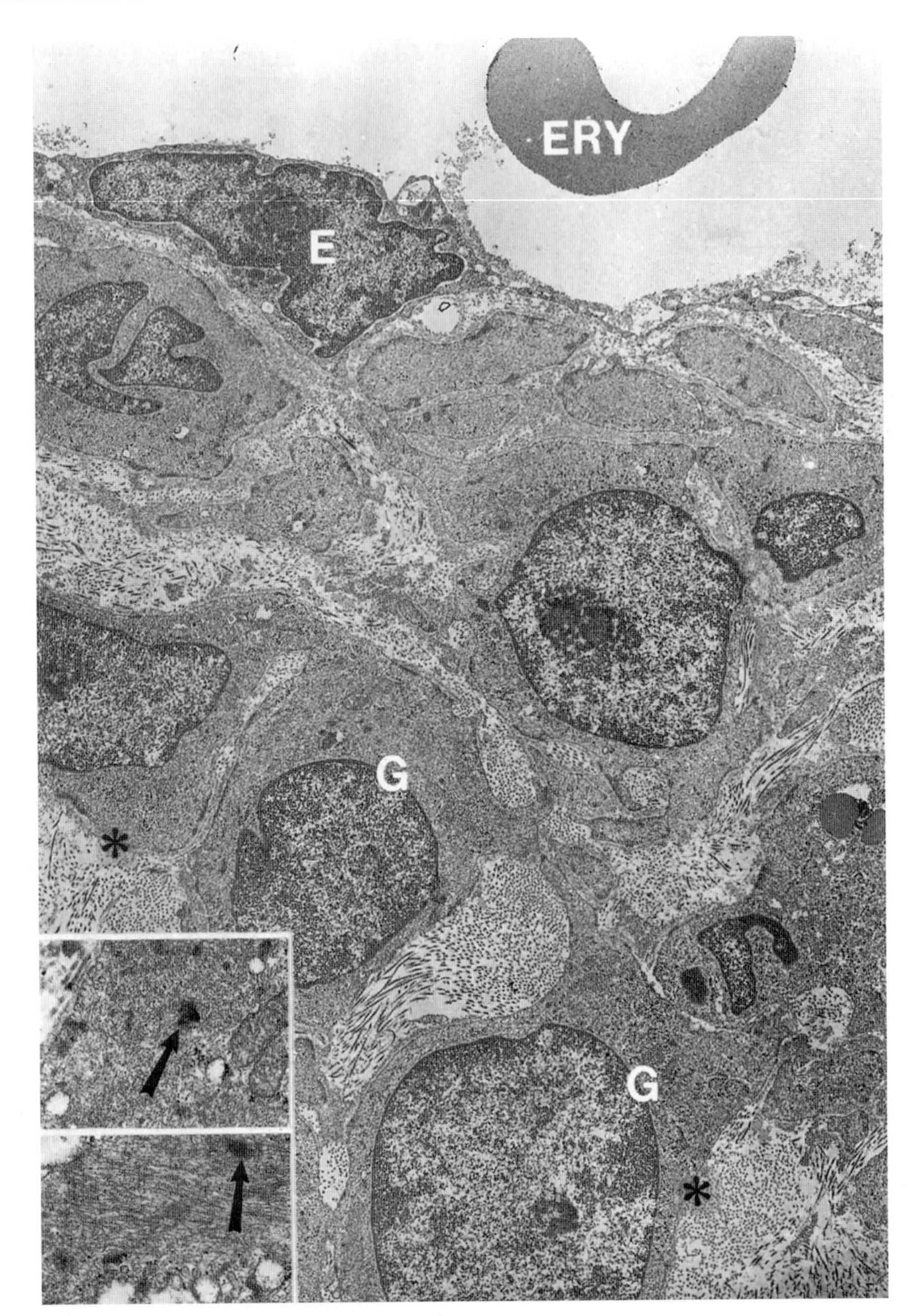

EM 21. Glomus tumor, (Inset) Myofilaments
The glomus cells are smooth muscle cells. Each glomus cell is surrounded by a basal lamina (*asterisk*). *E,* endothelial cell of capillary; *G,* glomus cell; *ERY,* erythrocyte within capillary lumen. (*Insets*) The *upper* inset shows the myofilaments in cross section, the *lower* inset in longitudinal section. *Arrows* point to so-called dense bodies.

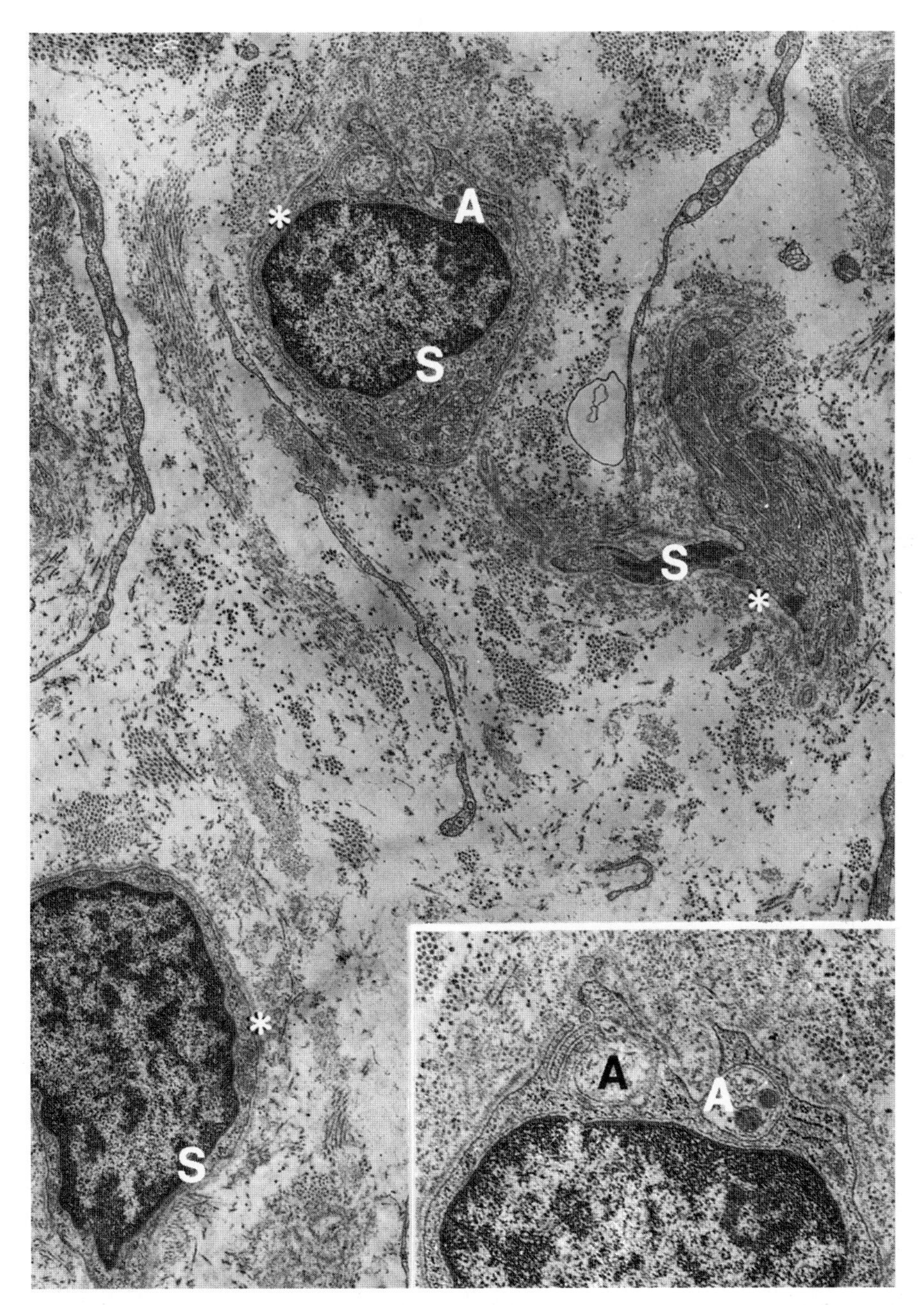

EM 22. Neurofibroma, (Inset) Axons in Schwann cell
The main cell type is the Schwann cell (*S*). Each cell is surrounded by a basal lamina (*asterisks*). Schwann cells contain axons (*A*) in their cytoplasm. (*Inset*) Two axons (*A*) of the upper Schwann cell are shown at higher magnification.

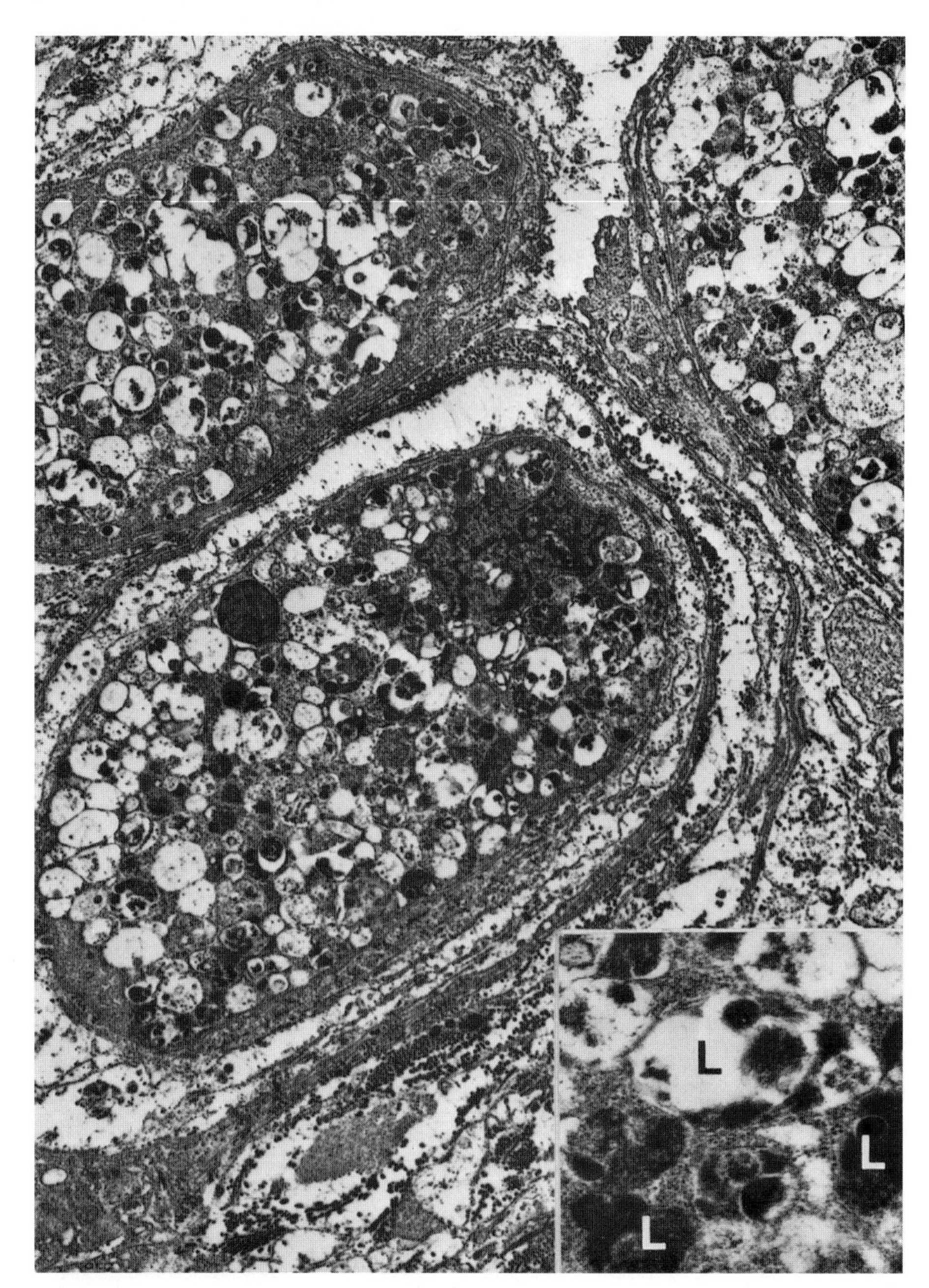

EM 23. Granular cell tumor, (Inset) Cytoplasmic granules
The cells contain numerous cytoplasmic granules, which are lysosomes. (*Inset*) The lysosomes (*L*) are shown at higher magnification.

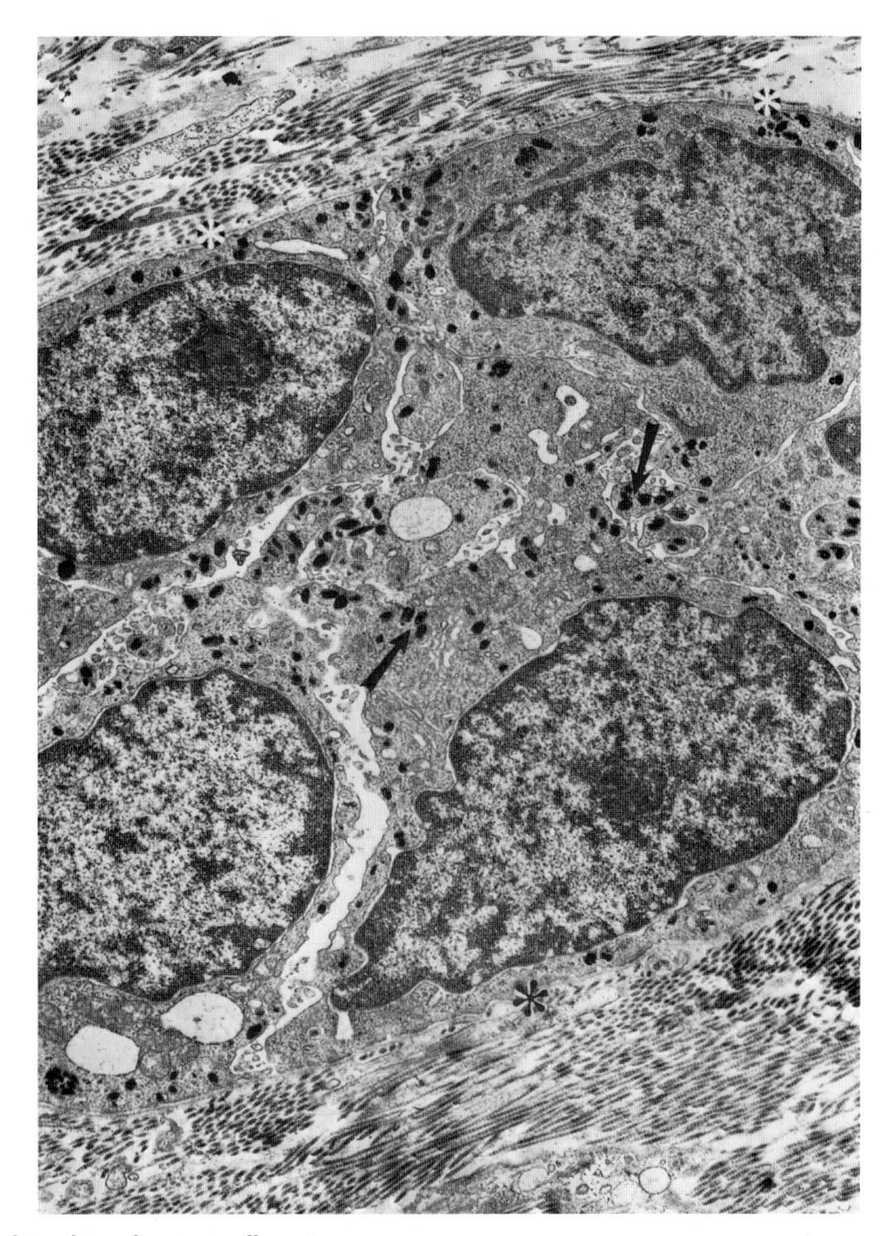

EM 24. Intradermal nevus cell nest
The nevus cell nest is surrounded by a basal lamina (*asterisk*). There are no desmosomes between adjacent nevus cells. The nevus cells contain numerous melanosomes (*arrows*).

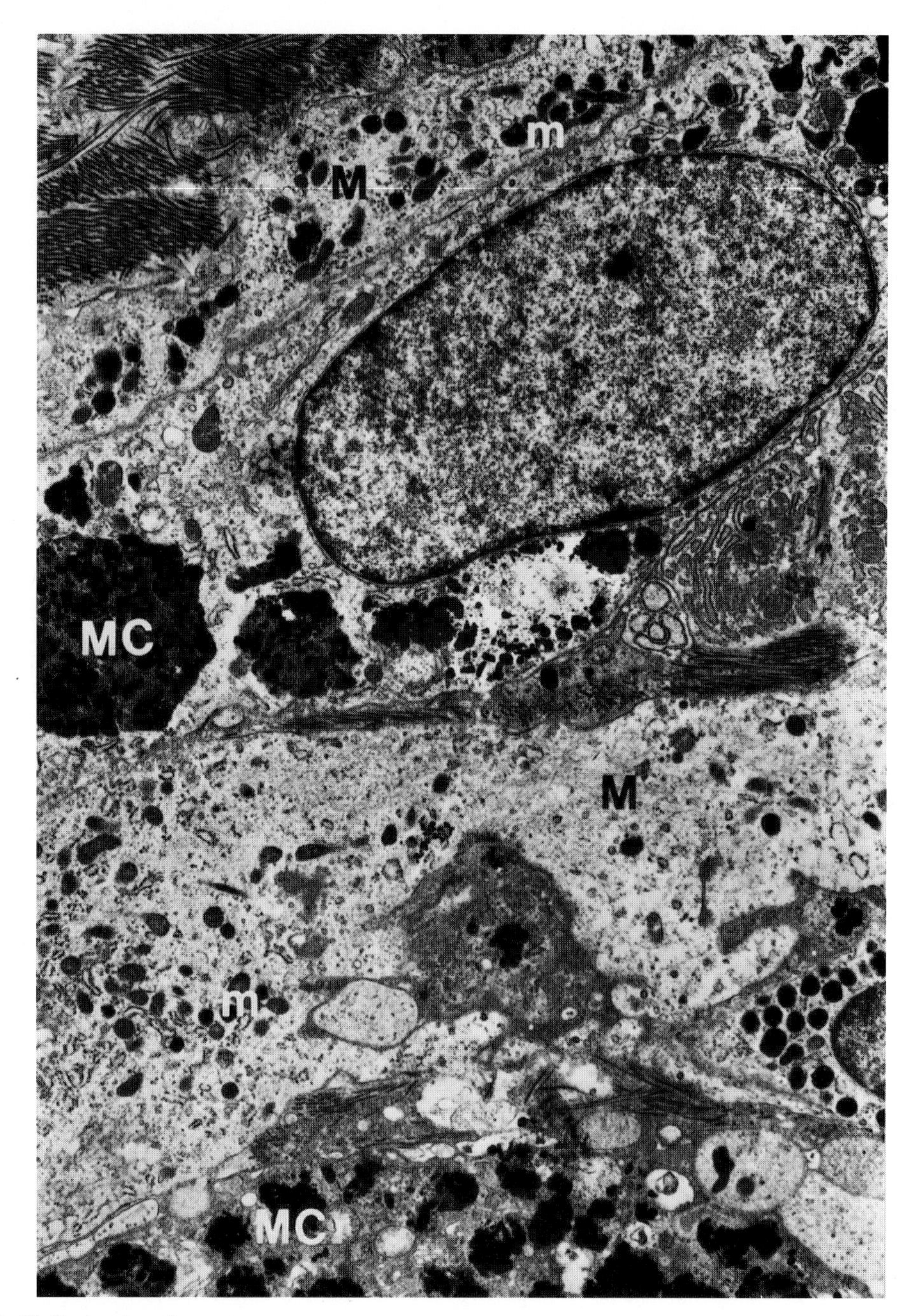

EM 25. Malignant melanoma
In addition to malignant spindle-shaped melanocytes (*M*) containing an abundance of melanosomes (*m*), melanophages with melanosome complexes (*MC*) are found.

Index

Numbers followed by an f *indicate a figure;* t *following a page number indicates tabular material.*